NEWMAN AND CARRANZA'S

CLINICAL PERIODONTOLOGY AND IMPLANTOLOGY

NEWMAN AND CARRANZA'S

CLINICAL PERIODONTOLOGY AND IMPLANTOLOGY

4TH SOUTH ASIA EDITION

MICHAEL G. NEWMAN, DDS, FACD
Professor Emeritus, Periodontics, University of California, Los Angeles School of Dentistry, Los Angeles, California
Editor-in-Chief, Practice Update Clinical Dentistry, American Dental Association, Chicago, Illinois
Past President, American Academy of Periodontology, Chicago, Illinois

PERRY R. KLOKKEVOLD, DDS, MS, FACD
Professor of Clinical Dentistry Emeritus, Section of Periodontics University of California, Los Angeles School of Dentistry, Los Angeles, California
Private Practice, PermaDent, Torrance, California

SATHEESH ELANGOVAN, BDS, DSC, DMSC
Professor Emeritus, Department of Periodontics, The University of Iowa College of Dentistry and Dental Clinics, Iowa City, Iowa
Adjunct Professor, Department of Periodontics and Dental Hygiene, University of Texas Health Science Center at Houston School of Dentistry, Houston, Texas

YVONNE L. HERNANDEZ-KAPILA, DDS, PHD
Felix and Mildred Yip Endowed Chair in Dentistry, Professor and Associate Dean for Research, Periodontics, Biosystems and Function, University of California, Los Angeles School of Dentistry, Los Angeles, California

Editors Emeriti

FERMIN A. CARRANZA, DR. ODONT, FACD
Professor Emeritus, Periodontics, University of California, Los Angeles School of Dentistry, Los Angeles, California

HENRY H. TAKEI, DDS, MS
Distinguished Clinical Professor Emeritus, Section of Periodontics, University of California, Los Angeles School of Dentistry;
Consultant, Periodontics, Veterans Administration Hospital Los Angeles, Los Angeles, California

ADAPTATION EDITORS

CD DWARAKANATH, MDS
Professor Emeritus
Department of Periodontics and Implantology
Vishnu Dental College
Bhimavaram, India

N AMBALAVANAN, MDS
Professor Emeritus
Department of Periodontics
Faculty of Dentistry
Meenakshi Academy of Higher Education and Research (Deemed to be University)
Chennai, India

DG NAIK, MDS
Pro Vice Chancellor MAHE, Mangalore Campus
Former Professor
Department of Periodontology
Manipal College of Dental Sciences, Mangalore
Manipal Academy of Higher Education
Manipal, India

A UPPOOR, MDS
Professor and Dean
Department of Periodontology
Manipal College of Dental Sciences, Mangalore
Manipal Academy of Higher Education
Manipal, India

A JAIN, MDS, PhD
Principal-cum-Professor
Dr HS Judge Institute of Dental Sciences
Panjab University
Chandigarh, India

ELSEVIER

ELSEVIER

RELX India Pvt. Ltd.
Registered Office: 818, Indraprakash Building, 8th Floor, 21, Barakhamba Road, New Delhi-110001, India
Corporate Office: 14th Floor, Building No. 10B, DLF Cyber City, Phase II, Gurgaon-122002, Haryana, India

Newman and Carranza's Clinical Periodontology and Implantology: 14th Edition, Michael G. Newman, Perry R. Klokkevold, Satheesh Elangovan, Yvonne L. Hernandez-Kapila

Publisher's note: Elsevier takes a neutral position with respect to territorial disputes or jurisdictional claims in its published content, including in maps and institutional affiliations.

ISBN: 978-0-323-87887-6

Previous editions copyrighted 2019, 2015, 2012, 2006.

This adaptation of Newman and Carranza's Clinical Periodontology and Implantology: 14th Edition, by Michael G. Newman, Perry R. Klokkevold, Satheesh Elangovan, Yvonne L. Hernandez-Kapila was undertaken by RELX India Private Limited and is published by arrangement with Elsevier, Inc.

Newman and Carranza's Clinical Periodontology and Implantology: 4th South Asia Edition
Adaptation Editors: CD Dwarakanath, N Ambalavanan, DG Naik, A Uppoor, A Jain

Adaptation ISBN: 978-81-312-6933-6

Previous editions copyrighted 2019, 2016, 2012.

First Printed in India 2024, Reprinted 2025

Content Strategist: Priyanka Raina Dhar
Content Project Manager: Anand K Jha
Sr Production Executive: Dhan Singh
Sr Cover Designer: Milind Majgaonkar

Printed in India by Balaji Art, Mumbai.

CONTRIBUTORS

Alfredo Aguirre, DDS, MS
Professor
Department of Oral Diagnostic Sciences
School of Dental Medicine
University at Buffalo
The State University of New York
Buffalo, New York

Edward P Allen, DD, PhD
Private Practice
Dallas, Texas

Robert R Azzi, DDS
Department of Periodontology
University of Paris, VII
Paris, France

Janet G Bauer, DDS
Advanced Education Services
Center for Dental Research
Loma Linda University School of Dentistry
Loma Linda, California
Professor Emerita
School of Dentistry
University of California, Los Angeles
Los Angeles, California

Mitchell J Bloom, DMD
Clinical Associate Professor
Ashman Department of Periodontology and Implant Dentistry
New York University College of Dentistry
Private Practice
Periodontology and Implant Dentistry
New York, New York

Jaime Bulkacz, DR ODONT, PhD
Lecturer
Section of Periodontics
School of Dentistry
University of California, Los Angeles
Los Angeles, California

Bobby Butler, BS, DDS
Affiliate Faculty, Periodontics
School of Dentistry
University of Washington
Seattle, Washington

Paulo M Camargo, DDS, MS, MBA, FACD
Professor and Tarrson Family Endowed Chair in Periodontics
Section of Periodontics
School of Dentistry
University of California, Los Angeles
Los Angeles, California

Fermin A Carranza, DR ODONT, FACD
Professor Emeritus
Section of Periodontics
School of Dentistry
University of California, Los Angeles
Los Angeles, California

Ana B Castro, DDS, MSc
Periodontology Section
University Hospitals Leuven
Department of Oral Health Services
KU Leuven
Leuven, Belgium

Frank Celenza, DDS
Associate Clinical Professor
Postgraduate Orthodontics
Rutgers School of Dental Medicine
Newark, New Jersey

Leandro Chambrone, DDS, MSc, PhD
Associate Professor
Unit of Basic Oral Investigation
School of Dentistry
El Bosque University
Bogota, Colombia
Professor
Master of Science Dentistry Program
Ibirapuera University
São Paulo, Brazil

Ting-Ling Chang, DDS
Clinical Professor
Chair of the Section of Prosthodontics
School of Dentistry
University of California, Los Angeles
Los Angeles, California

Yu-Cheng Chang, DDS, MS
Instructor
Department of Periodontics
The Robert Schattner Center
School of Dental Medicine
University of Pennsylvania
Philadelphia, Pennsylvania

Sang Choon Cho, DDS
Clinical Assistant Professor
Periodontology and Implant Dentistry
New York University College of Dentistry
New York, New York

Chih-Hung Chou, PhD
Manager
Molecular Biology Department
WuXi AppTec
Philadelphia, Pennsylvania

Evelyn Chung, DDS
Clinical Professor
Residency Program Director, GPR
Section of Hospital Dentistry
School of Dentistry
University of California, Los Angeles
Los Angeles, California

Sebastian G Ciancio, DDS
Distinguished Service Professor and Chair
Department of Periodontics and Endodontics
University at Buffalo
The State University of New York
Buffalo, New York

David L Cochran, DDS, MS, PhD, MMSci
Chair and Professor
Department of Periodontics
School of Dentistry
UT Health San Antonio
San Antonio, Texas

Joseph P Cooney, BDS, MS
Clinical Professor Emeritus
Restorative Dentistry
University of California, Los Angeles
Los Angeles, California

Simone Cortellini, DDS, MSc
Periodontology Section
University Hospitals Leuven
Department of Oral Health Services
KU Leuven
Leuven, Belgium

J David Cross, DDS
Private Practice
Springfield, Illinois

Sophie De Geest, DDS, MSc
Clinical Consultant
Periodontology Section
University Hospitals Leuven
Department of Oral Health Services
KU Leuven
Leuven, Belgium

Charlotte De Hous, DDS, MSc
Clinical Resident in Dentistry
Periodontology Section
University Hospitals Leuven
Department of Oral Health Services
KU Leuven
Leuven, Belgium

Christel Dekeyser, DDS
Head of Periodontology Section
Periodontology Section
University Hospitals Leuven
Department of Oral Health Services
KU Leuven
Leuven, Belgium

Raymond R Derycke, DDS
CEO, Haptitude

Scott R Diehl, BS, PhD
Professor
Department of Oral Biology
Rutgers School of Dental Medicine
Professor
Department of Health Informatics
Rutgers School of Health Professions
Newark, New Jersey

Jonathan H Do, DDS
Assistant Clinical Professor
Section of Periodontics
School of Dentistry
University of California, Los Angeles
Los Angeles, California
Private Practice Limited to Periodontics and Implant Surgery
Poway, California

Henrik Dommisch, DDS, PhD
Professor
Periodontology and Synoptic Dentistry
Charité—Universitätsmedizin Berlin
Berlin, Germany
Associate Professor
Oral Health Sciences
University of Washington
Seattle, Washington

Donald F Duperon, DDS, MSc
Professor Emeritus
Section of Pediatric Dentistry
School of Dentistry
University of California, Los Angeles
Los Angeles, California

Satheesh Elangovan, BDS, DSc, DMSc
Professor
Department of Periodontics
University of Iowa College of Dentistry and Dental Clinics
Iowa City, Iowa

Daniel H Etienne, DDS, MS
Honorary Associate Professor in Periodontology
Pitié-Salpêtrière Hospital
Denis Diderot University
Paris, France

Richard D Finkelman, DDS, PhD
Senior Clinical Pharmacology Medical Director
Clinical Pharmacology and Pharmacokinetics
Shire
Lexington, Massachusetts

Joseph P Fiorellini, DMD, DMSc
Professor
Department of Periodontics
The Robert Schattner Center
School of Dental Medicine
University of Pennsylvania
Philadelphia, Pennsylvania

Jane L Forrest, BSDH, MS, EdD
Professor of Clinical Dentistry
Dental Public Health and Pediatric Dentistry
Herman Ostrow School of Dentistry
University of Southern California
Los Angeles, California

Marcelo Freire, DDS, PhD, DMSc
Associate Professor
Department of Genomic Medicine and Infectious Disease
J. Craig Venter Institute
La Jolla, California

Scott H Froum, DDS
Clinical Assistant Professor
Department of Peiodontology
School of Dental Medicine
Stony Brook University
Stony Brook, New York
Private Practice
New York, New York

Stuart J Froum, DDS
Clinical Professor and Director of Clinical Research
Periodontology and Implant Dentistry
New York University College of Dentistry
New York, New York

Ying Gu, DDS, PhD
Associate Professor
General Dentistry
School of Dental Medicine
Stony Brook University
Stony Brook, New York

Thomas J Han, DDS, MS
Clinical Professor
Department of Periodontics
Herman Ostrow School of Dentistry
University of Southern California
Los Angeles, California

M Cenk Haytac, DDS, PhD
Professor
Department of Periodontology
Faculty of Dentistry
Cukurova University
Adana, Turkey

James E Hinrichs, DDS, MS
Professor
Department of Developmental and Surgical Sciences
Division of Periodontology
School of Dentistry
University of Minnesota
Minneapolis, Minnesota

Eva L Hogan, MD, DDS, MS
Lecturer
Section of Periodontics
School of Dentistry
University of California, Los Angeles
Los Angeles, California

Richard Holliday, BDS (Hons), MFDS RCSEd, MFDS an eundem RCSEng, MClinRes, MPerio RCSEd
NIHR Doctoral Research Fellow/Specialty Registrar in Restorative Dentistry
Newcastle Dental Hospital
Newcastle upon Tyne, United Kingdom

Ching-Yu Huang, PhD
Assistant Professor
Department of Computer Science
Kean University
Union, New Jersey

Philippe P Hujoel, DDS, MS, MSD, PhD
Professor, Oral Health Sciences
Adjunct Professor, Epidemiology
School of Dentistry
University of Washington
Seattle, Washington

Carol A Jahn, RDH, MS
Director Professional Relations and Education
Water Pik, Inc.
Fort Collins, Colorado

Nicholas Jakubovics, BSc, PhD
Senior Lecturer in Oral Microbiology
Centre for Oral Health Research, School of Dental Sciences
Newcastle University
Newcastle upon Tyne, United Kingdom

Mo K Kang, DDS, PhD
Professor and Chairman
Jack A. Weichman Endowed Chair
Section of Endodontics
Division of Constitutive and Regenerative Sciences
School of Dentistry
University of California, Los Angeles
Los Angeles, California

Alpdogan Kantarci, DDS, PhD
Associate Staff Member
Applied Oral Sciences
Forsyth Institute
Cambridge, Massachusetts
Associate Professor
Cellular and Molecular Biology
Henry M. Goldman School of Dental Medicine
Boston University
Lecturer
Harvard School of Dental Medicine
Boston, Massachusetts

Richard T Kao, DDS, PhD
Private Practice
Cupertino, California
Clinical Professor
Division of Periodontology
School of Dentistry
University of California, San Francisco
Adjunct Clinical Professor
Department of Periodontology
Arthur A. Dugoni School of Dentistry
University of the Pacific
San Francisco, California

Moritz Kebschull, DMD
Associate Professor
Department of Periodontology, Restorative and Preventive
University Hospital Bonn
Bonn, Germany
Adjunct Associate Professor of Dental Medicine
Division of Periodontics
Section of Oral, Diagnostic, and Rehabilitation Sciences
Columbia University College of Dental Medicine
New York, New York

David M Kim, DDS, DMSc
Associate Professor
Department of Oral Medicine, Infection, and Immunity
Harvard School of Dental Medicine
Boston, Massachusetts

Keith L Kirkwood, DDS, PhD
Professor and Chair
Craniofacial Biology
Medical University of South Carolina
Charleston, South Carolina

Perry R Klokkevold, DDS, MS, FACD
Associate Professor
Program Director, Periodontics Residency
Section of Periodontics
School of Dentistry
University of California, Los Angeles
Los Angeles, California

†Vincent G Kokich, DDS, MSD
Department of Orthodontics
School of Dentistry
University of Washington
Seattle, Washington
†Deceased.

Olga A Korczeniewska, PhD
Research Associate I
Department of Diagnostic Sciences
Rutgers School of Dental Medicine
Newark, New Jersey

Georgios A Kotsakis, DDS, MS
Assistant Professor
Department of Periodontics
School of Dentistry
University of Washington
Seattle, Washington

Fengshen Kuo, PhD, MS
Bioinformatics Engineer III
Memorial Sloan Kettering Cancer Center
New York, New York

Isabelle Laleman, DDS, MSc
Periodontologist
Periodontology Section
University Hospitals Leuven
Department of Oral Health Services
KU Leuven
Leuven, Belgium

Clarice S Law, DMD, MS
Associate Clinical Professor
Pediatric Dentistry and Orthodontics
Section of Pediatric Dentistry
School of Dentistry
University of California, Los Angeles
Los Angeles, California

Yasmin Mair, DDS, MS
Visiting Assistant Professor
Department of Oral Diagnostic Sciences
School of Dental Medicine
University at Buffalo
The State University of New York
Buffalo, New York
Assistant Professor
Oral Diagnostic Sciences
King Abdulaziz University
Jeddah, Saudi Arabia

Sanjay M Mallya, BDS, MDS, PhD
Associate Professor, Program Director, and Chair
Section of Oral and Maxillofacial Radiology
School of Dentistry
University of California, Los Angeles
Los Angeles, California

Angelo J Mariotti, DDS, PhD
Chair and Professor
Division of Periodontology
College of Dentistry
The Ohio State University
Columbus, Ohio

Michael J McDevitt, DDS
Visiting Faculty
Periodontics
College of Dental Medicine
Augusta, Georgia
Private Practice of Periodontics
Atlanta, Georgia

Adriana McGregor, DDS
Private Practice
Westlake Village, California

Brian L Mealey, DDS, MS
Professor and Graduate Program Director
Department of Periodontics
University of Texas Health Science Center at San Antonio
San Antonio, Texas

Shebli Mehrazarin, DDS, PhD
Resident
Division of Periodontics
Section of Oral, Diagnostic, and Rehabilitation Sciences
Columbia University College of Dental Medicine
New York, New York

Philip R Melnick, DMD
Lecturer
Section of Periodontics
School of Dentistry
University of California, Los Angeles
Los Angeles, California

Robert L Merin, DDS, MS
Private Practice
Woodland Hills, California

Greg W Miller, DDS
Private Practice
Deer Park, Washington

Syrene A Miller, BA
Project Manager
National Center for Dental Hygiene Research and Practice
Culver City, California

Ian Needleman, BDS, MSc, PhD
Professor of Restorative Dentistry and Evidence-Based Healthcare
Department of Periodontology
UCL Eastman Dental Institute
London, United Kingdom

Michael G Newman, DDS, FACD
Professor Emeritus
Section of Periodontics
School of Dentistry
University of California, Los Angeles
Los Angeles, California

Karen F Novak, DDS, MS, PhD
Clinical Professor
Department of Periodontics and Dental Hygiene
Special Assistant to the Dean
School of Dentistry
Health Science Center at Houston
University of Texas
Houston, Texas

M John Novak, BDS, LDS, MS, PhD
Professor of Periodontics, Retired
Director, Delta Dental of Kentucky Clinical Research Center
University of Kentucky College of Dentistry
Lexington, Kentucky

Chad M Novince, DDS, MSD, PhD
Assistant Professor
Oral Health Sciences
Medical University of South Carolina
Charleston, South Carolina

Joan Otomo-Corgel, DDS, MPH
Associate Clinical Professor
Section of Periodontics
School of Dentistry
University of California, Los Angeles
Los Angeles, California

Kwang-Bum Park, DDS
Director
MINEC Institute of Clinical Periodontics and Implantology
Lecturer in Oral Anatomy and Histology
Kyung-Pook National University
Taegu, South Korea

Anna M Pattison, BS, MS
Co-Director
Pattison Institute
Los Angeles, California

Gordon L Pattison, DDS
Private Practice
Co-Director
Pattison Institute
Los Angeles, California

Dorothy A Perry, RDH, PhD, MS
Professor Emeritus
School of Dentistry
University of California, San Francisco
San Francisco, California

Nelson R Pinto, DDS
Periodontology and Implant Dentistry
University of Los Andes
Las Condes
Santiago, Chile

Flavia Q Pirih, DDS, PhD
Associate Professor
Section of Periodontics
School of Dentistry
University of California, Los Angeles
Los Angeles, California

Alan M Polson, DDS
Professor
Department of Periodontics
The Robert Schattner Center
School of Dental Medicine
University of Pennsylvania
Philadelphia, Pennsylvania

Philip M Preshaw, BDS, FDS RCSEd, FDS (Rest Dent) RCSEd, PhD
Professor of Periodontology
School of Dental Sciences
Institute of Cellular Medicine
Newcastle University
Newcastle upon Tyne, United Kingdom

Marc Quirynen, DDS, PhD
Professor
Periodontology Section
University Hospitals Leuven
Department of Oral Health Services
KU Leuven
Leuven, Belgium

Terry D Rees, DDS, MSD
Professor
Department of Periodontics
Baylor College of Dentistry
Texas A&M University
Dallas, Texas

Carlos Rossa, Jr, DDS, MSc, PhD
Associate Professor
Diagnosis and Surgery
School of Dentistry at Araraquara-Univ Estadual Paulista
Sao Paulo, Brazil

Maria Emanuel Ryan, DDS, PhD
Vice President and Chief Dental Officer
Colgate Palmolive Company
Piscataway, New Jersey

Hector L Sarmiento, DMD, MSc
Assistant Clinical Professor
Department of Periodontics
The Robert Schattner Center
School of Dental Medicine
University of Pennsylvania
Philadelphia, Pennsylvania

E Todd Scheyer, DDS, MS
Private Practice
Houston, Texas

Titus Schleyer, DMD, PhD
Professor of Biomedical Informatics
Indiana University School of Medicine
Research Scientist
Center for Biomedical Informatics
Regenstrief Institute
Indianapolis, Indiana

Todd R Schoenbaum, DDS, FACD
Associate Clinical Professor
Director of Continuing Dental Education
School of Dentistry
University of California, Los Angeles
Los Angeles, California

Dennis A Shanelec, DDS
Private Practice
Santa Barbara, California

Kitetsu Shin, DDS, PhD
Professor of Periodontology
Meikai University School of Dentistry
Sakado, Saitama, Japan

†Gerald Shklar, DDS
Department of Oral Medicine and Diagnostic Sciences
Harvard School of Dental Medicine
Boston, Massachusetts
†Deceased.

Daniela R Silva, DDS, MS
Chair and Residency Program Director
Associate Clinical Professor
Section of Pediatric Dentistry
School of Dentistry
University of California, Los Angeles
Los Angeles, California

Thomas N Sims, BS, DDS
Senior Lecturer
Section of Periodontics
School of Dentistry
University of California, Los Angeles
Los Angeles, California

Sue S Spackman, DDS
Division of General Dentistry
Center for Dental Research
Loma Linda University School of Dentistry
Loma Linda, California

Frank M Spear, DDS, MSD
Founder and Director
Spear Education
Scottsdale, Arizona

Panagiota G Stathopoulou, DDS
Assistant Professor
Department of Periodontics
The Robert Schattner Center
School of Dental Medicine
University of Pennsylvania
Philadelphia, Pennsylvania

Corey Stein, DMD, MS
College of Dental Medicine
Western University of Health Sciences
Pomona, California

Henry H Takei, DDS, MS, FACD
Distinguished Clinical Professor
Section of Periodontics
School of Dentistry
University of California, Los Angeles
Los Angeles, California

Dennis P Tarnow, DDS
Clinical Professor
Director of Implant Education
Columbia University College of Dental Medicine
New York, New York

Andy Temmerman, DDS, MSc, PhD
Assistant Professor
Periodontology Section
University Hospitals Leuven
Department of Oral Health Services
KU Leuven
Leuven, Belgium

Sotirios Tetradis, DDS, PhD
Professor and Senior Associate Dean
Section of Oral and Maxillofacial Radiology
School of Dentistry
University of California, Los Angeles
Los Angeles, California

Wim Teughels, DDS, PhD
Professor
Periodontology Section
University Hospitals Leuven
Department of Oral Health Services
KU Leuven
Leuven, Belgium

Vivek Thumbigere-Math, BDS, PhD
Guest Researcher
National Institutes of Health
Bethesda, Maryland

Thankam P Thyvalikakath, DMD, MDS, PhD
Associate Professor and Director of Dental Informatics Core
Department of Cariology, Operative Dentistry, and Dental Public Health
Indiana University School of Dentistry
Research Scientist
Center for Biomedical Informatics
Regenstrief Institute
Indianapolis, Indiana

Leonard S Tibbetts, DDS, MSD
Private Practice
Arlington, Texas

Kenneth C Trabert, DDS, MEd
Clinical Professor Emeritus
Section of Endodontics
Division of Constitutive and Regenerative Sciences
School of Dentistry
University of California, Los Angeles
Los Angeles, California

Onur Ucak Turer, DDS, PhD
Associate Professor
Department of Periodontology
Faculty of Dentistry
Cukurova University
Adana, Turkey

Istvan A Urban, DMD, MD, PhD
Assistant Professor
Graduate Implant Dentistry
Loma Linda University
Loma Linda, California
Associate Professor
Periodontology
University of Szeged
Szeged, Hungary
Private Practice
Budapest, Hungary

Jose Luis Tapia Vazquez, DDS, MS
Assistant Professor
Department of Oral Diagnostic Sciences
School of Dental Medicine
University of Buffalo
The State University of New York
Buffalo, New York

Giuseppe Vercellotti, PhD
Adjunct Assistant Professor
School of Health and Rehabilitation Sciences
Division of Health Sciences
The Ohio State University
Columbus, Ohio

Tomas Vercellotti, DDS, MS
Honorary Professor and Faculty Member
University College of London
London, United Kingdom
Private Practice
Genoa, Italy

Keisuke Wada, DDS, PhD, DMSc, DMD
Associate Professor and Program Director
Kornberg School of Dentistry
Temple University
Philadelphia, Pennsylvania

Michael Whang, DDS
Lecturer
Section of Periodontics
School of Dentistry
University of California, Los Angeles
Los Angeles, California

Adrian K Zacher, MBA
Founder and Managing Director
Snorer.com
Oxford, United Kingdom

CONTRIBUTORS TO THE ADAPTATION EDITION

N Ambalavanan, MDS
Professor Emeritus
Department of Periodontics
Faculty of Dentistry
Meenakshi Academy of Higher Education and Research
(Deemed to be University)
Chennai, India

CD Dwarakanath, MDS
Professor Emeritus
Department of Periodontics and Implantology
Vishnu Dental College
Bhimavaram, India

A Jain, MDS, PhD
Principal-cum-Professor
Dr HS Judge Institute of Dental Sciences
Panjab University
Chandigarh, India

DG Naik, MDS
Pro Vice Chancellor MAHE, Mangalore Campus
Former Professor
Department of Periodontology
Manipal College of Dental Sciences, Mangalore
Manipal Academy of Higher Education
Manipal, India

A Uppoor, MDS
Professor and Dean
Department of Periodontology
Manipal College of Dental Sciences
Mangalore
Manipal Academy of Higher Education
Manipal, India

S U Nayak
Associate Professor
Department of Periodontology
Manipal College of Dental Sciences
Mangalore
Manipal Academy of Higher Education
Manipal, Karnataka, India

Vishakha Grover, MDS, PhD
Associate Professor
Department of Periodontology and Oral Implantology
Dr H.S.J. Institute of Dental Sciences Panjab University, India

Joann Pauline George, MDS
Professor
Dept of Periodontology
Krishnadevarya College of Dental Sciences
Bangalore, India

ABOUT THE ADAPTATION EDITORS

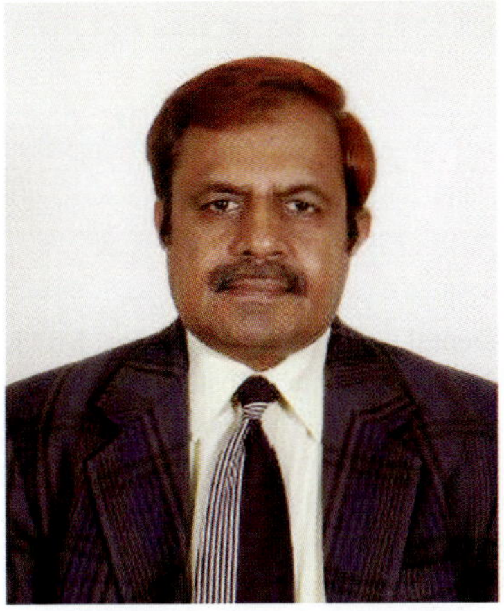

Dr C D Dwarakanath obtained his Bachelor's degree in Dentistry from Government Dental College, Bangalore in the year 1975 and Master's degree in Periodontics from Tamilnadu Government Dental College, Chennai in 1980. Being totally dedicated to academics he taught in India and abroad for 35 years until he retired from active service. At present he is the Professor Emeritus, Department of Periodontics and Implantology, Vishnu Dental College, Bhimavaram and Senior Consultant Periodontist in Bangalore. He has lectured extensively throughout India. He has conducted a number of Teachers training programs and has been a former President of the Indian Society of Periodontology.

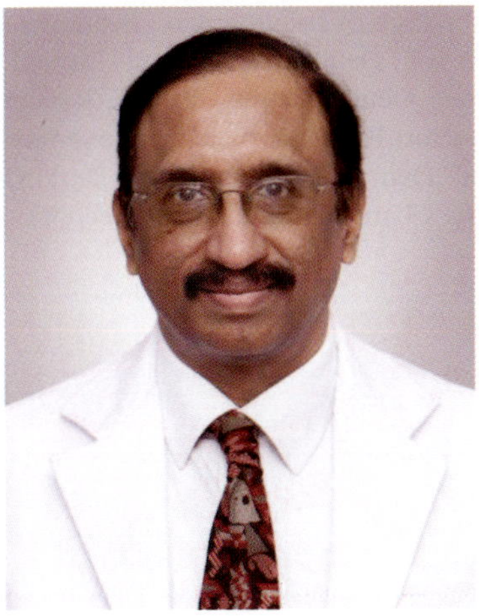

Dr N Ambalavanan obtained his BDS degree in 1981 and MDS degree in 1985 from Madras University. Being an active academician, he has been teaching both UG and PG students for more than 35 years. At present he is Professor Emeritus, Department of Periodontics – Faculty of Dentistry – Meenakshi Academy of Higher Education and Research. He is a life member of Indian Society of Periodontology. He is also a life member of Indian Dental Association and has served as President for its Madras branch. He has been a research guide for many Postgraduate students and has numerous scientific publications to his credit.

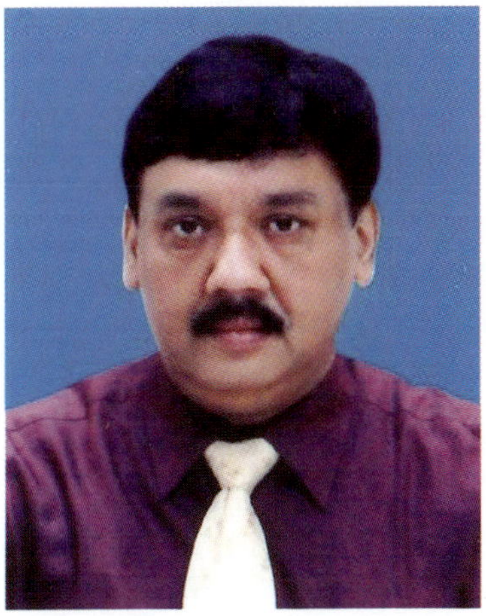

Dr Dilip G Naik obtained his BDS in 1983 and MDS in Periodontology in 1986 from Manipal College of Dental Sciences, Manipal. He is a founder staff of Manipal College of Dental Sciences, Mangalore, having joined in 1987. At present, he is the Pro Vice Chancellor MAHE, Mangalore Campus, Former Professor, Department of Periodontology, Manipal College of Dental Sciences, Mangalore; Manipal Academy of Higher Education (MAHE). He had a stint of 8 years at the Al-Arab Medical University, Benghazi, Libya. He obtained a certificate in Oral Implantology from Manipal University in the year 2000. He has undergone training in Oral Implantology at Germany. He has been a keynote speaker at several national and international conferences. He has over 40 national and international publications to his credit. He has conducted 12 national and international multicentric clinical trials. He was the Vice President of Indian Society of Periodontology for 2 consecutive years.

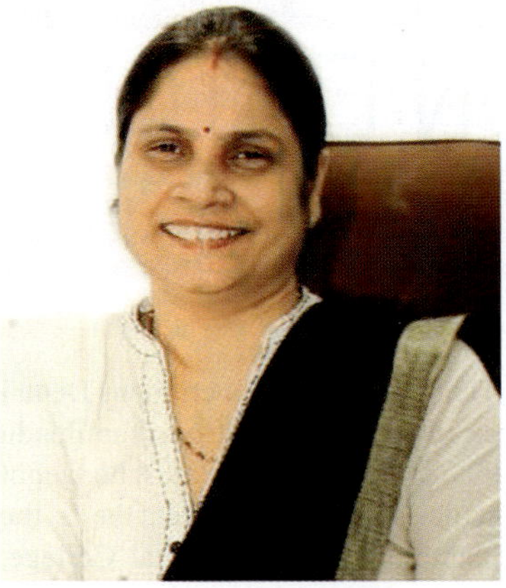

Dr Ashita Uppoor graduated from Nair Dental College, Bombay in 1988 and went on to do her MDS in Periodontology in 1994 from Manipal College of Dental Sciences, Manipal. Later, she joined Manipal College of Dental Sciences, Mangalore Manipal Academy of Higher Education (MAHE) as an assistant professor. At present she is the Dean and Professor of Periodontology in the same institution. She has been teaching both UG and PG students for past 28 years. She has to her credit publications in both national and international journals. She was also the editor-in-chief of *Journal of Interdisciplinary Dentistry*.

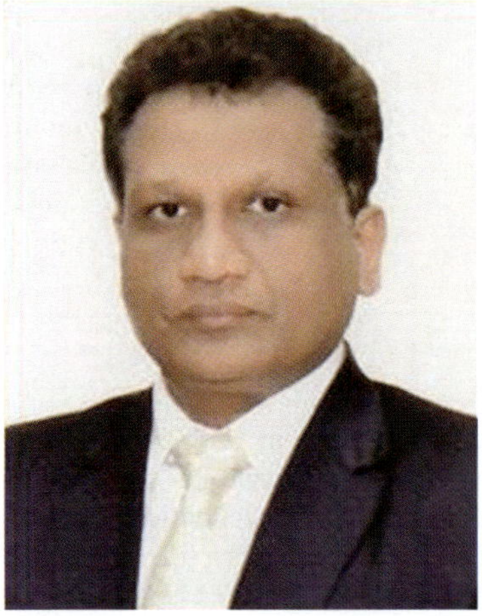

Dr Ashish Jain did his Masters in Periodontology from Nair Dental College, Bombay. Post MDS, he did a Post Doctoral Fellowship at Goldman School of Dental Medicine, Boston University. He did another Fellowship in Implant Dentistry from Harvard School of Dental Medicine, Harvard University, USA. Dr Jain is recipient of Global Scholarship from ITI, Switzerland. He is also an Adjunct Associate Research Investigator at Forsyth Institute, Harvard University and has been an Adjunct Associate Professor at Boston University. Dr Jain has held the post of President, Indian Society of Periodontology. He was Assistant Editor of *Journal of ISP* and Founder Vice-President of Academy of Oral Implantologists. Dr Jain has been Editor of *Dentistry India*, official publication of Dental Council of India. He has been awarded Dr ML Soni Memorial Award in 2004 by International College of Dentists. He has more than 100 publications and lectures extensively at various national and international platforms and has delivered more than 150 lectures so far. He has unique distinction of heading two government dental colleges as Principal – Dr Harvansh Singh Judge Institute of Dental Sciences and Hospital, Panjab University, Chandigarh (2010–2017) and Government Dental Institute, RIMS, Ranchi (2022–23). Dr Ashish Jain is presently working as Director IQAC at Panjab University, Chandigarh. Currently, he is serving as Professor and Head, Dept of Periodontology, Dr. HSJ Institute of Dental Sciences and Hospital, Panjab University, Chandigarh and as the Secretary, Indian Society of Periodontology.

PREFACE TO THE FOURTH SOUTH ASIA EDITION

Ever since the first edition of this classic book authored by Late Dr Irving Glickman was published in 1952, it has remained the "*numero uno*" textbook in Periodontology. Successive editions have been updated in line with the advances in all aspects of periodontal diseases and their management. The current paradigm of Periodontal pathogenesis, reconstruction and regeneration of periodontal tissues, periodontal esthetics, and dental implants have been extensively covered in the newer editions.

The 3rd South Asian edition, which was an adaptation of the 13th edition of Carranza's Clinical Periodontology published in 2019, was a huge success, being widely followed by both undergraduate and postgraduate students in India and other South Asian countries. Apart from very positive feedback, a lot of constructive and valuable suggestions were received which has immensely helped us to improve this edition. This new edition, which is an adaptation of the original 14th edition, is a sincere effort to meet the requirements of the students and faculty within the ambit of the philosophy of the original "Glickman and Carranza."

As an improvement to the third South Asia edition, we have presented this adaptation in a compact printed edition. Additional reading material, newer chapters, references, etc. are available in the online platform associated with this book.

We sincerely hope that this new edition would continue to be the preferred textbook on Periodontology maintaining the tradition of the older editions.

CD Dwarakanath
N Ambalavanan
DG Naik
A Uppoor
A Jain

ACKNOWLEDGMENTS TO THE FOURTH SOUTH ASIA EDITION

It is with immense gratitude I acknowledge the invaluable assistance provided by Dr. Kumari Abhilasha, Consultant Periodontist, in preparing and editing the manuscript files and proof reading prior to the final submission of my chapters in this edition. Besides being extremely talented in computers her deep knowledge of the subject and critical thinking were commendable.

My heartfelt appreciation to my dear friend Dr A V Ramesh, Director, Dental Health Clinic, Bangalore for providing free access to his Library to prepare the manuscript.

Special thanks to my former colleague Dr Joanne Pauline George for her contribution as a co-author for the chapter on Periodontal Plastic and Esthetic surgery.

I am grateful to my former students and now great academicians Drs. Salika Sheikh and Fouzia Tarannum for their constant help in all my academic endeavours.

My wife Rajashree Dwarakanath who has been my life partner for the past 38 years continues to be my pillar of strength with her unselfish love, understanding and care.

My sons Rahul and Rohit, daughter in law Sabrina Rahul and grandson Kiaan are my support and mainstay as I step into my seventies.

CD Dwarakanath

I would like to thank my parents, my wife Ponni and my son Dr Vikram and also express my gratitude to the teaching faculty of the Department of Periodontics, Faculty of Dentistry, Meenakshi Academy of Higher Education and Research (Deemed to be University) for their encouragement. Special thanks to Dr Vijayalakshmi Rajaram and Dr K Anitha Logaranjani for their support and assistance in the editing of relevant chapters.

N Ambalavanan

We wish to acknowledge and express our gratitude to Dr Sangeeta Nayak, Dr Priyanka P Sahu and Dr Vimarsha Achar for their help and support throughout the preparation of the manuscript. We wholeheartedly thank our university Manipal Academy of Higher Education (MAHE) for their unstinted support and encouragement in all our academic endeavors.

DG Naik
A Uppoor

This work like any other, this life, this belonging—DAD only because you gave. In your feet as always and ever. I know you are watching; I know you are blessing. Till we meet again.

A Jain

CONTENTS

†Deceased.

PART 3 ORAL IMPLANTOLOGY

CHAPTER 1

Gingiva

JP Fiorellini | PG Stathopoulou | DG Naik | A Uppoor

CHAPTER OUTLINE

Definition and Scope of Periodontology

Definition: Periodontology is the scientific study of periodontium in health and disease.

Scope: Periodontology has experienced many exciting scientific developments related to inflammation and systemic health, demonstrating that inflammation may link periodontal diseases to other chronic conditions (e.g., heart disease, diabetes). In addition, periodontology continues to bring clinical advancements in reconstruction of oral hard and soft tissue as well as continued development of dental implants to the profession.

Periodontal Phenotype: The term periodontal biotype was first defined by Seibert in 1989 to categorize periodontium into "thin-scalloped," "thick-flat," and "thick-scalloped" biotypes. Other terms such as "gingival biotype," "periodontal morphotype," "gingival morphotype," and "gingival phenotype" were also widely used to refer to the clinical variations in the gingival thickness, the amount of the keratinized tissue width, bone morphotypes, the shape of the tooth, and other morphological characteristics of the gingiva and the periodontium. The 2017 World Workshop on the Classification of Periodontal and Peri-Implant Diseases and Conditions recommended the adoption of the term "periodontal phenotype" to describe the combination of gingival phenotype (three-dimensional gingival volume and the width of the keratinized tissue) and bone morphotype. This classification system categorizes periodontal phenotype into "thin-scalloped," "thick-scalloped," and "thick-flat." Periodontal phenotype is considered as the combination of the gingival phenotype and bone morphotype. Phenotype is influenced by a combination of genetic traits and environmental factors. It is important to know that the periodontal phenotype changes over time due to environmental factors or by phenotype modification therapy. The periodontal phenotype may play an important role in disease progressions such as gingival recession and bone resorption. However, further studies are needed to evaluate the correlation between the periodontal phenotype and the therapy outcome.

Oral Mucosa

The *oral mucosa* consists of the following three zones:

1. The gingiva and the covering of the hard palate, termed the *masticatory mucosa*.
2. The dorsum of the tongue, covered by *specialized mucosa*.
3. The oral mucous membrane lining the remainder of the oral cavity.

The periodontium (in Greek "peri" means "around" and "odontos" means "tooth") is a dynamic structure composed of the tissues supporting and investing the teeth. It comprises four principal components which have been divided into two parts:

- Gingiva whose main function is protection of the underlying tissues.
- Periodontal ligament, cementum, and alveolar bone, which comprises the attachment apparatus.

Each of these periodontal components is distinct in its location, tissue architecture, biochemical composition, and chemical composition, but all of these components function together as a single unit. Recent research has revealed that the extracellular matrix components of one periodontal compartment can influence the cellular activities of adjacent structures. Therefore, the pathologic changes that occur in one periodontal component may have significant ramifications for the maintenance, repair, or regeneration of other components of the periodontium.

This section first discusses the structural components of the normal periodontium; it then describes their development, vascularization, innervation, and functions.

Gingiva

The *gingiva* is the part of the oral mucosa that covers the alveolar processes of the jaws and surrounds the necks of the teeth.

Clinical Features

In an adult, normal gingiva covers the alveolar bone and tooth root to a level just coronal to the cementoenamel junction. The gingiva is divided anatomically into *marginal*, *attached*, and *interdental areas*. Although each type of gingiva exhibits considerable variation in differentiation, histology, and thickness according to its functional demands, all types are specifically structured to function appropriately against mechanical and microbial damage. In other words, the specific structure of different types of gingiva reflects each one's effectiveness as a barrier to the penetration by microbes and noxious agents into the deeper tissue.

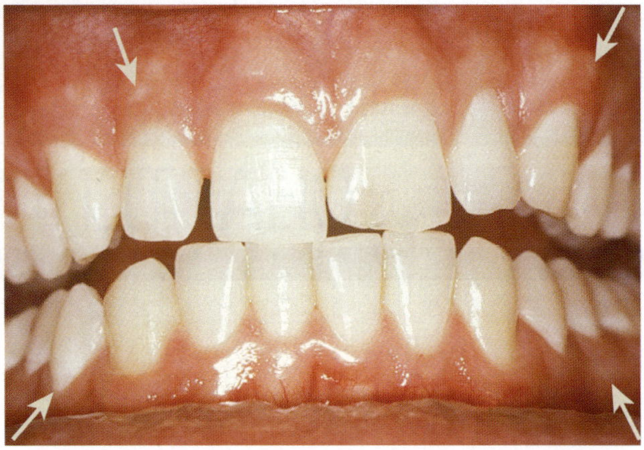

Fig. 1.1 Normal gingiva in a young adult. Note the demarcation (mucogingival line) *(arrows)* between the attached gingiva and the darker alveolar mucosa.

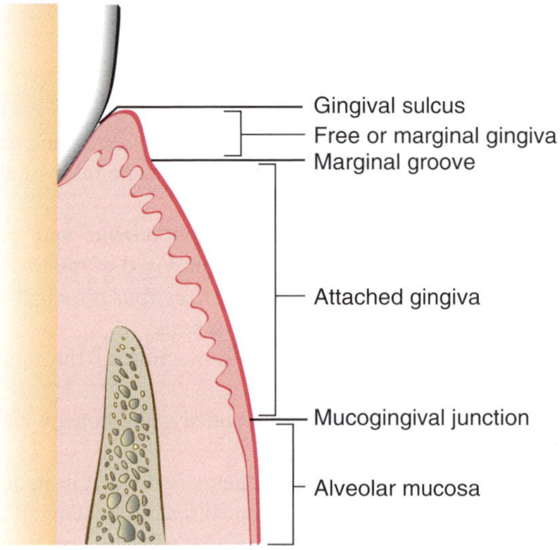

Fig. 1.2 Diagram showing the anatomic landmarks of the gingiva.

Marginal Gingiva

The marginal or unattached gingiva is the terminal edge or border of the gingiva that surrounds the teeth in collar-like fashion (Figs. 1.1 and 1.2). In about 50% of cases, it is demarcated from the adjacent attached gingiva by a shallow linear depression called the *free gingival groove*. The marginal gingiva is usually about 1 mm wide, and it forms the soft-tissue wall of the gingival sulcus. It may be separated from the tooth surface with a periodontal probe. The most apical point of the marginal gingival scallop is called the *gingival zenith*. Its apicocoronal and mesiodistal dimensions vary between 0.06 and 0.96 mm.

Gingival Sulcus

The gingival sulcus is the shallow crevice or space around the tooth bounded by the surface of the tooth on one side and the epithelium lining the free margin of the gingiva on the other side. It is V-shaped, and it barely permits the entrance of a periodontal probe. The clinical determination of the depth of the gingival sulcus is an important diagnostic parameter. Under absolutely normal or ideal conditions, the depth of the gingival sulcus is 0 mm or close to 0 mm. These strict conditions of normalcy can be produced experimentally only in germ-free animals or after intense and prolonged plaque control.

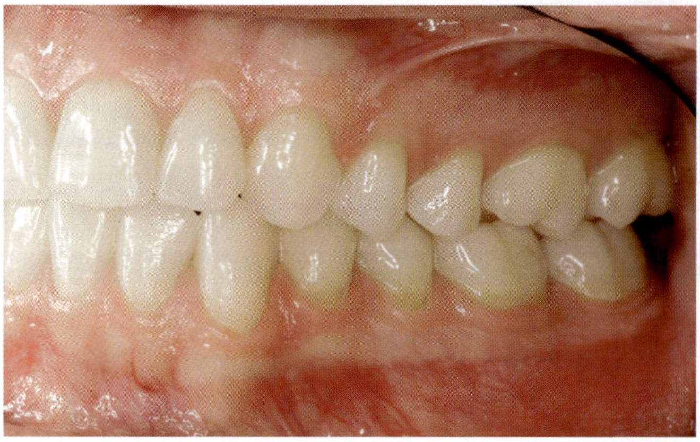

Fig. 1.3 Mean width of the attached gingiva in the human permanent dentition.

In clinically healthy human gingiva, a sulcus of some depth can be found. The depth of this sulcus, as determined in histologic sections, has been reported as 1.8 mm, with variations from 0 to 6 mm; other studies have reported 1.5 and 0.69 mm. The clinical evaluation used to determine the depth of the sulcus involves the introduction of a metallic instrument (i.e., the periodontal probe) and the estimation of the distance it penetrates (i.e., the probing depth). The histologic depth (biologic depth) of a sulcus does not need to be exactly equal to the depth of penetration of the probe. The penetration of the probe depends on several factors, such as probe diameter, probing force, and the level of inflammation. Consequently, the probing depth is not necessarily exactly equal to the histologic depth of the sulcus. The so-called probing depth of a clinically normal gingival sulcus in humans is 2–3 mm. The visibility of the periodontal probe through the gingiva during probing is also a commonly used technique to measure gingiva thickness. If the periodontal probe through the gingiva during probing is also commonly used as a technique to measure gingiva thickness. If the periodontal probe is visible through the gingiva after being inserted in the sulcus, the periodontal phenotype is considered as thin.

Attached Gingiva

The attached gingiva is continuous with the marginal gingiva. It is firm, resilient, and tightly bound to the underlying periosteum of alveolar bone. The facial aspect of the attached gingiva extends to the relatively loose and movable alveolar mucosa; it is demarcated by the *mucogingival junction* (Fig. 1.2).

The *width of the attached gingiva* is another important clinical parameter. It is the distance between the mucogingival junction and the projection on the external surface of the bottom of the gingival sulcus or the periodontal pocket. It should not be confused with the *width of the keratinized gingiva* although this also includes the marginal gingiva (Fig. 1.2).

The width of the attached gingiva on the facial aspect differs in different areas of the mouth. It is generally greatest in the incisor region (i.e., 3.5–4.5 mm in the maxilla, 3.3–3.9 mm in the mandible) and narrower in the posterior segments (i.e., 1.9 mm in the maxillary first premolars and 1.8 mm in the mandibular first premolars) (Fig. 1.3).

Because the mucogingival junction remains stationary throughout adult life, changes in the width of the attached gingiva are caused by modifications in the position of its coronal portion. The width of the attached gingiva increases by the age of 4 years and in supraerupted teeth. On the lingual aspect of the mandible, the attached gingiva terminates at the junction of the lingual alveolar mucosa, which is continuous with the mucous membrane that lines the floor of the mouth. The palatal surface of the attached gingiva in the maxilla blends imperceptibly with the equally firm and resilient palatal mucosa.

Interdental Gingiva

The interdental gingiva occupies the gingival embrasure, which is the interproximal space beneath the area of tooth contact. The interdental gingiva can be pyramidal, or it can have a "col" shape. In the former, the tip of one papilla is located immediately beneath the contact point; the latter presents a valley-like depression that connects a facial and lingual papilla and that conforms to the shape of the interproximal contact (Figs. 1.4 and 1.5). The shape of the gingiva in a given interdental space depends on the presence or absence of a contact point between the adjacent teeth, the distance between the contact point and the osseous crest, and the presence or absence of some degree of recession. Fig. 1.6 depicts the variations in normal interdental gingiva.

The facial and lingual surfaces are tapered toward the interproximal contact area, whereas the mesial and distal surfaces are slightly concave. The lateral borders and tips of the interdental papillae are formed by the marginal gingiva of the adjoining teeth. The intervening portion consists of attached gingiva (Fig. 1.7). If a diastema is present, the gingiva is firmly bound over the interdental bone to form a smooth, rounded surface without interdental papillae (Fig. 1.8).

Microscopic Features

Microscopic examination reveals that gingiva is composed of the overlying stratified squamous epithelium and the underlying central core of connective tissue. Although the epithelium is predominantly cellular in nature, the connective tissue is less cellular and composed primarily of collagen fibers and ground substance. These two tissues are considered separately.

Gingival Epithelium

General Aspects of Gingival Epithelium Biology

Historically, the epithelial compartment was thought to provide only a physical barrier to infection and the underlying gingival attachment. However, we now believe that epithelial cells play an active role in innate host defense by responding to bacteria in an interactive manner, which means that the epithelium participates actively in responding to infection, in signaling further host reactions, and in integrating innate and acquired immune responses. For example, epithelial cells may respond to bacteria by increased proliferation, the alteration of cell-signaling events, changes in differentiation and cell death, and, ultimately, the alteration of tissue homeostasis. To understand this new perspective of the epithelial innate defense responses and the role of epithelium in gingival health and disease, it is important to understand its basic structure and function (Box 1.1).

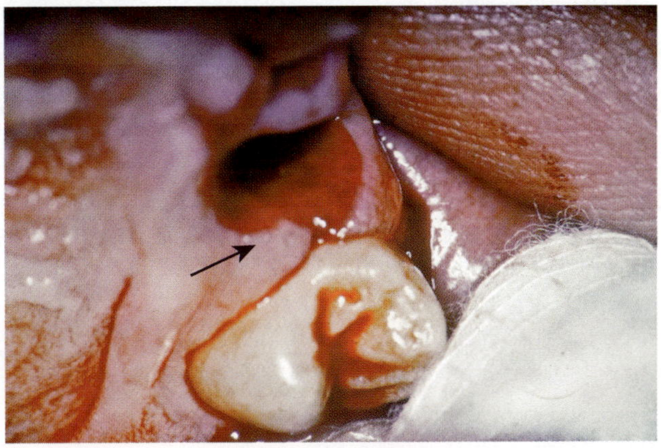

Fig. 1.4 Site of extraction showing the facial and palatal interdental papillae and the intervening col *(arrow).*

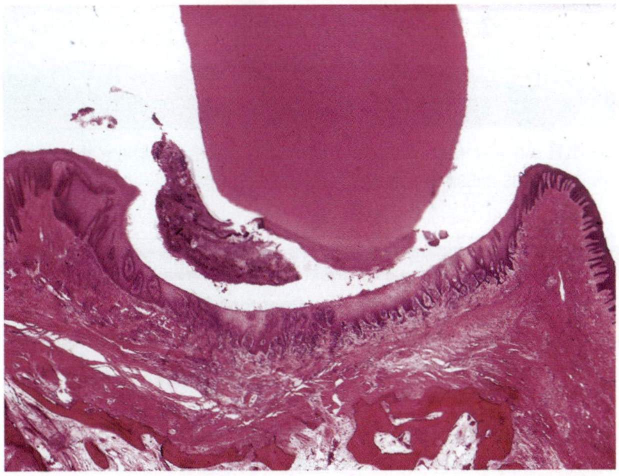

Fig. 1.5 Faciolingual section of a monkey showing the col between the facial and lingual interdental papillae. The col is covered with nonkeratinized stratified squamous epithelium.

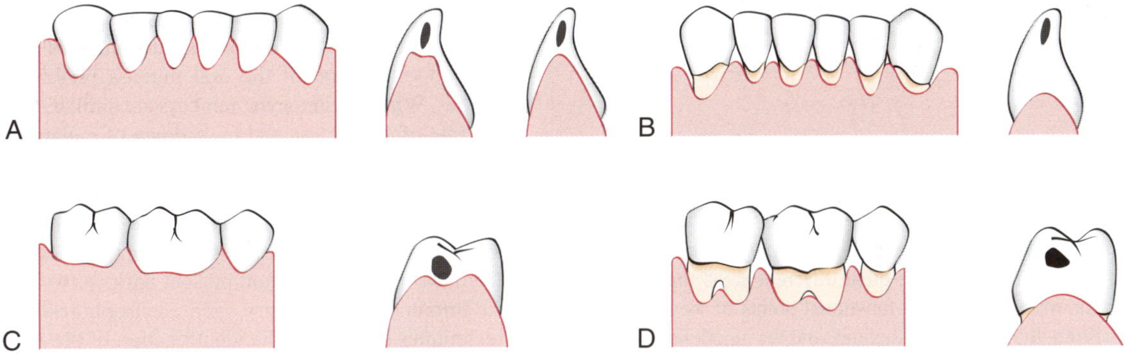

Fig. 1.6 A diagram that compares anatomic variations of the interdental col in the normal gingiva *(left side)* and after gingival recession *(right side).* A and B, Mandibular anterior segment, facial and buccolingual views, respectively. C and D, Mandibular posterior region, facial and buccolingual views, respectively. Tooth contact points are shown with *black marks* in the lower individual teeth.

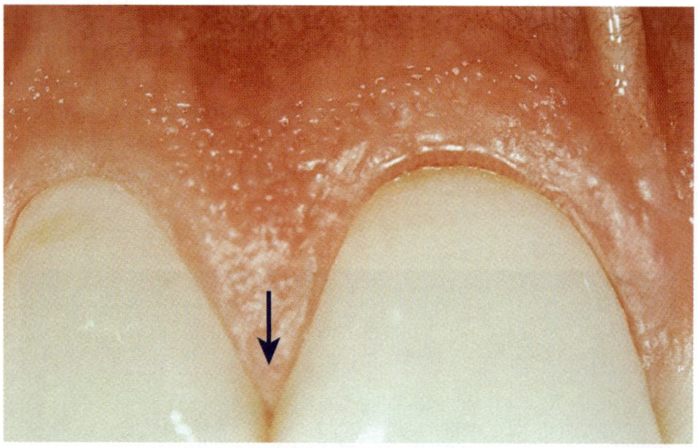

Fig. 1.7 Interdental papillae *(arrow)* with a central portion formed by the attached gingiva. The shape of the papillae varies according to the dimension of the gingival embrasure. *(Courtesy: Dr Osvaldo Costa.)*

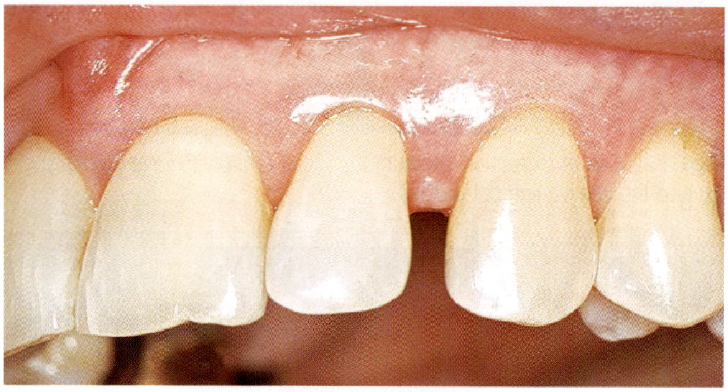

Fig. 1.8 An absence of interdental papillae and col where the proximal tooth contact is missing. *(Courtesy: Dr Osvaldo Costa.)*

BOX 1.1 Functions and Features of Gingival Epithelium

Functions
Mechanical, chemical, water, and microbial barrier
Signaling functions

Architectural Integrity
Cell–cell attachments
Basal lamina
Keratin cytoskeleton

Major Cell Type
Keratinocyte

Other Cell Types
Langerhans cells
Melanocytes
Merkel cells

Constant Renewal
Replacement of damaged cells

Cell–Cell Attachments
Desmosomes
Adherens junctions
Tight junctions
Gap junctions

Cell–Basal Lamina
Synthesis of basal lamina components
Hemidesmosome

Modified from Dale BA: *Periodontol 2000* 30:71, 2002.

The gingival epithelium consists of a continuous lining of stratified squamous epithelium. There are three different areas that can be defined from the morphologic and functional points of view: the oral or outer epithelium, the sulcular epithelium, and the junctional epithelium.

The principal cell type of the gingival epithelium—as well as of other stratified squamous epithelia—is the *keratinocyte*. Other cells found in the epithelium are the clear cells or nonkeratinocytes, which include the Langerhans cells, the Merkel cells, and the melanocytes.

The keratinocyte receives its name because it can synthesize keratin. It constitutes about more than 90% of the cell population.

The main function of the gingival epithelium is to protect the deep structures while allowing for a selective interchange with the oral environment. This is achieved via the proliferation and differentiation of the keratinocytes. The *proliferation* of keratinocytes takes place by mitosis in the basal layer and less frequently in the suprabasal layers, in which a small proportion of cells remains as a proliferative compartment while a larger number begin to migrate to the surface.

Differentiation involves the process of keratinization, which consists of progressions of biochemical and morphologic events that occur in the cell as they migrate from the basal layer (Fig. 1.9). The main morphologic changes include the following: (1) the progressive flattening of the cell with an increasing prevalence of tonofilaments; (2) the couple of intercellular junctions with the production of keratohyalin granules; and (3) the disappearance of the nucleus.

Three types of surface keratinization can occur in the gingival epithelium:

1. Keratinization. A complete keratinization process leads to the production of an *orthokeratinized* superficial horny layer similar to that of the skin, with no nuclei in the stratum corneum and a well-defined stratum granulosum provided by the keratohyaline granules. When the lipid content of the keratohyaline granules merges with the plasma membrane of the cell in the keratinized layer, the granules are no longer present intracellularly (Fig. 1.10). Only some areas of the outer gingival epithelium are orthokeratinized. The other gingival areas are covered by parakeratinized or nonkeratinized epithelium and are considered to be at the intermediate stages of keratinization. These areas can progress to maturity or dedifferentiate under different physiologic or pathologic conditions.
2. Parakeratinization. It is considered to be an intermediate stage of keratinization and is the most prevalent surface area of the gingival epithelium. These areas can progress to maturity or dedifferentiate under different physiologic or pathologic conditions.

In *parakeratinized epithelia*, the stratum corneum retains pyknotic nuclei, and the keratohyalin granules are dispersed rather than giving rise to a stratum granulosum.

3. Nonkeratinization. The *nonkeratinized epithelium* (although cytokeratins are the major component as in all epithelia) has neither granulosum nor corneum strata, whereas superficial cells have viable nuclei.

Nonkeratinocyte cells are present in the gingival epithelium as in other nonkeratinizing epithelia. Melanocytes are cells with dendritic processes and are located in the basal and spinous layers of the gingival epithelium between keratinocytes. They store melanin in organelles called premelanosomes or melanosomes. The color pigmentation of the oral mucosa presents a wide range of shades. While melanocyte numbers are similar, the differences lie in the rate of production and breakdown of melanin.

Langerhans cells are dendritic cells that contain elongated granules (Birbeck granules) and are located among keratinocytes at all suprabasal levels. They belong to the mononuclear phagocyte system (reticuloendothelial system) as modified monocytes derived from the bone marrow and present antigens to lymphocytes.

Immunohistochemistry, gel electrophoresis, and immunoblot techniques have made the identification of the characteristic pattern of cytokeratins possible in each epithelial type. The keratin proteins are composed of different polypeptide subunits characterized by their isoelectric points and molecular weights. They are numbered in a sequence that is contrary to their molecular weight. In general,

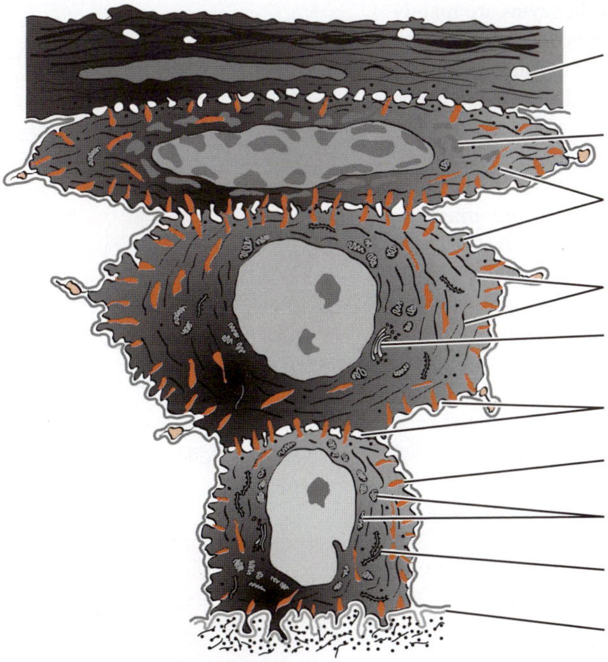

Fig. 1.9 Diagram showing representative cells from the various layers of stratified squamous epithelium as seen by electron microscopy. *(Modified from Weinstock A: In Ham AW, editor: Histology, ed 7, Philadelphia, 1974, Lippincott.)*

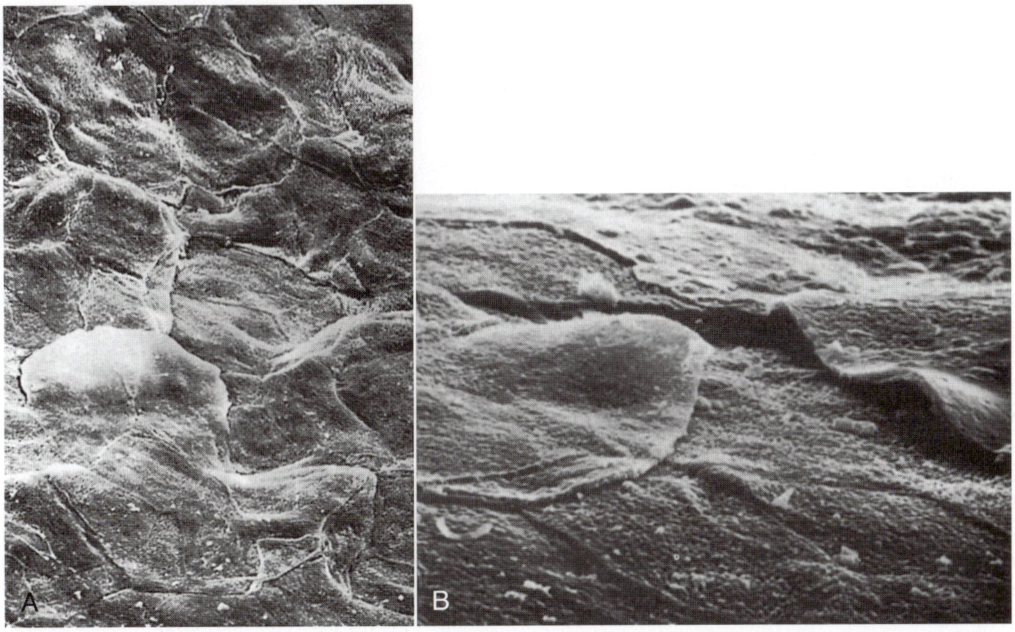

Fig. 1.10 A, Scanning electron micrograph of keratinized gingiva showing the flattened keratinocytes and their boundaries on the surface of the gingiva (×1000). B, Scanning electron micrograph of the gingival margin at the edge of the gingival sulcus showing several keratinocytes about to be exfoliated (×3000). *(From Kaplan GB, Pameijer CH, Ruben MP: J Periodontol 48:446, 1977.)*

basal cells begin synthesizing lower-molecular-weight keratins [e.g., K19 (40 kD)], and they express other higher-molecular-weight keratins as they migrate to the surface. K1 keratin polypeptide (68 kD) is the main component of the stratum corneum.

Cytokeratins are expressed in pairs of acidic and neutral or basic pH and lower and higher molecular weight. Cytokeratins provide shape and structure to individual cells by constituting the cytoskeleton and to cell layers by assembling them into tonofilaments that connect to desmosomes and hemidesmosomes.

Other proteins unrelated to keratins are synthesized during the maturation process. The most extensively studied are *keratolinin* and *involucrin*, which are precursors of a chemically resistant structure (the envelope) located below the cell membrane, and *filaggrin*, which has precursors that are packed into the keratohyalin granules. At the sudden transition to the horny layer, the keratohyalin granules disappear and give rise to filaggrin, which forms the matrix of the most differentiated epithelial cell, the *corneocyte*.

Thus in the fully differentiated state, the corneocytes are mainly formed by bundles of keratin tonofilaments embedded in an amorphous matrix of filaggrin and surrounded by a resistant envelope under the cell membrane. The immunohistochemical patterns of the different keratin types, envelope proteins, and filaggrin change under normal or pathologic stimuli, thereby modifying the keratinization process.

Electron microscopy reveals that keratinocytes are interconnected by structures on the cell periphery called *desmosomes*. These desmosomes have a typical structure that consists of two dense attachment plaques into which tonofibrils insert and an intermediate, electron-dense line in the extracellular compartment. Tonofilaments, which are the morphologic expression of the cytoskeleton of keratin proteins, radiate in brush-like fashion from the attachment plaques into the cytoplasm of the cells. The space between the cells shows cytoplasmic projections that resemble microvilli and that extend into the intercellular space and often interdigitate.

Less frequently observed forms of epithelial cell connections are tight junctions (*zonae occludens*), in which the membranes of the adjoining cells are thought to be fused. They are found in the oral gingival epithelium in the uppermost layers. Tight junctions are formed by claudin and occluding proteins and seal the epithelium from the passage of fluids and solubles. Gap junctions are small pores that exist between cells that allow ions and small molecules to pass from one cell to another. Connexin is found in prickle cells of the sulcular epithelium, oral gingival epithelium, and junctional epithelium. The most frequent type of cell–cell connection in the gingiva are adherens junctions (zonula adherens) through homodimers of E-cadherin, P-cadherin, and α-catenin. Evidence suggests that these structures allow ions and small molecules to pass from one cell to another.

Cytoplasmic organelle concentration varies among different epithelial strata. Mitochondria are more numerous in deeper strata and decrease toward the surface of the cell.

Accordingly, the histochemical demonstration of succinic dehydrogenase, nicotinamide adenine dinucleotide, cytochrome oxidase, and other mitochondrial enzymes reveals a more active tricarboxylic cycle in basal and parabasal cells, in which the proximity of the blood supply facilitates energy production through aerobic glycolysis.

Conversely, enzymes of the pentose shunt (an alternative pathway of glycolysis), such as glucose-6-phosphatase, increase their activity toward the surface. This pathway produces a larger amount of intermediate products for the production of ribonucleic acid (RNA), which in turn can be used for the synthesis of keratinization proteins. This histochemical pattern is in accordance with the increased volume and the amount of tonofilaments observed in cells reaching the surface; the intensity of the activity is proportional to the degree of differentiation.

The uppermost cells of the stratum spinosum contain numerous dense granules called *keratinosomes* or *Odland bodies*, which are modified lysosomes. They contain a large amount of acid phosphatase, an enzyme involved in the destruction of organelle membranes, which occurs suddenly between the granulosum and corneum strata and during the intercellular cementation of cornified cells. Thus, acid phosphatase is another enzyme that is closely related to the degree of keratinization. Nonkeratinocyte cells are present in gingival epithelium as in other malpighian epithelia. *Melanocytes* are dendritic cells located in the basal and spinous layers of the gingival epithelium. They synthesize melanin in organelles called *premelanosomes* or *melanosomes* (Fig. 1.11). These contain tyrosinase, which hydroxylates tyrosine to dihydroxyphenylalanine (dopa), which in turn is progressively converted to melanin. Melanin granules are phagocytozed and contained within other cells of the epithelium and connective tissue called melanophages or melanophores.

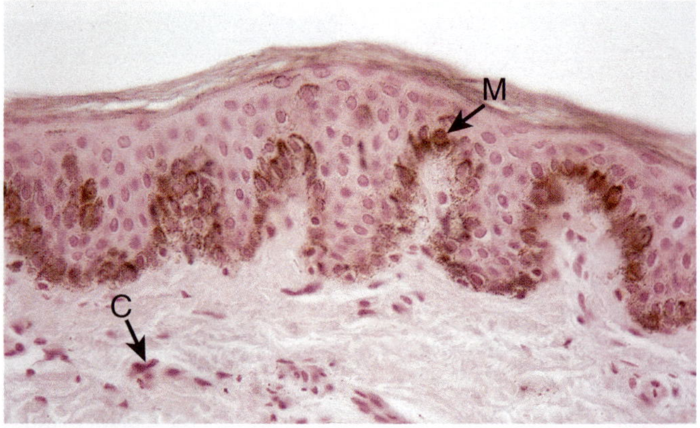

Fig. 1.11 Pigmented gingiva of dog showing melanocytes *(M)* in the basal epithelial layer and melanophores *(C)* in the connective tissue (Glucksman technique).

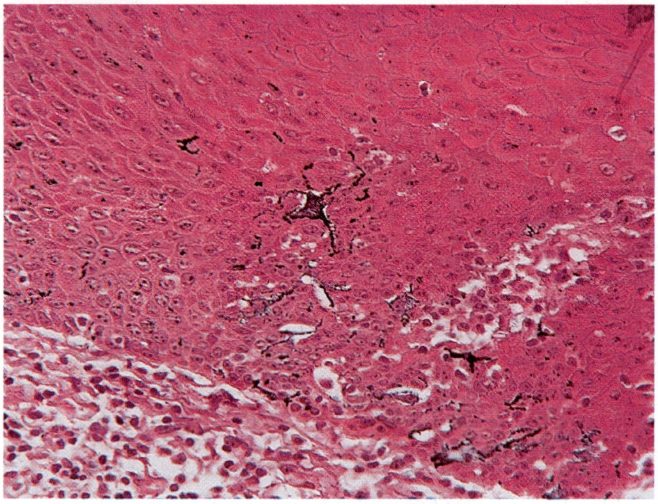

Fig. 1.12 Human gingival epithelium, oral aspect. Immunoperoxidase technique showing Langerhans cells.

Langerhans cells are dendritic cells located among keratinocytes at all suprabasal levels (Fig. 1.12). They belong to the mononuclear phagocyte system (reticuloendothelial system) as modified monocytes derived from the bone marrow. They contain elongated granules, and they are considered macrophages with possible antigenic properties. Langerhans cells have an important role in the immune reaction as antigen-presenting cells for lymphocytes. They contain g-specific granules (Birbeck granules), and they have marked adenosine triphosphatase activity. They are found in the oral epithelium of normal gingiva and in smaller amounts in the sulcular epithelium; they are probably absent from the junctional epithelium of normal gingiva.

Merkel cells are located in the deeper layers of the epithelium; they harbor nerve endings, and they are connected to adjacent cells by desmosomes. They have been identified as tactile perceptors.

The epithelium is joined to the underlying connective tissue by a *basal lamina* 300–400 Å thick and lying approximately 400 Å beneath the epithelial basal layer. The terms "basal lamina" and "basement membrane" refer to the same structure. "Basal lamina" is used in conjunction with electron microscopy and "basement membrane" with light microscopy. The functions of this sheet-like structure are to connect tissues that would be separated otherwise and to control the exchange of molecules between tissues. The basal

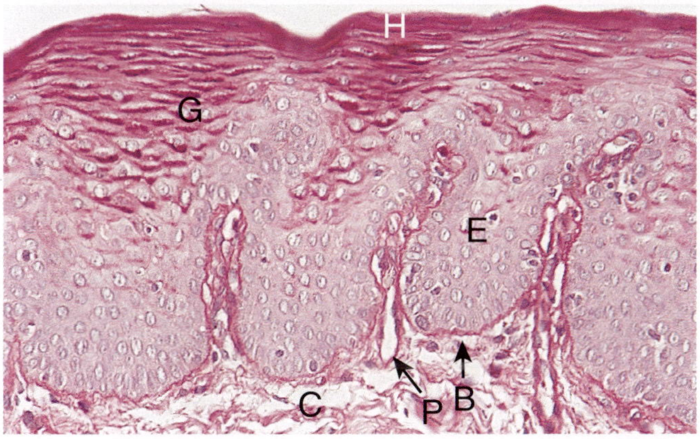

Fig. 1.13 Normal human gingiva stained with the periodic acid–Schiff histochemical method. The basement membrane *(B)* is seen between the epithelium *(E)* and the underlying connective tissue *(C)*. In the epithelium, glycoprotein material occurs in cells and cell membranes of the superficial hornified *(H)* and underlying granular layers *(G)*. The connective tissue presents a diffuse, amorphous ground substance and collagen fibers. The blood vessel walls stand out clearly in the papillary projections of the connective tissue *(P)*.

lamina consists of lamina lucida and lamina densa. The lamina lucida is the zone where integrin $\alpha4\beta6$ interacts with the glycoprotein, laminin (formerly laminin-5). Hemidesmosomes are electron-dense structures embedded in the plasma membrane of epithelial cells, positioned next to the extracellular matrix. Their primary function is to anchor epithelial cells to the basal lamina and to transmit signals from the matrix to the cell. The basal lamina is composed of two layers: the lamina lucida and the lamina densa. Hemidesmosomes of basal epithelial cells are in contact with the lamina lucida, which is primarily made up of the glycoprotein laminin. The lamina densa, on the other hand, is composed of type IV collagen.

The basal lamina, which is clearly distinguishable at the ultrastructural level, is connected to a reticular condensation of the underlying connective tissue fibrils (mainly collagen type IV) by the anchoring fibrils. Anchoring fibrils have been measured at 750 nm in length from their epithelial end to their connective tissue end, where they appear to form loops around collagen fibers. The complex of basal lamina and fibrils is the periodic acid–Schiff–positive and argyrophilic line observed at the optical level (Fig. 1.13). The basal lamina is permeable to fluids, but it acts as a barrier to particulate matter.

Structural and Metabolic Characteristics of Different Areas of Gingival Epithelium

The epithelial component of the gingiva shows regional morphologic variations that reflect tissue adaptation to the tooth and alveolar bone. These variations include the oral epithelium, the sulcular epithelium, and the junctional epithelium. Whereas the oral epithelium and the sulcular epithelium are largely protective in function, the junctional epithelium serves many more roles and is of considerable importance in the regulation of tissue health. It is now recognized that epithelial cells are not "passive bystanders" in the gingival tissues; rather, they are metabolically active and capable of reacting to external stimuli by synthesizing a number of cytokines, adhesion molecules, growth factors, and enzymes.

The degree of gingival keratinization diminishes with age and the onset of menopause, but it is not necessarily related to the different phases of the menstrual cycle. Keratinization of the oral mucosa varies in different areas in the following order: palate (most keratinized), gingiva, ventral aspect of the tongue, and cheek (least keratinized).

Keratins K1, K2, and K10 through K12, which are specific to epidermal-type differentiation, are immunohistochemically expressed with high intensity in orthokeratinized areas and with less intensity in parakeratinized areas. K6 and K16, which are characteristic of highly proliferative epithelia, and K5 and K14, which are stratification-specific cytokeratins, are also present. Parakeratinized areas express K19, which is usually absent from orthokeratinized normal epithelia.

In keeping with the complete or almost-complete maturation, histoenzyme reactions for acid phosphatase and pentose-shunt enzymes are very strong.

Glycogen can accumulate intracellularly when it is not completely degraded by any of the glycolytic pathways. Thus, its concentration in normal gingiva is inversely related to the degree of keratinization and inflammation.

Oral (Outer) Epithelium

The oral or outer epithelium covers the crest and outer surface of the marginal gingiva and the surface of the attached gingiva. On average, the oral epithelium is 0.2–0.3 mm in thickness. It is keratinized or parakeratinized, or it may present various combinations of these conditions (Fig. 1.14). The prevalent surface, however, is parakeratinized. The oral epithelium is composed of four layers: stratum basale (basal layer), stratum spinosum (prickle cell layer), stratum granulosum (granular layer), and stratum corneum (cornified layer).

Sulcular Epithelium

The sulcular epithelium lines the gingival sulcus (Fig. 1.15). It is a thin, nonkeratinized stratified squamous epithelium without rete pegs, and it extends from the coronal limit of the junctional epithelium to the crest of the gingival margin (Fig. 1.16). It usually shows many cells with hydropic degeneration.

As with other nonkeratinized epithelia, the sulcular epithelium lacks granulosum and corneum strata and K1, K2, and K10 through K12 cytokeratins, but it contains K4 and K13, the so-called "esophageal-type cytokeratins." It also expresses K19, and it normally does not contain Merkel cells.

Histochemical studies of enzymes have consistently revealed a lower degree of activity in the sulcular than in the outer epithelium, particularly in the case of enzymes related to keratinization. Glucose-6-phosphate dehydrogenase expresses a faint and homogeneous reaction in all strata, unlike the increasing gradient toward the surface observed in cornified epithelia. Acid phosphatase staining is negative although lysosomes have been described in exfoliated cells.

Despite these morphologic and chemical characteristics, the sulcular epithelium has the potential to keratinize if it is reflected and exposed to the oral cavity or if the bacterial flora of the sulcus is totally eliminated. Conversely, the outer epithelium loses its keratinization when it is placed in contact with the tooth. These findings suggest that the local irritation of the sulcus prevents sulcular keratinization.

The sulcular epithelium is extremely important; it may act as a semipermeable membrane through which injurious bacterial products pass into the gingiva and through which tissue fluid from the gingiva seeps into the sulcus. Unlike the junctional epithelium, however, the sulcular epithelium is not heavily infiltrated by polymorphonuclear neutrophil leukocytes, and it appears to be less permeable.

Junctional Epithelium

The junctional epithelium consists of a collar-like band of stratified squamous nonkeratinizing epithelium. It is 3–4 layers thick in early life, but the number of layers increases with age to 10 or even

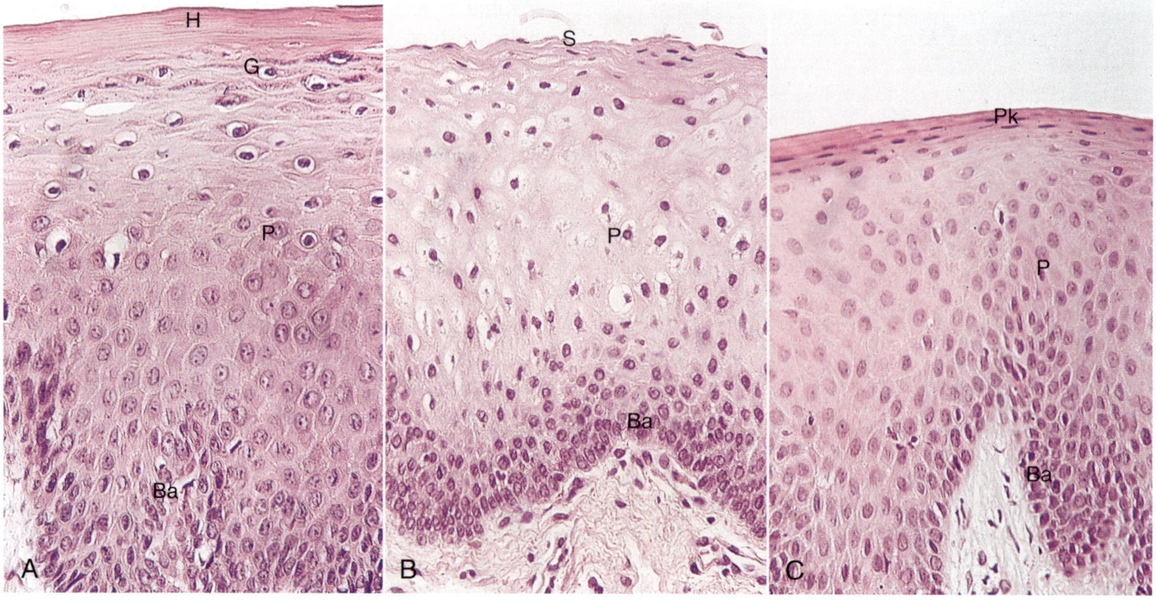

Fig. 1.14 Variations in the gingival epithelium. A, Keratinized. B, Nonkeratinized. C, Parakeratinized. Horny layer *(H)*, granular layer *(G)*, prickle cell layer *(P)*, basal cell layer *(Ba)*, flattened surface cells *(S)*, and parakeratotic layer *(Pk)*.

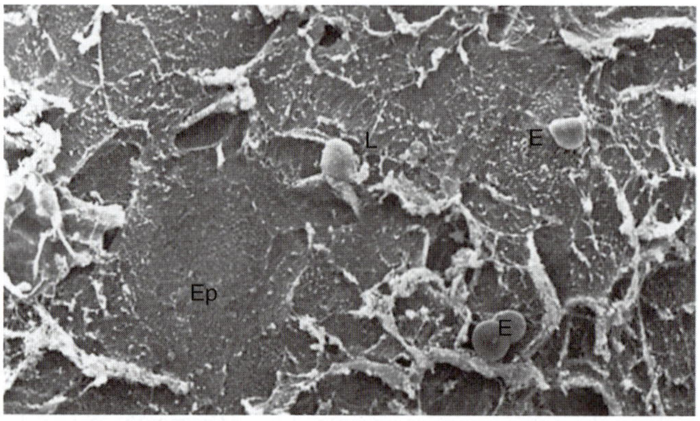

Fig. 1.15 Scanning electron microscopic view of the epithelial surface facing the tooth in a normal human gingival sulcus. The epithelium *(Ep)* shows desquamating cells, some scattered erythrocytes *(E)*, and a few emerging leukocytes *(L)* (×1000).

20 layers. In addition, the junctional epithelium tapers from its coronal end, which may be 10–29 cells wide to 1–2 cells wide at its apical termination, which is located at the cementoenamel junction in healthy tissue. These cells can be grouped in two strata: the basal layer that faces the connective tissue and the suprabasal layer that extends to the tooth surface. The length of the junctional epithelium ranges from 0.25 to 1.35 mm (0.97–1.14 mm).

The junctional epithelium is formed by the confluence of the oral epithelium and the reduced enamel epithelium during tooth eruption. However, the reduced enamel epithelium is not essential for its formation; in fact, the junctional epithelium is completely restored after pocket instrumentation or surgery, and it forms around an implant.

The junctional epithelium is attached to the tooth surface (epithelial attachment) by means of an internal basal lamina. It is attached to the gingival connective tissue by an external basal lamina that has the same structure as other epithelial–connective tissue attachments elsewhere in the body. The internal basal lamina consists of a lamina densa (adjacent to the enamel) and a lamina lucida to which hemidesmosomes are attached. Hemidesmosomes are

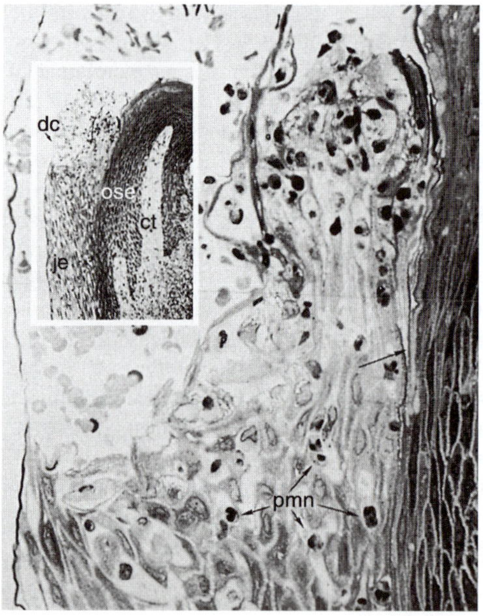

Fig. 1.16 Epon-embedded human biopsy specimen showing a relatively normal gingival sulcus. The soft-tissue wall of the gingival sulcus is made up of the oral sulcular epithelium *(ose)* and its underlying connective tissue *(ct)*, whereas the base of the gingival sulcus is formed by the sloughing surface of the junctional epithelium *(je)*. The enamel space is delineated by a dense cuticular structure *(dc)*. A relatively sharp line of demarcation exists between the junctional epithelium and the oral sulcular epithelium *(arrow)*, and several polymorphonuclear leukocytes *(pmn)* can be seen traversing the junctional epithelium. The sulcus contains red blood cells that resulted from the hemorrhage that occurred at the time of biopsy (×391; inset ×55). *(From Schluger S, Youdelis R, Page RC: Periodontal disease, ed 2, Philadelphia, 1990, Lea SaloniAndamp; Febiger.)*

integrated into the plasma membrane of epithelial cells facing the internal basal lamina and attach the junctional epithelium to the internal basal lamina on the tooth surface. Hemidesmosomes recognize signals from the basal lamina and relay them to the cell for the regulation of gene expression, cell proliferation, and cell differentiation. Hemidesmosomes contain integrin $\alpha 4\beta 6$ receptors that span the membrane as heterodimers and bind laminin-332 with the β6 domain. Hemidesmosomes connect to keratin filaments through plectin, BP230, and Keratins K1, K2, and K10 through K12, which are specific to epidermal-type differentiation, are immunohistochemically expressed with high intensity in orthokeratinized areas, and with less intensity in parakeratinized areas. K6 and K16, which are characteristic of highly proliferative epithelia, and K5 and K14, which are stratification-specific cytokeratins, also are present. Parakeratinized areas express K19, which is usually absent from orthokeratinized normal epithelia. As with other nonkeratinized epithelia, the sulcular epithelium lacks granulosum and corneum strata and K1, K2, and K10 through K12 cytokeratins, but it contains K4 and K13, the so-called esophageal-type cytokeratins. It also expresses K19, and it normally does not contain Merkel cells. Histochemical studies of enzymes have consistently revealed a lower degree of activity in the sulcular than in the outer epithelium, particularly in the case of enzymes related to keratinization. Glucose-6-phosphate dehydrogenase expresses a faint and homogeneous reaction in all strata, unlike the increasing gradient toward the surface observed in cornified epithelia. Acid phosphatase staining is negative, although lysosomes have been described in exfoliated cells.

Cell layers that are not juxtaposed to the tooth exhibit numerous free ribosomes, prominent membrane-bound structures (e.g., Golgi complexes), and cytoplasmic vacuoles that are presumably phagocytic. Lysosome-like bodies also are present, but the absence of keratinosomes (Odland bodies) and histochemically demonstrable acid phosphatase, which are correlated with the low degree of differentiation, may reflect a low-defense power against microbial plaque accumulation in the gingival sulcus. Similar morphologic findings have been described in the gingiva of germ-free rats. Polymorphonuclear neutrophil leukocytes are found routinely in the junctional epithelium of both conventional rats and germ-free rats. Research has shown that, although numerous migrating polymorphonuclear neutrophil leukocytes are evident and present around healthy junctional epithelium, a considerable increase in polymorphonuclear neutrophil leukocyte numbers can be expected with the accumulation of dental plaque and gingival inflammation.

The different keratin polypeptides of the junctional epithelium have a particular histochemical pattern. Junctional epithelium expresses K19, which is absent from keratinized epithelia, and the stratification-specific cytokeratins K5 and K14. Morgan et al. reported that reactions to demonstrate K4 or K13 reveal a sudden change between sulcular and junctional epithelia; the junctional area is the only stratified nonkeratinized epithelium in the oral cavity that does not synthesize these specific polypeptides. Another particular behavior of junctional epithelium is the lack of expression of K6 and K16, which is usually linked to highly proliferative epithelia, although the turnover of the cells is very high.

Similar to sulcular epithelium, junctional epithelium exhibits lower glycolytic enzyme activity than outer epithelium, and it also lacks acid phosphatase activity.

The lamina densa of the internal basal lamina lacks type IV collagen. Recently, basement membrane proteins of the secreted calcium-binding phosphoproteins were identified to attach to the junctional epithelium. The secreted calcium-binding phosphoproteins are a cluster of genes on human chromosome 4 that arose through multiple gene duplication. In the developing tooth, ODAM (odontogenic ameloblast-associated) and amelotin are expressed in maturation stage ameloblasts and form the basement membrane for the maturing enamel. After tooth eruption, the *reduced enamel epithelium* (REE) contributes to the junctional epithelium, and the secretion of basement membrane proteins continues, now serving as the internal basal lamina for the junctional epithelium. ODAM, amelotin, and SCPPPQ1 form a network and create an attachment, specific for interfacing the tooth at the internal basal lamina. The epithelial attachment is mediated by the combination of hemidesmosomes and internal basal lamina. The basal lamina is permeable to fluids, but it acts as a barrier to particulate matter. The external basal lamina is clearly distinguishable at the ultrastructural level and at the optical level as periodic acid–Schiff–positive and by argyrophilic lines. The main difference between the internal basal lamina and lamina densa is in the composition of proteins. Collagen type IV forms a network from tetramers resembling chicken wire. Nidogen and perlecan bind to this network, as well as to laminin-332, to interconnect lamina lucida and lamina densa. The lamina reticularis underneath the lamina densa contains anchoring fibrils (collagen type VII). Anchoring fibrils have been measured to be 750 nm in length from their epithelial end to their connective tissue end, where they appear to form loops around collagen fibers (type I and III) by interacting with type IV collagen. The proteins of the internal and external basal lamina interact within the lamina lucida, lamina densa, lamina reticularis, and the tooth surface to create attachment across different tissues. The attachment of the junctional epithelium to the tooth is reinforced by the gingival fibers, which brace the marginal gingiva against the tooth surface. For this reason, the junctional epithelium and the gingival fibers are considered together as a functional unit referred to as the dentogingival unit. In conclusion, it is usually accepted that the junctional epithelium exhibits several unique structural and functional features that contribute to preventing pathogenic bacterial flora from colonizing the subgingival tooth surface. First, junctional epithelium is firmly attached to the tooth surface, thereby forming an epithelial barrier against plaque bacteria. Second, it allows access of gingival fluid, inflammatory cells, and components of the immunologic host defense to the gingival margin. Third, junctional epithelial cells exhibit rapid turnover, which contributes to the host–parasite equilibrium and the rapid repair of damaged tissue.

The junctional epithelium is attached to the tooth surface (epithelial attachment) by means of an internal basal lamina. It is attached to the gingival connective tissue by an external basal lamina that has the same structure as other epithelial–connective tissue attachments elsewhere in the body.

The internal basal lamina consists of a lamina densa (adjacent to the enamel) and a lamina lucida to which hemidesmosomes are attached. Hemidesmosomes have a decisive role in the firm attachment of the cells to the internal basal lamina on the tooth surface.

Recent data suggest that the hemidesmosomes may also act as specific sites of signal transduction and thus may participate in the regulation of gene expression, cell proliferation, and cell differentiation. Organic strands from the enamel appear to extend into the lamina densa. The junctional epithelium attaches to afibrillar cementum that is present on the crown (usually restricted to an area within 1 mm of the cementoenamel junction) and root cementum in a similar manner.

Three zones have been described in the junctional epithelium: apical, middle, and coronal. The apical zone shows cells with germinative characteristics, the middle zone is of major adhesiveness, and the coronal zone is one of greater permeability.

Histochemical evidence for the presence of neutral polysaccharides in the zone of the epithelial attachment has been reported. Data also have shown that the basal lamina of the junctional epithelium resembles that of endothelial and epithelial cells in its laminin content but differs in its internal basal lamina, which has no type IV collagen. These findings indicate that the cells of the junctional epithelium are involved in the production of laminin and play a key role in the adhesion mechanism.

The attachment of the junctional epithelium to the tooth is reinforced by the gingival fibers, which brace the marginal gingiva against the tooth surface. For this reason, the junctional epithelium and the gingival fibers are considered together as a functional unit referred to as the *dentogingival unit*.

In conclusion, the junctional epithelium has several unique structural and functional characteristics that help prevent pathogenic bacteria from colonizing the subgingival tooth surface. Firstly, the junctional epithelium is firmly attached to the tooth surface, forming a barrier against plaque bacteria. Secondly, it allows gingival fluid, inflammatory cells, and components of the immune system to access the gingival margin. Thirdly, the cells of the junctional epithelium exhibit rapid turnover, which supports the balance between host and parasite and enables quick repair of damaged tissue. Additionally, some researchers have suggested that the cells of the junctional epithelium possess an endocytic capacity similar to that of macrophages and neutrophils, which may provide a protective function.

Development of Gingival Sulcus

After enamel formation is complete, the enamel is covered with REE, which is attached to the tooth by a basal lamina and hemidesmosomes. When the tooth penetrates the oral mucosa, the REE unites with the oral epithelium and transforms into the junctional epithelium. As the tooth erupts, this united epithelium condenses along the crown, and the ameloblasts, which form the inner layer of the REE (Fig. 1.17), gradually become squamous epithelial cells. The transformation of the REE into a junctional epithelium proceeds in an apical direction without interrupting the attachment to the tooth. According to Schroeder and Listgarten, this process takes between 1 and 2 years.

The junctional epithelium is a continually self-renewing structure, with mitotic activity occurring in all cell layers. The regenerating epithelial cells move toward the tooth surface and along it in a coronal direction to the gingival sulcus, where they are shed (Fig. 1.18). The migrating daughter cells provide a continuous attachment to the tooth surface. The strength of the epithelial attachment to the tooth has not been measured.

The gingival sulcus is formed when the tooth erupts into the oral cavity. At that time, the junctional epithelium and the REE form a broad band that is attached to the tooth surface from near the tip of the crown to the cementoenamel junction. The gingival sulcus is the shallow, V-shaped space or groove between the tooth and the gingiva that encircles the newly erupted tip of the crown. In the fully erupted tooth, only the junctional epithelium persists. *The sulcus consists of the shallow space that is coronal to the attachment of the junctional epithelium and bounded by the tooth on one side and the sulcular epithelium on the other. The coronal extent of the gingival sulcus is the gingival margin.*

Renewal of Gingival Epithelium

The oral epithelium undergoes continuous renewal. Its thickness is maintained by a balance between new cell formation in the basal and spinous layers and the shedding of old cells at the surface. The mitotic activity exhibits a 24-h periodicity, with the highest and lowest rates occurring in the morning and evening, respectively. The mitotic rate is higher in nonkeratinized areas and increased in gingivitis, without significant gender differences. Opinions differ with regard to whether the mitotic rate gets increased or decreased with age.

The mitotic rate in experimental animals varies among different areas of the oral epithelium in descending order: buccal mucosa, hard palate, sulcular epithelium, junctional epithelium, outer surface of the marginal gingiva, and attached gingiva. The following have been reported as turnover times for different areas of the oral epithelium in experimental animals: palate, tongue, and cheek, 5–6 days; gingiva, 10–12 days, with the same or more time required with age; and junctional epithelium, 1–6 days.

With regard to junctional epithelium, it was previously thought that only epithelial cells facing the external basal lamina were

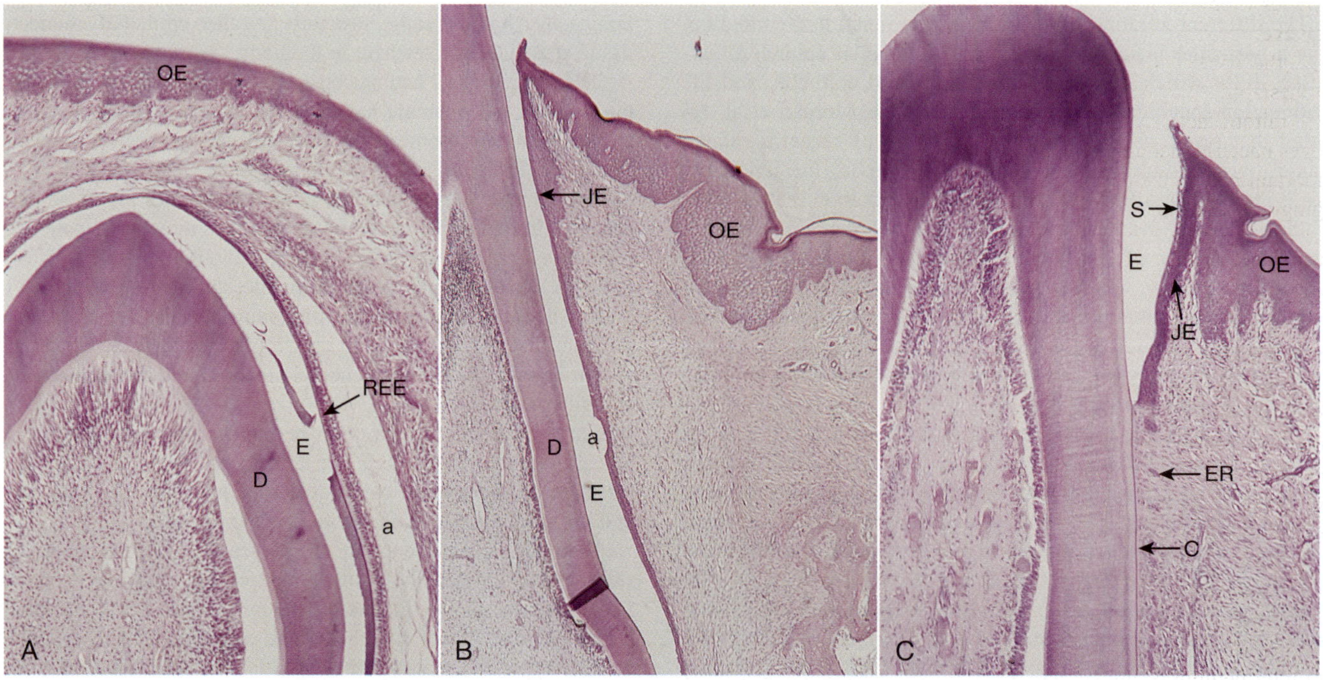

Fig. 1.17 Eruption process in cat's tooth. A, Unerupted tooth. Dentin *(D)*, remnants of enamel matrix *(E)*, reduced enamel epithelium *(REE)*, oral epithelium *(OE)*, and artifact *(a)*. B, Erupting tooth forming junctional epithelium *(JE)*. C, Completely erupted tooth. Sulcus with epithelial debris *(S)*, cementum *(C)*, and epithelial rests *(ER)*.

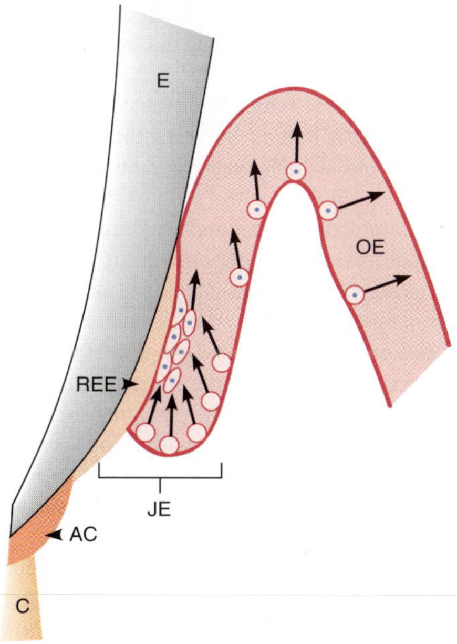

Fig. 1.18 Junctional epithelium on an erupting tooth. The junctional epithelium *(JE)* is formed by the joining of the oral epithelium *(OE)* and the reduced enamel epithelium *(REE)*. Afibrillar cementum *(AC)* is sometimes formed on enamel after the degeneration of the REE. The *arrows* indicate the coronal movement of the regenerating epithelial cells, which multiply more rapidly in the JE than in the OE. *E*, enamel; *C*, root cementum. A similar cell turnover pattern exists in the fully erupted tooth. *(Modified from Listgarten MA: J Can Dent Assoc 36:70, 1970.)*

rapidly dividing. The rapid addition of cells effectively removes bacteria that adhere to the epithelial cells and therefore is an important part of the antimicrobial defense mechanisms at the dentogingival junction. In addition to the role of epithelial cells in microbial shedding, the gingiva produces and secretes small antimicrobial peptides, known as defensins, to maintain bacterial homeostasis. However, evidence indicates that a significant number of the cells (e.g., the basal cells along the connective tissue) are capable of synthesizing deoxyribonucleic acid (DNA), thereby demonstrating their mitotic activity. The rapid shedding of cells effectively removes bacteria that adhere to the epithelial cells and therefore is an important part of the antimicrobial defense mechanisms at the dentogingival junction.

Cuticular Structures on the Tooth

The term *cuticle* describes a thin acellular structure with a homogeneous matrix that is sometimes enclosed within clearly demarcated linear borders.

Listgarten has classified cuticular structures into coatings of developmental origin and acquired coatings. *Acquired coatings* include those of exogenous origin such as saliva, bacteria, calculus, and surface stains. *Coatings of developmental origin* are those that are normally formed as a part of tooth development. They include the REE, the coronal cementum, and the dental cuticle.

After enamel formation is completed, the ameloblastic epithelium is reduced to one or two layers of cells that remain attached to the enamel surface by hemidesmosomes and a basal lamina. This REE consists of postsecretory ameloblasts and cells from the stratum intermedium of the enamel organ. In some animal species, the REE disappears entirely and very rapidly, thereby placing the enamel surface in contact with the connective tissue. Connective tissue cells then deposit a thin layer of cementum known as *coronal cementum* on the enamel. In humans, thin patches of afibrillar cementum sometimes may be seen in the cervical half of the crown.

Electron microscopy has demonstrated a dental cuticle that consists of a layer of homogeneous organic material of variable thickness (approximately 0.25 μm) overlying the enamel surface. It is nonmineralized, and it is not always present. In some cases, near the cementoenamel junction, it is deposited over a layer of afibrillar cementum, which in turn overlies enamel. The cuticle may be present between the junctional epithelium and the tooth. Ultrastructural histochemical studies have shown that the dental cuticle is proteinaceous, and it may be an accumulation of tissue fluid components.

Gingival Fluid (Sulcular Fluid)

The value of the gingival fluid is that it can be represented as either a transudate or an exudate. The gingival fluid contains a vast array of biochemical factors, thereby offering its potential use as a diagnostic or prognostic biomarker of the biologic state of the periodontium in health and disease. It also contains components of connective tissue, epithelium, inflammatory cells, serum, and microbial flora that inhabit the gingival margin or the sulcus (pocket).

In the healthy sulcus, the amount of gingival fluid is very small. During inflammation, however, the gingival fluid flow increases, and its composition starts to resemble that of an inflammatory exudate. The main route of the gingival fluid diffusion is through the basement membrane, through the relatively wide intercellular spaces of the junctional epithelium, and then into the sulcus. The gingival fluid is believed to do the following: (1) cleanse material from the sulcus; (2) contain plasma proteins that may improve adhesion of the epithelium to the tooth; (3) possess antimicrobial properties; and (4) exert antibody activity to defend the gingiva.

Gingival Connective Tissue

The major components of the gingival connective tissue are collagen fibers (about 60% by volume), fibroblasts (5%), vessels, nerves, and matrix (about 35%). The connective tissue of the gingiva is known as the *lamina propria*, and it consists of two layers: (1) a *papillary layer* subjacent to the epithelium that consists of papillary projections between the epithelial rete pegs; and (2) a *reticular layer* that is contiguous with the periosteum of the alveolar bone.

Connective tissue has a cellular compartment and an extracellular compartment composed of fibers and ground substance. Thus, the gingival connective tissue is largely a fibrous connective tissue that has elements that originate directly from the oral mucosal connective tissue as well as some fibers (dentogingival) that originate from the developing dental follicle.

The *ground substance* fills the space between fibers and cells; it is amorphous, and it has a high water content. It is composed of proteoglycans (mainly hyaluronic acid and chondroitin sulfate) and glycoproteins (mainly fibronectin). Glycoproteins account for the faint periodic acid–Schiff–positive reaction of the ground substance. Fibronectin binds fibroblasts to the fibers and many other components of the intercellular matrix, thereby helping to mediate cell adhesion and migration. Laminin, which is another glycoprotein found in the basal lamina, serves to attach it to epithelial cells.

The three types of connective tissue fibers are collagen, reticular, and elastic. Collagen type I forms the bulk of the lamina propria and provides the tensile strength to the gingival tissue. Type IV collagen (argyrophilic reticulum fiber) branches between the collagen type I bundles, and it is continuous with fibers of the basement membrane and the blood vessel walls.

The elastic fiber system is composed of oxytalan, elaunin, and elastin fibers distributed among collagen fibers. Therefore, densely packed collagen bundles that are anchored into the acellular extrinsic fiber cementum just below the terminal point of the junctional epithelium form the connective tissue attachment. The stability of this attachment is a key factor in the limitation of the migration of junctional epithelium.

Gingival Fibers

The connective tissue of the marginal gingiva is densely collagenous, and it contains a prominent system of collagen fiber bundles called the *gingival fibers*. These fibers consist of type I collagen. The gingival fibers have the following functions:

1. To brace the marginal gingiva firmly against the tooth.
2. To provide the rigidity necessary to withstand the forces of mastication without being deflected away from the tooth surface.
3. To unite the free marginal gingiva with the cementum of the root and the adjacent attached gingiva.

The gingival fibers are arranged in three groups: gingivodental, circular, and transseptal.

The *gingivodental fibers* are those on the facial, lingual, and interproximal surfaces. They are embedded in the cementum just beneath the epithelium at the base of the gingival sulcus. On the facial and lingual surfaces, they project from the cementum in a fan-like conformation toward the crest and outer surface of the marginal gingiva where they terminate short of the epithelium (Figs. 1.19 and 1.20). They also extend externally to the periosteum of the facial and lingual alveolar bones, terminating in the attached gingiva or blending with the periosteum of the bone. Interproximally, the gingivodental fibers extend toward the crest of the interdental gingiva.

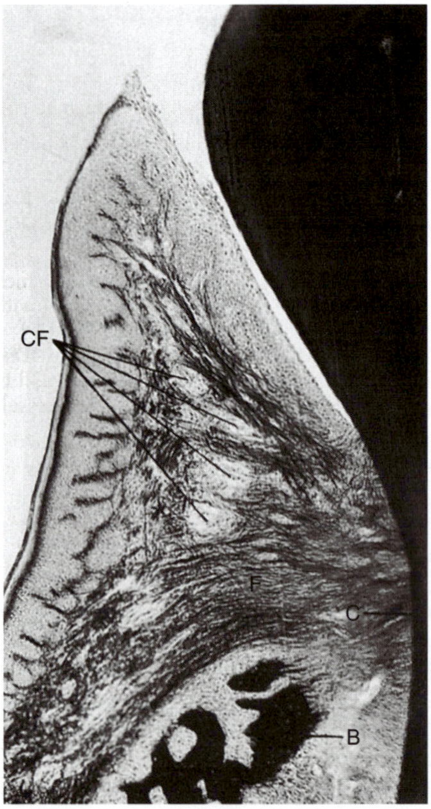

Fig. 1.19 Faciolingual section of marginal gingiva showing gingival fibers *(F)* that extend from the cementum *(C)* to the crest of the gingiva, to the outer gingival surface, and external to the periosteum of the bone *(B)*. Circular fibers *(CF)* are shown in cross-section between the other groups. *(Courtesy: Sol Bernick.)*

The *circular fibers* course through the connective tissue of the marginal and interdental gingivae and encircle the tooth in ring-like fashion.

The *transseptal fibers*, which are located interproximally, form horizontal bundles that extend between the cementum of the approximating teeth into which they are embedded. They lie in the area between the epithelium at the base of the gingival sulcus and the crest of the interdental bone, and they are sometimes classified with the principal fibers of the periodontal ligament.

A group of *semicircular fibers* that attach at the proximal surface of a tooth immediately below the cementoenamel junction go around the facial or lingual marginal gingiva of the tooth and attach on the other proximal surface of the same tooth; another group of *transgingival fibers* that attach in the proximal surface of one tooth, traverse the interdental space diagonally, go around the facial or lingual surface of the adjacent tooth, again traverse the interdental space diagonally, and then attach in the proximal surface of the next tooth.

Tractional forces in the extracellular matrix produced by fibroblasts are believed to be the forces responsible for generating tension in the collagen. This keeps the teeth tightly bound to each other and to the alveolar bone.

Cellular Elements

The preponderant cellular element in the gingival connective tissue is the *fibroblast*. Numerous fibroblasts are found between the fiber bundles. Fibroblasts are of mesenchymal origin and play a major role in the development, maintenance, and repair of gingival connective tissue. As with connective tissue elsewhere in the body, fibroblasts synthesize collagen and elastic fibers as well as the glycoproteins and glycosaminoglycans of the amorphous intercellular substance. Fibroblasts also regulate collagen degradation through phagocytosis and the secretion of collagenases.

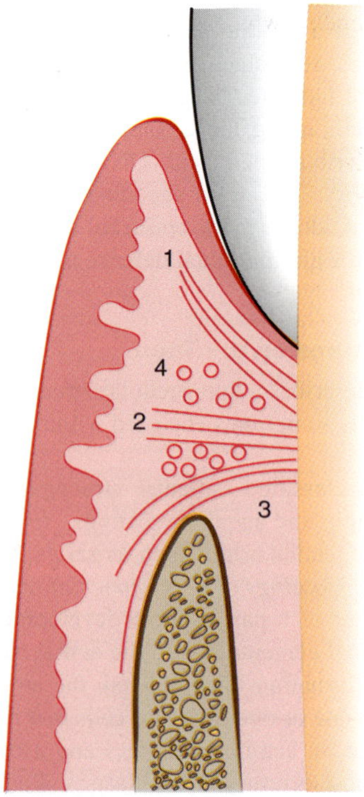

Fig. 1.20 Diagram of the gingivodental fibers that extend from the cementum *(1)* to the crest of the gingiva, *(2)* to the outer surface, and *(3)* external to the periosteum of the labial plate. Circular fibers *(4)* are shown in cross-section.

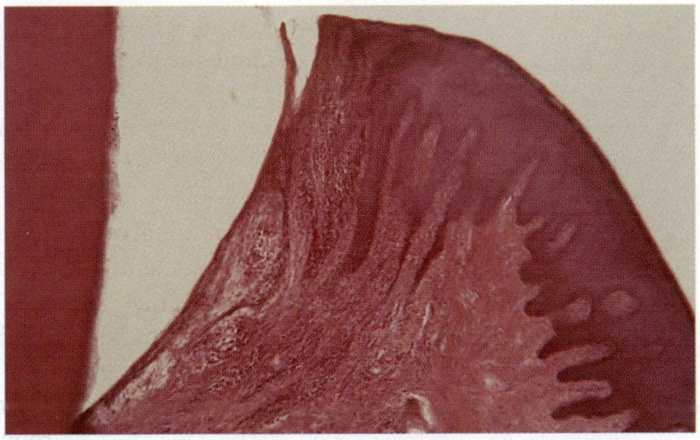

Fig. 1.21 Section of clinically normal gingiva showing some degree of inflammation, which is almost always present near the base of the sulcus.

Fibroblast heterogeneity is now a well-established feature of fibroblasts in the periodontium. Although the biologic and clinical significance of such heterogeneity is not yet clear, it seems that this is necessary for the normal functioning of tissues in health, disease, and repair.

Mast cells, which are distributed throughout the body, are numerous in the connective tissue of the oral mucosa and the gingiva. *Fixed macrophages* and *histiocytes* are present in the gingival connective tissue as components of the mononuclear phagocyte system (reticuloendothelial system) and are derived from blood monocytes. *Adipose cells* and *eosinophils*, although scarce, are also present in the lamina propria.

In clinically normal gingiva, small foci of plasma cells and lymphocytes are found in the connective tissue near the base of the sulcus (Fig. 1.21). Neutrophils can be seen in relatively high numbers in both the gingival connective tissue and the sulcus. These inflammatory cells are usually present in small amounts in clinically normal gingiva.

Speculations about whether small amounts of leukocytes should be considered a normal component of the gingiva or an incipient inflammatory infiltrate without clinical expression are of theoretic rather than practical importance. Lymphocytes are absent when gingival normalcy is judged by strict clinical criteria or under special experimental conditions, but they are practically constant in healthy, normal gingiva, even before complete tooth eruption.

Immunohistochemical studies involving monoclonal antibodies have identified the different lymphocyte subpopulations. The infiltrate in the area below the junctional epithelium of healthy gingiva in newly erupted teeth in children is mainly composed of T lymphocytes (helper, cytotoxic, suppressor, and natural killer) and thus could be interpreted as a normal lymphoid tissue involved in the early defense recognition system. As time elapses, B lymphocytes and plasma cells appear in greater proportions to elaborate specific antibodies against already-recognized antigens that are always present in the sulcus of clinically normal gingiva.

Repair of Gingival Connective Tissue

Because of the high turnover rate, the connective tissue of the gingiva has remarkably good healing and regenerative capacity. Indeed, it may be one of the best healing tissues in the body, and it generally shows little evidence of scarring after surgical procedures. This is likely caused by the rapid reconstruction of the fibrous architecture of the tissues. However, the reparative capacity of gingival connective tissue is not as great as that of the periodontal ligament or the epithelial tissue.

Blood Supply, Lymphatics, and Nerves

Microcirculatory tracts, blood vessels, and lymphatic vessels play an important role in the drainage of tissue fluid and in the spread of inflammation. In individuals with gingivitis and periodontitis, the microcirculation and vascular formation change greatly in the vascular network directly under the gingival sulcular epithelium and the junctional epithelium.

Blood vessels are easily evidenced in tissue sections by means of immunohistochemical reactions against proteins of endothelial cells (i.e., factor VIII and adhesion molecules). Before these techniques were developed, vascularization patterns of periodontal tissues had been described using histoenzymatic reactions for alkaline phosphatase and adenosine triphosphatase because of the great activity of these enzymes in endothelial cells.

In experimental animals, perfusion with India ink also was used to study vascular distribution. The injection and subsequent demonstration of peroxidase allow for blood vessel identification and permeability studies. The periodic acid–Schiff reaction also outlines vascular walls by revealing a positive line in the basal membrane. Endothelial cells express 5-nucleotidase activity as well. Scanning electron microscopy can be used after the injection of plastic into the vessels through the carotid artery, which is followed by the corrosion of the soft tissues. In addition, laser Doppler flow measurement provides a noninvasive means for the observation of blood flow modifications related to disease. Speculations about whether small amounts of leukocytes should be considered a normal component of the gingiva or an incipient inflammatory infiltrate without clinical expression are of theoretic rather than practical importance. Lymphocytes are absent when gingival normalcy is judged by strict clinical criteria or under special experimental conditions, but they are practically constant in healthy, normal gingiva, even before complete tooth eruption. Immunohistochemical studies involving monoclonal antibodies have identified the different lymphocyte subpopulations. The infiltrate in the area below the junctional epithelium of healthy gingiva in newly erupted teeth in children is mainly composed of T lymphocytes (helper, cytotoxic, suppressor, and natural killer) and thus could be interpreted as a normal lymphoid tissue involved in the early defense recognition system. As time elapses, B lymphocytes and plasma cells appear in greater proportions to elaborate specific antibodies against already-recognized antigens that are always present in the sulcus of clinically normal gingiva. Blood vessels are easily evidenced in tissue sections by means of immunohistochemical reactions against proteins of endothelial cells (i.e., factor VIII and adhesion molecules). Before these techniques were developed, vascularization patterns of periodontal tissues had been described using histoenzymatic reactions for alkaline phosphatase and adenosine triphosphatase because of the great activity of these enzymes in endothelial cells. In experimental animals, perfusion with India ink also was used to study vascular distribution. The injection and subsequent demonstration of peroxidase allow for blood vessel identification and permeability studies. The periodic acid–Schiff reaction also outlines vascular walls by revealing a positive line in the basal membrane. Endothelial cells express 5-nucleotidase activity as well. Scanning electron microscopy can be used after the injection of plastic into the vessels through the carotid artery, which is followed by the corrosion of the soft tissues. In addition, laser Doppler flow measurement provides a noninvasive means for the observation of blood flow modifications related to disease.

Three sources of blood supply to the gingiva are as follows (Figs. 1.22 and 1.23):

1. *Supraperiosteal arterioles* along the facial and lingual surfaces of the alveolar bone from which capillaries extend along the

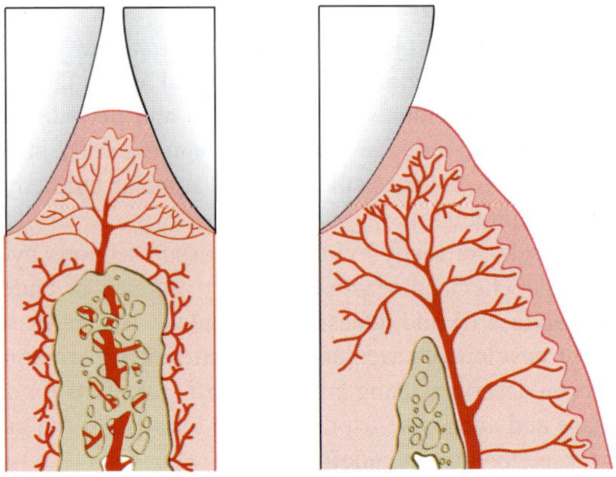

Fig. 1.22 Diagram of an arteriole penetrating the interdental alveolar bone to supply the interdental tissues *(left)* and a supraperiosteal arteriole overlying the facial alveolar bone, sending branches to the surrounding tissue *(right)*.

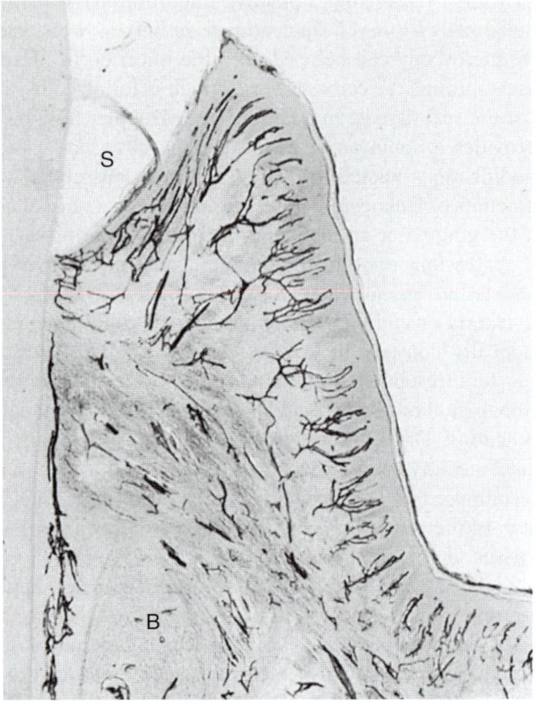

Fig. 1.23 Blood supply and peripheral circulation of the gingiva. Tissues perfused with India ink. Note the capillary plexus parallel to the sulcus *(S)* and the capillary loops in the outer papillary layer. Note also the supraperiosteal vessels external to the bone *(B)*, which supply the gingiva, and a periodontal ligament vessel anastomosing with the sulcus plexus. *(Courtesy: Sol Bernick.)*

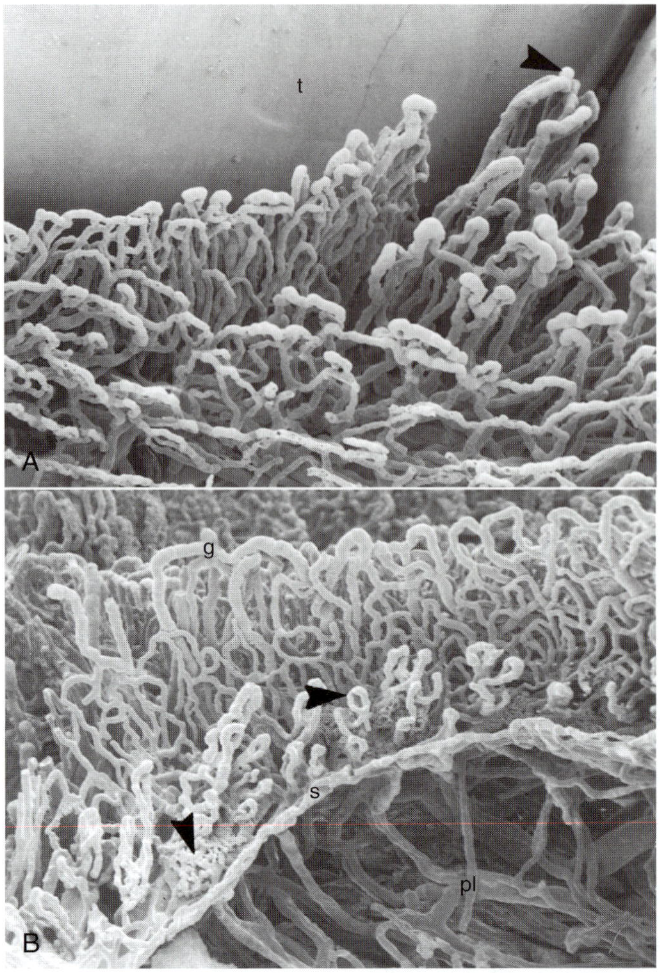

Fig. 1.24 Scanning electron microscopic view of the gingival tissues of rat molar palatal gingiva after the vascular perfusion of plastic and the corrosion of soft tissue. A, Oral view of gingival capillaries: *t*, tooth; interdental papilla *(arrowhead)* (×180). B, View from the tooth side. Note the vessels of the plexus next to the sulcular and junctional epithelium. The *arrowheads* point to vessels in the sulcus area with mild inflammatory changes. *g*, Crest of the marginal gingiva; *s*, bottom of the gingival sulcus; *pl*, periodontal ligament vessels (×150*). (Courtesy: NJ Selliseth and K Selvig, University of Bergen, Norway.)*

sulcular epithelium and between the rete pegs of the external gingival surface. Occasional branches of the arterioles pass through the alveolar bone to the periodontal ligament or run over the crest of the alveolar bone.

2. *Vessels of the periodontal ligament*, which extend into the gingiva and anastomose with capillaries in the sulcus area.
3. *Arterioles*, which emerge from the crest of the interdental septa and extend parallel to the crest of the bone to anastomose with vessels of the periodontal ligament, with capillaries in the gingival crevicular areas and vessels that run over the alveolar crest.

Beneath the epithelium on the outer gingival surface, capillaries extend into the papillary connective tissue between the epithelial rete pegs in the form of terminal hairpin loops with efferent and afferent branches, spirals, and varices (Figs. 1.23 and 1.24). The loops are sometimes linked by cross-communications, and flattened capillaries serve as reserve vessels when the circulation is increased in response to irritation.

Along the sulcular epithelium, capillaries are arranged in a flat, anastomosing plexus that extends parallel to the enamel from the base of the sulcus to the gingival margin. In the col area, a mixed pattern of anastomosing capillaries and loops occurs.

As mentioned previously, anatomic and histologic changes have been shown to occur in the gingival microcirculation of individuals with gingivitis. Prospective studies of the gingival vasculature in animals have demonstrated that, in the absence of inflammation, the vascular network is arranged in a regular, repetitive, and layered pattern. By contrast, the inflamed gingival vasculature exhibits an irregular vascular plexus pattern, with the microvessels exhibiting a looped, dilated, and convoluted appearance.

Microvessels

The role of the lymphatic system in removing excess fluids, cellular and protein debris, microorganisms, and other elements is important for controlling diffusion and the resolution of inflammatory processes. The *lymphatic drainage of the gingiva* brings in the lymphatics of the connective tissue papillae. It progresses into the collecting network external to the periosteum of the alveolar process and then moves to the regional lymph nodes, particularly the submaxillary group. In addition, lymphatics just beneath the junctional epithelium extend into the periodontal ligament and accompany the blood vessels.

Neural elements are extensively distributed throughout the gingival tissues. Within the gingival connective tissues, most nerve fibers are myelinated and closely associated with the blood vessels. *Gingival innervation* is derived from fibers that arise from nerves in the periodontal ligament and from the labial, buccal, and palatal nerves. The following nerve structures are present in the connective tissue: a meshwork of terminal argyrophilic fibers, some of which extend into the epithelium; Meissner-type tactile corpuscles; Krause-type end bulbs, which are temperature receptors; and encapsulated spindles.

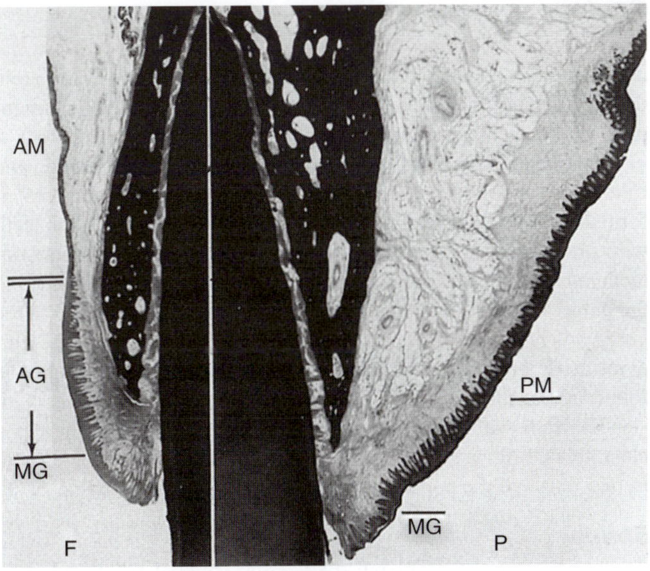

Fig. 1.26 Oral mucosa, facial, and palatal surfaces. The facial surface *(F)* shows the marginal gingiva *(MG)*, the attached gingiva *(AG)*, and the alveolar mucosa *(AM)*. The *double line* marks the mucogingival junction. Note the differences in the epithelium and the connective tissue in the attached gingiva and the alveolar mucosa. The palatal surface *(P)* shows the marginal gingiva *(MG)* and the thick, keratinized palatal mucosa *(PM)*.

Correlation of Clinical and Microscopic Features

An understanding of the normal clinical features of the gingiva requires the ability to interpret them in terms of the microscopic structures that they represent.

Color

The color of the attached and marginal gingiva is generally described as "coral pink"; it is produced by the vascular supply, the thickness and degree of keratinization of the epithelium, and the presence of pigment-containing cells. The color varies among different persons and appears to be correlated with the cutaneous pigmentation. It is lighter in blond individuals with fair complexions than in swarthy, dark-haired individuals (Fig. 1.25).

The attached gingiva is demarcated from the adjacent alveolar mucosa on the buccal aspect by a clearly defined mucogingival line. The alveolar mucosa is red, smooth, and shiny rather than pink and stippled. A comparison of the microscopic structure of the attached gingiva with that of the alveolar mucosa provides an explanation for the difference in appearance. The epithelium of the alveolar mucosa is thinner and nonkeratinized, and it contains no rete pegs (Fig. 1.26). The connective tissue of the alveolar mucosa is loosely arranged, and the blood vessels are more numerous.

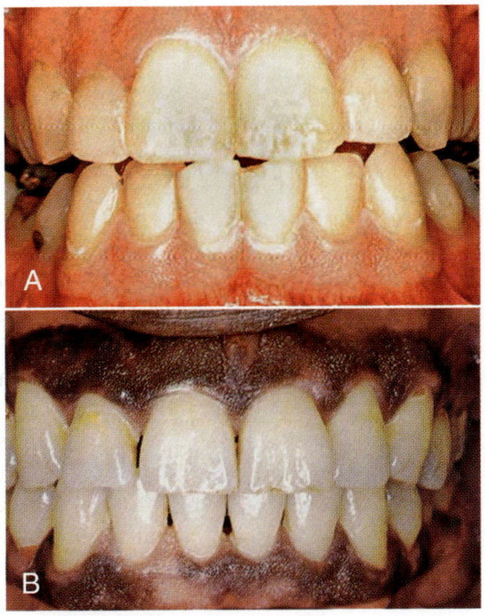

Fig. 1.25 A, Clinically normal gingiva in a young adult. B, Heavily pigmented (melanotic) gingiva in a middle-aged adult. *(From Glickman I, Smulow JB: Periodontal disease: clinical, radiographic, and histopathologic features, Philadelphia, 1974, Saunders.)*

Physiologic Pigmentation (Melanin)

Melanin is a nonhemoglobin-derived brown pigment with the following characteristics:

- Melanin is responsible for the normal pigmentation of the skin, the gingiva, and the remainder of the oral mucous membrane.
- Melanin is present in all normal individuals (often not in sufficient quantities to be detected clinically), but it is absent or severely diminished in albinos.
- Melanin pigmentation in the oral cavity is prominent in black individuals (Fig. 1.25).
- Ascorbic acid directly downregulates melanin pigmentation in gingival tissues.

According to Dummett, the distribution of oral pigmentation in black individuals is as follows: gingiva, 60%; hard palate, 61%; mucous membrane, 22%; and tongue, 15%. Gingival pigmentation occurs as a diffuse, deep-purplish discoloration, or as irregularly shaped brown and light-brown patches. It may appear in the gingiva as early as 3 h after birth, and it is often the only evidence of pigmentation.

Oral repigmentation refers to the clinical reappearance of melanin pigment after a period of clinical depigmentation of the oral mucosa as a result of chemical, thermal, surgical, pharmacologic, or idiopathic factors. Information about the repigmentation of oral tissues after surgical procedures is extremely limited, and no definitive treatment is offered at this time.

Size

The size of the gingiva corresponds with the sum total of the bulk of cellular and intercellular elements and their vascular supply. Alteration in size is a common feature of gingival disease.

Contour

The contour or shape of the gingiva varies considerably and depends on the shape of the teeth and their alignment in the arch, the location and size of the area of proximal contact, and the dimensions of the facial and lingual gingival embrasures.

The marginal gingiva envelops the teeth in collar-like fashion and follows a scalloped outline on the facial and lingual surfaces. It forms a straight line along teeth with relatively flat surfaces. On teeth with pronounced mesiodistal convexity (e.g., maxillary canines) or teeth in labial version, the normal arcuate contour is accentuated, and the gingiva is located farther apically. On teeth in lingual version, the gingiva is horizontal and thickened (Fig. 1.27). In addition, the gingival tissue biotype varies significantly. A thin and clear gingiva is found in one-third of the population and primarily in females with slender teeth with a narrow zone of keratinized tissue, whereas a clear, thick gingiva with a broad zone of keratinized tissue is present in two-thirds of the population and primarily in males.

Shape

The shape of the interdental gingiva is governed by the contour of the proximal tooth surfaces and the location and shape of the gingival embrasures.

When the proximal surfaces of the crowns are relatively flat faciolingually, the roots are close together, the interdental bone is thin mesiodistally, and the gingival embrasures and interdental gingiva are narrow mesiodistally. Conversely, with proximal surfaces that flare away from the area of contact, the mesiodistal diameter of the interdental gingiva is broad (Fig. 1.28). The height of the interdental gingiva varies with the location of the proximal contact. Thus in the anterior region of the dentition, the interdental papilla is pyramidal in form, whereas the papilla is more flattened in a buccolingual direction in the molar region.

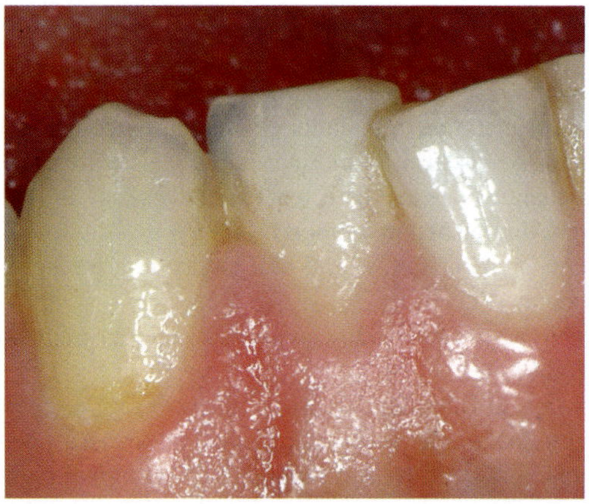

Fig. 1.27 A thickened, shelf-like contour of gingiva on a tooth in lingual version aggravated by local irritation caused by plaque accumulation.

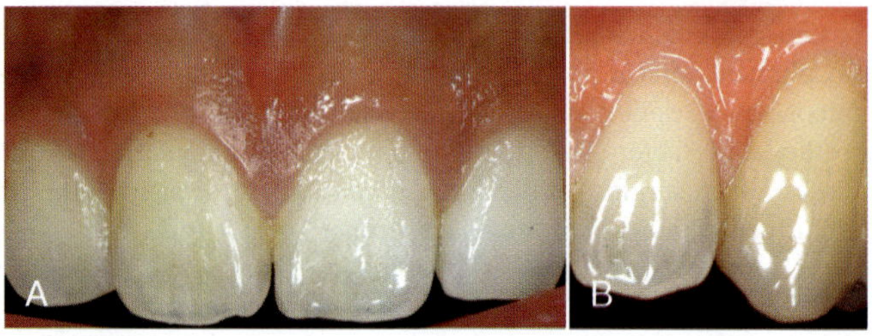

Fig. 1.28 Shape of the interdental gingival papillae correlated with the shape of the teeth and the embrasures. A, Broad interdental papillae. B, Narrow interdental papillae.

Consistency

The gingiva is firm and resilient and, with the exception of the movable free margin, tightly bound to the underlying bone. The collagenous nature of the lamina propria and its contiguity with the mucoperiosteum of the alveolar bone determine the firmness of the attached gingiva. The gingival fibers contribute to the firmness of the gingival margin.

Surface Texture

The gingiva presents a textured surface similar to that of an orange peel and is referred to as *stippled* (Fig. 1.25 and see Fig. 13.12). Stippling is best viewed by drying the gingiva. *The attached gingiva is stippled; the marginal gingiva is not.* The central portion of the interdental papillae is usually stippled, but the marginal borders are smooth. The pattern and extent of stippling vary among individuals and among different areas of the same mouth. Stippling is less prominent on lingual than facial surfaces and may be absent in some persons.

Stippling varies with age. It is absent during infancy, it appears in some children at about 5 years of age, it increases until adulthood, and it frequently begins to disappear during old age.

Microscopically, stippling is produced by alternate rounded protuberances and depressions in the gingival surface. The papillary layer of the connective tissue projects into the elevations, and the elevated and depressed areas are covered by stratified squamous epithelium (Fig. 1.29). The degree of keratinization and the prominence of stippling appear to be related.

Scanning electron microscopy has shown considerable variation in shape but a relatively constant depth of stippling. At low magnification, a rippled surface is seen, and this is interrupted by irregular depressions that are 50 μm in diameter. At higher magnification, cell micropits are seen.

Stippling is a form of adaptive specialization or reinforcement for function. It is a feature of healthy gingiva, and the reduction or loss of stippling is a common sign of gingival disease. When the gingiva is restored to health after treatment, the stippled appearance returns.

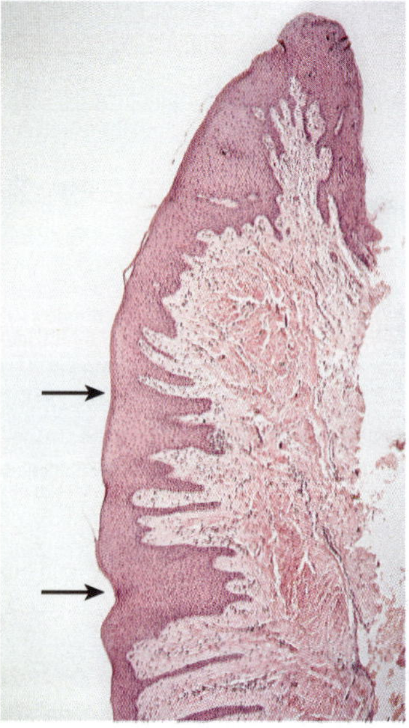

Fig. 1.29 Gingival biopsy of the patient shown in Fig. 2.7 demonstrating alternate elevations and depressions *(arrows)* in the attached gingiva that are responsible for the stippled appearance.

The surface texture of the gingiva is also related to the presence and degree of epithelial keratinization. Keratinization is considered a protective adaptation to function. It increases when the gingiva is stimulated by toothbrushing. However, research on free gingival grafts has shown that, when connective tissue is transplanted from a keratinized area to a nonkeratinized area, it becomes covered by a keratinized epithelium. This finding suggests a connective tissue-based genetic determination of the type of epithelial surface.

Position

The *position* of the gingiva is the level at which the gingival margin is attached to the tooth. When the tooth erupts into the oral cavity, the margin and sulcus are at the tip of the crown; as eruption progresses, they are seen closer to the root. During this eruption process, as described previously, the junctional epithelium, the oral epithelium, and the reduced enamel epithelium undergo extensive alterations and remodeling while maintaining the shallow physiologic depth of the sulcus. Without this remodeling of the epithelia, an abnormal anatomic relationship between the gingiva and the tooth would result.

Continuous Tooth Eruption

According to the concept of continuous eruption, eruption does not cease when the teeth meet their functional antagonists; rather, it continues throughout life. Eruption consists of an active phase and a passive phase. *Active eruption* is the movement of the teeth in the direction of the occlusal plane, whereas *passive eruption* is the exposure of the teeth via apical migration of the gingiva.

This concept distinguishes between the anatomic crown (i.e., the portion of the tooth covered by enamel) and the anatomic root (i.e., the portion of the tooth covered by cementum) and between the clinical crown (i.e., the part of the tooth that has been denuded of its gingiva and projects into the oral cavity) and the clinical root (i.e., the portion of the tooth covered by periodontal tissues). When the teeth reach their functional antagonists, the gingival sulcus and the junctional epithelium are still on the enamel, and the clinical crown is approximately two-thirds of the anatomic crown.

Gottlieb and Orban believed that active and passive eruption proceed together. Active eruption is coordinated with attrition; the teeth erupt to compensate for tooth substance that has been worn away by attrition. Attrition reduces the clinical crown and prevents it from becoming disproportionately long in relation to the clinical root, thus avoiding excessive leverage on the periodontal tissues. Ideally, the rate of active eruption keeps pace with tooth wear, thereby preserving the vertical dimension of the dentition.

As teeth erupt, cementum is deposited at the apices and furcations of the roots, and bone is formed along the fundus of the alveolus and at the crest of the alveolar bone. In this way, part of the tooth substance lost by attrition is replaced by lengthening of the root, and the socket depth is maintained to support the root.

Although originally thought to be a normal physiologic process, passive eruption is now considered a pathologic process. Passive eruption is divided into the following four stages (Fig. 1.30):

Stage 1: The teeth reach the line of occlusion. The junctional epithelium and the base of the gingival sulcus are on the enamel.

Stage 2: The junctional epithelium proliferates so that part is on the cementum and part is on the enamel. The base of the sulcus is still on the enamel.

Stage 3: The entire junctional epithelium is on the cementum, and the base of the sulcus is at the cementoenamel junction. As the junctional epithelium proliferates from the crown onto the root, it does not remain at the cementoenamel junction any longer than at any other area of the tooth.

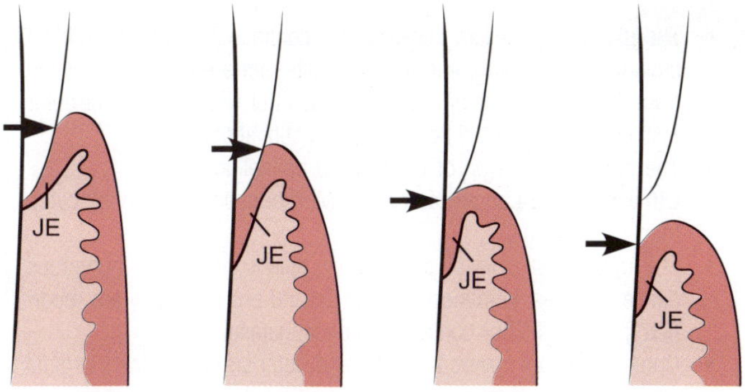

Fig. 1.30 Diagrammatic representation of the four steps of passive eruption according to Gottlieb and Orban. 1, The base of the gingival sulcus *(arrow)* and the junctional epithelium *(JE)* are on the enamel. 2, The base of the gingival sulcus *(arrow)* is on the enamel, and part of the junctional epithelium is on the root. 3, The base of the gingival sulcus *(arrow)* is at the cementoenamel line, and the entire junctional epithelium is on the root. 4, The base of the gingival sulcus *(arrow)* and the junctional epithelium are on the root.

Stage 4: The junctional epithelium has proliferated farther on the cementum. The base of the sulcus is on the cementum, a portion of which is exposed. Proliferation of the junctional epithelium onto the root is accompanied by degeneration of the gingival and periodontal ligament fibers and their detachment from the tooth. The cause of this degeneration is not understood. At present, it is believed to be the result of chronic inflammation and therefore a pathologic process.

As noted, apposition of bone accompanies active eruption. The distance between the apical end of the junctional epithelium and the crest of the alveolus remains constant throughout continuous tooth eruption (i.e., 1.07 mm).

Exposure of the tooth via the apical migration of the gingiva is called *gingival recession* or *atrophy*. According to the concept of continuous eruption, the gingival sulcus may be located on the crown, the cementoenamel junction, or the root, depending on the age of the patient and the stage of eruption. Therefore, some root exposure with age would be considered normal and referred to as *physiologic recession*. Again, this concept is not accepted at present. Excessive exposure is termed *pathologic recession.*

Key points

- The gingiva is the part of the oral mucosa that covers the alveolar processes of the jaws and surrounds the necks of the teeth.
- Gingiva is divided anatomically into marginal, attached, and interdental gingiva.
- Gingival sulcus is the shallow crevice or space around the tooth bounded by the surfaces of the tooth on one side and the epithelium lining the free gingival margin of the gingiva on the other side.
- The clinical determination of the depth of the gingival sulcus is an important diagnostic parameter. The so-called probing depth of a clinically normal gingival sulcus in humans is 2–3 mm.
- Attached gingiva is continuous with marginal gingiva, and it is firm and tightly bound to the underlying periosteum of alveolar bone.
- Width of attached gingiva is the greatest in the incisor region, –3.5 to 4.5 mm in maxilla and 3.3 to 3.9 mm in mandible. It is narrower in posterior segment, –1.9 mm in maxillary and 1.8 mm in mandibular first premolar region.
- Mucogingival junction remains stationary throughout adult life; changes in the width of the attached gingiva are caused by modifications in the position of its coronal portion.

- The gingival epithelium consists of a continuous lining of stratified squamous epithelium, and the three different areas can be defined from the morphologic and functional point of view. The oral or outer epithelium, sulcular epithelium, and junctional epithelium.
- The principal cell type of the gingival epithelium are keratinocytes. Other cells are Langerhans cells, Merkel cells, and melanocytes (nonkeratinocytes).
- The uppermost cells of the stratum spinosum contain numerous dense granules, keratinosomes, or Odland bodies, which are modified lysosomes. They contain acid phosphatase.
- Outer epithelium covers the crest and outer surface of the marginal gingiva and the surface of the attached gingiva. On an average it is 0.2–0.3 mm thick. It can be keratinized or parakeratinized.
- Various layers of stratified squamous epithelium as seen in electron microscopy are stratum basale, stratum spinosum, stratum granulosum, and stratum corneum.
- Sulcular epithelium lines the gingival sulcus. It is thin, nonkeratinized stratified squamous epithelium without rete pegs.
- The sulcular epithelium is very important because it may act as a semipermeable membrane through which injurious bacterial products pass into gingiva.
- Junctional epithelium consists of a collar-like band of stratified squamous nonkeratinized epithelium. It is 3–4 layers thick in early life and increases with age to 10–20 layer thickness. The length of the junctional epithelium ranges from 0.25 to 1.35 mm.
- The junctional epithelium and the gingival fibers are considered as a functional unit, referred to as the dentogingival unit.
- The major components of the gingival connective tissue are collagen fibers, fibroblasts, vessels, nerves, and matrix.
- The types of connective tissue fibers are collagen, reticular, and elastic.
- Gingival fibers mainly contain type I collagen. The different gingival fibers are gingivodental fibers, circular fibers, and transseptal fibers.
- Blood supply of gingiva is mainly by supraperiosteal arterioles, vessels of periodontal ligament, and arteriole, which emerge from the crest of the interdental septa.
- The normal color of the gingiva is "coral pink."
- Stippling is an orange peel appearance. The attached gingiva and core of the interdental papilla have stippling.

Suggested Readings

Ainamo J, Löe H: Anatomical characteristics of gingiva: a clinical and microscopic study of the free and attached gingiva, *J Periodontol* 37:5, 1966.

Bernick S: Innervation of the teeth and periodontium, *Dent Clin North Am* 503:185–205, 1959.

Carranza FA, Carranza FA Jr: The management of the alveolar bone in the treatment of the periodontal pocket, *J Periodontol* 27:29, 1956.

Gottlieb B: Biology of the cementum, *J Periodontol* 13:13, 1942.

Grant D, Bernick S: Formation of the periodontal ligament, *J Periodontol* 43:17, 1972.

Listgarten MA: The ultrastructure of human gingival epithelium, *Am J Anat* 114:49, 1964.

Orban B: Tissue changes in traumatic occlusion, *J Am Dent Assoc* 15:2090, 1928.

Schroeder HE, Listgarten MA: The gingival tissues: the architecture of periodontal protection, *Periodontol 2000* 13:91, 1997.

Selvig KA: The fine structure of human cementum, *Acta Odontol Scand* 23:423, 1965.

Tarnow DP, Magner AW, Fletcher P: The effect of the distance from the contact point to the crest of bone on the presence or absence of the interproximal dental papilla, *J Periodontol* 63:995, 1992.

Ten Cate AR: The development of the periodontium. In Melcher AH, Bowen WH, editors: *Biology of the periodontium*, New York, 1969, Academic Press.

The American Academy of Periodontology: *Glossary of periodontal terms*, ed 4, Chicago, IL, 2001, The American Academy of periodontology, p. 40.

Turesky S, Glickman I, Litwin T: A histochemical evaluation of normal and inflamed human gingivae, *J Dent Res* 30:792, 1951.

Weinmann JP, Sicher H: *Bone and bones: fundamentals of bone biology*, ed 2, St Louis, 1955, Mosby.

Zander HA, Hurzeler B: Continuous cementum apposition, *J Dent Res* 37:1035, 1958.

References

References and MCQs with answers for the chapter are available on www.medenact.com.

CHAPTER 2

Tooth Supporting Structures

JP Fiorellini | PG Stathopoulou | DG Naik | A Uppoor

CHAPTER OUTLINE

Development of the Attachment Apparatus

After the crown has formed, the stratum intermedium and the stellate reticulum of the enamel organ disappear. The outer and inner epithelia of the enamel organ remain and form reduced enamel epithelium (REE). The apical portion of this constitutes the Hertwig epithelial root sheath, which will continue to grow apically and which determines the shape of the root. Before the beginning of root formation, the root sheath bends horizontally at the future cementoenamel junction, thereby narrowing the cervical opening and forming the epithelial diaphragm. The epithelial diaphragm separates the dental follicle from the dental papilla.

After root dentin formation begins, the Hertwig root sheath breaks up and partially disappears; the remaining cells form the epithelial clusters or strands known as the *epithelial rests of Malassez* (Fig. 2.7A). In multirooted teeth, the epithelial diaphragm grows in such a way that tongue-like extensions develop horizontally, thereby leaving spaces for each of the future roots to form.

The role of the Hertwig epithelial root sheath in root development, especially as it relates to the initiation of cementogenesis, has become a focus of research. On the basis of various studies, it is now generally accepted that there is a transient period of the secretion of proteins (e.g., bone sialoprotein, osteopontin, amelin) by the cells of the Hertwig epithelial root sheath. In addition, research shows that growth and differentiation factors may play roles in the development of the attachment apparatus of periodontal tissues. Pluripotent dental follicle cells have been shown to differentiate into osteoblasts, cementoblasts, and periodontal fibroblasts.

Periodontal Ligament

It is a specialized fibrous connective tissue that surrounds and attaches roots of teeth to the alveolar bone. It is also known as *Periodontal* membrane. The periodontal ligament is composed of a complex vascular and highly cellular connective tissue that surrounds the tooth root and connects it to the inner wall of the alveolar bone. It is continuous with the connective tissue of the gingiva, and it communicates with the marrow spaces through vascular channels in the bone. Although the average width of the periodontal ligament space is documented to be about 0.2 mm, considerable variation exists. The periodontal space is diminished around teeth that are not in function and in unerupted teeth, but it is increased in teeth that have been subjected to hyperfunction.

Development of the Periodontal Ligament

Once the root formation begins and outer dentinal layer of root is formed, the periodontal ligament develops. The external and internal enamel epithelia proliferate from the cervical loop of the dental organ to form a Hertwig epithelial root sheath. This sheath is double layered. Due to growth changes, the root sheath is stretched and then it fragments to form discrete clusters of the epithelial cells called "epithelial rests of Malassez." The enamel organ and Hertwig epithelial root sheath are surrounded by a dental sac that is formed by condensed cells. A thin layer of these cells lies adjacent to the dental (enamel) organ. This is known as dental follicle. The cells of the dental follicle divide and differentiate into the cementoblasts, fibroblasts, and osteoblasts. The fibroblasts synthesize the fibers and ground substance of the periodontal ligament. These fibers of the periodontal ligament then get embedded at one end into the newly formed cementum laid down by cementocytes and at the other end into the bone laid down by osteoblasts. When tooth erupts in the oral cavity, these fibers get oriented in a characteristic manner. The fiber bundles of the periodontal ligament gradually thicken after the teeth have been in function for sometime.

As the crown approaches the oral mucosa during tooth eruption, these fibroblasts become active and start producing collagen fibrils. They initially lack orientation, but they soon acquire an orientation that is oblique to the tooth. The first collagen bundles then appear in the region immediately apical to the cementoenamel junction and give rise to the gingivodental fiber groups. As tooth eruption progresses, additional oblique fibers appear and become attached to the newly formed cementum and bone. The transseptal and alveolar crest fibers develop when the tooth merges into the oral cavity. Alveolar bone deposition occurs simultaneously with periodontal ligament organization.

Studies of the squirrel monkey have shown that, during eruption, cemental Sharpey fibers appear first, followed by Sharpey fibers emerging from the bone. Sharpey fibers are fewer in number and more widely spaced than those that emerge from the cementum. At a later stage, alveolar fibers extend into the middle zone to join the lengthening cemental fibers and to attain their classic orientation, thickness, and strength when occlusal function is established.

Early investigators suggested that the individual fibers, rather than being continuous, consisted of two separate parts spliced together midway between the cementum and the bone in a zone called the intermediate plexus. The plexus has been reported in the periodontal ligament of continuously growing incisors but not in the posterior teeth of rodents or in actively erupting human and monkey teeth and not after teeth reach occlusal contact. The rearrangement of the fiber ends in the plexus is supposed to accommodate tooth eruption without necessitating the embedding of new fibers into the tooth and the bone. The existence of such a plexus, however, has not been confirmed by radioautographic data and other studies, and it is considered a microscopic artifact.

The developing periodontal ligament and the mature periodontal ligament contain undifferentiated stem cells that retain the potential to differentiate into osteoblasts, cementoblasts, and fibroblasts.

The structural components of periodontal ligament:

Cellular Elements

1. Synthesizing cells: fibroblasts, cementoblasts, osteoblasts
2. Resorptive cells: fibroblasts, cementoclasts, osteoclasts
3. Epithelial cell rests of Malassez, pregenitor cells, defense cells, such as mast cells and macrophages

Periodontal Fibers

1. *Principal fibers*
   Alveolar crest fibers, horizontal fibers, oblique fibers, apical fibers, interradicular fibers
2. *Other fibers*
   Oxytalan fibers, elaunin fibers, *Ground substance*
   1. Glycosaminoglycans
      a. Hyaluronic acid
      b. Proteoglycans
   2. Glycoproteins
      a. Water
      b. Fibronectin
      c. Laminin

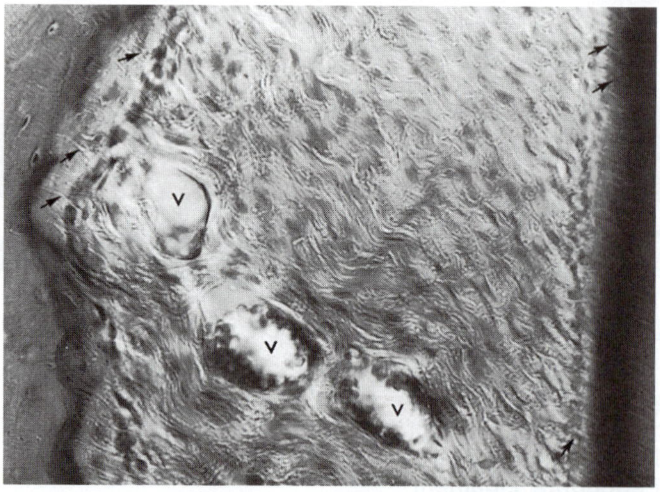

Fig. 2.1 Principal fibers of the periodontal ligament follow a wavy course when sectioned longitudinally. The formative function of the periodontal ligament is illustrated by the newly formed osteoid and osteoblasts along a previously resorbed bone surface (left) and the cementoid and cementoblasts (right). Note the fibers embedded in the forming calcified tissues (*arrows*). *V,* Vascular channels.

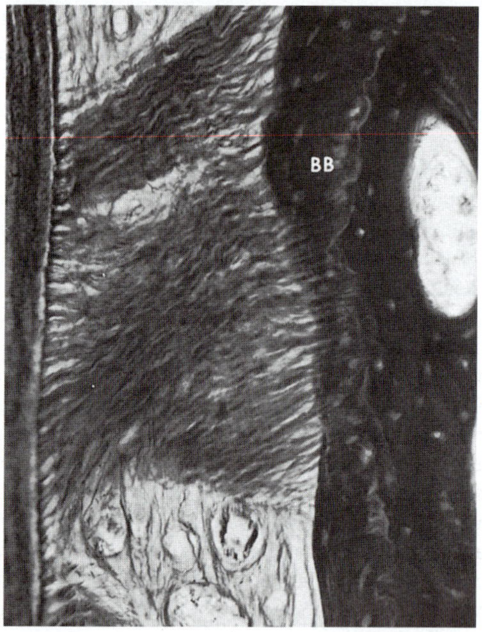

Fig. 2.2 Collagen fibers embedded in the cementum (left) and the bone (right) (silver stain). Note the Sharpey fibers within the bundle bone (*BB*) overlying the lamellar bone.

Periodontal Fibers

The most important elements of the periodontal ligament are the *principal fibers,* which are collagenous and arranged in bundles and which follow a wavy course when viewed in a longitudinal section (Fig. 2.1). The terminal portions of the principal fibers that are inserted into the cementum and bone are termed *Sharpey fibers* (Fig. 2.2). The principal fiber bundles consist of individual fibers that form a continuous anastomosing network between tooth and bone. Once embedded in the wall of the alveolus or in the tooth, Sharpey fibers calcify to a significant degree. They are associated with abundant noncollagenous proteins that are typically found in bone, and they have also recently been identified in tooth cementum. Notable among these proteins are osteopontin and bone sialoprotein. These proteins are thought to contribute to the regulation of mineralization and to tissue cohesion at sites of increased biomechanical strain.

Collagen is a protein that is composed of different amino acids, the most important of which are glycine, proline, hydroxylysine, and hydroxyproline. The amount of collagen in a tissue can be determined by its hydroxyproline content. Collagen is responsible for the maintenance of the framework and the tone of tissue, and it exhibits a wide range of diversity. There are at least 19 recognized collagen species encoded by at least 25 separate genes dispersed among 12 chromosomes.

Collagen biosynthesis occurs inside the fibroblasts to form tropocollagen molecules. These aggregate into microfibrils that are packed together to form fibrils. Collagen fibrils have a transverse striation with a characteristic periodicity of 64 μm; this striation is caused by the overlapping arrangement of the tropocollagen molecules. In collagen types I and III, these fibrils associate to form fibers; in collagen type I, the fibers associate to form bundles (Fig. 2.3).

Collagen is synthesized by fibroblasts, chondroblasts, osteoblasts, odontoblasts, and other cells. The several types of collagen are all distinguishable by their chemical composition, distribution, function, and morphology. The principal fibers are composed mainly of collagen type I, whereas reticular fibers are composed of collagen type III. Collagen type IV is found in the basal lamina. The

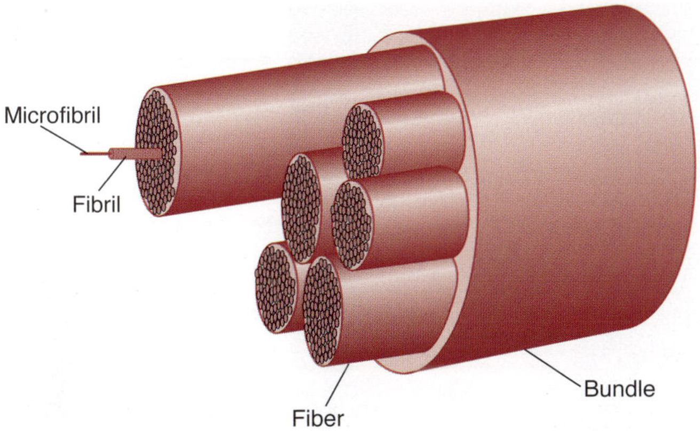

Fig. 2.3 Collagen microfibrils, fibrils, fibers, and bundles.

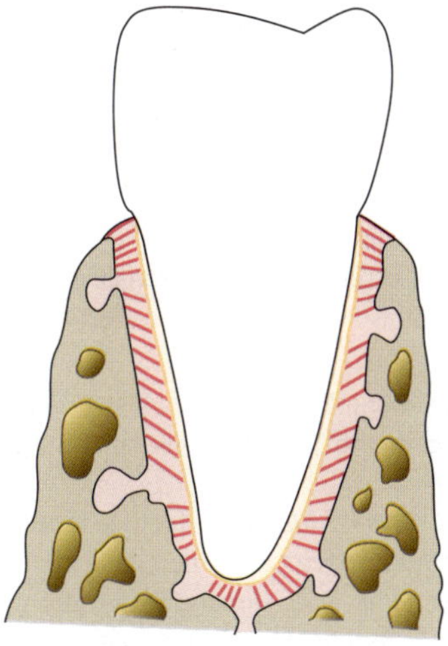

Fig. 2.4 Diagram of the principal fiber groups.

expression of type XII collagen during the tooth development is timed with the alignment and organization of periodontal fibers and is limited in tooth development to cells within the periodontal ligament. Type VI collagen has also been immunolocalized in the periodontal ligament and the gingiva.

The molecular configuration of collagen fibers provides them with a tensile strength that is greater than that of steel. Consequently, collagen imparts a unique combination of flexibility and strength to the tissues.

The principal fibers of the periodontal ligament are arranged in six groups that develop sequentially in the developing root: the transseptal, alveolar crest, horizontal, oblique, apical, and interradicular fibers (Fig. 2.4).

Transseptal fibers extend interproximally over the alveolar bone crest and are embedded in the cementum of adjacent teeth (Fig. 2.5). They are reconstructed even after destruction of the alveolar bone that results from periodontal disease. These fibers may be considered as belonging to the gingiva because they do not have osseous attachment.

Alveolar crest fibers extend obliquely from the cementum just beneath the junctional epithelium to the alveolar crest (Fig. 2.6). Fibers also run from the cementum over the alveolar crest and to the fibrous layer of the periosteum that covers the alveolar bone. The alveolar crest fibers prevent the extrusion of the tooth and resist lateral tooth movements. The incision of these fibers during periodontal surgery does not increase tooth mobility unless significant attachment loss has occurred.

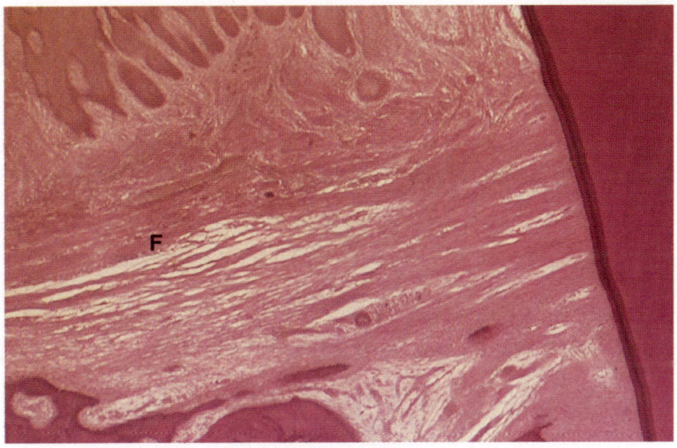

Fig. 2.5 Transseptal fibers (*F*) at the crest of the interdental bone.

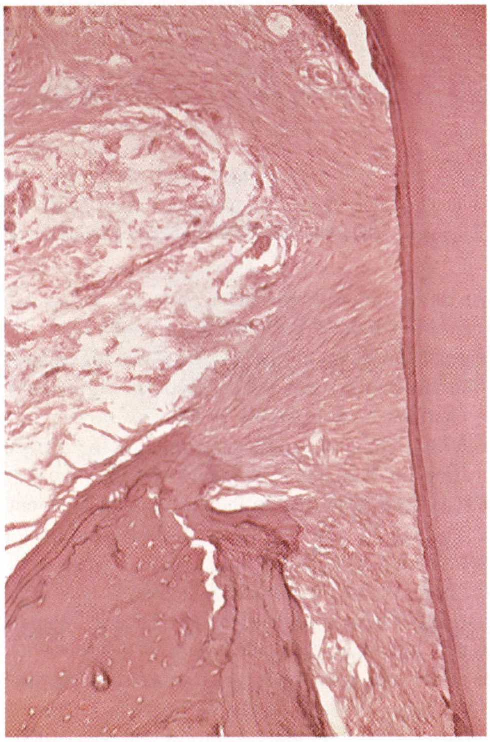

Fig. 2.6 Rat molar section showing alveolar crest fibers radiating coronally.

Horizontal fibers extend at right angles to the long axis of the tooth from the cementum to the alveolar bone. They prevent lateral tooth movement. *Oblique fibers,* which comprise the largest group in the periodontal ligament, extend from the cementum in a coronal direction obliquely to the bone (see Fig. 2.4). They bear the brunt of vertical masticatory stresses and transform such stresses into tension on the alveolar bone.

The *apical fibers* radiate in a rather irregular manner from the cementum to the bone at the apical region of the socket. They do not occur on incompletely formed roots. They prevent tooth tipping, resist forces of luxation, and protect blood, lymph, and nerve supply.

The *interradicular fibers* fan out from the cementum to the tooth in the furcation areas of multirooted teeth. They resist tipping of tooth, forces of luxation and rotation.

Other well-formed fiber bundles interdigitate at right angles or splay around and between regularly arranged fiber bundles. Less regularly arranged collagen fibers are found in the interstitial

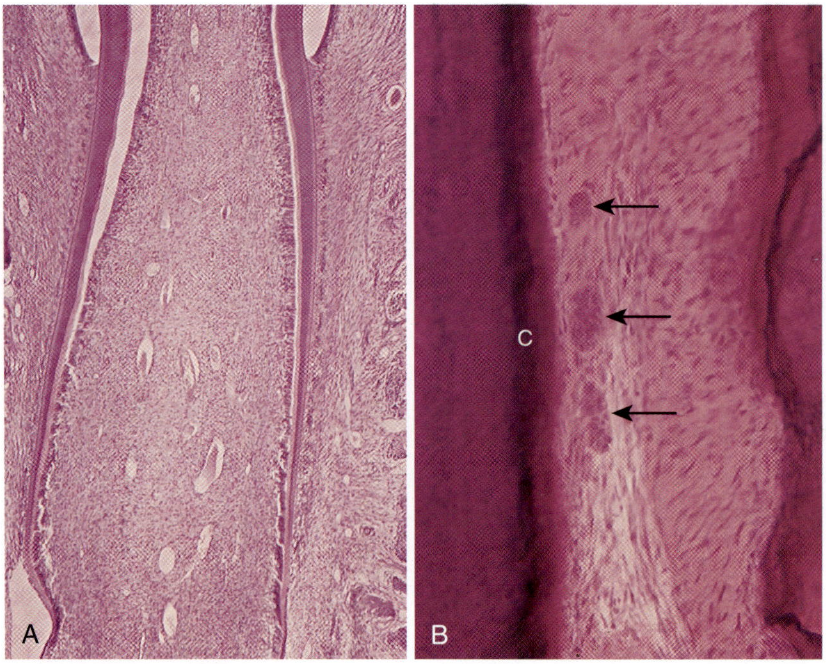

Fig. 2.7 Epithelial rests of Malassez. A, Erupting tooth in a cat. Note the fragmentation of the Hertwig epithelial root sheath giving rise to epithelial rests located along and close to the root surface. B, Human periodontal ligament with rosette-shaped epithelial rests (*arrows*) lying close to the cementum (*C*).

connective tissue between the principal fiber groups; this tissue contains the blood vessels, lymphatics, and nerves.

Although the periodontal ligament does not contain mature elastin, two immature forms are found: oxytalan and elaunin. The so-called oxytalan fibers run parallel to the root surface in a vertical direction and bend to attach to the cementum in the cervical third of the root. They are thought to regulate vascular flow. An elastic meshwork has been described in the periodontal ligament as being composed of many elastin lamellae with peripheral oxytalan fibers and elaunin fibers. Oxytalan fibers have been shown to develop de novo in the regenerated periodontal ligament.

The principal fibers are remodeled by the periodontal ligament cells to adapt to physiologic needs and in response to different stimuli. In addition to these fiber types, small collagen fibers associated with the larger principal collagen fibers have been described. These fibers run in all directions and form a plexus called the *indifferent fiber plexus.*

Cellular Elements

Four types of cells have been identified in the periodontal ligament: connective tissue cells, epithelial rest cells, immune system cells, and cells associated with neurovascular elements.

Connective tissue cells include fibroblasts, cementoblasts, and osteoblasts. Fibroblasts are the most common cells in the periodontal ligament; they appear as ovoid or elongated cells oriented along the principal fibers, and they exhibit pseudopodia-like processes. These cells synthesize collagen and possess the capacity to phagocytose "old" collagen fibers and degrade them via enzyme hydrolysis. Thus, collagen turnover appears to be regulated by fibroblasts in a process of intracellular degradation of collagen that does not involve the action of collagenase.

Phenotypically distinct and functionally different subpopulations of fibroblasts exist in the adult periodontal ligament. They appear to be identical at both the light and electron microscopic levels, but they may have different functions, such as the secretion of different collagen types and the production of collagenase.

Osteoblasts, cementoblasts, osteoclasts, and odontoclasts are also seen in the cemental and osseous surfaces of the periodontal ligament.

The *epithelial rests of Malassez* form a latticework in the periodontal ligament and appear as either isolated clusters of cells or interlacing strands (Fig. 2.7), depending on the plane in which the microscopic section is cut. Continuity with the junctional epithelium has been suggested in experimental animals. The epithelial rests are considered remnants of the Hertwig root sheath, which disintegrates during root development (Fig. 2.7A).

Epithelial rests are distributed close to the cementum throughout the periodontal ligament of most teeth; they are most numerous in the apical area and the cervical area. They diminish in number with age by degenerating and disappearing or by undergoing calcification to become cementicles. The cells are surrounded by a distinct basal lamina, they are interconnected by hemidesmosomes, and they contain tonofilaments.

Although their functional properties are still considered to be unclear, the epithelial rests are reported to contain keratinocyte growth factors, and they have been shown to be positive for tyrosine kinase A neurotrophin receptor. In addition, epithelial rests proliferate when stimulated, and they participate in the formation of periapical cysts and lateral root cysts.

The *defense cells* in the periodontal ligament include neutrophils, lymphocytes, macrophages, mast cells, and eosinophils. These cells, as well as those associated with neurovascular elements, are similar to the cells found in other connective tissues.

Ground Substance

The periodontal ligament also contains a large proportion of ground substance that fills the spaces between fibers and cells. This substance consists of two main components: *glycosaminoglycans,* such as hyaluronic acid and proteoglycans, and *glycoproteins,* such as fibronectin and laminin. It also has a high water content (i.e., 70%).

The cell surface proteoglycans participate in several biologic functions, including cell adhesion, cell–cell and cell–matrix interactions,

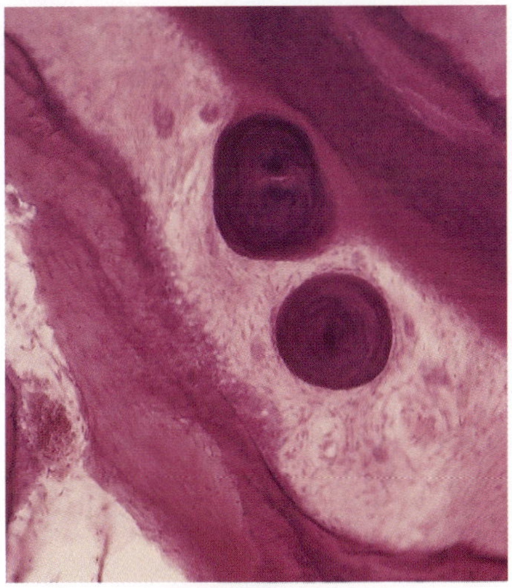

Fig. 2.8 Cementicles in the periodontal ligament. One is lying free and the other is adherent to the tooth surface.

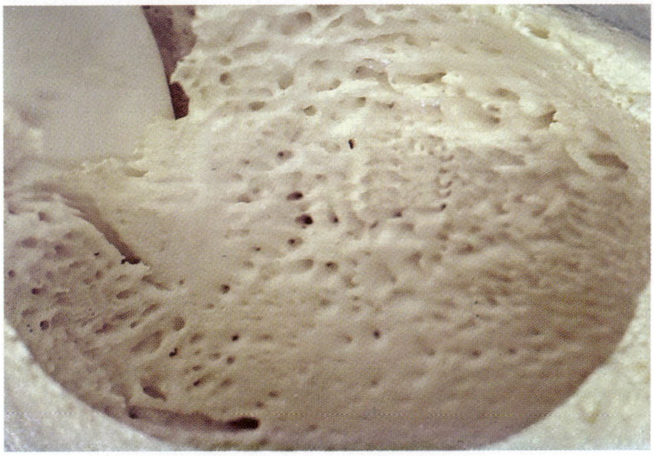

Fig. 2.9 Foramina perforating the lamina dura of a dog jaw.

binding to various growth factors as coreceptors, and cell repair. For example, fibromodulin (a small proteoglycan rich in keratan sulfate and leucine) has been identified in bovine periodontal ligament. The most comprehensive study of the proteoglycans in periodontal ligament was performed with the use of fibroblast cultures of human ligament.

The periodontal ligament may also contain calcified masses called *cementicles*, which are adherent to or detached from the root surfaces (Fig. 2.8).

Cementicles may develop from calcified epithelial rests around small spicules of cementum or alveolar bone traumatically displaced into the periodontal ligament; from calcified Sharpey fibers; and from calcified, thrombosed vessels within the periodontal ligament.

Functions of Periodontal Ligament

The functions of the periodontal ligament are categorized as physical, formative and remodeling, nutritional, and sensory.

Physical Functions

The physical functions of the periodontal ligament entail the following:

1. Provision of a soft-tissue "casing" to protect the vessels and nerves from injury by mechanical forces.
2. Transmission of occlusal forces to the bone.
3. Attachment of the teeth to the bone.
4. Maintenance of the gingival tissues in their proper relationship to the teeth.
5. Resistance to the impact of occlusal forces (i.e., shock absorption).

Resistance to Impact of Occlusal Forces (Shock Absorption)

Two theories pertaining to the mechanism of tooth support have been considered: the tensional theory and the viscoelastic system theory.

The tensional theory of tooth support states that the principal fibers of the periodontal ligament are the major factors in supporting the tooth and transmitting forces to the bone. When a force is applied to the crown, the principal fibers first unfold and straighten, and they then transmit forces to the alveolar bone, thereby causing an elastic deformation of the bony socket. Finally, when the alveolar bone has reached its limit, the load is transmitted to the basal bone. Many investigators find this theory insufficient to explain the available experimental evidence.

The viscoelastic system theory states that the displacement of the tooth is largely controlled by fluid movements, with fibers having only a secondary role. When forces are transmitted to the tooth, the extracellular fluid passes from the periodontal ligament into the marrow spaces of the bone through the foramina in the cribriform plate. These perforations of the cribriform plate link the periodontal ligament with the cancellous portion of the alveolar bone; they are more abundant in the cervical third than in the middle and apical thirds (Fig. 2.9).

After the depletion of tissue fluids, the fiber bundles absorb the slack and tighten. This leads to a blood vessel stenosis. Arterial back pressure causes ballooning of the vessels and passage of the blood ultrafiltrates into the tissues, thereby replenishing the tissue fluids.

Transmission of Occlusal Forces to Bone

The arrangement of the principal fibers is similar to that of a suspension bridge or a hammock. When an axial force is applied to a tooth, a tendency toward displacement of the root into the alveolus occurs. The oblique fibers alter their wavy, untensed pattern, assume their full length, and sustain the major part of the axial force. When a horizontal or tipping force is applied, two phases of tooth movement occur. The first is within the confines of the periodontal ligament, and the second produces a displacement of the facial and lingual bony plates. The tooth rotates about an axis that may change as the force is increased.

The apical portion of the root moves in a direction that is opposite to the coronal portion. In areas of tension, the principal fiber bundles are taut rather than wavy. In areas of pressure, the fibers are compressed, the tooth is displaced, and a corresponding distortion of bone exists in the direction of root movement.

In single-rooted teeth, the axis of rotation is located in the area between the apical third and the middle third of the root (Fig. 2.10A). The root apex and the coronal half of the clinical root have been suggested as other locations of the axis of rotation. The periodontal ligament, which has an hourglass shape, is narrowest in the region of the axis of rotation (Table 2.1). In multirooted teeth, the axis of rotation is located in the bone between the roots (Fig. 2.11). In compliance with the physiologic mesial migration of the teeth, the periodontal ligament is thinner on the mesial root surface than on the distal surface.

Formative and Remodeling Function

Periodontal ligament and alveolar bone cells are exposed to physical forces in response to mastication, parafunction, speech, and orthodontic tooth movement. Cells of the periodontal ligament

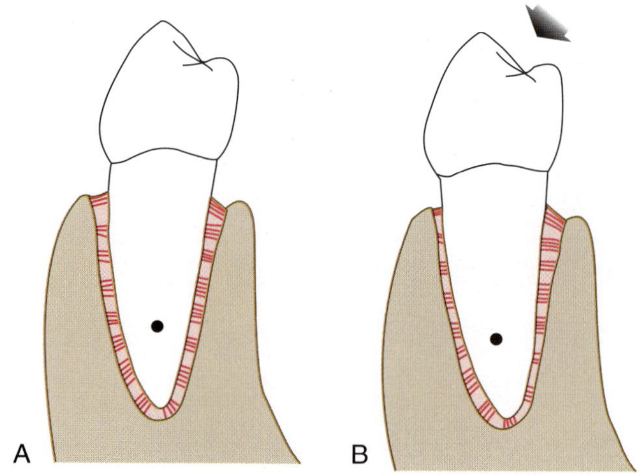

Fig. 2.10 A, Diagram of a mandibular premolar in a resting state. B, When a force is exerted on the tooth—in this case, in faciolingual direction (*arrow*)—the tooth rotates around the fulcrum or axis of rotation (*black circle on root*). The periodontal ligament is compressed in areas of pressure and distended in areas of tension.

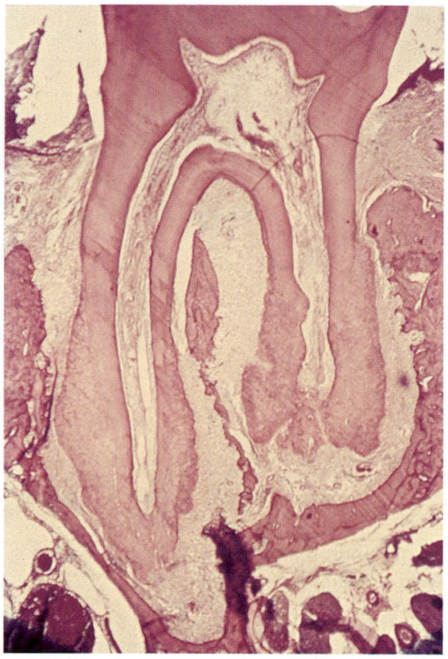

Fig. 2.11 Microscopic view of a rat molar subjected to occluso horizontal forces. Note the alternating widened and narrowed areas of the periodontal ligament as the tooth rotates around its axis of rotation. The axis of rotation is in the interradicular space.

participate in the formation and resorption of cementum and bone, which occur during physiologic tooth movement, during the accommodation of the periodontium to occlusal forces, and during the repair of injuries.

Variations in cellular enzyme activity are correlated with the remodeling process. Although applied loads may induce vascular and inflammatory reactive changes in periodontal ligament cells, current evidence suggests that these cells have a mechanism to respond directly to mechanical forces via the activation of various mechanosensory signaling systems, including adenylate cyclase, stretch-activated ion channels, and via changes in cytoskeletal organization.

Cartilage formation in the periodontal ligament, although unusual, may represent a metaplastic phenomenon in the repair of this ligament after injury.

The periodontal ligament is constantly undergoing remodeling. Old cells and fibers are broken down and replaced by new ones, and mitotic activity can be observed in the fibroblasts and the endothelial cells. Fibroblasts form the collagen fibers, and the residual mesenchymal cells develop into osteoblasts and cementoblasts. Therefore, the rate of formation and the differentiation of osteoblasts, cementoblasts, and fibroblasts affect the rate of formation of collagen, cementum, and bone.

Radioautographic studies with radioactive thymidine, proline, and glycine indicate a high turnover rate of collagen in the periodontal ligament. The rate of collagen synthesis is twice as fast as that in the gingiva and four times as fast as that in the skin, as established in the rat molar. A rapid turnover of sulfated glycosaminoglycans in the cells and amorphous ground substance of the periodontal ligament also occurs. It should be noted that most of these studies have been performed in rodents and that information about primates and humans is scarce.

Nutritional and Sensory Functions

The periodontal ligament supplies nutrients to the cementum, bone, and gingiva by way of the blood vessels, and it also provides lymphatic drainage as discussed later in this chapter. In relation to other ligaments and tendons, the periodontal ligament is a highly vascularized tissue; almost 10% of its volume in the rodent molar is blood vessels. This relatively high blood vessel content may provide hydrodynamic damping to applied forces as well as high perfusion rates to the periodontal ligament.

The periodontal ligament is abundantly supplied with sensory nerve fibers that are capable of transmitting tactile, pressure, and pain sensations via the trigeminal pathways. Nerve bundles pass into the periodontal ligament from the periapical area and through channels from the alveolar bone that follow the course of the blood vessels. The bundles divide into single myelinated fibers, which ultimately lose their myelin sheaths and end in one of four types of neural termination: (1) free endings, which have a tree-like configuration and carry pain sensation; (2) Ruffini-like mechanoreceptors, which are located primarily in the apical area; (3) coiled Meissner

TABLE 2.1 Thickness of the Periodontal Ligaments of 172 Teeth From 15 Human Subjects

	Average of Alveolar Crest (mm)	Average of Midroot (mm)	Average of Apex (mm)	Average of Tooth (mm)
Ages 11 through 16 years (83 teeth from 4 jaws)	0.23	0.17	0.24	0.21
Ages 32 through 50 years (36 teeth from 5 jaws)	0.20	0.14	0.19	0.18
Ages 51 through 67 years (35 teeth from 5 jaws)	0.17	0.12	0.16	0.15
Age 24 years (1 case; 18 teeth from 1 jaw)	0.16	0.09	0.15	0.13

(Modified from Coolidge ED: *J Am Dent Assoc* 24:1260, 1937.)

corpuscles and mechanoreceptors, which are found mainly in the midroot region; and (4) spindle-like pressure and vibration endings, which are surrounded by a fibrous capsule and located mainly in the apex.

Regulation of Periodontal Ligament Width

Some of the most interesting features of the periodontal ligament in animals are its adaptability to rapidly changing applied force and its capacity to maintain its width at constant dimensions throughout its lifetime. These are important measures of periodontal ligament homeostasis that provide insight into the function of the biologic mechanisms that tightly regulate the metabolism and spatial locations of the cell populations involved in the formation of bone, cementum, and periodontal ligament fibers. In addition, the ability of periodontal ligament cells to synthesize and secrete a wide range of regulatory molecules is an essential component of tissue remodeling and periodontal ligament homeostasis.

Cementum

Cementum is the calcified, avascular mesenchymal tissue that forms the outer covering of the anatomic root.

Development of Cementum

The rupture of the Hertwig root sheath allows the mesenchymal cells of the dental follicle to contact the dentin where they start forming a continuous layer of cementoblasts.

On the basis of immunochemical and ultrastructural studies, Thomas and others have speculated that cementoblasts can be of epithelial origin (i.e., the Hertwig root sheath), having undergone an epithelial mesenchymal transformation.

Cementum formation begins with the deposition of a meshwork of irregularly arranged collagen fibrils sparsely distributed in a ground substance or matrix called *precementum* or *cementoid.* This is followed by a phase of matrix maturation, which subsequently mineralizes to form cementum. Cementoblasts, which are initially separated from the cementum by uncalcified cementoid, sometimes become enclosed within the matrix and are trapped. After they are enclosed, they are referred to as *cementocytes*, and they will remain viable in a manner similar to that of osteocytes.

A layer of connective tissue known as the dental sac surrounds the enamel organ and includes the epithelial root sheath as it develops. The zone that is immediately in contact with the dental organ and continuous with the ectomesenchyme of the dental papilla is called the dental follicle, and it consists of undifferentiated fibroblasts.

Types and Composition

The two main types of cementum are acellular (*primary*) and cellular (*secondary*) cementum. Both consist of a calcified interfibrillar matrix and collagen fibrils.

The two main sources of collagen fibers in cementum are Sharpey fibers (*extrinsic*), which are the embedded portion of the principal fibers of the periodontal ligament and which are formed by the fibroblasts, and fibers that belong to the cementum matrix *(intrinsic)*, which are produced by the cementoblasts. Cementoblasts also form the noncollagenous components of the interfibrillar ground substance, such as proteoglycans, glycoproteins, and phosphoproteins. Proteoglycans are most likely to play a role in regulating cell–cell and cell–matrix interactions, both during normal development and during the regeneration of the cementum. In addition, immunohistochemical studies have shown that the distribution of proteoglycans is closely associated with the cementoblasts and the cementocytes.

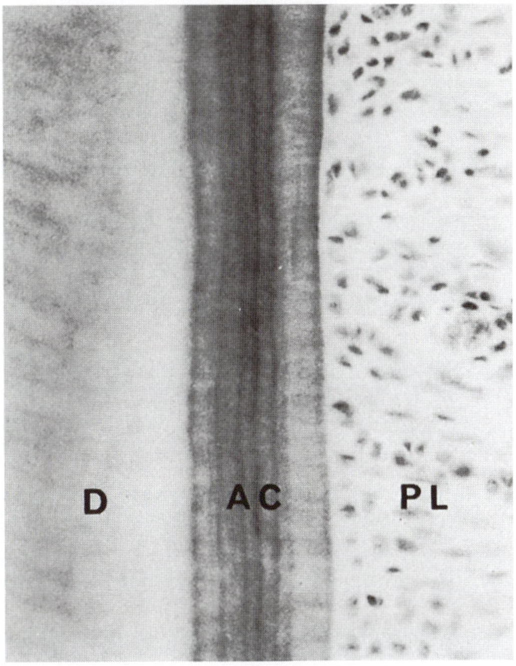

Fig. 2.12 Acellular cementum (*AC*) showing incremental lines running parallel to the long axis of the tooth. These lines represent the appositional growth of cementum. Note the *thin, light lines* running into the cementum perpendicular to the surface; these represent the Sharpey fibers of the periodontal ligament (*PL*). *D*, Dentin (×300).

The major proportion of the organic matrix of cementum is composed of type I (90%) and type III (about 5%) collagens. Sharpey fibers, which constitute a considerable proportion of the bulk of cementum, are composed of mainly type I collagen. Type III collagen appears to coat the type I collagen of the Sharpey fibers.

Acellular cementum is the first cementum formed; it covers approximately the cervical third or half of the root, and it does not contain cells (Fig. 2.12). This cementum is formed before the tooth reaches the occlusal plane, and its thickness ranges from 30 to 230 μm. Sharpey fibers make up most of the structure of acellular cementum, which has a principal role in supporting the tooth. Most fibers are inserted at approximately right angles into the root surface and penetrate deep into the cementum but others enter from several different directions. Their size, number, and distribution increase with function. Sharpey fibers are completely calcified, with the mineral crystals oriented parallel to the fibrils as in dentin and bone, except in a 10–50-μm–wide zone near the cementodentinal junction where they are only partially calcified. The peripheral portions of Sharpey fibers in actively mineralizing cementum tend to be more calcified than the interior regions, according to evidence obtained by scanning electron microscopy. Acellular cementum also contains intrinsic collagen fibrils that are calcified and irregularly arranged or parallel to the surface.

Cellular cementum, which is formed after the tooth reaches the occlusal plane, is more irregular and contains cells (cementocytes) in individual spaces (lacunae) that communicate with each other through a system of anastomosing canaliculi (Fig. 2.13). Cellular cementum is less calcified than the acellular type. Sharpey fibers occupy a smaller portion of the cellular cementum and are separated by other fibers that are arranged either parallel to the root surface or at random. Sharpey fibers may be completely or partially calcified, or they may have a central, uncalcified core surrounded by a calcified border.

Both acellular cementum and cellular cementum are arranged in lamellae separated by incremental lines parallel to the long axis of

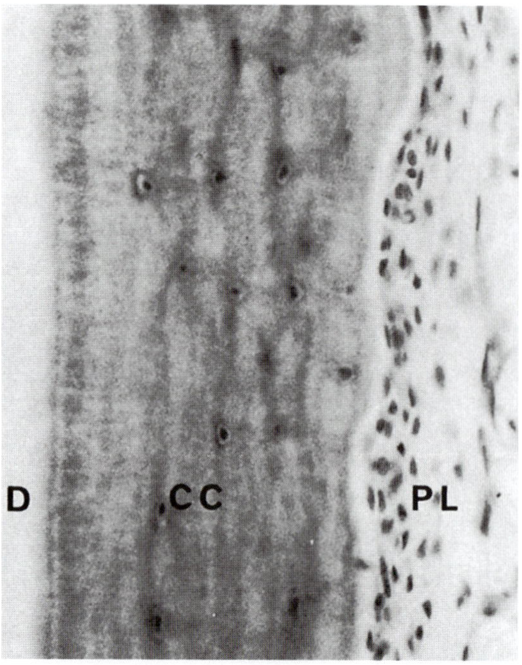

Fig. 2.13 Cellular cementum (*CC*) showing cementocytes lying within the lacunae. Cellular cementum is thicker than acellular cementum (see Fig. 2.15). The evidence of incremental lines also exists, but they are less distinct than in the acellular cementum. The cells adjacent to the surface of the cementum in the periodontal ligament (*PL*) space are cementoblasts. *D*, Dentin (×300).

the root (see Figs. 2.12 and 2.13). These lines represent "rest periods" in cementum formation, and they are more mineralized than the adjacent cementum. In addition, the loss of the cervical part of the reduced enamel epithelium at the time of tooth eruption may place portions of mature enamel in contact with the connective tissue, which then will deposit an acellular and afibrillar type of cementum over the enamel.

On the basis of these findings, *Schroeder* has classified cementum as follows:

- *Acellular afibrillar cementum* contains neither cells nor extrinsic or intrinsic collagen fibers, except for a mineralized ground substance. Acellular afibrillar cementum is a product of cementoblasts and found as coronal cementum in humans, with a thickness of 1–15 μm.
- *Acellular extrinsic fiber cementum* is composed almost entirely of densely packed bundles of Sharpey fibers and lacks cells. Acellular extrinsic fiber cementum is a product of fibroblasts and cementoblasts. It is found in the cervical third of roots in humans, but it may extend farther apically. Its thickness is between 30 and 230 μm.
- *Cellular mixed stratified cementum* is composed of extrinsic (Sharpey) and intrinsic fibers, and it may contain cells. Cellular mixed stratified cementum is a coproduct of fibroblasts and cementoblasts. In humans, it appears primarily in the apical third of the roots and apices and in furcation areas. Its thickness ranges from 100 to 1000 μm.
- *Cellular intrinsic fiber cementum* contains cells but no extrinsic collagen fibers. Cellular intrinsic fiber cementum is formed by cementoblasts, and, in humans, it fills the resorption lacunae.

Intermediate cementum is a poorly defined zone near the cementodentinal junction of certain teeth that appear to contain cellular remnants of the Hertwig sheath embedded in calcified ground substance.

Inorganic content of cementum (hydroxyapatite; $Ca_{10}[Po_4]_6[OH]_2$) is 45%–50%, which is less than that of bone (65%), enamel (97%), or dentin (70%). Opinions differ with regard to whether the microhardness increases or decreases with age, and no relationship has been established between aging and the mineral content of cementum.

It is well known that the protein extracts of mature cementum promote cell attachment and cell migration and stimulate the protein synthesis of gingival fibroblasts and periodontal ligament cells. Studies of cementum have identified adhesion proteins with arginyl–glycyl–aspartic acid sequences: bone sialoprotein, osteopontin, and osteonectin. Bone sialoprotein and osteopontin are expressed during early tooth root development by cells along the root surface, and they are thought to play a major role in the differentiation of the cementoblast progenitor cells to the cementoblasts.

Some of the molecules unique to the cementum have been described. Recent work has investigated the role of *cementum attachment protein,* which is a collagenous cementum-derived protein. Cementum attachment protein has been shown to promote the adhesion and spreading of mesenchymal cell types, with osteoblasts and periodontal ligament fibroblasts showing better adhesion than gingival fibroblasts and keratinocytes. In addition, Ikezawa and coworkers described the characterization of *cementum-derived growth factor*, which is an insulin-like, growth factor-I–like molecule. Cementum-derived growth factor has been shown to enhance the proliferation of gingival fibroblasts and periodontal ligament cells.

Permeability of Cementum

In very young animals, acellular cementum and cellular cementum are very permeable and permit the diffusion of dyes from the pulp and the external root surface. In cellular cementum, the canaliculi in some areas are contiguous with the dentinal tubuli. The permeability of cementum diminishes with age.

Cementoenamel Junction

The cementum at and immediately subjacent to the *cementoenamel junction* is of particular clinical importance in root-scaling procedures. Three types of relationships involving the cementum may exist at the cementoenamel junction. In about 60%–65% of cases, cementum overlaps the enamel (Fig. 2.14). This occurs when the enamel epithelium degenerates at its cervical termination permitting the connective tissue to come in direct contact with the enamel surface; in about 30%, an edge-to-edge butt joint exists; and in 5%–10%, the cementum and enamel fail to meet. This occurs when enamel epithelium in the cervical portion of the root is delayed in its separation from dentin. In this case, gingival recession may result in accentuated sensitivity as a result of exposed dentin.

Cementodentinal Junction

The terminal apical area of the cementum where it joins the internal root canal dentin is known as the *cementodentinal junction.* When root canal treatment is performed, the obturating material should be at the cementodentinal junction. There appears to be no increase or decrease in the width of the cementodentinal junction with age; its width appears to remain relatively stable. Scanning electron microscopy of the human teeth reveals that the cementodentinal junction is 2–3 μm wide. The fibril-poor layer contains a significant amount of proteoglycans, and fibrils intermingle between the cementum and the dentin.

Thickness of Cementum

Cementum deposition is a continuous process that occurs at varying rates throughout life. Cementum formation is most rapid in the

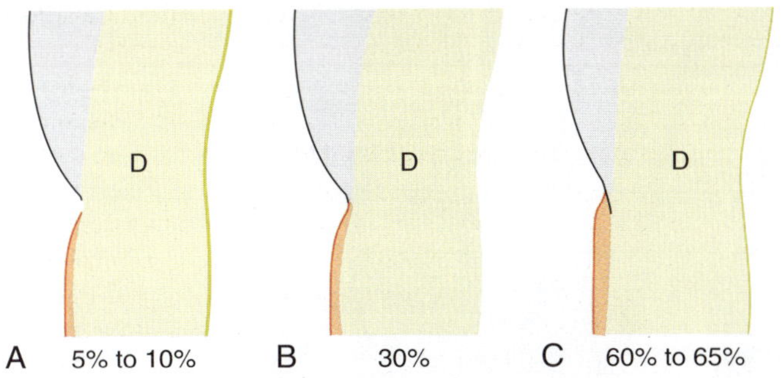

Fig. 2.14 Normal variations in tooth morphology at the cementoenamel junction. A, Space between the enamel and the cementum with the dentin (*D*) exposed. B, End-to-end relationship of enamel and cementum. C, Cementum overlapping the enamel.

apical regions where it compensates for tooth eruption, which itself compensates for attrition.

The thickness of cementum on the coronal half of the root varies from 16 to 60 μm, which is about the thickness of a hair. It attains its greatest thickness (≤150–200 μm) in the apical third and in the furcation areas. It is thicker in distal surfaces than in mesial surfaces, probably because of functional stimulation from mesial drift over time. Between the ages of 11 and 70 years, the average thickness of the cementum increases threefold, with the greatest increase seen in the apical region. Average thicknesses of 95 μm at the age of 20 years and of 215 μm at the age of 60 years have been reported.

Abnormalities in the thickness of cementum may range from an absence or paucity of cellular cementum (i.e., cemental aplasia or hypoplasia) to an excessive deposition of cementum (i.e., cemental hyperplasia or hypercementosis).

The term *hypercementosis* refers to a prominent thickening of the cementum. It is largely an age-related phenomenon, and it may be localized to one tooth or affect the entire dentition. As a result of considerable physiologic variation in the thickness of cementum among different teeth in the same person and also among different persons, distinguishing between hypercementosis and the physiologic thickening of cementum is sometimes difficult. Nevertheless, the excessive proliferation of cementum may occur with a broad spectrum of neoplastic and nonneoplastic conditions, including benign cementoblastoma, cementifying fibroma, periapical cemental dysplasia, florid cemento-osseous dysplasia, and other benign fibro-osseous lesions.

Hypercementosis occurs as a generalized thickening of the cementum, with nodular enlargement of the apical third of the root. It also appears in the form of spike-like excrescences (i.e., cemental spikes) created by either the coalescence of cementicles that adhere to the root or the calcification of periodontal fibers at the sites of insertion into the cementum.

Radiographically, the radiolucent shadow of the periodontal ligament and the radiopaque lamina dura are always seen on the outer border of an area of hypercementosis, enveloping it as it would in normal cementum. On the other hand, from a diagnostic standpoint, periapical cemental dysplasia, condensing osteitis, and focal periapical osteopetrosis may be differentiated from hypercementosis because all of these entities are located outside of the shadow of the periodontal ligament and the lamina dura.

The cause of hypercementosis varies and is not completely understood. The spike-like type of hypercementosis generally results from excessive tension caused by orthodontic appliances or occlusal forces. The generalized type occurs in a variety of circumstances. In teeth without antagonists, hypercementosis is interpreted as an effort to keep pace with excessive tooth eruption. In teeth that are subject to low-grade periapical irritation that arises from pulp disease, it is considered compensation for the destroyed fibrous attachment to the tooth. The cementum is deposited adjacent to the inflamed periapical tissue. Hypercementosis of the entire dentition may occur in patients with Paget disease. Other systemic disturbances that may lead to or may be associated with hypercementosis include acromegaly, arthritis, calcinosis, rheumatic fever, and thyroid goiter.

Hypercementosis itself does not require treatment. It could pose a problem if an affected tooth requires extraction. In a multirooted tooth, sectioning of the tooth may be required before extraction.

Cementum Resorption and Repair

Permanent teeth do not undergo physiologic resorption as primary teeth do. However, the cementum of erupted (as well as unerupted) teeth is subject to resorptive changes that may be of microscopic proportion or sufficiently extensive to present a radiographically detectable alteration in the root contour.

Microscopic cementum resorption is extremely common; in one study, it occurred in 236 of 261 teeth (90.5%). The average number of resorption areas per tooth was 3.5. Of the 922 areas of resorption, 708 (76.8%) were located in the apical third of the root, 177 (19.2%) in the middle third, and 37 (4.0%) in the gingival third. Approximately 70% of all resorption areas were confined to the cementum without involving the dentin.

Cementum resorption may be caused by local or systemic factors, or it may occur without apparent etiology (i.e., idiopathic). Local conditions that cause cementum resorption include trauma from occlusion (Fig. 2.15); orthodontic movement; pressure from malaligned erupting teeth, cysts, and tumors; teeth without functional antagonists; embedded teeth; replanted and transplanted teeth; periapical disease; and periodontal disease. Systemic conditions that are cited as predisposing an individual to or inducing cemental resorption include calcium deficiency, hypothyroidism, hereditary fibrous osteodystrophy, and Paget disease.

Cementum resorption appears microscopically as bay-like concavities in the root surface. (Fig. 2.16). Multinucleated giant cells and large mononuclear macrophages are generally found adjacent to the cementum that is undergoing active resorption (Fig. 2.17). Several sites of resorption may coalesce to form a large area of destruction. The resorptive process may extend into the underlying dentin and even into the pulp, but it is usually painless. Cementum resorption is not necessarily continuous and may alternate with periods of repair and the deposition of new cementum. The newly formed cementum is demarcated from the root by a deeply staining irregular line termed a *reversal line*, which delineates the border of the previous resorption. A recent study showed that the reversal lines of human teeth contain a few collagen fibrils and highly accumulated proteoglycans with mucopolysaccharides (glycosaminoglycans) and that fibril intermingling occurs only in some places between reparative cementum and resorbed dentin or cementum. Embedded fibers of the periodontal ligament reestablish a functional relationship in the new cementum.

Cementum repair requires the presence of a viable connective tissue. If epithelium proliferates into an area of resorption, repair will not take place. Cementum repair can occur in devitalized as well as vital teeth.

Histologic evidence demonstrates that cementum formation is critical for the appropriate maturation of the periodontium, both during development and during the regeneration of lost periodontal tissues. In other words, a variety of macromolecules present in the extracellular matrix of the periodontium are likely to play a regulatory role in cementogenesis.

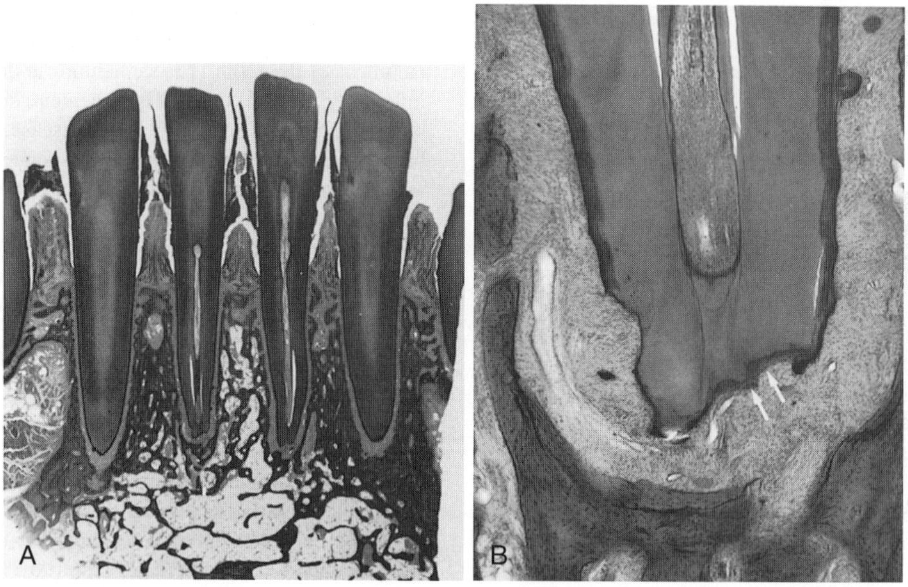

Fig. 2.15 **Cemental resorption associated with excessive occlusal forces.** A, Low-power histologic section of the mandibular anterior teeth. B, High-power micrograph of the apex of the left central incisor shortened by the resorption of cementum and dentin. Note the partial repair of the eroded areas (*arrows*) and the cementicle at the upper right.

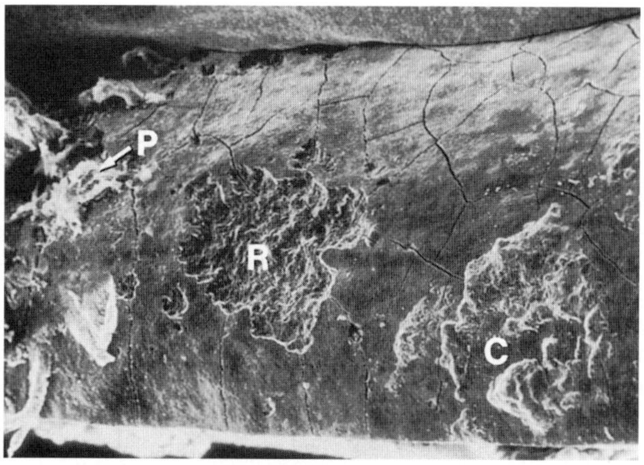

Fig. 2.16 **Scanning electron micrograph of a root exposed by periodontal disease showing a large resorption bay (*R*).** Remnants of the periodontal ligament (*P*) and calculus (*C*) are visible. Cracking of the tooth surface occurs as a result of the preparation technique (×160). *(Courtesy Dr John Sottosanti, La Jolla, CA.)*

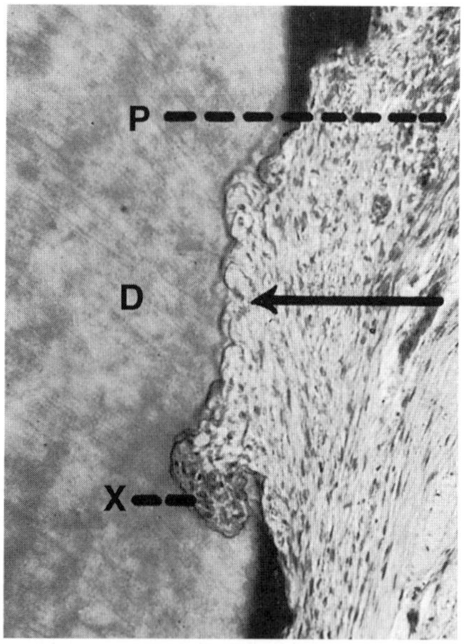

Fig. 2.17 **Resorption of cementum and dentin.** A multinuclear osteoclast in seen (*X*). The direction of resorption is indicated by the *arrow.* Note the scalloped resorption front in the dentin (*D*). The cementum is the darkly stained band at the upper and lower right. *P*, Periodontal ligament.

The regeneration of cementum requires cementoblasts, but the origin of the cementoblasts and the molecular factors that regulate their recruitment and differentiation are not fully understood. However, recent research provides a better understanding; for example, the epithelial cell rests of Malassez are the only odontogenic epithelial cells that remain in the periodontium after the eruption of teeth, and they may have some function in cementum repair and regeneration under specific conditions. The rests of Malassez may be related to cementum repair by activating their potential to secrete matrix proteins that have been expressed in tooth development, such as amelogenins, enamelins, and sheath proteins. Several growth factors have been shown to be effective in cementum regeneration, including members of the transforming growth factor superfamily (i.e., bone morphogenetic proteins), platelet-derived growth factor, insulin-like growth factor, and enamel matrix derivatives (Fig. 2.18).

Ankylosis

Fusion of the cementum and the alveolar bone with obliteration of the periodontal ligament is termed *ankylosis.* Ankylosis occurs in teeth with cemental resorption, which suggests that it may represent a form of abnormal repair. Ankylosis may also develop after chronic periapical inflammation, tooth replantation, and occlusal trauma and around embedded teeth. This condition is relatively uncommon, and it occurs most frequently in the primary dentition.

Ankylosis results in the resorption of the root and its gradual replacement by bone tissue. For this reason, reimplanted teeth that ankylose will lose their roots after 4–5 years and will be exfoliated.

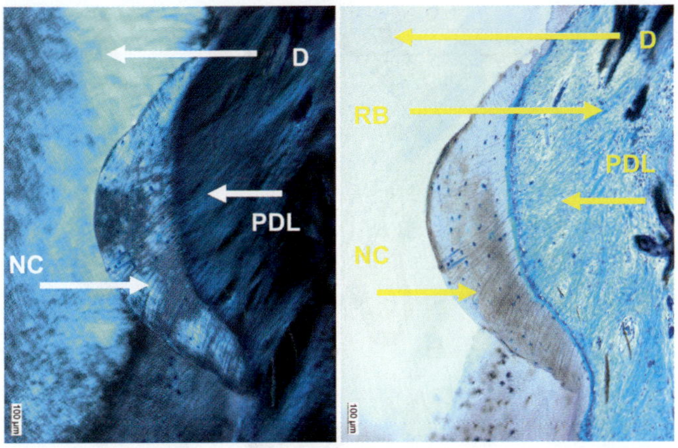

Fig. 2.18 A clinical human histology shows that new cementum and new periodontal ligament fiber formed at a previous periodontal defect treated with recombinant human platelet-derived growth factor-BB with β-tricalcium phosphate. *(Courtesy Dr Daniel WK Kao, Philadelphia, PA.)*

Clinically, ankylosed teeth lack the physiologic mobility of normal teeth, which is one diagnostic sign for ankylotic resorption. In addition, these teeth usually have a special metallic percussion sound; if the ankylotic process continues, they will be in infraocclusion. However, the clinical diagnosis of ankylosis by mobility and percussion tests alone is only reliable when at least 20% of the root surface is affected.

As the periodontal ligament is replaced with bone during ankylosis, proprioception is lost because pressure receptors in the periodontal ligament are deleted or do not function correctly. Furthermore, the physiologic drifting and eruption of teeth can no longer occur, and thus the ability of the teeth and periodontium to adapt to altered force levels or directions of force is greatly reduced. Radiographically, resorption lacunae are filled with bone, and the periodontal ligament space is missing.

Since no definitive causes can be found in ankylotic root resorption, no predictable treatment can be suggested. Treatment modalities range from a conservative approach, such as restorative intervention, to the surgical extraction of the affected tooth.

When titanium implants are placed in the jaw, healing results in bone that is formed in direct apposition to the implant without an intervening connective tissue. This may be interpreted as a form of ankylosis. Since resorption of the metallic implant cannot occur, the implant remains indefinitely "ankylosed" to the bone. In addition, a true periodontal pocket will not form; the apical proliferation of the epithelium along the root, which is a key element of pocket formation, is not possible because of the ankylosis.

Exposure of Cementum to the Oral Environment

Cementum becomes exposed to the oral environment in cases of gingival recession and as a result of the loss of attachment in pocket formation. The cementum is sufficiently permeable to be penetrated in these cases by organic substances, inorganic ions, and bacteria. Bacterial invasion of the cementum occurs frequently in individuals with periodontal disease, and cementum caries can develop.

Alveolar Process

The alveolar process is the portion of the maxilla and mandible that forms and supports the tooth sockets (alveoli). It forms when the tooth erupts to provide the osseous attachment to the forming periodontal ligament; it disappears gradually after the tooth is lost.

Development of Alveolar Bone

The alveolar bone develops around each tooth follicle during odontogenesis. When a deciduous tooth is shed, its alveolar bone is resorbed. The succedaneous permanent tooth moves into place and develops its own alveolar bone from its own dental follicle. As the tooth root forms and the surrounding tissues develop and mature, alveolar bone merges with the separately developing basal bone, and the two become one continuous structure. Although alveolar bone and basal bone have different intermediate origins, both are ultimately derived from neural crest ectomesenchyme.

Mandibular basal bone begins mineralization at the exit of the mental nerve from the mental foramen, whereas the maxillary basal bone begins at the exit of the infraorbital nerve from the infraorbital foramen.

Just before mineralization, osteoblasts start producing matrix vesicles. These vesicles contain enzymes (e.g., alkaline phosphatase) that help to jump start the nucleation of hydroxyapatite crystals. As these crystals grow and develop, they form coalescing bone nodules, which, with fast-growing nonoriented collagen fibers, are the substructure of woven bone and the first bone formed in the alveolus. Later, through bone deposition, remodeling, and the secretion of oriented collagen fibers in sheets, mature lamellar bone is formed.

The hydroxyapatite crystals are generally aligned with their long axes parallel to the collagen fibers, and they appear to be deposited on and within the collagen fibers in mature lamellar bone. In this way, bone matrix is able to withstand the heavy mechanical stresses applied to it during function.

Since the alveolar processes develop and undergo remodeling with tooth formation and eruption, they are tooth-dependent bony structures. Therefore, the size, shape, location, and function of the teeth determine their morphology. Interestingly, although the growth and development of the bones of the jaw determine the position of the teeth, a certain degree of repositioning of the teeth can be accomplished through occlusal forces and in response to orthodontic procedures that rely on the adaptability of the alveolar bone and the associated periodontal tissues.

Parts of the Alveolar Process

The alveolar process consists of the following:

1. An external plate of cortical bone is formed by haversian bone and compacted bone lamellae.
2. The inner socket wall of thin, compact bone called the *alveolar bone proper* is seen as the lamina dura in radiographs. Histologically, it contains a series of openings (i.e., the *cribriform plate*) through which neurovascular bundles link the periodontal ligament with the central component of the alveolar bone: the cancellous bone.
3. Cancellous trabeculae between these two compact layers act as supporting alveolar bone. The *interdental septum* consists of cancellous supporting bone enclosed within a compact border (Fig. 2.19).

In addition, the bones of the jaw include the basal bone, which is the portion of the jaw located apically but unrelated to the teeth (Fig. 2.20).

The alveolar process is divisible into separate areas on an anatomic basis, but it functions as a unit, with all parts interrelated in the support of the teeth. Figures 2.21 and 2.22 show the relative proportions of cancellous bone and compact bone that form the alveolar process. Most of the facial and lingual portions of the sockets are formed by compact bone alone; cancellous bone surrounds the lamina dura in apical, apicolingual, and interradicular areas.

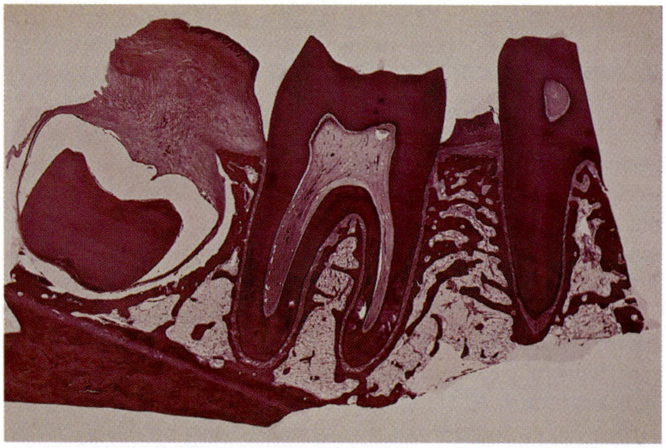

Fig. 2.19 Mesiodistal section through the mandibular molars of a 17-year-old girl obtained at autopsy. Note the interdental bony septa between the first and second molars. The dense cortical bony plates represent the alveolar bone proper (i.e., the cribriform plates) and are supported by cancellous bony trabeculae. The third molar is still in the early stages of root formation and eruption.

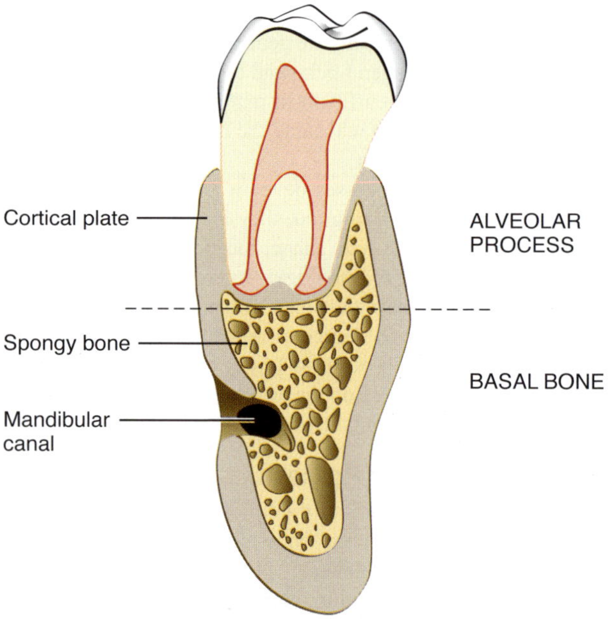

Fig. 2.20 Section through a human jaw with a tooth in situ. The *dotted line* indicates the separation between the basal bone and the alveolar bone. *(Redrawn from Ten Cate AR: Oral histology: development, structure, and function, ed 4, St Louis, 1994, Mosby.)*

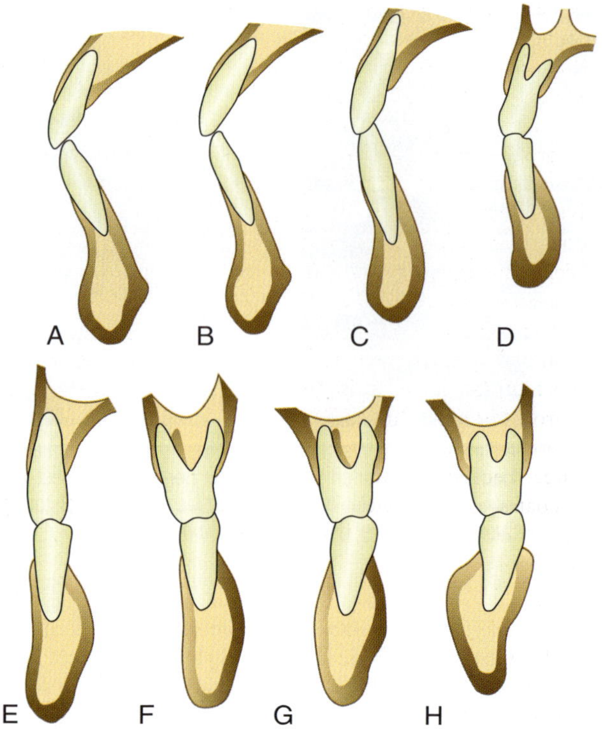

Fig. 2.21 Relative proportions of cancellous bone and compact bone in a longitudinal faciolingual section of, A, mandibular molars; B, lateral incisors; C, canines; D, first premolars; E, second premolars; F, first molars; G, second molars; and H, third molars.

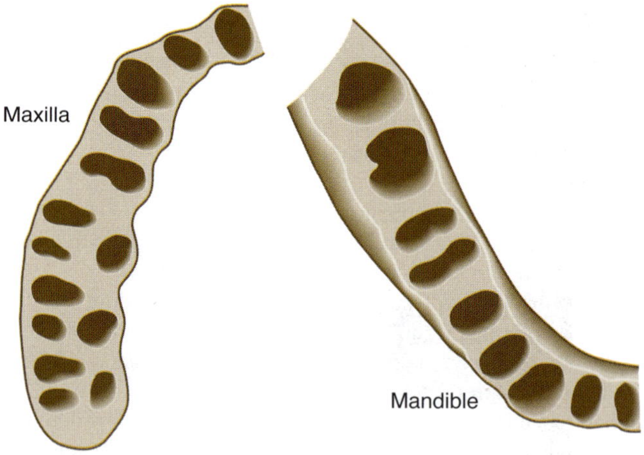

Fig. 2.22 The shape of the roots and the surrounding bone distribution in a transverse section of maxilla and mandible at the midroot level.

Composition of Alveolar Bone

Bone consists of two-thirds inorganic matter and one-third organic matrix. The inorganic matter is composed principally of the minerals calcium and phosphate along with hydroxyl, carbonate, citrate, and trace amounts of other ions such as sodium, magnesium, and fluorine. The mineral salts are in the form of hydroxyapatite crystals of ultramicroscopic size and constitute approximately two-thirds of the bone structure.

The organic matrix consists mainly of collagen type I (90%), with small amounts of noncollagenous proteins such as osteocalcin, osteonectin, bone morphogenetic protein, phosphoproteins, and proteoglycans. Osteopontin and bone sialoprotein are cell-adhesion proteins that appear to be important for the adhesion of both osteoclasts and osteoblasts. In addition, paracrine factors, including cytokines, chemokines, and growth factors, have been implicated in the local control of mesenchymal condensations that occur at the onset of organogenesis. These factors probably play a prominent role in the development of the alveolar processes.

Although the alveolar bone tissue is constantly changing its internal organization, it retains approximately the same form from childhood through adult life. Bone deposition by osteoblasts is balanced by resorption by osteoclasts during tissue remodeling and renewal. It is well known that the number of osteoblasts decreases with aging; however, no remarkable change in the number of osteoclasts has ever been reported.

Remodeling is the major pathway of bony changes in shape, resistance to forces, repair of wounds, and calcium and phosphate homeostasis in the body. Indeed, the coupling of bone resorption with bone formation constitutes one of the fundamental principles by which bone is necessarily remodeled throughout its life. Bone remodeling involves the coordination of activities of cells from two distinct lineages, the osteoblasts and the osteoclasts, which form and resorb the mineralized connective tissues of bone.

The regulation of bone remodeling is a complex process that involves hormones and local factors acting in an autocrine and a paracrine manner on the generation and activity of differentiated bone cells. Bone contains 99% of the body's calcium ions and therefore is the major source for calcium release when the calcium blood levels decrease; this is monitored by the parathyroid gland. A decrease in blood calcium is mediated by receptors on the chief cells of the parathyroid glands, which then release parathyroid hormone. Parathyroid hormone stimulates osteoblasts to release interleukin-1 and interleukin-6, which stimulate monocytes to migrate into the bone area. Leukemia-inhibiting factor, which is secreted by osteoblasts, coalesces monocytes into multinucleated osteoclasts, which then resorb bone, thereby releasing calcium ions from hydroxyapatite into the blood. This release normalizes the blood level of calcium. A feedback mechanism for normal blood levels of calcium turns off the secretion of parathyroid hormone. Meanwhile, osteoclasts have resorbed organic matrix along with hydroxyapatite. The breakdown of collagen from the organic matrix releases various osteogenic substrates, which are covalently bound to collagen. This in turn stimulates the differentiation of osteoblasts, which ultimately deposit bone. This interdependency of osteoblasts and osteoclasts in remodeling is called coupling.

The bone matrix that is laid down by osteoblasts is nonmineralized osteoid. While new osteoid is being deposited, the older osteoid located below the surface becomes mineralized as the mineralization front advances.

Bone resorption is a complex process that is morphologically related to the appearance of eroded bone surfaces (i.e., Howship lacunae) and large, multinucleated cells (osteoclasts) (Fig. 2.23). Osteoclasts originate from hematopoietic tissue and are formed by the fusion of mononuclear cells of asynchronous populations. When osteoclasts are active rather than resting, they possess an elaborately developed ruffled border from which hydrolytic enzymes are thought to be secreted. These enzymes digest the organic portion of the bone. The activity of osteoclasts and the morphology of the ruffled border can be modified and regulated by hormones such as parathyroid hormone (indirectly) and calcitonin, which has receptors on the osteoclast membrane.

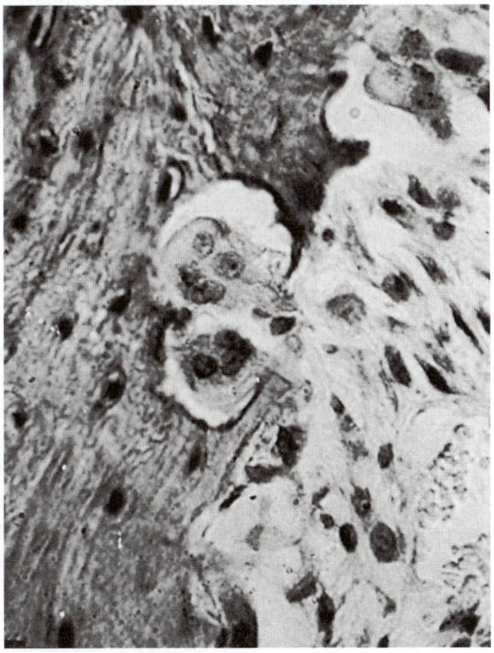

Fig. 2.23 **Rat alveolar bone.** This histologic view shows two multinucleated osteoclasts in the Howship lacuna.

Another mechanism of bone resorption involves the creation of an acidic environment on the bone surface, thereby leading to the dissolution of the mineral component of bone. This event can be produced by different conditions, including a proton pump through the cell membrane of the osteoclast, bone tumors, and local pressure translated through the secretory activity of the osteoclast.

Ten Cate described the sequence of events in the resorptive process as follows:

1. Attachment of osteoclasts to the mineralized surface of bone.
2. Creation of a sealed acidic environment through the action of the proton pump, which demineralizes bone and exposes the organic matrix.
3. Degradation of the exposed organic matrix to its constituent amino acids via the action of released enzymes (e.g., acid phosphatase, cathepsin).
4. Sequestering of mineral ions and amino acids within the osteoclast.

Notably, the cellular and molecular events involved in bone remodeling have a strong similarity to many aspects of inflammation and repair. The relationships among matrix molecules (e.g., osteopontin, bone sialoprotein, SPARC [secreted protein, acidic, rich in cysteine], osteocalcin), blood clotting, and wound healing are clearly evident.

Cells and Intercellular Matrix

Osteoblasts, which are the cells that produce the organic matrix of bone, are differentiated from pluripotent follicle cells. Alveolar bone is formed during fetal growth by intramembranous ossification, and it consists of a calcified matrix with osteocytes enclosed within spaces called *lacunae.* The osteocytes extend processes into *canaliculi* that radiate from the lacunae. The canaliculi form an anastomosing system through the intercellular matrix of the bone, which brings oxygen and nutrients to the osteocytes through the blood and removes metabolic waste products. Blood vessels branch extensively and travel through the periosteum. The endosteum lies adjacent to the marrow vasculature. Bone growth occurs via the apposition of an organic matrix that is deposited by osteoblasts. Haversian systems (i.e., *osteons*) are the internal mechanisms that bring a vascular supply to bones that are too thick to be supplied only by surface vessels. These are found primarily in the outer cortical plates and the alveolar bone proper.

Socket Wall

The socket wall consists of dense, lamellated bone, some of which is arranged in haversian systems and bundle bone. *Bundle bone* is the term given to the bone adjacent to the periodontal ligament that contains a great number of Sharpey fibers (Fig. 2.24). It is characterized by thin lamellae arranged in layers parallel to the root, with intervening appositional lines (Fig. 2.25). Bundle bone is localized within the alveolar bone proper. Some Sharpey fibers are completely calcified, but most contain an uncalcified central core within a calcified outer layer. Bundle bone is not unique to the jaws; it occurs throughout the skeletal system wherever ligaments and muscles are attached.

The cancellous portion of the alveolar bone consists of trabeculae that enclose irregularly shaped marrow spaces lined with a layer of thin, flattened endosteal cells. Wide variation occurs in the

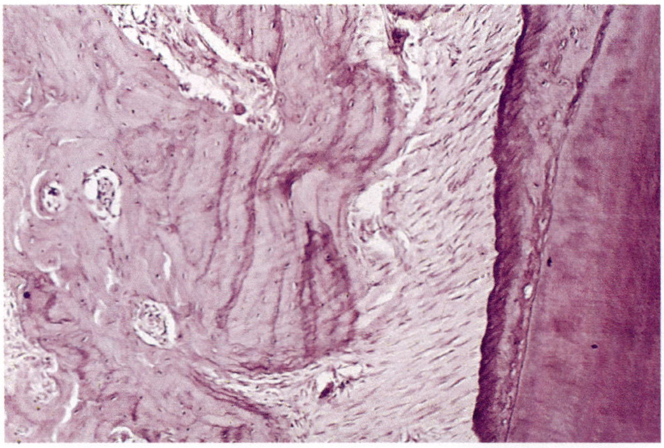

Fig. 2.24 Deep penetration of Sharpey fibers into bundle bone of a rat molar.

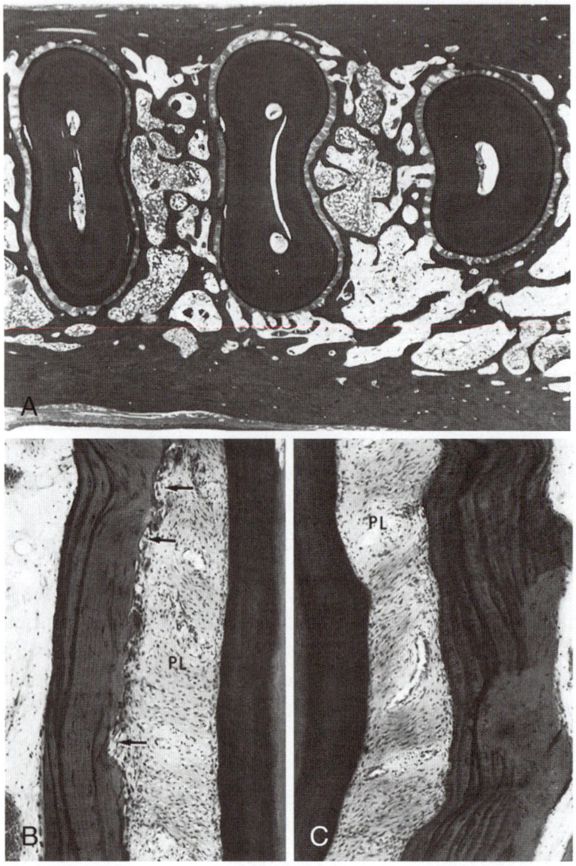

Fig. 2.25 **Bundle bone associated with the physiologic mesial migration of the teeth.** A, Horizontal section through the molar roots during the process of mesial migration (left, mesial; right, distal). B, Mesial root surface showing osteoclasis of bone (*arrows*). C, Distal root surface showing bundle bone that has been partially replaced with dense bone on the marrow side. *PL*, Periodontal ligament.

trabecular pattern of cancellous bone, which is affected by occlusal forces. The matrix of the cancellous trabeculae consists of irregularly arranged lamellae separated by deeply staining incremental and resorption lines indicative of previous bone activity, with an occasional haversian system.

Cancellous bone is found predominantly in the interradicular and interdental spaces and in limited amounts facially or lingually, except in the palate. In the adult human, more cancellous bone exists in the maxilla than in the mandible.

Bone Marrow

In the embryo and the newborn, the cavities of all bones are occupied by red hematopoietic marrow. The red marrow gradually undergoes a physiologic change to the fatty or yellow inactive type of marrow. In the adult, the marrow of the jaw is normally of the latter type, and red marrow is found only in the ribs, sternum, vertebrae, skull, and humerus. However, foci of the red bone marrow are occasionally seen in the jaws, often accompanied by the resorption of bony trabeculae. Common locations are the maxillary tuberosity, the maxillary and mandibular molar and premolar areas, and the mandibular symphysis and ramus angle, which may be visible radiographically as zones of radiolucency.

Periosteum and Endosteum

Layers of differentiated osteogenic connective tissue cover all of the bone surfaces. The tissue that covers the outer surface of bone is termed *periosteum*, whereas the tissue that lines the internal bone cavities is called *endosteum*.

The periosteum consists of an *inner layer* composed of osteoblasts surrounded by osteoprogenitor cells, which have the potential to differentiate into osteoblasts, and an *outer layer* rich in blood vessels and nerves and composed of collagen fibers and fibroblasts. Bundles of periosteal collagen fibers penetrate the bone, thereby binding the periosteum to the bone. The endosteum is composed of a single layer of osteoblasts and sometimes a small amount of connective tissue. The inner layer is the osteogenic layer, and the outer layer is the fibrous layer.

Cellular events at the periosteum modulate bone size throughout an individual's life span, and a change in bone size is probably the result of the balance between periosteal osteoblastic and osteoclastic activities. Little is currently known about the control of periosteal osteoblastic activity or the clinical importance of variations in periosteal bone formation. Moreover, the nature and impact of periosteal bone resorption are virtually unexplored.

Interdental Septum

The interdental septum consists of cancellous bone that is bordered by the socket wall cribriform plates (i.e., lamina dura or alveolar bone proper) of approximating teeth and the facial and lingual cortical plates (Fig. 2.26). If the interdental space is narrow, the septum may consist of only the cribriform plate. In one study, for example, the space between the mandibular second premolars and first molars consisted of cribriform plate and cancellous bone in 85% of the cases and of only cribriform plate in the remaining 15%. If the roots are too close together, an irregular "window" can appear in the bone between adjacent roots (Fig. 2.27). Between maxillary molars, the septum consisted of cribriform plate and cancellous bone in 66.6% of the cases; it was composed of only cribriform plate in 20.8%, and it had a fenestration in 12.5%.

Determining root proximity radiographically is important. The mesiodistal angulation of the crest of the interdental septum usually parallels a line drawn between the cementoenamel junctions of the approximating teeth. The distance between the crest of the alveolar bone and the cementoenamel junction in young adults varies between 0.75 and 1.49 mm (average, 1.08 mm). This distance increases with age to an average of 2.81 mm. However, this phenomenon may not be as much a function of age as of periodontal disease.

The mesiodistal and faciolingual dimensions and shape of the interdental septum are governed by the size and convexity of the crowns of the two approximating teeth as well as by the position of the teeth in the jaw and their degree of eruption.

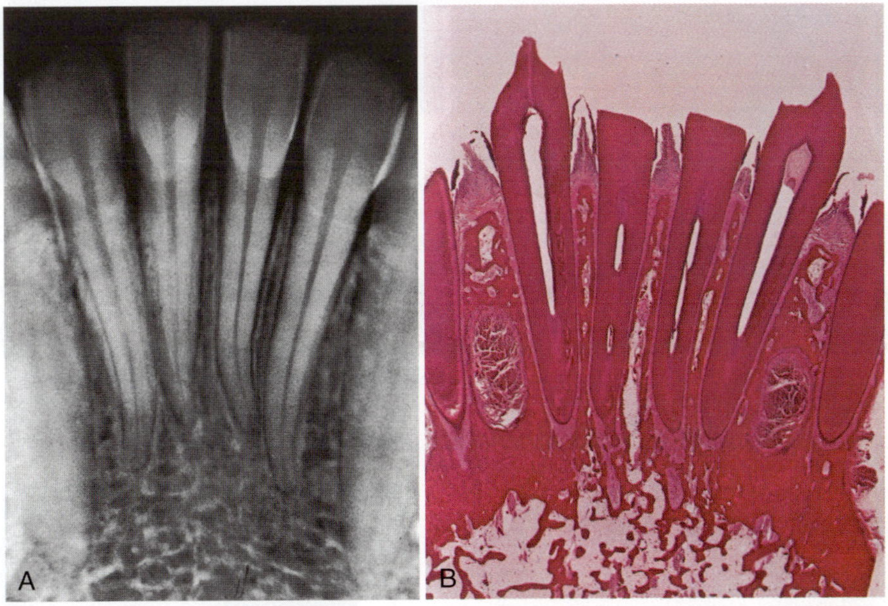

Fig. 2.26 Interdental septa. A, Radiograph of the mandibular incisor area. Note the prominent lamina dura. B, Interdental septa between the mandibular anterior teeth shown in A. There is a slight reduction in bone height with widening of the periodontal ligament in the coronal areas. The central cancellous portion is bordered by the dense bony cribriform plates of the socket, which form the lamina dura around the teeth in the radiograph. Attachments for the mentalis muscle are seen between the canine and lateral incisors. *(From Glickman I, Smulow J: Periodontal disease: clinical, radiographic, and histopathologic features, Philadelphia, 1974, Saunders.)*

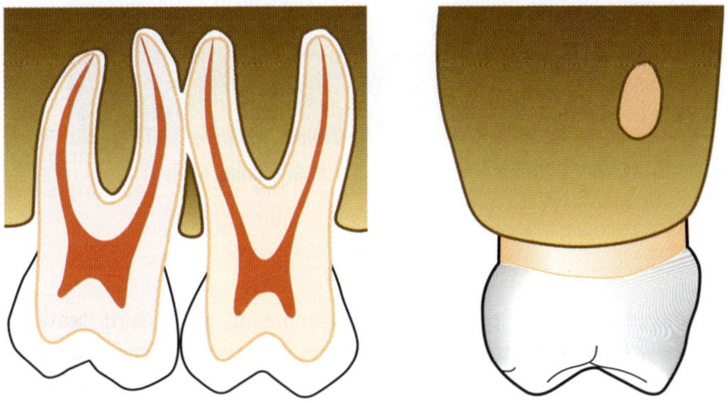

Fig. 2.27 Boneless "window" between adjoining close roots of molars.

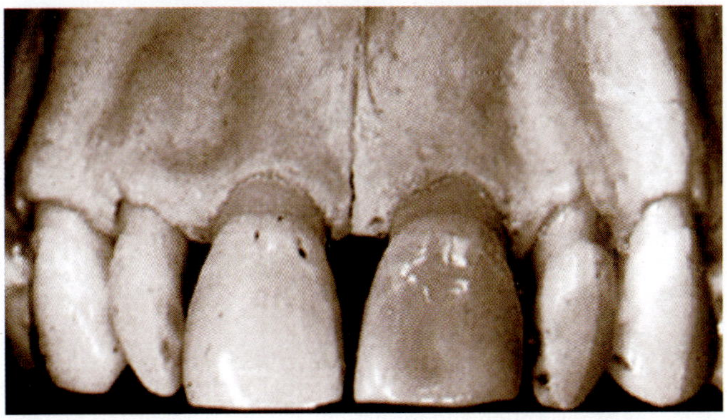

Fig. 2.28 Normal bone contour conforms to the prominence of the roots.

Osseous Topography

The bone contour normally conforms to the prominence of the roots, with intervening vertical depressions that taper toward the margin (Fig. 2.28). Alveolar bone anatomy varies among patients and has important clinical implications. The height and thickness of the facial and lingual bony plates are affected by the alignment of the teeth, the angulation of the root to the bone, and occlusal forces.

On teeth in labial version, the margin of the labial bone is located farther apically than it is on teeth that are in proper alignment. The bone margin is thinned to a knife edge, and it presents an accentuated arc in the direction of the apex. On teeth in lingual version, the facial bony plate is thicker than normal. The margin is blunt, rounded, and horizontal rather than arcuate. The effect of the root-to-bone angulation on the height of alveolar bone is most noticeable on the palatal roots of the maxillary molars. The bone margin is located farther apically on the roots, and it forms relatively acute angles with the palatal bone. The cervical portion of the alveolar plate is sometimes considerably thickened on the facial surface, apparently as reinforcement against occlusal forces (Fig. 2.29).

Fenestration and Dehiscence

Isolated areas in which the root is denuded of bone and the root surface is covered only by periosteum and overlying gingiva are termed *fenestrations*. In these areas, the marginal bone is intact. When the denuded areas extend through the marginal bone, the defect is called a *dehiscence* (Fig. 2.30).

Such defects occur on approximately 20% of the teeth; they occur more often on the facial bone than on the lingual bone, they are more common on anterior teeth than on posterior teeth, and they are frequently bilateral. Microscopic evidence of lacunar resorption may be present at the margins. The cause of these defects is not clear. Prominent root contours, malposition, and labial protrusion of the root in combination with a thin bony plate are predisposing factors. Fenestration and dehiscence are important because they may complicate the outcome of periodontal surgery.

Remodeling of Alveolar Bone

In contrast with its apparent rigidity, alveolar bone is the least stable of the periodontal tissues because its structure is in a constant state

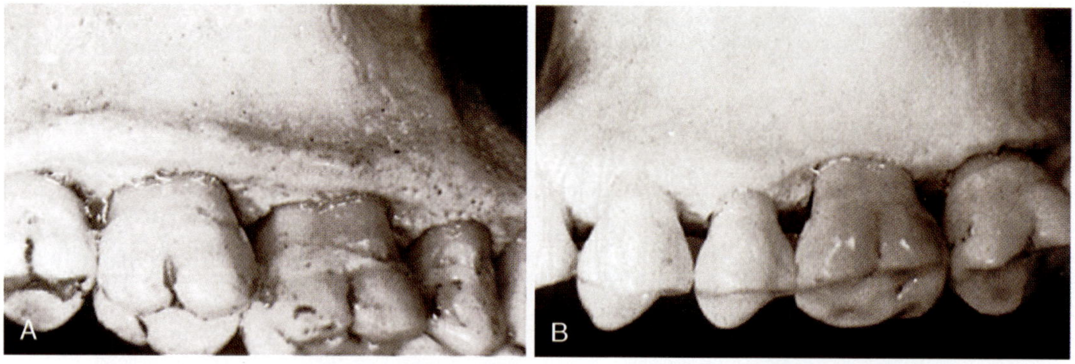

Fig. 2.29 **Variations in the cervical portion of the buccal alveolar plate.** A, Shelf-like conformation. B, Comparatively thin buccal plate.

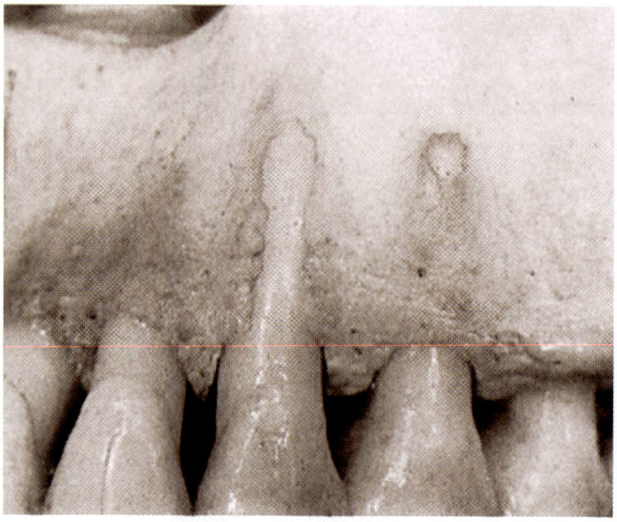

Fig. 2.30 Dehiscence on the canine and fenestration of the first premolar.

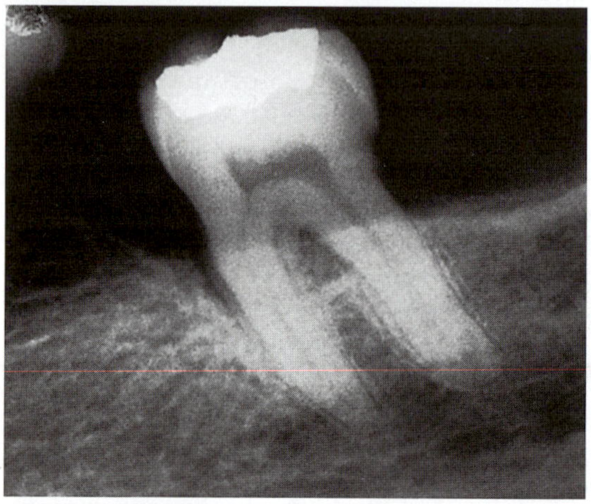

Fig. 2.31 Bony trabeculae realigned perpendicular to the mesial root of a tilted molar.

of flux. A considerable amount of internal remodeling takes place by means of resorption and formation, and this is regulated by local and systemic influences. Local influences include functional requirements on the tooth and age-related changes in bone cells. Systemic influences are probably hormonal (e.g., parathyroid hormone, calcitonin, vitamin D_3).

The remodeling of the alveolar bone affects its height, contour, and density and is manifested in the following three areas: adjacent to the periodontal ligament, in relation to the periosteum of the facial and lingual plates, and along the endosteal surface of the marrow spaces.

Clinical Considerations

Physiologic Migration of the Teeth

Tooth movement does not end when active eruption is completed and the tooth is in functional occlusion. With time and wear, the proximal contact areas of the teeth are flattened, and the teeth tend to move mesially. This is referred to as *physiologic mesial migration.* By the age of 40 years, this process results in a reduction of about 0.5 cm in the length of the dental arch from the midline to the third molars. Alveolar bone is reconstructed in compliance with the physiologic mesial migration of the teeth. Bone resorption is increased in areas of pressure along the mesial surfaces of the teeth, and new layers of bundle bone are formed in areas of tension on the distal surfaces (see Fig. 2.25).

External Forces and the Periodontium

The periodontium exists for the purpose of supporting teeth during function, and it depends on the stimulation that it receives from function for the preservation of its structure. Therefore, a constant and sensitive balance is present between external forces and the periodontal structures.

Alveolar bone undergoes constant physiologic remodeling in response to external forces, particularly occlusal forces. Bone is removed from areas where it is no longer needed and added to areas where it is presently needed.

The socket wall reflects the responsiveness of alveolar bone to external forces. Osteoblasts and newly formed osteoid line the socket in areas of tension; osteoclasts and bone resorption occur in areas of pressure. Forces exerted on the tooth also influence the number, density, and alignment of cancellous trabeculae. The bony trabeculae are aligned in the path of the tensile and compressive stresses to provide maximal resistance to the occlusal force with a minimum of bone substance (Fig. 2.31). When forces are increased, the cancellous bony trabeculae increase in number and thickness, and bone may be added to the external surface of the labial and lingual plates.

A study has shown that the presence of antagonists of occlusal force and the severity of periodontal disease increase the extension of periodontal tissue resorption.

The periodontal ligament also depends on the stimulation provided by function to preserve its structure. Within physiologic limits, the periodontal ligament can accommodate increased function with an increase in width (Table 2.2), a thickening of its fiber bundles, and an increase in the diameter and number of Sharpey fibers. Forces that exceed the adaptive capacity of the periodontium produce injury called *trauma from occlusion.* Since trauma from occlusion can only be confirmed histologically, the clinician is challenged to use clinical and radiographic surrogate indicators in an attempt to facilitate and assist with its diagnosis.

When occlusal forces are reduced, the number and thickness of the trabeculae are reduced. The periodontal ligament also atrophies and appears thinned; the fibers are reduced in number and density, disoriented, and ultimately arranged parallel to the root surface (Fig. 2.32). This phenomenon is termed *disuse atrophy* or *functional atrophy.* With this condition, the cementum is either unaffected or thickened, and the distance from the cementoenamel junction to the alveolar crest is increased.

Decreased occlusal function causes changes in the periodontal microvasculature, such as the occlusion of blood vessels and a decrease in the number of blood vessels. For example, Murrell and coworkers reported that the application and removal of orthodontic force produced significant changes in blood vessel number and density; however, no evidence-based explanation exists for why the force stimulated such changes in the number of blood vessels.

Orthodontic tooth movement is thought to result from site-specific bone remodeling in the absence of inflammation. It is well recognized that tensional forces will stimulate the formation and activity of osteoblastic cells, whereas compressive forces promote osteoclastic activity.

TABLE 2.2 Comparison of Periodontal Width of Functioning and Functionless Teeth in a 38-Year-Old Man

	AVERAGE WIDTH OF PERIODONTAL SPACE		
	Entrance of Alveolus (mm)	Middle of Alveolus (mm)	Fundus of Alveolus (mm)
Heavy function	0.35	0.28	0.30
Left upper second bicuspid			
Light function	0.14	0.10	0.12
Left lower first bicuspid			
Functionless	0.10	0.06	0.06
Left upper third molar			

(Modified from Kronfeld R: *J Am Dent Assoc* 18:1242, 1931.)

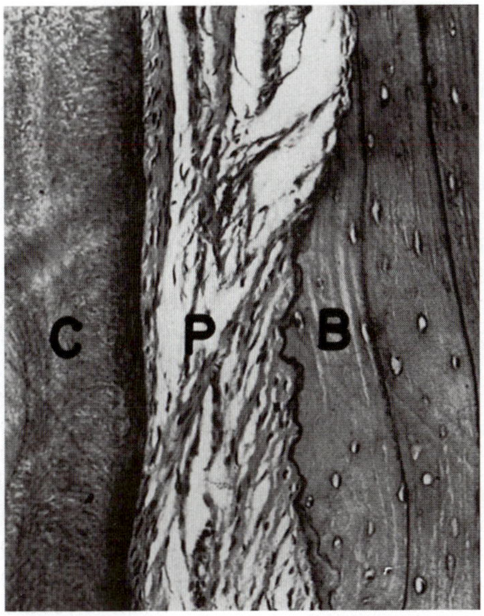

Fig. 2.32 Atrophic periodontal ligament *(P)* of a tooth devoid of function. Note the scalloped edge of the alveolar bone (*B*), which indicates that resorption has occurred. *C*, Cementum.

Vascularization of the Supporting Structures

The blood supply to the supporting structures of the tooth is derived from the inferior and superior alveolar arteries to the mandible and maxilla, and it reaches the periodontal ligament from three sources: apical vessels, penetrating vessels from the alveolar bone, and anastomosing vessels from the gingiva.

The branches of the apical vessels supply the apical region of the periodontal ligament before the vessels enter the dental pulp. The transalveolar vessels are branches of the intraseptal vessels that perforate the lamina dura and enter the ligament. The intraseptal vessels continue to vascularize the gingiva; these gingival vessels in turn anastomose with the periodontal ligament vessels of thc ccrvical region.

The vessels within the periodontal ligament are contained in the interstitial spaces of loose connective tissue between the principal fibers, and they are connected in a netlike plexus that runs longitudinally and closer to the bone than the cementum (Figs. 2.33 and 2.34).

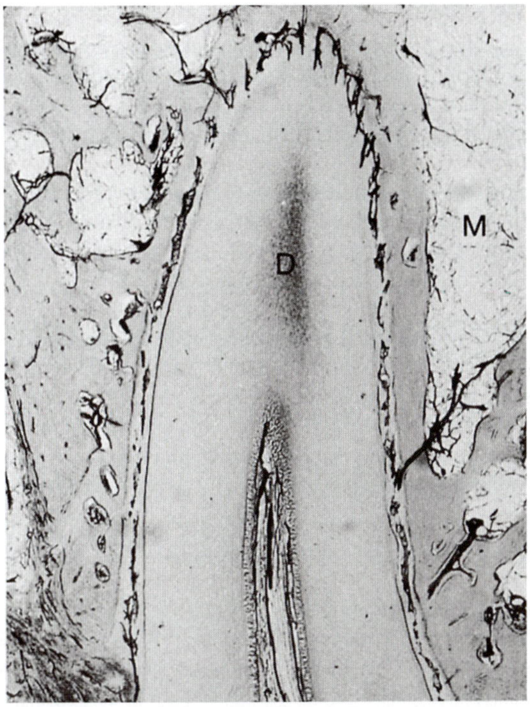

Fig. 2.33 Vascular supply of a monkey periodontium perfused with India ink. Note the longitudinal vessels in the periodontal ligament and the alveolar arteries passing through channels between the bone marrow (*M*) and the periodontal ligament. *D*, Dentin. *(Courtesy: Dr Sol Bernick, Los Angeles.)*

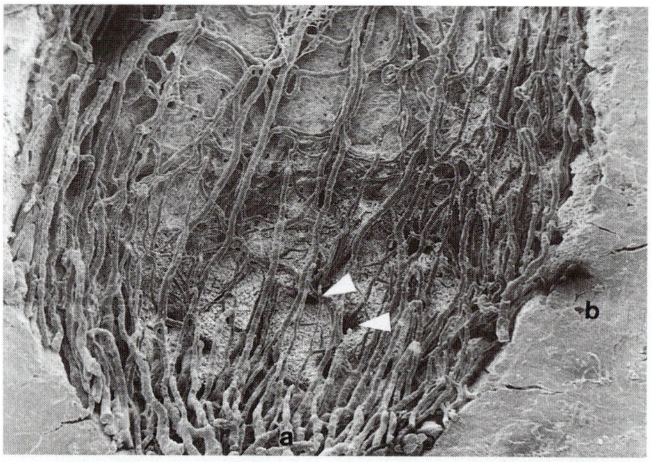

fig. 2.34 vascular supply to the periodontal ligament in a rat molar as viewed by scanning electron microscopy after perfusion with plastic and tissue corrosion. Middle and apical areas of the periodontal ligament are shown with longitudinal blood vessels from the apex (below) to the gingiva (above), perforating vessels entering the bone (*b*), and many transverse connections (*arrowheads*). Apical vessels (*a*) form a cap that connects with the pulpal vessels. *(Courtesy: NJ selliseth and K Selvig, University of Bergen, Norway.)*

The blood supply increases from the incisors to the molars; it is greatest in the gingival third of single-rooted teeth, less in the apical third, and least in the middle; it is equal in the apical and middle thirds of multirooted teeth; it is slightly greater on the mesial and distal surfaces than on the facial and lingual surfaces; and it is greater on the mesial surfaces of the mandibular molars than on the distal surfaces.

The vascular supply to the bone enters the interdental septa through nutrient canals together with veins, nerves, and lymphatics. Dental arterioles, which also branch off of the alveolar arteries, send tributaries through the periodontal ligament, and some small branches enter the marrow spaces of the bone through the perforations in the cribriform plate. Small vessels that emanate from the facial and lingual compact bone also enter the marrow and spongy bone.

The *venous drainage* of the periodontal ligament accompanies the arterial supply. Venules receive blood through the abundant capillary network. In addition, arteriovenous anastomoses bypass the capillaries and are seen more frequently in apical and interradicular regions; their significance is unknown.

Lymphatics supplement the venous drainage system. Lymphatic channels that drain the region just beneath the junctional epithelium pass into the periodontal ligament and accompany the blood vessels into the periapical region. From there, they pass through the alveolar bone to the inferior dental canal in the mandible or the infraorbital canal in the maxilla and then go on to the submaxillary lymph nodes.

Key points

Periodontal Ligament

- The normal periodontium provides the support necessary to maintain teeth in function. The principal components are gingiva, periodontal ligament, cementum, and alveolar bone. Each of these components are distinct in their location, tissue architecture, biochemical composition, and composition, but all these function together as a single unit.
- The periodontal ligament is composed of a complex vascular and highly cellular connective tissue that surrounds the tooth root and connects it to the inner wall of alveolar bone.
- The average width of periodontal ligament space is documented to be about 0.2 mm, considerable variation exists.
- The space diminishes around the teeth which are not in function, and in unerupted teeth, it is increased in teeth subjected to hyperfunction.
- The principal fibers of periodontal ligament are re-arranged in six groups that develop sequentially in the developing root: transeptal, alveolar crest, horizontal, oblique, apical, and interradicular fibers.
- The terminal portion of the principal fibers that are inserted into cementum and bone are called Sharpey fibers.
- The functions of the periodontal ligament are grouped into physical, formative and remodeling, nutritional and sensory functions.

Cementum

- It is a calcified, avascular mesenchymal tissue that forms the outer covering of the anatomic root.
- The main two types of cementum are acellular (primary) and cellular (secondary) cementum. Acellular cementum is the first cementum formed and covers approximately the cervical third or half of the root and does not contain any cells.
- This cementum is formed before the tooth reaches the occlusal plane and its thickness ranges from 30 to 230 μm.
- Cellular cementum is formed after the tooth reaches the occlusal plane. It is more regular and contains cells in individual spaces that communicate with each other through a system of anastomosing canaliculi.
- Cementum attachment protein, a collagenous role of cementum-derived protein along with cementum-derived growth factor and insulin-like growth factor I are present in cementum.
- The permeability of cementum diminishes with age.
- Three types of CEJ are present—overlapping, edge to edge, and gap type of joints. The gap-type junction can cause gingival recession and accentuated sensitivity because of exposed dentin.
- Abnormalities in the thickness of cementum may range from an absence or paucity of cellular cementum (cemental aplasia or hypercementosis).
- Fusion of the cementum and alveolar bone with obliteration of the periodontal ligament is termed as ankylosis.

Alveolar Process

- The alveolar process is the portion of the maxilla and mandible that forms and supports the tooth sockets.
- The inner socket wall of thin and compact bone is called alveolar bone proper, which is termed as lamina dura in radiographs.
- The interdental septum consists of cancellous supporting bone enclosed within a compact border.
- The osteoblasts decreases with aging.
- Remodeling is the major pathway of bony changes in shape, resistance to forces, repair of wounds, and calcium and phosphate homeostasis in the body. Coupling of bone resorption with bone formation constitutes one of the fundamental principles by which bone is necessarily remodeled throughout its life.

Suggested Readings

Ainamo J, Löe H: Anatomical characteristics of gingiva: a clinical and microscopic study of the free and attached gingiva, *J Periodontol* 37: 5, 1966.

Bernick S: Innervation of the teeth and periodontium, *Dent Clin North Am* July: 503, 1959.

Carranza FA, Carranza FA Jr: The management of the alveolar bone in the treatment of the periodontal pocket, *J Periodontol* 27: 29, 1956.
Gottlieb B: Biology of the cementum, *J Periodontol* 13: 13, 1942.
Grant D, Bernick S: Formation of the periodontal ligament, *J Periodontol* 43: 17, 1972.
Listgarten MA: The ultrastructure of human gingival epithelium, *Am J Anat* 114: 49, 1964.
Orban B: Tissue changes in traumatic occlusion, *J Am Dent Assoc* 15: 2090, 1928.
Schroeder HE, Listgarten MA: The gingival tissues: the architecture of periodontal protection, *Periodontol 2000* 13: 91, 1997.
Selvig KA: The fine structure of human cementum, *Acta Odontol Scand* 23: 423, 1965.
Tarnow DP, Magner AW, Fletcher P: The effect of the distance from the contact point to the crest of bone on the presence or absence of the interproximal dental papilla, *J Periodontol* 63: 995, 1992.
Ten Cate AR: The development of the periodontium. In Melcher AH, Bowen WH, editors: *Biology of the periodontium*, New York, 1969, Academic Press.
Turesky S, Glickman I, Litwin T: A histochemical evaluation of normal and inflamed human gingivae, *J Dent Res* 30: 792, 1951.
Weinmann JP, Sicher H: *Bone and bones: fundamentals of bone biology*, ed 2, St Louis, 1955, Mosby.
Zander HA, Hurzeler B: Continuous cementum apposition, *J Dent Res* 37: 1035, 1958.

References

References for this chapter are found on www.medenact.com.

CHAPTER 3

Defense Mechanisms of the Gingiva

J Bulkacz | FA Carranza | DG Naik | A Uppoor

CHAPTER OUTLINE

The gingival tissue is constantly subjected to mechanical and bacterial aggressions. The saliva, the epithelial surface, and the initial stages of the inflammatory response provide resistance to these actions. Section 1 reviews the role of the epithelium, including its degree of keratinization and its turnover rate. This chapter describes the permeability of the junctional and sulcular epithelia and the role of the sulcular fluid, leukocytes, and saliva.

Sulcular Fluid

The presence of sulcular fluid, or *gingival crevicular fluid* (GCF), has been known since the 19th century, but its composition and its possible role in oral defense mechanisms were elucidated by the pioneering work of Waerhaug, Brill, and Krasse during the 1950s. The latter investigators introduced filter paper into the gingival sulci of dogs that had previously been injected intramuscularly with fluorescein; within 3 min, the fluorescent material was recovered on the paper strips. This indicated the passage of fluid from the bloodstream through the tissues and the exiting of fluid via the gingival sulcus.

In subsequent studies, Brill confirmed the presence of GCF in humans and considered it as a "transudate." However, others demonstrated that GCF is an inflammatory exudate rather than a continuous transudate. In strictly normal gingiva, little or no fluid can be collected.

More recently, interest in the development of tests for the detection or prediction of periodontal disease has resulted in numerous research papers about the components, origin, and function of GCF. Potential markers from crevicular fluid are now used as diagnostic tools for the activity of periodontal diseases and a return to homeostasis, with potential for the evaluation of systemic markers.

Methods of Collection

The most difficult hurdle to overcome when collecting GCF is the scarcity of material that can be obtained from the sulcus. Many collection methods have been tried. These methods include the use of *absorbing paper strips, the placement of twisted threads around and into the sulcus, and techniques involving micropipettes and intracrevicular washings*. There are limitations to the techniques, including fluid collection, collection time, flow rate, contamination, and reproducibility.

The *absorbing paper strips* are placed within the sulcus (intrasulcular method) or at its entrance (extrasulcular method) (Fig. 3.1). The placement of the filter paper strip in relation to the sulcus or pocket is important. The Brill technique involves inserting it into the pocket until resistance is encountered (Fig. 3.1A). This method produces some degree of irritation of the sulcular epithelium that by itself can trigger the flow of fluid.

To minimize this irritation, Löe and Holm-Pedersen placed the filter paper strip just at the entrance of the pocket or over the pocket entrance (Fig. 3.1B and C). In this way, fluid that seeps out is picked up by the strip, but the sulcular epithelium is not in contact with the paper.

Preweighed twisted threads were used by Weinstein and colleagues. The threads were placed in the gingival crevice around the tooth, and the amount of fluid collected was estimated by weighing the sample thread.

The use of micropipettes permits the collection of fluid by capillarity. *Capillary tubes* of known internal diameter are inserted into the entrance of the gingival crevice. Isolation and drying of a site is done first. GCF gets collected by capillary action. Since the internal diameter is known, the volume of fluid collected can be accurately determined by measuring the distance which the GCF has migrated. This technique appears to be ideal as it provides an undiluted sample of "native" GCF whose volume can be accurately assessed. However, it is difficult to collect an adequate volume of GCF in a short period atraumatically. A further complication of this technique is the difficulty of removing the complete sample from the tubing.

Crevicular washings can be used to study GCF from clinically normal gingiva. One method involves the use of an appliance that consists of a hard acrylic plate that covers the maxilla, with soft borders and a groove that follows the gingival margins; it is connected to four collection tubes. The washings are obtained by rinsing the crevicular areas from one side to the other with the use of a peristaltic pump.

A modification of the previous method involves the use of two injection needles that have been fitted one within the other so that, during sampling, the inside (ejection) needle is at the bottom of the pocket and the outside (collecting) needle is at the gingival margin. The collection needle is drained into a sample tube via continuous suction.

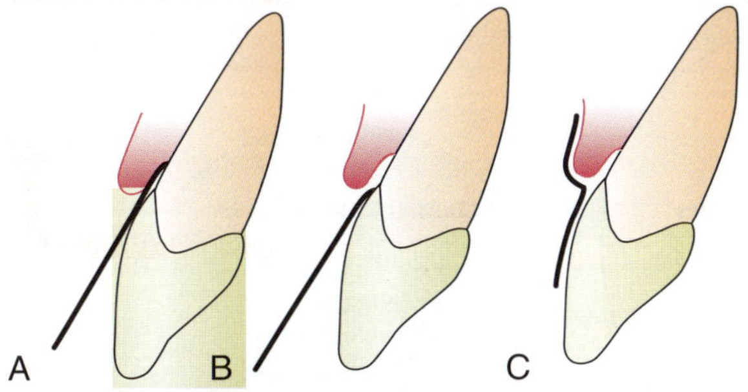

Fig. 3.1 Placement of a filter strip in the gingival sulcus for the collection of fluid. A, Intrasulcular method. B and C, Extrasulcular methods.

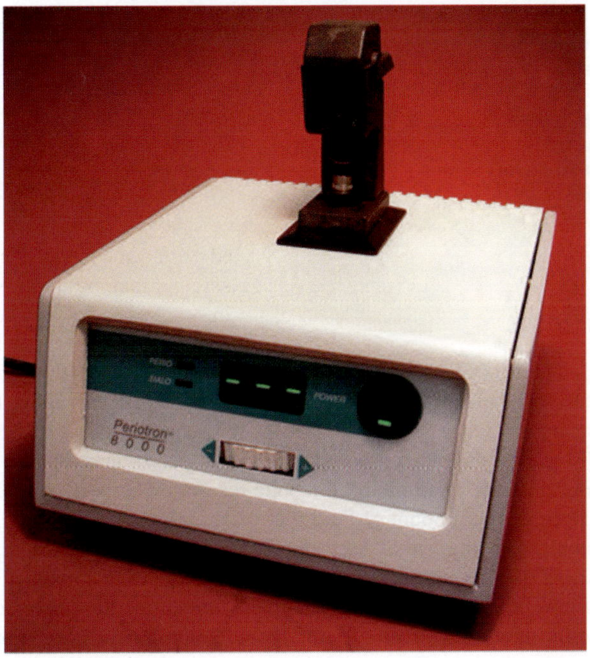

Fig. 3.2 Electronic device for measuring the amount of fluid collected on filter paper.

Permeability of Junctional and Sulcular Epithelia

The initial studies by Brill and Krasse involving the use of fluorescein were later confirmed with substances such as India ink and saccharated iron oxide. Substances that have been shown to penetrate the sulcular epithelium include albumin, endotoxin, thymidine, histamine, phenytoin, and horseradish peroxidase. These findings indicate permeability to substances with a molecular weight of up to 1000 kD.

Squier and Johnson reviewed the mechanisms of penetration through an intact epithelium. The intercellular movement of molecules and ions along with intercellular spaces appears to be a possible mechanism. Substances that take this route do not traverse the cell membranes.

Amount

The amount of GCF collected on a paper strip can be evaluated in a variety of ways. The wetted area can be made more visible by staining with ninhydrin; it is then measured planimetrically on an enlarged photograph or with a magnifying glass or a microscope.

An electronic method has been devised for measuring the fluid collected on a "blotter" (Periopaper) with the use of an electronic transducer (Periotron, Harco Electronics, Winnipeg, Manitoba, Canada) (Fig. 3.2). The wetness of the paper strip affects the flow of an electronic current and provides a digital readout. Three models of Periotron have been produced (the 600, 6000, and now the 8000), and each one has been shown to be an efficient means of measuring the volume of fluid collected on filter paper strips. One of the limitations of the Periotron has its inability to measure volumes of GCF greater than 1.0 μL.

A comparison of the ninhydrin-staining method and the electronic method performed in vitro revealed no significant differences between the two techniques.

The amount of GCF collected is extremely small. Measurements performed by Cimasoni showed that a strip of paper 1.5-mm wide and inserted 1 mm within the gingival sulcus of a slightly inflamed gingiva absorbs about 0.1 mg of GCF in 3 min. Challacombe used an isotope dilution method to measure the amount of GCF present in a particular space at any given time. His calculations for human volunteers with mean gingival indices of less than 1 showed that the mean GCF volume in the proximal spaces from the molar teeth ranged from 0.43 to 1.56 μL.

Problems with GCF collection and data interpretation are as follows:

Contamination: The major sources of contamination of GCF samples would be blood, saliva, or plaque.

Sample time: The problem with prolonged collection times is that the nature of the GCF sample collected is likely to change with the composition concentration (protein, IGM).

Volume determination: Evaporation is considered to be a significant problem in accurate volume determination of GCF samples.

Recovery from the strips: Conflicting results have been described between different research groups, possibly because of entrapment within or binding of GCF proteins to the filter papers. Complete recovery of the content is difficult.

Composition

The components of GCF can be characterized according to individual proteins, specific antibodies, antigens, and enzymes of several specificities. The GCF also contains cellular elements.

Many research efforts have attempted to use GCF components to detect or diagnose active disease or to predict patients who are at risk for periodontal disease. So far, more than 40 compounds found in GCF have been analyzed, but their origin is not known with certainty. These compounds can be derived from the host or produced by the bacteria in the gingival crevice, but their source can be difficult to elucidate; examples include β-glucuronidase, which is a lysosomal enzyme, and lactic acid dehydrogenase, which is a cytoplasmic enzyme. The sources of collagenases may be fibroblasts or polymorphonuclear leukocytes [PMNs (neutrophils)], or collagenases may be secreted by bacteria. Phospholipases are lysosomal and cytoplasmic enzymes, but they are also produced by microorganisms. The majority of GCF elements detected thus far have been enzymes, but there are nonenzymatic substances as well.

Cellular Elements

Cellular elements found in GCF include bacteria, desquamated epithelial cells, and leukocytes (i.e., PMNs, lymphocytes, and monocytes/macrophages), which migrate through the sulcular epithelium.

Electrolytes

Potassium, sodium, and calcium have been studied in the GCF. Most studies have demonstrated a positive correlation of calcium and sodium concentrations with the sodium/potassium ratio seen with inflammation.

Organic Compounds

Both carbohydrates and proteins have been investigated. Glucose hexosamine and hexuronic acid are two of the compounds that are

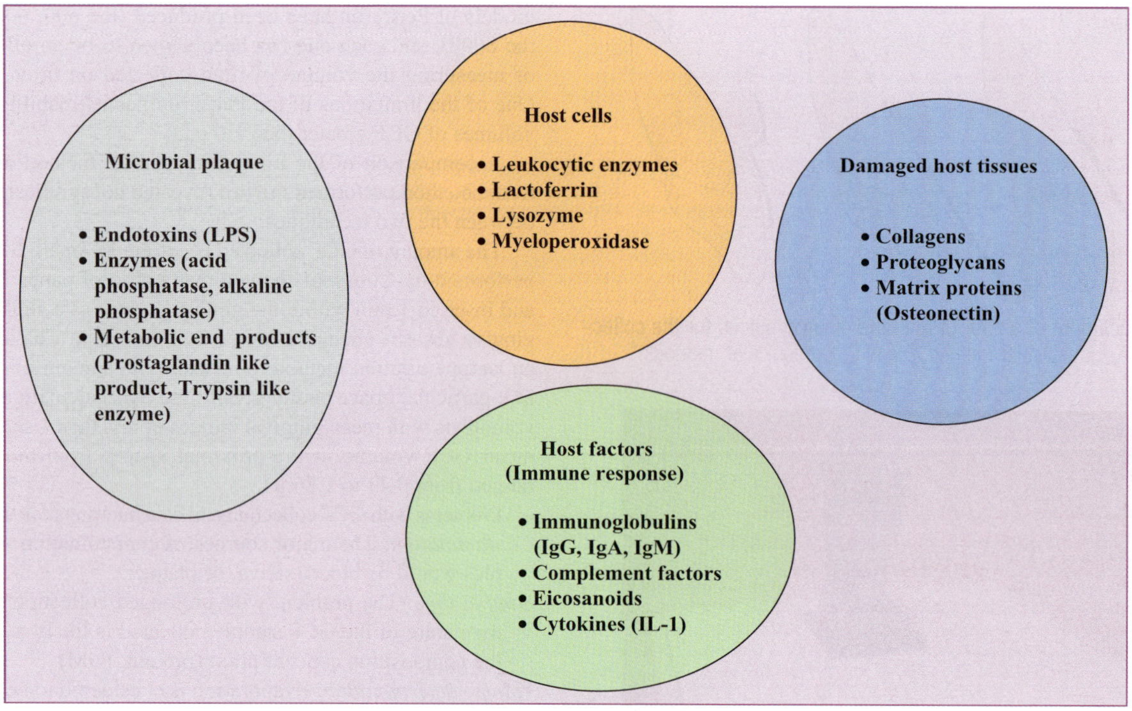

Fig. 3.3 Composition of GCF.

found in GCF. Blood glucose levels do not correlate with GCF glucose levels; glucose concentration in GCF is three to four times greater than that in serum. This is interpreted not only as a result of the metabolic activity of adjacent tissues but also as a function of the local microbial flora.

The total protein content of GCF is much less than that of serum. No significant correlations have been found between the concentration of proteins in GCF and the severity of gingivitis, pocket depth, or extent of bone loss.

Metabolic and bacterial products identified in GCF include lactic acid, urea, hydroxyproline, endotoxins, cytotoxic substances, hydrogen sulfide, and antibacterial factors.

Many enzymes have also been identified (Fig. 3.3).

The methodology used for the analysis of GCF components is as varied as the diversity of those components. Examples include fluorometry for the detection of metalloproteinases; enzyme-linked immunosorbent assays to detect enzyme levels and interleukin-1β (IL-1β); radioimmunoassays for the detection of cyclooxygenase derivatives and procollagen III; high-pressure liquid chromatography to detect timidazole; and direct and indirect immunodot tests for the detection of acute-phase proteins.

Cellular and Humoral Activity in Gingival Crevicular Fluid

Monitoring periodontal disease is a complicated task because very few noninvasive procedures can follow the initiation and progress of the disease. The analysis of GCF constituents in health and disease may be extremely useful as a result of GCF's simplicity and because GCF can be obtained with noninvasive methods.

The analysis of GCF has identified cell and humoral responses in both healthy individuals and in those with periodontal disease. The cellular immune response includes the appearance of cytokines in GCF, but there is no clear evidence of a relationship between cytokines and disease. However, IL-1α and IL-1β are known to increase the binding of PMNs and monocytes/macrophages to endothelial cells, stimulate the production of prostaglandin E_2 and the release of lysosomal enzymes, and stimulate bone resorption. Preliminary evidence also indicates the presence of interferon-α in GCF, which may have a protective role in periodontal disease because of its ability to inhibit the bone resorption activity of IL-1β.

Because the amount of fluid recoverable from gingival crevices is small, only the use of very sensitive immunoassays permits the analysis of the specificity of antibodies. A study that compared antibodies in different crevices with serum antibodies directed at specific microorganisms did not provide any conclusive evidence regarding the significance of the presence of antibodies in GCF among individuals with periodontal disease.

Although the role of antibodies in the gingival defense mechanisms is difficult to ascertain, the consensus is that, in a patient with periodontal disease, a reduction in antibody response is detrimental, and an antibody response plays a protective role.

Clinical Significance

As mentioned previously, GCF is an inflammatory exudate. Its presence in clinically normal sulci can be explained because gingiva that appears clinically normal invariably exhibits inflammation when it is examined microscopically.

CLINICAL CORRELATION

- Novel diagnostics tools allow evaluations of biomarkers from tissue and oral biofluids.
- Drug delivery targeting oral tissues has optimal absorption and bioavailability.
- Gingival fluid and saliva are biologic fluids that can provide information on human genomics and metagenomics (microbiome, transcriptome, metabolome, and proteome).
- Oral immunity is activated through rapid response from innate immune components (fluids, mucosal surfaces, epithelium, cell mediators, molecules, host–bacterial interactions).

The amount of GCF is greater when inflammation is present, and it is sometimes proportional to the severity of inflammation. GCF production is not increased by trauma from occlusion, but it is increased by the mastication of coarse foods, toothbrushing and gingival massage, ovulation, hormonal contraceptives, prosthetic appliances, and smoking. Other factors that influence the amount of GCF are circadian periodicity and periodontal therapy.

Circadian Periodicity

There is a gradual increase in the amount of GCF from 6:00 am to 10:00 pm and a decrease thereafter.

Sex Hormones

Female sex hormones increase GCF flow, probably because they enhance vascular permeability. Pregnancy, ovulation, and hormonal contraceptives, all increase GCF production.

Mechanical Stimulation

Chewing and vigorous gingival brushing stimulate the flow of GCF. Even the minor stimuli represented by the intrasulcular placement of paper strips increases the production of fluid.

Smoking

Smoking produces an immediate transient but marked increase in GCF flow.

Periodontal Therapy

There is an increase in GCF production during the healing period after periodontal surgery.

Drugs in Gingival Crevicular Fluid

Drugs that are excreted through the GCF may be used advantageously in periodontal therapy. Bader and Goldhaber demonstrated in dogs that tetracyclines are excreted through the GCF; this finding triggered extensive research that showed a concentration of tetracyclines in GCF as compared to the serum. Metronidazole is another antibiotic that has been detected in human GCF.

Leukocytes in the Dentogingival Area

Leukocytes have been found in clinically healthy gingival sulci in humans and experimental animals. The leukocytes found are predominantly PMNs. They appear in small numbers extravascularly in the connective tissue adjacent to the bottom of the sulcus; from there, they travel across the epithelium to the gingival sulcus where they are expelled (Figs. 3.4 and 3.5).

Leukocytes are present in sulci even when histologic sections of adjacent tissue are free of inflammatory infiltrate. Differential counts of leukocytes from clinically healthy human gingival sulci have shown 91.2%–91.5% PMNs and 8.5%–8.8% mononuclear cells.

Mononuclear cells were identified as 58% B lymphocytes, 24% T lymphocytes, and 18% mononuclear phagocytes. The ratio of T lymphocytes to B lymphocytes was found to be reversed from the normal ratio of about 3:1 found in peripheral blood to about 1:3 in GCF.

Leukocytes are attracted by different plaque bacteria, but they can also be found in the dentogingival region of germ-free adult animals. Leukocytes were reported in the gingival sulcus in nonmechanically irritated (resting) healthy gingiva, thereby indicating that their migration may be independent of an increase in vascular permeability. The majority of these cells are viable and have phagocytic and killing capacity. Therefore, leukocytes constitute a major protective mechanism against the extension of plaque into the gingival sulcus.

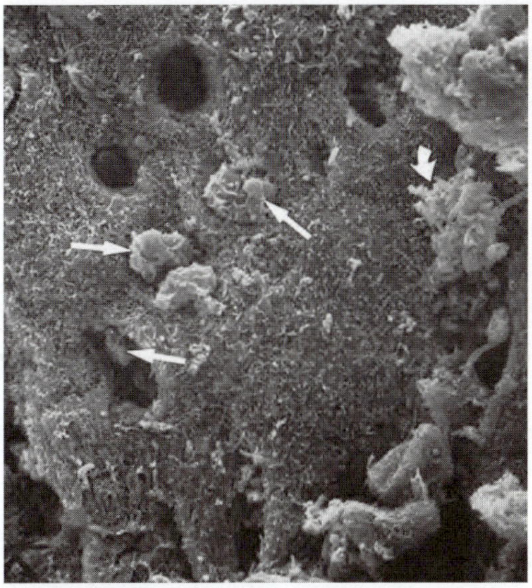

Fig. 3.4 Scanning electron microscope view of the periodontal pocket wall. Several leukocytes are emerging (*straight arrows*), some of which are partially covered by bacteria (*curved arrow*). Empty holes correspond to tunnels through which leukocytes have emerged.

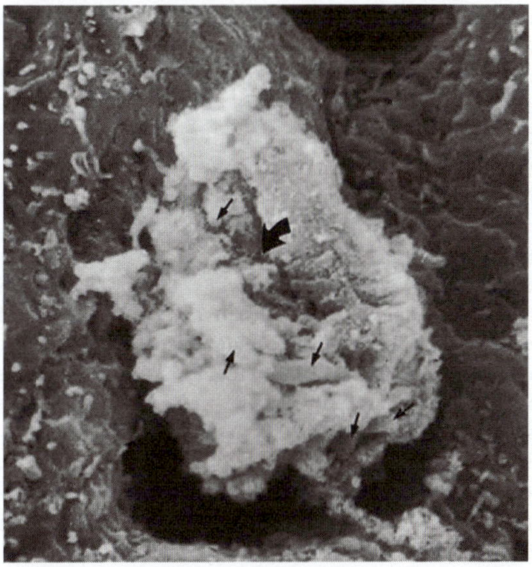

Fig. 3.5 Scanning electron microscope view at higher magnification than shown in Fig. 3.4. A leukocyte emerging from the pocket wall is covered with bacteria (*small arrows*). The large, curved arrow points to a phagosomal vacuole through which bacteria are being engulfed.

Leukocytes are also found in saliva; this is discussed later in this chapter. The main port of entry of leukocytes into the oral cavity is the gingival sulcus.

Saliva

Salivary secretions are protective in nature because they maintain the oral tissues in a physiologic state (Table 3.1). Saliva exerts a major influence on plaque by mechanically cleansing the exposed oral surfaces, by buffering acids produced by bacteria, and by controlling bacterial activity. Saliva is now considered a main biologic fluid for diagnosis of human health and diseases. Systemic and local disease markers are available through saliva. Available tests allow the individual to measure multiomics outputs. Functional and static assays are now available as biosensors of health and disease.

TABLE 3.1 Role of Saliva in Oral Health

Function	Salivary Components	Probable Mechanism
Lubrication	Glycoproteins, mucoids	Coating similar to gastric mucin
Physical protection	Glycoproteins, mucoids	Coating similar to gastric mucin
Cleansing	Physical flow	Clearance of debris and bacteria
Buffering	Bicarbonate and phosphate	Antacids
Tooth integrity maintenance	Minerals	Maturation, remineralization
	Glycoprotein pellicle	Mechanical protection
Antibacterial action	Immunoglobulin A	Control of bacterial colonization
	Lysozyme	Breaks bacterial cell walls
	Lactoperoxidase	Oxidation of susceptible bacteria

Antibacterial Factors

Saliva contains numerous inorganic and organic factors that influence bacteria and their products in the oral environment. Inorganic factors include ions and gases, bicarbonate, sodium, potassium, phosphates, calcium, fluorides, ammonium, and carbon dioxide. Organic factors include lysozyme, lactoferrin, myeloperoxidase, lactoperoxidase, and agglutinins such as glycoproteins, mucins, β2-macroglobulins, fibronectins, and antibodies.

Lysozyme is a hydrolytic enzyme that cleaves the linkage between structural components of the glycopeptide muramic acid-containing region of the cell wall of certain bacteria in vitro. Lysozyme works on both Gram-negative and Gram-positive organisms; its targets include *Veillonella* species and *Actinobacillus actinomycetemcomitans.* It probably repels certain transient bacterial invaders of the mouth.

The *lactoperoxidase–thiocyanate system* in saliva has been shown to be bactericidal to some strains of *Lactobacillus* and *Streptococcus* by preventing the accumulation of lysine and glutamic acid, both of which are essential for bacterial growth. Another antibacterial finding is lactoferrin, which is effective against *Actinobacillus* species.

Myeloperoxidase, which is an enzyme that is similar to salivary peroxidase, is released by leukocytes; it is bactericidal for *Actinobacillus*, but it has the added effect of inhibiting the attachment of *Actinomyces* strains to hydroxyapatite.

Salivary Antibodies

As with GCF, saliva contains antibodies that are reactive with indigenous oral bacterial species. Although immunoglobulins G (IgG) and M (IgM) are present, the preponderant immunoglobulin found in saliva is *immunoglobulin A* (IgA). However, IgG is more prevalent in GCF. Major and minor salivary glands contribute all of the secretory IgA and lesser amounts of IgG and IgM. GCF contributes most of the IgG, complement, and PMNs that, in conjunction with IgG or IgM, inactivate or opsonize bacteria.

Salivary antibodies appear to be synthesized locally because they react with strains of bacteria that are indigenous to the mouth but not with organisms that are characteristic of the intestinal tract. Many bacteria found in saliva have been shown to be coated with IgA, and the bacterial deposits on teeth contain both IgA and IgG in quantities that are greater than 1% of their dry weight. It has been shown that IgA antibodies present in parotid saliva can inhibit the attachment of oral *Streptococcus* species to epithelial cells. Gibbons and colleagues suggested that antibodies in secretions may impair the ability of bacteria to attach to mucosal or dental surfaces.

FLASH BACK

Saliva was known to have protective actions against infection through immunoglobulins only. Now it is clear that enzymes, cytokines, nucleotides, and live cells are part of the host armamentarium.

Enzymes

The *enzymes* that are normally found in the saliva are derived from the salivary glands, bacteria, leukocytes, oral tissues, and ingested substances; the major enzyme is parotid amylase. Certain salivary enzymes have been reported in increased concentrations in periodontal disease: hyaluronidase and lipase, β-glucuronidase and chondroitin sulfatase, aspartate aminotransferase and alkaline phosphatase, amino acid decarboxylases, catalase, peroxidase, and collagenase.

Proteolytic enzymes in the saliva are generated by both the host and oral bacteria. These enzymes have been recognized as contributors to the initiation and progression of periodontal disease. To combat these enzymes, saliva contains antiproteases that inhibit cysteine proteases such as cathepsins and antileukoproteases that inhibit elastase. Another antiprotease, which has been identified as a tissue inhibitor of matrix metalloproteinase, has been shown to inhibit the activity of collagen-degrading enzymes.

High-molecular-weight mucinous glycoproteins in saliva bind specifically to many plaque-forming bacteria. The glycoprotein–bacteria interactions facilitate bacterial accumulation on the exposed tooth surface. The specificity of these interactions has been demonstrated. The interbacterial matrix of human plaque appears to contain polymers that are similar to salivary glycoproteins and that may aid in the maintenance of the integrity of plaque. In addition, these glycoproteins selectively adsorb to the hydroxyapatite to make up part of the acquired pellicle. Other salivary glycoproteins inhibit the sorption of some bacteria to the tooth surface and to epithelial cells of the oral mucosa. This activity appears to be associated with the glycoproteins that possess blood group reactivity. Another effect of mucin is the deletion of bacterial cells from the oral cavity via aggregation with mucin-rich films.

Glycoproteins and a glycolipid that is present on mammalian cell surfaces appear to serve as receptors for the attachment of some viruses and bacteria. Thus, the close similarity between the glycoproteins of salivary secretions and the components of the epithelial cell surface suggests that the secretions can competitively inhibit antigen sorption and that they therefore may limit pathologic alterations.

Salivary Buffers and Coagulation Factors

The maintenance of the physiologic hydrogen ion concentration (pH) at the mucosal epithelial cell surface and the tooth surface is an important function of salivary buffers. The primary effect of these buffers has been studied in relationship to dental caries. In saliva, the most important salivary buffer is the bicarbonate–carbonic acid system.

Saliva also contains coagulation factors (i.e., factors VIII, IX, and X; plasma thromboplastin antecedent; and Hageman factor) that hasten blood coagulation and that protect wounds from bacterial invasion. An active fibrinolytic enzyme may also be present.

Leukocytes

In addition to desquamated epithelial cells, the saliva contains all forms of leukocytes, of which the principal cells are PMNs. Whole-blood PMNs are naïve and not activated, whereas the cells found in saliva have interacted with multiple antigens from the microbiome. The number of PMNs varies from person to person at different times of the day, and it is increased in the presence of gingivitis. PMNs reach the oral cavity by migrating through the lining of the gingival sulcus. Living PMNs in saliva are sometimes referred to as *orogranulocytes*, and their rate of migration into the oral cavity is termed the *orogranulocytic migratory rate.* Some investigators think that the rate of migration correlates with the severity of gingival inflammation and that it is therefore a reliable index for the assessment of gingivitis.

CLINICIAN'S CORNER

What is the clinical importance of saliva?

Saliva has several important properties, including mechanical, chemical, biologic, and immunologic. It is a viscous, clear, watery fluid secreted from salivary glands. It is a major biologic fluid for diagnosis and "omics" research. Diagnosing local and systemic conditions is possible through salivary markers. Low saliva is a risk factor for caries and periodontal disease. Xerostomia is defined as dry mouth resulting from reduced or absent saliva flow. Xerostomia is a symptom of various medical conditions, and it is a side effect of radiation to the head and neck and a wide variety of medications.

Role in Periodontal Pathology

Saliva exerts a major influence on plaque initiation, maturation, and metabolism. Salivary flow and composition also influence calculus formation, periodontal disease, and caries. The removal of the salivary glands in experimental animals significantly increases the incidence of dental caries and periodontal disease in addition to delaying wound healing.

In humans, an increase in inflammatory gingival diseases, dental caries, and rapid tooth destruction that is associated with cervical or cemental caries is partially a consequence of decreased salivary gland secretion (xerostomia). Xerostomia may result from sialolithiasis, sarcoidosis, Sjögren syndrome, Mikulicz disease, irradiation, the surgical removal of the salivary glands, and other factors.

FLASH BACK

- Gingival tissue is constantly challenged by external factors.
- Epithelial surface, crevicular fluid, saliva, epithelial surfaces, immune cells, and mediators provide oral immunity.
- Oral diseases, including caries and periodontal diseases, benefit from oral immune components.

Key points

- The presence of GCF or sulcular fluid has been known since 19th century and its composition and possible role in oral defense mechanisms were elucidated by the pioneering work of Waerhaug, Brill, and Krasse.
- It acts as transudate or exudate based on clinical tissue condition.
- In strictly normal gingiva, little or no fluid can be collected.
- GCF can be collected by the intrasulcular method and the extrasulcular method.
- GCF can be collected using absorbing paper strips, twisted threads, micropipettes, and intracrevicular washings.
- The amount of GCF collected on a paper strip can be evaluated in a variety of ways. It can be done using ninhydrin dye and electronic method by periotron.
- The composition of GCF include specific antibodies, antigens and enzymes, and cellular elements.
- GCF production is not increased by trauma from occlusion but increased by mastication of coarse foods, toothbrushing and gingival massage, ovulation, hormonal contraceptives, and smoking. Other factors are circadian periodicity and periodontal therapy.
- Tetracycline and Metronidazole are detected in GCF.
- Saliva secretions are protective in nature because they maintain the oral tissues in physiologic state.
- It has antibacterial, lubricating, cleansing, and buffering action. It also helps in physical protection and tooth integrity maintenance.
- The preponderant immunoglobulin found in saliva is IgA, and in GCF, it is IgG.
- The lactoperoxidase–thiocyanate system in saliva has been shown to be bactericidal to some strains of *Lactobacillus* and *Streptococcus.*

Suggested Readings

Bader HJ, Goldhaber P: The passage of intravenously administered tetracycline in the gingival sulcus of dogs, *J Oral Ther* 2: 324, 1966.

Brill N, Krasse B: The passage of tissue fluid into the clinically healthy gingival pocket, *Acta Odontol Scand* 16: 223, 1958.

Bulkacz J: Enzymatic activities in gingival fluid with special emphasis on phospholipases, *J West Soc Periodontol Periodontal Abstr* 36: 145, 1986.

Egelberg J: Cellular elements in gingival pocket fluid, *Acta Odontol Scand* 21: 283, 1963.

Egelberg J: Gingival exudate measurements for evaluation of inflammatory changes of the gingiva, *Odont Rev* 15: 381, 1964.

Griffiths J: Formation, collection, and significance of gingival crevice fluid, *Periodontol 2000* 31: 32–42, 2003.

Lamster IB, Novak MJ: Host mediators in gingival crevicular fluid: implications for the pathogenesis of periodontal disease, *Crit Rev Oral Biol Med* 3: 31, 1992.

Skougaard MR, Bay I, Klinkhamer JM: Correlation between gingivitis and orogranulocytic migratory rate, *J Dent Res* 48: 716, 1994.

References

References for this chapter are found on www.medenact.com.

CHAPTER 4

Aging and the Periodontium

I Needleman | DG Naik | A Uppoor

CHAPTER OUTLINE

Classification of Elderly Population

Aging is a natural process. Old age should be regarded as a normal, inevitable biological phenomenon. The gradual changes taking place in the dental tissues after the teeth are fully formed and are referred to as age changes.

The "Elderly" Segment of the Population

1. People aged 65–74 years are the new or young elderly who tend to be relatively healthy and active.
2. People aged 75–84 years are the old or mid-old, who vary from those being healthy and active to those managing an array of chronic diseases.
3. People of 85 years and older are the oldest-old, who tend to be physically frailer. This last group is the fastest-growing segment of the older adult population.

Increased health awareness and improvements in preventive dentistry have led to decreasing tooth loss for all age groups. The effects of this shift in tooth retention need to be considered carefully. In particular, increased life expectancy and greater health expectations may lead to changes in demand from older individuals for periodontal treatment and potentially a substantial increase in supportive periodontal therapy. Therefore, an understanding of the impact of aging on the periodontium is critical. This chapter will first review the literature concerning the fundamental aspects of aging on the periodontal tissues; broader aspects of aging will then be examined and their possible effects on treatment outcomes discussed.

The evidence base is not without problems, many of which make it difficult to draw conclusions about the effects of aging. Some of these problems include inconsistency with regard to the definition of a true "older" group, the inadequate exclusion of adults with systemic diseases that can modify study findings, and attempts to extrapolate results from animal research. For the purposes of this chapter, the effects of aging are limited to a narrow review of possible biologic and microbiologic changes. (For further information on the effects of aging on the dental and periodontal patient, the reader should consult Holm-Pedersen P, Walls AW, Ship JA: *Textbook of geriatric dentistry*, ed 3, Oxford, UK, 2015, Wiley-Blackwell.) The reader should be fully aware that this narrower scope excludes many important age-associated phenomena, including reductions in an individual's cognitive or motor function skills, which may have a direct impact on periodontal management. These issues are discussed more fully in Chapter 42. Several studies have reported associations between periodontitis and cognitive impairment and aging, although whether these findings reflect causation or simply association remains unclear. These links are difficult to entangle because "*chronic inflammation is a prominent feature of aging and of age-related diseases.*"

CLINICAL CORRELATION

For a full understanding of aging and managing periodontal health, in addition to this chapter on biology, readers should understand aging more broadly, including cognitive and motor function effects that could affect oral hygiene, for instance.

The volume of new research into aging and the periodontium has not increased substantially. Highly sensitive molecular and genomic techniques have been employed in related laboratory research, and these are starting to provide insight into age-associated effects. These approaches will likely prove fruitful in the future. Despite the limited data directly related to the periodontium, much effort and many resources have been used to research questions at least partially related to this topic. These include the effect of periodontal infection on general health and the impact of osteoporosis on periodontal status.

Effects of Aging on the Periodontium

Gingival Epithelium

Thinning and decreased keratinization of the gingival epithelium have been reported with age. The significance of these findings could mean an increase in epithelial permeability to bacterial antigens, a decreased resistance to functional trauma, or both. If so, such changes may influence long-term periodontal outcomes. However, other studies have found no age-related differences in the gingival epithelium of humans or dogs. Other reported changes with aging include the flattening of rete pegs and altered cell density. Conflicting data regarding the surgical regeneration times

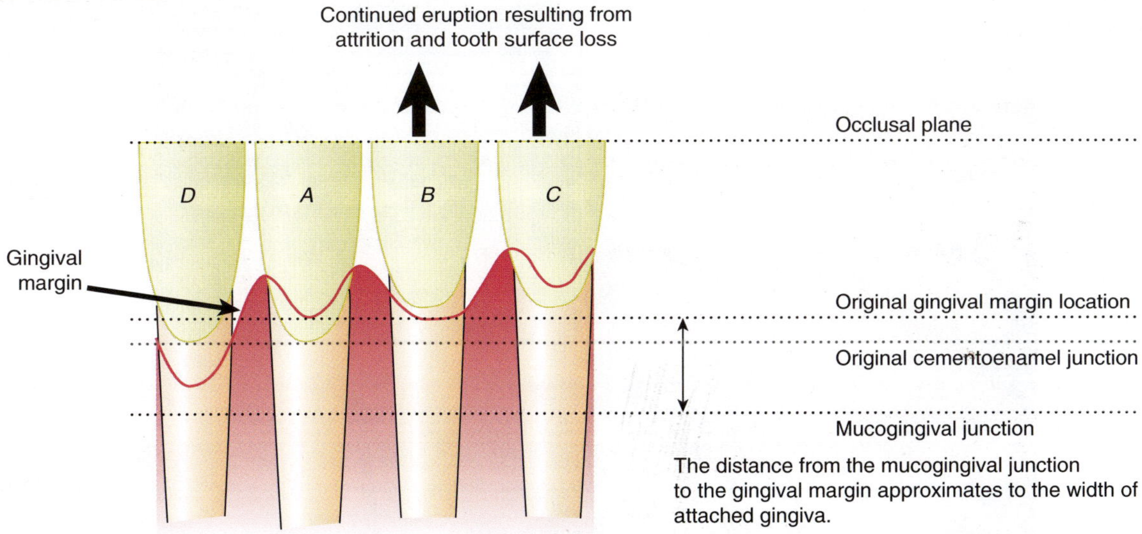

Fig. 4.1 Diagram showing the relationship of the gingival margin with the crown and root surface. A, Normal relationship with the gingival margin 1–2 mm above the cementoenamel junction. B, Wear of the incisal edge and continued tooth eruption. The gingival margin remains in the same position as shown in A. Therefore, the root surface is exposed, and clinical recession is evident. The width of the attached gingiva has not changed. C, Wear of the incisal edge and continued tooth eruption. The gingival margin has moved with the tooth; therefore, the entire dentogingival complex has moved coronally, with a resulting increase in the width of the attached gingiva. D, No wear of incisal edge is evident. The gingiva has moved apically, and clinical recession is evident. The width of attached gingiva is reduced.

for gingival epithelium have been ascribed to problems with research methodology.

The effect of aging on the location of the junctional epithelium has been the subject of much speculation. Some reports show migration of the junctional epithelium from its position in healthy individuals (i.e., on the enamel) to a more apical position on the root surface with accompanying gingival recession. However, in other animal studies, no apical migration has been noted. With continuing gingival recession, the width of the attached gingiva would be expected to decrease with age, but the opposite appears to be true. This is attributed to the eruptive movement of the teeth rather than to the intrinsic aging phenomenon. The migration of the junctional epithelium to the root surface could be caused by the tooth erupting through the gingiva in an attempt to maintain occlusal contact with its opposing tooth (passive eruption) as a result of tooth surface loss from attrition (Fig. 4.1).

The consensus is that gingival recession is not an inevitable physiologic process of aging but rather it can be explained by the cumulative effects of inflammation or trauma on the periodontium (Fig. 4.2); this is discussed in more detail later in this chapter. Changes in the apoptotic gene expression of gingival tissue with age have recently been reported in nonhuman primates. This finding requires further research to understand its potential impact on gingival homeostasis and the pathogenesis of periodontal diseases.

KEY FACT

Gingival recession is not an inevitable consequence of aging but is the cumulative result of trauma or periodontitis.

Gingival Connective Tissue

Increasing age results in coarser and denser gingival connective tissues. Qualitative and quantitative changes to collagen have been reported. These include an increased rate of conversion of soluble to insoluble collagen, increased mechanical strength, and increased denaturing temperature. These results indicate increased collagen stabilization caused by changes in the macromolecular conformation. Not surprisingly, an increased collagen content has been found in the gingivae of older animals, despite a lower rate of collagen synthesis decreasing with age.

Periodontal Ligament

Changes in the periodontal ligament that have been reported with aging include decreased number of fibroblasts and a more irregular structure, thus paralleling the changes seen in the gingival connective tissues. Other findings include decreased organic matrix production, epithelial cell rests, and increased amounts of elastic fiber. Conflicting results have been reported for changes in the width of the periodontal ligament in human and animal models. Although true variation may exist, this finding probably reflects the functional status of the teeth in the studies: the width of the space will decrease if the tooth is unopposed (i.e., hypofunction) or increase with excessive occlusal loading. Both scenarios can be anticipated as a result of tooth loss in this population. These effects may also explain the variability in studies that have reported qualitative changes within the periodontal ligament.

KEY FACT

- Findings comparing periodontal ligament cells in older individuals (i.e., >60 years old) with those of younger individuals (i.e., 15–20 years old) have suggested greater gene expression for proinflammatory cytokines such as IL 1 and IL 6.
- In addition to increased IL-1 and IL-6 expression, osteoprotegerin (OPG) was also increased, which suggests that increased OPG may be a homeostatic response to the upregulation of inflammation.
- Periodontal ligament cell proliferation is decreased with age, thereby suggesting an impairment in repair potential.

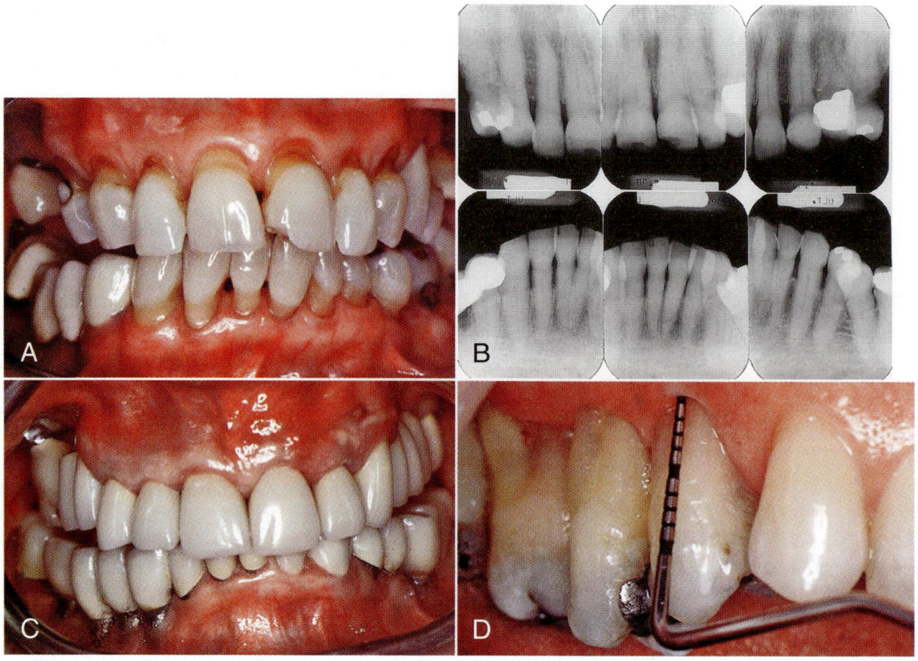

Fig. 4.2 Three scenarios illustrating the variation of the position of the gingival margin with age. A, Overeruption with recession in an older individual (i.e., a 68-year-old woman) with generalized recession and a history of previously treated periodontitis. Note some overeruption of the lower anterior teeth and wear of teeth related to oral hygiene measures. B, Radiographs of the patient shown in A. C, Overeruption without recession in an older individual (i.e., a 72-year-old woman) with no periodontitis but marked lower incisor tooth wear and overeruption. Note how the gingival margin has migrated coronally with the erupting teeth. D, Extensive recession in a younger individual (i.e., a 32-year-old man) with marked recession and no history of periodontitis. The recession has resulted from a combination of anatomically thin tissues and toothbrush-related trauma.

Cementum

Some consensus regarding the effect of aging on cementum exists. An increase in cemental width is a common finding; this increase may be 5–10 times with increasing age. This finding is not surprising because deposition continues after tooth eruption. The increase in width is greater apically and lingually. Although cementum has limited capacity for remodeling, an accumulation of resorption bays explains the finding of increasing surface irregularity.

Alveolar Bone

Reports of morphologic changes in alveolar bone mirror age-related changes in other bony sites. Specific to the periodontium are findings of a more irregular periodontal surface of bone and the less-regular insertion of collagen fibers. Although age is a risk factor for the bone mass reductions in individuals with osteoporosis, it is not causative and therefore should be distinguished from physiologic aging processes. Overriding the diverse observations of bony changes with age is the important finding that the healing rate of bone in extraction sockets appears to be unaffected by increasing age. Indeed, the success of osseointegrated dental implants, which relies on intact bone healing responses, does not appear to be age-related. However, balancing this view is the recent observation that bone graft preparations (i.e., decalcified freeze-dried bone) from donors who were more than 50 years old possessed significantly less osteogenic potential than graft material from younger donors. The possible significance of this phenomenon for normal healing responses needs to be investigated.

Tooth–Periodontium Relationship

There is loss of tooth substance due to attrition leading to reduction in cuspal height and inclination due to wear.

The degree of attrition is influenced by the musculature, consistency of food, tooth hardness, occupational factors, and habits such as grinding and clenching. The rate of attrition may be coordinated with other age-related changes such as continuous tooth eruption and gingival recession. As the tooth erupts, cementum is usually deposited in the apical region of the root.

The reduction in bone height that occurs with aging is not necessarily related to occlusal wear. Bone loss results in an increase in crown to root ratio. Wear of teeth also occurs on the proximal surfaces accompanied by mesial migration of teeth. Proximal wear reduces the anteroposterior length of the dental arch by approximately 0.5 cm by age 40. Progressive attrition and proximal wear result in a maxillary–mandibular overjet in the molar area and an edge-to-edge bite anteriorly.

Bacterial Plaque

Dentogingival plaque accumulation has been suggested to increase with age. This might be explained by the increase in hard-tissue surface area as a result of gingival recession and the surface characteristics of the exposed root surface as a substrate for plaque formation as compared to enamel. Other studies have shown no difference in plaque quantity with age. This contradiction might reflect the different age ranges of experimental groups as variable degrees of gingival recession and root surface exposure. For supragingival plaque, no real qualitative differences have been shown for plaque composition. With regard to subgingival plaque, one study has shown subgingival flora to be similar to normal flora, whereas another study reported increased numbers of enteric rods and pseudomonads in older adults. Mombelli suggests caution when interpreting this finding because of the increased oral carriage of these species among older adults. It has been speculated that a shift occurs in the importance of certain periodontal pathogens with age, specifically including an increased role for *Porphyromonas gingivalis* and a decreased role for *Aggregatibacter actinomycetemcomitans*. However, differentiating true age effects from the changes in ecologic determinants for periodontal bacteria will be difficult.

Another approach to investigating microbiology consists of conducting intervention studies and examining the impact on the microflora. Among individuals who were 60–75 years old, the prevalence of *P. gingivalis, Treponema forsythia, Treponema denticola, A. actinomycetemcomitans*, and *Prevotella intermedia* was high and was not clearly related to probing depth. The finding of high levels of the organisms could have been related to the sample of individuals: the participants were mostly those with low incomes and with no recent dental care. Long-term use (i.e., 5 years) of a 0.12% chlorhexidine mouthrinse did not promote reductions in the proportions of the organisms in individuals experiencing alveolar bone loss as compared to the placebo mouthrinse, possibly because the mouthrinse routine may have been less frequent than daily.

Immune and Inflammatory Responses

Recent advances in the study of the effects of aging on the immune response (i.e., immunosenescence) have altered the understanding of this phenomenon. In particular, more recent studies have set tighter controls on excluding individuals with systemic conditions known to affect the immune response. As a result, age has been recognized as having much less effect on the alteration of the host response than previously thought. Differences between younger and older individuals can be demonstrated for T and B cells, cytokines, and natural killer cells but not for polymorphonuclear cells and macrophage activity. (Differences between younger and older individuals can be demonstrated for T and B cells, cytokines, and natural killer cells, with increased inflammatory-type (M1) macrophage subset gene expression (in a nonhuman primate model) but not for polymorphonuclear cells.) McArthur concluded the following: "Measurement of indicators of immune and inflammatory competency suggested that, within the parameters tested, there was no evidence for age-related changes in host defenses correlating with periodontitis in an elderly (65 to 75 years) group of individuals, with and without disease." Recent laboratory studies have shown age-related changes in the expression of proinflammatory mediators and innate immunity with the potential to alter the pathology of periodontal diseases or antimicrobial function. However, the relevance of these findings to the clinical situation has not been demonstrated. Age-related differences in the inflammatory response among individuals with gingivitis have been clearly demonstrated and are discussed later in this textbook.

In relation to systematic inflammatory responses, C-reactive protein (CRP) is an acute phase protein that is widely regarded as a marker of inflammatory burden and response to bacterial infection. When investigating serum CRP levels among individuals who are 60–75 years old and comparing individuals with progressive periodontitis with those with stable disease, CRP levels were increased in those with progressive periodontitis and no other systemic conditions. This may indicate that inflammatory burden can be investigated with the use of CRP although there is growing evidence that CRP alone may not be as reliable a marker in older people.

A further modulator of the immune and inflammatory responses is nutrition. Interest in this field is increasing rapidly as part of both medicine and periodontology. Nutrition has been studied extensively in geriatric medicine as a result of the nutritional intake changes that occur with age. The impact of nutrition as a potential risk factor for periodontal diseases and their progression is therefore of interest. Emerging data suggest a negative association of serum folate with periodontitis. After controlling for major known confounders, lower serum folate levels in dentate adults who are more than 60 years old are associated with greater levels of periodontitis. These cross-sectional data cannot demonstrate causality alone, but the recognized relationship between folate protection and chronic inflammatory diseases (e.g., cardiovascular disease) offers biologic plausibility to a potential relationship that merits further investigation with prospective studies.

Although many contradictions exist, a survey of the literature demonstrates that some age-related changes are evident in the periodontium and the host response. Whether these changes are significant in the alteration of the progression of periodontal diseases or the response of an older adult to periodontal treatment will be examined next.

Effects of Aging on the Progression of Periodontal Diseases

In a classic experimental gingivitis study, subjects were rendered free of plaque and inflammation through frequent professional cleaning. After this was achieved, the subjects abstained from oral hygiene measures for a period of 3 weeks to allow gingivitis to develop. In this experimental model, a comparison of developing gingivitis between younger and older individuals demonstrated a greater inflammatory response in older subjects, both in humans and in dogs. In the older age group (i.e., 65–80 years), the findings included a greater amount of infiltrated connective tissue, increased gingival crevicular fluid flow, and an increased gingival index. Other studies have not demonstrated differences between subjects; this may be related to smaller differences between the ages of the younger and older experimental groups. Intriguingly, even at the baseline level of excellent gingival health before the commencement of plaque accumulation, differences may exist between groups, with older individuals demonstrating more inflammation.

The phrase *getting long in the tooth* expresses a widespread belief that age is inevitably associated with an increased loss of connective tissue attachment. However, this observation may equally well reflect cumulative exposure to a number of potentially destructive processes. These exposures may include plaque-associated periodontitis, chronic mechanical trauma from toothbrushing, and iatrogenic damage from unfavorable restorative dentistry or repeated scaling and root planing. The effects of these exposures act in one direction only (i.e., an increased loss of attachment).

In an attempt to differentiate the effects of age from these other processes, several studies have been designed to eliminate confounding issues and to address more clearly the question of age as a risk factor for periodontitis. The conclusions from these studies are strikingly consistent and show that the effect of age is either nonexistent or provides a small and clinically insignificant increased risk of loss of periodontal support. Indeed, in a study, comparison with the odds ratio of 20.52 for poor oral hygiene status and periodontitis, the odds ratio for age was only 1.24, and smoking was much more influential than age. Therefore, age has been suggested to be not a true risk factor but rather a background or associated factor for periodontitis. In addition, the clarification of a genetic basis for susceptibility to severe forms of periodontitis underlines the overriding importance of plaque, smoking, and susceptibility in explaining most of the variations in periodontal disease severity among individuals. Nevertheless, a longitudinal study of essentially untreated periodontitis in an older adult (≥70 years old) Japanese population indicated that 296 of 394 individuals (75%) had a least

1 site with 3 mm or more loss of attachment over a 2-year period. Smoking and a baseline attachment level of 6 mm or more were significantly associated with disease progression. A more recent study modeling the transition of periodontal health states over a 2-year period estimated that the risk of transitioning from health to gingivitis was overall reduced by 3% with age. Each year of age increase was associated with a 2% decreased risk of such a transition. Furthermore, increased age was not statistically associated with an increased risk of transitioning from health or gingivitis to periodontitis.

Aging and the Response to Treatment of the Periodontium

The successful treatment of periodontitis requires both meticulous home plaque control by the patient and meticulous supragingival and subgingival debridement by the therapist. Unfortunately, only a few studies have directly compared such an approach among patients of different age groups. The few studies that have done so clearly demonstrate that, despite the histologic changes in the periodontium with aging, no differences in response to nonsurgical or surgical treatment have been shown for periodontitis. However, if plaque control is not ideal, the continued loss of attachment is inevitable. Furthermore, without effective periodontal therapy, the progression of disease may be faster with increasing age. Attempts to increase plaque control by chemical means have also been reported.

A purely biologic or physiologic review indicates that aging has some impact on the structure and function of the periodontium as well as on the immune response and the nature of either supragingival or subgingival plaque. However, these changes have a negligible impact on an individual's responsiveness to treatment. Aging may affect other aspects of the management of periodontal health like root caries, and the resulting difficulties should not be underestimated. Interestingly, a recent study has identified greater compliance with supportive maintenance among older individuals as compared to younger patients.

KEY FACT

The biologic effects of aging have either no impact or a minimal impact on an individual's response to periodontal treatment. However, other factors may have a profound impact, including cognitive and motor skills as well as medical history.

Key points

- Thinning and decreased keratinization of the gingival epithelium have been reported with age.
- Changes in the periodontal ligament reported with aging include decreased numbers of fibroblasts and a more irregular structure, paralleling the changes in the gingival connective tissues.
- There is increase in the amount of elastic fibers.
- An increase in cemental width is a common finding with an increase in age. This increase may be 5–10 times increasing with age.
- Dentogingival plaque accumulation has been suggested to increase with age.
- The successful treatment of periodontitis requires both meticulous plaque control by the patient at home and professionally.

Suggested Readings

Amler MH, Amler MH: Age factor in human alveolar bone repair, *J Oral Implantol* 19: 138–142, 1993.

Benatti BB, Silvqrio KG, Casati MZ, et al: Inflammatory and bone-related genes are modulated by aging in human periodontal ligament cells, *Cytokine* 46: 176–181, 2009.

Bryant SR, Zarb GA, Bryant SR, et al: Osseointegration of oral implants in older and younger adults, *Int J Oral Maxillofac Implants* 13: 492–499, 1998.

Burt BA, Burt BA: Periodontitis and aging: reviewing recent evidence, *J Am Dent Assoc* 125: 273–279, 1994.

Chung HY, Lee EK, Choi YJ, et al: Molecular inflammation as an underlying mechanism of the aging process and age-related diseases, *J Dent Res* 90: 830–840, 2011.

Garcia RI, Nunn ME, Dietrich T: Risk calculation and periodontal outcomes, *Periodontol* 2000 (50): 65–77, 2009.

Hajishengallis G: Too old to fight? Aging and its toll on innate immunity, *Mol Oral Microbiol* 25: 25–37, 2010.

Holm-Pedersen IC, Loe T: *Textbook of geriatric changes in the teeth with aging*, London, 1997, Wiley.

Needleman I, Suvan J, Moles DR, et al: A systematic review of professional mechanical plaque removal for prevention of periodontal diseases, *J Clin Periodontol* 32 (Suppl 6): 229–282, 2005.

Newman MG, Grinenco V, Weiner M, et al: Predominant microbiota associated with periodontal health in the aged, *J Periodontol* 49: 553–559, 1978.

Ostan R, Bucci L, Capri M, et al: Immunosenescence and immunogenetics of human longevity, *Neuroimmunomodulation* 15: 224–240, 2008.

References

References for this chapter are found on www.medenact.com.

CHAPTER 5

Classification of Diseases and Conditions Affecting the Periodontium

JE Hinrichs | G Kotsakis | DG Naik | A Uppoor

CHAPTER OUTLINE

Our understanding of the causes and pathogenesis of oral diseases and conditions is continually changing with an increase in scientific knowledge. In light of this, a classification can be most consistently defined by the differences in the clinical manifestations of diseases and conditions; they are clinically consistent and require little (if any) clarification by scientific laboratory testing. The current classification of periodontal diseases is based on their extent (generalized vs localized), severity (slight, moderate, or severe), rate of progression (aggressive vs chronic), and localization (i.e., contained within the gingiva, as in gingivitis, or further involving periodontal bone loss, as in periodontitis). The existing definitions encompass the best available way to universally define a spectrum of diseases affecting the periodontal tissues and to guide therapeutic approaches. Nonetheless, the disease state is dynamic, and the appropriate diagnosis for an individual can change over time. For instance, a patient diagnosed with existing periodontitis who undergoes successful periodontal therapy may be classified as having a healthy but reduced periodontium (with slight, moderate, or severe attachment loss) at the reevaluation. Subsequently, if the same individual presents with gingival inflammation without signs of further attachment loss at a future appointment, the appropriate diagnosis would be "gingivitis on a reduced periodontium." Depending on their future compliance with home care and maintenance visits, patients may progress to periodontitis or maintain a healthy but reduced periodontium. If a case of gingivitis on a reduced periodontium relapses into periodontitis, the prognosis of the affected teeth will depend on the preexisting attachment loss.

The classification presented in this chapter is based on the internationally accepted consensus opinions of the diseases and conditions that affect the tissues of the periodontium; it was presented and discussed at the 1999 International Workshop for the Classification of the Periodontal Diseases organized by the American Academy of Periodontology (AAP). Box 5.1 presents the overall classification system, and each disease or condition is discussed where clarification is needed. In each case, the reader is referred to pertinent reviews on the subject and specific chapters within this book that discuss the topics in more detail.

> An updated classification system, which was recently published jointly by the American Academy of Periodontology (AAP) and the European Federation of Periodontology (EFP). The goal of this effort is to address some of the shortcomings that exist with the current classification system (discussed in this chapter), including diagnostic inaccuracy and significant overlap of disease entities. Several working groups were created to focus on specific disease entities using the currently available scientific evidence, resulting in the most substantial update to the classification system since 1999.

To view the **updated AAP/EFP 2018 classification system,** visit the companion website www.expertconsult.com.

Gingival Diseases

Dental Plaque-Induced Gingival Diseases

Gingivitis that is associated with dental-plaque formation is the most common form of gingival disease (Fig. 5.1). Box 5.2 outlines the classifications of gingival diseases. Gingivitis has been previously characterized by the presence of clinical signs of inflammation that are confined to the gingiva and associated with teeth showing no attachment loss. Gingivitis has also been observed to affect the gingiva of periodontitis-affected teeth that have previously lost attachment but that have received periodontal therapy to stabilize any further attachment loss. In these treated cases, plaque-induced gingival inflammation may recur but without any evidence of further attachment loss.

From this evidence, it has been concluded that plaque-induced gingivitis may occur on a periodontium with no attachment loss or

BOX 5.1 Classification of Periodontal Diseases and Conditions

Gingival Diseases
Plaque-induced gingival diseases[a]
Nonplaque-induced gingival lesions

Chronic Periodontitis[b]
Localized
Generalized

Aggressive Periodontitis
Localized
Generalized

Periodontitis as a Manifestation of Systemic Disease

Necrotizing Periodontal Diseases
Necrotizing ulcerative gingivitis
Necrotizing ulcerative periodontitis

Abscesses of the Periodontium
Gingival abscess
Periodontal abscess
Pericoronal abscess

Periodontitis Associated With Endodontic Lesions
Endodontic–periodontal lesion
Periodontal–endodontic lesion
Combined lesion

Developmental or Acquired Deformities and Conditions
Localized tooth-related factors that predispose an individual to plaque-induced gingival diseases or periodontitis
Mucogingival deformities and conditions around the teeth
Mucogingival deformities and conditions on edentulous ridges
Occlusal trauma

[a]These diseases may occur on a periodontium with no attachment loss or on a periodontium with attachment loss that is stable and not progressing.
[b]Chronic periodontitis can be further classified on the basis of its extent and severity. As a general guide, extent can be characterized as localized (<30% of sites involved) or generalized (>30% of sites involved). Severity can be characterized on the basis of the amount of clinical attachment loss (CAL) as follows: slight, 1 or 2 mm CAL; moderate, 3 or 4 mm CAL; and severe, ≥5 mm CAL.
Data from Armitage GC: *Ann Periodontol* 4:1, 1999.

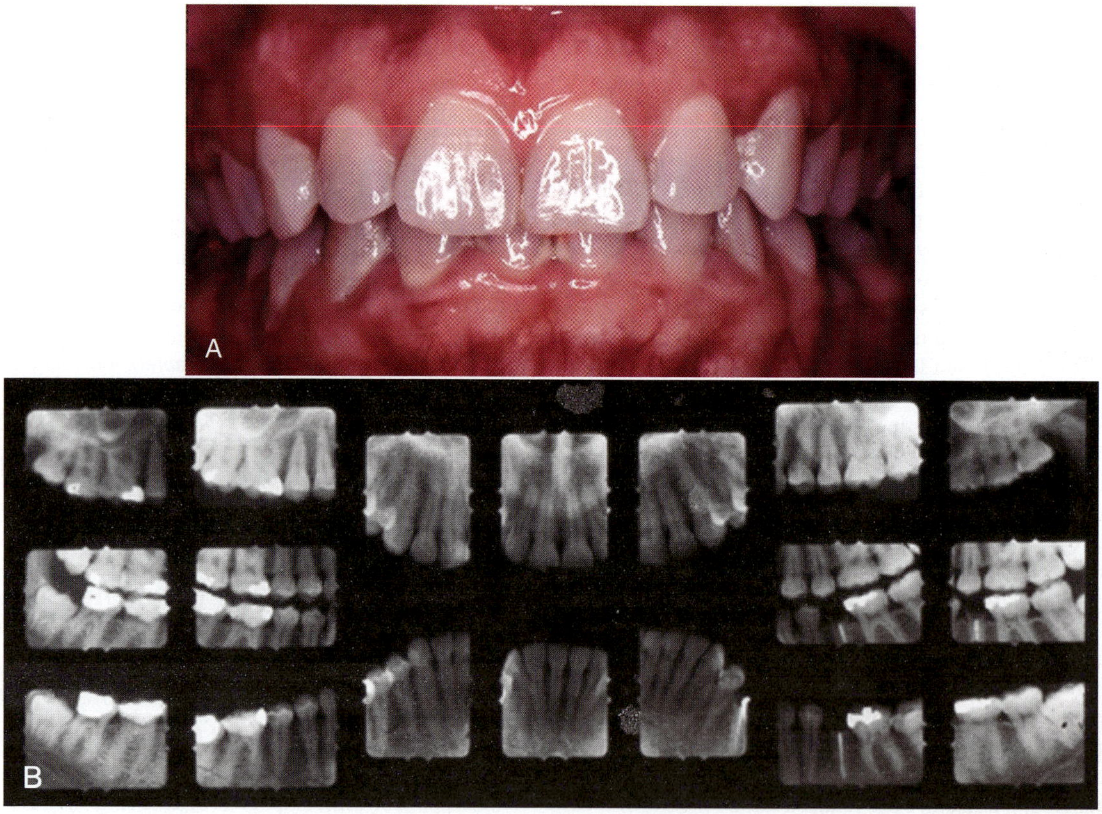

Fig. 5.1 Plaque-related gingivitis and marginal and papillary inflammation, with 1–4 mm probing depths and generalized zero clinical attachment loss, except for the recession seen with mandibular right first premolar.

on a periodontium with previous attachment loss that is stable and not progressing. This implies that gingivitis may be the diagnosis for inflamed gingival tissues associated with a tooth with no previous attachment loss or with a tooth that has previously undergone attachment and bone loss (i.e., with reduced periodontal support) but that is not currently losing attachment or bone even though gingival inflammation is present (Fig. 5.2). For this diagnosis to be made, longitudinal records of periodontal status, including clinical attachment levels, should be available.

KEY FACT

Gingivitis may be the diagnosis for inflamed gingival tissues associated with a tooth without previous attachment loss or with a tooth that has previously undergone attachment and bone loss (i.e., with reduced periodontal support) but is not currently losing attachment, even though gingival inflammation is present. In the latter case, the appropriate definition would be "gingivitis on a reduced periodontium."

BOX 5.2 Gingival Diseases

Dental Plaque-Induced Gingival Diseases

These diseases may occur on a periodontium with no attachment loss or on a periodontium with attachment loss that is stable and not progressing.

- I. Gingivitis associated with dental plaque only
  - A. Without local contributing factors
  - B. With local contributing factors (see Box 5.4)
- II. Gingival diseases modified by systemic factors
  - A. Associated with the endocrine system
    - 1. Puberty-associated gingivitis
    - 2. Menstrual cycle-associated gingivitis
    - 3. Pregnancy-associated conditions
      - a. Gingivitis
      - b. Pyogenic granuloma
    - 4. Diabetes mellitus-associated gingivitis
  - B. Associated with blood dyscrasias
    - 1. Leukemia-associated gingivitis
    - 2. Other
- III. Gingival diseases modified by medications
  - A. Drug-influenced gingival diseases
    - 1. Drug-influenced gingival enlargements
    - 2. Drug-influenced gingivitis
      - a. Oral contraceptive-associated gingivitis
      - b. Other
- IV. Gingival diseases modified by malnutrition
  - A. Ascorbic acid-deficiency gingivitis
  - B. Other

Nonplaque-Induced Gingival Lesions

- I. Gingival diseases of specific bacterial origin
  - A. *Neisseria gonorrhoeae*
  - B. *Treponema pallidum*
  - C. *Streptococcus* species
  - D. Other
- II. Gingival diseases of viral origin
  - A. Herpes virus infections
    - 1. Primary herpetic gingivostomatitis
    - 2. Recurrent oral herpes
    - 3. Varicella zoster
  - B. Other
- III. Gingival diseases of fungal origin
  - A. *Candida* species infections: generalized gingival candidiasis
  - B. Linear gingival erythema
  - C. Histoplasmosis
  - D. Other
- IV. Gingival lesions of genetic origin
  - A. Hereditary gingival fibromatosis
  - B. Other
- V. Gingival manifestations of systemic conditions
  - A. Mucocutaneous lesions
    - 1. Lichen planus
    - 2. Pemphigoid
    - 3. Pemphigus vulgaris
    - 4. Erythema multiforme
    - 5. Lupus erythematosus
    - 6. Drug-induced conditions
    - 7. Other
  - B. Allergic reactions
    - 1. Dental restorative materials
      - a. Mercury
      - b. Nickel
      - c. Acrylic
      - d. Other
    - 2. Reactions attributable to the following:
      - a. Toothpastes or dentifrices
      - b. Mouth rinses or mouthwashes
      - c. Chewing-gum additives
      - d. Foods and additives
    - 3. Other
- VI. Traumatic lesions (factitious, iatrogenic, or accidental)
  - A. Chemical injury
  - B. Physical injury
  - C. Thermal injury
- VII. Foreign-body reactions
- VIII. Not otherwise specified

Data from Holmstrup P: *Ann Periodontol* 4:20, 1999; and Mariotti A: *Ann Periodontol* 4:7, 1999.

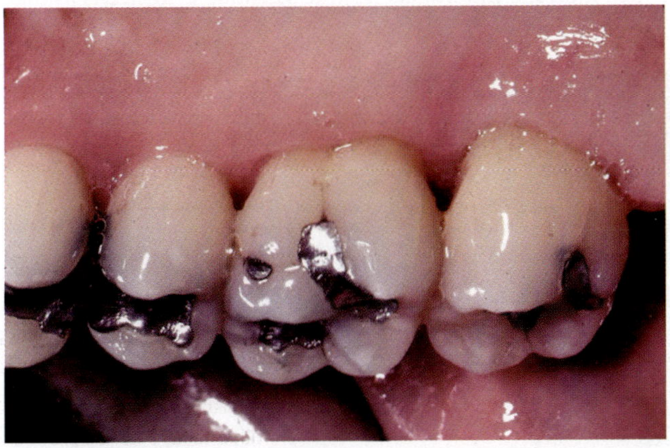

Fig. 5.2 The maxillary second molar exhibits mild inflammation at the mesial–palatal surface. However, the clinical attachment loss has been stable for 15 years after the placement of an apically positioned flap and periodontal maintenance. The diagnosis is a history of moderate periodontitis, but the case is in remission.

Gingivitis Associated With Dental Plaque Only

Plaque-induced gingival disease is the result of an interaction between the microorganisms found in the dental-plaque biofilm, the tissues, and inflammatory cells of the host. The plaque–host interaction can be altered by the effects of local factors, systemic factors, medications, and malnutrition, all of which can influence the severity and duration of the response. Local factors may contribute to gingivitis formation in addition to plaque-retentive calculus formation on the crown and root surfaces. These factors are contributory because of their ability to retain plaque microorganisms and to inhibit the removal of those microorganisms via patient-initiated plaque-control techniques.

A cause-and-effect relationship between microbial plaque and gingivitis has been elegantly demonstrated by a classic experiment demonstrating that the cessation of oral hygiene consistently leads to the manifestation of gingivitis within 2–3 weeks in healthy adults. Clinical gingivitis is histologically characterized by a dense infiltrate of lymphocytes and other mononuclear cells, fibroblast alterations, increased vascular permeability, and continuing loss of collagen in response to the microbial challenge. However, the alveolar bone is not affected. Microbial plaque is thus considered to be the primary etiologic factor for gingivitis. The severity and duration of the inflammatory response interaction can be altered by the modifying local or systemic modifying factors. Gingivitis is fully reversible in otherwise healthy persons within weeks following the removal of local factors and reduction of the microbial load around the teeth. As noted earlier, gingivitis is rapidly established in cases of generalized or localized inefficient plaque removal. Therefore, it is crucial that patients are instructed in oral hygiene to maintain long-term gingival health.

Gingival Diseases Modified by Systemic Factors

Systemic factors that contribute to gingivitis—such as the endocrine changes associated with puberty (Fig. 5.3), the menstrual cycle, pregnancy (Fig. 5.4), and diabetes—may be exacerbated as a result of alterations in the gingival inflammatory response to plaque.

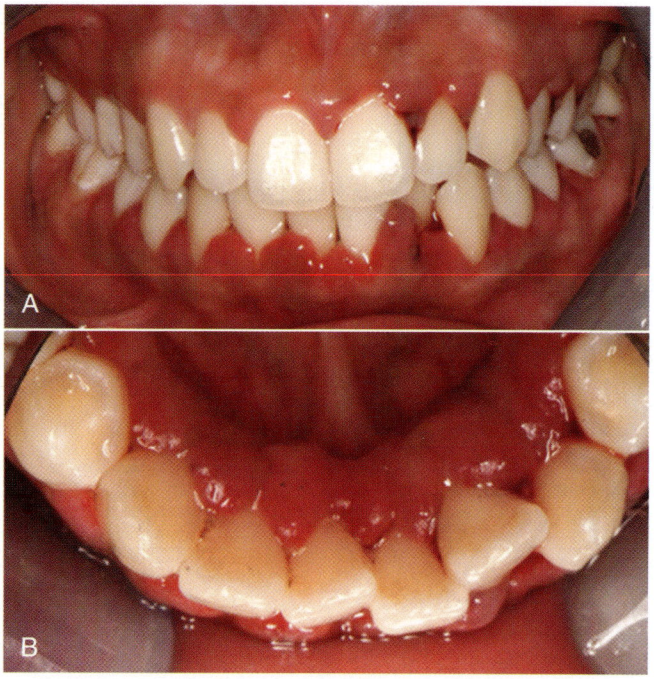

Fig. 5.3 A 13-year-old girl with hormone-exaggerated marginal and papillary inflammation, with 1–4 mm probing depths yet minimal clinical attachment loss. A, Facial view; B, lingual view.

This altered response appears to result from the effects of systemic conditions on the host's cellular and immunologic functions. These changes are most apparent during pregnancy, when the prevalence and severity of gingival inflammation may increase, even in the presence of low levels of plaque. Blood dyscrasias (e.g., leukemia) may alter immune function by disturbing the normal balance of the immunologically competent white blood cells that supply the periodontium. Gingival enlargement and bleeding are common findings that may be associated with the swollen, spongy gingival tissues caused by the excessive infiltration of blood cells (Fig. 5.5).

CLINICAL CORRELATION

Increased estrogen and progesterone levels in pregnant women during their third trimester have been associated with increased severity of gingivitis via substituting nutrient needs for certain oral bacteria and stimulating their proliferation. One species that has been specifically associated with gingivitis during pregnancy is *Prevotella intermedia.*

Gingival Diseases Modified by Medications

Gingival diseases that are modified by medications are increasingly prevalent as a result of the increased use of drugs known to induce gingival enlargement. These include anticonvulsant drugs, such as phenytoin, immunosuppressive drugs, such as cyclosporine (Fig. 5.6), and calcium-channel blockers, such as nifedipine (Fig. 5.7), verapamil, diltiazem, and sodium valproate. The development and severity of gingival enlargement in response to medications are patient-specific and may be influenced by uncontrolled plaque accumulation, as well as by elevated hormonal levels. The increased use of oral contraceptives by premenopausal women has also been previously associated with a higher incidence of gingival inflammation and gingival enlargement. Although this fact stood true for earlier contraceptive formulations, existing contraceptives that include more modest doses of active ingredients are not commonly associated with gingival inflammation.

Gingival Diseases Modified by Malnutrition

Gingival diseases modified by malnutrition have received attention because of clinical descriptions of bright red, swollen, and bleeding gingiva associated with severe ascorbic acid (vitamin C) deficiency or scurvy. Nutritional deficiencies are known to affect immune function, and they may alter the host's ability to protect himself or herself against some of the detrimental effects of cellular products, such as oxygen radicals. Unfortunately, little scientific evidence is available

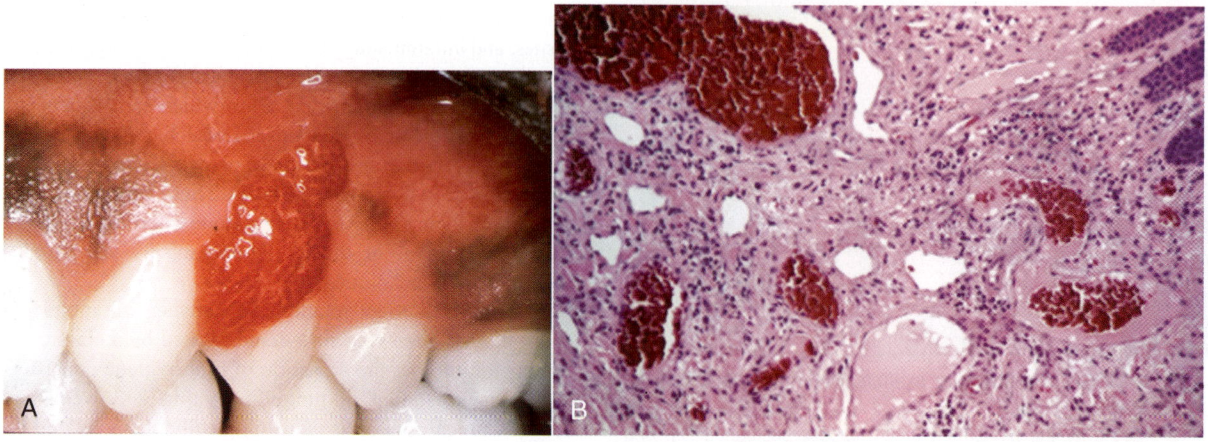

Fig. 5.4 Clinical image of pyogenic granuloma in a 27-year-old pregnant woman.

to support the role for specific nutritional deficiencies in the development or severity of gingival inflammation or periodontitis in humans. Various nutrients, such as long chain omega-3 fatty acids, have been found to have immunomodulatory properties, whereas others act to ameliorate the destructive effects of reactive oxygen species (ROS) functioning as ROS scavengers. Nonetheless, the available evidence to support a clinically impactful role for mild nutritional deficiencies in the development or severity of gingival inflammation in humans is limited. Data have shed light on the implication of increased dietary carbohydrate intake on gingivitis, in addition to its known causal role on the occurrence of dental caries.

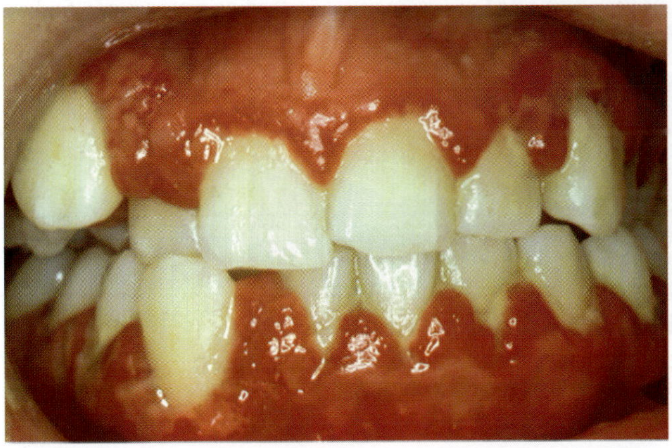

Fig. 5.5 A 12-year-old girl with a primary medical diagnosis of leukemia who exhibits swollen and spongy gingiva.

Nonplaque-Induced Gingival Lesions

Oral manifestations of systemic conditions that produce lesions in the tissues of the periodontium are rare. These effects are observed more frequently among lower socioeconomic groups, in developing countries, and in immunocompromised individuals. This category mainly encompasses lesions of autoimmune or idiopathic etiology that can manifest in the gingiva. Benign mucous membrane pemphigoid is an example of a nonplaque-induced lesion without socioeconomic implications. Sloughing gingival tissues leaves painful ulcerations of the gingiva (Fig. 5.8A and B). Autoimmune antibodies are targeted at the basement membrane and cleave it from the underlying connective tissue (Fig. 5.8C and D).

Gingival Diseases of Specific Bacterial Origin

Gingival diseases of specific bacterial origin are increasing in prevalence, especially as a result of sexually transmitted diseases, such as gonorrhea (*Neisseria gonorrhoeae*), and to a lesser degree, syphilis (*Treponema pallidum*). Oral lesions may be a result of

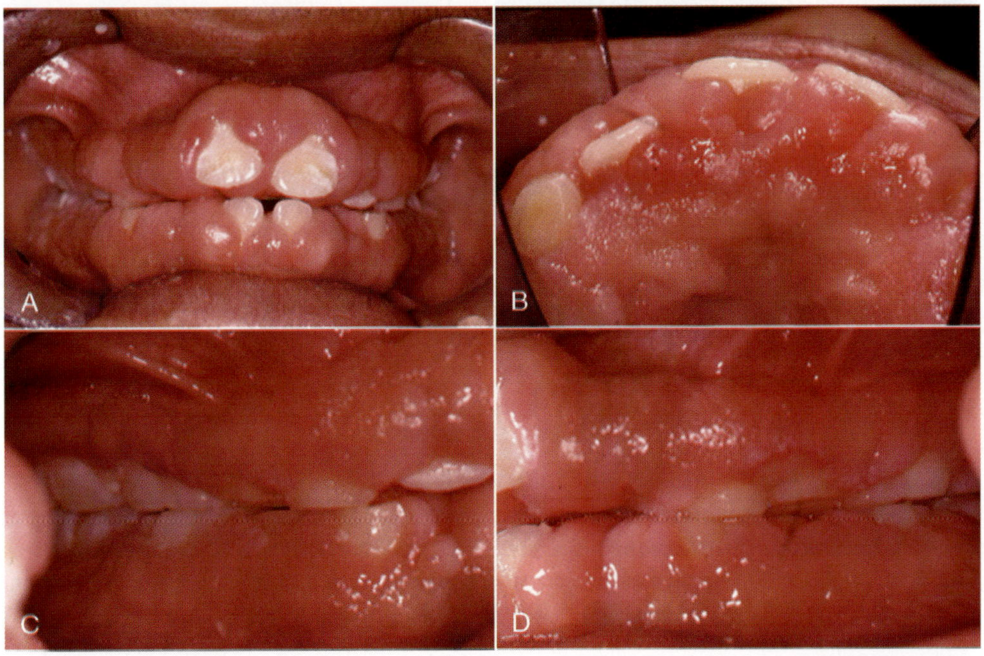

Fig. 5.6 Clinical images of a 9-year-old boy with severe gingival overgrowth as a result of a heart transplant and cyclosporine therapy.

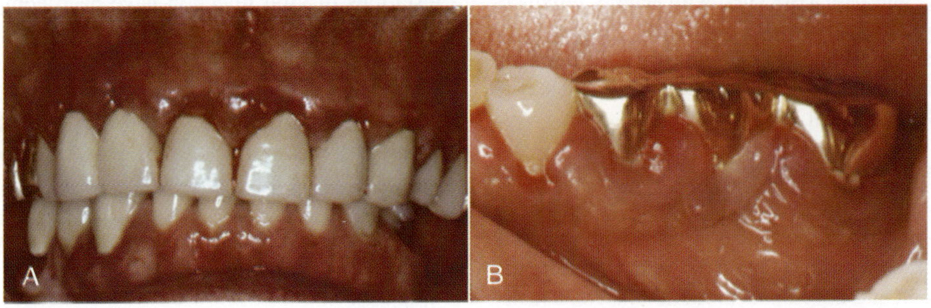

Fig. 5.7 Clinical images of gingival overgrowth after the use a of calcium-channel blocker to control hypertension.

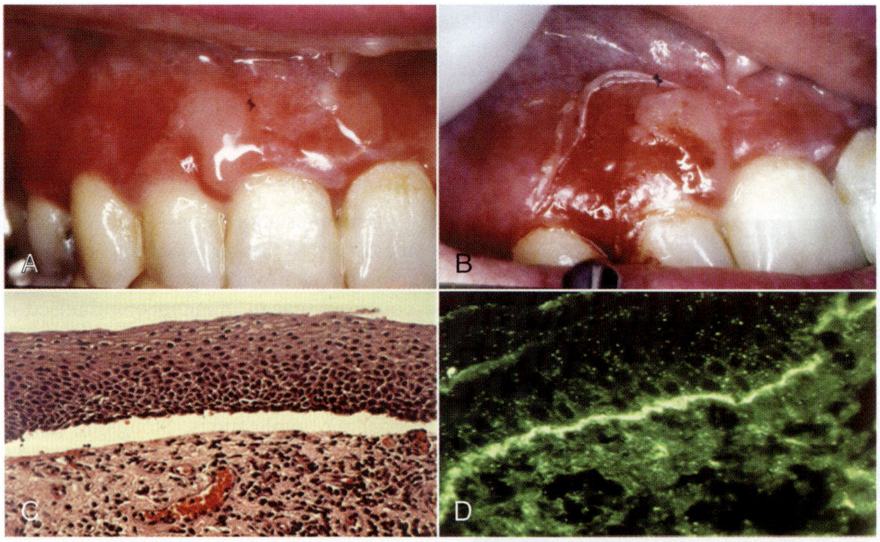

Fig. 5.8 **A 62-year-old woman with benign mucous membrane pemphigoid.** A and B, Clinical images with sloughing of the epithelial surface. C, Hematoxylin–eosin stain depicting the separation of the epithelium from the connective tissue. D, Immunofluorescent-labeled antibodies in the basement membrane.

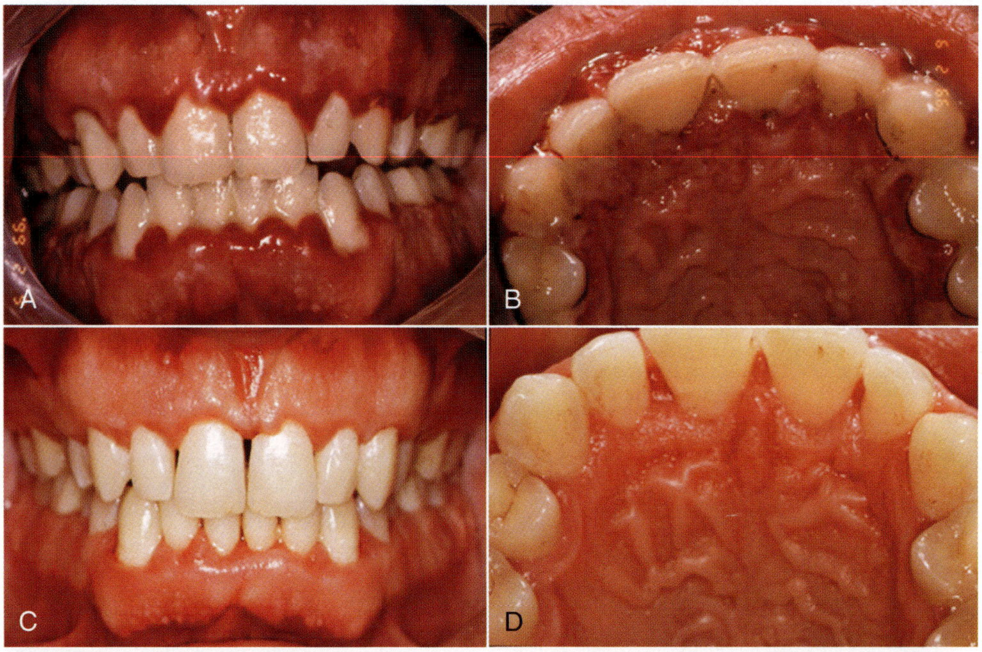

Fig. 5.9 **A and B, A 29-year-old man with primary herpetic infection and severe gingival inflammation.** C and D, Six weeks after treatment with systemic acyclovir.

systemic infection or direct infection. Streptococcal gingivitis or gingivostomatitis is a rare entity that may present as an acute condition with fever, malaise, and pain associated with acutely inflamed, diffuse, red, and swollen gingiva with increased bleeding and occasional gingival abscess formation. The gingival infections are usually preceded by tonsillitis and they have been associated with group A β-hemolytic Streptococcal infections.

Gingival Diseases of Viral Origin

Gingival diseases of viral origin may be caused by a variety of deoxyribonucleic acid- and ribonucleic-acid viruses, with the most common being the herpes viruses (Fig. 5.9A and B). Herpetic lesions are not uncommon and develop as intraoral blisters, usually grouped together, that quickly burst, leaving minuscule ulcerations. Lesions are frequently related to the reactivation of latent viruses, especially as a result of reduced immune function. The oral manifestations of viral infection have been comprehensively reviewed. Viral gingival diseases are treated with topical or systemic antiviral drugs (Fig. 5.9C and D).

CLINICAL CORRELATION

Unlike other herpetic recurrences, varicella zoster virus (VZV) usually manifests with a prodrome of tingling, itching, burning, or a unilateral numbness at the affected dermatome. These symptoms are followed by moderate to severe pain shortly after initiation and are very important for differential diagnosis.

Gingival Diseases of Fungal Origin

Gingival diseases of fungal origin are relatively uncommon in immunocompetent individuals, but they occur more frequently in immunocompromised individuals and in those with normal oral flora that has been disturbed by the long-term use of broad-spectrum antibiotics. The most common oral fungal infection is candidiasis, which is caused by infection with *Candida albicans*; it can also be seen under prosthetic devices, in individuals using topical steroids, and in individuals with decreased salivary flow, increased salivary glucose, or decreased salivary pH. A generalized candidal infection may manifest as white patches on the gingiva, tongue, or oral mucous membrane that can be removed with gauze and that leave a red, bleeding surface. In individuals with human immunodeficiency virus (HIV), candidal infection may present as erythema of the attached gingiva; this has been referred to as *linear gingival erythema* or *HIV-associated gingivitis*.

The diagnosis of candidal infection can be made by culture, smear, or biopsy. Less common fungal infections have also been described.

Gingival Diseases of Genetic Origin

Gingival diseases of genetic origin may involve the tissues of the periodontium and have been described in detail. One of the most clinically evident conditions is *hereditary gingival fibromatosis*, which exhibits autosomal-dominant or (rarely) autosomal recessive modes of inheritance. The gingival enlargement may completely cover the teeth, delay eruption, and present as an isolated finding; alternatively, it may be associated with several more generalized syndromes.

Gingival Manifestations of Systemic Conditions

Gingival manifestations of systemic conditions may appear as desquamative lesions, ulcerations of the gingiva, or both. Allergic reactions that manifest with gingival changes are uncommon but have been observed in association with several restorative materials (Fig. 5.10A), toothpastes, mouthwashes, chewing gums (Fig. 5.11), and foods (Box 5.2). The diagnosis of these conditions may prove difficult and may require an extensive history and the selective elimination of potential causes. Conjoint assessment with an allergologist is indicated, and percutaneous tests are often recommended. Histologic traits of biopsies from gingival allergic reactions include a dense infiltrate of eosinophilic cells (Fig. 5.10B and C).

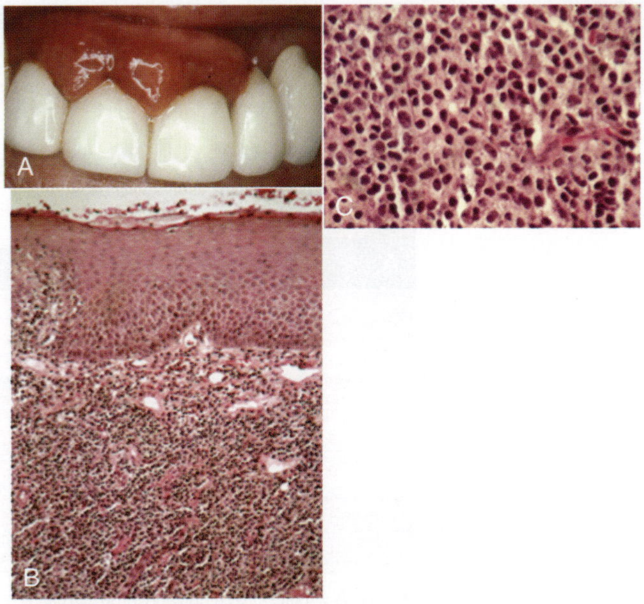

Fig. 5.10 A, Localized pronounced gingival inflammation in response to a nickel allergy. B and C, Biopsy of a dense infiltrate of plasma cells.

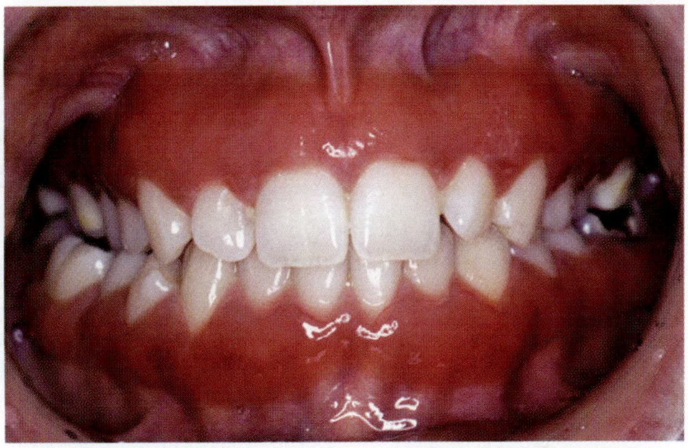

Fig. 5.11 A generalized severe allergic response of the gingiva in response to an additive in chewing gum.

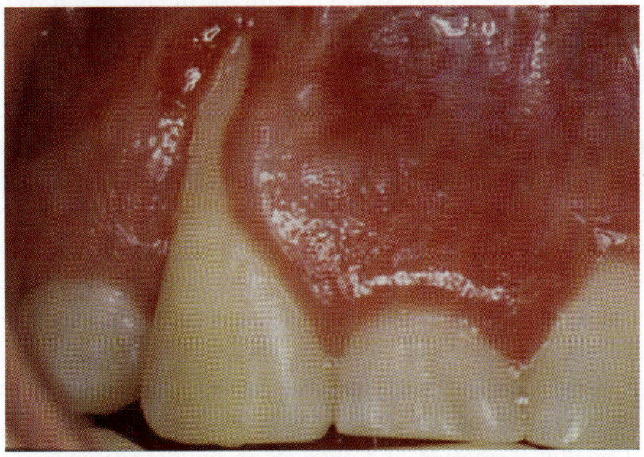

Fig. 5.12 Self-inflicted gingival dehiscence induced via the patient's fingernail.

Traumatic Lesions

Traumatic lesions may be self-inflicted and *factitious* in origin, which means that they are produced by intentional or unintentional artificial means (Fig. 5.12). Other examples of traumatic lesions include toothbrush trauma that results in gingival ulceration, recession, or both. *Iatrogenic trauma* (i.e., induced by the dentist or health professional) to the gingiva can be caused by the induction of orthodontic cement or preventive or restorative materials (Fig. 5.13A). Peripheral ossifying fibroma may develop in response to the embedment of a foreign body, Fig. 5.13B and C and the complete resolution after 4 weeks after excisional biopsy (Fig 5.13D). Alternatively, *accidental damage* to the gingiva may occur as a result of minor burns from hot foods and drinks.

CLINICAL CORRELATION

Individuals who perform aggressive horizontal brushing are often found to have gingival recession or cervical abrasion on the teeth quadrants contralateral to their dominant hand.

Foreign-Body Reactions

Foreign-body reactions lead to localized inflammatory conditions of the gingiva and are caused by the introduction of foreign material into the gingival connective tissues through breaks in the epithelium. Common examples include the introduction of amalgam into the gingiva during the placement of a restoration, the extraction

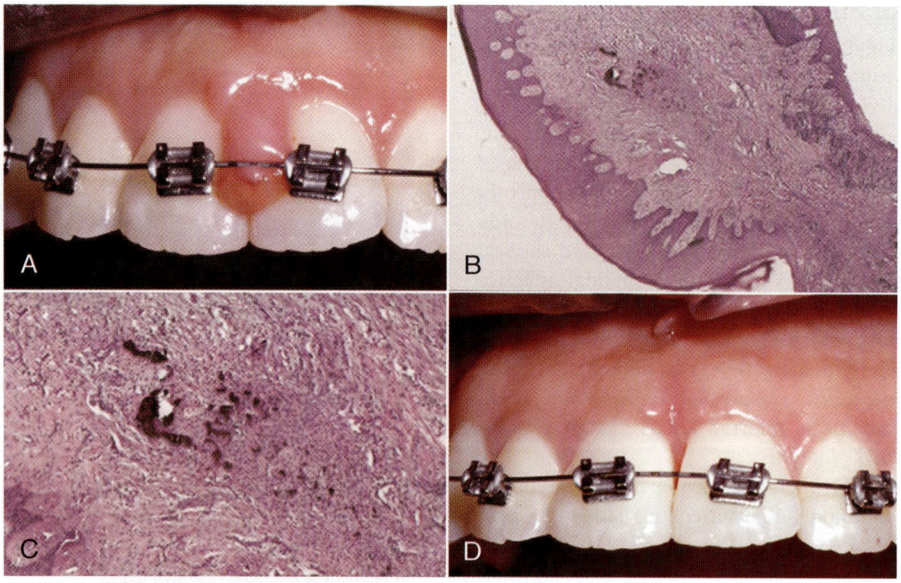

Fig. 5.13 A, Proliferative gingival overgrowth as a result of the impaction of foreign body. B, Histology of peripheral ossifying fibroma. C, Higher magnification of the image shown in B. D, Four weeks after excisional biopsy.

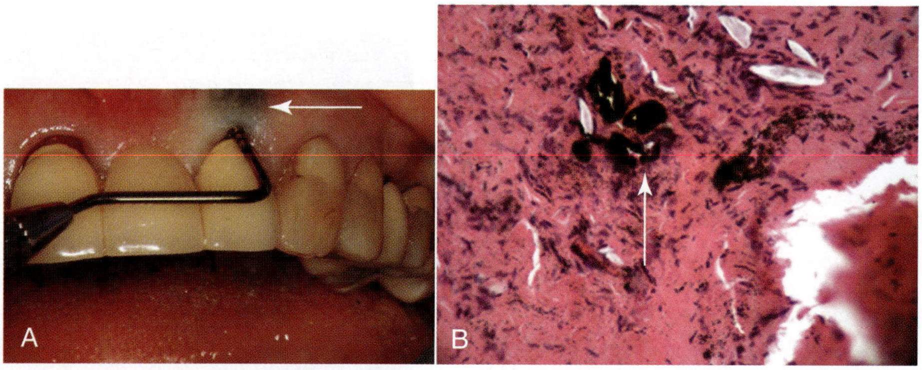

Fig. 5.14 A, Gingival pigmentation associated with previous apicoectomy and amalgam retrofill. B, Biopsy depicting metal fragments.

of a tooth, or an endodontic apicoectomy with retrofill leaving an amalgam tattoo (Fig. 5.14A), with resultant metal fragment observed during biopsies (Fig. 5.14B); abrasives may also be introduced during polishing procedures.

Periodontitis

Periodontitis is defined as "an inflammatory disease of the supporting tissues of the teeth caused by specific microorganisms or groups of specific microorganisms, resulting in progressive destruction of the periodontal ligament and alveolar bone with increased probing depth formation, recession, or both." The clinical feature that distinguishes periodontitis from gingivitis is the presence of clinically detectable attachment loss. This loss is often accompanied by periodontal pocket formation and changes in the density and height of the subjacent alveolar bone. In some cases, recession of the marginal gingiva may accompany attachment loss, thereby masking ongoing disease progression if only probing depth measurements are taken without measurements of clinical attachment levels. Clinical signs of inflammation—such as changes in color, contour, and consistency, as well as bleeding with probing—may not always be positive indicators of ongoing attachment loss. However, the presence of continued bleeding with probing during sequential visits has proved to be a reliable indicator of the presence of inflammation and the potential for subsequent attachment loss at the bleeding site. The attachment loss associated with periodontitis has been shown to progress either continuously or in episodic bursts of disease activity. However, the available clinical instruments for detecting disease are not sensitive enough to capture the cycles of attachment loss and repair that occur during disease activity and remission, respectively (i.e., the periodontal probe is graded in 1 mm increments).

KEY FACT

Probing depth measurement alone is inadequate for an assessment of periodontitis. Clinical attachment loss is usually assessed by adding the extent of gingival recession to the probing depth measurement to estimate the total extent of tissue loss from the cementoenamel junction (CEJ) of the tooth. However, when recession is not visible, it is essential that height of the marginal gingiva coronal to the CEJ be determined and that measurement subtracted from the probing depth to establish the extent of clinical attachment loss. The measurement of clinical attachment around a tooth provides insights on the history and extent of periodontal destruction around the tooth. One common pitfall of clinical periodontal examination is the direct translation of probing depths as clinical attachment levels when the gingival margin lies above the cementoenamel junction, leading to an overestimation of attachment levels.

KEY FACT

In the AAP/EFP 2018 classification of periodontal diseases, a multidimensional staging and grading system is introduced to subclassify periodontitis disease entities. The severity of periodontal disease at the time of presentation and the complexity of disease management dictates the staging, while grading offers additional information, including the rate of past progression of the disease and the risk for future progression.

Although many classifications of the different clinical manifestations of periodontitis have been presented over the past 20 years, consensus workshops in North America in 1989 and in Europe in 1993 identified that periodontitis may present in early-onset, adult-onset, and necrotizing forms (Table 5.1). In addition, the AAP consensus concluded that periodontitis may be associated with systemic conditions (e.g., diabetes, HIV) and that some forms of periodontitis may be refractory to conventional therapy. Early-onset disease was distinguished from adult-onset disease by the age of onset (35 years of age was set as an arbitrary separation of diseases), the rate of disease progression, and the presence of alterations in host defenses. The early-onset diseases were more aggressive, occurred in individuals younger than 35 years old, and were associated with defects in host defenses; alternatively, adult forms of disease were slowly progressive, became clinically more evident during the fourth decade of life, and were not associated with defects in host defenses. In addition, early-onset periodontitis was subclassified into prepubertal, juvenile, and rapidly progressive forms with localized or generalized disease distributions.

Extensive clinical and basic scientific research involving these disease entities has been performed in many countries, and some disease characteristics that were outlined 10 years ago no longer stand up to rigid scientific scrutiny. In particular, supporting evidence was lacking for the distinct classifications of adult periodontitis, refractory periodontitis, and the various different forms of early-onset periodontitis as outlined by the AAP Workshop for the International Classification of Periodontal Diseases in 1999 (Table 5.1).

It has been observed that chronic periodontal destruction caused by the accumulation of local factors (e.g., plaque, calculus) can occur before the age of 35 years and that the aggressive disease seen in young patients may be independent of age and instead have a familial (genetic) association. With respect to refractory periodontitis, little evidence supports that this condition is indeed a distinct clinical entity; the causes of continued loss of clinical attachment and alveolar bone after periodontal therapy are currently poorly defined and apply to many disease entities. The clinical and causative manifestations of the different diseases outlined in North America in 1989 and in Europe in 1993 were not consistently observed in different countries around the world and did not always fit the models presented. In addition, clinical data from the medical community emerged to support the belief that forms of periodontitis that were collectively referred to as prepubertal periodontitis were in fact representing periodontitis as a manifestation of distinct systemic diseases, such as in leukocyte adhesion deficiency syndromes. As a result, the AAP held an International Workshop for the Classification of Periodontal Diseases in 1999 to further refine the classification system with the use of current clinical and scientific data. The resulting classification of the different forms of periodontitis was simplified to describe three general clinical manifestations of periodontitis: chronic periodontitis, aggressive periodontitis, and periodontitis as a manifestation of systemic disease (Table 5.1 and Box 5.3).

Since the establishment of the currently accepted 1999 classification, a taskforce commissioned by the AAP proposed an update to the existing classification scheme in 2015. The update focused on suggestions to address the challenges in clinical documentation of attachment level changes and the distinction between chronic

TABLE 5.1 Classification of the Various Forms of Periodontitis

Classification	Forms of Periodontitis	Disease Characteristics
American Academy of Periodontology World Workshop in Clinical Periodontics, 1989	Adult periodontitis	Age of onset >35 years, slow rate of disease progression, no defects in host defenses
Early-onset periodontitis (may be prepubertal, juvenile, or rapidly progressive)	Age of onset <35 years, rapid rate of disease progression, defects in host defenses, associated with specific microflora	
Periodontitis associated with systemic disease	Systemic diseases that predispose to rapid rates of periodontitis; diseases: diabetes, Down syndrome, HIV infection, PLS	
Necrotizing ulcerative periodontitis	Similar to acute necrotizing ulcerative gingivitis but with associated clinical attachment loss	
Refractory periodontitis	Recurrent periodontitis that does not respond to treatment	
European Workshop in Periodontology, 1993	Adult periodontitis	Age of onset: fourth decade of life, slow rate of disease progression, no defects in host response
Early-onset periodontitis	Age of onset <40 years, rapid rate of disease progression, defects in host defense	
Necrotizing periodontitis	Tissue necrosis with attachment and bone loss	
American Academy of Periodontology International Workshop for Classification of Periodontal Diseases, 1999	Chronic periodontitis, aggressive periodontitis, periodontitis as a manifestation of systemic disease, necrotizing periodontitis	See Box 5.3

BOX 5.3 Periodontitis

The disease periodontitis can be subclassified into the following three major types on the basis of clinical, radiographic, historical, and laboratory characteristics.

Chronic Periodontitis

The following characteristics are common to patients with chronic periodontitis:

- Prevalent in adults but can occur in children
- Amount of destruction consistent with local factors
- Associated with a variable microbial pattern
- Subgingival calculus frequently found
- Slow to moderate rate of progression with possible periods of rapid progression
- Possibly modified by or associated with the following:
- Systemic diseases (e.g., diabetes mellitus, HIV)
- Local factors that predispose an individual to periodontitis
- Environmental factors (e.g., cigarette smoking, emotional stress)

Chronic periodontitis may be further subclassified into localized and generalized forms and characterized as slight, moderate, or severe on the basis of the common features described previously and the following specific features:

- Localized form: <30% of sites involved
- Generalized form: >30% of sites involved
- Slight: 1–2 mm of clinical attachment loss
- Moderate: 3–4 mm of clinical attachment loss
- Severe: ≥5 mm of clinical attachment loss

Aggressive Periodontitis

The following characteristics are common to patients with aggressive periodontitis:

- Otherwise clinically healthy patient
- Rapid attachment loss and bone destruction
- Amount of microbial deposits inconsistent with disease severity
- Familial aggregation of diseased individuals

The following characteristics are common but not universal:

- Diseased sites infected with *Aggregatibacter actinomycetemcomitans*
- Abnormalities in phagocyte function
- Hyperresponsive macrophages that produce increased levels of prostaglandin E_2 and interleukin-1β
- In some cases, self-arresting disease progression

Aggressive periodontitis may be further classified into localized and generalized forms on the basis of the common features described here and the following specific features:

Localized Form

- Circumpubertal onset of disease
- Localized first molar or incisor disease with proximal attachment loss on at least two permanent teeth, one of which is a first molar
- Robust serum-antibody response to infecting agents

Generalized Form

- Usually (but not always) affects people who are <30 years old
- Generalized proximal attachment loss that affects at least three teeth other than the first molars and incisors
- Pronounced episodic nature of periodontal destruction
- Poor serum-antibody response to infecting agents

Periodontitis as a Manifestation of Systemic Diseases

Periodontitis may be observed as a manifestation of the following systemic diseases:

1. Hematologic disorders
   a. Acquired neutropenia
   b. Leukemia
   c. Other
2. Genetic disorders
   a. Familial and cyclic neutropenia
   b. Down syndrome
   c. Leukocyte adhesion deficiency syndromes
   d. PLS
   e. Chédiak–Higashi syndrome
   f. Histiocytosis syndromes
   g. Glycogen storage disease
   h. Infantile genetic agranulocytosis
   i. Cohen syndrome
   j. Ehlers–Danlos syndrome (types IV and VIII, autosomal dominant)
   k. Hypophosphatasia
   l. Other
3. Not otherwise specified

Data from Flemmig TF: *Ann Periodontol* 4:32, 1999; Kinane DF: *Ann Periodontol* 4:54, 1999; and Tonetti MS, Mombelli A: *Ann Periodontol* 4:39, 1999.

and aggressive periodontitis. In particular, the AAP task force recommended the consideration of probing depth levels, in addition to attachment levels, in determining the severity of periodontitis to avoid overestimation. The classification of diseases and conditions of the periodontium discussed in this chapter will focus on the currently accepted 1999 classification with references to the AAP update when appropriate.

Chronic Periodontitis

Chronic periodontitis is the most common form of periodontitis; Box 5.3 includes the characteristics of this form of periodontitis. Chronic periodontitis is most prevalent in adults, but it can also be observed in children; therefore, the age range of more than 35 years that had been previously designated for the classification of this disease has been discarded. Different classification schemes have confirmed or discarded the age range of more than 35 years to separate chronic versus aggressive periodontitis. According to the existing definition, persons younger than 35 years may exhibit a rate of progression of disease consistent with the definition of chronic periodontitis. Nonetheless, epidemiologic evidence supports the suggestion that persons younger than 25 years at disease onset are likely to exhibit aggressive periodontitis. Intraoral radiographs along with periodontal charting records are of paramount importance to the documentation of disease onset and rate of progression. Chronic periodontitis is associated with the accumulation of plaque and calculus; it generally has a slow to moderate rate of disease progression, but periods of more rapid destruction may also be observed. Increases in the rate of disease progression may be caused by the impact of local, systemic, or environmental factors that may influence the normal host–bacteria interaction. Local factors may influence plaque accumulation (Box 5.4); systemic diseases (e.g., diabetes mellitus, HIV) may influence the host's defenses; and environmental factors (e.g., cigarette smoking, stress) may also influence the response of the host to plaque accumulation. Chronic periodontitis may occur as a localized disease in which less than 30% of evaluated sites demonstrate attachment and bone loss, or it

BOX 5.4 Developmental or Acquired Deformities and Conditions

Localized Tooth-Related Factors That Modify or Predispose Individuals to Plaque-Induced Gingival Diseases or Periodontitis

1. Tooth anatomic factors
2. Dental restorations and appliances
3. Root fractures
4. Cervical root resorption and cemental tears

Mucogingival Deformities and Conditions Around the Teeth

1. Gingival or soft-tissue recession
   a. Facial or lingual surfaces
   b. Interproximal (papillary)
2. Lack of keratinized gingiva
3. Decreased vestibular depth
4. Aberrant frenum or muscle position
5. Gingival excess
   a. Pseudopocket
   b. Inconsistent gingival margin
   c. Excessive gingival display
   d. Gingival enlargement (see Box 5.2)
   e. Abnormal color

Mucogingival Deformities and Conditions of the Edentulous Edges

1. Vertical or horizontal ridge deficiency
2. Lack of gingiva or keratinized tissue
3. Gingival or soft-tissue enlargements
4. Aberrant frenum or muscle position
5. Decreased vestibular depth
6. Abnormal color

Occlusal Trauma

1. Primary occlusal trauma
2. Secondary occlusal trauma

Data from Blieden TM: *Ann Periodontol* 4:91, 1999; Halmon WW: *Ann Periodontol* 4:102, 1999; and Pini Prato GP: *Ann Periodontol* 4:98, 1999.

may occur as a more generalized disease in which more than 30% of sites are affected. The disease may also be described by the severity of disease as slight (1–2 mm of loss; Fig. 5.15), moderate (3–4 mm of loss; Fig. 5.16), or severe (≥5 mm of loss; Fig. 5.17) on the basis of the amount of clinical attachment loss (Box 5.3).

KEY FACT

Chronic periodontitis is classified by extent and severity of disease, such as generalized (extent), moderate (severity), and chronic periodontitis.

Clinical attachment levels provide important benefits over probing depth alone to monitor disease progression using the CEJ as a fixed reference point. In fact, probing depth levels only have poor to moderate sensitivity for predicting attachment level changes over time. Nonetheless, clinical experience has revealed that oftentimes measurement of clinical attachment levels in practice may prove to be erroneous. The most common error occurs in the case of sites without gingival recession, whereby the location of the gingival margin is coronal to the CEJ. If the clinician in such a case only records the probing depth without charting the location of the CEJ (often charted as "positive recession" in electronic periodontal charts), the resulting attachment levels will be erroneously recorded as being equal to the probing depth. To prevent such an overestimate of disease, it has been suggested that clinicians consider that mild periodontitis be associated with probing depths of <4 mm, moderate periodontitis with probing depths of 5–6 mm, and severe periodontitis with probing depths of ≥7 mm. However, probing depths alone should not be used to classify periodontitis without simultaneous consideration of clinical attachment levels and radiographic bone loss.

KEY FACT

In the AAP/EFP 2018 classification of periodontal diseases, both chronic and aggressive periodontitis disease entities are grouped together and simply called *periodontitis*.

Aggressive Periodontitis

Aggressive periodontitis differs from the chronic form primarily by the rapid rate of disease progression seen in an otherwise healthy individual (Figs. 5.18 and 5.19); the absence of large accumulations of plaque and calculus; and the presence of a family history of aggressive disease that is suggestive of a genetic trait (Box 5.3). This form of periodontitis was previously classified as early-onset periodontitis (Table 5.1) and therefore still includes many of the characteristics previously identified with the localized and generalized forms of early-onset periodontitis. Although the clinical presentation of aggressive disease appears to be universal, the causative factors involved are not always consistent. Box 5.3 outlines additional clinical, microbiologic, and immunologic characteristics of aggressive disease that may be present. As was previously described for early-onset disease, aggressive forms of periodontitis usually affect young individuals during or shortly after puberty and may be observed during the second and third decades of life (i.e., 10–30 years of age). The disease may be localized as previously described for localized juvenile periodontitis or generalized as previously described for generalized juvenile periodontitis and rapidly progressive periodontitis (Table 5.1). Box 5.3 provides the common features of the localized and generalized forms of aggressive periodontitis.

FLASH BACK

Recall that chronic periodontitis is also categorized by the extent of *localized* or *generalized* disease according to the percentage of teeth involved with 30% of teeth being the cutoff between the two categories. Importantly, there is a distinct difference in the use of these definitions in the context of aggressive periodontitis. For aggressive periodontitis, the localized form is recognized to have a specific clinical phenotype, which is typically limited to incisor and first molar teeth.

Periodontitis as a Manifestation of Systemic Disease

Several hematologic and genetic disorders have been associated with the development of periodontitis in affected individuals (Box 5.3). The majority of these observations of effects on the periodontium are the result of case reports, and few research studies have been performed to investigate the exact nature of the effect of the specific condition on the tissues of the periodontium. It is speculated that the major effect of these disorders is through

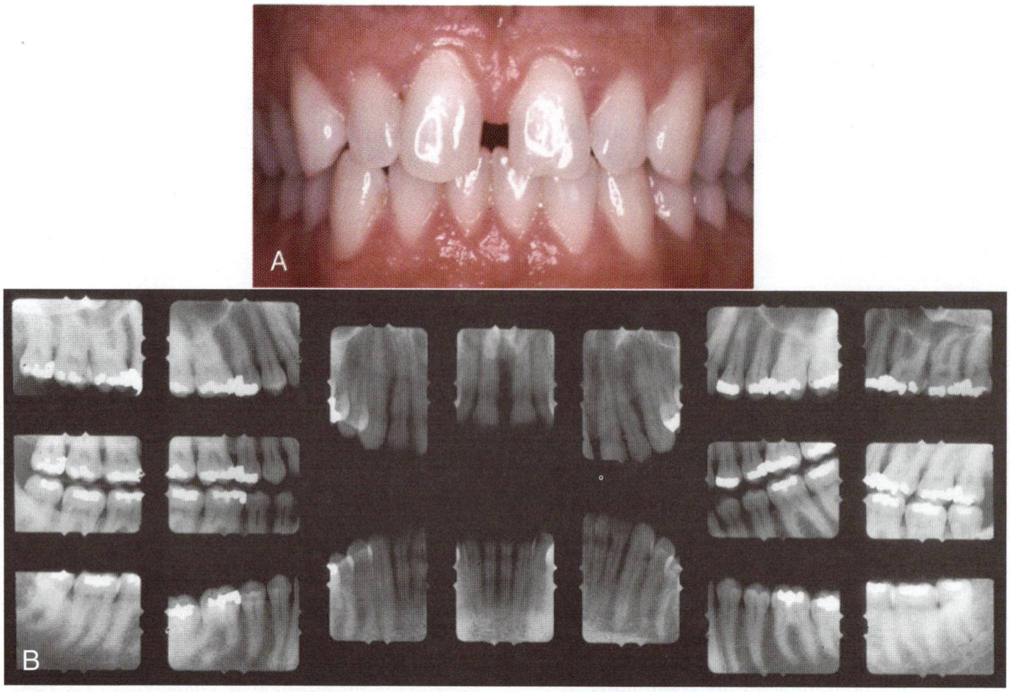

Fig. 5.15 A, Clinical image of plaque-related slight early chronic periodontitis with 1–2 mm of clinical attachment loss in a 40-year-old woman. B, Radiographic images of the patient.

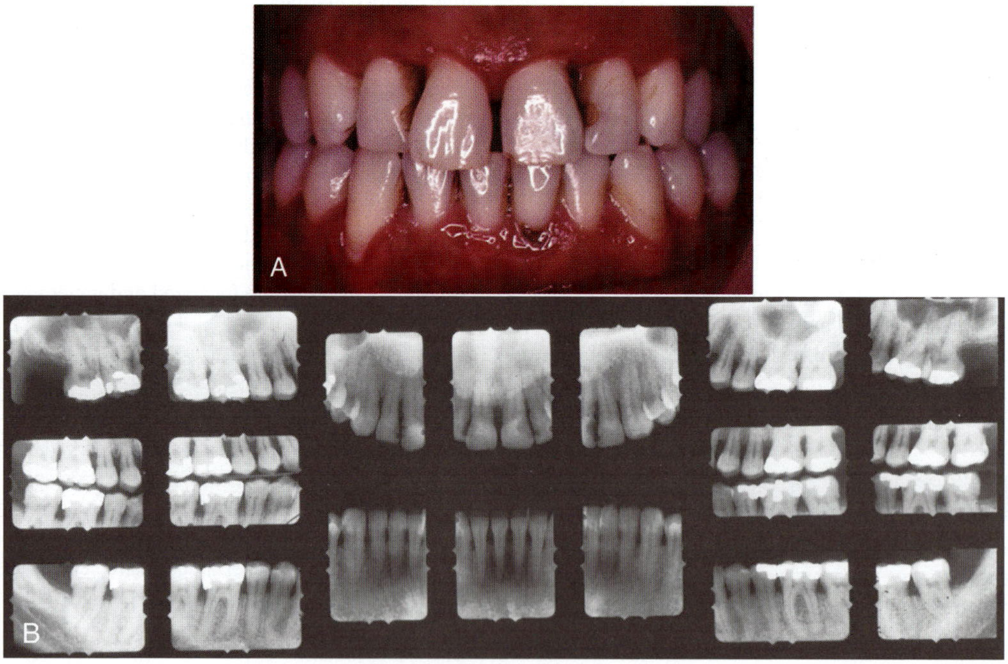

Fig. 5.16 A, Clinical image of plaque-related moderate chronic periodontitis with 3–4 mm of clinical attachment loss in a 53-year-old man who smokes. B, Radiographic images of the patient.

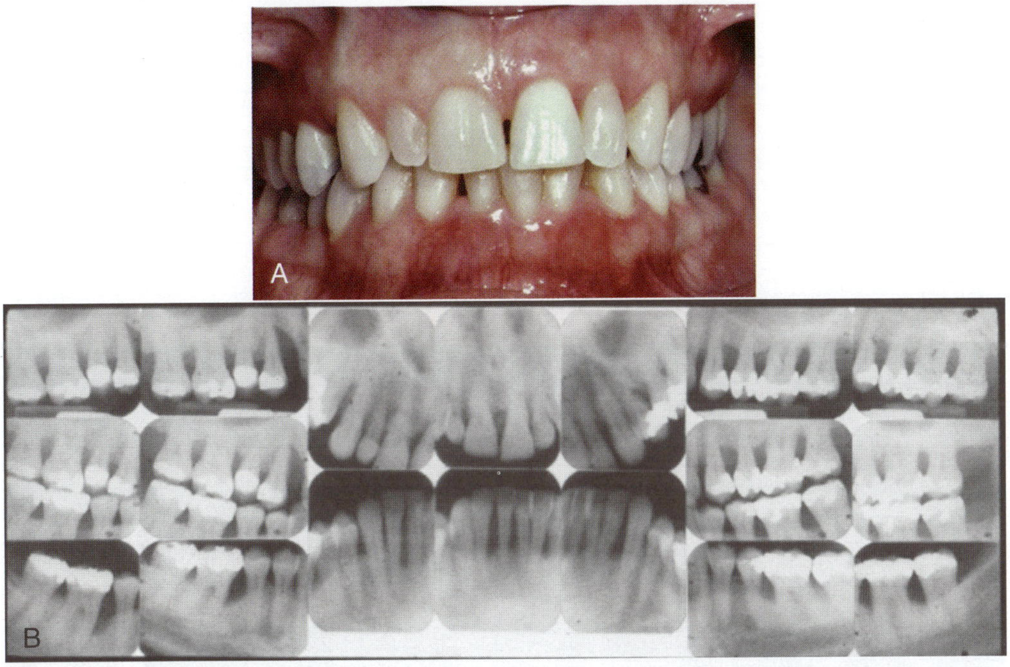

Fig. 5.17 A, Clinical image of plaque-related severe advanced chronic periodontitis with >5 mm of clinical attachment loss in a 47-year-old woman. B, Radiographic images of the patient.

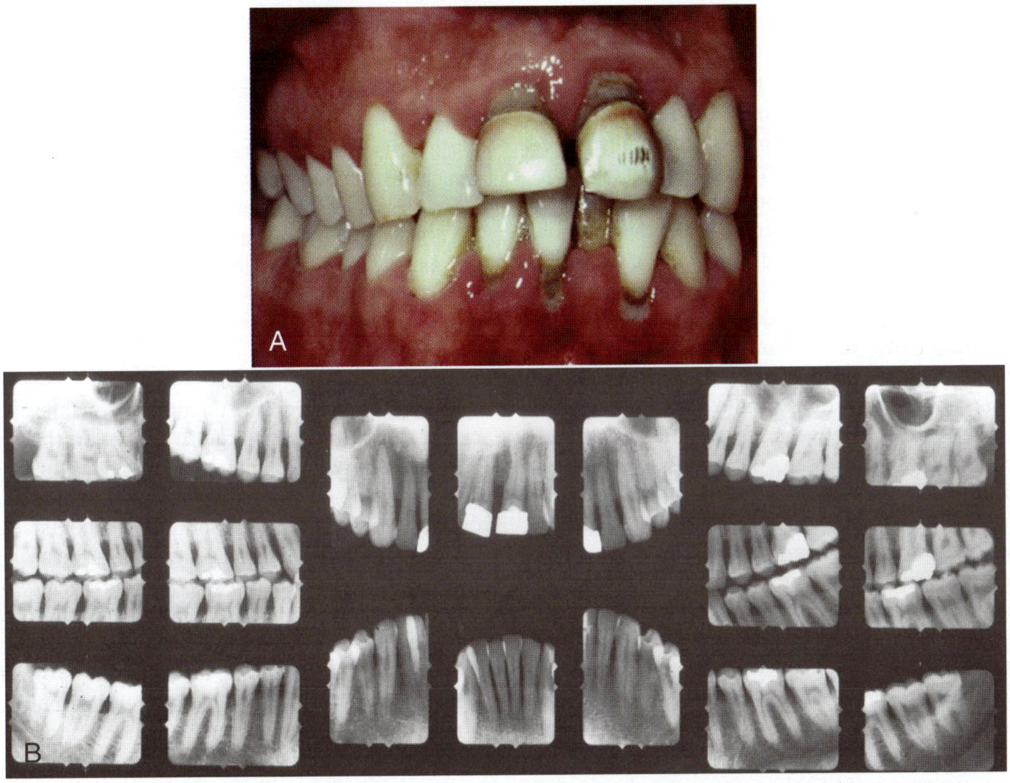

Fig. 5.18 A, Clinical image of plaque-related aggressive moderate periodontitis with 1–7 mm of PD and 3–4 mm of clinical attachment loss in a 31-year-old man. B, Radiographic images of the patient.

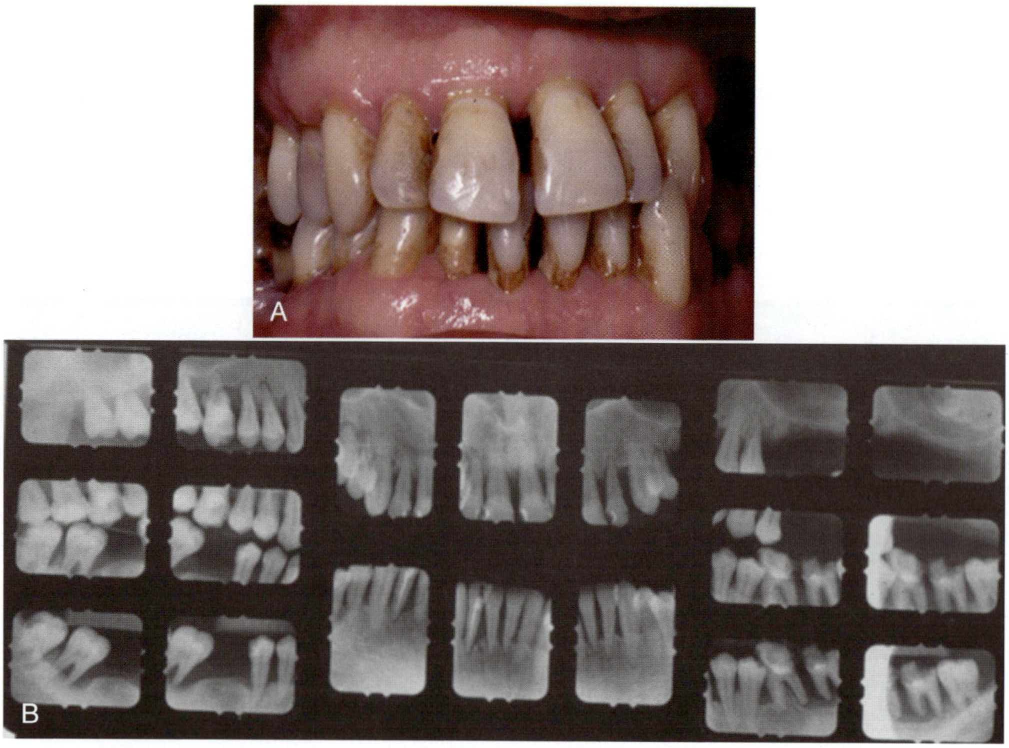

Fig. 5.19 A, Clinical image of plaque-related aggressive severe periodontitis with 3–13 mm of PD and 7–15 mm of clinical attachment loss in a 32-year-old man. B, Radiographic images of the patient.

alterations in host–defense mechanisms that have been clearly described for disorders (e.g., neutropenia, leukocyte adhesion deficiencies) but that are less well understood for multifaceted syndromes. The clinical manifestation of many of these disorders appears at an early age and may be confused with aggressive forms of periodontitis with rapid attachment loss and the potential for early tooth loss. This was one of the drivers for the transition from the term early-onset periodontitis, which characterized a heterogeneous group of diseases, to the definitions of aggressive periodontitis and periodontitis as a manifestation of systemic diseases. With the introduction of this form of periodontitis in this and previous classification systems (Table 5.1), the potential exists for overlap and confusion between periodontitis as a manifestation of systemic disease and both, the aggressive and the chronic form of disease, when a systemic component is suspected. At present, *periodontitis as a manifestation of systemic disease* is the diagnosis to be used when the systemic condition is the major predisposing factor and when local factors (e.g., large quantities of plaque and calculus) are not clearly evident. In the case in which periodontal destruction is clearly the result of local factors but has been exacerbated by the onset of conditions, such as diabetes mellitus (Figs. 5.20 and 5.21) or HIV infection, the diagnosis should be *chronic periodontitis modified by the systemic condition.*

Papillon–Lefèvre syndrome (PLS) is an autosomal-recessive disorder caused by mutations in the cathepsin C gene located on chromosome 11q14. The clinical manifestations of the syndrome include severe aggressive periodontitis and diffuse keratoderma on the palms and on the soles, the knees, or both (Figs. 5.22 and 5.23). The consanguinity of the parents is a common finding in approximately one-third of the cases (Fig. 5.24).

CLINICAL CORRELATION

When monogenic diseases are encountered, consanguinity can be a common finding particularly in certain ethnic cultures where it is socially acceptable. Appropriate genetic counseling is advisable. In addition, when the diagnosis for the proband (the first offspring for whom disease is noted) is established, it is crucial that the siblings are carefully examined for prompt diagnosis of additional cases.

Impaired neutrophil function is considered to be the primary cause of PLS that eventually results in the deregulation of the polymorphonuclear leukocyte response to microbial infection. Although the subgingival microflora associated with PLS is diverse, opportunistic periodontal pathogens such as *Aggregatibacter actinomycetemcomitans*, *Porphyromonas gingivalis*, *Tannerella forsythia*, *Fusobacterium nucleatum*, and *Prevotella intermedia* are frequently identified among plaque samples from PLS patients.

Sarcoidosis is a chronic disease that is expressed as a cell-mediated, delayed-type hypersensitivity that primarily affects the lungs, lymph nodes, skin, eyes, liver, spleen, and small bones of the hands and feet. Sarcoidosis rarely affects the oral cavity, with incidence of occurrence in descending order noted in the lymph nodes, lips, soft palate, buccal mucosa, gingiva, tongue, and bone. Fig. 5.25 depicts the pretreatment pattern of bone loss and recession associated with sarcoidosis, with pulmonary parenchymal fibrous infiltrate being noted in the lungs as depicted by a white lacy pattern on a chest radiograph (Fig. 5.25C). Histologic features of sarcoidosis include the presence of an intense chronic inflammatory infiltrate with focal

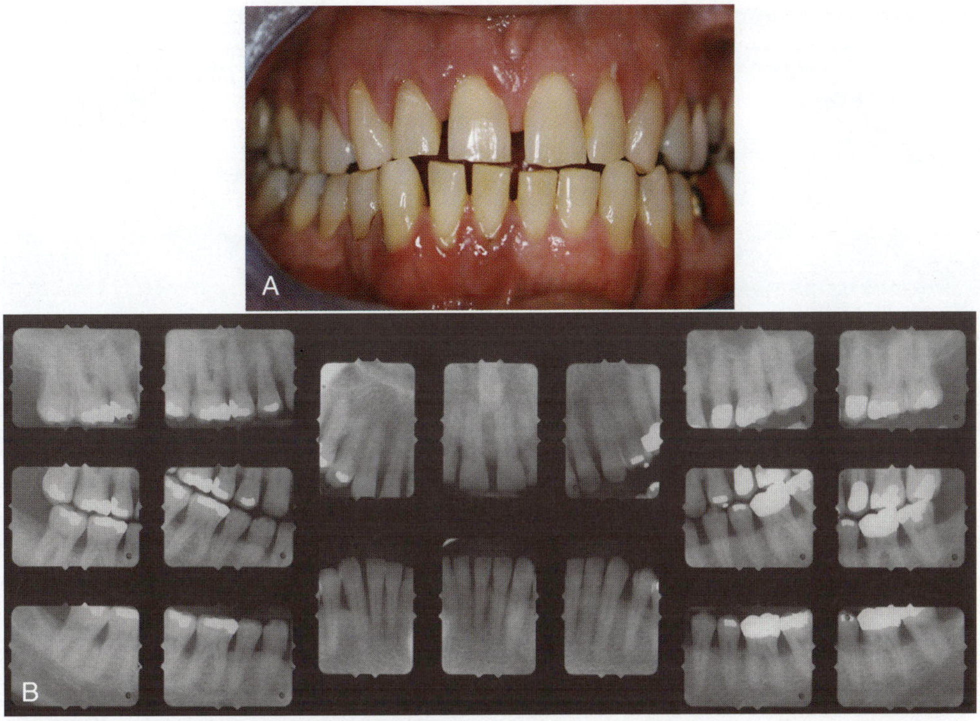

Fig. 5.20 A, Clinical image of plaque-related showing severe aggressive periodontitis in a 53-year-old man who smokes and who has diabetes and a hemoglobin A_{1c} level of 10.7. B, Radiographic images of the patient.

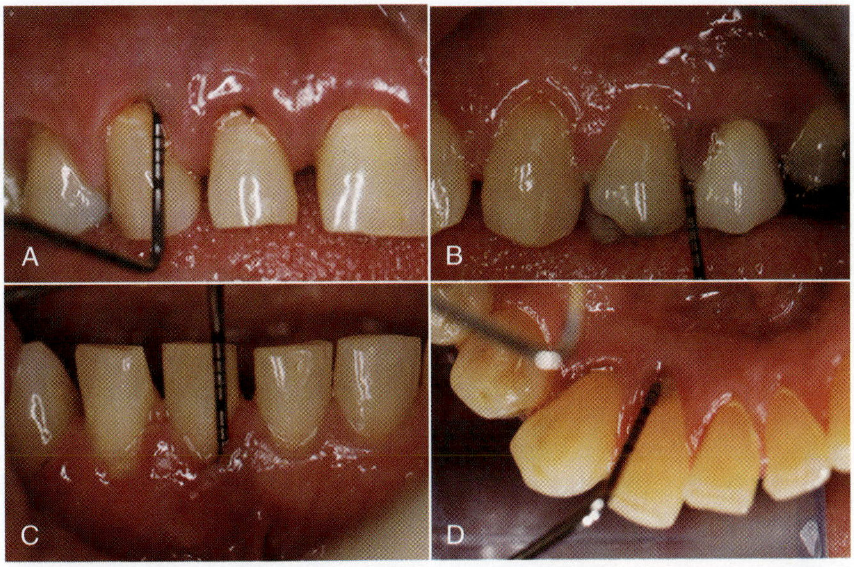

Fig. 5.21 Selective probing depths of the same 53-year-old diabetic patient shown in Fig. 5.20 with severe aggressive periodontitis.

areas of noncaseating granulomas and a positive Kveim test (Fig. 5.26C). The remineralization of alveolar bone is noted on radiographs obtained 1 year after the systemic administration of steroids (e.g., prednisone) (Fig. 5.26A).

Medication-Related Osteonecrosis of the Jaw

Medication-related osteonecrosis of the jaw (MRONJ) is an updated term that has replaced the phrase bisphosphonate-related osteonecrosis of the jaw (BRONJ). Bisphosphonates (BPs) are pyrophosphate analogs with a high affinity for hydroxyapatite crystals. They inhibit osteoclast-mediated bone resorption and play a key role in the management of osteolytic bone disorders, including osteoporosis, Paget disease, bone metastasis, and multiple myeloma. However, their prolonged use is associated with bisphosphonate-related osteonecrosis of the jaw (BRONJ).

The American Association of Oral and Maxillofacial Surgeons defines MRONJ as "exposed bone in the maxillofacial area occurring in the absence of head and neck irradiation and showing no evidence of healing for at least 8 weeks after identification in patients treated with BP therapy" (Figs. 5.27 and 5.28). To date, the true incidence of, causes of, and risk factors for the development of MRONJ are largely unknown. An overwhelming proportion

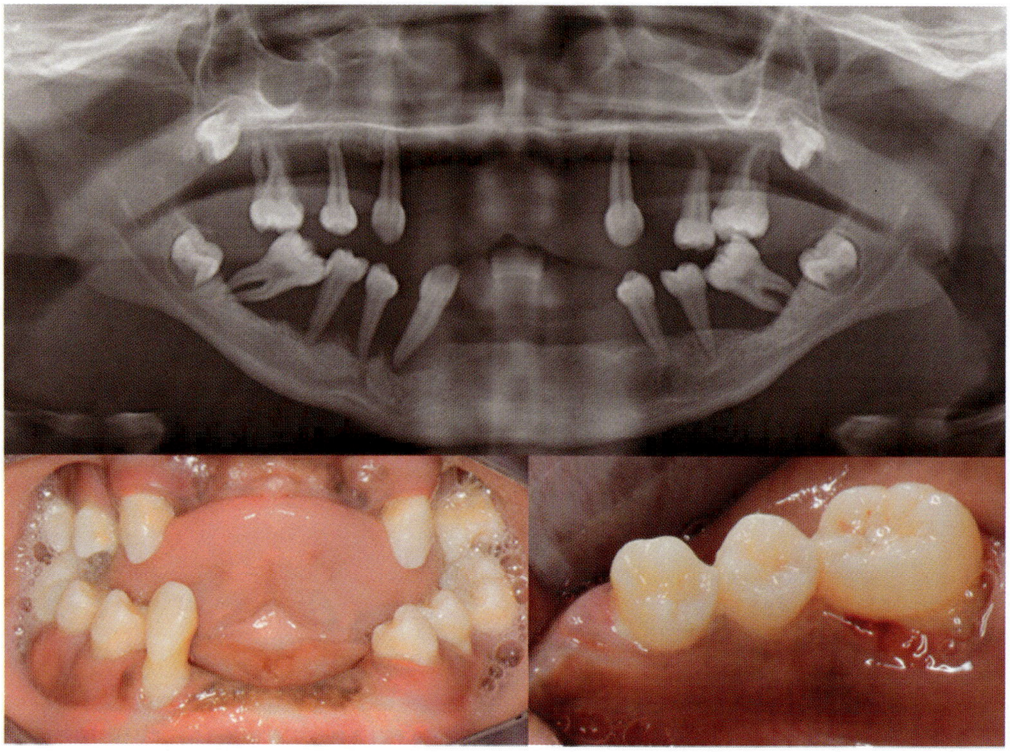

Fig. 5.22 Panoramic radiograph and clinical photographs of a 13-year-old girl with PLS. *(Courtesy Dr Georgios Kotsakis, Minneapolis, MN.)*

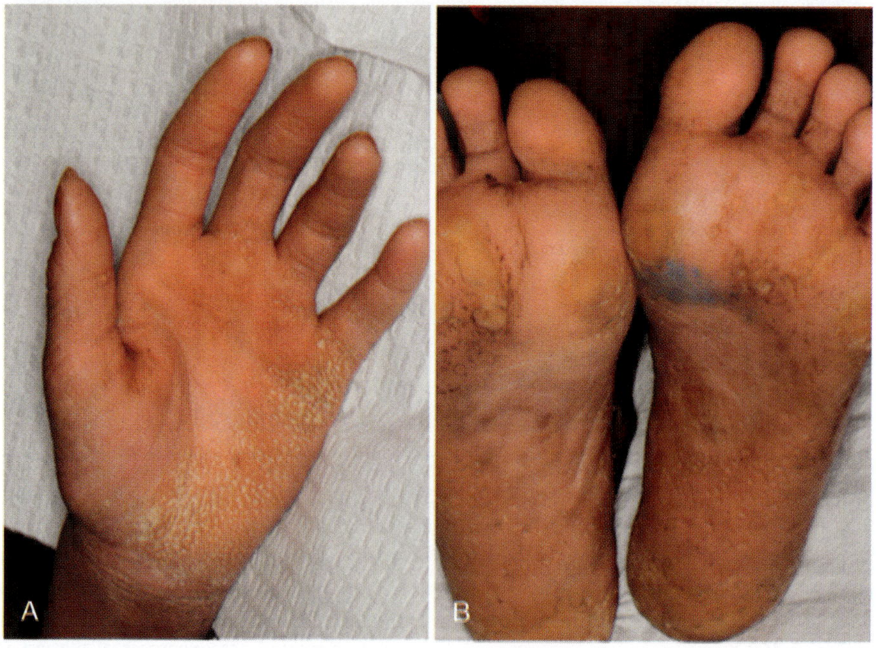

Fig. 5.23 Patient with PLS exhibiting hyperkeratosis on the palms of the hands and the soles of the feet. *(Courtesy Dr Georgios Kotsakis, Minneapolis, MN.)*

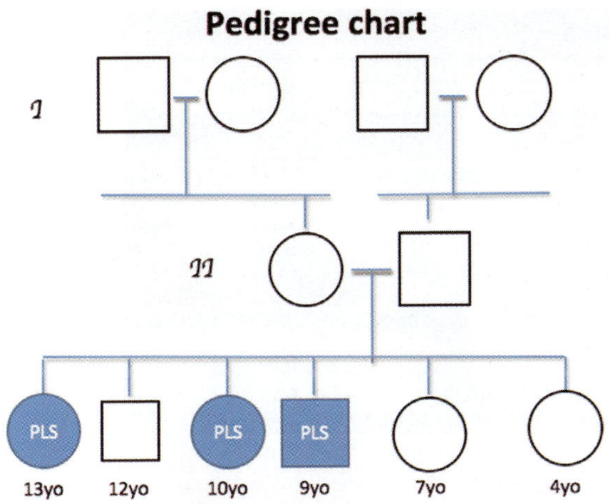

Fig. 5.24 No history of consanguinity was reported in this case. However, approximately one-third of diagnosed PLS cases descend from the same ancestor. Offsprings III1, III3, and III4 display a PLS phenotype. All siblings should be thoroughly examined by a periodontist after a case of PLS has been diagnosed. *(Courtesy Dr Georgios Kotsakis, Minneapolis, MN.)*

(i.e., 97%) of the reported cases are related to the high-dose intravenous BP given to patients with cancer. However, a small fraction (i.e., 3%) has been reported in patients with osteoporosis and patients with Paget disease who are receiving oral BP. The estimated incidence of MRONJ in patients with osteoporosis who are receiving oral BP is around 0.7 per 100,000 persons/years of exposure. The incidence of MRONJ among patients with cancer who are receiving intravenous BP ranges from 0.72% to 7.4%.

MRONJ lesions may be asymptomatic, or they may be present with pain, purulent discharge, swelling, tooth mobility, and paresthesia, thereby culminating in a reduced ability to eat and speak. MRONJ occurs most frequently in the mandible (65%), followed by the maxilla (26%), and both jaws (95%). The frequency of MRONJ is higher in the posterior region of the jaw. Among patients who develop MRONJ, approximately 60% of cases occur after an invasive dental procedure (e.g., tooth extraction), whereas 40% develop spontaneously. Radiographic evaluation is usually inconclusive for early lesions; in advanced cases, a poorly defined moth-eaten radiolucency is noted with radiopaque sequestra.

Currently, there is no effective treatment for MRONJ. The discontinuance of BP is not helpful because BPs tend to reside in the bone for very long periods of time. Radical surgical intervention often exacerbates the condition, and the merit of hyperbaric oxygen treatment for the management of MRONJ is not conclusive. Patients are typically treated via minimally invasive conservative debridement, antibiotics, and chlorhexidine mouth rinses to limit the extent of the damage and to facilitate wound healing. The American Dental Association suggests that an oral health program that consists of sound hygiene practices and regular dental care is a valuable approach to lowering the risk of developing MRONJ. Practitioners are encouraged to use atraumatic surgical techniques and to minimize the extent of dentoalveolar manipulation. Communication with the patient's physician and proper risk assessment are fundamental to the successful management of patients who are receiving BP therapy.

The use of the term MRONJ was introduced to capture the rising number of osteonecrosis cases of the jaw that are associated with new types of medication, such as other antiresorptive (denosumab) and antiangiogenic therapies, by the American Association of Oral and Maxillofacial Surgeons (AAOMS) in their 2014 update. Readers are referred to the position paper by the AAOMS for additional information on MRONJ.

Necrotizing Periodontal Diseases

The clinical characteristics of necrotizing periodontal diseases may include (but are not limited to) ulcerated and necrotic papillary and marginal gingiva covered by a yellowish–white or grayish slough or pseudomembrane, blunting and cratering of the papillae, bleeding on provocation or spontaneous bleeding, pain, and fetid breath.

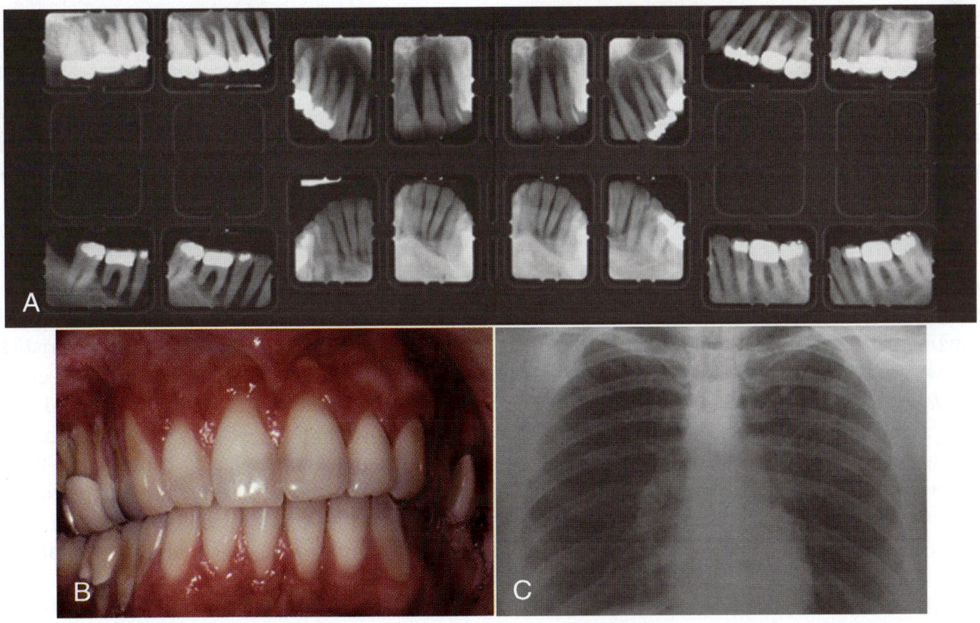

Fig. 5.25 **Sarcoidosis pretreatment.** A, The intraoral radiographs depict more extensive bone loss than clinical attachment loss for the anterior teeth. B, Extensive recession plus clinical attachment loss. C, Pulmonary parenchymal fibrous infiltrate.

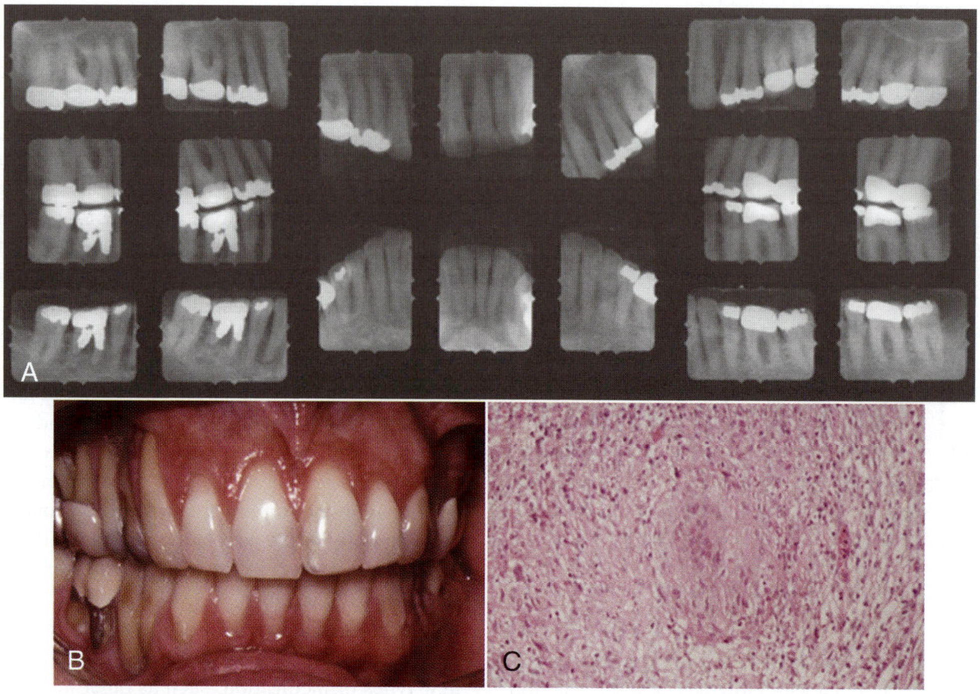

Fig. 5.26 **Sarcoidosis after treatment with prednisone.** A, Intraoral radiographs depict the remineralization of bone. B, Reduction in gingival inflammation while extensive recession and clinical attachment loss persist. C, Pretreatment biopsy.

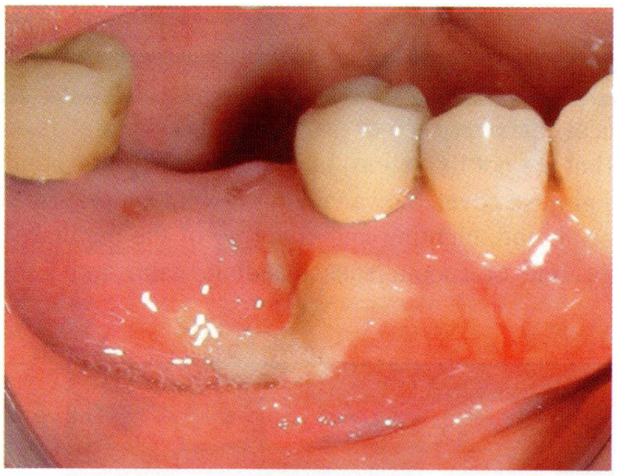

Fig. 5.27 Exposed bone on the buccal lower premolar and molar in a patient with BP-associated osteonecrosis of the jaw after extraction of the first molar. *(Courtesy Dr Vivek Thumbigere Math, Minneapolis, MN.)*

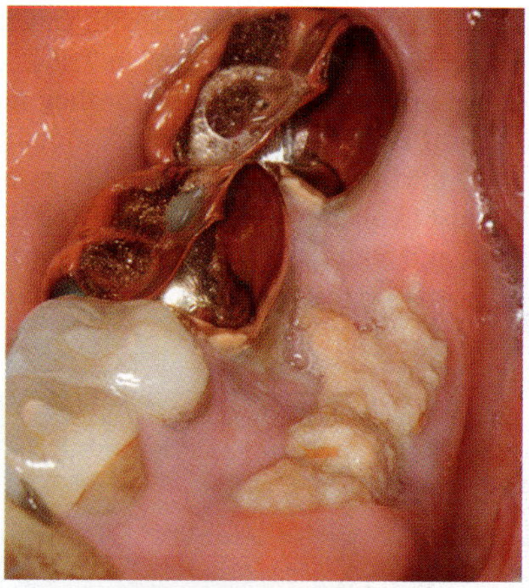

Fig. 5.28 Patient with BP-associated osteonecrosis of the jaw with exposed bone on the lingual aspect of the lower premolar and molar after root canal treatment. *(Courtesy Dr Vivek Thumbigere Math, Minneapolis, MN.)*

These diseases may be accompanied by fever, malaise, and lymphadenopathy although these characteristics are not consistent. Two forms of necrotizing periodontal disease have been described; *necrotizing ulcerative gingivitis* (NUG) (Fig. 5.29) and *necrotizing ulcerative periodontitis* (NUP) (Fig. 5.30). NUG has been previously classified as "gingival disease" or "gingivitis" because clinical attachment loss is not a consistent feature; NUP has been classified as a form of "periodontitis" because attachment loss is present. Recent reviews of the causative and clinical characteristics of NUG and NUP have suggested that the two diseases represent clinical manifestations of the same disease, except that distinct features of NUP are clinical attachment and bone loss. Nonetheless, NUP cases are almost exclusively reported in immunocompromised persons. As a result, both NUG and NUP have been determined to comprise a separate group of diseases that have *tissue necrosis* as a primary clinical feature (Box 5.1).

Necrotizing Ulcerative Gingivitis

The clinical and causative characteristics of NUG are described in detail in Chapter 20. The defining characteristics of NUG are its bacterial cause, necrotic lesion, and predisposing factors, such as psychologic stress, smoking, and immunosuppression. In addition, malnutrition may be a contributing factor in developing countries. NUG is usually seen as an acute lesion that responds well to antimicrobial therapy in combination with professional plaque and calculus removal as well as improved oral hygiene.

Necrotizing Ulcerative Periodontitis

NUP differs from NUG in that the loss of clinical attachment and alveolar bone is a consistent feature originating from the proximal region. The characteristics of NUP are described in detail in Chapter 29. NUP may be observed among HIV seropositive individuals with

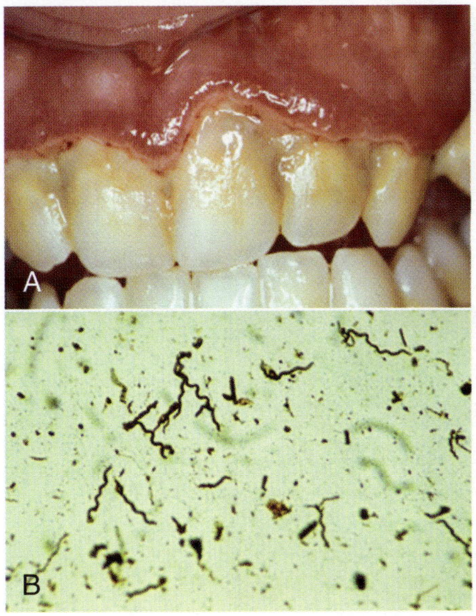

Fig. 5.29 A, Ulcerative gingivitis illustrating the sloughing of the marginal gingiva. B, Phase-contrast microscopy reveals Spirochetes in the subgingival plaque sample.

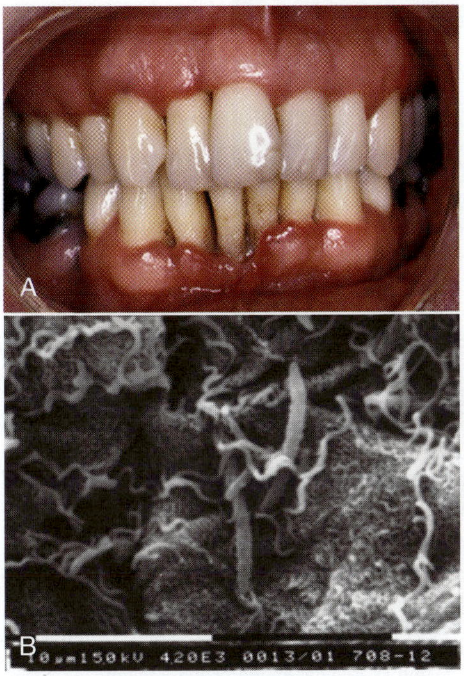

Fig. 5.30 A, Necrotizing ulcerative periodontitis with severe clinical attachment loss in a 28-year-old man with human immunodeficiency virus. B, Spirochetes are noted on the surface of sloughed epithelial cells.

low CD4 counts. Clinical manifestations include local ulceration and the necrosis of gingival tissue with the exposure and rapid destruction of underlying bone as well as spontaneous bleeding and severe pain. HIV+ persons with NUP are 20.8 times more likely to have CD^{4+} cell counts of less than 200 cells/mm^3 of peripheral blood as compared to those without NUP, which suggests that immunosuppression is a major contributing factor. NUP has also been associated with severe malnutrition in developing countries. More aggressive cases of necrotizing stomatitis exhibit tissue necrosis beyond the confines of the periodontium to include other oral tissues, such as the hard palate.

KEY FACT

Necrotizing stomatitis is a serious inflammatory condition that develops in systemically compromised individuals and is characterized by soft tissue necrosis that extends beyond the gingiva, with potential bony sequestrum formation. This disease entity is now included in the AAP/EFP 2018 classification of periodontal disease.

Abscesses of the Periodontium

A periodontal abscess is a localized purulent infection of periodontal tissues, and it is classified by its tissue of origin. The clinical, microbiologic, immunologic, and predisposing characteristics are discussed in Chapter xx on abscesses of the periodontium.

Periodontitis Associated With Endodontic Lesions

The classification of lesions that affect the periodontium and the pulp is based on the sequence of the disease process.

Endodontic–Periodontal Lesions

In endodontic–periodontal lesions, pulpal necrosis precedes periodontal changes. A periapical lesion that originates with pulpal infection and necrosis may drain to the oral cavity through the periodontal ligament, thereby resulting in the destruction of the periodontal ligament and the adjacent alveolar bone. This may be present clinically as a localized, deep, periodontal probing depth that extends to the apex of the tooth (Fig. 5.31A). A resultant extensive alveolar ridge defect (Fig. 5.31B and C) may necessitate reconstructive surgery (Fig. 5.31D) before the placement of implants and prostheses (Fig. 5.32) to reestablish a functional and esthetic outcome. Pulpal infection may also drain through accessory canals, especially in the area of the furcation, and this may lead to furcal involvement through the loss of clinical attachment and alveolar bone.

CLINICAL CORRELATION

In early stages of primary endodontic lesions, root canal therapy may be the only treatment necessary to restore the periodontal apparatus.

Periodontal–Endodontic Lesions

It is more uncommon for periodontal disease to lead to endodontic disease than vice versa. In periodontal–endodontic lesions, bacterial infection from a periodontal pocket associated with a loss of attachment and root exposure may spread through the accessory canals to the pulp, thereby resulting in pulpal necrosis. In the case of advanced periodontal disease, the infection may reach the pulp through the apical foramen. Scaling and root planing remove cementum and underlying dentin, which may lead to chronic pulpitis through the bacterial penetration of dentinal tubules. However, many teeth that have been affected by periodontitis that have been scaled and root planed show no evidence of pulpal involvement.

Combined Lesions

Combined lesions occur when pulpal necrosis and a periapical lesion occur on a tooth that is also periodontally involved. An angular intrabony defect that communicates with a periapical lesion of pulpal origin results in a combined periodontal–endodontic lesion.

In all cases of periodontitis associated with endodontic lesions, the endodontic infection should be controlled before the definitive

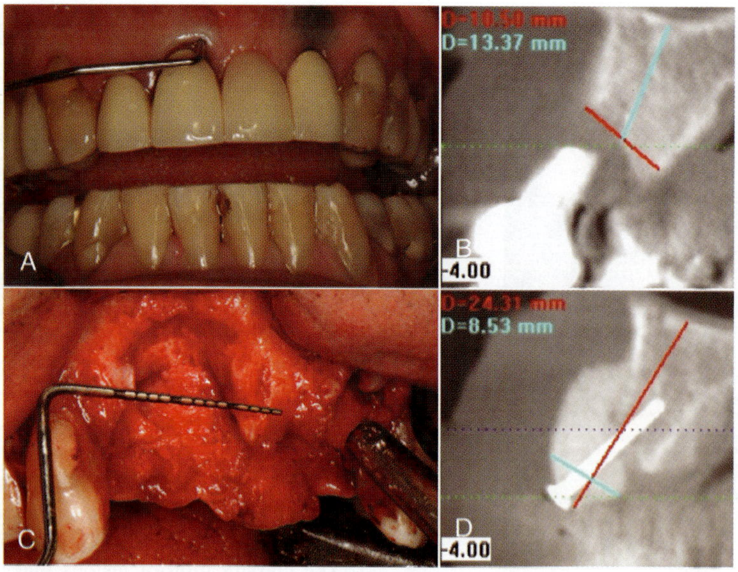

Fig. 5.31 A and C, Clinical images of extensive loss of the alveolar ridge as a result of a periapical endodontic lesion. B, A computed tomography image that depicts alveolar bone loss. D, A computed tomography image of a ridge that was regenerated with the use of allogenic bone graft and a tenting screw and membrane.

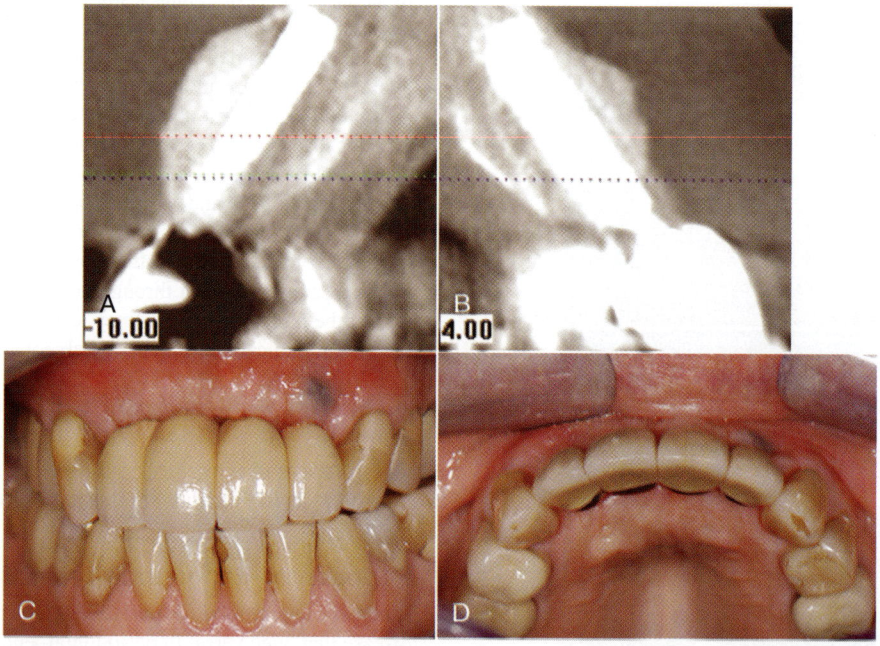

Fig. 5.32 The same patient who was depicted in Fig. 5.31. A and B, A computed tomography image of a regenerated ridge, with implants placed in areas #7, #9, and #10. C and D, Clinical image of the implant-supported bridge.

management of the periodontal lesion is begun, especially when regenerative or bone-grafting techniques are planned. Tooth prognosis in combined lesions highly depends on the outcome of the periodontal treatment.

Developmental or Acquired Deformities and Conditions

Localized Tooth-Related Factors That Modify or Predispose Individuals to Plaque-Induced Gingival Diseases or Periodontitis

In general, these localized tooth-related factors contribute to the initiation and progression of periodontal disease through the enhancement of plaque accumulation or the prevention of effective plaque removal via normal oral-hygiene measures. These factors fall into the four subgroups outlined in Box 5.4.

Tooth Anatomic Factors

Tooth anatomic factors are associated with malformations of tooth development or tooth location. Anatomic factors (e.g., cervical enamel projections, enamel pearls) have been associated with clinical attachment loss, especially in furcation areas. Cervical enamel projections are found on 15%–24% of mandibular molars and on 9%–25% of maxillary molars, and strong associations have been observed with furcation involvement. Palatogingival grooves, which are found primarily on maxillary incisors, are observed in

8.5% of individuals, and they are associated with increased plaque accumulation, clinical attachment, and bone loss. Proximal root grooves on incisors and maxillary premolars also predispose individuals to plaque accumulation, inflammation, and the loss of clinical attachment and bone.

Tooth location is considered important for the initiation and development of disease. Malaligned teeth predispose individuals to plaque accumulation with resultant inflammation in children, and they may predispose adults to clinical attachment loss, especially when they are associated with poor oral-hygiene habits. In addition, open contacts have been associated with an increased loss of alveolar bone, most likely through food impaction.

Dental Restorations and Appliances

Dental restorations or appliances are frequently associated with the development of gingival inflammation, especially when they are located subgingivally. This may apply to subgingivally placed onlays, crowns, fillings, and orthodontic bands. Restorations may impinge on the biologic width by being placed deep in the sulcus or within the junctional epithelium. This may promote inflammation and the loss of clinical attachment and bone, with apical migration of the junctional epithelium, and the reestablishment of the attachment apparatus at a more apical level. Contour of a complete crown restoration can affect plaque retention with flat surfaces being more hygienic as compared to convex restorations exhibiting increased bulk of material at the cervical region.

Root Fractures

Root fractures that are caused by traumatic forces or by restorative or endodontic procedures (Fig.5.33A–C) may lead to periodontal involvement through the apical migration of plaque along the fracture when the fracture originates coronal to the clinical attachment and is exposed to the oral environment, with a resulting alveolar ridge defect (Fig. 5.33D).

FLASH BACK

Vertical root fractures involving both the pulp and PDL are true combined endodontic–periodontal lesions.

Cervical Root Resorption and Cemental Tears

Cervical root resorption (as noted on the computed tomography scans shown in Fig. 5.34A and B) and cemental tears may lead to periodontal destruction when the lesion communicates with the oral cavity and allows bacteria to migrate subgingivally. Avulsed teeth that are reimplants frequently develop ankylosis and cervical resorption many years after reimplantation. If the patient is still in the phase of skeletal growth, decoronation may be the treatment of choice for ridge preservation. In adults with completed skeletal growth, atraumatic removal of such ankylosed teeth, followed by ridge reconstruction and placement of implants and prosthesis, is a viable treatment option in adults (Fig. 5.35).

Mucogingival Deformities and Conditions Around the Teeth

Mucogingival deformity is a generic term used to describe the mucogingival junction and its relationship to the gingiva (Fig. 5.36), the alveolar mucosa, and frenula muscle attachments. A *mucogingival deformity* is a significant departure from the normal shape of the gingiva and the alveolar mucosa, and it may involve the underlying alveolar bone. Mucogingival surgery and periodontal plastic and esthetic surgery correct defects in the morphology, position, or amount of gingiva. The surgical correction of mucogingival deformities may be performed for esthetic reasons, to enhance function, or to facilitate oral hygiene.

Mucogingival Deformities and Conditions of the Edentulous Ridges

Mucogingival deformities, such as a lack of stable keratinized gingiva between the vestibular fornices and the floor of the mouth (Fig. 5.37A), may require soft-tissue grafting and vestibular deepening before prosthodontic reconstruction (Fig. 5.37B–D). Alveolar bone defects in edentulous ridges (Fig. 5.38A and B) usually require corrective surgery (Fig. 5.38C and D) to restore form and function before the placement of implants and prostheses to replace missing teeth (Fig. 5.37–5.39).

Occlusal Trauma

The causes of trauma from occlusion and the effect of this trauma on the periodontium are discussed in detail in Chapter xx on periodontal response to external forces.

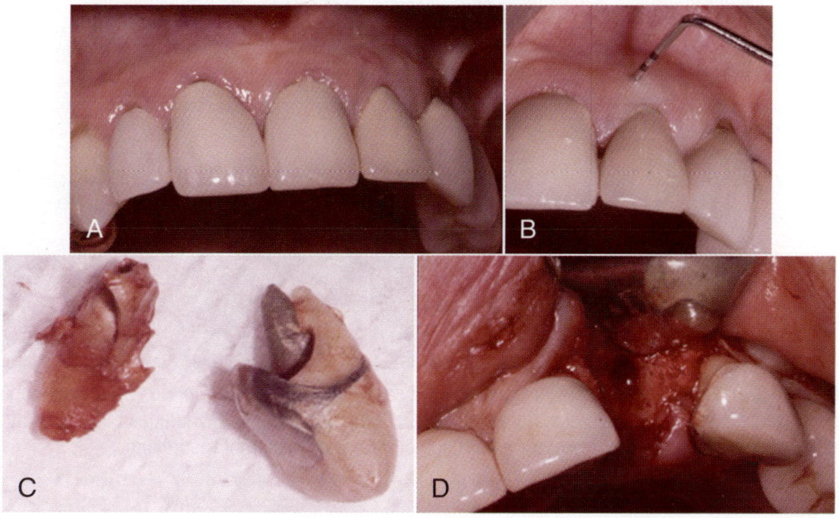

Fig. 5.33 A and B, Clinical images of a fistula tract. C, Root fracture. D, Resultant alveolar ridge defect.

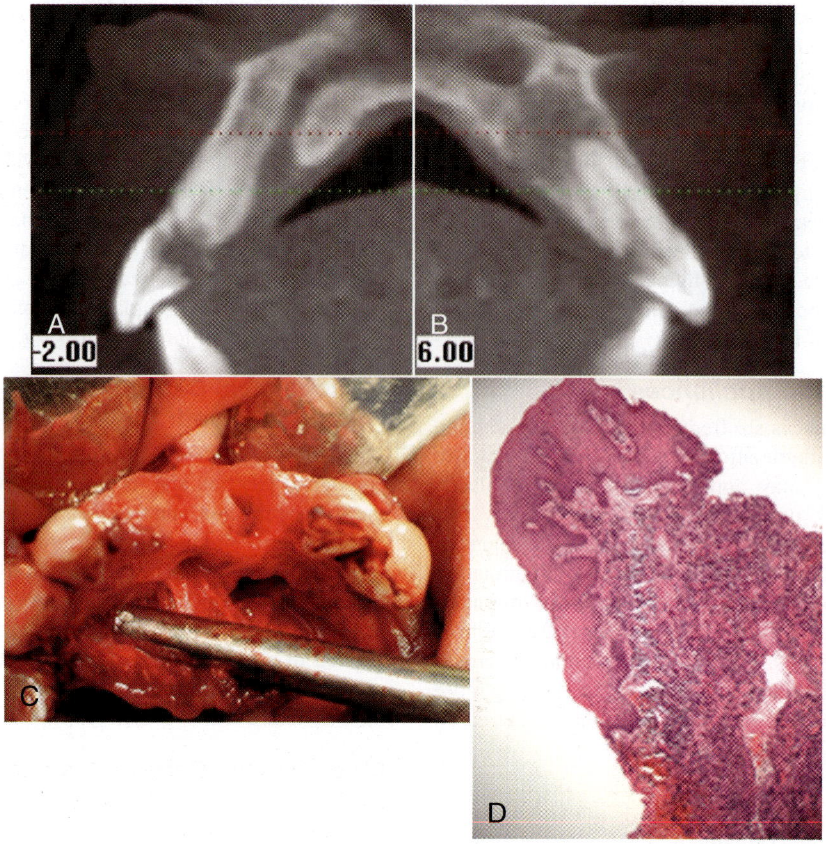

Fig. 5.34 A and B, Computed tomography scanning reveals severe cervical root resorption of the maxillary central incisors and periapical abscess. C, Crowns fractured as a result of resorption. D, Biopsy of soft tissue from the resorption.

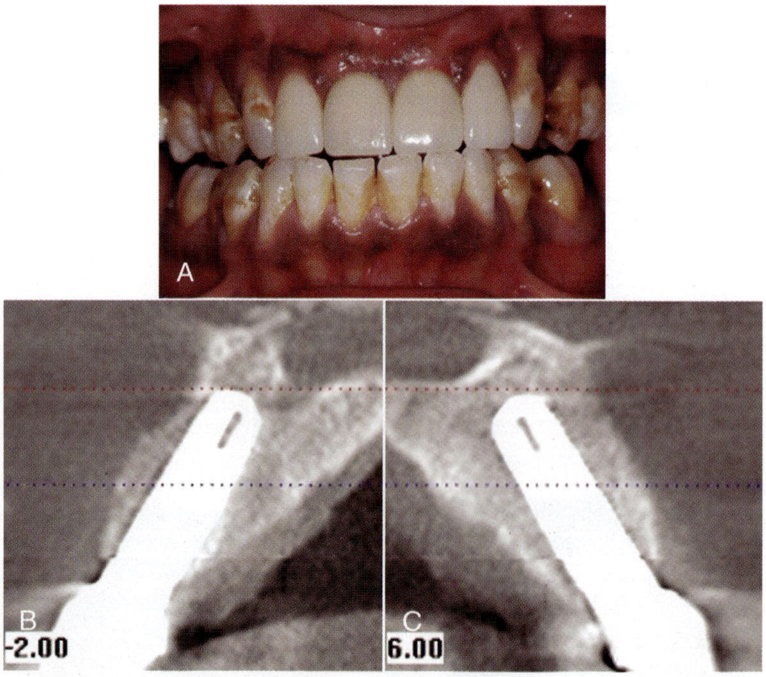

Fig. 5.35 A, Posttreatment clinical image of the same patient depicted in Fig. 5.34 with implant-supported crowns and veneers on the lateral surfaces. B and C, Computed tomography images of bone grafts and implants replacing central incisors that were lost as a result of severe cervical root resorption.

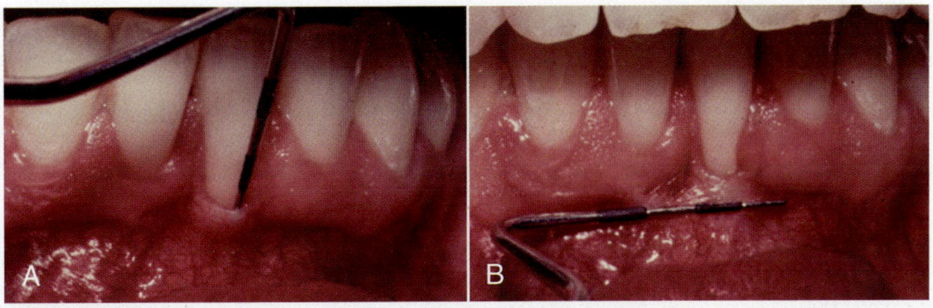

Fig. 5.36 A, Mucogingival defect depicted by recession. B, Defects extend into the alveolar mucosa which lack keratinized gingiva.

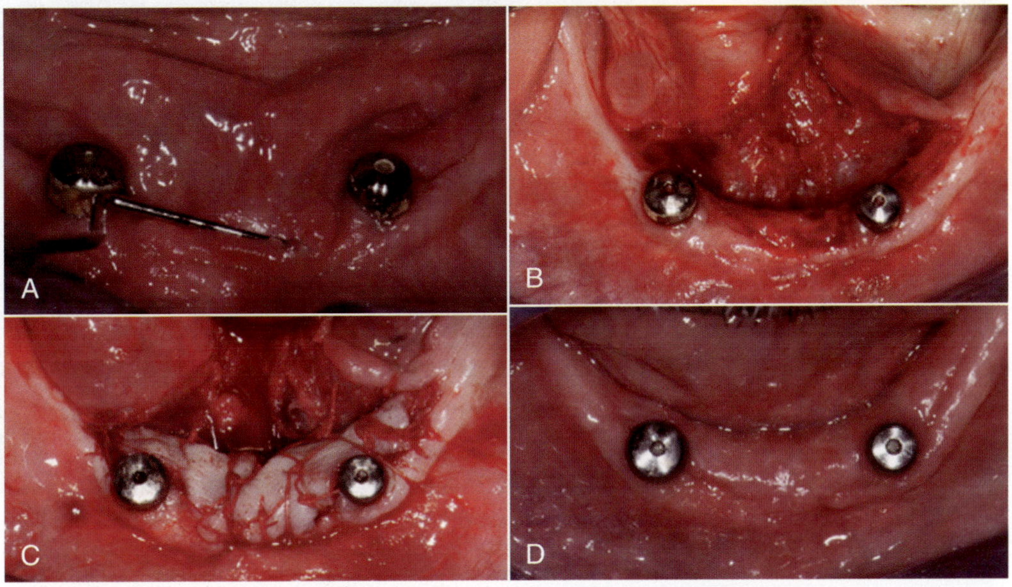

Fig. 5.37 A, Mucogingival ridge defect from the floor of the mouth to the vestibular fornix. B, A partial-thickness flap with vestibular deepening. C, The placement of free gingival graft. D, The reestablishment of vestibular depth and keratinized attached gingiva.

Key points

- A classification can be most consistently defined by the differences in the clinical manifestations of diseases and conditions; they are clinically consistent and require little (if any) clarification by scientific laboratory testing.
- Plaque-induced gingivitis may occur on a periodontium with no attachment loss or on a periodontium with previous attachment loss that is stable and not progressing. This suggests that gingivitis may be the diagnosis for inflamed gingival tissues associated with a tooth with no previous attachment loss or with a tooth that has previously undergone attachment and bone loss (i.e., with reduced periodontal support) but that is not currently losing attachment or bone even though gingival inflammation is present.
- Systemic factors such as the endocrine changes associated with puberty, the menstrual cycle, pregnancy, and diabetes—may be exacerbated as a result of alterations in the gingival inflammatory response to plaque. This altered response appears to result from the effects of systemic conditions on the host's cellular and immunologic functions.
- Medications like anticonvulsant drugs, such as phenytoin, immunosuppressive drugs, such as cyclosporine, and calcium-channel blockers, such as nifedipine, verapamil, diltiazem, and sodium valproate. The development and severity of gingival enlargement in response to medications are patient-specific and may be influenced by uncontrolled plaque accumulation, as well as by elevated hormonal levels.
- Gingival disease can have bacterial, fungal, or viral origin as the etiology.
- In endodontic–periodontal lesions, pulpal necrosis precedes periodontal changes. A periapical lesion that originates with pulpal infection and necrosis may drain to the oral cavity through the periodontal ligament, thereby resulting in the destruction of the periodontal ligament and the adjacent alveolar bone.
- Pulpal infection may also drain through accessory canals, especially in the area of the furcation, and this may lead to furcal involvement through the loss of clinical attachment and alveolar bone.
- In periodontal–endodontic lesions, bacterial infection from a periodontal pocket associated with a loss of attachment and root exposure may spread through the accessory canals to the pulp, thereby resulting in pulpal necrosis.
- Combined lesions occur when pulpal necrosis and a periapical lesion occur on a tooth that is also periodontally involved. An angular intrabony defect that communicates with a periapical lesion of pulpal origin results in a combined periodontal–endodontic lesion.

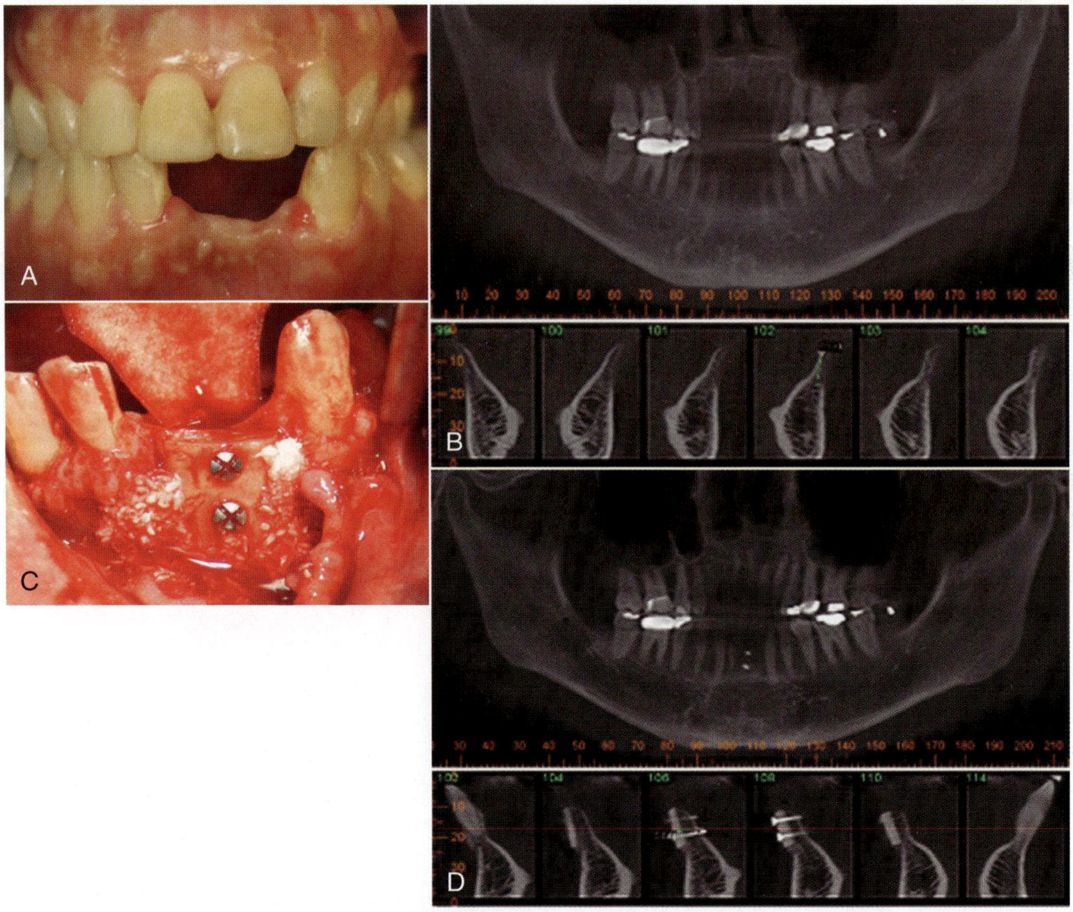

Fig. 5.38 A, Clinical image of an edentulous ridge defect. B, Pretreatment computed tomography image of the defect. C, Ridge that was reconstructed with the use of a ramus block graft. D, Computed tomography scan of the grafted site.

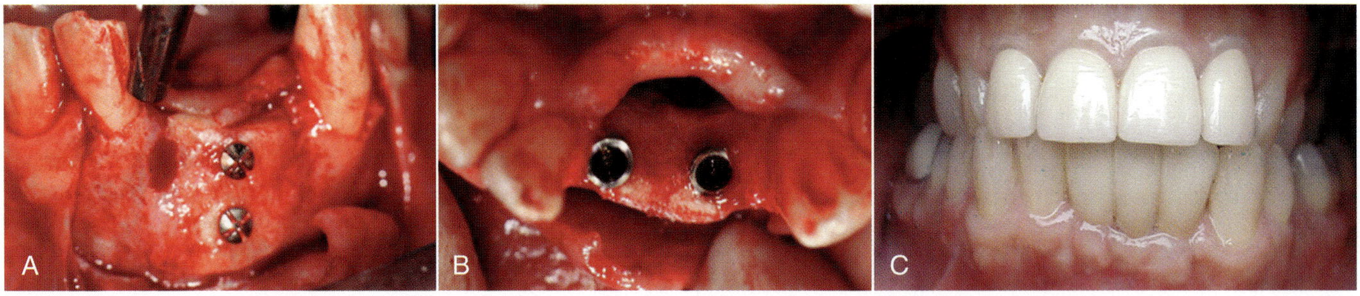

Fig. 5.39 A, Clinical image of the ridge 6 months after grafting. B, Placement of implants in the areas of teeth #23 and #25. C, Porcelain-fused-to-metal crowns for the maxillary incisors and an implant-supported bridge from teeth #23 through #25.

Suggested Readings

American Association of Oral and Maxillofacial: Surgeons position paper on bisphosphonate-related osteonecrosis of the jaws. *J Oral Maxillofac Surg* 65:369–376, 2007.

Armitage GC: Development of a classification system for periodontal diseases and conditions, *Ann Periodontol* 4: 1, 1999.

Attstrom R, Vander Velden U: Summary of session 1. In Lang N, Karring T, editors: In *Proceedings of the 1st European Workshop in Periodontology*, Berlin, 1993, Quintessence.

Caton J: Periodontal diagnosis and diagnostic aids: consensus report. *Proceedings of the World Workshop in Clinical Periodontics*, Chicago, 1989, American Academy of Periodontology.

Hellstein JW, Adler RA, Edwards B, et al: Managing the care of patients receiving antiresorptive therapy for prevention and treatment of osteoporosis: executive summary of recommendations from the American Dental Association Council on Scientific Affairs, *J Am Dent Assoc* 142: 1243-1251, 2011.

Kinane DF: Periodontitis modified by systemic factors, *Ann Periodontol* 4: 54, 1999.

Mariotti A: Dental plaque-induced gingival diseases, *Ann Periodontol* 4: 7, 1999.

Pini Prato GP: Mucogingival deformities, *Ann Periodontol* 4: 98, 1999.

Tonetti MS, Mombelli A: Early-onset periodontitis, *Ann Periodontol* 4: 39, 1999.

Woo SB, Hellstein JW, Kalmar JR: Narrative [corrected] review: bisphosphonates and osteonecrosis of the jaws, *Ann Intern Med* 144: 753-761, 2006.

References

References for this chapter are found on www.medenact.com.

CHAPTER 6

Epidemiology of Gingival and Periodontal Diseases

VW Spolsky | DG Naik | A Uppoor

CHAPTER OUTLINE

Epidemiologic surveys conducted throughout the world point to the almost universal distribution of caries and periodontal disease. Progress in the study of the epidemiology of periodontal diseases has been slower than that in the study of dental caries because of several important factors that do not exist in the study of dental caries. The pathologic changes of dental caries involve hard, calcified tissues, whereas periodontal disease involves soft and hard tissues. Unlike dental caries, periodontal disease does not lend itself easily to objective measurement because the signs of periodontal pathologic alteration involve color changes in the soft tissues, swelling, bleeding, and bone changes that are reflected in crevice depth changes or pathologic pockets, as well as loss of tooth function because of tooth mobility. Therefore, examining the teeth for the signs of dental caries is far easier than evaluating the pathologic variables used to define periodontal diseases.

Dental epidemiology is the study of the pattern (distribution) and dynamics of dental diseases in a human population. "Pattern" implies that certain people are affected by a disease and that the association between the disease and the affected population can be described by variables such as age, sex, racial or ethnic group, occupation, social characteristics, place of residence, susceptibility, and exposure to specific agents. The term *dynamics* refers to a temporal pattern (distribution) and is concerned with trends, cyclic patterns, and the time that elapses between the exposure in citing factors and the onset of the specific disease. Russell defined dental epidemiology as "not so much the study of disease as a process as it is a study of the condition of the people in whom the disease occurs."

The purpose or objective of epidemiology is to increase the understanding of the disease process (i.e., to identify the risk factors or determinants of disease), thereby leading to the development of methods of control and prevention. In addition, epidemiology attempts to discover populations at high and low risk, to define the specific problem under investigation, and to determine trends in disease patterns.

The design, conduct, and interpretation of clinical trials of preventive and curative measures are also within its purview. Ainamo has astutely described the significance of epidemiologic research to the understanding of periodontal disease. Epidemiologic research has clarified the prevalence of periodontal disease, provided new insights on its pathogenesis through controlled clinical trials, and focused attention on assessing treatment needs for improving the periodontal health of the public.

Epidemiologic Study Designs

The essence of epidemiology and clinical epidemiology is to relate measures of disease occurrence to suspected causes or interventions. Can the dramatic drop in destructive periodontal disease prevalence in India be attributed to a change in smoking prevalence? Can the presence of particular microbiologic species around a tooth be related to the risk of future tooth loss? Can the rate of tooth loss in a sample of elderly patients be related to the use of an antimicrobial rinse? With an evidence-based approach, these questions can be most reliably answered by three epidemiologic study designs. These study designs (in order of decreasing reliability) are the randomized controlled trial, the cohort study, and the case–control study.

Randomized Controlled Trials

Randomized controlled trials in periodontics typically assign patients or some teeth within a patient randomly to a treatment. Patients are then monitored, and subsequent outcomes are assessed.

The randomized controlled trial is the only study design that can provide a probabilistic basis for the making of a causal inference between an intervention and an outcome. Reliable inference regarding the causality of associations can be obtained if the delicate machinery of clinical trial design and analysis is strictly respected. For example, there needs to be a pretrial hypothesis that specifies the endpoint, the treatments to be compared, the patient population, and the degree of required precision. Other factors that are important for obtaining reliable answers include a secure randomization process, the masking of patients and clinicians, the presence of an independent data and safety monitoring board, and strict adherence to the pretrial hypothesis, which must include an intent-to-treat analysis. Trials with exquisite attention to detail are referred to as *definitive trials*, and they are rare in any field, including periodontal research. Definitive trials are required to provide reliable answers about treatment efficacy. Most of the trials published in the literature are in the category of exploratory trials. These trials typically do not report a pretrial hypothesis, and they conclude that the intervention was successful when compared to the control. These are almost always false-positive conclusions

Cohort Studies

Cohort studies can also be referred to as *exposure-based study designs.* Subjects who are free of the disease of interest are classified with respect to an exposure (e.g., cigarette smoking, diabetes) and followed longitudinally for the assessment of periodontal outcomes.

Cohorts can be defined by a geographic area, records, exposure status, or a combination of different criteria. In one study of the causal factors of edentulism, the population of interest was defined as the inhabitants of the town of Tecumseh, Michigan. Persons within this community were examined in 1959 as part of a community-wide health study. Twenty-eight years later, a subset of these patients was reexamined to study the risk factors for edentulism. Some natural disease history studies of destructive periodontal disease have been conducted on the basis of geographic location. Examples include the Norwegian Longitudinal Study, the Veterans Administration Longitudinal Study, and the Sri Lanka study. A cohort can be defined by records (e.g., schools, health insurance plans, unions, industries, professional organizations). Many cohort studies of periodontal disease outcomes are performed in patients who belong to a particular dental insurance company or to a professional group. Finally, cohorts can be defined on the basis of a specific exposure. For example, different levels of fluoride concentrations in the water supply have been used for the definition of cohorts.

Case–Control Studies

Case–control studies are typically referred to as *outcome-based study designs.* Persons with a condition or outcome of interest (i.e., cases) are compared to persons without a condition of interest (i.e., controls) with respect to the history of the suspected causal factors. Many people intuitively think along the lines of a case–control study when evaluating disease causes. For example, if an individual suffers from food poisoning after a party, he or she is likely to compare past food intake with those individuals who did *not* experience food poisoning. Similarly, if one is diagnosed with a serious illness, a common reaction is to ask, "Why me?" This is usually followed by a comparison of one's history of exposures with those of other individuals who did *not* develop the serious illness. The primary goal of a case–control study is to find out what *past* exposures or factors are different between patients with a disease versus those without the disease.

The case–control study is a challenging type of study to conduct. Trying to minimize the role of bias in case–control studies requires careful planning, conduct, and analysis. Even when everything is done perfectly, one can come to the wrong conclusions in case–control studies. A review of the quality of periodontal case–control studies suggested that they are frequently inadequately conducted and reported

Two important elements of the case–control study design are the definitions of the terms *case* and *control.* A *case* is a person in the population or study group who has been identified as having a particular disease, health disorder, or condition. The case definition should be rigorous to minimize bias and misclassification; it can be based on symptoms, signs, or the results of diagnostic tests. For example, the case definition for a myocardial infarction in a case–control study of the relationship between dental health and acute myocardial infarction was as follows:

1. Symptoms start within 36 hours before the admission.
2. No prior myocardial infarction.
3. Residing in Helsinki or an immediate neighborhood.
4. Age <60 years for men and <65 years for women.
5. Blood samples available at admission and at 4 weeks.

In a case–control study, the *controls* should be at risk for developing the investigated disease and come from the same population that generated the cases. For example, if the investigated disease is root caries, the controls should be at risk for developing root caries (i.e., have exposed root surfaces) and originate from the same population that generated the cases that have root caries.

Epidemiologic Indices

One of the most valuable techniques employed in dental epidemiology is the epidemiologic index. *Epidemiologic indices are attempts to quantitate clinical conditions on a graduated scale, thereby facilitating comparison among populations examined by the same criteria and methods.* Unlike the absolute or definitive diagnosis that can be made of disease in a solitary patient, an epidemiologic index (which is a numerical value) estimates only the relative prevalence or occurrence of the clinical condition.

Prevalence is the proportion of persons affected by a disease at a specific point in time, as determined by a cross-sectional survey.

Incidence is defined as the rate of occurrence of a new disease in a population during a given interval of time.

In general, indices are actually underestimates of the true clinical condition.

A good epidemiologic index must be easy to use, permit the examination of many people in a short period of time, define clinical conditions objectively, be highly reproducible in assessing a clinical condition when used by one or more examiners, be amenable to statistical analysis, and be strongly related numerically to the clinical stages of the specific disease under investigation. Calibration or standardization in reference to the use of an index's criteria by an examiner or examiners is imperative to ensure the reliability of the data.

In general, there are *two types* of dental indices.

The first type of index measures the number or proportion of people in a population with or without a specific condition at a specific point in time or interval of time.

The second type of dental index measures the number of people affected and the severity of the specific condition at a specific time or interval of time.

More explicitly, the second type of index not only helps to identify the person in the population affected with a specific condition but also assesses the condition under study on a graduated scale. Most of the indices described in this chapter are of the second type.

Indices Used to Study Periodontal Problems

Although there are many indices for recording and quantitating the entities that make up periodontal disease, space limitations only permit the inclusion of indices that have historically contributed to the understanding of periodontal diseases or are currently in frequent use. A scholarly overview of epidemiologic research in periodontal disease is provided by Ainamo. The indices that are discussed in this chapter can, for the purpose of convenience and reason, be divided according to the following measured variables:

1. The degree of inflammation of gingival tissues.
2. The degree of periodontal destruction.
3. The amount of plaque accumulated.
4. The amount of calculus present.

In addition, indices developed to assess treatment needs will be discussed.

Indices Used to Assess Gingival Inflammation

Papillary-Marginal-Attachment Index

Originally, the Papillary-Marginal-Attachment (PMA) index was used to count the number of gingival units affected with gingivitis. This approach was predicated on the belief that the number of units affected correlated with the degree or severity of gingival inflammation. The facial surface of the gingiva around a tooth was divided into three gingival scoring units: the mesial dental papilla (P), the gingival margin (M), and the attached gingiva (A). The presence or absence of inflammation on each gingival unit was recorded as 1 or 0, respectively. The P, M, and A numerical values for all teeth were totaled separately and then added together to express the PMA Index score per person. Although all of the facial tissues surrounding all of the teeth could be assessed in this manner, usually only the maxillary and mandibular incisors, the canines, and the premolars are examined. The developers of this index eventually added a severity component for assessing gingivitis; the papillary units (P) were scored on a scale of 0–5 and the marginal (M) and attached (A) gingivae were scored on a scale of 0–3.

The value of this index lies in its broad application to epidemiologic surveys and clinical trials and in its capacity for use in individual patients. The criteria for and approach to assessing gingival inflammation developed by Schour and Massler served as the basis for many other indices. Examples of indices that are based on modifications of the PMA Index are those developed by Mühlemann and Mazor, Lobene, and Suomi and Barbano.

Periodontal Index

The Periodontal Index (PI) was intended to estimate the extent of deeper periodontal disease that the PMA Index could measure by determining the presence or absence of gingival inflammation and its severity, pocket formation, and masticatory function. The criteria given in Table 6.1 are used to assess all of the gingival tissues circumscribing each tooth (i.e., all of the tissue circumscribing a tooth is considered a scoring or gingival unit). Since the PI measures both reversible and irreversible aspects of periodontal disease, it is an epidemiologic index with a true biologic gradient. A PI score for an individual is determined by adding all of the tooth scores and dividing by the number of teeth examined. Since only a mouth mirror and no calibrated probes or radiographs are used when performing a PI examination, the results tend to underestimate the true level of periodontal disease, especially early bone loss, in a population. The number of periodontal pockets without obvious supragingival calculus is also underestimated in the PI.

TABLE 6.1 The Periodontal Index

Score	Criteria and Scoring for Field Studies	Additional Criteria Followed in the Clinical Test
0	*Negative.* There is neither overt inflammation in the investing tissues nor loss of function owing to destruction of supporting tissues.	Radiographic appearance is essentially normal.
1	*Mid Gingivitis.* There is an overt area of inflammation in the free gingivae, but this area does not circumscribe the tooth.	
2	*Gingivitis.* Inflammation completely circumscribes the tooth, but there is no apparent break in the epithelial attachment.	
4	(Used when radiographs are available.)	There is early, notch-like resorption of the alveolar crest.
6	*Gingivitis with pocket formation.* The epithelial attachment has been broken, and there is a pocket (not merely a deepened gingival crevice as a result of swelling in free gingivae). There is no interference with normal masticatory function; the tooth is firm and has not drifted.	There is horizontal bone loss involving the entire alveolar crest, up to half of the length of the tooth root.
8	*Advanced destruction with loss of masticatory function.* The tooth may be loose, may have drifted, may sound dull on percussion with a metallic instrument, or may be depressible in its socket.	There is advanced bone loss involving more than one-half of the length of the tooth root or a definite infrabony pocket with widening of the periodontal ligament. There may be root resorption or rarefaction at the apex.
Rule: When in Doubt, Assign the Lesser Scores		
	Periodontal index score per person =	Sum of individual scores
		Number of teeth present
Clinical Condition	*Group PI Scores*	Stage of Disease
Clinically normal supportive tissues	0–0.2	
Simple gingivitis	0.3–0.9	Reversible
Beginning destructive periodontal disease	0.7–1.9	
Established destructive periodontal disease	1.6–5.0	Irreversible
Terminal disease	3.8–8.0	

(Modified from Russell AL: The periodontal index. *J Periodontal* 38:585, 1967.)

Gingivitis Component of the Periodontal Disease Index

The Periodontal Disease Index (PDI) is similar to the PI in that both are used to measure the presence and severity of periodontal disease. The PDI does so by combining the assessments of gingivitis and gingival sulcus depth on six selected teeth (teeth # 16, 21, 24, 36, 41, and 46). This group of teeth, frequently referred to as the *Ramfjord teeth*, have been tested as reliable indicators for the various regions of the mouth. Calculus and plaque are also examined to assist in formulating a comprehensive assessment of periodontal status and are described in the following discussions.

The criteria used to assess the tissue circumscribing the Ramfjord teeth combine elements of the PMA Index and the PI and appear in Table 6.2. A numerical score for the gingival status component of the PDI (i.e., the Gingivitis Index score per person) [see Section "Gingival Index (Loe and Silness)"] is obtained by adding the value for all of the gingival units and dividing by the number of teeth present. The PDI has been used in epidemiologic surveys, longitudinal studies of periodontal disease, and clinical trials of therapeutic or preventive procedures.

Gingival Index (Loe and Silness)

The Gingival Index (GI) was developed solely for the purpose of assessing the severity of gingivitis and its location in four possible areas. The tissues surrounding each tooth are divided into four gingival scoring units: the distofacial papilla, the facial margin, the mesiofacial papilla, and the entire lingual gingival margin. To minimize examiner variability in scoring, the lingual surface is not subdivided because it will most likely be viewed indirectly with a mouth mirror. A blunt instrument, such as a periodontal pocket probe, is used to assess the bleeding potential of the tissues. Each of the four gingival units is assessed according to the criteria shown in Table 6.3.

Totaling the scores around each tooth yields the GI score for the area. If the scores around each tooth are totaled and divided by four, the GI score for the tooth is obtained. Totaling all of the scores per tooth and dividing by the number of teeth examined provides the GI score per person. The GI may also be used to evaluate a segment of the mouth or group of teeth.

The numerical scores of the GI are associated with varying degrees of clinical gingivitis as follows:

Gingival Scores	Degree of Gingivitis
0.1–1.0	Mild
1.1–2.0	Moderate
2.1–3.0	Severe

TABLE 6.2 Criteria for Several Components of the Periodontal Disease Index

Gingival Status (Gingivitis Index)

0 = Absence of signs of inflammation

1 = Mid to moderate inflammatory gingival changes, not extending around the tooth

2 = Mild to moderately severe gingivitis extending all around the tooth

3 = Severe gingivitis characterized by marked redness, swelling, tendency to bleed, and ulceration

Crevicular Measurements

A. If the gingival margin is on the enamel, measure from the gum margin to the cementoenamel junction and record the measurement. If the epithelial attachment is on the crown and the cementoenamel junction cannot be felt by the probe, record the depth of the gingival sulcus on the crown. Then record the distance from the gingival margin to the bottom of the pocket if the probe can be moved apically to the cementoenamel junction without resistance or pain. The distance from the cementoenamel junction to the bottom of the pocket can then be found by subtracting the first from the second measurement.

B. If the gingival margin is on the cementum, record the distance from the cementoenamel junction to the gingival margin as a minus value. Then record the distance from the cementoenamel junction to the bottom of the gingival sulcus as plus value. Both loss of attachment and actual sulcus depth can easily be assessed from the scores.

Periodontal Disease Index (PDI) Criteria for Surveys

If the gingival sulcus in none of the measured areas extended apically to the cementoenamel junction, the recorded score for gingivitis is the PDI score for the tooth. If the gingival sulcus in any of the two measured areas extended apically to the cementoenamel junction but not more than 3 mm (including 3 mm in any area), the tooth is assigned a PDI score of 4. The score for gingivitis is then disregarded in the PDI score for that tooth. If the gingival sulcus in either of the two recorded areas of the tooth extends apically to from 3 to 6 mm (including 6 mm) in relation to the cemntoenamel junction, the tooth is assigned a PDI score of 5 (again, the gingivitis score is disregarded). Whenever the gingival sulcus extends more than 6 mm apically to the cementoenamel junction in any of the measured areas of the tooth, the score of 6 is assigned as the PDI score for that tooth (again disregarding the gingivitis score).

Shick–Ash Modification of Plaque Criteria

0 = Absence of dental plaque

1 = Dental plaque in the interproximal area or at the gingival margin covering less than one-third of the gingival half of the facial or lingual surface of the tooth

2 = Dental plaque covering more than one-third but less than two-thirds of the gingival half of the facial or lingual surface of the tooth

3 = Dental plaque covering two-thirds or more of the gingival half of the facial or gingival surface of the tooth

Calculus Criteria

0 = Absence of calculus

1 = Supragingival calculus extending only slightly below the free gingival margin (not more than 1 mm)

2 = Moderate amount of supragingival and subgingival calculus or subgingival calculus alone

3 = An abudance of supragingival and subgingival calculus

TABLE 6.3 Criteria for the Gingival Index, the Plaque Index, and the Modified Gingival Index

Gingival Index (GI)

0 = Normal gingiva
1 = Mild inflammation, slight change in color, slight edema, *no bleeding on palpation*
2 = Moderate inflammation, redness, edema, and glazing; *bleeding on probing*[a]
3 = Severe inflammation, market redness and edema, ulcerations; *tendency to spontaneous bleeding*

Plaque Index (PI)

0 = No plaque in the gingival area
1 = A film of plaque adhering to the free gingival margin and adjacent area of the tooth. The plaque may be recognized only by running a probe across the tooth surface
2 = Moderate accumulation of soft deposits within the gingival pocket and on the gingival margin and/or adjacent tooth surface that can be seen by the naked eye
3 = Abundance of soft matter within the gingival pocket and/or on the gingival margin and adjacent tooth surface

Modified Gingival Index (MGI)

0 = Absence of inflammation
1 = Mild inflammation; slight change in color, little change in texture of portion of the marginal or papillary gingival unit
2 = Mild inflammation; criteria as mentioned earlier but involving the entire marginal or papillary gingival unit
3 = Moderate inflammation; glazing, redness, edema, and/or hypertrophy of the marginal or papillary gingival unit
4 = Severe inflammation; marked redness, edema, and/or hypertrophy of the marginal or papillary gingival unit, spontaneous bleeding, congestion, or ulceration

[a]A periodontal probe is drawn horizontally along the soft tissue wall of the entrance to the gingival sulcus.

The index can be used to determine the prevalence and severity of gingivitis in both epidemiologic surveys and in an individual. This latter attribute has contributed to making the GI the index of choice in controlled clinical trials of preventive or therapeutic agents.

Lobene and coworkers created the modified GI (MGI) by eliminating the bleeding criterion, making the MGI a noninvasive index. By redefining the criteria for mild and moderate inflammation, the MGI increases sensitivity in the lower portion of the scoring scale. The criteria for the MGI are given in Table 6.3.

Indices of Gingival Bleeding

Two indices that combine the clinical estimates of inflammation and bleeding have been described. The Sulcus Bleeding Index (SBI) of Mühlemann and Mazor uses bleeding on gentle probing as the first criterion for indicating gingival inflammation. In 1971, Mühlemann and Son added an additional category to the original criteria, resulting in a 0–5 scale for assessing inflammation or sulcular bleeding.

Several years later Mühlemann assessed sulcus bleeding on probing at the interdental papilla. This Papillary Bleeding Index (PBI) used a scale of 0–4. A timing component was added to the PBI by Barnett and coworkers in an effort to make the PBI more sensitive than the GI in assessing gingival changes.

All of Mühlemann indices are predicated on an understanding of sulcular bleeding as a precursor of gingival inflammation and as the first sign of inflammation. The GI of Löe and Silness, however, uses the presence of a slight color change and the absence of bleeding when a blunt instrument is used to palpate the soft tissue wall at the gingival margin to indicate initial gingival inflammation. Although the correlation between the two variables (inflammation and bleeding) is not perfect, the histologic evidence for associating inflammation with the GI criteria is stronger than that for associating gingival fluid flow and the SBI. From the epidemiologic viewpoint, it is better to measure single elements than to measure a combination of several. The MGI illustrated how the signs of inflammation and bleeding in the GI were separated.

Several other indices are worthy of mention. The Bleeding Points Index was developed to assess a patient's oral hygiene performance. It determines the presence or absence of gingival bleeding interproximally and on the facial and lingual surface of each tooth. A periodontal probe is drawn horizontally through the gingival crevice of a quadrant, and the gingiva is examined for bleeding after 30 s.

The Gingival Bleeding Index also assesses the presence or absence of gingival bleeding, but only at the interproximal spaces and using unwaxed dental floss. The floss is thought to assess a larger area more quickly than a periodontal probe, and it can be used by both the professional and the patient when the latter is instructed to perform self-evaluation in control program.

The Interdental Bleeding Index, also referred to as the Eastman Interdental Bleeding Index, utilizes a triangle-shaped toothpick made of soft, pliable wood to stimulate the interproximal gingival tissue. The presence or absence of bleeding with a specific stimulus permits the dentist and, perhaps more important, the patient to monitor interproximal gingival health. The interproximal cleaner is inserted horizontally between the teeth from the facial surface, depressing the interproximal papilla by up to 2 mm. The wooden cleaner is inserted and removed four times, and the presence or absence of bleeding within 15 s is noted. The Interdental Bleeding Index score is determined by dividing the number of bleeding sites by the number of sites evaluated.

The Gingival Bleeding Index (GBI) of Ainamo and Bay was developed as an easy and suitable way for the practitioner to assess a patient's progress in plaque control. The presence or absence of gingival bleeding is determined by gentle probing of the gingival crevice with a periodontal probe. The appearance of bleeding within 10 s indicates a positive score, which is expressed as a percentage of the total number of gingival margins examined.

Gingival Index Used by the National Institute of Dental Research

The dichotomous criteria used by the National Institute of Dental Research (NIDR) to assess gingival inflammation (Table 6.4) are the presence or absence of bleeding. Two sites per tooth (mesial-buccal interproximal and mid-buccal on all teeth *excluding* the molars; and mesial-buccal interproximal and mid-buccal of the

TABLE 6.4 Criteria Used by the NIDR to Assess Gingival Inflammation and Calculus

Gingival Inflammation (Bleeding Index)

0 = No bleeding present

1 = Bleeding results after probe is placed in gingival sulcus up to 2 mm and drawn along the inner surface of the gingival sulcus

Calculus Assessment (Calculus Index)

0 = Calculus is absent

1 = Supragingival calculus,[a] but no subgingival calculus is present

2 = Supragingival and subgingival calculus, or subgingival calculus only is present

[a]Supragingival calculus includes calculus located on the exposed crown and root of the tooth and extending to 1 mm below the free gingival margin.

mesial root of molars) on one-half of the maxillary arch and the contralateral half of the mandibular arch are assessed after excess moisture is dried with air. The decision of starting at either the right or left half of the maxillary arch is decided randomly. The NIDR probe (a periodontal probe that is graduated in 2-mm increments, with alternating increments colored in yellow) is gently inserted up to 2 mm into the gingival sulcus at the midpoint of the buccal and then drawn gently into the mesial-buccal interproximal area. After all the sites in both halves of the arches are probed (i.e., the gingival sulcus is palpated), the bleeding sites are counted. This number is divided by the total number of sites assessed and then multiplied by 100 to yield the percentage of sites with gingival bleeding.

In conclusion, the use of gingival bleeding indices is desirable because bleeding is a more objective indicator than early gingival color changes and provides evidence of recent plaque exposure. In general, the indices that utilize apical probing (i.e., probing to the bottom of the gingival sulcus or pocket) (Palpation refers to the gentle touching of the surface gingival tissue with the blunt end of a periodontal probe and/or the gentle sweeping of the probe in a horizontal direction along the inner surface of the gingival sulcus *without* apical pressure.), however, are more suitable for diagnosing periodontitis and for assessing the effects of subgingival pocket therapy.

Indices Used to Measure Periodontal Destruction

The destruction of bone is still the most important criterion for assessing the severity of periodontal disease. Some of the approaches to measuring bone loss that are discussed are gingival crevice measurements, radiographic evaluations of bone loss, and assessments of gingival recession and tooth mobility.

Gingival Sulcus Measurement Component of the PDI

The technique developed by Ramfjord for determining gingival sulcus depth with a calibrated periodontal probe involves measuring the distance from the cement-enamel junction to the free gingival margin and the distance from the free gingival margin to the bottom of the gingival sulcus or pocket. The difference between the two measurements yields the clinical attachment level. This is considered the most important clinical measurement (i.e., the "gold standard") in determining the status of the periodontium. Ramfjord technique is considered useful in epidemiologic surveys, longitudinal studies of periodontal disease, and clinical trials of preventive and therapeutic agents.

The first measurement in this two-step process may be used in assessing gingival loss (recession) or gain. It is considered more accurate and reliable in clinical trials than the Gingival Recession Index used in epidemiologic surveys.

The criteria developed by Ramfjord for making sulcus depth determinations are shown in Table 6.2. The Ramfjord criteria are most applicable to longitudinal studies of periodontal disease and clinical trials of preventive or therapeutic agents. Either the six teeth used by Ramfjord (teeth) (teeth 16, 21, 24, 36, 41, and 44) or other teeth appropriate to the objective of the study may be assessed. Quadrants of teeth or all teeth should be considered in longitudinal studies.

In an epidemiologic survey (e.g., a cross-sectional survey) in which the purpose is to determine the prevalence of total periodontal disease, only the six index teeth should be used. The set of criteria for a cross-sectional survey is the PDI (see Table 6.2). The PDI score for the individual is obtained by totaling the scores of the teeth and dividing by the number of teeth examined (a maximum of six).

Extent and Severity Index

The Extent and Severity Index (ESI) was developed because of a lack of satisfaction with pervious indices of periodontal disease and because of the emergence of a newer conceptual model of periodontal disease pathogenesis developed by Socransky and coworkers. The older model, the PI, was based on the concept of periodontal disease as a slowly progressing, continuous disease process; it dealt with gingivitis as part of the biological gradient that extended from health to advanced periodontal disease. In the newer model, periodontal disease is viewed as a chronic process with intermittent periods of activity and remission that affects individual teeth and sites around teeth at different rates within the same mouth. Unlike the PI, which uses a mouth mirror only, the ESI uses a periodontal probe (the NIDR periodontal probe) to determine attachment levels.

The ESI score is a bivariate statistic. It expresses the percentage of sites that exhibit disease (E for Extent) and measures mean attachment loss in millimeters (S for Severity). Hence the ESI = (E, S). Disease is defined arbitrarily as any site with more than 1 mm of attachment loss. Unlike the PI, which examines the tissues surrounding all teeth present, the ESI is based on probe measurements (at the mesiobuccal interproximal and mid-buccal locations on all teeth *excluding* molars and at the mesiobuccal interproximal and mid-buccal of the mesial root of molars) at 14 sites in half of the maxillary arch and at 14 sites in the contralateral mandibular arch. The decision to start at either the right or left half of the maxillary arch is made randomly. Attachment level measurements are made using the criteria of Ramfjord (see Table 6.2). Carlos and coworkers found that interexaminer agreement on site scores was within 1 mm more than 95% of the time. Unlike the PI or PDI, the ESI describes the distribution (extent) of disease. Currently, the NIDR diagnostic criterion includes the methodology of the ESI but has modified the definition of disease to be more than 3 mm of attachment loss.

Radiographic Approaches to Measuring Bone Loss

In general, the use of radiographs in the study of the epidemiology of periodontal disease would appear to overcome some of the criticisms of the more subjective clinical measurements. Radiographs present a permanent objective record of interdental bone levels; in longitudinal studies, they may ensure less variability than poorly standardized evaluations by dental examiners, and they offer the only method available for making crown and root measurements. Their disadvantages are that they are not useful in the buccal or lingual assessment of bone level, they do not provide adequate information on soft tissue attachment, and their value may be lost if improper angulation is used. Furthermore, obtaining radiographs of survey participants, without the intent of providing treatment if needed, is unethical.

Only a few indices have been specifically designed to evaluate the radiographic assessment of periodontal disease, but other more precise techniques for making reasonably accurate measurements from radiographs have been developed.

Of historical interest are indices developed by Dunning and Leach (the Gingival–Bone Count Index), which records the gingival condition on a scale of 0–3 and the level of the crest of the alveolar bone, and a similar index by Sheiham and Striffer. The strength of each of these radiographic indices is in epidemiologic surveys in which evaluation time is limited because of large study populations.

The Periodontitis Severity Index (PSI) assesses the presence or absence of periodontitis as the product of clinical inflammation (CIS) and interproximal bone loss (BLS) determined radiographically using a modified Schei ruler. Due to the need for periapical radiographs, the PSI is limited to longitudinal studies and lacks validation.

Indices Used to Measure Plaque Accumulation

In general, most of the indices used to measure plaque accumulation utilize a numerical scale to measure the extent of the surface area of a tooth covered by plaque. For these purposes, plaque is defined as a soft, nonmineralized tooth deposit, which includes debris and materia alba.

Plaque Component of the PDI

The first index that attempted to use a numerical scale to assess the extent of plaque covering the surface area of a tooth was developed by Ramfjord. The plaque component of the PDI is used on the six teeth selected by Ramfjord (teeth #3, 9, 12, 19, 25, and 28) (teeth 16, 21, 24, 36, 41, and 46) after staining with Bismarck brown solution. The criteria measure the presence and extent of plaque on a scale of 0–3, looking specifically at all interproximal facial and lingual surfaces of the index teeth. The criteria are suitable for longitudinal studies of periodontal disease. Even though the plaque component is not a part of the PDI score, it is helpful in a total assessment of periodontal status.

Shick and Ash modified the original criteria of Ramfjord by excluding consideration of the interproximal areas of the teeth and "restricting the scoring of plaque to the gingival half" of the facial and lingual surfaces of the index teeth. The criteria for the Shick–Ash modification of the Ramfjord plaque criteria are shown in Table 6.2.

The plaque score per person is obtained by totaling all of the individual tooth scores and dividing by the number of teeth examined. These modified plaque criteria are suitable for clinical trials of preventive or therapeutic agents.

Simplified Oral Hygiene Index

Greene and Vermillion developed the Oral Hygiene Index (OHI) in 1960 and later simplified it to include only six tooth surfaces that were representative of all anterior and posterior segments of the mouth. This modification was called the Simplified OHI (OHI-S). The OHI-S measures the surface area of the tooth that is covered by debris and calculus. The imprecise term *debris* was used because it was not practical to distinguish among plaque, debris, and materia alba. In addition, the practicality of determining the weight and thickness of the soft deposits prompted the assumption that the dirtier the mouth is, the greater is the tooth surface area covered by debris. This assumption also implied a time factor, because the longer oral hygiene practices are neglected, the greater the likelihood that the surface area of the tooth will be covered by debris.

The OHI-S consists of two components: a Simplified Debris Index (DI-S) and a Simplified Calculus Index (CI-S). Each component is assessed on a scale of 0–3. Only a mouth mirror and a shepherd crook or sickle-type dental explorer and no disclosing agent are used for the examination. The six teeth surfaces examined in the OHI-S are the facial surfaces of teeth # 16, 11, 26, and 31 and the lingual surfaces of teeth # 36 and 46.

TABLE 6.5 Criteria for Scoring the Oral Debris (DI-S) and Calculus (CI-S) Components of the Simplified Oral Hygiene Index (OHI-S)

Score	Criteria
Oral Debris Index (DI-S)	
0	No debris or stain present
1	Soft debris covering not more than one-third of the tooth surface or the presence of extrinsic stains without other debris, regardless of surface area covered
2	Soft debris covering more than one-third but not more than two-thirds of the exposed tooth surface
3	Soft debris covering more than two-thirds of the exposed tooth surface
Calculus Index (CI-S)	
0	No calculus present
1	Supragingival calculus covering not more than one-third of the exposed tooth surface
2	Supragingival calculus covering more than one-third but not more than two-thirds of the exposed tooth surface or the presence of individual flecks of subgingival calculus around the cervical portion of the tooth, or both
3	Supragingival calculus covering more than two-thirds of the exposed tooth surface or a continuous heavy band of subgingival calculus around the cervical portion of the tooth, or both

Each tooth surface is divided horizontally into gingival, middle, and incisal thirds. For the DI-S, a dental explorer is placed on the incisal third of the tooth and moved toward the gingival third according to the criteria in Table 6.5. The DI-S score per person is obtained by totaling the debris score per tooth surface and dividing by the number of surfaces examined.

The CI-S assessment is performed by gently placing a dental explorer into the distal gingival crevice and drawing the explorer into the distal gingival crevice and drawing it subgingivally from the distal contact area to the mesial contact area (one-half of a tooth's circumference is considered a scoring unit). The criteria for scoring the calculus component of the OHI-S are given in Table 6.5. The CI-S score per person is obtained by totaling the calculus scores per tooth surface and dividing by the number of surfaces examined. The OHI-S score per person is the total of the DI-S and CI-S scores per person.

The clinical levels of oral cleanliness for debris that can be associated with group DI-S scores are as follows:

Good 0.0–0.6
Fair 0.7–1.8
Poor 1.9–3.0

The clinical levels of oral hygiene that can be associated with group OHI-S scores are as follows:

Good 0.0–1.2
Fair 1.3–3.0
Poor 3.1–6.0

The importance of the OHI-S is that, like the PI of Russell, it has been used extensively throughout the world and has contributed greatly to the understanding of periodontal disease. It was also used in the Ten-State Nutrition Survey 1 NHS, NHANES I, and HHANES. The high degree of correlation ($r = 0.82$) between the OHI-S and tin PI makes it possible, if one of the two scores is known, to calculate the other score with regression analysis. The major strength of the OHI-S is its use in epidemiologic surveys and

TABLE 6.6 Turesky–Gilmore–Glickman Modification of the Quigley–Hein Plaque Index

0	= No plaque
1	= Separate flecks of plaque at the cervical margin of the tooth
2	= A thin continuous band of plaque (up to 1 mm) at the cervical margin
3	= A band of plaque wider than 1 mm but covering less than one-third of the crown
4	= Plaque covering at least one-third but less than two-thirds of the crown
5	= Plaque covering two-thirds or more of the crown

in evaluation of dental health education programs (longitudinal studies). It can also evaluate an individual's level of oral cleanliness and can, to a more limited extent, be used in clinical trials. The index is easy to use because the criteria are objective, the examination may be performed quickly, and a high level of reproducibility is possible with a minimum of training sessions.

Turesky–Gilmore–Glickman Modification of the Quigley–Hein Plaque Index

In 1962, Quigley and Hein reported a plaque measurement that focused on the gingival third of the tooth surface. They examined only the facial surfaces of the anterior teeth, using a basic fuchsin mouthwash as a disclosing agent and a numerical scoring system of 0–5. Turesky and coworkers strengthened the objectivity of the Quigley–Hein criteria by redefining the scores of the gingival third area. The Turesky–Gilmore–Glickman modification of the Quigley–Hein criteria appears in Table 6.6. Plaque was assessed on the facial and lingual surfaces of all of the teeth after using a disclosing agent. A plaque score per person was obtained by totaling all of the plaque scores and dividing by the number of surfaces examined. This system of scoring plaque is relatively easy to use because of the objective definitions of each numerical score. The strength of this plaque index is its application to longitudinal studies and clinical trials of preventive and therapeutic agents. The Turesky–Gilmore–Glickman modification of the Quigley–Hein criteria is considered one of the two indices of choice when assessing plaque in clinical trials.

Plaque Index

The Plaque Index (PII) is unique among the indices described so far because it ignores the coronal extent of plaque on the tooth surface area and assesses only the thickness of plaque at the gingival area of the tooth. Since it was developed as a component to parallel the GI of Löe and Silness, it examines the same scoring units of the teeth: distofacial, facial, mesiofacial, and lingual surfaces. A mouth mirror and a dental explorer are used after air drying of the teeth to assess plaque. Unlike most indices, the PII does not exclude or substitute for teeth with gingival restorations or crowns. Either all or only selected teeth may be used in the PII. The criteria for the PII of Silness and Löe are given in Table 6.3.

The PII score for the area is obtained by totaling the four plaque scores per tooth. If the sum of the PII scores per tooth is divided by four, the PII score for the tooth is obtained. The PII score per person is obtained by adding the PII scores per tooth and dividing by the number of teeth examined. The PII may be obtained for a segment of the mouth or a group of teeth in a similar manner.

The strength of the PII is in its application to longitudinal studies and clinical trials. In spite of the studies that have been conducted to ensure the reliability of PII data, the assessment of plaque thickness is so subjective that obtaining valid data requires highly trained and experienced examiners.

Other Plaque Indices

The Modified Navy Plaque Index records the presence or absence of plaque with a score of 1 or 0, respectively, on nine areas of each tooth surface of the six index teeth used by Ramfjord like the Patient Hygiene Performance (PHP) Index of Podshadley and Haley, the Modified Navy Plaque Index is of value in assessing health education programs and the ability of individuals to perform oral hygiene practices.

A variation of the Modified Navy Plaque Index is the Distal Mesial Plaque Index (DMPI), which places more emphasis on the gingival and interproximal areas of a tooth. Plaque is one of the two factors measured in the Irritants Index, which is a component of the Gingival Periodontal Index (GPI) of O'Leary and coworkers. The presence and coronal extent of plaque are scored on a scale of 0–3. Other factors that contribute to the Irritants Index are supragingival and subgingival calculus and subgingival irritants, such as overhanging or deficient restorations.

PHP Index

Patient Hygiene Performance index (PHP) by Podshadley and Haley was the first index developed for the sole purpose of assessing an individual's performance in removing debris after toothbrushing instruction. It records the presence or absence of debris as 1 or 0, respectively, using the six surface of the six OHI-S teeth. The PHP Index is more sensitive than the OHI-S because it divides each tooth surface into five areas: three longitudinal thirds, with the middle third subdivided horizontally into thirds. Scoring is preceded by the use of a disclosing agent. The index is easy to use because its criteria are dichotomous and it can be performed quickly. Its value lies chiefly in its application to individual patient education.

Two other indices with a similar purpose that also use dichotomous criteria are the Plaque Control Record and the plaque portion of the Bleeding Points Index.

Bjorby and Löe developed a Retention Index that not only examined supragingival and subgingival calculus but also grossly assessed dental caries and the quality of the margins of restorations. Collectively, all of these variables were scored on a numerical scale of 0–3.

Indices Used to Measure Calculus

In general, the indices used to assess calculus may be conveniently divided into those that are most appropriate to epidemiologic surveys; those that are appropriate to longitudinal studies, with an examination every 3–6 months; and those that are used in short-term clinical studies, usually no longer than 6 weeks.

Calculus Component of the Simplified Oral Hygiene Index

The Simplified Calculus Index (CI-S) component of the OHI-S was previously discussed with indices used to measure plaque accumulation because it is less separable from the combined scoring system than are any of the other indices that include several component measures. The value of the CI-S component is its application to epidemiologic surveys and longitudinal studies of periodontal disease. Table 6.5 presents the specific criteria of the OHI-S used to assess calculus.

Calculus Component of the Periodontal Disease Index

The calculus component of the PDI assesses the presence and extent of calculus on the facial and lingual surfaces of Ramfjord's six index teeth (i.e., teeth #16, 21, 36, 41, 44, and 46) on a numerical scale of 0–3. A mouth mirror and a dental explorer and/or a periodontal probe are used in the examination. The criteria for assigning a score to each tooth surface for the calculus component of the PDI are given in Table 6.2.

The calculus scores per tooth are totaled and then divided by the number of teeth examined to yield the calculus score per person. Like the CI-S of the OHI-S, the calculus component of the PDI has a high degree of examiner reproducibility, can be performed quickly, and has its best application in epidemiologic surveys and longitudinal studies.

Probe Method of Calculus Assessment

The Probe Method of Calculus Assessment was developed for longitudinal studies of the quantity of supragingival calculus formed. A periodontal probe graduated in millimeter divisions is used to measure the deposits of calculus on the lingual surfaces of the six mandibular anterior teeth. The Probe Method of Calculus Assessment has been shown to possess a high degree of inter- and intraexaminer reproducibility. However, extensive training under an experienced investigator is required to master it.

Calculus Surface Index

The Calculus Surface Index (CSI) is one of two indices that are used in short-term (e.g., less than 6 weeks) clinical trials of calculus-inhibiting agents. The objective of this type of study is to determine rapidly whether a specific agent has any effect on reducing or preventing supragingival or subgingival calculus. The CSI assesses the presence or absence of supragingival and/or subgingival calculus on the four mandibular incisors. The index has also been applied to the six mandibular anterior teeth. The presence or absence of calculus is determined by visual examination or by tactile examination using a mouth mirror and a sickle-type dental explorer.

A companion index to the CSI is the Calculus Surface Severity Index (CSSI). The CSSI measures the quantity of calculus present on the surfaces examined for the CSI.

Marginal Line Calculus Index

A second index that is frequently used in short-term clinical trials of anticalculus agents is the Marginal Line Calculus Index (MLCI). This index was developed to assess the accumulation of supragingival calculus on the gingival third of the tooth or, more specifically, supragingival calculus along the margin of the gingiva.

Calculus Index Used by NIDR

The NIDR uses a three-point ordinal scale for the assessment of calculus (see Table 6.4). Unlike the NIDR gingival assessment, the Calculus Index assigns only one score per tooth, after examining both the mid-buccal and mesial-bussal interproximal sites, on one-half of the maxillary and one-half of the contralateral mandibular arch. As in the gingival assessment, the decision to start at either the right or left half of the maxillary is made randomly. Both sites are examined for the presence and extent of calculus (with either the NIDR periodontal probe or a no. 17 dental explorer) after all of the teeth in one-half of an arch are air dried. The Calculus index score is obtained by dividing the score for each tooth by the number of teeth examined.

Indices Used to Assess Treatment Needs

Interpretations of the indices described in this section are to be viewed with caution because of the difficulty that exists concerning the estimation of treatment need. Without knowing the response of the periodontal tissues to phase 1 or initial therapy, any estimate of treatment needs may be subject to over- or underestimation of what is clinically prudent.

GPI

The GPI is a modification of the PDI of Ramfjord for the purpose of screening persons to determine who needs periodontal treatment. The GPI assesses three components of periodontal disease: gingival status, periodontal status (crevice depth); and, collectively materia alba, calculus, and overhanging restorations. The latter triad is independently called the Irritation Index. Only the criteria for the gingival status component are described.

The maxillary and mandibular arches are each divided into three segments: the six anterior teeth, the left posterior teeth, and the right posterior teeth. The primary objective in using the index is to determine the tooth or surrounding tissues with the severest condition within each of the six segments. Each segment is assessed for each of the three components of periodontal disease described previously. The specific criteria for the gingival status component of the GPI are as follows:

0 = tissue tightly adapted to the teeth; firm consistency with physiologic architecture.
1 = slight to moderate inflammation, as indicated by changes in color and consistency, involving one or more teeth in the same segment but not completely surrounding any one tooth.
2 = the aforementioned changes either singly or combined completely encircling one or more teeth in a segment.
3 = marked inflammation, as indicated by loss of surface continuity (ulceration), spontaneous hemorrhage, loss of faciolingual continuity or any interdental papilla, marked deviation from normal contour (such as gross thickening or enlargement covering more than one-third of the anatomic crown), recession, and clefts.

The area with the highest score determines the gingival score for the entire segment, and the gingival status for the mouth is obtained by dividing the sum of the gingival scores by the number of segments.

The GPI has been used extensively in military populations. Unlike the traditional indices used in epidemiology (which attempt primarily to assess the status of a specific disease condition, with only the crudest suggestion of determining treatment needs), the GPI was developed for the specific purpose of detecting periodontal disease early so that treatment may be instituted promptly.

Periodontal Treatment Need System

The next index to evolve with the purpose of assessing treatment needs was the Periodontal Treatment Need System (PTNS), which has been used with interesting results. It attempts to place individuals into one of four classes based on treatment procedures relative to time requirements. It considers the presence or absence of gingivitis and plaque and the presence of pockets 5 mm or deeper in each quadrant of the mouth, as shown in Table 6.7.

Community Periodontal Index of Treatment Needs

In 1977, the WHO appointed an expert committee to review the methods available to review periodontal status and treatment needs. The index that resulted after extensive field testing by investigators from the WHO and the International Dental Federation (FDI) was called the *Community Periodontal Index of Treatment Needs* (CPITN). The CPITN was "primarily designed: assess periodontal treatment needs rather than pet status." Combining elements of the GPI and PTNS CPITN assesses the presence or absence of gingival bleeding on gentle probing; the presence or absence of supragingival or subgingival calculus; and the presence or absence of periodontal pockets, subdivided into shallow and deep. A specially designed periodontal probe with a 0.5-mm ball tip and gradations corresponding to shallow and deep pocket was developed to probe for bleeding and calculus and to determine

TABLE 6.7 Criteria for the Periodontal Treatment Need System (PTNS) Classification

PTNS Classification	Unit	Plaque	Calculus and/or Overhangs	Inflammation	Pocket Depth
Class 0	Mouth	No	No	No	Not considered
Class A	Mouth	Yes	No	Yes	≤5 mm
Class B	Quadrant	Yes	Yes	Yes	<5 mm
Class C	Quadrant	Yes	Yes	Yes	>5 mm

(Adapted from Johansen JR, Gjermo P, Bellini HT: A system to classify the need for periodontal treatment. *Acta Odontol Scand* 31: 297, 1973, by permission of Scandinavian University Press.)

pocket depth. In epidemiologic surveys, 10 index teeth are examined, but only the worst finding from the index teeth is recorded of individual patients, only the worst finding from all of the teeth in a sextant is recorded, resulting in six scores. The CPITN criteria for determining periodontal status and the corresponding treatment needs to appear in Table 6.8. Each subject or sextant of teeth is classified according to one of the treatment needs.

The value of the CPITN is that it permits rapid examination of a population to determine periodontal treatment needs. However, a lot of effort is expended and a great deal of useful information is lost when only the worst score per sextant is recorded.

Community Periodontal Index

This index is a modification of the CPITN. The modification is done by the inclusion of measurement of "loss of attachment" and elimination of the "treatment needs" category. A mouth mirror along with Community Periodontal Index (CPI) probe (WHO probe) is used for the recording.

Selection of Teeth

Teeth are selected as:

- Index teeth (up to 19 years)—16, 11, 26, 36, 31, 46.
- Index teeth (aged 20 years or more)—17, 16, 11, 26, 27, 37, 36, 31, 46, 47.

Loss of Attachment

Information on loss of attachment may be collected from index teeth. The most reliable way of examining loss of attachment in each sextant is to record this immediately after recording the CPI score for that particular sextant. The highest scores for CPI and loss of attachment may not necessarily be found on the same tooth in a sextant.

Loss of attachment should not be recorded for children under the age of 15.

When the CEJ is not visible and the highest CPI score for a sextant is less than 4 (probing depth less than 6 mm), any loss of attachment for that sextant is estimated to be less than 4 mm (loss of attachment score = 0). The extent of loss of attachment is recorded using the following codes (Table 6.9).

To ensure the reliability of periodontal indices, all studies should incorporate measures of reliability into the study design. Since there is no agreement as to the best statistical method for describing reliability, several methods should be used.

TABLE 6.8 Criteria for the Community Periodontal Index of Treatment Needs

Periodontal Status	Treatment Needs
0 = Healthy periodontium	0 = No treatment needed
1 = Bleeding observed, directly or by using mouth mirror, after sensing	I = Oral hygiene needs improvement II = I + professional scaling
2 = Calculus felt during probing, but the entire black area[a] of the probe is visible	II = I + profession scaling III = I + II + complex treatment[b]
3 = Pocket 4 or 5 mm (giving margin is situated on black area[a] of probe)	
4 = Pocket >6 mm (black area[a] of probe not visible)	

[a]Portion of probe between 3.5 and 5.5 mm.
[b]Complex treatment may require scaling and root planning under local anesthesia, with or without surgical exposure for access.

TABLE 6.9 Codes and Criteria for Community Periodontal Index

Code	Criteria for Periodontal Status	Code	Criteria for Loss of Attachment
0	Healthy	0	Loss of attachment 0–3 mm (CEJ not visible and CPI score 0–3)
1	Bleeding observed, directly or by using a mouth mirror, after probing	1	Loss of attachment 4–5 mm (CEJ within the black band)
2	Calculus detected during probing, but all of the black band on the probe visible	2	Loss of attachment 6–8 mm (CEJ between the upper limit of the black band and the 8.5 mm ring)
3	Pocket 4–5 mm (gingival margin within the black band on the probe)	3	Loss of attachment 9–11 mm (CEJ between the 8.5 and 11.5 mm rings)
4	Pocket 6 mm or more (black band on the probe not visible)	4	Loss of attachment 12 mm or more
X	Excluded sextant (less than two teeth present)	X	Excluded sextant (<2 teeth)
9	Not recorded	9	Not recorded (CEJ neither visible nor detectable)

TABLE 6.10 Studies on Prevalence of Periodontal Diseases in India

Author	Year	Place	Observation	Conclusion
Marshall-Day and Shourie	1949	Punjab Province	568 people from 9 to 60 years of age	Periodontosis present in about 35% of the cases.
Mehta et al	1953	Bombay and Ratnagiri district	2219 male subjects of low socioeconomic level in the age group 19–55 years	Periodontal disease is very high among this population.
Sanjana MK and Mehta FS	1956	Bombay	Residents including 1445 population in age group of 16–50 years	83.2% generalized periodontal disease.
S. Ramfjord	1957–1963	Bombay and Bassein (present "Vasai") region	1677 urban and rural population using Ramfjord periodontal disease index	Prevalence of periodontal disease was close to 100% and starts after age 15; and at 17 years, 10% of Indian boys had periodontitis.
Greene JC	1960	Bombay and Bassein (Vasai) region	1676 urban plus rural population using Russells' periodontal index	97% of the 11- to 17-year-old persons examined, had high prevalence of periodontal disease.
S. Rao and S. Tewani	1968	Bombay	1200 males and females	6.83% population were suffering from periodontosis.
Anil S and Hari S	1990	Trivandrum (Kerala)	2756 subjects	36% population was having periodontal disease.
Mathur B and Talwar as a part of National Oral Health Survey aided by Dental Council of India, New Delhi	2002–2003	A three-stage sampling design was adopted to select 210 rural and 110 urban subjects in each of the age groups, viz., 5, 12, 15, 35–44, 65–74 years, from each homogeneous region comprising of a number of districts of each state and on the basis of geographical factors used by the Planning Commission. CPI index was used for disease assessment.		The prevalence reported was 57%, 67.7%, 89.6%, and 79.9% in the age groups 12, 15, 35–44, and 65–74 years, respectively.
Shah N et al, A multicentric study under the Directorate General of Health and as a collaborative program between World Health Organization and Ministry of Health and Family Welfare, Government of India.	2005	3200 samples of age group 12, 15, 35–44 and 65–74 years from total of 22,400 persons in rural and urban areas of the selected districts of Arunachal Pradesh, Delhi, Maharashtra, Puducherry, Rajasthan, Orissa, and Uttar Pradesh.	The highest prevalence in 65–74 years group was recorded in Maharashtra (96%), followed by Orissa (90%), Delhi (85.5%), Rajasthan (75%), Uttar Pradesh (68%), and Puducherry (55%)	

Prevalence of Periodontal Diseases in India

The studies on the prevalence of periodontal disease in different populations are useful for not only determining the extent and severity of the disease but also describing the rate of progression of the underlying condition and identifying the possible etiological factors of the disease.

A number of epidemiological studies were performed in the 1950s in India to assess periodontal disease in different parts of the subcontinent (Table 6.10). The earliest epidemiological study was by Marshall Day in 1941. It was also found that no prevalence studies have been carried out in few North and North Eastern states and Union Territories of India. Due to nonavailability of same age groups in selected studies an overall prevalence rate may be difficult to interpret. However, it was observed that few areas of states In North India have reported a prevalence rate of periodontal disease of more than 85% in their general population.

Suggested Readings

Burt BA, Eklund SA: *Dentistry, dental practice and the community*, ed 6, Philadelphia, 2005, Elsevier.

Carter HG, Barnes GP: The gingival bleeding index, *J Periodontol* 45:801, 1974.

Loe H, Silness P: Periodontal disease in pregnancy, *Acta Odontol Scand* 21: 533, 1963.

Loe H: The gingival index the plaque index and the retention index systems, *J Periodontol* 38:610–616, 1967.

Massler M: The P-M-A index for assessment of ginigivitis, *J Periodontol* 38: 592, 1967.
Muhlemann HR, Son S: Gingival sulcus bleeding—a leading symptom in initial gingivitis, *Helvetia Odontologica Acta* 15: 107, 1971.
Ramfjord SP: The periodontal disease index, *J Periodontol* 38: 602, 1967.
Turesky S, Gilmore ND, Glickman I: Reduced plaque formation by the chloromethyl analogue of Vitamin C, *J Periodontol* 41: 41–43, 1970.
Volpe AR: Indices for measurement of hard deposits in clinical studies of oral hygiene and periodontal disease, *J Periodontal Res* 9 (Suppl 14): 31, 1974.
World Health Organization: *Oral health surveys, Basic methods*, ed 4, Gerneva, 1997, WHO.

References

References and MCQs with answers for the chapter are available on www.medenact.com.

CHAPTER 7

Periodontal Disease Pathogenesis

PM Preshaw | Kai Soo Tan | N Ambalavanan

CHAPTER OUTLINE

Periodontal disease is complex in nature. It is a multifactorial disease, which is largely influenced by genetic, environmental, and microbial factors. Pathogenesis is defined as "the origination and development of a disease." Knowledge of pathogenesis helps us to understand about the processes that lead to the development of this disease and consequently the changes it produces in the structure and function of the periodontium. In broad terms, the pathogenesis of a disease is the mechanism by which a causative factor or factors cause the disease.

Periodontal disease results from a complex interplay between the subgingival biofilm and the host immune–inflammatory events that develop in the gingival and periodontal tissues in response to the challenge presented by the bacteria. The tissue damage that results from the immune–inflammatory response is recognized clinically as periodontitis. Gingivitis precedes periodontitis, but it is clear that not all cases of gingivitis progress to periodontitis. In gingivitis, the inflammatory lesion is confined to the gingiva; however, with periodontitis, the inflammatory processes extend to additionally affect the periodontal ligament and the alveolar bone. The net result of these inflammatory changes is the breakdown of the fibers of the periodontal ligament, resulting in clinical loss of attachment together with resorption of the alveolar bone.

Periodontal disease is therefore a unique clinical entity. It is not an infection in the classic sense of the word. With many infections, a single infective organism causes the disease (e.g., human immunodeficiency virus, syphilis, tuberculosis), and the identification of that organism can provide the basis for the diagnosis. With periodontal disease, many species are identifiable in the periodontal pocket, and it is impossible to conclude that a single species or even a group of species causes periodontal disease. Many of the species that are considered important in periodontal pathogenesis may predominate in deep pockets because the pocket is a favorable environment in which they can survive (i.e., it is warm, moist, and anaerobic, with a ready supply of nutrients). Many of the unique features of periodontitis are derived from the anatomy of the periodontium, in which a hard, nonshedding surface (the tooth) is partly embedded within the body (within connective tissue), crosses an epithelial surface, and is partly exposed to the outside world (within the confines of the mouth). The bacteria that colonize this surface are effectively outside of the body (although they are in the gingival crevice or pocket), yet the inflammatory response that develops is located within the body (i.e., within the tissues). These factors add complexity to our understanding of the role of the biofilm and the immune–inflammatory responses that are part of periodontal tissue breakdown.

Histopathology of Periodontal Disease

To understand periodontal pathogenesis better, it is important to have an appreciation of the histology of clinically healthy tissues, as well as of inflamed gingival and periodontal tissues. Even gingival tissues that clinically would be considered to be noninflamed and healthy always have evidence of inflammatory responses occurring at the microscopic level. This is normal given the chronic low-grade challenge presented by the subgingival biofilm. The low-grade inflammatory response that results is not detectable macroscopically at the clinical level, but it is an essential protective mechanism for combating the microbial challenge and for preventing bacteria and their products from infiltrating tissues and causing tissue damage. In clinically healthy tissues, this steady-state equilibrium between low-grade inflammation in the tissues and the continual presence of the bacterial biofilm may persist for many years or indeed for the lifetime of the individual. Overt clinical signs of gingivitis (i.e., redness, swelling, and bleeding on probing) do not develop because of several innate and structural defense mechanisms, including the following:

- The maintenance of an intact epithelial barrier (the junctional and sulcular epithelium).
- The outflow of GCF from the sulcus (dilution effect and flushing action).
- The sloughing of surface epithelial cells of the junctional and sulcular epithelium.
- The presence of neutrophils and macrophages in the sulcus that phagocytose bacteria.
- The presence of antibodies in the GCF.

Our current understanding of susceptibility to periodontitis suggests that individuals who are susceptible to the disease mount an excessive or dysregulated immune–inflammatory response for a given bacterial challenge that leads to increased tissue breakdown as compared to those individuals who have a more normal inflammatory response.

(For a more complete understanding of Histopathology of Gingivitis and Periodontitis refer to Chapter 12 on Gingival Inflammation.)

Inflammatory Responses in the Periodontium

It is now clear that the great majority of the tissue breakdown in periodontal disease results from the host's inflammatory processes. The bacteria are important because they initiate and perpetuate the inflammation, but they are only directly responsible for a relatively small proportion of the tissue damage that occurs.

The molecules that play a role in the pathogenesis of periodontitis can be broadly divided into two main groups: those derived from the subgingival bacteria (i.e., microbial virulence factors) and those derived from the host immune–inflammatory response. In terms of the relative importance of each, it is clear that most of the tissue breakdown results from the host inflammatory processes.

Microbial Virulence Factors

The subgingival biofilm initiates and perpetuates inflammatory responses in the gingival and periodontal tissues. The subgingival bacteria also contribute directly to tissue damage by the release of noxious substances, but their primary importance in periodontal pathogenesis is that of activating immune–inflammatory responses that, in turn, result in tissue damage, which may well be beneficial to the bacteria located within the periodontal pocket by providing nutrient sources.

Microbial virulence factors that are important in these processes are as follows:

Lipopolysaccharide

Lipopolysaccharides (LPSs) are large molecules composed of a lipid component (lipid A) and a polysaccharide component. They are found in the outer membrane of gram-negative bacteria, they act as endotoxins (LPS is frequently referred to as *endotoxin*), and they elicit strong immune responses in animals. LPSs are highly conserved in gram-negative bacterial species, a finding that reflects their importance in maintaining the structural integrity of the bacterial cells. LPS is of key importance for initiating and sustaining inflammatory responses in the gingival and periodontal tissues (Box 7.1).

Lipoteichoic Acid

Lipoteichoic acid (LTA), a major component of cell walls of gram positive bacteria, also stimulates immune responses, although less potently than LPS. Both LPS and LTA are released from the bacteria present in the biofilm and stimulate inflammatory responses in the tissues, thereby resulting in increased vasodilation and vascular permeability, the recruitment of inflammatory cells by chemotaxis, and the release of proinflammatory mediators by the leukocytes that are recruited to the area.

A component of gram-positive cell walls, lipoteichoic acid, also stimulates immune responses, although less potently than LPS. Lipoteichoic acid signals through TLR-2. Both LPS and lipoteichoic acid are released from the bacteria present in the biofilm and stimulate inflammatory responses in the tissues, thereby resulting in increased vasodilation and vascular permeability, the recruitment of inflammatory cells by chemotaxis, and the release of proinflammatory mediators by the leukocytes that are recruited to the area.

BOX 7.1 Biologic Properties of Lipopolysaccharide

- Located in the outer membrane of gram-negative bacteria.
- Fundamental for maintaining structural integrity of the bacteria.
- Elicits a strong response from animal immune systems.
- Interacts with the CD14/TLR-4/MD-2 receptor complex on immune cells, such as macrophages, monocytes, dendritic cells, and B cells, with resulting release of proinflammatory mediators such as cytokines from these cells.

Exotoxins

Exotoxins are heat-labile proteins secreted by both gram-positive and gram-negative bacteria. In periodontitis, exotoxins produced by bacteria primarily cause cell/tissue destruction or cause dysregulation of host inflammatory immune responses, facilitating the survival of bacteria. Plaque bacteria produce proteases, which are capable of breaking down structural proteins of the periodontium, such as collagen, elastin, and fibronectin. Bacteria produce these proteases to digest proteins and, thereby, provide peptides for bacterial nutrition. Bacterial proteases disrupt host responses, compromise tissue integrity, and facilitate the microbial invasion of the tissues. P. gingivalis produces two classes of cysteine proteases that have been implicated in periodontal pathogenesis. These are known as gingipains, and they can modulate the immune system and disrupt immune–inflammatory responses, thus potentially leading to increased tissue breakdown.

Aggregatibacter actinomycetemcomitans, a gram-negative capnophilic bacterium associated with rapidly progressing forms of periodontitis, produces two exotoxins, namely leukotoxin (Ltx) and cytolethal-distending toxin (Cdt). Ltx specifically targets leukocytes and at the cellular level, triggers the rapid degranulation of lysosomal enzymes of neutrophils, causes apoptosis of T-cells, and stimulates the activation and secretion of the pro-inflammatory cytokines (Box 7.1).

A component of gram-positive cell walls, lipoteichoic acid, also stimulates immune responses, although less potently than LPS. Lipoteichoic acid signals through TLR-2. Both LPS and lipoteichoic acid are released from the bacteria present in the biofilm and stimulate inflammatory responses in the tissues, thereby resulting in increased vasodilation and vascular permeability, the recruitment of inflammatory cells by chemotaxis, and the release of proinflammatory mediators by the leukocytes that are recruited to the area.

Bacterial Enzymes and Noxious Products

Plaque bacteria produce several metabolic waste products that contribute directly to tissue damage. These include noxious agents such as ammonia (NH_3) and hydrogen sulfide (H_2S), as well as short-chain carboxylic acids such as butyric acid and propionic acid. These acids are detectable in GCF and are found in increasing concentrations as the severity of periodontal disease increases. These substances have profound effects on host cells.

Plaque bacteria produce proteases, which are capable of breaking down structural proteins of the periodontium such as collagen, elastin, and fibronectin. Bacteria produce these proteases to digest proteins and thereby provide peptides for bacterial nutrition. Bacterial proteases disrupt host responses, compromise tissue integrity, and facilitate the microbial invasion of the tissues.

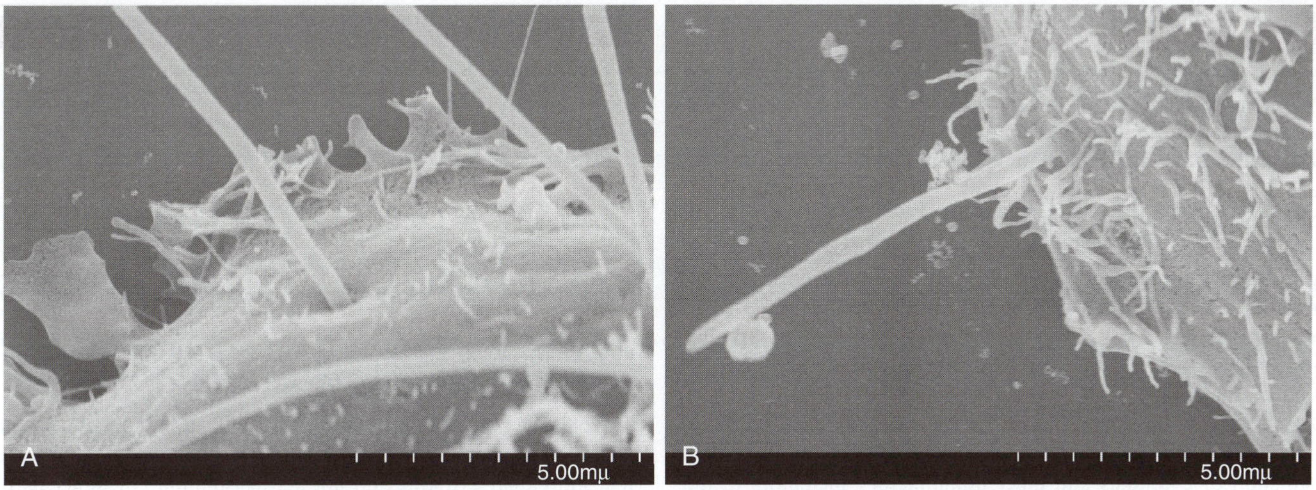

Fig. 7.1 Invasion of epithelial cells by *Fusobacterium nucleatum.* In both images, a single epithelial cell is shown being penetrated by invading *F. nucleatum* bacteria; three or four bacteria are evident in (A), and one bacterium is evident in (B). A, The ruffled surface of the epithelial cells (multiple small fingerlike projections that are much smaller than the *F. nucleatum* bacteria) is likely to be an artifact. B, *F. nucleatum* may facilitate the colonization of epithelial cells by bacteria that are unable to adhere or invade directly as evidenced by the single coccoid bacterium (*Streptococcus cristatus*) that has coaggregated with the *F. nucleatum* bacterium as it penetrates the epithelial cell. *(A and B, Courtesy: Dr. A.E. Edwards, Imperial College, London, UK; Dr. J.D. Rudney, Bath University, Bath, UK; and Dr. T.J. Grossman, the University of Minnesota, Minneapolis, Minn.)*

Microbial Invasion

Microbial invasion of the periodontal tissues has long been a contentious topic. In histologic specimens, bacteria (including cocci, filaments, and rods) have been identified in the intercellular spaces of the epithelium. Periodontal pathogens such as *P. gingivalis* and *Aggregatibacter actinomycetemcomitans* have been reported to invade the gingival tissues, including the connective tissues. *Fusobacterium nucleatum* can invade oral epithelial cells, and bacteria that routinely invade host cells may facilitate the entry of noninvasive bacteria by coaggregating with them (Fig. 7.1). It has also been shown that *A. actinomycetemcomitans* can invade epithelial cells and persist intracellularly. The clinical relevance of these various findings is unclear, however, and more recent studies have reported that although species such as *P. gingivalis* can be found located within the tissues, they are mainly within the epithelium, and it is unusual for the bacteria to reach the connective tissue until extensive tissue destruction has occurred, and even then it is as a result of inflammation rather than "invading" bacteria.

Reports of bacteria present in the tissues have sometimes been used to justify the use of antibiotics for treatment of periodontitis as a means to try to eliminate those organisms that are located in the tissues and that are therefore "protected" from mechanical disruption by root surface debridement. Also the bacteria in the tissues may represent a "reservoir for reinfection after nonsurgical management.

Fimbriae

The fimbriae of certain bacterial species, particularly *P. gingivalis*, may also play a role in periodontal pathogenesis. *P. gingivalis* fimbriae stimulate immune responses, such as IL-6 secretion, leading to sustained inflammation. Bacterial fimbriae are therefore important for modifying and stimulating immune responses in the periodontium.

Bacterial Deoxyribonucleic Acid and Extracellular Deoxyribonucleic Acid

Bacterial DNA stimulates immune cells. Extracellular DNA (eDNA) is a ubiquitous constituent of all biofilms and of particular interest in biofilms associated with chronic diseases, such as periodontitis. eDNA is derived from the genomic DNA of bacteria in biofilms, and the majority of eDNA is released after bacterial cell lysis. However, evidence also indicates that eDNA secretion may occur from bacterial cells by mechanisms that are independent of cell lysis. The presence of naked pieces of DNA extracellularly may be taken up by competent bacteria in plaque biofilm increasing genetic diversity and facilitate the spread of antibiotic resistance genes. More importantly, it is becoming increasingly clear that eDNA plays a number of important roles in biofilm formation and maintenance of structural integrity of the biofilm slime layer on hard and soft tissues in the oral cavity.

Host-Derived Inflammatory Mediators

The inflammatory and immune processes that develop in the periodontal tissues in response to the long-term presence of the subgingival biofilm are protective by intent but can result in considerable tissue damage. This has sometimes been referred to as *bystander damage*, which denotes that the host response is mainly responsible for the tissue damage that occurs, thereby leading to the clinical signs and symptoms of periodontal disease.

Having understood that the majority of the tissue damage in periodontitis is derived from the excessive and dysregulated production of a variety of inflammatory mediators and destructive enzymes in response to the presence of the subgingival plaque bacteria, it is important to review the key types of mediators that orchestrate the host responses. These can be broadly divided into the cytokines, the prostanoids, and the matrix metalloproteinases (MMPs).

Cytokines

Cytokines play a fundamental role in inflammation, and they are key inflammatory mediators in periodontal disease. They are soluble proteins, and they act as messengers to transmit signals from one cell to another. Cytokines are effective in very low concentrations, they are produced transiently in the tissues, and they primarily act locally in the tissues in which they are produced. Cytokines are able to induce their own expression in either an autocrine or paracrine fashion, and they have pleiotropic effects (i.e., multiple biologic activities) on a large number of cell types. (Autocrine signaling means that the autocrine agent [in this case cytokines] binds to receptors on the cell that secreted the agent, whereas paracrine signaling affects other nearby cells.) Simply put, cytokines bind to cell surface receptors and trigger a sequence of intracellular events that lead ultimately to the production of protein by the target cell that alters that cell's behavior and could result in, for example, the increased secretion of more cytokines in a positive feedback loop that leads to inflammation.

Cytokines are produced by a large number of cell types, including infiltrating inflammatory cells (e.g., neutrophils, macrophages, lymphocytes), as well as resident cells in the periodontium (e.g., fibroblasts, epithelial cells). Cytokines signal, broadcast, and amplify immune responses, and they are fundamentally important for regulating immune–inflammatory responses and for combating infections. They have profound biologic effects that also lead to tissue damage with chronic inflammation; the prolonged and excessive production of cytokines and other inflammatory mediators in the periodontium leads to tissue damage that characterizes the clinical signs of the disease. For example, cytokines mediate connective tissue and alveolar bone destruction through the induction of fibroblasts and osteoclasts to produce proteolytic enzymes (i.e., MMPs) that break down structural components of these connective tissues.

Cytokines play a key role at all stages of the immune response in periodontal diseases. Some of the important proinflammatory cytokines are IL-1α, IL-1β, IL-6, and TNF-α. These cytokines play a key role in the initiation, regulation, and perpetuation of innate immune responses in the periodontium, thereby resulting in vascular changes and the migration of effector cells such as neutrophils into the periodontium as part of a normal immune response to the presence of subgingival bacteria (Box 7.2).

BOX 7.2 Properties of Key Types of Inflammatory Mediators in Periodontitis

Cytokines	Proteins that transmit signals from one cell to another. Bind to cell surface receptors to trigger production of protein by the cell. There are proinflammatory and antiinflammatory cytokines. A key proinflammatory cytokine is interleukin-1β, which upregulates inflammatory responses and is produced by multiple cell types in the periodontium.
Prostaglandins	Lipid compounds derived from arachidonic acid. Prostaglandin E_2 (PGE_2) is a key inflammatory mediator, stimulating production of other inflammatory mediators and cytokine production. PGE_2 also stimulates bone resorption and plays a key role in periodontitis progression.
Matrix metalloproteinases (MMPs)	A group of enzymes that break down structural proteins of the body MMPs include collagenases, which break down collagen. Key MMPs in periodontitis include MMP-8 and MMP-9, which are produced by neutrophils as they migrate through the periodontal tissues, thus contributing to periodontal tissue breakdown.

BOX 7.3 Proinflammatory and Antiinflammatory Cytokines

Proinflammatory Cytokines	Antiinflammatory Cytokines
IL-1α, IL-1β	IL-10
IL-6	TGF-β
PGE_2	IL-1Ra
TNF-α	IL-1F5
MMPs	IL-1F10

Antiinflammatory Cytokines

The balance between proinflammatory and antiinflammatory events is crucial for determining disease progression, and it is now clear that individual cytokines do not act in isolation but rather as part of complex networks of mediators that have different functional activities (Box 7.3).

Prostaglandins

The prostaglandins (PGs) are a group of lipid compounds derived from arachidonic acid, a polyunsaturated fatty acid found in the plasma membrane of most cells. Arachidonic acid is metabolized by cyclooxygenase-1 and 2 (COX-1 and COX-2) to generate a series of related compounds called the *prostanoids*, which include the PGs, the thromboxanes, and the prostacyclins. PGs are important mediators of inflammation, particularly prostaglandin E_2 (PGE_2), which results in vasodilation and induces cytokine production by a variety of cell types. COX-2 is upregulated by IL-1β, TNF-α, and bacterial LPS, thus resulting in increased production of PGE_2 in inflamed tissues. PGE_2 is produced by various types of cells and most significantly in the periodontium by macrophages and fibroblasts. PGE_2 results in the induction of MMPs and osteoclastic bone resorption, and it has a major role in contributing to the tissue damage that characterizes periodontitis.

Matrix Metalloproteinases

MMPs are a family of proteolytic enzymes that degrade extracellular matrix molecules such as collagen, gelatin, and elastin. They are produced by a variety of cell types, including neutrophils, macrophages, fibroblasts, epithelial cells, osteoblasts, and osteoclasts. The names and functions of key MMPs are shown in Table 7.1. MMPs can be divided into collagenases, gelatinases/type IV collagenases, stromelysins, matrilysins, membrane-type metalloproteinases, and others.

Key inhibitors of MMPs found in the serum include the glycoprotein α_1-antitrypsin and α_2-macroglobulin, a large plasma protein produced by the liver that is capable of inactivating a wide variety of proteinases. Inhibitors of MMPs that are found in the tissues include the tissue inhibitors of metalloproteinases (TIMPs), which are produced by many cell types; the most important in periodontal disease is TIMP-1.

MMPs are also inhibited by the tetracycline class of antibiotics, which has led to the development of a subantimicrobial formulation of doxycycline as an adjunctive systemic drug treatment for periodontitis that exploits the anti-MMP properties of this molecule.

Chemokines

Chemokines are cytokine-like molecules that are characterized by their chemotactic activity. This activity gave rise to the term *chemokine* (i.e., they are chemotactic cytokines). Chemokines orchestrate

TABLE 7.1 Biologic Activities of Selected Matrix Metalloproteinases Relevant to Periodontal Disease

MMP Type	Enzyme	Biologic Activity
Collagenases	All	Degrade interstitial collagens (types I, II, and III)
		Digest ECM and non-ECM molecules
	MMP-1	Keratinocyte migration and re-epithelialization
		Platelet aggregation
	MMP-13	Osteoclast activation
Gelatinases	All	Degrade denatured collagens and gelatin
	MMP-2	Differentiation of mesenchymal cells with inflammatory phenotype
		Epithelial cell migration
		Increased bioavailability of MMP-9
Stromelysins	All	Digest ECM molecules
	MMP-3	Activate pro-MMPs
		Disrupted cell aggregation
		Increased cell invasion
Matrilysins	MMP-7	Disrupted cell aggregation
		Increased cell invasion
Membrane-type MMPs	All	Digest ECM molecules
		Activate pro-MMP-2 (except MT4-MMP)
	MT1-MMP	Epithelial cell migration
		Degrade collagen types I, II, and III

ECM, Extracellular matrix; *MMPs*, matrix metalloproteinases; *MT*, membrane type.
Adapted from Hannas AR, Pereira JC, Granjeiro JM, et al: The role of matrix metalloproteinases in the oral environment. *Acta Odontol Scand* 65:1–13, 2007.

leukocyte recruitment in physiologic and pathologic conditions, so they are important for periodontal pathogenesis, which results in the chemotactic migration of neutrophils through the periodontal tissues toward the site of the bacterial challenge in the periodontal pocket. Chemokines play a key role in neutrophil recruitment and the recruitment of other adaptive and innate immune cells to the site of immune and inflammatory responses. The chemokine IL-8, has been demonstrated to be localized in the gingival tissues in areas of plaque accumulation and in the presence of neutrophilic infiltration, and it has also been found in GCF.

It is becoming clear that chemokines also play an important role in macrophage migration, and play a role in T-cell migration in inflamed periodontal tissues. Chemokines therefore play important roles in immune responses, repair, and inflammation, and they regulate osteoclast activity by influencing myeloid cell differentiation into osteoclasts, which may be of particular importance in the context of periodontitis.

Linking Pathogenesis to Clinical Signs of Disease

Advanced forms of periodontal disease are characterized by the symptoms of tooth mobility, tooth loss, and tooth migration. These result from the loss of attachment between the tooth and its supporting tissues after the breakdown of the inserting fibers of the periodontal ligament and the resorption of alveolar bone.

When the bacterial challenge persists, the cellular and fluid infiltrate continues to develop, and neutrophils and other inflammatory cells soon occupy a significant volume of the inflamed gingival tissues. Neutrophils are key components of the innate immune system, and they play a fundamental role in maintaining periodontal health, despite the constant challenge presented by the plaque biofilm. Neutrophils are protective leukocytes that phagocytose and kill bacteria, and deficiencies in neutrophil functioning result in increased susceptibility to infections in general, as well as periodontal disease. Neutrophils also release large quantities of destructive enzymes (e.g., MMPs) as they migrate through the tissues (particularly MMP-8 and MMP-9), a process that results in the breakdown of structural components of the periodontium and the development of collagen-depleted areas. Neutrophils also release their potent lysosomal enzymes, cytokines, and reactive oxygen species (ROS) extracellularly, thereby causing further tissue damage. Neutrophil hyperactivity in periodontitis has also been suggested, which leads to the overproduction of damaging ROS and other mediators. Patients with periodontitis have been reported to have neutrophils that demonstrate enhanced enzymatic activity and that produce increased levels of ROS.

The very first steps in the development of the pocket result from a combination of factors, including the detachment of cells at the coronal aspect of the junctional epithelium, whereas cells at the apical aspect migrate apically into the collagen-depleted areas; intraepithelial cleavage occurs within the junctional epithelium. Epithelial tissues do not have their own blood supply and must rely on the diffusion of nutrients from the underlying connective tissues. Thus, as the epithelium proliferates and thickens, necrosis of epithelial cells that are more distant from the connective tissues can lead to intraepithelial clefts and splits, which also contribute to the early stages of pocket formation.

A cycle of chronic inflammation is therefore established in which the presence of subgingival bacteria drives inflammatory responses in the periodontal tissues; this is characterized by infiltration by leukocytes, the release of inflammatory mediators and destructive enzymes, connective tissue breakdown, and the breakdown and proliferation of the epithelium in an apical direction. The junctional and pocket epithelia become thin and ulcerated and bleed more readily, a condition that results in bleeding on probing. The bacteria in the pocket are never fully eliminated because they are effectively outside the body, but their continued presence drives the destructive inflammatory response in the periodontal tissues. Attempts at effective oral hygiene are rendered more difficult by the deepening of the pocket, and the cycle continues.

Alveolar Bone Resorption

As the advancing inflammatory front approaches the alveolar bone, osteoclastic bone resorption commences. This is a protective mechanism to prevent bacterial invasion of the bone, but it ultimately leads to tooth mobility and even tooth loss. The resorption of alveolar bone occurs simultaneously with the breakdown of the periodontal ligament in the inflamed periodontal tissues.

Histologic studies have confirmed that the bone resorbs so that a width of noninfiltrated connective tissue of about 0.5–1.0 mm overlying the bone is always present. It has also been demonstrated that bone resorption ceases when at least a 2.5-mm distance is present between the site of bacteria in the pocket and the bone. Osteoclasts are stimulated by proinflammatory cytokines and other mediators of inflammation to resorb the bone, and the alveolar bone "retreats" from the advancing inflammatory front. Osteoclasts are multinucleated cells that are formed from osteoclast progenitor cells and macrophages, and osteoclastic bone resorption is activated by a variety of mediators (e.g., IL-1β, TNF-α, IL-6, PGE_2).

Receptor Activator of Nuclear Factor-κB Ligand and Osteoprotegerin

A key system for controlling bone turnover is the receptor activator of nuclear factor-κB (RANK)/RANK ligand (RANKL)/osteoprotegerin (OPG) system. RANK is a cell surface receptor expressed by osteoclast progenitor cells, as well as by mature osteoclasts. RANKL is a ligand that binds to RANK and is produced as either a membrane-bound or secreted protein by a range of cells, including fibroblasts, osteoblasts, mesenchymal cells, and T- and B-lymphocytes. OPG is the inhibitor of RANKL and functions as a decoy receptor—that is, it binds to RANKL and prevents it from interacting with RANK. OPG is secreted primarily by osteoblasts, fibroblasts, and bone marrow stromal cells. The binding of RANKL to RANK results in osteoclast differentiation and activation, and thus bone resorption (Fig 7.2). The balance between RANKL and OPG activity (often referred to as the *RANKL:OPG ratio*) can therefore determine bone resorption or bone formation (Box 7.4).

IL-1β and TNF-α regulate the expression of RANKL and OPG, and T cells express RANKL, which binds directly to RANK on the surfaces of osteoclast progenitors and osteoclasts, thereby resulting in cell activation and differentiation to form mature osteoclasts. In individuals with periodontitis, elevated levels of proinflammatory cytokines (e.g., IL-1β, TNF-α) and increasing numbers of infiltrating T cells result in the activation of osteoclasts by RANK, which results in alveolar bone loss. It has been reported that levels of RANKL are higher and that levels of OPG are lower in sites with active periodontal breakdown as compared with sites with healthy gingiva. In addition, GCF RANKL/OPG ratios are higher in periodontitis than in healthy tissue. It is clear that alterations in the relative levels of these key regulators of osteoclasts play a key role in the bone loss that characterizes periodontal disease.

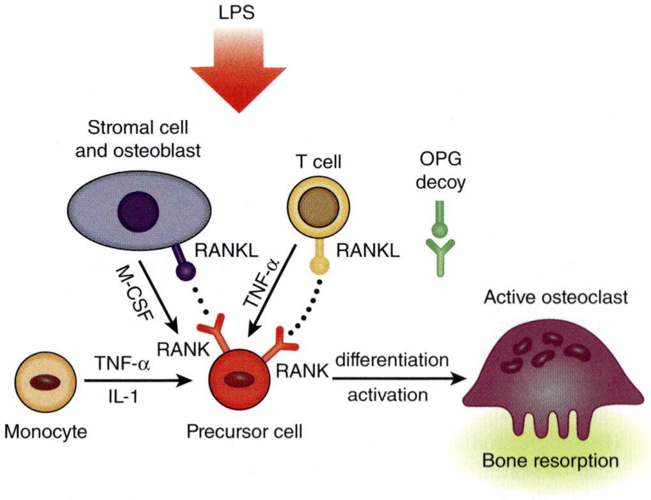

Fig 7.2 Stimuli factors regulating osteoclast formation and function: Cytokines such as interleukin-1 (IL-1), tumor necrosis factor alpha (TNF-α), and macrophage colony stimulating factor (M-CSF), produced by bone marrow stromal cells, osteoblasts, monocytes, and T cells are key regulators on this process. Osteoprotegerin (OPG) acts as a decoy receptor that prevents RANKL from binding to its receptor RANK on precursor cells and downregulate the osteoclastogenesis.

BOX 7.4 RANK/RANKL/OPG System

RANK (receptor activator of nuclear factor-κB)	Cell surface receptor on osteoclast progenitor cells
RANKL (RANK ligand)	Cytokine-like molecule that is the ligand for RANK (i.e., binds to RANK) and causes maturation into fully differentiated osteoclasts
OPG (osteoprotegerin)	Cytokine-like molecule that binds to RANKL and inhibits the interaction between RANKL and RANK

The RANK/RANKL/OPG signaling pathway plays a key role in regulating bone resorption. RANKL binds to RANK and stimulates osteoclast differentiation and activation. OPG antagonizes this action by binding to RANKL and preventing it from binding to RANK. The ratio of RANKL to OPG is important, with studies reporting higher levels of RANKL and lower levels of OPG in patients with advanced periodontitis compared to healthy controls.

Resolution of Inflammation

Inflammation is an important defense mechanism to combat the threat of bacterial infection, but inflammation also results in tissue damage associated with the development and progression of most chronic diseases associated with aging, including periodontal disease. It is becoming evident that the resolution of inflammation (i.e., "turning off" inflammation) is an active process that is regulated by specific mechanisms that restore homeostasis (see Chapter 10). It is possible that controlling or augmenting these mechanisms may lead to the development of new treatment strategies for managing chronic diseases such as periodontitis. The resolution of inflammation is an active process that results in a return to homeostasis, and it is mediated by specific molecules, including a class of endogenous, proresolving lipid mediators that includes the lipoxins, resolvins, and protectins. These molecules are actively synthesized during the resolution phases of acute inflammation; they are antiinflammatory, and they inhibit neutrophil infiltration.

Immune Responses in Periodontal Pathogenesis

Immune responses are categorized as either innate or adaptive. Innate immune responses may adapt with exposure to the same pathogen but subside once the threat has been eliminated. An example of innate immunity is phagocytic cells (i.e., monocytes, macrophages, neutrophils), which possess a number of inherently antimicrobial peptides and proteins that kill many different pathogens rather than one specific pathogen. In contrast, the specific immune responses will increase after exposure to a pathogen and usually maintain higher levels for years. Lymphocytes (e.g., T cells, B cells) are important in the fundamental form of specific adaptive immunity referred to as the specific immune response. The ability of T cells and B cells to recognize specific oligomeric structures on a pathogen and generate progeny that also recognize the structure enables the immune system to respond more rapidly and effectively when re-exposed to that same pathogen.

Cells of Immunity and Inflammation

Cells of the immune system that are important in inflammation and host defenses include mast cells, dermal dendrocytes (histiocytes),

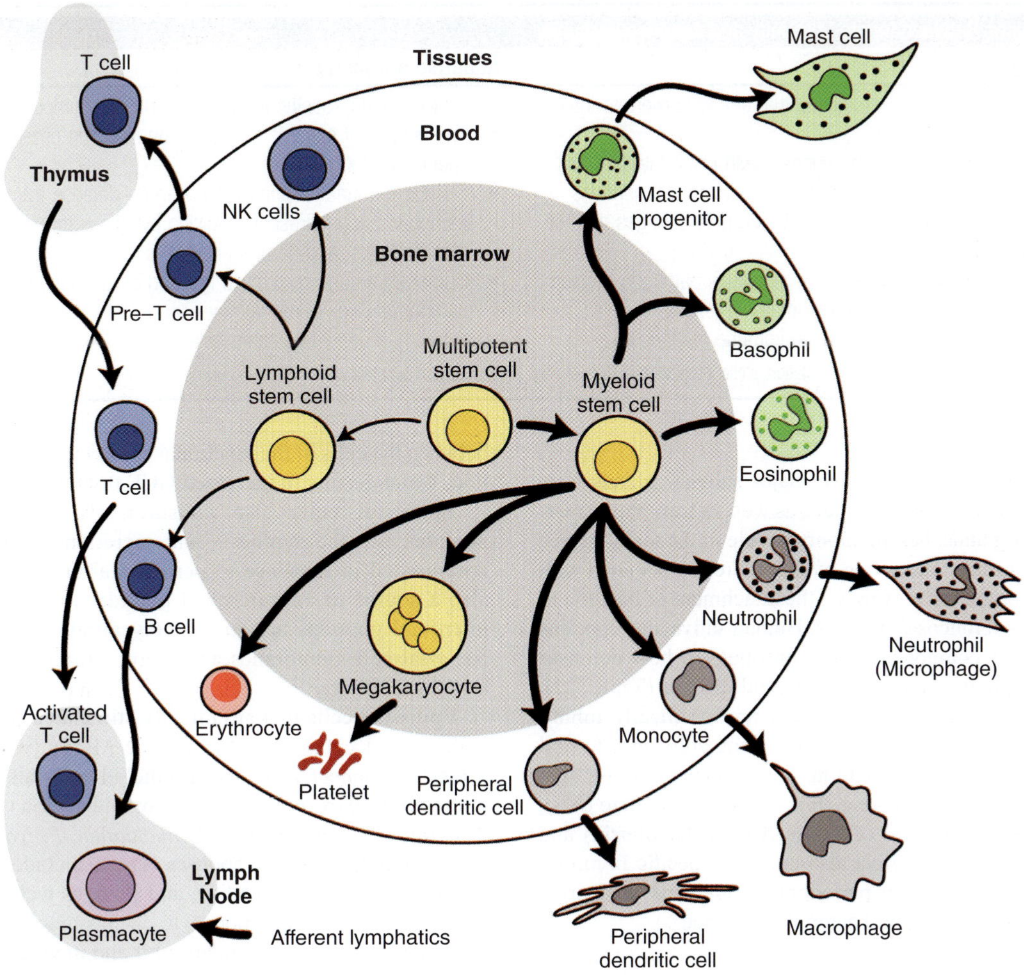

Fig 7.3 The main cells of the immune system are derived from lymphoid and myeloid arms of the hematopoietic system.

peripheral dendritic cells, neutrophils, monocytes/macrophages, T cells, B cells, and natural killer (NK) cells (Fig. 7.3). Other hematopoietic leukocytes, including basophils, eosinophils, erythrocytes, and platelets, also participate in certain forms of inflammation or immune function.

Cells possess receptors, which are molecules on the cell surfaces that enable the cell to interact with other molecules or cells. Receptors reflect and dictate the function of cells. Historically, the names given to receptors are often related to function. In addition to these common names, a systematic nomenclature known as the CD (cluster of differentiation) has been developed.

The immune system is essential for the maintenance of periodontal health, and it is central to the host response to periodontal pathogens. However, if the immune response is dysregulated, inappropriate, persistent, or excessive in some way, then damaging chronic inflammatory responses such as those observed in periodontal disease can ensue. It is now widely appreciated that immune responses are complex biologic networks in which pathogen recognition, innate immunity, and adaptive immunity are integrated and mutually dependent.

We need to understand how the polymicrobial biofilm (as opposed to individual species of periodontal pathogens) interacts with host immune defenses. We also need to appreciate specific immunologic properties that relate to the unique anatomy of the periodontium, to understand how immune responses contribute to the dynamic aspects of periodontal disease and its various clinical courses, and to gain a comprehension of how elements of host immunity contribute to tissue destruction, resolution, repair, and regeneration.

Innate Immunity

Defenses against infection include a wide range of mechanical, chemical, and microbiologic barriers that prevent pathogens from invading the cells and tissues of the body. Saliva, GCF, and the epithelial keratinocytes of the oral mucosa all protect the underlying tissues of the oral cavity and the periodontium. The commensal microbiota (e.g., in dental biofilm) may also be important for providing protection against infection by pathogenic microorganisms through effective competition for resources and ecologic niches and also by stimulating protective immune responses.

The term *innate immunity* refers to the elements of the immune response that are determined by inherited factors (and therefore "innate"), that have limited specificity, and that are "fixed" in that they do not change or improve during an immune response or as a result of previous exposure to a pathogen. The recognition of pathogenic microorganisms and the recruitment of effector cells (e.g., neutrophils) and molecules (e.g., the complement system) are central to effective innate immunity. Innate immune responses are orchestrated by a broad range of cytokines, chemokines, and cell surface receptors, and the stimulation of innate immunity leads to a state of inflammation. If innate immune responses fail to eliminate infection, then the effector cells of adaptive immune responses (lymphocytes) are activated (Box 7.5).

BOX 7.5 Differences Between Innate Immunity and Adaptive Immunity

Innate Immunity	Adaptive Immunity
Refers to nonspecific defense mechanisms that act as barriers to infection. Components include: • Barriers to infection such as skin, mucosa, acid pH in the stomach • Antimicrobial molecules such as lysozyme, antimicrobial peptides • Immune system cells such as neutrophils and macrophages that kill infecting organisms • Receptors (e.g., Toll-like receptors) that recognize pathogen-derived molecules and activate immune–inflammatory responses • Antigen presentation to activate adaptive immune responses	Refers to antigen-specific immune responses. Components include: • Recognition of specific molecules on infecting organisms at the species and strain level • Cellular immune responses focused on defense from intracellular pathogens (e.g., viruses), involving cytokines from T helper cells, macrophages, and natural killer cells • Humoral immune responses focused on defense from extracellular pathogens (e.g., bacteria), involving B cells that differentiate into antibody-producing plasma cells

Innate and adaptive immunity do not function in isolation; close integration exists between the innate and adaptive arms of the immune response.

Saliva

Saliva that is secreted from the three major salivary glands (i.e., parotid, submandibular, and sublingual), as well as from the numerous minor salivary glands, has an important role in the maintenance of oral and dental health. The action of shear forces associated with saliva flow is important for preventing the attachment of bacteria to the dentition and oral mucosal surfaces. Human saliva also contains numerous molecular components that contribute to host defenses against bacterial colonization and periodontal disease (Table 7.2). These components include molecules that nonspecifically inhibit the formation of the plaque biofilm by inhibiting adherence to oral surfaces and promoting agglutination (e.g., mucins), those that inhibit specific virulence factors (e.g., histatins that neutralize LPS), and those that inhibit bacterial cell growth (e.g., lactoferrin) and that may induce cell death. Saliva also contains specific immunoglobulin A (IgA) antibodies to periodontal pathogens that target specific antigens and that inhibit bacterial adherence.

Epithelial Tissues

The epithelial tissues play a key role in host defense because they are the main site of the initial interactions between plaque bacteria and the host, and they are also the site of the invasion of microbial pathogens. The keratinized epithelium of the sulcular and gingival epithelial tissues provides protection for the underlying periodontal tissue in addition to acting as a barrier against bacteria and their products. By contrast, the junctional epithelium has significant intercellular spaces, it is not keratinized, and it exhibits a higher cellular turnover rate. These properties render the junctional epithelium permeable, thereby allowing for the inward movement of microbes and their products and the outward movement of GCF and the cells and molecules of innate immunity. Furthermore, the spaces between the cells of the junctional epithelium widen with inflammation, which results in increased GCF flow.

Epithelial cells also constitutively express antimicrobial peptides and the synthesis and secretion of these molecules is upregulated in response to periodontal bacteria. Neutrophils are also a source of antimicrobial peptides (i.e., α-defensins). Antimicrobial peptides are small, polycationic peptides that disrupt bacterial cell membranes and thereby directly kill bacteria with broad specificity.

Epithelial cells that are directly stimulated with bacterial components and cytokines can produce MMPs, which contribute to a loss of connective tissue. Epithelial cells also secrete a range of cytokines in response to periodontal bacteria (e.g., *P. gingivalis*, *A. actinomycetemcomitans*, *F. nucleatum*, *Prevotella intermedia*), which signal immune responses. These include the proinflammatory cytokines IL-1β, TNF-α, and IL-6, as well as the chemokine IL-8 (CXCL8) and the monocyte chemoattractant protein-1 (MCP-1), which serve to signal neutrophil and monocyte migration from the vasculature into the periodontal tissue.

TABLE 7.2 Constituents of Saliva That Contribute to Innate Immunity

Saliva Constituent	Host Defense Function
Antibodies (e.g., immunoglobulin A)	Inhibit bacterial adherence, promote agglutination
Histatins	Neutralize lipopolysaccharides, inhibit destructive enzymes
Cystatins	Inhibit bacterial growth
Lactoferrin	Inhibits bacterial growth
Lysozyme	Lyses bacterial cell walls
Mucins	Inhibits bacterial adherence, promotes agglutination
Peroxidase	Neutralizes bacterial hydrogen peroxide

Gingival Crevicular Fluid

GCF originates from the postcapillary venules of the gingival plexus. It has a flushing action in the gingival crevice, but it also likely functions to bring the blood components (e.g., neutrophils, antibodies, complement components) of the host defenses into the sulcus. The flow of GCF increases in inflammation, and neutrophils are an especially important component of GCF in periodontal health and disease.

Pathogen Recognition and Activation of Cellular Innate Responses

If plaque bacteria and their products penetrate the periodontal tissues, specialized "sentinel cells" of the immune system recognize their presence and signal protective immune responses. These cells include macrophages and dendritic cells, which express a range of pattern recognition receptors (PRRs) that interact with microbe-associated molecular patterns (MAMPs). The activation of PRRs activates innate immune responses to provide immediate protection, and adaptive immunity is also activated with the aim of establishing a sustained antigen-specific defense. Excessive and inappropriate or dysregulated immune responses lead to chronic inflammation and the concomitant tissue destruction associated with periodontal disease.

Neutrophil Function

When there is inflammation neutrophils perform the following functions:

Margination and diapedesis:

Neutrophils adhere to the luminal surface of the vascular endothelium (rolling, margination) and migrate across the endothelium (diapedesis, interendothelial transmigration). There are two phases of leukocyte-endothelium adherence: the selectin-dependent phase (primarily involved in rolling) and the integrin-dependent phase (primary involved in diapedesis).

Chemotaxis:

Once the leukocyte enters the connective tissue, it must be able to locate and migrate to the site of insult. This is accomplished by chemotaxis, which depends on the leukocyte's ability to sense a chemical gradient across its cell body and migrate in the direction of increasing concentration. To migrate toward a target, leukocytes assume an asymmetric or polarized shape rather than the rounded morphology evident in blood. Even under ideal experimental conditions, neutrophil migration has been observed to be primarily random until the neutrophil is one to two body lengths (10–20 μm) away from a recognizable target particle.

Phagocytosis:

Phagocytosis is the process by which cells ingest particles of a size visible to light microscopy. Neutrophils and monocytes/macrophages are the only cells efficient enough at phagocytosis to be considered "professional phagocytes." Phagocytosis results in the eventual containment of a pathogen within a membrane-delimited structure, the phagosome. The mechanisms of coating the pathogen with a few recognizable ligands (IgG, C3b which are referred to as opsonins) enable the phagocyte to bind to and ingest the pathogen. This is referred to as opsonization.

Phagocytes kill bacteria through two broad categories of killing mechanisms. One category is based on the reduction of oxygen and is referred to as "oxidative." Oxidative mechanisms require (1) the presence of oxygen and (2) an oxidation: potential, Eh, at or above –160 mV. In the presence of oxygen, phagocytes possess mechanisms of oxidative killing. In particular, neutrophils exert intense microbicidal activity by forming toxic, reduced-oxygen metabolites such as superoxide anion (O_2-) using the NADPH oxidase system. The superoxide anion also contributes to the formation of hydrogen peroxide (H_2O_2), which is capable of diffusing across membranes. Inside a target cell, H_2O_2 may be further reduced to the hydroxyl radical, which can cause DNA damage.

Neutrophils also possess capabilities for the second category of killing mechanisms, the nonoxidative mechanisms as they do not require oxygen for energy and can function under anaerobic conditions. Nonoxidative killing requires phagosome-lysosome fusion. This process involves the movement toward and subsequent membrane fusion of the lysosome with the phagosome, which forms a phagolysosome. This results in the secretion of antimicrobial lysosomal components into the phagolysosome leading to lysis of ingested bacteria.

Neutrophil functional deficiencies could lead to periodontal breakdown (Box 7.6).

Neutrophils are the "professional" phagocytes that are critical to the clearance of bacteria that invade host tissues. Neutrophils are present in clinically healthy gingival tissues, and they migrate through the intercellular spaces of the junctional epithelium into the sulcus. This is part of a "low-grade defense" against plaque bacteria, and it is necessary to prevent infection and periodontal tissue damage. The importance of neutrophils to the maintenance of periodontal health is demonstrated clinically by the observations of severe periodontitis in patients with neutrophil defects.

A small proportion (1%–2%) of the intercellular spaces in healthy junctional epithelium is occupied by neutrophils (and other leukocytes at various stages of differentiation), but this can increase to 30% with even modest inflammation. Neutrophils migrate from the gingival plexus to the extravascular connective tissue and then into the junctional epithelium through the basement membrane. The presence of a layer of neutrophils in the junctional epithelium forms a host defense barrier between subgingival biofilm and the gingival tissue. At the molecular level, the interaction of adhesion molecules (e.g., ICAM-1) on endothelial and epithelial cells with $\beta 2$ integrins on neutrophils facilitates neutrophil migration. Indeed, evidence from immunohistochemistry studies indicate the existence of gradients of IL-8 (a "chemotactic gradient"), as well as gradients of ICAM-1, which direct the neutrophils from the vasculature into the tissues and toward the junctional epithelium. The migration of neutrophils contributes to the disruption of the junctional epithelium by the degradation of the basement membrane through protease release and the action of ROS.

BOX 7.6 Neutrophil Disorders Associated With Periodontal Disease

1. Leukocyte adhesion deficiency (LAD1 and LAD2)
2. Hyperimmunoglobulinemia E (Jobs syndrome)
3. Chediak–Higashi syndrome
4. Chronic and cyclic neutropenia
5. Agranulocytosis
6. Chronic granulomatous disease
7. Specific granule deficiency

Adaptive Immunity

Adaptive immunity has evolved to provide a focused and intense defense against infections that overwhelm innate immune responses.

Adaptive immunity contrasts with innate immunity with regard to the dynamic of the underlying cellular and molecular responses: adaptive immunity is slower and reliant on complex interactions between APCs and T and B lymphocytes. A key element is the antigen specificity of the responses that facilitates the specific targeting of a diverse range of effector elements, including cytotoxic T cells and antibodies. Another facet is the ability of adaptive immune responses to improve during exposure to antigen and on subsequent reinfection events. The importance of adaptive immune responses in periodontal pathogenesis is endorsed by histologic studies of established lesions in periodontal disease. The population of leukocytes in the periodontium in gingivitis (i.e., the early stages of responses to the plaque biofilm) and in stable periodontal lesions (i.e., those in which tissue destruction is apparently not progressing) has been reported to be dominated by T cells, and these cells are clustered mainly around blood vessels. Cell surface marker studies suggest that these cells are activated but not proliferating. In addition, a predominance of the helper T-cell subset (i.e., CD4-expressing T cells) over the cytotoxic T-cell subset (i.e., CD8-expressing T cells) is observed. These T cells are considered to be proactively maintaining tissue homeostasis in the presence of the microbial challenge of the plaque biofilm. By contrast, in active (progressing) periodontitis, B cells and plasma cells predominate and are associated with pocket formation and the progression of disease.

Antigen-Presenting Cells

APCs are sentinel cells in mucosal tissues such as the periodontium. APCs detect and take up microorganisms and their antigens, after which they may migrate to lymph nodes and interact with T cells to present antigen. The periodontium is often compared to other mucosal tissues and the skin in terms of its repertoire of immune cells, and it contains a number of "professional" APCs, including B cells, macrophages, and at least two types of dendritic cells (i.e., dermal dendritic cells and Langerhans cells). These cells naturally express the major histocompatibility complex class II molecules necessary for antigen presentation to T-cell receptors, and they may take up specific antigens and transport them to local lymph nodes, thereby facilitating the activation of specific effector T cells and the generation of an antigen-specific immune response to periodontal pathogens.

T Cells

Several different subsets of thymic lymphocytes (i.e., T cells) develop in the bone marrow and thymus and migrate to the peripheral tissues to participate in adaptive immune responses. The expression of the cell surface molecules (CD4 or CD8) or particular T-cell antigen receptors ($\alpha\beta$ or $\gamma\delta$) broadly defines functional T-cell subsets that emerge from the thymus. The role of T cells in periodontal disease has been established through immunohistologic studies of diseased tissues. $CD4^+$ helper T cells are the predominant phenotype in the stable periodontal lesion, and it is thought that alterations in the balance of effector T-cell subsets within the $CD4^+$ population may lead to progression toward a destructive, B-cell–dominated lesion.

B Cells

B cells help control extracellular antigens such as bacteria, fungal, yeast, and virions. B cells recognize diverse antigens using the *B-cell antigen receptor* (BCR). The high affinity interaction between the BCR and antigen enables the B cell to bind and ingest the antigen. Ingested antigen is degraded and presented to T cells. After antigen presentation, some B cells differentiate to produce *plasma cells* dedicated to the production and secretion of antibodies.

Antibodies

Specific antibodies are produced in response to the bacterial challenge in periodontal disease and are the endpoint of B-cell activation. Circulating antibodies may be more important than locally produced antibodies. Even so, these generally appear in a high titer but have low biologic activity, so there is some doubt as to their effectiveness. Commensurate with the appearance of antibodies against bacterial antigens is the appearance of differentiated plasma cells. High levels of antibodies appear in GCF (in addition to those in the circulation), and these are produced locally by plasma cells in periodontal tissues. Antibodies to periodontal pathogens are primarily IgG, with few IgM or IgA types produced.

Many species of oral bacteria elicit a polyclonal B-cell response (with the consequent production of specific antibodies against those bacteria). However, these responses augment responses against nonoral bacteria and may lead to the production of autoantibodies (e.g., antibodies against collagen and connective tissue proteins), which may contribute to tissue destruction in periodontal disease. The incidence and levels of specific serum and GCF IgG antibodies are raised in chronic periodontitis, a finding suggesting that local and peripheral generation of antibodies may be important in the immune response to periodontal pathogens. Antibodies (i.e., IgA) to periodontal pathogens are also found in saliva. Variations in the levels of specific antibodies to different species in different clinical presentations suggest differences in pathogenesis. For example, antibodies to *A. actinomycetemcomitans* of the IgG_2 subclass predominate in aggressive periodontitis.

P. gingivalis molecules (i.e., fimbriae and hemagglutinin) also act as antigens. Specific antibodies are also generated by serotype-specific carbohydrate antigens (e.g., capsular polysaccharide of *P. gingivalis*, carbohydrate of *A. actinomycetemcomitans* LPS).

The significance of antibodies in periodontitis is not clear. It is not known whether these antibodies have a protective function or whether they participate in disease pathogenesis. Although some evidence indicates a correlation between clinical parameters of disease and titers of specific antibodies to periodontal pathogens, other studies report an inverse correlation of antibody levels and avidity with periodontal destruction. In addition, specific antibodies to periodontal pathogens are found in healthy individuals, as well as in persons with periodontal disease.

Complement Systems

In cases of periodontal disease, the host defense also is dependent on a functional complement system, which coordinates the recruitment and activation of inflammatory cells, bacterial opsonization, phagocytosis, and lysis. The complement system is critical to the linking of innate and adaptive immunity by regulating the activation of both B cells and T cells, either directly or through effects on antigen-presenting cells (APCs).

The activation of the complement cascade involves the sequential activation and proteolytic cleavage of a series of serum proteins via three distinct mechanisms, namely the classical, lectin, and alternative. Classical pathway activation occurs in response to antigen–antibody complexes that are recognized by the C1q subunit of C1. However, the lectin pathway is triggered through the interaction of a secreted pattern-recognition receptor (mannose-binding lectin) with specific carbohydrate groups on the surface of a variety of microorganisms. Both the classical and the lectin pathways then proceed through C4 and C2 cleavage for the generation of the classical/lectin C3 convertase (C4bC2b). The alternative pathway is initiated by the hydrolysis of C3 to $C3(H_2O)$, which is a C3b analog that forms the initial alternative pathway for C3 convertase, or through bacterial lipopolysaccharide and lipooligosaccharide molecules in concert with microbial-derived properdin. The alternative pathway also serves as a positive feedback loop for the classical and lectin pathways. All three pathways converge at the third component of complement (C3), which upon activation by pathway-specific C3 convertases leads to the generation of key effector molecules. These include the C3a and C5a anaphylatoxins, which activate specific G-protein–coupled receptors and which mediate the mobilization and activation of leukocytes. Also important are the C3b opsonins, which promote phagocytosis through complement receptors, and the C5b-9 membrane attack complex, which can lyse targeted pathogens.

The complement systems have also been shown to provide a barrier against the spread of bacterial infections; to facilitate clotting mechanisms; to mobilize hematopoietic stem cells and progenitor cells from the bone marrow; to help replenish new leukocytes; and to activate the differentiation of specific T-cell subsets. The dysregulation of complement activities may lead to a failure to protect the host against pathogens and amplify inflammatory tissue damage. In the context of periodontal inflammation, complement subversion appears to play a major role in periodontal pathogenesis.

Activated complement components are found in the gingival crevicular fluid of patients with chronic periodontitis as compared to healthy sites. Virtually all of the complement components have been detected in chronically inflamed gingiva or in the gingival crevicular fluid of patients as compared to healthy control samples. Finally, local complement activation may promote periodontal inflammation predominantly via C5a-induced vasodilation, increased vascular permeability and flow of inflammatory exudate, and chemotactic recruitment of inflammatory cells, especially neutrophils.

Concept of Host Susceptibility

The immune and inflammatory processes that result from the challenge presented by the subgingival biofilm are complex and are mediated by a large number of proinflammatory and antiinflammatory

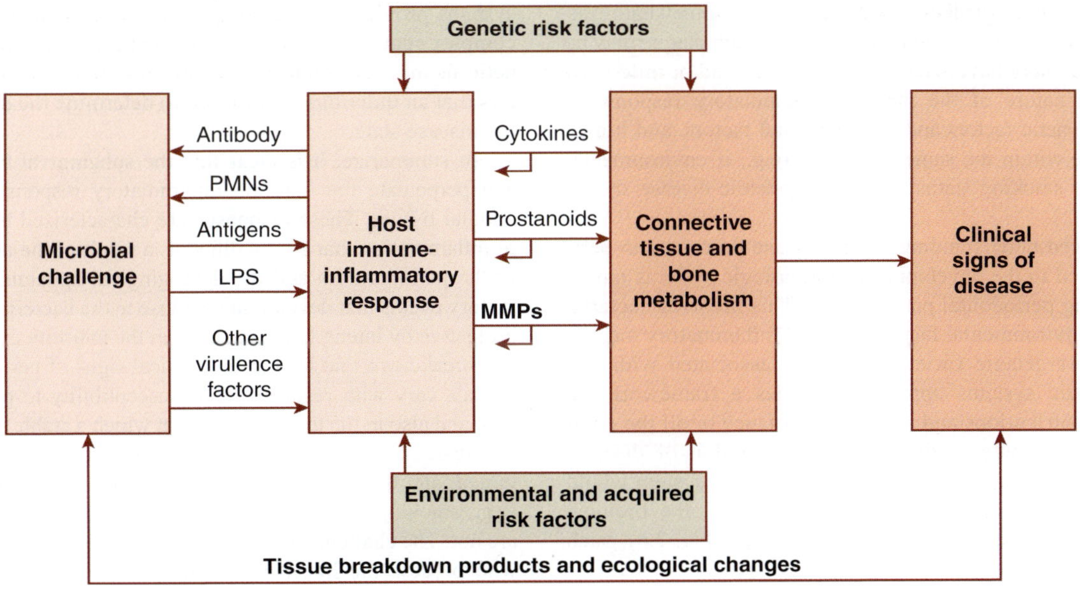

Fig 7.4 Schematic illustration of the pathogenesis of periodontitis. The microbial challenge presented by subgingival plaque bacteria results in an upregulated host immune-inflammatory response in the periodontal tissues that is characterized by the excessive production of inflammatory cytokines (e.g., interleukins, tumor necrosis factor), prostanoids (e.g., prostaglandin E2), and enzymes, including the matrix metalloproteinases (*MMPs*). These proinflammatory mediators are responsible for the majority of periodontal breakdown that occurs, leading to the clinical signs and symptoms of periodontitis. The process is modified by environmental (e.g., tobacco use) and acquired risk factors (e.g., systemic diseases) and genetic susceptibility. *PMNs*, Polymorphonuclear leukocytes; *LPS*, lipopolysaccharide. *(Modified from Kornman KS: ClinInfect Dis 28:520, 1999.)*

cytokines and enzymes that function as a network of mediators with overlapping roles and activity. Immune responses to the bacterial challenge do not occur in isolation but rather take place in the context of other host and environmental factors that influence these responses and thereby determine the progression of disease (Fig. 7.4). Certain risk factors increase susceptibility to periodontal disease, particularly smoking and diabetes; these are considered elsewhere in this book.

A feature of human development and evolution has been that quantitative and qualitative differences exist in immune responses among individuals. Indeed, infectious agents (e.g., bacteria) exert evolutionary selection pressures on the species that they infect. This may be relevant in periodontal disease, and some studies have confirmed that immune cells from patients with periodontal disease secrete higher quantities of proinflammatory cytokines than do cells from persons who are periodontally healthy. Cytokine profiles are also different in those individuals with immune-mediated diseases as compared to healthy control subjects.

These observations have led to the concept of the "hyperinflammatory" or "hyperresponsive" trait in which certain individuals possess a hyperinflammatory phenotype that accounts for their increased susceptibility to chronic inflammatory conditions such as periodontitis. Such a trait may also underpin shared susceptibility between conditions such as periodontitis and cardiovascular disease or diabetes. However, at present, it is not possible to identify with certainty those patients who are hyperresponders. The hyperresponder concept was originally proposed in the context of the responsiveness of monocytes to LPS challenge; this suggests that patients with disease possess an individual hyperresponsive monocytic trait. Fig. 7.5 is a schematic illustration of how increasing bacterial challenge can result in differing levels of inflammatory response according to the response profile of an individual patient. Most individuals would be considered normal, and for a given bacterial challenge, they would produce a certain level of inflammatory mediators in the periodontal tissues. For those who are hyperresponders, the same bacterial challenge results in a greater inflammatory response, which over time would result in increased tissue breakdown, earlier presentation of the clinical signs of disease, and a clinical interpretation of having increased susceptibility to periodontitis. Those individuals who are hyporesponsive produce lower

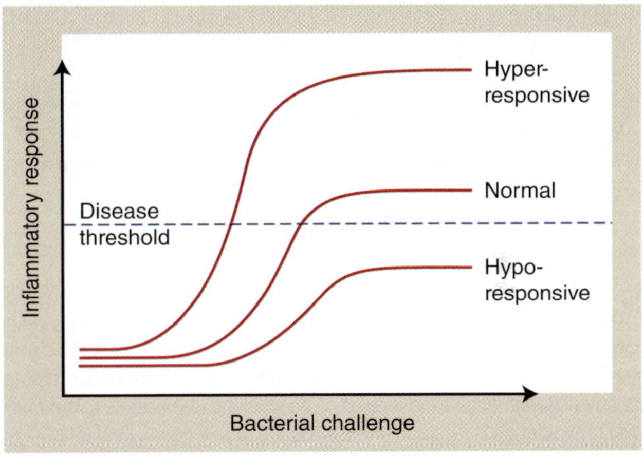

Fig. 7.5 **Inflammatory response characteristics in relation to bacterial challenge.** A given bacterial challenge results in differing levels of inflammatory response according to the response profile of an individual. Most people are close to normal and produce a certain level of inflammatory mediators for a given challenge. Those who are hyperresponders generate an excessive inflammatory response for the same bacterial challenge and cross the threshold into active disease at an earlier stage. Those who are hyporesponsive produce lower levels of inflammatory mediators and, despite a significant bacterial challenge, may never develop advanced periodontitis. *(Modified from Champagne CM, Buchanan W, Reddy MS, et al: Potential for gingival crevice fluid measures as predictors of risk for periodontal diseases. Periodontol 2000 31:167–180, 2003.)*

levels of inflammatory mediators and are therefore somewhat resistant to the development of periodontitis, even though plaque may be present and they may have widespread gingivitis and/or mild periodontitis. The nature of the immune–inflammatory response is governed by genetic factors and environmental factors, and it may vary over time within the same individual (e.g., if environmental factors such as smoking status, stress, or systemic disease should change).

Our improved understanding of the disease processes in periodontitis has led to the development of a biologic systems model for representing periodontal pathogenesis. This involves bacterial components, environmental factors, specific inflammatory mechanisms, and host–genetic variations that are associated with disease. A biologic systems approach provides a framework for viewing the contributions and relative importance of all the components that contribute to the clinical presentation of disease. Thus, in the context of periodontal disease, such a system would include a person level, a genetic/epigenetic level, the biologic phenotype, and, ultimately, the clinical phenotype (Fig. 7.6). Such systems provide a more comprehensive view of the disease as a complex regulatory network in which aspects of the specific genetic factors, environmental exposures, and other modifying factors that an individual is exposed to determine the development of the disease state.

To summarize, it is clear that the subgingival bacteria initiate and perpetuate the immune–inflammatory responses in the periodontal tissues. These responses are characterized by classic signs of inflammation that are modified as a result of the unique anatomy of the periodontium and the dentogingival apparatus. The inflammatory events that develop in response to the bacterial challenge are protective by intent, but they result in the majority of tissue damage and breakdown that lead to the clinical signs of periodontitis. Individuals vary with regard to their susceptibility to periodontal disease and also in the threshold level at which a stable periodontal site progresses to an active site. Such variations are genetically determined, and they are also influenced by environmental risk factors (e.g., smoking), some of which are modifiable and some of which are not. The challenge for the future is to identify at-risk individuals who possess the hyperinflammatory trait so that disease can be prevented by careful management strategies before tissue loss has occurred.

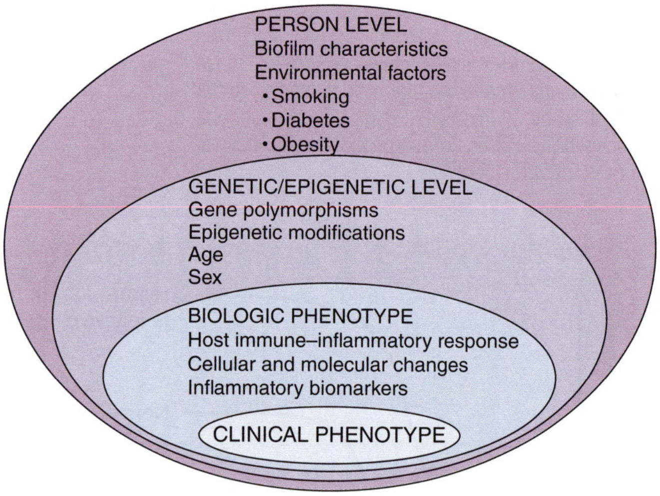

Fig. 7.6 **A biologic systems model of periodontitis.** The outermost level of this model is the *Person Level*, which represents an individual's unique characteristics as they are related to periodontitis. These include the compositional characteristics of the subgingival biofilm, as well as known risk factors and environmental exposures such as smoking and diabetes. The *Person Level* characteristics interact with the *Genetic/Epigenetic Level* characteristics, which include nonmodifiable factors such as age, sex, and genetic composition. Gene polymorphisms are known to be associated with periodontal disease, and epigenetics refers to changes in phenotype (i.e., clinical disease expression) caused by mechanisms other than changes in the underlying DNA sequence. Epigenetics can be defined as all the meiotically and mitotically inherited changes in gene expression that are not encoded in the DNA sequence itself. Epigenetic modifications are important permissive and suppressive factors for controlling the expressed genome through gene transcription. Two major epigenetic mechanisms are the posttranslational modification of histone proteins in chromatin and the methylation of DNA. The *Genetic/Epigenetic Level* characteristics influence the *Biologic Phenotype*, which is characterized by the specific immune–inflammatory responses (i.e., cellular and molecular events and the production of inflammatory mediators) that are associated with the *Clinical Phenotype* (i.e., the clinical presentation of the disease). This model reflects how different individuals with the same presentation (e.g., periodontitis) may have very different predisposing and risk factors. The model depicts the different biologic factors that underpin the development of periodontal disease in different individuals and that ultimately may be used to classify disease by the contribution provided to the clinical phenotype at each level. *(Modified from Offenbacher S, Barros SP, Beck JD: Rethinking periodontal inflammation. J Periodontol 79:1577–1584, 2008.)*

Key points

- Clinical signs of gingivitis are redness, swelling, and bleeding on probing.
- Defense mechanisms of gingiva include intact epithelial barrier, outflow of GCF, sloughing of surface epithelial cells, presence of antibodies in the GCF, presence of neutrophils and macrophages.
- Lipopolysacchride as endotoxins, which activate the immune–inflammatory response resulting in tissue damage.
- Bacteria produce proteases to digest proteins, disrupt host responses, compromise tissue integrity, and facilitate the microbial invasion of the tissues.
- *Porphyromonas gingivalis* and *Aggregatibacter actinomycetemcomitans* are putative periodontal pathogens which invade the tissues.
- Key inflammatory mediators are cytokines, prostanoids, and matrix metalloproteinases (MMPs).
- Important proinflammatory cytokines are IL-1α, IL-1β, IL-6, and TNF-α.
- Chemokines are small peptide cytokines that result in the chemotactic migration of neutrophils.
- Neutrophils are protective leukocytes that phagocytose and kill bacteria, and deficiencies in neutrophil functioning result in increased susceptibility to infections in general, as well as periodontal disease
- Neutrophils release large quantities of destructive enzymes (e.g., MMPs), which result in the breakdown of structural components of the periodontium.
- Immune cells that are involved in inflammation and host defenses include mast cells, dermal dendrocytes (histiocytes), peripheral dendritic cells, neutrophils, monocytes/macrophages, T cells, B cells, and natural killer (NK) cells.
- Antigen presenting cells detect microorganisms and their antigens, and migrate to lymph nodes and interact with T cells to present antigen.
- The inflammatory events that develop in response to the bacterial challenge are protective by intent but they result in the majority of tissue damage and breakdown resulting in clinical signs of periodontitis.

Suggested Readings

Champagne CM, Buchanan W, Reddy MS, et al: Potential for gingival crevice fluid measures as predictors of risk for periodontal diseases, *Periodontol 2000* 31:167–180, 2003.

Gemmell E, Seymour GJ: Immunoregulatory control of Th1/Th2 cytokine profiles in periodontal disease, *Periodontol 2000* 35:21–41, 2005.

Gemmell E, Yamazaki K, Seymour GJ: The role of T cells in periodontal disease: homeostasis and autoimmunity, *Periodontol 2000* 43:14–40, 2007.

Kinane DF, Preshaw PM, Loos BG: Host-response: understanding the cellular and molecular mechanisms of host-microbial interactions–consensus of the Seventh European Workshop on Periodontology, *J Clin Periodontol* 38(Suppl 11):44–48, 2011.

Kornman KS: Mapping the pathogenesis of periodontitis: a new look, *J Periodontol* 79:1560–1568, 2008.

Offenbacher S, Barros SP, Beck JD: Rethinking periodontal inflammation, *J Periodontol* 79:1577–1584, 2008.

Preshaw PM, Taylor JJ: How has research into cytokine interactions and their role in driving immune responses impacted our understanding of periodontitis? *J Clin Periodontol* 38(Suppl 11):60–84, 2011.

References

References and MCQs with answers for the chapter are available on www.medenact.com.

CHAPTER 8

Biofilm and Periodontal Microbiology

W Teughels | M Feres | SM Ganesan | NS Jakubovics | MD Gidley | YL Hernandez-Kapila | N Ambalavanan

CHAPTER OUTLINE

As the human fetus inside the uterus passes through the birth canal, it acquires vaginal and fecal microorganisms. Within 2 weeks, a nearly mature *microbiota* is established in the gut of the newborn baby. After weaning (>2 years), the entire human microbiota is formed and comprises a very complex collection of hundreds of different types of bacteria with approximately 10^{14} microbial cells. From this moment onwards, our body contains *1.3–10 times more bacteria* than human cells. It has been estimated that, for a normal and healthy human being, the bacterial population comprises 2 kg of the total body weight. This is fascinating if one realizes that the average human brain weighs only about 1.4 kg.

The colonization of the oral cavity also starts close to the time of birth. Within hours after birth, the sterile oral cavity is colonized by low numbers of mainly facultative and aerobic bacteria. At that time, the oral microbiota of newborns closely resembles the mother's vaginal microbiota or, for newborns delivered by cesarean section, the mother's skin microbiota. From the second day, anaerobic bacteria can be detected in the infant's edentulous mouth. The number of oral bacteria increases gradually as a result of exposure to external environmental microbial sources. *Streptococcus salivarius* and *Streptococcus mitis* have been identified as the first and most dominant oral microbes to colonize the oral cavity of newborn infants. *Veillonella* spp., *Neisseria* spp., *Actinomyces* spp., and *Staphylococcus* spp. are also among the first colonizers of the oral cavity. After tooth eruption, a more complex oral microbiota is established. The species that colonize the teeth after eruption include *Streptococcus sanguinis*, *Lactobacillus* spp., and *Streptococcus oralis*. Oral streptococci, including *S. oralis, Streptococcus anginosus*, mutans streptococci (*Streptococcus mutans* and *Streptococcus sobrinus*), and *Streptococcus gordonii*, are commonly reported to be present after the first year of life. In addition, anaerobes, including *Fusobacterium* spp. and *Prevotella* spp., can also be detected in young children. In later childhood, the bacterial diversity and numbers in the oral cavity increase as more teeth erupt and provide more areas for the adherence and retention of bacteria.

It is estimated that the oral bacterial microbiome of adults encompasses approximately 700 commonly occurring species, approximately half of which can be present at any time in any individual. However, most oral bacteria are harmless commensals under normal circumstances. This means that this microbiota lives in harmony with its host but, under specific conditions (i.e., increased mass and/or pathogenicity, suppression of commensal or beneficial bacteria, and/or reduced host response), disease can occur. The importance of the commensal microbiota is clearly illustrated by the development of *Candida* infections when the normal oral microbiota is reduced, such as after a longer period of systemic antibiotic usage. It is obvious that the periodontal microbiota is extremely complex. Because it both affects and is affected by the host, the oral environment, and periodontal treatment, a profound knowledge of periodontal microbiology is necessary.

The Oral Cavity From a Microbe's Perspective

With the exception of those microorganisms that are present in feces and in secretory fluids, all bacteria maintain themselves within their host by adhering to a surface. This principle also applies to the oral cavity. From an ecologic viewpoint, the oral cavity, which communicates with the pharynx, should be considered as an "open growth system" with an uninterrupted ingestion and removal of microorganisms and their nutrients.

The oral cavity is an extremely varied landscape which forms a dynamic ecosystem with a range of ecological niches that microorganisms are able to colonize. It is an entry point for microbes through dietary intake, direct contact, inhalation, open-mouth breathing, and host-to-host contact. Colonization of the oral cavity is a selective process and not all microbes are well-adapted to thrive in this environment. The intraoral environment is subject to significant changes in the prevailing conditions at different times and at different sites within the oral cavity. The composition and diversity of the microbial community is therefore impacted by physical gradients of temperature, humidity, nutrient content, salivary flow, oxygen tension and n and pH, as well as shear forces due to mastication.

In order to persist in the oral cavity, microbes need to adhere to either the soft or hard tissues in order to avoid removal forces such as washing out by the salivary and crevicular flow, swallowing, frictional removal by diet and tongue and masticatory movements, and through oral hygiene regime. Surface features of distinct intraoral habitats providing opportunities for adhesion, therefore, have an impact on microbial colonization and distribution.

One of the major distinctions between intraoral environments colonized by microbes is whether microbial communities are formed on shedding (oral mucosa) or nonshedding surfaces (teeth, dental restorations, dental implants, or dental prostheses). The rapid turnover of oral lining epithelia (shedding three times per day) provides an effective mechanism to reduce bacterial adhesion to the soft tissues; the rapid turnover would allow less time for microbial communities to form. Nonshedding surfaces, such as the enamel surface of teeth, dental implants, and dental appliances, such as dentures and orthodontic appliances, are potentially susceptible to microbial colonization. Within each ecological niche, a number of physical and chemical factors have a selective effect on microbial communities at any one time, including salivary or gingival crevicular fluid (GCF) flow rates, pH and redox potential, and aspects of the host immune response.

Hard Tissues

In the human body, teeth and nails are the only naturally occurring nonshedding surfaces. From a microbiological viewpoint, teeth and implants are unique for two reasons: (1) they provide a hard, nonshedding surface that allows for the development of extensive structured bacterial deposits; and (2) they form a unique ectodermal interruption. A special seal of epithelium (junctional epithelium) and connective tissue is present between the external environment and the internal parts of the body.

The accumulation and metabolism of bacteria on these hard surfaces are considered the primary causes of caries, gingivitis, periodontitis, peri-implantitis, and, sometimes, bad breath. The teeth provide hard, smooth, nonshedding surfaces that are accessible to microbial colonization both above the gum line (supragingival) and below the gum line (subgingival) and have been reported to account for approximately 20% of the total surface area of the oral cavity. The teeth are bathed in saliva which enables dispersal of microbes over the surfaces of the teeth. Areas of the teeth such as pits and fissures and proximal surfaces are more protected from salivary flow and also from the activity of the tongue. The rate of saliva flow, therefore, varies over individual tooth surfaces and varies based on tooth position, and these variations in saliva flow rate and saliva clearance can directly impact the physiology and ecology of microbial communities.

In patients suffering from the onset of periodontitis, the formation of periodontal pockets creates a subgingival ecological niche. Periodontal pocket formation leads to an increase in surface area for microbial colonization on the root surface of teeth leading to the development of a subgingival microbial biofilm. A periodontal pocket has a subgingival tooth surface available for colonization and also the gingival tissue forming one side of the pocket. The increased surface area available for colonization by microorganisms can lead to a significant increase in microbial load between periodontal health and periodontitis. Deeper periodontal pockets lead to the development of low-oxygen microhabitats which favor colonization by anaerobic bacteria. Localized inflammation results from increased microbial colonization of this subgingival environment, leading to increases in temperature and GCF flow rate. The increased flow of GCF provides proteins and glycoproteins that can be used as substrates for bacterial metabolism.

The environmental parameters of the subgingival region differ from those of the supragingival region. The gingiva surrounding the teeth provide a keratinized stratified squamous epithelium and the juncture with the teeth creates a nutrient-rich crevice. The gingival crevice or pocket is bathed by the flow of crevicular fluid, which is derived from serum and contains many substances that bacteria may use as nutrients. There can be variations in temperature in the gingival sulcus, depending on whether the gingival tissues are in a state of health or disease. Host inflammatory cells and mediators are likely to have considerable influence on the establishment and growth of bacteria in the subgingival region. Studies of subgingival biofilm reveal distinctions between the tooth-associated regions and the soft tissue-associated regions of subgingival dental biofilms (Fig. 8.2A–C). In periodontal pockets, there are high numbers of bacteria attached to pocket epithelial cells in vivo. Areas of gingival inflammation are characterized by an increased number of adhering bacteria. These adhering bacteria can also infiltrate the pocket wall in relatively large numbers and reach the underlying stroma. In general, a positive correlation exists between the adhesion rate of pathogenic bacteria to different epithelia and the susceptibility of the affected patient to certain infections.

Soft Tissues

The dorsum of the tongue, especially where covered with papillae, creates an environment with crevices with low oxygen tension suitable for anaerobic bacteria. The hard palate comprises a firmer keratinized epithelium. The flexible lining mucosa of the floor of the mouth, buccal mucosa, soft palate, and labial mucosa lacks keratinization. The buccal mucosa is characterized by a high oxygen concentration, lubrication by saliva, and has a high rate of desquamation of epithelial cells. Mucosal surfaces are covered in a pellicle that is distinct from the enamel pellicle. While it is also a subset of salivary proteins, the mucosal pellicle is thought to be composed mainly of large molecular weight glycoproteins such as salivary mucins. Evidence suggests it has a protective role involved in lubrication of the oral epithelia and moisture retention and also protects against excessive bacterial colonization.

Tooth surfaces and oral epithelia are likely to provide different receptors to enable bacterial adhesion and would also most likely be associated with different antagonistic and synergistic species interactions which would exert influence on microbial colonization.

In health, a core set of microorganisms is almost universally present in these ecosystems. This core microbiome includes members of the phyla Firmicutes (*Streptococcus* spp., *Veillonella* spp., and *Granulicatella* spp.), Proteobacteria (*Neisseria* spp., *Campylobacter* spp., and *Haemophilus* spp.), Actinobacteria (*Corynebacterium* spp., *Rothia* spp., and *Actinomyces* spp.), Bacteroidetes (*Prevotella* spp., *Capnocytophaga* spp., and *Porphyromonas* spp.), and Fusobacteria (*Fusobacterium* spp.).

In the periodontal pocket, different strategies contribute to bacterial survival, such as adhesion to the pocket epithelium and, when dentin is encountered, the colonization of the dentinal tubules. The crevicular fluid with its constant outflow does not favor the maintenance of unattached bacteria in the periodontal pocket.

Investigators have suggested that teeth are the primary habitat for periodontopathogens because soon after a full-mouth tooth extraction in patients with severe periodontitis, key pathogens such as *Aggregatibacter actinomycetemcomitans* and *Porphyromonas gingivalis* disappear from the oral cavity, as determined by bacterial culturing techniques. *Prevotella intermedia* and other black-pigmented *Prevotella* spp. remain but at lower detection frequencies and numbers.

The same applies to edentulous infants and wearers of full dentures in whom significant proportions of periodontopathogens have been recorded, with the exception of *A. actinomycetemcomitans* and *P. gingivalis*. Therefore, teeth were considered as a port of entry for periodontopathogens.

Bacteria and their Biofilm Mode of Living

Biofilms are composed of microbial cells encased within a matrix of extracellular polymeric substances, such as polysaccharides, proteins, and nucleic acids.

Biofilm bacteria are often up to 1000 times more resistant to antimicrobial agents than their planktonic counterparts. Bacteria that grow in multispecies biofilms interact closely with neighboring cells. Sometimes these interactions are mutually beneficial, as is the case when one organism removes another organism's waste products and uses them as an energy source.

In other instances, bacteria compete with their neighbors by secreting antibacterial molecules, such as inhibitory peptides (bacteriocins) or hydrogen peroxide (H_2O_2). In addition, the biofilm mode of growth facilitates cell–cell signaling and deoxyribonucleic acid (DNA) exchange between bacteria. It is clear that microbial ecology within biofilm communities is highly complex and that, in many cases, knowledge is only emerging at this point.

Biofilms are heterogeneous: variations in biofilm structure exist within individual biofilms, between different types of biofilms, and between individuals. However, some structural features that are common to many biofilms have been noted. For example, biofilms frequently contain microcolonies of bacterial cells. Water channels are commonly found in biofilms, and these can form a primitive circulatory system that removes waste products and brings fresh nutrients to the deeper layers of the film. The bacteria exist and proliferate within the intercellular matrix through which the channels run. The matrix confers a specialized environment that distinguishes the bacteria that exist within the biofilm from those that are free floating; this is the so-called planktonic state in solutions such as saliva or crevicular fluid. The biofilm matrix functions as a barrier. Substances produced by bacteria within the biofilm are retained and concentrated, which fosters metabolic interactions among the different bacteria.

Dental Plaque Biofilm

Dental plaque is composed primarily of microorganisms encased within an extracellular matrix. One gram of plaque (wet weight) contains approximately 10^{11} bacteria. The number of bacteria in supragingival plaque on a single tooth surface can exceed 10^9 cells. In a periodontal pocket, counts can range from 10^3 bacteria in a healthy crevice to more than 10^8 bacteria in a deep pocket. It has been estimated that more than 500 distinct microbial phylotypes can be present as natural inhabitants of dental plaque.

Any individual may harbor 150 or more different species. Nonbacterial microorganisms that are found in plaque include archaea, yeasts, protozoa, and viruses.

The intercellular matrix consists of organic and inorganic materials derived from saliva, GCF, and bacterial products.

Organic constituents of the matrix include polysaccharides, proteins, glycoproteins, lipid material, and DNA. Albumin, which probably originates from crevicular fluid, has been identified as a component of the plaque matrix. The lipid material consists of debris from the membranes of disrupted bacterial and host cells, bacterial vesicles, and possibly food debris. *Glycoproteins* from the saliva are important components of the pellicle that initially coats a clean tooth surface, but they also become incorporated into the developing plaque biofilm. Polysaccharides produced by bacteria also contribute to the organic portion of the matrix. They play a major role in maintaining the integrity of the biofilm.

The *inorganic components* of plaque are predominantly calcium and phosphorus, with trace amounts of other minerals such as sodium, potassium, and fluoride. The source of inorganic constituents of supragingival plaque is primarily saliva. As the mineral content increases, the plaque mass becomes calcified to form calculus. Calculus is frequently found in areas of the dentition adjacent to salivary ducts (e.g., the lingual surface of the mandibular incisors and canines, the buccal surface of the maxillary first molars), and this reflects the high concentration of minerals available from saliva in those regions. The inorganic components of subgingival plaque are derived from crevicular fluid (a serum transudate). The calcification of subgingival plaque also results in calculus formation. Subgingival calculus is typically dark green or dark brown, which probably reflects the presence of blood products that are associated with subgingival hemorrhage.

Structure of a Mature Dental Plaque Biofilm

Dental plaque (see Fig. 8.1) is defined clinically as a structured, resilient, yellow-grayish substance that adheres tenaciously to the intraoral hard surfaces, including removable and fixed restorations. The tough extracellular matrix makes it impossible to remove plaque by rinsing or with the use of sprays. Plaque can thus be differentiated from other deposits that may be found on the tooth surface, such as materia alba and calculus. *Materia alba* refers to soft accumulations of bacteria, food matter, and tissue cells that lack the organized structure of dental plaque and that are easily displaced with a water spray. *Calculus* is a hard deposit that forms via the mineralization of dental plaque and that is generally covered by a layer of unmineralized plaque (Table 8.1).

Dental plaque is broadly classified as supragingival or subgingival on the basis of its position on the tooth surface toward the gingival margin.

- *Supragingival plaque* is found at or above the gingival margin; when in direct contact with the gingival margin, it is referred to as *marginal plaque.*
- *Subgingival plaque* is found below the gingival margin, between the tooth, and the gingival pocket epithelium.

Supragingival plaque typically demonstrates the stratified organization of a multilayered accumulation of bacterial morphotypes.

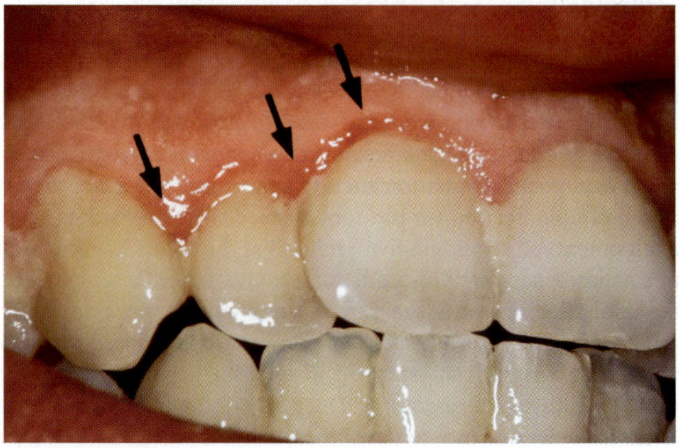

Fig. 8.1 Clinical picture of a 10-day-old supragingival plaque. The first signs of gingival inflammation (*arrows*) are becoming visible.

TABLE 8.1 Differences Between Tooth Deposits

Materia Alba	Dental Plaque	Calculus
• White, cheese-like accumulation	• Resilient clear to yellow-grayish substance	• Hard deposit that forms via the mineralization of dental plaque
• Soft accumulation of salivary proteins, some bacteria, many desquamated epithelial cells, and occasional disintegrating food debris	• Primarily composed of bacteria in a matrix of salivary glycoproteins and extracellular polysaccharides	• Generally covered by a layer of unmineralized dental plaque
• Lacks an organized structure and is therefore not as complex as dental plaque	• Considered to be a biofilm	
• Easily displaced with a water spray	• Impossible to remove by rinsing or with the use of sprays	

Gram-positive cocci and short rods predominate at the tooth surface, whereas gram-negative rods, filaments, and spirochetes predominate in the outer surface of the mature plaque mass.

In general, the subgingival microbiota differs in composition from the supragingival plaque, primarily because of the local availability of blood products and a low reduction–oxidation (redox) potential, which characterizes the anaerobic environment.

The environmental parameters of the subgingival region differ from those of the supragingival region. The gingival crevice or pocket is bathed by the flow of crevicular fluid, which contains many substances that bacteria may use as nutrients. Host inflammatory cells and mediators are likely to have considerable influence on the establishment and growth of bacteria in the subgingival region. Both morphologic and microbiologic studies of subgingival plaque reveal distinctions between the tooth-associated regions and the soft tissue-associated regions of subgingival plaque (see Fig. 8.2A–D).

The tooth-associated cervical plaque that adheres to the root cementum does not markedly differ from that observed in gingivitis. At this location, filamentous microorganisms dominate, but cocci and rods also occur. This plaque is dominated by gram-positive rods and cocci, including *S. mitis*, *S. sanguinis*, *Actinomyces oris*, *Actinomyces naeslundii*, and *Eubacterium* spp. However, in the deeper parts of the pocket, the filamentous organisms become fewer in number; in the apical portion, they seem to be virtually absent. Instead, the microbiota is dominated by smaller organisms without a particular orientation. The apical border of the plaque mass is separated from the junctional epithelium by a layer of host leukocytes, and the bacterial population of this apical tooth-associated region shows an increased concentration of gram-negative rods.

The layers of microorganisms that face the soft tissue lack a definite intermicrobial matrix and contain primarily gram-negative rods and cocci, as well as large numbers of filaments, flagellated rods, and spirochetes. Studies of plaque associated with crevicular epithelial cells indicate a predominance of species such as *S. oralis*, *Streptococcus intermedius*, *Parvimonas micra* (formerly *Micromonas micros* and *Peptostreptococcus micros*), *P. gingivalis*, *P. intermedia*, *Tannerella forsythia*, and *Fusobacterium nucleatum*. Host–tissue cells (e.g., white blood cells, epithelial cells) may also be found in this region. Bacteria are also found within the host tissues, such as in the soft tissues, and within epithelial cells, as well as in the dentinal tubules.

The composition of the subgingival plaque depends on the pocket depth. The apical part is more dominated by spirochetes, cocci, and rods, whereas in the coronal part, more filaments are observed.

The site specificity of plaque is significantly associated with diseases of the periodontium. Marginal plaque, for example, is of prime importance during the initiation and development of gingivitis. Supragingival plaque and tooth-associated subgingival plaque are critical in calculus formation and root caries, whereas tissue-associated subgingival plaque is important in the tissue destruction that characterizes different forms of periodontitis. Biofilms also establish on artificial surfaces exposed to the oral environment, such as prostheses and implants.

Formation of Dental Plaque Biofilm

The process of plaque formation can be divided into following several phases: (1) the formation of the pellicle on the tooth surface, (2) the initial adhesion/attachment of bacteria, and (3) colonization/plaque maturation.

Formation of the Pellicle

All surfaces in the oral cavity, including the hard and soft tissues, are coated with a layer of organic material known as the acquired pellicle. The pellicle on tooth surfaces consists of more than 180 peptides, proteins, and glycoproteins, including keratins, mucins, proline-rich proteins, phosphoproteins (e.g., statherin), histidine-rich proteins, and other molecules that can function as adhesion sites (receptors) for bacteria. The salivary pellicle can be detected on clean enamel surfaces within 1 min after their introduction into the mouths of volunteers. By 2 h, the pellicle is essentially in equilibrium between adsorption and detachment, although further pellicle maturation can be observed for several hours.

Consequently, bacteria that adhere to tooth surfaces do not contact the enamel directly but interact with the acquired enamel pellicle. However, the pellicle is not merely a passive adhesion matrix. Many proteins retain enzymatic activity when they are incorporated into the pellicle, and some of these, such as peroxidases, lysozyme, and α-amylase, may affect the physiology and metabolism of adhering bacterial cells.

Initial Adhesion/Attachment of Bacteria

The initial steps of transport and interaction with the surface are essentially nonspecific (i.e., they are the same for all bacteria). The specific interactions between microbial cell surface "adhesin" molecules and receptors in the salivary pellicle determine whether a bacterial cell will remain associated with the surface. Only a relatively small proportion of oral bacteria possess adhesins that interact with receptors in the host pellicle, and these organisms are generally the most abundant bacteria in biofilms on tooth enamel shortly after cleaning. Over the first 4–8 h, the genus *Streptococcus* tends to dominate, usually accounting for >20% of bacteria present. Other bacteria that commonly present at this time include species that cannot survive without oxygen (obligate aerobes), such

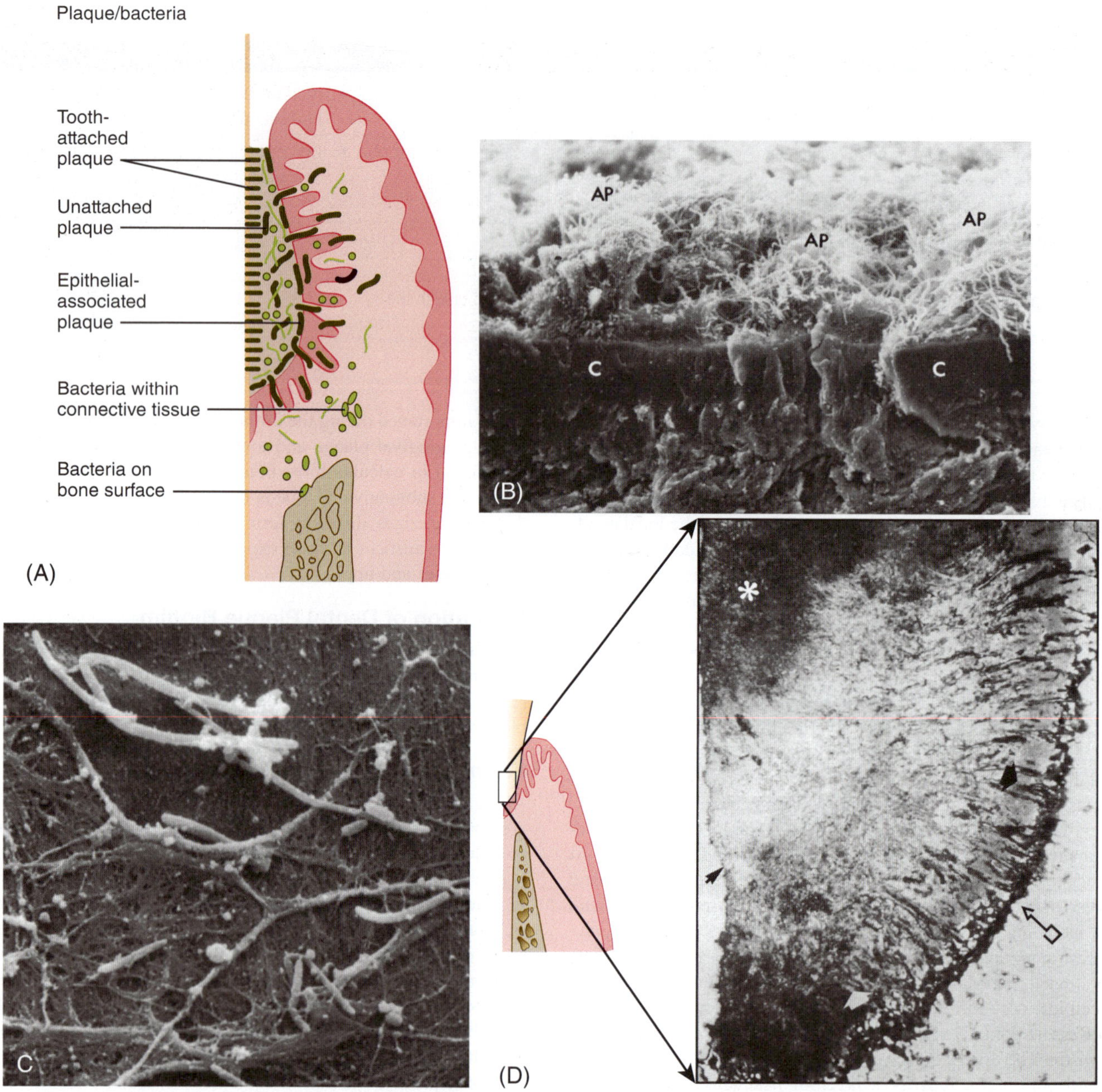

Fig. 8.2 A, Diagram depicting the plaque–bacteria association between the tooth surface and the periodontal tissues. B, Scanning electron photomicrograph of a cross-section of cementum (*C*) with attached subgingival plaque (*AP*). The area shown is within a periodontal pocket. C, Scanning electron micrograph of cocci and filaments associated with the surface of pocket epithelium in a case of marginal gingivitis (×3000). D, *Left*, Diagrammatic representation of the histologic structure of subgingival plaque. *Right*, Histologic section of subgingival plaque. *Arrow with box*, Sulcular epithelium. *White arrow*, Predominantly gram-negative unattached zone. *Black arrow*, Tooth surface. *Asterisk, Predominantly gram-positive attached zone. (B, Courtesy: Dr J. Sottosanti, La Jolla, CA.)*

as *Haemophilus* spp. and *Neisseria* spp., as well as organisms that can grow in the presence or absence of oxygen (facultative anaerobes) including *Actinomyces* spp. and *Veillonella* spp. These species are considered the "primary colonizers" of tooth surfaces. The primary colonizers provide new binding sites for adhesion by other oral bacteria. The metabolic activity of the primary colonizers modifies the local microenvironment in ways that can influence the ability of other bacteria to survive in the dental plaque biofilm. For example, by removing oxygen, the primary colonizers provide conditions of low oxygen tension that permit the survival and growth of obligate anaerobes.

Colonization and Plaque Maturation

The primary colonizing bacteria (Table 8.2) adhered to the tooth surface provide new receptors for attachment by other bacteria as part of a process known as *coadhesion*. Together with the growth of adherent microorganisms, coadhesion leads to the development of microcolonies and eventually to a mature biofilm.

When many genetically distinct bacteria adhere to each other and form clumps, it is referred to as *coaggregation.* Coaggregation is a direct interaction; it is distinct from agglutination, which occurs when cells are stuck together by molecules in solution. At least 18 genera from the oral cavity have shown some form of coaggregation.

TABLE 8.2 Overview of Primary and Secondary Colonizers in Dental Plaque

Primary colonizers	*Streptococcus gordonii* *Streptococcus intermedius* *Streptococcus mitis* *Streptococcus oralis* *Streptococcus sanguinis* *Actinomyces gerencseriae* *Actinomyces israelii* *Actinomyces naeslundii* *Actinomyces oris* *Aggregatibacter actinomycetemcomitans* serotype a *Capnocytophaga gingivalis* *Capnocytophaga ochracea* *Capnocytophaga sputigena* *Eikenella corrodens* *Actinomyces odontolyticus* *Veillonella parvula*
Secondary colonizers	*Campylobacter gracilis* *Campylobacter rectus* *Campylobacter showae* *Eubacterium nodatum* *Aggregatibacter actinomycetemcomitans* serotype b *Fusobacterium nucleatum* spp. *nucleatum* *Fusobacterium nucleatum* spp. *vincentii* *Fusobacterium nucleatum* spp. *polymorphum* *Fusobacterium periodonticum* *Parvimonas micra* *Prevotella intermedia* *Prevotella loescheii* *Prevotella nigrescens* *Streptococcus constellatus* *Tannerella forsythia* *Porphyromonas gingivalis* *Treponema denticola*

All oral bacteria possess surface molecules that foster some sort of cell–cell interaction (Fig. 8.6).

Different species—or even different strains of a single species—have distinct sets of coaggregation partners. Fusobacteria coaggregate with all other human oral bacteria, whereas *Veillonella* spp., *Capnocytophaga* spp., and *Prevotella* spp. bind with streptococci and/or actinomyces. Each newly accreted cell becomes itself a new surface and therefore may act as a coaggregation bridge to the next potentially accreting cell type that passes by.

Well-characterized interactions of secondary colonizers (see Table 8.2) with early colonizers include the coaggregation of *F. nucleatum* with *S. sanguinis*, *Prevotella loescheii* with *A. oris,* and *Capnocytophaga ochracea* with *A. oris.*

Secondary colonizers (see Table 8.2) such as *P. intermedia*, *P. loescheii*, *Capnocytophaga* spp., *F. nucleatum*, and *P. gingivalis* do not initially colonize clean tooth surfaces but rather adhere to bacteria that are already in the plaque mass. The transition from early supragingival dental plaque to mature plaque growing below the gingival margin involves a shift in the microbial population from primarily gram-positive organisms to high numbers of gram-negative bacteria. Therefore, during the later stages of plaque formation, coaggregation among different gram-negative species is likely to predominate. Examples of these types of interactions are the coaggregation of *F. nucleatum* with *P. gingivalis* or *Treponema denticola.*

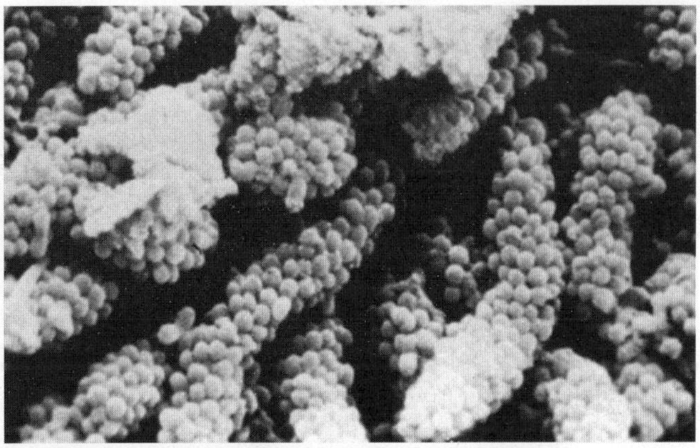

Fig. 8.3 Long-standing supragingival plaque near the gingival margin demonstrates a "corn cob" arrangement. A central gram-negative filamentous core supports the outer coccal cells that are firmly attached by interbacterial adherence or coaggregation.

The idea that coaggregation is important during the formation of oral biofilms opens new perspectives, especially for the use of probiotics. Special examples of coaggregations are the corn cob formation (Fig. 8.3), in which streptococci adhere to filaments of *Corynebacterium matruchotii* or *Actinomyces* spp., and the test-tube brush formation, composed of filamentous bacteria to which gram-negative rods adhere.

An analysis of more than 13,000 plaque samples that looked for 40 subgingival microorganisms using a DNA-hybridization methodology defined color-coded "complexes" of periodontal microorganisms that tend to be found together in health or disease. The composition of the different complexes was based on the frequency with which different clusters of microorganisms were recovered, and the complexes were color-coded for easy conceptualization (Fig. 8.4). Interestingly, the early colonizers are either independent of defined complexes (*A. naeslundii, A. oris*) or members of the yellow (*Streptococcus* spp.) or purple complexes (*Actinomyces odontolyticus*). The microorganisms primarily considered secondary colonizers fell into the green, orange, and red complexes. The green complex includes *Eikenella corrodens*, *A. actinomycetemcomitans* serotype a, and *Capnocytophaga* spp. The orange complex includes *Fusobacterium* spp., *Prevotella* spp., and *Campylobacter* spp. The green and orange complexes include species recognized as pathogens in periodontal and nonperiodontal infections. The red complex consists of *P. gingivalis*, *T. forsythia*, and *T. denticola.* This complex is of particular interest because it is associated with bleeding on probing. The existence of complexes of species in plaque is another reflection of bacterial interdependency in the biofilm environment.

Factors That Affect Supragingival Dental Plaque Formation

Clinically, early undisturbed plaque formation on teeth follows an exponential growth curve when measured planimetrically. During the first 24 h when starting with a clean tooth surface, plaque growth is negligible from a clinical viewpoint (i.e., $<3\%$ coverage of the vestibular tooth surface, which is an amount nearly undetectable clinically). This "lag time" is a result of the fact that the microbial population must reach a certain size before it can easily be detected by a clinician. During the following 3 days, coverage progresses rapidly to the point at which, after 4 days, an average of 30% of the total coronal tooth area will be covered with plaque.

The microbial composition of the dental plaque will change, with a shift toward a more anaerobic and a more gram-negative

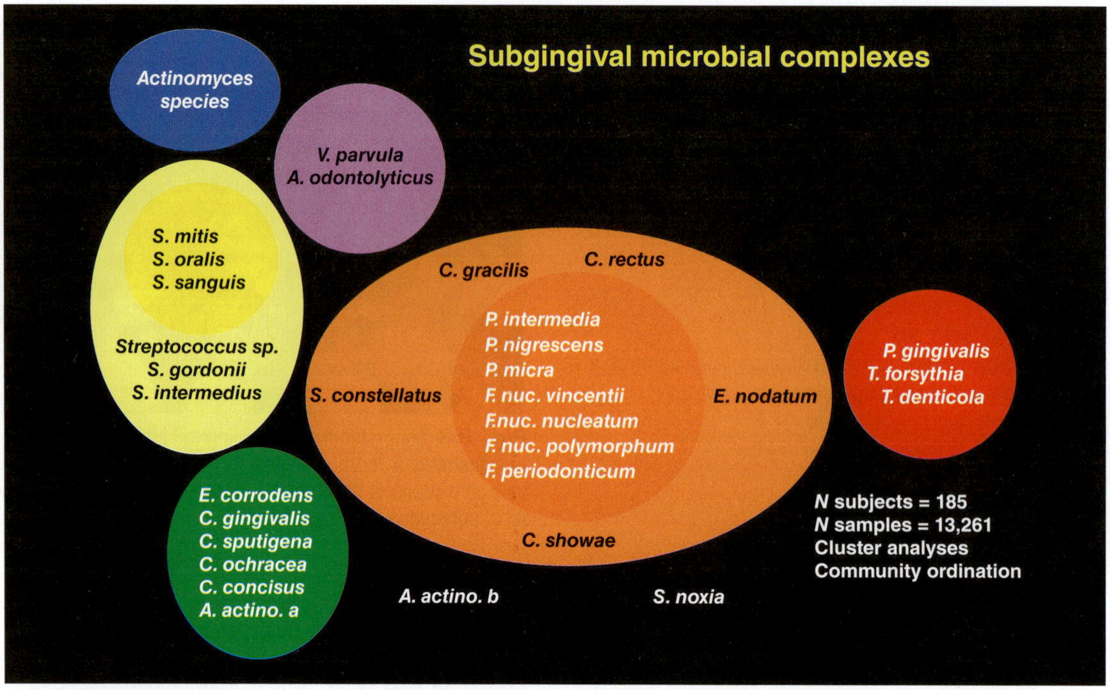

Fig. 8.4 A diagram of the association among subgingival species. The data were derived from 13,261 subgingival plaque samples taken from the mesial aspect of each tooth in 185 adult subjects. Each sample was individually analyzed for the presence of 40 subgingival species with the use of checkerboard DNA–DNA hybridization. Associations were sought among species via cluster analysis and community ordination techniques. The complexes to the left comprised species that are thought to colonize the tooth surface and to proliferate at an early stage. The orange complex becomes numerically dominant later; it is thought to bridge the early colonizers and the red complex species, which become numerically more dominant during the later stages of plaque development. *(Adapted from Socransky SS, Haffajee AD, Cugini MA, et al: J Clin Periodontol 25:134, 1998.)*

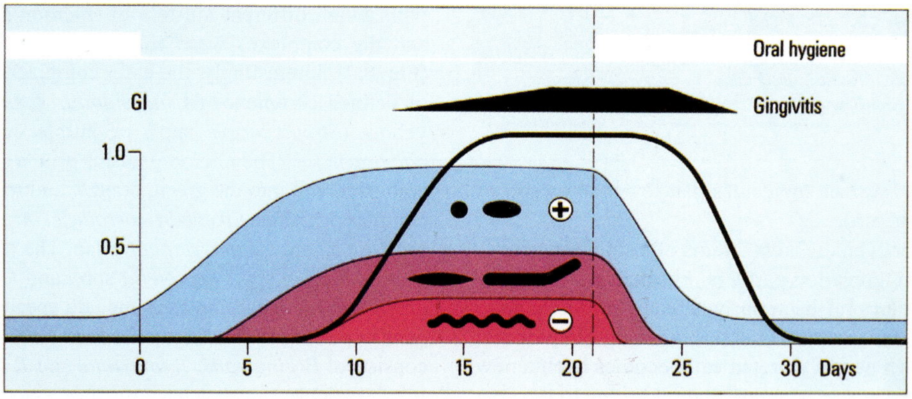

Fig. 8.5 Artistic impression of the 1965 published classic experimental proof of the bacterial etiology of gingivitis using the experimental gingivitis model. In plaque-free subjects with clinically noninflamed gingiva, plaque will slowly develop on the teeth when all mechanical plaque control is stopped. With time, the plaque composition changes. During the first few days, the plaque is mainly composed of gram-positive (+) cocci and rods. Later on, the composition is shifted toward more gram-negative species and more rods and filaments; finally, gram-negative (−) spirochetes appear (see morphotypes in *black*). Within a few days, mild gingivitis ensues (*black line*; gingival index [GI] of 1 according to Löe and Silness). From the moment that proper plaque control is re-established (*vertical line*), the plaque composition returns to the initial situation, and the symptoms of gingivitis disappear. *(From Löe H, Theilade E, Jensen SB: Experimental gingivitis in man. J Periodontol 36:177, 1965.)*

flora, including an influx of fusobacteria, filaments, spiral forms, and spirochetes (Fig. 8.5). This was clearly illustrated in experimental gingivitis studies. With this ecologic shift within the biofilm, a transition occurs from the early aerobic environment, which is characterized by gram-positive facultative species, to a highly oxygen-deprived environment, in which gram-negative anaerobic microorganisms predominate. Bacterial growth in older plaque is much slower than in newly formed dental plaque, presumably because nutrients become limiting for much of the plaque biomass.

Topography of Supragingival Plaque

Early plaque formation on teeth follows a typical topographic pattern, with initial growth along the gingival margin and from the interdental spaces (i.e., the areas protected from shear forces).

Later, a further extension in the coronal direction can be observed. This pattern may change severely when the tooth surface contains irregularities that offer a favorable growth path.

By multiplication, the bacteria subsequently spread out from these starting-up areas as a relatively even monolayer. Surface irregularities are also responsible for the so-called individualized plaque growth pattern, which is reproduced in the absence of optimal oral hygiene. This phenomenon illustrates the importance of surface roughness in plaque growth, which should lead to proper clinical treatment options.

Surface Microroughness

Rough intraoral surfaces (e.g., crown margins, implant abutments, denture bases) accumulate and retain more plaque and calculus in terms of thickness, area, and colony-forming units. Ample plaque also reveals an increased maturity or pathogenicity of its bacterial components, which is characterized by an increased proportion of motile organisms and spirochetes and/or a denser packing of them. Smoothing an intraoral surface decreases the rate of plaque formation.

Individual Variables That Influence Plaque Formation

The rate of plaque formation differs significantly among subjects, and these differences may overrule surface characteristics. A distinction is often made between "heavy" (fast) and "light" (slow) plaque formers.

A multiple regression analysis showed that the clinical wettability of the tooth surfaces, the saliva-induced aggregation of oral bacteria, and the relative salivary flow conditions around the sampled teeth explained 90% of the variation.

Variation Within the Dentition

Within a dental arch, large differences in plaque growth rate can be detected. In general, early plaque formation occurs faster: in the lower jaw (as compared to the upper jaw); in molar areas; on the buccal tooth surfaces (as compared to palatal sites, especially in the upper jaw); and in the interdental regions (as compared to the buccal or lingual surfaces).

Impact of Gingival Inflammation and Saliva

Several studies clearly indicate that early in vivo plaque formation is more rapid on tooth surfaces facing inflamed gingival margins than on those adjacent to healthy gingivae. These studies suggest that the increase in crevicular fluid production enhances plaque formation. Probably some substances from this exudate (e.g., minerals, proteins, carbohydrates) favor both the initial adhesion and/or the growth of the early colonizing bacteria. In addition, it is known that, during the night, the plaque growth rate is reduced by some 50%. This seems surprising because one would expect that reduced plaque removal and the decreased salivary flow at night would enhance plaque growth. The fact that the supragingival plaque obtains its nutrients mainly from the saliva appears to be of greater significance than the antibacterial activity of saliva.

Impact of Patient's Age

There are various factors that may influence dental biofilm formation in more elderly patients. Various studies have reported that more elderly patients have reduced salivary flow rates and changes in salivary composition. This may be due to the effects of medication, associated with medical conditions, or as a result of age-related physiological changes. A reduction in salivary flow bathing the oral tissues may impact on the ability to wash away oral bacteria and food debris and this may affect the formation of supragingingival dental biofilms. Elderly patients may also have reduced manual dexterity, which could affect the ability to effectively perform an adequate oral hygiene regime to mechanically disrupt and remove dental biofilms.

BOX 8.1 Properties of Plaque Biofilm

- It is composed of microbial cells encased within a matrix of extracellular polymeric substances, such as polysaccharides, proteins, and nucleic acids.
- The presence of voids or water channels which permits passage of nutrients and acts as a primitive circulatory system.
- Biofilm bacteria are 1000–1500 times resistant to antibiotics than planktonic bacteria.
- Exchange of genetic information among bacteria.
- In biofilm, quorum sensing is the capacity of bacteria to communicate with each other.

Characteristics of Biofilm Bacteria (Box 8.1)

Metabolism of Dental Plaque Bacteria

Most nutrients for dental plaque bacteria originate from saliva or GCF, although the host diet provides an occasional but nevertheless important food supply. The transition from gram-positive to gram-negative microorganisms observed in the structural development of dental plaque is paralleled by a physiologic transition in the developing plaque.

The early colonizers (e.g., *Streptococcus* and *Actinomyces* spp.) use oxygen and lower the redox potential of the environment, which then favors the growth of anaerobic species. Many of the gram-positive early colonizers use sugars as an energy source. The bacteria that predominate in mature plaque are anaerobic and asaccharolytic (i.e., they do not break down sugars), and they use amino acids and small peptides as energy sources.

Laboratory studies have demonstrated many metabolic interactions among the different bacteria found in dental plaque (Fig. 8.6). For example, lactate and formate are byproducts of the metabolism of streptococci and *Actinomyces* spp.; they may be used in the metabolism of other plaque microorganisms, including *Veillonella* spp. and *A. actinomycetemcomitans*.

The growth of *P. gingivalis* is also enhanced by metabolic byproducts produced by other microorganisms, such as succinate from *C. ochracea* or *T. denticola* and protoheme from *Campylobacter rectus*. In turn, *P. gingivalis* provides isobutyric acid that stimulates growth of *T. denticola*. Overall, the total plaque population is more efficient than any one constituent organism at releasing energy from the available substrates.

Metabolic interactions also occur between the host and the plaque microorganisms. The bacterial enzymes that degrade host proteins mediate the release of ammonia, which may be used by bacteria as a nitrogen source. Hemin iron from the breakdown of host hemoglobin may be important in the metabolism of *P. gingivalis*. Increases in steroid hormones are associated with significant increases in the proportions of *P. intermedia* found in subgingival plaque. These nutritional interdependencies are probably critical to the growth and survival of microorganisms in dental plaque, and they may partly explain the evolution of the highly specific structural interactions observed among bacteria in plaque.

Communication Between Biofilm Bacteria

Bacterial cells do not exist in isolation. In a biofilm, bacteria have the capacity to communicate with each other. One example of this is *quorum sensing*, in which bacteria secrete a signaling molecule

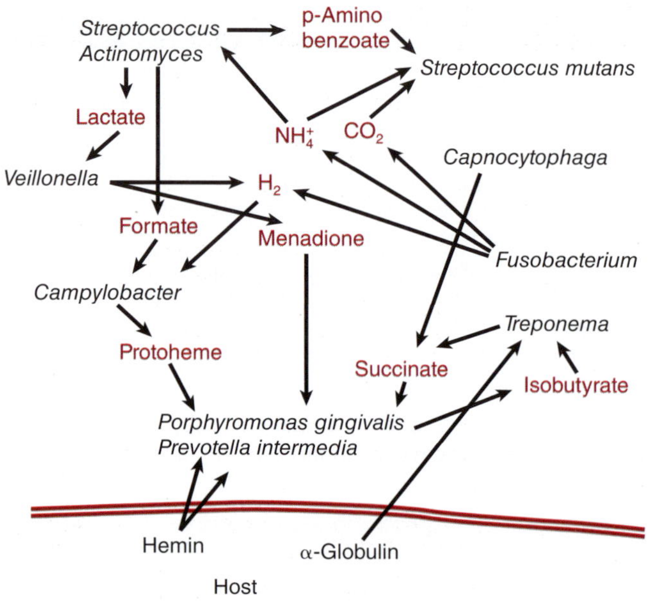

Fig. 8.6 Schematic illustration of metabolic interactions among different bacterial species found in plaque and between the host and the plaque bacteria. These interactions are likely to be important to the survival of bacteria in the periodontal environment. *CO_2*, Carbon dioxide; *H_2*, hydrogen; *$NH^{!}_4$*, ammonium. *(Data from Carlsson J: Microbiology of plaque associated periodontal disease. In Lindhe J, editor: Textbook of clinical periodontology, Munksgrd, 1983, Munksgrd International Publishers; Grenier D: Nutritional interactions between two suspected periodontopathogens, Treponema denticola and Porphyromonas gingivalis. Infect Immun 60:5298, 1992; Loesche WJ: Importance of nutrition in gingival crevice microbial ecology. Periodontics 6:245, 1968; and Walden WC, Hentges DJ: Differential effects of oxygen and oxidation-reduction potential on the multiplication of three species of anaerobic intestinal bacteria. Appl Microbiol 30:781, 1975.)*

that accumulates in the local environment and triggers a response such as a change in the expression of specific genes once they reach a critical threshold concentration. The threshold concentration is reached only at a high cell density, and therefore bacteria sense that the population has reached a critical mass or quorum.

Quorum sensing appears to play diverse roles in, for example, modulating the expression of genes for antibiotic resistance, encouraging the growth of beneficial species in the biofilm, and discouraging the growth of competitors.

Biofilms and Antimicrobial Resistance

Bacteria growing in microbial communities adherent to a surface do not "behave" the same way as bacteria growing suspended in a liquid environment (i.e., in a planktonic or unattached state). For example, the resistance of bacteria to antimicrobial agents is dramatically increased in the biofilm. Almost without exception, organisms in a biofilm are 1000–1500 times more resistant as compared to antibiotics in their planktonic state. The mechanisms of this increased resistance differ from species to species, from antibiotic to antibiotic, and for biofilms growing in different habitats.

An important mechanism of resistance appears to be the slower rate of growth of bacterial species in a biofilm, which makes them less susceptible to many but not all antibiotics. The biofilm matrix, although not a significant physical barrier to the diffusion of antibiotics, does have certain properties that can retard antibiotic penetration. For example, strongly charged or chemically highly reactive agents can fail to reach the deeper zones of the biofilm because the biofilm acts as an ion-exchange resin that removes such molecules from solution.

In addition, extracellular enzymes such as β-lactamases, formaldehyde lyase, and formaldehyde dehydrogenase may become trapped and concentrated in the extracellular matrix and as such inactivate some antibiotics (especially positively charged hydrophilic antibiotics).

Some antibiotics, such as the macrolides, which are positively charged but hydrophobic, are unaffected by this process.

"Superresistant" bacteria were identified within a biofilm. These cells have multidrug resistance pumps that can extrude antimicrobial agents from the cell. Because these pumps place the antibiotics outside of the outer membrane, the process offers protection against antibiotics that target, for example, cell wall synthesis. The penetration and efficacy of antimicrobials against biofilm bacteria are critical issues for the treatment of periodontal infections.

Antibiotic resistance may be spread through a biofilm via the intercellular exchange of DNA. The high density of bacterial cells in a biofilm facilitates the exchange of genetic information among cells of the same species and across species and even across genera. Conjugation (i.e., the exchange of genes through a direct interbacteria connection formed by a sex pilus), transformation (i.e., the movement of small pieces of DNA from the environment into the bacterial chromosome), plasmid transfer, and transposon transfer have all been shown to occur in biofilms.

Bacterial Transmission and Translocation

The transmission of pathogens from one *locus* to another is an important aspect of infectious diseases. In theory, such transmission may jeopardize the outcome of periodontal therapy; in addition, the transmission of pathogens from one person to another may be important in terms of disease transmission. The significance of such an intraoral transmission or of a vertical or horizontal transmission is, however, difficult to prove or to quantify.

Molecular fingerprinting techniques have clearly illustrated that periodontal pathogens are transmissible within members of a family.

The existence of an "intraoral" translocation of bacteria (i.e., from one niche to another) has been investigated more thoroughly.

Previously noninfected pockets may get colonized with *A. actinomycetemcomitans* via a single course of probing with a probe that had been previously inserted in an infected pocket of the same patient.

Quirynen and coworkers used a treatment strategy called "one-stage, full-mouth disinfection" to investigate the impact of intraoral translocation on the outcome of nonsurgical periodontal therapy. This strategy attempted to suppress the translocation of periodontopathogens from all of their intraoral habitats (i.e., mucous membranes, tongue, and saliva) to root-planed periodontal pockets. Several comparative studies between the one-stage, full-mouth approach and the standard therapy (i.e., root planing per quadrant with 2-week intervals that allow for translocation) have shown that one-stage full-mouth disinfection leads to gain in attachment, pocket-depth reduction, and significantly lower pathogenic microorganisms (refer Chapter 30).

Role of Viruses in the Pathogenesis of Periodontitis

Viruses are important ulcerogenic and tumorigenic agents of the human mouth. The finding of an abundance of mammalian viruses in periodontitis lesions may suggest a role for viruses in more oral diseases than previously recognized. Bacteria are recognized as indispensable for the development of periodontitis, and the current hypotheses regarding the pathogenic mechanisms of periodontitis emphasize the importance of assessing bacterial and host factors collectively. Sole bacterial–host interactions appear insufficient to explain the clinical characteristics of the disease. The localized distribution and intermittent exacerbations of periodontal breakdown and other issues remain a riddle. In response, the involvement of *herpesviruses* in the etiology of periodontitis has been suggested on the basis of their increased presence in inflamed gingival tissue, crevicular fluid, and subgingival plaque in periodontally diseased sites and their potential to induce proinflammatory cytokines. However, it remains unclear whether herpesvirus activation occurs spontaneously or as a result of concurrent infection, stress, or other immunosuppressive factors. Several risk factors for periodontitis also have the potential to reactivate herpesviruses. Bacterioviral synergism may play an important role in the onset and progression of periodontitis. However, the hypothesis that herpesviruses are involved in the etiology of periodontitis is still controversial. No doubt exists that herpesviruses are present in the periodontal pocket. Next to herpesviruses, many other viruses have been detected in periodontal pockets. Papillomaviruses, HIV, human T-lymphotropic virus type I, hepatitis B and C viruses, and torque teno virus can all inhabit periodontitis lesions. In addition, the inflamed periodontium may constitute the major oral reservoir for EBV, CMV, papillomaviruses, and hepatitis C virus.

Microbiologic Specificity of Periodontal Diseases

Nonspecific Plaque Hypothesis

During the mid-1900s, periodontal diseases were thought to result from an accumulation of plaque over time, eventually in conjunction with a diminished host response and increased host susceptibility with age. This theory, which is called the *nonspecific plaque hypothesis*, was supported by epidemiologic studies that correlated both age and the amount of plaque with evidence of periodontitis.

According to the nonspecific plaque hypothesis, periodontal disease results from the "elaboration of noxious products by the entire plaque flora." When only small amounts of plaque are present, the noxious products are neutralized by the host. Similarly, large amounts of plaque would cause a higher production of noxious products, which would essentially overwhelm the host's defenses.

Several observations contradicted these conclusions. First, some individuals with considerable amounts of plaque and calculus, as well as gingivitis, never developed destructive periodontitis. Furthermore, individuals who did present with periodontitis demonstrated considerable site specificity with regard to the pattern of disease. Some sites were unaffected, whereas advanced disease was found in adjacent sites. In the presence of a uniform host response, these findings were inconsistent with the concept that all plaque was equally pathogenic. Recognition of the differences in plaque at sites of different clinical status (i.e., disease versus health) led to a renewed search for specific pathogens in periodontal diseases and a conceptual transition from the nonspecific to the specific plaque hypothesis.

Inherent in the nonspecific plaque hypothesis is the concept that the control of periodontal disease depends on the reduction of the total amount of plaque. The current standard treatment of periodontitis by debridement (nonsurgical or surgical) and oral hygiene measures still focuses on the removal of plaque and its products. Although the nonspecific plaque hypothesis has been discarded in favor of other etiologic hypotheses, most of the therapeutic interventions are still based on the basic principles of the nonspecific plaque hypothesis.

Specific Plaque Hypothesis

The specific plaque hypothesis underlines the importance of the qualitative composition of the resident microbiota. The pathogenicity of dental plaque depends on the presence of or an increase in specific microorganisms. This concept encapsulates that plaque that harbors specific bacterial pathogens may provoke periodontal disease because key organisms produce substances that mediate the destruction of host tissues. The association of specific bacterial species with disease came about during the early 1960s, when the microscopic examination of plaque revealed that different bacterial morphotypes were found in healthy versus periodontally diseased sites. At about the same time, major advances were made in the techniques used to isolate and identify periodontal microorganisms. These included improvements in procedures to sample subgingival plaque, in the handling of samples to prevent killing the bacteria, and in the media used to grow the bacteria in the laboratory. The results were a tremendous increase in the ability to isolate periodontal microorganisms and considerable refinement in bacterial taxonomy. Acceptance of the specific plaque hypothesis was spurred by the recognition of *A. actinomycetemcomitans* as a pathogen in localized aggressive periodontitis. These advances led to a series of association studies focused on identifying specific periodontal pathogens by examining the microbiota associated with states of health and disease in cross-sectional and longitudinal studies.

Criteria for the Identification of Periodontopathogens

During the 1870s, Robert Koch developed the classic criteria by which a microorganism can be judged to be a causative agent in human infections. These criteria, known as Koch's postulates, stipulate that the causative agent must do the following:

1. Be routinely isolated from diseased individuals.
2. Be grown in pure culture in the laboratory.
3. Produce a similar disease when inoculated into susceptible laboratory animals.
4. Be recovered from lesions in a diseased laboratory animal.

Difficulties exist with regard to the application of these criteria to polymicrobial diseases, and the applicability of Koch's postulates has been increasingly challenged. In the case of periodontitis, three primary problems exist: (1) the inability to culture all of the organisms that have been associated with disease (e.g., many of the oral spirochetes), (2) the difficulties inherent in defining and culturing sites of active disease, and (3) the lack of a good animal model system for the study of periodontitis. In fact, if the ecologic plaque hypothesis proves correct, it must be inherently impossible to fulfill Koch's postulates because no single organism or group of organisms is responsible for all cases of disease.

Sigmund Socransky, a researcher at the Forsyth Dental Center in Boston, proposed criteria by which periodontal microorganisms may be judged to be potential pathogens. According to these criteria, a potential pathogen must do the following:

1. Be associated with disease, as evidenced by increases in the number of organisms at diseased sites.
2. Be eliminated or decreased in sites that demonstrate the clinical resolution of disease with treatment.
3. Induce a host response in the form of an alteration in the host cellular or humoral immune response.
4. Be capable of causing disease in experimental animal models.
5. Produce demonstrable virulence factors that are responsible for enabling the microorganism to cause the destruction of the periodontal tissues.

These criteria support the role of *A. actinomycetemcomitans* as a periodontal pathogen in the pathogenesis of localized aggressive periodontitis.

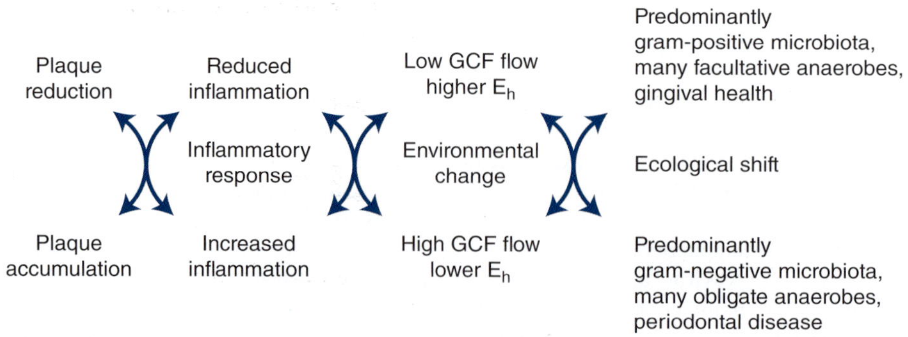

Fig. 8.7 Ecologic plaque hypothesis in relation to periodontal diseases: gingivitis and periodontitis. The accumulation of plaque causes the inflammation of adjacent tissues (gingivitis) and other environmental changes that favor the growth of gram-negative anaerobes and proteolytic species, including periodontopathogens. The increased proportions of such species result in the destruction of periodontal tissues (i.e., periodontitis). *E_h*, Redox potential; *GCF*, gingival crevicular fluid. *(Adapted from Marsh PD: Microbial ecology of dental plaque and its significance in health and disease. Adv Dent Res 8:263, 1994.)*

Ecologic Plaque Hypothesis

During the 1990s, Marsh and coworkers developed the "ecologic plaque hypothesis" as an attempt to unify the existing theories regarding the role of dental plaque in oral disease (Fig. 8.7). According to the ecologic plaque hypothesis, both the total amount of dental plaque and the specific microbial composition of plaque may contribute to the transition from health to disease. The health-associated dental plaque microbiota is considered to be relatively stable over time and in a state of dynamic equilibrium or "microbial homeostasis." The host controls subgingival plaque to some extent by a tempered immune response and low levels of GCF flow. Perturbations to the host response may be brought about by an excessive accumulation of nonspecific dental plaque, by plaque-independent host factors [e.g., the onset of an immune disorder, changes in hormonal balance (e.g., during pregnancy)], or by environmental factors (e.g., smoking, diet).

Changes in the host status, such as inflammation, tissue degradation, and/or high GCF flow, may lead to a shift in the microbial population in plaque. As a result of microenvironmental changes, the number of beneficial species may decrease, whereas the number of potentially pathogenic species increases. This gradual shift in the entire microbial community, known as *dysbiosis*, may result in a chronic disease state such as periodontitis. The ecologic plaque hypothesis is entirely consistent with observations that disease-associated organisms are minor components of the oral microbiota in health; these organisms are kept in check by interspecies competition during microbial homeostasis. Disease is associated with the overgrowth of specific members of the dental plaque biofilm when the local microenvironment changes, but it is not necessarily the same species in each case. An important consideration of the ecologic plaque hypothesis is that therapeutic intervention can be useful on a number of different levels. Eliminating the etiologic stimulus—whether it is microbial, host, or environmental—will help to restore microbial homeostasis. Targeting specific microorganisms may be less effective because the conditions for disease will remain.

Keystone Pathogen Hypothesis and Polymicrobial Synergy and Dysbiosis Model

The keystone pathogen hypothesis indicates that certain low-abundance microbial pathogens can orchestrate inflammatory disease by remodeling a normally benign microbiota into a dysbiotic one. It may provide a novel conceptual basis for the development of targeted diagnostic and treatment modalities for complex dysbiotic diseases.

Some evidence indicates that certain pathogens may trigger the disruption of microbial homeostasis, thereby leading to the development of periodontal disease, even when they are present only in low numbers. *P. gingivalis* can be considered as a "keystone" pathogen as it is often an organism that is central to the disease process, even when it is at a relatively low abundance.

The Transition From Health to Disease

The oral microbial ecology is dynamic. The presence and numbers of particular microorganisms, even as a part of a community colonizing a niche in a human being, are controlled by the type and quantity of nutrients present (nutritional determinant), their ability to tolerate the specific physicochemical factors (physicochemical determinants), and their ability to cope with antimicrobial compounds (biologic determinants) or mechanical removal forces (mechanical determinants). Although these determinants are well defined from a theoretical point of view, in practice they overlap each other, especially in more complex environments (i.e., multispecies environments). Inherent to their biologic nature, bacteria interact with each other, with their environment, and vice versa. Therefore, the microbial ecology will change its composition or the composition of the microbial ecology will be changed when transitioning from a healthy status to a diseased status or vice versa. A change in the composition of a bacterial community as the result of external, nonmicrobial factors is termed *allogenic succession.* Smoking is a good example of such interaction. In *autogenic succession* (i.e., a change in the composition of a microbial community that arises from microbial activities), interbacterial and viral–bacterial interactions are involved.

Early microscopic studies clearly demonstrated that the number and proportions of different subgingival bacterial morphotypes differ between healthy and diseased sites (Fig. 8.8). The total number of bacteria, which was determined by microscopic counts per gram of plaque, was twice as high in periodontally diseased sites as compared to healthy sites. Because considerably more plaque is found at diseased sites, this suggests that, in general, the total bacterial load in diseased sites is greater than that of healthy sites. Fewer coccal cells and more motile rods and spirochetes are found in diseased sites as compared to healthy sites. Culturing has shown that the microbiota in periodontally healthy sites consists predominantly of gram-positive facultative rods and cocci (approximately 75%). The recovery of this group of microorganisms is decreased proportionally in gingivitis (44%) and periodontitis (10%–13%). These

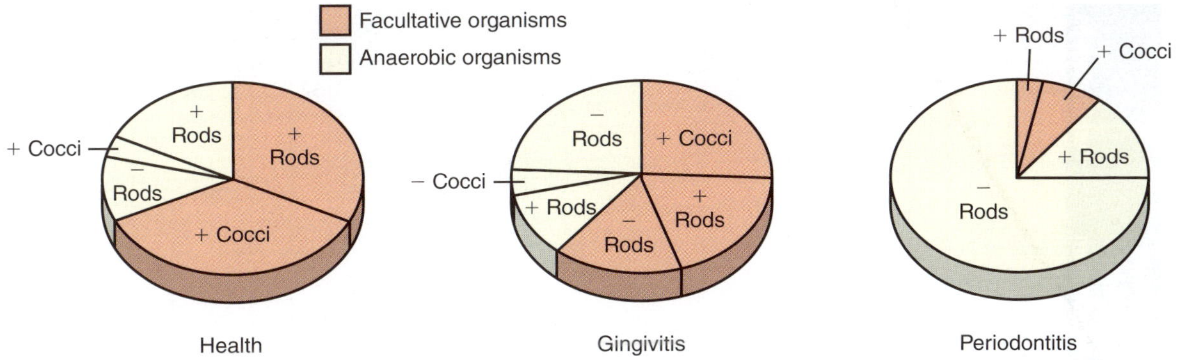

Fig. 8.8 Pie charts based on culturing studies that represent the relative proportion of different morphotypes in subgingival samples in cases of periodontal health, gingivitis, and periodontitis. A clear distinction is made between facultative species and obligate anaerobic species. Spirochetes are not included. +, gram-positive; −, gram-negative.

decreases are accompanied by increases in the proportions of gram-negative rods, from 13% in health to 40% in gingivitis and 74% in advanced periodontitis.

The current concept regarding the etiology of periodontal diseases considers three groups of factors that determine whether active periodontal destruction will occur in a subject: a susceptible host, the presence of pathogenic species, and the absence or small proportion of so-called beneficial bacteria. The clinical manifestations of periodontal destruction will result from a complex interplay among these etiologic agents. In general, small amounts of bacterial plaque can be controlled by the body's defense mechanisms without destruction; however, when dysbiosis happens (e.g., as a result of increased susceptibility, high bacterial load, or pathogenic infections), periodontal destruction could occur.

When comparing the microbiota among conditions of health, gingivitis, and periodontitis, the following microbial shifts can be identified as health progresses to periodontitis:

- From gram-positive to gram-negative.
- From cocci to rods (and, at a later stage, to spirochetes).
- From nonmotile to motile organisms.
- From facultative anaerobes to obligate anaerobes.
- From fermenting to proteolytic species.

Periodontal Health

The recovery of microorganisms from periodontally healthy sites is lower as compared to diseased sites (Table 8.3). The bacteria associated with periodontal health are primarily gram-positive facultative species and members of the genera *Streptococcus* and *Actinomyces* (e.g., *S. sanguinis*, *S. mitis*, *A. oris*, *Actinomyces israelii*, *Actinomyces gerencseriae*, *Actinomyces viscosus*, *A. naeslundii*). Small proportions of gram-negative species are also found, most frequently *P. intermedia*, *F. nucleatum*, *F. nucleatum* spp. polymorphum, *Fusobacterium periodonticum*, *Capnocytophaga* spp. (*C. gingivalis*, *C. ochracea*, and *C. sputigena*), *Neisseria* spp., and *Veillonella* spp. Microscopic analyses indicate that a few spirochetes and motile rods may also be present.

Certain bacterial species have been proposed to be protective or beneficial to the host, including *S. sanguinis*, *Veillonella parvula*, and *C. ochracea.* They are typically found in high numbers at periodontal sites that do not demonstrate attachment loss (inactive sites) but in low numbers at sites where active periodontal destruction occurs. These species probably function to prevent the colonization or proliferation of pathogenic microorganisms. Clinical studies have shown that sites with high levels of *C. ochracea* and *S. sanguinis* are associated with a greater gain in attachment after therapy, thereby further supporting this concept. A better understanding of plaque ecology and the interactions between bacteria and their products in plaque will undoubtedly reveal many other examples.

Gingivitis

The development of gingivitis has been extensively studied in a model system referred to as *experimental gingivitis* and initially described by Löe and coworkers. Periodontal health is first established in human subjects via cleaning and rigorous oral hygiene measures that are followed by abstinence from oral hygiene for 21 days. After 8 h without oral hygiene, bacteria may be found at concentrations of 10^3–10^4 per square millimeter of tooth surface, and they will increase in number by a factor of 100–1000 during the next 24-h period. After 36 hours, the plaque becomes clinically visible. The initial microbiota of experimental gingivitis (see Fig. 8.5) consists of gram-positive rods, gram-positive cocci, and gram-negative cocci. The transition to gingivitis is evidenced by inflammatory changes; it is accompanied first by the appearance of gram-negative rods and filaments and then by spirochetal and motile microorganisms.

The subgingival microbiota of dental plaque-induced gingivitis (chronic gingivitis) differs from that of both health and chronic periodontitis. It consists of roughly equal proportions of gram-positive (56%) and gram-negative (44%) species as well as facultative (59%) and anaerobic (41%) microorganisms. It should be noted that the majority of predominant species in chronic periodontitis are already present in the gingivitis state but mostly in small numbers.

Predominant gram-positive species include *Streptococcus* spp. (*S. sanguinis*, *S. mitis*, *S. intermedius*, *S. oralis*, *S. anginosus*), *Actinomyces* spp. (*A. oris*, *A. naeslundii*), *Eubacterium nodatum*, and *P. micra.* The gram-negative microorganisms are predominantly *Capnocytophaga* spp., *Fusobacterium* spp., *Prevotella* spp., *Campylobacter gracilis*, *Campylobacter concisus*, *V. parvula*, *Haemophilus* spp., and *E. corrodens.*

Pregnancy-associated gingivitis is an acute inflammation of the gingival tissues that is associated with pregnancy. This condition is accompanied by increases in steroid hormones in the crevicular fluid and dramatic increases in the levels of *P. intermedia* and *C. rectus*, which use the steroids as growth factors.

Chronic Periodontitis

The microscopic examination of plaque from sites with chronic periodontitis has consistently revealed elevated proportions of spirochetes. The cultivation of plaque microorganisms from sites of chronic periodontitis reveals high percentages of anaerobic (90%) gram-negative (75%) bacterial species (Table 8.3).

TABLE 8.3 Summary of Bacterial Species Significantly Associated With Different Clinical Conditions Based on Culture, Polymerase Chain Reaction, and Checkerboard Data

Bacterial Species	Health	Gingivitis	Chronic Periodontitis	Localized Aggressive Periodontitis	Generalized Aggressive Periodontitis	Necrotizing Periodontal Diseases	Abscesses of the Periodontium	Peri-Implantitis
Actinomyces gerencseriae	X							
Actinomyces israelii	X							
Actinomyces naeslundii	X	X						
Actinomyces oris	X							
Actinomyces viscosus	X	X						
Aggregatibacter actinomycetemcomitans								X
Aggregatibacter actinomycetemcomitans high (leukotoxin clone)				X				
Aggregatibacter actinomycetemcomitans serotype a		X						
Aggregatibacter actinomycetemcomitans serotype b			X		X			
Campylobacter concisus		X						
Campylobacter gracilis					X			
Campylobacter rectus		X	X	X				X
Campylobacter showae					X			
Capnocytophaga gingivalis	X							
Capnocytophaga ochracea	X							
Capnocytophaga spp.	X	X		X				X
Capnocytophaga sputigena	X							
Eikenella corrodens		X	X	X				
Enterobacter spp.			X					X
Eubacterium nodatum		X	X	X	X			
Eubacterium saburreum	X							
Fusobacterium nucleatum		X	X	X		X	X	X
Fusobacterium periodonticum	X							
Fusobacterium polymorphum	X							
Haemophilus spp.		X						
Leptotrichia buccalis			X	X				

Neisseria spp.	X							
Parvimonas micra		X	X				X	X
Prevotella intermedia			X	X	X	X	X	X
Prevotella intermedia spirochetes		X						
Porphyromonas gingivalis			X	X	X		X	X
Prevotella nigrescens			X		X			
Propionibacterium acnes	X							
Pseudomonas aeruginosa								X
Selenomonas noxia			X					
Spirochetes			X	X	X	X	X	X
Staphylococcus aureus								X
Staphylococcus epidermidis								X
Streptococcus anginosus	X	X						
Streptococcus gordonii	X							
Streptococcus intermedius		X						
Streptococcus mitis	X	X						
Streptococcus oralis	X	X						
Streptococcus sanguinis	X	X						
Tannerella forsythia			X	X	X			X
Treponema denticola			X	X	X			X
Treponema spp.		X	X	X	X	X		X
Veillonella parvula	X	X						

In patients with chronic periodontitis, the bacteria that are most often detected at high levels include *P. gingivalis*, *T. forsythia*, *P. intermedia*, *Prevotella nigrescens*, *C. rectus*, *E. corrodens*, *F. nucleatum*, *A. actinomycetemcomitans* (often serotype b), *P. micra*, *E. nodatum*, *Leptotrichia buccalis*, *Treponema* (*T. denticola*), *Selenomonas* spp. (*S. noxia*), and *Enterobacter* spp. When periodontally active sites (i.e., with recent attachment loss) were examined in comparison with inactive sites (i.e., with no recent attachment loss), concentrations of *C. rectus*, *P. gingivalis*, *P. intermedia*, *F. nucleatum*, and *T. forsythia* were found to be elevated in the active sites. Furthermore, detectable levels of *P. gingivalis*, *P. intermedia*, *T. forsythia*, *C. rectus*, and *A. actinomycetemcomitans* are associated with disease progression, and their elimination via therapy is associated with an improved clinical response. Both *P. gingivalis* and *A. actinomycetemcomitans* are known to invade host tissue cells, which may be significant in aggressive forms of periodontitis.

Studies have documented an association between chronic periodontitis and viral microorganisms of the herpesviruses group, most notably EBV-1 and human cytomegalovirus (hCMV). Furthermore, the presence of subgingival EBV-1 and hCMV are associated with high levels of putative bacterial pathogens, including *P. gingivalis*, *T. forsythia*, *P. intermedia*, and *T. denticola*. These data support the hypothesis that viral infection may contribute to periodontal pathogenesis, but the potential role of viral agents remains to be determined.

Localized Aggressive Periodontitis

The microbiota associated with localized aggressive periodontitis is predominantly composed of gram-negative, capnophilic (i.e., CO_2 requiring), anaerobic rods (see Table 8.3). Microbiologic studies indicate that almost all localized juvenile periodontitis sites harbor *A. actinomycetemcomitans*, which may comprise as much as 90% of the total cultivable microbiota. Other organisms found in significant levels include *P. gingivalis, E. corrodens, C. rectus, F. nucleatum, Bacteroides capillus, Eubacterium brachy*, and *Capnocytophaga* spp. and spirochetes. Checkerboard DNA–DNA hybridization studies have also shown high proportions of *E. nodatum*, *P. intermedia*, *Treponema* spp. (*T. denticola*), *L. buccalis*, and *T. forsythia*. In addition, herpesviruses, including EBV-1 and hCMV, have also been associated with localized aggressive periodontitis.

A. actinomycetemcomitans is generally accepted as the primary etiologic agent in most but not all cases of localized aggressive periodontitis. A high leukotoxic clone, known as JP2, is uniquely associated with aggressive forms of periodontitis. Mechanical debridement in combination with systemic antibiotic treatment is necessary to control the levels of *A. actinomycetemcomitans* associated with this disease. The failure of mechanical therapy alone may relate to the ability of this organism to invade host tissues.

Generalized Aggressive Periodontitis

It is a severe form of periodontitis that occurs at a relatively young age (i.e., between 20 and 40 years). It is characterized by severe gingivitis, a large number of deepened pockets, and a high tendency for bleeding on probing. In relation to the patient's age, bone destruction is extensive. It is sometimes considered a generalized form of localized aggressive periodontitis. From a microbiologic point of view, it has many similarities with localized aggressive periodontitis (see Table 8.3). However, aggressive periodontitis is clearly dominated more by *P. gingivalis*, *P. intermedia*, *T. forsythia*, and *Treponema* spp. (*T. denticola*) and less by *A. actinomycetemcomitans*. Checkerboard DNA–DNA hybridization studies also indicate high proportions of *E. nodatum, C. gracilis, Campylobacter showae*, and *P. nigrescens*.

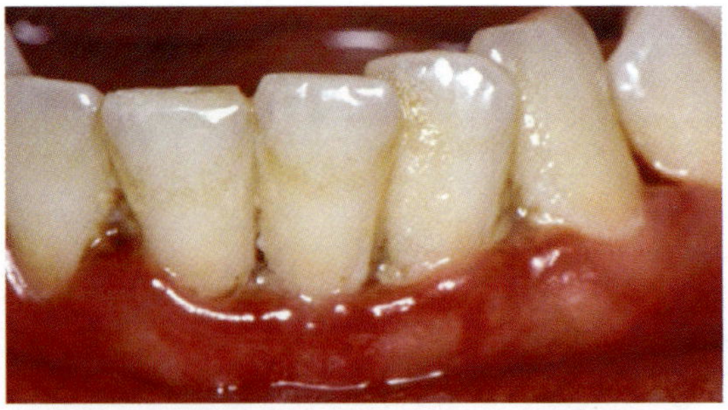

Fig. 8.9 Clinical picture of lower front teeth with necrotizing gingivitis.

Necrotizing Periodontal Diseases

Necrotizing periodontal diseases (Fig. 8.9) manifest as acute inflammation of the gingival and periodontal tissues that is characterized by the necrosis of the marginal gingival tissue and the interdental papillae. Clinically, these conditions are often associated with stress or HIV infection. They may be accompanied by malodor and pain and possibly systemic symptoms, including lymphadenopathy, fever, and malaise. Microbiologic studies on necrotizing periodontal diseases indicate that they are associated with high levels of spirochetes, fusiform bacteria, and *P. intermedia*.

Abscesses of the Periodontium

Investigations reveal that bacteria recognized as periodontal pathogens are commonly found in significant numbers in periodontal abscesses. The microbial composition of periodontal abscesses is similar to that observed in periodontitis. Classical periodontal pathogens are commonly found in significant numbers/proportion in this lesion, including *P. gingivalis, P. intermedia, P. melaninogenica, F. nucleatum, T. forsythia*, Treponema species, Campylobacter species, Capnocytophaga species, *A. actinomycetemcomitans*, or gram-negative enteric rods. In addition, the role of viruses has been proposed but with less evidence.

Endo-Periodontal Lesions

Endo-periodontal lesions are acute or chronic clinical conditions involving both the pulp and periodontal tissues. The two main signs and symptoms associated with a tooth affected by an endo-periodontal lesion are deep periodontal pockets reaching or close to the apex and negative or altered response to pulp tests. In addition, other signs and symptoms have been reported, such as bone resorption, spontaneous pain or pain on palpation and percussion, purulent exudate, tooth mobility, sinus tract, crown, and gingival color alterations. Studies on microbiological composition of endo-periodontal lesions have identified classical periodontal pathogens such as *P. gingivalis*, *T. forsythia*, or *P. micra* and species from the genera *Fusobacterium*, *Prevotella*, and *Treponema*. In addition, studies using "open-ended" molecular techniques have observed a higher microbial diversity and identified fewer common taxa, such as *F. alocis*, *Enterococcus faecalis*, and species from the genera *Desulfobulbus*, *Dialister*, *Fretibacterium*, or *Rothia*. Overall, no major differences exist between the microorganisms found in the endodontic and periodontal lesions or a specific microbial profile associated with the endo-periodontal lesions

Peri-Implantitis

The term *peri-implantitis* refers to an inflammatory process that affects the tissues around an already osseointegrated implant and that results in the loss of supporting bone. Healthy peri-implant pockets are characterized by high proportions of coccoid cells, a low ratio of anaerobic-to-aerobic species, a low number of gram-negative anaerobic species, and low detection frequencies for periodontopathogens. Implants with peri-implantitis reveal a microbiota that encompasses conventional periodontal pathogens (see Table 8.3), as well as the cariogenic bacterium *S. mutans*. Species such as *A. actinomycetemcomitans, P. gingivalis, T. forsythia, P. micra, C. rectus, F. nucleatum, P. intermedia, T. denticola*, and *Capnocytophaga* are often isolated from failing sites, but they can also be detected around healthy peri-implant sites. Other species, such as *Pseudomonas aeruginosa*, *Enterobacter* spp., *Candida albicans*, and staphylococci, are also frequently detected around implants.

Biofilm and Microbiome Modulation by Different Periodontal Treatments

The recognition that the entire oral cavity is in dysbiosis in subjects affected by periodontitis indicates that effective periodontal treatment would require a striking ecological shift in the oral environment. Not only deep pockets, but all oral niches would require antiinfective treatment in order to achieve a new biofilm climax community compatible with periodontal health and, consequently, reestablish homeostasis. The gold standard scaling and root planing procedure produces a deep beneficial change in the composition of the subgingival including a reduction in pathogens and an increase in Actinomyces species.

The clinical and microbiological effects of adjunctive treatment targeting specific oral habitats, such as antimicrobials locally delivered to deep periodontal pockets, were not found to be particularly promising. The most consolidated adjunctive treatment to mechanical debridement is systemic antibiotics, followed by probiotics/prebiotics and host-modulators.

Probiotics

The use of probiotics is a new developing field in oral health care. Probiotics have been defined as living micro-organisms that, when administered in adequate amounts, confer a health benefit to the host. The effects of probiotics are both local and systemic, presumably by interfering with the host immune system. The clinical benefits of the use of probiotics for oral and periodontal health have been well-documented in several clinical trials. The benefits of using probiotics as adjuncts to standard periodontal therapies have also been demonstrated in several clinical studies, with improvements in important periodontal clinical parameters, such as periodontal pocket depth, clinical attachment loss, gingival index, plaque index, and bleeding on probing.

One study reported stronger reductions in *P. gingivalis* numbers in saliva, supra- and subgingival samples for the scaling and root planing + probiotic group compared to the scaling and root planing alone group. Patients with chronic periodontitis and treated with a *Bacillus subtilis*-containing mouthrinse showed significantly decreased abundances of the "red complex" periodontal pathogens (*P. gingivalis*, *T. denticola*, and *T. forsythia*), indirectly measured as changes in the proteolytic activity of these anaerobes, compared to treatment with a classical mouthrinse. In healthy volunteers without severe periodontitis, the oral administration of *Lactobacillus salivarius* (now reclassified as *Ligilactobacillus salivarius*) WB21-containing tablets resulted in a significantly reduced total count of five periodontal pathogens (*A. actinomycetemcomitans*, *P. gingivalis*, *P. intermedia*, *T. forsythia*, and *T. denticola*) in subgingival biofilm samples 4 weeks posttreatment but not 8 weeks posttreatment.

Prebiotics

In light of the continuous search for novel preventive or therapeutic strategies, the modulation of the commensal oral microbiota by means of prebiotics is increasingly gaining attention. Prebiotics are substrates that are selectively utilized by host microorganisms conferring a health benefit. From this definition, it is evident that the utilization of the prebiotic by the commensal microbiota results in a health benefit to the host. This health benefit can be due to microbiological changes, like stimulation of the growth and abundance of certain species, but also due to metabolic changes, such as the stimulation of certain metabolic activities. Over the past years, several other in vitro and in vivo studies have investigated the potential use of prebiotics for oral health. With increasing knowledge of the pathogenesis of oral diseases, these studies have been focusing on substrates that stimulate bacterial species with inhibitory activities on oral pathogens and/or modify environmental conditions that contribute to disease onset and progression such as environmental pH. Sensitivity of periodontal pathogens to H_2O_2 suggests that arginine could be used in the prevention or treatment of periodontal diseases. Recently, nitrate was also suggested as a potential prebiotic substrate for oral health. However, the use of potential prebiotics should consider individual factors such as disease susceptibility and the specific composition of the commensal oral microbiota.

Biofilm Modulation in Peri-Implantitis

Nonsurgical treatment of peri-implantitis does not seem very promising in controlling the disease, even in association with other adjunctive treatments. Decontamination of dental implant surfaces by means of mechanical, chemical, and physical methods has been tested in various clinical trials. The main target of all decontamination methods is primarily to decontaminate the implant surface and to remove the inflammatory peri-implant soft tissues. Adjunctive use of metronidazole and amoxicillin debridement did not show benefits in the treatment of severe peri-implantitis. This lack of effectiveness may be due to mechanical difficulties in decontaminating the implant threads, mainly in deeper pockets. Thus, it could be hypothesized that effective treatment of peri-implantitis would require open flap debridement. There is some clinical evidence that metronidazole and amoxicillin adjunct to open flap surgery would be an effective protocol to treat peri-implantitis. The effects of this treatment in changing the peri-implant biofilm composition have not been determined.

Virulence Factors of Periodontopathogens

Virulence factors of periodontal microorganisms can be subdivided as follows: (1) factors that promote colonization (adhesins), (2) toxins and enzymes that degrade host tissues, and (3) mechanisms that protect pathogenic bacteria from the host.

Adhesive Surface Proteins and Fibrils

To colonize the periodontal pocket, bacteria must adhere to cells or tissues in the region, such as teeth, the existing microbial biofilm, or the pocket epithelium. Bacterial cell surface structures provide the points of contact. Often these structures extend some distance from the cell surface. Fimbriae or pili are polymeric fibrils that are composed of repeating subunits that can extend several micrometers from the cell membrane. Pili were once thought to be unique to gram-negative bacteria, but they have now been identified in several gram-positive organisms, including streptococci and actinomyces. Strains of *P. gingivalis* produce two types of fimbriae, which are known as the major fimbriae and the minor fimbriae.

Several nonpilus proteins from periodontopathogens have been shown to interact with host or bacterial receptors, as well as, in some cases, with both. A relatively well-studied example is the major sheath protein (Msp) of *T. denticola*. Msp is a 53- to 64-kDa protein that was originally thought to assemble into a hexagonal array in the outer sheath. However, careful analysis by electron microscopy indicated that Msp is predominantly a periplasmic protein and that some regions are exposed on the cell surface. Purified Msp interacts with the host extracellular matrix proteins fibrinogen, fibronectin, and laminin. In addition, Msp recognizes receptors on *P. gingivalis* and *F. nucleatum* and mediates coaggregation. Therefore, Msp is a multifunctional adhesin that promotes binding to host and bacterial receptors.

Tissue Destruction-Promoting Factors

Many bacterial proteins that interact with host cells are recognized by the immune system, and they may trigger immune responses. Fimbriae of *P. gingivalis* and *A. actinomycetemcomitans* are highly antigenic. Inflammation is a major contributor to tissue destruction in periodontal disease. However, some bacterial products directly promote tissue destruction in addition to modulating host immunity, with extracellular proteolytic enzymes being the most notable. Most of the tissue destruction in periodontal pockets is actually caused by host matrix metalloproteinases, but bacterial proteases play important roles in activating the host enzymes.

Trypsin-like proteases are produced by *P. gingivalis*, *T. denticola*, and *T. forsythia.* Proteases supply nutrition in the form of peptides or amino acids to the bacteria that produce them. During this process, they may cause the extensive degradation of host extracellular proteins. However, the bulk of the host tissue-degrading activity is restricted to a small number of these enzymes. In the case of *P. gingivalis*, three enzymes known as gingipains are responsible for at least 85% of the total proteolytic activity of the bacterium. The gingipains belong to the cysteine protease family, and they use an active-site cysteine residue for catalysis. Gingipains are classed as "Arg-gingipains" (RgpA and RgpB) or "Lys-gingipains" (Kgp) on the basis of their ability to cleave Arg-X or Lys-X peptide bonds (X represents any amino acid). Gingipains are multifunctional proteins that play important roles in adhesion, tissue degradation, and the evasion of host responses.

Proteases are produced by *A. actinomycetemcomitans*, but these appear to be less important for the virulence of this organism than the leukotoxin (LtxA). LtxA is a member of the repeats-in-toxin family of proteins. These toxins act by delivering an adenylate cyclase domain into cells, which catalyzes the uncontrolled conversion of adenosine triphosphate to cyclic adenosine monophosphate.

Most strains of *A. actinomycetemcomitans* produce low levels of LtxA. However, some strains are regarded as hyperleukotoxic because they express high levels of the transcript from the *ltxA* gene, thereby encoding LtxA.

Strategies for Evading Host Immunity

Pathogenic bacteria have many and varied strategies for evading or subverting the host immune system, including the following: (1) the production of an extracellular capsule, (2) the proteolytic degradation of host innate or acquired immunity components, (3) the modulation of host responses by binding serum components on the bacterial cell surface, and (4) the invasion of gingival epithelial cells. Six different antigenic capsule types have been described on the basis of the differences in the polysaccharide K antigen. In a mouse model, capsular strains of *P. gingivalis* produced a spreading type of infection, whereas acapsular strains tended to form more localized abscesses. Most *P. gingivalis* isolates from periodontitis patients are encapsulated. It is hypothesized that the capsule protects cells from the host immune system. Several periodontopathogens are resistant to complement-mediated phagocytosis, and it is thought that the proteolysis of complement components contributes to resistance to some extent. *P. gingivalis* gingipains have been shown to degrade complement components C3, C4, C5, and factor B. More recently, a cysteine protease of *P. intermedia* called interpain A has also been shown to degrade C3. In vitro, interpain A acts synergistically with gingipains to decrease the deposition of complement C3b. These data fit with the hypothesis that periodontal disease processes are mediated by polymicrobial consortia rather than by individual periodontopathogens.

Periodontal pathogens are notoriously difficult to eradicate completely. Despite aggressive antibacterial attacks from the host defenses and from clinical treatments, it is often impossible to prevent reinfection. One potential reservoir for periodontopathogens is inside gingival epithelial cells. *P. gingivalis* and *A. actinomycetemcomitans*, for example, can invade epithelial cells in vitro. In vivo, *P. gingivalis*, *T. forsythia*, *P. intermedia*, *T. denticola*, and *A. actinomycetemcomitans* can be detected within the gingival epithelial cells of patients with periodontitis before and after periodontal therapy. Adhesion to host cells is critical for invasion. However, it has been suggested that some factors may specifically control the ability of bacteria to invade cells. In *A. actinomycetemcomitans*, a screen for invasion-associated genes identified two loci, encoding ApiA and ApiBC, which are related to known bacterial invasion proteins (invasins). The ability of bacteria to invade cells may be influenced by their interactions with other organisms in the gingival sulcus. Thus, the coinfection of an epithelial cell line with *P. gingivalis* and a coaggregating strain of *F. nucleatum* resulted in increased invasion by *P. gingivalis* as compared to a monoculture control. Coaggregation with *F. nucleatum* is mediated by the *P. gingivalis* capsular polysaccharide and lipopolysaccharide; therefore, these molecules may indirectly contribute to invasion.

Key points

- After weaning (>2 years), the entire human microbiota is formed and comprises a very complex collection of hundreds of different types of bacteria that totals to approximately 10^{14} microbial cells.
- Dental plaque is composed primarily of microorganisms encased within an extracellular matrix. One gram of plaque (wet weight) contains approximately 10^{11} bacteria.
- *Organic constituents* of the matrix include polysaccharides, proteins, glycoproteins, lipid material, and DNA. The *inorganic components* of plaque are predominantly calcium and phosphorus, with trace amounts of other minerals, such as sodium, potassium, and fluorine.
- Dental plaque is defined clinically as a structured, resilient, yellow-grayish substance that adheres tenaciously to the intraoral hard surfaces, including removable and fixed restorations.
- *Materia alba* refers to soft accumulations of bacteria, food matter, and tissue cells that lack the organized structure of dental plaque and that are easily displaced with a water spray.
- Dental plaque is broadly classified as supragingival or subgingival. *Supragingival plaque* is found at or above the gingival margin; *Subgingival plaque* is found below the gingival margin.
- The process of plaque formation can be divided into three main phases: (1) formation of the pellicle on the tooth surface, (2) initial adhesion/attachment of bacteria, and (3) secondary colonization/plaque maturation.
- When many genetically distinct bacteria adhere to each other and form clumps, it is referred to as coaggregation.
- Special examples of coaggregations are the corn cob formation, in which *Streptococci* adhere to filaments of *Corynebacterium matruchotii* or *Actinomyces* spp., and the test-tube brush formation, composed of filamentous bacteria to which gram-negative rods adhere.
- In a biofilm, bacteria have the capacity to communicate with each other which is called *quorum sensing.*
- Organisms in a biofilm are 1000–1500 times more resistant to antibiotics as compared to their planktonic state.

- According to the nonspecific plaque hypothesis, periodontal disease results from the "elaboration of noxious products by the entire plaque flora." According to the specific plaque hypothesis, pathogenicity of dental plaque depends on the presence of or an increase in specific microorganisms.
- Ecological plaque hypothesis states that both the total amount of dental plaque, as well as the specific microbial composition of plaque may contribute to the transition from health to disease.
- The keystone pathogen hypothesis indicates that certain low-abundance microbial pathogens can orchestrate inflammatory disease by remodeling a normally benign microbiota into a dysbiotic one.

Suggested Readings

Berezow AB, Darveau RP: Microbial shift and periodontitis, *Periodontol 2000* 55:36–47, 2011.
Bergquist R: Parasitic infections affecting the oral cavity, *Periodontol 2000* 49:96–105, 2009.
Griffen AL, Beall CJ, Campbell JH, et al: Distinct and complex bacterial profiles in human periodontitis and health revealed by 16S pyrosequencing, *ISME J* 6:1176–1185, 2012.
Hajishengallis G, Darveau RP, Curtis MA: The keystone-pathogen hypothesis, *Nat Rev Microbiol* 10:717–725, 2012.
Jakubovics NS, Palmer RJ: *Oral microbial ecology: current research and new perspectives*, Caister Academic Press, 2013, p. 1.
Samaranayake LP, Keung LW, Jin L: Oral mucosal fungal infections, *Periodontol 2000* 49:39–59, 2009.
Slots J: Oral viral infections of adults, *Periodontol 2000* 49:60–86, 2009.
Teles RP, Haffajee AD, Socransky SS: Microbiological goals of periodontal therapy, *Periodontol 2000* 42:180, 2006.
Zijnge V, van Leeuwen MB, Degener JE, et al: Oral biofilm architecture on natural teeth, *PLoS ONE* 5 (2): e9321, 2010.

References

References and MCQs with answers for the chapter are available on www.medenact.com.

CHAPTER 9

Smoking and Periodontal Disease

PM Preshaw | L Chambrone | R Holliday | N Ambalavanan

CHAPTER OUTLINE

The Smoking Epidemic

Smoking is highly prevalent and can be considered an epidemic in both developed and developing nations. In India 28.6% (266.8 million) of adults—aged 15 and above are smokers and 3.7% (34.4 million) are occasional users. The prevalence of tobacco users include people who currently have either smoked or chewed tobacco. Among the adults 24.9% (232.4 million) are daily tobacco users; tobacco users among men and women are 42.4% and 14.2%, respectively. According to the Global Adult Tobacco Survey 2 (GATS 2), every third adult in rural areas and every fifth adult in urban areas use tobacco in some form or the other.

Smoking rates, however, have seen marked declines since the 1980s. Global estimated daily tobacco smoking prevalence rates (in individuals >5 years old) reduced from 41.2% in 1980 to 31.1% in 2012 for men and from 10.6% (1980) to 6.2% (2012) for women. Despite this development, with population growth, the number of daily smokers worldwide has actually increased to just short of a billion people in 2012, upholding tobacco smoking's position as a major public health threat (Box 9.1).

Smoking is harmful to almost every organ in the body and is associated with multiple diseases that reduce life expectancy and quality of life. Diseases associated with smoking include lung cancer, heart disease, stroke, emphysema, bronchitis, and cancers of the oral cavity, bladder, kidney, stomach, liver, and cervix. Approximately half of long-term smokers will die early as a result of smoking, and those who die before the age of 70 years will lose an average of 20 years of life. Most deaths from smoking are due to lung cancer, chronic obstructive pulmonary disease, and coronary heart disease. Tobacco use is responsible for 14% of all noncommunicable disease deaths in people aged 30 years and older worldwide and for 9.5% (1 million) of all deaths in India.

BOX 9.1 A Global Perspective

- As many as 6.25 trillion cigarettes are smoked annually across the globe.
- Tobacco kills 6 million people each year.
- Only 30% of people worldwide have access to smoking cessation services.
- Only 22% of people worldwide are protected by smoke-free laws.

Tobacco smoke contains thousands of noxious chemicals, and it comprises a gaseous phase and a solid (particulate) phase. The gas phase contains carbon monoxide, ammonia, formaldehyde, hydrogen cyanide, and many other toxic and irritant compounds, including more than 60 known carcinogens such as benzo(a)pyrene and dimethyl nitrosamine. The particulate phase includes nicotine, "tar" (itself made up of many toxic chemicals), benzene, and benzo(a)pyrene. Tar is inhaled with the smoke. In its condensate form, it is the sticky brown substance that stains fingers and teeth yellow and brown. Nicotine, which is an alkaloid, is found within the tobacco leaf and evaporates when the cigarette is lighted. It is quickly absorbed in the lungs, and it reaches the brain within 10–19 s. Nicotine is highly addictive. It causes a rise in blood pressure, increased heart and respiratory rates, and peripheral vasoconstriction.

All dental patients must be asked about their smoking status or tobacco usage. Current smoking status is the minimal information that must be recorded (e.g., "Patient is currently smoking *X* cigarettes per day"), but the importance of cumulative exposure to cigarette smoke means that it is more appropriate to record pack-years of smoking (Box 9.2). Biochemical tests can also be used to assess smoking status, including exhaled carbon monoxide and the measurement of cotinine (the major metabolite of nicotine) in serum, saliva, or urine. Cotinine is measured in preference to nicotine because the half-life of nicotine is short (≈1–2 h), whereas that of cotinine is approximately 20 h.

Smoking is a major risk factor for periodontitis, and it affects the prevalence, extent, and severity of disease. In addition, smoking has an adverse impact on the clinical outcome of nonsurgical and surgical therapy as well as the long-term success of implant placement.

BOX 9.2 Challenge of Assessing Smoking Status

Current Smokers

Ask about current smoking and past smoking. Many smokers are trying to quit, and therefore simply asking how many cigarettes they are smoking today may not give an accurate assessment of their lifetime exposure (e.g., a patient who is currently smoking 5 cigarettes per day may have been smoking 40 cigarettes per day until yesterday, when he or she decided to cut down). Try to get an indication of the patient's approximate level of smoking (e.g., the average number of cigarettes per day for a certain number of years). It can also be useful to calculate the number of pack-years:

$$\text{Pack-years} = \text{Number of packs smoked per day} \times \text{Number of years of smoking}$$

In other words, 1 pack-year is the cumulative exposure that corresponds with the smoking of 1 pack of 20 cigarettes per day for 1 year. For example, a smoker who has smoked 20 cigarettes per day for 15 years has 15 pack-years of smoking.

Former Smokers

Ask patients about their past smoking. Patients with periodontitis may have a significant smoking history that has had an impact on their periodontal status, even if they no longer smoke. Former smokers should always be congratulated for their achievement in quitting, but it is also very important to document the following:

- How much they used to smoke
- How many years they smoked
- When they quit

Is the Patient's Response Accurate?

The inaccurate or false reporting of smoking status is common; patients will tell you what they think you want to hear, or they may be embarrassed because they have not managed to cut down yet. Many patients report smoking 20 cigarettes per day, because this is the number of cigarettes in a pack in most countries, so 20 may be a convenient response rather than an accurate response. Cultural factors may also influence responses.

When Is a Smoker Not a Smoker?

- Smokers have smoked ≥100 cigarettes in their lifetime and currently smoke.
- Former smokers have smoked ≥100 cigarettes in their lifetime and do not currently smoke.
- Nonsmokers have not smoked ≥100 cigarettes in their lifetime and do not currently smoke.

It must be noted that many periodontal research studies have not used these definitions, and this can sometimes make it difficult to interpret the studies, particularly in the context of what constitutes a former smoker. For example, from an exposure point of view, there is a big difference between someone who smoked 5 cigarettes per day for 10 years and who quit 30 years ago as compared to someone who smoked 40 cigarettes per day for 20 years and quit 6 months ago. It is always best in clinical practice to gather full information about each patient's smoking history.

Effects of Smoking on the Prevalence and Severity of Periodontal Diseases

Gingivitis

Controlled clinical studies have demonstrated that, in human models of experimental gingivitis, the development of inflammation in response to plaque accumulation is reduced in smokers as compared to nonsmokers (Table 9.1). In addition, cross-sectional studies have consistently demonstrated that smokers present with less gingival inflammation than nonsmokers. These data suggest that smokers have a decreased expression of clinical inflammation in the presence of plaque accumulation as compared to nonsmokers.

TABLE 9.1 Effects of Smoking on Gingivitis and Periodontitis

Periodontal Disease	Effects of Smoking
Gingivitis	↓ Gingival inflammation and bleeding on probing
Periodontitis	↑ Prevalence and severity of periodontal destruction
	↑ Pocket depth, attachment loss, and bone loss
	↑ Rate of periodontal destruction
	↑ Prevalence of severe periodontitis
	↑ Tooth loss
	↑ Prevalence with increased number of cigarettes smoked per day
	↓ Prevalence and severity with smoking cessation

↓, Decreased; ↑, increased.

Periodontitis

Although gingival inflammation in smokers appears to be reduced in response to plaque accumulation as compared to nonsmokers, an overwhelming body of evidence points to smoking as a major risk factor for increasing the prevalence and severity of periodontal destruction. Multiple cross-sectional and longitudinal studies have demonstrated that pocket depth, attachment loss, and alveolar bone loss are more prevalent and severe in patients who smoke as compared to nonsmokers. On average, smokers were four times as likely to have periodontitis as compared to persons who had never smoked after adjusting for age, gender, race/ethnicity, education, and income/poverty ratio. Former smokers were 1.7 times more likely to have periodontitis than persons who had never smoked. This study also demonstrated a dose–response relationship between cigarettes smoked per day and the odds of having periodontitis. In subjects smoking nine or fewer cigarettes per day, the odds for having periodontitis were 2.8, whereas subjects who smoked 31 or more cigarettes per day were almost six times more likely to have periodontitis. In former smokers, the odds of having periodontitis declined with the number of years since quitting.

Older adult smokers are approximately three times more likely to have severe periodontal disease, and the number of years of tobacco use is a significant factor in tooth loss, coronal root caries, and periodontal disease.

Smoking has also been shown to affect periodontal disease severity in younger individuals. Cigarette smoking is associated with increased severity of generalized aggressive periodontitis in young adults, and those who smoke are 3.8 times more likely to have periodontitis as compared to nonsmokers. In addition, smokers are more than six times as likely as nonsmokers to demonstrate continued attachment loss. Over a 10-year period, bone loss has been reported to be twice as rapid in smokers as in nonsmokers and to proceed more rapidly even in the presence of excellent plaque control.

Less information is available about the effects of cigar and pipe smoking, but it appears that effects similar to those of cigarette smoking are observed with these forms of tobacco use. The prevalence of moderate and severe periodontitis and the percentage of teeth with more than 5 mm of attachment loss were most severe in

BOX 9.3 Helping Your Patients to Quit Smoking

Smoking cessation must be an integral part of the management of dental patients who smoke, and it is the responsibility of all dental health professionals to address this issue with their patients. The dental team is well placed to provide this treatment because they see patients on a regular basis as part of ongoing routine dental management. Furthermore, interventions to help patients quit smoking in dental practices are effective, with quit rates of 15%–20% as compared to approximately 5% in control groups. The whole dental team should therefore be involved in smoking cessation, but this is not always the case. Why? Some of the barriers to providing smoking cessation counseling in the dental practice are shown. Various methods for helping patients to quit smoking in the dental environment have been described, and these are typically referred to as *brief intervention programs.* One such program is known as the 5 A's:

ASK Ask the patient about his or her smoking status (see Box 9.2).
This should be part of the medical history.

ADVISE Advise smokers of the associations between oral disease and smoking.
Be informative, honest, and helpful but not judgmental. The patient's response to this information will reveal his or her interest in quitting.

ASSESS Assess the patient's interest in and readiness to attempt smoking cessation.
Patients may not yet be in an action phase when it comes to quitting smoking, which is why it is always important to make these assessments every time you see the patient.

ASSIST Assist the patient with his or her quit attempt.
If you are trained, there are many techniques that can be used. Alternatively, assist the patient with seeking the help that he or she needs (see Box 9.4).

ARRANGE Arrange for a follow-up visit or a referral to professional smoking cessation services.
The most important aspect of this strategy is to keep in regular contact, particularly around the quit date and during the immediate period after the patient quits.

A simplified version of this is the 3 A's. This is a *very brief intervention* and can be particularly useful for the dental team. The intervention is designed to be used at every clinical contact, and its very brief nature may help overcome some of the barriers presented by dental practices (the duration is <30 s). The focus is taken away from advising smokers to stop and shifts to offering support. The "advise" step deliberately leaves out the health benefits of stopping smoking or the harms of smoking. This minimizes the duration of the intervention and helps to avoid a defensive reaction or developing anxiety in the patient. The 3 A's technique is as follows:

ASK and record smoking status.

ADVISE how to stop.

ACT on the patient's response (prescribe, monitor, or refer).
Clearly, for the patient undergoing a comprehensive course of periodontal therapy, over several visits, there may be more opportunity to focus on the harms of smoking and the personal benefits of quitting.

current cigarette smokers, but cigar and pipe smokers showed a severity of disease that was intermediate between that of current cigarette smokers and nonsmokers. Tooth loss is also increased among cigar and pipe smokers as compared to nonsmokers.

Former smokers have less risk for periodontitis than current smokers but more risk than nonsmokers, and the risk for periodontitis decreases with the increasing number of years since quitting smoking. This suggests that the negative effects of smoking on the host are reversible with smoking cessation and therefore that smoking cessation programs must be an integral component of periodontal education and therapy (Box 9.3). Several tobacco intervention approaches can be used when helping the patient deal with the physiologic factors (i.e., nicotine withdrawal symptoms) and the psychological factors associated with smoking cessation (Box 9.4). Electronic cigarettes have also emerged and are being used by many smokers to help them quit (Box 9.5). However, the effects on oral health are yet to be established.

Effects of Smoking on the Etiology and Pathogenesis of Periodontal Disease

The increased prevalence and severity of periodontal destruction associated with smoking suggests that the host–bacterial interactions normally seen with chronic periodontitis are altered, resulting in more extensive periodontal breakdown (Table 9.2). This imbalance between bacterial challenge and host response may be caused by changes in the composition of the subgingival biofilm (e.g., increases in the numbers and virulence of pathogenic organisms), changes in the host response to the bacterial challenge, or a combination of both.

Microbiology

A study of 798 subjects with different smoking histories found that smokers had significantly higher levels of *Tannerella forsythia* and that smokers were 2.3 times more likely to harbor *T. forsythia* as compared to nonsmokers and former smokers. Of interest were observations that smokers did not respond to mechanical therapy as well as nonsmokers did; this was associated with increased levels of *T. forsythia*, *Aggregatibacter actinomycetemcomitans*, and *Porphyromonas gingivalis* remaining in the pockets after therapy in the smoking group as compared to nonsmokers. A study sampled subgingival biofilm from all teeth with the exception of third molars in 272 adult subjects, including 50 current smokers, 98 former smokers, and 124 nonsmokers. Using checkerboard DNA–DNA hybridization technology to screen for 29 different subgingival species, it was found that members of the orange and red complex species—including *Eikenella nodatum*, *Fusobacterium nucleatum* ss *vincentii*, *Prevotella intermedia*, *Peptostreptococcus micros*, *Prevotella nigrescens*, *T. forsythia*, *P. gingivalis*, and *Treponema denticola*—were significantly more prevalent in current smokers than in nonsmokers and former smokers. The increased prevalence of these periodontal pathogens was caused by an increased colonization of shallow sites (pocket depth ≤4 mm), with no differences among smokers, former smokers, and nonsmokers in pockets 4 mm or greater. In addition, these pathogenic bacteria were more prevalent in the maxilla than the mandible. These data suggest that smokers have a greater extent of colonization by periodontal pathogens than nonsmokers or former smokers, which may increase the risk of periodontal disease progression.

Contemporary studies have drawn similar conclusions, analysis of periodontally healthy smokers demonstrating a highly diverse,

BOX 9.4 Overview of Smoking Cessation Approaches

Willpower Alone
This is the least effective method of smoking cessation, with only 3% of smokers managing to quit after 12 months.

Self-Help Materials
The provision of self-help materials can increase quit rates compared to no intervention, although only by a small amount. When included with any other intervention, there was no additional benefit.

Brief Intervention Program in Primary Care
A brief advice intervention delivered by a physician or dentist can increase the rate of quitting (12 months) by 40%–90%. Assuming an unassisted quit rate of 3%, a brief intervention by a dentist could increase the quit rates to around 4.5%–6%. Although this cessation rate may seem low, if the dental team gave this brief advice to most of their smoking patients, a significant number of smokers in the whole population would be assisted to quit each year.

Nicotine Replacement Therapy
Nicotine replacement therapy (NRT) can increase the rate of quitting (12 months) by 50%–70%. For example, in primary care settings in which brief advice is given, 12-month success rates can increase from around 5% to around 8% if NRT is also used. In an intensive setting such as a smoker's clinic, success rates increase from around 10% to up to 16%. NRT is not a magic cure, but it helps with cravings and withdrawal when a person quits smoking. Although NRT products do contain nicotine, they do not contain the toxic products such as tar and carbon monoxide that are found in cigarette smoke. NRT products include the following:

- Patches (available in different doses and worn for 16–24 h/day).
- Lozenges and gum (available in different flavors; should be chewed slowly to allow the nicotine to be absorbed through the mouth).
- Nasal spray (delivers nicotine solution via the nasal passages).
- Inhalator (a plastic mouthpiece with a supply of nicotine cartridges that fit on the end; nicotine is absorbed in the mouth by drawing on the inhalator like a cigarette).

Varenicline
A course of varenicline, at standard dose, can increase the rate of quitting (12 months) by 100%–150%. Varenicline is a nicotine receptor partial agonist, and it aims to reduce both withdrawal symptoms and the pleasure people usually experience when they smoke.

Bupropion
Bupropion can increase the rate of quitting (12 months) by 50%–80%. This medication is used as an antidepressant at higher doses, but it is effective for smoking cessation at lower doses. It is usually prescribed to be started 1–2 weeks before the quit date. There are serious potential drug interactions and unwanted effects.

Other Methods
Whatever works for the patient is good! In addition to combinations of the methods listed here, techniques for smoking cessation can include intensive counseling, motivational interviewing, cognitive behavioral therapy, hypnosis, and acupuncture. Many smokers are now also using e-cigarettes to help to quit smoking.

pathogen-rich, commensal-poor, anaerobic microbiome that is more similar to the microbiome observed in patients with advanced periodontitis.

Immune–Inflammatory Responses

The immune response of the host to biofilm accumulation is essentially protective. In periodontal health, a balance exists between the bacterial challenge of the biofilm and the immune–inflammatory responses in the gingival tissues, with no resulting loss of periodontal support. By contrast, periodontitis is associated with an alteration in the host–bacterial balance that may be initiated by changes in the bacterial composition of the subgingival biofilm, changes in the host responses, other environmental changes, or a combination of these.

Smoking exerts a major effect on the immune–inflammatory response that results in an increase in the extent and severity of periodontal destruction. The deleterious effects of smoking appear to result from alterations in the immune–inflammatory response to bacterial challenge. The neutrophil is an important component of the host response to the bacterial challenge, and alterations in

BOX 9.5 Smoking Cessation Aids

Beyond E-Cigarettes
The popularity of e-cigarettes took most people by surprise. But what's next?

"Heat-Not-Burn" Tobacco Products
These products heat tobacco to 500°C, producing an inhalable aerosol. Although not a new idea, they have received recent attention. One manufacturer introduced a product into the Japanese market in 2015, which has been popular, with the media reporting sales outstripping demand.

Water Pipes (Hookah, Shisha)
Popular in some communities, these are likely to carry significant negative health risks. A good summary is produced by the National Center for Smoking Cessation and Training (NCSCT).

Nicotine Gels
These gels allow nicotine to be absorbed through the skin. Currently they are not very popular.

Oral Nicotine Pouches
A range of products have been marketed since 2018. Typically, users hold the pouch between the upper lip and gum while the nicotine is released.

TABLE 9.2 Effects of Smoking on the Etiology and Pathogenesis of Periodontal Disease

Etiologic Factor	Effects of Smoking
Microbiology	Increased complexity of the microbiome and colonization of periodontal pockets by periodontal pathogens
Immune–inflammatory response	Altered neutrophil chemotaxis, phagocytosis, and oxidative burst ↑ Tumor necrosis factor-α and prostaglandin E_2 in gingival crevicular fluid ↑ Neutrophil collagenase and elastase in gingival crevicular fluid ↑ Production of prostaglandin E_2 by monocytes in response to lipopolysaccharide
Physiology	↓ Gingival blood vessels with ↑ inflammation ↓ Gingival crevicular fluid flow and bleeding on probing with ↑ inflammation ↓ Subgingival temperature ↑ Time needed to recover from local anesthesia

↓, Decreased; ↑, increased.

neutrophil number or function may result in localized and systemic infections. Critical functions of neutrophils include *chemotaxis* (directed locomotion from the bloodstream to the site of infection), *phagocytosis* (internalization of foreign particles such as bacteria), and *killing* via oxidative and nonoxidative mechanisms.

Neutrophils obtained from the peripheral blood, oral cavity, or saliva of smokers or exposed in vitro to whole tobacco smoke or nicotine have demonstrated functional alterations in chemotaxis, phagocytosis, and the oxidative burst. In vitro studies of the effects of tobacco products on neutrophils have shown detrimental effects on cell movement as well as on the oxidative burst. In addition, levels of antibody to the periodontal pathogens essential for phagocytosis and killing of bacteria, specifically immunoglobulin G_2, have been reported to be reduced in smokers as compared to nonsmokers with periodontitis, thereby suggesting that smokers may have reduced protection against periodontal bacteria. By contrast, elevated levels of tumor necrosis factor-α have been demonstrated in the gingival crevicular fluid of smokers, and elevated levels of prostaglandin E_2, neutrophil elastase, and matrix metalloproteinase-8 have also been found. These data suggest that smoking alters the response of neutrophils to the bacterial challenge such that there are increases in the release of tissue-destructive enzymes, causing increased periodontal tissue destruction.

Physiology

Previous studies have shown that certain clinical signs of inflammation (e.g., gingival redness, gingival bleeding) are less pronounced in smokers than in nonsmokers. This may result from alterations in the vascular response of the gingival tissues. Although no significant differences in the vascular density of healthy gingiva have been observed between smokers and nonsmokers, the response of the microcirculation to biofilm accumulation appears to be altered in smokers as compared to nonsmokers. With developing inflammation, increases in gingival crevicular fluid flow, bleeding on probing, and gingival blood vessels are lower in smokers than in nonsmokers. In addition, the oxygen concentration in healthy gingival tissues appears to be lower in smokers than in nonsmokers, although this condition is reversed in the presence of moderate inflammation. Subgingival temperatures are lower in smokers than nonsmokers, and recovery from the vasoconstriction caused by local anesthetic administration takes longer in smokers. These data suggest that significant alterations are present in the gingival microvasculature of smokers as compared to nonsmokers and that these changes lead to decreased blood flow and decreased clinical signs of inflammation. This explains the long-observed phenomenon of a transient increase in gingival bleeding when a smoker quits; patients need to be warned about this phenomenon.

Effects of Smoking on the Response to Periodontal Therapy

Nonsurgical Therapy

Numerous studies have indicated that current smokers do not respond as well to periodontal therapy as nonsmokers or former smokers do (Table 9.3). Most clinical research supports the observation that probing depth reductions are generally greater in nonsmokers than in smokers after nonsurgical periodontal therapy. In addition, gains in clinical attachment as a result of nonsurgical treatment are less pronounced in smokers than in nonsmokers. When a higher level of oral hygiene was achieved as part of nonsurgical care, the differences in the resolution of 4- to 6-mm pockets between nonsmokers and smokers became clinically less significant.

TABLE 9.3 Effects of Smoking on the Response to Periodontal Therapy

Therapy	Effects of Smoking
Nonsurgical	↓ Clinical response to root surface debridement ↓ Reduction in probing depth ↓ Gain in clinical attachment levels ↓ Negative impact of smoking with ↑ level of plaque control
Surgery and implants	↓ Probing depth reduction and ↓ gain in clinical attachment levels after access flap surgery ↑ Deterioration of furcations after surgery ↓ Gain in clinical attachment levels, ↓ bone fill, ↑ recession, and ↑ membrane exposure after guided tissue regeneration ↓ Root coverage after grafting procedures for localized gingival recession ↓ Probing depth reduction after bone graft procedures ↑ Risk for implant failure and peri-implantitis
Maintenance care	↑ Probing depth and attachment loss during maintenance therapy ↑ Disease recurrence in smokers ↑ Need for retreatment in smokers ↑ Tooth loss in smokers after surgical therapy

↓, Decreased; ↑, increased.

It can be concluded that smokers respond less well to nonsurgical therapy than do nonsmokers. With excellent plaque control, these differences may be minimized, but the emphasis is on truly excellent plaque control. When comparing current smokers with former smokers and nonsmokers, the former and nonsmoking subjects appear to respond equally well to nonsurgical care, thereby reinforcing the need for patients to be informed of the benefits of smoking cessation.

Surgical Therapy and Implants

The less favorable response of the periodontal tissues to nonsurgical therapy that is observed in current smokers is also observed after surgical therapy. In a longitudinal comparative study of the effects of four different treatment modalities (coronal scaling, root planing, modified Widman flap surgery, and osseous resection surgery), smokers (with "heavy" defined as ≥20 cigarettes/day and "light" defined as ≤19 cigarettes/day) consistently showed less pocket reduction and less gain in clinical attachment as compared to nonsmokers or former smokers. These differences were evident immediately after the completion of therapy and continued throughout 7 years of supportive periodontal therapy. During the 7 years, deterioration at furcation areas was greater in heavy and light smokers than in former smokers and nonsmokers. Smoking has also been shown to have a negative impact on the outcomes of guided tissue regeneration and the treatment of infrabony defects by bone grafts. By 12 months after guided tissue regeneration therapy at deep infrabony defects, smokers demonstrated less than half the attachment gain that was observed in nonsmokers (2.1 mm vs 5.2 mm). In a second study, 73 smokers also showed less attachment gain than nonsmokers (1.2 mm vs 3.2 mm), more gingival recession, and less bone infill of the defect. Similarly, after the use of bone grafts for the treatment of infrabony defects, smokers showed less reduction in probing depths as compared to nonsmokers.

Open flap access surgery without regenerative or grafting procedures is a common surgical procedure used for accessing the root and bone surfaces. By 6 months after this procedure, smokers showed significantly less reduction of deep pockets (≥7 mm) than nonsmokers (3 mm for smokers vs 4 mm for nonsmokers) and significantly less gain in clinical attachment (1.8 mm for smokers vs 2.8 mm for nonsmokers), even though all of the patients received supportive periodontal therapy every month for 6 months.

Tobacco smoking also affects the outcomes of periodontal plastic surgery. For instance, a systematic review assessed the influence of smoking on the outcomes achieved by root coverage procedures. This review identified that significantly greater root coverage and greater gains in clinical attachment levels were recorded for nonsmokers as compared to smokers after the treatment of gingival recession defects by subepithelial connective-tissue grafts. Furthermore, smokers showed significantly fewer sites with complete root coverage than were seen in the nonsmokers.

In patients who had undergone implant therapy, smoking increases the risk of implant failure. Overall, the risk for implant failure in smokers appears to be approximately double the risk for failure in nonsmokers, and the risks appear to be higher in maxillary implants and when implants are placed in poor-quality bone. Recent evidence from human histologic clinical trials evaluating transitional implants showed that smoking had: (1) a detrimental impact on peri-implant bone healing (reduced bone-to-implant contact, bone density in the threaded area, and bone density outside the threaded area); and (2) reduced survival rates, especially for maxillary implants.

Smoking has also been shown to be a risk factor for peri-implantitis, with a majority of studies showing a significant increase in peri-implant bone loss as compared to nonsmokers. Collectively, these data indicate that implant failure is more common among smokers than nonsmokers. However, because numerous factors can influence implant success, further controlled clinical trials are needed to address the role of smoking as an independent variable in implant failure. Given the current evidence, all patients who are considering implant therapy should be informed about the benefits of smoking cessation and the risks of smoking for the development of peri-implantitis and implant failure.

Maintenance Therapy

The detrimental effect of smoking on treatment outcomes appears to be long lasting and independent of the frequency of maintenance therapy. After four modalities of therapy (scaling, scaling and root planing, modified Widman flap surgery, and osseous surgery), maintenance therapy was performed by a hygienist every 3 months for 7 years. Smokers consistently had deeper pockets than nonsmokers and less gain in attachment when evaluated each year for the 7-year period. Even with more intensive maintenance therapy given every month for 6 months after flap surgery, smokers had deeper and more residual pockets than nonsmokers, although no significant differences in plaque or bleeding on probing scores were found. These data suggest that the effects of smoking on the host response and the healing characteristics of the periodontal tissues may have a long-term effect on pocket resolution in smokers, possibly requiring more intensive management during the maintenance phase. Smokers also tend to experience more periodontal breakdown than nonsmokers after therapy. In studies of patients who failed to respond to periodontal therapy, approximately 90% of these poorly responding patients were smokers.

Tobacco smoking was positively associated with tooth loss even when regular recall maintenance care was performed (overall, smokers had a risk of losing their teeth that was up to 380% higher than that of nonsmokers). Similarly, smoking has a detrimental effect on peri-implant tissue status, even when patients are under strict peri-implant preventive maintenance care.

It is clear from these studies that (1) smokers may present with periodontal disease at an early age, (2) they may be difficult to treat effectively with the conventional therapeutic strategies; (3) they may continue to have progressive or recurrent periodontitis; and (4) they may be at an increased risk of tooth loss or peri-implant bone loss, even when adequate maintenance control is established. For these reasons, smoking cessation counseling must be a cornerstone of periodontal therapy in smokers.

Effects of Smoking Cessation on Periodontal Treatment Outcomes

Periodontal treatment outcomes have been assessed in smokers, former smokers, and nonsmokers. Collectively, these studies have demonstrated that smokers have significantly worse periodontal status than either former smokers or nonsmokers and usually have poorer treatment outcomes. The periodontal status of former smokers is intermediate to that of current smokers and nonsmokers, and it appears to usually be closer to that of nonsmokers. Smoking cessation positively influenced periodontal treatment outcomes. When patients received nonsurgical therapy as treatment for their periodontitis, in addition to smoking cessation counseling for a period of 12 months, those individuals who successfully quit smoking for the entire 12 months of the study had the best response to the periodontal treatment.

The benefit of smoking cessation on the periodontium is likely to be mediated through various pathways, such as a shift toward a less-pathogenic microbiome, the recovery of the gingival microcirculation, and improvements in certain aspects of the immune–inflammatory responses. In conclusion, smoking is a major risk factor for periodontitis, and smoking cessation should be an integral part of periodontal therapy among patients who smoke. Smoking cessation should be considered a priority for the management of periodontitis in smokers.

Key points

- The gas phase of tobacco smoke contains carbon monoxide, ammonia, formaldehyde, hydrogen cyanide, and toxic compounds such as benzo(a)pyrene and dimethylnitrosamine.
- The particulate phase of tobacco smoke includes nicotine, tar, benzene, and benzo(a)pyrene.
- Nicotine is quickly absorbed in the lungs, and it reaches the brain within 10–19 seconds.
- Nicotine causes a rise in blood pressure, increased heart and respiratory rates, and peripheral vasoconstriction.
- Smokers have reduced gingival inflammation and bleeding on probing.
- In smokers, even shallow periodontal pockets are colonized by periodontal pathogens.
- Smokers were four times as likely to have periodontitis as compared to persons who had never smoked.
- Former smokers were 1.7 times more likely to have periodontitis.
- Smoking reduces positive response to both nonsurgical and surgical periodontal therapy.
- Tobacco smoking was positively associated with tooth loss even when regular recall maintenance care was performed.
- Smoking cessation positively influenced periodontal treatment outcomes.

Suggested Readings

Chambrone L, Chambrone D, Lima LA, et al: Predictors of tooth loss during long-term periodontal maintenance: a systematic review of observational studies, *J Clin Periodontol* 37:675–684, 2010.

Chambrone L, Preshaw PM, Rosa EF, et al: Effects of smoking cessation on the outcomes of non-surgical periodontal therapy: a systematic review and individual patient data meta-analysis, *J Clin Periodontol* 40:607–615, 2013.

Heasman L, Stacey F, Preshaw PM, et al: The effect of smoking on periodontal treatment response: a review of clinical evidence, *J Clin Periodontol* 33:241–253, 2006.

Preshaw PM, Heasman L, Stacey F, et al: The effect of quitting smoking on chronic periodontitis, *J Clin Periodontol* 32:869–879, 2005.

Rosa EF, Corraini P, de Carvalho VF, et al: A prospective 12-month study of the effect of smoking cessation on periodontal clinical parameters, *J Clin Periodontol* 38:562–571, 2011.

Tomar SL, Asma S: Smoking-attributable periodontitis in the United States: findings from NHANES III. National Health and Nutrition Examination Survey, *J Periodontol* 71:743-751, 2000.

Warnakulasuriya S, Dietrich T, Bornstein MM, et al: Oral health risks of tobacco use and effects of cessation, *Int Dent J* 60:7–30, 2010.

References

References and MCQs with answers for the chapter are available on www.medenact.com.

CHAPTER 10

Role of Dental Calculus and Other Predisposing Factors

JE Hinrichs | V Thumbigere-Math | Olga A. Korczeniewska | SR Diehl | N Ambalavanan

CHAPTER OUTLINE

The primary cause of gingival inflammation is bacterial plaque. Other predisposing factors include calculus, faulty restorations, complications associated with orthodontic therapy, self-inflicted injuries, and the use of tobacco. These will be discussed in turn.

Calculus

Calculus consists of mineralized bacterial plaque that forms on the surfaces of natural teeth and dental prostheses.

Supragingival and Subgingival Calculus (Table 10.1)

Supragingival calculus is located coronal to the gingival margin and therefore is visible in the oral cavity. It is usually white or whitish yellow in color; hard, with a clay-like consistency; and easily detached from the tooth surface. After removal, it may rapidly recur, especially in the lingual area of the mandibular incisors. The color is influenced by contact with substances such as tobacco and food pigments. It may be localized on a single tooth or group of teeth, or it may be generalized throughout the mouth.

The two most common locations for the development of supragingival calculus are the buccal surfaces of the maxillary molars (Fig. 10.1) and the lingual surfaces of the mandibular anterior teeth (Fig. 10.2).

Saliva from the parotid gland flows over the facial surfaces of the upper molars via the parotid duct, whereas the submandibular duct and the lingual duct empty onto the lingual surfaces of the lower incisors from the submaxillary and sublingual glands, respectively. In extreme cases, calculus may form a bridge-like structure over the interdental papilla of adjacent teeth or cover the occlusal surface of teeth that are lacking functional antagonists.

Subgingival calculus is located below the crest of the marginal gingiva and therefore is not visible on routine clinical examination. The location and the extent of subgingival calculus may be evaluated by careful tactile perception with a delicate dental instrument such as an explorer. Subgingival calculus is typically hard and dense; it frequently appears to be dark brown or greenish black in color (Fig. 10.3), and it is firmly attached to the tooth surface. Supragingival calculus and subgingival calculus generally occur together, but one may be present without the other. Microscopic studies demonstrate that deposits of subgingival calculus usually extend nearly to the base of periodontal pockets in individuals with chronic periodontitis but do not reach the junctional epithelium.

When the gingival tissues recede, subgingival calculus becomes exposed and is therefore reclassified as supragingival (Fig. 10.4A). Thus, supragingival calculus can be composed of both the initial supragingival calculus and previous subgingival calculus. A reduction in gingival inflammation and probing depths with a gain in clinical attachment can be observed after the removal of subgingival plaque and calculus (see Fig. 10.4B).

Prevalence

The formation of supragingival calculus was observed early in life in individuals, probably shortly after the teeth erupted. The first areas to exhibit calculus deposits were the facial aspects of maxillary molars and the lingual surfaces of mandibular incisors. The deposition of supragingival calculus continued as individuals aged, and it reached a maximal calculus score when the affected individuals were 25–30 years old.

At this time, most of the teeth were covered by calculus, although the facial surfaces had less calculus than the lingual or palatal surfaces. Calculus accumulation appeared to be symmetric, and by the age of 45 years, these individuals had only a few teeth (typically the premolars) without calculus deposits. Subgingival calculus appeared first either independently or on the interproximal aspects of areas where supragingival calculus already existed. By the age of 30 years, all surfaces of all teeth had subgingival calculus without any pattern of predilection.

Both supragingival calculus and subgingival calculus may be seen on radiographs. Highly calcified interproximal calculus deposits are readily detectable as radiopaque projections that protrude into the interdental spaces (Fig. 10.5). However, the sensitivity level of detecting calculus by radiographs is inconsistent. The location of calculus does not indicate the bottom of the periodontal pocket because the most apical plaque is not sufficiently calcified to be visible on radiographs.

Composition

Inorganic Content

Dental calculus is primarily composed of inorganic components (70%–90%) and the organic components constitute the rest. The

TABLE 10.1 Differences Between Supragingival and Subgingival Calculus

Supragingival Calculus	Subgingival Calculus
Located coronal to the gingival margin—visible in the oral cavity	Located below the crest of the marginal gingiva—not visible on routine clinical examination
White or whitish yellow in color	Dark brown or greenish black in color
Hard with clay-like consistency	Hard and dense
Easily detached from the tooth surface	Firmly attached to the tooth surface

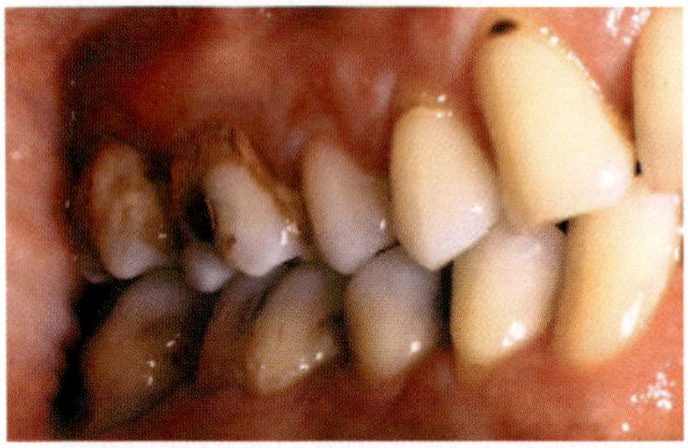

Fig. 10.1 Supragingival calculus is depicted on the buccal surfaces of maxillary molars adjacent to the orifice for the parotid duct.

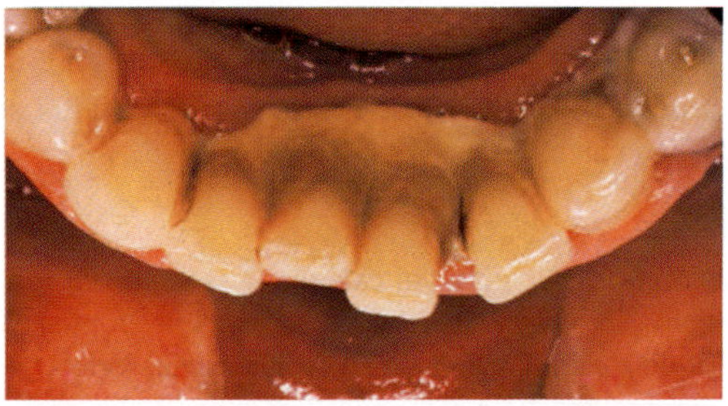

Fig. 10.2 Extensive supragingival calculus is present on the lingual surfaces of the lower anterior teeth.

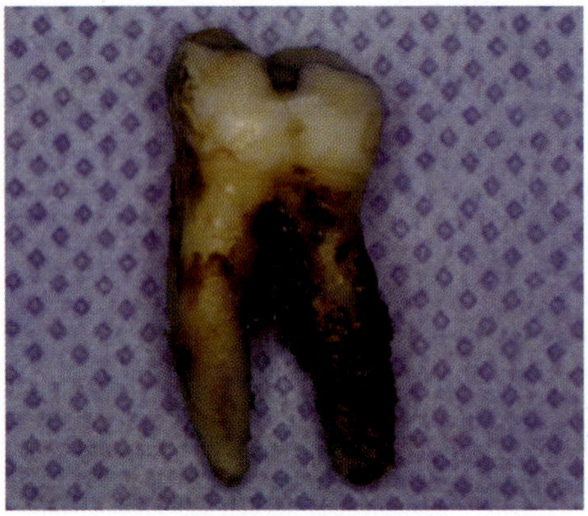

Fig. 10.3 Dark pigmented deposits of subgingival calculus are shown on the distal root of an extracted lower molar.

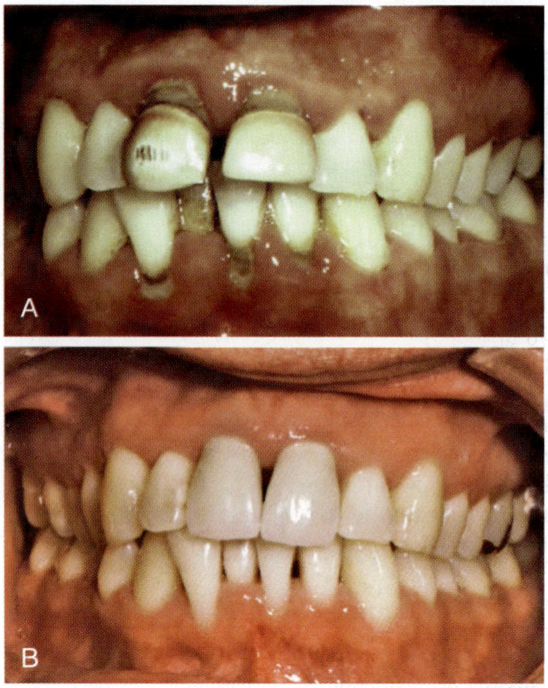

Fig. 10.4 A, A 31-year-old man with extensive supragingival and subgingival calculus deposits throughout his dentition. B, 1 year after receiving thorough scaling and root planing to remove supragingival and subgingival calculus deposits, followed by restorative care. Note the substantial reduction in gingival inflammation.

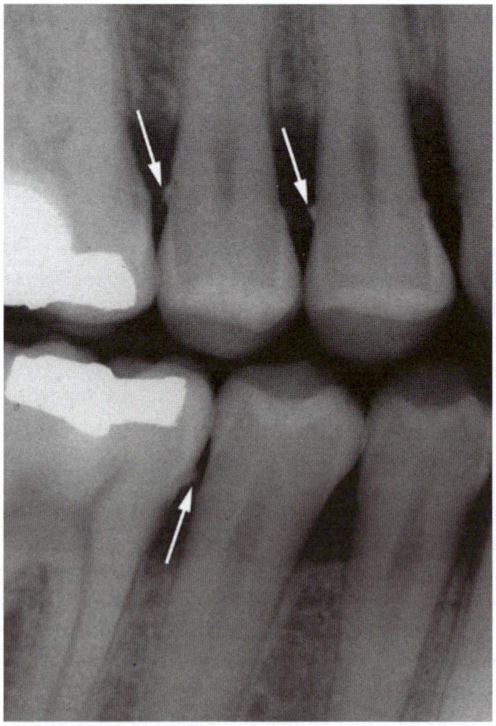

Fig. 10.5 A bitewing radiograph illustrating subgingival calculus deposits that are depicted as interproximal spurs (*arrows*).

major inorganic proportions of calculus are approximately 76% calcium phosphate ($Ca_3[PO_4]_2$), 3% calcium carbonate ($CaCO_3$), 4% magnesium phosphate ($Mg_3[PO_4]_2$), 2% carbon dioxide, and traces of other elements such as sodium, zinc, strontium, bromine, copper, manganese, tungsten, gold, aluminum, silicon, iron, and fluorine. The percentage of inorganic constituents in calculus is similar to that of other calcified tissues of the body (Table 10.2).

At least two-thirds of the inorganic component is crystalline in structure. The four main crystal forms and their approximate percentages are as follows: hydroxyapatite, 58%; magnesium whitlockite, 21%; octacalcium phosphate, 12%; and brushite, 9%.

TABLE 10.2 Calculus Versus Other Oral Hard Tissues

Structure	Inorganic Content (%)[a]
Dental calculus	70–90
Enamel	96
Dentin	45
Bone	60–70

[a]Organic components and water constitute the rest.

Two or more crystal forms are typically found in a sample of calculus. Hydroxyapatite and octacalcium phosphate are detected most frequently (i.e., in 97%–100% of all supragingival calculus) and constitute the bulk of the specimen. Brushite is more common in the mandibular anterior region, and magnesium whitlockite is found in the posterior areas. The incidence of the four crystal forms varies with the age of the deposit.

Organic Content

The organic component of calculus consists of a mixture of protein–polysaccharide complexes, desquamated epithelial cells, leukocytes, and various types of microorganisms.

Between 1.9% and 9.1% of the organic component is carbohydrate, which consists of galactose, glucose, rhamnose, mannose, glucuronic acid, galactosamine, and sometimes arabinose, galacturonic acid, and glucosamine. All of these organic components are present in salivary glycoprotein, with the exception of arabinose and rhamnose. Salivary proteins account for 5.9%–8.2% of the organic component of calculus and include most amino acids. Lipids account for 0.2% of the organic content in the form of neutral fats, free fatty acids, cholesterol, cholesterol esters, and phospholipids.

The composition of subgingival calculus is similar to that of supragingival calculus, with some differences (Table 10.3). It has the same hydroxyapatite content but more magnesium whitlockite and less brushite and octacalcium phosphate. The ratio of calcium to phosphate is higher in subgingival calculus, and the sodium content increases with the depth of periodontal pockets. These altered compositions may be attributed to the fact that the origin of subgingival calculus is plasma, whereas supragingival calculus is partially composed of salivary constituents. Salivary proteins present in supragingival calculus are not found in subgingival calculus. Dental calculus, salivary duct calculus, and calcified dental tissues are similar in inorganic composition.

TABLE 10.3 Composition of Supragingival and Subgingival Calculus

Supragingival Calculus	Subgingival Calculus
Inorganic content Calcium phosphate—75.9% Calcium carbonate—3.1% Traces of magnesium phosphate	Ratio of calcium to phosphate is higher subgingivally
Two-thirds of inorganic content is crystalline in structure: • Hydroxyapatite—58% • Magnesium whitlockite—21% • Octacalcium phosphate—12% • Brushite—9%	• Similar hydroxyapatite content • More magnesium whitlockite compared to supragingival calculus • Less brushite and octacalcium phosphate than supragingival calculus
Organic content Consists of a mixture of protein–polysaccharide complexes, desquamated epithelial cells, leukocytes, and various types of microorganisms	
Carbohydrates: 1.9%–9.1% Salivary proteins: 5.9%–8.2% Lipids: 0.2%	Salivary proteins not found subgingivally

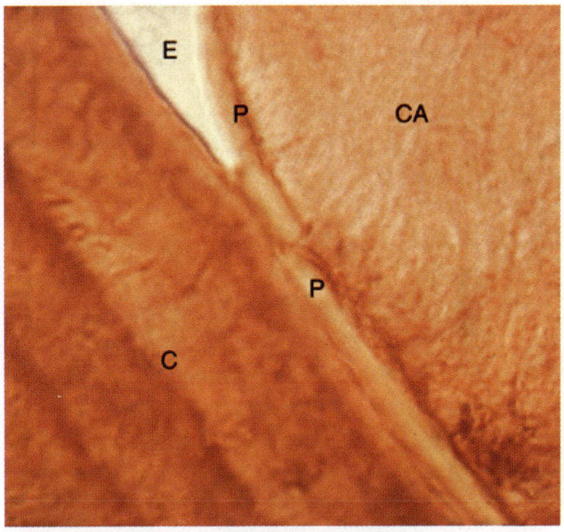

Fig. 10.6 Calculus attached to the pellicle on the enamel surface and the cementum. An enamel void *(E)* has been created during the preparation of the specimen. *C*, Cementum; *CA*, calculus; *P*, pellicle.

Attachment to the Tooth Surface

Differences in the manner in which calculus is attached to the tooth surface affect the relative ease or difficulty encountered during its removal. Four modes of attachment have been described. (1) Attachment by means of an organic pellicle on cementum is depicted in Fig. 10.6, and attachment on enamel is shown in Fig. 10.7. (2) Mechanical locking into surface irregularities, such as caries lesions or resorption lacunae. (3) Close adaptation of the undersurface of calculus to depressions or gently sloping mounds of the unaltered cementum surface is shown in Fig. 10.8. (4) Penetration of bacterial calculus into cementum.

Formation

Calculus is *mineralized dental plaque.* The soft plaque is hardened by the precipitation of mineral salts, which usually starts between the 1st and 14th days of plaque formation. Calcification has been reported to occur within as little as 4–8 h. Calcifying plaques may become 50% mineralized in 2 days and 60%–90% mineralized in 12 days. All plaque does not necessarily undergo calcification. Early plaque contains a small amount of inorganic material, which increases as the plaque develops into calculus. Plaque that does not develop into calculus reaches a plateau of maximal mineral content within 2 days. Microorganisms are not always essential in calculus formation because calculus readily occurs in germ-free rodents.

Saliva is the primary source of mineralization for supragingival calculus, whereas the serum transudate called *gingival crevicular fluid* furnishes the minerals for subgingival calculus. The calcium concentration or content in plaque is 2–20 times higher than in saliva. Early plaque of heavy calculus formers contains more calcium, three times more phosphorus, and less potassium than that of noncalculus formers, suggesting that phosphorus may be more critical than calcium for plaque mineralization. Calcification entails the

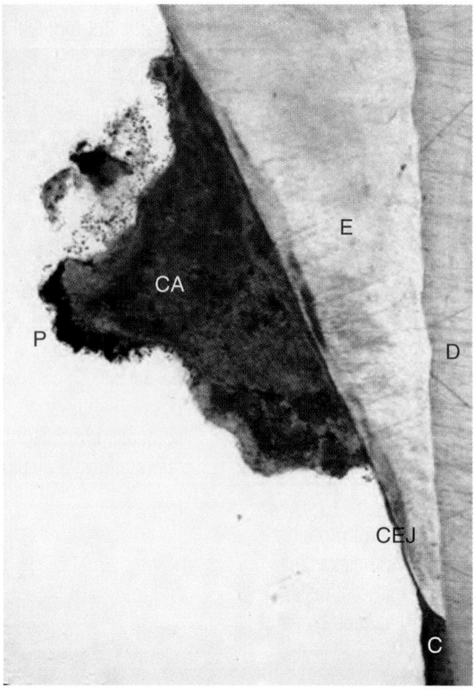

Fig. 10.7 Nondecalcified specimen with calculus *(CA)* attached to enamel *(E)* surface just coronal to the cementoenamel junction *(CEJ)*. Note plaque *(P)* on the surface of the calculus; dentin *(D)* and cementum *(C)* are also identified. *(Courtesy: Dr. Michael Rohrer, Minneapolis, MN.)*

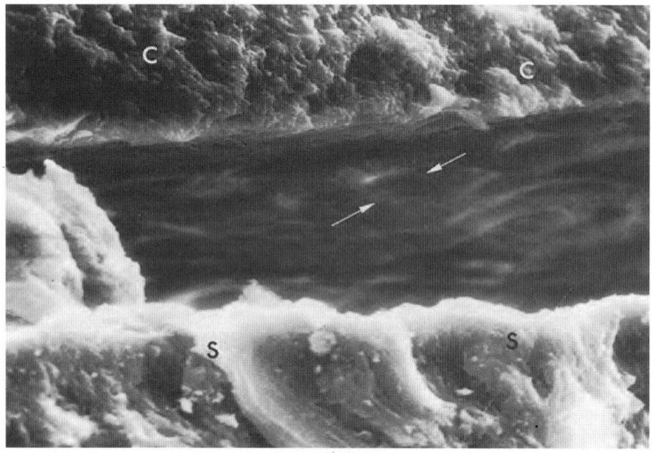

Fig. 10.8 Undersurface of subgingival calculus *(C)* previously attached to the cementum surface *(S)*. Note the impression of cementum mounds in the calculus (*arrows*). *(Courtesy: Dr. John Sottosanti, La Jolla, CA.)*

binding of calcium ions to the carbohydrate–protein complexes of the organic matrix and the precipitation of crystalline calcium phosphate salts. Crystals form initially in the intercellular matrix and on the bacterial surfaces and finally within the bacteria.

The calcification of supragingival plaque and the attached component of subgingival plaque begins along the inner surface adjacent to the tooth structure. Separate foci of calcification increase in size and coalesce to form solid masses of calculus. For the initial mineralization process to occur, calcium phosphate supersaturation, certain membrane-associated components, and regulation of nuclear inhibitors are required. Calcification may be accompanied by alterations in the bacterial content and staining qualities of the plaque. As calcification progresses, the number of filamentous bacteria increases, and the foci of calcification change from basophilic to eosinophilic. Calculus is formed in layers, which are often separated by a thin cuticle that becomes embedded in the calculus as calcification progresses.

The initiation of calcification and the rate of calculus accumulation vary among individuals, among tooth variety in the same dentition, and at different times in the same person. On the basis of these differences, persons may be classified as *heavy*, *moderate*, or *slight* calculus formers or as noncalculus formers. The average daily increment in calculus formers is from 0.10%–0.15% of dry weight calculus. Calculus formation continues until it reaches a maximum, after which it may be reduced in amount. The time required to reach the maximal level has been reported to be between 10 weeks and 6 months.

The decline from maximal calculus accumulation, which is referred to as the *reversal phenomenon*, may be explained by the vulnerability of bulky calculus to mechanical wear from food and from the cheeks, lips, and tongue movement.

Theories Regarding the Mineralization of Calculus

The theoretical mechanisms by which plaque becomes mineralized can be stratified into two categories.

1. Mineral precipitation results from a local rise in the degree of saturation of calcium and phosphate ions, which may be brought about in several ways:
   - *A rise in the pH of the saliva causes the precipitation of calcium phosphate salts by lowering the precipitation constant.* The pH may be elevated by the loss of carbon dioxide and the formation of ammonia by dental plaque bacteria or by protein degradation during stagnation.
   - *Colloidal proteins in saliva bind calcium and phosphate ions and maintain a supersaturated solution with respect to calcium phosphate salts.* With the stagnation of saliva, colloids settle out, and the supersaturated state is no longer maintained, thereby leading to the precipitation of calcium phosphate salts.
   - *Phosphatase liberated from dental plaque, desquamated epithelial cells, or bacteria precipitates calcium phosphate by hydrolyzing organic phosphates in saliva, thereby increasing the concentration of free phosphate ions. Esterase* is another enzyme that is present in the cocci and filamentous organisms, leukocytes, macrophages, and desquamated epithelial cells of dental plaque. Esterase may initiate calcification by hydrolyzing fatty esters into free fatty acids. The fatty acids form soaps with calcium and magnesium that are later converted into the less-soluble calcium phosphate salts.
2. Seeding agents induce small foci of calcification that enlarge and coalesce to form a calcified mass. This concept has been referred to as the *epitactic concept* or, more appropriately, as *heterogeneous nucleation.* The seeding agents in calculus formation are not known, but it is suspected that the intercellular matrix of plaque plays an active role. The carbohydrate–protein complexes may initiate calcification by removing calcium from the saliva (chelation) and binding with it to form nuclei that induce the subsequent deposition of minerals.

Role of Microorganisms in the Mineralization of Calculus

Mineralization of plaque generally starts extracellularly around both gram-positive and gram-negative organisms, but it may also start intracellularly. Filamentous organisms, diphtheroids, and *Bacterionema* and *Veillonella* species have the ability to form intracellular apatite crystals. Mineralization spreads until the matrix and the bacteria are calcified.

Bacterial plaque may actively participate in the mineralization of calculus by forming phosphatases, which change the pH of the plaque and induce mineralization, but the prevalent opinion is that these bacteria are only passively involved and are simply calcified with other plaque components. The occurrence of calculus-like deposits in germ-free animals supports this opinion. However, other experiments suggest that transmissible factors are involved in calculus formation and that penicillin in the diets of some of these animals reduces calculus formation.

Etiologic Significance

Distinguishing between the effects of calculus and plaque on the gingiva is difficult because calculus is always covered with a nonmineralized layer of plaque. A positive correlation between the presence of calculus and the prevalence of gingivitis exists, but this correlation is not as great as that between plaque and gingivitis. The initiation of periodontal disease in young people is closely related to plaque accumulation, whereas calculus accumulation is more prevalent in chronic periodontitis found in older adults.

The incidence of calculus, gingivitis, and periodontal disease increases with age. It is extremely rare to find periodontal pockets in adults without at least some subgingival calculus being present, although the subgingival calculus may be of microscopic proportions.

Calculus does not contribute directly to gingival inflammation, but it provides a fixed nidus for the continued accumulation of bacterial plaque and its retention in close proximity to the gingiva.

Subgingival calculus is likely to be the product rather than the cause of periodontal pockets. Plaque initiates gingival inflammation, which leads to pocket formation, and the pocket in turn provides a sheltered area for plaque and bacterial accumulation. The increased flow of gingival crevicular fluid associated with gingival inflammation provides the minerals that mineralize the continually accumulating plaque, resulting in the formation of subgingival calculus. Aggressive periodontitis areas with detectable subgingival calculus were much more likely to experience a loss of periodontal attachment than sites that did not initially exhibit subgingival calculus.

Although the bacterial plaque that coats the teeth is the main etiologic factor in the development of periodontal disease, the removal of subgingival plaque and calculus constitutes the cornerstone of periodontal therapy. Calculus plays an important role in maintaining and accentuating periodontal disease by keeping plaque in close contact with the gingival tissue and by creating areas where plaque removal is impossible. Therefore, the clinician must not only possess the clinical skill to remove the plaque and calculus, but he or she must also be very conscientious about performing this task.

Materia Alba, Food Debris, and Dental Stains

Materia alba is an accumulation of microorganisms, desquamated epithelial cells, leukocytes, and a mixture of salivary proteins and lipids, with few or no food particles; it lacks the regular internal pattern observed in plaque. It is a yellow or grayish-white, soft, sticky deposit, and it is somewhat less adherent than dental plaque. The irritating effect of materia alba on the gingiva is caused by bacteria and their products.

Most food debris is rapidly liquefied by bacterial enzymes and cleared from the oral cavity by salivary flow and the mechanical action of the tongue, cheeks, and lips. The rate of clearance from the oral cavity varies with the type of food and the individual. Aqueous solutions are typically cleared within 15 minutes, whereas sticky foods may adhere for more than 1 hour. Dental plaque is not a derivative of food debris, and food debris is not an important cause of gingivitis.

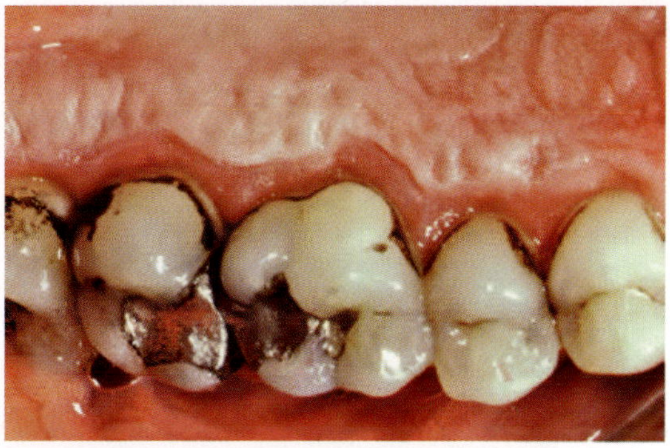

Fig. 10.9 Tobacco stains on the apical third of the clinical crown caused by cigarette smoking.

Pigmented deposits on the tooth surface are called *dental stains*. Stains are primarily an esthetic problem and do not cause inflammation of the gingiva. The use of tobacco products (Fig. 10.9), coffee, tea, certain mouthrinses, and pigments in foods can contribute to stain formation.

Other Predisposing Factors

Iatrogenic Factors

Deficiencies in the quality of dental restorations or prostheses are contributing factors to gingival inflammation and periodontal destruction. Inadequate dental procedures that contribute to the deterioration of the periodontal tissues are referred to as *iatrogenic factors*. Iatrogenic endodontic complications that can adversely affect the periodontium include root perforations, vertical root fractures, and endodontic failures that may necessitate tooth extraction. Immediate implant placement in conjunction with extraction can contribute to an excessive labial and apical position of the implant, whereby the blood supply of surrounding osseous and gingival tissues is compromised, yielding to gingival fenestration or dehiscence (Fig. 10.10). In order to mitigate the risk of dental implant complications, practitioners should consider cone-beam computed tomography for dental implant treatment planning.

Characteristics of dental restorations and removable partial dentures that are important to the maintenance of periodontal health include the location of the gingival margin for the restoration, the space between the margin of the restoration and the unprepared tooth, the contour of the restorations, the occlusion, the materials used in the restoration, the restorative procedure itself, and the design of the removable partial denture. These characteristics are described in this chapter as they relate to the etiology of periodontal disease. A more comprehensive review with special emphasis on the interrelationship between restorative procedures and the periodontal status is presented in Chapter 54.

Margins of Restorations

Overhanging margins of dental restorations contribute to the development of periodontal disease by (1) changing the ecologic balance of the gingival sulcus to an area that favors the growth of disease-associated organisms (predominantly gram-negative anaerobic species) at the expense of the health-associated organisms (predominantly gram-positive facultative species) and (2) inhibiting the patient's access to remove accumulated plaque.

The frequency of overhanging margins on proximal restorations has varied in different studies from 16.5% to 75%. A highly significant statistical relationship has been reported between marginal defects and reduced bone height. The removal of overhangs allows

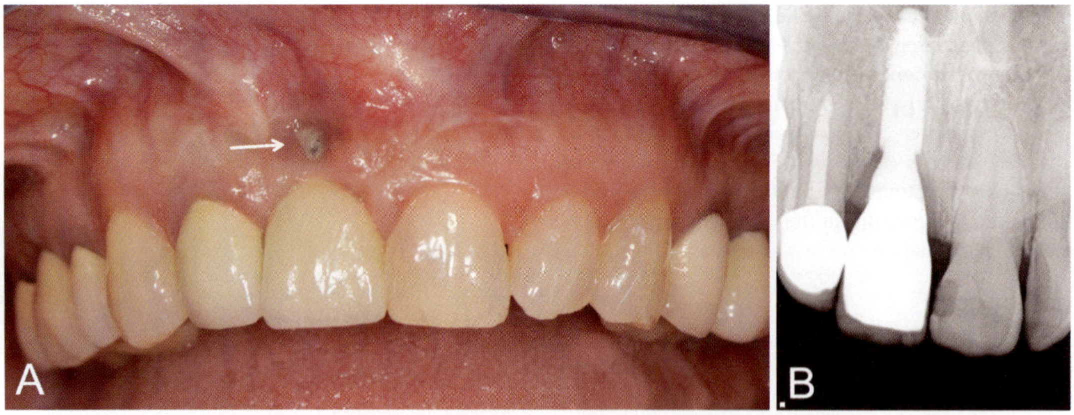

Fig. 10.10 A, A fenestration defect (*arrow*) is noted after placement of a dental implant too far labial and apical, yielding inadequate bone and blood supply to support the surrounding gingiva. B, Radiograph of the malpositioned dental implant.

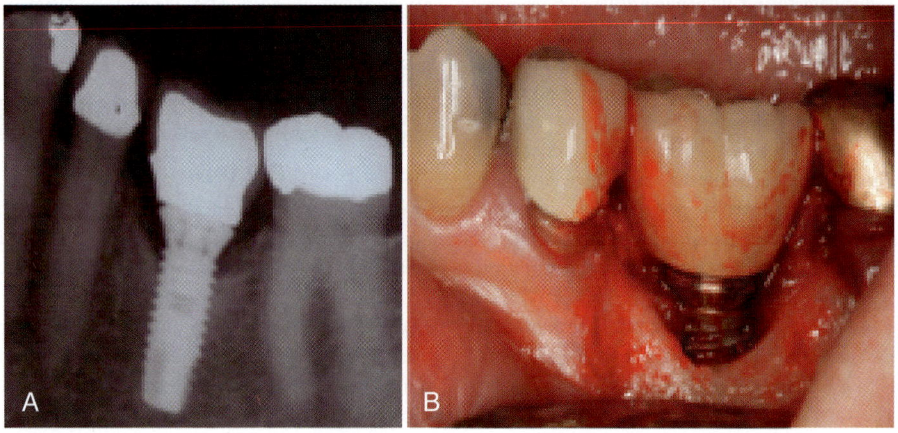

Fig. 10.11 A, Radiograph of a moat-like bony defect at a peri-implantitis site associated with retained cement and a crown that is not fully seated. B, Moat-like bony defect and retained excessive cement. *(Courtesy Dr. Emilie Vachon, Minneapolis, MN.)*

for the more effective control of plaque, thereby resulting in a reduction of gingival inflammation and a small increase in radiographic alveolar bone support.

The location of the gingival margin of a restoration is directly related to the health status of the adjacent periodontal tissues. Numerous studies have shown a positive correlation between restoration margins located apical to the marginal gingiva and the presence of gingival inflammation. Subgingival margins are associated with large amounts of plaque, more severe gingivitis, deeper pockets, and a change in the composition of the subgingival microflora that closely resembles the microflora noted in chronic periodontitis. Even high-quality restorations with clinically perfect margins, if placed subgingivally, will increase plaque accumulation, gingival inflammation, and the rate of gingival crevicular fluid flow. Margins placed at the level of the gingival crest induce less severe inflammation, whereas supragingival margins are associated with a degree of periodontal health similar to that seen with nonrestored interproximal surfaces.

Roughness in the subgingival area is considered to be a major contributing factor to plaque buildup and subsequent gingival inflammation. The subgingival zone is composed of the margin of the restoration, the luting material, and the prepared and unprepared tooth surfaces. Sources of marginal roughness include grooves and scratches in the surface of acrylic resin, porcelain, or gold restorations; separation of the restoration margin and the luting material from the cervical finish line, thereby exposing the rough surface of the prepared tooth; dissolution and disintegration of the luting material between the preparation and the restoration, thereby leaving a space; and inadequate marginal fit of the restoration. Subgingival margins typically have a gap of 20–40 µm between the margin of the restoration and the unprepared tooth. Colonization of this gap by bacterial plaque undoubtedly contributes to the detrimental effect of margins placed in a subgingival environment.

Retained Cement and Peri-Implantitis

Peri-implantitis is an inflammatory disease of the tissues around dental implants resulting in progressive bone loss (Fig. 10.11A and B), whereas peri-implant mucositis is a reversible inflammatory change of the soft tissues around implants without bone loss. The prevalence of peri-implantitis among implant-supported prostheses/restorations ranges from 28% to 56%. The early diagnosis of this condition and its proper management are critical to the longevity of the implant and the supported prosthesis.

Local factors such as retained residual cement or inadequate seating of the implant abutment or prosthesis can lead to bone loss around an implant. In a retrospective study, Wilson found that 81% of the implants diagnosed with peri-implantitis had residual cement associated with their cement-retained restorations. The surgical removal of the residual cement resolved the infection and halted the peri-implantitis in 74% of the implants. A deeper crown margin makes it more difficult to remove excess cement. The greatest amount of residual cement was noted when the crown margin was 2 or 3 mm below the gingival margin.

The possible adverse effect of traumatic occlusion on implants has been correlated with early implant failures. However, the relationship between traumatic occlusion and peri-implantitis is, to date, a controversial issue. In vivo experiments have shown that, in the absence of peri-implant inflammation, the application of excessive occlusal stress leads to only minor alterations in the marginal bone level. Alternatively, the application of excessive occlusal forces in the presence of plaque-induced inflammation can significantly increase the rate of bone loss around implant-supported restorations.

Contours and Open Contacts

Overcontoured crowns and restorations tend to accumulate plaque and handicap oral hygiene measures in addition to possibly preventing the self-cleaning mechanisms of the adjacent cheek, lips, and tongue (Fig. 10.12A and B). Restorations that fail to reestablish adequate interproximal embrasure spaces are associated with papillary inflammation. Undercontoured crowns that lack a protective height of contour do not retain as much plaque as overcontoured crowns and therefore may not be as detrimental during mastication as once thought.

The contour of the occlusal surface as established by the marginal ridges and related developmental grooves normally serves to deflect food away from the interproximal spaces. The optimal cervico-occlusal location for a posterior contact is at the longest mesiodistal diameter of the tooth, which is generally just apical to the crest of the marginal ridge. The integrity and location of the proximal contacts along with the contour of the marginal ridges and developmental grooves typically prevent interproximal food impaction. *Food impaction* is the forceful wedging of food into the periodontium by occlusal forces. As the teeth wear down, their originally convex proximal surfaces become flattened, and the wedging effect of the opposing cusp is exaggerated. Cusps that tend to forcibly wedge food into interproximal embrasures are known as *plunger cusps*. The interproximal plunger cusp effect may also be observed when missing teeth are not replaced and the relationship between the proximal contacts of adjacent teeth is altered. An intact proximal contact precludes the forceful wedging of food into the interproximal embrasure space, whereas a light or open contact is conducive to impaction.

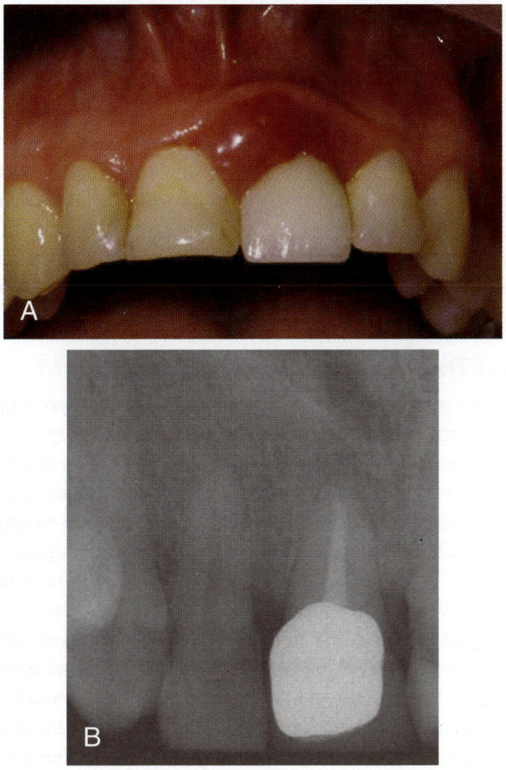

Fig. 10.12 A, Inflamed marginal and papillary gingiva adjacent to an overcontoured porcelain-fused-to-metal crown on the maxillary left central incisor. B, Radiograph of an ill-fitting porcelain-fused-to-metal crown.

The classic analysis of the factors that lead to food impaction was made by Hirschfeld, who recognized the following factors: uneven occlusal wear, opening of the contact point as a result of loss of proximal support or from extrusion, congenital morphologic abnormalities, and improperly constructed restorations.

The presence of the previously mentioned abnormalities does not necessarily lead to food impaction and periodontal disease. A study of interproximal contacts and marginal ridge relationships in three groups of periodontally healthy males revealed that 4.9%–62.5% of the proximal contacts were defective and that 33.5% of adjacent marginal ridges were uneven. However, greater probing depth and a loss of clinical attachment have been reported for sites that exhibited both an open contact and food impaction as compared to contralateral control sites without open contacts or food impaction. Excessive anterior overbite is a common cause of food impaction on the lingual surfaces of the maxillary anterior teeth and the facial surfaces of the opposing mandibular teeth. These areas may be exemplified by attachment loss with gingival recession.

Materials

In general, restorative materials are not in themselves injurious to the periodontal tissues. One exception to this may be self-curing acrylics.

Plaque that forms at the margins of restorations is similar to that found on adjacent nonrestored tooth surfaces. The composition of plaque formed on all types of restorative materials is similar, with the exception of that formed on silicate. Although surface textures of restorative materials differ with regard to their capacity to retain plaque, all can be adequately cleaned if they are polished and accessible to methods of oral hygiene. The undersurface of pontics in fixed bridges should barely touch the mucosa. Access for oral hygiene is inhibited with excessive pontic-to-tissue contact, thereby contributing to plaque accumulation that will cause gingival inflammation and possibly the formation of pseudopockets.

Design of Removable Partial Dentures

Several investigations have shown that after the insertion of partial dentures, mobility of the abutment teeth, gingival inflammation, and periodontal pocket formation all increase. This is because partial dentures favor the accumulation of plaque, particularly if they cover the gingival tissue. Partial dentures that are worn during both night and day induce more plaque formation than those worn only during the daytime. These observations emphasize the need for careful and personalized oral hygiene instruction to avoid the harmful effects of partial dentures on the remaining teeth and the periodontium. The presence of removable partial dentures induces not only quantitative changes in dental plaque but also qualitative changes, thereby promoting the emergence of spirochetal microorganisms.

Restorative Dentistry Procedures

The use of rubber dam clamps, matrix bands, and burs in such a manner as to lacerate the gingiva results in varying degrees of mechanical trauma and inflammation. Although such transient injuries generally undergo repair, they are needless sources of discomfort to the patient. The forceful packing of a gingival retraction cord into the sulcus to prepare the subgingival margins of a tooth or for the purpose of obtaining an impression may mechanically injure the periodontium and leave behind impacted debris that is capable of causing a foreign body reaction.

Malocclusion

The irregular alignment of teeth as found in cases of malocclusion may facilitate plaque accumulation and make plaque control more difficult. Several authors have found a positive correlation between crowding and periodontal disease, whereas other investigators did not find such a correlation. Uneven marginal ridges of contiguous posterior teeth have been found to have a low correlation with pocket depth, loss of attachment, plaque, calculus, and gingival inflammation. Roots of teeth that are prominent in the arch (Fig. 10.13A and B)—such as in a buccal or lingual version or that are associated with a high frenal attachment and small quantities of attached gingiva—frequently exhibit recession.

The failure to replace missing posterior teeth may have adverse consequences on the periodontal support for the remaining teeth. The following hypothetical scenario illustrates the possible ramifications of not replacing a missing posterior tooth. When the mandibular first molar is extracted, the initial change is a mesial drifting and tilting of the mandibular second and third molars with extrusion of the maxillary first molar. As the mandibular second molar tips mesially, its distal cusps extrude and act as plungers. The distal cusps of the mandibular second molar wedge between the maxillary first and second molars and open the contact by deflecting the maxillary second molar distally. Subsequently, food impaction may occur and may be accompanied by gingival inflammation with the eventual loss of the interproximal bone between the maxillary first and second molars. This example does not occur in all cases in which mandibular first molars are not replaced. However, the drifting and tilting of the remaining teeth with an accompanying alteration of the proximal contacts is generally a consequence of not replacing posterior teeth that have been extracted.

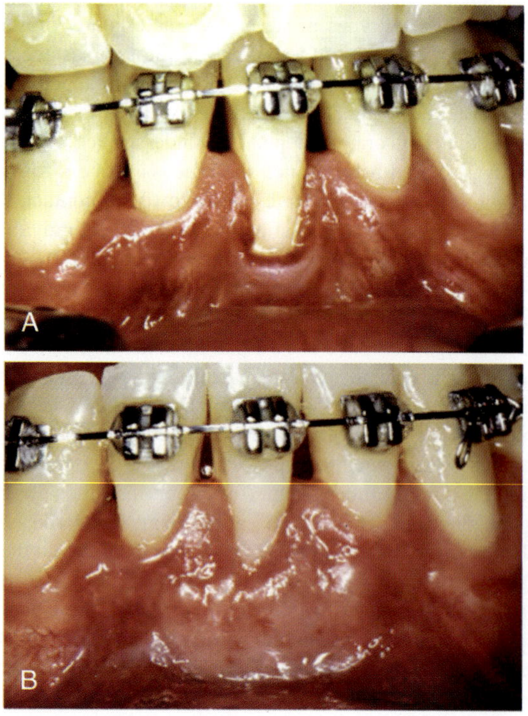

Fig. 10.13 A, Lower incisor showing a prominent root with gingival recession and a lack of attached gingiva. B, Appearance 3 months after the placement of a free gingival graft, which resulted in a gain in attached gingiva and a reduction in gingival recession.

Tongue thrusting exerts excessive lateral pressure on the anterior teeth, which may result in the spreading and tilting of the anterior teeth (Fig. 10.14A and B). Tongue thrusting is an important contributing factor to tooth migration and the development of an anterior open bite. Mouth breathing may be observed in association with a habit of tongue thrusting and an anterior open bite. Marginal and papillary gingivitis is frequently encountered in the maxillary anterior sextant in cases that involve an anterior open bite with mouth breathing.

Several case reports of gingival hyperplasia have been associated with mouth breathing. Although considered as inflammatory, the exact mechanism of gingival overgrowth in mouth breathers is unclear. It is thought to be due to alternate wetting and drying of the gingival surface. A diagnostic feature of this type of enlargement is the presence of significant overgrowth in the maxillary and mandibular anterior regions without any involvement of posterior regions.

Restorations that do not conform to the occlusal pattern of the mouth result in occlusal disharmonies that may cause injury to the supporting periodontal tissues. More issues involving deeper initial probing depths, worse prognoses, and greater mobility have been observed for teeth with occlusal discrepancies as compared to teeth without initial occlusal discrepancies.

Periodontal Complications Associated With Orthodontic Therapy

Orthodontic therapy may affect the periodontium by favoring plaque retention, by directly injuring the gingiva as a result of overextended bands, and by creating excessive forces, unfavorable forces, or both on the tooth and its supporting structures.

Plaque Retention and Composition

Orthodontic appliances tend to retain bacterial plaque and food debris, thereby resulting in gingivitis (Fig. 10.15), and they are also capable of modifying the gingival ecosystem. An increase in *Prevotella melaninogenica*, *Prevotella intermedia*, and *Actinomyces odontolyticus* and a decrease in the proportion of facultative microorganisms were detected in the gingival sulcus after the placement of orthodontic bands. More recently, *Aggregatibacter actinomycetemcomitans* was found in at least one site in 85% of children who were wearing orthodontic appliances. By contrast, only 15% of unbanded control subjects were positive for *A. actinomycetemcomitans*.

Gingival Trauma and Alveolar Bone Height

Orthodontic treatment is often started soon after the eruption of the permanent teeth, when the junctional epithelium is still adherent to the enamel surface. Orthodontic bands should not be forcefully placed beyond the level of attachment because this will detach the gingiva from the tooth and result in the apical proliferation of the junctional epithelium with an increased incidence of gingival recession.

The mean alveolar bone loss per patient for adolescents who underwent 2 years of orthodontic care during a 5-year observation period ranged between 0.1 and 0.5 mm. This small magnitude of alveolar bone loss was also noted in the control group and therefore is considered to be of little clinical significance. However, the degree of bone loss during adult orthodontic care may be higher than that observed in adolescents, especially if the periodontal condition is not treated before the initiation of orthodontic therapy..Therefore, orthodontic treatment should not be commenced in the presence of uncontrolled periodontal disease.

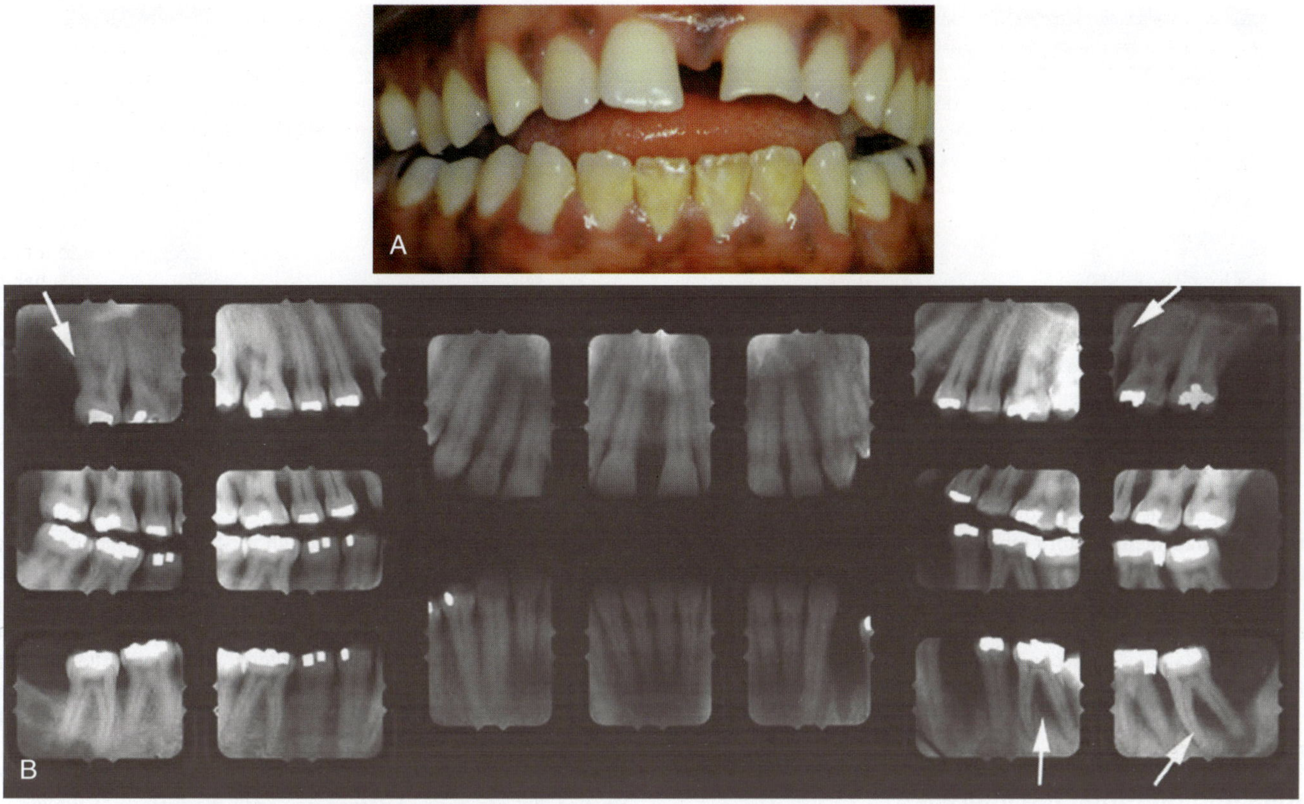

Fig. 10.14 A, Anterior open bite with flared incisors as observed in association with a habit of tongue thrusting. B, Radiographs show severe periodontal destruction (*arrows*) in the molar regions.

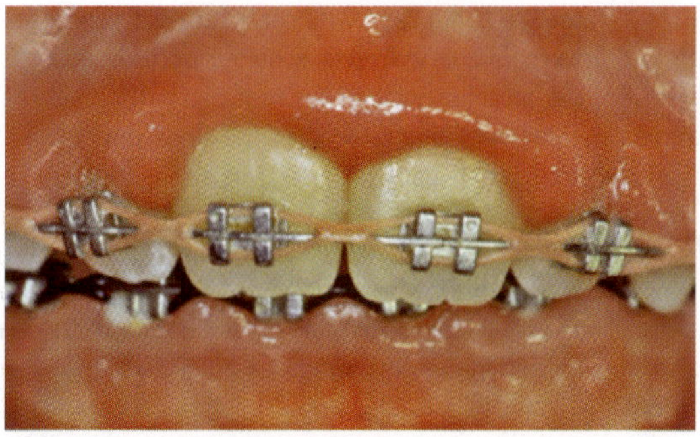

Fig. 10.15 Gingival inflammation and enlargement associated with an orthodontic appliance and poor oral hygiene.

Tissue Response to Orthodontic Forces

Orthodontic tooth movement is possible because the periodontal tissues are responsive to externally applied forces. Alveolar bone is remodeled by osteoclasts that induce bone resorption in areas of pressure and by osteoblasts that form bone in areas of tension. Although moderate orthodontic forces ordinarily result in bone remodeling and repair, excessive force may produce necrosis of the periodontal ligament and the adjacent alveolar bone. Excessive orthodontic forces also increase the risk of apical root resorption. The prevalence of severe root resorption (i.e., resorption of more than one-third of the root length) during orthodontic therapy in adolescents has been reported to be 3%. The incidence of moderate to severe root resorption for incisors among adults aged 20–45 years has been reported to be 2% before treatment and 24.5% after treatment. Risk factors associated with root resorption during orthodontic treatment include the duration of treatment, the magnitude of the force applied, the direction of the tooth movement, and the continuous versus intermittent application of forces.

The use of elastics to close a diastema may result in severe attachment loss with possible tooth loss as the elastics migrate apically along the root surface. The surgical exposure of impacted teeth and orthodontic-assisted eruption has the potential to compromise periodontal attachment on adjacent teeth. However, the majority of impacted teeth that are surgically exposed and aided in their eruption by orthodontic treatment subsequently exhibited more than 90% of their attachment as being intact.

It has been reported that the dentoalveolar gingival fibers that are located within the marginal and attached gingiva are stretched when teeth are rotated during orthodontic therapy. The surgical severing or removal of these gingival fibers in combination with a brief period of retention may reduce the incidence of relapse after orthodontic treatment that is intended to realign rotated teeth.

Extraction of Impacted Third Molars

Numerous clinical studies have reported that the extraction of impacted third molars often results in the creation of vertical defects distal to the second molars. This iatrogenic effect is unrelated to flap design, and it appears to occur more often when third molars are extracted from individuals who are more than 25 years old. Other factors that appear to play a role in the development of lesions on the distal surface of second molars—particularly in those who are more than 25 years old—include the presence of visible plaque, bleeding on probing, root resorption in the contact area between the second and third molars, the presence of a pathologically widened follicle, the inclination of the third molar, and the close proximity of the third molar to the second molar. Other potential iatrogenic adverse consequences of the removal of third molars include permanent paresthesia (i.e., numbness of the lip, tongue, and cheek),

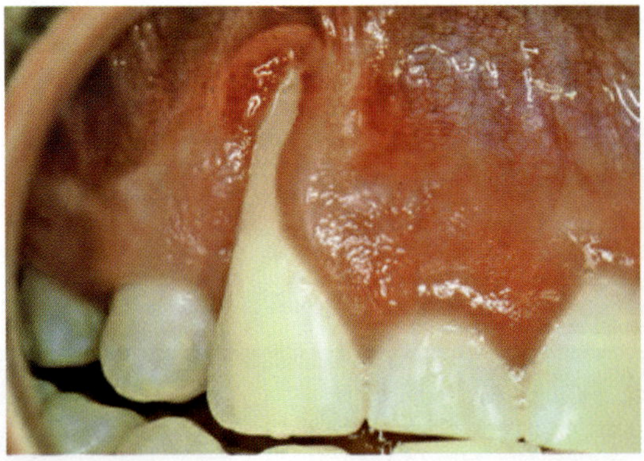

Fig. 10.16 Gingival recession on a maxillary canine caused by self-inflicted trauma from the patient's fingernail.

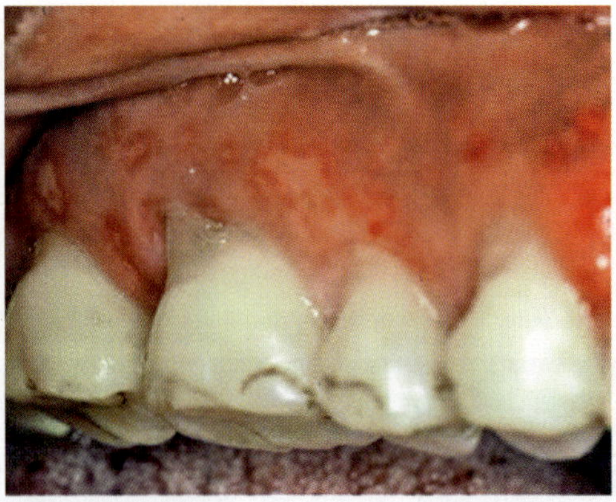

Fig. 10.17 The overzealous use of a toothbrush resulted in denudation of the gingival epithelial surface and exposure of the underlying connective tissue as a painful ulcer.

damage to adjacent teeth, mandibular fracture, maxillary tuberosity fracture, displacement of third molars and root tips, oroantral communications or fistula, and temporomandibular joint complications. Permanent paresthesia occurs at a frequency of approximately 1 of every 100,000 wisdom teeth removed in the United States. The incidence of damage to second molar as a consequence of third molar extraction has been estimated to be 0.3%–0.4%. Although the incidence of mandibular fracture during or after third molar removal is low.

Habits and Self-Inflicted Injuries

Patients may not be aware of their self-inflicted injurious habits that may be important to the initiation and progression of their periodontal disease. Mechanical forms of trauma can stem from the improper use of a toothbrush, the wedging of toothpicks between the teeth, the application of fingernail pressure against the gingiva (Fig. 10.16), pizza burns, and other causes. Sources of chemical irritation include the topical application of caustic medications such as aspirin or cocaine, allergic reactions to toothpaste or chewing gum, the use of chewing tobacco, and concentrated mouthrinses. Accidental and iatrogenic gingival injuries may be caused by a variety of chemical, physical, and thermal sources, yet they are generally self-limited. Iatrogenic injuries are often acute, whereas factitious injuries tend to be more chronic in nature.

Trauma Associated With Oral Jewelry

The use of piercing jewelry in the lip or tongue has become more common among teenagers and young adults. However, piercings are associated with potential complications including gingival injury or recession; damage to teeth, restorations, and fixed porcelain prostheses; increased salivary flow; interference with speech, mastication, or deglutition; scar tissue formation; and development of metal hypersensitivities.

The incidence of lingual recession with pocket formation and radiographic evidence of bone loss was 50% among subjects with a mean age of 22 years who wore lingual "barbells" for 2 years or longer. Chipped lower anterior teeth were noted in 47% of the patients who wore tongue-piercing jewelry for 4 years or longer. Patients need to be informed of the risks of wearing oral jewelry and cautioned against such practices.

Toothbrush Trauma

Abrasions of the gingiva as well as alterations in tooth structure may result from aggressive tooth brushing in a horizontal or rotary fashion. The deleterious effect of excessively forceful brushing is accentuated when highly abrasive dentifrices are used. The gingival changes that are attributable to toothbrush trauma may be acute or chronic. The acute changes vary with regard to their appearance and duration, from scuffing of the epithelial surface to denudation of the underlying connective tissue with the formation of a painful gingival ulcer (Fig. 10.17). Diffuse erythema and denudation of the attached gingiva throughout the mouth may be a striking result of overzealous brushing. Signs of acute gingival abrasions are frequently noted when the patient first uses a new brush. Puncture lesions may be produced when heavy pressure is applied to firm bristles that are aligned perpendicular to the surface of the gingiva. A forcibly embedded toothbrush bristle can be retained in the gingiva and cause an acute gingival abscess.

Chronic toothbrush trauma results in gingival recession with denudation of the root surface. Interproximal attachment loss is generally a consequence of bacteria-induced periodontitis, whereas buccal and lingual attachment loss is frequently the result of toothbrush abrasion. The improper use of dental floss may result in lacerations of the interdental papilla.

Chemical Irritation

Acute gingival inflammation may be caused by chemical irritation that results from either sensitivity or nonspecific tissue injury. In allergic inflammatory states, the gingival changes range from simple erythema to painful vesicle formation and ulceration. Severe reactions to ordinarily innocuous mouthwashes, dentifrices, and denture materials are often explainable on this basis.

Acute inflammation with ulceration may be produced by the nonspecific injurious effect of chemicals on the gingival tissues. The indiscriminate use of strong mouthwashes, the topical application of corrosive drugs such as aspirin (Fig. 10.18) or cocaine, and accidental contact with drugs such as phenol or silver nitrate are common examples of chemical exposures that cause irritation of the gingiva. A histologic view of an aspirin-induced chemical burn shows vacuoles with serous exudates and an inflammatory infiltrate in the connective tissue.

Smokeless Tobacco

Snuff and chewing tobacco constitute the two main forms of smokeless tobacco. Snuff is a fine-cut form of tobacco that is available loosely packed or in small sachets. Chewing tobacco is a more coarse-cut tobacco that is available in the form of loose leaves, a solid block, a plug, or a twist of dried leaves. Chewing tobacco is typically placed in the mandibular buccal vestibule for several hours, during which time saliva and dilute tobacco are periodically expectorated. The nicotine uptake of smokeless tobacco is similar

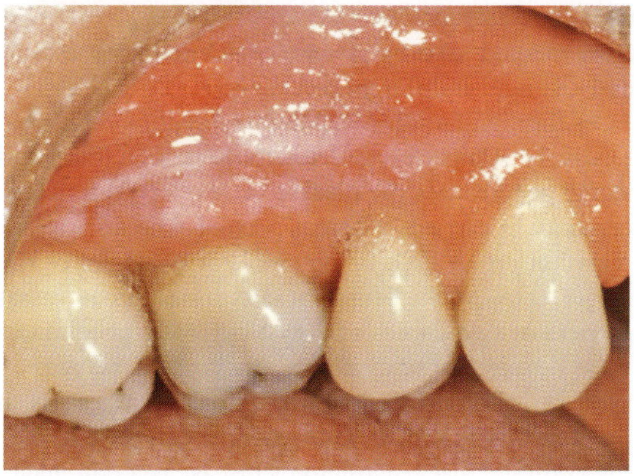

Fig. 10.18 Chemical burn caused by aspirin; note the sloughing gingival tissue and the resultant recession.

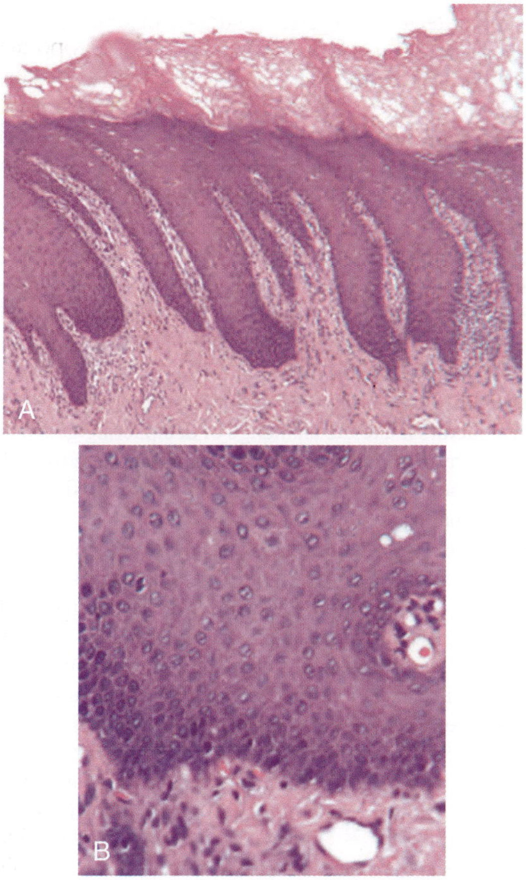

Fig. 10.19 A, Histologic features of oral leukoplakia associated with smokeless tobacco. Note the chevron-like pattern of hyperkeratosis with focal areas of inflammation. B, Hyperplasia in the basal cell layer.

to that of smoking cigarettes in that the consumption of a 34-g container of smokeless tobacco is approximately equal to 1.5 packs of cigarettes. Histologic features of oral leukoplakia associated with smokeless tobacco include (1) a chevron-like pattern of hyperkeratosis with focal areas of inflammation and (2) hyperplasia in the basal cell layer (Fig. 10.19A and B). Increased incidences of gingival recession, cervical root abrasion, and root caries have been reported with the use of smokeless tobacco (Fig. 10.20).

The incidence of gingival recession among adolescents who use smokeless tobacco has been reported to be 42%, compared to 17% among nonusers.

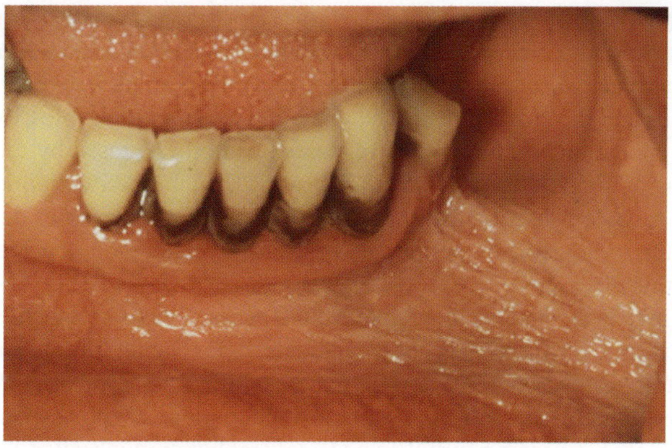

Fig. 10.20 Oral leukoplakia, recession, and clinical attachment loss associated with the use of smokeless tobacco.

Radiation Therapy

Radiation therapy has cytotoxic effects on both normal cells and malignant cells. A typical total dose of radiation for head and neck tumors is in the range of 5000–8000 centigray (cGy); 1 cGy is equal to 1 radiation absorbed dose (rad) and equivalent to 50–80 Sieverts (Sv). The total dose of radiation is usually given in partial incremental doses, and this is referred to as *fractionation.* Fractionation helps to minimize the adverse effects of radiation while maximizing the death rate for the tumor cells. Fractionated doses are typically administered in the range of 100–1000 cGy or 1–10 Sv per week.

Radiation treatment induces an obliterative endarteritis that results in soft tissue ischemia and fibrosis; irradiated bone becomes hypovascular and hypoxic. Adverse effects of head and neck radiation therapy include dermatitis and mucositis of the irradiated area as well as muscle fibrosis and trismus, which may restrict access to the oral cavity. The mucositis typically develops 5–7 days after radiation therapy is initiated. Saliva production is permanently impaired when salivary glands that are located within the portal of radiation receive 6000 cGy (60 Sv) or more. Xerostomia results in greater plaque accumulation and a reduced buffering capacity of saliva. Effective oral hygiene, professional dental prophylactic cleanings, fluoride applications, and frequent dental examinations are essential to control caries and periodontal disease. The use of customized trays appears to be a more effective method for fluoride application compared to the toothbrush.

Among cancer patients who were treated with high-dose unilateral radiation, periodontal attachment loss and tooth loss were reported to be greater on the irradiated site compared to the nonradiated control side of the dentition. Patients who are diagnosed with oral cancer and who require radiation therapy should ideally be assessed for dental needs (i.e., mucositis, xerostomia, faulty restorations, periapical lesion, coronal and cervical decay, and periodontal status) before the initiation of radiation treatment. The treatment and prevention of trismus, oral fungal infections, odontogenic infections, osteoradionecrosis, decay, and periodontal disease are critical to minimize oral morbidity for these patients. Dental and periodontal infections have the potential to be severe risks for patients who have been treated with head and neck radiation. The risk of osteoradionecrosis for oncology patients can be minimized by evaluating their oral status, providing dental care, and allowing time for tissue repair before the commencement of radiotherapy.

The risk of osteoradionecrosis must be evaluated before the performance of atraumatic extractions or limited periodontal surgical procedures in previously irradiated sites. Therefore, the dentist may choose to consult with the patient's oncologist before the initiation of dental therapy.

Genetic Susceptibility to Periodontal Disease

Periodontal diseases occur due to complex interplay between the genes and the environment, both playing very important roles. With the exception of a handful of very rare syndromes caused by mutations of single genes, evidence indicates that inherited variation in DNA has a role roughly equal to that of the environment in determining who remains periodontally healthy versus who is affected by this disease.

In genetic studies, more than 23,000 genes need to be considered as potential hypotheses or "candidates" for being disease risk factors. Depending on the gene's size and the frequency of genetic recombination in the gene's chromosomal region, scientists need to evaluate between a handful or up to several hundred inherited DNA variants in each gene as potential "biomarkers" of disease risk. Each one of these variants essentially amounts to a test of the hypothesis as to whether the variant is associated with disease risk. Furthermore, many complex diseases have been found to be very strongly associated with DNA variation in parts of the human genome where no genes are known to exist but where the genetic material may have important functional effects nonetheless.

Only by carefully studying the genetics of disease in populations and pedigrees can we hope to begin to unearth the complex interactions between genes and the environment that underlie individual differences in disease susceptibility. This field of research is known as *genetic epidemiology.*

Genetic Study Designs

1. Familial aggregation and relative risk:
   Many diseases run in families, and the degree of clustering within the family can be estimated by comparing the number of disease cases in relatives of patients to the risk of disease in the general population. Difficulties with this approach relate to the fact that, in addition to having many genes in common, family members also share many aspects of a common environment (e.g., diet, nutrition, smoking, infectious organisms, shared socioeconomic factors).
2. Twin studies:
   The comparison of disease occurrence or severity in identical (monozygotic) versus nonidentical (dizygotic) twins is a very powerful method for distinguishing between effects caused by variation in genes versus factors in the environment. This requires us to make what is usually a reasonable assumption that the environments of pairs of identical twins are no more or less similar than the environments shared by pairs of nonidentical twins. If variation among individuals in disease susceptibility or severity is caused entirely by factors in the environment, then we expect pairs of identical twins to be no more similar to each other than pairs of nonidentical twins. All twins (whether identical or nonidentical) are expected to be more similar to their cotwins, on average, than to unrelated members of their local population because they were raised in the same family environment, with similar diets, microbial exposures, and so on. However, if genetic variation plays an important role in determining a certain trait, then genetically identical twin pairs will be more similar to each other than nonidentical twin pairs. This is because identical twins share 100% of the same genes, whereas nonidentical twin pairs share only 50% of their parents' genes on average. Genetic epidemiologists calculate a measure called *heritability* that is based on these correlations and that estimates the portion of all variation in the trait that is attributable to inherited genetic variation.
3. Segregation analysis:
   Another method used by genetic epidemiologists to understand and distinguish different mechanisms of transmission of diseases through families is called *segregation analysis.* This is relatively straightforward for traits in which mutation in a single gene causes the disease to develop with nearly 100% certainty in carriers, whereas persons who do not inherit the mutation are at little or no risk. For example, carriers of a single copy of the Huntington's disease gene mutation or carriers of two copies of a cystic fibrosis gene mutation always develop these diseases if they reach the ages at which symptoms of these conditions normally emerge. By tracking the transmission of these diseases in families, it is obvious, for example, that Huntington's disease is a dominant single-gene disorder: it is transmitted with 50% probability to offspring of affected individuals and thus it is often found occurring across many generations of large pedigrees. By contrast, parents of children with cystic fibrosis are very rarely affected themselves, and 25% of siblings are affected by cystic fibrosis when the disease is present in a nuclear family. This pattern of transmission is expected if a disease is recessive (i.e., it requires the inheritance of a mutated gene copy from both parents, who themselves have one normal and one mutated copy and so are not affected). For most common "complex" diseases, however, having a high-risk gene does not automatically lead to development of the disease; this phenomenon is called *reduced penetrance.* Furthermore, several genes or even dozens of different genes may influence disease susceptibility; this is known as *oligogenic inheritance* and *genetic heterogeneity.* Environmental exposures are also important modifiers of disease risk. Such highly complex combinations of multiple genetic and environmental risk factors make the challenge of deciphering genetic mechanisms by merely observing transmission patterns in families using the segregation analysis approach unfeasible.
4. Linkage analysis:
   One method that has been highly successful for finding molecular defects related to simple genetic diseases caused by the mutation of a single gene, such as cystic fibrosis and Huntington's disease, is *linkage analysis.* This gene-mapping strategy requires families with one or more members affected by the disease to be recruited and clinically and molecularly evaluated for a relatively small number of genetic markers. Investigators usually try to recruit families with two or more close relatives, such as sibling pairs, who are affected by the disease as well as parents and other siblings who may be unaffected.
5. Association analysis:
   Another approach is called *association analysis* although this had been relegated to studies of Human Leukocyte Antigen (HLA) and a few other markers of special interest during the prime of linkage approaches. Association analyses are sometimes referred to as *case–control studies* although this is only one of several sampling methods that can be used (including studies of families). Genotype frequencies of an inherited DNA variant for a group of periodontitis cases are statistically compared to the frequencies of the variant in a matched group of periodontally healthy control subjects. If the genotype frequencies differ so greatly that the results are very unlikely to occur by chance, then we conclude that the genotype that is more common in the cases as compared to the controls is "associated with" increased disease risk. The good news is now clearly in: association studies have been

a boon for the discovery of inherited genetic variation important for a wide range of complex diseases, including diabetes, cardiovascular disease, metabolic disorders, obesity, and mental illnesses.

6. Candidate gene approach:

A gene-mapping approach tests whether one allele of a gene occurs more often in patients with the disease than in subjects without the disease. These methods are also referred to as *association analyses*, and they aim to identify which genes are associated with the disease. Candidate genes are chosen on the basis of their known or presumed function (i.e., they have some plausible role in the disease process, such as producing a protein that is important in the disease pathogenesis).

Inherited Variation and Risk of Periodontitis

As a result of the appropriate focus on the role of bacterial infections in the disease pathogenesis of periodontitis, inherited human genetic variation is often referred to as *host defense* or, somewhat more broadly, *host response*. However, these terms cover only a small portion of the range of gene functions that may be important for periodontitis risk. Many additional biologic processes that are not directly related to defenses against or responses to infection by microbial pathogens are also likely to play important roles in determining an individual's susceptibility to this disease.

Periodontitis in Genetic Syndromes

A number of extremely rare conditions consistently include periodontitis among the array of clinical manifestations that define a syndrome. Many genetic syndromes involve mutations of single genes or larger chromosomal regions. Some of the syndromes that include periodontitis are caused by mutations in specific genes. For example, mutations in the cathepsin C gene have been shown to cause both Papillon–Lèfevre syndrome and Haim–Munk syndrome as well as some forms of nonsyndromic prepubertal periodontitis, and they may also be associated with a risk of aggressive periodontitis. Periodontitis frequently occurs with some subtypes of Ehlers–Danlos syndrome, Kindler syndrome, Down syndrome (trisomy 21), leukocyte adhesion deficiencies, hypophosphatasia, two types of neutropenia, and aplasia of the lacrimal and salivary glands.

Nonsyndromic Aggressive and Chronic Periodontitis

Finding evidence for the association of inherited genetic variation with aggressive and chronic periodontitis for cases that present without the cooccurrence of anomalies or disorders of other parts of the body is classified as *nonsyndromic periodontitis*. The elevated risk of periodontitis that is associated with metabolic conditions (e.g., diabetes, which is addressed elsewhere in this book) is more appropriately considered comorbidity rather than being a cause for the designation of a syndrome.

Twin studies have shown that chronic periodontitis has very substantial heritability, and we know that aggressive periodontitis aggregates strongly in families. Neither segregation analyses nor gene-mapping linkage studies are capable of providing reliable information about the genetic etiology of a highly complex disease such as periodontitis. However, during the past decade, several hundred papers have reported associations of nonsyndromic aggressive and chronic periodontitis with polymorphisms in a number of candidate genes.

Association tests involve the evaluation of candidate genes that were selected on the basis of known or postulated mechanisms of disease pathogenesis.

For example, when bacteria challenge gingival tissue, CD14 binds lipopolysaccharide, and TLR4 plays a key role in pathogen recognition and the activation of innate immunity. Lactotransferrin plays an antimicrobial role as the first line of host defense, and it can also neutralize endotoxin and inhibit the induction of nuclear factor-$\kappa\beta$ (NF-$\kappa\beta$) in monocytes in response to lipopolysaccharides. Myeloperoxidase is an oxidative enzyme expressed in polymorphonuclear leukocytes. It is involved in the defense against periodontal bacteria and is also able to mediate inflammatory tissue destruction in periodontal disease. Glutathione S-transferase mu 1 (GSTM1) and *N*-acetyltransferase 2 (NAT2) genes are responsible for the detoxification of a wide range of chemicals, including tobacco carcinogens. HLA complex genes play a central role in the immune system by presenting extracellular peptides that are important for either self-recognition or initiating immune responses to foreign pathogens. The Fcγ receptor genes (FcγRS) encode receptors for the Fc portion of immunoglobulin G, and they are involved in the removal of antigen–antibody complexes from the circulation as well as other antibody-dependent responses. Formyl peptide receptor (FPR1) is a G protein-coupled receptor of phagocytic cells that interacts with bacterial peptides and that mediates chemotaxis, degranulation, and superoxide production involved in inflammation. Cytokines such as the interleukins (IL-1, IL-2, IL-4, IL-6, IL-10), tumor necrosis factor (TNF), and lymphotoxin-alpha (LTA) play a number of important roles in the immunopathology of periodontal disease. Various studies have shown mild to moderate genetic association for the above mechanisms involved in the pathogenesis of periodontal diseases.

In dentistry, a test based on genetic variations of the IL-1α and IL-1β cytokine and receptor antagonist genes to predict the progression and severity of periodontitis has been commercialized and is offered today although it does not appear to be widely used. A number of reviews of the large number of studies of the IL-1 gene polymorphisms indicate that genetic variation at these loci may be associated with a modest effect on disease risk.

Epigenetic Control

Epigenetic changes are heritable changes that do not depend on changes in DNA sequence. Epigenetic mechanisms are essential for regulation of transcription and provide a dynamic, reversible, and mechanistic framework that could explain the way in which environmental and behavioral factors interact with the genome to alter disease risk.

Epigenetic factors play an important role in chronic inflammatory conditions by allowing microbial persistence to play a role in the infectious mechanism, resulting in pathogen interference with the host genome. Thus, periodontal pathogens containing lipopolysaccharides can be a cause of epigenetic modifications affecting expression of inflammatory mediators in periodontal tissue, and low-grade chronic inflammation present in periodontal disease has been shown to promote DNA methylation. Periodontal disease is closely linked with diabetes mellitus complications, which are related to epigenetic changes.

Key points

- Calculus is mineralized bacterial plaque that forms on the surfaces of natural teeth and dental prostheses.
- Supragingival calculus is located coronal to the gingival margin and therefore is visible in the oral cavity. Subgingival calculus is located below the crest of the marginal gingiva and therefore is not visible on routine clinical examination.

- At least two-thirds of the inorganic component of calculus is crystalline in structure. The four main crystal forms are hydroxyapatite, 58%; magnesium whitlockite, 21%; octacalcium phosphate, 12%; and brushite, 9%.
- Modes of attachment of calculus: Attachment by means of an organic pellicle on cementum and on enamel, mechanical locking to surface irregularities, close adaptation of the undersurface of calculus to depressions or gently sloping mounds of the unaltered cementum surface, and the penetration of bacterial calculus into cementum.
- Saliva is the source of mineralization for supragingival calculus, whereas the serum transudate called gingival crevicular fluid furnishes the minerals for subgingival calculus.
- Theories of mineralization of calculus: (1) Mineral precipitation resulting from a local rise in the degree of saturation of calcium and phosphate ions. (2) Seeding agents induce small foci of calcification that enlarge and coalesce to form a calcified mass. This concept has been referred to as the epitactic concept or heterogeneous nucleation.
- Calculus does not contribute directly to gingival inflammation, but it provides a fixed nidus for the continued accumulation of plaque and its retention in close proximity to the gingiva.
- Margins of restorations placed at the level of the gingival crest induce less severe inflammation, whereas supragingival margins are associated with better periodontal health.
- Cusps that tend to forcibly wedge food into interproximal embrasures are known as plunger cusps.
- Orthodontic treatment should not be commenced in the presence of uncontrolled periodontal disease.

Suggested Readings

Albandar J, Kingman A, Brown L, et al: Gingival inflammation and subgingival calculus as determinants of disease progression in early-onset periodontitis, *J Clin Periodontol* 25:231, 1998.

Anerud A, Löe H, Boysen H: The natural history and clinical course of calculus formation in man, *J Clin Periodontol* 18:160, 1991.

Frazer KA, Murray SS, Schork NJ, et al: Human genetic variation and its contribution to complex traits, *Nat Rev Genet* 10(4):241–251, 2009.

Jeffcoat M, Howell T: Alveolar bone destruction due to overhanging amalgam in periodontal disease, *J Periodontol* 51:599, 1980.

Kinane DF, Shiba H, Hart TC: The genetic basis of periodontitis, *Periodontol 2000* 39:91–117, 2005.

Kugelberg C: Third molar surgery, *Curr Opin Dent* 2:9, 1992.

Lupi J, Handelman C, Sadowsky C: Prevalence and severity of apical root resorption and alveolar bone loss in orthodontically treated adults, *Am J Orthod Dentofacial Orthop* 109:28, 1996.

Sorensen J, Larsen I, Jorgensen K: Gingival and alveolar bone response to marginal fit of subgingival crown margins, *Scand J Dent Res* 94:109, 1986.

Wilson TG Jr: The positive relationship between excess cement and peri-implant disease: a prospective clinical endoscopic study, *J Periodontol* 80:1388–1392, 2009.

Zander H: The attachment of calculus to root surfaces, *J Periodontol* 24:16, 1953

References

References and MCQs with answers for the chapter are available on www.medenact.com.

CHAPTER 11

Influence of Systemic Conditions on the Periodontium

PR Klokkevold | BL Mealey | YL Hernandez-Kapila | N Ambalavanan

CHAPTER OUTLINE

Many systemic diseases, disorders, and conditions have been implicated as risk indicators or risk factors in periodontal disease. Clinical and basic science research over the past several decades has led to an improved understanding of and appreciation for the complexity and pathogenesis of periodontal diseases. Perhaps the most significant advance in our understanding of the pathogenesis of periodontitis is that the host response varies among individuals and that an altered, deficient, or exaggerated host immune response to bacterial pathogens may lead to more severe forms of the disease. In other words, the individual host immune response to periodontal pathogens is very important and likely explains many of the differences in disease severity observed from one individual to the next. Furthermore, systemic diseases, disorders, and conditions alter host tissues and physiology, which may impair the host's barrier function and immune defense against periodontal pathogens, thereby creating the opportunity for destructive periodontal disease to progress.

The relationships between periodontal infections and host defense are complex. A number of environmental, physical, and psychosocial factors have the potential to alter periodontal tissues and the host immune response, thereby resulting in more severe periodontal disease expression. It is important to recognize that the systemic diseases, disorders, or conditions themselves do not cause periodontitis; rather, they may predispose, accelerate, or otherwise increase the disease's progression. This chapter discusses important systemic diseases, disorders, and conditions that have the potential to influence periodontal health.

Endocrine Disorders and Hormonal Changes

Endocrine diseases such as diabetes and hormonal fluctuations that are associated with puberty and pregnancy are well-known examples of systemic conditions that adversely affect the condition of the periodontium. Endocrine disturbances and hormone fluctuations affect the periodontal tissues directly, modify the tissue response to local factors, and produce anatomic changes in the gingiva that may favor plaque accumulation and disease progression.

Diabetes Mellitus

Diabetes mellitus is an extremely important disease from a periodontal standpoint. It is a complex metabolic disorder characterized by chronic hyperglycemia. Diminished insulin production, impaired insulin action, or a combination of both result in the inability of glucose to be transported from the bloodstream into the tissues, which in turn results in high blood glucose levels and the excretion of sugar in the urine. Lipid and protein metabolism are altered in diabetes as well. Uncontrolled diabetes (chronic hyperglycemia) is associated with several long-term complications, including microvascular diseases (retinopathy, nephropathy, or neuropathy), macrovascular diseases (cardiovascular and cerebrovascular conditions), increased susceptibility to infections, and poor wound healing.

There are two major types of diabetes, type 1 and type 2, with several less common secondary types. *Type 1 diabetes mellitus*, which was formerly known as *insulin-dependent diabetes mellitus*, is caused by a cell-mediated autoimmune destruction of the insulin-producing beta cells of the islets of Langerhans in the pancreas, which results in insulin deficiency. Type 1 diabetes accounts for 5%–10% of all cases of diabetes and most often occurs in children and young adults. This type of diabetes results from a lack of insulin production, and it is very unstable and difficult to control. It has a marked tendency toward ketosis and coma, it is not preceded by obesity, and it requires the injection of insulin to be controlled. Patients with type 1 diabetes mellitus present with the symptoms that are traditionally associated with diabetes, including polyphagia, polydipsia, polyuria, and predisposition to infections.

Type 2 diabetes mellitus, which was formerly known as *noninsulin-dependent diabetes mellitus*, is caused by peripheral resistance to insulin action, impaired insulin secretion, and increased glucose production in the liver. The insulin-producing beta cells in the pancreas are not destroyed by cell-mediated autoimmune reaction. It typically begins as insulin resistance, which leads to the reduced pancreas production of insulin as the demand increases. Type 2 diabetes is the most common form of diabetes, and it accounts for 90%–95% of all diagnosed cases in adults. Individuals are often not aware they have the disease until severe symptoms or complications occur. Type 2 diabetes generally occurs in obese individuals, and it can often be controlled by diet and oral hypoglycemic agents. Ketosis and coma are uncommon. Type 2 diabetes can manifest with the same symptoms as type 1 diabetes but typically in a less-severe form.

An additional category of diabetes is *hyperglycemia* secondary to other diseases or conditions. A prime example of this type of hyperglycemia is gestational diabetes associated with pregnancy. *Gestational diabetes* develops in 2%–10% of all pregnancies but disappears after delivery. Women who have had gestational diabetes are at increased risk of developing type 2 diabetes. Other secondary types of diabetes are those associated with diseases that involve the pancreas and the destruction of the insulin-producing cells. Endocrine diseases (e.g., acromegaly, Cushing syndrome), tumors, pancreatectomy, and drugs or chemicals that cause altered insulin levels are included in this group. Experimentally induced types of diabetes generally belong in this category rather than in the categories of type 1 or 2 diabetes mellitus.

Oral Manifestations

Numerous oral changes have been described in patients with diabetes, including cheilosis, mucosal drying and cracking, burning mouth and tongue, diminished salivary flow, and alterations in the flora of the oral cavity, with greater predominance of *Candida albicans*, hemolytic streptococci, and staphylococci. An increased rate of dental caries has also been observed in patients with poorly controlled diabetes. It is important to note that these changes are not always present, that they are not specific, and that they are not pathognomonic for diabetes. Furthermore, these changes are less likely to be observed in patients with well-controlled diabetes. Individuals with controlled diabetes have a normal tissue response, a normally developed dentition, a normal defense against infections, and no increase in the incidence of caries (Table 11.1).

The influence of diabetes on the periodontium has been thoroughly investigated. Although it is difficult to make definitive conclusions about the specific effects of diabetes on the periodontium, a variety of changes have been described, including a tendency toward an enlarged gingiva, sessile or pedunculated gingival polyps, polypoid gingival proliferations, abscess formation, periodontitis, and loosened teeth (Fig. 11.1A–E). Perhaps the most striking changes in patients with uncontrolled diabetes are the reductions in the defense mechanisms and the increased susceptibility to infections, which lead to destructive periodontal disease. In fact, periodontal disease is considered to be the sixth complication of diabetes. Periodontitis in patients with type 1 diabetes appears to start after the age of 12 years, and it has a fivefold increased prevalence in teenagers. The prevalence of periodontitis has been reported as 9.8% in 13- to 18-year-old patients, and it increases to 39% in those who are 19 years old and above.

TABLE 11.1 Oral and Periodontal Changes in Patients With Diabetes

Oral Changes in Patients With Diabetes
Cheilosis
Mucosal drying and cracking
Burning mouth and tongue
Diminished salivary flow
Alterations in the flora of the oral cavity
Increased rate of dental caries
Periodontal Changes in Patients With Diabetes
Enlarged gingiva
Sessile or pedunculated gingival polyps
Polypoid gingival proliferations
Abscess formation
Periodontitis and loosened teeth

The extensive literature on this subject and the overall impression of clinicians indicate that *periodontal disease in patients with diabetes follows no consistent or distinct pattern.* Severe gingival inflammation, deep periodontal pockets, rapid bone loss, and frequent periodontal abscesses often occur in patients with poorly controlled diabetes and poor oral hygiene. Children with type 1 diabetes tend to have more destruction around the first molars and incisors, but this destruction becomes more generalized at older ages. In patients with juvenile diabetes, extensive periodontal destruction often occurs as a consequence of having more severe disease at a younger age.

Investigators have reported that the rate of periodontal destruction appears to be similar for those with diabetes and those without diabetes up to the age of 30 years. Older patients with diabetes have a greater degree of periodontal destruction, possibly related to more disease destruction over time. Patients who have had overt diabetes for more than 10 years have a greater loss of periodontal support than those with a diabetic history of less than 10 years. This destruction may also be related to the diminished tissue integrity, which continues to deteriorate over time (see Altered Collagen Metabolism).

Majority of well-controlled studies show a higher prevalence and severity of periodontal disease in individuals with diabetes compared to nondiabetic persons with similar local factors. Findings include a greater loss of attachment, increased bleeding on probing, and increased tooth mobility. Adults who are 45 years of age or older with poorly controlled diabetes (i.e., with a glycated hemoglobin level >9%) were 2.9 times more likely to have severe periodontitis than those without diabetes. The likelihood was even greater (4.6 times) among smokers with poorly controlled diabetes. As with other systemic conditions associated with periodontitis, diabetes mellitus does not cause gingivitis or periodontitis, but evidence indicates that it alters the response of the periodontal tissues to local factors, thereby hastening bone loss and delaying postsurgical healing. Frequent periodontal abscesses appear to be an important feature of periodontal disease in patients with diabetes.

Bacterial Pathogens

The glucose content of gingival fluid and blood is higher in individuals with diabetes than in those without diabetes with similar plaque and gingival index scores. The increased glucose in the gingival fluid and blood of patients with diabetes could change the environment of the microflora, thereby inducing qualitative changes in bacteria that may contribute to the severity of periodontal disease observed in those with poorly controlled diabetes.

Patients with type 1 diabetes mellitus and periodontitis have been reported to have a subgingival flora that is composed mainly of *Capnocytophaga*, anaerobic vibrios, and *Actinomyces* species. *Porphyromonas gingivalis*, *Prevotella intermedia*, and *Aggregatibacter actinomycetemcomitans*, which are common in periodontal lesions of individuals without diabetes, are present in low numbers in those with the disease. However, other studies have found scarce *Capnocytophaga* and abundant *A. actinomycetemcomitans* and black-pigmented *Bacteroides* as well as *P. intermedia*, *Prevotella melaninogenica*, and *Campylobacter rectus*. Black-pigmented species—especially *P. gingivalis*, *P. intermedia*, and *C. rectus*—are prominent in severe periodontal lesions of Pima Indians with type 2 diabetes. Although these results may suggest an altered flora in the periodontal pockets of patients with diabetes, the exact role of these microorganisms has not been determined. To date, there is insufficient evidence to support the role of a specific altered microflora that is responsible for periodontal disease destruction in patients with diabetes.

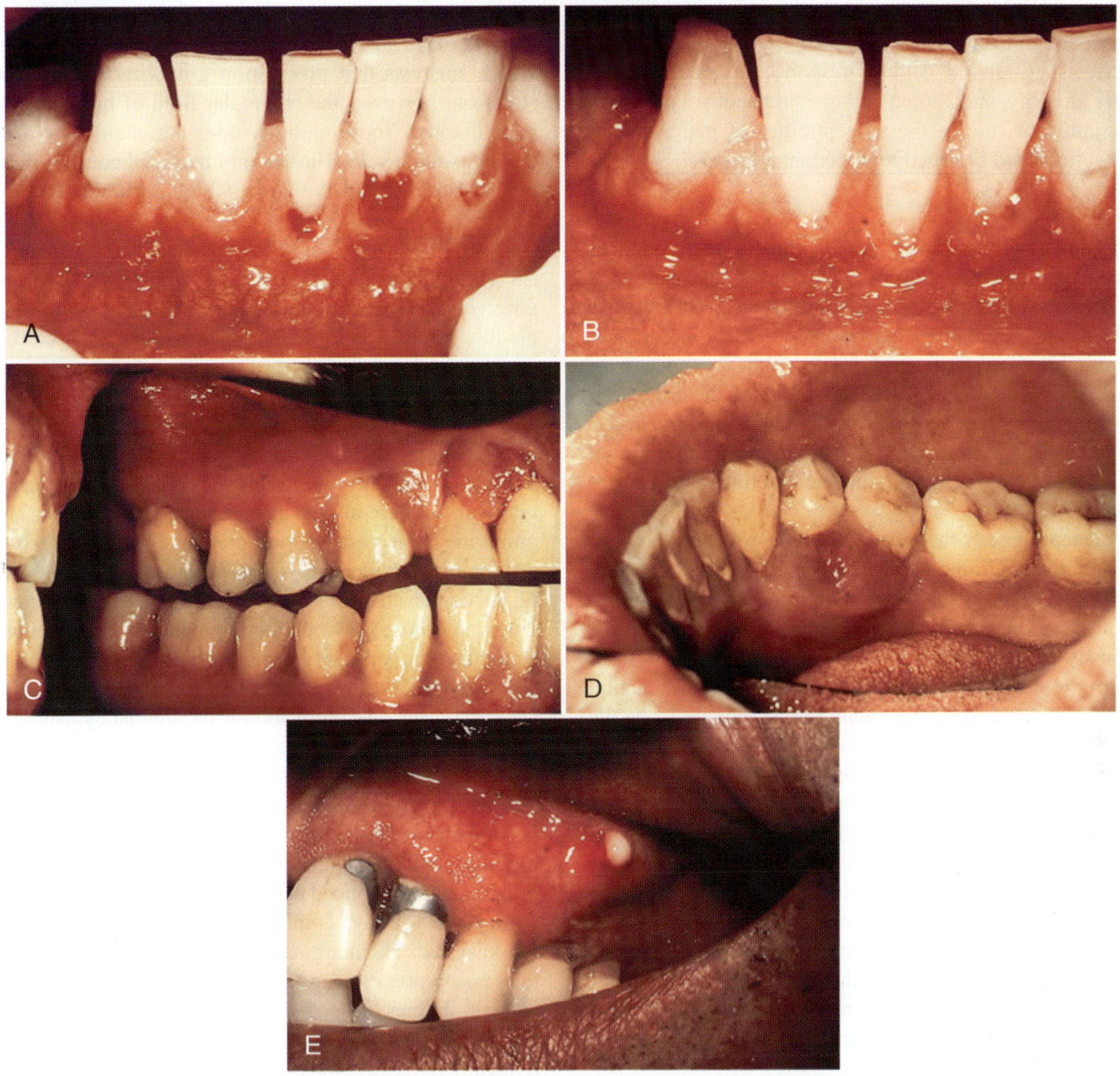

Fig. 11.1 Periodontal condition in patients with diabetes. A, Adult with diabetes (blood glucose level >400 mg/dL). Note the gingival inflammation, spontaneous bleeding, and edema. B, The same patient as shown in A. Improved control of diabetes was noted after 4 days of insulin therapy (blood glucose level <100 mg/dL). The clinical periodontal condition has improved without local therapy. C, Adult patient with uncontrolled diabetes. Note the enlarged, smooth, erythematous gingival margins and papilla in the anterior area. D, The same patient as shown in C. This is a lingual view of the right mandibular area. Note the inflamed and swollen tissues in the anterior and premolar areas. E, Adult patient with uncontrolled diabetes. There is a suppurating abscess on the buccal surface of the maxillary premolars.

Polymorphonuclear Leukocyte Function

The increased susceptibility of patients with diabetes to infection has been hypothesized as being caused by polymorphonuclear leukocyte (PMN) deficiencies that result in impaired chemotaxis, defective phagocytosis, or impaired adherence. In patients with poorly controlled diabetes, the functions of PMNs, monocytes, and macrophages are impaired. As a result, the primary defense mounted by PMNs against periodontal pathogens is diminished, and bacterial proliferation is more likely. No alteration of immunoglobulin A (IgA), G (IgG), or M (IgM) has been found in patients with diabetes.

Altered Collagen Metabolism

Chronic hyperglycemia impairs collagen structure and function, which may directly impact the integrity of the periodontium. Decreased collagen synthesis, osteoporosis, and a reduction in alveolar bone height have been demonstrated in diabetic animals. Chronic hyperglycemia adversely affects the synthesis, maturation, and maintenance of collagen and extracellular matrix. In the hyperglycemic state, numerous proteins and matrix molecules undergo a nonenzymatic glycosylation, thereby resulting in *accumulated glycation end-products* (AGEs). The formation of AGEs occurs at normal glucose levels as well; however, in hyperglycemic environments, AGE formation is excessive. Many types of molecules are affected, including proteins, lipids, and carbohydrates. Collagen is cross-linked by AGE formation, which makes the collagen less soluble and less likely to be normally repaired or replaced. Cellular migration through cross-linked collagen is impeded, and, perhaps more importantly, tissue integrity is impaired as a result of damaged collagen that remains in the tissues for longer periods (i.e., collagen is not renewed at a normal rate). As a result, collagen in the tissues of patients with poorly controlled diabetes is older and more susceptible to pathogenic breakdown (i.e., less resistant to destruction by periodontal infections).

Poor glycemic control, with the associated increase in AGEs, renders the periodontal tissues more susceptible to destruction. The cumulative effects of altered cellular response to local factors, impaired tissue integrity, and altered collagen metabolism undoubtedly play a significant role in the susceptibility of patients with diabetes to infections and destructive periodontal disease.

Metabolic Syndrome

Obesity is a global concern with serious health consequences including diabetes mellitus and cardiovascular disease. It is believed that the condition of excess adipose tissue contributes to an increased systemic proinflammatory response in these individuals. Metabolic syndrome is a term used to describe a condition of abdominal obesity combined with two or more of the following metabolic disturbances: hypertension, dyslipidemia, and hyperglycemia. Individuals diagnosed with metabolic syndrome are at increased risk for developing type 2 diabetes mellitus and cardiovascular disease.

Recent evidence suggests that obesity, obesity-related characteristics, and metabolic syndrome in particular may be risk indicators for the severity and progression of periodontitis. Previous studies have documented the relationship between obesity and periodontitis as well as obesity-related characteristics such as body mass index and future progression of periodontal disease. The association between periodontitis and metabolic syndrome is thought to be the result of systemic oxidative stress and an increased inflammatory response. It may be explained by common risk factors such as obesity and obesity-related habits including diet, exercise, and poor oral hygiene. Obesity is associated with increased cytokine production as well as T-cell and monocyte/macrophage dysfunction, factors known to contribute to periodontitis. The proinflammatory cytokines interleukin-6 (IL-6) and tumor necrosis factor alpha (TNF-α), which are elevated in obese individuals, are thought to be produced by activated macrophages that have infiltrated adipose tissue. Although these associations are highly suggestive, the specific mechanisms and relationship between metabolic syndrome and periodontitis remain unknown.

Female Sex Hormones

Gingival alterations during puberty, pregnancy, and menopause are associated with physiologic hormonal changes in the female patient. During puberty and pregnancy, these changes are characterized by nonspecific inflammatory reactions with a predominant vascular component, which leads clinically to a marked hemorrhagic tendency. Oral changes during menopause may include thinning of the oral mucosa, gingival recession, xerostomia, altered taste, and burning mouth.

Puberty

Puberty is often accompanied by an exaggerated response of the gingiva to plaque. Pronounced inflammation, edema, and gingival enlargement result from local factors that might ordinarily elicit a comparatively mild gingival response. As adulthood approaches, the severity of the gingival reaction diminishes, even when local factors persist. However, complete return to normal health requires the removal of these factors. Although the prevalence and severity of gingival disease are increased during puberty, gingivitis is not a universal occurrence for all adolescents. With good oral hygiene, it can be prevented.

Menstruation

During the menstrual period, the prevalence of gingivitis increases. Some patients may complain of bleeding gums or a bloated, tense feeling in the gums during the days preceding menstrual flow. The exudate from inflamed gingiva is increased during menstruation, which suggests that preexisting gingivitis is aggravated by menstruation; however, the crevicular fluid of normal, healthy gingiva is unaffected. Tooth mobility does not change significantly during the menstrual cycle. The salivary bacterial count is increased during menstruation and at ovulation, which occurs up to 14 days earlier.

Pregnancy

As with other systemic conditions, *pregnancy itself does not cause gingivitis*. Gingivitis during pregnancy is caused by bacterial plaque, just as it is in nonpregnant women. The hormonal changes of pregnancy accentuate the gingival response to plaque and modify the resultant clinical picture (Fig. 11.2). *No notable changes occur in the gingiva during pregnancy in the absence of local factors.*

Pregnancy affects the severity of previously inflamed areas, but it does not alter healthy gingiva. Tooth mobility, pocket depth, and gingival fluid are also increased during pregnancy. The severity of gingivitis is increased during pregnancy beginning in the second or third month. Patients with mild chronic gingivitis that attracted no particular attention before the pregnancy become aware of the gingiva because previously inflamed areas become enlarged, edematous, and more notably discolored (Fig. 11.2A–C).

Gingivitis becomes more severe by the eighth month and decreases during the ninth month of pregnancy. Some investigators report that the greatest severity is between the second and third trimesters. Partial reduction in the severity of gingivitis occurs by 2 months postpartum, and after 1 year, the condition of the gingiva is comparable to that of patients who have not been pregnant. Tooth mobility, pocket depth, and gingival fluid are also reduced after pregnancy. Pronounced ease of bleeding is the most striking clinical feature. The gingiva is inflamed and varies in color from bright red to bluish red. The marginal and interdental gingivae are edematous; they pit on pressure, appear smooth and shiny, are soft and pliable, and sometimes have a raspberry-like appearance. The extreme redness results from marked vascularity, and there is an increased tendency to bleed. The gingival changes are usually painless unless they are complicated by acute infection. In some cases, the inflamed gingiva forms discrete tumor-like masses, which are referred to as *pregnancy tumors* (see Fig. 11.2D).

Microscopically, gingival disease during pregnancy appears as nonspecific, vascularizing, and proliferative inflammation. Marked inflammatory cellular infiltration occurs, with edema and degeneration of the gingival epithelium and connective tissue. The epithelium is hyperplastic, with accentuated rete pegs, reduced surface keratinization, and various degrees of intracellular and extracellular edema and infiltration by leukocytes. Newly formed, engorged capillaries are present in abundance.

Bacterial–hormonal interactions may change the composition of plaque and lead to gingival inflammation. Subgingival flora changes to a more anaerobic flora as pregnancy progresses. *P. intermedia* appears to be the only microorganism that increases significantly during pregnancy. This increase appears to be associated with elevations in systemic levels of estradiol and progesterone and to coincide with the peak in gingival bleeding. The aggravation of gingivitis during pregnancy has been attributed principally to the increased level of progesterone, which produces dilation and tortuosity of the gingival microvasculature, circulatory stasis, and increased susceptibility to mechanical irritation, all of which favor the leakage of fluid into the perivascular tissues. A marked increase in estrogen and progesterone occurs during pregnancy, with a reduction after parturition. The severity of gingivitis varies with the hormonal levels of pregnancy.

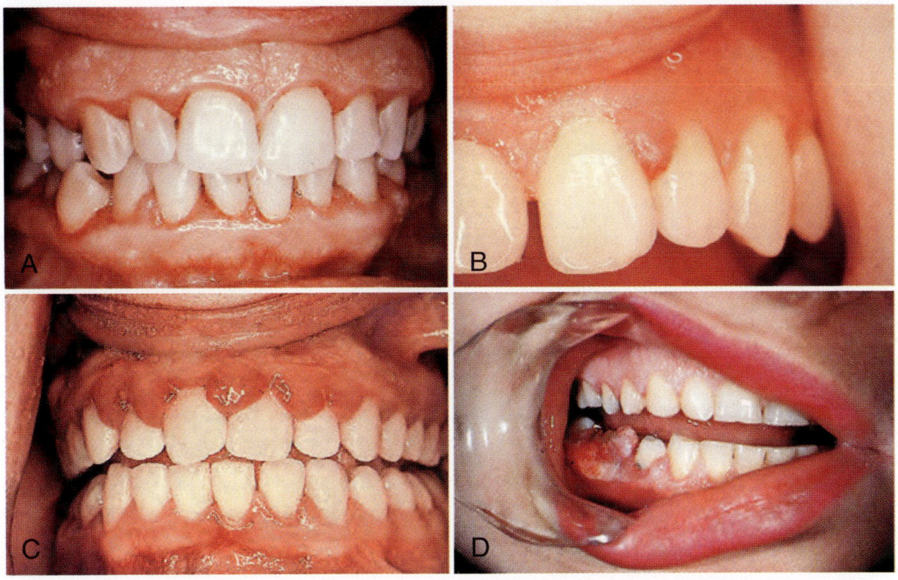

Fig. 11.2 Periodontal condition during pregnancy. A, Marginal erythema and easily bleeding gingiva in a woman who is 5 months pregnant. B, Localized incipient gingival enlargement between the maxillary central and lateral incisors in a woman who is 4 months pregnant. C, Generalized gingival enlargement of the interdental papilla and gingival margins on the facial surface of the maxillary incisors in a pregnant woman. D, Extensive gingival enlargement localized on the buccal surface of the mandibular premolars in a pregnant woman. These lesions are often referred to as "pregnancy tumors."

It has also been suggested that the accentuation of gingivitis during pregnancy has two peaks: during the first trimester, when there is an overproduction of gonadotropins, and during the third trimester, when estrogen and progesterone levels are highest. The destruction of gingival mast cells by the increased sex hormones and the resultant release of histamine and proteolytic enzymes may also contribute to the exaggerated inflammatory response to local factors.

Hormonal Contraceptives

Hormonal contraceptives aggravate the gingival response to local factors in a manner similar to that seen during pregnancy; when these drugs are taken for longer than 1.5 years, there is an increase in periodontal destruction. Although some brands of oral contraceptives produce more dramatic changes than others, no correlation has been found to exist on the basis of differences in the progesterone or estrogen content of various brands. Cumulative exposure to oral contraceptives apparently has no effect on gingival inflammation or oral debris index scores.

Menopause

During menopause, the usual rhythmic hormonal fluctuations of the female cycle are ended as estradiol ceases to be the major circulating estrogen. As a result, women can develop a gingivostomatitis. This condition occurs during menopause or during the postmenopausal period. Mild signs and symptoms sometimes appear, and these are associated with the earliest menopausal changes. Menopausal gingivostomatitis is not a common condition.

The gingiva and the remaining oral mucosa are dry and shiny, they vary in color from abnormal paleness to redness, and they bleed easily. Fissuring occurs in the mucobuccal fold in some women, and comparable changes may occur in the vaginal mucosa. Microscopically, the gingiva exhibits atrophy of the germinal and prickle cell layers of the epithelium and, in some patients, areas of ulceration. The patient complains of a dry, burning sensation throughout the oral cavity that is associated with extreme sensitivity to thermal changes; abnormal taste sensations described as "salty," "peppery," or "sour"; and difficulty with removable partial prostheses. The signs and symptoms of menopausal gingivostomatitis are somewhat comparable to those of chronic desquamative gingivitis (see Chapter 16). Signs and symptoms similar to those of menopausal gingivostomatitis occasionally occur after ovariectomy or sterilization by radiation in the treatment of malignant neoplasms.

Hyperparathyroidism

Parathyroid hypersecretion produces generalized demineralization of the skeleton, increased osteoclasis with proliferation of the connective tissue in the enlarged marrow spaces, and the formation of bone cysts and giant cell tumors. The disease is called *osteitis fibrosa cystica* or *von Recklinghausen bone disease.* Loss of the lamina dura and giant cell tumors in the jaws are late signs of hyperparathyroid bone disease, which in itself is uncommon. The complete loss of the lamina dura does not occur often, and clinicians may attach too much diagnostic significance to it. The loss of lamina dura may also occur with Paget disease, fibrous dysplasia, and osteomalacia.

Reports have suggested that 25%–50% of patients with hyperparathyroidism have associated oral changes. These changes include malocclusion and tooth mobility, radiographic evidence of alveolar osteoporosis with closely meshed trabeculae, widening of the periodontal ligament space, absence of the lamina dura, and radiolucent cyst-like spaces (Fig. 11.3). Bone cysts become filled with fibrous tissue with abundant hemosiderin-laden macrophages and giant cells. These cysts have been called *brown tumors*, but they are not tumors. More accurately, they are reparative giant cell granulomas. In some cases, these lesions appear in the periapical region of teeth, and they can lead to a misdiagnosis of a lesion of endodontic origin.

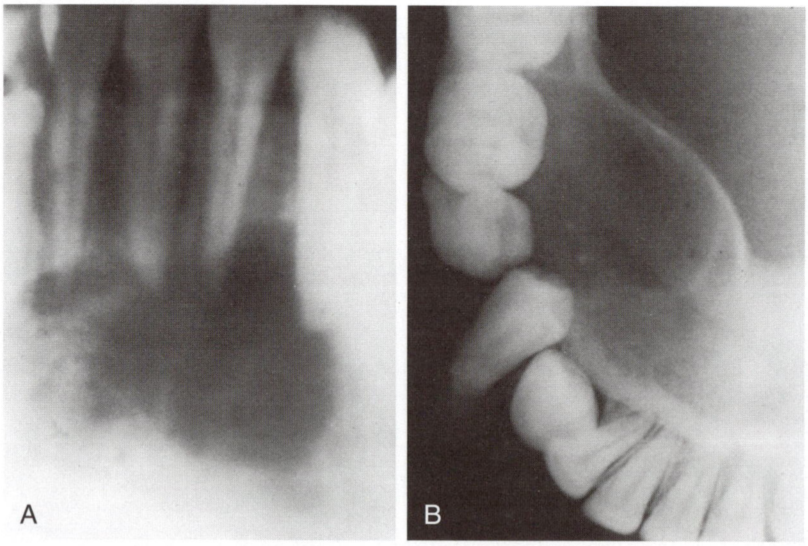

Fig. 11.3 A, Periapical radiograph of a brown tumor in a patient with hyperparathyroidism. B, Occlusal radiographic view of the brown tumor. Note the expansion of the lingual cortical plate and the movement of the premolar. *(Courtesy: Dr. L. Roy Eversole, San Francisco, CA.)*

Hematologic Disorders and Immune Deficiencies

All blood cells play an essential role in the maintenance of a healthy periodontium. White blood cells (WBCs) are involved in inflammatory reactions, and they are responsible for cellular defense against microorganisms as well as for proinflammatory cytokine release. Red blood cells (RBCs) are responsible for gas exchange and nutrient supply to the periodontal tissues and platelets, and they are necessary for normal hemostasis as well as for the recruitment of cells during inflammation and wound healing. Consequently, disorders of any blood cells or blood-forming organs can have a profound effect on the periodontium.

Certain oral changes (e.g., hemorrhage) may suggest the existence of a blood dyscrasia. However, a specific diagnosis requires a complete physical examination and a thorough hematologic study. Comparable oral changes occur in more than one form of blood dyscrasia, and secondary inflammatory changes produce a wide range of variation in the oral signs.

Hemorrhagic tendencies occur when the normal hemostatic mechanisms are disturbed. Abnormal bleeding from the gingiva or other areas of the oral mucosa that is difficult to control is an important clinical sign that suggests a hematologic disorder. Petechiae and ecchymosis (Fig. 11.4), observed most often in the soft palate area, are signs of an underlying bleeding disorder. It is essential to diagnose the specific etiology to appropriately address any bleeding or immunologic disorder.

Deficiencies in the host immune response may lead to severely destructive periodontal lesions. These deficiencies may be primary (inherited) or secondary (acquired) and may be caused by either immunosuppressive drug therapy or the pathologic destruction of the lymphoid system. Leukemia, Hodgkin disease, lymphomas, and multiple myeloma may result in secondary immunodeficiency disorders.

Leukocyte (Neutrophil) Disorders

Disorders that affect the production or function of leukocytes may result in severe periodontal destruction. PMNs (i.e., neutrophils) in particular play a critical role in bacterial infections, because PMNs are the first line of defense (see Chapter 7). A quantitative deficiency of leukocytes (e.g., neutropenia, agranulocytosis) is typically associated with a more generalized periodontal destruction that affects all teeth.

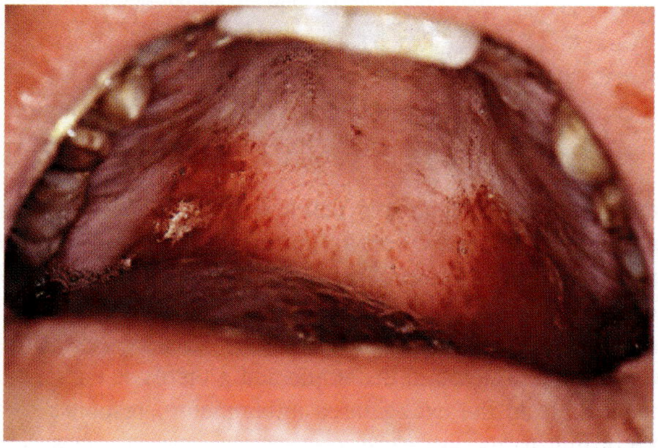

Fig. 11.4 Ecchymosis that is evident on the lateral aspects of the soft palate and tonsillar pillars of a patient with chemotherapy-induced thrombocytopenia.

Neutropenia

Neutropenia is a blood disorder that results in low levels of circulating neutrophils. It is a serious condition that may be caused by diseases, medications, chemicals, infections, idiopathic conditions, or hereditary disorders. It may be chronic or cyclic and severe or benign. It affects as many as one in three patients who are receiving chemotherapy for cancer. An absolute neutrophil count (ANC) of 1000–1500 cells/μL is diagnostic for mild neutropenia. An ANC of 500–1000 cells/μL is considered moderate neutropenia and an ANC of <500 cells/μL indicates a severe neutropenia. Infections are sometimes difficult to manage and may be life threatening, particularly with severe neutropenia.

Agranulocytosis

Agranulocytosis is a more severe neutropenia that involves not only neutrophils but also basophils and eosinophils. It is defined as an ANC of <100 cells/μL. It is characterized by a reduction in the number of circulating granulocytes, and it results in severe infections, including ulcerative necrotizing lesions of the oral mucosa, the skin, and the gastrointestinal and genitourinary tracts. Less severe forms of the disease are called *neutropenia* or *granulocytopenia.*

Drug idiosyncrasy is the most common cause of agranulocytosis, but, in some cases, its cause cannot be explained. Agranulocytosis has been reported after the administration of drugs such as aminopyrine, barbiturates and their derivatives, benzene ring derivatives, sulfonamides, gold salts, and arsenical agents. It generally occurs as an acute disease. It may be chronic or periodic, with recurring neutropenic cycles (e.g., cyclic neutropenia).

The onset of disease is accompanied by fever, malaise, general weakness, and sore throat. Ulceration in the oral cavity, the oropharynx, and the throat is characteristic. The mucosa exhibits isolated necrotic patches that are black and gray and that are sharply demarcated from the adjacent uninvolved areas. The absence of a notable inflammatory reaction caused by a lack of granulocytes is a striking feature. The gingival margin may or may not be involved. Gingival hemorrhage, necrosis, increased salivation, and fetid odor are accompanying clinical features. With cyclic neutropenia, the gingival changes recur with recurrent exacerbation of the disease. The occurrence of generalized aggressive periodontitis has been described in patients with cyclic neutropenia.

Because infection is a common feature of agranulocytosis, the differential diagnosis involves consideration of such conditions as necrotizing ulcerative gingivitis, noma, acute necrotizing inflammation of the tonsils, and diphtheria. Definitive diagnosis depends on the hematologic findings of pronounced leukopenia and the almost complete absence of neutrophils.

Leukemia

Leukemia is an important disease to understand and appreciate because of its seriousness and periodontal manifestations. The leukemias are malignant neoplasias of WBC precursors that are characterized by the following: (1) diffuse replacement of the bone marrow with proliferating leukemic cells, (2) abnormal numbers and forms of immature WBCs in the circulating blood, and (3) widespread infiltrates in the liver, spleen, lymph nodes, and other body sites.

According to the cell type involved, leukemias are classified as *lymphocytic* or *myelogenous*. A subgroup of the *myelogenous* leukemias are the *monocytic* leukemias. The term *lymphocytic* indicates that the malignant change occurs in cells that normally form lymphocytes. The term *myelogenous* indicates that the malignant change occurs in cells that normally form RBCs, some types of WBCs, and platelets. According to their evolution, leukemias can be *acute* (which is rapidly fatal), *subacute*, or *chronic.* In acute leukemia, the primitive blast cells released into the peripheral circulation are immature and nonfunctional; in chronic leukemia, the abnormal cells tend to be more mature and to have normal morphologic characteristics and functions when released into the circulation.

All leukemias tend to displace normal components of the bone marrow elements with leukemic cells, thereby resulting in the reduced production of normal RBCs, WBCs, and platelets, which leads to anemia, *leukopenia* (a reduction in the number of *nonmalignant* WBCs), and thrombocytopenia. Anemia results in poor tissue oxygenation, which makes tissues more friable and susceptible to breakdown. A reduction of normal WBCs in the circulation leads to a poor cellular defense and an increased susceptibility to infections. *Thrombocytopenia* leads to bleeding tendency, which can occur in any tissue but which in particular affects the oral cavity, especially the gingival sulcus. Some patients may have normal blood counts while leukemic cells reside primarily in the bone marrow. This type of disease is called *aleukemic leukemia*.

The Periodontium in Leukemic Patients

Oral and periodontal manifestations of leukemia may include leukemic infiltration, bleeding, oral ulcerations, and infections. The expression of these signs is more common with acute and subacute forms of leukemia than with chronic forms.

Leukemic Infiltration

Leukemic cells can infiltrate the gingiva and, less frequently, the alveolar bone. Gingival infiltration often results in *leukemic gingival enlargement* (see Chapter 14).

A study of 1076 adult patients with leukemia showed that 3.6% of the patients with teeth had leukemic gingival proliferative lesions, with the highest incidence seen in patients with acute monocytic leukemia (66.7%), followed by those with acute myelocytic–monocytic leukemia (18.7%) and acute myelocytic leukemia (3.7%). It should be noted, however, that monocytic leukemia is an extremely rare form of the disease. Leukemic gingival enlargement is not found in edentulous patients or in patients with chronic leukemia, suggesting that it represents the accumulation of immature leukemic blast cells in the gingiva adjacent to tooth surfaces with bacterial plaque. Leukemic gingival enlargement consists of a basic infiltration of the gingival corium by leukemic cells that increases the gingival thickness and creates gingival pockets in which bacterial plaque accumulates, thereby initiating a secondary inflammatory lesion that contributes to the enlargement of the gingiva. It may be localized to the interdental papilla area (Fig. 11.5), or it may expand to include the marginal gingiva and partially cover the crowns of the teeth (Fig. 11.6C and D). Clinically, the gingiva appears bluish red and cyanotic, with a rounding and tenseness of the gingival margin. The abnormal accumulation of leukemic cells in the dermal and subcutaneous connective tissue is called *leukemia cutis*, and it forms elevated and flat macules and papules (see Fig. 11.6A and B).

Microscopically, the gingiva exhibits a dense, diffuse infiltration of predominantly immature leukocytes in the attached and marginal gingiva. Occasionally, mitotic figures indicative of ectopic hematopoiesis may be seen. The normal connective tissue components of the gingiva are displaced by the leukemic cells (Fig. 11.7). The nature of the cells depends on the type of leukemia. The cellular accumulation is denser in the entire reticular connective tissue layer. In almost all cases, the papillary layer contains comparatively few leukocytes. The blood vessels are distended and contain predominantly leukemic cells, and the RBCs are reduced in number. The epithelium shows a variety of changes, and it may be thinned or hyperplastic. Common findings include degeneration associated with intercellular and intracellular edema and leukocytic infiltration with diminished surface keratinization.

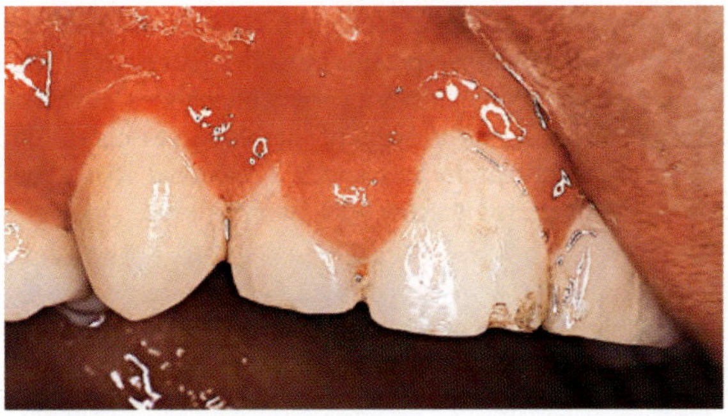

Fig. 11.5 Leukemic infiltration that causes localized gingival swelling of the interdental papillae between the maxillary lateral and central incisors. Note the tense induration of the area.

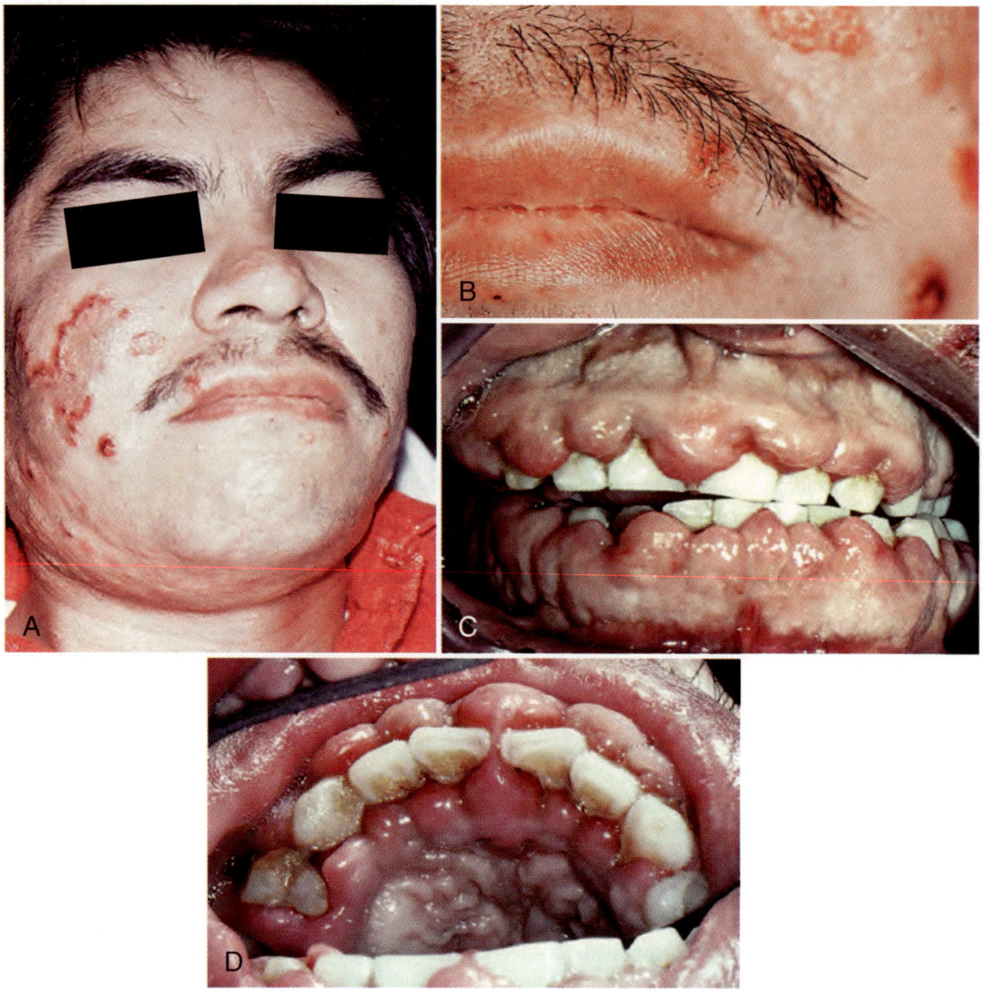

Fig. 11.6 Adult male with acute myelocytic leukemia. A, A view of the patient's face. Note the elevated, flat macules and papules (leukemia cutis) on the right cheek. B, Close-up view of skin lesions. C, An intraoral view showing pronounced gingival enlargements of the entire gingival margin and interdental papilla areas of both arches. D, Occlusal view of the maxillary anterior teeth. Note the marked enlargement in both the facial and the palatal aspects. *(Courtesy: Dr. Spencer Woolfe, Dublin, Ireland.)*

The microscopic picture of the marginal gingiva differs from that of other gingival locations in that it usually exhibits a notable inflammatory component in addition to the leukemic cells. Scattered foci of plasma cells and lymphocytes with edema and degeneration are common findings. The inner aspect of the marginal gingiva is usually ulcerated, and marginal necrosis with pseudomembrane formation may also be seen.

The periodontal ligament and alveolar bone may also be involved in acute and subacute leukemia. The periodontal ligament may be infiltrated with mature and immature leukocytes. The marrow of the alveolar bone exhibits a variety of changes, such as localized areas of necrosis, thrombosis of the blood vessels, infiltration with mature and immature leukocytes, occasional RBCs, and the replacement of the fatty marrow with fibrous tissue.

Bleeding

Gingival hemorrhage is a common finding in leukemic patients even in the absence of clinically detectable gingivitis. Bleeding gingiva can be an early sign of leukemia. It is caused by the thrombocytopenia that results from the replacement of bone marrow cells with leukemic cells and from the inhibition of normal stem cell function by leukemic cells or their products. This bleeding tendency

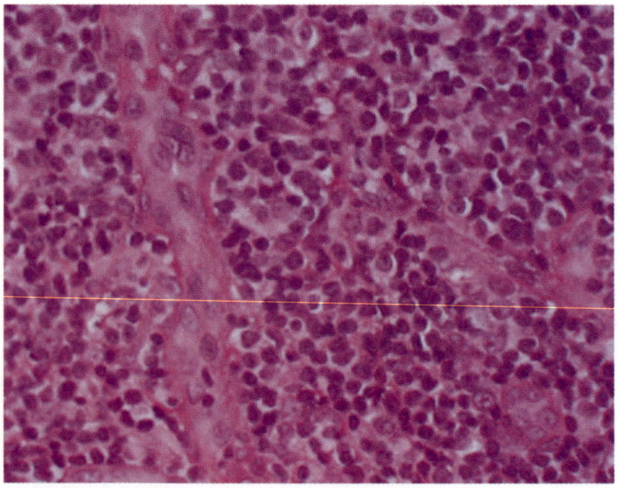

Fig. 11.7 Human histologic appearance of leukemic infiltrate with dense diffuse infiltration of predominantly immature leukocytes. The normal connective tissue components of the gingiva are displaced by the leukemic cells. The cellular accumulation is denser in the entire reticular connective tissue layer. *(Courtesy: Dr. Russell Christensen, University of California, Los Angeles, CA.)*

can also manifest in the skin and throughout the oral mucosa, where petechiae are often found, with or without leukemic infiltrates. A more diffuse submucosal bleeding manifests as ecchymosis (see Fig. 11.4). Oral bleeding has been reported as a presenting sign in 17.7% of patients with acute leukemia and in 4.4% of patients with chronic leukemia. Bleeding may also be a side effect of the chemotherapeutic agents used to treat leukemia.

Oral Ulceration and Infection

In patients with leukemia, the response to bacterial plaque or other local irritation is altered. The cellular component of the inflammatory exudate differs both quantitatively and qualitatively from that found in nonleukemic individuals in that there is a pronounced infiltration of immature leukemic cells in addition to the usual inflammatory cells. As a result, the normal inflammatory response may be diminished.

Granulocytopenia (diminished WBC count) results from the displacement of normal bone marrow cells by leukemic cells, which increases the host susceptibility to opportunistic microorganisms and leads to ulcerations and infections. Discrete, punched-out ulcers that penetrate deeply into the submucosa and are covered by a firmly attached white slough can be found on the oral mucosa. These lesions occur in sites of trauma (e.g., the buccal mucosa) in relation to the line of occlusion or on the palate. Patients with a history of herpesvirus infection may develop recurrent herpetic oral ulcers (often in multiple sites) and large atypical forms, especially after chemotherapy is instituted.

A gingival (bacterial) infection in leukemic patients can be the result of an exogenous bacterial infection or an existing bacterial infection (e.g., gingival or periodontal disease). Acute gingivitis and lesions that resemble necrotizing ulcerative gingivitis are more frequent and more severe in patients with terminal cases of acute leukemia. The inflamed gingiva in patients with leukemia differs clinically from that found in nonleukemic individuals. The gingiva is a peculiar bluish red, it is sponge-like and friable, and it bleeds persistently on the slightest provocation or even spontaneously in leukemic patients. This greatly altered and degenerated tissue is extremely susceptible to bacterial infection, which can be so severe as to cause acute gingival necrosis with pseudomembrane formation or bone exposure. These are secondary oral changes that are superimposed on the oral tissues that have been altered by the blood dyscrasia. They produce associated disturbances that may be a source of considerable difficulty to the patient, such as systemic toxic effects, loss of appetite, nausea, blood loss from persistent gingival bleeding, and constant gnawing pain. Eliminating or reducing local factors (e.g., bacterial plaque) can minimize the severe oral changes associated with leukemia. In some patients with severe acute leukemia, symptoms may be relieved only by treatment that leads to the remission of the disease.

In those with chronic leukemia, oral changes that suggest a hematologic disturbance are rare. The microscopic changes of chronic leukemia may consist of replacing the normal fatty marrow of the jaws with islands of mature lymphocytes or lymphocytic infiltration of the marginal gingiva without dramatic clinical manifestations.

The existence of leukemia is sometimes revealed by a gingival biopsy performed to clarify the nature of a troublesome gingival condition. In such cases, the gingival findings must be corroborated by medical examination and hematologic study. In patients with diagnosed leukemia, gingival biopsy may indicate the extent to which leukemic infiltration is responsible for the altered clinical appearance of the gingiva. *Although such findings are of interest, their benefit to the patient is insufficient to warrant routine gingival biopsy studies in patients with leukemia.* Furthermore, it is important to note that the absence of leukemic involvement in a gingival biopsy specimen does not rule out the possibility of leukemia. A gingival biopsy in a patient with chronic leukemia may reveal typical gingival inflammation without any suggestion of a hematologic disturbance.

Anemia

Anemia is a deficiency in the quantity or quality of the blood as manifested by a reduction in the number of erythrocytes and in the amount of hemoglobin. Anemia may be the result of blood loss, defective blood formation, or increased RBC destruction. Anemias are classified according to cellular morphology and hemoglobin content as follows: (1) macrocytic hyperchromic anemia (pernicious anemia), (2) microcytic hypochromic anemia (iron deficiency anemia), (3) sickle cell anemia, and (4) normocytic–normochromic anemia (hemolytic or aplastic anemia).

Pernicious anemia results in tongue changes in 75% of patients. The tongue appears red, smooth, and shiny as a result of atrophy of the papillae (Fig. 11.8). There is also marked pallor of the gingiva (Fig. 11.9). *Iron deficiency anemia* induces similar tongue and gingival changes. A syndrome that consists of glossitis and ulceration of the oral mucosa and oropharynx and that induces dysphagia (Plummer–Vinson syndrome) has been described in patients with iron deficiency anemia. *Sickle cell anemia* is a hereditary form of

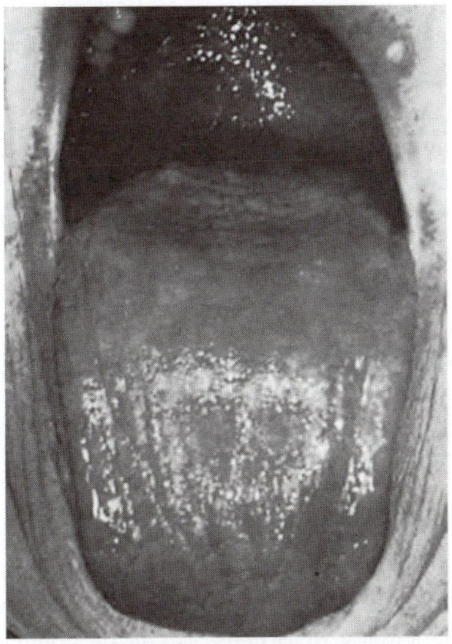

Fig. 11.8 A smooth tongue in a patient with pernicious anemia.

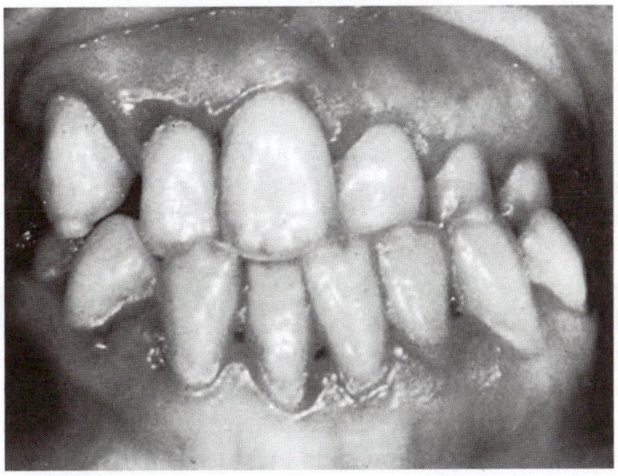

Fig. 11.9 The diffuse pallor of the gingiva in a patient with anemia. The discolored and inflamed gingival margin stands out in sharp contrast to the adjacent pale and attached gingiva.

chronic hemolytic anemia that occurs almost exclusively in blacks. It is characterized by pallor, jaundice, weakness, rheumatoid manifestations, and leg ulcers. Oral changes include generalized osteoporosis of the jaws, with a peculiar stepladder alignment of the trabeculae of the interdental septa, along with pallor and yellowish discoloration of the oral mucosa. Periodontal infections may precipitate sickle cell crisis. *Aplastic anemia* results from a failure of the bone marrow to produce erythrocytes. The etiology is usually the effect of toxic drugs on the marrow or the displacement of RBCs by leukemic cells. Oral changes include pale discoloration of the oral mucosa and increased susceptibility to infection because of the concomitant neutropenia.

Thrombocytopenia

Thrombocytopenia is a term that is used to describe the condition of a reduced platelet count that results from either a lack of platelet production or an increased loss of platelets. *Purpura* refers to the purplish appearance of the skin or mucous membranes where bleeding has occurred as a result of decreased platelets. *Thrombocytopenic purpura* may be idiopathic (i.e., of unknown etiology, as with Werlhof disease), or it may occur secondary to some known etiologic factor that is responsible for a reduced amount of functioning marrow and a resultant reduction in the number of circulating platelets. Such etiologic factors include aplasia of the marrow, displacement of the megakaryocytes in the marrow (as with leukemia), replacement of the marrow by tumor, and destruction of the marrow by irradiation or radium or by drugs such as benzene, aminopyrine, or arsenical agents.

Thrombocytopenic purpura is characterized by a low platelet count, a prolonged clot retraction and bleeding time, and a normal or slightly prolonged clotting time. There is spontaneous bleeding into the skin or from the mucous membranes. Petechiae and hemorrhagic vesicles occur in the oral cavity, particularly in the palate, the tonsillar pillars, and the buccal mucosa. The gingivae are swollen, soft, and friable. Bleeding occurs spontaneously or with the slightest provocation, and it is difficult to control. *Gingival changes represent an abnormal response to local irritation.* The severity of the gingival condition is dramatically alleviated by removal of the local factors.

Antibody Deficiency Disorders

Agammaglobulinemia, or hypogammaglobulinemia, is an immune deficiency that results from inadequate antibody production caused by a deficiency in B cells. It can be congenital (X-linked or Bruton agammaglobulinemia) or acquired (common variable immunodeficiency).

T-cell function remains normal in individuals with agammaglobulinemia. The disease, whether congenital or acquired, is characterized by recurrent bacterial infections, especially ear, sinus, and lung infections. Patients are also susceptible to periodontal infections. Periodontitis, stage 3 or 4, grade C (aggressive periodontitis) is a common finding in children who are diagnosed with agammaglobulinemia.

Genetic Disorders

Systemic conditions that are associated with or that predispose an individual to periodontal destruction include genetic disorders that result in an inadequate number or reduced function of circulating neutrophils. This underscores the importance of the neutrophil in the protection of the periodontium against infection. Severe periodontitis has been observed in individuals with primary neutrophil disorders such as neutropenia, agranulocytosis, Chédiak–Higashi syndrome, and lazy leukocyte syndrome. In addition, severe periodontitis has been observed in individuals who exhibit secondary neutrophil impairment, such as those with Down syndrome, Papillon–Lefèvre syndrome, and inflammatory bowel disease.

Chédiak–Higashi Syndrome

Chédiak–Higashi syndrome is a rare disease that affects the production of organelles found in almost every cell. It affects mostly the melanocytes, platelets, and phagocytes. It causes partial albinism, mild bleeding disorders, and recurrent bacterial infections. Neutrophils contain abnormal, giant lysosomes that can fuse with the phagosome, but their ability to release their contents is impaired. As a result, the killing of ingested microorganisms is delayed. Patients with Chédiak–Higashi syndrome are susceptible to repeated infections that can be serious and life threatening. Aggressive periodontitis has been described in these patients.

Lazy Leukocyte Syndrome

Lazy leukocyte syndrome is characterized by susceptibility to severe microbial infections, neutropenia, defective chemotactic response by neutrophils, and an abnormal inflammatory response. Those who are diagnosed with lazy leukocyte syndrome are susceptible to aggressive periodontitis with destruction of bone and early tooth loss.

Leukocyte Adhesion Deficiency

Leukocyte adhesion deficiency (LAD) is a very rare genetic disorder; only a few hundred cases have been diagnosed. Because LAD is an inherited disease, it is categorized as a primary immunodeficiency that is most often diagnosed at birth. Many children with LAD do not survive.

LAD results from an inability to produce or a failure to normally express an important cell surface integrin (CD18), which is necessary for leukocytes to adhere to the vessel wall at the site of infection. When leukocytes cannot effectively adhere to the vessel wall near the site of infection, they cannot migrate to the infection. As a result, bacterial infections are able to continue to destroy host tissues unimpeded by the normal host immune response. Infections act similarly to those observed in neutropenic patients, because phagocytes are unable to reach the site of infection.

Cases of periodontal disease that are attributed to LAD are rare. They begin during or immediately after the eruption of the primary teeth. Extremely acute inflammation and proliferation of the gingival tissues with rapid destruction of the bone are found. Profound defects in peripheral blood neutrophils and monocytes and an absence of neutrophils in the gingival tissues have been noted in patients with LAD. These patients also have frequent respiratory tract infections and sometimes otitis media. Both the primary and the permanent teeth are affected, often resulting in early tooth loss.

Papillon–Lefèvre Syndrome

Papillon–Lefèvre syndrome, which was first described by French physicians Papillon and Lefèvre in 1924, is a very rare inherited condition that appears to follow an autosomal-recessive pattern. Parents are not affected, and both must carry the autosomal genes for the syndrome to appear in their offspring.

The syndrome is characterized by hyperkeratotic skin lesions, severe destruction of the periodontium, and, in some cases, calcification of the dura. The cutaneous and periodontal changes usually appear together when the patient is between the ages of 2 and 4 years. The skin lesions consist of hyperkeratosis and ichthyosis of localized areas on the palms, soles, knees, and elbows (Fig. 11.10A and B).

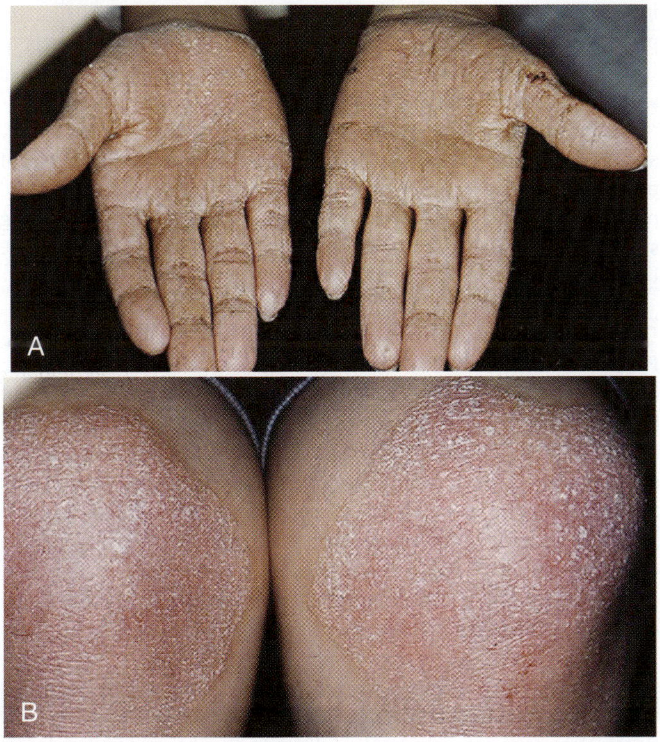

Fig. 11.10 This intraoral clinical view of a 17-year-old boy with Papillon–Lefèvre syndrome shows early tooth loss and severe bone loss around the remaining teeth as evidenced by gingival recession. The missing teeth were exfoliated.

Periodontal involvement consists of early inflammatory changes that lead to bone loss and exfoliation of teeth. The primary teeth are lost by 5 or 6 years of age. The permanent dentition then erupts normally, but within a few years, the permanent teeth are also lost as a result of destructive periodontal disease. At a very early age (usually 15–20 years), patients are often edentulous except for the third molars. These may be lost as well a few years after eruption. Tooth extraction sites heal uneventfully.

The microscopic changes reported include marked chronic inflammation of the lateral wall of the pocket with a predominantly plasma cell infiltrate, considerable osteoclastic activity with an apparent lack of osteoblastic activity, and an extremely thin cementum. Bacterial flora studies of plaque in a patient with Papillon–Lefèvre syndrome revealed a similarity to bacterial flora in patients with chronic periodontitis. Spirochete-rich zones in the apical portion of the pockets as well as spirochete adherence to the cementum and microcolony formation of *Mycoplasma* species have been reported with Papillon–Lefèvre syndrome. Gram-negative cocci and rods appear at the apical border of the plaque. This syndrome may be associated with neutrophil defects as a contributing factor.

Down Syndrome

Down syndrome (mongolism, trisomy 21) is a congenital disease caused by a chromosomal abnormality and is characterized by mental deficiency and growth retardation. The prevalence of periodontal disease in patients with Down syndrome is high, occurring in almost 100% of patients who are younger than 30 years of age. Although plaque, calculus, and local irritants (e.g., diastemata, crowding of teeth, high frenum attachments, malocclusion) are present and oral hygiene is poor, the severity of periodontal destruction exceeds that explainable by local factors alone.

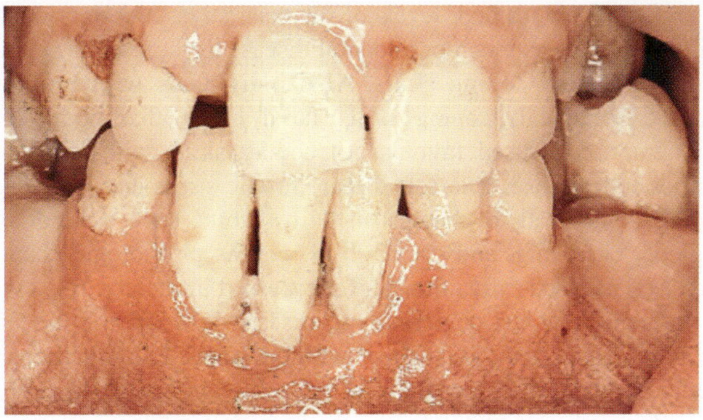

Fig. 11.11 Severe periodontal destruction in a 14-year-old patient with Down syndrome. Note the extensive loss of periodontal support around the mandibular incisors as evidenced by severe gingival recession. Moderate to heavy bacterial plaque is associated with moderate gingival inflammation in the area.

Periodontal disease in those with Down syndrome is characterized by the formation of deep periodontal pockets associated with substantial plaque accumulation and moderate gingivitis (Fig. 11.11). These findings are usually generalized, although they tend to be more severe in the lower anterior region. Moderate recession is sometimes seen in this region as well. The disease progresses rapidly. The high prevalence and increased severity of periodontal destruction associated with Down syndrome is most likely explained by poor PMN chemotaxis, phagocytosis, and intracellular killing.

Stress and Psychosomatic Disorders

Psychologic conditions, particularly psychosocial stress, have been implicated as risk indicators for periodontal disease. The most notable example is the documented relationship between stress (e.g., experienced by soldiers at war or by students during examinations) and acute necrotizing ulcerative gingivitis (see Chapters 15 and 21). The presence of necrotizing ulcerative gingivitis among soldiers stressed by wartime conditions in the trenches led to one of the early diagnostic terms used to describe this condition: "trench mouth." Despite this well-known association between stress and necrotizing ulcerative gingivitis, confirming the connection between psychologic conditions and other forms of periodontal disease (e.g., chronic periodontitis) has been elusive. These relationships are difficult to elucidate, because, as with many common diseases, the etiology and pathogenesis of periodontal disease is multifactorial, and the role of individual risk factors is difficult to define.

Psychosocial Stress, Depression, and Coping

Several clinical studies and a systematic review of the subject have documented a positive relationship between psychosocial stress and chronic forms of periodontal disease.

All individuals experience stress, but these events do not invariably result in destructive periodontitis. The types of stress that lead to periodontal destruction appear to be more chronic or long term and less likely to be controlled by the individual. Life events such as the loss of a loved one (e.g., spouse, family member), a failed relationship, loss of employment, and financial difficulties are examples of stressful life events that are typically not controllable by the individual or not perceived by the individual as being under his or her control, thereby resulting in a feeling of helplessness. The duration of the stressful life event also has an influence on the total impact of the stress-induced disease destruction.

Individuals with high levels of financial stress and poor coping skills had twice as much periodontal disease as those with minimal stress and good coping skills. Also individuals with problem-focused (practical) coping skills fared better than individuals with emotion-focused (avoidance) coping skills with respect to periodontal disease. It is found that chronic stress and inadequate coping could lead to changes in daily habits, such as poor oral hygiene, clenching, and grinding, as well as physiologic changes such as decreased saliva flow and suppressed immunity.

Influence of stress on periodontal disease destruction is the manner in which the individual copes with the stress. Emotional coping methods appear to render the host more susceptible to the destructive effects of periodontal disease than do practical coping methods.

Stress-Induced Immunosuppression

Stress and psychosomatic disorders most likely impact periodontal health via changes in the individual's behavior and through complex interactions among the nervous, endocrine, and immune systems. Individuals under stress may have poorer oral hygiene, they may start or increase the clenching and grinding of their teeth, and they may smoke more frequently. All of these behavioral changes increase their susceptibility to periodontal disease destruction. Likewise, individuals who are under stress may be less likely to seek professional care.

In addition to the many behavioral changes that may influence periodontal disease destruction, psychosocial stress may also impact the disease through alterations in the immune system. The influence of stress on the immune system and systemic health conditions (e.g., cardiovascular disease) is well known. Stress-related immune system changes clearly have the potential to affect the pathogenesis of periodontal disease as well. One possible mechanism involves the production of cortisol. Stress increases cortisol production from the adrenal cortex by stimulating an increase in the release of adrenocorticotropic hormone from the pituitary gland. Increased cortisol suppresses the immune response directly through the suppression of neutrophil activity, immunoglobulin G production, and salivary IgA secretion. All of these immune responses are critical for the normal immunoinflammatory response to periodontal pathogens (see Chapter 7). The resulting stress-induced immunosuppression increases the potential for destruction by periodontal pathogens. Stress may also affect the cellular immune response directly through an increased release of neurotransmitters, including epinephrine, norepinephrine, neurokinin, and substance P, which interact directly with lymphocytes, neutrophils, monocytes, and macrophages via receptors that cause an increase in their tissue-destructive function. Thus, in a manner similar to cortisol production, the stress-induced release of these neurotransmitters results in an upregulated immune response that increases the potential for destruction by the cellular response to periodontal pathogens.

It is important to remember that, although stress may predispose an individual to more destruction from periodontitis, the presence of periodontal pathogens remains as the essential etiologic factor. In other words, stress alone does not cause or lead to periodontitis in the absence of periodontal pathogens.

Influence of Stress on Periodontal Therapy Outcomes

Psychologic conditions such as stress and depression may also influence the outcome of periodontal therapy. Depression might have a negative effect on periodontal treatment outcomes.

A study investigating the relationship between psychologic stress and wound repair in patients after routine surgery (in this case, inguinal hernia open incision repair) revealed that stress impairs the inflammatory response and matrix degradation. Greater psychologic stress was significantly associated with lower levels of IL-1 and MMP-9 (Matrix Metalloproteinases) as well as with a significantly more painful, poorer, and slower recovery.

Both stressful life events and the individual's personality and coping skills are factors to consider when assessing the risk of periodontal disease destruction and the potential for successful periodontal therapy. If patients with emotional or defensive coping skills are identified, care should be taken to ensure that they receive information in a manner that does not elicit a defensive reaction.

Psychiatric Influence of Self-Inflicted Injury

Psychosomatic disorders may result in harmful effects to the health of tissues in the oral cavity through the development of habits that are injurious to the periodontium. Neurotic habits such as grinding or clenching the teeth, nibbling on foreign objects (e.g., pencils, pipes), nail biting, and excessive use of tobacco are all potentially injurious to the teeth and the periodontium. Self-inflicted gingival injuries, such as gingival recession, have been described in both children and adults. However, these types of self-inflicted, factitious injuries do not appear to be common among psychiatric patients.

Nutritional Influences

Some clinicians enthusiastically adhere to the theory in periodontal disease that assigns a key role to nutritional deficiencies and imbalances. Previous research did not support this view, but numerous problems in experimental design and data interpretation could be responsible for making these research findings inadequate. The majority of opinions and research findings regarding the effects of nutrition on oral and periodontal tissues point to the following:

1. *There are no nutritional deficiencies that by themselves can cause gingivitis or periodontitis.* However, nutritional deficiencies can affect the condition of the periodontium and thereby may accentuate the deleterious effects of plaque-induced inflammation in susceptible individuals. Theoretically, one may presume that an individual with a nutritional deficiency is less able to defend against a bacterial challenge as compared to a nutritionally competent individual.
2. *There are nutritional deficiencies that produce changes in the oral cavity.* These changes include alterations of the tissues of the lips, oral mucosa, gingiva, and bone. These alterations are considered to be the periodontal and oral manifestations of nutritional disease.

The role of nutrition in periodontal disease may be related to the effect of nutrition on inflammation. A 2009 review of the literature evaluating the effect of nutritional factors on inflammation demonstrated that subtle shifts in nutritional status are associated with the prevalence of periodontitis. More specifically, the authors reported that the results of contemporary animal and human studies have demonstrated the role of specific micronutrients in the modulation of the host's inflammatory response by reducing inflammatory biomarkers, which may in turn be responsible for periodontal destruction. The evidence for the effect of nutrition on inflammation is significant. Data suggest that diets that contain foods rich in antioxidants are beneficial, whereas foods that contain high levels of refined carbohydrates are detrimental to the inflammatory process.

Fat-Soluble Vitamin Deficiency

Vitamins A, D, and E are fat-soluble vitamins that are required in the human diet.

Vitamin A Deficiency

A major function of vitamin A is to maintain the health of the epithelial cells of the skin and mucous membranes. A deficiency of vitamin A results in dermatologic, mucosal, and ocular manifestations. In the absence of vitamin A, degenerative changes occur in epithelial tissues, thereby resulting in a keratinizing metaplasia. Because epithelial tissues provide a primary barrier function to protect against invading microorganisms, vitamin A may play an important role in protecting against microbial invasion by maintaining epithelial integrity.

Little information is available regarding the effects of vitamin A deficiency on the oral structures in humans. Several epidemiologic studies have failed to demonstrate any relationship between this vitamin and periodontal disease in humans.

Vitamin D Deficiency

Vitamin D or calciferol is essential for the absorption of calcium from the gastrointestinal tract and for the maintenance of the calcium–phosphorus balance. A deficiency of vitamin D and an imbalance in calcium–phosphorus intake result in rickets in young children and osteomalacia in adults. No studies have demonstrated a relationship between vitamin D deficiency and periodontal disease.

Vitamin E Deficiency

Vitamin E serves as an antioxidant to limit free-radical reactions and to protect cells from lipid peroxidation. Cell membranes, which are high in polyunsaturated lipids, are the major site of damage in patients with vitamin E deficiency. No relationship has been demonstrated between deficiencies in vitamin E and oral disease, but systemic vitamin E appears to accelerate gingival wound healing in the rat.

Water-Soluble Vitamin Deficiency

Vitamins B and C are water-soluble vitamins that are required in the human diet.

B-Complex Deficiency

The vitamin B complex includes thiamin, riboflavin, niacin, pyridoxine (B_6), biotin, folic acid, and cobalamin (B_{12}). Oral disease is rarely caused by a deficiency in just one component of the B-complex group; the deficiency is generally multiple.

Oral changes that are common to B-complex deficiencies are gingivitis, glossitis, glossodynia, angular cheilitis, and inflammation of the entire oral mucosa. The gingivitis in individuals with vitamin B deficiencies is nonspecific because it is caused by bacterial plaque rather than by the deficiency; however, gingivitis is subject to the deficiency's modifying effect.

The human manifestations of **thiamin deficiency**, called *beriberi*, are characterized by paralysis; cardiovascular symptoms, including edema; and loss of appetite. Frank beriberi is rare in the United States. Oral disturbances that have been attributed to thiamin deficiency include hypersensitivity of the oral mucosa; minute vesicles (simulating herpes) on the buccal mucosa, under the tongue, or on the palate; and erosion of the oral mucosa.

The symptoms of **riboflavin deficiency** (*ariboflavinosis*) include glossitis, angular cheilitis, seborrheic dermatitis, and a superficial vascularizing keratitis. The glossitis is characterized by a magenta discoloration and atrophy of the papillae. In mild-to-moderate cases, the dorsum exhibits a patchy atrophy of the lingual papillae and engorged fungiform papillae, which project as pebble-like elevations. With severe deficiency, the entire dorsum is flat, with a dry and often fissured surface. Changes observed in riboflavin-deficient monkeys include severe lesions of the gingiva, the periodontal tissues, and the oral mucosa, including noma.

Angular cheilitis begins as an inflammation of the commissure of the lips, and this is followed by erosion, ulceration, and fissuring. Riboflavin deficiency is not the only cause of angular cheilitis. A loss of vertical dimension, together with the drooling of saliva into the angles of the lips, may produce a condition similar to angular cheilitis. Candidiasis may develop in the commissures of debilitated persons; this lesion has been termed *perlèche.* Supplemental riboflavin is ineffective to resolve cases of glossitis and angular cheilitis that are not caused by vitamin deficiency.

Niacin deficiency results in *pellagra*, which is characterized by symptoms of dermatitis, gastrointestinal disturbances, neurologic and mental disturbances (dermatitis, diarrhea, or dementia), glossitis, gingivitis, and generalized stomatitis. This condition is rare, but it may occasionally result from malabsorption or alcoholism. Glossitis and stomatitis may be the earliest clinical signs of niacin deficiency. The gingiva may be involved in *aniacinosis* with or without tongue changes. The most common finding is necrotizing ulcerative gingivitis, usually in areas of local irritation.

Oral manifestations of vitamin B complex and niacin deficiency in experimental animals include black tongue and gingival inflammation with destruction of the gingiva, the periodontal ligament, and the alveolar bone. Necrosis of the gingiva and other oral tissues as well as leukopenia are terminal features of niacin deficiency in experimental animals.

Folic acid deficiency results in macrocytic anemia with megaloblastic erythropoiesis accompanied by oral changes, gastrointestinal lesions, diarrhea, and intestinal malabsorption. Folic acid-deficient animals demonstrate necrosis of the gingiva, the periodontal ligament, and the alveolar bone without inflammation. The absence of inflammation is the result of deficiency-induced granulocytopenia. In humans with sprue and other folic acid deficiency states, generalized stomatitis occurs, which may be accompanied by ulcerated glossitis and cheilitis. Ulcerative stomatitis is an early indication of the toxic effect of the folic acid antagonists (e.g., methotrexate) used for the treatment of leukemia.

There is a significant reduction of gingival inflammation after the systemic or local use of folic acid as compared to placebo. This reduction occurred with no change in plaque accumulation. The authors also postulated that the gingival changes associated with pregnancy and oral contraceptives may be partly related to suboptimal levels of folic acid in the gingiva.

Vitamin C Deficiency

Severe vitamin C (ascorbic acid) deficiency in humans results in scurvy, a disease that is characterized by hemorrhagic diathesis and delayed wound healing. Vitamin C is required in the diet of humans as well as other primates, guinea pigs, and some rare flying mammals. Because vitamin C is abundant in fruits and vegetables, scurvy is uncommon in developed countries. It may occur in infants during their first year of life if infant formulas are not fortified with vitamins and in older persons, especially those living alone and with restricted diets. Malnutrition associated with alcoholism may predispose an individual to scurvy.

Scurvy results in the defective formation and maintenance of collagen, the impairment or cessation of osteoid formation, and impaired osteoblastic function. Vitamin C deficiency is also characterized by increased capillary permeability, susceptibility to traumatic hemorrhages, hyporeactivity of the contractile elements of the peripheral blood vessels, and sluggishness of blood flow. Clinical manifestations of scurvy include hemorrhagic lesions into the muscles of the extremities, the joints, and sometimes the nail beds; petechial hemorrhages, often around the hair follicles; increased susceptibility to infections; and impaired wound healing.

Bleeding, swollen gingiva, and loosened teeth are common features of scurvy.

Possible Etiologic Factors

Ascorbic acid may play a role in periodontal disease through one or more of the following suggested mechanisms:

1. Low levels of ascorbic acid influence the metabolism of collagen within the periodontium, thereby affecting the ability of the tissue to regenerate and repair itself. No experimental evidence supports this view of the role of ascorbic acid. Furthermore, it has been shown that collagen fibers in the periodontal ligament of scorbutic monkeys are the last to be affected before the death of the animals.
2. Ascorbic acid deficiency interferes with bone formation and leads to the loss of periodontal bone. Changes that do occur in alveolar bone and other bones as a result of failure of the osteoblasts to form osteoid take place very late in the deficiency state. Osteoporosis of alveolar bone in scorbutic monkeys results from increased osteoclastic resorption; it is not associated with periodontal pocket formation.
3. Ascorbic acid deficiency increases the permeability of the oral mucosa to tritiated endotoxin and tritiated inulin and of normal human crevicular epithelium to tritiated dextran. Optimal levels of vitamin C would therefore maintain the epithelium's barrier function to bacterial products.
4. Increasing levels of ascorbic acid enhance the chemotactic and migratory actions of leukocytes without influencing their phagocytic activity. Megadoses of vitamin C seem to impair the bactericidal activity of leukocytes. The significance of these findings for the pathogenesis and treatment of periodontal diseases is not understood.
5. An optimal level of ascorbic acid is apparently required to maintain the integrity of the periodontal microvasculature as well as the vascular response to bacterial plaque and wound healing.
6. Depletion of vitamin C may interfere with the ecologic equilibrium of bacteria in plaque and thus increase its pathogenicity. However, no evidence demonstrates this effect.

Gingivitis

The legendary association of severe gingival disease with scurvy led to the presumption that vitamin C deficiency is an etiologic factor in gingivitis, which is common at all ages. Gingivitis with enlarged, hemorrhagic, bluish-red gingiva is described as one of the classic signs of vitamin C deficiency, but *gingivitis is not caused by vitamin C deficiency.* Vitamin C-deficient patients do not necessarily have gingivitis. Acute vitamin C deficiency does not cause or increase the incidence of gingival inflammation, but it does increase its severity. Gingivitis in vitamin C-deficient patients is caused by bacterial plaque. Vitamin C deficiency may aggravate the gingival response to plaque and worsen the edema, enlargement, and bleeding. In addition, although correcting the deficiency may reduce the severity of the disorder, gingivitis will remain as long as bacterial factors are present.

Periodontitis

Changes in the supporting periodontal tissues and gingiva in individuals with vitamin C deficiency have been documented extensively in experimental animals. Acute vitamin C deficiency results in edema and hemorrhage in the periodontal ligament, osteoporosis of the alveolar bone, and tooth mobility; hemorrhage, edema, and degeneration of the collagen fibers occur in the gingiva. Vitamin C deficiency also impairs gingival healing. The periodontal fibers that are least affected by vitamin C deficiency are those just below the junctional epithelium and above the alveolar crest, which explains the infrequent apical downgrowth of the epithelium.

Vitamin C deficiency alone does not cause periodontal destruction. Local bacterial factors are required for increased probing depth and attachment loss to occur. However, acute vitamin C deficiency accentuates the destructive effect of gingival inflammation on the underlying periodontal ligament and alveolar bone.

Analysis of the literature indicates that the microscopic signs of vitamin C deficiency are quite different from those that occur with plaque-induced periodontal disease in humans. Patients with acute or chronic vitamin C-deficient states and no plaque accumulation demonstrate minimal (if any) changes in their gingival health status.

Protein Deficiency

Protein depletion results in hypoproteinemia with many pathologic changes, including muscular atrophy, weakness, weight loss, anemia, leukopenia, edema, impaired lactation, decreased resistance to infection, slow wound healing, lymphoid depletion, and reduced ability to form certain hormones and enzyme systems. Protein deprivation has been shown to cause changes in the periodontium of experimental animals. The following observations have been made in protein-deprived animals: degeneration of the connective tissue of the gingiva and the periodontal ligament, osteoporosis of the alveolar bone, impaired deposition of the cementum, delayed wound healing, and atrophy of the tongue epithelium. Similar changes occur in the periosteum and bone in nonoral areas. Osteoporosis results from the reduced deposition of osteoid, a reduction in the number of osteoblasts, and impairment in the morphodifferentiation of connective tissue cells to form osteoblasts rather than from increased osteoclastic activity.

These observations are of interest in that they reveal a loss of alveolar bone that results from the inhibition of normal bone-forming activity rather than from the introduction of destructive factors. Protein deficiency also accentuates the destructive effects of bacterial plaque and occlusal trauma on the periodontal tissues, but the initiation of gingival inflammation and its severity depend on the bacterial plaque. In other words, protein deprivation results in periodontal tissues that lack integrity and that, as a result, are more vulnerable to breakdown when challenged by bacteria.

Medications

Bisphosphonates

Bisphosphonate medications are primarily used to treat cancer (via intravenous administration) and osteoporosis (via oral administration). They act by inhibiting osteoclastic activity, which leads to less bone resorption, less bone remodeling, and less bone turnover. The use of bisphosphonates in cancer treatment is aimed at preventing the often lethal imbalance of osteoclastic activity. During the treatment of osteoporosis, the goal is simply to harness osteoclastic activity to minimize or prevent bone loss and, in many cases, to increase bone mass by creating an advantage for osteoblastic activity. The major differences in the use of bisphosphonates for cancer versus osteoporosis are the potency and route of administration of the specific bisphosphonate medication used. Potency is influenced by the chemical properties as well as by the binding and release pharmacokinetic properties of these agents as they apply to bone. Specifically, the strength of binding and the ease of release of bisphosphonates with hydroxyapatite make these drugs more or less potent.

Bisphosphonates and Periodontal Bone Loss

The bone-preserving action of bisphosphonates has been studied and advocated for use in the prevention of bone loss from periodontal disease. Several animal studies have shown that bisphosphonates, either applied topically or administered systemically, have the potential to prevent the alveolar bone loss caused by periodontitis. The use of bisphosphonates for bone regeneration has been proposed as well.

Corticosteroids

In humans, the systemic administration of cortisone and adrenocorticotropic hormone appears to have no effect on the incidence or severity of gingival and periodontal disease. However, renal transplantation patients receiving immunosuppressive therapy (either prednisone or methylprednisone combined with either azathioprine or cyclophosphamide) have significantly less gingival inflammation than control subjects with similar amounts of plaque.

Other Systemic Conditions

Osteoporosis

Osteoporosis is a disease that is characterized by low bone mass and structural deterioration leading to an increased risk of bone fracture. It affects approximately 10 million people in the United States. The condition has a higher predilection for females (80%) compared to males (20%). An additional 34 million individuals in the United States are estimated to have osteopenia or low bone density. The loss of bone mass and the incidence of osteoporosis increase with age for both men and women, with women being affected earlier than men. The rate of bone loss is greatest for women during the perimenopausal years, when estrogen levels decrease.

A bone mineral density (BMD) test is used to measure an individual's bone mass. BMD is measured with the use of a dual-energy x-ray absorptiometry (DEXA) scan. The DEXA value or T-score is a comparison of the patient's BMD with that of a healthy 30-year-old adult with peak bone mass. The World Health Organization defines osteoporosis and osteopenia by measures of standard deviation rather than comparison with a normal, healthy, young adult. Thus, a T-score between +1 and −1 is considered normal, whereas a T-score between −1 and −2.5 indicates low bone density or osteopenia and a T-score of less than −2.5 (i.e., more than 2.5 standard deviations below normal) is diagnostic for osteoporosis (Table 11.2).

One of the most significant consequences of osteoporosis is the increased risk of bone fracture. All bones affected by osteoporosis are susceptible to fracture, but fractures of the pelvis and vertebrae carry the most serious risk of morbidity and mortality. Although it is logical to surmise a relationship between osteoporosis and periodontitis, it has been a challenging hypothesis to prove. One of the difficulties is the fact that both osteoporosis and periodontitis are chronic, multifactorial diseases that result in bone loss, and bone loss in each condition is exacerbated by local and systemic factors. Gender, genetic predisposition, inactivity, deficient diets (e.g., deficient in calcium or vitamin D), alcohol, smoking, hormones, and medications put individuals at risk for osteoporosis, with some of these factors putting them at risk for the progression of periodontitis as well. Estrogen deficiency and osteopenia or osteoporosis together are risk factors for alveolar bone loss in postmenopausal women with a history of periodontitis. Estrogen deficiency may play a significant role in the progression of periodontitis in osteopenic or osteoporotic women. In patients with periodontal disease and concomitant postmenopausal osteoporosis, the possibility exists that the lack of estrogen influences the activities of bone cells and immune cells in such a way that the progression of alveolar bone loss is enhanced. In fact, there are numerous studies that report less risk for tooth loss and improved oral health among postmenopausal women receiving hormone replacement therapy.

TABLE 11.2 Definitions of Osteoporosis and Osteopenia Indicated by T-Scores[a]

T-Score	Bone Mineral Density Category
≥−1	Normal
−1 to −2.5	Low (osteopenia)
≤−2.5	Osteoporosis

[a]Ranges of T-scores are based on standard deviations from the normal value, which is based on the bone mineral density of a healthy 30-year-old adult.

(Adapted from World Health Organization Scientific Group on the Assessment of Osteoporosis at Primary Health Care Level: *Summary Meeting Report*, Brussels, May 5–7, 2004.)

Congenital Heart Disease

Congenital heart disease occurs in about 1% of live births. Approximately 40% of individuals born with heart defects would die without treatment. However, the prognosis has been dramatically improved with advances in cardiac surgery. Cardiac defects can involve the heart, the adjacent vessels, or a combination of both. The most striking feature of congenital heart disease is cyanosis caused by the shunting of deoxygenated blood from the right to the left, which results in the return of poorly oxygenated blood to the systemic circulation. In severe cases, cyanosis is obvious at birth, particularly in the presence of tetralogy of Fallot. Chronic hypoxia causes impaired development, compensatory polycythemia (i.e., an increase in RBCs and hemoglobin), and clubbing edema of toes and fingers. Polycythemia is significant because it can result in hemorrhagic or thrombotic tendencies. Patients with congenital heart defects are often at risk for infective endocarditis as a result of turbulent blood flow in the heart and the associated cardiovascular defects. The need for prophylactic antibiotics should be evaluated before dental therapy.

In addition to the obvious cyanosis of the lips and the oral mucosa, oral abnormalities associated with cyanotic congenital heart disease include delayed eruption of both primary and permanent dentitions, increased positional abnormalities, and enamel hypoplasia. The teeth often have a bluish-white appearance with an increased pulp vascular volume. Gingival disease and other oral symptoms have been reported in children with congenital heart disease. Reports seem to indicate more severe caries and periodontal disease in patients with cyanotic congenital heart defects. However, the apparent increase in dental disease may be attributed to poor oral hygiene and a general lack of dental care rather than a disease-related etiology.

Tetralogy of Fallot

As its name implies, tetralogy of Fallot is characterized by four cardiac defects: (1) ventricular septal defect, (2) pulmonary stenosis, (3) malposition of the aorta to the right, and (4) compensatory right ventricular enlargement. Clinical features include severe cyanosis, audible heart murmurs, and breathlessness. Cyanosis and breathlessness cause cerebral anoxia and syncope. Oral changes include a purplish-red discoloration of the lips and the gingiva. Severe marginal gingivitis and periodontal destruction have been reported. The discoloration of the lips and the gingiva corresponds to the general degree of cyanosis and returns to normal after corrective heart surgery. The tongue appears coated, fissured, and edematous, and there is extreme reddening of the fungiform and filiform papillae. The number of subepithelial capillaries is increased, but this also returns to normal after heart surgery.

Eisenmenger Syndrome

Among patients with ventricular septal defects, about half of those with large defects (i.e., >1.5 cm in diameter) develop Eisenmenger syndrome. This syndrome is distinguished by a greater blood flow from the stronger left ventricle to the right ventricle (backward flow) through the septal defect. This causes increased pulmonary blood flow, which in turn leads to progressive pulmonary fibrosis, small vessel occlusion, and high pulmonary vascular resistance. With increasing pulmonary resistance, the right ventricle hypertrophies, the shunt becomes bidirectional, and ultimately blood flow is reversed (i.e., it flows from right to left). The increased vascular resistance builds pressure in the right ventricle, thereby causing right ventricular hypertrophy and a reversal in the direction of the blood flow, which results in a right-to-left shunt.

The natural history of a patient with untreated Eisenmenger syndrome is a gradual increase in cyanosis over many years that eventually leads to cardiac failure. Cyanosis of the lips, cheeks, and buccal mucous membranes is observed in these patients, but it is much less severe than in those with tetralogy of Fallot. Severe, generalized periodontitis has been reported in patients with Eisenmenger syndrome. However, as in patients with other types of congenital heart disease, the incidence of periodontal disease reported in those with Eisenmenger syndrome may be related more to poor oral hygiene and a general lack of dental care than to any specific, syndrome-related etiology.

Hypophosphatasia

Hypophosphatasia is a rare familial skeletal disease that is characterized by rickets, poor cranial bone formation, craniostenosis, and the premature loss of the primary teeth, particularly the incisors. Patients have a low level of serum alkaline phosphatase, and phosphoethanolamine is present in serum and urine.

Teeth are lost with no clinical evidence of gingival inflammation, and they show reduced cementum formation. In patients with minimal bone abnormalities, the premature loss of the deciduous teeth may be the only symptom of hypophosphatasia. In adolescents, this disease resembles localized juvenile (aggressive) periodontitis.

Metal Intoxication

The ingestion of metals such as mercury, lead, and bismuth in medicinal compounds and through industrial contact may result in oral manifestations caused by either intoxication or absorption without evidence of toxicity.

Bismuth Intoxication

Chronic bismuth intoxication is characterized by gastrointestinal disturbances, nausea, vomiting, and jaundice as well as by an ulcerative gingivostomatitis, generally with pigmentation and accompanied by a metallic taste and burning sensation of the oral mucosa. The tongue may be sore and inflamed. Urticaria, different types of exanthematous eruptions, bullous and purpuric lesions, herpes zoster-like eruptions, and pigmentation of the skin and mucous membranes are among the dermatologic lesions attributed to bismuth intoxication. Acute bismuth intoxication, which is seen less frequently, is accompanied by methemoglobin formation, cyanosis, and dyspnea.

Bismuth pigmentation in the oral cavity usually appears as a narrow, bluish-black discoloration of the gingival margin in areas of preexisting gingival inflammation (Fig. 11.12). Such pigmentation results from the precipitation of particles of bismuth sulfide associated with vascular changes in inflammation; it is not evidence of intoxication but simply indicates the presence of bismuth in the bloodstream. Bismuth pigmentation in the oral cavity also occurs in cases of intoxication; it assumes a linear form if the marginal gingiva is inflamed.

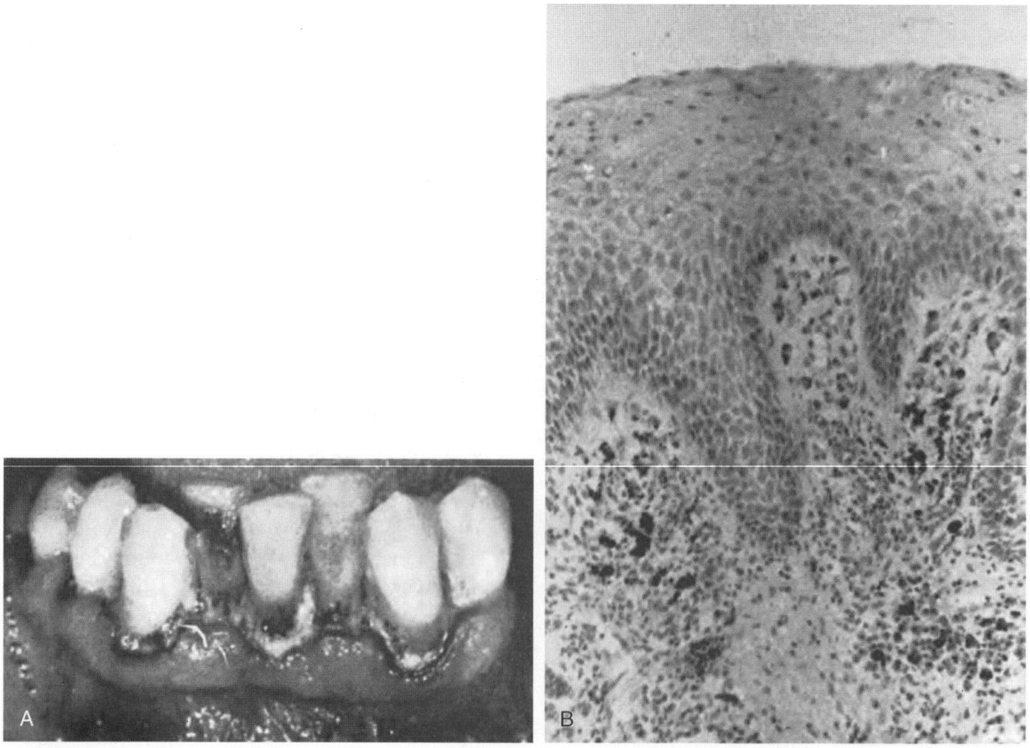

Fig. 11.12 Bismuth line. Linear discoloration of the gingiva in relation to local irritation in a patient receiving bismuth therapy.

Lead Intoxication

Lead is slowly absorbed, and toxic symptoms are not particularly definitive when they do occur. There is a pallor of the face and lips and gastrointestinal symptoms that consist of nausea, vomiting, loss of appetite, and abdominal colic. Peripheral neuritis, psychologic disorders, and encephalitis have been reported. Oral signs include salivation, coated tongue, a peculiar sweetish taste, gingival pigmentation, and ulceration. Gingival pigmentation is linear (Burtonian line), steel gray, and associated with local inflammation. Oral signs may occur without toxic symptoms.

Mercury Intoxication

Mercury intoxication is characterized by headache, insomnia, cardiovascular symptoms, pronounced salivation (ptyalism), and a metallic taste. Gingival pigmentation in linear form results from the deposition of mercuric sulfide. The chemical also acts as an irritant, which accentuates the preexisting inflammation and often leads to notable ulceration of the gingiva and the adjacent mucosa as well as the destruction of the underlying bone. Mercurial pigmentation of the gingiva also occurs in areas of local irritation in patients without symptoms of intoxication.

Other Chemicals

Other chemicals (e.g., phosphorus, arsenic, chromium) may cause necrosis of the alveolar bone, with loosening and exfoliation of the teeth. Inflammation and ulceration of the gingiva are usually associated with the destruction of the underlying tissues. Benzene intoxication is accompanied by gingival bleeding and ulceration with the destruction of the underlying bone.

Key points

- Oral changes in diabetic patients include cheilosis, mucosal drying and cracking, burning mouth and tongue, diminished salivary flow, and alterations in the flora.
- Effects of diabetes on periodontium include enlarged gingiva, sessile or pedunculated gingival polyps, polypoid gingival proliferations, abscess formation, periodontitis, and loosened teeth.
- Periodontal disease is considered to be the sixth complication of diabetes.
- Impaired PMNs observed in diabetes leads to decreased defense against periodontal pathogens.
- Chronic hyperglycemia impairs collagen structure and function, which impacts the integrity of the periodontium.
- Proteins and matrix molecules undergo a nonenzymatic glycosylation in hyperglycemic state, resulting in *accumulated glycation endproducts* (AGEs).
- Metabolic syndrome is a condition of abdominal obesity combined with two or more metabolic disturbances such as hypertension, dyslipidemia, and hyperglycemia.
- Oral changes during menopause include thinning of the oral mucosa, gingival recession, xerostomia, altered taste, and burning mouth.
- In menopause, patient complains of dry burning sensation, extreme sensitivity to thermal changes, abnormal taste sensations, and difficulty with removable partial prostheses.
- During pregnancy, gingivitis becomes more severe between the second and third trimester.
- *Prevotella intermedia* is the predominant periodontal pathogen that increases significantly during pregnancy.
- Oral changes in hyperparathyroidism include malocclusion and tooth mobility, radiographic evidence of alveolar osteoporosis with closely meshed trabeculae, widening of the periodontal ligament space, absence of the lamina dura, and radiolucent cyst-like spaces.
- Severe periodontitis has been observed in individuals with neutrophil disorders such as neutropenia, agranulocytosis, Chédiak–Higashi syndrome, lazy leukocyte syndrome, Down syndrome, Papillon–Lefèvre syndrome.
- Severe vitamin C deficiency in humans results in scurvy, which may aggravate the gingival response to plaque and worsen the edema, enlargement, and bleeding.
- Estrogen deficiency may play a significant role in the progression of periodontitis in osteopenic or osteoporotic women.
- In hypophosphatasia, teeth are lost with no clinical evidence of gingival inflammation, and they show reduced cementum formation.

Suggested Readings

Genco RJ, Ho AW, Grossi SG, et al: Relationship of stress, distress and inadequate coping behaviors to periodontal disease, *J Periodontol* 70: 711–723, 1999.

Geurs NC, Lewis CE, Jeffcoat MK: Osteoporosis and periodontal disease progression, *Periodontol 2000* 32:105–110, 2003.

Iacopino AM: Periodontitis and diabetes interrelationships: role of inflammation, *Ann Periodontol* 6:125–137, 2001.

Loe H: Periodontal disease. The sixth complication of diabetes mellitus, *Diabetes Care* 16:329–334, 1993.

Mealey BL, Moritz AJ: Hormonal influences: effects of diabetes mellitus and endogenous female sex steroid hormones on the periodontium, *Periodontol 2000* 32:59–81, 2003.

Ruggiero SL, Dodson TB, Assael LA, et al: American Association of Oral and Maxillofacial Surgeons position paper on bisphosphonate-related osteonecrosis of the jaws—2009 update, *J Oral Maxillofac Surg* 67 (Suppl 5):2–12, 2009.

Schmidt AM, Weidman E, Lalla E, et al: Advanced glycation endproducts (AGEs) induce oxidant stress in the gingiva: a potential mechanism underlying accelerated periodontal disease associated with diabetes, *J Periodontal Res* 31:508–515, 1996.

Solomon DH, Mercer E, Woo SB, et al: Defining the epidemiology of bisphosphonate-associated osteonecrosis of the jaw: prior work and current challenges, *Osteoporos Int* 24 (1):237–244, 2013.

Wimmer G, Janda M, Wieselmann-Penkner K, et al: Coping with stress: its influence on periodontal disease, *J Periodontol* 73:1343–1351, 2002.

References

References and MCQs with answers for the chapter are available on www.medenact.com

CHAPTER 12

Gingival Inflammation

JP Fiorellini | DM Kim | PG Stathopoulou | DG Naik | A Uppoor

CHAPTER OUTLINE

Pathogenesis can be defined as the unfolding of a disease process or the sequence of events in the development of a disease from its earliest beginnings. The natural history of inflammatory gingival and periodontal disease is not understood completely, and important aspects of its pathogenesis remain obscure. The sequence of events culminating in clinically apparent gingivitis has been separated into the initial, early, and established stages, and periodontitis has been designated as the advanced stage. In spite of extensive research, we still cannot distinguish definitively between the normal gingival tissue and the initial stage of gingivitis. The factors comprising this transition are not well understood.

Pristine gingiva: Normal gingiva that is free from "significant" accumulation of inflammatory cells histologically may be described as prestine gingiva or a state of superhealth (Fig. 12.1).

Clinically healthy gingiva: It looks clinically similar to prestine gingiva but histologically features an inflammatory infiltrate with predominantly neutrophils associated with junctional epithelium and lymphocytes in the subjacent connective tissue.

Page and Schroeder in 1976 classified progression of gingival and periodontal inflammation on the basis of clinical and histopathological evidence. The descriptions of the initial and early lesion were intended to characterize the histopathology of clinically healthy gingiva and early stages of gingivitis while the established lesion featured "chronic" gingivitis (Table 12.1).

Stage I Gingival Inflammation: The Initial Lesion (Fig. 12.2)

The first manifestations of gingival inflammation are vascular changes that consist of dilated capillaries and increased blood flow. These initial inflammatory changes occur in response to the microbial activation of resident leukocytes and the subsequent stimulation of endothelial cells. Clinically, this initial response of the gingiva to bacterial plaque (i.e., subclinical gingivitis) is not apparent.

> Microscopically, some classic features of acute inflammation can be seen in the connective tissue beneath the junctional epithelium. Changes in blood vessel morphologic features (e.g., the widening of small capillaries or venules) and the adherence of neutrophils to vessel walls (margination) occur within 1 week and sometimes as early as 2 days after plaque has been allowed to accumulate. Leukocytes—mainly polymorphonuclear neutrophils (PMNs)—leave the capillaries by migrating through the walls via diapedesis and emigration. They can be seen in increased quantities in the connective tissue, the junctional epithelium, and the gingival sulcus. The exudation of fluid from the gingival sulcus and extravascular proteins are present.

However, these findings are not accompanied by manifestations of tissue damage that are perceptible at the light microscopic or ultrastructural level; they do not form an infiltrate, and their presence is not considered to indicate pathologic change.

Subtle changes can also be detected in the junctional epithelium and the perivascular connective tissue at this early stage. For example, the perivascular connective tissue matrix becomes altered, and there is exudation and deposition of fibrin in the affected area. In addition, lymphocytes soon begin to accumulate. The increase in the migration of leukocytes and their accumulation within the gingival sulcus may be correlated with an increase in the flow of gingival fluid into the sulcus.

The character and intensity of the host response determine whether this *initial lesion* resolves rapidly, with the restoration of the tissue to a normal state; alternatively, it may evolve into a chronic inflammatory lesion. If the latter occurs, an infiltrate of macrophages and lymphoid cells appears within a few days.

Stage II Gingival Inflammation: The Early Lesion (Fig. 12.3)

The *early lesion* evolves from the *initial lesion* within about 1 week after the beginning of plaque accumulation. Clinically, the early lesion may appear as early gingivitis, and it overlaps with and evolves from the initial lesion with no clear-cut dividing line. As time goes on, clinical signs of erythema may appear, mainly because of the proliferation of capillaries and the increased formation of capillary loops between rete pegs or ridges. Bleeding on probing may also be evident. Gingival fluid flow and the numbers of

TABLE 12.1 Stages of Gingivitis

Stage	Time (Days)	Blood Vessels	Junctional and Sulcular Epithelia	Predominant Immune Cells	Collagen	Clinical Findings
I. Initial lesion	2–4	Vascular dilation Vasculitis	Infiltration by PMNs	PMNs	Perivascular loss	Gingival fluid flow
II. Early lesion	4–7	Vascular proliferation	Same as stage I Rete pegs Atrophic areas	Lymphocytes	Increased loss around infiltrate	Erythema Bleeding on probing
III. Established lesion	14–21	Same as stage II, plus blood stasis	Same as stage II but more advanced	Plasma cells	Continued loss	Changes in color, size, texture, and so on

PMNs, Polymorphonuclear leukocytes (neutrophils).

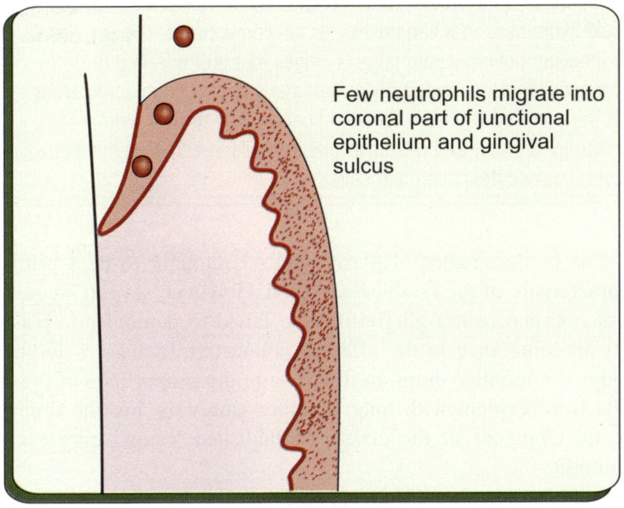

Fig. 12.1 Pristine gingiva.

transmigrating leukocytes reach their maximum between 6 and 12 days after the onset of clinical gingivitis.

> Microscopic examination of the gingiva reveals leukocyte infiltration in the connective tissue beneath the junctional epithelium, which consists mainly of lymphocytes (75%, with the majority being T cells) but that also includes some migrating neutrophils as well as macrophages, plasma cells, and mast cells. All of the changes seen in the initial lesion continue to intensify with the early lesion. The junctional epithelium becomes densely infiltrated with neutrophils, as does the gingival sulcus, and the junctional epithelium may begin to show the development of rete pegs or ridges.

The amount of collagen destruction also increases; 70% of the collagen is destroyed around the cellular infiltrate. The main fiber groups that are affected appear to be the circular and dentogingival fiber assemblies. Alterations in blood vessel morphologic features and vascular bed patterns have also been described.

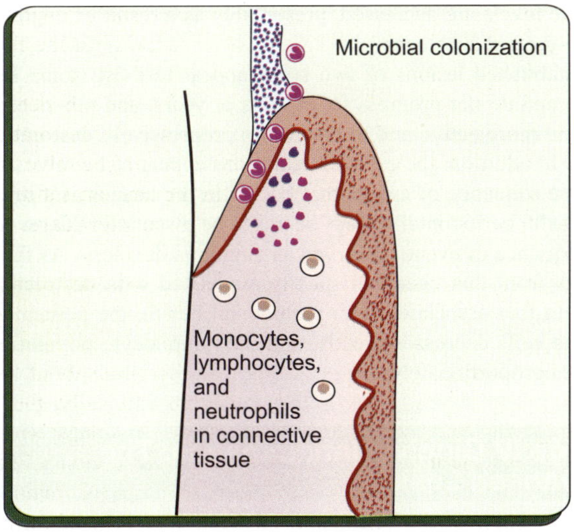

Fig. 12.2 Healthy gingiva.

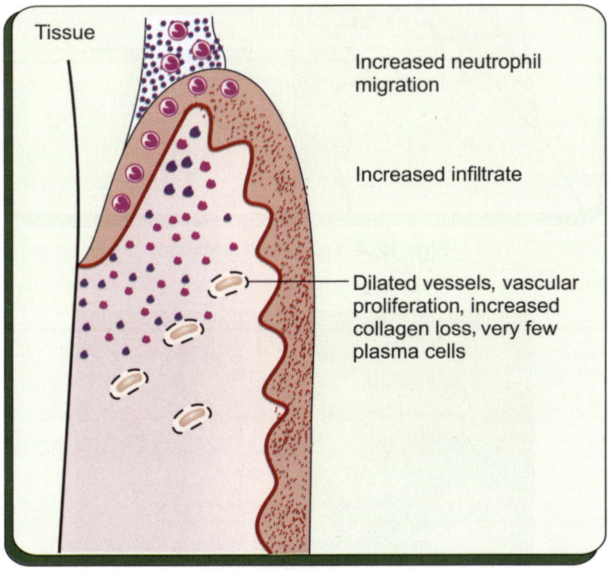

Fig. 12.3 Early gingivitis.

Polymorphonuclear neutrophils (PMNs) leave the blood vessels in response to chemotactic signals from plaque components. They travel to the epithelium, cross the basement membrane, and are found in the epithelial tissue, emerging in the pocket area. PMNs are attracted to bacteria and engulf them through the process of phagocytosis. PMNs release their lysosomes in association with the ingestion of bacteria. Fibroblasts show cytotoxic alterations, with a decreased capacity for collagen.

Meanwhile, on the opposite side of molecular events, collagen degradation is related to matrix metalloproteinases (MMPs). Different MMPs are responsible for extracellular matrix remodeling within 7 days of inflammation, which is directly related to MMP-2 and MMP-9 production and activation.

Stage III Gingival Inflammation: The Established Lesion (Fig. 12.4)

Over time, the *established lesion* evolves. It is characterized by a predominance of plasma cells and B lymphocytes, and it is probably in conjunction with the creation of a small gingival pocket lined with a pocket epithelium. The B cells that are found in the established lesion are predominantly of the immunoglobulin G1 and G3 subclasses.

With chronic gingivitis, which occurs 2–3 weeks after the beginning of plaque accumulation, the blood vessels become engorged and congested, venous return is impaired, and the blood flow becomes sluggish (Fig. 12.5). The result is localized gingival *anoxemia*, which superimposes a somewhat bluish hue on the reddened gingiva. The extravasation of erythrocytes into the connective tissue and the breakdown of hemoglobin into its component pigments can also deepen the color of the chronically inflamed gingiva. The established lesion can be described as moderately to severely inflamed gingiva.

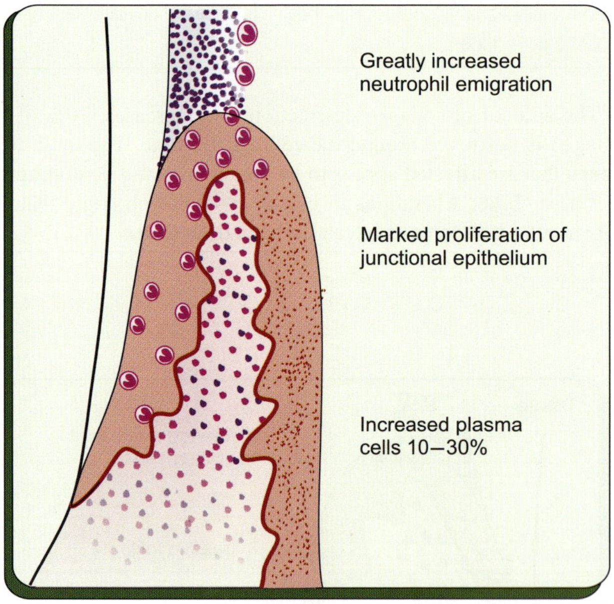

Fig. 12.4 Established gingivitis.

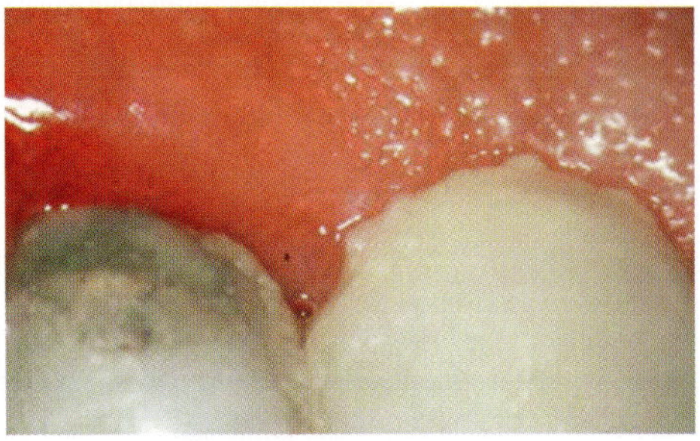

Fig. 12.5 Marginal supragingival plaque and gingivitis.

In histologic sections, an intense and chronic inflammatory reaction is observed. Several detailed cytologic studies have been performed on chronically inflamed gingiva. A key feature that differentiates the established lesion is the increased number of plasma cells, which become the preponderant inflammatory cell type. Plasma cells invade the connective tissue not only immediately below the junctional epithelium but also deep into the connective tissue, around the blood vessels, and between the bundles of collagen fibers. The junctional epithelium reveals widened intercellular spaces that are filled with granular cellular debris, including lysosomes derived from disrupted neutrophils, lymphocytes, and monocytes. The lysosomes contain acid hydrolases that can destroy tissue components. The junctional epithelium develops rete pegs or ridges that protrude into the connective tissue, and the basal lamina is destroyed in some areas. In the connective tissue, collagen fibers are destroyed around the infiltrate of intact and disrupted plasma cells, neutrophils, lymphocytes, monocytes, and mast cells.

The predominance of plasma cells is thought to be a primary characteristic of the established lesion. However, several studies of human experimental gingivitis have failed to demonstrate plasma cell predominance in the affected connective tissues, including a study of 6 months' duration. Increase in the proportions of plasma cells were evident with long standing gingivitis, but the time for the development of the classic "established lesion" may exceed 6 months.

An inverse relationship appears to exist between the number of intact collagen bundles and the number of inflammatory cells. Collagenolytic activity is increased in inflamed gingival tissue by the enzyme collagenase. Collagenase is normally present in gingival tissues; it is produced by some oral bacteria and by PMNs.

Enzyme histochemistry studies have shown that chronically inflamed gingivae have elevated levels of acid and alkaline phosphatase, β-glucuronidase, β-glucosidase, β-galactosidase, esterases, aminopeptidase, and cytochrome oxidase. Neutral mucopolysaccharide levels are decreased, presumably as a result of degradation of the ground substance.

Established lesions of two types appear to exist; some remain stable and do not progress for months or years, and others seem to become more active and to convert to progressively destructive lesions. In addition, the established lesions appear to be reversible in that the sequence of events that occurs in the tissues as a result of successful periodontal therapy seems to be essentially the reverse of the sequence of events observed as gingivitis develops. As the flora reverts from that characteristically associated with destructive lesions to that associated with periodontal health, the percentage of plasma cells decreases greatly, and the lymphocyte population increases proportionately.

Stage IV Gingival Inflammation: The Advanced Lesion

The extension of the lesion into alveolar bone characterizes the fourth stage, which is known as the *advanced lesion* or *phase of periodontal breakdown.*

Microscopically, there will be continuous loss of collagen subjacent to the pocket epithelium with fibrosis at more distant sites. The junctional epithelium migrates apically from the cementoenamel junction. The pocket epithelium is more permeable to the passage of substances into and out of the underlying connective tissues and temporarily ulcerated in many places. Alveolar bone loss occurs. There are widespread manifestations of inflammatory and immunopathologic tissue damage. At the advanced stage, the presence of plasma cells dominates the connective tissue, and neutrophils continue dominating the junctional epithelium.

Patients with experimental gingivitis had significantly more plaque accumulation, higher interleukin-1β levels, and lower interleukin-8 concentrations at 28 days.

Gingivitis will progress to periodontitis only in individuals who are susceptible. Patients who had sites with consistent bleeding (gingival index = 2) had 70% more attachment loss as compared to sites that were not inflamed consistently (gingival index = 0). Teeth with noninflamed sites consistently had a 50-year survival rate of 99.5%, whereas teeth with consistently inflamed gingiva had a 63.4% survival rate over 50 years. On the basis of this longitudinal study of the natural history of periodontitis in a well-maintained male population, persistent gingivitis represents a risk factor for periodontal attachment loss and for tooth loss. However, whether periodontitis can occur without a precursor of gingivitis is not known at this time.

Key points

- Gingival inflammation—can be classified as
  Stage I gingivitis—The initial lesion
  Stage II gingivitis—The early stage
  Stage III gingivitis—The established lesion
  Stage IV gingivitis—The advanced lesion
- Clinical features are bleeding on probing change in color, gingival crevicular fluid, size, texture, etc.
- Predominant immune cells—PMNs, lymphocytes, plasma cells.
- Clinically the initial response of gingiva to bacterial plaque—subclinical gingivitis where clinical features are not apparent.

Suggested Readings

Deinzer R, Weik U, Kolb-Bachofen V, et al: Comparison of experimental gingivitis with persistent gingivitis: differences in clinical parameters and cytokine concentrations, *J Periodontal Res* 2 (4):318–324, 2007.

Lang NP, Schätzle MA, Löe H: Gingivitis as a risk factor in periodontal disease, *J Clin Periodontol* 36 (Suppl 10):3–8, 2009.

Listgarten MA, Hellden L: Relative distribution of bacteria at clinically healthy and periodontal diseased sites in humans, *J Clin Periodontol* 5:115, 1978.

Lorencini M, Silva JA, de la Hoz CL, et al: Changes in MMPs and inflammatory cells in experimental gingivitis, *Histol Histopathol* 24 (2): 157–166, 2009.

Page RC, Schroeder HE: Pathogenesis of inflammatory periodontal disease: a summary of current work, *Lab Invest* 34:235, 1976.

References

References and MCQs with answers for the chapter are available on www.medenact.com.

CHAPTER 13

Clinical Features of Gingivitis

JP Fiorellini | PG Stathopoulou | DG Naik | A Uppoor

CHAPTER OUTLINE

Experimental gingivitis studies provided the first empiric evidence that the accumulation of microbial biofilm on clean tooth surfaces results in the development of an inflammatory process around gingival tissue. Research has also shown that the local inflammation will persist as long as the microbial biofilm is present adjacent to the gingival tissues and that the inflammation may resolve subsequently to a meticulous removal of the biofilm.

The prevalence of gingivitis is evident worldwide. Epidemiologic studies indicate that more than 82% of adolescents in the United States have overt gingivitis and signs of gingival bleeding. A similar or higher prevalence of gingivitis is reported for children and adolescents in other parts of the world. A significant percentage of adults also shows signs of gingivitis; more than half of the US adult population is estimated to exhibit gingival bleeding, and other populations have even higher levels of gingival inflammation. Whereas plaque remains the primary etiological factor that causes gingivitis, other factors may affect the development of periodontal diseases. Recent experimental gingivitis studies suggest an important role of the host response in the development and degree of gingival inflammation.

In general, the clinical signs of inflammation in the gingival tissue reflect the classic signs of inflammation—rubor (redness), tumor (swelling), calor (warmth), and dolor (pain). This is characterized by the presence of any of the following clinical signs—redness and sponginess of the gingival tissue, bleeding on provocation, changes in contour, and the presence of calculus or plaque with no radiographic evidence of crestal bone loss. The histologic examination of inflamed gingival tissue reveals ulcerated epithelium. The presence of inflammatory mediators negatively affects its epithelial function as a protective barrier. Repair of this ulcerated epithelium depends on the proliferative or regenerative activity of the epithelial cells. Removal of the etiologic agents that triggers the gingival breakdown is essential.

Oral Microbiome

Approximately, 800 bacterial species have been identified and the Human ORAL Microbiome Database (eHOMD: homd.org) is one of the most comprehensive repository databases for the oral and nasal cavities. To unravel the complex microbiome, new approaches have been employed. Novel technology 16S rRNAgene (16S) sequence has allowed elucidation of commensals and pathobionts. *Pophyromonas gingivalis* was the first oral microbe to have its complete genome sequenced by Sanger sequencing. Subsequently, Bik and colleagues employed sequencing to determine the oral microbiome of 10 healthy individuals and discovered species-level data. This was followed by 454 and shotgun sequencing, in which oral metagenomic studies became more common and these sequences now reveal the landscape of the human oral microbiome. Sequencing is key to the field of oral microbiology because it allows the discovery of organisms that are not cultivable, and it enables the dissection of the polymicrobial community.

The scale and magnitude of the oral interface suggest that the host–microbe interactions impact disease susceptibility, microbial metabolism, and host immune responses. Tooth eruption and interactions with the oral microbiome impact periodontal niches (sulcular, gingival fluid, and periodontal pocket). There are differences in the biofilm attached to the tooth and root surfaces even millimeters apart. The human microbiome harbors thousands of pathways that control metabolites and secrete molecules responsible for producing the signature that the host response interacts with. Metatranscriptomic studies of the healthy to gingivitis transition revealed a network of regulatory genes in proteolytic and nucleolytic processes that are key for microbial virulence. The diversity of the 16S rRNA revealed that samples cluster according to disease severity and oral hygiene status. With the advent of metabolomics and proteomics, a new level of resolution is now possible, providing details on the function of microbes versus only their compositions. The transition from a commensal (habitant and healthy) microbiome to pathobionts (opportunistic and pathogenic) relates to nutritional backgrounds, genetic variations, niche anatomy, immune exposures, and other environmental factors. The biofilm members (composition) and the microbiome-derived metabolism (function) impact the salivary planktonic ecology, which in turn, impacts the host immune cell migration and sulcus permeability initiating a host response.

Course and Duration

Gingivitis can occur with a sudden onset for a short duration and can be painful. A less severe phase of this condition can also occur.

Chronic gingivitis is slow in onset and of long duration. It is painless, unless it is complicated by acute or subacute exacerbations,

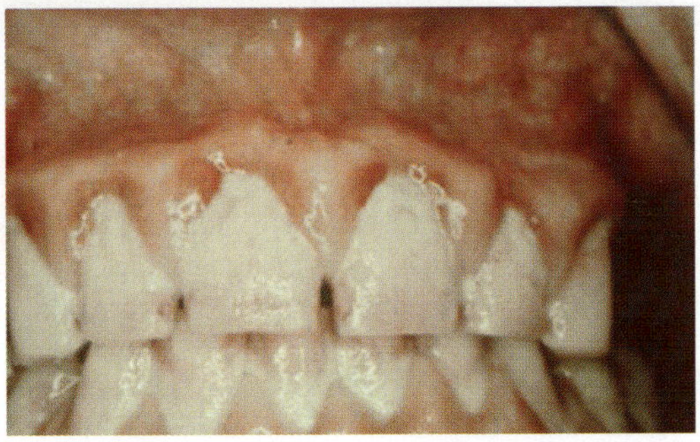

Fig. 13.1 **Chronic gingivitis.** The marginal and interdental gingivae are smooth, edematous, and discolored. Isolated areas of acute response are seen.

and it is the type that is most often encountered (Fig. 13.1). Chronic gingivitis is a fluctuating disease in which inflammation persists or resolves and normal areas become inflamed.

Recurrent gingivitis reappears after having been eliminated by treatment or disappearing spontaneously.

Description

Localized gingivitis is confined to the gingiva of a single tooth or group of teeth, whereas *generalized gingivitis* involves the entire mouth.

Marginal gingivitis involves the gingival margin and may include a portion of the contiguous-attached gingiva. *Papillary gingivitis* involves the interdental papillae and it often extends into the adjacent portion of the gingival margin. Papillae are involved more frequently than the gingival margin, and the earliest signs of gingivitis often occur in the papillae. *Diffuse gingivitis* affects the gingival margin, the attached gingiva, and the interdental papillae. Gingival disease in individual cases is described by combining the preceding terms as follows:

- *Localized marginal gingivitis* is confined to one or more areas of the marginal gingiva (Fig. 13.2).
- *Localized diffuse gingivitis* extends from the margin to the mucobuccal fold in a limited area (Fig. 13.3).
- *Localized papillary gingivitis* is confined to one or more interdental spaces in a limited area.
- *Generalized marginal gingivitis* involves the gingival margins in relation to all the teeth. The interdental papillae are usually affected (Fig. 13.4).
- *Generalized diffuse gingivitis* involves the entire gingiva. The alveolar mucosa and the attached gingiva are affected, so the mucogingival junction is sometimes obliterated (Fig. 13.5). Systemic conditions can be involved in the cause of generalized-diffuse gingivitis and should be evaluated if they are suspected as an etiologic cofactor.

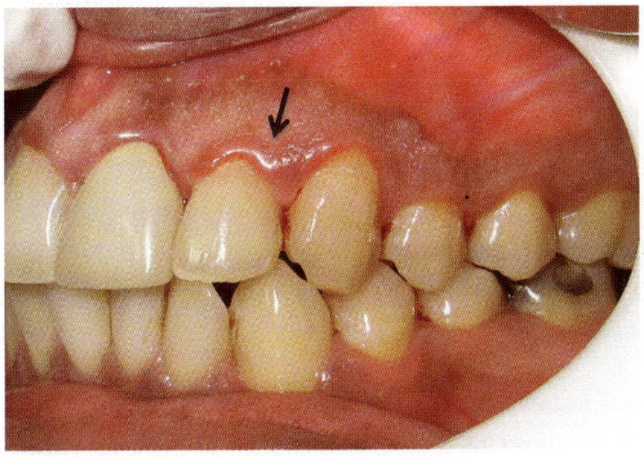

Fig. 13.2 Localized marginal gingivitis in the maxillary anterior region.

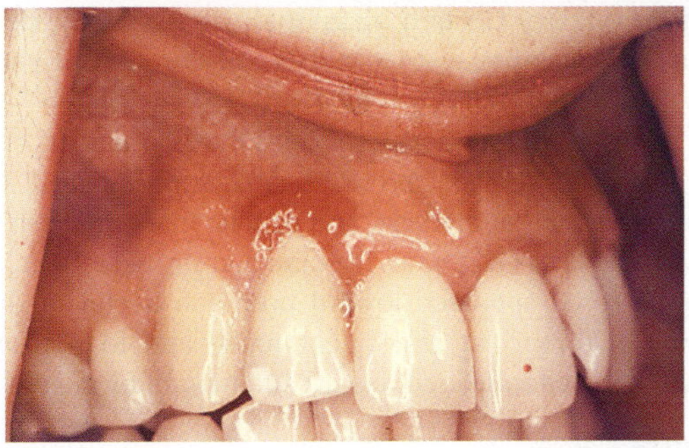

Fig. 13.3 Localized, diffuse, intensely red area on the facial surface of maxillary right lateral incisor and dark-pink marginal changes in the remaining anterior teeth.

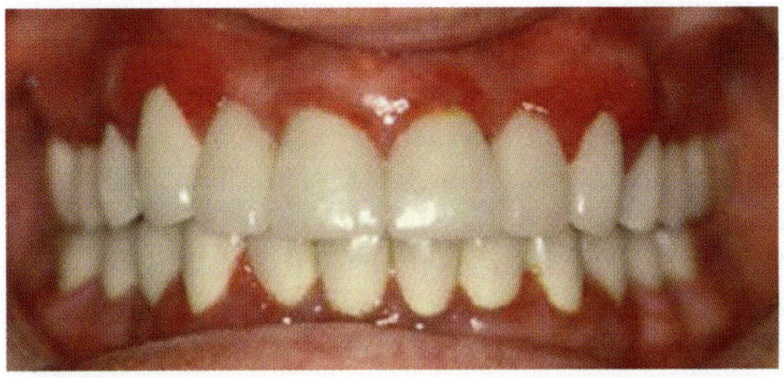

Fig. 13.4 Generalized marginal gingivitis in the upper jaw with areas of diffuse gingivitis.

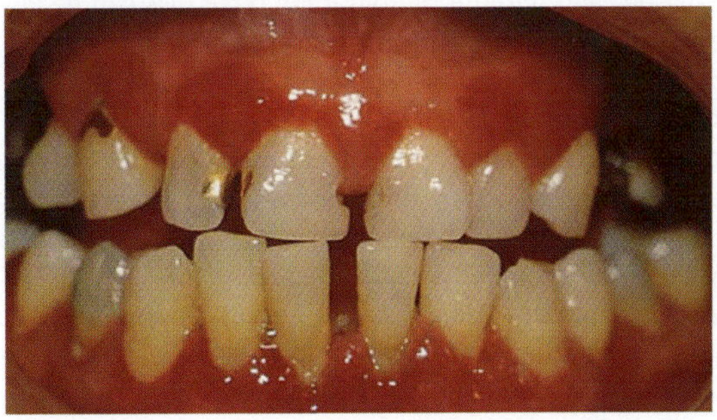

Fig. 13.5 Generalized diffuse gingivitis involves the marginal, papillary, and attached gingivae.

Hallmarks of Gingivitis

Feature	Healthy Gingiva	Gingivitis
Color	Coral pink	Red
Contour	Knife-edged and scalloped	Rolled with bulbous papillae
Consistency and texture	Firm and resilient with stippling of the attached gingiva	Edematous and with loss of stippling

2017 World Workshop Definition and Grading

A dental plaque biofilm-induced gingivitis site (GS) is defined as an inflammatory lesion, resulting from interactions between the dental plaque biofilm and the host's immune-inflammatory response. The 2017 World Workshop has recognized plaque biofilm-induced gingivitis as either a GS or a gingivitis case (GC). The definitions are based on a comprehensive analysis of the clinical parameters (gingival crevicular fluid, gingival index, and gingival bleeding indices) and specific biomarkers in oral fluids (gingival crevicular fluid proteomics, salivary proteomics, microbiological markers, systemic inflammation markers, and genetic markers). Differentiating between GS and GC allows the clinician-provider to incorporate a patient-centered approach toward precision dental medicine, to develop the appropriate assessment tools, and to reinforce oral home care instruction geared toward attaining clinical health.

Gingivitis Case

Intact Periodontium

The grading system for GC can be objectively identified by using the BOP score (BOP %) and further classified into categories of an intact periodontium, reduced periodontium, and having localized severity or generalized severity. The intact periodontium will present without clinical attachment loss or radiographic bone loss. Localized gingivitis in the intact periodontium can have a BOP % score ≥10% and ≤30%, noting that patients may or may not potentially report symptoms of bleeding gums during routine oral home care. Although generalized gingivitis in the intact periodontium can also present without clinical attachment loss and radiographic bone loss, the typical BOP % grading score is greater than 30%. These patients typically self-report bleeding gums during routine care. After clinical examination, a periodontal assessment of an intact periodontium with less than 10% BOP measurements (minimal inflammation) and without radiographic bone loss can be appropriately assigned a status of clinical health.

Reduced Periodontium

The reduced periodontium patient can be broadly categorized as either not having a history of periodontitis or having completed periodontal therapy while maintaining a state of periodontal stability. As reported by Trombelli and colleagues (2017), the GC on a reduced periodontium can typically present as gingival recession, or crown lengthening with BOP % ≥ 10%. Localized severity is defined as BOP ≥ 10% and ≤30%. Generalized severity shows as BOP greater than 30%. This grading system also considers the reduced periodontium patient who has been successfully treated for periodontitis and presenting with probing attachment loss, possible radiographic bone loss, and BOP % ≥ 10%. The most significant consideration presenting without BOP in any site probing is ≥ 4 mm. Furthermore, while clinical periodontal health is defined as a state free from inflammatory periodontal disease, clinical gingival health on a reduced periodontium incorporates multiple factors under the new grading system. This is specifically characterized by an absence of BOP, erythema, edema in the presence of reduced clinical attachment, and possible reduced bone levels.

Clinical Findings

A *systematic* approach is required for the evaluation of the clinical features of gingivitis. The clinician should focus on subtle tissue alterations because these may be of diagnostic significance. A systematic clinical approach requires an orderly examination of the gingiva for color, contour, consistency, position, and ease and severity of bleeding and pain. This section discusses these clinical characteristics and the microscopic changes that are responsible for each.

Gingival Bleeding on Probing

The two earliest signs of gingival inflammation that precede established gingivitis are as follows:

1. Increased gingival crevicular fluid production rate.
2. Bleeding from the gingival sulcus on gentle probing (Fig. 13.6).

Gingival bleeding varies with regard to severity, duration, and ease of provocation. Bleeding on probing is easily detected clinically and therefore is of value for the early diagnosis and prevention of more advanced gingivitis. It has been shown that bleeding on probing appears earlier than a change in color or other visual signs of inflammation. In addition, the use of bleeding, rather than color changes to diagnose early gingival inflammation, is advantageous as bleeding is a more objective sign that requires less subjective estimation by the examiner.

Probing pocket-depth measurements by themselves are of limited value for the assessment of the extent and severity of gingivitis. For example, gingival recession may result in a reduction of the probing depth and thus cause an inaccurate assessment of the periodontal status. Therefore, bleeding on probing is widely used by clinicians and epidemiologists to measure disease prevalence and progression, outcomes of treatment, and to motivate patients to perform necessary home care. Several gingival indices that are based on bleeding have been developed. In general, gingival bleeding on probing indicates an inflammatory lesion both in the epithelium and in the connective tissue that exhibits specific histologic differences as compared to healthy gingiva. Even though gingival bleeding on probing may not be a good diagnostic indicator for clinical attachment loss, its absence is an excellent negative predictor of future attachment loss. Therefore, the absence of gingival bleeding on probing is desirable and implies a low risk of future clinical attachment loss. Longitudinal findings revealed that sites with consistent bleeding (gingival index = 2) had 70% more attachment loss than sites that were noninflamed over a 26-year period in 565 males. Thus, persistent gingivitis can be considered as a risk factor for periodontal attachment loss that may lead to tooth loss.

Interestingly, numerous studies have shown that current cigarette smoking suppressed the gingival inflammatory response, and smoking was found to exert a strong, chronic, dose-dependent suppressive effect on gingival bleeding with probing in the Third National Health and Nutrition Examination Survey. In addition,

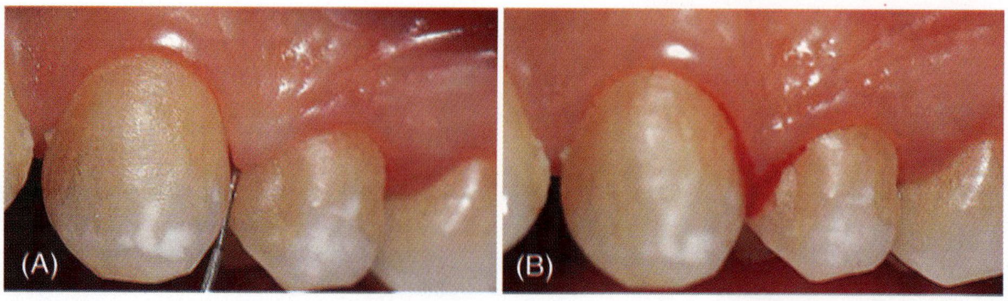

Fig. 13.6 Bleeding on probing. A, Mild edematous gingivitis; a probe has been introduced to the bottom of the gingival sulcus. B, Bleeding appears after a few seconds.

recent research reveals an increase in gingival bleeding with probing in patients who quit smoking. Thus, people who are committed to a smoking-cessation program should be informed about the possibility of an increase in gingival bleeding associated with smoking cessation.

Gingival Bleeding Caused by Local Factors

Factors that contribute to plaque retention and that may lead to gingivitis include anatomic and developmental tooth variations, caries, frenum pull, iatrogenic factors, malpositioned teeth, mouth breathing, overhangs, partial dentures, lack of attached gingiva, and recession. In addition, orthodontic treatment and fixed retainers were associated with increased plaque retention and increased bleeding on probing.

Chronic and Recurrent Bleeding

The most common cause of abnormal gingival bleeding on probing is chronic inflammation. The bleeding is chronic or recurrent, and it is provoked by mechanical trauma (e.g., from toothbrushing, toothpicks, or food impaction) or by biting into solid foods (e.g., apples).

In gingival inflammation, histopathologic alterations that result in abnormal gingival bleeding include dilation and engorgement of the capillaries and thinning or ulceration of the sulcular epithelium (Fig. 13.7). The capillaries become engorged and move closer to the surface. At the same time, the thinned, degenerated epithelium offers less protection. As a result, normally harmless stimuli can cause the capillaries to rupture, leading to gingival bleeding.

Sites that bleed on probing have a greater area of inflamed connective tissue (i.e., cell-rich, collagen-poor tissue) than sites that do not bleed. In most cases, the cellular infiltrate of sites that bleed on probing is predominantly lymphocytic, which is a characteristic of stage II (early) gingivitis.

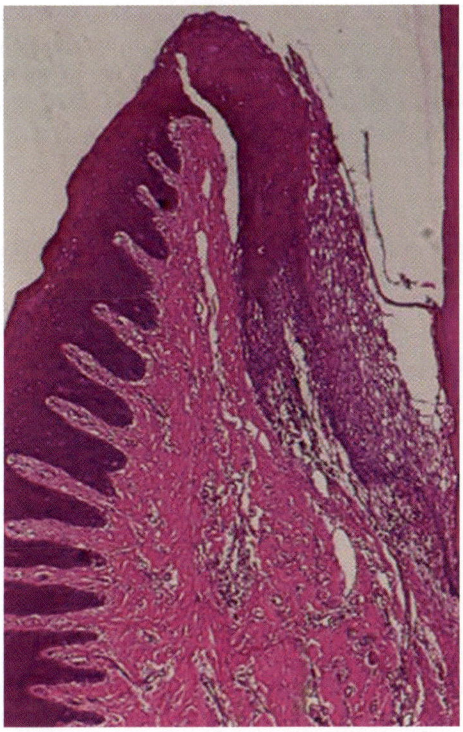

Fig. 13.7 Microscopic view of the interdental space in a human autopsy specimen. Note the inflammatory infiltrate and the thinned epithelium in the area adjacent to the tooth as well as the collagenous tissue in the outer half of the section.

Histologic evaluations of animal specimens have revealed that during the early stages of gingivitis, expression of the cytokines [i.e., matrix metalloproteinases (MMPs)] that are responsible for connective tissue breakdown is ubiquitous. Different MMPs play roles in this breakdown at different stages (e.g., a decrease of MMP-14 activity at day 7 of inflammation; immediate increase in MMP-2, especially with fibroblastic stimulation). MMP-9 expression peaked 5 days after gingivitis occurrence, which was also regulated by macrophages and neutrophils. Extracellular matrix remodeling was regulated with MMP-2 and MMP-9 production and activation by the host inflammatory response.

The severity of bleeding and the ease of its provocation depend on the intensity of the inflammation. After the vessels are damaged and ruptured, interrelated mechanisms induce hemostasis. The vessel walls contract, blood flow diminishes, blood platelets adhere to the edges of the tissue, and a fibrous clot is formed that contracts and results in approximation of the edges of the injured area. Bleeding recurs when the area is irritated.

In cases of moderate or advanced periodontitis, the presence of bleeding on probing is considered as a sign of active tissue destruction.

KEY FACT

Medications and Gingival Bleeding

- Drugs such as antiplatelet medications (e.g., aspirin) or anticoagulants (e.g., warfarin) that are prescribed for specific medical indications also increase the bleeding tendencies of gingival tissues.
- Women taking oral contraceptives are significantly more prone to gingivitis and therefore to gingival bleeding.

Acute Bleeding

Acute episodes of gingival bleeding are caused by injury, and they can occur spontaneously in patients with acute gingival disease. Laceration of the gingiva by toothbrush bristles during aggressive toothbrushing or by sharp pieces of hard food can cause gingival bleeding even in the absence of gingival disease. Gingival burns from hot foods or chemicals increase the ease of gingival bleeding.

Spontaneous bleeding or bleeding on slight provocation can occur with acute necrotizing ulcerative gingivitis. With this condition, engorged blood vessels in the inflamed connective tissue are exposed via the ulceration of the necrotic surface epithelium.

Gingival Bleeding Associated With Systemic Changes

With some systemic disorders, gingival hemorrhage occurs spontaneously or after irritation and it is excessive and difficult to control. These hemorrhagic diseases represent a wide variety of conditions that vary with regard to etiologic factors and clinical manifestations. Such conditions have the common feature of a hemostatic mechanism failure and result in abnormal bleeding in the skin, the internal organs, and other tissues, including the oral mucosa.

The hemorrhagic tendency may be due to failure of one or more of the hemostatic mechanism. Hemorrhagic disorders in which abnormal gingival bleeding is encountered include vascular abnormalities [vitamin C deficiency, allergy (e.g., Henoch–Schönlein purpura)], platelet disorders (thrombocytopenic purpura), hypoprothrombinemia (vitamin K deficiency), other coagulation defects (hemophilia, leukemia, and Christmas disease), deficient platelet thromboplastic factor as a result of uremia, multiple myeloma, and postrubella purpura. The effects of hormonal replacement therapy, oral contraceptives, pregnancy, and the menstrual cycle are also reported to affect gingival bleeding. In women, long-term depression-related stress exposure may increase concentrations of interleukin-6 in gingival crevicular fluid and worsen periodontal conditions, producing elevated levels of gingival inflammation and increased pocket depths.

KEY FACT

Pregnancy-Associated Gingivitis: Pregnancy-associated gingivitis affects many pregnant women and is primarily caused by the hormonal imbalances associated with pregnancy. It is characterized by mild to severe gingival inflammation along with pain and, in some cases, significant hyperplasia and bleeding. In most patients, the condition normally resolves by itself after delivery, when the hormonal levels return to normal.

In addition, changes in androgenic hormones have long been established as significant modifying factors in gingivitis, especially among adolescents. Several reports have shown notable effects of fluctuating estrogen and progesterone levels on the periodontium, starting as early as puberty. Among pathologic endocrine changes, diabetes is an endocrine condition with a well-characterized effect on gingivitis. In diabetes, marked inflammation affects both the epithelial and connective tissues, which leads to the degeneration of the dermal papilla, an increase in the number of inflammatory cells, the destruction of reticulin fibers, and an accumulation of dense collagen fibers that causes fibrosis.

Several medications have also been found to have adverse effects on the gingiva. For example, anticonvulsants, antihypertensive calcium-channel blockers, and immunosuppressant drugs are known to cause gingival enlargement which secondarily can cause gingival bleeding. The American Heart Association has recommended over-the-counter aspirin as a therapeutic agent for cardiovascular disease. Aspirin is often prescribed for rheumatoid arthritis, osteoarthritis, rheumatic fever, and other inflammatory joint diseases. Thus, it is important to consider aspirin's effect on bleeding during a routine dental examination to avoid false-positive readings, which could result in an inaccurate patient diagnosis (Table 13.1).

Color Changes in the Gingiva

The color of the gingiva is determined by several factors, including the number and size of blood vessels, the epithelial thickness, the quantity of keratinization, and the pigments within the epithelium.

TABLE 13.1 Causes of Gingival Bleeding

- Gingivitis
- Poor oral hygiene
- Inadequate plaque removal
- Calculus accumulation
- Periodontitis
- Anticoagulants such as coumarin and heparin
- Self-inflicted trauma such as improper flossing and toothbrushing
- Bleeding and coagulation disorders
- Vitamin C deficiency
- Vitamin K deficiency
- Hormonal changes during pregnancy
- Chemical irritants, such as aspirin
- Leukemia
- Placement of new denture leading to denture sores/irritation

Color Changes With Gingivitis

Change in color is an important clinical sign of gingival disease. The normal gingival color is "coral pink," and it is produced by the tissue's vascularity and modified by the overlying epithelial layers. For this reason, the gingiva becomes red when vascularization increases or when the degree of epithelial keratinization reduces or disappears. The color becomes pale when vascularization is reduced (in association with fibrosis of the corium) or when epithelial keratinization increases. Thus, chronic inflammation intensifies the red or bluish-red color as a result of vascular proliferation and reduced keratinization. In addition, venous stasis will contribute a bluish hue. The gingival color changes with increasing chronicity of the inflammatory process. The changes start in the interdental papillae and the gingival margin and then spread to the attached gingiva.

Proper diagnosis and treatment require an understanding of the tissue changes that alter the color of the gingiva at the clinical level.

Color changes in acute gingival inflammation differ with regard to both nature and distribution from those in patients with chronic gingivitis. The color changes may be marginal, diffuse, or patch-like, depending on the underlying acute condition. With acute necrotizing ulcerative gingivitis, the involvement is marginal; with herpetic gingivostomatitis, it is diffuse; and with acute reactions to chemical irritation, it is patch-like or diffuse.

KEY FACT

Mouth breathing and gingival inflammation gingivitis in the maxillary buccal area of the oral cavity is a common finding in patients who are mouth breathers. The affected gingiva typically appears red, shiny, and edematous, which is thought to be related to the surface dehydration caused by mouth breathing.

Color changes vary with the intensity of the inflammation. Initially, there is an increase in erythema. If the condition does not worsen, this is the only color change until the gingiva reverts to normal. With severe acute inflammation, the red color gradually becomes a dull, whitish-gray. The gray discoloration produced by tissue necrosis is demarcated from the adjacent gingiva by a thin, and sharply defined erythematous zone.

Metallic Pigmentation

Heavy metals (i.e., bismuth, arsenic, mercury, lead, and silver) that are absorbed systemically as a result of therapeutic use or occupational or household environments may discolor the gingiva and other areas of the oral mucosa. These changes are rare, but they should still be ruled out in suspected cases.

Metals typically produce a black or bluish line in the gingiva that follows the contour of the margin (Fig. 13.8). The pigmentation may also appear as isolated black blotches involving the interdental marginal and attached gingiva. This differs from the tattooing produced by the accidental embedding of amalgam or other metal fragments (Fig. 13.9).

Gingival pigmentation from systemically absorbed metals results from the perivascular precipitation of metallic sulfides in the subepithelial connective tissue. Gingival pigmentation is not a result of systemic toxicity. It occurs only in areas of inflammation in which the increased permeability of irritated blood vessels permits the seepage of the metal into the surrounding tissue. In addition to inflamed gingiva, mucosal areas that are irritated by biting or abnormal chewing habits (e.g., inner surface of lips, cheek at level of occlusal line, and lateral border of tongue) are common sites of pigmentation. Pigmentation can be eliminated by treating the inflammatory changes without necessarily discontinuing the metal-containing medication.

Color Changes Associated With Systemic Factors

Many systemic diseases may cause color changes in the oral mucosa, including the gingiva. In general, these abnormal pigmentations are nonspecific, and they should stimulate further diagnostic efforts or referral to the appropriate specialist.

Endogenous oral pigmentations can be caused by melanin, bilirubin, or iron. *Melanin* oral pigmentations can be normal physiologic pigmentations and they are often found in highly pigmented ethnic groups. Diseases that increase melanin pigmentation include the following:

- *Addison disease* is caused by adrenal dysfunction, and it produces isolated patches of discoloration that vary from bluish-black to brown.
- *Peutz-Jeghers syndrome* produces intestinal polyposis and melanin pigmentation in the oral mucosa and the lips.
- *Albright syndrome (polyostotic fibrous dysplasia)* and *von Recklinghausen disease (neurofibromatosis)* produce areas of oral melanin pigmentation.

The skin and the mucous membranes can also be stained by *bile pigments*. Jaundice is best detected via the examination of the sclera, but the oral mucosa may also acquire a yellowish color. The deposition of *iron* in hemochromatosis may produce a blue-gray pigmentation of the oral mucosa. Several endocrine and metabolic disturbances, including diabetes and pregnancy, may result in color changes. Blood dyscrasias, such as anemia, polycythemia, and leukemia, may also induce color changes.

Exogenous factors that are capable of producing color changes in the gingiva include atmospheric irritants, such as coal and metal dust, and coloring agents in food or lozenges. Tobacco causes hyperkeratosis of the gingiva, and it may also induce a significant increase in melanin pigmentation of the oral mucosa. Localized bluish-black areas of pigment are often caused by amalgam implanted in the mucosa (Fig. 13.9).

During recent years, the need for esthetics in dentistry has increased, with a growing demand for a pleasing smile. This has made many individuals more aware of their gingival pigmentation, which may be apparent during smiling and speech. Traditionally, gingival depigmentation has been carried out with the use of nonsurgical and surgical procedures, including chemical, cryosurgical, and electrosurgical techniques (electrocautery, laser, and scalpel). However, those techniques were met with skepticism because of their varying degrees of success. More recently, lasers have been used to ablate cells that produce the melanin pigment; a nonspecific laser beam destroys the epithelial cells, including those at the basal layer. In addition, selective ablation with the use of a laser beam with a wavelength that is specifically absorbed in melanin effectively destroys the pigmented cells without damaging the nonpigmented cells. In both cases, radiation energy is transformed into ablation energy, thereby resulting in cellular rupture and vaporization with minimal heating of the surrounding tissue.

Changes in the Consistency of the Gingiva

Both chronic and acute inflammations produce changes in the normal firm and resilient consistency of the gingiva. As previously noted, in patients with chronic gingivitis, both destructive (edematous) and reparative (fibrotic) changes coexist; and the consistency of the gingiva is determined by their relative predominance (Figs. 13.10 and 13.11). Table 13.2 summarizes the clinical alterations in the consistency of the gingiva and the microscopic changes that produce them.

Calcified Masses in the Gingiva

Calcified microscopic masses may be found in the gingiva. These can occur alone or in groups, and they vary with regard to size, location, shape, and structure. Such masses may be calcified material that has been removed from the tooth and traumatically displaced into the gingiva during scaling, root remnants, cementum fragments, or cementicles. Chronic inflammation and fibrosis, an occasional

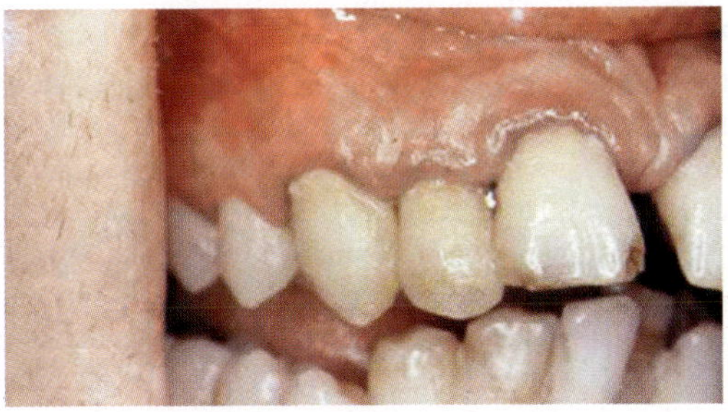

Fig. 13.8 Bismuth gingivitis. Note the linear black discoloration of the gingiva in a patient who is receiving bismuth therapy.

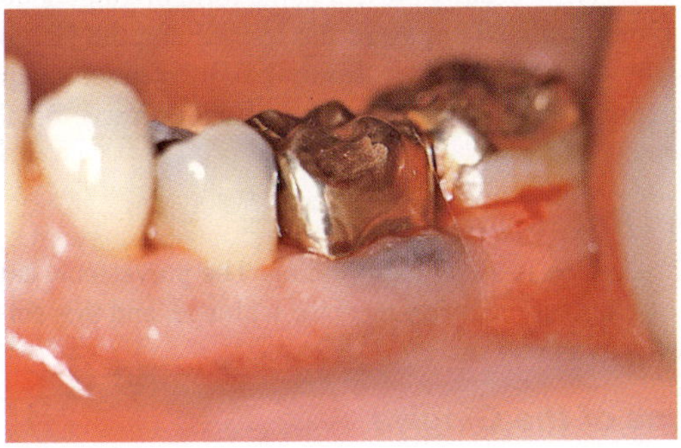

Fig. 13.9 Discoloration of the gingiva caused by embedded metal particles (amalgam).

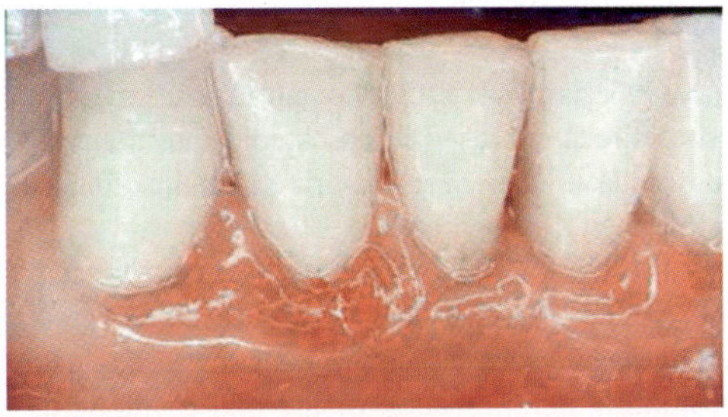

Fig. 13.10 Chronic gingivitis. Swelling, loss of stippling, and discoloration occur when inflammatory exudate and edema are the predominant microscopic changes. The gingiva is soft and friable and bleeds easily.

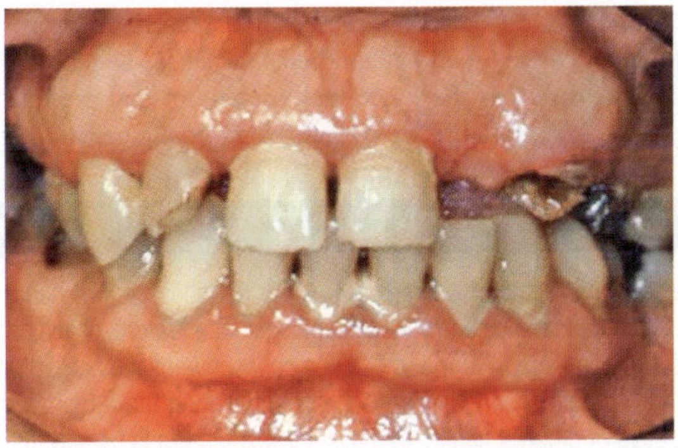

Fig. 13.11 Chronic gingivitis. Firm gingiva is produced when fibrosis predominates in the inflammatory process.

TABLE 13.2 Clinical and Histopathologic Changes in Gingival Consistency

Clinical Changes	Underlying Microscopic Features
Chronic gingivitis	
1. Soggy puffiness that pits on pressure	1. Infiltration by fluid and cells of inflammatory exudate
2. Marked softness and friability, with ready fragmentation on exploration with probe and pinpoint surface areas of redness and desquamation	2. Degeneration of connective tissue and epithelium associated with injurious substances that provoke the inflammation and the inflammatory exudate; change in the connective tissue–epithelium relationship, with inflamed, engorged connective tissue expanding to within a few epithelial cells of the surface; thinning of epithelium and degeneration associated with edema and leukocyte invasion, separated by areas in which rete pegs are elongated to connective tissue
3. Firm, leathery consistency	3. Fibrosis and epithelial proliferation associated with long-standing chronic inflammation
Acute forms of gingivitis	
1. Diffuse puffiness and softening	1. Diffuse edema of acute inflammatory origin; fatty infiltration in xanthomatosis
2. Sloughing with grayish, flake-like particles of debris adhering to eroded surface	2. Necrosis with formation of pseudomembrane composed of bacteria, polymorphonuclear leukocytes, and degenerated epithelial cells in fibrinous meshwork
3. Vesicle formation	3. Intercellular and intracellular edema with degeneration of nucleus and cytoplasm and rupture of cell wall

foreign body, and giant cell activity occur in relation to these masses. They are sometimes enclosed in an osteoid-like matrix. Crystalline foreign bodies have also been described in the gingiva, but their origin has not been determined.

Toothbrushing

Toothbrushing has various effects on the consistency of the gingiva, such as promoting keratinization of the oral epithelium, enhancing capillary gingival circulation, and thickening alveolar bone. In animal studies, mechanical stimulation by toothbrushing was found to increase the proliferative activity of the junctional basal cells in dog gingiva by 2.5 times as compared to the use of a scaler. These findings may indicate that toothbrushing causes an increased turnover rate and desquamation of the junctional epithelial surfaces. This process may repair small breaks in the junctional epithelium and prevent direct access to the underlying tissue by periodontal pathogens.

KEY FACT

Stippling and Its Clinical Importance: Healthy, attached gingiva has a pitted orange-peel appearance on its surface. This surface feature, called stippling, is an external reflection of the underlying connective tissue projections into the overlying epithelium. The presence of stippling in the attached gingiva is indicative of gingival health, and this surface feature is usually lost when the tissue is edematous.

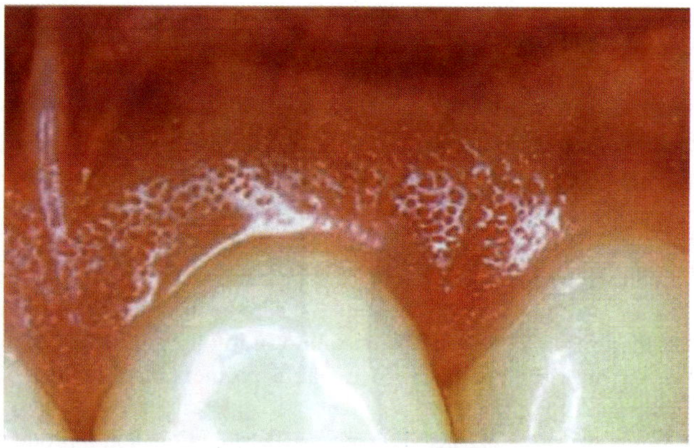

Fig. 13.12 Stippling seen on attached gingiva.

Changes in the Surface Texture of the Gingiva

The surface of normal gingiva usually exhibits numerous small depressions and elevations that give the tissue an *orange-peel* appearance referred as *stippling.* Stippling is restricted to the attached gingiva and predominantly localized to the subpapillary area; but it extends to a variable degree into the interdental papilla (Fig. 13.12). Although the biologic significance of gingival stippling is not known, some investigators conclude that the loss of stippling is an early sign of gingivitis. However, clinicians must take into consideration that its pattern and extent vary in different mouth areas, among patients, and with age.

In patients with chronic inflammation, the gingival surface is either smooth and shiny or firm and nodular, depending on whether the dominant changes are exudative or fibrotic. Smooth surface texture is also produced by epithelial atrophy in atrophic gingivitis, and peeling of the surface occurs with chronic desquamative gingivitis. Hyperkeratosis results in a leathery texture and drug-induced gingival overgrowth produces a nodular surface.

Changes in the Position of the Gingiva

Traumatic Lesions

One of the unique features of the most recent gingival disease classification is the recognition of nonplaque-induced traumatic gingival lesions as distinct gingival conditions. Traumatic lesions—whether they are chemical, physical, or thermal—are among the most common lesions in the mouth. Sources of chemical injuries include aspirin, hydrogen peroxide, silver nitrate, phenol, and endodontic materials. Physical injuries can include lip, oral, and tongue piercings, which can result in gingival recession. Thermal injuries can result from hot drinks and foods. In acute cases, the appearance of slough (necrotizing epithelium), erosion, ulceration, and the accompanying erythema are common features. In chronic cases, permanent gingival defects are usually present in the form of gingival recession. Typically, the localized nature of the lesions and the lack of symptoms readily eliminate them from the differential diagnosis of systemic conditions that may be present with erosive or ulcerative oral lesions.

Gingival Recession

Gingival recession is a common finding. The prevalence, extent, and severity of gingival recession increase with age, and this condition is more prevalent among males.

Positions of the Gingiva

By clinical definition, recession is the exposure of the root surface by an apical shift in the position of the gingiva. To understand recession, it is important to distinguish between the actual and apparent positions of the gingiva. The *actual position* is the level of the coronal end of the epithelial attachment on the tooth, whereas the *apparent position* is the level of the crest of the gingival margin (Fig. 13.13). *The severity of recession is determined by the actual position of the gingiva and not by its apparent position.* For example, in periodontal disease, the inflamed pocket wall covers part of the denuded root; thus some of the recession is hidden, and some may be visible. The total amount of recession is the sum of the two.

Recession refers to the location of the gingiva rather than to its condition. Receded gingiva can be inflamed, but it may be normal except for its position (Fig. 13.14). Recession may be localized to one tooth or to a group of teeth or it may be generalized throughout the mouth.

Gingival recession increases with age; the incidence varies from 8% in children to 100% after the age of 50 years. This has led some investigators to assume that recession may be a physiologic process related to aging. However, no convincing evidence has been presented for a physiologic shift of the gingival attachment. The gradual apical shift is most likely the result of the cumulative effect of minor

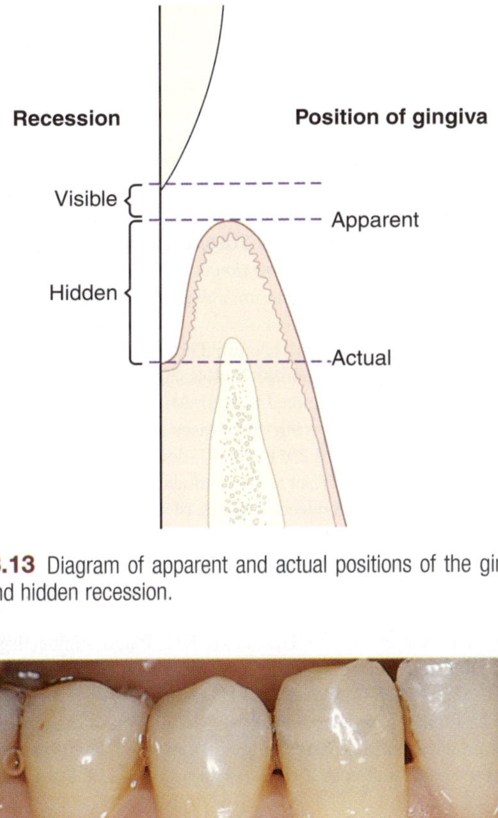

Fig. 13.13 Diagram of apparent and actual positions of the gingiva and visible and hidden recession.

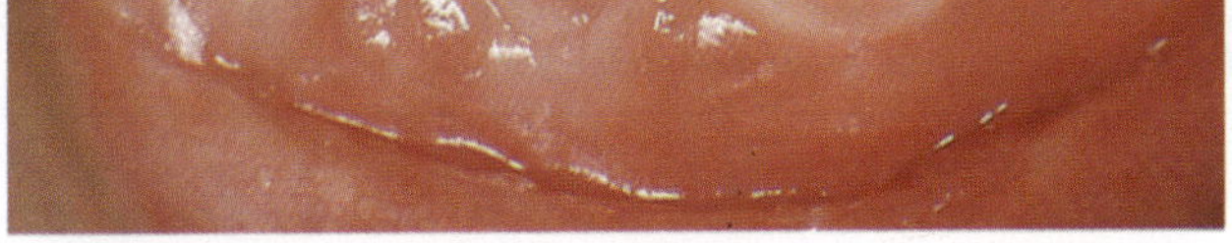

Fig. 13.14 Different degrees of recession. Recession is slight in mandibular right lateral incisor and second premolar and marked in mandibular right canine and first premolar. The change in gingival contour and the recession as seen in mandibular right first premolar is referred to as *Stillman's cleft.*

pathologic involvement and repeated minor direct trauma to the gingiva. In some populations without access to dental care, recession, however, may be the result of increasing periodontal disease.

The following etiologic factors have been implicated in gingival recession: faulty toothbrushing technique (gingival abrasion), tooth malposition, friction from the soft tissues (gingival ablation), gingival inflammation, abnormal frenum attachment, and iatrogenic dentistry. Trauma from occlusion has been suggested in the past, but its mechanism of action has never been demonstrated. For example, a deep overbite has been associated with gingival inflammation and recession. Excessive incisal overlap may result in a traumatic injury to the gingiva. Orthodontic movement in a labial direction in monkeys has been shown to result in the loss of marginal bone and connective tissue attachment, as well as in gingival recession.

Standard oral hygiene procedures, whether they involve toothbrushing or flossing, may lead to frequent transient and minimal gingival injury. Although toothbrushing is important for gingival health, faulty toothbrushing technique or brushing with hard bristles may cause significant injury. This type of injury may present as lacerations, abrasions, keratosis, and recession, with the facial marginal gingiva being the most affected. Thus, in these cases, recession tends to be more frequent and severe in patients with clinically healthy gingiva, little bacterial plaque, and good oral hygiene.

Susceptibility to recession is also influenced by the position of teeth in the arch, the root–bone angle, and the mesiodistal curvature of the tooth surface. On rotated, tilted, or facially displaced teeth, the bony plate is thinned or reduced in height. Pressure from mastication or moderate toothbrushing damages the unsupported gingiva and produces recession. The effect of the angle of the root in the bone with recession is often observed in the maxillary molar area. If the lingual inclination of the palatal root is prominent or if the buccal roots flare outward, the bone in the cervical area is thinned or shortened, then recession results from repeated trauma of the thin marginal gingiva.

The health of the gingival tissue also depends on properly designed and placed restorative materials. Pressure from a poorly designed partial denture, such as an ill-fitting denture clasp, can cause gingival trauma and recession. Overhanging dental restorations have long been viewed as a contributing factor to gingivitis because of plaque retention. In addition, there is a general agreement that placing restorative margins within the biologic width frequently leads to gingival inflammation, clinical attachment loss, and, eventually, bone loss. Clinically, the violation of biologic width typically manifests as gingival inflammation, deepened periodontal pockets, and gingival recession.

A relationship may exist between smoking and gingival recession. The multifactorial mechanisms may include reduced gingival blood flow and altered immune response but they are not as yet conclusive.

Clinical Significance

Several aspects of gingival recession make it clinically significant. Exposed root surfaces are susceptible to caries. Abrasion or erosion of the cementum exposed by recession leaves an underlying dentinal surface that can be sensitive. Hyperemia of the pulp and associated symptoms may also result from the excessive exposure of the root surface. Interproximal recession creates oral hygiene problems and resulting plaque accumulation.

Changes in Gingival Contour

Changes in gingival contour are primarily associated with gingival enlargement, but such changes may also occur with other conditions. Of historical interest are the descriptions of indentations of the gingival margin referred to as *Stillman clefts* (Fig. 13.14) and the *McCall festoons*. The term *Stillman clefts* has been used to describe a specific type of gingival recession that consists of a narrow, triangular-shaped gingival recession. As the recession progresses apically, the cleft becomes broader, thereby exposing the cementum of the root surface. When the lesion reaches the mucogingival junction, the apical border of oral mucosa is usually inflamed because of the difficulty with maintaining adequate plaque control at this site.

The term *McCall festoons* has been used to describe a rolled, thickened band of gingiva that is usually seen adjacent to the cuspids when recession approaches the mucogingival junction. Initially, Stillman clefts and McCall festoons were attributed to traumatic occlusion and the recommended treatment was occlusal adjustment. However, this association was never proved, and these indentations merely represent peculiar inflammatory changes of the marginal gingiva.

Key points

- Gingivitis can be classified based on duration as acute, chronic, and recurrent gingivitis.
- Based on the involvement of teeth, it can be classified as localized and generalized gingivitis.
- Based on the location, gingivitis can be classified as marginal, attached, and papillary gingivitis.
- Gingival disease in individual cases can be described by combining location and involved teeth.
- Bleeding on probing is easily detected clinically and, therefore, is of value for the early diagnosis and prevention of more advanced gingivitis. Bleeding is a more objective sign that requires less subjective estimation by the examiner.
- Gingival bleeding can occur due to various local and systemic causes.
- The color of the gingiva is "coral pink."
- The factors responsible for color of gingiva are number and size of blood vessels, epithelial thickness, quantity of keratinization, and pigments within the epithelium.
- Gingival pigmentation from systemically absorbed metals results from perivascular precipitation of metallic sulfides in the subepithelial connective tissue. It is not a result of systemic toxicity.
- Color changes are associated with systemic factors. Endogenous pigmentations can be seen in certain diseases like Addison's disease, Peutz–Jeghers syndrome, and Albright's syndrome.
- Exogenous factors capable of producing color changes in the gingiva include atmospheric irritants, such as coal and metal dust, and coloring agents in food or lozenges. Tobacco causes hyperkeratosis of the gingiva and also may induce a significant increase in melanin pigmentation of the oral mucosa.
- Normal consistency of gingiva is firm and resilient. In acute condition, it becomes soft and edematous and in chronic condition, it becomes firm and fibrotic.
- Stippling of orange peel appearance. It is present in attached gingiva and core of the interdental papilla.
- Stippling pattern and extent vary in different mouth areas, among patients, and with age.
- Changes in position of the gingiva—recession is exposure of the root surface by an apical shift in the gingiva.
- The actual position of gingiva is the level of the epithelial attachment on the tooth.
- Apparent position is the level of the crest of the gingival margin.
- The severity of recession is determined by the actual position of the gingiva, not by its apparent position.
- Recession can be occurred due to aging, tooth positioning, gingival inflammation, iatrogenic dentistry, abnormal frenal attachment, faulty toothbrushing, etc.
- Exposed roots are susceptible to root caries, sensitivity, esthetic problems, and plaque accumulation.

Suggested Readings

Albandar JM, Tinoco EM. Global epidemiology of periodontal diseases in children and young persons. Periodontol 2000. 2002;29:153-176. doi:10.1034/j.1600-0757.2002.290108.x

Chapple ILC, Mealey BL, Van Dyke TE, et al. Periodontal health and gingival diseases and conditions on an intact and a reduced periodontium: Consensus report of workgroup 1 of the 2017 World Workshop on the Classification of Periodontal and Peri-Implant Diseases and Conditions. *J Periodontol*. 2018;89 Suppl 1:S74-S84. doi:10.1002/JPER.17-0719

Bergström J: The topography of papillary gingiva in health and early gingivitis, *J Clin Periodontol* 11:423, 1984.

Danser MM, Timmerman MF, Ijzerman Y, et al: Evaluation of the incidence of gingival abrasion as a result of toothbrushing, *J Clin Periodontol* 25:701, 1998.

Dietrich T, Bernimoulin JP, Glynn RJ: The effect of cigarette smoking on gingival bleeding, *J Periodontol* 75:16, 2004.

Greenstein G: The role of bleeding upon probing in the diagnosis of periodontal disease: a literature review, *J Periodontol* 55:684, 1984.

Lang NP, Adler R, Joss A, et al: Absence of bleeding upon probing: an indicator of periodontal stability, *J Clin Periodontol* 17:714, 1990.

Löe H, Theilade E, Jensen SB: Experimental gingivitis in man, *J Periodontol* 36:177, 1965.

Machtei EE, Mahler D, Sanduri H, et al: The effect of menstrual cycle on periodontal health, *J Periodontol* 75:408, 2004.

Nowicki EM, Shroff R, Singleton JA, et al. Microbiota and Metatranscriptome Changes Accompanying the Onset of Gingivitis. *mBio*. 2018; 9(2):e00575-18. Published 2018 Apr 17. doi:10.1128/mBio.00575-18

Silva JA, Lorencini M, Reis JR, et al: The influence of type I diabetes mellitus in periodontal disease induced changes of the gingival epithelium and connective tissue, *Tissue Cell* 40:283, 2008.

Tal H, Oegiesser D, Tal M: Gingival depigmentation by erbium: YAG laser: clinical observations and patient responses, *J Periodontol* 74:1660, 2003.

Trombelli L, Farina R, Silva CO, Tatakis DN. Plaque-induced gingivitis: Case definition and diagnostic considerations. *J Clin Periodontol*. 2018;45 Suppl 20:S44-S67. doi:10.1111/jcpe.12939

Trombelli L, Tatakis DN, Scapoli C, et al: Modulation of clinical expression of plaque-induced gingivitis. II. Identification of "high-responder" and "low-responder" subjects, *J Clin Periodontol* 31:239, 2004.

References

References and MCQs with answers for the chapter are available on www.medenact.com.

CHAPTER 14

Gingival Enlargement

FA Carranza | EL Hogan | DG Naik | A Uppoor

CHAPTER OUTLINE

Inflammation of the periodontal tissues results in three outcomes: complete resolution of inflammation and restoration of tissue integrity (i.e., homeostasis), destruction of periodontal tissues, and loss of attachment (i.e., periodontitis) or fibrosis. A change in the dimensions of gingival tissue is always a pathologic event. Gingival enlargement can be transient and reversible or can be chronic and irreversible. Enlargement of the keratinized gingiva, a distinct group of pathologies leading to the overgrowth of the gingival structures and collectively known as "gingival enlargement," can manifest with various clinical characteristics. Fibrosis is mechanistically analogous to defense mechanisms at play against the progression of periodontal inflammation. During this process, fibroblasts stimulated by the presence of fibrin, growth factors, and cytokines may generate excessive amounts of collagen and noncollagenous proteins of the extracellular matrix. If this excessive matrix deposition is not sufficiently balanced by the enzymatic degradation of the matrix composition (e.g., collagen type I) by the matrix metalloproteinases (MMPs) and their tissue inhibitors (TIMPs), it can result in fibrotic changes of the soft tissues. In contrast to other tissues in which fibrosis is observed, gingival lesions present with clinical inflammation due to biofilm accumulation. In addition, maintenance of optimal oral hygiene is impaired due to disrupted tissue architecture. Thus, the gingival overgrowth lesions involve complex infecto-inflammatory pathogenetic mechanisms and are unique in their clinical manifestations. Pathologic enlargements of gingival tissues were identified and linked to systemic conditions as early as the 18th century. Most common forms of gingival enlargement result from systemic use of medications. The first scientific report on drug-induced gingival overgrowth (DIGO) was published in 1939 when the anticonvulsant diphenylhydantoin was associated with gingival enlargement. Later studies provided significant insights into the complex molecular and cellular mechanisms underlying gingival enlargement. Because many forms of gingival enlargement are related to systemic factors and conditions, understanding the pathogenesis of these clinical conditions is essential for designing better approaches to management, treatment, and optimizing care. This chapter discusses the clinical, etiologic, and pathologic aspects of gingival enlargement that are used to develop novel and targeted approaches to therapy. Neoplastic enlargements of gingival tissues associated with benign or malignant oral cancers are not covered in depth because this emerging field of oral pathology has evolved beyond the scope of this chapter and can be found in oral pathology textbooks that provide extensive coverage of oral tumors.

Terminology and Classification

An increase in size of the gingiva is a common feature of gingival disease. The accepted current terms for this condition are *gingival enlargement (GE)* and *gingival overgrowth (GO)*. These are strictly clinical descriptive terms and they avoid the erroneous pathologic connotations of terms used in the past, such as *hypertrophic gingivitis* and *gingival hyperplasia. Hyperplasia is an increase in the number of cells in tissues that results in increased tissue volume. Hypertrophy refers to increased tissue size and volume resulting from increased cell size.* Although their pathogenetic mechanisms are different, hyperplasia and hypertrophy usually occur simultaneously when cellular involvement in hyperplasia most likely triggers the overgrowth.

The two processes are closely linked. Fibrosis refers to a pathologic process in which disrupted wound healing is associated with defective cell proliferation, cell-to-cell interactions, cell-to-matrix interactions, and matrix deposition and with an impaired immune system response. In this regard, fibrosis can be defined as a pathologic lesion, whereas hyperplasia and hypertrophy can be viewed as pathologic processes.

All of these terms refer to different pathogenetic states. In gingival tissues, they are associated with various phases of inflammation. Hyperplastic, hypertrophic, and fibrotic changes are observed during gingival enlargement and cannot be accurately differentiated.

The many types of gingival enlargement can be classified according to etiologic factors and pathologic changes as follows:

1. Inflammatory enlargement
   a. Chronic
   b. Acute
2. Drug-induced enlargement
   a. Anticonvulsants
   b. Immunosuppressants
   c. Calcium-channel blockers

3. Enlargements associated with systemic diseases or conditions
   a. Conditioned enlargement
      1) Pregnancy
      2) Puberty
      3) Vitamin C deficiency
      4) Plasma cell gingivitis
      5) Nonspecific conditioned enlargement (pyogenic granuloma)
   b. Systemic diseases that cause gingival enlargement
      1) Leukemia
      2) Granulomatous diseases (e.g., Wegener granulomatosis and Sarcoidosis)
4. Neoplastic enlargement (gingival tumors)
   a. Benign tumors
   b. Malignant tumors
5. False enlargement
   a. Underlying osseous lesions
   b. Underlying dental tissues

Diagnosis

Because GE is frequently associated with systemic conditions, the general health of the patient and his or her drug use should be carefully managed. GE is one of the most serious pathologies in periodontal medicine, and it requires a meticulous differential diagnosis for selecting a therapeutic approach tailored to the patient's systemic status.

Accurate diagnosis requires a thorough review of the medical history of the patient. With the use of the criteria of location and distribution, gingival enlargement is designated as follows:

- *Localized:* Limited to the gingiva adjacent to a single tooth or group of teeth.
- *Generalized:* Involving the gingiva throughout the mouth.
- *Marginal:* Confined to the marginal gingiva.
- *Papillary:* Confined to the interdental papilla.
- *Diffuse:* Involving the marginal and attached gingivae and papillae.
- *Discrete:* An isolated sessile or a pedunculated, tumor-like enlargement.

But, it is sometimes difficult to differentiate between diffuse and discrete enlargements. However, these categorizations can be critical for determining the correct cause of the pathology.

In periodontal tissues, indices are important for quantification of the extent and severity of GE. Various indices have been proposed. For example, the degree of gingival enlargement can be scored as follows:

- *Grade 0:* No signs of gingival enlargement.
- *Grade I:* Enlargement confined to interdental papilla.
- *Grade II:* Enlargement involves papilla and marginal gingiva.
- *Grade III:* Enlargement covers three quarters or more of the crown.

In addition to clinical determination of the degree of severity, a more accurate assessment of GE can be made by models cast on the impressions. A technique developed by Seymour and colleagues has been validated by others and can be a valuable tool for precise determination of the severity and extent of GE, especially for research purposes and long-term follow-up. Other indices used to assess the severity of GE include those developed by Angelopoulos and Goaz and Pernu and coworkers. Three-dimensional scanning can be used to measure GE and compare the treatment outcomes with baseline values.

Regardless of the method used for measuring the extent and severity of GE lesions, an accurate assessment is critical for identifying the inflammatory and fibrotic components. Indices should be chosen based on practicality of the data acquired to allow clinicians to select the method of therapy (e.g., gingivectomy and gingivoplasty vs nonsurgical treatment measures) and plan the maintenance phase.

Inflammatory Enlargement

Gingival enlargement may result from chronic or acute inflammatory changes although chronic changes are much more common. In addition, inflammatory enlargements are usually a secondary complication of any of the other types of enlargement, thereby creating a combined gingival enlargement. In these cases, it is important to understand the double etiology and to treat both causes adequately.

Chronic Inflammatory Enlargement

Clinical Features

Chronic inflammatory gingival enlargement originates as a slight ballooning of the interdental papilla and marginal gingiva. In the early stages, it produces a life preserver-shaped bulge around the involved teeth. This bulge can increase in size until it covers part of the crowns. The enlargement may be localized or generalized; it progresses slowly and painlessly unless it is complicated by acute infection or trauma (Figs. 14.1 and 14.2).

Occasionally, chronic inflammatory gingival enlargement occurs as a discrete sessile or pedunculated mass that resembles a tumor. It may be interproximal or on the marginal or attached gingiva. The lesions are slow-growing masses and are usually painless. They may undergo a spontaneous reduction in size that is followed by exacerbation and continued enlargement. Painful ulceration sometimes occurs in the fold between the mass and the adjacent gingiva.

Histopathology

Chronic inflammatory gingival enlargements show the exudative and proliferative features of chronic inflammation (Fig. 14.3). Lesions that are clinically deep red or bluish-red are soft and friable with a smooth, shiny surface, and they bleed easily. They also have a preponderance of inflammatory cells and fluid, with vascular engorgement, new capillary formation, and associated degenerative changes. Lesions that are relatively firm, resilient, and pink have a greater fibrotic component with an abundance of fibroblasts and collagen fibers.

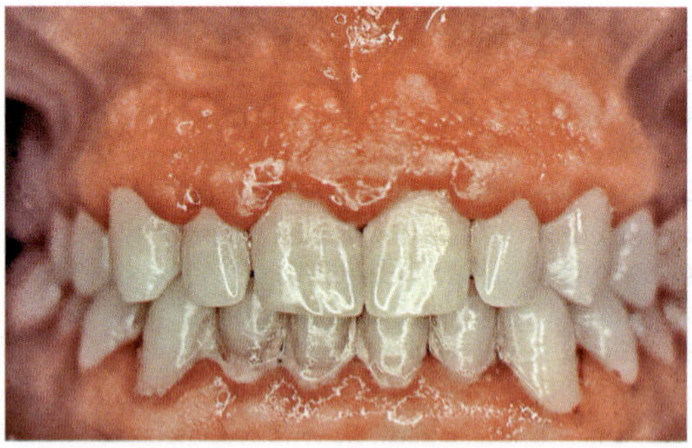

Fig. 14.1 Chronic inflammatory gingival enlargement localized to the anterior region.

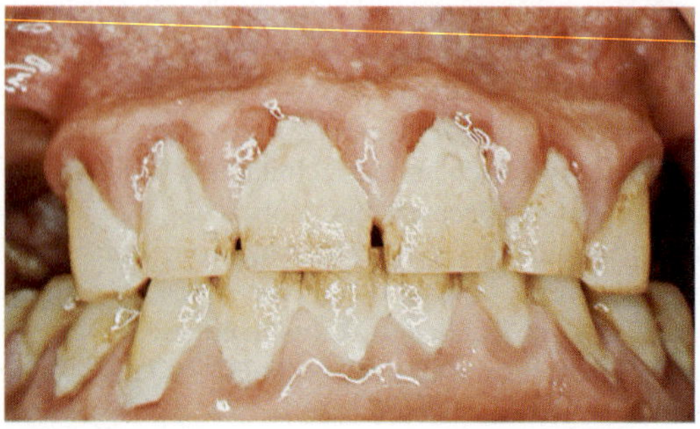

Fig. 14.2 Chronic inflammatory gingival enlargement.

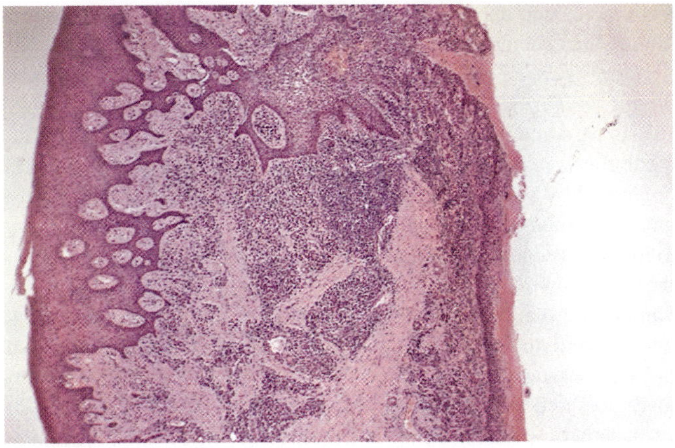

Fig. 14.3 Survey section of chronic inflammatory gingival enlargement showing the inflamed connective tissue core and strands of proliferating epithelium.

Etiology

Chronic inflammatory gingival enlargement is caused by prolonged exposure to dental plaque. Factors that favor plaque accumulation and retention include poor oral hygiene, irritation by anatomic abnormalities, and improper restorative and orthodontic appliances.

KEY FACT

The main etiological factor for acute inflammatory gingival enlargement is trauma. Traumatic lesions occur when a foreign substance (e.g., toothbrush bristle) is forcefully embedded into the gingiva and the situation is complicated by the presence of microbial pathogens. Trauma-induced injuries result in a chronic process characterized by granulation tissue formation and fibrosis. Because nerve tissue does not proliferate, pain is uncommon.

Gingival Changes Associated With Mouth Breathing

Gingivitis and gingival enlargement are often seen in patients who are mouth breathers. The gingiva appears red and edematous, with a diffuse surface shininess of the exposed area. The maxillary anterior region is the common site of such involvement. In many cases, the altered gingiva is clearly demarcated from the adjacent unexposed normal gingiva (Fig. 14.4). The exact manner in which mouth breathing affects gingival changes has not been demonstrated. Its harmful effect is generally attributed to irritation from surface dehydration. However, comparable changes could not be produced by air drying the gingiva of experimental animals.

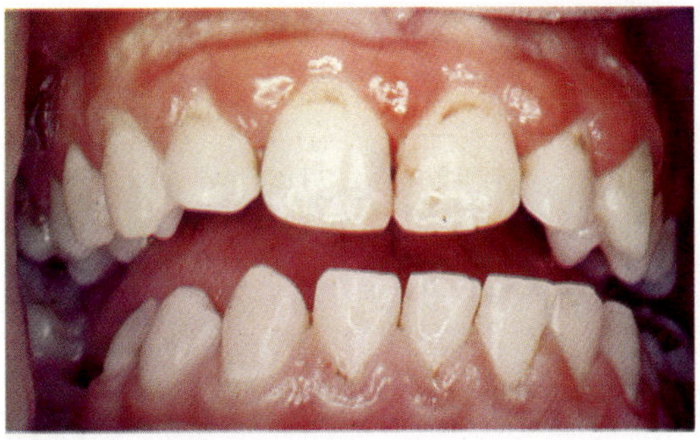

Fig. 14.4 Gingival enlargement in a mouth breather. Note the lesion that is sharply circumscribed to the anterior marginal and papillary areas.

Acute Inflammatory Enlargement

Gingival Abscess

Periodontal Abscess

Please find detailed description in Chapter 18.

Drug-Induced Gingival Enlargement

Gingival enlargement is a well-known consequence of the administration of some anticonvulsants, immunosuppressants, and calcium-channel blockers. The condition may create speech, mastication, tooth eruption, and esthetic problems.

Clinical and microscopic features of the enlargements caused by the different drugs are similar. These are presented first, followed by a description of the particular features of each drug.

General Information

Clinical Features

The growth starts as a painless, bead-like enlargement of the interdental papilla that then extends to the facial and lingual gingival margins (Fig. 14.5A and B). As the condition progresses, the marginal and papillary enlargements unite, and they may develop into a massive tissue fold that covers a considerable portion of the crowns; this may interfere with occlusion (Fig. 14.6).

When uncomplicated by inflammation, the lesion is mulberry-shaped, firm, pale-pink, and resilient, with a minutely lobulated surface and no tendency to bleed. The enlargement characteristically appears to project from beneath the gingival margin from which it is separated by a linear groove. However, the presence of the enlargement makes plaque control difficult, often resulting in a secondary inflammatory process that complicates the gingival overgrowth caused by the drug.

The resultant enlargement then becomes a combination of the increase in size caused by the drug and the complicating inflammation caused by bacteria. Secondary inflammatory changes not only add to the size of the lesion caused by the drug but also produce

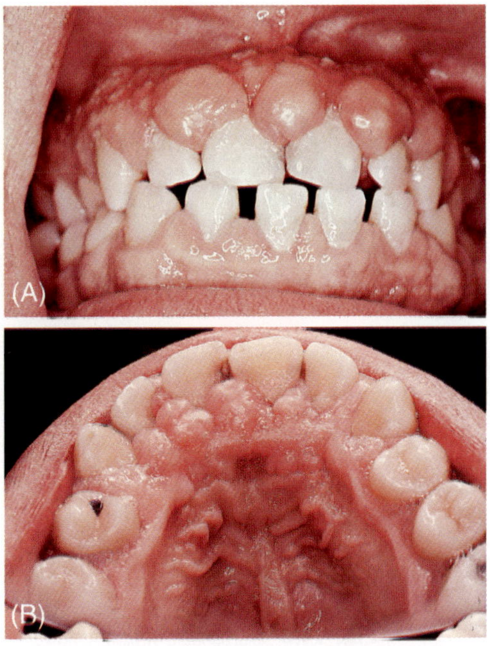

Fig. 14.5 Gingival enlargement associated with phenytoin therapy. A, Facial view. Note the prominent papillary lesions and the firm, nodular surface. B, Occlusal view of the upper jaw.

a red or bluish-red discoloration, obliterate the lobulated surface demarcations, and increase bleeding tendency (Fig. 14.7).

The enlargement is usually generalized throughout the mouth but it is more severe in the maxillary and mandibular anterior regions. It occurs in areas in which teeth are present (not in edentulous spaces), and the enlargement disappears in areas from which teeth have been extracted. Hyperplasia of the mucosa in edentulous mouths has been reported but is rare.

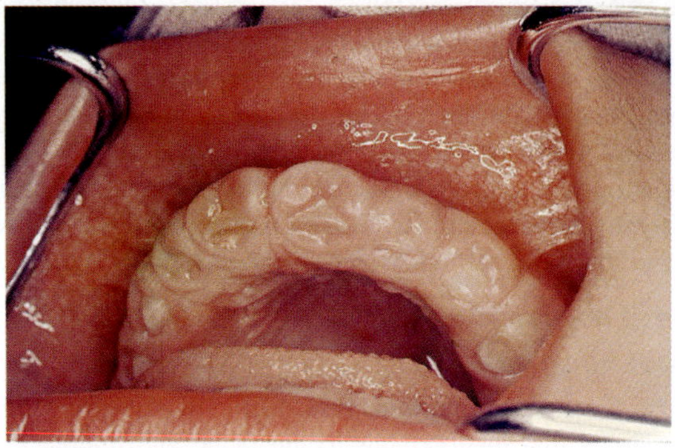

Fig. 14.6 Phenytoin gingival enlargement in a 5-year-old child covering most of the clinical crowns of the teeth.

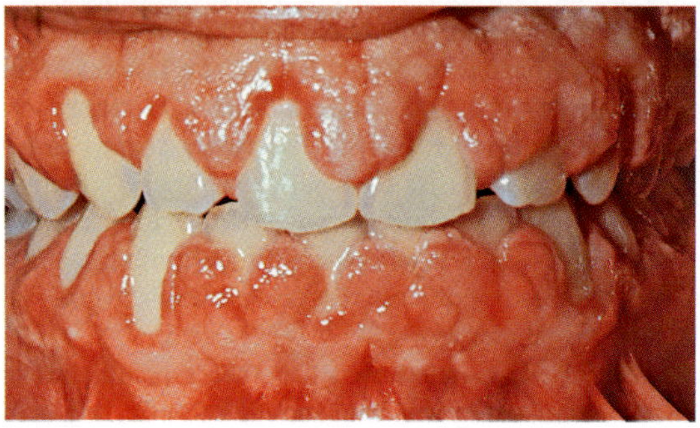

Fig. 14.7 Combined gingival enlargement resulting from the inflammatory involvement of a phenytoin-induced overgrowth.

Drug-induced enlargement may occur in mouths with little or no plaque and it may be absent in mouths with abundant deposits. However, some investigators believe that inflammation is a prerequisite for development of the enlargement, which therefore could be prevented by plaque removal and fastidious oral hygiene. Oral hygiene by means of toothbrushing or the use of a chlorhexidine toothpaste reduces the inflammation but does not lessen or prevent the overgrowth. Hassell et al. have hypothesized that, in noninflamed gingiva, fibroblasts are less active or even quiescent and do not respond to circulating phenytoin, whereas fibroblasts within inflamed tissue are in an active state as a result of the inflammatory mediators and the endogenous growth factors that are present.

A genetic predisposition is a suspected factor for determining whether a person treated with phenytoin will develop gingival enlargement.

The enlargement is chronic and it slowly increases in size. Even if it is surgically removed, it recurs. Spontaneous disappearance occurs within a few months after the discontinuation of the drug.

Histopathology

Drug-induced gingival enlargement (DIGE) consists of a pronounced hyperplasia of the connective tissue and epithelium (Fig. 14.8A and B). There is acanthosis of the epithelium and elongated rete pegs extend deep into the connective tissue, which exhibits densely arranged collagen bundles with an increase in the number of fibroblasts and new blood vessels. An abundance of amorphous ground substance has also been reported. Structural changes in the outer epithelial cell surface have been reported with cyclosporine-induced enlargements.

The enlargement begins as a hyperplasia of the connective tissue core of the marginal gingiva and increases by its proliferation and expansion beyond the crest of the gingival margin. An inflammatory infiltrate may be found at the bottom of the sulcus or pocket. Cyclosporine enlargements usually involve more highly vascularized

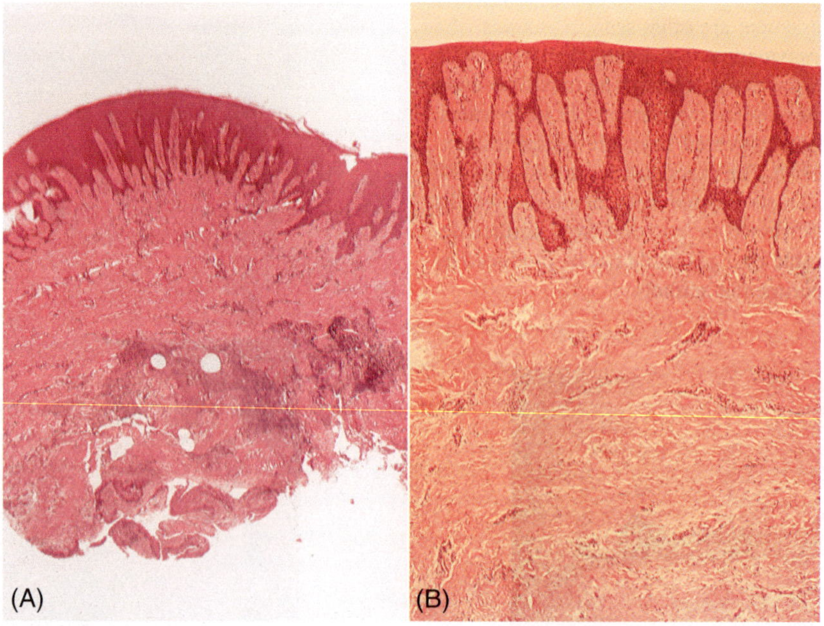

Fig. 14.8 Microscopic view of gingival enlargement associated with phenytoin therapy. A, Hyperplasia and acanthosis of the epithelium and densely collagenous connective tissue, with evidence of inflammation in the area adjacent to the gingival sulcus (pocket). B, High-power view showing the extension of deep rete pegs into the connective tissue.

connective tissue with foci of chronic inflammatory cells (particularly plasma cells).

The "mature"-phenytoin enlargement has a fibroblast-to-collagen ratio that is equal to that of normal gingiva from normal individuals, which suggests that, at some point in the development of the lesion, fibroblastic proliferation must have been abnormally high. Recurring phenytoin enlargements appear as granulation tissue composed of numerous young capillaries and fibroblasts and irregularly arranged collagen fibrils with occasional lymphocytes.

KEY FACT

Different types of DIGE lesions demonstrate a thick, stratified squamous epithelium with long, thin rete pegs extending deep into the connective tissue. Fibrosis is a common finding in patients with phenytoin-induced GE. Histologic characteristics of GE induced by calcium channel blockers are similar to those of phenytoin-induced lesions, including epithelial thickness, rete peg formation, and excessive matrix accumulation. Cyclosporin A-induced GE lesions have more inflammatory infiltration and increased vascularization compared to GE caused by phenytoin or calcium channel blockers.

Anticonvulsants

The first DIGE reported were those produced by phenytoin (Dilantin). Dilantin is a hydantoin that was introduced by Merritt and Putnam in 1938 for the treatment of all forms of epilepsy except petit mal seizures. Shortly thereafter, its relationship with gingival enlargement was reported.

Other hydantoins that are known to induce gingival enlargement are ethotoin (Peganone) and mephenytoin (Mesantoin). Other anticonvulsants that have the same side effect are the succinimides [ethosuximide (Zarontin), methsuximide (Celontin)] and valproic acid (Depakene).

Gingival enlargement occurs in about 50% of patients receiving the drug although different authors have reported incidences from 3% to 84.5%. It occurs more often in younger patients. Its occurrence and severity are not necessarily related to the dosage after a threshold level has been exceeded. Phenytoin appears in the saliva. There is no consensus, however, regarding whether the severity of the overgrowth is related to the levels of phenytoin in plasma or saliva. Some reports indicate a relationship between the drug dosage and the degree of gingival overgrowth.

Tissue-culture experiments indicate that phenytoin stimulates the proliferation of fibroblast-like cells and epithelium. Two analogs of phenytoin (1-allyl-5-phenylhydantoinate and 5-methyl-5-phenylhydantoinate) have a similar effect on fibroblast like cells. Fibroblasts from a phenytoin-induced gingival overgrowth show increased synthesis of sulfated glycosaminoglycans in vitro. Phenytoin may induce a decrease in collagen degradation as a result of the production of an inactive fibroblastic collagenase.

In experimental animals, phenytoin causes gingival enlargement that is independent of local inflammation. In cats, one of the metabolic products of phenytoin is 5-(parahydroxyphenyl)-5-phenylhydantoin; the administration of this metabolite to cats also induces gingival enlargement in some cases. This led Hassell et al. to hypothesize that gingival enlargement may result from the genetically determined ability or inability of the host to deal effectively with the prolonged administration of phenytoin.

The systemic administration of phenytoin accelerates the healing of gingival wounds in nonepileptic humans and increases the tensile strength of healing abdominal wounds in rats. The administration of phenytoin may precipitate megaloblastic anemia and folic-acid deficiency.

In conclusion, the pathogenesis of gingival enlargement induced by phenytoin is not known, but some evidence links it to a direct effect on specific, genetically predetermined subpopulations of fibroblasts, the inactivation of collagenase, and plaque-induced inflammation.

Immunosuppressants

Cyclosporine is a potent immunosuppressive agent that is used to prevent organ-transplant rejection and to treat several diseases of autoimmune origin. Its exact mechanism of action is not well-known, but it appears to selectively and reversibly inhibit helper T cells, which play a role in cellular and humoral immune responses. Cyclosporine A (Sandimmune and Neoral) is administered intravenously or by mouth and dosages of more than 500 mg/day have been reported to induce gingival overgrowth.

Cyclosporine-induced gingival enlargement is more vascularized than phenytoin enlargement (Figs. 14.9 and 14.10). Its occurrence varies according to different studies from 25% to 70%. It affects children more frequently, and its magnitude appears to be related more to the plasma concentration than to the patient's periodontal status. Gingival enlargement is greater in patients who are medicated with both cyclosporine and calcium-channel blockers, such as nifedipine.

The microscopic finding of many plasma cells plus the presence of an abundant amorphous extracellular substance has suggested that the enlargement is a hypersensitivity response to the cyclosporine.

In experimental animals (rats), the oral administration of cyclosporine was also reported to induce the abundant formation of new cementum.

In addition to gingival enlargement, cyclosporine induces other major side effects, such as, nephrotoxicity, hypertension, and

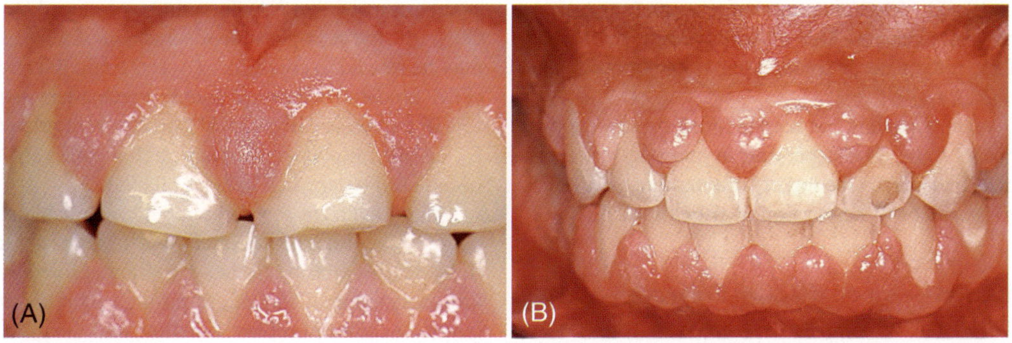

Fig. 14.9 Cyclosporine-associated gingival enlargement. A, Mild involvement located particularly on the papillae between upper central and lateral incisors. B, Advanced generalized enlargement.

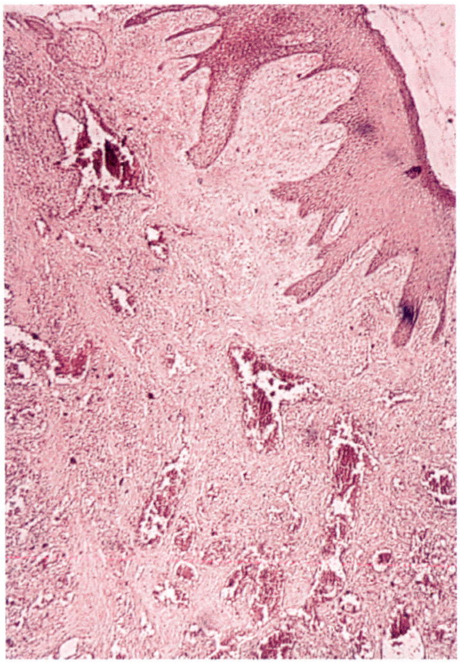

Fig. 14.10 Microscopic view of cyclosporine-associated gingival enlargement. Note the epithelial hyperplasia and fibrous stroma with abundant vascularization.

hypertrichosis. Another immunosuppressive drug, tacrolimus, has been used effectively; it is also nephrotoxic, but it results in much less severe hypertension, hypertrichosis, and gingival overgrowth.

Calcium-Channel Blockers

Calcium-channel blockers are drugs that were developed for the treatment of cardiovascular conditions, such as hypertension, angina pectoris, coronary artery spasms, and cardiac arrhythmias. They inhibit calcium-ion influx across the cell membrane of heart and smooth muscle cells, thereby blocking the intracellular mobilization of calcium. This induces the direct dilation of the coronary arteries and arterioles and improves oxygen supply to the heart muscle; it also reduces hypertension by dilating the peripheral vasculature.

These drugs are the *dihydropyridine derivatives* [amlodipine (Lotrel and Norvasc), felodipine (Plendil), nicardipine (Cardene), nifedipine (Adalat and Procardia)]; the *benzothiazine derivatives* [diltiazem (Cardizem, Dilacor XR, and Tiazac)]; and the *phenylalkylamine derivatives* [verapamil (Calan, Isoptin, Verelan, and Covera HS)].

Some of these drugs can induce gingival enlargement. Nifedipine, which is one of the most often used, induces gingival enlargement in 20% of patients. Diltiazem, felodipine, nitrendipine, and verapamil also induce gingival enlargement. The dihydropyridine derivative isradipine can replace nifedipine in some cases; it does not induce gingival overgrowth.

Nifedipine gingival enlargement has been induced experimentally in rats where it appears to be dose-dependent in humans; however, this dose dependency is not clear. One report indicates that nifedipine increases the risk of periodontal destruction in patients with type 2 diabetes mellitus.

Pathogenesis of Drug-Induced Gingival Enlargement

The pathogenesis of DIGE is complex. The main mechanism is mediated through defective function of gingival fibroblasts. Because gingival fibroblasts are responsible for the matrix deposition of gingival tissues, extensive research has focused on these key cells and their function. Study findings vary, some pathways have not been validated in humans, and data are limited to in vitro and animal studies, but collectively, the findings suggest that DIGE-associated medications affect the extracellular matrix metabolism by decreasing collagenase activity and increasing the production of matrix proteins.

Gingival fibroblasts from phenytoin-induced GE are characterized by elevated levels of collagen synthesis. It has been suggested that fibroblasts may be susceptible to the development of DIGE. Gingival fibroblasts from nifedipine-induced GE lesions have defective collagen production due to decreased levels of collagenase activity, which can result in collagen deposition. Through interference with calcium metabolism, calcium channel blockers decrease calcium levels in gingival fibroblasts and T cells, thereby affecting T-cell proliferation or activation and collagen biosynthesis.

Cyclosporin A directly impairs collagen synthesis by gingival fibroblasts, with a concomitant rise in the levels of type I collagen. Cyclosporin A also decreases expression of matrix metalloproteinase-1 (MMP-1) and MMP-3. In addition to collagen, which is the major extracellular matrix component of gingival tissues, noncollagenous matrix is affected by the medications that result in DIGE. Glycosaminoglycan metabolism is impaired in patients with phenytoin-induced GE and in response to cyclosporin A treatment of gingival fibroblasts.

In addition to fibroblast metabolism and function, inflammatory regulation of tissue turnover is a major factor in DIGE pathogenesis. Fibroblast functions such as proliferation, differentiation, and production of extracellular matrix are affected by levels of cytokines and growth factors. GE lesions are characterized by increased levels of interleukin-6 (IL-6), IL-1β, platelet-derived growth factor subunit B (PDGFB), fibroblast growth factor 2 (FGF2), transforming growth factor-β (TGF-β), and connective tissue growth factor (CTGF). Macrophages are the main source of these cytokines.

The TGF-β1–CTGF axis has been characterized in detail and is an essential mechanism leading to DIGE. TGF-β1 regulates cell proliferation and differentiation and can activate gene expression for the synthesis of extracellular matrix components, including collagen in cyclosporin A-induced GE. TGF-β1 induces CTGF mRNA and protein expression in human gingival fibroblasts; the TGF-β1–CTGF pathway directly regulates fibrosis, gingival fibroblast lysyl oxidase, and collagen generation. CTGF expression is increased in all forms of DIGE, with the highest levels occurring in phenytoin-induced GE, which also has the highest levels of fibrosis.

CTGF expression is not limited to the connective tissue. It also is demonstrated in the gingival epithelium, predominantly in the basal epithelial cells close to the connective tissue border. In vitro studies showed that CTGF could be produced by gingival epithelial cells, illustrating a possible mechanism of fibrosis in gingiva, which may be related to crosstalk between epithelial and connective tissue cells. Studies revealed a unique mechanism for TGF-β1-induced CTGF expression in gingival fibroblasts regulated by prostaglandin E_2, cAMP, mitogen-activated protein kinases (MAPKs), and activation of Jun N-terminal kinases (JNKs).

A key event in the pathogenetic mechanism of DIGE is some degree of epithelial-mesenchymal transition induced by medications. Highly fibrotic tissues are characterized by increased epithelial-mesenchymal transition, through which epithelial cells in the gingiva acquire fibroblast function, and the process is regulated by CTGF. The molecular pathways of DIGE have been reviewed elsewhere.

KEY FACT

DIGO cannot be prevented, but it can be alleviated by eliminating local factors, plaque control, and regular periodontal maintenance. The most effective treatment for drug-induced gingival overgrowth is withdrawal or substitution of the medication. Nonsurgical treatment results in the elimination of the inflammatory component of DIGO. Surgical elimination of DIGO lesions involves gingivectomy and gingivoplasty. Unfortunately, the recurrence rate is high. Maintenance should include oral hygiene instructions, periodontal prophylaxis, and removal of calculus as needed.

Idiopathic Gingival Enlargement

Idiopathic gingival enlargement is a rare condition of undetermined cause. It has been designated by terms, such as gingivostomatosis, elephantiasis, idiopathic fibromatosis, hereditary gingival hyperplasia, and congenital familial fibromatosis.

General Information

Clinical Features

The enlargement affects the attached gingiva, as well as the gingival margin and the interdental papillae. This is in contrast with phenytoin-induced overgrowth, which is often limited to the gingival margin and the interdental papillae (Fig. 14.5). The facial and lingual surfaces of the mandible and maxilla are generally affected but the involvement may be limited to either jaw. The enlarged gingiva is pink, firm, and almost leathery in consistency, and it has a characteristic minutely pebbled surface (Fig. 14.11A and B). In severe cases, the teeth are almost completely covered and the enlargement projects into the oral vestibule. The jaws appear distorted as a result of the bulbous enlargement of the gingiva. Secondary inflammatory changes are common at the gingival margin.

Histopathology

Idiopathic gingival enlargement shows a bulbous increase in the amount of connective tissue that is relatively avascular and that consists of densely arranged collagen bundles and numerous fibroblasts. The surface epithelium is thickened and acanthotic with elongated rete pegs.

Etiology

The cause is unknown and thus the condition is designated as "idiopathic." Some cases have a hereditary basis but the genetic mechanisms involved are not well understood. A study of several families found the mode of inheritance to be autosomal recessive in some cases and autosomal dominant in others. In some families, the gingival enlargement may be linked to the impairment of physical development. The enlargement usually begins with the eruption of the primary or secondary dentition and it may regress after extraction, which suggests that the teeth (or the plaque attached to them) may be initiating factors. The presence of bacterial plaque is a complicating factor.

Gingival enlargement has been described in tuberous sclerosis, which is an inherited condition characterized by a triad of epilepsy, mental deficiency, and cutaneous angiofibromas.

KEY FACT

The genetic basis of hereditary gingival fibromatosis is well established. In some families, gingival enlargement is linked to impairment of physical development. Other syndromes can coexist with gingival fibromatosis. Idiopathic forms of gingival fibromatosis have not been linked to any specific genes.

Enlargements Associated With Systemic Diseases or Conditions

Many systemic diseases can develop oral manifestations that may include gingival enlargement. These diseases and conditions can affect the periodontium via two different mechanisms:

1. *The magnification of an existing inflammation initiated by dental plaque.* This group of diseases, which are discussed in the "conditioned enlargements" section, includes some hormonal conditions (e.g., pregnancy and puberty), some nutritional diseases (e.g., vitamin C deficiency), and some cases in which the systemic influence is not identified (i.e., nonspecific conditioned enlargement).
2. *The manifestation of the systemic disease independently of the inflammatory status of the gingiva.* These mechanisms are described in the "Systemic Diseases that Cause Gingival Enlargement" section and the "Neoplastic Enlargement (Gingival Tumors)" section.

Conditioned Enlargements

Conditioned enlargements occur when the systemic condition of the patient exaggerates or distorts the usual gingival response to dental plaque. The specific manner in which the clinical picture of conditioned gingival enlargement differs from that of chronic gingivitis depends on the nature of the modifying systemic influence. *Bacterial plaque is necessary for the initiation of this type of enlargement.* However, plaque is not the sole determinant of the nature of the clinical features.

The three types of conditioned gingival enlargement are *hormonal* (pregnancy and puberty), *nutritional* (associated with vitamin C deficiency), and *allergic*. Nonspecific conditioned enlargement is also seen.

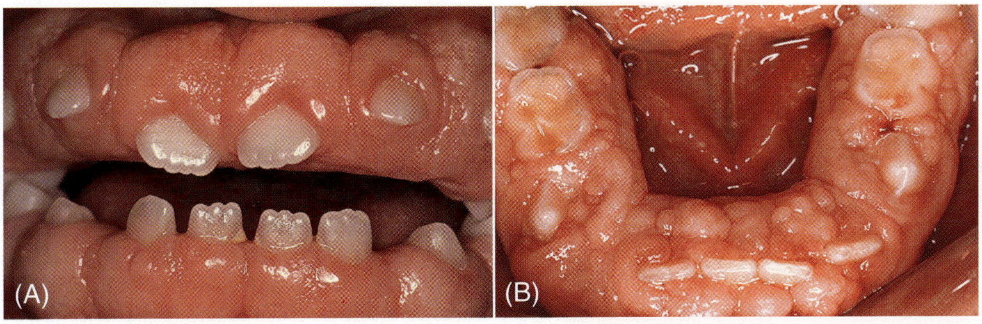

Fig. 14.11 Idiopathic gingival enlargement in a 14-year-old white male patient. A, Facial view. The gingiva is firm, with a nodular, pebbled surface and partially covering the crowns of the teeth. B, Occlusal view of the lower jaw.

Enlargement in Pregnancy

Pregnancy gingival enlargement may be marginal and generalized; or it may occur as a single mass or multiple tumor-like masses.

During pregnancy, there is an increase in levels of both progesterone and estrogen, which by the end of the third trimester reach levels 10- and 30 times the levels present during the menstrual cycle, respectively. These hormonal changes induce changes in vascular permeability, which leads to gingival edema and an increased inflammatory response to dental plaque. The subgingival microbiota may also undergo changes, including an increase in *Prevotella intermedia.*

Marginal Enlargement

Marginal gingival enlargement during pregnancy results from the aggravation of previous inflammation and its incidence has been reported between 10% and 70%. Sometimes, the lesions can be observed as single enlargements, which are referred to as pregnancy tumors. Pregnancy tumors are not neoplasms; they represent an inflammatory response to microbial plaque modified by the patient's condition. It usually appears after the third month of pregnancy, but it may occur earlier. The reported incidence is 1.8%–5%.

The clinical picture varies considerably. The enlargement is usually generalized, and it tends to be more prominent interproximally than on the facial and lingual surfaces. The enlarged gingiva is bright red or magenta, soft, and friable and has a smooth, shiny surface. Bleeding occurs spontaneously or on slight provocation.

Tumor-Like Gingival Enlargement

The so-called pregnancy tumor is not a neoplasm; it is an inflammatory response to bacterial plaque and it is modified by the patient's condition. It usually appears after the third month of pregnancy but it may occur earlier. The reported incidence is 1.8%–5%.

The lesion appears as a discrete, mushroom-like, flattened spherical mass that protrudes from the gingival margin or more often from the interproximal space, and it is attached by a sessile or pedunculated base (Fig. 14.12). It tends to expand laterally, and pressure from the tongue and the cheek perpetuates its flattened appearance. It is generally dusky-red or magenta in color; it has a smooth, glistening surface that often exhibits numerous deep-red, pinpoint markings. It is a superficial lesion that usually does not invade the underlying bone. The consistency varies; the mass is usually semifirm, but it may have varying degrees of softness and friability. It is usually painless unless its size and shape foster the accumulation of debris under its margin or interfere with occlusion, in which case painful ulceration may occur.

Although the microscopic findings are characteristic of gingival enlargement during pregnancy, they are not pathognomonic because they cannot be used to differentiate pregnant and nonpregnant patients.

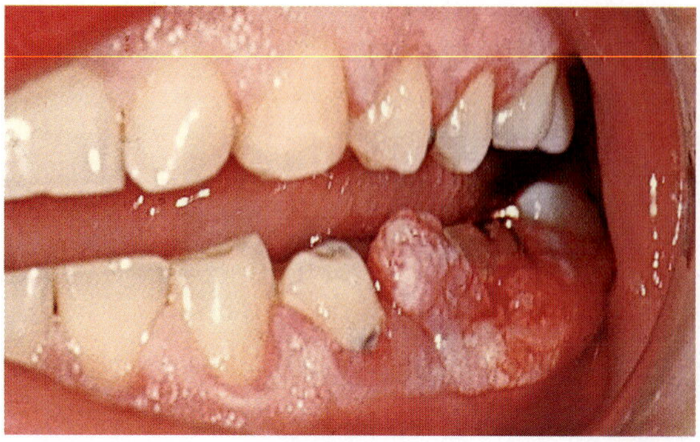

Fig. 14.12 Localized gingival enlargement in a 27-year-old pregnant patient.

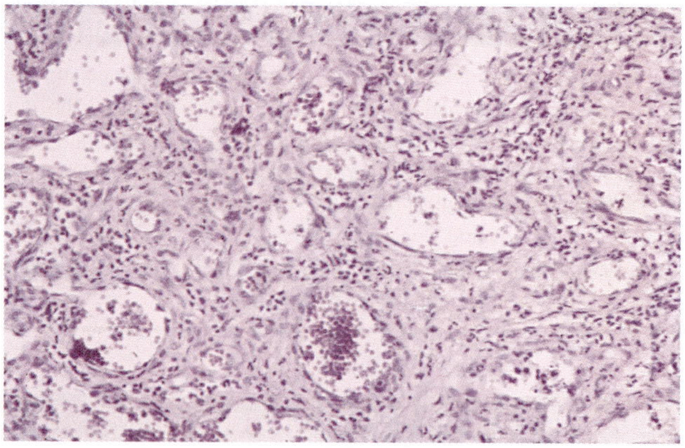

Fig. 14.13 Microscopic view of gingival enlargement in pregnant patient showing an abundance of blood vessels and interspersed inflammatory cells.

Histopathology

Gingival enlargement in pregnancy is called *angiogranuloma.* Both marginal and tumor-like enlargements consist of a central mass of connective tissue, with numerous diffusely arranged, newly formed, and engorged capillaries lined by cuboid endothelial cells (Fig. 14.13), as well as a moderately fibrous stroma with varying degrees of edema and chronic inflammatory infiltrate. The stratified squamous epithelium is thickened with prominent rete pegs and some degree of intracellular and extracellular edema, prominent intercellular bridges, and leukocytic infiltration.

Most gingival disease during pregnancy can be prevented by the removal of plaque and calculus, as well as by the institution of fastidious oral hygiene at the outset. During pregnancy, treatment of the gingiva that is limited to the removal of tissue without the complete elimination of local irritants is followed by the recurrence of gingival enlargement. Although spontaneous reduction in the size of gingival enlargement typically follows the termination of pregnancy, complete elimination of the residual inflammatory lesion requires the removal of all plaque deposits and factors that favor its accumulation.

Treatment

Like other forms of gingival changes associated with hormonal variations during pregnancy, GO lesions can be prevented by good oral hygiene in most cases. Therefore, oral care in pregnant women should be meticulous, and patients should be treated by removing calculus and biofilm. Severe cases may require surgical excision during the second trimester; however, removing the GO lesions without establishing an optimal oral hygiene regimen will likely lead to the recurrence of gingival enlargement. Although the spontaneous reduction in the size of gingival enlargement typically follows the termination of pregnancy, complete elimination of the residual inflammatory lesion and GO requires removal of all plaque deposits, elimination of factors that favor its accumulation, and in some fibrotic cases, surgical intervention after the pregnancy.

Enlargement in Puberty

Enlargement of the gingiva is sometimes seen during puberty. It occurs in both male and female adolescents and appears in areas of plaque accumulation.

The size of the gingival enlargement greatly exceeds that, which is usually seen in association with comparable local factors. It is marginal and interdental and is characterized by prominent bulbous interproximal papillae (Fig. 14.14). Often, only the facial gingivae are enlarged and the lingual surfaces are relatively unaltered; the

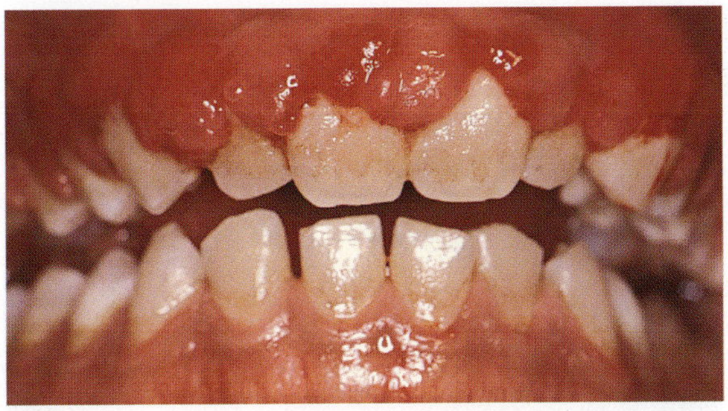

Fig. 14.14 Conditioned gingival enlargement during puberty in a 13-year-old boy.

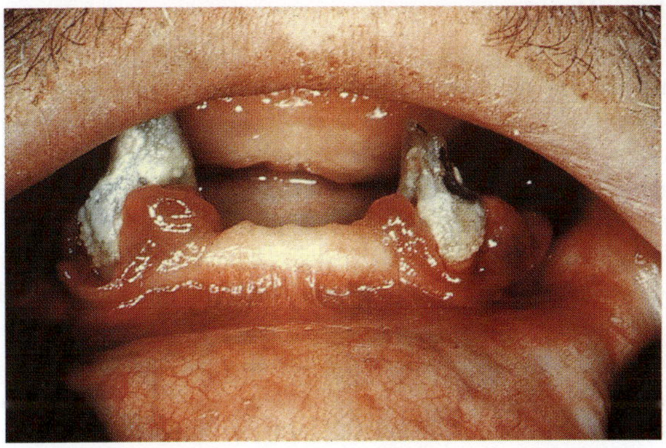

Fig. 14.15 Gingival enlargement in a patient with vitamin C deficiency. Note the prominent hemorrhagic areas. *(Courtesy: Dr Gerald Shklar, Boston, MA.)*

mechanical action of the tongue and the excursion of food prevent a heavy accumulation of local irritants on the lingual surface.

Gingival enlargement during puberty has all of the clinical features that are generally associated with chronic inflammatory gingival disease. It is the degree of enlargement and its tendency to recur in the presence of relatively scant plaque deposits that distinguish pubertal gingival enlargement from uncomplicated chronic inflammatory gingival enlargement. After puberty, the enlargement undergoes spontaneous reduction but does not disappear completely until the plaque and calculus are removed.

A longitudinal study of the subgingival microbiota of children between the ages of 11 and 14 years and their association with clinical parameters implicated the *Capnocytophaga* species in the initiation of pubertal gingivitis. Other studies have reported that hormonal changes coincide with an increase in the proportion of *P. intermedia* and *P. nigrescens.*

Histopathology

The microscopic appearance of gingival enlargement during puberty is chronic inflammation with prominent edema and associated degenerative changes.

Treatment

After puberty, enlargement undergoes spontaneous reduction, but it may not disappear completely until the plaque and calculus are removed.

Enlargement in Vitamin C Deficiency

The enlargement of the gingiva is generally included in classic descriptions of scurvy. Acute vitamin C deficiency itself does not cause gingival inflammation but it does cause hemorrhage, collagen degeneration, and edema of the gingival connective tissue. These changes modify the response of the gingiva to plaque to the extent that the normal defensive delimiting reaction is inhibited and the extent of the inflammation is exaggerated, thereby resulting in the massive gingival enlargement seen in patients with scurvy (Fig. 14.15).

Gingival enlargement with vitamin C deficiency is marginal; the gingiva is bluish-red, soft, and friable and has a smooth, shiny surface. Hemorrhage that occurs either spontaneously or on slight provocation as well as surface necrosis with pseudomembrane formation are common features.

Histopathology

In patients with vitamin C deficiency, the gingiva has a chronic inflammatory cellular infiltration with a superficial acute response. There are scattered areas of hemorrhage with engorged capillaries. Marked diffuse edema, collagen degeneration, and a scarcity of collagen fibrils and fibroblasts are striking findings.

Treatment

Nutrition-associated GO lesions are rare. Changes in nutrition accompanied by nonsurgical treatment and good oral hygiene usually result in complete resolution of the pathology. However, in rare cases, surgical removal may be indicated.

Plasma Cell Gingivitis

Plasma cell gingivitis consists of a mild marginal gingival enlargement that extends to the attached gingiva. The gingiva appears red, friable, and sometimes granular; and it bleeds easily; usually does not induce a loss of attachment (Fig. 14.16A and B). This lesion is located in the oral aspect of the attached gingiva and therefore differs from plaque-induced gingivitis.

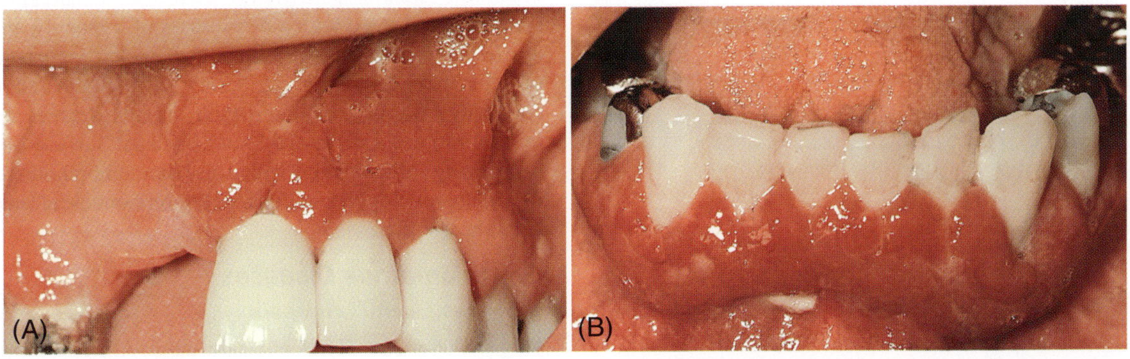

Fig. 14.16 Plasma cell gingivitis. A, Diffuse lesions on the facial surface of the anterior maxilla. B, Mandibular lesions. (Courtesy: Dr Kim D. Zussman, Thousand Oaks, CA.)

Histopathology

In patients with plasma cell gingivitis, the oral epithelium shows spongiosis and infiltration with inflammatory cells; ultrastructurally, there are signs of damage in the lower spinous layers and the basal layers. The underlying connective tissue contains a dense infiltrate of plasma cells that also extends to the oral epithelium, thereby inducing a dissecting type of injury.

An associated cheilitis and glossitis have been reported. Plasma cell gingivitis is thought to be allergic in origin and possibly related to components of chewing gum, dentifrices, or various diet components. The cessation of exposure to the allergen brings resolution of the lesion.

In rare instances, marked inflammatory gingival enlargements with a predominance of plasma cells can appear; these are associated with rapidly progressive periodontitis.

A solitary plasma cell tumor or *plasmocytoma* has been described in the nasopharynx and rarely in the oral mucosa. It is a slow-growing pedunculated tumor with a pink and smooth surface and is composed of normal plasma cells. It is usually benign; however, in rare cases, it can be an oral manifestation of multiple myeloma, which is a malignant tumor of the bone marrow.

Nonspecific Conditioned Enlargement (Pyogenic Granuloma)

Pyogenic granuloma is a tumor-like gingival enlargement that is considered an exaggerated conditioned response to minor trauma (Fig. 14.17). The exact nature of the systemic conditioning factor has not been identified. Pyogenic granuloma is similar in clinical and microscopic appearance to the conditioned gingival enlargement seen during pregnancy. The differential diagnosis is based on the patient's history.

Treatment consists of the removal of the lesions plus the elimination of irritating local factors. The recurrence rate is about 15%.

Gingival Fibromatosis

Gingival fibromatosis (GF) can be hereditary or idiopathic. These lesions are rare and occur in highly fibrotic forms of GO. Hereditary gingival fibromatosis is the most common form, and it has been linked to several genetic loci, including mutations of the Son-of-Sevenless 1 (SOS1) and REI-silencing transcription factor (REST) (genes 8, 26, 43, 44, 95, 111, 112). Idiopathic gingival fibromatosis is a rare condition of undetermined cause, likely driven by yet to be discovered genetic defects or physiologic. In all forms of GF, the enlargement is highly fibrotic with minimal clinical inflammation.

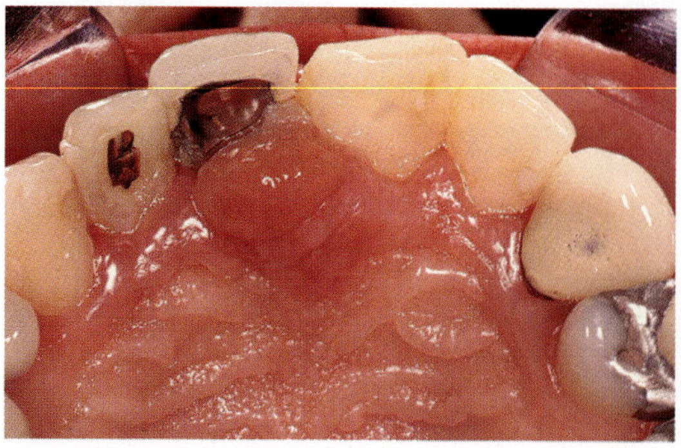

Fig. 14.17 Pyogenic granuloma. *(Courtesy: Dr Silvia Oreamuno, San José, Costa Rica.)*

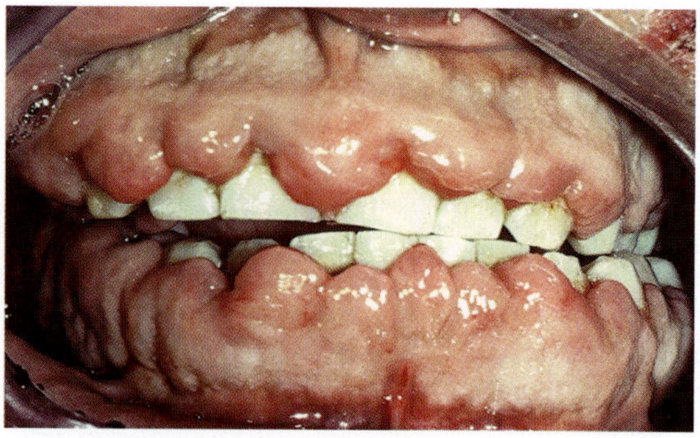

Fig. 14.18 Leukemic gingival enlargement (acute myelocytic leukemia). *(Courtesy: Dr Spencer Wolfe, Dublin, Ireland.)*

Systemic Diseases That Cause Gingival Enlargement

Several systemic diseases may result in gingival enlargement by different mechanisms. These are uncommon cases and are only briefly discussed.

Leukemia

Leukemic gingival enlargement may be diffuse or marginal and localized or generalized. It may appear as a diffuse enlargement of the gingival mucosa, an oversized extension of the marginal gingiva (Fig. 14.18), or a discrete tumor-like interproximal mass.

Clinical Features

In patients with leukemic enlargement, the gingiva is generally bluish-red and has a shiny surface. The consistency is moderately firm but there is a tendency toward friability and hemorrhage that occur either spontaneously or with slight irritation. Acute painful necrotizing ulcerative inflammatory involvement may occur in the crevice formed at the junction of the enlarged gingiva and the contiguous tooth surfaces.

Patients with leukemia may also have a simple chronic inflammation without the involvement of leukemic cells, and they may be present with the same clinical and microscopic features seen in patients without the systemic disease. Most cases, however, reveal features of both simple chronic inflammation and leukemic infiltrate.

True leukemic enlargement often occurs with acute leukemia but may also be seen with subacute leukemia. It seldom occurs with chronic leukemia.

Histopathology

Gingival enlargements in leukemic patients show various degrees of chronic inflammation. Mature leukocytes and areas of connective tissue are infiltrated with a dense mass of immature and proliferating leukocytes; the specific nature of which varies with the type of leukemia. Engorged capillaries, edematous and degenerated connective tissue, epithelium with various degrees of leukocytic infiltration, and edema are found. Isolated surface areas of acute necrotizing inflammation with a pseudomembranous meshwork of fibrin, necrotic epithelial cells, polymorphonuclear leukocytes, and bacteria are often seen.

Granulomatous Diseases

Wegener Granulomatosis

Wegener granulomatosis is a rare disease that is characterized by acute granulomatous necrotizing lesions of the respiratory tract, including nasal and oral defects. Renal lesions develop and acute

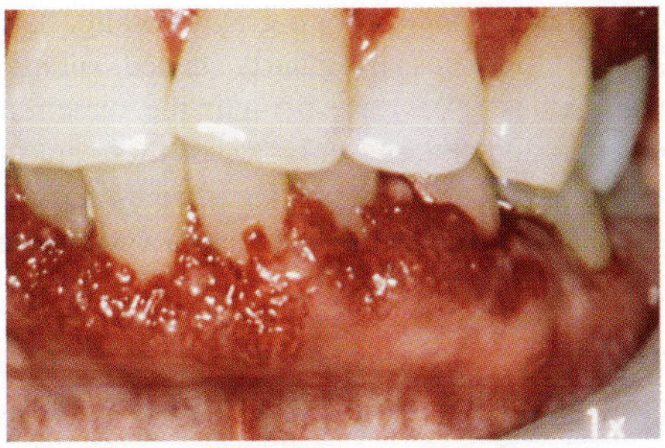

Fig. 14.19 Wegener granulomatosis affecting the gingival tissues. The classic "strawberry gums" appearance of the mandibular gingiva is seen in this patient. A slight resemblance with desquamative gingivitis is also evident.

necrotizing vasculitis affects the blood vessels. The initial manifestations of Wegener granulomatosis may involve the orofacial region and include oral mucosal ulceration, gingival enlargement, abnormal tooth mobility, exfoliation of teeth, and delayed healing response.

The granulomatous papillary enlargement is reddish-purple and bleeds easily on stimulation (Fig. 14.19).

Histopathology

Chronic inflammation involves scattered giant cells, foci of acute inflammation, and microabscesses covered by a thin, acanthotic epithelium. Vascular changes have not been described with gingival enlargement in patients with Wegener granulomatosis (Fig. 14.19), probably because of the small size of the gingival blood vessels.

The cause of Wegener granulomatosis is unknown but the condition is considered to be an immunologically mediated tissue injury. At one time, the usual outcome for patients with this condition was death from kidney failure within a few months; but more recently, the use of immunosuppressive drugs has produced prolonged remissions in more than 90% of patients.

Sarcoidosis

Sarcoidosis is a granulomatous disease of unknown etiology. It starts in individuals during their 20s or 30s, it predominantly affects blacks, and it can involve almost any organ, including the gingiva, in which a red, smooth, painless enlargement may appear.

Histopathology

Sarcoid granulomas consist of discrete, noncaseating whorls of epithelioid cells and multinucleated, and foreign body-type giant cells with peripheral mononuclear cells.

Neoplastic Enlargement (Gingival Tumors)

This section provides only a brief description of some of the more common neoplastic and pseudoneoplastic lesions of the gingiva. The reader is referred to oral pathology texts for more comprehensive coverage.

Benign Tumors of the Gingiva

Epulis is a generic term that is used clinically to designate all discrete tumors and tumor-like masses of the gingiva. It serves to locate the tumor but not to describe it. Most lesions referred to by this term are inflammatory rather than neoplastic.

Neoplasms account for a comparatively small proportion of gingival enlargements and they make up a small percentage of the total number of oral neoplasms. In a survey of 257 oral tumors, approximately 8% occurred on the gingiva. In another study of 868 growths of the gingiva and palate (of which 57% were neoplastic and the remainder inflammatory), the following incidences of tumors were noted: carcinoma, 11.0%; fibroma, 9.3%; giant-cell tumor, 8.4%; papilloma, 7.3%; leukoplakia, 4.9%; mixed tumor (salivary-gland type), 2.5%; angioma, 1.5%; osteofibroma, 1.3%; sarcoma, 0.5%; melanoma, 0.5%; myxoma, 0.45%; fibropapilloma, 0.4%; adenoma, 0.4%; and lipoma, 0.3%.

Fibroma

Fibromas of the gingiva arise from the gingival connective tissue or from the periodontal ligament. They are slow-growing spherical tumors that tend to be firm and nodular but that may be soft and vascular. Fibromas are usually pedunculated. Hard fibromas of the gingiva are rare; most of the lesions that are diagnosed clinically as "fibromas" are inflammatory enlargements.

Histopathology

Fibromas are composed of bundles of well-formed collagen fibers with scattered fibrocytes and variable vascularity.

The so-called giant-cell fibroma contains multinucleated fibroblasts. In another variant, mineralized tissue (bone, cementum-like material, and dystrophic calcifications) may be found; this type of fibroma is called *peripheral ossifying fibroma.*

Papilloma

Papillomas are benign proliferations of surface epithelium that are, in many (but not all) cases, associated with the human papillomavirus (HPV). Gingival papillomas appear as solitary wart-like or cauliflower-like protuberances (Fig. 14.20). They may be small and discrete, or they may be broad, hard elevations with minutely irregular surfaces.

Histopathology

The papilloma lesion consists of finger-like projections of stratified squamous epithelium that are often hyperkeratotic with central cores of fibrovascular connective tissue.

Peripheral Giant-Cell Granuloma

Giant-cell lesions of the gingiva arise interdentally or from the gingival margin; they occur most frequently on the labial surface and they may be sessile or pedunculated. They vary in appearance from smooth, regularly outlined masses to irregularly shaped, multilobulated protuberances with surface indentations (Fig. 14.21). The ulceration of the margin is occasionally seen. The lesions are painless, vary in size, and cover several teeth. They may be firm or spongy, and their color varies from pink to deep red or purplish-blue. There are no pathognomonic clinical features whereby these lesions can be differentiated from other forms of gingival enlargement. Microscopic examination is required for definitive diagnosis.

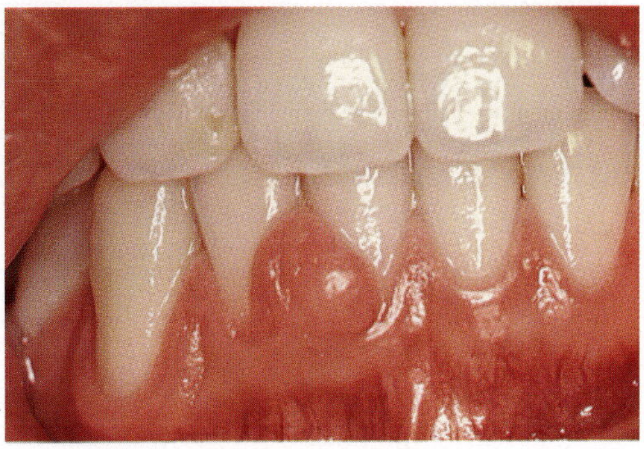

Fig. 14.20 Papilloma of the gingiva in a 26-year-old man.

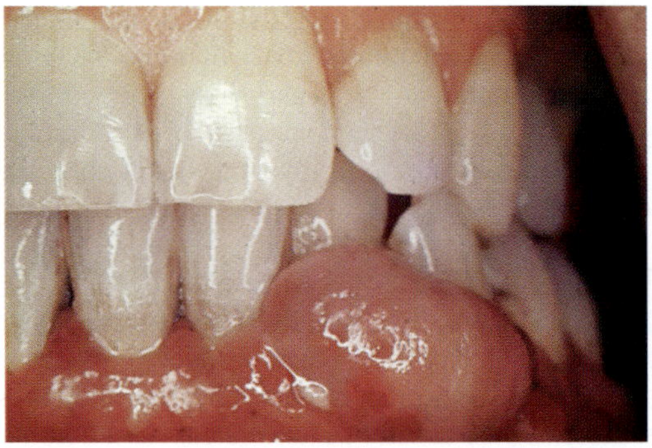

Fig. 14.21 Gingival giant-cell granuloma.

The prefix *peripheral* is needed to differentiate them from comparable lesions that originate within the jawbone (i.e., central giant-cell granulomas).

In some cases, the giant-cell granuloma of the gingiva is locally invasive and causes destruction of the underlying bone (Fig. 14.22). Complete removal leads to uneventful recovery.

Histopathology

The giant-cell granuloma has numerous foci of multinuclear giant cells and hemosiderin particles in a connective tissue stroma (Fig. 14.22A and B). Areas of chronic inflammation are scattered throughout the lesion with acute involvement occurring at the surface. The overlying epithelium is usually hyperplastic with ulceration at the base. Bone formation occasionally occurs within the lesion (Fig. 14.23).

Central Giant-Cell Granuloma

Giant-cell lesions arise within the jaws and produce central cavitation. They occasionally create a deformity of the jaw that makes the gingiva appear enlarged.

Mixed tumors, salivary gland types of tumors, and plasmacytomas of the gingiva have also been described but are not often seen.

Leukoplakia

Leukoplakia is a strictly clinical term defined by the World Health Organization as a white patch or plaque that does not rub off and that cannot be diagnosed as any other disease. The cause of leukoplakia remains obscure although it is associated with the use of tobacco (smoke or smokeless). Other probable factors are *Candida albicans*, HPV-16 and HPV-18, and trauma. Leukoplakia of the gingiva varies in appearance from a grayish white, flattened, scaly lesion (Fig. 14.24) to a thick, irregularly shaped, keratinous plaque.

Most leukoplakias (80%) are benign; the remaining 20% are malignant or premalignant, and only 3% of these are invasive carcinomas. The biopsy of all leukoplakias is necessary, with the most suspicious area being selected, to arrive at a correct diagnosis and to then institute a proper therapy.

Histopathology

Leukoplakia exhibits hyperkeratosis and acanthosis. Premalignant and malignant cases have a variable degree of atypical epithelial changes that may be mild, moderate, or severe, depending on the extent of involvement of the epithelial layers. When dysplastic changes involve all layers, it is diagnosed as a *carcinoma in situ*, and this may become invasive carcinoma when the basement membrane is breached. Inflammatory involvement of the underlying connective tissue is a common associated finding.

Gingival Cyst

Gingival cysts of microscopic proportions are common but they seldom reach a clinically significant size. When they do, they appear as localized enlargements that may involve the marginal and attached gingiva. The cysts occur in the mandibular canine and premolar areas; most often on the lingual surface. They are painless but, with expansion, they may cause erosion of the surface of the alveolar bone. The gingival cyst should be differentiated from the lateral periodontal cyst (see Chapter 20), which arises within the alveolar bone adjacent to the root and which is developmental in origin. Gingival cysts develop from odontogenic epithelium or from surface or sulcular epithelium traumatically implanted in the area. Removal is followed by uneventful recovery.

Histopathology

A gingival cyst cavity is lined by a thin, flattened epithelium with or without localized areas of thickening. Less frequently, the following types of epithelium can be found: unkeratinized stratified squamous epithelium, keratinized stratified squamous epithelium, and parakeratinized epithelium with palisading basal cells.

Other Benign Masses

Other benign tumors have also been described as rare or infrequent findings in the gingiva. They include nevus, myoblastoma, hemangioma, neurilemoma, neurofibroma, mucus-secreting cysts (mucoceles), and ameloblastoma.

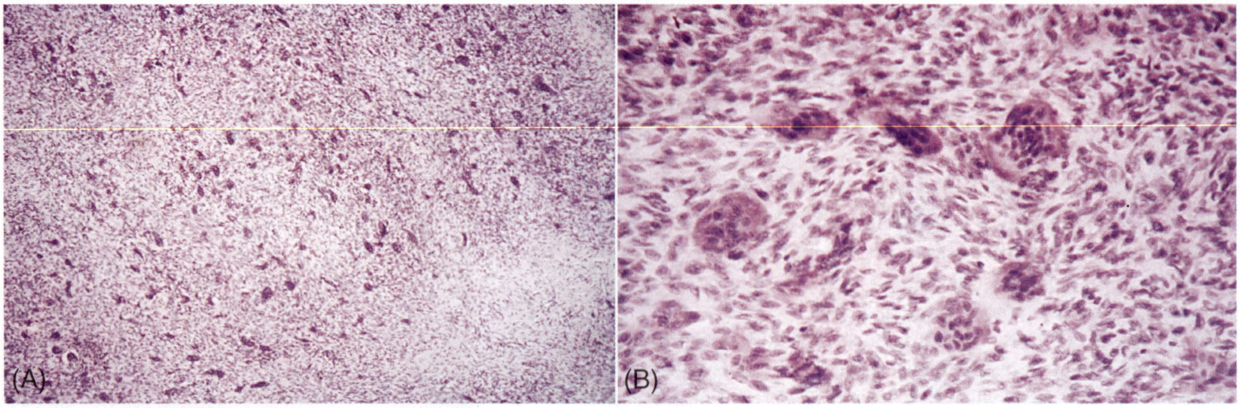

Fig. 14.22 A, Microscopic survey of a peripheral giant-cell granuloma. B, High-power study of the lesion demonstrating the giant cells and the intervening stroma that make up the major portion of the mass.

Malignant Tumors of the Gingiva

Carcinoma

Oral cancer accounts for less than 3% of all malignant tumors in the body but it is the sixth most common cancer in males and the 12th most common in females. The gingiva is not a frequent site of oral malignancy, accounting for only 6% of oral cancers.

Squamous cell carcinoma is the most common malignant tumor of the gingiva. It may be *exophytic*, presenting as an irregular outgrowth, or *ulcerative*, appearing as flat, erosive lesions. It is often symptom-free, going unnoticed until complicated by inflammatory changes that may mask the neoplasm but cause pain; sometimes it becomes evident after tooth extraction. These masses are locally invasive and they involve the underlying bone and periodontal ligament of adjoining teeth and the adjacent mucosa (Fig. 14.25A and B). Metastasis is usually confined to the region above the clavicle; however, more extensive involvement may include the lung, liver, or bone.

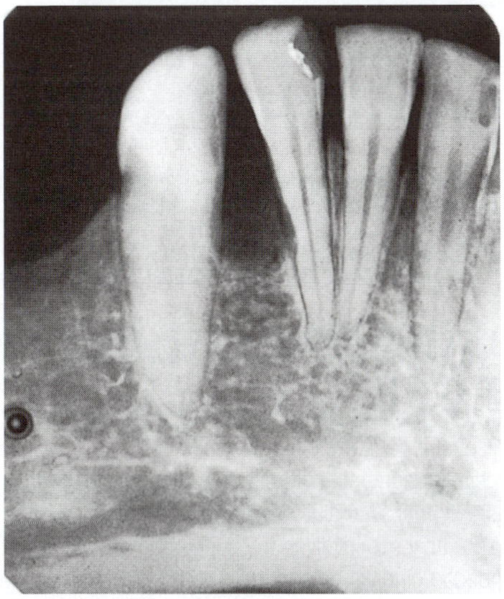

Fig. 14.23 Bone destruction in the interproximal space between the canine and lateral incisor caused by the extension of a peripheral giant-cell reparative granuloma of the gingiva. *(Courtesy: Dr Sam Toll.)*

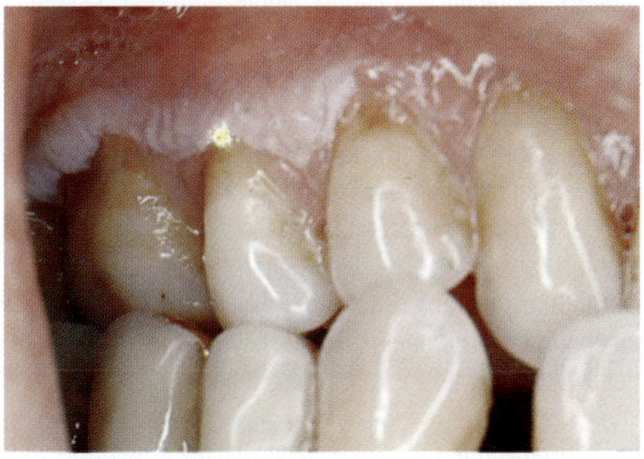

Fig. 14.24 Leukoplakia of the gingiva.

Malignant Melanoma

Malignant melanoma is a rare oral tumor that tends to occur in the hard palate and maxillary gingiva of older persons. It is usually darkly pigmented and is often preceded by localized pigmentation. It may be flat or nodular, and it is characterized by rapid growth and early metastasis. It arises from melanoblasts in the gingiva, cheek, or palate. Infiltration into the underlying bone and metastasis to cervical and axillary lymph nodes are common.

Sarcoma

Fibrosarcoma, lymphosarcoma, and reticulum-cell sarcoma of the gingiva are rare; only isolated cases have been described in the literature. Kaposi's sarcoma often occurs in the oral cavity of patients with acquired immunodeficiency syndrome, particularly in the palate and the gingiva.

Metastasis

Tumor metastasis to the gingiva occurs infrequently. Such metastasis has been reported with various tumors, including adenocarcinoma of the colon, lung carcinoma, melanoma, renal-cell carcinoma, hypernephroma, chondrosarcoma, and testicular tumor.

The low incidence of oral malignancy should not mislead the clinician. Ulcerations that do not respond to therapy in the usual manner, as well as all gingival tumors and tumor-like lesions, must be biopsied and submitted for microscopic diagnosis.

False Enlargement

False enlargements are not true enlargements of the gingival tissues but may appear as such as a result of increases in the size of the underlying osseous or dental tissues. The gingiva usually presents with no abnormal clinical features except the massive increase in the size of the area.

Underlying Osseous Lesions

Enlargement of the bone subjacent to the gingival area occurs most often with tori and exostoses but it can also occur with Paget disease, fibrous dysplasia, cherubism, central giant-cell granuloma, ameloblastoma, osteoma, and osteosarcoma. Figure 14.26A and B

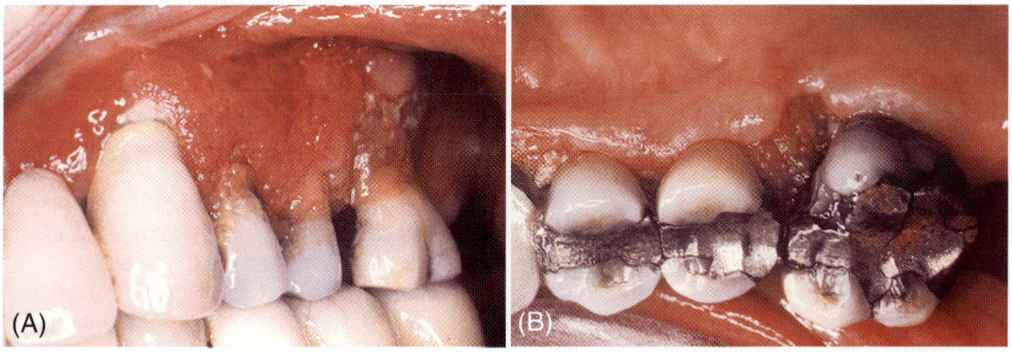

Fig. 14.25 Squamous cell carcinoma of the gingiva. A, Facial view. Note the extensive verrucous involvement. B, Palatal view. Note the mulberry-like tissue emerging between the second premolar and the first molar.

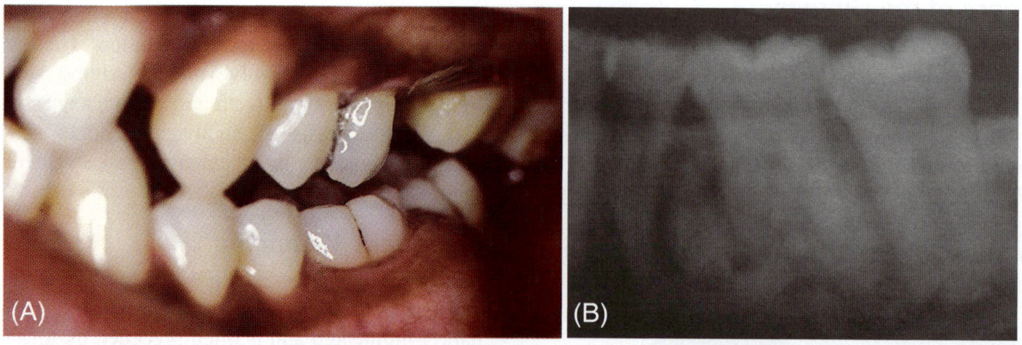

Fig. 14.26 A, Apparent gingival enlargement associated with bone augmentation in a patient with fibrous dysplasia. B, Radiograph of the case shown in A, depicting a ground-glass, mottled pattern.

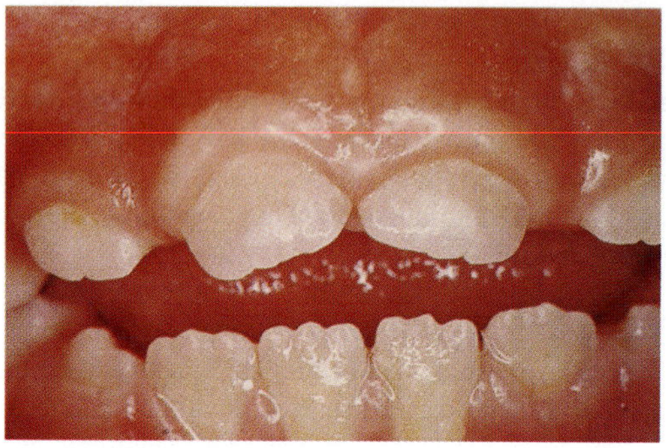

Fig. 14.27 Developmental gingival enlargement. The normal bulbous contour of the gingiva around the incompletely erupted anterior teeth is accentuated by chronic inflammation.

shows fibrous dysplasia (florid-type) in a 38-year-old black woman that induced an osseous enlargement in the mandibular molar area that appeared to be a gingival enlargement. The gingival tissue can appear normal or it may have unrelated inflammatory changes.

Underlying Dental Tissues

During the various stages of eruption, particularly of the primary dentition, the labial gingiva may show a bulbous marginal distortion caused by the superimposition of the bulk of the gingiva on the normal prominence of the enamel in the gingival half of the crown. This enlargement has been called *developmental enlargement* and often persists until the junctional epithelium has migrated from the enamel to the cementoenamel junction.

In a strict sense, developmental gingival enlargements are physiologic and they usually present no problems. However, when such enlargement is complicated by marginal inflammation, the composite picture gives the impression of extensive gingival enlargement (Fig. 14.27). Treatment to alleviate the marginal inflammation—rather than resection of the enlargement—is sufficient for these patients.

NOTE: Refer online resource Atlas of Periodontal Diseases available for numerous examples of gingival enlargements.

Key points

- Increase in size of the gingiva is a common feature of gingival disease.
- Gingival enlargement can be classified according to etiologic factors and pathologic changes.
- Chronic inflammatory gingival enlargement originates as a slight ballooning of the interdental papilla and marginal gingiva.
- Prolonged exposure to dental plaque can lead to chronic inflammatory enlargement.
- In mouth breather, the gingiva appears red and edematous, with a diffuse surface shininess of the exposed area. Maxillary anterior region is the common site of such involvement.
- A gingival abscess is a localized, painful, rapidly expanding lesion that is usually of sudden onset. Acute inflammatory gingival enlargement results from bacteria carried deep into the tissues when a foreign substance like tooth brush bristle, piece of apple core, and lobster shell fragment is forcefully embedded into the gingiva. It involves only marginal gingiva.
- Periodontal abscess involves the supporting periodontal tissue.
- Drug-induced gingival enlargement is a well-known consequence of the administration of some anticonvulsants, immune suppressants, and calcium channel blockers.
- Usually in drug-induced gingival enlargement, the growth starts as a painless, bead-like enlargement of the interdental papilla and extends to the facial and lingual gingival margins. As the condition progresses, the marginal and papillary enlargement unite; they may progress to massive tissue fold covering a considerable portion of the crowns and may interfere with occlusion.
- The enlargement is usually generalized throughout the mouth but is more severe in maxillary and mandibular anterior regions.
- Gingival enlargement occurs in areas in which teeth are present, not in edentulous spaces. The enlargement disappears in areas from which teeth are extracted.
- Cyclosporine enlargements usually have more highly vascularized connective tissue with foci of chronic inflammatory cells, particularly plasma cells.
- The first drug-induced gingival enlargements reported were those produced by phenytoin. Dilantin is a hydantoin, introduced by Merritt and Putnam in 1938.
- Dosage of more than 500 mg/day of cyclosporine A, administered intravenously or by mouth has been reported to induce gingival enlargement.
- Nifedipine is one the most commonly used calcium channel blockers which induces gingival enlargement.
- Idiopathic gingival enlargement is a rare condition of undetermined cause. It has been labeled by such terms as gingivomatosis, elephantiasis, idiopathic fibromatosis, hereditary gingival hyperplasia, and congenital familial fibromatosis. It affects the attached gingiva, marginal gingiva, and interdental papillae.
- Usually, facial or lingual surfaces of the upper and lower jaw get involved but the involvement may be limited to either jaw.
- Tuberous sclerosis is an inherited condition characterized by a triad of epilepsy, mental deficiency, and cutaneous angiofibromas.

- Conditioned enlargement occurs when the systemic condition of the patient exaggerates or distorts the usual gingival response to dental plaque. The three types of conditioned gingival enlargement are hormonal (pregnancy, puberty), nutritional (associated with vitamin C deficiency), and allergic. Nonspecific conditioned enlargement is also seen.
- In pregnancy, subgingival microbiota also undergoes changes. *Prevotella intermedia* number also increases.
- Pregnancy tumor is not a neoplasm; it is an inflammatory response to bacterial plaque and is modified by the patient's condition. It usually appears after the third month of pregnancy but may occur earlier.
- Gingival enlargement in pregnancy is called angiogranuloma.
- In scurvy (vitamin C deficiency), gingival enlargement is seen. Deficiency itself does not cause gingival inflammation, but it does cause hemorrhage, collagen degeneration, and edema of the gingival connective tissue. These changes modify the response of the gingiva to plaque to the extent that the normal defensive delimiting reaction is inhibited, and the extent of the inflammation is exaggerated, resulting in the massive gingival enlargement seen in scurvy.
- Plasma cell gingivitis is also called as atypical gingivitis and plasma cell gingivostomatitis. This is associated with cheilitis and glossitis. Plasma cell gingivitis is thought to be allergic in origin, possibly related to components of chewing gum, dentifrices, or various diet components. Cessation of exposure to the allergen brings resolution of the lesion.
- Nonspecific conditioned enlargement—pyogenic granuloma—it is a tumor-like gingival enlargement that is considered an exaggerated conditioned response to minor trauma.
- Pyogenic granuloma is similar in clinical and microscopic appearance to the conditioned gingival enlargement seen in pregnancy. Differential diagnosis is based on the patient's history.
- Leukemic enlargement may be diffused or marginal and localized or generalized. In acute leukemia, usually, gingival enlargement is seen.
- Granulomatous diseases such as Wegener's granulomatosis, sarcoidosis, and gingival enlargement are seen.
- Epulis, fibroma, papilloma, peripheral giant cell granuloma, central giant cell granuloma, gingival cyst, mucocele, ameloblastoma, myoblastoma, and hemangioma are the few benign conditions of gingival enlargement.
- Squamous cell carcinoma is the most common malignant tumor of the gingiva.
- Malignant melanoma is a rare oral tumor that tends to occur in the hard palate and maxillary gingiva of older individuals.
- Kaposi sarcoma often occurs in the oral cavity of patients with AIDS, particularly in the palate and the gingiva.
- False enlargements are not true enlargements of the gingival tissues but may appear as such as a result of an increase in size of the underlying osseous or dental tissues.
- Enlargement of the bone subjacent to the gingiva occurs commonly in tori and exostoses. It can also occur in Paget's disease, fibrous dysplasia, cherubism, and ameloblastoma.

Suggested Readings

Aas E: *Hyperplasia gingivae diphenylhydantoinea*, Oslo, 1963, Universitetsforlaget.

Fowler CB: Benign and malignant neoplasms of the periodontium, *Periodontol 2000* 21:33, 1999.

Hallmon WW, Rossmann JA: The role of drugs in the pathogenesis of gingival overgrowth, *Periodontol 2000* 21:176, 1999.

Kuffer R, Lombardi T: Premalignant lesions of the oral mucosa. A discussion about the place of oral intraepithelial neoplasia (OIN), *Oral Oncol* 38:125, 2002.

Nuki K, Cooper SH: The role of inflammation in the pathogenesis of gingival enlargement during the administration of diphenylhydantoin sodium in cats, *J Periodontal Res* 7:91, 1972.

Rees TD: Drugs and oral disorders, *Periodontol 2000* 18:21, 1998.

Sapp JP, Eversole LR, Wysocki GP: *Contemporary oral and maxillofacial pathology*, ed 2, Mosby, 2004, Elsevier.

Seymour RA, Thomason JM, Ellis JS: The pathogenesis of drug-induced gingival overgrowth, *J Clin Periodontol* 23:165, 1996.

References

References and MCQs with answers for the chapter are available on www.medenact.com.

CHAPTER 15

Acute Gingival Infections

PR Klokkevold | FA Carranza | DG Naik | A Uppoor

CHAPTER OUTLINE

Necrotizing Ulcerative Gingivitis
Primary Herpetic Gingivostomatitis
Pericoronitis

Acute gingival infections often present with painful intraoral or perioral lesions. Patients presenting with acute infections require urgent treatment to relieve symptoms and to resolve the infection. However, determining the most effective treatment depends identifying on the etiology and making the proper diagnosis. It is critically important to conduct a careful assessment and to accurately diagnose each case based on the presenting signs and symptoms. It is also important to identify any contributing risk factors that may increase susceptibility to the acute gingival infection. This chapter reviews the presenting history, signs, symptoms, clinical features, and expected clinical course of acute gingival infections, including necrotizing ulcerative gingivitis, primary herpetic gingivostomatitis, and pericoronitis. Factors used to differentiate between one acute infection and another, which may present with similar symptoms, are described.

Necrotizing Ulcerative Gingivitis

Necrotizing ulcerative gingivitis (NUG) is a microbial disease of the gingiva in the context of an impaired host response. It is characterized by the necrosis and sloughing of gingival tissue, and it presents with characteristic signs and symptoms.

In the past, it was also referred to as Vincent's infection, acute ulceromembranous gingivitis, Trench mouth, ulcerative gingivitis, Vincent stomatitis, Plaut–Vincent stomatitis, stomatitis ulcerosa, fedid stomatitis, fusospirillary gingivitis, and putrid stomatitis.

Historical Background

NUG was recognized as far back as the 4th century B.C. by Xenophon, who mentioned that Greek soldiers were affected with "sore mouth" and foul smelling breath. John Hunter, in 1778, described the clinical findings and differentiated it from scurvy and chronic destructive periodontal disease. NUG occurred in epidemic form in the French army in 19th century, and, in 1886, Hersch discussed some features associated with the disease, such as lymph node enlargement, fever, malaise, and increased salivation. In the 1890s, Plaut and Vincent described the disease and attributed its origin to fusiform bacilli and spirochetes.

Clinical Features

Although the acronym ANUG (acute necrotizing ulcerative gingivitis) is frequently used, it is a misnomer. Historically, NUG has been identified as an acute disease. However, the term acute is used as a clinical descriptor rather than a diagnostic term because chronic forms of the disease do not exist. The term acute has not been used in diagnosis since 1999. Furthermore, a summary of acute periodontal lesions advocated the more simplified term necrotizing gingivitis rather than NUG, but the latter term continues to be used in this chapter.

More advanced forms of necrotizing ulcerative disease can include destruction of the periodontal attachment apparatus, including bone, especially in patients with long-standing disease or severe immunosuppression. When periodontal attachment and bone loss occur, the condition is called necrotizing ulcerative periodontitis (NUP).

History

NUG is characterized by its sudden onset, sometimes after an episode of debilitating disease or acute respiratory tract infection. A change in living habits, protracted work without adequate rest, poor nutrition, tobacco use, and psychological stress are frequent features of the patient's history.

Oral Signs

Characteristic lesions are *punched-out, crater-like depressions at the crest of the interdental papillae* that subsequently extend to the marginal gingiva and rarely to the attached gingiva and oral mucosa. The surface of the gingival craters is covered by a *gray, pseudomembranous slough* that is demarcated from the remainder of the gingival mucosa by a pronounced *linear erythema* (Fig. 15.1A). In some cases, the lesions are denuded of the surface pseudomembrane, thereby exposing the gingival margin, which is red, shiny, and hemorrhagic. The characteristic lesions may progressively destroy the gingiva and the underlying periodontal tissues (Fig. 15.1B).

Spontaneous gingival hemorrhage or pronounced bleeding after the slightest stimulation are additional characteristic clinical signs (Fig. 15.1B and C). Other signs that are often found include a fetid odor and increased salivation.

NUG can occur otherwise in disease-free mouths, or it can be superimposed on chronic gingivitis or periodontal pockets. However, NUG or NUP does not usually lead to periodontal pocket formation because the necrotic changes involve the junctional epithelium; a viable junctional epithelium is needed for pocket deepening. It is rare in edentulous mouths, but isolated spherical lesions occasionally occur in the soft palate.

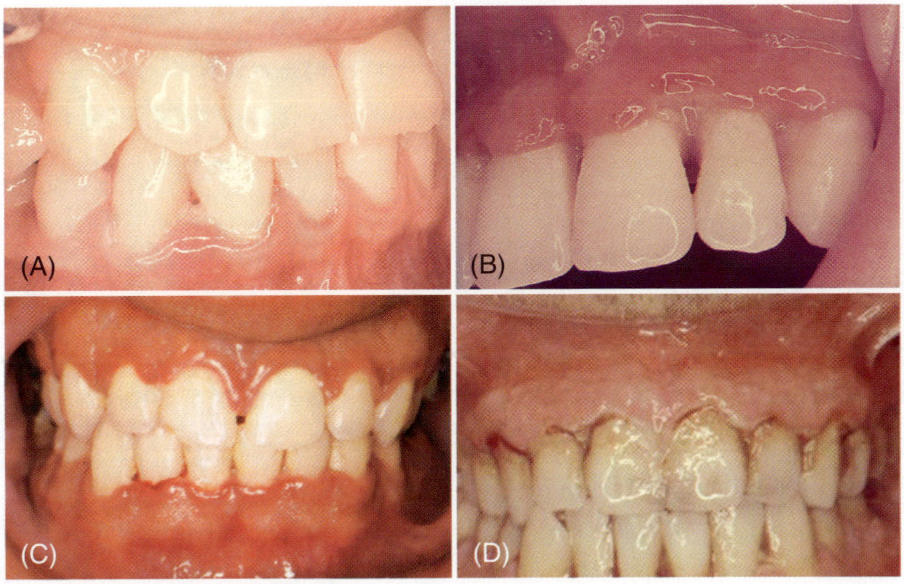

Fig. 15.1 **Necrotizing ulcerative gingivitis.** A, Typical punched-out papilla between the mandibular canine and the lateral incisor, covered by a grayish-white pseudomembrane. B, More advanced case showing the destruction of the papillae, which results in an irregular marginal contour. C, Typical lesions with spontaneous hemorrhage. D, Generalized involvement of the papillae and the marginal gingiva, with whitish necrotic lesions.

KEY FACT

Necrotizing ulcerative gingivitis can be superimposed on chronic periodontitis with pockets, but it does not usually lead to pocket formation because the necrotic changes involve the gingival and junctional epithelium.

Oral Symptoms

The lesions are *extremely sensitive to touch*, and the patient often complains of a constant radiating, gnawing pain that is intensified by eating spicy or hot foods and chewing. There is a "metallic" foul taste, and the patient is conscious of an excessive amount of "pasty" saliva.

Extraoral and Systemic Signs and Symptoms

Patients are usually ambulatory and have a minimum of systemic symptoms. Local lymphadenopathy and a slight elevation in temperature are common features of the mild and moderate stages of the disease. In severe cases, there may be high fever, increased pulse rate, leukocytosis, loss of appetite, and general lassitude. Systemic reactions are more severe in children. Insomnia, constipation, gastrointestinal disorders, headache, and mental depression sometimes accompany the condition.

In very rare cases, severe sequelae such as gangrenous stomatitis and noma have been described. These patients are almost exclusively encountered in populations in developing countries, especially children with systemic disease or malnutrition.

Clinical Course

The clinical course can vary. If untreated, NUG may lead to NUP where in there is a progressive destruction of the periodontium as well as gingival recession accompanied by an increase in the severity of systemic complications.

Stages in progression of NUG are described by Pindborg and coworkers.

The lesion starts as:

1. Erosion of the tip of the interdental papilla.
2. The lesion involving all of the papilla and also involving the marginal gingiva.
3. The attached gingiva also gets involved.
4. Exposure of the bone with complete loss of interdental papilla, marginal gingiva, and the attached gingiva.

Horning and Cohen extended the staging as follows:

- Stage 1: necrosis of the tip of the interdental papilla (93%).
- Stage 2: necrosis of the entire papilla (19%).
- Stage 3: necrosis extending to the marginal gingiva (21%).
- Stage 4: necrosis of the attached gingiva (1%).
- Stage 5: necrosis involving the buccal and labial mucosa (6%).
- Stage 6: necrosis exposing alveolar bone (1%).
- Stage 7: necrosis perforating skin of the cheek (0%).

According to Horning and Cohen, Stage 1 is NUG, Stage 2 may be either NUG or NUP because attachment loss may have occurred, Stages 3 and 4 would correspond to NUP, Stages 5 and 6 would correspond to necrotizing stomatitis, and Stage 7 would be noma.

Histopathology

Microscopically, the NUG lesion is a nonspecific acute necrotizing inflammation of the gingival margin that involves both the stratified squamous epithelium and the underlying connective tissue. The surface epithelium is destroyed and replaced by a meshwork of fibrin, necrotic epithelial cells, polymorphonuclear leukocytes (neutrophils) (PMNs), and various types of microorganisms (Fig. 15.2). This is the zone that appears clinically as the surface pseudomembrane. At the immediate border of the necrotic pseudomembrane, the epithelium is edematous, and the individual cells exhibit varying degrees of hydropic degeneration. In addition, there is an infiltration of PMNs in the intercellular spaces.

The underlying connective tissue is markedly hyperemic, with numerous engorged capillaries and a dense infiltration of PMNs. This acutely inflamed zone appears clinically as the linear erythema beneath the surface pseudomembrane. Numerous plasma cells may appear in the periphery of the infiltrate; this is interpreted as an area of established chronic gingivitis on which the acute lesion became superimposed.

The epithelium and connective tissue alterations decrease as the distance from the necrotic gingival margin increases, blending gradually with the uninvolved gingiva.

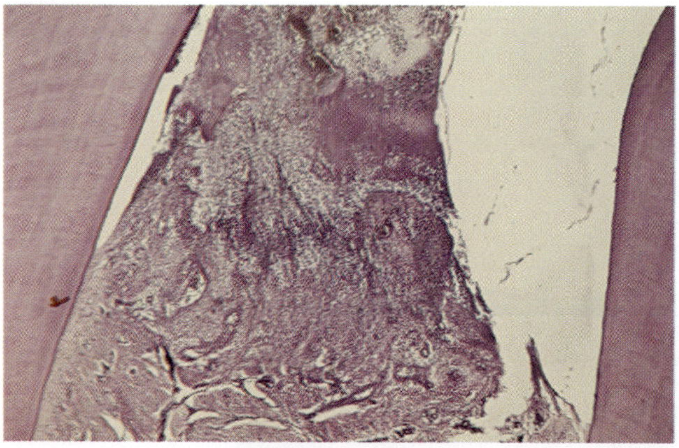

Fig. 15.2 Survey section of interdental papilla in a patient with necrotizing ulcerative gingivitis. The top portion of the section shows the necrotic tissue that forms the gray marginal pseudomembrane. In the lower portion, note the ulceration and the accumulation of leukocytes and fibrin.

It is noteworthy that the microscopic appearance of NUG is nonspecific. Comparable changes result from trauma, chemical irritation, or the application of caustic medications.

Relation of Bacteria to the Necrotizing Ulcerative Gingivitis Lesion

Light and electron microscopy have been used to study the relationship of bacteria to the characteristic lesion of NUG. Light microscopy shows that the exudate on the surface of the necrotic lesion contains microorganisms that morphologically resemble cocci, fusiform bacilli, and spirochetes. The layer between the necrotic and living tissue contains enormous numbers of fusiform bacilli and spirochetes in addition to leukocytes and fibrin. Spirochetes and other bacteria invade the underlying living tissue.

Lisgarten described the following four zones, which blend with each other and may not all be present in every case:

Zone 1: bacterial zone, the most superficial, consists of varied bacteria, including a few spirochetes of small, medium, and large type.

Zone 2: neutrophil rich zone contains numerous leukocytes, preponderant neutrophils with bacteria, including many spirochetes of various types between the leukocytes.

Zone 3: necrotic zone consists of disintegrated tissue cells, fibrillar material, remnants of collagen fibers, and numerous intermediate and large spirochetes with few other organisms.

Zone 4: zone of spirocheteal infiltration consists of well-preserved tissue infiltrated with intermediate and large spirochetes without other organisms.

Spirochetes have been found as deep as 300 μm from the surface. The majority of spirochetes in the deeper zones are morphologically different from cultivated strains of *Treponema microdentium.* They occur in nonnecrotic tissue before other types of bacteria, and they may be present in high concentrations intercellularly in the epithelium adjacent to the ulcerated lesion and in the connective tissue.

Smears from the lesions (Fig. 15.3) show scattered bacteria (predominantly spirochetes and fusiform bacilli), desquamated epithelial cells, and occasional PMNs. Spirochetes and fusiform bacteria are usually seen with other oral spirochetes, vibrios, and filaments.

Diagnosis

Diagnosis is based on clinical findings of gingival pain, ulceration, and bleeding. A bacterial smear is not necessary or definitive because the bacterial picture is not appreciably different from that of

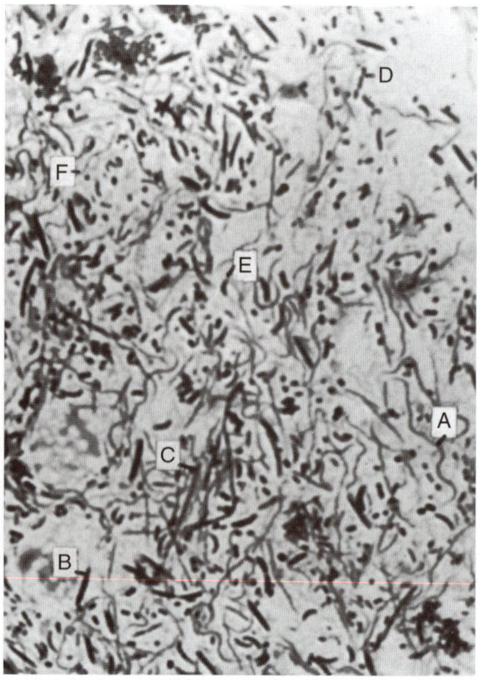

Fig. 15.3 Bacterial smear from a lesion in a patient with necrotizing ulcerative gingivitis. A, Spirochete. B, *Bacillus fusiformis.* C, Filamentous organism (*Actinomyces* or *Leptotrichia*). D, *Streptococcus.* E, *Vibrio.* F, *Treponema microdentium.*

patients with marginal gingivitis, periodontal pockets, pericoronitis, or primary herpetic gingivostomatitis. However, bacterial studies are useful for the differential diagnosis of NUG and specific infections of the oral cavity (e.g., diphtheria, thrush, actinomycosis, streptococcal stomatitis).

The microscopic examination of a biopsy specimen is not sufficiently specific to be diagnostic. It can be used to differentiate NUG from specific infections (e.g., tuberculosis) or from neoplastic disease, but it does not differentiate between NUG and other necrotizing conditions of nonspecific origin, such as those produced by trauma or caustic medications.

KEY FACT

A bacterial smear or culture is not necessary or definitive in the diagnosis of NUG because the bacterial flora is not appreciably different from that of patients with other common inflammatory conditions (e.g., gingivitis, periodontitis). However, bacterial studies are useful for the differential diagnosis of NUG when specific infections of the oral cavity (e.g., diphtheria, thrush, actinomycosis, streptococcal stomatitis) are suspected.

Differential Diagnosis

NUG should be differentiated from other conditions that resemble it in some respects, such as herpetic gingivostomatitis (Table 15.1); chronic periodontitis; desquamative gingivitis (Table 15.2); streptococcal gingivostomatitis; aphthous stomatitis; gonococcal gingivostomatitis; diphtheritic and syphilitic lesions (Table 15.3); tuberculous gingival lesions; candidiasis, agranulocytosis, and dermatoses (pemphigus, erythema multiforme, and lichen planus); and stomatitis venenata. Treatment options for these diseases vary dramatically, and improper treatment may exacerbate the condition. In the case of primary herpetic gingivostomatitis, early diagnosis may result in treatment with antiviral drugs that would be ineffective for NUG, whereas

TABLE 15.1 Differentiation Between Necrotizing Ulcerative Gingivitis and Primary Herpetic Gingivostomatitis

Necrotizing Ulcerative Gingivitis	Primary Herpetic Gingivostomatitis
Etiology: interaction between host and bacteria, most probably fusospirochetes	Specific viral etiology
Necrotizing condition	Diffuse erythema and vesicular eruption
Punched-out gingival margin; pseudomembrane that peels off and leaves raw areas	Vesicles rupture and leave slightly depressed oval or spherical ulcer
Marginal gingiva affected; other oral tissues rarely affected	Diffuse involvement of gingiva; may include buccal mucosa and lips
Uncommon in children	Occurs more frequently in children
No definite duration	Duration of 7–10 days
No demonstrated immunity	Acute episode results in some degree of immunity
Contagion not demonstrated	Contagion

TABLE 15.2 Differentiation Among Necrotizing Ulcerative Gingivitis, Chronic Desquamative Gingivitis, and Chronic Periodontal Disease

Necrotizing Ulcerative Gingivitis	Desquamative Gingivitis	Chronic Destructive Periodontal Disease
Bacterial smears show fusospirochetal complex	Bacterial smears reveal numerous epithelial cells and few bacterial forms	Bacterial smears variable
Marginal gingiva affected	Diffuse involvement of marginal and attached gingivae and other areas of oral mucosa	Marginal gingiva affected
Acute history	Chronic history	Chronic history
Painful	May or may not be painful	Painless if uncomplicated
Pseudomembrane	Patchy desquamation of gingival epithelium	Generally no desquamation, but purulent material may appear from pockets
Papillary and marginal necrotic lesions	Papillae do not undergo necrosis	Papillae do not undergo noticeable necrosis
Affects adults of both genders and occasionally affects children	Affects adults, most often women	Generally found in adults, occasionally found in children
Characteristic fetid odor	No odor	Some odor present but not strikingly fetid

TABLE 15.3 Differentiation Among Necrotizing Ulcerative Gingivitis, Diphtheria, and Secondary Stage of Syphilis

Necrotizing Ulcerative Gingivitis	Diphtheria	Secondary Stage of Syphilis (Mucous Patch)
Etiology: interaction between host and bacteria, most probably fusospirochetes	Specific bacterial etiology: *Corynebacterium diphtheriae*	Specific bacterial etiology: *Treponema pallidum*
Affects marginal gingiva	Rarely affects marginal gingiva	Rarely affects marginal gingiva
Membrane removal easy	Membrane removal difficult	Membrane not detachable
Painful condition	Less painful	Minimal pain
Marginal gingivae affected	Throat, fauces, and tonsils affected	Any part of mouth affected
Serologic findings normal	Serologic findings normal	Serologic findings abnormal[a]
Immunity not conferred	Immunity conferred by an attack	Immunity not conferred
Doubtful contagiousness	Contagion	Only direct contact will communicate disease
Antibiotic therapy relieves symptoms	Antibiotic treatment has minimal effect	Antibiotic therapy has excellent results

[a]Wassermann, Kahn, Venereal Disease Research Laboratories.

the treatment of a case of herpes with the debridement required for NUG could exacerbate the herpes.

Streptococcal gingivostomatitis is a rare condition that is characterized by a diffuse erythema of the gingiva and other areas of the oral mucosa. In some cases, it is confined as a marginal erythema with marginal hemorrhage. Necrosis of the gingival margin is not a feature of this disease, and there is no notable fetid odor. Bacterial smears show a preponderance of streptococcal forms, which were identified as *Streptococcus viridans*, but other studies report findings of group A β-hemolytic streptococcus.

Agranulocytosis is characterized by a marked decrease in the number of circulating PMNs, lesions of the throat and other mucous membranes, and ulceration and necrosis of the gingiva that may resemble that of NUG and that occurs most commonly after chemotherapy in cancer patients or in patients with leukemia. The oral condition of patients with agranulocytosis is primarily necrotizing, but it lacks the severe inflammatory reaction seen with NUG. Blood studies serve to differentiate between NUG and the gingival necrosis associated with agranulocytosis.

Vincent angina is a fusospirochetal infection of the oropharynx and throat as distinguished from NUG, which affects the marginal gingiva. Patients with Vincent's angina have a painful membranous ulceration of the throat, with edema and hyperemic patches breaking down to form ulcers that are covered with pseudomembranous material. The process may extend to the larynx and the middle ear.

NUG in the patient with *leukemia* is not produced by leukemia itself, but it may result from the reduced host defense mechanisms seen with leukemia. In addition, NUG may be superimposed on the gingival tissue alterations caused by leukemia. The differential diagnosis consists not of distinguishing between NUG and leukemic gingival changes but rather of determining whether leukemia is a predisposing factor in the mouth of a patient with NUG. For example, if a patient with necrotizing involvement of the gingival margin also has generalized diffuse discoloration and edema of the attached gingiva, the possibility of an underlying systemically induced gingival change should be considered. Leukemia is one of the conditions that would need to be ruled out.

NUG in the patient with *human immunodeficiency virus infection* has the same clinical features, although it often follows an extremely destructive course that leads to NUP, with a loss of soft tissue and bone and the formation of bony sequestra.

KEY FACT

A serious systemic disease or condition, such as leukemia or acquired immunodeficiency syndrome (AIDS), that renders the host immunocompromised can be the predisposing causative factor leading to acute gingival disease.

Etiology

Role of Bacteria

Plaut, in 1894, and Vincent, in 1896, postulated that NUG was caused by specific bacteria: fusiform bacillus and a spirochetal organism.

Opinions still differ with regard to whether bacteria are the primary causative factors of NUG. Several observations support this concept, including that spirochetal organisms and fusiform bacilli are always found in patients with the disease, with other organisms also involved. Rosebury et al. described a fusospirochetal complex that consists of *T. microdentium*, intermediate spirochetes, vibrios, fusiform bacilli, and filamentous organisms in addition to several *Borrelia* species.

Loesche et al. described a predominant constant flora and a variable flora associated with NUG. The constant flora is composed of *Prevotella intermedia* in addition to *Fusobacterium*, *Treponema*, and *Selenomonas* species. The variable flora consists of a heterogeneous array of bacterial types.

Treatment with metronidazole results in a significant reduction of *Treponema* species, *P. intermedia*, and *Fusobacterium*, with resolution of the clinical symptoms. The antibacterial spectrum of this drug provides evidence for the anaerobic members of the flora as etiologic agents.

These bacteriologic findings have been supported by immunologic data that demonstrated increased immunoglobulin G and M antibody titers for medium-sized spirochetes and *P. intermedia* in patients with NUG as compared to titers in those patients with chronic gingivitis and healthy controls.

Role of the Host Response

Regardless of whether specific bacteria are implicated in the etiology of NUG, the presence of these organisms appears to be insufficient to cause the disease.

In the first place, the fusiform–spirochete flora is frequently found in patients who do not have NUG. In addition, exudates from NUG lesions produce fusospirochetal abscesses rather than typical NUG when such exudates are inoculated subcutaneously into experimental animals.

The role of an impaired host response in NUG has long been recognized. Even in the early descriptions of the disease, NUG was associated with physical and emotional stress as well as decreased resistance to infection. NUG has not been produced experimentally in humans or animals by only the inoculation of bacterial exudates from the lesions. In the animal model, local or systemic immunosuppression with glucocorticoids (e.g., ketoconazole) results in more characteristic lesions of NUG in infected animals. Furthermore, NUG is not found in well-nourished individuals with a fully functional immune system. All of the predisposing factors for NUG are associated with immunosuppression. Cogen et al. described a depression in host defense mechanisms, particularly in PMN chemotaxis and phagocytosis, in patients with NUG.

It is essential for the clinician to determine the predisposing factors that lead to immunodeficiency in patients with NUG to address the continued susceptibility of the patient and to determine whether an underlying systemic disease is present. Immunodeficiency may be related to varying levels of nutritional deficiency, fatigue caused by chronic sleep deprivation, other health habits (e.g., alcohol or drug abuse), psychosocial factors, or systemic disease. Importantly, NUG may be the presenting symptom for patients with immunosuppression related to human immunodeficiency virus infection.

Local Predisposing Factors

Preexisting gingivitis, injury to the gingiva, and smoking are important predisposing factors. Although NUG may appear in an otherwise disease-free mouth, it most often occurs superimposed on preexisting chronic gingival disease and periodontal pockets. Deep periodontal pockets and pericoronal flaps are particularly vulnerable areas because they offer a favorable environment for the proliferation of anaerobic fusiform bacilli and spirochetes. Areas of the gingiva that are traumatized by opposing teeth in malocclusion (e.g., the palatal surface behind the maxillary incisors, the labial gingival surface of the mandibular incisors) may predispose an individual to the development of NUG.

The relationship between NUG and *smoking* has often been mentioned in the literature. Pindborg reported that 98% of his patients with NUG were smokers and that the frequency of this disease increases with increasing exposure to tobacco smoke. The effect of smoking on periodontal disease in general has been the subject of numerous studies during the past two decades, and smoking has been established as a high risk factor for disease.

Systemic Predisposing Factors

NUG is not found in a well-nourished individual with a fully functional immune system. Therefore, it is important for the clinician to determine the predisposing factors that lead to immunodeficiency. Again, immunodeficiency may be related to varying levels of nutritional deficiency; fatigue caused by chronic sleep deficiency; other health habits (e.g., alcohol or drug abuse); and systemic disease (e.g., diabetes, debilitating infection).

Nutritional Deficiency

Necrotizing gingivitis has been produced in animals by giving them nutritionally deficient diets. Several researchers found an increase in the fusospirochetal flora in the mouths of the experimental animals, but the bacteria were regarded as opportunists that proliferate only when the tissues were altered by the deficiency. A poor diet has been cited as a predisposing factor for NUG and its sequelae in developing African countries although the effects appear primarily to diminish the effectiveness of the immune response.

Nutritional deficiencies (e.g., vitamin C, vitamin B_2) accentuate the severity of the pathologic changes induced when the fusospirochetal bacterial complex is injected into animals.

Debilitating Disease

Debilitating systemic disease may predispose patients to the development of NUG. Such systemic disturbances include chronic diseases (e.g., syphilis, cancer), severe gastrointestinal disorders (e.g., ulcerative colitis), blood dyscrasias (e.g., leukemia, anemia), and acquired immunodeficiency syndrome. Nutritional deficiency that results from debilitating disease may be an additional predisposing factor. Experimentally induced leukopenia in animals may produce ulcerative gangrenous stomatitis. Ulceronecrotic lesions appear in the gingival margins of hamsters that are exposed to total body irradiation; these lesions can be prevented with systemic antibiotics.

Psychosomatic Factors

Psychologic factors appear to be important in the etiology of NUG. The disease often occurs in association with stressful situations (e.g., induction into the armed forces, school examinations). Psychologic disturbances as well as increased adrenocortical secretion are also common in patients with the disease.

A significant correlation between disease incidence and two personality traits—dominance and abasement—suggests the presence of a NUG-prone personality. Data from a study evaluating the relationship between personality traits and stress with gingival inflammation and soft tissue pathology in military recruits found that gingival inflammation correlated significantly with personality traits (e.g., tolerance to change, anxiety).

The mechanisms whereby psychologic factors create or predispose an individual to gingival damage have not been established, but alterations in digital and gingival capillary responses that suggest increased autonomic nervous activity have been demonstrated in patients with NUG.

It can be concluded that opportunistic bacteria are the primary etiologic agents of NUG in patients who demonstrate immunosuppression. Stress, smoking, and preexisting gingivitis are common predisposing factors.

Epidemiology and Prevalence

The prevalence of NUG appears to have been rather low in the United States and Europe before 1914. During World Wars I and II, numerous "epidemics" broke out among the Allied troops, but German soldiers did not seem to have been similarly affected. Epidemic-like outbreaks have also occurred among civilian populations. A study at a dental clinic in Prague, Czech Republic, reported the incidence of NUG as 0.08% among patients between the ages of 15 and 19 years old, 0.05% among those 20–24 years old, and 0.02% among those 25–29 years old.

NUG occurs in individuals of all ages, with the highest incidence reported in patients between the ages of 15 and 30 years. It is not common among children in the United States, Canada, and Europe, but it has been reported in children from low socioeconomic groups in underdeveloped countries. In India, 54% and 58% of patients in two studies were less than 10 years old.

In a random school population in Nigeria, NUG occurred in 11.3% of children between the ages of 2 and 6 years old. In a Nigerian hospital population, it was present in 23% of children who were less than 10 years old. It has been reported in several members of the same family in low socioeconomic groups. NUG is more common among children with Down syndrome than among other children with mental deficiencies.

Opinions differ with regard to whether NUG is more common during the winter, summer, or fall and whether there is a peak seasonal incidence.

Communicability

NUG often occurs in groups in an epidemic pattern. At one time, NUG was considered contagious and involved required reporting to the community health department, but it was later concluded not to be communicable. A distinction must be made between "communicability" and "transmissibility" when referring to the characteristics of disease. The term *transmissible* denotes a capacity for the maintenance of an infectious agent in successive passages through a susceptible animal host. The term *communicable* signifies a capacity for the maintenance of infection by natural modes of spread, such as direct contact through drinking water, food, and eating utensils; via the airborne route; or by means of arthropod vectors. A disease that is communicable is described as *contagious.* It has been demonstrated that disease associated with the fusospirochetal bacterial complex is transmissible; however, *it has not been shown to be communicable or contagious.*

Attempts have been made to spread NUG from human to human without success. King traumatized an area in his gingiva and introduced debris from a patient with a severe case of NUG. There was no response until he happened to fall ill shortly thereafter; subsequent to his illness, he observed the characteristic lesion in the experimental area. It may be inferred with reservation from this experiment that systemic debility is a prerequisite for the contagion of NUG.

It is a common impression that, because NUG often occurs among groups that use the same kitchen facilities, the disease is spread by bacteria on eating utensils. However, the growth of fusospirochetal organisms requires carefully controlled conditions and an anaerobic environment; they do not ordinarily survive on eating utensils.

The occurrence of NUG in epidemic-like outbreaks does not necessarily mean that it is contagious. The affected groups may be afflicted by the disease as a result of common predisposing factors rather than because of its spread from person to person. In all likelihood, both a predisposed immunocompromised host and the presence of appropriate bacteria are necessary for the production of this disease.

KEY FACT

Although certain bacteria (e.g., fusospirochetal complex) are likely responsible for the lesions observed in necrotizing ulcerative gingivitis, immunocompromise appears to be a necessary predisposing condition for the disease.

Primary Herpetic Gingivostomatitis

Primary herpetic gingivostomatitis is an infection of the oral cavity caused by herpes simplex virus (HSV) type 1. It occurs most often among infants and children who are less than 6 years old, but it is also seen in adolescents and adults. It occurs with equal frequency in male and female patients. In most individuals, however, the primary infection is asymptomatic.

As part of the primary infection, the virus ascends through the sensory and autonomic nerves, where it persists as latent HSV in neuronal ganglia that innervate the site. In approximately one-third of the world's population, secondary manifestations or recurrent

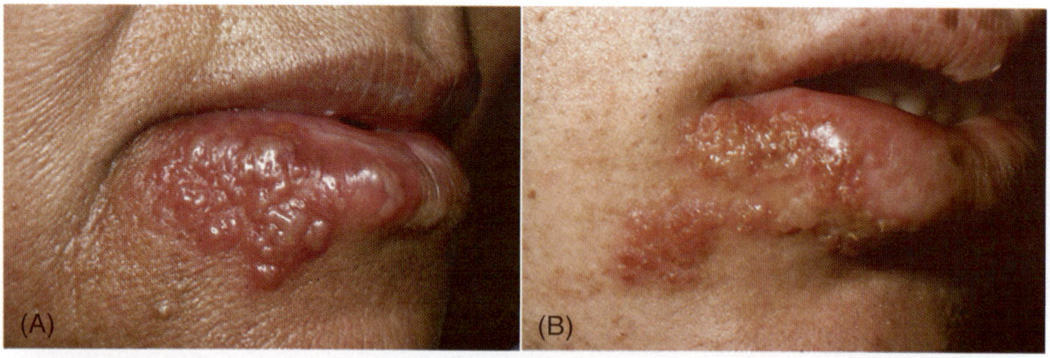

Fig. 15.4 Recurrent herpetic vesicles in the lip. A, early stage and B, late stage showing brownish crusted lesions. *(From Sapp JP, Eversole, LR, Wysocki GP:* Contemporary oral and maxillofacial pathology, *ed 2, St Louis, 2002, Mosby.)*

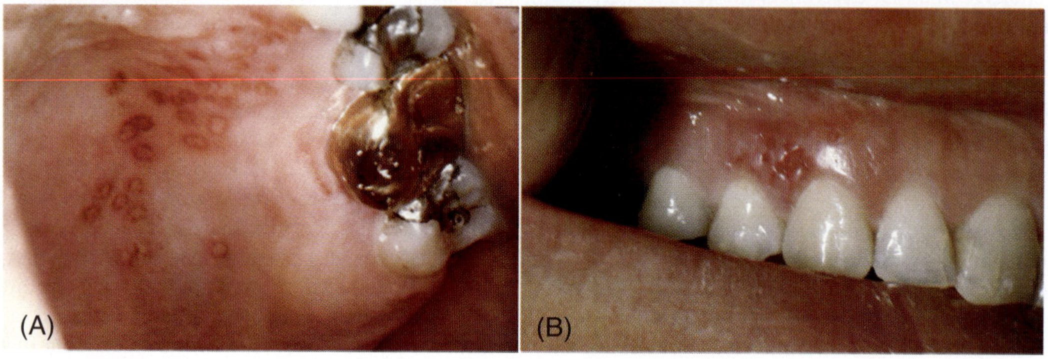

Fig. 15.5 Recurrent intraoral herpetic vesicles, A, in the palate and B, in the gingiva. The latter location is rare. *(From Sapp JP, Eversole, LR, Wysocki GP:* Contemporary oral and maxillofacial pathology, *ed 2, St Louis, 2002, Mosby.)*

herpetic episodes will occur. These recurrent outbreaks may be precipitated by dental treatment, respiratory infection, sunlight exposure, fever, trauma, exposure to chemicals, or emotional stress in individuals with a history of herpes virus infection. Secondary manifestations include (Fig. 15.4) herpes labialis, herpetic stomatitis, herpes genitalis, ocular herpes, and herpetic encephalitis. Secondary herpetic stomatitis can occur on the palate, on the gingiva (Fig. 15.5), or on the mucosa as a result of dental treatment that traumatizes or stimulates the latent virus in the ganglia that innervates the area. It may manifest as pain away from the site of treatment 2 to 4 days later. Careful inspection for characteristic vesicles can be diagnostic

Clinical Features

Oral Signs

Primary herpetic gingivostomatitis appears as a diffuse, erythematous, shiny involvement of the gingiva and the adjacent oral mucosa, with varying degrees of edema and gingival bleeding. During its initial stage, it is characterized by the presence of discrete, spherical gray vesicles, which may occur on the gingiva, the labial and buccal mucosae, the soft palate, the pharynx, the sublingual mucosa, and the tongue (Fig. 15.6). After approximately 24 h, the vesicles rupture and form painful small ulcers with red, elevated, halo-like margins and depressed yellowish or grayish-white central portions. These occur either in widely separated areas or in clusters where confluence occurs (Fig. 15.7).

Occasionally, primary herpetic gingivitis may occur without overt vesiculation. The clinical picture consists of diffuse, erythematous, shiny discoloration, and edematous enlargement of the gingivae with a tendency toward bleeding.

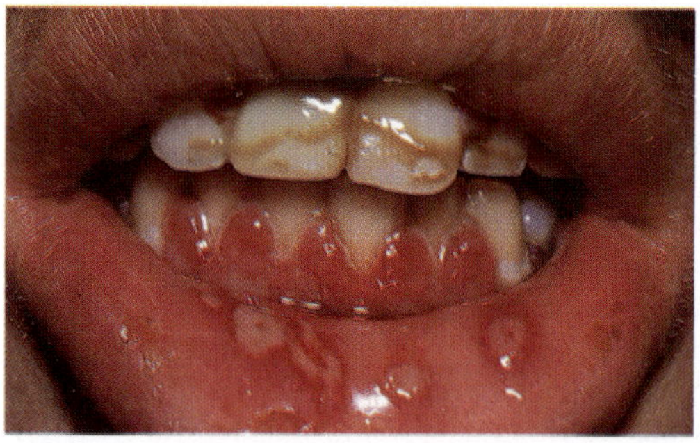

Fig. 15.6 Primary herpetic gingivostomatitis in a 12-year-old boy, with diffuse erythematous involvement of the gingiva and a spherical gray vesicle in the lip. *(Courtesy: Dr Heddie Sedano, University of California, Los Angeles, and University of Minnesota.)*

The course of the disease is limited to 7–10 days. The diffuse gingival erythema and edema that appear early during the course of the disease persist for several days after the ulcerative lesions have healed. Scarring does not occur in the areas of healed ulcerations.

Oral Symptoms

The disease is accompanied by generalized "soreness" of the oral cavity, which interferes with eating, drinking, and oral hygiene. The ruptured vesicles are the focal sites of pain; they are particularly sensitive to touch, thermal changes, foods such as condiments and fruit juices, and the action of coarse foods. In infants, the disease is marked by irritability and refusal to take food.

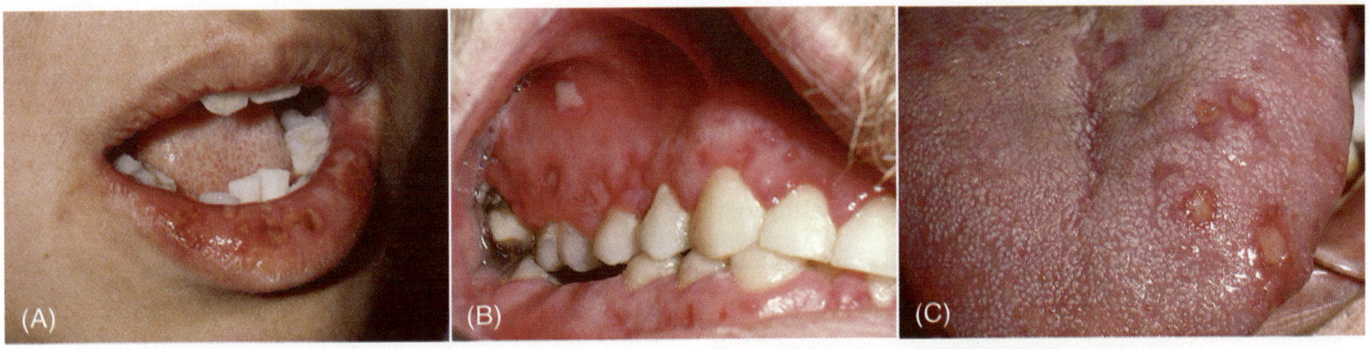

Fig. 15.7 A–C, Involvement of the lip, gingiva, and tongue in primary herpetic gingivostomatitis. *(From Sapp JP, Eversole, LR, Wysocki GP:* Contemporary oral and maxillofacial pathology, *ed 2, St Louis, 2002, Mosby.)*

Extraoral and Systemic Signs and Symptoms

Cervical adenitis, fever as high as 101°F–105°F (38°C–40.6°C), and generalized malaise are common.

History

Primary herpetic gingivostomatitis is the result of an acute infection by HSV, and it has an acute onset.

Histopathology

The virus targets the epithelial cells, which show "ballooning degeneration" that consists of acantholysis, nuclear clearing, and nuclear enlargement. These cells are called *Tzanck cells.* Infected cells fuse to form multinucleated cells, and intercellular edema leads to the formation of intraepithelial vesicles that rupture and develop a secondary inflammatory response with a fibropurulent exudate (Fig. 15.8). Discrete ulcerations that result from the rupture of the vesicles have a central portion of acute inflammation, with varying degrees of purulent exudate surrounded by engorged blood vessels.

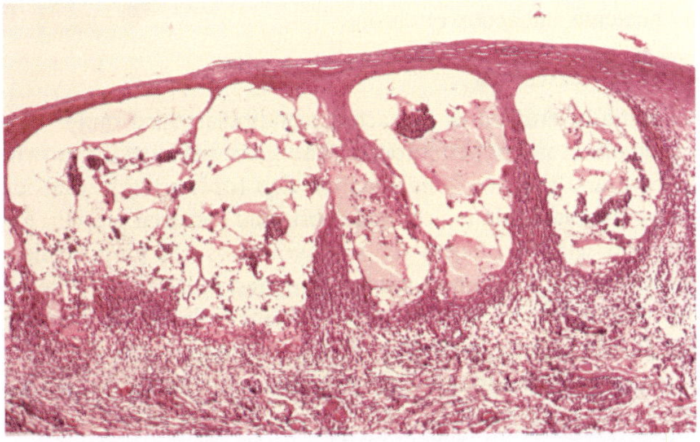

Fig. 15.8 Biopsy showing intraepithelial viral vesicles that contain fluid and debris, with a large number of viruses and virally altered epithelial cells (i.e., Tzanck cells). *(Courtesy: Dr Heddie Sedano, University of California, Los Angeles, and University of Minnesota.)*

Diagnosis

It is critical to arrive at a diagnosis as early as possible in a patient with a primary herpetic infection. Treatment with antiviral medications can dramatically alter the course of the disease by reducing symptoms and potentially reducing recurrences. The diagnosis is usually established from the patient's history and the clinical findings. Material may be obtained from the lesions and submitted to the laboratory for confirmatory tests, including virus culture and immunologic tests that involve the use of monoclonal antibodies or deoxyribonucleic acid hybridization techniques. This should not delay treatment if strong clinical evidence exists for primary gingivostomatitis.

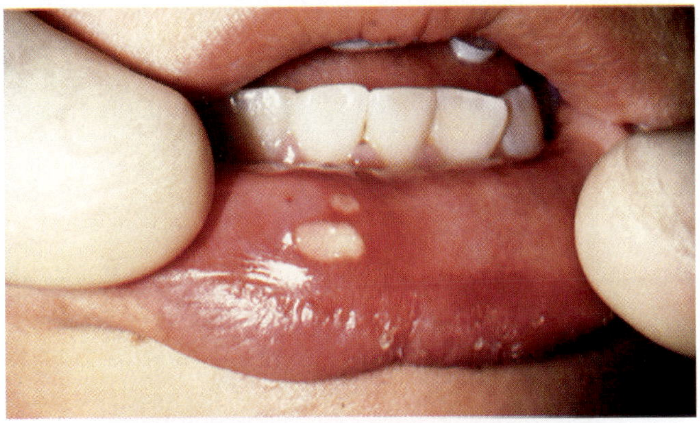

Fig. 15.9 Aphthous lesion in the lip. The depressed gray center is surrounded by an elevated red border. *(From Sapp JP, Eversole, LR, Wysocki GP:* Contemporary oral and maxillofacial pathology, *ed 2, St Louis, 2002, Mosby.)*

Differential Diagnosis

Primary herpetic gingivostomatitis should be differentiated from several conditions.

Lesions of *recurrent aphthous stomatitis* (RAS) range from occasionally small (0.5–1 cm in diameter), well-defined, round or ovoid shallow ulcers with a yellowish-gray central area surrounded by an erythematous halo, which heal in 7–10 days without scarring, to larger (1–3 cm in diameter) oval or irregular ulcers, which persist for weeks and heal with scarring (Fig. 15.9). The cause is unknown although immunopathologic mechanisms appear to play a role. RAS is a different clinical entity from primary herpetic gingivostomatitis. The ulcerations may look the same for the two conditions, but diffuse erythematous involvement of the gingiva and acute toxic systemic symptoms do not occur with RAS. A history of previous episodes of painful mucosal ulcerations suggests RAS rather than primary HSV.

Communicability

Primary herpetic gingivostomatitis is contagious. Most adults have developed immunity to HSV as a result of infection during childhood, which, in most cases, is subclinical. For this reason, acute herpetic gingivostomatitis usually occurs in infants and children. Recurrent herpetic gingivostomatitis has been reported although it is not often clinically significant unless immunity is destroyed by debilitating systemic disease. Studies that have demonstrated HSV in periodontal pockets suggest more recurrence of viral replication than has previously been recognized. Secondary herpetic infection of the skin, such as herpes labialis, does recur.

KEY FACT

Acute herpetic gingivostomatitis usually occurs in infants and children because most adults have developed immunity to herpes simplex virus from childhood exposure, often with mild or no symptoms.

Pericoronitis

The term *pericoronitis* refers to inflammation of the gingiva in relation to the crown of an incompletely erupted tooth (Fig. 15.10). It occurs most often in the mandibular third molar area. Pericoronitis may be acute, subacute, or chronic.

Clinical Features

The partially erupted or impacted mandibular third molar is the most common site of pericoronitis. The space between the crown of the tooth and the overlying gingival flap (operculum) is an ideal area for the accumulation of food debris and bacterial growth. Even in patients with no clinical signs or symptoms, the gingival flap is often chronically inflamed and infected, and it has varying degrees of ulceration along its inner surface. Acute inflammatory involvement is a constant possibility; it may be exacerbated by trauma, occlusion, or a foreign body trapped underneath the tissue flap (e.g., popcorn husk and nut fragment).

Acute pericoronitis is identified by varying degrees of inflammatory involvement of the pericoronal flap and adjacent structures as well as by systemic complications. The inflammatory fluid and cellular exudate increase the bulk of the flap, which then may interfere with complete closure of the jaws and which can be traumatized by contact with the opposing jaw, thereby aggravating the inflammatory involvement.

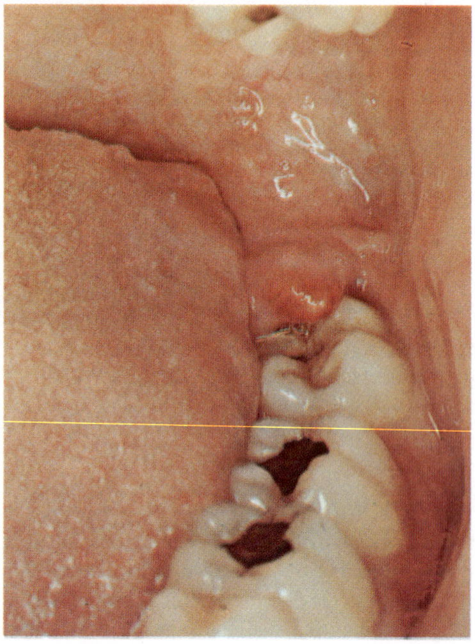

Fig. 15.10 Pericoronitis. An inflamed coronal flap is covering the disto-occlusal surface of the impacted mandibular third molar. Note the swelling and redness. *(From Glickman I, Smulow J:* Periodontal disease: clinical, radiographic and histopathologic features, *Philadelphia, 1974, Saunders.)*

The resultant clinical picture is a red, swollen, suppurating lesion that is exquisitely tender, with radiating pains to the ear, the throat, and the floor of the mouth. The patient is extremely uncomfortable as a result of pain, a foul taste, and an inability to close the jaws. Swelling of the cheek in the region of the angle of the jaw and lymphadenitis are common findings. Trismus may also be a presenting complaint. In addition, the patient may have systemic complications such as fever, leukocytosis, and malaise.

Complications

Involvement may be localized in the form of a pericoronal abscess. It may spread posteriorly into the oropharyngeal area and medially to the base of the tongue, thereby making it difficult for the patient to swallow. Depending on the severity and extent of the infection, there may be involvement of the submaxillary, posterior cervical, deep cervical, and retropharyngeal lymph nodes. Peritonsillar abscess formation, cellulitis, and Ludwig's angina are infrequent but potential sequelae of acute pericoronitis.

Conclusion

Acute gingival diseases are similar in that they typically manifest with painful intraoral or perioral lesions and there is a need for urgent treatment to relieve symptoms. However, each case requires careful assessment and an accurate diagnosis, including identification of risk factors. In many cases, there are systemic risk factors that increase susceptibility to acute gingival disease.

Key points

- Necrotizing ulcerative gingivitis (NUG) can cause tissue destruction involving the periodontal attachment apparatus, mainly in patients with long-standing disease or severe immunosuppression. When it involves bone loss, the condition is termed as "nectrotizing ulcerative periodontitis (NUP)."
- Characteristic lesions are punched-out crater-like depressions at the crest of the interdental papillae, subsequently extending to the marginal, attached gingiva and oral mucosa.
- Gray, pseudomembranous slough covers the gingival craters.
- Spontaneous gingival hemorrhage or pronounced bleeding after the slightest stimulation is an additional characteristic clinical sign of NUG. Fetid odor, metallic taste, and increased pasty salivation are also noticed.
- NUG or NUP does not lead to periodontal pocket formation because the necrotic changes involve the marginal gingiva.
- Extraoral and systemic signs and symptoms include elevation of temperature, loss of appetite, headache, and mental depression.
- Light microscopy shows cocci, fusiform bacilli, and spirochetes.
- Diagnosis is based on clinical finishing of gingival pain, ulceration, and bleeding.
- Primary herpetic gingivostomatitis is an infection of the oral cavity caused by the herpes simplex virus type I. It often occurs in infants and children younger than 6 years of age but is also seen in adolescents and adults.
- As a part of the primary infection, the virus ascends through sensory and autonomic nerves, where it persists as latent HSV in neuronal ganglia that innervate the site.
- In histologic view, the virus targets the epithelial cells, which show "ballooning degeneration" consisting of acantholysis, nuclear clearing, and nuclear enlargement. The cells are called "Tzanck cells."
- The term pericoronitis refers to inflammation of the gingiva in relation to the crown of an incompletely erupted tooth. It occurs mostly in mandibular molars.

Suggested Readings

Horning GM, Cohen ME: Necrotizing ulcerative gingivitis, periodontitis and stomatitis: clinical staging and predisposing factors, *J Periodontol* 66:990, 1995.

Johnson BD, Engel D: Acute necrotizing gingivitis. A review of diagnosis, etiology and treatment, *J Periodontol* 7:141, 1986.

Listgarten MA, Lewis DW: The distribution of spirochetes in the lesion of acute necrotizing ulcerative gingivitis: an electron microscopic and statistical survey, *J Periodontol* 38:379, 1967.

Loesche WJ, Syed SA, Langhorn BE, et al: The bacteriology of acute necrotizing ulcerative gingivitis, *J Periodontol* 53:223, 1982.

McCarthy PL, Shklar G: *Diseases of the oral mucosa*, ed 2, Philadelphia, 1980, Lea & Febiger.

Sapp JP, Eversole LR, Wysocki GP: *Contemporary oral and maxillofacial pathology*, ed 2, St. Louis, 2004, Mosby.

Shannon IL, Kilgore WG, Leary TJ: Stress as a predisposing factor in necrotizing ulcerative gingivitis, *J Periodontol* 40:240, 1969.

References

References and MCQs with answers for the chapter are available on www.medenact.com.

CHAPTER 16

Desquamative Gingivitis

A Aguirre | JLT Vazquez | Y Mair | CD Dwarakanath

CHAPTER OUTLINE

Desquamative Gingivitis

Desquamative gingival lesions are unusual disorders which have been recognized for over a century. They were called by various names and different etiological factors were proposed like nutritional deficiency, degeneration, and hormonal derangement. Tomes and Tomes reported this in 1894, Goodby mentioned in his book in 1923, and the term chronic diffuse desquamative gingivitis was given by Prinz in 1932. Merrit and Sorin published articles in 1933, whereas Schour and Massler gave the term "gingivosis" in anemic hospitalized children of postwar Italy in 1947. But the classic description and classification were provided by McCarthy and others in 1960, followed by inputs from Glickman and Smulow and Ziskin and Zegareli.

Definition

Desquamative gingivitis is defined as an unusual, unique, nonplaque associated gingivitis, characterized by intense diffuse erythema and desquamation (peeling) of the surface epithelium. It is often associated with ulceration of the marginal and attached gingiva. It is not a specific disease entity but a clinical manifestation of a variety of conditions.

Classification

Based on the etiological considerations, desquamative gingival lesions are classified as under.

This is a modification of the original classification formulated by McCarthy and others.

Dermatoses:

1. Lichen planus (Fig. 16.1)
2. Benign mucous membrane phemphigoid (cicatricial phemphigoid)
3. Bullous phemphigoid
4. Pemphigus vulgaris (Fig. 16.2)
5. Psoriasis
6. Linear immunoglobulin A disease
7. Dermatitis herptiformis
8. Lupus erythematosus
9. Erythema multiforme

Endocrinal imbalance:

1. Estrogen deficiency in females (menopause, following hysterectomy and oopharectomy)
2. Testosterone deficiency in males

Chronic infections:

1. Tuberculosis
2. Chronic candidiasis
3. Histoplasmosis

Idiopathic

Drug reactions (lichenoid reactions):

1. Toxic antimetabolites
2. Allergic barbiturates, antibiotics, and certain dental materials (Fig. 16.3)

Others (conditions which mimic desquamative gingivitis):

1. Crohn's disease
2. Chronic ulcerative stomatitis
3. Plasma cell gingivitis (Fig. 16.4)
4. Graft versus host disease
5. Factitious lesions
6. Kindler syndrome
7. Wegener's granulomatosis
8. Foreign body gingivitis

Upon perusal of the above list, it becomes clear that the exact diagnosis of the condition resulting in desquamative gingivitis is very vital to establish a correct therapeutic approach for effective management. Despite the use of clinical and laboratory parameters, including histopathologic and immunofluorescence studies, the cause of desquamative gingivitis cannot be elucidated in up to one-third of the cases. However, a majority of the cases seen in the clinical practice belong to lichen planus, mucous membrane pemphigoid, and pemphigus.

Clinical Features of Desquamative Gingivitis

It is important that the clinician is familiar with the various terms used to describe mucosal and skin lesions. A few of them have been defined below:

- A "**Macule**" is a circumscribed flat area less than 1 cm of discoloration without elevation or depression of relative surface. For example, erythema multiforme, hemangiomas, Koplik spots.

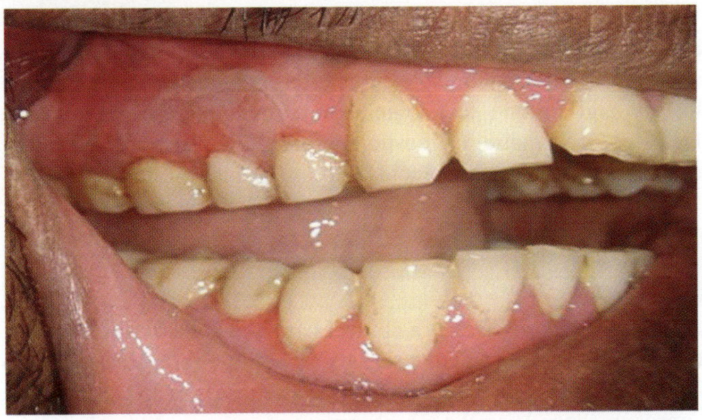

Fig. 16.1 Desquamative gingivitis with lichen planus.

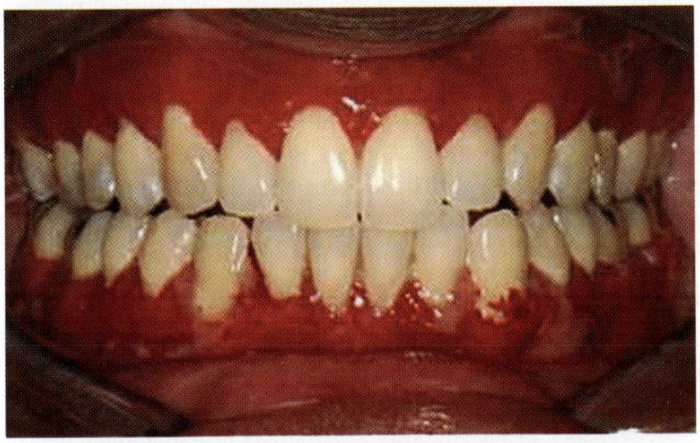

Fig. 16.2 Desquamtive gingivitis with pemphigus vulgaris.

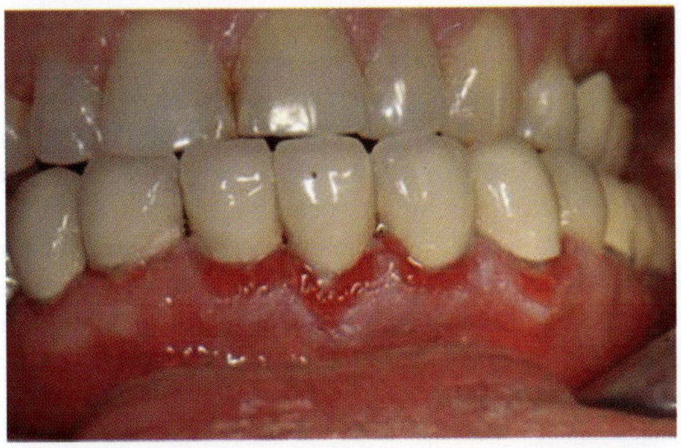

Fig. 16.3 Lichenoid reaction due to allergy to acrylic crowns.

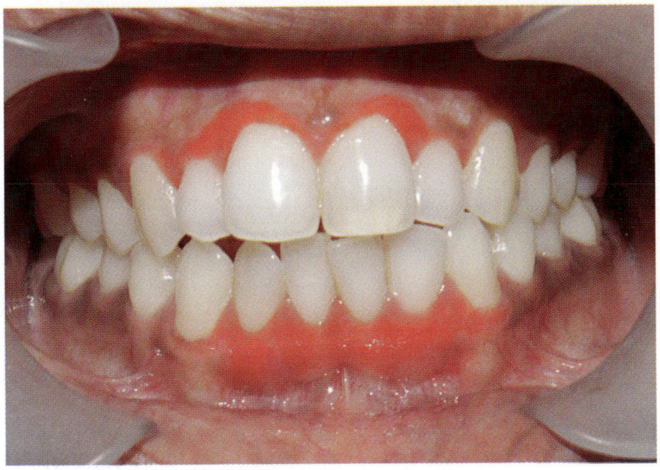

Fig. 16.4 Plasma cell gingivitis.

- A "**Papule**" is a circumscribed, elevated solid lesion less than 1 cm in diameter. For example, papilloma.
- A "**Patch**" is a circumscribed flat area more than 1 cm. For example, secondary syphilitic mucosal patch.
- A "**Vesicle**" is a small superficial circumscribed elevated lesion less than 0.5 cm that contains serous fluid. For example, herpetic gingivitis, erythema multiforme.
- A "**Bulla**" is a bigger vesicle (>0.5 cm).
- A "**Nodule**" is a palpable, solid lesion greater than 1 cm in diameter found in the skin (e.g., xanthoma).
- A "**Pustule**" is an elevated, circumscribed lesion that contains pus. For example, anthrax.
- An "**Ulcer**" is a break in the continuity of the epithelium due to molecular disintegration.
- A "**Purpura**" is a reddish to purple flat lesion caused by blood from vesicles leaking into submucosal tissue. Does not blanch when pressed. Classified as petechiae or ecchymosis depending on the size.
- **Nikolsky's sign** refers to the ability to induce peeling of a bulla as a consequence of applying lateral pressure to the border of an intact bulla. It is used to identify suprabasal or intraepithelial splits in the lesion. It is found in pemphigus.
- **Auspitz sign** is the appearance of punctate bleeding spots when a psoriasis lesion is scrapped off.
- **Tzanck cell** is a degenerated cell from the epithelium disconnected from adjacent cells caused by acantholysis seen in pemphigus.
- **Acantholysis** is the loss of intercellular connection such as desmosomes, resulting in loss of cohesion between kertinocytes. It is present in pemphigus vulgaris but absent in bullous pemphigoid.

Desquamative gingival lesions are seen in about 1.5%–2.5% of population with females being more affected than males. It is most common in the third or fourth decade of life but can be seen in younger individuals. Patients may be asymptomatic; when symptomatic their complaints range from burning sensation to severe pain. Approximately 50% of the cases are confined to gingiva but other intraoral and dermatological involvement may be found. Lesions such as pemphigus vulgaris have systemic impact, which transcends the boundaries of the oral cavity and results in significant morbidity and even mortality.

Glickman and Smulow have described three forms of desquamative gingivitis, viz. mild, moderate, and severe.

Mild form (Fig. 16.5):

1. Diffuse erythema.
2. Condition is usually painless.
3. Some blanching may be seen.
4. Patients may complain of intolerance to hot and spicy foods.

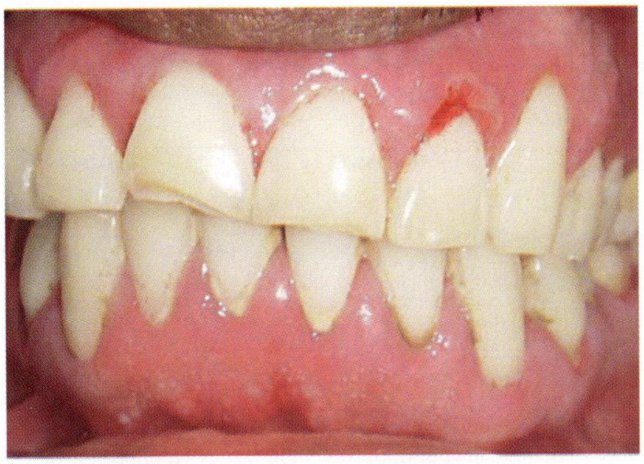

Fig. 16.5 Mild form of desquamative gingivitis.

Moderate form (Fig. 16.6):

1. Patchy distribution of bright red and gray areas.
2. Smooth, shiny, soft gingiva.
3. Burning sensation, sensitivity to temperature.
4. Inhalation of air may be painful.
5. Massaging the gingiva results in peeling of the epithelium with bleeding on brushing.
6. Intolerance to spicy foods, citrus fruits, and drinks.
7. Brushing is highly discomforting.

Severe form (Fig. 16.7):

1. Wide areas of the oral cavity involved.
2. Surface epithelium appears shredded.
3. Blowing of air causes a bubble in gingival epithelium.
4. Very painful.
5. Constant dry, burning sensation.

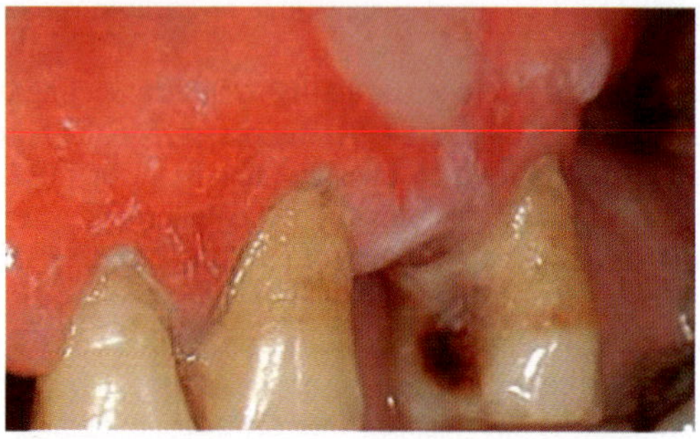

Fig. 16.6 Moderate form of desquamative gingivitis.

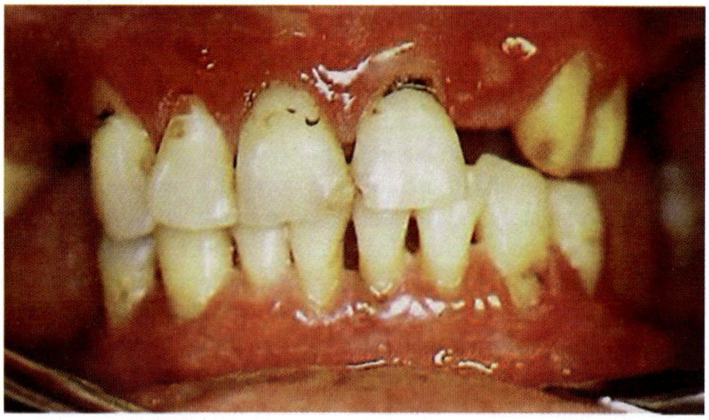

Fig 16.7 Severe form of desquamative gingivitis.

It is important to ascertain the disease responsible for desquamative gingivitis to establish the appropriate therapeutic approach. To achieve this goal, a clinical examination is coupled with a thorough history and routine histologic and immunofluorescence studies. Despite a systematic diagnostic approach, the cause of desquamative gingivitis cannot be elucidated in up to one-third of cases.

Diagnosis of Desquamative Gingivitis: A Systematic Approach

Desquamative gingivitis is a clinical term and not a diagnosis. After the condition is identified, a series of laboratory procedures should be used to arrive at a final diagnosis. The success of any therapeutic approach depends on the establishment of an accurate final diagnosis. The following sections describe a systematic approach to determining the disease that triggers desquamative gingivitis (Fig. 16.8).

History

A thorough history is mandatory to begin the assessment of desquamative gingivitis. Data regarding the symptoms associated with this condition and its historical aspects (e.g., lesion onset, whether it has worsened, habits that exacerbate it) provide the foundation for a thorough examination. Information about previous therapy to alleviate the condition should be documented.

Clinical Examination

The distribution pattern of the lesions (e.g., focal or multifocal, with or without confinement to gingival tissues) provides information that can begin to narrow the differential diagnosis. A simple clinical maneuver such as the Nikolsky's sign offers insight into the plausibility of a vesiculobullous disorder.

Biopsy

Given the extent and number of lesions that may be present in an individual, an incisional biopsy is the best strategy for beginning the microscopic and immunologic evaluation. An important consideration is the selection of the biopsy site. A perilesional incisional biopsy should avoid areas of ulceration because necrosis and epithelial denudation severely hamper the diagnostic process.

After the tissue is excised from the oral cavity, the specimen can be bisected and then submitted for microscopic examination. Buffered formalin (10%) should be used to fix the tissue for conventional hematoxylin and eosin (H&E) evaluation. Michel's

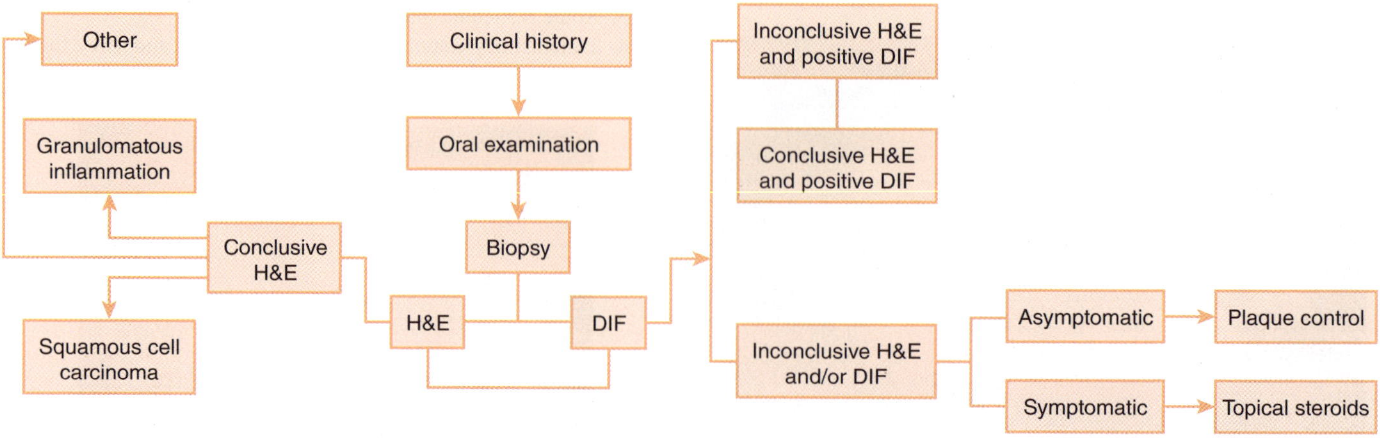

Fig. 16.8 The diagnostic approach for desquamative gingivitis includes hematoxylin and eosin (H&E) and direct immunofluorescence (DIF) evaluation of biopsy specimens.

buffer (i.e., ammonium sulfate buffer, pH 7.0) is used as the transport solution for immunofluorescence assessment. An incisional biopsy of uninvolved (normal) mucosa typically shows the same immunofluorescent findings as the biopsy of the perilesional tissue. However, there are notable exceptions, such as lichen planus and chronic cutaneous lupus erythematosus, in which only the lesional tissue exhibits the corresponding immunologic markers (Table 16.1).

Microscopic Examination

Sections of approximately 5 μm of formalin-fixed, paraffin-embedded tissue stained with conventional H&E are obtained for light microscopy examination.

Immunofluorescence

For *direct* immunofluorescence, unfixed frozen sections are incubated with a variety of fluorescein-labeled, antihuman serum

TABLE 16.1 Diagnostic Findings for Conditions That Can Manifest as Desquamative Gingivitis

		DIRECT IMMUNOFLUORESCENCE		INDIRECT IMMUNOFLUORESCENCE
Disease	**Histopathology**	**Biopsy of Perilesional Mucosa**	**Biopsy of Uninvolved Mucosa**	**Serum**
Pemphigus	Intraepithelial clefting above the basal cell layer; basal cells have a characteristic tombstone appearance; acantholysis	Intercellular deposits in epithelium IgG in all cases and C3 in most cases	Same as for perilesional mucosa	Intercellular antibodies (IgG) in ≥90% of cases
Cicatricial pemphigoid	Subepithelial clefting with epithelial separation from the underlying lamina propria, leaving an intact basal layer	Linear deposits of C3 with or without IgG at the basement membrane zone in most cases	Same as for perilesional mucosa	Basement membrane zone antibodies (IgG) in 10% of cases
Bullous pemphigoid	Subepithelial clefting with epithelial separation from the underlying lamina propria, leaving an intact basal layer	Linear deposits of C3 with or without IgG at the basement membrane zone in most cases	Same as for perilesional mucosa	Basement membrane zone in 40%–70% of cases
Epidermolysis bullosa acquisita	Similar to bullous and cicatricial pemphigoid	Linear deposits of IgG and C3 at the basement membrane zone in most cases	Same as for perilesional mucosa	Basement membrane zone antibodies (IgG) in 25% of cases
Lichen planus	Hyperkeratosis, hydropic degeneration of the basal layer, and sawtooth rete pegs; lamina propria exhibits dense, bandlike infiltrate, primarily of T lymphocytes; colloid bodies	Fibrillar deposits of fibrin at the dermal–epidermal junction	Negative	Negative
Chronic ulcerative stomatitis	Similar to erosive lichen planus; hyperkeratosis, acanthosis, basal cell layer liquefaction, subepithelial clefting, and lymphohistiocytic chronic infiltrate in a bandlike configuration	IgG deposits in the nuclei of the basal layer of epithelial cells	Same as for perilesional mucosa	ANA specific for basal cells of stratified squamous epithelium
Linear IgA disease	Similar to erosive lichen planus	Linear deposits of IgA at the basement membrane zone	Same as for perilesional mucosa	IgA basement membrane zone antibodies (IgA) in 30% of cases
Dermatitis herpetiformis	Collection of neutrophils, eosinophils, and fibrin in the connective tissue papillae	IgA deposits in the dermal papillae in 85% of cases	IgA deposits in dermal papillae in 100% of cases	IgA endomysial antibodies in 70% of cases; gliadin antibodies in 30% of cases
Systemic lupus erythematosus	Hyperkeratosis, basal cell degeneration, epithelial atrophy, and perivascular inflammation	IgG or IgM with or without C3 deposits at the dermal–epidermal junction	Same as for perilesional mucosa	ANA in >95% of cases; DNA and ENA antibodies in >50% of cases
Chronic cutaneous erythematosus	Hyperkeratosis, basal cell degeneration, epithelial atrophy, and perivascular inflammation	IgG or IgM with or without C3 deposits at the dermal–epidermal junction	Negative	Usually negative

Continued

TABLE 16.1 Diagnostic Findings for Conditions That Can Manifest as Desquamative Gingivitis—cont'd

		DIRECT IMMUNOFLUORESCENCE		INDIRECT IMMUNOFLUORESCENCE
Disease	**Histopathology**	**Biopsy of Perilesional Mucosa**	**Biopsy of Uninvolved Mucosa**	**Serum**
Subacute lupus erythematosus	Less inflammatory cell infiltrate than systemic and chronic cutaneous forms but with similar microscopic features	IgG or IgM with or without C3 deposits at the dermal-epidermal junction in 60% of cases; granular IgG deposits in basal cell cytoplasm in 30% of cases	Same as for perilesional mucosa	ANA in 60%–90% of cases; Ro (SSA) in 80% of cases; RF in 30% of cases; anti-RNP in 10% of cases

ANA, Antinuclear antibodies; *C3*, complement 3; *DNA*, deoxyribonucleic acid; *ENA*, extractable nuclear antigens; *IgA*, immunoglobulin A; *IgG*, immunoglobulin G; *IgM*, immunoglobulin M; *RF*, rheumatoid factor; *RNP*, ribonucleoprotein.

Adapted from Rinaggio J, Neiders ME, Aguirre A, Kumar V. Using immunofluorescence in the diagnosis of chronic ulcerative lesions of the oral mucosa. *Compend Contin Educ Dent.* 1999;20:943–944, 947–948, 950 passim quiz 962. PubMed PMID: 10650375.

(i.e., anti-IgG, anti-IgA, anti-IgM, antifibrin, and anti-C3). For *indirect* immunofluorescence, unfixed frozen sections of oral or esophageal mucosa from an animal, such as a monkey, are first incubated with the patient's serum to enable attachment of serum antibodies to the mucosal tissue. The tissue is then incubated with fluorescein-labeled antihuman serum. Immunofluorescence tests are positive if a fluorescent signal is observed in the epithelium, its associated basement membrane, or the underlying connective tissue (see Table 16.1).

Management

After the diagnosis is established, the dentist must choose the optimal management strategy. The choice depends on the practitioner's experience, the systemic impact of the disease, and the systemic complications of the medications. A detailed consideration of these factors dictates three scenarios.

In the first scenario, the dental practitioner takes direct and exclusive responsibility for the treatment of the patient. This occurs with conditions such as erosive lichen planus, which is responsive to topical steroids (Fig. 16.9).

In the second scenario, the dentist collaborates with another health care provider to evaluate and treat a patient concurrently. The classic example is seen with cicatricial pemphigoid, in which dentists and ophthalmologists work together to provide treatment (Fig. 16.10). Although the dentist addresses the oral lesions, the ophthalmologist monitors the integrity of the ocular conjunctiva.

In the third scenario, the patient is immediately referred to a dermatologist for further evaluation and treatment. This occurs with conditions for which the systemic impact of the disease transcends the boundaries of the oral cavity and results in significant morbidity or mortality. Pemphigus vulgaris is an example of a condition that, after diagnosis by the dentist, requires immediate referral to a dermatologist (Fig. 16.11). The complications (e.g., diabetes mellitus, osteoporosis, methemoglobinemia) of chronically administered systemic medications that are indicated for the management of diseases, such as pemphigus vulgaris or nonresponsive mucous membrane pemphigoid (MMP), warrant referral to a dermatologist or a specialist in internal medicine.

It is important that patients diagnosed with DG should practice optimal oral hygiene since dental biofilm can aggravate the clinical features. Soft toothbrushes with gentle pressure is advocated as lesions can be very painful and may discourage patients from toothbrushing. The use of strong mouthwashes should be discouraged. Oral treatment begins with topical application of steroids such as 0.1% Triamcinolone acetonide. However, severe conditions require systemic administration of steroids such as Prednisolone 5–10 mg daily. Often, a combination of drugs may be required. When oral treatment is provided, periodic evaluation is needed to monitor the patient's response to therapy. Initially, the patient should be evaluated at 2–4 weeks after beginning treatment to ensure that the condition is under control. Observation should continue until the patient is free of discomfort. Appointments every 3–6 months are then appropriate. Medication dosages are usually adjusted during this interval. Recurrence after discontinuation of steroid therapy is not uncommon. Hence, a judicious approach in managing such patients is warranted.

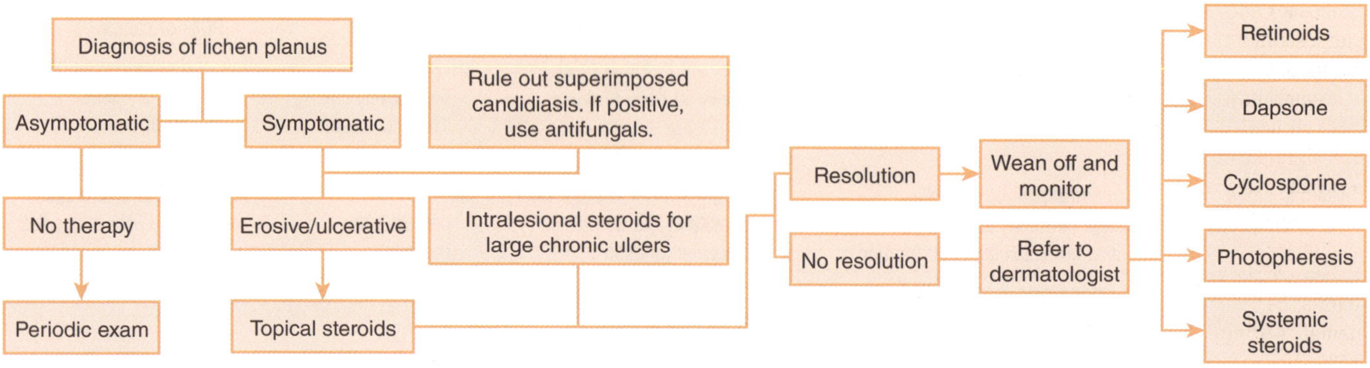

Fig. 16.9 Algorithm for the treatment of lichen planus.

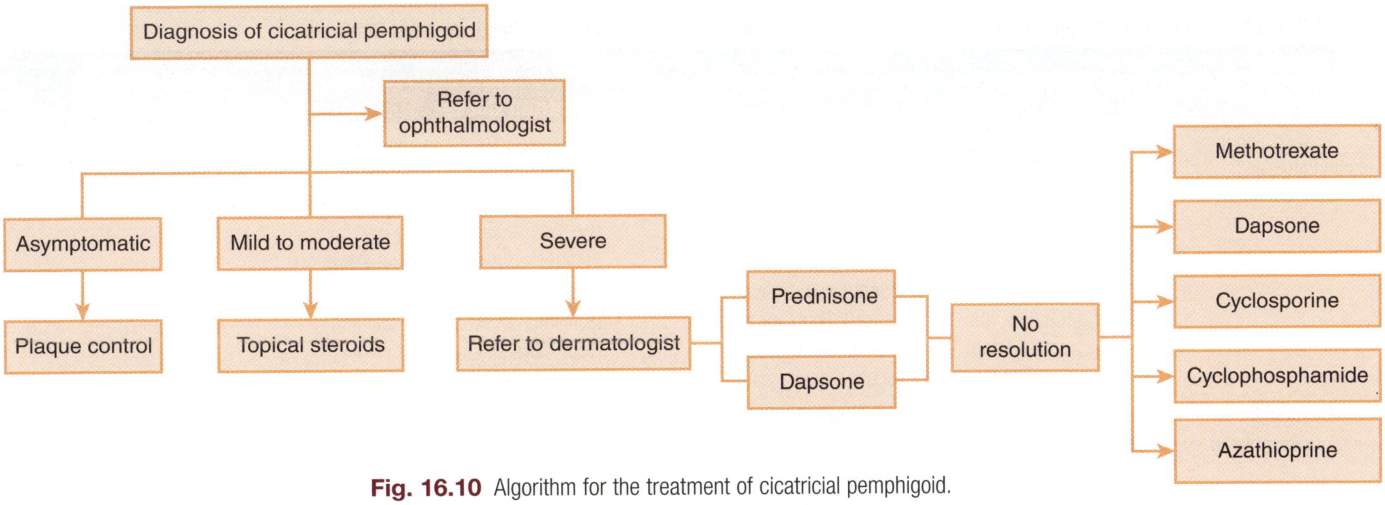

Fig. 16.10 Algorithm for the treatment of cicatricial pemphigoid.

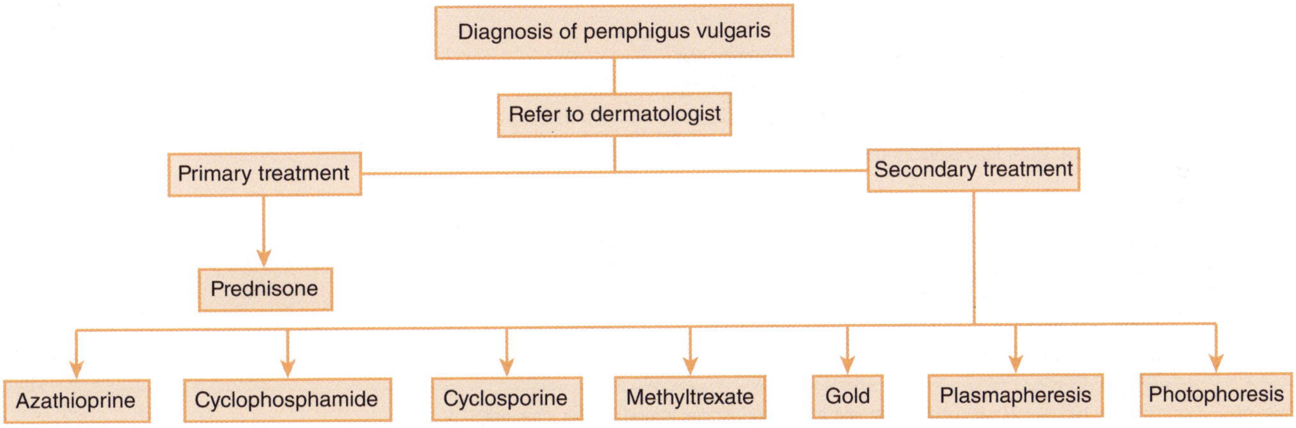

Fig. 16.11 Algorithm for the treatment of pemphigus vulgaris.

Table 16.2 summarizes suggested contemporary therapeutic approaches that can be used to treat selected conditions that can manifest as desquamative gingivitis.

Diseases That Can Manifest as Desquamative Gingivitis

Lichen Planus

Lichen planus is an inflammatory mucocutaneous disorder that can involve the mucosal surfaces (e.g., oral cavity, genital tract, or other mucosae) and the skin, including the scalp and the nails. Evidence suggests that lichen planus is an immunologically mediated mucocutaneous disorder in which host T lymphocytes play a central role. Although the oral cavity can have lichen planus lesions with a distinct clinical configuration and distribution, the clinical presentation can simulate other mucocutaneous disorders. Oral lichen planus has a broad differential diagnosis.

Numerous epidemiologic studies have found that oral lichen planus occurs in 0.1%–4% of the population. Most patients with oral lichen planus are middle-aged or older women; the disorder occurs with a 2:1 ratio of women to men. Children are rarely affected. In a dental setting, cutaneous lichen planus is observed in about 15%–30% of patients diagnosed with oral lichen planus. Two-thirds of patients seen in dermatologic clinics exhibit oral lichen planus.

Oral Lesions

Although there are several clinical forms of oral lichen planus (i.e., reticular, papular, patch, atrophic, erosive, and bullous), the most common are the reticular and erosive subtypes. The typical reticular lesions are asymptomatic and bilateral, and they consist of interlacing white lines on the posterior region of the buccal mucosa. The lateral border and dorsum of the tongue, the hard palate, the alveolar ridge, and the gingiva may also be affected. The reticular lesions can have an erythematous background, which is a feature associated with coexisting candidiasis. Oral lichen planus lesions follow a chronic course and have alternating, unpredictable periods of quiescence and flare-ups.

The erosive subtype of lichen planus is often associated with pain. It manifests as atrophic, erythematous, and often ulcerated areas. Fine, white radiating striations are observed bordering the atrophic and ulcerated zones. These areas may be sensitive to heat, acid, and spicy foods (Fig. 16.12).

Gingival Lesions

Approximately 7%–10% of patients with oral lichen planus have lesions restricted to the gingival tissue. They may occur as one or more types of the following four distinctive patterns:

1. *Keratotic lesions.* The raised, white lesions can manifest as groups of individual papules, linear or reticular lesions, or plaque-like configurations.

TABLE 16.2 Therapeutic Approaches for Treating Selected Conditions That Manifest as Desquamative Gingivitis

	THERAPY		
Disease	**Mild Cases**	**Recalcitrant Cases**	**Severe or Refractory Cases**
Erosive lichen planus	Delivery of therapeutic agent is enhanced with use of vacuum-formed custom trays **Rx:** Lidex (0.05% fluocinonide) gel **Disp:** One tube (15 g) **Sig:** Apply to affected area pc and hs Monitoring of patient's oral cavity warranted because candidiasis may develop after a few weeks of topical steroid use; concomitant use of antifungal may be necessary **Rx:** Clotrimazole 10-mg troches **Disp:** 90 **Sig:** Dissolve in mouth tid, then expectorate for 30 consecutive days	**Rx:** Protopic (0.1% tacrolimus) ointment **Disp:** One tube (30 g) **Sig:** Apply to affected area bid **Rx:** Tacrolimus (0.1 mg per 100 mL of distilled water) **Disp:** Dilute one 0.5-mg capsule of tacrolimus in 500 mL of distilled water **Sig:** Rinse mouth with 15 mL for 2 min qid	Refer to dermatologist for management with systemic corticosteroids
Cicatricial pemphigoid	**Rx:** Lidex (0.05% fluocinonide) gel **Disp:** One tube (15 g) **Sig:** Apply to affected area pc and hs **Rx:** Temovate (0.05% clobetasol propionate) **Disp:** One tube (15 g) **Sig:** Apply to affected area qid		Refer to dermatologist for management with prednisone (20–30 mg/day); concomitant use of azathioprine may be needed; dapsone, sulfonamide, and tetracycline are other alternatives
Pemphigus	Refer to dermatologist for management with prednisone (20–30 mg/day); concomitant use of azathioprine may be needed		
Chronic ulcerative stomatitis	**Rx:** Lidex (0.05% fluocinonide) gel **Disp:** One tube (15 g) **Sig:** Apply to affected area qid **Rx:** Temovate (0.05% clobetasol propionate) **Disp:** One tube (15 g) **Sig:** Apply to affected area qid	Refer to dermatologist for management with hydroxychloroquine **Disp:** 200 mg tablets **Sig:** Take 200–400 mg a day	

bid, Twice daily; *g*, grams; *hs*, at bedtime; *IU*, international units; *mg*, milligrams; *pc*, after meals; *qid*, four times daily.

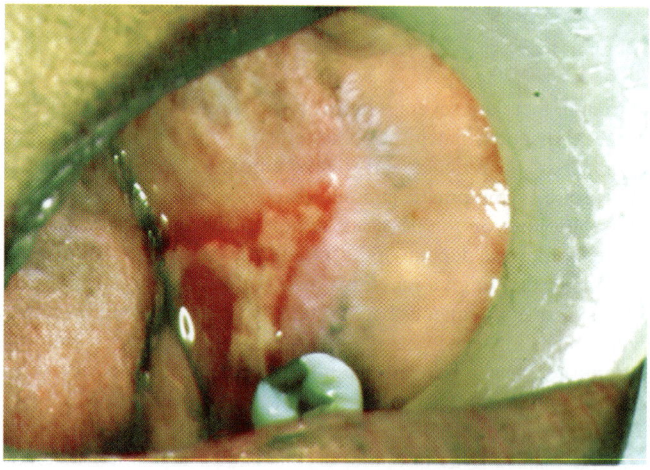

Fig. 16.12 In a case of erosive lichen planus, the large ulcerative lesion on the left buccal mucosa exhibits bordering erythema. The typical white striations of lichen planus are evident in the periphery of the ulcer.

2. *Erosive or ulcerative lesions.* The extensive erythematous areas with a patchy distribution can manifest as focal or diffuse hemorrhagic areas. The lesions are exacerbated by slight trauma (e.g., toothbrushing) (Fig. 16.13).
3. *Vesicular or bullous lesions.* The raised, fluid-filled lesions are uncommon and short lived on the gingiva, quickly rupturing and leaving ulcerations.

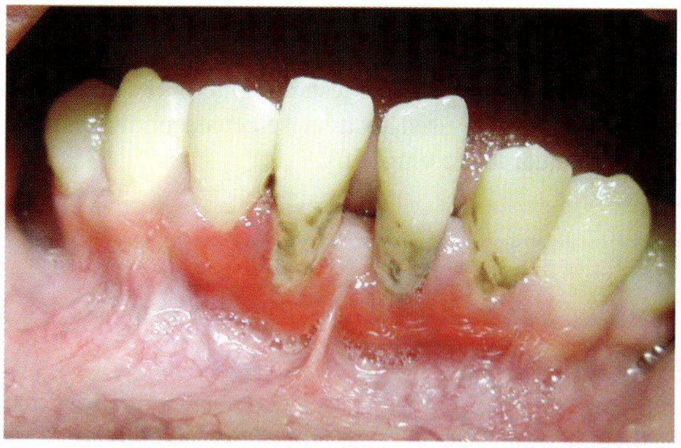

Fig. 16.13 Erosive lichen planus can manifest as desquamative gingivitis. The gingival tissues are erythematous, ulcerated, and painful. *(Courtesy: Dr. Luis Gaitan, Oral Pathology Laboratory, Faculty of Odontology, National Autonomous University of Mexico, Mexico City, Mexico.)*

4. *Atrophic lesions.* Atrophy of the gingival tissues with ensuing epithelial thinning results in erythema that is confined to the gingiva.

Histopathology

Microscopically, three main features characterize oral lichen planus: (1) hyperkeratosis or parakeratosis; (2) hydropic degeneration of the basal layer; and (3) a dense, bandlike infiltrate, consisting primarily of T lymphocytes, in the lamina propria (Fig. 16.14).

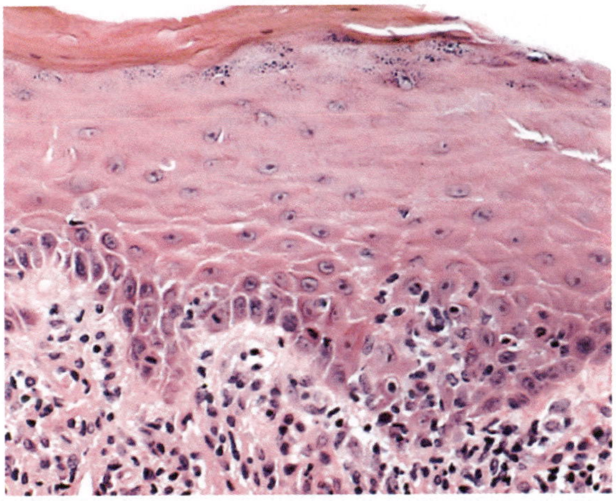

Fig. 16.14 Microscopic appearance of lichen planus. The biopsy specimen from a gingival lesion shows hyperkeratosis and mild hypergranulosis, along with focal basal cell degeneration, lymphocytic exocytosis, and thickening of the basement membrane. The rete pegs exhibit a slight serrated configuration. The papillary lamina propria shows a bandlike infiltrate of lymphohistiocytic chronic inflammatory cells. Hematoxylin and eosin stain; original magnification ×100.

Classically, the epithelial rete ridges have a sawtooth configuration. Hydropic degeneration of the basal layer of the epithelium can be sufficiently extensive that the epithelium becomes thin and atrophic or detaches from the underlying connective tissue and produces a subepithelial vesicle or an ulcer. Colloid bodies (i.e., Civatte bodies) are often seen at the epithelium—connective tissue interface.

The microscopic diagnosis of oral lichen planus is straightforward for the keratotic lesions, and biopsy specimens should be obtained from these areas if possible. However, classic histologic features may be obscured in areas of ulceration, making a conclusive diagnosis of oral lichen planus difficult if it is based solely on conventional microscopy. Electron microscopy studies indicate that separation of the basal lamina from the basal cell layer is an early manifestation of lichen planus.

The pattern of oral lesions of lichen planus can change, and in unusual cases, a second or third biopsy may be necessary to arrive at a definitive diagnosis. Controversy exists regarding the malignant potential of oral lichen planus. A meta-analysis and systematic review cited an average rate of 1.09% of oral cancer emerging in oral lichen planus. Other researchers reject or question the connection between oral lichen planus and oral cancer. Despite this controversy, biopsy and close follow-up are warranted for these patients.

Immunopathology

Direct immunofluorescence of lesional and perilesional oral lichen planus biopsy specimens reveals linear fibrillar (i.e., shaggy) deposits of fibrin in the basement membrane zone (Fig. 16.15), along with scattered immunoglobulin-staining cytoid bodies in the upper areas of the lamina propria (Fig. 16.16). Results of serum tests involving the use of indirect immunofluorescence are negative for patients with lichen planus (see Table 16.1).

Differential Diagnosis

The classic clinical presentation of oral lichen planus can be simulated by other conditions, mainly by lichenoid mucositis. If oral lichen planus is confined to the gingival tissues (i.e., erosive oral lichen planus), the identification of fine, white radiating striations

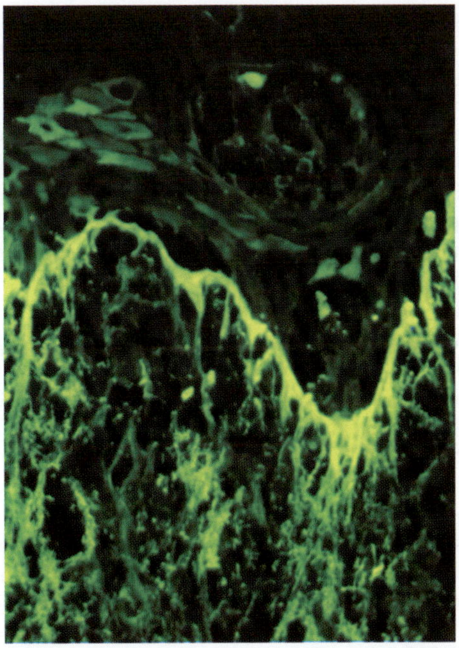

Fig. 16.15 Direct immunofluorescence staining of lichen planus. Fibrin deposits along the basement membrane of the epithelium exhibit a shaggy configuration.

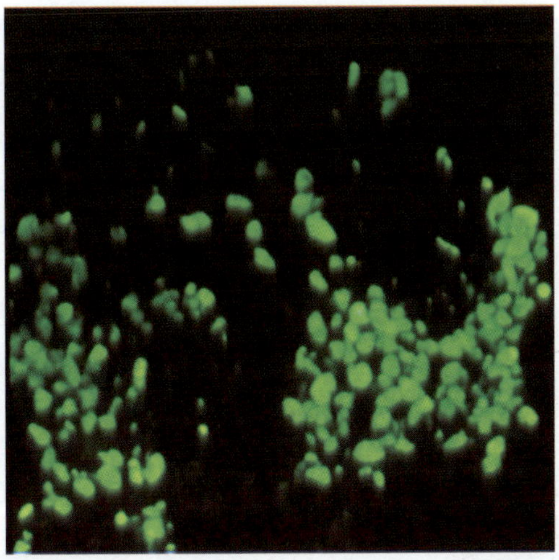

Fig. 16.16 Direct immunofluorescence staining of lichen planus. Clusters of cytoid bodies exhibit immunoglobulin M deposits in the lamina propria.

bordering the erosive areas support a diagnosis of oral lichen planus. If the white striations are absent, the differential diagnosis should primarily include MMP and pemphigus vulgaris. Less common possibilities include linear immunoglobulin A disease (LAD), lichen planus pemphigoides, and chronic ulcerative stomatitis.

Treatment

The keratotic lesions of oral lichen planus are asymptomatic and do not require treatment after the microscopic diagnosis has been established. However, evaluation of the patient every 6–12 months is warranted to monitor suspicious clinical changes and to look for the emergence of an erosive component.

The erosive, bullous, or ulcerative lesions of oral lichen planus are treated with high-potency topical steroids, such as 0.05% fluocinonide gel (Lidex, three times daily). Lidex can also be mixed 1:1 with carboxymethylcellulose (Orabase) paste or another adhesive ointment. A gingival tray can be used to deliver 0.05% fluocinonide ointment or gel or 0.05% clobetasol propionate with 100,000 IU/mL of nystatin in Orabase (Fig. 16.17).

Three daily 5-min applications of the mixture appear to be effective for controlling erosive lichen planus. Intralesional injections of triamcinolone acetonide (10–20 mg) or short-term regimens of 40 mg of prednisone daily for 5 days, followed by 10–20 mg daily for an additional 2 weeks, have also been used in more severe cases. Because of the potential side effects, systemic steroids should be administered and monitored by a dermatologist.

Other treatment modalities (e.g., retinoids, hydroxychloroquine, cyclosporine, azathioprine, cyclophosphamide, free gingival grafts) have been used. In recalcitrant cases, tacrolimus (0.1% Protopic ointment, twice daily) can be effective for controlling the lesions of erosive lichen planus. Topical tacrolimus may also be indicated in patients with diabetes mellitus where the continuous use of corticosteroids may result in hyperglycemia.

Because candidiasis is often associated with symptomatic oral lichen planus, and because topical steroid therapy promotes fungal growth, treatment should also include a topical antifungal agent.

Pemphigoid

The term *pemphigoid* applies to several cutaneous, immune-mediated, subepithelial bullous diseases that are characterized by a separation of the basement membrane zone, including bullous pemphigoid, MMP, and pemphigoid (herpes) gestationis. Among these conditions, bullous pemphigoid and MMP (i.e., benign MMP or cicatricial pemphigoid) have received considerable attention. Molecular findings for these two diseases indicate that they are separate entities. However, considerable histologic and immunopathologic overlap exists between them, and differentiation may be impossible on the basis of the two criteria.

In many cases, the clinical findings are probably the best way to discriminate between them. Accordingly, the term *bullous pemphigoid* is preferred when the disease is nonscarring and mainly affects the skin. The term *cicatricial pemphigoid* is favored when scarring occurs, and the disease is mainly confined to mucous membranes, although scarring may be absent with some subtypes of MMP. Until more research allows a better understanding of this family of diseases, bullous pemphigoid and MMP are discussed separately.

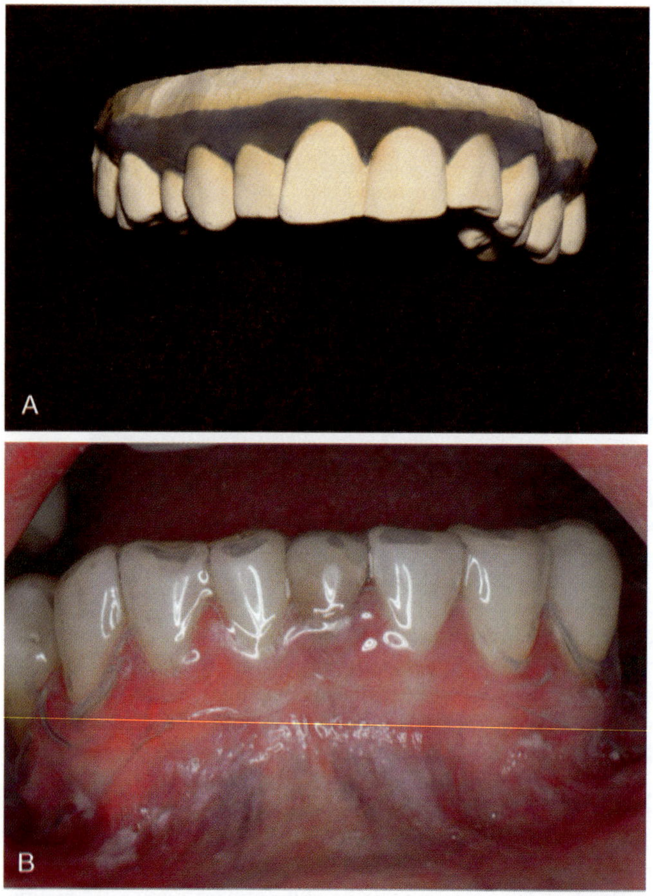

Fig. 16.17 A, An alginate impression is obtained to create a stone model. A thin layer of block-out resin is applied on the gingival and alveolar mucosal areas with desquamative gingivitis to create a space to carry the medication. A trimmed maxillary stone model shows the block-out resin in place (*blue area*). B, A mandibular gingival tray is in place. Soft sheet material for vacuum-forming trays is prepared and trimmed to conform to the local anatomy.

Bullous Pemphigoid

Bullous pemphigoid (BP) is a chronic, autoimmune, subepidermal bullous disease with tense cutaneous bullae that rupture and become flaccid (Fig. 16.18). Recently, it has been suggested that some cases of BP can be drug-induced (i.e., checkpoint inhibitors and antihyperglycemic agents such as DPP4-inhibitors). Although the skin lesions of bullous pemphigoid clinically resemble those of pemphigus, the microscopic picture is quite distinct.

Histopathology

There is no evidence of acantholysis in bullous pemphigoid, and the developing vesicles are subepithelial rather than intraepithelial. The epithelium separates from the underlying connective tissue at the basement membrane zone. Electron microscopic studies show horizontal splitting or replication of the basal lamina. The separating epithelium remains relatively intact, and the basal layer appears to be regular. The two major antigenic determinants of bullous pemphigoid are the 230-kDa protein plaque known as *bullous pemphigoid 1 (BP1)* and the 180-kDa collagen-like transmembrane protein known as *bullous pemphigoid 2 (BP2)*.

Immunofluorescence

Immunologically, bullous pemphigoid is characterized by immunoglobulin G (IgG) and complement 3 (C3) immune deposits along the epithelial basement membranes and circulating IgG antibodies to the epithelial basement membrane. Direct immunofluorescence studies are positive for 90%–100% of these patients, whereas indirect

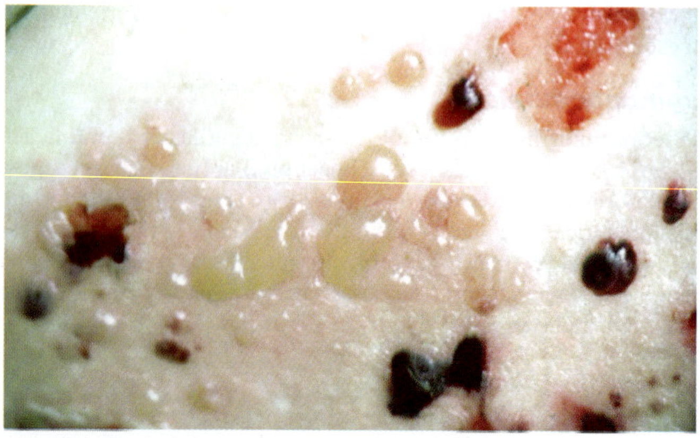

Fig. 16.18 Coalescing cutaneous bullae are seen in a case of bullous pemphigoid, and some of them are hemorrhagic. Rupture of the bullae leads to the formation of serpiginous ulcers.

immunofluorescence studies are positive for 60%–90% of affected patients (see Table 16.1).

Oral Lesions

Oral lesions of bullous pemphigoid have been reported to occur secondarily in about one-third of cases. The clinical presentation includes an erosive or desquamative gingivitis and occasional vesicular or bullous lesions.

Treatment

Because the etiologic factors of bullous pemphigoid are unknown, treatment is designed to control its signs and symptoms. The primary treatment is a moderate dose of systemic prednisone. Steroid-sparing strategies (i.e., prednisone plus other immunomodulatory drugs) are used when high doses of steroids are needed or when the steroid alone fails to control the disease. The chimeric monoclonal antibody Rituximab has shown high rates of remission with an excellent safety profile. For localized lesions of bullous pemphigoid, high-potency topical steroids or tetracycline with or without nicotinamide can be effective.

Mucous Membrane Pemphigoid

MMP (i.e., cicatricial pemphigoid) is a chronic vesiculobullous autoimmune disorder of unknown cause that predominantly affects women during the fifth decade of life. It has rarely been reported in young children. An undesirable side effect of anti-PD-1 checkpoint inhibitors is the development of MMP in some patients.

Cicatricial pemphigoid involves the oral cavity, the conjunctiva, and the mucosa of the nose, vagina, rectum, esophagus, and urethra. In about 20% of patients, the skin may also be involved.

Investigations suggest that cicatricial pemphigoid encompasses a group of heterogeneous conditions with distinct clinical and molecular features. An elaborate cascade of events is involved in the pathogenesis of cicatricial pemphigoid. Initially, antigen–antibody complexing occurs at the basement membrane zone, which is followed by complement activation and subsequent leukocyte recruitment. Proteolytic enzymes are then released and dissolve or cleave the basement membrane zone, usually at the level of the lamina lucida.

The two major antigenic determinants for cicatricial pemphigoid are BP1 and BP2. Most cases of cicatricial pemphigoid are the result of an immune response directed against BP2; less often, this response is mounted against BP1, epiligrin (i.e., laminin 5, a lamina lucida protein in the basement membrane of stratified epithelium), and β_4 integrins.

There is strong evidence of the existence of at least five subtypes of cicatricial pemphigoid: oral pemphigoid, antiepiligrin pemphigoid, anti-BP antigen mucosal pemphigoid, ocular pemphigoid, and multiple-antigen pemphigoid. The sera of ocular pemphigoid patients recognize the β_4 integrin subunit, whereas the sera of patients with oral pemphigoid recognize the α_6 unit.

Ocular Lesions

Among patients (mainly those with desquamative gingivitis) who first see a dentist, ocular involvement may later occur in approximately 25%. In contrast, among patients who first see a dermatologist, 66% have conjunctival lesions; in ophthalmic studies, 100% of patients have ocular involvement.

The initial lesion is characterized by unilateral conjunctivitis that becomes bilateral within 2 years. Subsequently, adhesions of the eyelid to the eyeball (i.e., symblepharon) may form (Fig. 16.19). Adhesions at the edges of the eyelids (i.e., ankyloblepharon) may lead to a narrowing of the palpebral fissure. Small vesicular lesions may develop on the conjunctiva, which can eventually produce scarring, corneal damage, and blindness.

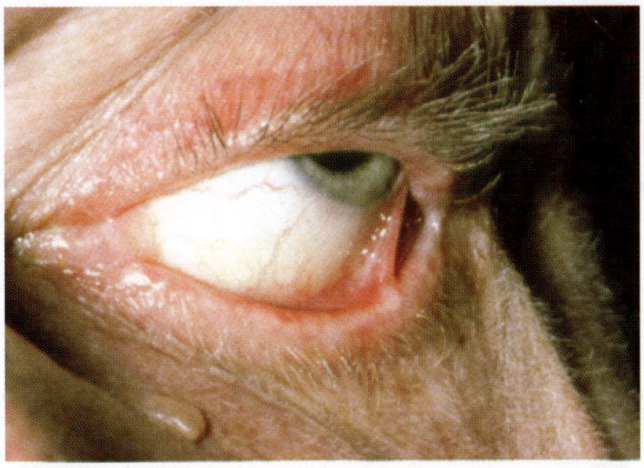

Fig. 16.19 In a patient with mucous membrane pemphigoid (i.e., cicatricial pemphigoid), the characteristic ocular lesion is a symblepharon, an adhesion of the eyelid to the eyeball. *(Courtesy: Dr. Carl Allen, The Ohio State University, Columbus, OH.)*

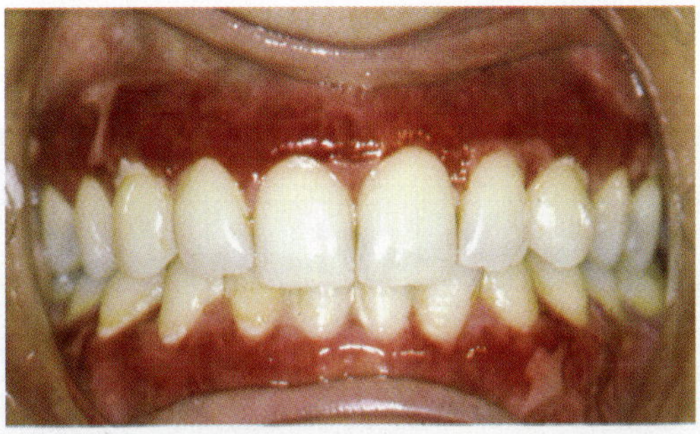

Fig. 16.20 When mucous membrane pemphigoid is confined to the gingival tissues, a typical desquamative gingivitis appearance is observed. *(Courtesy: Dr. Stuart L. Fischman, State University of New York at Buffalo, Buffalo, NY.)*

Oral Lesions

The most characteristic feature of oral involvement is desquamative gingivitis, typically with areas of erythema, desquamation, ulceration, and vesiculation of the attached gingiva (Fig. 16.20). Vesiculobullous lesions can occur elsewhere in the mouth. The bullae tend to have a relatively thick roof and rupture in 2–3 days after formation, leaving irregularly shaped areas of ulceration. Healing of these lesions can take up to 3 weeks or longer.

Histopathology

The microscopic appearance of the oral lesions, although not completely diagnostic of MMP, is sufficiently distinctive that a tentative diagnosis can be considered. A striking subepithelial vesiculation with the epithelium separated from the underlying lamina propria leaves an intact basal layer (Fig. 16.21). Separation of the epithelium and the connective tissue occurs at the basement membrane zone. Electron microscopic studies demonstrate a split in the basal lamina. A mixed inflammatory infiltrate (i.e., lymphocytes, plasma cells, neutrophils, and scarce eosinophils) is observed in the underlying fibrous connective tissue.

Immunofluorescence

Positive findings along the basement membrane area have been reported with the use of direct and indirect immunofluorescence. In

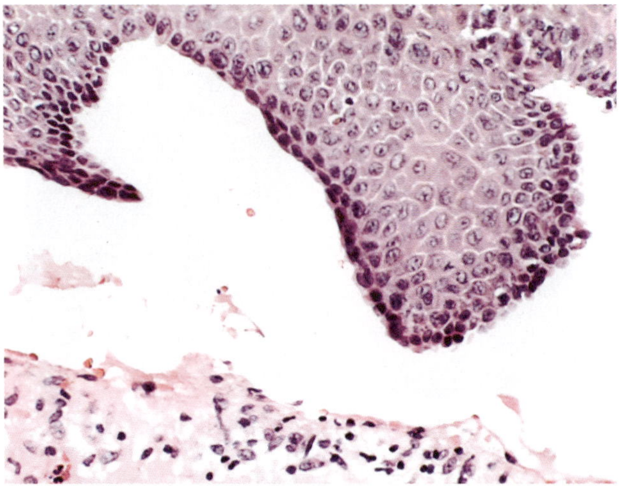

Fig. 16.21 Microscopic features of oral mucous membrane pemphigoid show a separation of the epithelium from the subjacent connective tissue (i.e., subepithelial clefting). An intact basal cell layer remains attached to the epithelium. Hematoxylin and eosin stain; original magnification ×100.

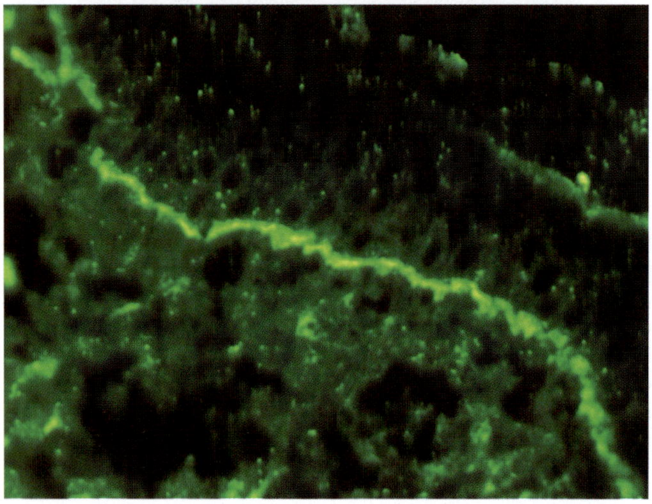

Fig. 16.22 Direct immunofluorescence staining of mucous membrane pemphigoid shows C3 deposits confined along the basement membrane.

biopsy tests using direct immunofluorescence, the main immunoreactants are IgG and C3, which are confined to the basement membrane (Fig. 16.22). Some studies indicate that a positive indirect immunofluorescence result is rare (<25%) for these patients. The lack of indirect immunofluorescence findings may reflect an earlier diagnosis of MMP, thereby resulting in the identification of patients with less extensive disease. In any event, circulating autoantibodies do not appear to play a role in the pathogenesis of the disease.

Differential Diagnosis

Several disease entities manifest with similar clinical and histologic (i.e., subepithelial bulla) features. They include bullous pemphigoid, bullous lichen planus, DH, LAD, erythema multiforme (EM), herpes gestationis, and epidermolysis bullosa acquisita.

Pemphigus may be confined to the oral cavity during its early stage, and the vesicular and ulcerative lesions may resemble those of MMP. An erosive or desquamative gingivitis also can be seen in pemphigus as a rare manifestation. Biopsy studies can quickly rule out pemphigus by revealing the absence or presence of acantholytic changes.

In EM, there are obvious vesiculobullous lesions. However, the onset is usually acute rather than chronic, labial involvement is severe, and the gingivae are usually not affected. Desquamative gingivitis is an unusual finding in EM, although occasional vesicular lesions can develop. A biopsy study of an oral lesion reveals an unusual degeneration of the upper stratum spinosum that is characteristically seen in oral EM lesions.

Cicatricial pemphigoid must be differentiated from epidermolysis bullosa acquisita, which can manifest with similar histopathologic and immunopathologic features. When the biopsy is treated with salt to separate the dermis from the epidermis, basement membrane immunodeposits occur on the epidermal side with pemphigoid and on the dermal side with epidermolysis bullosa acquisita.

Treatment

Topical steroids are the mainstay of treatment for MMP, particularly when lesions are localized. Fluocinonide (0.05%) and clobetasol propionate (0.05%) in an adhesive vehicle can be used three times daily for up to 6 months. When the oral lesions of MMP are confined to the gingival tissues, topical corticosteroids are effectively delivered with vacuum-formed custom trays or veneers. Optimal oral hygiene is essential because local irritants on the tooth surface result in an exaggerated gingival inflammatory response. Gingival irritation from a dental prosthesis should be minimized.

If the disease is not severe and symptoms are mild, systemic corticosteroids may be omitted. If ocular involvement exists, systemic corticosteroids are indicated.

When lesions do not respond to steroids, systemic dapsone (4-4'-diaminodiphenylsulfone) has proved to be effective. Because of the systemic side effects of dapsone, including hemolysis and methemoglobinemia (particularly in patients with glucose-6-phosphate dehydrogenase deficiency), referral to a dermatologist is often indicated. Systemic steroids can be combined with azathioprine or cyclophosphamide.

Biologic agents such as Rituximab (i.e., anti-CD20 monoclonal antibody) combined with an immunosuppressant (i.e., dapsone and/or sulfasalazine) have shown promising results in severe, refractory cases. Some investigators advocate sulfonamides and tetracycline. Although surgery is not a treatment for MMP, it is used for some patients to prevent blindness and for esophageal and upper airways stenosis. Connective tissue grafting to alleviate root surface sensitivity and to improve aesthetics has been used with success to manage gingival recession in a patient with cicatricial pemphigoid.

Pemphigus Vulgaris

The pemphigus diseases are a group of autoimmune bullous disorders that produce cutaneous and mucous membrane blisters (Figs. 16.23 and 16.24). Pemphigus vulgaris is the most common of the pemphigus diseases, which also include pemphigus foliaceus, pemphigus vegetans, and pemphigus erythematosus. Pemphigus vulgaris is a potentially lethal chronic condition with a 10% mortality rate and a worldwide annual incidence of 0.1–0.5 cases per 100,000 individuals. A predilection for women, usually after the fourth decade of life, has been observed. However, pemphigus vulgaris has also been reported in unusually young children and even in newborns.

The epidermal and mucous membrane blisters occur when the cell-to-cell adhesion structures are damaged by the action of circulating autoantibodies and by the in vivo binding of the autoantibodies to the pemphigus vulgaris antigens, which are cell surface

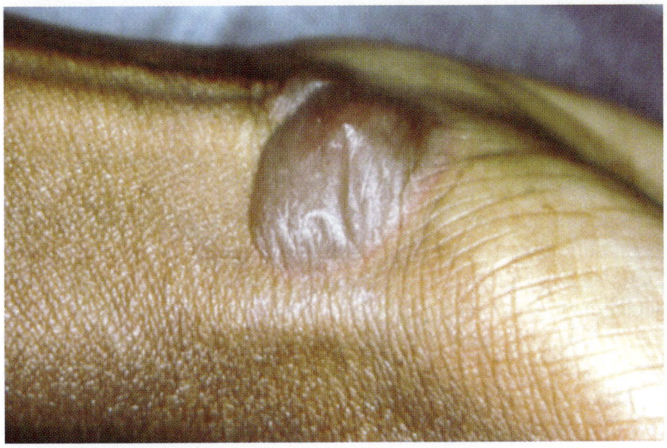

Fig. 16.23 Patient with pemphigus vulgaris exhibiting a large bulla on the flexor surface of the wrist.

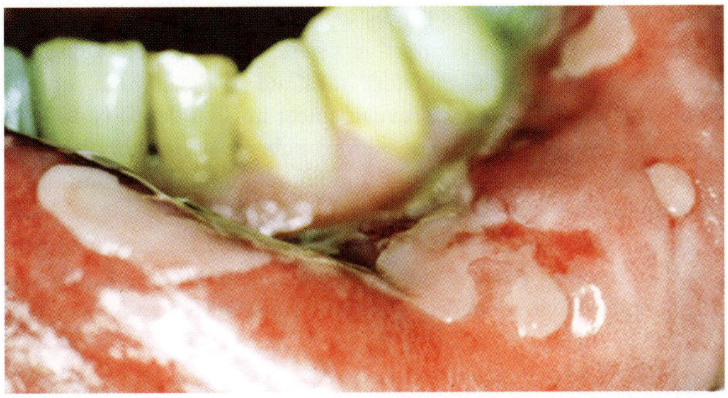

Fig. 16.24 Patient with pemphigus vulgaris of the oral cavity presenting multiple and coalescent areas of ulceration covered by pseudomembranes of necrotic epithelium. The patient had large ulcers on the labial mucosa, tongue, and soft palate.

glycoproteins on keratinocytes. The pemphigus vulgaris glycoproteins are members of the desmoglein (DSG) subfamily of the cadherin superfamily of cell–cell adhesion molecules, which occur in desmosomes. Whereas high levels of desmoglein 3 (DSG3) autoantibodies correlate with the severity of oral disease in patients with pemphigus vulgaris, elevated levels of desmoglein 1 (DSG1) autoantibodies are associated with severity of cutaneous disease. Evidence suggests that DSG3, which is the gene that codes for pemphigus vulgaris, is located on chromosome 18.

Most cases of pemphigus vulgaris are idiopathic. However, medications such as penicillamine and captopril can produce drug-induced pemphigus, which is usually reversible after withdrawal of the causative drug. Other triggering factors include UV radiation exposure, hepatitis B infection, dietary factors such as garlic, and vitamin D. Paraneoplastic pemphigus is antigenically distinct from pemphigus vulgaris, and it is associated with underlying malignancies.

In approximately 60% of patients with pemphigus vulgaris, the oral lesions are the first sign of the disease. The lesions may herald the dermatologic involvement by a year or more.

Oral Lesions

Oral lesions can range from small vesicles to large bullae. When the bullae rupture, they leave extensive areas of ulceration (Fig. 16.25). Virtually any region of the oral cavity can be involved, but multiple

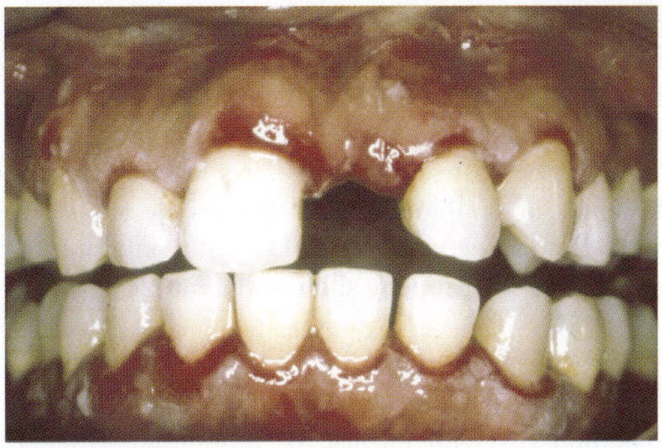

Fig. 16.25 Patient with pemphigus vulgaris confined to the gingivae. Clinically diagnosed as consistent with desquamative gingivitis. *(Courtesy: Dr. Beatriz Aldape, Faculty of Odontology, National Autonomous University of Mexico, Mexico City, Mexico.)*

lesions often develop at sites of irritation or trauma. The soft palate is most often involved (80%), followed by the buccal mucosa (46%), the ventral aspect or dorsum of the tongue (20%), and the lower labial mucosa (10%). Oral lesions of pemphigus vulgaris are confined less often to the gingival tissues. In these patients, erosive gingivitis or desquamative gingivitis is the sole manifestation of oral pemphigus.

Histopathology

The lesions of pemphigus demonstrate a characteristic intraepithelial separation that occurs above the basal cell layer. The intraepithelial vesiculation begins as a microscopic alteration (Fig. 16.26) and gradually results in a grossly visible, fluid-filled bulla. Occasionally, the entire superficial layers of epithelium are lost, leaving behind only the basal cells attached to the underlying lamina propria and conferring a characteristic tombstone appearance to the epithelial cells.

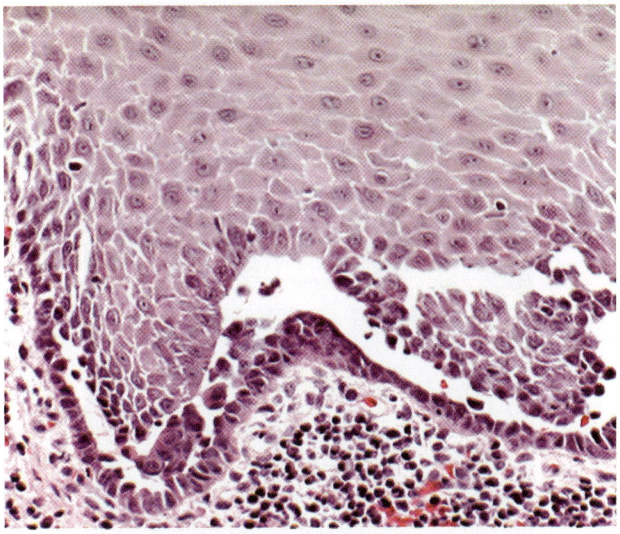

Fig. 16.26 Microscopic features of pemphigus vulgaris include typical intraepithelial clefting with a tombstone appearance of the basal cells, which remain attached to the subjacent basement membrane and fibrous connective tissue. Acantholysis of epithelial cells with the formation of Tzanck cells is seen in the intraepithelial cleft. (Hematoxylin and eosin stain; original magnification ×100.)

Acantholysis, which involves the separation of the epithelial cells of the lower stratum spinosum, takes place. It is characterized by round rather than polyhedral epithelial cells. The intercellular bridges are lost, and the nuclei are large and hyperchromatic. The underlying connective tissue usually has a mild to moderate, chronic inflammatory cell infiltrate. As the vesicle or bulla ruptures, the ulcerated lesion becomes infiltrated with polymorphonuclear leukocytes, and the surface may show suppuration.

Immunofluorescence

Autoantibodies can be demonstrated in the oral mucosa of patients with oral pemphigus with the use of immunofluorescence techniques. For direct immunofluorescence, perilesional unfixed frozen sections are incubated with fluorescein-labeled human anti-IgG. For indirect immunofluorescence, unfixed frozen sections of oral or esophageal mucosa from an animal such as a monkey are first incubated with the patient's serum to allow attachment of serum antibodies to the mucosal tissue. The tissue is then incubated with fluorescein-labeled antihuman IgG serum. The test result is positive if immunofluorescence is observed in the intercellular spaces of the stratified squamous epithelium of the mucosa (Fig. 16.27).

The indirect technique is less sensitive than the direct technique, and it may be negative during the early stages of the disease, particularly in its localized forms (see Table 16.1). In most cases, however, the indirect immunofluorescence titers are helpful for monitoring of disease activity, and they have prognostic value.

Differential Diagnosis

The oral lesions of pemphigus vulgaris may be similar to those seen in EM. In patients with EM, however, recurrent active episodes of comparatively short duration are followed by long intervals that are free of skin and oral lesions. EM affects the lips with considerable severity. Microscopic examination with conventional H&E and direct immunofluorescence can discriminate between the oral lesions of pemphigus and those of EM. Pemphigus vulgaris shows characteristic intraepithelial clefting at the basal–spinous cell layers and interface with acantholysis, whereas EM shows microvesiculation of the superficial epithelial layers and numerous necrotic keratinocytes. Pemphigus vulgaris shows an intercellular and intraepithelial signal with direct immunofluorescence; EM exhibits negative immunofluorescence.

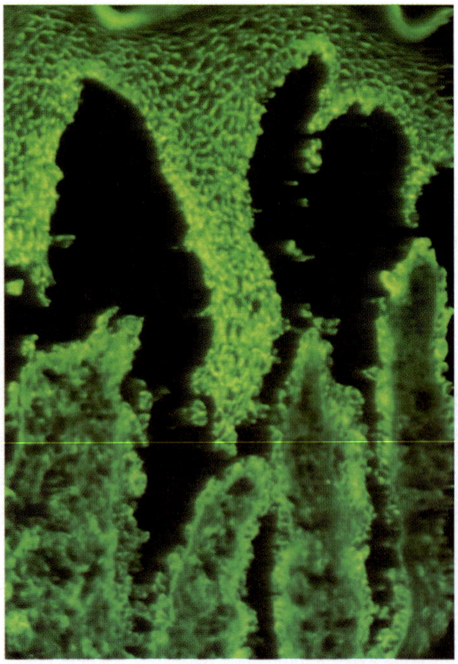

Fig. 16.27 Direct immunofluorescence staining of an oral pemphigus specimen shows the positive intercellular signal for immunoglobulin G deposits in keratinocytes of the stratified squamous epithelium.

Pemphigoid may clinically resemble pemphigus. Microscopic examination and direct immunofluorescence studies are needed to establish a correct diagnosis. Bullous pemphigoid and MMP exhibit detachment of the epithelium from the underlying connective tissue (i.e., lifting off) rather than the acantholytic lesion characteristic of pemphigus.

Bullous lichen planus must also be considered during the differential diagnosis. The primary lesion of pemphigus may have a bullous character, and this may be followed by erosion, with its associated pain and discomfort. In patients with lichen planus, the characteristic reticular lesions are invariably associated with the bullae. Microscopic examination and direct immunofluorescence studies are necessary to differentiate this condition from pemphigus. Bullous lichen planus shows separation of the epithelium from the underlying fibrous connective tissue, sawtooth rete pegs, and a bandlike chronic inflammatory infiltrate in the lamina propria. Direct immunofluorescence reveals linear fibrillar deposits of fibrin in the basement membrane of bullous lichen planus, whereas pemphigus vulgaris has intercellular immunoglobulin deposition in the epithelium.

If the oral lesions of pemphigus vulgaris are restricted to the gingival tissues, erosive lichen planus, pemphigoid, LAD, and chronic ulcerative stomatitis should be ruled out.

Treatment

Guidelines for the treatment of pemphigus vulgaris are available. The main therapy for pemphigus vulgaris is systemic corticosteroids with or without the addition of other immunosuppressive agents. If the patient responds well to corticosteroids, the dosage can be gradually reduced, but a low maintenance dosage is usually necessary to prevent or minimize the recurrence of lesions. Many dermatologists monitor the dose of steroids by periodic evaluation of the titers of DSG3 and DSG1 antibodies. Increasing titers are often associated with an impending exacerbation and warrant an increase of the steroid dose. A decrease in titer justifies a reduction of the steroid dose.

In patients who are not responsive to corticosteroids or who gradually adapt to them, steroid-sparing therapies are used. They are combinations of steroids plus other medications (e.g., azathioprine, cyclophosphamide, cyclosporine, dapsone, gold, methotrexate), as well as photoplasmapheresis and plasmapheresis. The biologic Rituximab is used as an adjunct to treat pemphigus vulgaris. However, when used in early stages of the disease, it may induce complete remission.

The maintenance phase aims to control the disease with the lowest dose of medication. To minimize the risk of morbidity associated with the long-term use of steroids, alternate-day steroid therapy, steroid-sparing drugs, and topical steroids can be combined. Because topical steroids may promote the development of candidiasis, topical antifungal medication may also be needed.

Minimization of oral irritation is important for patients with oral pemphigus vulgaris. Optimal oral hygiene is essential because there is usually widespread involvement of the marginal and attached gingivae and of other areas of the mouth, which can be exacerbated by plaque-associated gingivitis and periodontitis. Periodontal care is an important issue in the overall management of patients with pemphigus vulgaris. To prevent flare-ups, patients in the maintenance phase should receive prednisone before professional oral prophylaxis and periodontal surgery. The fit and design of removable prosthetic appliances should receive special attention because even slight irritation from these prostheses can cause severe inflammation with vesiculation and ulceration.

Chronic Ulcerative Stomatitis

Chronic ulcerative stomatitis, which was first reported in 1990, manifests with chronic oral ulcerations and has a predilection for women in the fourth decade of life. The erosions and ulcerations occur predominantly in the oral cavity, with only a few cases exhibiting cutaneous lesions. Circulating specific IgG autoantibodies to ΔNp63α, an epithelial nuclear transcription factor that modulates epithelial cell growth, have been demonstrated.

Oral Lesions

Painful, solitary, small blisters, and erosions with surrounding erythema occur mainly on the buccal mucosae followed by the gingiva, tongue, labial mucosa, and the hard palate. Because of the magnitude and clinical features of the gingival lesions, a diagnosis of desquamative gingivitis is considered (Fig. 16.28).

Histopathology

The microscopic features of chronic ulcerative stomatitis are similar to those observed in erosive lichen planus. Hyperkeratosis, acanthosis, and liquefaction of the basal cell layer with areas of subepithelial clefting are prominent features of the epithelium. The underlying lamina propria exhibits an admixture of T lymphocytes and plasma cells in a band-like configuration.

Immunofluorescence

Direct immunofluorescence of normal and perilesional tissues reveals typical stratified epithelium-specific antinuclear antibodies (SES-ANA). They are nuclear deposits of IgG with a speckled pattern, and they are found mainly in the basal and parabasal cell layers of the normal epithelium (Fig. 16.29). Deposition of complement 3 has been reported in some cases. Fibrin deposits are visualized at the epithelial tissue-connective tissue interface. Indirect immunofluorescence studies involving the use of an esophageal substrate also reveal stratified epithelium-specific antinuclear antibodies.

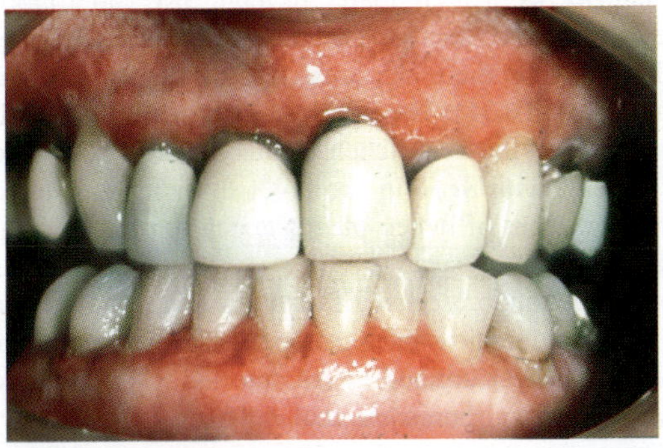

Fig. 16.28 Erythema and ulceration of the gingiva are consistent with a clinical diagnosis of chronic desquamative gingivitis. Direct and indirect immunofluorescence studies demonstrate stratified epithelium-specific antinuclear antibodies. *(Courtesy: Dr. Douglas Damm, University of Kentucky, Lexington, KY.)*

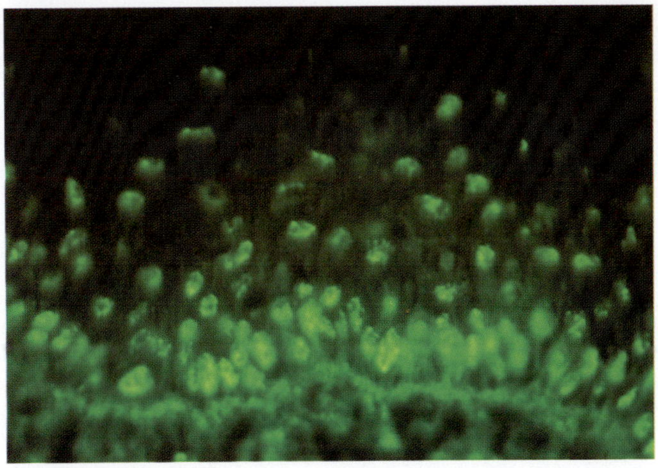

Fig. 16.29 Direct immunofluorescence study of chronic ulcerative stomatitis shows nuclear deposits of immunoglobulin G that are prominent in the basal cell layer and fade toward the superficial layers. *(Courtesy: Dr. Douglas Damm, University of Kentucky, Lexington, KY.)*

Diagnosis

Chronic ulcerative stomatitis is clinically similar to erosive lichen planus. Pemphigus vulgaris, MMP, LAD, bullous pemphigoid, and lupus erythematosus also have to be included in the differential diagnosis. Microscopic examination usually reduces the number of possibilities to chronic ulcerative stomatitis, LAD, and erosive lichen planus. Direct and indirect immunofluorescence studies are needed to arrive at the correct diagnosis. An enzyme-linked immunosorbent assay (ELISA) has been developed, which may allow correlation of antibody titers with treatment response.

Treatment

For mild cases, topical steroids (e.g., fluocinonide, clobetasol propionate) and topical tetracycline can produce clinical improvement, but recurrences are common. For severe cases, a high dose of a systemic corticosteroid is needed to achieve remission. Unfortunately, reduction of the corticosteroid dose results in relapse of the lesions. Hydroxychloroquine sulfate at a dosage of 200–400 mg/day seems to be the treatment of choice to produce complete, long-lasting remission. However, a long-term follow-up study demonstrated that combined therapy (i.e., small doses of corticosteroids and chloroquine) might be required because the initial good response to chloroquine ceases after several months or years of treatment.

Linear Immunoglobulin A Disease

LAD (i.e., linear IgA dermatosis) is an uncommon mucocutaneous disorder with a predilection for women. The etiopathogenic aspects of LAD are not fully understood, although drug-induced LAD triggered by angiotensin-converting enzyme inhibitors and angioimmunoblastic T-cell lymphoma associated with LAD have been reported.

LAD manifests as a pruritic vesiculobullous rash, usually during middle age or later, although younger individuals may also be affected. Characteristic plaques or crops with an annular manifestation surrounded by a peripheral rim of blisters affect the skin of the upper and lower trunk, the shoulders, the groin, and the lower limbs. The face and perineum may also be affected. Mucosal involvement, including that of the oral mucosa, ranges from 50% to 100% of the cases published.

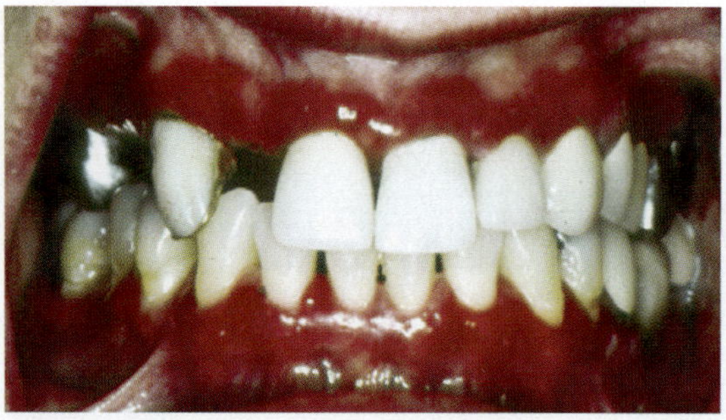

Fig. 16.30 In a patient with linear immunoglobulin A disease, intense erythema and ulceration of the gingiva are consistent with a diagnosis of desquamative gingivitis.

LAD can mimic lichen planus clinically and histologically. Immunofluorescence studies are needed to establish the correct diagnosis.

Oral Lesions

Oral manifestations of LAD consist of vesicles, painful ulcerations or erosions, and erosive gingivitis or cheilitis. The hard and soft palates are affected more often; the tonsillar pillars, buccal mucosa, tongue, and gingiva follow in frequency. Rarely, oral lesions may be the only manifestation of LAD for several years before cutaneous lesions occur. The oral lesions of LAD have been clinically reported as desquamative gingivitis (Fig. 16.30).

Histopathology

The microscopic features of LAD are similar to those observed with erosive lichen planus.

Immunofluorescence

Linear deposits of IgA are observed at the epithelial tissue-connective tissue interface. They are different from the granular pattern that is observed with DH.

Differential Diagnosis

The differential diagnosis of LAD includes erosive lichen planus, chronic ulcerative stomatitis, pemphigus vulgaris, bullous pemphigoid, and lupus erythematosus. Microscopic examination and immunofluorescence studies are necessary to establish the correct diagnosis.

Treatment

The primary treatment of LAD involves a combination of sulfones and dapsone. Small amounts of prednisone (10–30 mg/day) can be added if the initial response is inadequate. Alternatively, tetracycline (2 g/day) in combination with nicotinamide (1.5 g/day) has shown promising results. Mycophenolate (500 mg twice daily) in combination with prednisolone (30 mg/day) resulted in the resolution of the refractory ulcerations associated with LAD.

Dermatitis Herpetiformis

DH is a chronic condition characterized by severe pruritus in the skin resulting from an inflammatory response to gluten ingestion. DH usually develops in young adults between the ages of 20 and 30 years, and it has a slight predilection for men. Evidence indicates that DH is a cutaneous manifestation of celiac disease, a gluten sensitivity enteropathy. Approximately 25% of patients with celiac disease have DH. The cause of celiac disease is obscure, but tissue transglutaminase seems to be the predominant autoantigen in the intestine, the skin, and sometimes the mucosae. Tissue transglutaminase (TG3) immunoglobulin A targets tissue transglutaminases TG3 (papillary dermis of DH patients) and TG-2 (celiac disease patients) to form deposits in the skin and small bowel. Circulating antibodies are also present in these patients. Gluten enteropathy can be severe in about two-thirds of patients, and it is mild or subclinical in the remaining one-third. In severe cases, patients may complain of dysphagia, weakness, diarrhea, and weight loss. Autoimmune thyroiditis, Sjogren's syndrome, and bullous pemphigoid have also been associated with DH.

Clinically, DH manifests with bilateral and symmetric pruritic papules or vesicles that are primarily restricted to the extensor surfaces of the extremities. The sacrum, the buttocks, and occasionally the face and oral cavity can be affected.

The term herpetic is derived from the initial manifestation of the disease, in which clusters of vesicles or papules arise on the skin. These vesicles or papules eventually resolve and are followed by hyperpigmentation of the skin, which ultimately wanes. The oral lesions of DH range from painful ulcerations preceded by the collapse of ephemeral vesicles or bullae to erythematous lesions.

Histopathology

Microscopic examination of the initial lesions of DH reveals focal aggregates of neutrophils and eosinophils among deposits of fibrin at the apices of the dermal pegs.

Immunofluorescence

Direct immunofluorescence demonstrates IgA and C3 at the dermal papillary apices in both perilesional tissue and normal, uninvolved tissue. In contrast, biopsies taken from lesional sites may fail to exhibit IgA or C3, producing false-negative results. Although no circulating autoantibodies to epithelial basement membrane occur in DH, almost 80% of patients have antiendomysial and gliadin antibodies.

Treatment

A gluten-free diet is essential for the treatment of celiac disease and DH. Oral dapsone is usually needed for patients with newly detected DH to alleviate symptoms promptly.

Lupus Erythematosus

Lupus erythematosus is an autoimmune disease with three clinical presentations: systemic, chronic cutaneous, and subacute cutaneous.

Systemic Lupus Erythematosus

Systemic lupus erythematosus (SLE) is a severe disease with a 10:1 predilection for women compared to men. SLE can affect the kidneys, heart, skin, and mucosa. The classic cutaneous lesions characterized by a rash on the malar area with a butterfly distribution are uncommon (Fig. 16.31). The oral lesions of SLE are usually ulcerative or similar to those of lichen planus. Oral ulcerations occur in 36% of patients with SLE. In about 4% of patients, hyperkeratotic plaques reminiscent of lichen planus appear on the buccal mucosa and palate.

Direct immunofluorescence of the perilesional and normal tissue reveals immunoglobulins and C3 deposits at the dermal-epidermal interface. Antinuclear antibodies are detected in more than 95% of cases, whereas deoxyribonucleic acid and extractable nuclear antigen antibodies are found in more than 50% of patients (see Table 16.1).

Chronic Cutaneous Lupus Erythematosus

Chronic cutaneous lupus erythematosus usually has no systemic signs or symptoms; lesions are limited to the skin or the mucosal surfaces. The skin lesions are referred to as discoid lupus erythematosus

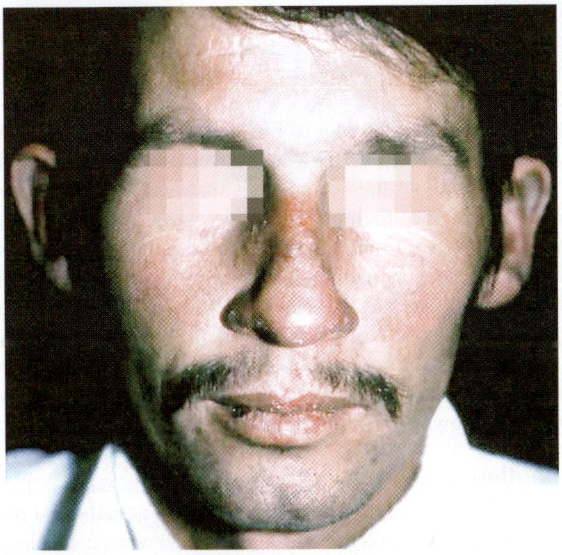

Fig. 16.31 Systemic lupus erythematosus produces erythema on the bridge of the nose with a butterfly pattern. *(Courtesy: Department of Dermatology, Hospital General Manuel Gea González, Mexico City, Mexico.)*

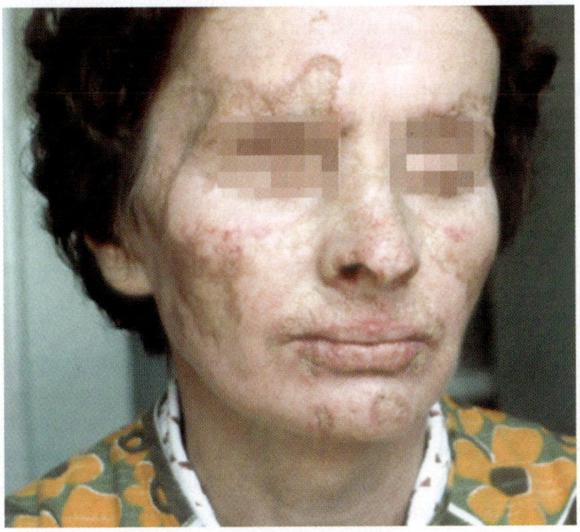

Fig. 16.32 In a patient with chronic cutaneous lupus erythematosus, there are multiple facial lesions with irregular hyperpigmented borders, some of which exhibit central scarring with cutaneous atrophy. Other lesions consist of hyperpigmented cutaneous patches.

(DLE). DLE describes the chronic scarring, atrophy-producing lesion that may develop into hyperpigmentation or hypopigmentation of the healing area (Fig. 16.32). In the oral cavity, about 9% of patients with chronic cutaneous lupus erythematosus have lichen-planus-like plaques on the palate and the buccal mucosa. The gingiva may be affected, and the condition can manifest as desquamative gingivitis (Fig. 16.33).

Histopathology

The histopathology of the oral lesions of chronic cutaneous lupus erythematosus consists of hyperkeratosis, alternating acanthosis and atrophy, and hydropic degeneration of the basal layer of the epithelium. The lamina propria exhibits a chronic inflammatory cell infiltrate similar to that observed with lichen planus. However, a more diffuse and deeper inflammatory infiltrate with a perivascular pattern is typically observed.

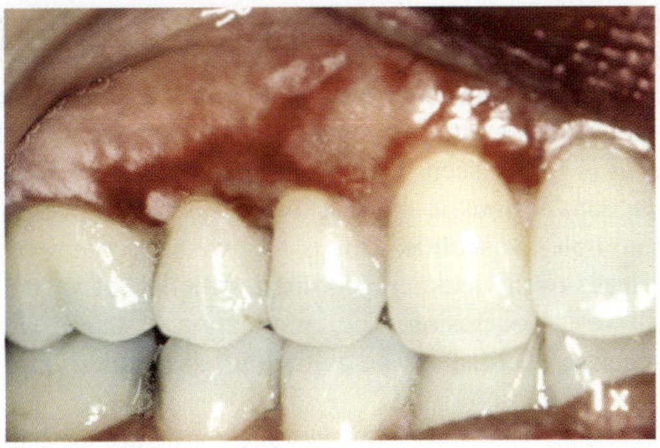

Fig. 16.33 Lupus erythematosus of the oral cavity can manifest as desquamative gingivitis. Intense erythema with ulceration is bordered by white radial lines. *(Courtesy: Dr. Stuart L. Fischman, State University of New York at Buffalo, NY.)*

Immunofluorescence

Direct immunofluorescence study of lesional tissue reveals immunoglobulins and C3 deposits at the dermal-epidermal junction of the lesional or perilesional tissue but not in normal tissue. This seems to differentiate SLE from DLE. The indirect immunofluorescence method reveals antinuclear antibodies in more than 95% of patients, whereas deoxyribonucleic acid and extractable nuclear antigen circulating antibodies are found in more than 50% of patients.

Subacute Cutaneous Lupus Erythematosus

Patients with subacute cutaneous lupus erythematosus have cutaneous lesions that are similar to those of DLE but that lack the development of scarring and atrophy. Arthritis and arthralgia, low-grade fever, malaise, and myalgia can occur in up to 50% of patients with subacute cutaneous lupus erythematosus.

Direct immunofluorescence reveals immunoglobulins and C3 deposits at the dermal-epidermal junction in 60% of cases and granular IgG deposits in the cytoplasm of basal cells in 30% of cases. About 80% of patients with subacute cutaneous lupus erythematosus have Ro (SSA) antibodies to nuclear antigens, whereas 25%–30% have La (SSB) antibodies to nuclear antigens. The test result for rheumatoid factor is positive in about 30% of these patients, positive for antinuclear antibodies in 60%–90%, and positive for antiribonucleoprotein antibodies to nuclear antigens in 10% (see Table 16.1).

Differential Diagnosis

Erosive lichen planus, EM, and pemphigus vulgaris can simulate the lesions observed in patients with lupus erythematosus. The diagnosis of DLE confined to the oral cavity is difficult to make, but microscopic studies may suggest the characteristic histopathology. Biopsy studies (i.e., H&E and direct immunofluorescence) help to differentiate lupus erythematosus from other erosive diseases.

Treatment

Therapy for SLE depends on the severity and extent of the disease. It can range from topical steroids to nonsteroidal antiinflammatory drugs to moderate to high doses of prednisone for severe systemic organ involvement. Immunosuppressive drugs (e.g., cytotoxic agents such as cyclophosphamide and azathioprine) and plasmapheresis alone or with steroids can be useful. Rituximab has produced dramatic, long-term remissions. For chronic cutaneous lupus erythematosus, topical steroids are effective to manage the cutaneous and oral lesions. For patients whose disease is resistant to topical therapy, systemic antimalarial drugs can be used with good results.

Erythema Multiforme

EM is an acute bullous and macular inflammatory mucocutaneous disease that affects mainly young adults between the ages of 20 and 40 years; it is rarely seen in children (≤20%). The genesis of the mucocutaneous lesions is thought to reside in the development of immune complex vasculitis. This is followed by complement fixation that leads to the leukocytoclastic destruction of vascular walls and small vessel occlusion. The culmination of these events produces ischemic necrosis of the epithelium and underlying connective tissue.

Target (i.e., iris) lesions with central clearing are the hallmark of EM. It can be a mild (i.e., EM minor) or a severe and possibly life-threatening condition (i.e., EM major or Stevens–Johnson syndrome). An underdiagnosed type of EM is recurrent oral erythema multiforme (ROEM), with which most patients have chronic or recurrent oral lesions only.

EM minor lasts approximately 4 weeks and exhibits moderate cutaneous and mucosal involvement. Stevens–Johnson syndrome can last a month or longer. It involves the skin, conjunctiva, oral mucosa, and genitalia, and it requires more aggressive therapy than EM minor. Some researchers consider toxic epidermal necrolysis to be the most severe form of EM, but other investigators think they are unrelated entities.

The two most common etiologic factors for the development of EM are herpes simplex infection and drug reactions. Recent reports documented EM major and EM-like lesions in adult and pediatric individuals infected with COVID-19. The most common causative drugs of EM are sulfonamides, penicillins, quinolones, chlormezanone, barbiturates, oxicam nonsteroidal antiinflammatory drugs, anticonvulsant drugs, protease inhibitors, and allopurinol.

Oral lesions in patients with EM are common, and they occur in more than 70% of patients with skin involvement. In rare instances, EM is confined to the mouth. The oral lesions consist of multiple, large, shallow, painful ulcers with an erythematous border. They affect the entire oral mucosa in approximately 20% of patients with EM. The lesions are so painful that chewing and swallowing are impaired (Fig. 16.34). The buccal mucosa and the tongue are the most frequently affected sites, followed by the labial mucosa. Areas that are less often affected include the floor of the mouth, the hard and soft palates, and the gingiva. EM is rarely confined exclusively to the gingival tissues, prompting a clinical diagnosis of desquamative gingivitis. Hemorrhagic crusting of the vermilion border of the lips may occur, which is helpful for arriving at a clinical diagnosis of EM.

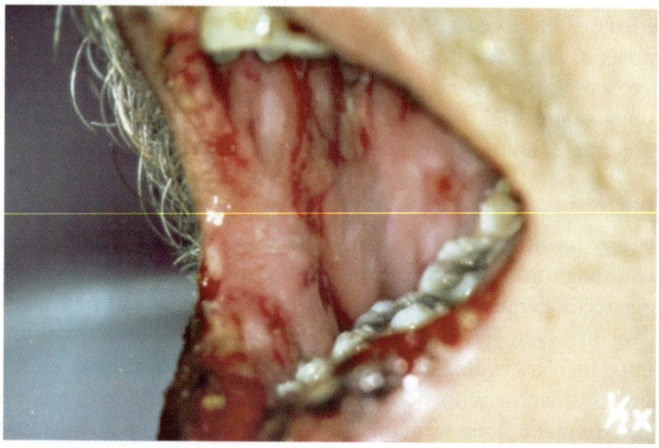

Fig. 16.34 In a patient with erythema multiforme, large, shallow, and painful ulcers involve the labial and buccal mucosae. Hemorrhagic crusting of the mandibular vermilion border of the lips is observed. *(Courtesy: Dr. Stuart L. Fischman, State University of New York at Buffalo, NY.)*

Histopathology

Common microscopic findings of EM include the liquefaction degeneration of the upper epithelium and development of intraepithelial microvesicles without the acantholysis that occurs with pemphigus. Acanthosis, pseudoepitheliomatous hyperplasia, and necrotic keratinocytes are observed in the epithelium. Degenerative changes also occur in the basement membrane. In some cases, the junction between the epithelium and the lamina propria is indistinct because of a dense inflammatory cell infiltrate. Edema of the lamina propria, vascular dilation, and congestion also occur. Deeper layers of the connective tissue stroma exhibit a perivascular chronic inflammatory cell infiltrate. However, neutrophils and eosinophils may also be seen.

Immunofluorescence

The immunofluorescence examination result is negative for patients with EM. Its value resides in ruling out other vesiculobullous and ulcerative disorders.

Treatment

There is no specific treatment for EM. For mild symptoms, systemic and local antihistamines, topical anesthetics, and debridement of lesions with an oxygenating agent are adequate. In patients with bullous or ulcerative lesions and severe symptoms, corticosteroids are considered the drug of choice, although their use is controversial and not completely accepted.

Drug-Related Eruptions

An increase in the incidence of skin and oral manifestations of hypersensitivity to drugs occurred with the advent of sulfonamides, barbiturates, and various antibiotics. The cutaneous and oral lesions are attributed to the drug acting as an allergen that sensitizes the tissues.

Eruptions in the oral cavity that result from sensitivity to drugs that have been taken orally or parenterally are called stomatitis medicamentosa. The local reaction from the use of a medicament in the oral cavity (e.g., stomatitis resulting from topical penicillin use) is referred to as stomatitis venenata or contact stomatitis. In many cases, skin eruptions accompany the oral lesions.

Most drug eruptions in the oral cavity are multiform. Vesicular and bullous lesions occur most often, but pigmented or nonpigmented macular lesions are also frequently observed. Erosions, which are often followed by deep ulceration with purpuric lesions, can occur. The lesions are seen in different areas of the oral cavity, with the gingiva often being affected.

The development of gingival lesions caused by contact allergy to the mercurial compounds in dental amalgam has been documented. Because of financial considerations, biopsy and patch testing may be indicated before the indiscriminate replacement of dental amalgam restorations. Similarly, desquamative gingivitis has been reported with the use of tartar control toothpaste. Pyrophosphates and flavoring agents have been identified as the main causative agents of this unusual condition. Oral reactions to cinnamon compounds (i.e., cinnamon oil, cinnamic acid, or cinnamic aldehyde) that are used to mask the taste of pyrophosphates in tartar control toothpaste include an intense erythema of the attached gingival tissues that is characteristic of plasma cell gingivitis (Fig. 16.35).

A thorough clinical history usually discloses the source of gingival disturbance. Elimination of the offending agent (i.e., tartar control toothpaste) leads to resolution of the gingival lesions within a week, and challenge with the offending agent leads to recurrence of the oral lesions. If removal of the offending medication is not

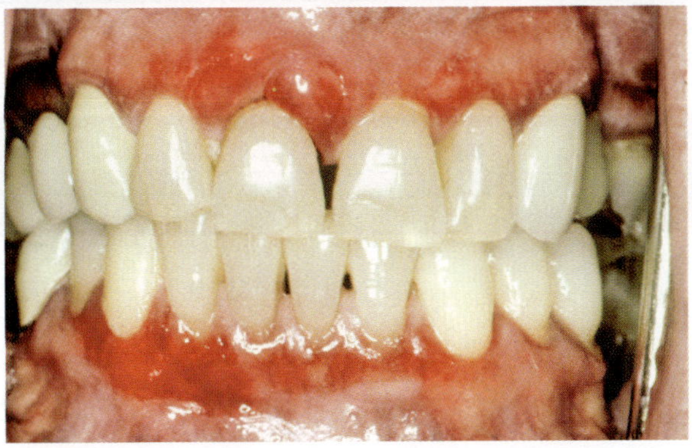

Fig. 16.35 **Plasma cell gingivitis.** The gingiva presents a band of moderate to severe inflammation that is reminiscent of desquamative gingivitis.

possible, topical corticosteroids and topical tacrolimus can be used to treat the lesions.

Clinical Correlation

Diseases That Mimic Desquamative Gingivitis

- Squamous cell carcinoma
- Wegener granulomatosis (strawberry gingivitis)
- Candidiasis
- Graft-versus-host disease
- Crohn's disease
- Foreign body gingivitis

Miscellaneous Conditions That Mimic Desquamative Gingivitis

Another group of heterogeneous conditions may masquerade as desquamative gingivitis. Factitious lesions, candidiasis, graft-versus-host disease, Wegener granulomatosis, foreign body gingivitis, Kindler syndrome, and squamous cell carcinoma can divert the attention of the clinician and provide a diagnostic challenge.

Factitious lesions are injuries that are consciously and intentionally produced without a clear motive, although guilt, seeking sympathy, or monetary compensation can be the driving forces for this abnormal behavior. Factitious desquamative gingivitis has been reported in the literature; it may be difficult to diagnose, and it may become apparent only after extensive and costly laboratory tests fail to reveal the genesis of the lesions.

Candidiasis is rarely limited to the gingival tissues and can simulate desquamative gingivitis. Linear gingival erythema is a Candida-associated lesion in individuals who are infected with human immunodeficiency virus. It manifests as a ribbon-like red band of the gingival margins and is reminiscent of desquamative gingivitis.

Graft-versus-host disease can occur in recipients of allogenic bone marrow transplants. The associated oral lesions occasionally resemble desquamative gingivitis.

Wegener granulomatosis is a systemic disease that can manifest with striking alterations that are confined to the gingival tissues. Classically, the gingival tissues exhibit erythema and enlargement, and they are typically described as strawberry gums.

Foreign body gingivitis is clinically characterized by red or red and white chronic lesions that can be painful and that are reminiscent of desquamative gingivitis. This condition is more common among women approaching the fifth decade of life. Microscopic analysis reveals small (<5 μm in diameter) foreign bodies associated with a chronic inflammatory cell response that can exhibit granulomatous and lichenoid characteristics. Energy-dispersive radiographic microanalysis revealed that most of these foreign bodies originate from dental materials (i.e., abrasives and restorative materials).

Kindler syndrome, which involves cutaneous neonatal bullae, poikiloderma, photosensitivity, and acral atrophy, can manifest with oral lesions that are clinically consistent with desquamative gingivitis.

A clinical diagnosis of desquamative gingivitis requires a series of diagnostic steps before a precise diagnosis can be obtained. The steps include a comprehensive clinical history, clinical-pathologic correlation, microscopic examination (e.g., H&E), and direct immunofluorescence studies. The failure to systematically evaluate a patient with a clinical condition that is consistent with desquamative gingivitis can produce poor outcomes. This is particularly true when therapy for a putative desquamative gingivitis is established before a biopsy of the lesional tissue is obtained. Every year, in our laboratory, we see at least two examples of clinically diagnosed desquamative gingivitis for which microscopic and immunofluorescence studies were not performed to rule out the cause of the gingival lesions. The patients were monitored or prescribed topical steroids for several months before the lack of response of the gingival lesions impelled the clinician to obtain a biopsy, which revealed squamous cell carcinoma. Clinicians should be alert to the possibility of squamous cell carcinoma of the gingival tissues with lesions that initially manifest as desquamative gingivitis.

Key points

- Desquamative gingivitis is not a specific disease entity but a manifestation of several disorders.
- Approximately 75% of the cases have dermatologic genesis. Intense erythema and peeling of the surface epithelium involving marginal and attached gingiva are the main features. Symptoms vary from mild discomfort to severe burning sensation and pain.
- Lichen planus, mucous membrane pemphigoid and pemphigus are the most common conditions leading to desquamative gingivitis.
- Careful history, clinical examination and biopsy including immunofluorescence tests are needed to establish diagnosis.
- A variety of drugs from topical and systemic steroids, immunosuppressants like azothioprine, cyclosporine and tetracycline, dapsone are employed in the treatment.

Suggested Reading

Nisengard RJ, Neiders M: Desquamative lesions of the gingiva. *J Periodontol* 52:500, 1981.

Michael Glick, Martin Greenberg et al.(eds), *Burket's Oral Medicine*, 13th edition, (2021) Wiley Blackwell.

CHAPTER 17

The Periodontal Pocket

FA Carranza | PM Camargo | DG Naik | A Uppoor

CHAPTER OUTLINE

The periodontal pocket, which is defined as a pathologically deepened gingival sulcus, is one of the most important clinical features of periodontal disease. All different types of periodontitis share histopathologic features, such as tissue changes in the periodontal pocket, mechanisms of tissue destruction, and healing mechanisms. However, they differ with regard to their etiology, natural history, progression, and response to therapy.

Classification

Deepening of the gingival sulcus may occur as a result of coronal movement of the gingival margin, apical displacement of the gingival attachment, or a combination of the two processes (Fig. 17.1). Pockets can be classified as follows:

- *Gingival pocket* (also called "pseudo-pocket") is formed by gingival enlargement without destruction of the underlying periodontal tissues. The sulcus is deepened because of the increased bulk of the gingiva (Fig. 17.2A).
- Periodontal pocket is formed by loss of periodontal attachment, which can lead to loosening and exfoliation of the teeth. The remainder of this chapter refers to this type of pocket.

Based on the location of the base of the pocket in relation to the underlying bone, periodontal pockets can be classified into the following types:

- *Suprabony* (*supracrestal* or *supraalveolar*) occurs when the bottom of the pocket is coronal to the underlying alveolar bone (Fig. 17.2B).
- *Intrabony* (*infrabony*, *subcrestal*, or *intraalveolar*) occurs when the bottom of the pocket is apical to the level of the adjacent alveolar bone. With this second type, the lateral pocket wall lies between the tooth surface and the alveolar bone (Fig. 17.2C).

Pockets can also be classified according to the involved tooth surface as (Fig. 17.3):

- Pockets can involve one, two, or more tooth surfaces, and they can be of different depths and types on different surfaces of the same tooth and on proximal surfaces of the same interdental space. Pockets can also be spiral (i.e., originating on one tooth surface and twisting around the tooth to involve one or more additional surfaces). These types of pockets are most common in furcation areas.

Clinical Features

Signs

- Enlarged bluish-red marginal gingiva with rolled-out edge separated from the tooth surface.
- Reddish-blue vertical zone from the gingival margin to attached gingiva/alveolar mucosa.
- Break in faciolingual continuity of interdental gingiva.
- Shiny discolored puffy gingiva.
- Gingival bleeding.
- Purulent exudate from the gingival margin in response to digital pressure.
- Looseness, extrusion, and migration of teeth.
- Development of diastema where none had previously existed.
- The only reliable method of locating periodontal pockets and determining their extent is careful probing of the gingival margin along each surface (Fig. 17.4).

Symptoms

- Localized pain or sensation of pressure after eating, which gradually diminishes.
- Foul taste in localized areas.
- Tendency to suck material in the interdental areas.
- Radiating pain deep in the bone.
- Gnawing feeling or itching in the gingiva and urge to dig a pointed instrument into the gums and relief obtained from resultant bleeding.
- Food sticks in between the teeth or teeth feel loose.
- Sensitivity to heat and cold.
- Toothache in absence of caries.

KEY FACT

Sulcus Versus Periodontal Pocket

Gingival sulcus is the space between the neck of the tooth and the circumferential gingival tissue. Sulcus, when it deepens (as in periodontal disease) due to the apical migration of junctional epithelium, accompanied by attachment loss, it is referred to as a *periodontal pocket*.

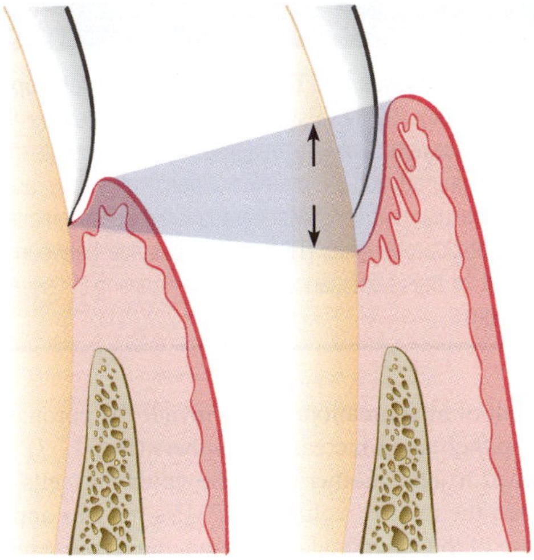

Fig. 17.1 Illustration of pocket formation that indicates expansion in two directions *(arrows)* from the normal gingival sulcus *(left)* to the periodontal pocket *(right)*.

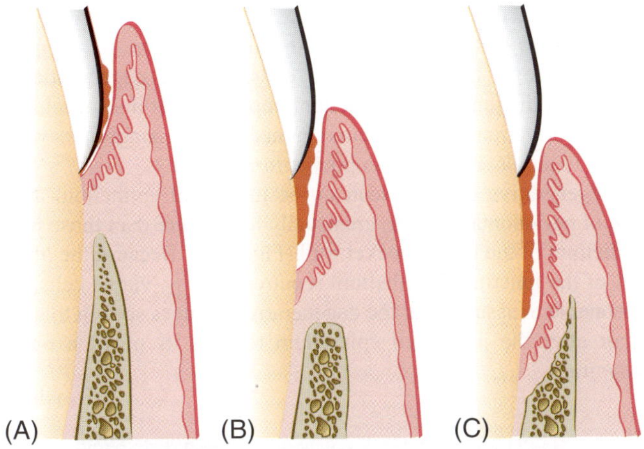

Fig. 17.2 Different types of periodontal pockets. (A), Gingival pocket. There is no destruction of the supporting periodontal tissues. (B), Suprabony pocket. The base of the pocket is coronal to the level of the underlying bone. Bone loss is horizontal. (C), infrabony pocket. The base of the pocket is apical to the level of the adjacent bone. Bone loss is vertical.

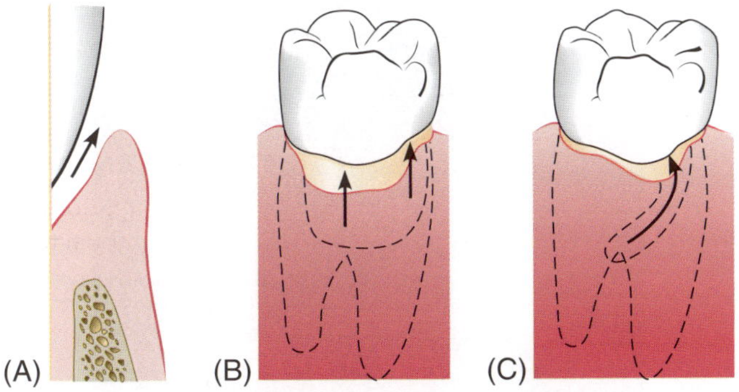

Fig. 17.3 Classification of pockets according to involved tooth surfaces. A, Simple pocket. B, Compound pocket. C, Complex pocket.

Pathogenesis

The initial lesion in the development of periodontitis is the inflammation of the gingiva in response to a bacterial challenge. Changes involved in the transition from the normal gingival sulcus to the pathologic periodontal pocket are associated with different proportions of bacterial cells in dental plaque. Healthy gingiva is associated with few microorganisms, mostly coccoid cells and straight rods. Diseased gingiva is associated with increased numbers of Spirochetes and motile rods. However, the microbiota of diseased sites cannot be used as a predictor of future attachment or bone loss because their presence alone is not sufficient for disease to start or progress.

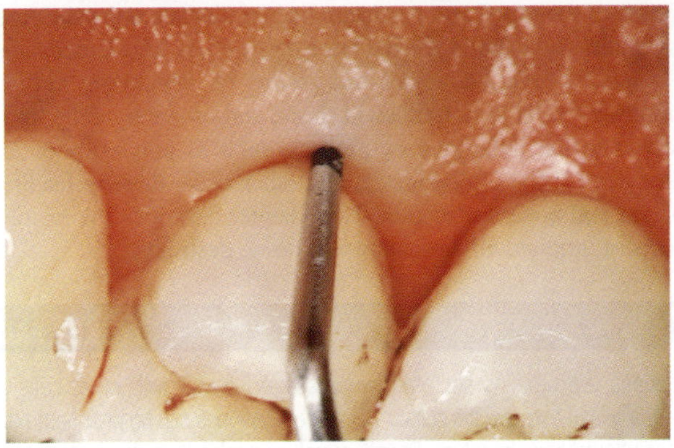

Fig. 17.4 Probing of a deep periodontal pocket. The entire length of the periodontal probe has been inserted to the base of the pocket in the palatal surface of the first premolar.

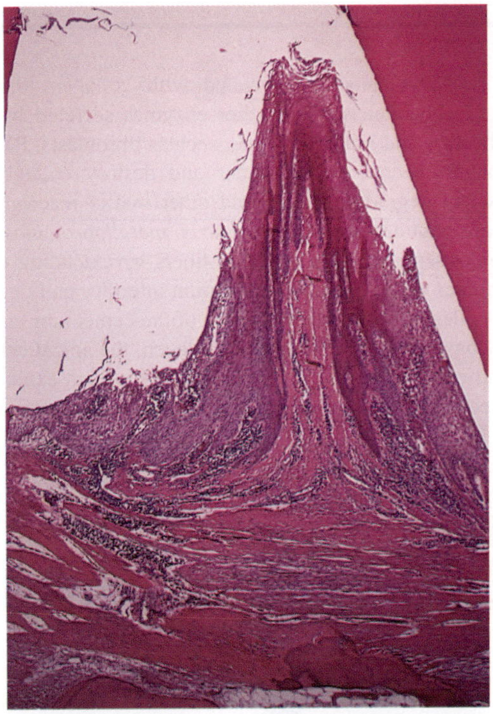

Fig. 17.5 Interdental papilla with suprabony pockets on proximal tooth surfaces. Note the densely inflamed connective tissue with the infiltrate extending between the collagen fibers and the proliferating and ulcerated pocket epithelium.

Pocket formation starts as an inflammatory change in the connective tissue wall of the gingival sulcus. The cellular and fluid inflammatory exudate causes degeneration of the surrounding connective tissue, including the gingival fibers. Just apical to the junctional epithelium, collagen fibers are destroyed, and the area is occupied by inflammatory cells and edema (Fig. 17.5).

Early concepts assumed that, after the initial bacterial attack, periodontal tissue destruction continued to be linked to bacterial action. More recently, it was established that the host's immunoinflammatory response to the initial and persistent bacterial attack unleashes mechanisms that lead to collagen and bone destruction. These mechanisms are related to various cytokines, some of which are produced normally by cells in noninflamed tissue and others by cells that are involved in the inflammatory process, such as polymorphonuclear leukocytes (PMNs), monocytes, and other cells, thereby leading to collagen and bone destruction. This chapter describes the histologic aspects of gingival inflammation and tissue destruction.

KEY FACT

Cytokines are proteins secreted by cells that interact with other cells and eventually lead to a specific cellular response. Cytokines can be proinflammatory or antiinflammatory in nature. Proinflammatory cytokines such as interleukin-1 (IL-1) and tumor necrosis factor-alpha (TNF-α) are implicated strongly in the pathogenesis of periodontal disease progression. Antiinflammatory cytokines such as IL-4 and IL-10 counteract the effects of proinflammatory cytokines.

The two mechanisms associated with collagen loss are as follows: (1) collagenases and other enzymes secreted by various cells in healthy and inflamed tissue, such as fibroblasts, PMNs, and macrophages, become extracellular and destroy collagen (these enzymes that degrade collagen and other matrix macromolecules into small peptides are called *matrix metalloproteinases*); and (2) fibroblasts phagocytize collagen fibers by extending cytoplasmic processes to the ligament–cementum interface and degrade the inserted collagen fibrils and the fibrils of the cementum matrix.

As a consequence of the loss of collagen, the apical cells of the junctional epithelium proliferate along the root and extend finger-like projections that are two or three cells in thickness (Fig. 17.6).

KEY FACT

Matrix Metalloproteinases and Tissue Inhibitors of Metalloproteinases

Matrix metalloproteinases (MMPs) are a group of proteases that play an important role in several biologic processes. Like any protease, they are involved in the degradation of proteins. Specifically, they are important players in extracellular matrix (ECM) degradation and are inhibited by tissue inhibitors of metalloproteinases (TIMPs). The balance between MMPs and TIMPs is critical for the maintenance of ECM remodeling in tissues, including the periodontium.

As a result of inflammation, PMNs invade the coronal end of the junctional epithelium in increasing numbers (Fig. 17.7). The PMNs are not joined to one another or to the epithelial cells by desmosomes. When the relative volume of PMNs reaches approximately 60% or more of the junctional epithelium, the tissue loses cohesiveness and detaches from the tooth surface. Thus, the coronal portion of the junctional epithelium detaches from the root as the apical portion migrates, thereby resulting in its apical shift; the oral sulcular epithelium gradually occupies an increasing portion of the sulcus (then a pocket) lining.

Extension of the junctional epithelium along the root requires the presence of healthy epithelial cells. Marked degeneration or necrosis of the junctional epithelium impairs rather than accelerates pocket formation. (This occurs in necrotizing gingivitis, which results in an ulcer rather than pocket formation.)

Degenerative changes seen in the junctional epithelium at the base of periodontal pockets are usually less severe than those in the epithelium of the lateral pocket wall (Fig. 17.7). Because the migration of the junctional epithelium requires healthy, viable cells, it is reasonable to assume that the degenerative changes seen in this area occur after the junctional epithelium reaches its position on the cementum.

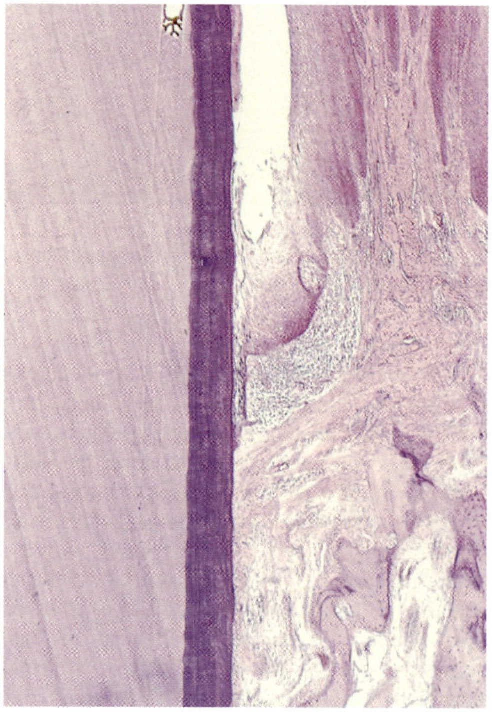

Fig. 17.6 Low-power view of the base of the periodontal pocket and apical area. Note the dense inflammatory infiltrate on the area of destroyed collagen fibers and the thin, finger-like extension of epithelium covering the cementum, which has been denuded of fibers.

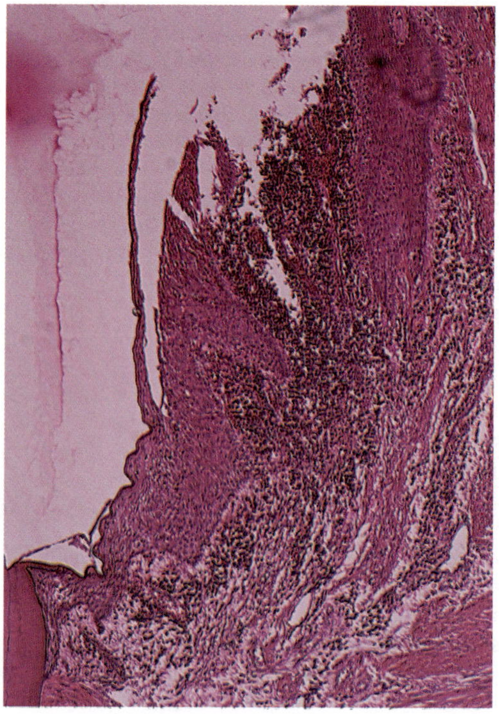

Fig. 17.7 View of the ulcerated lateral pocket wall of a periodontal pocket. Note the extension of epithelial cells and the dense accumulation of leukocytes within the epithelium and in the connective tissue.

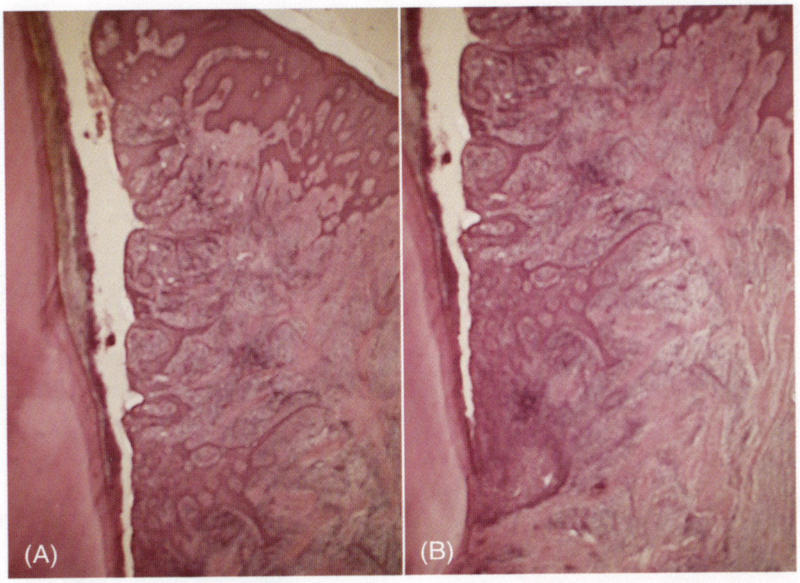

Fig. 17.8 A, Lateral wall of a periodontal pocket showing epithelial proliferative and atrophic changes as well as marked inflammatory infiltrate and the destruction of collagen fibers. B, Slightly apical view of the same patient showing the shortened junctional epithelium.

The degree of leukocyte infiltration of the junctional epithelium is independent of the volume of inflamed connective tissue; thus, this process may occur in gingiva with only slight signs of clinical inflammation.

With continued inflammation, the gingiva increases in bulk, and the crest of the gingival margin extends coronally. The apical cells of the junctional epithelium continue to migrate along the root; and its coronal cells continue to separate from it. The epithelium of the lateral wall of the pocket proliferates to form bulbous, cord-like extensions into the inflamed connective tissue. Leukocytes and edema from the inflamed connective tissue infiltrate the epithelium that lines the pocket, thereby resulting in various degrees of degeneration and necrosis.

The transformation of a gingival sulcus into a periodontal pocket creates an area in which plaque removal becomes impossible and a feedback mechanism is established. The rationale for pocket reduction is based on the need to eliminate areas of plaque accumulation.

Histopathology

Changes that occur during the initial stages of gingival inflammation are presented in the chapter on Gingival Inflammation. After the pocket is formed, several microscopic features are present, which will be discussed in this section.

Soft-Tissue Wall

The connective tissue is edematous and densely infiltrated with plasma cells (approximately 80%), lymphocytes, and a scattering of PMNs. The blood vessels are increased in number, dilated, and engorged, particularly in the subepithelial connective tissue layer. The connective tissue exhibits varying degrees of degeneration. Single or multiple necrotic foci are occasionally present. In addition to exudative and degenerative changes, the connective tissue shows proliferation of the endothelial cells, with newly formed capillaries, fibroblasts, and collagen fibers (Fig. 17.5).

The junctional epithelium at the base of the pocket is usually much shorter than that of a normal sulcus. Although marked variations are found with regard to the length, width, and condition of the epithelial cells, usually the coronoapical length of the junctional epithelium is reduced to only 50–100 μm. The cells may be well formed and in good condition, or they may exhibit slight to marked degeneration (Figs. 17.6 and 17.8).

The most severe degenerative changes in the periodontal pocket occur along the lateral wall (Fig. 17.7). The epithelium of the lateral wall of the pocket presents striking proliferative and degenerative changes. Epithelial buds or interlacing cords of epithelial cells project from the lateral wall into the adjacent inflamed connective tissue and may extend farther apically than the junctional epithelium (Figs. 17.8 and 17.9A and B). These epithelial projections, as well as the remainder of the lateral epithelium, are densely infiltrated by leukocytes and edema from the inflamed connective tissue. The cells undergo vacuolar degeneration and rupture to form vesicles. Progressive degeneration and necrosis of the epithelium lead to ulceration of the lateral wall, exposure of the underlying inflamed connective tissue, and suppuration. In some cases, acute inflammation is superimposed on the underlying chronic changes.

A comparative study of gingival changes in aggressive and chronic periodontitis revealed more pronounced degenerative changes in the epithelium of aggressive cases with more open intercellular spaces, including microclefts and necrotic areas.

The severity of the degenerative changes is not necessarily related to pocket depth. Ulceration of the lateral wall may occur in shallow pockets, and deep pockets are occasionally observed in which the lateral epithelium is relatively intact or shows only slight degeneration.

The epithelium at the gingival crest of a periodontal pocket is generally intact and thickened, with prominent rete pegs.

KEY FACT

Features of Junctional Epithelium

- It acts as a physical barrier against plaque bacteria.
- It is stratified squamous nonkeratinized in nature, which develops by the union of oral epithelium and reduced enamel epithelium during tooth eruption.
- It is attached to the tooth by internal basal lamina and to the connective tissue by external basal lamina.
- It exhibits higher permeability to cells, gingival fluid, and host–defense molecules to flow through.
- It has higher rate of cellular proliferation and turnover.

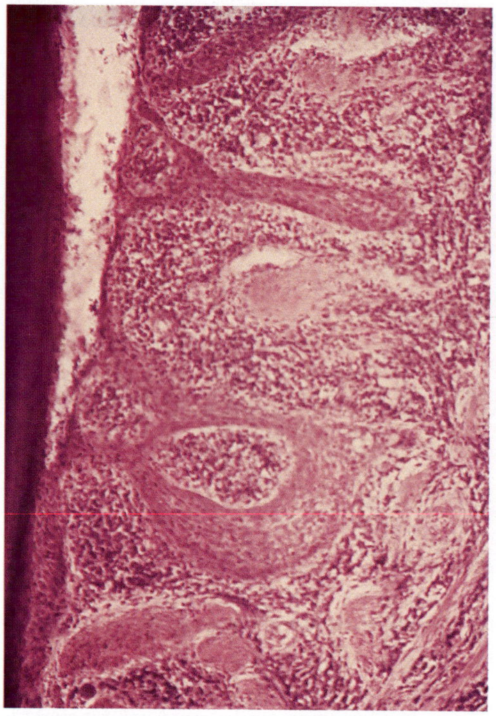

Fig. 17.9 Base of periodontal pocket showing extensive proliferation of lateral epithelium next to atrophic areas, dense inflammatory infiltrate, remnants of destroyed collagen fibers, and the junctional epithelium, which is apparently in a less altered state than the lateral pocket epithelium.

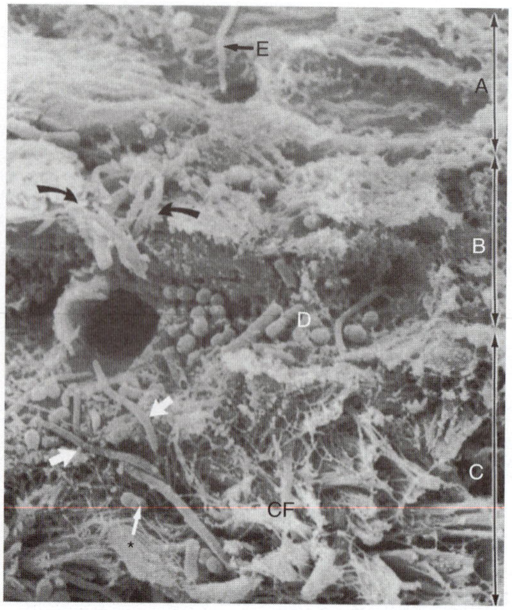

Fig. 17.10 Scanning electron micrograph of a section of pocket wall in advanced periodontitis in a human specimen showing bacterial penetration into the epithelium and connective tissue. Scanning electron microscope view of the surface of the pocket wall (A), sectioned epithelium (B), and sectioned connective tissue (C). *Curved arrows* point to areas of bacterial penetration into the epithelium. *Thick white arrows* point to bacterial penetration into the connective tissue through a break in the continuity of the basal lamina. *CF*, Connective tissue fibers; (D), accumulation of bacteria (rods, cocci, and filaments) on the basal lamina; (E), filamentous organism on the surface of the epithelium. The *asterisk* points to coccobacillus in the connective tissue.

Bacterial Invasion

Bacterial invasion of the apical and lateral areas of the pocket wall has been described in human chronic periodontitis. Filaments, rods, and coccoid organisms with predominant Gram-negative cell walls have been found in intercellular spaces of the epithelium. Hillmann et al. have reported the presence of *Porphyromonas gingivalis* and *Prevotella intermedia* in the gingiva of aggressive periodontitis cases. *Aggregatibacter actinomycetemcomitans* has also been found in the tissues.

Bacteria may invade the intercellular space under exfoliating epithelial cells, but they are also found between deeper epithelial cells, as well as accumulated on the basement lamina. Some bacteria traverse the basement lamina and invade the subepithelial connective tissue (Figs. 17.10 and 17.11).

The presence of bacteria in the gingival tissues has been interpreted by different investigators as bacterial invasion or as the "passive translocation" of plaque bacteria. This important point has significant clinicopathologic implications and has not yet been clarified.

Mechanisms of Tissue Destruction

The inflammatory response triggered by bacterial plaque unleashes a complex cascade of events aimed at destroying and removing bacteria, necrotic cells, and deleterious agents. However, this process is nonspecific; in an attempt to restore health, the host's cells (e.g., neutrophils, macrophages, fibroblasts, and epithelial cells) produce proteinases, cytokines, and prostaglandins that can damage or destroy the tissues.

Microtopography of the Gingival Wall

Scanning electron microscopy has permitted the description of several areas in the soft-tissue (gingival) wall of the periodontal pocket in which different types of activity take place. These areas are

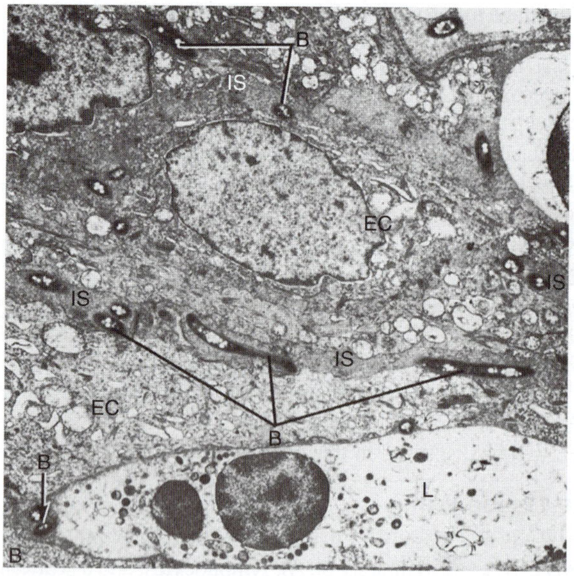

Fig. 17.11 Transmission electron micrograph of the epithelium in the periodontal pocket wall showing bacteria in the intercellular spaces. *B*, Bacteria; *EC*, epithelial cell; *IS*, intercellular space; *L*, leukocyte about to engulf bacteria (×8000).

irregularly oval or elongated and adjacent to one another, and they measure about 50–200 μm. These findings suggest that the pocket wall is constantly changing as a result of the interaction between the host and the bacteria. The following areas have been noted:

1. *Areas of relative quiescence*, showing a relatively flat surface with minor depressions and mounds and occasional shedding of cells (Fig. 17.12, area *A*).

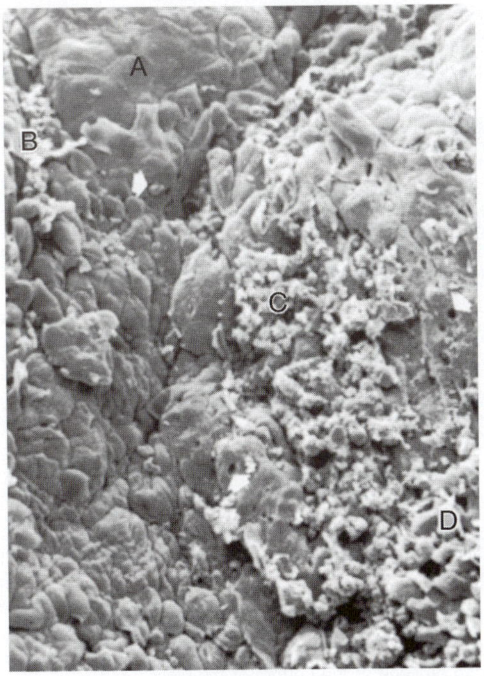

Fig. 17.12 Scanning electron frontal micrograph of the periodontal pocket wall. Different areas can be seen in the pocket wall surface. A, Area of quiescence; B, bacterial accumulation; C, bacterial–leukocyte interaction; D, intense cellular desquamation. *Arrows* point to emerging leukocytes and holes left by leukocytes in the pocket wall (×800).

2. *Areas of bacterial accumulation*, which appear as depressions on the epithelial surface, with abundant debris and bacterial clumps penetrating into the enlarged intercellular spaces. These bacteria are mainly cocci, rods, and filaments, with a few Spirochetes (Fig. 17.12, area *B*).
3. *Areas of emergence of leukocytes*, in which leukocytes appear in the pocket wall through holes located in the intercellular spaces (Fig. 17.13).
4. *Areas of leukocyte–bacteria interaction*, in which numerous leukocytes are present and covered with bacteria in an apparent process of phagocytosis. Bacterial plaque associated with the epithelium is seen either as an organized matrix covered by a fibrin-like material in contact with the surface of cells or as bacteria penetrating into the intercellular spaces (Fig. 17.12, area *C*).
5. *Areas of intense epithelial desquamation*, which consist of semi-attached and folded epithelial squames, which are sometimes partially covered with bacteria (Fig. 17.12, area *D*).
6. *Areas of ulceration*, with exposed connective tissue (Fig. 17.14).
7. *Areas of hemorrhage*, with numerous erythrocytes.

The transition from one area to another could result from bacteria accumulating in previously quiescent areas and triggering the emergence of leukocytes and the leukocyte–bacteria interaction. This would lead to intense epithelial desquamation and finally to ulceration and hemorrhage.

Periodontal Pockets as Healing Lesions

Periodontal pockets are chronic inflammatory lesions and thus are constantly undergoing repair. Complete healing does not occur because of the persistence of the bacterial attack, which continues to stimulate an inflammatory response, thereby causing degeneration of the new tissue elements formed during the continuous effort at repair.

The condition of the soft-tissue wall of the periodontal pocket results from the interplay of the destructive and constructive tissue

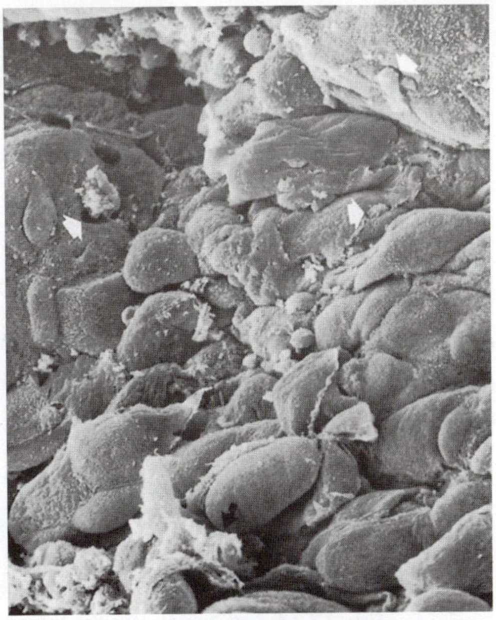

Fig. 17.13 Scanning electron micrograph of the periodontal pocket wall, frontal view, in a patient with advanced periodontitis. Note the desquamating epithelial cells and leukocytes *(white arrows)* emerging onto the pocket space. Scattered bacteria can also be seen *(black arrow)* (×1500).

changes. Their balance determines clinical features, such as color, consistency, and surface texture of the pocket wall. If the inflammatory fluid and cellular exudate predominate, the pocket wall is bluish-red, soft, spongy, and friable, with a smooth, shiny surface; at the clinical level, this is generally referred to as an *edematous pocket wall*. If there is a relative predominance of newly formed connective tissue cells and fibers, the pocket wall is more firm and pink and clinically referred to as a *fibrotic pocket wall* (Table 17.1). Edematous and fibrotic pockets represent opposite extremes of the same pathologic process rather than different disease entities. They are subject to constant modification, depending on the relative predominance of exudative and constructive changes.

Fibrotic pocket walls may be misleading because they do not necessarily reflect what is taking place throughout the pocket wall. The most severe degenerative changes in periodontal tissues occur adjacent to the tooth surface and the subgingival plaque. In some cases, inflammation and ulceration on the inside of the pocket are walled off by fibrous tissue on the outer aspect (Fig. 17.15). Externally the pocket appears pink and fibrotic, despite the inflammatory changes occurring internally.

Pocket Contents

Periodontal pockets contain debris that consists principally of microorganisms and their products (enzymes, endotoxins, and other metabolic products), gingival fluid, food remnants, salivary mucin, desquamated epithelial cells, and leukocytes. Plaque-covered calculus usually projects from the tooth surface (Fig. 17.16). Purulent exudate, if present in the patient, consists of living, degenerated, and necrotic leukocytes; living and dead bacteria; serum; and a scant amount of fibrin. The contents of periodontal pockets, when filtered free of organisms and debris, have been demonstrated to be toxic when injected subcutaneously into experimental animals.

Significance of Pus Formation

Pus is a common feature of periodontal disease but it is only a secondary sign. The presence of pus or the ease with which it can

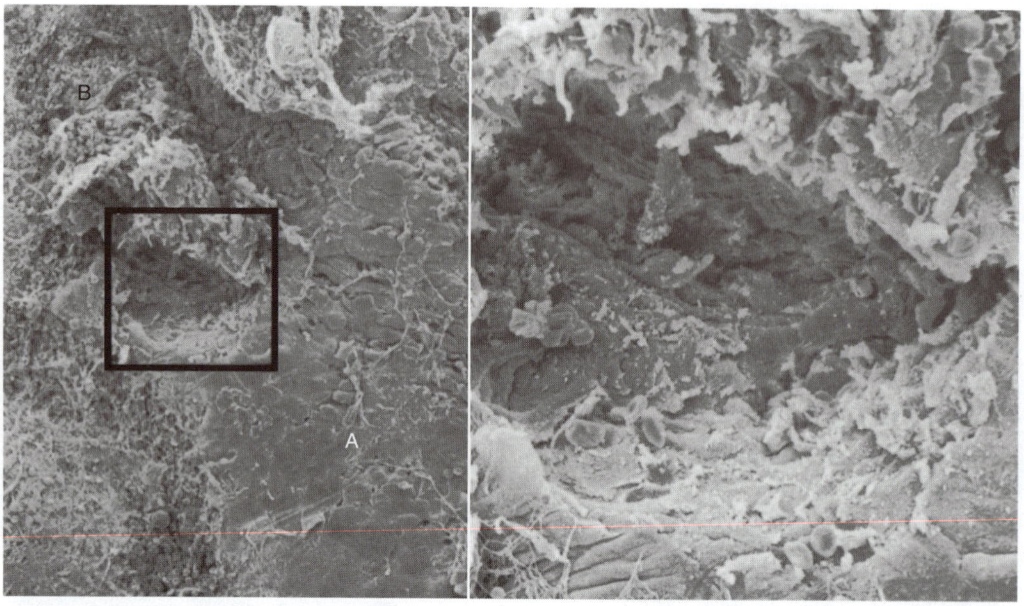

Fig. 17.14 *Left*, Area of ulceration in the lateral wall of a deep periodontal pocket in a human specimen (×800). A, Surface of pocket epithelium in a quiescent state; B, area of hemorrhage. *Right*, Scanning electron microscopy (×3000) of the square on the left. Connective tissue fibers and cells can be seen at the bottom of the ulcer.

TABLE 17.1 Correlation of Clinical and Histopathologic Features of the Periodontal Pocket

Clinical Features	Histopathologic Features
The gingival wall of the pocket presents various degrees of bluish-red discoloration; flaccidity; a smooth, shiny surface; and pitting on pressure.	The discoloration is caused by circulatory stagnation; the flaccidity by the destruction of gingival fibers and surrounding tissues; the smooth, shiny surface by atrophy of the epithelium and edema; and the pitting on pressure by edema and degeneration.
Less frequently, the gingival wall may be pink and firm.	In such cases, fibrotic changes predominate over exudation and degeneration, particularly in relation to the outer surface of the pocket wall. However, despite the external appearance of health, the inner wall of the pocket invariably presents some degeneration and is often ulcerated (see Fig. 17.15).
Bleeding is elicited by gently probing the soft-tissue wall of pocket.	Ease of bleeding results from increased vascularity, the thinning and degeneration of the epithelium, and the proximity of engorged vessels to the inner surface.
When explored with a probe, the inner aspect of the pocket is generally painful.	Pain on tactile stimulation is caused by the ulceration of the inner aspect of the pocket wall.
In many cases, pus may be expressed with the application of digital pressure.	Pus occurs in pockets with suppurative inflammation of the inner wall.

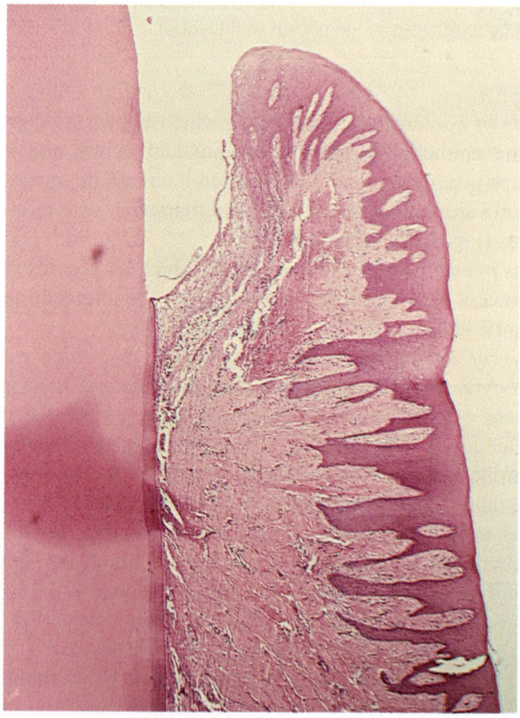

Fig. 17.15 Periodontal pocket wall. The inner half is inflamed and ulcerated; the outer half is densely collagenous.

be expressed from the pocket merely reflects the nature of the inflammatory changes in the pocket wall. It is not an indication of the depth of the pocket or the severity of the destruction of the supporting tissues. Extensive pus formation may occur in shallow pockets, whereas deep pockets may exhibit little or no pus. The localized accumulation of pus constitutes an abscess, which is discussed later in this chapter.

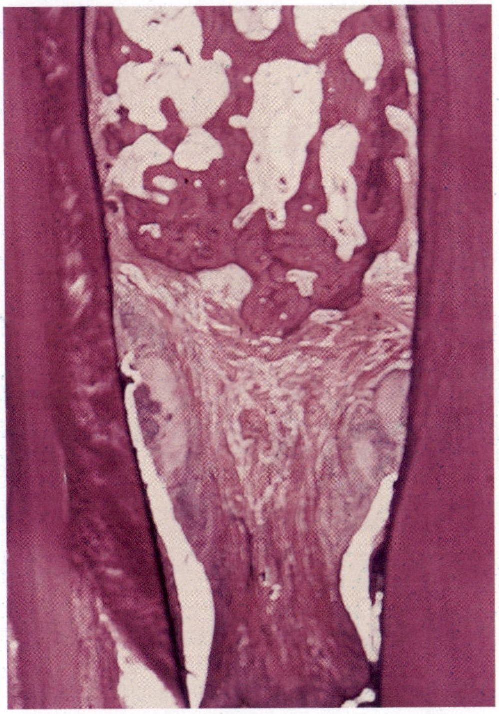

Fig. 17.16 Interdental papilla with ulcerated suprabony periodontal pockets on its mesial and distal aspects. Calculus is present on the approximal tooth surfaces and within the gingiva.

KEY FACT

Gingival Crevicular Fluid

Gingival crevicular fluid (GCF) is an ultrafiltrate of blood, present in the gingival sulcus space, that contains several molecular components like bacterial degradation products, host tissue degradation products, and inflammatory mediators. Due to the location and ease of collection, several human clinical studies have been and are currently exploring and validating biomarkers of periodontal disease in GCF. The implant equivalent of GCF is commonly referred to as peri-implant sulcular fluid (PISF).

Root Surface Walls

The root surface wall of periodontal pockets often undergoes changes that are significant because they may perpetuate the periodontal infection, cause pain, and complicate periodontal treatment.

As the pocket deepens, collagen fibers embedded in the cementum are destroyed, and cementum becomes exposed to the oral environment. Collagenous remnants of Sharpey's fibers in the cementum undergo degeneration, creating an environment favorable to the penetration of bacteria. Viable bacteria have been found in the roots of 87% of periodontally diseased noncarious teeth. Bacterial penetration into the cementum can be found as deep as the cementodentinal junction, and it may also enter the dentinal tubules. Penetration and the growth of bacteria lead to fragmentation and breakdown of the cementum surface and result in areas of necrotic cementum that are separated from the tooth by masses of bacteria.

Pathologic granules have been observed with light and electron microscopy, and they may represent areas of collagen degeneration or areas in which collagen fibrils have not been fully mineralized initially.

In addition, bacterial products (e.g., endotoxins) have also been detected in the cementum wall of periodontal pockets. When root fragments from teeth with periodontal disease are placed in tissue culture, they induce irreversible morphologic changes in the cells of the culture. Such changes are not produced by normal roots. Diseased root fragments also prevent the in vitro attachment of human gingival fibroblasts, whereas normal root surfaces allow the cells to attach freely. When placed in the oral mucosa of the patient, diseased root fragments induce an inflammatory response, even if they have been autoclaved.

KEY FACT

Bacterial Endotoxin

Endotoxins are lipopolysaccharide (LPS) in nature and are associated with the cell walls of gram-negative bacteria. LPS is highly immunogenic, which the innate immune system recognizes via Toll-like receptors (TLRs), leading to an immune response. LPS from *Porphyromonas gingivalis*, a key pathogen in periodontal disease, plays an important role in both triggering and sustaining inflammation in the periodontium.

These changes manifest clinically as softening of the cementum surface; this is usually asymptomatic, but it can be painful when a probe or explorer penetrates the area. They also constitute a possible reservoir for reinfection of the area after treatment. During the course of treatment, these necrotic areas are removed by root planing until a hard, smooth surface is reached. Cementum is very thin in the cervical areas, and scaling and root planing often remove it entirely, exposing the underlying dentin. Sensitivity to cold may result until the pulp tissue forms secondary dentin. Recent studies indicate that endotoxins are not tightly bound to cementum and can be easily removed using ultrasonic instrumentation without having to completely remove the entire cementum layer.

Decalcification and Remineralization of Cementum

Areas of *increased mineralization* are probably a result of an exchange of minerals and organic components at the cementum–saliva interface after exposure to the oral cavity. The mineral content of exposed cementum increases, and the minerals that are increased in diseased root surfaces include calcium, magnesium, phosphorus, and fluoride. Microhardness, however, remains unchanged. The development of a highly mineralized superficial layer may increase the tooth's resistance to decay.

The hypermineralized zones are detectable by electron microscopy, and they are associated with increased perfection of the crystal structure and organic changes that are suggestive of a subsurface cuticle. These zones have also been seen in microradiographic studies as a layer that is generally 10–20 mm thick, with areas as thick as 50 mm. No decrease in mineralization was found in deeper areas, indicating that increased mineralization does not come from adjacent areas. A loss of or reduction in the crossbanding of collagen near the cementum surface and a subsurface condensation of organic material of exogenous origin have also been reported.

Areas of demineralization are often related to root caries. Exposure to oral fluid and bacterial plaque results in proteolysis of the embedded remnants of Sharpey fibers; the cementum may be softened, and it may undergo fragmentation and cavitation. Unlike enamel caries, root surface caries tend to progress around rather than into the tooth. Active root caries lesions appear as well-defined yellowish or light brown areas; they are frequently covered by plaque, and they have a softened or leathery consistency on probing. Inactive lesions are well-defined darker lesions with a smooth surface and a harder consistency on probing.

The dominant microorganism in root surface caries is *Actinomyces viscosus*, although its specific role in the development of the lesion has not been established. Other bacteria, such as *Actinomyces naeslundii, Streptococcus mutans, Streptococcus salivarius, Streptococcus sanguinis,* and *Bacillus cereus*, have been found to produce root caries in animal models. Quirynen and colleagues reported that when plaque levels and pocket depths decrease after periodontal therapy (both nonsurgical and surgical), a shift in oral bacteria occurs, leading to a reduction in periodontal pathogens, an increase in *S. mutans*, and the development of root caries.

A prevalence rate study of root caries among 20- to 64-year-old individuals revealed that 42% had one or more root caries lesions and that these lesions tended to increase with age.

The tooth may not be painful, but exploration of the root surface reveals the presence of a defect, and penetration of the involved area with a probe causes pain. Caries of the root may lead to pulpitis, sensitivity to sweets and thermal changes, or severe pain. Pathologic exposure of the pulp occurs in severe cases. Root caries may be the cause of toothache in patients with periodontal disease and no evidence of coronal decay.

Caries of the cementum requires special attention when the pocket is treated. The necrotic cementum must be removed by scaling and root planing until firm tooth surface is reached, even if this entails extension into the dentin.

Areas of cellular resorption of cementum and dentin are common in roots that are unexposed by periodontal disease. These areas are of no particular significance because they are symptom free, and, as long as the root is covered by the periodontal ligament, they are likely to undergo repair. However, if the root is exposed by progressive pocket formation before repair occurs, these areas appear as isolated cavitations that penetrate into the dentin. These areas can be differentiated from caries of the cementum by their clear-cut outline and hard surface. They may be sources of considerable pain that require the placement of a restoration.

Surface Morphology of Tooth Wall

The following zones can be found in the bottom of a periodontal pocket (Fig. 17.17):

1. *Cementum covered by calculus*, in which all of the changes described in the preceding paragraphs can be found.
2. *Attached plaque*, which covers calculus and which extends apically from it to a variable degree (typically 100–500 μm).
3. The zone of *unattached plaque* that surrounds attached plaque and extends apically to it.
4. The zone of *attachment of the junctional epithelium to the tooth.* The extension of this zone, which in normal sulci is more than 500 μm, is usually reduced in periodontal pockets to less than 100 μm.
5. A zone of *semidestroyed connective tissue fibers* may be apical to the junctional epithelium (see the "Pathogenesis" section earlier in this chapter).

Zones 3, 4, and 5 make up the "plaque-free zone" seen in extracted teeth. The total width of the plaque-free zone varies according to the type of tooth (i.e., it is wider in the molars than in the incisors) and the depth of the pocket (i.e., it is narrower in deeper pockets). It is important to remember that the term *plaque-free zone* refers only to attached plaque because unattached plaque contains a variety of gram-positive and gram-negative morphotypes, including cocci, rods, filaments, fusiforms, and Spirochetes.

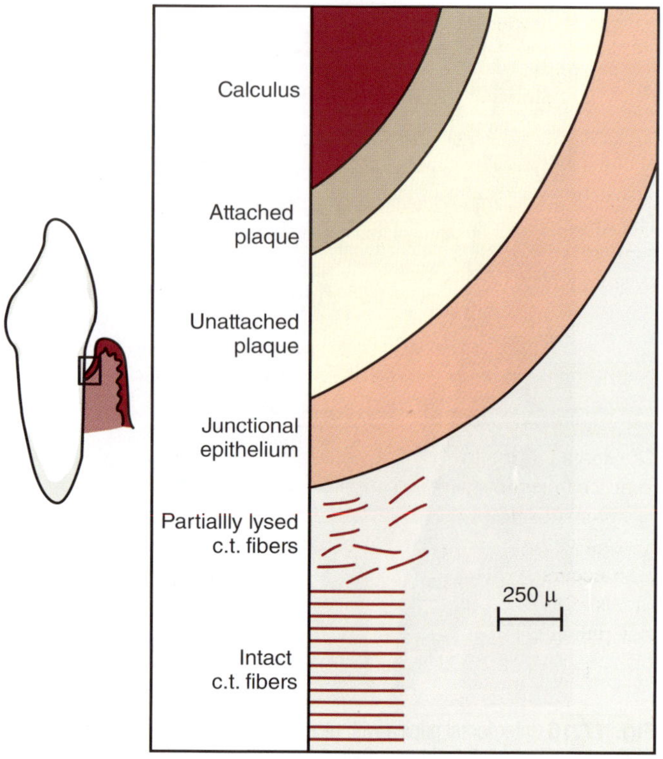

Fig. 17.17 Diagram of the area at the bottom of a pocket. *c.t.*, Connective tissue.

The most apical zone contains predominantly gram-negative rods and cocci.

Periodontal Disease Activity

For many years, the loss of attachment produced by periodontal disease was thought to be a slow but continuously progressive phenomenon. More recently, as a result of studies of the specificity of plaque bacteria, the concept of periodontal disease activity has evolved.

According to this concept, periodontal pockets go through periods of exacerbation and quiescence as a result of episodic bursts of activity followed by periods of remission. *Periods of quiescence* are characterized by a reduced inflammatory response and little or no loss of bone and connective tissue attachment. A buildup of unattached plaque, with its Gram-negative, motile, and anaerobic bacteria, starts a *period of exacerbation* during which bone and connective tissue attachment are lost and the pocket deepens. This period may last for days, weeks, or months, and it is eventually followed by a period of remission or quiescence during which gram-positive bacteria proliferate and a more stable condition is established. On the basis of a study of radioiodine I absorptiometry, it was confirmed that bone loss in patients with untreated periodontal disease occurs in an episodic manner.

These periods of quiescence and exacerbation are also known as *periods of inactivity* and *periods of activity.* Clinically, active periods show bleeding, either spontaneously or with probing, and greater amounts of gingival exudate. Histologically, the pocket epithelium appears thin and ulcerated, and an infiltrate composed predominantly of plasma cells, PMNs, or both is seen. Bacterial samples from the pocket lumen that are analyzed with dark-field microscopy show high proportions of motile organisms and Spirochetes.

Site Specificity

Periodontal destruction does not occur in all parts of the mouth at the same time; rather, it occurs on a few teeth at a time or even only on some aspects of some teeth at any given time. This is referred to as the *site specificity* of periodontal disease. Sites of periodontal destruction are often found next to sites with little or no destruction. Therefore, the severity of periodontitis increases with the development of new disease sites and with the increased breakdown of existing sites.

Pulp Changes Associated With Periodontal Pockets

The spread of infection from periodontal pockets may cause pathologic changes in the pulp. Such changes may give rise to painful symptoms or they may adversely affect the response of the pulp to restorative procedures. Involvement of the pulp in periodontal disease occurs through either the apical foramen or the lateral pulp canals after pocket infection reaches them. Atrophic and inflammatory pulpal changes occur in such cases.

Relationship of Attachment Loss and Bone Loss to Pocket Depth

The severity of the attachment loss in pocket formation is generally but not always correlated with the depth of the pocket. This is because the degree of attachment loss depends on the location of the base of the pocket on the root surface, whereas pocket depth is the distance between the base of the pocket and the crest of the gingival margin. Pockets of the same depth may be associated with different degrees of attachment loss (Fig. 17.18) and pockets of different depths may be associated with the same amount of attachment loss (Fig. 17.19).

The severity of bone loss is generally but not always correlated with pocket depth. Extensive attachment and bone loss may be associated with shallow pockets if the attachment loss is accompanied by recession of the gingival margin and slight bone loss can occur with deep pockets.

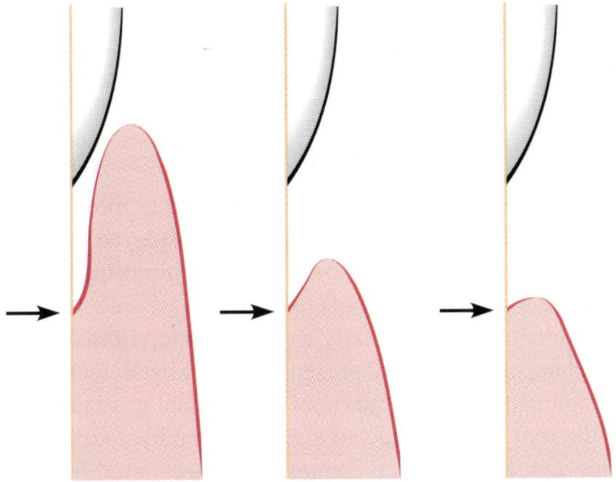

Fig. 17.18 Different pocket depths with the same amount of attachment loss. *Arrows* point to the bottom of the pocket. The distance between the arrow and the cementoenamel junction remains the same despite different pocket depths.

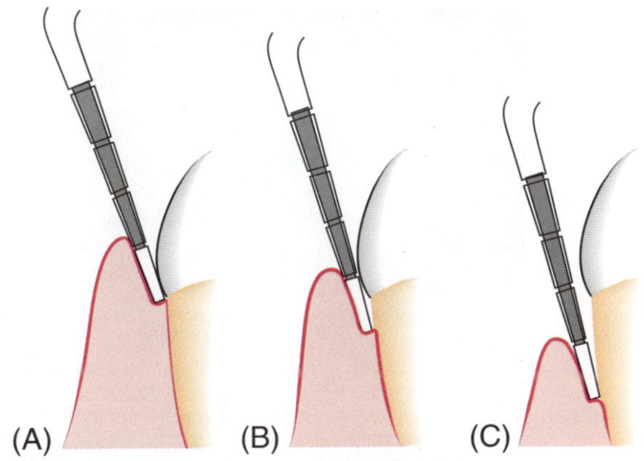

Fig. 17.19 Same pocket depth with different amounts of recession. A, Gingival pocket with no recession. B, Periodontal pocket of similar depth as shown in (A), but with some degree of recession. C, Pocket depth the same as shown in (A) and (B), but with still more recession.

Area Between Base of Pocket and Alveolar Bone

Normally, the distance between the apical end of the junctional epithelium and the alveolar bone is relatively constant. The distance between the apical extent of calculus and the alveolar crest in human periodontal pockets is most constant, having a mean length of 1.97 mm (±33.16%).

The distance from attached plaque to bone is never less than 0.5 mm and never more than 2.7 mm. These findings suggest that the bone-resorbing activity induced by the bacteria is exerted within these distances. However, the finding of isolated bacteria or clumps of bacteria in the connective tissue and on the bone surface may modify these considerations.

Relationship of Pocket to Bone

In infrabony pockets, the base of the pocket is apical to the crest of the alveolar bone and the pocket wall lies between the tooth and the bone. The bone loss is in most cases is vertical. Alternatively, in suprabony pockets, the base is coronal to the crest of the alveolar bone and the pocket wall lies coronal to the bone. This type of bone loss is always horizontal.

This creates some microscopic differences that have some therapeutic importance. They are the relationship of the soft-tissue wall of the pocket to the alveolar bone, the pattern of bone destruction, and the direction of the transseptal fibers of the periodontal ligament (Figs. 17.20–17.22).

In suprabony pockets, the alveolar crest gradually attains a more apical position in relation to the tooth but it retains its general morphology and architecture. The interdental fibers that run over the bone from one tooth to the other maintain their usual horizontal direction. In infrabony pockets, the morphology of the alveolar crest changes completely with the formation of an angular bony defect. The interdental fibers, in this case, run over the bone in an oblique direction between the two teeth of the interdental space. This may affect the function of the area and also necessitate a modification in treatment techniques. Table 17.2 summarizes the distinguishing features of suprabony and infrabony pockets.

Lateral Periodontal Cyst

The periodontal cyst, which is also called *lateral periodontal cyst*, is an uncommon lesion that produces localized destruction of the

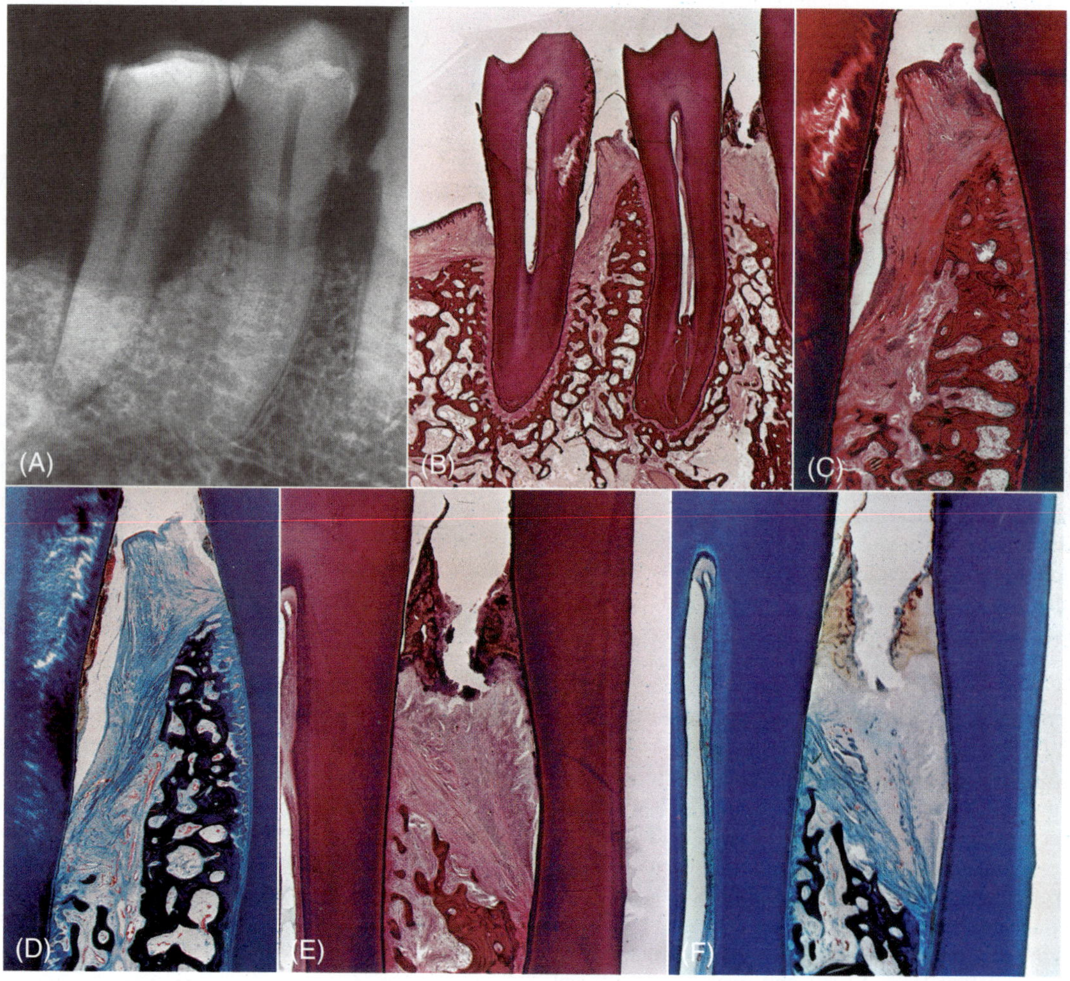

Fig. 17.20 Radiographic and microscopic features of infrabony pockets. A, Radiograph of a mandibular canine and premolar area showing angular bone loss mesial to the second premolar. The type of bone loss between the first premolar and the canine is not radiographically apparent. B, Mesiodistal histologic section of the teeth seen in (A), showing an infrabony pocket mesial to the second premolar, as well as suprabony pockets distal to the second premolar and mesial and distal to the first premolar. The mesial suprabony pocket of the first premolar appears to be coronal to a vertical bone loss. C, Higher-power view of the area between the premolars. Note the angular bone loss and the transseptal fibers that cover the bone. D, Higher-power view of the area between the premolars stained with Mallory connective tissue stain; clearly showing the direction of transseptal fibers. E, Higher-power view of the area between the first premolar and the canine. Note the abundant calculus, the dense leukocytic infiltration of the gingiva, and the angulation of the transseptal fibers and bone. The pocket is still suprabony. F, Mallory stain of a similar area to the one shown in E. Note the destruction of the gingival fibers caused by inflammation and the angular fibers formed over angular bone loss, which are less affected by the inflammation. Transseptal fibers extend from the distal surface of the premolar over the crest of the alveolar bone into the infrabony pocket. Note the leukocytic infiltration of the transseptal fibers. *(From Glickman I, Smulow J:* Periodontal disease: clinical, radiographic and histopathologic features, *Philadelphia, 1974, Saunders.)*

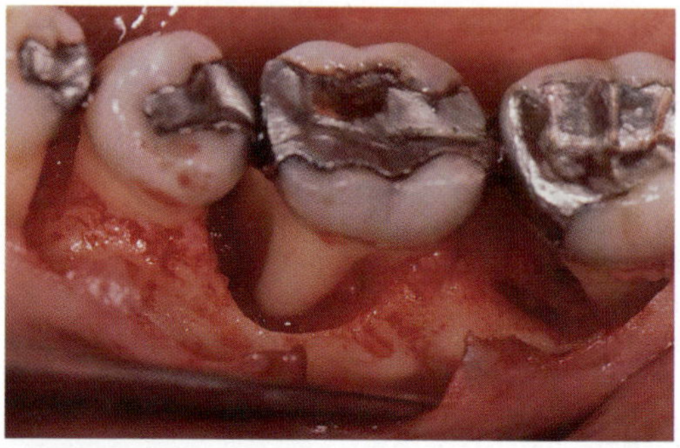

Fig. 17.21 After raising a flap for the treatment of the infrabony pockets, the vertical bone loss around the mesial roots of the mandibular first and second molars can be seen.

periodontal tissues along a lateral root surface, most often in the mandibular canine–premolar area. It is considered to be derived from the rests of Malassez or other proliferating odontogenic rests.

A periodontal cyst is usually asymptomatic without grossly detectable changes; but it may present as a localized, tender swelling. Radiographically, an interproximal periodontal cyst appears on the side of the root as a radiolucent area bordered by a radiopaque line. Its radiographic appearance cannot be differentiated from that of a periodontal abscess.

Microscopically, the cystic lining may be (1) a loosely arranged, thin, nonkeratinized epithelium, sometimes with thicker proliferating areas; or (2) an odontogenic keratocyst.

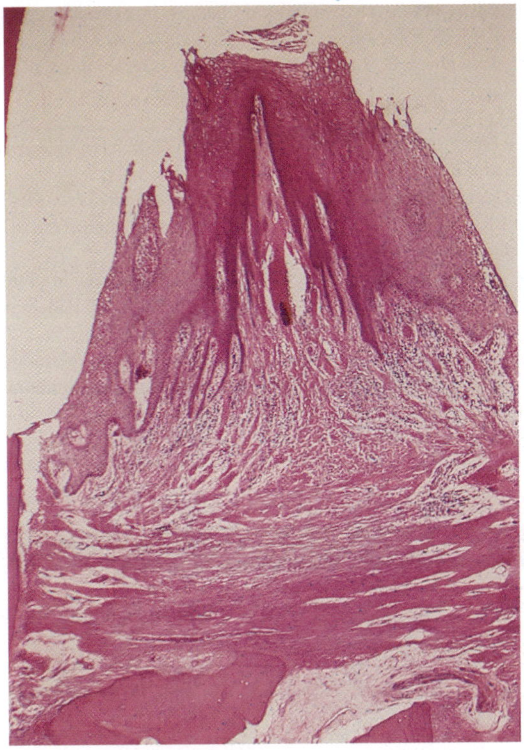

Fig. 17.22 Two suprabony pockets in an interdental space. Note the normal horizontal arrangement of the transseptal fibers.

TABLE 17.2 Distinguishing Features of Suprabony and Intrabony Periodontal Pockets

Suprabony Pocket	Infrabony Pocket
The base of the pocket is coronal to the level of the alveolar bone.	The base of the pocket is apical to the crest of the alveolar bone so that the bone is adjacent to the soft-tissue wall (see Fig. 17.2).
The pattern of destruction of the underlying bone is horizontal.	The pattern of bone destruction is vertical (angular) (see Figs. 17.20 and 17.21).
Interproximally, transseptal fibers that are restored during progressive periodontal disease are arranged horizontally in the space between the base of the pocket and the alveolar bone (see Fig. 17.22).	Interproximally, transseptal fibers are oblique rather than horizontal. They extend from the cementum beneath the base of the pocket along the alveolar bone and over the crest to the cementum of the adjacent tooth (see Fig. 17.20).
On the facial and lingual surfaces, periodontal ligament fibers beneath the pocket follow their normal horizontal–oblique course between the tooth and the bone.	On the facial and lingual surfaces, periodontal ligament fibers follow the angular pattern of the adjacent bone. They extend from the cementum beneath the base of the pocket along the alveolar bone and over the crest to join with the outer periosteum.

Key points

- Pathologically deepened gingival sulcus is called as periodontal pocket.
- It can be classified as gingival pocket and periodontal pocket.
- In periodontal pocket, it involves destruction of supporting periodontal tissue. Periodontal pocket is further classified as suprabony and infrabony pocket.
- Pocket can involve one or two more tooth surfaces and can be of different depths.
- Pocket can also be spiral and twisting around the tooth to involve one more additional surfaces.
- Clinical signs that suggest the presence of periodontal pockets include a bluish-red, thickend marginal gingiva and a bluish-red vertical zone from the gingival margin to the alveolar mucosa, gingival bleeding, suppuration, tooth mobility, diastema, and pain or localized pain.
- The initial lesion in the development of periodontitis is the inflammation of the gingiva in response to a bacterial challenge.
- Extension of the junctional epithelium along the root requires the presence of healthy epithelial cells. Marked degeneration or necrosis of the junctional epithelium retards rather than accelerates pocket formation.
- The most severe degenerative change in the periodontal pocket occurs along the lateral wall.
- The severity of the degenerative changes is not necessarily related to pocket depth. Ulceration of the lateral wall may occur in shallow pockets, and deep pockets are occasionally observed in which the lateral epithelium is relatively intact or shows only slight degeneration.
- Periodontal pockets are chronic inflammatory lesions and are constantly undergoing repair. Complete healing does not occur because of the persistence of the bacterial attack, which continues to stimulate an inflammatory response, causing degeneration of the new tissue elements formed in the continuous effort at repair.
- Pus is a common feature of periodontal disease, but it is only a secondary sign.
- The root surface wall of periodontal pockets often undergoes changes that are significant because they may perpetuate the periodontal infection, cause pain, and complicate the periodontal treatment.
- Pathologic granules have been observed with optical and electron microscopy and may represent area of collagen degeneration, and collagen fibrils have not been fully mineralized initially.
- Periodontal destruction does not occur in all parts of the mouth at the same time but rather on a few teeth at a time or even only some aspects of teeth at any given time. This is called as site specificity of the periodontal disease.
- A gingival abscess is defined as a localized purulent infection that involves the marginal gingiva or interdental papilla.
- A gingival abscess is characterized by a purulent focus in the connective tissue, surrounded by diffuse infiltration of polymorphonuclear leukocytes, edematous tissue, and vascular engorgement, with the surface epithelium showing varying degrees of intracellular and extracellular edema, leukocyte invasion, and occasionally ulceration.
- Diagnosing a periodontal abscess requires correlating the patient's history with clinical and radiographic findings; the dental history may reveal previous periodontal treatments, endodontic therapy, and abscesses, and clinical evidence includes ovoid gingival swelling, pain, tooth mobility and elevation, suppuration, and deep periodontal pockets.
- Radiographically, a periodontal abscess appears as a discrete area of radiolucency along the root's lateral aspect, although soft tissue lesions and those on facial or lingual surfaces may not produce distinct radiographic changes.

- A periapical abscess presents with sharp, intermittent, throbbing, severe, and diffuse pain that is often not localized, making it difficult for the patient to identify the offending tooth; the vitality test does not show vital pulp, and the tooth is painful to percussion or movement, with the abscess potentially associated with deep restorations. Swelling is typically present in the apical area with common sinus tract formation, and clinically, there may be no periodontal pocket or it probes as a narrow defect.
- A periodontal abscess is characterized by dull, steady, continuous, and localized pain, with the offending tooth easily identifiable by the patient, a vital pulp, and less pain upon percussion or movement. It is associated with a pre-existing periodontal pocket or caries, gingival tissue swelling with an uncommon fistula tract, and radiographic evidence of vertical or angular bone loss or furcation radiolucency.

Suggested Readings

Adriaens PA, DeBoever JA, Loesche WJ: Bacterial invasion in root cementum and radicular dentin of periodontally diseased teeth in humans: a reservoir of periodontopathic bacteria, *J Periodontol* 59:222, 1988.

Armitage GC, Christie TM: Structural changes in exposed cementum. I. Light microscopic observations, *J Periodontal Res* 8:343, 1973a.

Armitage GC, Christie TM: Structural changes in exposed cementum. II. Electronmicroscopic observations, *J Periodontal Res* 8:356, 1973b.

Lindhe J, Liljenberg B, Listgarten MA: Some microbiological and histopathological features of periodontal disease in man, *J Periodontol* 52:264, 1980.

Listgarten MA: Structure of the microbial flora associated with periodontal health and disease in man, *J Periodontol* 47:1, 1976.

Listgarten MA: Pathogenesis of periodontitis, *J Clin Periodontol* 13:418, 1986.

Newman MG, Sims TN: The predominant cultivable microbiota of the periodontal abscess, *J Periodontol* 50:350, 1979.

Page RC, Schroeder HH: Structure and pathogenesis. In Schluger S, Youdelis R, Page R, editors: *Periodontal disease*, Philadelphia, 1977, Lea & Febiger.

Quirynen M, Gizani S, Mongardini C, et al: The effect of periodontal therapy on the number of cariogenic bacteria in different intraoral niches, *J Clin Periodontol* 26:322, 1999.

Saglie FR, Newman MG, Carranza FA Jr, et al: Bacterial invasion of gingiva in advanced periodontitis in humans, *J Periodontol* 53:217, 1982.

References

References and MCQs with answers for the chapter are available on www.medenact.com.

CHAPTER 18

Abscesses of the Periodontium

SU Nayak | DG Naik | A Uppoor

CHAPTER OUTLINE

KEY FACT

The 1999 International workshop for the classification of periodontal diseases organized by AMERICAN ASSOCIATION OF PERIODONTOLOGY (AAP) has classified abscesses of the periodontium as gingival abscess, periodontal abscess, and pericoronal abscess.

Gingival Abscess

A gingival abscess is defined as a localized purulent infection that involves the marginal gingiva or interdental papilla (Fig. 18.1). The diagnosis of gingival abscess is uncomplicated as it is confined to only the gingival marginal tissues which are previously a nondiseased site. It is often an acute inflammatory response to the impaction of food material or a foreign body into the gingiva. The retrieval of the foreign body is thus often diagnostic.

In its early stages, it appears as a red swelling with a smooth, shiny surface. Within 24–48 h, the lesion usually becomes fluctuant and pointed, with a surface orifice from which a purulent exudate may be expressed. The adjacent teeth are often sensitive to percussion. If permitted to progress, the lesion generally ruptures spontaneously.

Histopathology

The gingival abscess consists of a purulent focus in the connective tissue surrounded by a diffuse infiltration of polymorphonuclear leukocytes, edematous tissue, and vascular engorgement. The surface epithelium has varying degrees of intracellular and extracellular edema, invasion by leukocytes, and sometimes ulceration.

Etiology

Acute inflammatory gingival enlargement results from bacteria carried deep into the tissues when a foreign substance (e.g., toothbrush bristle, piece of apple core, lobster shell fragment) is forcefully embedded into the gingiva. The lesion is confined to the gingiva and should not be confused with periodontal or lateral abscesses.

Pericoronal Abscess

The pericoronal abscess associated with the crown of a partially erupted tooth is one of the complications of pericoronitis. It may spread posteriorly into the oropharyngeal areas and medially to the base of the tongue, making it difficult for the patient to swallow.

Periodontal (Lateral) Abscess

A periodontal abscess is a localized purulent inflammation in the periodontal tissues (Fig. 18.2). It is also known as a *lateral abscess* or a *parietal abscess.* It is an infection located contiguous to the periodontal pocket and may result in destruction of the periodontal ligament and alveolar bone.

Classification of Periodontal Abscess

According to Location

1. Abscess in the supporting periodontal tissues along the lateral aspect of the root.
2. Abscess in the soft tissue wall of the deep periodontal pocket.

According to Onset or Course of Lesion

1. *Acute periodontal abscess:* It appears as a bright red ovoid elevation of the gingiva, which may be relatively firm or pointed and soft. In most instances, pus may be expressed from the gingival margin by gentle digital pressure. It is accompanied by symptoms such as throbbing, radiating pain, sensitivity to percussion, tooth mobility, and, in some cases, lymphadenopathy and systemic effects such as fever and malaise.
2. *Chronic periodontal abscess*: It usually presents a sinus that opens onto the gingival mucosa somewhere along the root length. It is usually asymptomatic. However, the patient may complain of intermittent exudation, dull gnawing pain, slight elevation of the tooth, and a desire to bite down on and grind the tooth (Box 18.1).

Acute lesions often subside but persist in the chronic state, whereas chronic lesions may exist without being acute. Chronic lesions frequently undergo acute exacerbation.

Depending on Number

1. *Single periodontal abscess:* They are usually related to local factors that contribute to the closure of the periodontal pocket.
2. *Multiple periodontal abscess:* They have been reported in diabetes mellitus and medically compromised patients.

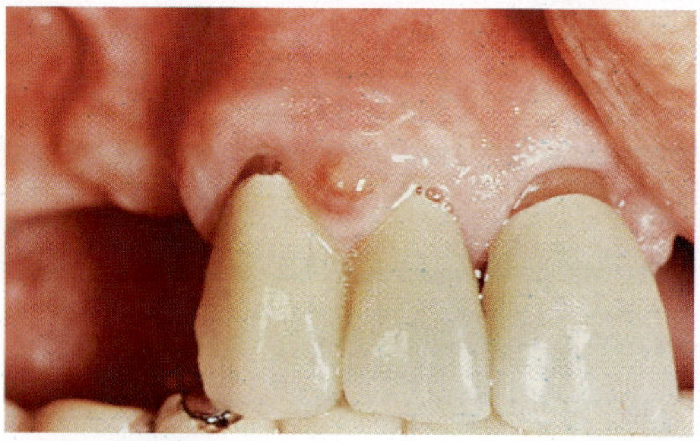

Fig. 18.1 Gingival abscess on the facial gingival surface in the space between the cuspid and the lateral incisor, unrelated to the gingival sulcus area.

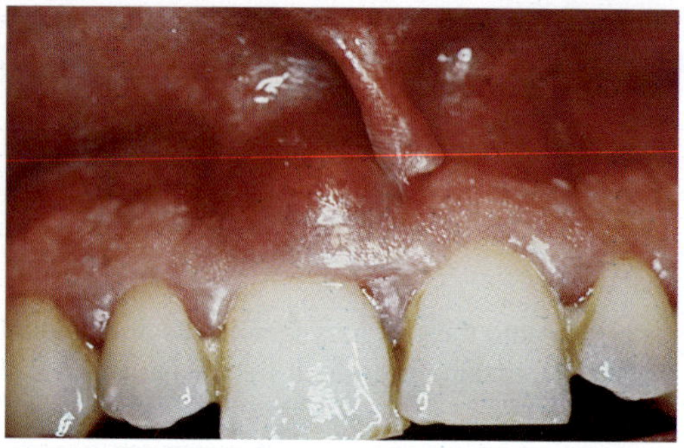

Fig. 18.2 Periodontal abscess on an upper right central incisor.

BOX 18.1 Signs and Symptoms of Periodontal Abscess

Acute Abscess
Mild to severe discomfort
Localized red, ovoid swelling
Periodontal pocket
Mobility
Tooth elevation in socket
Tenderness to percussion or biting
Exudation
Elevated temperature[a]
Regional lymphadenopathy[a]

Chronic Abscess
No pain or dull pain
Localized inflammatory lesion
Slight tooth elevation
Intermittent exudation
Fistulous tract often associated with a deep pocket
Usually without systemic involvement

[a]May indicate the need for systemic antibiotics.
Data from Dahlen G: Microbiology and treatment of dental abscesses and periodontal-endodontic lesions. *Periodontol 2000* 28:206, 2002; Meng HX: Periodontal abscess. *Ann Periodontol* 4:79, 1999; and Sanz M, Herrera D, van Winkelhoff AJ: The periodontal abscess. In Lindhe J, editor: *Clinical periodontology*, Copenhagen, 2000, Munksgaard.

Etiology

Periodontal abscesses have been associated either directly to periodontitis (periodontitis-related abscess) or to sites without the prior existence of a periodontal pocket (nonperiodontitis-related abscess).

1. *Periodontitis-Related Abscess*
   a. The existence of tortuous pockets, with cul-de-sac that eventually becomes isolated, may favor the formation of abscess.

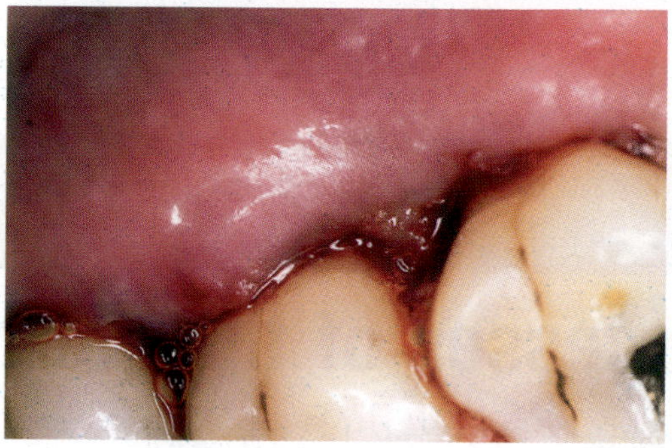

Fig. 18.3 Periodontal abscess due to incomplete removal of subgingival calculus.

   b. The marginal closure of the periodontal pocket may lead to an extension of infection into the surrounding periodontal tissues due to the pressure of suppuration inside the closed pocket.
   c. The development of periodontal abscess in periodontitis may occur at different stages during the course of the infection as an exacerbation of an untreated periodontitis, during periodontal therapy, in refractory periodontitis, or during periodontal maintenance. Also, fibrin secretions, leading to the local accumulation of pus, may favor the closure of gingival margin to the tooth surface.
   d. Changes in composition of the microflora, bacterial virulence, or in host defenses could also make the pocket lumen inefficient to drain the increased suppuration.
   e. Treatment with systemic antibiotics without subgingival debridement in patients with advanced periodontitis may also cause abscess formation.
   f. Abscess can form due to inadequate scaling, which will allow calculus to remain in the deepest pocket area, while the resolution of the inflammation at the coronal pocket area will occlude the normal drainage and entrapment of the subgingival flora in the deepest part of the pocket. Also calculus might get dislodged and pushed into the soft tissue after procedures like scaling (Fig. 18.3).
2. *Nonperiodontitis-Related Abscess*
   a. Impaction of foreign bodies, such as a toothbrush bristle, a piece of dental floss, orthodontic elastic, a dislodged cemental tear, food (such as fish bone) into the gingival tissue, and so on can result in abscess formation. Periodontal abscesses caused by foreign bodies, related with oral hygiene aids, have been named "oral hygiene abscesses."
   b. Lateral perforation of the root during endodontic therapy and trauma to the tooth.
   c. Local factors affecting morphology of roots such as cemental tears, external root resorption, invaginated tooth, and cracked tooth may predispose to periodontal abscess formation.

KEY FACT

Most periodontal abscesses are due to the incomplete removal of subgingival calculus in a periodontal pocket.

Pathogenesis and Histopathology

The entry of bacteria into the soft tissue pocket wall could be the first event to initiate the periodontal abscess. Inflammatory cells are then attracted by chemotactic factors released by the bacteria, and

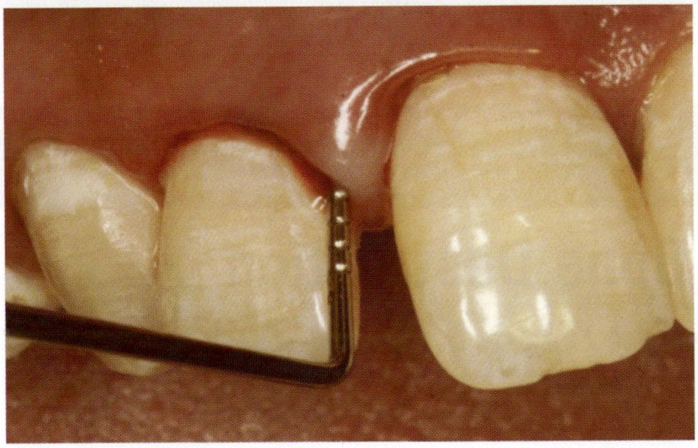

Fig. 18.4 Clinical view showing deep periodontal pocket in relation to upper right lateral incisor.

the concomitant inflammatory reaction leads to destruction of the connective tissues, the encapsulation of the bacterial infection, and the production of pus.

Histologically intact neutrophils are found surrounding a central area of soft tissue debris and destroyed leukocytes. At a later stage, a pyogenic membrane composed of macrophages and neutrophils is organized. An acute inflammatory reaction surrounds the purulent area, and the overlying epithelium exhibits intracellular and extracellular edema and invasion of leukocytes. Gram-negative bacteria may be seen invading the pocket epithelium and the altered connective tissue.

Diagnosis

The diagnosis of the periodontal abscess requires correlation of the history, and clinical and radiographic findings. The dental history can provide information about previous periodontal treatments, endodontic therapy, and previous abscesses.

The suspected area should be carefully probed (Fig. 18.4). Continuity of the lesion with the gingival margin serves as the clinical evidence that the abscess is periodontal. Other findings are ovoid swelling of the gingiva, pain, tooth mobility, tooth elevation, suppuration, either spontaneous or on digital pressure, and the presence of deep periodontal pockets. Radiographically, it appears as a discrete area of radiolucency along the lateral aspect of the root. However, lesions in the soft tissue wall of a periodontal pocket are less likely to produce radiographic changes than those deep in the supporting tissues. Similarly, abscesses on the facial or lingual surfaces are obscured by the radiopaucity of the root.

Differential Diagnosis

The differential diagnosis of periodontal abscesses should be made using different signs and symptoms, such as pulp vitality, the presence of dental caries versus periodontal pockets, the location of abscess, and a careful radiographic examination. It is differentiated from gingival abscess (Table 18.1) and periapical abscess (Table 18.2), which are the other abscesses found in the oral cavity that have similar appearance and symptomatology although their etiologies are different.

TABLE 18.1 Differentiation Between Gingival and Periodontal Abscess

Gingival Abscess	Periodontal Abscess
It is confined to the marginal gingiva	It involves the supporting periodontal structures
It often occurs in former disease-free areas	It occurs in the course of chronic destructive periodontitis
It is an acute inflammatory response that results when a foreign object (apple core, lobster fragment) is forcefully embedded into the gingiva	The occlusion of the orifice of a preexisting periodontal pocket prevents drainage of the purulent material leading to abscess formation
Treatment involves only drainage and irrigation	Treatment involves drainage, irrigation, and pocket elimination procedure

TABLE 18.2 Differentiation Between Periapical and Periodontal Abscess

Periapical Abscess	Periodontal Abscess
Pain may be sharp, intermittent, throbbing, severe, and diffuse	The pain is usually dull, steady, and continuous
Pain is not always localized, and the patient may not be able to locate the offending tooth	The pain is localized, and the patient usually can locate the offending tooth
Vitality test does not show vital pulp	Vitality test shows vital pulp
The tooth is painful to percussion or with movement	The tooth is usually not as painful to percussion or with movement
The abscess may be associated with deep restoration	The abscess is associated with a preexisting periodontal pocket, caries, or both
Swelling usually present in apical area and sinus tract formation is common	Swelling usually includes gingival tissue and fistula tract is uncommon
Clinically may have no periodontal pocket, or if present, probes as narrow defect	Clinically, there is the presence of periodontal pocket and radiographically, there is the presence of vertical or angular bone loss or furcation radiolucency

Suggested Readings

Corbet EF: Diagnosis of acute periodontal abscess, *Periodontol 2000* 34: 204, 2004.

Dahlen G: Microbiology and treatment of dental abscess and periodontic-endodontic lesions, *Periodontol 2000* 28: 206, 2002.

Gilette WB, van house RL: Ill effects of improper oral hygiene procedures, *J Am Dent Assoc* 101: 476-481, 1980.

MCQs

MCQs with answers for the chapter are available on www.medenact.com.

CHAPTER 19

Bone Loss and Patterns of Bone Destruction

FA Carranza | PM Camargo | HH Takei | DG Naik | A Uppoor

CHAPTER OUTLINE

This chapter discusses periodontal bone loss as a consequence of inflammation and as modified by other factors, such as trauma from occlusion. The inflammatory process develops as a response to the bacterial biofilm front and follows the path of the large blood vessels in the affected area. The average progression of bone loss in untreated periodontitis is 0.2–0.3 mm per year, but the range varies substantially depending on the individual's susceptibility to the disease. The destructive radius of action of the inflammatory process is estimated to be 1.5–2.5 mm.

Although periodontitis is an infectious disease of the gingival tissue, changes that occur in bone are crucial because the destruction of bone is responsible for tooth loss.

The height and density of the alveolar bone are normally maintained by an equilibrium, regulated by local and systemic influences, between bone formation and bone resorption. When resorption exceeds formation, both bone height and bone density may be reduced. The level of bone is the consequence of past pathologic experiences, whereas changes in the soft tissue of the pocket wall reflect the present inflammatory condition. Therefore, the degree of bone loss is not necessarily correlated with the depth of periodontal pockets, the severity of ulceration of the pocket wall, or the presence or absence of pus. As an example, a reduced periodontium may exist in areas where bone loss occurred in the past but that currently present with periodontal health (i.e., following periodontal treatment).

Bone Destruction Caused by the Extension of Gingival Inflammation

The most common cause of bone destruction in periodontal disease is the extension of inflammation from the marginal gingiva into the supporting periodontal tissues. The inflammatory invasion of the bone surface and the initial bone loss that follows mark the transition from gingivitis to periodontitis.

Periodontitis is always preceded by gingivitis, but not all gingivitis progresses to periodontitis. Some cases of gingivitis apparently never become periodontitis, and other cases go through a brief gingivitis phase and rapidly develop into periodontitis. The factors that are responsible for the extension of inflammation to the supporting structures, thereby initiating the conversion of gingivitis to periodontitis, are not clearly understood at this time.

The transition from gingivitis to periodontitis is associated with changes in the composition of bacterial plaque. In advanced stages of disease, the number of motile organisms and spirochetes increases, whereas the number of coccoid rods and straight rods decreases. The cellular composition of the infiltrated connective tissue also changes with increasing severity of the lesion. Fibroblasts and lymphocytes predominate in stage 1 gingivitis, whereas the number of plasma cells and blast cells increases gradually as the disease progresses. Seymour et al. have postulated a stage of "contained" gingivitis in which T lymphocytes are preponderant; they think that, as the lesion becomes a B-lymphocyte lesion, it becomes progressively destructive.

Heijl et al. were able to convert, in experimental animals, a confined, naturally occurring chronic gingivitis into a progressive periodontitis by placing a silk ligature into the sulcus and tying it around the neck of the tooth. This induced ulceration of the sulcular epithelium, a shift in the inflammatory infiltrate from predominantly plasma cells to predominantly polymorphonuclear leukocytes, and osteoclastic resorption of the alveolar crest. The recurrence of episodes of acute destruction over time may be one mechanism that leads to progressive bone loss in individuals with marginal chronic periodontitis.

The extension of inflammation to the supporting structures of a tooth may be modified by the pathogenic potential of plaque and the resistance of the host. The latter includes immunologic activity and other tissue-related mechanisms, such as the degree of fibrosis of the gingiva, probably the width of the attached gingiva, and the reactive fibrogenesis and osteogenesis that occur peripheral to the inflammatory lesion. Some studies suggest that the quality of the host response to a similar bacterial insult varies, resulting in some individuals being more susceptible to the destructive aspects of periodontitis than others.

Histopathology

Gingival inflammation extends along the collagen fiber bundles and follows the course of the blood vessels through the loosely arranged tissues around them into the alveolar bone (Fig. 19.1A and B). Although the inflammatory infiltrate is concentrated in the marginal periodontium, the reaction is a much more diffuse one, often reaching the bone and eliciting a response before evidence of crestal resorption or loss of attachment exists. In the upper molar region,

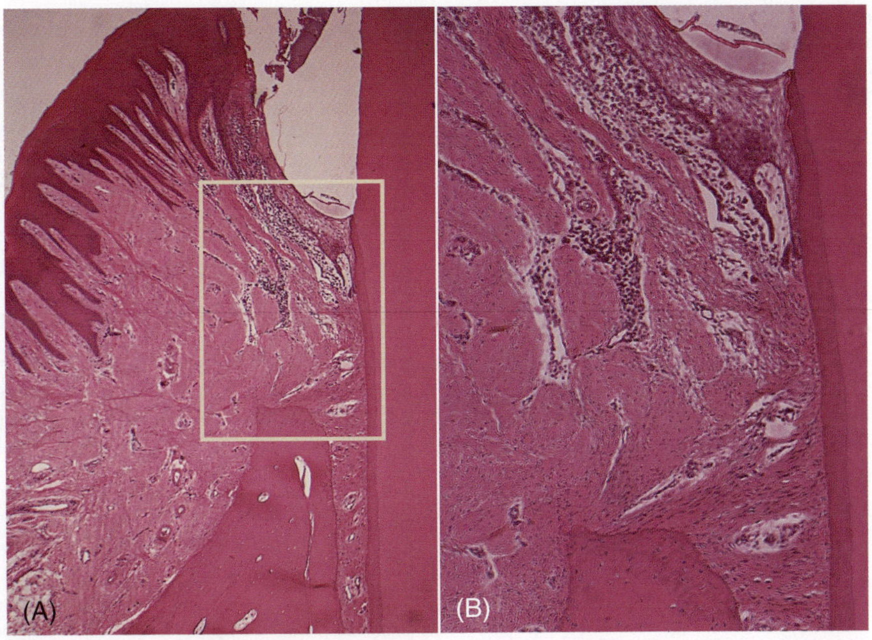

Fig. 19.1 A, An area of inflammation extending from the gingiva into the suprabony area. B, Extension of inflammation along the blood vessels and between collagen bundles.

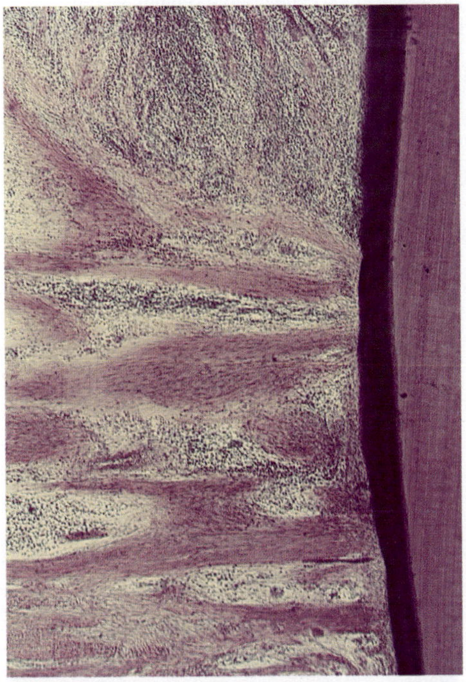

Fig. 19.2 Inflammation that extends from the pocket area *(top)* between the collagen fibers, which are partially destroyed.

inflammation can extend to the maxillary sinus, thereby resulting in thickening of the sinus mucosa.

Interproximally, inflammation spreads to the loose connective tissue around the blood vessels through the fibers and then into the bone through vessel channels that perforate the crest of the interdental septum at the center of the crest (Fig. 19.2), toward the side of the crest (Fig. 19.3A and B), or at the angle of the septum. In addition, inflammation may enter the bone through more than one channel. Less frequently, the inflammation spreads from the gingiva directly into the periodontal ligament and from there into the interdental septum (Fig. 19.4A).

Facially and lingually, inflammation from the gingiva spreads along the outer periosteal surface of the bone (Fig. 19.4B) and penetrates into the marrow spaces through vessel channels in the outer cortex.

Along its course from the gingiva to the bone, the inflammation destroys the gingival and transseptal fibers, reducing them to disorganized granular fragments interspersed among the inflammatory cells and edema. However, there is a continuous tendency to recreate transseptal fibers across the crest of the interdental septum farther along the root as the bone destruction progresses (Fig. 19.5). As a result, transseptal fibers are present even in cases of extreme periodontal bone loss.

The dense transseptal fibers form a firm covering over the bone that is encountered during periodontal flap surgery after the superficial granulation tissue is removed.

After inflammation reaches the bone via extension from the gingiva (Fig. 19.6), it spreads into the marrow spaces and replaces the marrow with a leukocytic and fluid exudate, new blood vessels, and proliferating fibroblasts (Fig. 19.7). Multinuclear osteoclasts and mononuclear phagocytes increase in number, and the bone surfaces appear to be lined with Howship's lacunae (Fig. 19.8).

In the marrow spaces, resorption proceeds from within and causes a thinning of the surrounding bony trabeculae and an enlargement of the marrow spaces; this is followed by the destruction of the bone and a reduction in bone height. Normally, fatty bone marrow is partially or totally replaced by a fibrous type of marrow in the vicinity of the resorption.

Bone destruction in periodontal disease is not a process of bone necrosis. It involves the activity of living cells along viable bone. When tissue necrosis and pus are present in periodontal disease, they occur in the soft-tissue walls of periodontal pockets rather than along the resorbing margin of the underlying bone.

The amount of inflammatory infiltrate correlates with the degree of bone loss but not with the number of osteoclasts. However, the distance from the apical border of the inflammatory infiltrate to the alveolar bone crest correlates with both the number of osteoclasts on the alveolar crest and the total number of osteoclasts. Similar findings have been reported in experimentally induced periodontitis in animals.

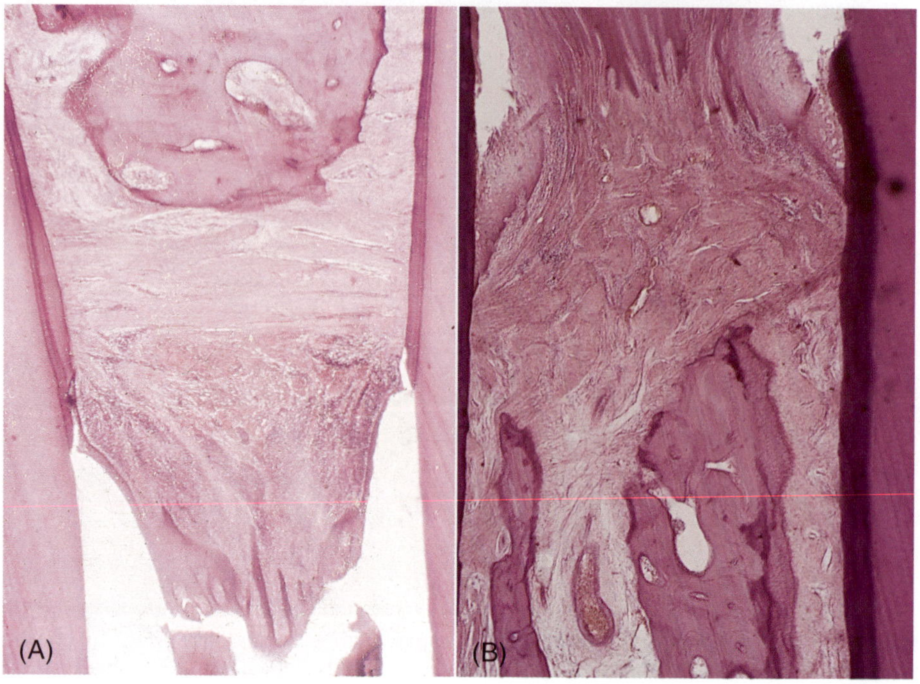

Fig. 19.3 A, Extension of inflammation into the center of the interdental septum. Inflammation from the gingiva penetrates the transseptal fibers and enters the bone around the blood vessel in the center of the septum. B, The cortical layer at the top of the septum has been destroyed, and the inflammation penetrates into the marrow spaces.

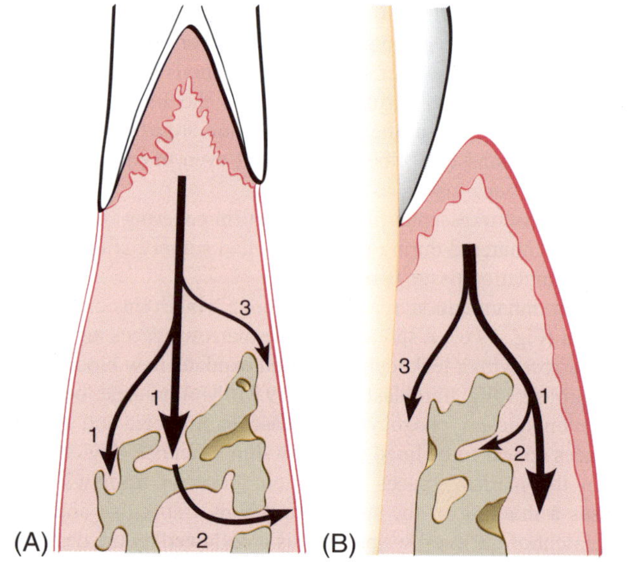

Fig. 19.4 Pathways of inflammation from the gingiva into the supporting periodontal tissues in a patient with periodontitis. A, Interproximally, from the gingiva into the bone *(1)*, from the bone into the periodontal ligament *(2)*, and from the gingiva into the periodontal ligament *(3)*. B, Facially and lingually, from the gingiva along the outer periosteum *(1)*, from the periosteum into the bone *(2)*, and from the gingiva into the periodontal ligament *(3)*.

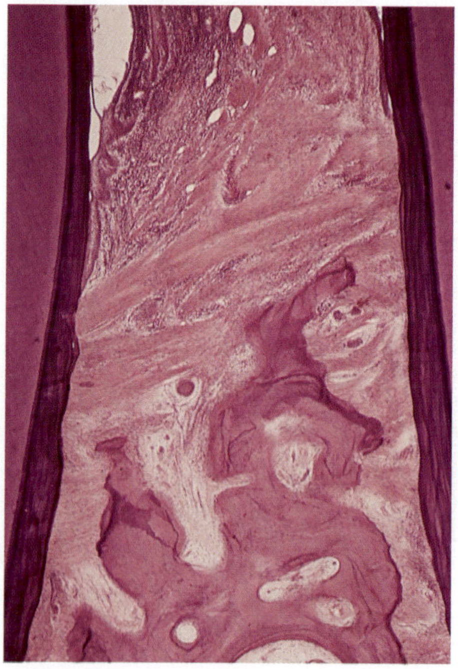

Fig. 19.5 Reformation of transseptal fibers. A mesiodistal section through the interdental septum shows gingival inflammation and bone loss. Recreated transseptal fibers can be seen above the bone margin, where they have been partially infiltrated by the inflammatory process.

Radius of Action

Garant and Cho suggested that locally produced bone resorption factors may need to be present in the proximity of the bone surface to exert their action. Page and Schroeder, on the basis of Waerhaug's measurements made on human autopsy specimens, postulated a range of effectiveness of about 1.5–2.5 mm in which bacterial plaque can induce loss of bone. Beyond 2.5 mm, there is no effect; interproximal angular defects can appear only in spaces that are wider than 2.5 mm because narrower spaces would be destroyed entirely. Tal corroborated this with measurements in human patients.

Large defects that greatly exceed a distance of 2.5 mm from the tooth surface (as described in aggressive types of periodontitis) may be caused by the presence of bacteria in the tissues.

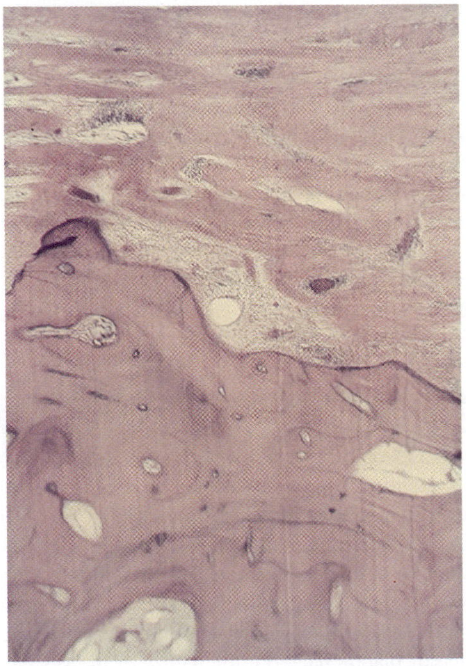

Fig. 19.6 Extension of inflammation has reached the crestal bone surface.

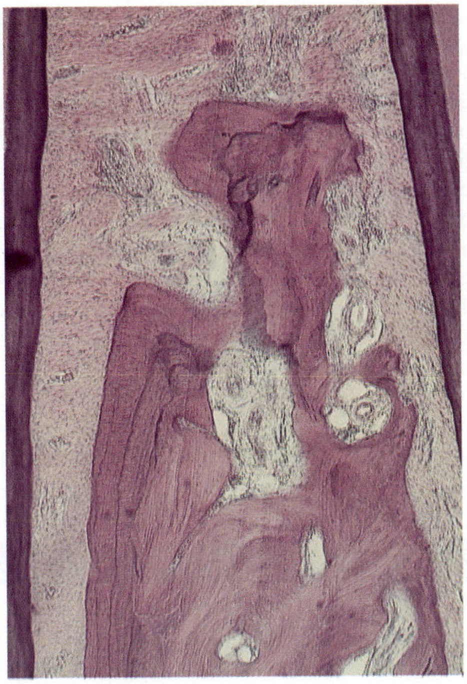

Fig. 19.7 Interdental septum in a human autopsy section. Extensive inflammatory infiltrate has invaded the marrow spaces, entering from both the mesial and distal aspects. Fatty bone marrow has been replaced by inflammatory cells and fibrous marrow.

Rate of Bone Loss

In a study of Sri Lankan tea laborers with no oral hygiene and no dental care, Löe et al. found the rate of bone loss to average about 0.2 mm/year for facial surfaces and about 0.3 mm/year for proximal surfaces when periodontal disease was allowed to progress untreated. However, the rate of bone loss may vary, depending on the type of disease present. Löe et al. also identified the following three subgroups of patients with periodontal disease on the basis of the interproximal loss of attachment and tooth mortality (loss of attachment can be equated with loss of bone although attachment loss precedes bone loss by about 6–8 months):

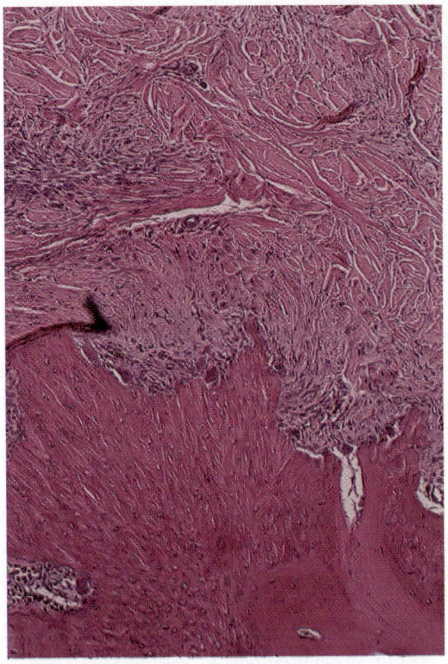

Fig. 19.8 Osteoclasts and Howship's lacunae in the resorption of crestal bone.

1. Approximately 8% of persons had a rapid progression of periodontal disease that was characterized by a yearly loss of attachment of 0.1–1.0 mm.
2. Approximately 81% of individuals had moderately progressive periodontal disease with a yearly loss of attachment of 0.05–0.5 mm.
3. The remaining 11% of persons had minimal or no progression of destructive disease with a yearly loss of attachment of 0.05–0.09 mm.

Periods of Destruction

Periodontal destruction occurs in an episodic, intermittent manner, with periods of inactivity or quiescence that alternate with destructive periods that result in the loss of collagen and alveolar bone and the deepening of the periodontal pocket.

Periods of destructive activity are associated with subgingival ulceration and an acute inflammatory reaction that results in the rapid loss of alveolar bone; it has been hypothesized that this coincides with the conversion of a predominantly T-lymphocyte lesion to one with a predominantly B-lymphocyte–plasma cell infiltrate. Microbiologically, these lesions are associated with an increase in the loose, unattached, motile, gram-negative, anaerobic pocket flora, whereas periods of remission coincide with the formation of a dense, unattached, nonmotile, gram-positive flora with a tendency to mineralize.

It has also been suggested that the onset of periods of destruction coincide with tissue invasion by one or several bacterial species and this is followed by an advanced local host defense that controls the attack.

KEY FACT

The dense network transseptal fiber that is attached interdentally from tooth to tooth is one of the barriers that protects the interdental bone from the inflammatory process. Even after these fibers are initially destroyed, they continually reform and are the fibers found during periodontal flap surgery.

Mechanisms of Bone Destruction

The factors involved in bone destruction in periodontal disease are bacterial and host mediated. Bacterial plaque products induce the differentiation of bone progenitor cells into osteoclasts and stimulate gingival cells to release mediators that have the same effect. Plaque products and inflammatory mediators can also act directly on osteoblasts or their progenitors, thereby inhibiting their action and reducing their numbers.

In addition, in patients with rapidly progressing diseases (e.g., aggressive periodontitis), bacterial microcolonies or single bacterial cells have been found between collagen fibers and over the bone surface, which suggests a direct effect.

Several host factors released by inflammatory cells are capable of inducing bone resorption in vitro, and they play a role in periodontal disease. These include host-produced prostaglandins and their precursors, interleukin-1 α, interleukin- β, and tumor necrosis factor-α.

When injected intradermally, prostaglandin E_2 induces the vascular changes that are seen with inflammation; when injected over a bone surface, prostaglandin E_2 induces bone resorption in the absence of inflammatory cells, with few multinucleated osteoclasts. In addition, nonsteroidal antiinflammatory drugs (e.g., flurbiprofen, ibuprofen) inhibit prostaglandin E_2 production, thereby slowing bone loss in naturally occurring periodontal disease in beagle dogs and humans. This effect occurs without changes in gingival inflammation, and it rebounds 6 months after the cessation of drug administration.

Bone Formation in Periodontal Disease

Areas of bone formation are also found immediately adjacent to sites of active bone resorption and along trabecular surfaces at a distance from the inflammation in an apparent effort to reinforce the remaining bone (i.e., buttressing bone formation). This osteogenic response is clearly found in experimentally produced periodontal bone loss in animals. In humans, it is less obvious, but it has been confirmed by histometric and histologic studies.

Autopsy specimens from individuals with untreated disease occasionally show areas in which bone resorption has ceased and new bone is being formed on previously eroded bone margins. This confirms the intermittent character of bone resorption in periodontal disease, and it is consistent with the varied rates of progression observed clinically in individuals with untreated periodontal disease.

The periods of remission and exacerbation (or inactivity and activity, respectively) appear to coincide with the quiescence or exacerbation of gingival inflammation as manifested by changes in the extent of bleeding, the amount of exudate, and the composition of bacterial plaque. The presence of bone formation in response to inflammation, even in those with active periodontal disease, has an effect on the outcome of treatment. The basic aim of periodontal therapy is the elimination of inflammation to remove the stimulus for bone resorption and therefore to allow the inherent constructive tendencies to predominate.

Bone Destruction Caused by Trauma From Occlusion

Another cause of bone destruction in periodontal disease is trauma from occlusion, which can occur in the absence or presence of inflammation.

In the absence of inflammation, the changes caused by trauma from occlusion vary from increased compression and tension of the periodontal ligament and increased osteoclasis of alveolar bone to necrosis of the periodontal ligament and bone and the resorption of bone and tooth structure. These changes are reversible in that they can be repaired if the offending forces are removed. However, persistent trauma from occlusion results in funnel-shaped widening of the crestal portion of the periodontal ligament with resorption of the adjacent bone. These changes, which may cause the bony crest to have an angular shape, represent adaptation of the periodontal tissues aimed at "cushioning" increased occlusal forces; however, the modified bone shape may weaken tooth support and cause tooth mobility.

When it is combined with inflammation, trauma from occlusion aggravates the bone destruction caused by the inflammation and results in bizarre bone patterns.

Bone Destruction Caused by Systemic Disorders

Local and systemic factors regulate the physiologic equilibrium of bone. When a generalized tendency toward bone resorption exists, bone loss initiated by local inflammatory processes may be magnified.

This systemic influence on the response of alveolar bone, as envisioned by Glickman during the early 1950s, considers a systemic regulatory influence in all cases of periodontal disease. In addition to the virulence of plaque bacteria, the nature of the systemic component rather than its presence or absence influences the severity of the periodontal destruction. This was called the bone factor concept. This concept of a role played by systemic defense mechanisms has been validated by the studies of immune deficiencies and host modulation in severely destructive types of periodontitis.

In recent years, interest has increased in the possible relationship between periodontal bone loss and osteoporosis. Osteoporosis is a physiologic condition of postmenopausal women that results in the loss of bone mineral content as well as structural bone changes. Periodontitis and osteoporosis share a number of risk factors (e.g., aging, smoking, certain diseases, medications that interfere with healing). Some studies show a relationship between skeletal density and oral bone density; between crestal height and residual ridge resorption; and between osteopenia and periodontitis, tooth mobility, and tooth loss.

Periodontal bone loss may also occur with generalized skeletal disturbances (e.g., hyperparathyroidism, leukemia, histiocytosis X) via mechanisms that may be totally unrelated to the usual periodontal problem.

KEY FACT

In the absence of inflammation, the localized bone loss caused by trauma from occlusion is reversible (can be repaired) if the offending forces are removed.

Factors Determining Bone Morphology in Periodontal Disease

Normal Variation in Alveolar Bone

Considerable normal variation exists within the morphologic features of alveolar bone, and this affects the osseous contours produced by periodontal disease. The anatomic features that substantially affect the bone-destructive pattern of periodontal disease include the following:

- Thickness, width, and crestal angulation of the interdental septa.
- Thickness of the facial and lingual alveolar plate.
- Presence of fenestrations and dehiscences.

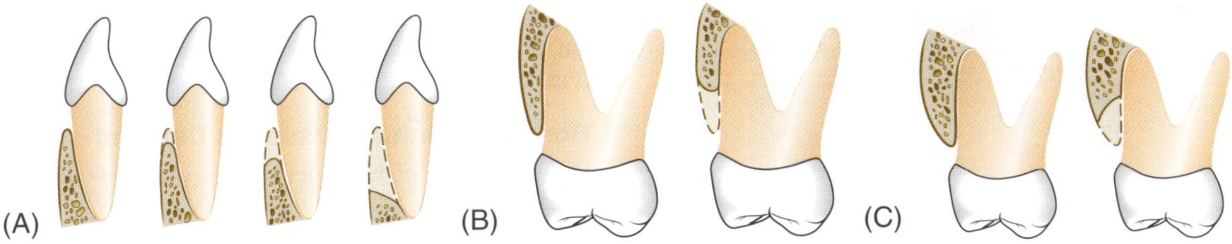

Fig. 19.9 A, Lower incisor with thin labial bone. Bone loss can become vertical only when it reaches thicker bone in apical areas. B, Upper molars with thin facial bone where only horizontal bone loss can occur. C, Upper molar with a thick facial bone that allows for vertical bone loss.

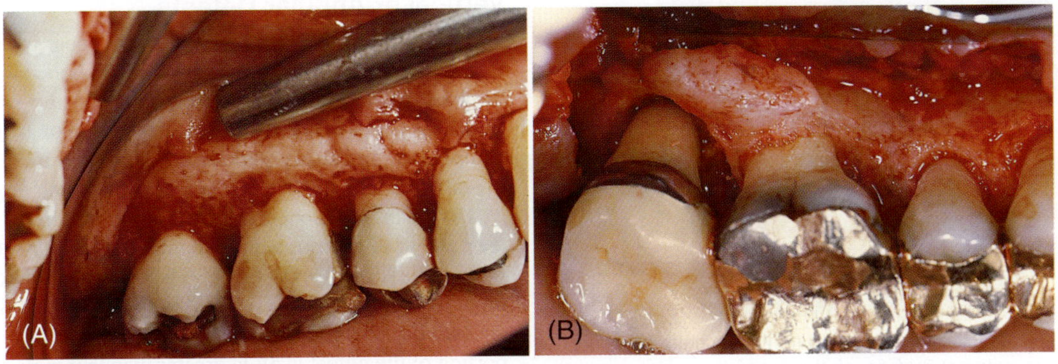

Fig. 19.10 A, Exostosis in the facial aspect of the upper second premolar and molars. B, Exostosis in the palatal aspect of the first and second molars. Note also the circumferential defect in the second molar *(left).*

- Alignment of the teeth.
- Root and root trunk anatomy.
- Root position within the alveolar process.
- Proximity with another tooth surface.

For example, angular osseous defects cannot form in thin facial or lingual alveolar plates, which have little or no cancellous bone between the outer and inner cortical layers. In such cases, the entire crest of the plate is destroyed and the height of the bone is reduced (Fig. 19.9A and B).

Exostoses

Exostoses are outgrowths of bone of varied size and shape. Palatal exostoses have been found in 40% of human skulls. They can occur as small nodules, large nodules, sharp ridges, spike-like projections, or any combination of these (Fig. 19.10A and B). Exostoses have been described in rare cases as developing after the placement of free gingival grafts.

Trauma From Occlusion

Trauma from occlusion may be a factor in determining the dimension and shape of bone deformities. It may cause a thickening of the cervical margin of alveolar bone or a change in bone morphology (e.g., angular defects, buttressing bone) on which inflammatory changes will later be superimposed.

KEY FACT

Angular osseous defects—as often seen in the interdental areas of the posterior dentition—cannot form in thin radicular, facial, or lingual alveolar bone. These areas have little or no cancellous bone between the outer and inner cortical layers. In these anatomic areas, the entire crest of the plate is destroyed, and the height of the bone is reduced in a horizontal fashion.

Buttressing Bone Formation

Bone formation sometimes occurs in an attempt to buttress bony trabeculae that are weakened by resorption. When it occurs within the jaw, it is termed *central buttressing bone formation.* When it occurs on the external surface, it is referred to as *peripheral buttressing bone formation.* The latter may cause bulging of the bone contour, which sometimes accompanies the production of osseous craters and angular defects (Fig. 19.11).

Food Impaction

Interdental bone defects often occur where proximal contact is abnormal or absent. Pressure and irritation from food impaction contribute to the inverted bone architecture. In some cases, the poor proximal relationship may result from a shift in tooth position as a result of extensive bone destruction that precedes food impaction. In such patients, food impaction is a complicating factor rather than the cause of the bone defect. Food impaction can be vertical—due to occlusal forces or lateral—due to pressure from the lips, cheeks, and tongue.

Aggressive Periodontitis

Aggressive periodontitis usually results in attachment and bone loss around incisors and first molars, particularly in cases where the disease is observed in teenagers. A vertical or angular pattern of alveolar bone destruction is found around the first molars in aggressive periodontitis. The cause of the localized bone destruction with this type of periodontal disease is unknown.

Periodontitis With Molar Incisor Pattern of Involvement

Periodontitis with molar incisor pattern usually results in attachment and bone loss around incisors and first molars, particularly in cases where the disease is observed in teenagers. Although such

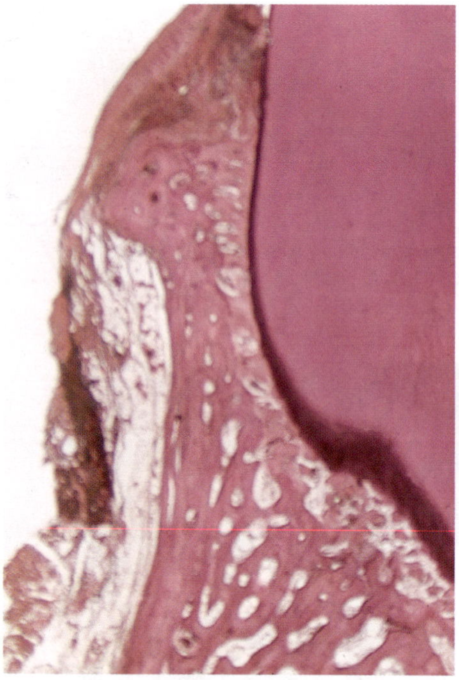

Fig. 19.11 Lipping of facial bone. There is a peripheral buttressing bone formation along the external surface of the facial bony plate and at the crest. Note the deformity in the bone produced by the buttressing bone formation and the bulging of the mucosa.

bone loss is usually horizontal in nature around incisors, a vertical or angular pattern of alveolar bone destruction is found around the first molars. The cause of the localized bone destruction associated with this type of periodontitis is unknown.

Bone Destruction Patterns in Periodontal Disease

Periodontal disease alters the morphologic features of the bone in addition to reducing bone height. An understanding of the nature and pathogenesis of these alterations is essential for effective diagnosis and treatment.

Horizontal Bone Loss

Horizontal bone loss is the most common pattern of bone loss in periodontal disease. The bone is reduced in height, but the bone margin remains approximately perpendicular to the tooth surface. The interdental septa and the facial and lingual plates are affected but not necessarily to an equal degree around the same tooth (Fig. 19.12A).

Bone Deformities (Osseous Defects)

Different types of bone deformities can result from periodontal disease. These usually occur in adults, but they have also been reported in human skulls with deciduous dentitions. Their presence may be suggested on radiographs, but careful probing and surgical exposure of the areas are required to determine their exact conformation and dimensions.

Vertical or Angular Defects

Vertical or angular defects are those that occur in an oblique direction, leaving a hollowed-out trough in the bone alongside the root; the base of the defect is located apical to the surrounding bone (Figs. 19.12B–19.14). In most instances, angular defects have accompanying infrabony periodontal pockets; infrabony pockets, on the other hand, must always have an underlying angular defect.

Goldman and Cohen classified angular defects on the basis of the number of osseous walls. Angular defects may have one, two, or three walls (Figs. 19.15–19.17). The continuous defects that involve more than one surface of a tooth, in a shape that is similar to trough, are called circumferential defects. The number of walls in the apical portion of the defect is often greater than that in its occlusal portion, in which case the term *combined osseous defect* is used (Figs. 19.18 and 19.19).

Vertical defects that occur interdentally can generally be seen on the radiograph although thick, bony plates may sometimes obscure them. Angular defects can also appear on facial and lingual or palatal surfaces, but these defects are not seen on radiographs. Surgical exposure is the only sure way to determine the presence and configuration of vertical osseous defects.

Vertical defects increase with age. Approximately 60% of persons with interdental angular defects have only a single defect. Vertical defects detected radiographically have been reported to appear most often on the distal and mesial surfaces. However, three-wall defects are more frequently found on the mesial surfaces of the upper and lower molars.

KEY FACT

The localized angular bone loss in aggressive periodontitis is usually located around the first molars and the incisors. These osseous lesions may be present in teenagers.

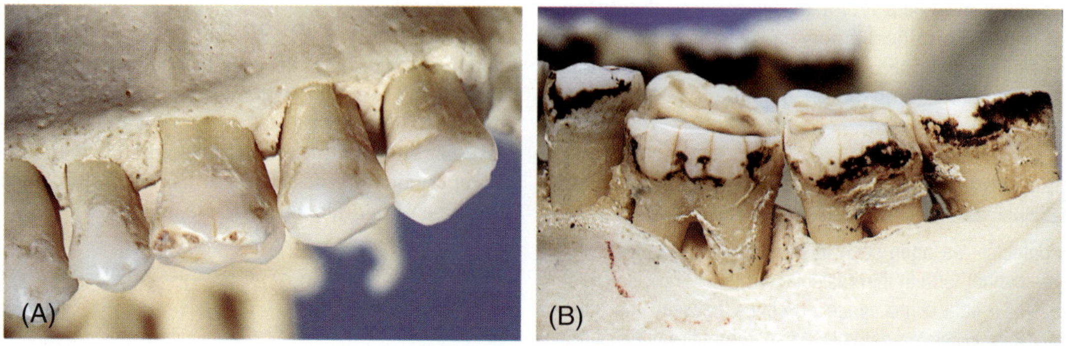

Fig. 19.12 A, Horizontal bone loss. Note the reduction in height of the marginal bone that exposes cancellous bone and reaches the furcation of the second molar. B, Vertical (angular) bone loss on the distal root of the first molar.

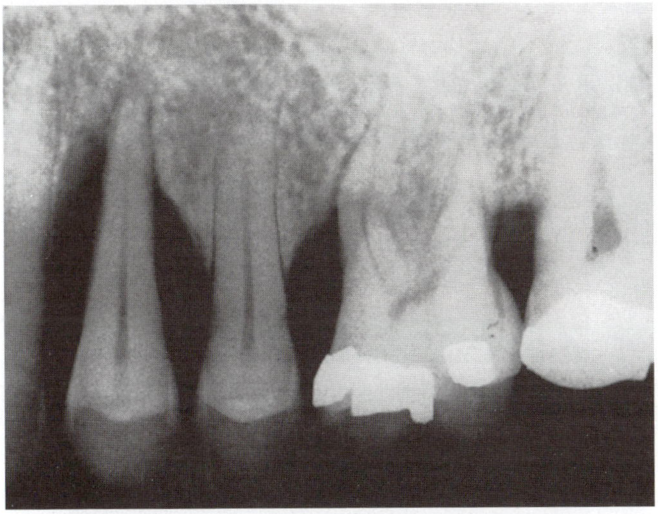

Fig. 19.13 Angular (vertical) defects of different depths.

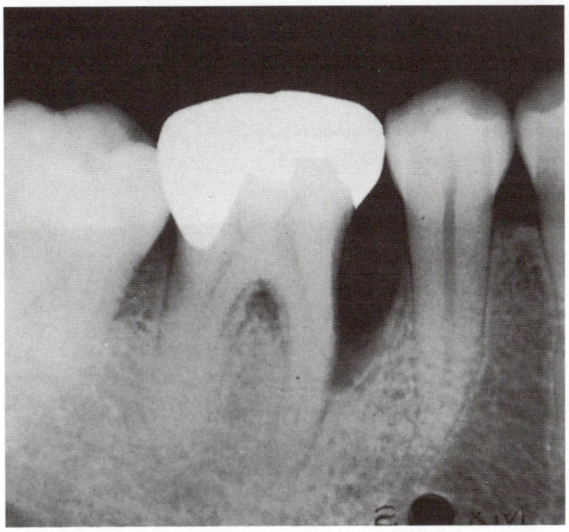

Fig. 19.14 Angular defect on the mesial surface of the first molar. Note also the furcation involvement.

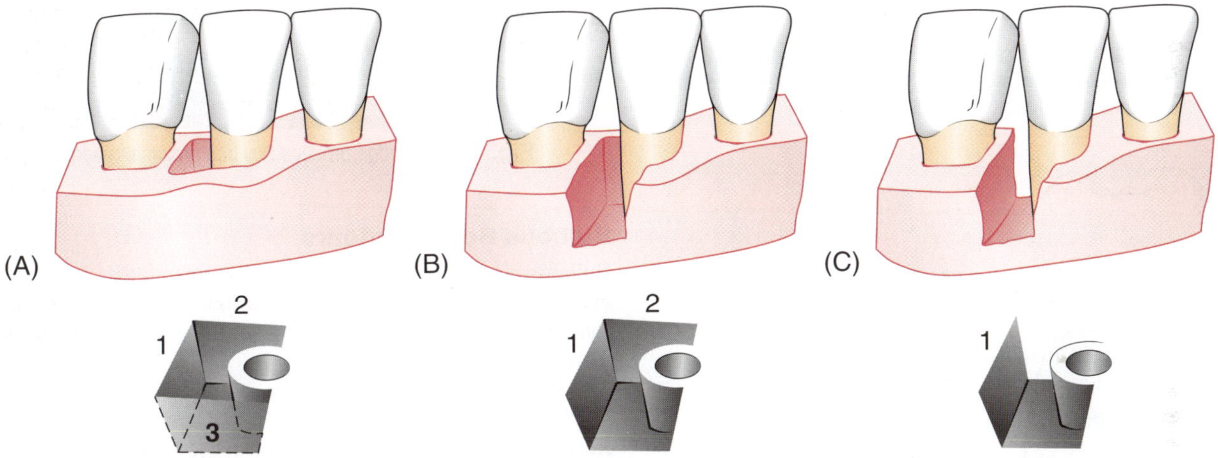

Fig. 19.15 One-, two-, and three-walled vertical defects on the right lateral incisor. A, Three bony walls: distal *(1)*, lingual *(2)*, and facial *(3)*. B, Two-wall defect: distal *(1)* and lingual *(2)*. (C), One-wall defect: distal wall only *(1)*.

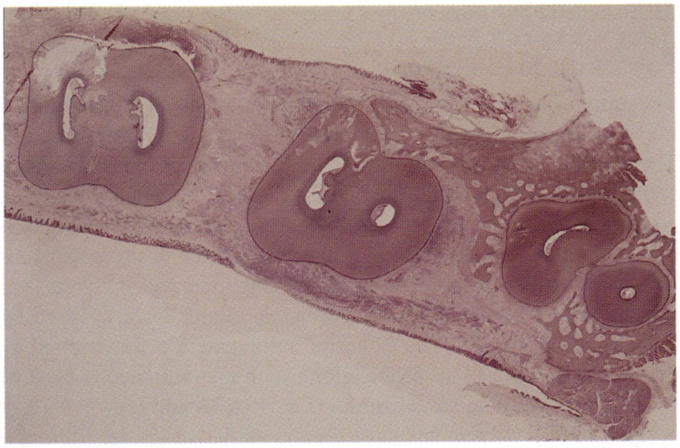

Fig. 19.16 Horizontal section of the lower molars at the midroot level showing a two-wall osseous defect distal to second molar.

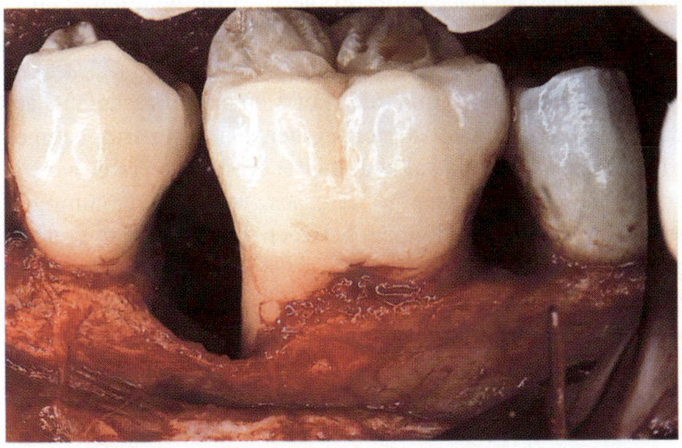

Fig. 19.17 One-wall vertical defect on the mesial surface of the lower first molar.

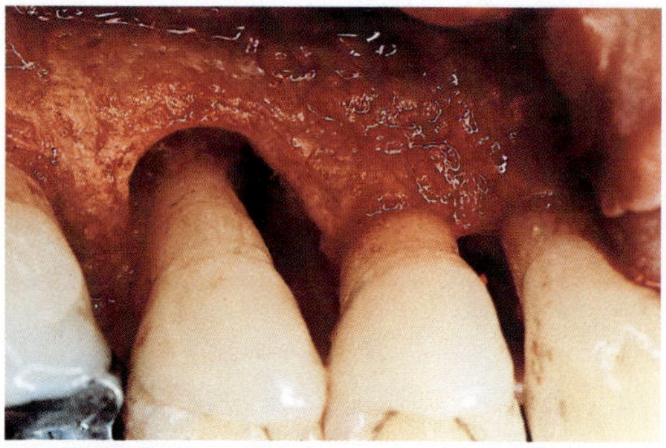

Fig. 19.18 Circumferential vertical defect in relation to the upper premolar.

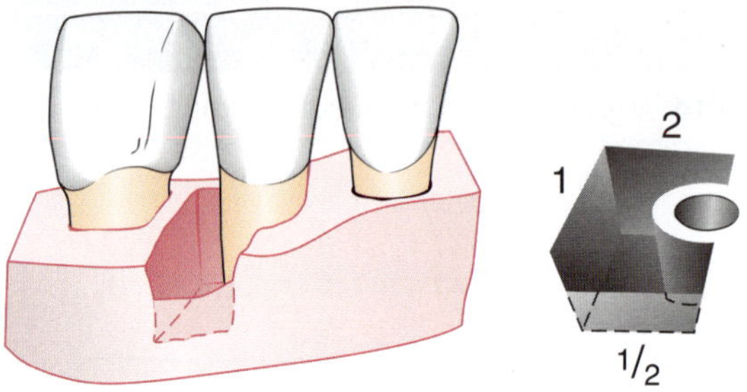

Fig. 19.19 Combined type of osseous defect. Since the facial wall is half the height of the distal *(1)* and lingual *(2)* walls, this is an osseous defect with three walls in its apical half and two walls in its occlusal half.

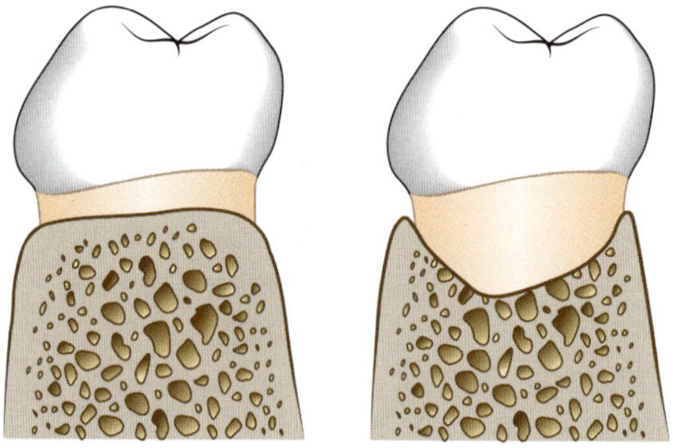

Fig. 19.20 Diagrammatic representation of an osseous crater in a faciolingual section between two lower molars. *Left,* Normal bone contour. *Right,* Osseous crater.

Osseous Craters

Osseous craters are concavities in the crest of the interdental bone that is confined within the facial and lingual walls (Fig. 19.20). Craters have been found to make up about one-third (35.2%) of all defects and about two-thirds (62%) of all mandibular defects and to occur twice as often in posterior segments as in anterior segments.

The heights of the facial and lingual crests of a crater have been found to be identical in 85% of cases, with the remaining 15% being almost equally divided between higher facial crests and higher lingual crests.

The following reasons for the high frequency of interdental craters have been suggested:

- The interdental area collects plaque and is difficult to clean.
- The normal flat or even slightly concave faciolingual shape of the interdental septum in the lower molars may favor crater formation.
- Vascular patterns from the gingiva to the center of the crest may provide a pathway for inflammation.

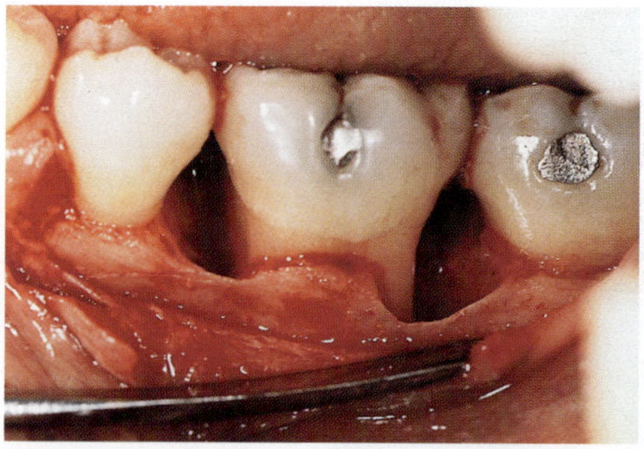

Fig. 19.21 Reversed architecture.The elevated flap shows the irregular bone margin.

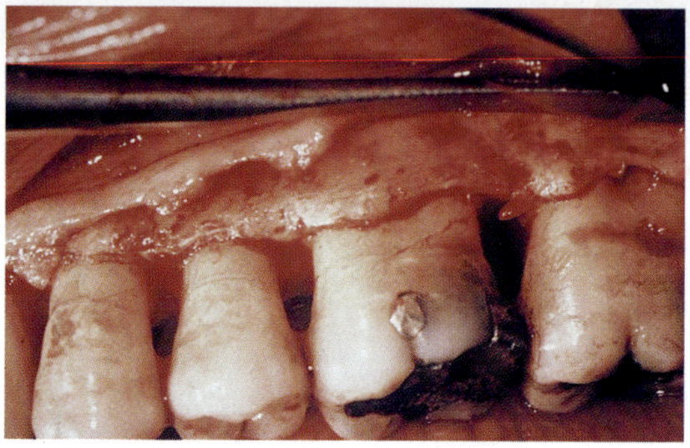

Fig. 19.22 Ledge produced by interproximal resorption.

Bulbous Bone Contours

Bulbous bone contours are bony enlargements that are caused by exostoses (Fig. 19.10), adaptation to function, or buttressing bone formation. They are found more frequently in the maxilla than in the mandible.

Reversed Architecture

Reversed architecture defects are produced by a loss of interdental bone, including the facial plates and the lingual plates, without a concomitant loss of radicular bone, thereby reversing the normal architecture (Fig. 19.21). This mostly occurs in necrotizing ulcerative periodontitis and are more common in the maxilla.

Ledges

Ledges are plateau-like bone margins that are caused by the resorption of thickened bony plates (Fig. 19.22).

Furcation Involvement

The term *furcation involvement* refers to the invasion of the bifurcation and trifurcation of multirooted teeth by periodontal disease. The prevalence of furcation-involved molars is not clear. Although some reports indicate that the mandibular first molars are the most common sites and that the maxillary premolars are the least common, other studies have found higher prevalence in the upper molars. The number of furcation involvements increases with age.

The denuded furcation may be visible clinically or covered by the wall of the pocket. The extent of involvement is determined by exploration with a blunt probe, along with a simultaneous blast of warm air to facilitate visualization (Fig. 19.23A and B).

Furcation involvements have been classified as grades I through IV according to the amount of tissue destruction. Grade I involves incipient bone loss; grade II involves partial bone loss (cul-de-sac);

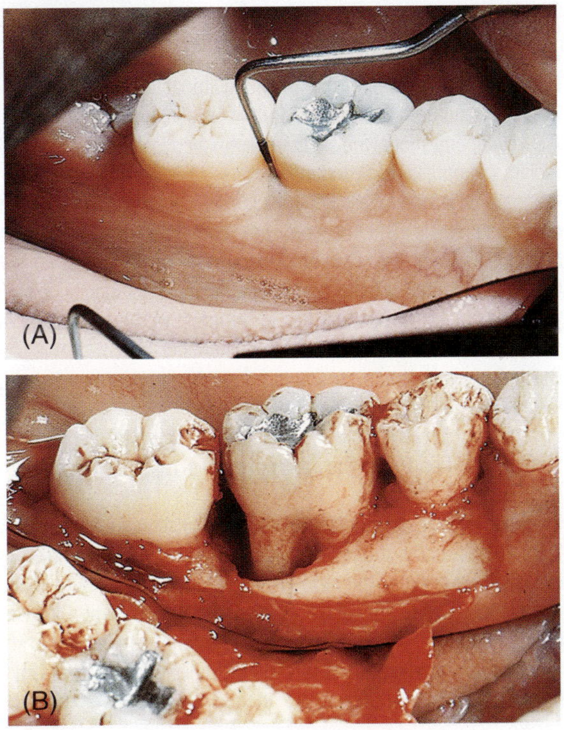

Fig. 19.23 A, A molar with slightly inflamed gingiva that is seen clinically; however, it has a deep distal pocket. B, Flap elevation reveals extensive bone loss and furcation involvement. *(Courtesy: Dr Terry Fiori, Palo Alto, CA.)*

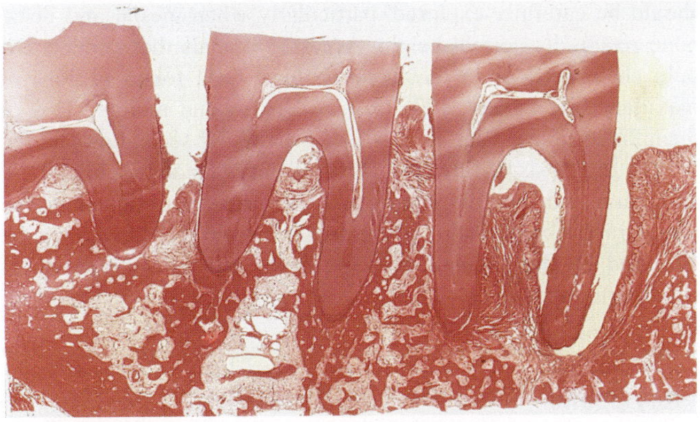

Fig. 19.24 Different degrees of furcation involvement in a human autopsy specimen. Furcation involvement is found in all three molars, with an advanced lesion in the second molar and an extremely severe lesion in the first molar that is exposing almost the entire mesial root.

and grade III involves total bone loss with a through-and-through opening of the furcation. Grade IV is similar to grade III but includes gingival recession that exposes the furcation to view.

Microscopically, furcation involvement presents no unique pathologic features. It is simply a phase in the rootward extension of the periodontal pocket. During its early stages, a widening of the periodontal space occurs with cellular and fluid inflammatory exudation, and this is followed by epithelial proliferation into the furcation area from an adjoining periodontal pocket. Extension of the inflammation into the bone leads to resorption and a reduction in bone height. The bone-destructive pattern may produce horizontal loss, or angular osseous defects associated with infrabony pockets may exist (Fig. 19.24). Plaque, calculus, and bacterial debris occupy the denuded furcation space.

The destructive pattern of a furcation involvement varies in different cases and with the degree of involvement. Bone loss around each individual root may be horizontal or angular, and frequently a crater develops in the interradicular area (Fig. 19.25A and B). Probing to determine the presence of these destructive patterns must be done horizontally and vertically around each involved root and in the crater area to establish the depth of the vertical component.

Furcation involvement is a stage of progressive periodontal disease, and it has its same etiology. The difficulty and sometimes the impossibility of controlling plaque in furcations are responsible for the presence of extensive lesions in this area.

The role of trauma from occlusion in the etiology of furcation lesions is controversial. Some assign a key role to trauma, thinking that furcation areas are most sensitive to injury from excessive occlusal forces. Others deny the initiating effect of trauma and consider that inflammation and edema caused by plaque in the furcation area tend to extrude the tooth, which then becomes traumatized and sensitive.

Other factors that may play a role are the presence of enamel projections into the furcation, which occurs in about 13% of multirooted teeth, and the proximity of the furcation to the cementoenamel junction, which occurs in about 75% of cases of furcation involvement.

The presence of accessory pulpal canals in the furcation area may extend pulpal inflammation to the furcation. This possibility

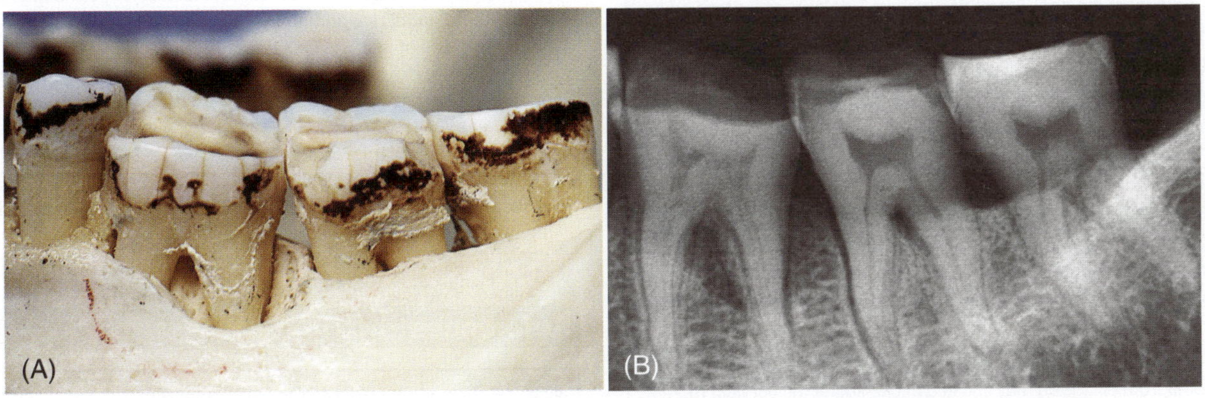

Fig. 19.25 A, Photograph and, B, radiograph of different degrees of bone loss in a skull. There are furcation involvements in the first and second molars; deep angular bone loss in the distal root of the first molar; and interradicular and interdental craters in the second molar and between the second and third molars, respectively.

should be carefully explored, particularly when mesial and distal bone retains its normal height. Accessory canals that connect the pulp chamber floor to the furcation have been found in 36% of maxillary first molars, 12% of maxillary second molars, 32% of mandibular first molars, and 24% of mandibular second molars.

The diagnosis of furcation involvement is made by clinical examination and careful probing with a specially designed probe. Radiographic examination of the area is helpful, but lesions can be obscured by the angulation of the beam and the radiopacity of neighboring structures.

Key points

- The height and density of the alveolar bone are normally maintained by an equilibrium, regulated by local and systemic influences between bone formation and bone resorption.
- The degree of bone loss is not necessarily correlated with the depth of periodontal pockets, the severity of ulceration of the pocket wall, or the presence or absence of pus.
- Periodontitis is always preceded by gingivitis, but not all gingivitis progresses to periodontitis.
- The transition from gingivitis to periodontitis is associated with changes in the composition of bacterial plaque.
- There is a continuous tendency to recreate transseptal fibers across the crest of the interdental septum farther along the root as the bone destruction progresses. As a result, transseptal fibers represent even in cases of extreme periodontal bone loss.
- Bone destruction in periodontal disease involves the activity of living cells along viable bone.
- Page and Schroeder, on the basis of Waerhaug's measurements made on human autopsy specimens, postulated a range of effectiveness of about 1.5–2.5 mm in which bacterial plaque can induce loss of bone beyond 2.5 mm, there is no effect; interproximal angular defect can appear only in spaces that are wider than 2.5 mm because narrower spaces would be destroyed completely.
- Period of destruction occurs in an episodic, intermittent manner, with period of inactivity or quiescence that alternate with destructive periods that result in the loss of collagen and alveolar bone and deepening of the periodontal pocket.
- Bone destruction in periodontal disease in presence or absence of inflammation is seen in trauma from occlusion.
- The persistent trauma from occlusion results in funnel-shaped widening of the crestal portion of the periodontal ligament with resorption of the adjacent bone.
- In addition to the virulence of plaque bacteria, the nature of the systemic component rather than its presence or absence influences the severity of the periodontal destruction. This concept is termed as bone factor concept.
- Osteoporosis is a physiologic condition of postmenopausal women that results in the loss of bone mineral content as well as structural bone changes.
- Periodontitis and osteoporosis share a number of risk factors. Aging, smoking, certain diseases, and medications that interfere with healing.
- Periodontal bone loss may also occur with generalized skeletal disturbances like hyperparathyroidism, leukemia, and histiocytosis X.
- Considerable normal variation exists within the morphologic features of alveolar bone, and this affects the osseous contours produced by periodontal disease.
- Exostoses are the outgrowths of bone of varied size and shape.
- Trauma from occlusion may cause a thickening of the cervical margin of alveolar bone or change in the bone morphology.
- Buttressing bone formation can be central buttressing bone formation or peripheral buttressing bone formation.
- Pressure and irritation from the food impaction contribute to the inverted bone architecture.
- A vertical pattern of alveolar bone destruction is seen around the first molars in aggressive periodontitis.
- Goldman and Cohen classified angular defects on basis of the number of osseous walls. They can be one-, two- or three-wall defects. In combined defect, the number of bony walls in the apical portion of the defect is often greater than in the occlusal portion.
- Osseous craters are concavities in the crest of the interdental bone that is confined within the facial and lingual walls.
- Bulbous bone contours are found frequently in upper jaw than in the lower jaw.
- Reverse architecture is seen in necrotizing ulcerative periodontitis.
- Plateau-like bone margins caused by the resorption of thickened bony plates.
- Furcation involvement is commonly seen in mandibular molars and least in maxillary premolars. Furcation involvements have been classified as grades I through IV according to the amount of tissue destruction. Grade I involves incipient bone loss, grade II involves partial bone loss, and grade III involves total bone loss with through and through opening of the furcation. Grade IV is similar to grade III but includes gingival recession.

Suggested Readings

Carranza FA Jr, Simes RJ, Mayo J, et al: Histometric evaluation of periodontal bone loss in rats. I. The effect of marginal irritation, systemic irradiation and trauma from occlusion, *J Periodont Res* 6:65, 1971.

Garant PR, Cho MJ: Histopathogenesis of spontaneous periodontal disease in conventional rats. I. Histometric and histologic study, *J Periodont Res* 14:297, 1979.

Glickman I: Inflammation and trauma from occlusion, co-destructive factors in chronic periodontal disease, *J Periodontol* 34:5, 1963.

Goldman HM, Cohen DW: The intrabony pocket: classification and treatment, *J Periodontol* 29:272, 1958.

Goodson JM, Haffajee AD, Socransky SS: The relationship between attachment level loss and alveolar bone loss, *J Clin Periodontol* 11:348, 1984.

Heijl L, Rifkin BR, Zander HA: Conversion of chronic gingivitis to periodontitis in squirrel monkeys, *J Periodontol* 47:710, 1976.

Kronfeld R: Condition of alveolar bone underlying periodontal pockets, *J Periodontol* 6:22, 1935.

Lindhe J, Liljenberg B, Listgarten MA: Some microbiological and histopathological features of periodontal disease in man, *J Periodontol* 51:264, 1980.

Löe H, Anerud A, Boysen H, et al: Natural history of periodontal disease in man. Rapid, moderate and no loss of attachment in Sri Lankan laborers 14 to 46 years of age, *J Clin Periodontol* 13:431, 1986.

Löe H, Anerud A, Boysen H, et al: The natural history of periodontal disease in man. The rate of periodontal destruction before 40 years of age, *J Periodontol* 49:607, 1978.

Page RC, Schroeder HE: Periodontitis in Man and Other Animals. A Comparative Review, Basel, 1982, Karger.

Waerhaug J: The furcation problem. Etiology, pathogenesis, diagnosis, therapy and prognosis, *J Clin Periodontol* 7:73, 1980.

References

References and MCQs with answers for the chapter are available on www.medenact.com.

CHAPTER 20

Periodontal Response to External Forces

FA Carranza | DG Naik | A Uppoor

CHAPTER OUTLINE

Adaptive Capacity of the Periodontium to Occlusal Forces

The periodontal ligament has a cushioning effect on forces applied to teeth as means to accommodate forces exerted on the crown. Due to the elastic nature of the periodontal ligament, all teeth with normal bone support present with physiologic mobility in all directions. Physiologic tooth mobility varies among individuals and within the dentition of the same individual. In the absence of excessive occlusal forces or the absence of reduced bone support induced by inflammatory periodontal disease, tooth mobility remains unchanged due to the fact that physiologic forces are not able to induce changes to the periodontal tissues.

The periodontium attempts to accommodate the forces exerted on the crown. This adaptive capacity varies in different persons and in the same person at different times. The effect of occlusal forces on the periodontium is influenced by the magnitude, direction, duration, and frequency of the forces.

When the *magnitude* of occlusal forces is increased, the periodontium responds with a widening of the periodontal ligament space, an increase in the number and width of periodontal ligament fibers, and an increase in the density of alveolar bone.

Changing the *direction* of occlusal forces causes a reorientation of the stresses and strains within the periodontium (Fig. 20.1). The principal fibers of the periodontal ligament are arranged so that they best accommodate occlusal forces along the long axis of the tooth. *Lateral* (horizontal) and *torque* (rotational) forces are more likely to injure the periodontium.

The response of alveolar bone is also affected by the *duration* and *frequency* of occlusal forces. Constant pressure on the bone is more injurious than intermittent forces. The more frequent the application of an intermittent force, the more injurious the force is to the periodontium.

KEY FACT

When there is an increase in occlusal forces, changes occur in the periodontium in order to accommodate for such forces. Changes in the periodontium depend on the magnitude, direction, duration, and frequency of increased occlusal forces.

Trauma From Occlusion

An inherent "margin of safety" that is common to all tissues permits some variation in occlusion without adversely affecting the periodontium. However, when occlusal forces exceed the adaptive capacity of the tissues, tissue injury results. The resultant injury is termed *trauma from occlusion*, which is also known as *traumatism* or *occlusal trauma*.

Thus, trauma from occlusion refers to the *tissue injury* rather than the *occlusal force*. An occlusion that produces such an injury is called a *traumatic occlusion*. Excessive occlusal forces may also disrupt the function of the masticatory musculature and cause painful spasms, injure the temporomandibular joints, or produce excessive tooth wear. However, the term *trauma from occlusion* is generally used in connection with injury in the periodontium.

KEY FACT

Trauma from occlusion refers to the *tissue injury* rather than the *occlusal force*. An occlusion that produces such an injury is called a *traumatic occlusion*.

The criterion that determines if an occlusion is traumatic is whether it produces periodontal injury; this criterion is *not* how the teeth occlude. Any occlusion that produces periodontal injury is traumatic. Malocclusion is not necessary to produce trauma; periodontal injury may occur when the occlusion appears normal. The dentition may be anatomically and esthetically acceptable but functionally injurious. Similarly, not all malocclusions are necessarily injurious to the periodontium. Traumatic occlusal relationships are referred to by terms such as *occlusal disharmony*, *functional imbalance*, and *occlusal dystrophy*. These terms refer to the effect of the occlusion on the periodontium rather than to the position of the teeth. Since trauma from occlusion refers to the tissue injury rather than the occlusion, an increased occlusal force is not traumatic if the periodontium can accommodate it.

Acute and Chronic Trauma

Trauma from occlusion may be acute or chronic. *Acute trauma* from occlusion results from an abrupt occlusal impact such as that

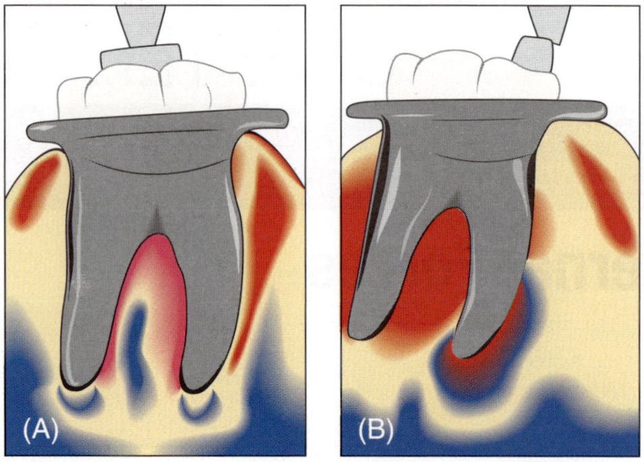

Fig. 20.1 Stress patterns around the roots changed by shifting the direction of occlusal forces (experimental model using photoelastic analysis). A, Buccal view of an ivorine molar subjected to an axial force. The *shaded fringes* indicate that the internal stresses are at the root apices. B, Buccal view of an ivorine molar subjected to a mesial tilting force. The *shaded fringes* indicate that the internal stresses are along the mesial surface and at the apex of the mesial root.

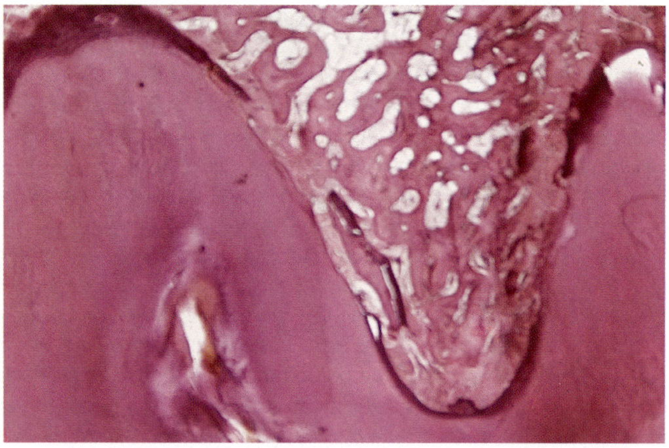

Fig. 20.2 Cemental tear, presumably caused by acute trauma from occlusion in a human autopsy specimen. Note the repair process depositing bone on the displaced, torn cementum and recreating a periodontal ligament.

produced by biting on a hard object (e.g., olive pit). Restorations or prosthetic appliances that interfere with or alter the direction of occlusal forces on the teeth may also induce acute trauma.

Acute trauma results in tooth pain, sensitivity to percussion, and increased tooth mobility. If the force is dissipated by a shift in the position of the tooth or by the wearing away or correction of the restoration, then the injury heals, and the symptoms subside. Otherwise, periodontal injury may worsen and develop into necrosis accompanied by periodontal abscess formation, or it may persist as a symptom-free chronic condition. Acute trauma can also produce cementum tears (Fig. 20.2).

KEY FACT

Acute trauma from occlusion refers to periodontal changes associated with an abrupt occlusal impact such as that produced by biting on a hard object (e.g., an olive pit). In addition, restorations or prosthetic appliances that interfere with or alter the direction of occlusal forces on the teeth may also induce acute trauma. Acute trauma results in tooth pain, sensitivity to percussion, and increased tooth mobility.

Chronic trauma from occlusion is more common than the acute form, and it is of greater clinical significance. It most often develops from gradual changes in occlusion produced by tooth wear, drifting movement, and extrusion of the teeth in combination with parafunctional habits (e.g., bruxism, clenching) rather than as a sequela of acute periodontal trauma. Chronic Trauma from Occlusion (TFO) is further classified as primary and secondary.

KEY FACT

Chronic trauma from occlusion refers to periodontal changes associated with gradual changes in occlusion produced by tooth wear, drifting movement, and extrusion of the teeth in combination with parafunctional habits (e.g., bruxism, clenching) rather than as a sequela of acute periodontal trauma. Chronic trauma from occlusion is more common than the acute form and of greater clinical significance.

Primary and Secondary Trauma From Occlusion

Trauma from occlusion may be caused by alterations in occlusal forces, a reduced capacity of the periodontium to withstand occlusal forces, or both. When trauma from occlusion is the result of alterations in occlusal forces, it is called *primary trauma from occlusion.* When it results from the reduced ability of the tissues to resist the occlusal forces, it is known as *secondary trauma from occlusion.*

Primary trauma from occlusion occurs if trauma from occlusion is considered the primary etiologic factor in periodontal destruction and if the only local alteration to which a tooth is subjected is a result of occlusion. Examples include periodontal injury produced around teeth with a previously healthy periodontium after the following: (1) the insertion of a "high filling"; (2) the insertion of a prosthetic replacement that creates excessive forces on abutment and antagonistic teeth; (3) the drifting movement or extrusion of the teeth into spaces created by unreplaced missing teeth; or (4) the orthodontic movement of teeth into functionally unacceptable positions. Most studies of the effect of trauma from occlusion involving experimental animals have examined the primary type of trauma. Changes produced by primary trauma do not alter the level of connective tissue attachment and do not initiate pocket formation. This is probably because the supracrestal gingival fibers are not affected and therefore prevent the apical migration of the junctional epithelium.

KEY FACT

Primary trauma from occlusion occurs if trauma from occlusion is considered the primary etiologic factor in periodontal destruction and if the only local alteration to which a tooth is subjected is a result of occlusion.

Secondary trauma from occlusion occurs when the adaptive capacity of the tissues to withstand occlusal forces is impaired by bone loss that results from marginal inflammation. This reduces the periodontal attachment area and alters the leverage on the remaining tissues. The periodontium becomes more vulnerable to injury, and previously well-tolerated occlusal forces become traumatic.

Fig. 20.3 depicts three different situations on which excessive occlusal forces can be superimposed:

1. Normal periodontium with normal height of bone.
2. Normal periodontium with reduced height of bone.
3. Marginal periodontitis with reduced height of bone.

The first case is an example of primary trauma from occlusion, whereas the last two represent secondary trauma from occlusion.

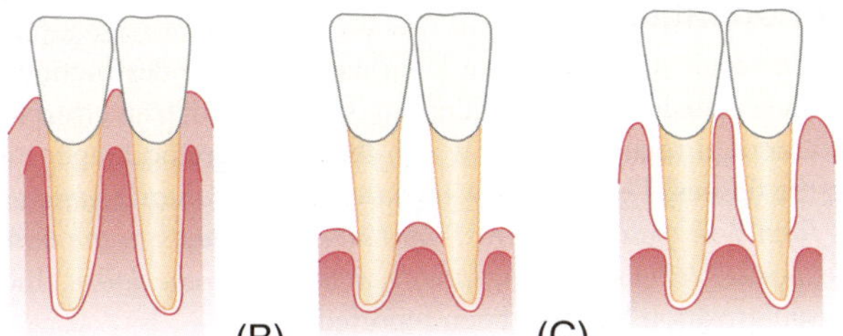

Fig. 20.3 Traumatic forces can occur on: A, normal periodontium with normal height of bone; B, normal periodontium with reduced height of bone; or C, marginal periodontitis with reduced height of bone.

The effects of trauma from occlusion in these different situations are analyzed in the following discussion.

It has been found in experimental animals that systemic disorders can reduce tissue resistance and that previously tolerable forces may become excessive. This could theoretically represent another mechanism by which tissue resistance to increased forces is lowered, thereby resulting in secondary trauma from occlusion.

Stages of Tissue Response to Increased Occlusal Forces

Tissue response occurs in three stages: injury, repair, and adaptive remodeling of the periodontium.

Stage I: Injury

Tissue injury is produced by excessive occlusal forces. The body then attempts to repair the injury and restore the periodontium. This can occur if the forces are diminished or if the tooth drifts away from them. If the offending force is chronic, however, the periodontium is remodeled to cushion its impact. The ligament is widened at the expense of the bone, which results in angular bone defects without periodontal pockets, and the tooth becomes loose.

Under the forces of occlusion, a tooth rotates around a fulcrum or axis of rotation, which in single-rooted teeth is located in the junction between the middle third and the apical third of the clinical root and in multirooted teeth in the middle of the interradicular bone. This creates areas of pressure and tension on opposite sides of the fulcrum (Fig. 20.4). Different lesions are produced by different degrees of pressure and tension. If jiggling forces are exerted, these different lesions may coexist in the same area.

Slightly excessive pressure stimulates resorption of the alveolar bone, with a resultant widening of the periodontal ligament space. *Slightly excessive tension* causes elongation of the periodontal ligament fibers and the apposition of alveolar bone. In areas of increased pressure, the blood vessels are numerous and reduced in size; in areas of increased tension, they are enlarged.

Greater pressure produces a gradation of changes in the periodontal ligament, starting with compression of the fibers, which produces areas of hyalinization. Subsequent injury to the fibroblasts and other connective tissue cells leads to necrosis of areas of the ligament. Vascular changes are also produced: within 30 min, impairment and stasis of blood flow occur; at 2–3 h, blood vessels appear to be packed with erythrocytes, which start to fragment; and between 1 and 7 days, disintegration of the blood vessel walls and release of the contents into the surrounding tissue occur. In addition, increased resorption of alveolar bone and resorption of the tooth surface occur.

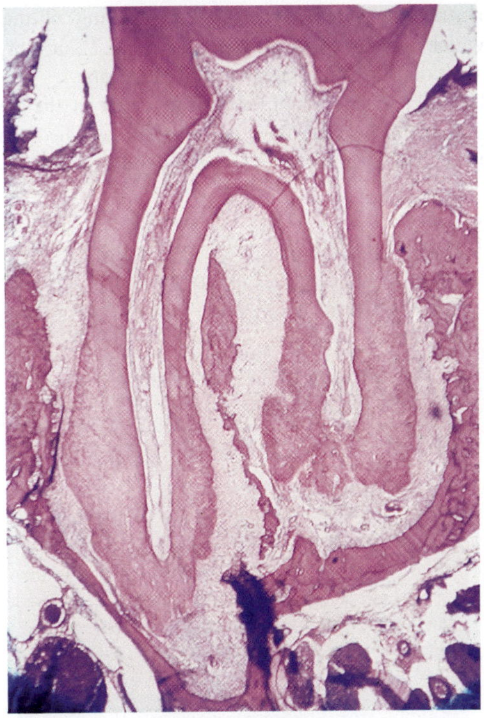

Fig. 20.4 Areas of tension and pressure in opposite sites of the periodontal ligament caused by experimentally induced orthodontic movement in a rat molar.

Severe tension causes widening of the periodontal ligament, thrombosis, hemorrhage, tearing of the periodontal ligament, and resorption of alveolar bone.

Pressure severe enough to force the root against bone causes necrosis of the periodontal ligament and bone. The bone is resorbed from viable periodontal ligament adjacent to necrotic areas and from marrow spaces; this process is called *undermining resorption.*

The areas of the periodontium that are most susceptible to injury from excessive occlusal forces are the furcations.

Injury to the periodontium produces a temporary depression in mitotic activity, in the rate of proliferation and differentiation of fibroblasts, in collagen formation, and in bone formation. These return to normal levels after the dissipation of the forces.

Stage II: Repair

Repair occurs constantly in the normal periodontium, and trauma from occlusion stimulates increased reparative activity.

The damaged tissues are removed, and new connective tissue cells and fibers, bone, and cementum are formed in an attempt to restore the injured periodontium (Fig. 20.5). Forces remain traumatic only as long as the damage produced exceeds the reparative capacity of the tissues.

When bone is resorbed by excessive occlusal forces, the body attempts to reinforce the thinned bony trabeculae with new bone (Fig. 20.6). This attempt to compensate for lost bone is called *buttressing bone formation*, and it is an important feature of the reparative process associated with trauma from occlusion. It also occurs when bone is destroyed by inflammation or osteolytic tumors.

Buttressing bone formation occurs within the jaw (central buttressing) and on the bone surface (peripheral buttressing). During *central buttressing*, the endosteal cells deposit new bone, which restores the bony trabeculae and reduces the size of the marrow spaces. *Peripheral buttressing* occurs on the facial and lingual surfaces of the alveolar plate. Depending on its severity, peripheral buttressing may produce a shelf-like thickening of the alveolar margin, which is referred to as *lipping* (Fig. 20.7), or a pronounced bulge in the contour of the facial and lingual bone.

Cartilage-like material sometimes develops in the periodontal ligament space as an aftermath of the trauma. The formation of crystals from erythrocytes has also been demonstrated.

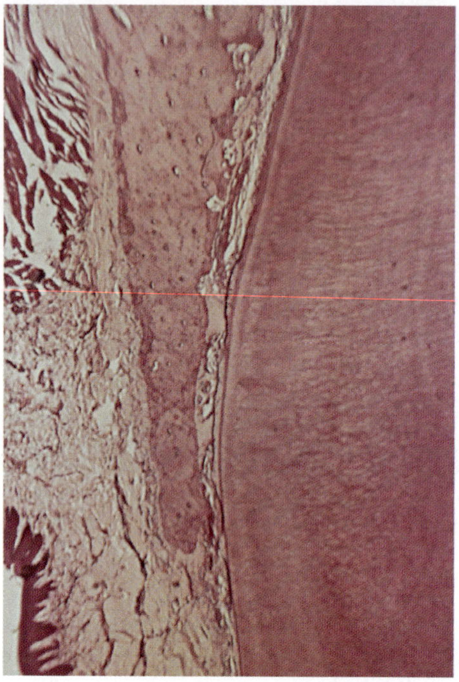

Fig. 20.5 Experimental occlusal trauma in rats. Note the area of necrosis of the marginal periodontal ligament and resorption and remodeling in the more apical periodontal sites.

Stage III: Adaptive Remodeling of the Periodontium

If the repair process cannot keep pace with the destruction caused by the occlusion, the periodontium is remodeled in an effort to create a structural relationship in which the forces are no longer injurious to the tissues. *This results in a widened periodontal ligament, which is funnel-shaped at the crest, and angular defects in the bone, with no pocket formation. The involved teeth become loose.* Increased vascularization has also been reported.

The three stages in the evolution of traumatic lesions have been differentiated histometrically by the relative amounts of periodontal bone surface undergoing resorption or formation (Fig. 20.8). The injury phase shows an increase in areas of resorption and a decrease

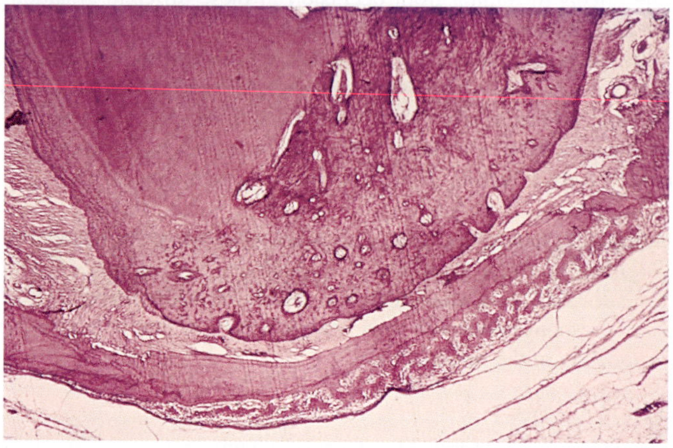

Fig. 20.6 Apical area of a premolar subjected to experimental occlusal trauma in a dog causing intrusion of the tooth and areas of necrosis in the periodontal ligament. Note the active bone formation on the outer aspect of the bone and the resorptive activity in the periphery of the necrotic site.

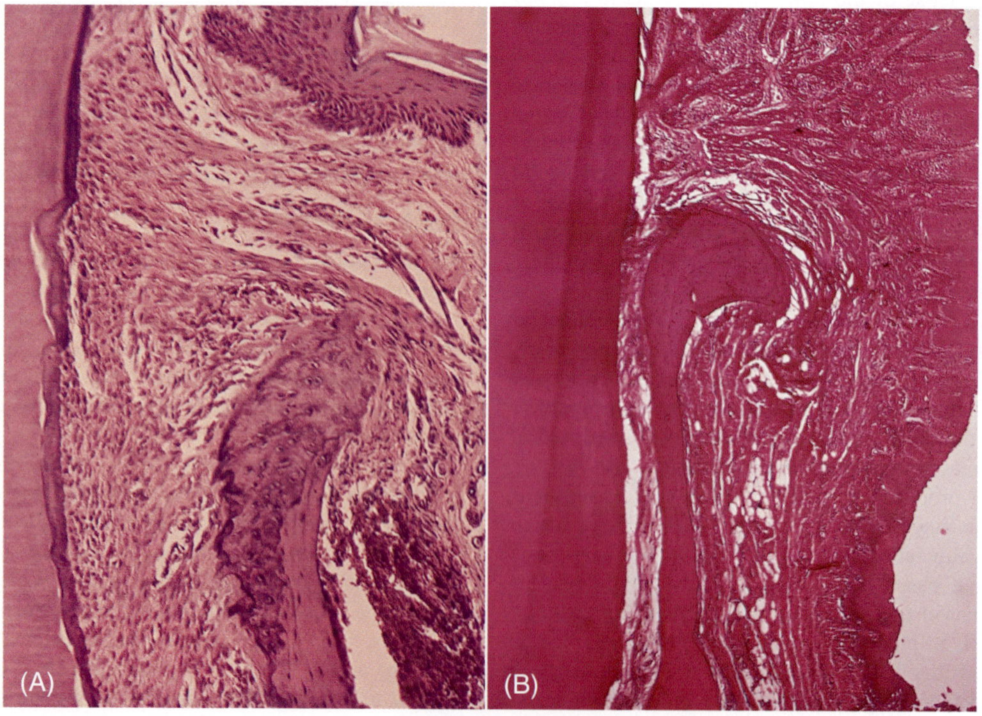

Fig. 20.7 A, Widening of the periodontal ligament space in the cervical area and a change in the shape of the marginal alveolar bone as a result of chronic prolonged trauma from occlusion in rats. B, Comparable changes in the shape of the marginal bone found in a human autopsy case.

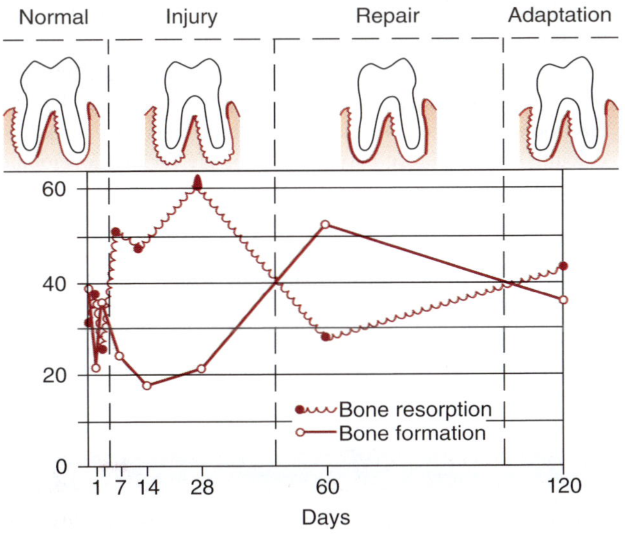

Fig. 20.8 Evolution of traumatic lesions as depicted experimentally in rats by variations in relative amounts of areas of bone formation and bone resorption in periodontal bone surfaces. The horizontal axis shows the number of days after the initiation of traumatic interference. The vertical axis shows the percentage of bone surface undergoing resorption or formation. The stages in the evolution of the lesions are represented in the top drawings, which show the average amount of bone activity for each group.

in bone formation, whereas the repair phase demonstrates decreased resorption and increased bone formation. After adaptive remodeling of the periodontium, resorption and formation return to normal.

Effects of Insufficient Occlusal Force

Insufficient occlusal force may also be injurious to the supporting periodontal tissues. Insufficient stimulation causes thinning of the periodontal ligament, atrophy of the fibers, osteoporosis of the alveolar bone, and a reduction in bone height. Hypofunction can result from an open-bite relationship, an absence of functional antagonists, or unilateral chewing habits that neglect one side of the mouth.

Reversibility of Traumatic Lesions

Trauma from occlusion is reversible. When trauma is artificially induced in experimental animals, the teeth move away or intrude into the jaw. When the impact of the artificially created force is relieved, the tissues undergo repair. Although trauma from occlusion is reversible under such conditions, it does not always correct itself, and therefore it is not always temporary or of limited clinical significance. The injurious force must be relieved for repair to occur. If conditions in humans do not permit the teeth to escape from or adapt to excessive occlusal force, periodontal damage persists and worsens.

The presence of inflammation in the periodontium as a result of plaque accumulation may impair the reversibility of traumatic lesions.

Effects of Excessive Occlusal Forces on Dental Pulp

The effects of excessive occlusal forces on the dental pulp have not been established. Some clinicians report the disappearance of pulpal symptoms after the correction of excessive occlusal forces. Pulpal reactions have been noted in animals subjected to increased occlusal forces, but these did not occur when the forces were minimal and occurred over short periods.

KEY FACT

Secondary trauma from occlusion occurs when the adaptive capacity of the tissues to withstand occlusal forces is impaired by bone loss that results from marginal inflammation. This reduces the periodontal attachment area and alters the leverage on the remaining tissues. The periodontium becomes more vulnerable to injury, and previously well-tolerated occlusal forces become traumatic.

Influence of Trauma From Occlusion on the Progression of Marginal Periodontitis

The clinical impressions of early investigators and clinicians assigned an important role to trauma from occlusion in the etiology of periodontal lesions. Since then, numerous studies have been performed that have attempted to determine the mechanisms by which trauma from occlusion may affect periodontal disease.

Initial studies involved the placement of high crowns or restorations on the teeth of dogs or monkeys, thereby resulting in a continuous or intermittent force in one direction. These investigations provided an orthodontic type of force and gave clear descriptions of changes that were occurring in pressure zones and tension zones. These procedures usually resulted in tooth displacement and consolidation in a new, nontraumatized position.

Trauma from occlusion in humans, however, is the result of forces that act alternatively in opposing directions. These were analyzed in experimental animals with "jiggling forces," which were usually produced by a high crown in combination with an orthodontic appliance that would bring the traumatized tooth back to its original position when the force was dissipated by separating the teeth. With another method, the teeth were separated by wooden or elastic material wedged interproximally to displace a tooth toward the opposite proximal side. After 48 h, the wedge was removed, and the procedure was repeated on the opposite side.

These studies resulted in a combination of changes produced by pressure and tension on both sides of the tooth, with an increase in the width of the ligament and increased tooth mobility. None of these methods caused gingival inflammation or pocket formation, and the results essentially represented different degrees of functional adaptation to increased forces.

To mimic the problem in humans more closely, studies were then conducted on the effect produced by jiggling trauma and simultaneous plaque-induced gingival inflammation.

The accumulation of bacterial plaque that initiates gingivitis and results in periodontal pocket formation affects the marginal gingiva, but trauma from occlusion occurs in the supporting tissues and does not affect the gingiva (Fig. 20.9). The marginal gingiva is unaffected by trauma from occlusion because its blood supply is not affected even when the vessels of the periodontal ligament are obliterated by excessive occlusal forces. It has been repeatedly proved that trauma from occlusion does not cause pockets or gingivitis and that it also does not increase gingival fluid flow. Furthermore, experimental trauma in dogs does not influence the bacterial repopulation of pockets after scaling and root planing. However, mobile teeth in humans harbor significantly higher proportions of *Campylobacter rectus* and *Peptostreptococcus micros* than nonmobile teeth.

As long as inflammation is confined to the gingiva, the inflammatory process is not affected by occlusal forces. When inflammation extends from the gingiva into the supporting periodontal tissues

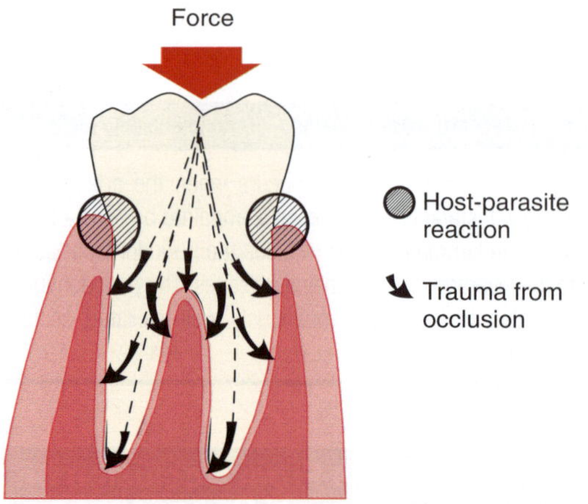

Fig. 20.9 The reaction between dental plaque and the host takes place in the gingival sulcus region. Trauma from occlusion appears in the tissues that are supporting the tooth.

(i.e., when gingivitis becomes periodontitis), plaque-induced inflammation enters the zone that is influenced by occlusion, which Glickman has called the *zone of codestruction.*

Two groups have studied this topic experimentally, with conflicting results, probably because of the different methods used. The Eastman Dental Center group in Rochester, NY, used squirrel monkeys, produced trauma by repetitive interdental wedging, and added mild to moderate gingival inflammation; experimental times were up to 10 weeks. They reported that the presence of trauma did not increase the loss of attachment induced by periodontitis. The University of Gothenburg group in Sweden used beagle dogs, produced trauma by placing cap splints and orthodontic appliances, and induced severe gingival inflammation; experimental times were up to 1 year. This group found that occlusal stresses increase the periodontal destruction induced by periodontitis.

When trauma from occlusion is eliminated, a substantial reversal of bone loss occurs, except in the presence of periodontitis. This indicates that inflammation inhibits the potential for bone regeneration. *Thus, it is important to eliminate the marginal inflammatory component in cases of trauma from occlusion because the presence of inflammation affects bone regeneration after the removal of the traumatizing contacts.* It has also been shown in experimental animals that trauma from occlusion does not induce progressive destruction of the periodontal tissues in regions that are kept healthy after the elimination of preexisting periodontitis.

Trauma from occlusion also tends to change the shape of the alveolar crest. The change in shape consists of a widening of the marginal periodontal ligament space, a narrowing of the interproximal alveolar bone, and a shelf-like thickening of the alveolar margin. Therefore, although trauma from occlusion does not alter the inflammatory process, it changes the architecture of the area around the inflamed site. *Thus, in the absence of inflammation, the response to trauma from occlusion is limited to adaptation to the increased forces. In the presence of inflammation, however, the changes in the shape of the alveolar crest may be conducive to angular bone loss, and existing pockets may become intrabony.*

Other theories that have been proposed to explain the interaction of trauma and inflammation include the following:

- Trauma from occlusion may alter the pathway of the extension of gingival inflammation to the underlying tissues. This may be favored by the reduced collagen density and the increased number of leukocytes, osteoclasts, and blood vessels in the coronal portion of increasingly mobile teeth. Inflammation may then proceed to the periodontal ligament rather than to the bone. Resulting bone loss would be angular, and pockets could become intrabony.
- Trauma-induced areas of root resorption uncovered by apical migration of the inflamed gingival attachment may offer a favorable environment for the formation and attachment of plaque and calculus and therefore may be responsible for the development of deeper lesions.
- Supragingival plaque can become subgingival if the tooth is tilted orthodontically or if it migrates into an edentulous area, which results in the transformation of a suprabony pocket into an intrabony pocket.
- Increased mobility of traumatically loosened teeth may have a pumping effect on plaque metabolites, thereby increasing their diffusion.

KEY FACT

Despite conflicting scientific data and speculations generated based on such data on the role of trauma from occlusion in periodontitis, two points are not contested: (1) changes related to trauma from occlusion (bone loss and tooth mobility) are reversible if they occurred in the absence of periodontitis; (2) in situations where both plaque-induced periodontitis and trauma from occlusion are present, elimination of the former will prevent further apical migration of the attachment unit, despite the presence of trauma from occlusion. Therefore, in terms of patient care, all facts support the priority that should be given to eliminate the bacterial plaque portion of the disease process.

Clinical and Radiographic Signs of Trauma From Occlusion Alone

The most common clinical sign of trauma to the periodontium is *progressive tooth mobility.* During the injury stage of trauma from occlusion, the destruction of periodontal fibers occurs, which increases tooth mobility. During the final stage, the accommodation of the periodontium to increased forces entails a widening of the periodontal ligament, which also leads to increased tooth mobility. Although this tooth mobility is greater than the so-called normal mobility, it cannot be considered pathologic because it is an adaptation and not a disease process. If it does become progressively worse, it can then be considered pathologic.

Other causes of increased tooth mobility include advanced bone loss, inflammation of the periodontal ligament of periodontal or periapical origin, and some systemic causes (e.g., pregnancy). The loss of adjacent alveolar bone, as seen in conditions like osteomyelitis or jaw tumors, can lead to heightened tooth mobility.

Radiographic signs of trauma from occlusion may include the following:

1. Increased width of the periodontal space, often with thickening of the lamina dura along the lateral aspect of the root, in the apical region, and in bifurcation areas. These changes do not *necessarily* indicate destructive changes because they may result from thickening and strengthening of the periodontal ligament and alveolar bone, thereby constituting a favorable response to increased occlusal forces.
2. A "vertical" rather than "horizontal" destruction of the interdental septum.
3. Radiolucency and condensation of the alveolar bone.
4. Root resorption.

In summary, trauma from occlusion does not initiate gingivitis or periodontal pockets, but it may constitute an additional risk factor for the progression and severity of the disease. An understanding of the effect of trauma from occlusion on the periodontium is useful during the clinical management of periodontal problems.

Pathologic Tooth Migration

Pathologic migration refers to tooth displacement that results when the balance among the factors that maintain physiologic tooth position is disturbed by periodontal disease. Pathologic migration is relatively common. It may be an early sign of disease, or it may occur in association with gingival inflammation and pocket formation as the disease progresses.

Pathologic migration occurs most frequently in the anterior region, but posterior teeth may also be affected. The teeth may move in any direction, and the migration is usually accompanied by mobility and rotation. Pathologic migration in the occlusal or incisal direction is termed *extrusion.* All degrees of pathologic migration are encountered, and one or more teeth may be affected (Fig. 20.10). It is important to detect migration during its early stages and to prevent more serious involvement by eliminating the causative factors. Even during the early stage, some degree of bone loss occurs.

Pathogenesis

Two major factors play a role in maintaining the normal position of the teeth: the health and normal height of the periodontal attachment apparatus and the forces exerted on the teeth. The latter includes the forces of occlusion and pressure from the lips, cheeks, and tongue. Factors that are important in relation to the forces of occlusion include the following: (1) tooth morphologic features and cuspal inclination; (2) the presence of a full complement of teeth; (3) a physiologic tendency toward mesial migration; (4) the nature and location of contact point relationships; (5) proximal, incisal, and occlusal attrition; and (6) the axial inclination of the teeth. Alterations in any of these factors start an interrelated sequence of changes in the environment of a single tooth or group of teeth that may result in pathologic migration. Thus, pathologic migration occurs under conditions that weaken the periodontal support, that increase or modify the forces exerted on the teeth, or both.

Weakened Periodontal Support

The inflammatory destruction of the periodontium in patients with periodontitis creates an imbalance between the forces that maintain the tooth in position and the occlusal and muscular forces the tooth ordinarily needs to bear. The tooth with weakened support is unable to maintain its normal position in the arch and moves away from the opposing force unless it is restrained by proximal contact. The force that moves the weakly supported tooth may be created by factors such as occlusal contacts or pressure from the tongue.

It is important to understand that the abnormality of pathologic migration rests with the weakened periodontium; the force itself is not necessarily abnormal. Forces that are acceptable to an intact periodontium become injurious when periodontal support is reduced as in the tooth with abnormal proximal contacts. Abnormally located proximal contacts convert the normal anterior component of force to a wedging force that moves the tooth occlusally or incisally. The wedging force, which can be withstood by the intact periodontium, causes the tooth to extrude when the periodontal support is weakened by disease. *As its position changes, the tooth is subjected to abnormal occlusal forces, which aggravate the periodontal destruction and the tooth migration.*

Pathologic migration may continue after a tooth no longer contacts its antagonist. Pressures from the tongue, the food bolus during mastication, and the proliferating granulation tissue provide the force.

Pathologic migration is also an early sign of localized aggressive periodontitis. Weakened by the loss of periodontal support, the maxillary and mandibular anterior incisors drift labially and extrude, thereby creating diastemata between the teeth.

Changes in the Forces Exerted on the Teeth

Changes in the magnitude, direction, or frequency of the forces exerted on the teeth can induce the pathologic migration of a tooth or group of teeth. These forces do not have to be abnormal to cause migration if the periodontium is sufficiently weakened. Changes in the forces may result from unreplaced missing teeth or other causes.

Unreplaced Missing Teeth

The drifting of teeth into the spaces created by unreplaced missing teeth often occurs. Drifting differs from pathologic migration in that it does not result from the destruction of the periodontal tissues. However, it usually creates conditions that lead to periodontal disease, and thus the initial tooth movement is aggravated by a loss of periodontal support (Fig. 20.11).

Drifting generally occurs in a mesial direction in combination with tilting or extrusion beyond the occlusal plane. The premolars frequently drift distally (Fig. 20.12). Although drifting is a common sequela when missing teeth are not replaced, it does not always occur (Fig. 20.13).

Failure to Replace First Molars

The pattern of changes that may follow the failure to replace missing first molars is characteristic. In extreme cases, it consists of the following:

1. The second and third molars tilt mesially, which results in a decrease in vertical dimension (Fig. 20.14).
2. The premolars move distally, and the mandibular incisors tilt or drift lingually. While drifting distally, the mandibular premolars lose their intercuspating relationship with the maxillary teeth, and they may tilt distally.
3. Anterior overbite is increased. The mandibular incisors strike the maxillary incisors near the gingiva or traumatize the gingiva.
4. The maxillary incisors are pushed labially and laterally (Fig. 20.15).
5. The anterior teeth extrude because the incisal apposition has largely disappeared.
6. Diastemata are created by the separation of the anterior teeth (Fig. 20.14).

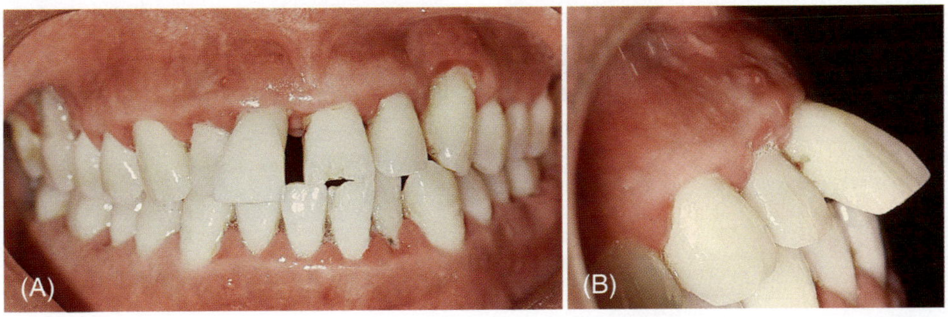

Fig. 20.10 Labial migration of the maxillary central incisors, especially the right incisor. A, Frontal view; B, lateral view.

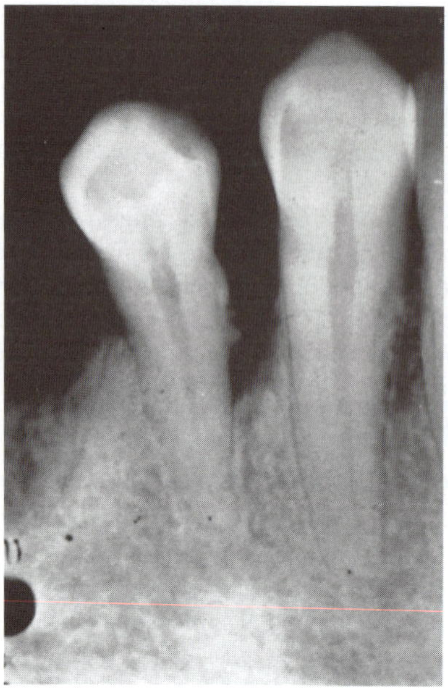

Fig. 20.11 Calculus and bone loss on the mesial surface of a canine that has drifted distally.

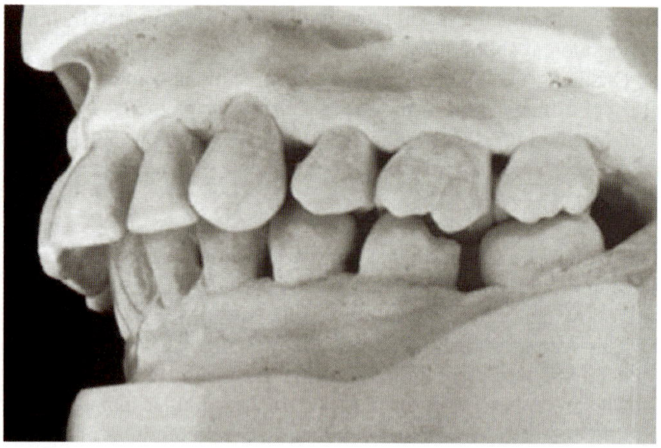

Fig. 20.12 Maxillary first molar that has tilted and extruded into the space created by a missing mandibular tooth.

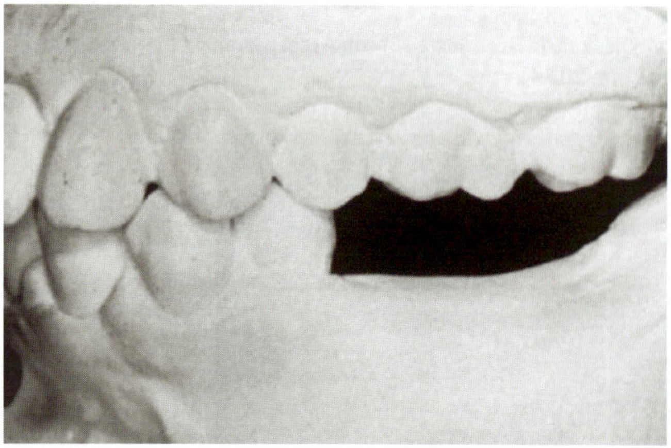

Fig. 20.13 No drifting or extrusion is present here, despite 4 years' absence of the mandibular teeth.

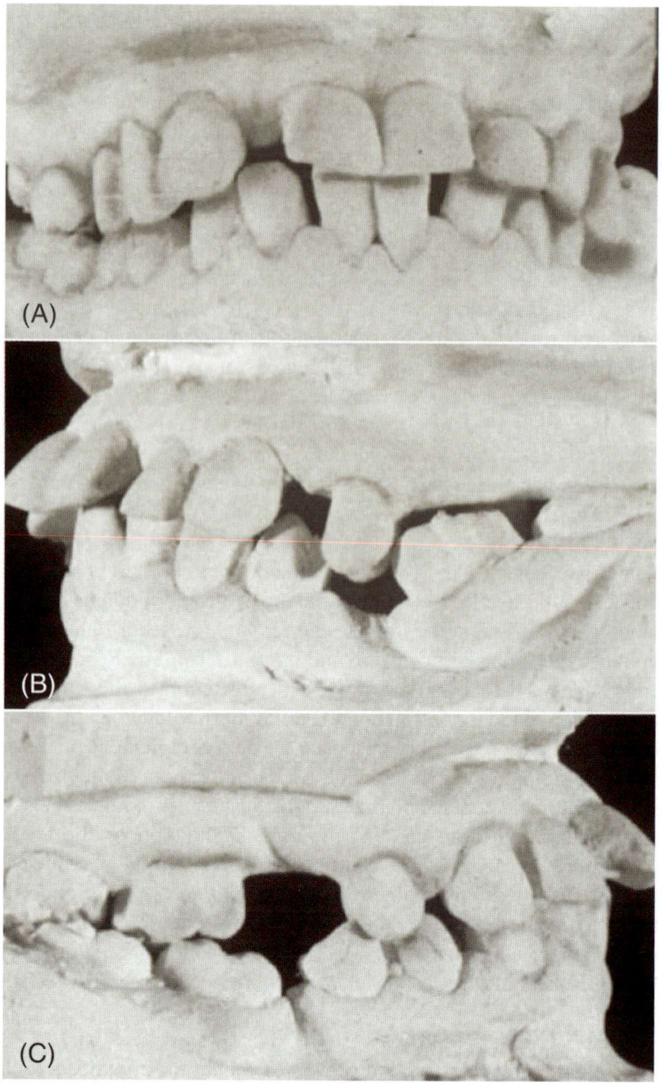

Fig. 20.14 Examples of the mutilation of occlusion associated with unreplaced missing teeth. Note: A, pronounced pathologic migration; B, disturbed proximal contacts; and C, functional relationships with closing of the bite.

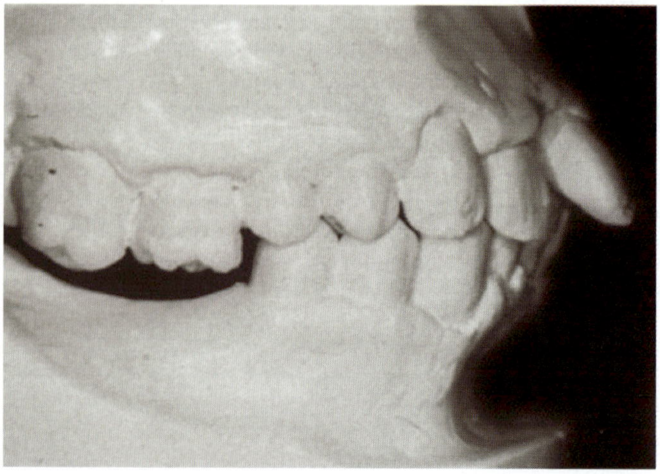

Fig. 20.15 Maxillary incisors pushed labially in a patient with bilateral unreplaced mandibular molars. Note the extrusion of the maxillary molars.

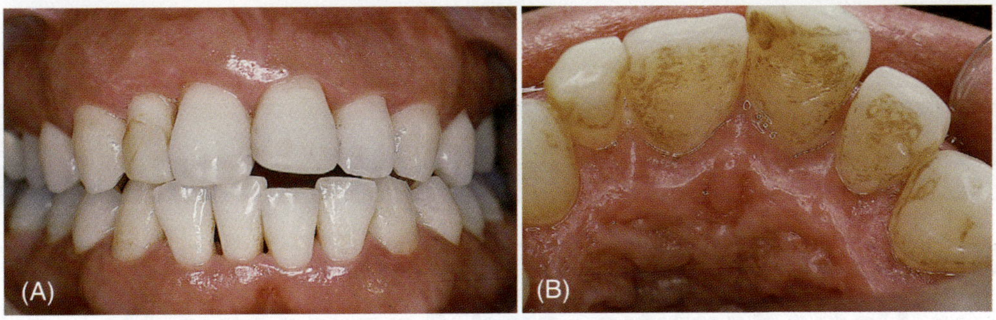

Fig. 20.16 Pathologic migration associated with tongue pressure. A, Facial view; B, palatal view.

The disturbed proximal contact relationships lead to food impaction, plaque accumulation that result in gingival inflammation, and pocket formation, which are followed by bone loss and tooth mobility. Occlusal disharmonies created by the altered tooth positions traumatize the supporting tissues of the periodontium and aggravate the destruction caused by the inflammation. The reduction in periodontal support leads to the further migration of the teeth and the mutilation of the occlusion.

Other Causes

Trauma from occlusion may cause a shift in tooth position either by itself or in combination with inflammatory periodontal disease. The direction of movement depends on the occlusal force.

Pressure from the tongue may cause drifting of the teeth in the absence of periodontal disease, or it may contribute to the pathologic migration of teeth with reduced periodontal support (Fig. 20.16).

When tooth support has been weakened by periodontal destruction, *pressure from the granulation tissue of periodontal pockets* has been mentioned as contributing to pathologic migration. The teeth may return to their original positions after the pockets are eliminated, but, if more destruction has occurred on one side of the tooth than on the other side.

Conclusion

It is important to understand the etiology of the changes that occur in the periodontal tissues from both the clinical and histologic perspectives. Whatever the etiology, the periodontal tissues have a tremendous adaptive ability to accommodate both the microbial and the traumatic occlusal factors within a certain limit. It is the combination of both and the patient's ability to resist these factors that may complicate the diagnosis and treatment plan of the clinical cases that are presented.

Key points

- The effect of occlusal forces on the periodontium is influenced by the magnitude, direction, duration, and frequency of the forces.
- When occlusal forces exceed the adaptive capacity of the tissues, tissue injury results. This resultant injury is called trauma from occlusion.
- The occlusion which causes the injury is called traumatic occlusion.
- Acute trauma from occlusion results from an abrupt occlusal impact, such as that produced by biting on a hard object or restoration/prosthesis which interferes with occlusion.
- Chronic trauma from occlusion is more common than acute form and it is of great clinical significance. It most often develops from gradual changes in the occlusion.
- Trauma from occlusion occurs as a result of alteration in occlusal forces and is termed as "primary trauma from occlusion."
- When trauma from occlusion occurs due to the reduced ability of the tissues to resist occlusal forces, it is called "secondary trauma from occlusion."
- The different stages of trauma from occlusion are stage I—injury, stage II—repair, and stage III—adaptive remodeling of the periodontium.
- The accumulation of bacterial plaque that initiates gingivitis and results in periodontal pocket formation affects marginal gingiva, but trauma from occlusion occurs in the supporting tissues and does not affect the gingiva.
- When inflammation extends from the gingiva into the supporting periodontal tissues, plaque-induced inflammation enters the zone influenced by occlusion.
- The most common clinical sign of trauma to the periodontium is increased tooth mobility.
- Radiographic signs of trauma from occlusion may include increased width of the periodontal space, often with thickening of the lamina dura along the lateral aspect of the root, in the apical region, and in bifurcation areas.
- Vertical bone loss is seen. Root resorption, radiolucence, and condensation of the alveolar bone are also seen.
- Pathologic migration refers to tooth displacement that results when the balance among the factors that maintain physiologic tooth position is disturbed by periodontal disease. It frequently occurs in anterior region. Pathological migration of tooth in occlusal or incisal direction is called extrusion.
- Pathologic migration may continue after a tooth no longer contacts its antagonist. Pressure from the tongue, the food bolus during mastication, and proliferating granulation tissue provide the force.
- Pathologic migration is an early sign of localized aggressive periodontitis.
- Changes in the forces may occur as a result of unreplaced missing teeth, failure to replace the first molar, or other causes.

Suggested Readings

Glickman I, Roeber F, Brion M, et al: Photoelastic analysis of internal stresses in the periodontium created by occlusal forces, *J Periodontol* 41:30, 1970.

Glickman I, Smulow JB: Adaptive alterations in the periodontium of the rhesus monkey in chronic trauma from occlusion, *J Periodontol* 39:101, 1968.

Lindhe J, Ericsson I: The influence of trauma from occlusion on reduced but healthy periodontal tissues in dogs, *J Clin Periodontol* 3:110, 1976.

Lindhe J, Svanberg G: Influence of trauma from occlusion on progression of experimental periodontitis in the beagle dog, *J Clin Periodontol* 1:3, 1974.

Meitner S: Co-destructive factors of marginal periodontitis and repetitive mechanical injury, *J Dent Res* 54:C78, 1975.

Polson AM: The relative importance of plaque and occlusion in periodontal disease, *J Clin Periodontol* 13:923, 1986.

Stahl SS: Accommodation of the periodontium to occlusal trauma and inflammatory periodontal disease, *Dent Clin North Am* 19:531, 1975.

References

References and MCQs with answers for the chapter are available on www.medenact.com.

CHAPTER 21

Periodontitis (Chronic Periodontitis, Necrotizing Ulcerative Periodontitis, and Aggressive Periodontitis)

H Dommisch | M Kebschull | PR Klokkevold | FA Carranza | DG Naik | A Uppoor

CHAPTER OUTLINE

Periodontitis

Definition of Periodontitis

Periodontitis is defined as a complex inflammatory disease that affects the tooth-supporting structures, including the periodontal ligament and alveolar bone. In this context, the word "complex" describes not only the fact that there are multiple clinical symptoms that account for the disease but also because of the multiple factors that lead to and influence periodontal inflammation. Periodontitis occurs most frequently in adults. Nonetheless, it may also be diagnosed in children and adolescents when associated with chronic plaque and calculus accumulation. Therefore, periodontitis should be understood as age-associated but not age-dependent, complex chronic inflammation of the periodontal tissues. As described below, systemic and/or environmental factors (e.g., diabetes mellitus, smoking) modify the host immune response to the dental biofilm so that the periodontal destruction becomes more progressive. Periodontitis is a highly prevalent progressing disease and is considered the sixth most common human disease which belongs to the group of chronic noncommunicable diseases. It affects approximately 10%, 5%, and up to 12% of the world population. In the past decade, it has been found that periodontitis exerts adverse effects on systemic health, and in this context, important pathological interdependencies with, for example, diabetes mellitus have been identified. Also, it is known that systemic inflammatory markers, such as the C-reactive protein (CRP), are elevated in patients with periodontitis. In general, periodontitis is considered a slowly progressing disease, but in the presence of severe systemic conditions and/or environmental factors, such as smoking, this inflammatory disease progresses more rapidly.

The former classification described two different major forms of periodontitis, aggressive and chronic periodontitis, with aggressive periodontitis being defined as a rapidly progressing entity in systemically healthy subjects with a familiar aggregation.

The classical definition reflected periodontitis as "an infectious disease resulting in inflammation within the supporting tissues of the teeth, progressive attachment loss, and bone loss." In the past decades, the etiopathologic factors that lead to periodontal inflammation, and subsequently, in the destruction of periodontal tissues, have been widely studied, and the interplay between the microbial environment and the individual host immune response gained attention in the scientific community.

Periodontitis represents major clinical and etiologic characteristics of this complex disease:

1. microbial biofilm formation (dental plaque),
2. periodontal inflammation (gingival swelling, bleeding on probing), and
3. attachment as well as alveolar bone loss.

Besides the local immune response to the dental biofilm, periodontitis may also be associated with a number of systemic disorders and defined syndromes. In most cases, patients with systemic diseases, which lead to impaired host immunity, may also show periodontal destruction. On the other hand, periodontitis is a disease not only limited to the area of the oral cavity but may be associated with severe systemic diseases such as cardiovascular disease, stroke, and diabetes mellitus.

General Characteristics and Symptoms

Characteristic clinical findings in patients with untreated periodontitis may include the following symptoms:

- Supragingival and subgingival plaque (and calculus).
- Gingival swelling, redness, and loss of gingival stippling.
- Altered gingival margins (rolled, flattened, cratered papillae, recessions).
- Pocket formation.
- Bleeding on probing.
- Attachment loss.
- Bone loss (angular or horizontal).
- Root furcation involvement.
- Increased tooth mobility.
- Change in tooth position.
- Tooth loss.

The aforementioned signs and symptoms may all be simultaneously present or not. However, the main symptom of periodontitis is the loss of attachment.

Periodontitis can be clinically revealed by means of periodontal screening (e.g., periodontal screening index; PSI), diagnosed by an assessment of the clinical attachment level, and therewith, the detection of inflammatory changes in the marginal gingiva. Measurements of periodontal probing pocket depth in combination with the location of the marginal gingiva allow conclusions regarding the loss of clinical attachment. Dental radiographs reveal the extent of bone loss indicated by the distance between the cementoenamel junction and the alveolar bone crest. Periodontitis is commonly a slowly progressive complex disease without pain experience. Therefore, most patients are unaware that they have developed a chronic disease. For the majority of patients, gingival bleeding during oral hygiene procedures or eating may be the first sign of disease occurrence. Areas with advanced periodontal inflammation may show pus emersion from the periodontal pocket. As a result of gingival recession, patients may notice black triangles between teeth and/or tooth sensibility in response to temperature changes (cold and heat). In addition, food impaction may occur in the space of interdental triangles leading to increased patient discomfort and bad breath. In cases with advanced attachment and bone loss, tooth mobility, tooth movement, fanned out or elongated front teeth, and, on rare occasions, tooth loss may be reported. In those cases with advanced disease progression, areas of localized dull pain or pain sensations radiating to other areas of the mouth and/or head may occur.

CHRONIC PERIODONTITIS

Chronic periodontitis is the most prevalent form of periodontitis, and it generally demonstrates the characteristics of a slowly progressing inflammatory disease. However, systemic and environmental factors (e.g., diabetes mellitus, smoking) may modify the host's immune response to the dental biofilm so that periodontal destruction becomes more progressive. Although chronic periodontitis is most frequently observed in adults, it can occur in children and adolescents in response to chronic plaque and calculus accumulation.

Chronic periodontitis has been defined as "an infectious disease resulting in inflammation within the supporting tissues of the teeth, progressive attachment loss, and bone loss." This definition outlines the major clinical and etiologic characteristics of the disease: (1) microbial biofilm formation (dental plaque); (2) periodontal inflammation (e.g., gingival swelling, bleeding on probing); and (3) attachment as well as alveolar bone loss.

In addition to the local immune response caused by the dental biofilm, periodontitis may also be associated with a number of systemic disorders and defined syndromes. In most cases, patients with systemic diseases that lead to impaired host immunity may also show periodontal destruction. Therefore, periodontitis is a disease that is not only limited to the area of the oral cavity; it is also associated with severe systemic diseases (e.g., cardiovascular disorders, diabetes mellitus).

This chapter discusses clinical features that have been described for chronic periodontitis. In addition, the disease's etiology is summarized with the use of categories that explain the known factors (i.e., microbiologic, immunologic, and genetic) involved in the pathology of chronic periodontitis.

Clinical Features

General Characteristics

Chronic periodontitis can be clinically revealed with periodontal screening and recording, which results in a PSI rating. The condition is diagnosed via the assessment of the clinical attachment level and the detection of inflammatory changes in the marginal gingiva

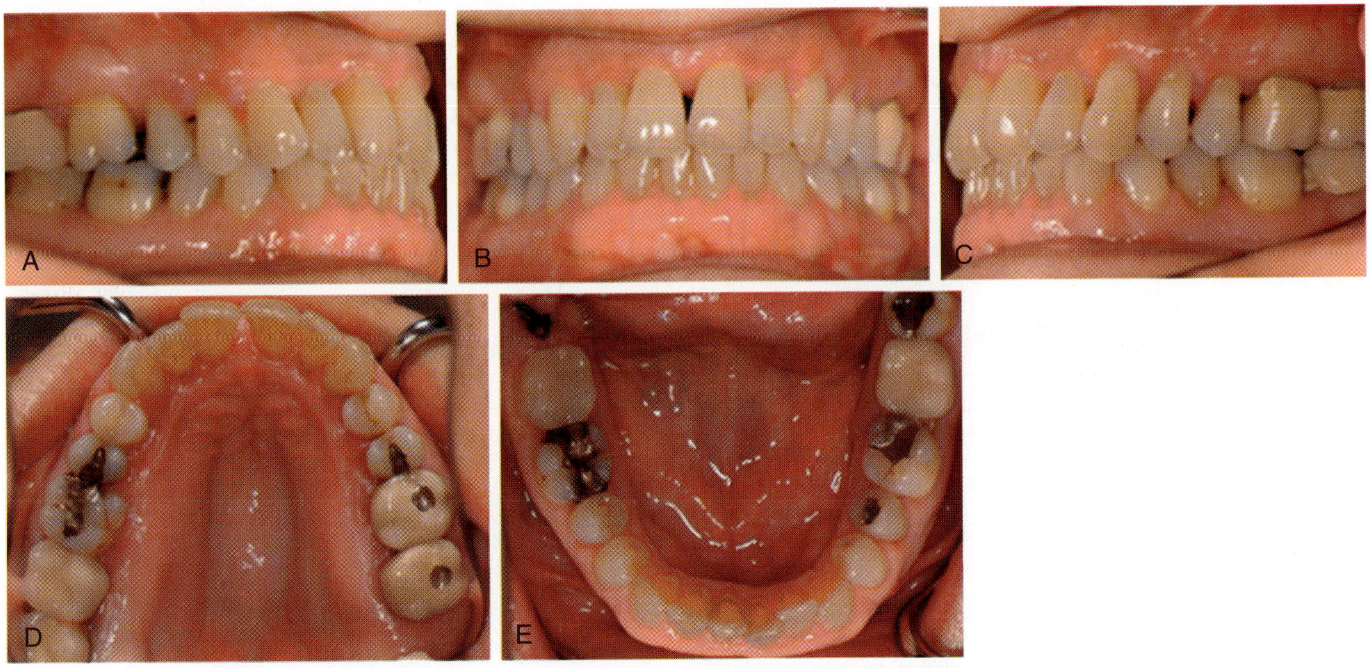

Fig. 21.1 Clinical features of generalized chronic periodontitis in a 49-year-old, medically healthy, male patient. The patient reported a smoking habit of 15 cigarettes per day. At the first visit, the periodontal photostatus displays untreated chronic periodontitis with abundant dental plaque and calculus deposits, gingival redness and swelling, and an alteration of the gingival texture (i.e., loss of gingival stippling). The patient noticed multiple recessions. In this case, recessions were the result of a loss of clinical attachment and alveolar bone. A, Right lateral view. B, Frontal view. C, Left lateral view. D, Maxillary view. E, Mandibular view. *(Reprinted from Kebschull and Dommisch, Thieme, 2012.)*

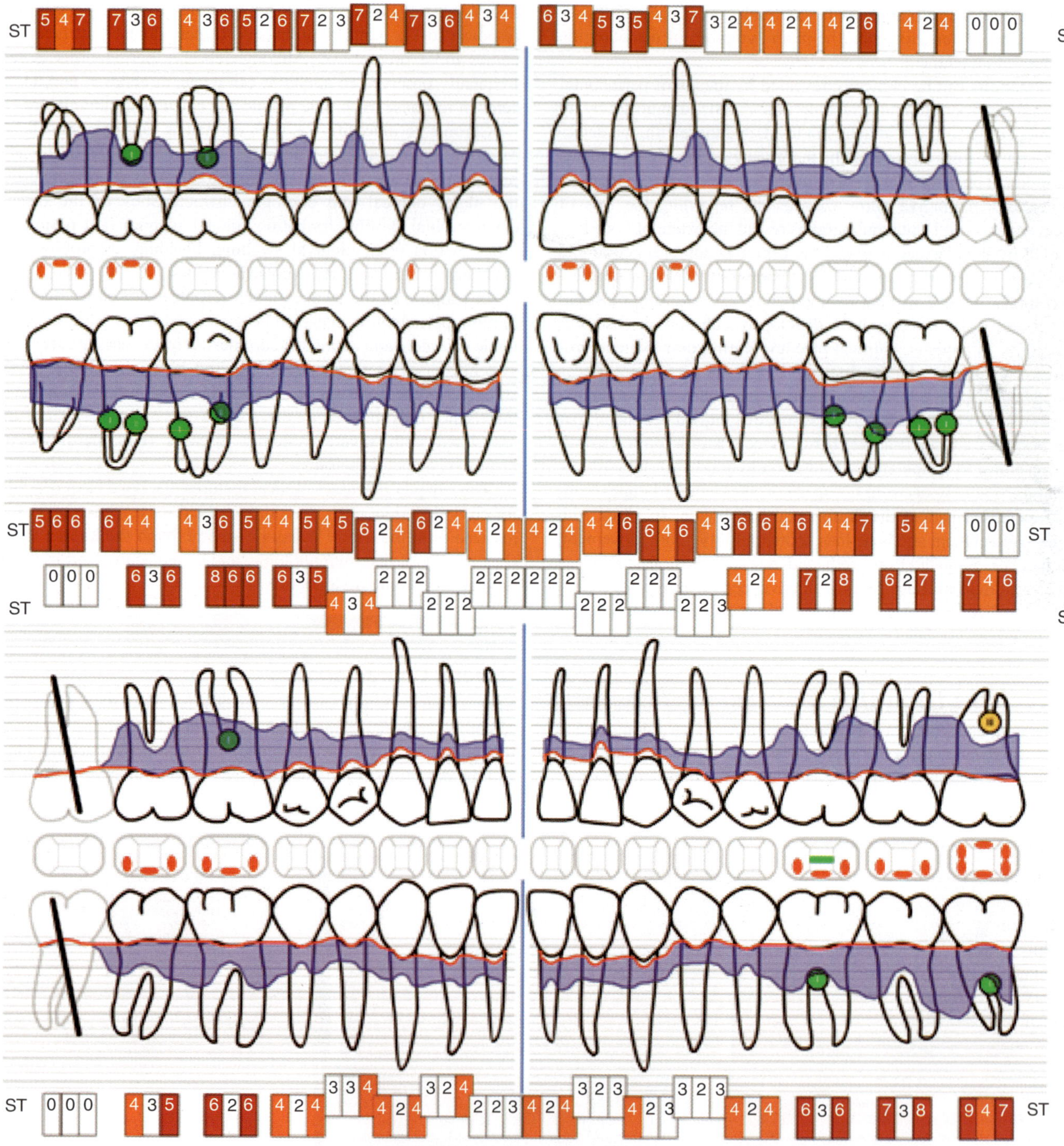

Fig. 21.2 Documentation of the periodontal attachment level in patient at the time of the first visit. The *red line* displays the gingival margin as it reflects the recessions. Clinical attachment loss is illustrated by the filled *(blue)* area on the root surfaces. The deepest periodontal pocket was measured at 9 mm. Class I *(green)* and Class II *(yellow)* furcation involvements were documented. Bleeding with periodontal probing (i.e., gingival inflammation) is reflected by *red dots.* As a result of the patient's history of smoking, the bleeding on probing score was relatively low, although the patient presented advanced attachment loss. Tooth mobility is indicated by the *green line* (tooth #19). *(Reprinted from Kebschull and Dommisch, Thieme, 2012.)*

(Fig. 21.1). Measurements of periodontal pocket depth in combination with the location of the marginal gingiva allow for conclusions to be drawn regarding the loss of clinical attachment (Figs. 21.2 and 21.3). Dental radiographs display the extent of bone loss, which is indicated by the distance between the cementoenamel junction and the alveolar bone crest (Fig. 21.3). The distinction between aggressive and chronic periodontitis is sometimes difficult because the clinical features may be similar at the time of the first examination. At later time points during treatment, aggressive and chronic periodontitis may be differentiated by the rate of disease progression over time, the familial nature of aggressive disease, the disease's resistance to periodontal antiinfective therapy, and the presence of local factors.

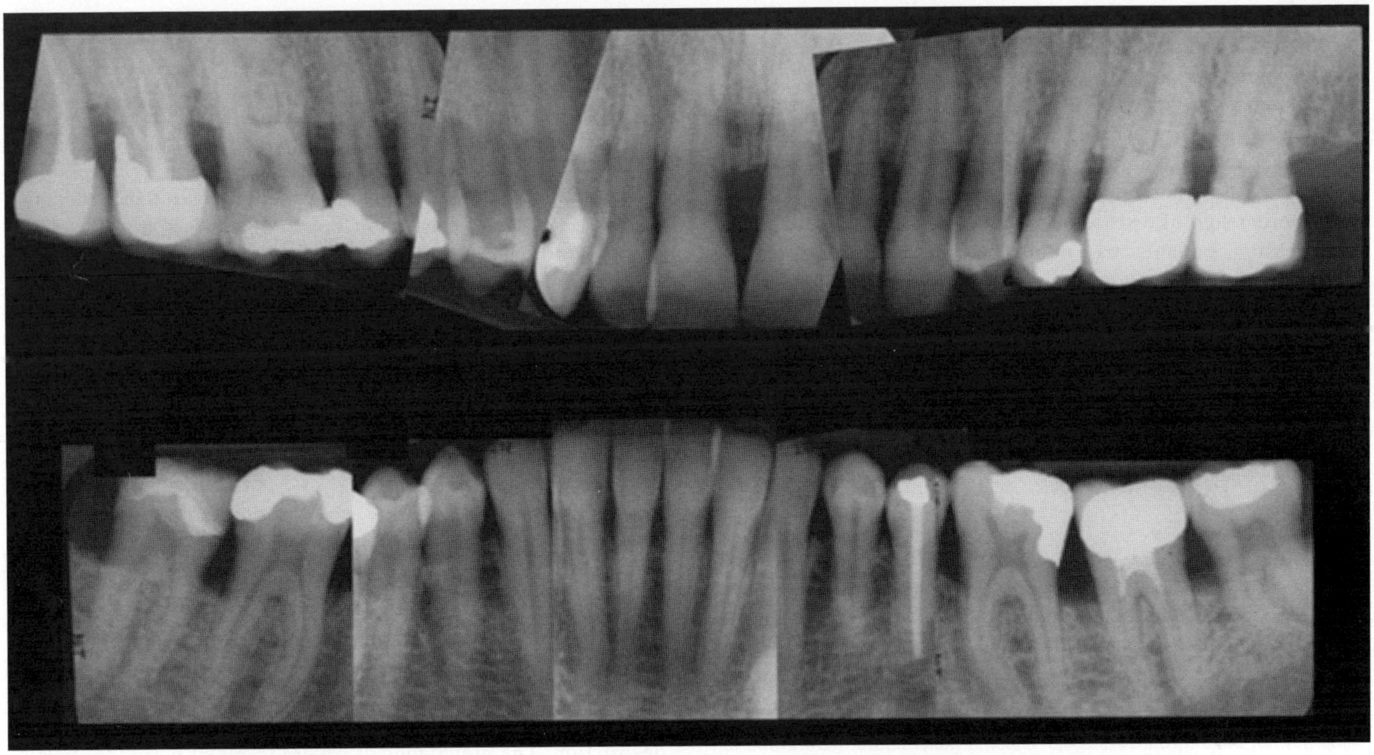

Fig. 21.3 Collage of a total of 11 radiographs showing the radiographic periodontal status at the time of diagnosis. Compare this with Figs. 21.1 and 21.2. Note the generalized horizontal and localized angular and vertical bone loss on the mesial and distal sites of the molars. The radiographs show deep subgingival restorations (teeth #2 and #19), overhanging margins of restorations (teeth #14 and #15), a carious lesion (tooth #14), and insufficient root canal treatment (tooth #18). *(Reprinted from Kebschull and Dommisch, Thieme, 2012.)*

Disease Distribution

Chronic periodontitis is considered a site-specific disease. Local inflammation, pocket formation, attachment loss, and bone loss are the consequences of direct exposure to the subgingival plaque (biofilm). As a result of this local effect, pocket formation and attachment as well as bone loss may occur on one surface of a tooth, whereas other surfaces maintain normal attachment levels. As a result of the site-specific nature, the number of teeth with clinical attachment loss classifies chronic periodontitis into the following types:

- *Localized chronic periodontitis:* Less than 30% of the sites (30% of the teeth) show attachment and bone loss.
- *Generalized chronic periodontitis:* 30% or more of the sites show attachment and bone loss.

During chronic periodontitis, the local inflammatory response may lead to different patterns of bone loss, including vertical (angular) and horizontal bone destruction. Although vertical bone loss is associated with intrabony pocket formation, horizontal bone loss is usually associated with suprabony (supraalveolar) pockets.

Key Differences Between Gingivitis and Chronic Periodontitis

Table 21.1 depicts key differences between gingivitis and chronic periodontitis.

Disease Severity

The severity of periodontal destruction that occurs as a result of chronic periodontitis is generally considered a function of time in combination with systemic disorders that impair or enhance host immune responses. With increasing age, attachment loss and bone loss become more prevalent and more severe as a result of an accumulation of destruction. Disease severity may be described as mild, moderate, or severe based on the amount of clinical attachment loss:

- *Mild chronic periodontitis:* when no more than 1–2 mm of clinical attachment loss has occurred.
- *Moderate chronic periodontitis:* when 3–4 mm of clinical attachment loss has occurred.
- *Severe periodontitis:* when 5 mm or more of clinical attachment loss has occurred.

TABLE 21.1 Differences Between Gingivitis and Chronic Periodontitis

Plaque-Induced Gingivitis	Chronic Periodontitis
Inflammation of the gingiva without attachment/bone loss.	Inflammation of periodontal apparatus with attachment/bone loss.
With optimal oral hygiene, this condition can be resolved completely (reversible).	The attachment loss is irreversible, in spite of successfully controlling the inflammation.
Not all sites with gingivitis progress to periodontitis.	All patients with chronic periodontitis must have experienced prior gingivitis.
The dental implant counterpart of gingivitis is peri-implant mucositis.	The dental implant counterpart of periodontitis is peri-implantitis.

Symptoms

Chronic periodontitis is commonly a slowly progressive disease that does not cause the affected individual to feel pain. Therefore, most patients are unaware that they have developed a chronic disease that is also associated with other systemic diseases (e.g., cardiovascular disease). For the majority of the patients, gingival bleeding during oral hygiene procedures or eating may be the first self-reported sign of disease occurrence. As a result of the gingival recession, patients may notice black triangles between the teeth or tooth sensitivity in response to temperature changes (i.e., cold and heat). In patients with advanced attachment and bone loss, tooth mobility, tooth movement, and, in rare occasions, tooth loss may be reported. In those individuals with advanced disease progression, areas of localized dull pain or pain sensations that radiate to other areas of the mouth or head may occur. The presence of areas of food impaction may add to the patient's discomfort. Gingival tenderness or "itchiness" may also be found.

KEY FACT

Site Specificity of Chronic Periodontitis

Not all sites in the mouth are equally prone to chronic periodontitis, and it exhibits site specificity. The progression of the disease occurs in certain sites but not uniformly. Interproximal sites, in general, are more prone to periodontal destruction, compared to buccal/facial sites.

Disease Progression

Patients appear to have the same susceptibility to plaque-induced chronic periodontitis throughout their lives. The rate of disease progression is usually slow, but it may be modified by systemic, environmental, and behavioral factors. Onset and the rate of disease progression, however, may be influenced by a number of modifiable (e.g., smoking, diet) and nonmodifiable (e.g., genetic disorders and risk issues) factors. In this context, patients who develop a metabolic disorder, such as diabetes mellitus, may exhibit a much higher progression rate of chronic periodontitis along with increased alveolar bone loss, periodontal bleeding, and pocketing. Thus, diabetes mellitus and the degree of blood sugar control belong to the most important systemic factors that are directly correlated with periodontal disease. The onset of chronic periodontitis can occur at any time, and the first signs may be detected during adolescence in the presence of chronic plaque and calculus accumulation. Due to its slow rate of progression, however, chronic periodontitis usually becomes clinically significant when a patient reaches his or her mid-30s or later.

Chronic periodontitis does not progress at an equal rate in all affected sites throughout the mouth. Some involved areas may remain static for long periods, whereas others may progress more rapidly. More rapidly progressive lesions occur most frequently in interproximal areas, and they may also be associated with areas of greater plaque accumulation and inaccessibility to plaque-control measures (e.g., furcation areas, overhanging margins of restorations, sites of malposed teeth, areas of food impaction).

Further factors that influence disease progression may be of systemic origin. Patients with poorly adjusted diabetes mellitus show a significantly higher risk of developing a severe progression of chronic periodontitis.

Several models have been proposed to describe the rate of disease progression. In these models, progression is measured by determining the amount of attachment loss during a given period as follows:

- The *continuous model* suggests that disease progression is slow and continuous, with affected sites showing a constantly progressive rate of destruction throughout the duration of the disease.
- The *random or episodic-burst model* proposes that periodontal disease progresses by short bursts of destruction followed by periods of no destruction. This pattern of disease is random with respect to the tooth sites affected and the chronology of the disease process.
- The *asynchronous, multiple-burst model* of disease progression suggests that periodontal destruction occurs around affected teeth during defined periods of life and that these bursts of activity are interspersed with periods of inactivity or remission. The chronology of these bursts of disease is asynchronous for individual teeth or groups of teeth.

Prevalence

Chronic periodontitis increases in prevalence and severity with age, and it generally affects both genders equally. Periodontitis is an age-associated (not an age-related) disease. Nonetheless, the prevalence of periodontitis increases with age so that 40% of patients who are 50 years old or older and almost 50% of patients who are 65 years old or older show moderate periodontal destruction. The prevalence of severe forms of periodontitis also increases with age. Up to 30% of patients develop severe periodontitis by the time they are 40 years old or older. Generally, 50% of the human population experiences at least one form of periodontal disease (Figs. 21.4 and 21.5).

Risk Factors for Disease

A number of different factors influence the etiopathology of chronic periodontitis. The composition of the oral microflora is a major etiologic factor that leads to periodontal destruction. In this context, the extent of the periodontal destruction depends on the host's immune competence as well as genetic predispositions that influence individual susceptibility to disease. In addition, both systemic diseases and environmental factors interfere with the development and progression of chronic periodontitis. The risk factors described in the following sections (microbiological, local, systemic, immunologic, genetic, environmental, and behavioral) may occur simultaneously, or a selection of factors is present in patients with chronic periodontitis. The degree of the individual risk factor contribution differs among patients, so it is worthwhile to not only identify the risk factors but also to specify each risk factor's degree of contribution.

The prior history of gingivitis and periodontitis should be considered as general predictors for the development or progression of chronic periodontitis. It is possible that the disease could not be successfully treated in the first place. The reason for an unsuccessful treatment outcome can be as simple as the patient's unwillingness (noncompliant patients) to understand the disease or perform proper oral hygiene. On the other hand, reasons for disease progression can also be more complex when nonmodifiable factors—such as genetic predispositions/syndromes, severe immunologic disorders, and other therapies (e.g., organ transplantations) that affect the patient's immune status, lack of dexterity, or other systemic diseases—are present. This highlights the complexity of not only the development but also the progression/reoccurrence of chronic periodontitis. Several risk factors that contribute to the patient's susceptibility to chronic periodontitis are discussed next.

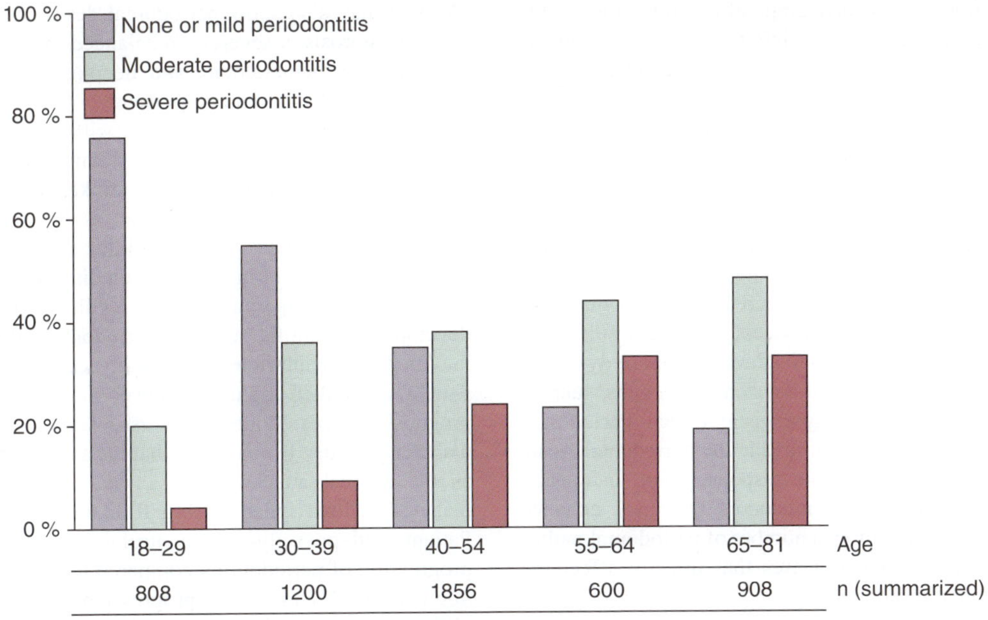

Fig. 21.4 Prevalence of periodontitis in the United States and Germany, 2007–2009. *(Eke PI, Dye BA, Wei L, et al: Prevalence of periodontitis in adults in the United States: 2009 and 2010. J Dent Res 91:914–920, 2012.)*

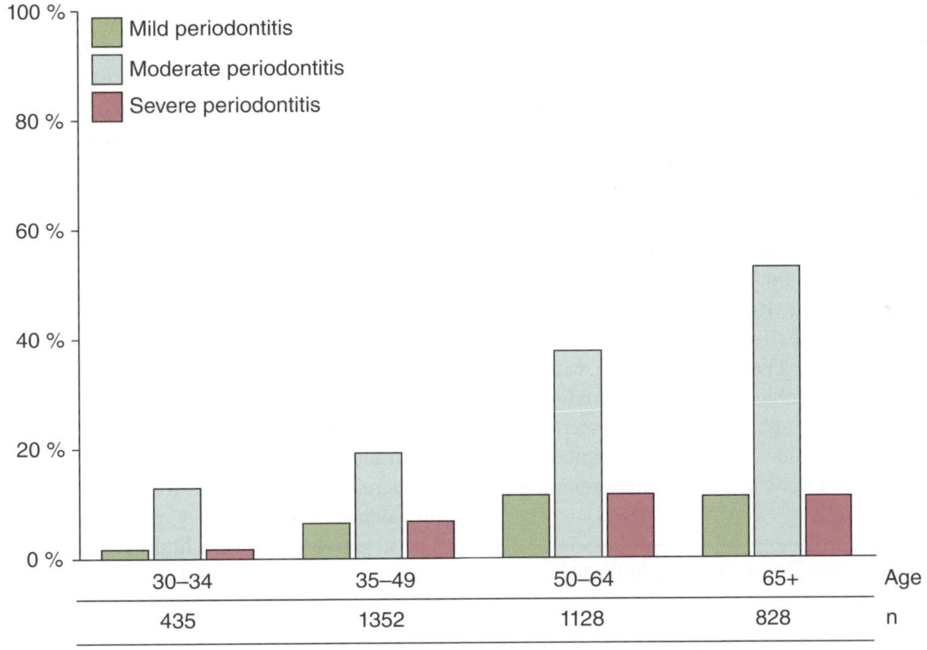

Fig. 21.5 Prevalence of periodontitis in the United States, 2009–2010. *(Eke PI, Dye BA, Wei L, et al: Prevalence of periodontitis in adults in the United States: 2009 and 2010. J Dent Res 91:914–920, 2012.)*

Microbiological Aspects

Plaque accumulation on the tooth and gingival surfaces at the dentogingival junction is considered the primary initiating agent in the etiology of gingivitis and chronic periodontitis. Attachment and bone loss are associated with an increase in the proportion of Gram-negative organisms in the subgingival biofilm, with specific increases in organisms that are known to be exceptionally pathogenic and virulent. *Porphyromonas gingivalis*, *Tannerella forsythia*, and *Treponema denticola*—otherwise known as the "red complex"—are frequently associated with ongoing attachment and bone loss in patients with chronic periodontitis. The development and progression of chronic periodontitis may not depend on the presence of one specific bacterium or bacterial complex alone. It is assumed that chronic periodontitis is the result of a multispecies infection with a number of different bacteria that influence the proinflammatory immune response of the host. Periodontal pathogens may invade the periodontal tissue and thus induce an immune response with increasing concentrations of proinflammatory mediators that may enhance periodontal breakdown. In addition, a number of periodontal pathogens are capable of producing proteases that directly influence tissue stability and host immune responses.

As the dental biofilm develops, early signs of an inflammatory reaction occur in the gingival margin (i.e., gingivitis), without actual attachment loss. Generally, optimal plaque control leads to the complete resolution of this early gingival inflammation. Alternatively, with neglected oral hygiene, inflammation will progress and eventually result in the loss of attachment around teeth. Although not all patients with gingivitis develop periodontitis, it is known that all patients with periodontitis experienced prior gingivitis. The occurrence of periodontitis depends on the individual immune response that modifies the onset and progression of the disease.

Furthermore, the concept of host–microbial interactions has gained scientific attention. It has been found that increased numbers of periodontal pathogens contribute to the development of a dysbiotic microbial environment, which is triggered by the inflammatory milieu in the periodontal pocket. This concept describes a shift from a symbiotic microbial environment to the development of dysbiosis within the biofilm involving so-called keystone pathogens, such as *P. gingivalis*, as a polymicrobial synergistic effect. Periodontal pathogens like *P. gingivalis* may then invade the periodontal tissue and therewith induce further immune responses with increasing concentrations of proinflammatory mediators that may enhance periodontal breakdown. In addition, a number of periodontal pathogens are capable of producing proteases that directly affect the tissues and host immune responses.

Local Factors

Plaque accumulation and biofilm development are the primary causes of periodontal inflammation and destruction. Therefore, factors that facilitate plaque accumulation or that prevent plaque removal by oral hygiene procedures can be detrimental to the patient. Plaque-retentive factors are important for the development and progression of chronic periodontitis because they retain microorganisms in proximity to the periodontal tissues, thereby providing an ecologic niche for biofilm maturation. Calculus is considered the most important plaque-retentive factor as a result of its ability to retain and harbor plaque bacteria on its rough surface as well as inside. As a consequence, calculus removal is essential for the maintenance of a healthy periodontium. In addition, tooth morphology may influence plaque retention. Roots may show grooves or concavities, and, in some instances, enamel projections on the surface or the furcation entrances. These morphologic variations may facilitate plaque retention, subgingival calculus formation, and disease progression. In addition, subgingival and overhanging margins of restorations, carious lesions that extend subgingivally, and furcations exposed by loss of bone promote plaque retention.

Common Retentive Local Factors That Contribute to Chronic Periodontitis

- Dental calculus
- Crown margins
- Restoration overhangs
- Furcation involvement
- Deep probing depths
- Anatomic grooves on the roots
- Subgingival caries or resorptive lesions

Systemic Factors

Chronic periodontitis is a complex disease that may not only be limited to the infection of local sites. In several instances, periodontitis is also associated with other systemic disorders, such as Haim–Munk syndrome, Papillon–Lefèvre syndrome, Ehlers–Danlos syndrome, Kindlers syndrome, and Cohen syndrome. Patients with diseases that impair the host immune response (e.g., human immunodeficiency virus [HIV], acquired immunodeficiency syndrome [AIDS]) may also show periodontal destruction. It is also known that osteoporosis, a severely unbalanced diet, and stress as well as dermatologic, hematologic, and neoplastic factors interfere with periodontal inflammatory responses.

In addition to being associated with defined syndromes, periodontitis also occurs with severe systemic diseases, such as diabetes mellitus, cardiovascular disorders, stroke, and lung disorders.

Periodontitis is now considered as the sixth complication of diabetes mellitus. For diabetes mellitus and periodontitis, there is a known interaction during which both diseases mutually correlate to each other. Patients with diabetes mellitus exhibit a higher risk to develop periodontitis, and the periodontal infection/inflammation may negatively interfere with the glycemic control of the diabetic patient. A number of studies showed that prevalence, severity, and prognosis of periodontitis are associated with the incidence of diabetes mellitus. It was found that the average pocket depth as well as the clinical attachment loss was increased in patients with diabetes mellitus (independently from the type of diabetes mellitus). Patients with poor glycemic control tend to experience more severe progression of periodontitis compared to patients with good glycemic control. Regarding the progression of severe periodontitis, no difference was found between patients with good glycemic control and nondiabetic patients. With diabetes mellitus, advanced glycation end products (AGEs) may arise, which lead to the release of free oxygen and proinflammatory mediators (cytokines). AGEs may also promote chemotaxis and adhesion of inflammatory cells to periodontal tissues, and increased apoptosis of fibroblasts and osteoblasts may occur. Furthermore, patients with diabetes mellitus tend to show a higher body mass index, and therefore increased concentrations of adipokines that directly influence inflammatory responses were found. Hyperglycemia per se leads to the release of proinflammatory mediators in the bloodstream, which in turn promote increased glucose concentration. Periodontal therapy may contribute to glycemic control of the diabetic patient. It was shown that the systematic therapy of chronic periodontitis leads to an at least short-term reduction of glycated hemoglobin (HbA1c) of approximately 0.3% up to 0.6%. Each therapy regimen that contributes to achieve reduction of glycated hemoglobin may decrease the risk of diabetes-related long-term consequences, such as myocardial infarction, microvascular complications, and many others.

In the context of diabetes mellitus, a number of patients exhibit an increased body weight (obesity), which also correlates with the prevalence and severity of periodontal attachment and bone loss. The negative effect of a high body mass index with regard to the outcome of periodontal therapy was comparable to the negative effect that has been described for smoking.

Immunologic Factors

Chronic periodontitis is a disease that is induced by bacteria organized in the dental biofilm. However, the onset, progression, and severity of the disease depend on the individual host's immune response. Patients may show alterations in their peripheral monocytes, which are related to the reduced reactivity of lymphocytes or an enhanced B-cell response. B-cells, macrophages, periodontal ligament cells, gingival fibroblasts, and epithelial cells synthesize proinflammatory mediators (e.g., interleukin-1β, interleukin-6, interleukin-8, prostaglandin E2, tumor necrosis factor-α) that modify innate and adaptive immune responses at periodontal sites. Proinflammatory mediators regulate synthesis and secretion of matrix-metalloproteinases (MMPs) and receptor-activator-of-NF-kappa B-ligand (RANKL). In periodontal lesions, MMPs contribute to soft and hard tissue degradation during active inflammatory processes. RANKL binds to its receptor RANK on the cell surface of premature osteoclasts, and therewith it initiates osteoclast differentiation leading to degradation of alveolar bone. Physiologically, osteoprotegerin (OPG) is an inhibitor of RANKL, and during periodontitis, an imbalance between OPG and RANKL promotes further bone degradation.

In addition, reduced counts in neutrophils (polymorphonuclear neutrophils [PMNs]) influence the degree of periodontal inflammation. Congenital neutropenia (Kostmann syndrome) leads not only to an increased susceptibility to infection in general but also to severe chronic periodontitis. Patients with Kostmann syndrome show reduced levels of antimicrobial peptides, such as the cathelicidin (LL-37) and neutrophil peptides (alpha defensins), which impair their innate immune response. LL-37 is an effective antimicrobial peptide that is synthesized from inactive precursors, and mutations in the cathepsin C gene hinder cleavage, and therewith activation, of LL-37. Those genetic alterations contribute to the severity and progression of chronic periodontitis (Papillon–Lefèvre syndrome, Haim–Munk syndrome).

Genetic Factors

Periodontitis is considered to be a multifactorial disease that is influenced by local, systemic, and immunologic factors, as described previously. Each factor is in turn directly related to individual genetic conditions. Genetic variations such as single nucleotide polymorphisms (SNPs) and genetic copy number variations may directly influence innate and adaptive immune responses as well as the structure of periodontal tissues. Periodontal destruction has been found among family members and across different generations within a family, thereby suggesting a genetic basis for the susceptibility to periodontal disease. In a number of studies, the prevalence of aggressive and chronic periodontitis has been investigated in families with a history of one or more family members with periodontitis. The data from those studies have demonstrated variable results, with a likelihood of heritability of up to 50%. Variations are mainly the result of different study designs as well as the number of evaluated individuals.

Studies of SNPs in the interleukin-1 gene led to early conclusions that alterations in sequences of immunologically relevant genes may explain the heritability of periodontitis.

Genome-wide association studies have revealed a significant association between periodontitis and coronary heart disease. Although four different genetic variations have been identified and validated, it is most likely that a higher number of genes require variations to result in the development of periodontitis.

Environmental and Behavioral Factors

In addition to microbial, immunologic, and genetic factors, the development and progression of chronic periodontitis are further influenced by environmental and behavioral factors, such as smoking and psychological stress. Smoking is a major risk factor for the development and progression of generalized chronic periodontitis. Periodontitis is influenced by smoking in a dose-dependent manner. The intake of more than 10 cigarettes per day tremendously increases the risk of disease progression as compared to nonsmokers and former smokers.

As compared to nonsmokers, the following features are found in smokers:

- Increased periodontal pocket depth of more than 3 mm.
- Increased attachment loss.
- More recessions.
- Increased loss of alveolar bone.
- Increased tooth loss.
- Fewer signs of gingivitis (e.g., less bleeding with probing).
- Greater incidence of furcation involvement.

As a result of the consumption of tobacco, reactive oxygen (i.e., radicals) is released that chemically irritates periodontal tissues via DNA damage, the lipid peroxidation of cell membranes, the damage of endothelial cells, and the induction of smooth muscle cell growth.

Psychological factors (e.g., stress, depression) also negatively influence the progression of chronic periodontitis. Patients with periodontitis often report the experience of family- or work-related stress. Positive correlations between cortisol levels and periodontal indices (e.g., plaque index, gingival index), bone loss, and missing teeth have been recorded. In addition, stress as an etiologic factor was even more strongly associated with periodontitis when patients were smokers as compared to nonsmokers.

Stress and Periodontal Disease: Potential Mechanisms

1. Immunosuppression via cortisol secretion
2. Poor oral hygiene compliance in patients with chronic stress
3. Patients with stress are less likely to seek professional care
4. Patients with stress may smoke more frequently

NECROTIZING ULCERATIVE PERIODONTITIS

Necrotizing ulcerative periodontitis (NUP) may be an extension of *necrotizing ulcerative gingivitis* (NUG) into the periodontal structures that leads to periodontal attachment and bone loss. Alternatively, NUP and NUG may be different diseases. To date, there is little evidence to support the progression of NUG to NUP or to establish a relationship between the two conditions as a single disease entity. However, numerous clinical descriptions and case reports of NUP clearly demonstrate many clinical similarities between the two conditions. Until a distinction between NUG and NUP can be proved or disproved, it has been suggested that NUG and NUP be classified together under the broader category of *necrotizing periodontal diseases*, although with differing levels of severity.

NUG has been recognized and described in the literature for centuries. The features of NUG are presented in Chapter 16.

The term *necrotizing ulcerative periodontitis* was first adopted at the 1989 World Workshop in Clinical Periodontics. It was changed from the 1986 term *necrotizing ulcerative gingivoperiodontitis*, which represented the condition of recurrent NUG that progresses to a chronic form of periodontitis that includes attachment and bone loss. The adoption of NUP as a disease entity occurred in 1989 when there was a heightened awareness and an increase in the number of necrotizing periodontitis cases being diagnosed and described in the literature. Specifically, more cases of NUP were being described among immunocompromised patients, especially those who were HIV positive or who had AIDS. In 1999, the subclassifications of NUG and NUP were included as separate diagnoses under the broader classification of "necrotizing ulcerative periodontal diseases."

Clinical Features

Similar to NUG, clinical cases of NUP are defined by necrosis and ulceration of the coronal portion of the interdental papillae and gingival margin, with a painful, bright-red marginal gingiva that bleeds easily.

The distinguishing feature of NUP is the *destructive progression* of the disease, which includes periodontal attachment and bone loss. Deep interdental osseous craters typify periodontal lesions of NUP (Fig. 21.6A–C). However, "conventional" periodontal pockets

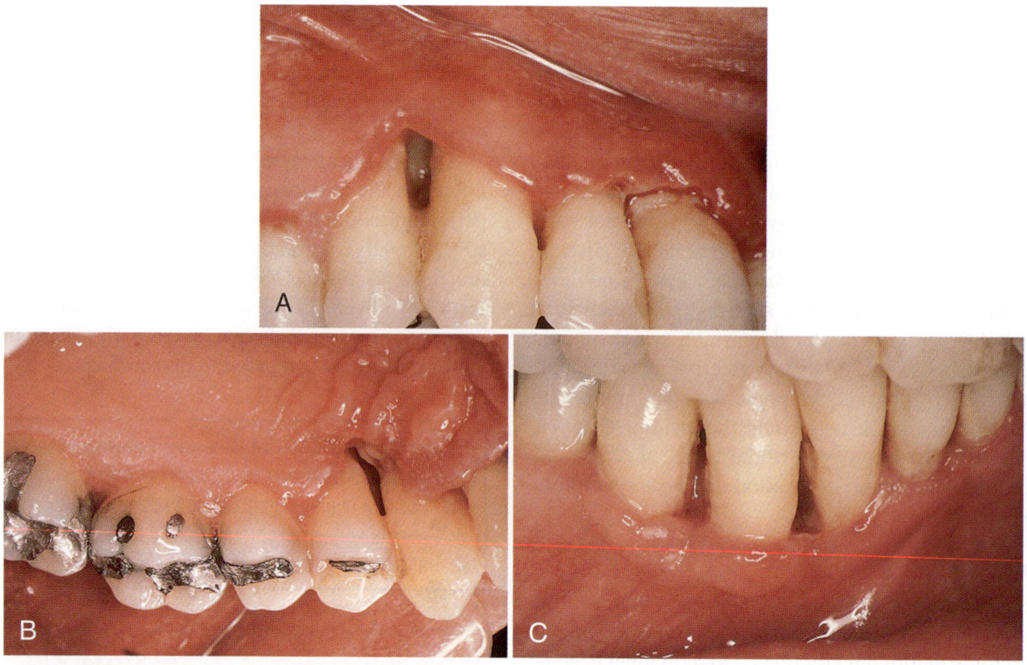

Fig. 21.6 Necrotizing ulcerative periodontitis in a 45-year-old, HIV-negative, white, male patient. A, Buccal view of the maxillary cuspid–bicuspid area. B, Palatal view of the same area shown in A. C, Buccal view of the mandibular anteriors. Note the deep craters associated with bone loss.

with deep probing depth are not found because the ulcerative and necrotizing nature of the gingival lesion destroys the marginal epithelium and connective tissue, thereby resulting in gingival recession. Periodontal pockets are formed because the junctional epithelial cells remain viable and can, therefore, migrate apically to cover areas of lost connective-tissue attachment. The necrosis of the junctional epithelium in patients with NUG and NUP creates an ulcer that prevents this epithelial migration, and a pocket cannot form. Advanced lesions of NUP lead to severe bone loss, tooth mobility, and ultimately tooth loss. In addition to these manifestations, as previously mentioned, patients with NUP may present with oral malodor, fever, malaise, or lymphadenopathy.

KEY FACT

Necrotizing ulcerative periodontitis (NUP) cases are defined by necrosis and ulceration of the coronal portion of the interdental papillae. Gingival margins are bright red and bleed easily. Lesions are painful. The feature that distinguishes NUP from NUG is the destructive progression of NUP, which includes periodontal attachment and bone loss.

Microscopic Findings

Necrotizing ulcerative periodontitis lesions found in patients with HIV or AIDS can present with features similar to those seen in HIV-negative patients. Alternatively, NUP lesions in patients with HIV or AIDS can be much more destructive and frequently result in complications that are extremely rare among patients without HIV or AIDS. For example, periodontal attachment and bone loss associated with NUP in an HIV-positive patient may be extremely rapid. Winkler and colleagues described cases of NUP in HIV-positive patients with teeth that lost more than 90% of periodontal attachment and 10 mm of bone over a 3- to 6-month period. Ultimately, many of these lesions resulted in tooth loss. Other complications reported in this population included the progression of the lesions to involve large areas of soft-tissue necrosis, with the exposure of bone and the sequestration of bone fragments. This type of severe, progressive lesion with extension into the vestibular area and the palate is referred to as *necrotizing ulcerative stomatitis*.

The reported prevalence of NUP among patients with HIV infection varies. Riley and colleagues described only two cases of NUP in 200 HIV-positive patients (1%), whereas Glick and colleagues found a prevalence of 6.3% for NUP cases in a prospective study of 700 HIV-positive patients. Variations in reported findings may be related to differences in the populations studied (e.g., intravenous drug users vs homosexuals versus patients with hemophilia) and differences in the immune statuses of the study subjects.

In a study involving the use of transmission electron microscopy and scanning electron microscopy of the microbial plaque overlying the necrotic gingival papillae, Cobb and coworkers demonstrated striking histologic similarities between NUP in HIV-positive patients and previous descriptions of NUG in HIV-negative patients. Microscopic examination revealed a surface biofilm composed of a mixed microbial flora with different morphotypes and a subsurface flora with dense aggregations of spirochetes (i.e., the bacterial zone). Below the bacterial layers were dense aggregations of polymorphonuclear leukocytes (PMNs) (i.e., the neutrophil-rich zone) and necrotic cells (necrotic zone). The biopsy technique used in this study did not allow for the observation of the deepest layer and thus was not able to identify the spirochetal infiltration zone, which is classically described in NUG lesions. In addition to the NUG-like microscopic features of NUP described in this study, high levels of yeasts and herpes-like viruses were observed. This latter finding is most likely indicative of the conditions afforded to opportunistic microbes in the immunocompromised host (i.e., HIV-positive patients).

Necrotizing forms of periodontitis appear to be more prevalent among patients with more severe immunosuppression. Case reports have depicted NUP as a progressive extension of HIV periodontitis (i.e., chronic to necrotic progression). Glick and coworkers found a high correlation between the diagnosis of NUP and immunosuppression in HIV-positive patients. Those patients who presented with NUP were 20.8 times more likely to have CD^{4+} counts of less than 200 cells/mm^3 as compared to HIV-positive patients without NUP. The authors consider a diagnosis of NUP to be a marker of immune deterioration and a predictor of the diagnosis of AIDS. Others have suggested that NUP may be used as an indicator of HIV infection in undiagnosed patients. Shangase and coworkers reported that a diagnosis of NUG or NUP in systemically healthy, asymptomatic South-African patients was strongly correlated with HIV infection. Of patients presenting with NUG or NUP, 39 of 56 (69.6%) were subsequently found to be infected with HIV.

Etiology of Necrotizing Ulcerative Periodontitis

The etiology of NUP has not been determined, although a mixed fusiform–spirochete bacterial flora appears to play a key role. Since bacterial pathogens are not solely responsible for causing the disease, some predisposing "host" factors may be necessary. Numerous predisposing factors have been attributed to NUG, including poor oral hygiene, preexisting periodontal disease, smoking, viral infections, immunocompromised status, psychosocial stress, and malnutrition.

NUG and NUP are more prevalent and more severe among patients with HIV. These patients require urgent treatment because untreated lesions can progress rapidly; within a few days, severe bone loss around affected teeth can be seen.

Smoking, malnutrition, and high plaque levels all increase the risk of NUG and need to be changed so that treatment success is obtained.

Clinicians should check all patients who present with NUP to ascertain their HIV status. NUP can progress rapidly and lead to tooth exfoliation, so treatment should include local debridement, local antiplaque agents, and systemic antibiotics. The early diagnosis and treatment of NUP are crucial because the osseous defects that occur during the late stages of the disease are extremely difficult to resolve.

Microbial Flora

Assessment of the microbial flora of NUP lesions is almost exclusively limited to studies involving patients with HIV or AIDS, with some conflicting evidence. Murray and coworkers reported that cases of NUP in HIV-positive patients demonstrated significantly greater numbers of the opportunistic fungus *Candida albicans* and a higher prevalence of *Aggregatibacter actinomycetemcomitans, Prevotella intermedia, P. gingivalis, Fusobacterium nucleatum,* and *Campylobacter* species as compared to HIV-negative controls. In addition, they reported a low or variable level of spirochetes, which is inconsistent with the flora associated with NUG. Citing differences in microbial flora, they refuted the notion that the destructive lesions seen in HIV-positive patients were related to NUG lesions; they suggested that the flora of NUP lesions in HIV-positive patients is comparable to that of chronic periodontitis lesions, thus supporting their concept that necrotizing periodontitis in the HIV-positive patient is an aggressive manifestation of chronic periodontitis in the immunocompromised host.

In contrast with these findings, Cobb and coworkers reported that the microbial composition of NUP lesions in HIV-positive patients was very similar to that of NUG lesions, as discussed previously. With the use of electron microscopy, the researchers described a mixed microbial flora with various morphotypes in 81.3% of specimens. The subsurface microbial flora featured dense aggregations of spirochetes in 87.5% of specimens. The authors also reported opportunistic yeasts and herpes-like viruses in 65.6% and 56.5% of NUP lesions, respectively. The differences between these reports may be explained by the limitations of obtaining viable cultures of spirochetes as compared to the more definitive electron microscopic observation of spirochetes.

In a recent review article, Feller and Lemmer suggested that spirochetes, herpesviruses, candida, and HIV all have potentially pathogenic roles in NUP lesions in the HIV-seropositive individual. Spirochetes have the ability to modulate the host's innate and adaptive immune responses and to stimulate host inflammatory reactions, which may reduce the local immune competence and facilitate the development of necrotizing disease. Activated herpesviruses have the capacity to deregulate the host's immune system, which may lead to an increase in the colonization and activity of other pathogenic microorganisms. *C. albicans* has been reported to produce eicosanoids, thereby leading to the release of proinflammatory mediators, which may facilitate spirochete colonization and invasion and promote the development of necrotizing periodontal diseases.

KEY FACT

Patients with NUP are more likely to be immunocompromised. Although a mixed fusiform–spirochete bacterial infection appears to play a key role in the etiology of NUP, bacterial pathogens are not solely responsible. Predisposing "host" factors appear to be necessary. Factors that have been attributed to NUG include poor oral hygiene, preexisting periodontal disease, smoking, viral infections, immunocompromised status, psychosocial stress, and malnutrition.

Immunocompromised Status

Clearly, both NUG and NUP lesions are more prevalent among patients with compromised or suppressed immune systems. Numerous studies—particularly those evaluating patients with HIV or AIDS—support the concept that a diminished host response is present in those individuals who have been diagnosed with necrotizing ulcerative periodontal diseases. Whereas a compromised immune system (i.e., "immune compromise") in the HIV-infected patient is driven by impaired T-cell function and altered T-cell ratios, evidence indicates that other forms of compromised immunity predispose individuals to NUG and NUP as well.

Cutler and colleagues described the impaired bactericidal activity of PMNs in two children with NUP. In a comparative assay of PMNs and periodontal pathogens, two brothers who were 9 and 14 years old showed significant depression of PMN phagocytosis and killing function as compared to gender- and age-matched controls. Furthermore, Batista and colleagues reported periodontal findings and NUP in an adolescent patient with a rare genetic disease (multifactorial congenital immunodeficiency) that causes the impaired secretion of immunoglobulin; the oral lesions resolved with the administration of intravenous immunoglobulin.

Psychologic Stress

Most studies evaluating the role of stress on necrotizing periodontal disease have involved subjects with NUG and thus have not specifically addressed the role of stress on NUP.

Patients with NUG have been found to have had significantly more anxiety, higher depression scores, a greater magnitude of recent stressful events, more overall distress and adjustments related to these events, and more negative life events. Although the role of stress in the development of NUP has not been reported specifically, the many similarities between NUG and NUP would suggest that similar relationships to stress may exist.

The mechanisms that predispose an individual with stress to necrotizing ulcerative periodontal diseases have not been established.

However, it is well known that stress increases the systemic cortisol levels, and sustained increases in cortisone have a suppressive effect on the immune response. In an investigation of 474 military personnel, Shannon and colleagues found that urinary levels of 17-hydroxycorticosteroid were higher among subjects with NUG than in all other subjects who had been diagnosed with periodontal health, gingivitis, or periodontitis. Experimentally, noma-like lesions have been produced in rats by administering cortisone and causing mechanical injury to the gingiva and in hamsters via total body irradiation. Thus, stress-induced immunosuppression may be one mechanism that impairs the host response and leads to necrotizing periodontal disease. The scientific evidence supporting an etiologic role of stress in chronic periodontitis is not as clear.

Malnutrition

Direct evidence of the relationship between malnutrition and necrotizing periodontal disease is limited to descriptions of necrotizing infections in severely malnourished children. Lesions resembling NUG but that progress to become *gangrenous stomatitis* or noma have been described in children with severe malnutrition in underdeveloped countries. Jimenez and Baer reported cases of NUG among malnourished children and adolescents between the ages of 2 and 14 years in Colombia. In the advanced stages, NUG lesions extended from the gingiva to other areas of the oral cavity, becoming gangrenous stomatitis (noma) and causing exposure, necrosis, and sequestration of the alveolar bone. Later, Jimenez and colleagues reported that 44 of the 45 cases of necrotizing disease (NUG = 29, NUP = 7, and noma = 9) documented from 1965 to 2000 were from a low socioeconomic group and that malnutrition was associated with nearly all of the necrotizing conditions (29/29 NUG cases, 6/7 NUP cases, and 9/9 noma cases). In a study of socioeconomically deprived Nigerian children with NUG (153 cases), Enwonwu and colleagues confirmed malnutrition by measuring circulating micronutrients. As compared to neighborhood counterparts, the children with NUG and micronutrient deficiencies demonstrated dysregulated cytokine production with a complex interplay of elevated proinflammatory and antiinflammatory mediators.

A possible explanation is that malnutrition, particularly when extreme, contributes to a diminished host resistance to infection and necrotizing disease. It is well documented that many of the host defenses—including phagocytosis; cell-mediated immunity; and complement, antibody, and cytokine production and function—are impaired in malnourished individuals. The depletion of nutrients to cells and tissues results in immunosuppression and increases disease susceptibility. Thus, it is reasonable to conclude that malnutrition can predispose an individual to opportunistic infections or intensify the severity of existing oral infections.

KEY FACT

A fusiform–spirochete infection along with weakened host immune system seem to play a major role in the pathogenesis of necrotizing ulcerative periodontitis.

KEY FACT

Necrotizing ulcerative periodontitis (NUP) is classified among necrotizing periodontal diseases in the 2017 World Workshop classification, due to its similarities in etiology, clinical features, treatment approaches, and potential progression to more severe forms like necrotizing stomatitis (NS). The elimination of the term "ulcerative" from the classification is justified by considering ulceration as a consequence rather than a primary feature of the necrotic process. These diseases, including NUG, NUP, and NS, are different stages of the same pathological spectrum. They share common characteristics, such as tissue necrosis, inflammation, and microbial involvement. Treatment strategies for these conditions typically involve meticulous debridement, antimicrobial therapy, and supportive care to control infection and promote tissue healing. Understanding the continuum from NUG, NUP, to NS underscores the importance of early intervention and comprehensive management to prevent disease progression and optimize patient outcomes.

AGGRESSIVE PERIODONTITIS

Aggressive periodontitis is characterized by swift degradation of periodontal attachment and supportive tooth bone in patients who are otherwise in good health.

The divergent literature on aggressive periodontitis highlights several key concerns. Firstly, the prevailing classification system is considered overly encompassing, potentially failing to adequately capture the nuances of the disease. Secondly, there exists a notable gap in research investigating aggressive periodontitis from its initial stages, hindering a comprehensive understanding of its progression and development. Finally, the limited availability of longitudinal studies encompassing various timeframes and populations further complicates efforts to discern the intricate dynamics of this condition. Addressing these issues is crucial for advancing our comprehension of aggressive periodontitis and refining approaches to diagnosis and treatment.

Historical Background

In 1923, Gottlieb described a patient with a fatal case of epidemic influenza and a disease that he called "diffuse atrophy of the alveolar bone." This disease was characterized by a loss of collagen fibers in the periodontal ligament and their replacement by loose connective tissue and extensive bone resorption, which resulted in a widened periodontal space. The gingiva apparently was not involved. In 1928, Gottlieb attributed this condition to the inhibition of continuous cementum formation, which he considered essential for the maintenance of the periodontal fibers. At that time, he called the disease "deep cementopathia," and he hypothesized that this was a "disease of eruption" and that the cementum initiated a foreign-body response. As a result, it was postulated that the host attempted to exfoliate the tooth, thereby resulting in the observed bone resorption and pocket formation.

In 1938, Wannenmacher described incisor and first molar involvement and called the disease "parodontitis marginalis progressiva." Several explanations have evolved for the etiology and pathogenesis of this type of disease. Many authors considered this to be a degenerative, noninflammatory disease process and therefore gave it the name *periodontosis*. Other investigators denied the existence of a degenerative type of periodontal disease and attributed the changes observed to trauma from occlusion. Finally, in 1966, the World Workshop in Periodontics concluded that the concept of periodontosis as a degenerative entity was unsubstantiated and that the term should be eliminated from periodontal nomenclature. However, the committee did recognize that a clinical entity different from adult periodontitis may occur among adolescents and young adults.

The term *juvenile periodontitis* was introduced by Chaput et al. in 1967 and by Butler in 1969. In 1971, Baer defined it as "a disease of the periodontium occurring in an otherwise healthy adolescent which is characterized by a rapid loss of alveolar bone about more than one tooth of the permanent dentition. The amount of destruction manifested is not commensurate with the amount of local irritants." In 1989, the World Workshop in Clinical Periodontics categorized this disease as localized juvenile periodontitis and as a subset of the broad classification of early-onset periodontitis. Under this classification system, age of onset and distribution of lesions were of primary importance when making a diagnosis of this condition.

In 1999, the World Workshop in Periodontics introduced a novel classification that was meant to eliminate the shortcomings of earlier endeavors to classify periodontal disease. Most importantly, the new 1999 classification sought "to discard classification terminologies that were age-dependent or required knowledge of rates of progression." In the new classification scheme, several rapidly progressing periodontitis forms were united under the term *aggressive periodontitis*.

A new World Workshop in Periodontics was jointly planned by the European Federation of Periodontology and the American Academy of Periodontology for November 2017 in order to further refine the classification of periodontal diseases. From a pathophysiologic point of view, both LAgP and CP have a common end result. The loss of bone and disorientation of the attachment apparatus results from disruption in homeostatic balance between deposition and resorption of bone. Initially identified as a noninflammatory condition (termed periodontosis), it is now clear that both LAgP and CP are entities resulting from inflammatory responses to a biofilm starting point, which results in bone loss. However, overall, it is clear that LAgP demonstrates a unique phenotype, but a more in-depth understanding of the differences among events leading up to bone loss in LAgP as compared to CP needs to wait for a more exacting definition of early events.

TABLE 21.2 Diagnostic Criteria to Distinguish Chronic and Aggressive Periodontitis

Criterion	Aggressive Periodontitis	Chronic Periodontitis
Rate of progression	Rapid	Slow but rapid episodes are possible
Familiar aggregation	Typical	Can be present when families share imperfect oral hygiene habits
Presence of etiological factors (e.g., plaque, calculus, and overhanging restorations)	Often minimal	Often commensurate with observed periodontal destruction
Age	Often in young patients (i.e., <35 years old) but can be found in all age groups	Often in older patients (i.e., >55 years old) but can be found in all age groups
Clinical inflammation signs	Sometimes lacking (especially in patients with localized aggressive periodontitis)	Commensurate with amount of etiological factors present

Considerations When Redefining Aggressive Periodontitis

Any new definition should be based on the (1) age of the subject, (2) location of lesions, and (3) extent of disease (stages). The first diagnosis could be in (1) childhood (prepubertal), (2) adolescence (puberty), and (3) early adulthood (postadolescence). The definition of disease in addition to age could include (1) the location of the lesion and the stage or extent of disease (one, two, or three or more teeth). This staged approach would signify the severity of disease (i.e., one tooth is less severe than two teeth, etc.). This staged approach would also enable the practitioner and researcher to identify the "burned out" or contained disease (i.e., a disease confined to one tooth or two teeth, etc.). In its simplest form, the staged definition could be categorized as Stage 1, a disease limited to one tooth, Stage 2 limited to two teeth, Stage 3 limited to three teeth (molars and incisors), and Stage 4 the classic Löe and Brown definition of disease. To prevent confusion with trauma or other noninfectious disease initiators, a diseased tooth would be defined as having proximal attachment loss but would not be based on buccal or lingual recession. This staged definition would be helpful to examine microbial initiators, host-response elements, and pathophysiologic changes.

Classification and Clinical Characteristics

Features

The 1999 International Workshop for the Classification of Periodontal Diseases and Conditions defined the entity of aggressive periodontitis as being characterized by three primary features (Table 21.2):

1. *The rapid loss of attachment and tooth-supporting bone.*

   With aggressive periodontitis, as compared to the more common variant chronic periodontitis, the loss of attachment progresses significantly faster. To evaluate this rapid course of destruction, the evaluation of clinical or radiographic data from earlier points in time is necessary, which helps in making an estimate of the start of the disease. Note that the age of the patient per se is not a primary criterion for the diagnosis of aggressive periodontitis. Since earlier clinical records are often not available, many clinicians argue that a severe loss of attachment in young patients may conceivably be the result of a rapid course of disease progression. However, this is not generally true; the neglect of all oral hygiene in a periodontitis-susceptible individual over a decade will lead to severe attachment loss even with a slow rate of progression. On the other hand, severe attachment loss in an older individual is not necessarily the result of long-lasting, slowly progressing disease. It is therefore inappropriate to use the age of an affected individual as a primary diagnostic criterion for the distinction of aggressive and chronic periodontitis. Note that, with chronic periodontitis, there are reportedly periods of rapid disease progression that can by themselves be misinterpreted as aggressive periodontitis.

2. *The subject is otherwise healthy (i.e., not suffering from any systemic disease or condition that could be responsible for the present periodontitis).*

   There are systemic diseases that lead to severely altered host defenses against periodontal pathogens, often resulting in the rapid loss of attachment and tooth loss at early age. This disease is designated "periodontitis as a manifestation of systemic disease." Note that the specific properties or abnormalities of some types of immune cells, listed later in this chapter and reported to be often associated with the diagnosis of aggressive periodontitis, do not themselves qualify for the aforementioned diagnosis.

3. *The presence of familiar aggregation.*
   The familiar aggregation of aggressive periodontitis cases is a feature that can be evaluated via medical and dental history questionnaires and by interviewing the patient. However, it is advisable to verify similar cases in the family, if possible, because many individuals may not be fully aware of their diagnoses. Many cases of "bad teeth that run in the family" turn up to be caries related or likely due to chronic periodontitis.

In addition, the Workshop defined several secondary features that are generally found in aggressive periodontitis cases but that are not universally necessary to diagnose the disease entity:

1. Inconsistency of the low amounts of present etiological factors (i.e., plaque) and the observed pronounced tissue destruction.
2. Strong colonization by *A. actinomycetemcomitans* (*Aa*) and, in some populations, *P. gingivalis*.
3. Immunological differences that do not entail the diagnosis of periodontitis as a manifestation of systemic disease.
   a. Hyperresponsive macrophages
   b. Abnormalities of neutrophil function
4. Self-limiting disease.

Subgroups

Aggressive periodontitis can be subclassified into localized and generalized forms. The diagnosis of the subcategory is based on clinical, radiographic, and historic data. These include the age of onset, the involvement of teeth other than first molars and incisors (i.e., the first permanent teeth to erupt), and the presence of a systemic antibody response against periodontal pathogens (Table 21.3).

Generalized Aggressive Periodontitis

Generalized aggressive periodontitis (GAP) is the subgroup of periodontal disease that is characterized by the highest severity and extent of disease and also by its large heterogeneity.

TABLE 21.3 Diagnostic Criteria for Localized and Generalized Aggressive Periodontitis

Criterion	Localized Aggressive Periodontitis	Generalized Aggressive Periodontitis
Age of onset	Circumpubertal	Most often <30 years of age but can also occur in older individuals
Serum-antibody response against infecting agents	Robust	Poor
Destruction pattern	Localized attachment loss at incisors and first molars; interproximal attachment loss at two or more permanent teeth, one of which is a first molar, and involvement of two or fewer teeth other than the first molars and incisors	Generalized interproximal attachment loss at three or more permanent teeth other than the first molars and incisors
Additional		Episodic nature of attachment loss

Clinically, GAP is characterized by "generalized interproximal attachment loss affecting at least three permanent teeth other than first molars and incisors."

The diagnosis of GAP encompasses the diseases that were previously classified as generalized juvenile periodontitis and rapidly progressive periodontitis.

Two gingival tissue responses can be found in cases of GAP (Figs. 21.7 and 21.8). One involves severe, acutely inflamed tissue that is often proliferating, ulcerated, and fiery red. Bleeding may occur spontaneously or with slight stimulation, and suppuration may be an important feature. This tissue response is thought to occur during the destructive stage in which attachment and bone are actively lost.

In other cases, the gingival tissues may appear pink, free of inflammation, and occasionally with some degree of stippling, although stippling may be absent. However, despite the apparently mild clinical appearance, deep pockets can be demonstrated by probing. Page and Schroeder thought that this tissue response coincides with periods of quiescence in which the bone level remains stationary.

Prevalence and Distribution by Age and Gender

Among the young Israeli army recruits, it was found that 1.8% suffered from GAP. When using extrapolation, as proposed by Demmer and Papapanou, a prevalence of about 1% to a maximum of 15% in individuals aged 25–35 years was found, depending on the study.

Specifically, data from the German Study of Health in Pomerania indicated an extrapolated prevalence within different age groups of 13% (≤29 years) and 7% (30–39 years), whereas the highest extrapolated prevalence was found in the Erie County Study, with up to 15% of individuals aged 25–35 years being affected.

Radiographic Findings

Radiographic picture in GAP can range from severe bone loss associated with a minimal number of teeth to advanced bone loss affecting the majority of teeth in the dentition.

Localized Aggressive Periodontitis

Localized aggressive periodontitis (LAP) is usually found in younger individuals than GAP (Figs. 21.9 and 21.10). Clinically, "it is characterized as having localized first molar/incisor presentation with interproximal attachment loss on at least two permanent teeth, one of which is a first molar, and involving no more than two teeth other than first molars and incisors."

The localized distribution of lesions in LAP is unexplained, but the following reasons have been suggested:

1. After initial colonization of first permanent teeth to erupt (first molars and incisors), *Aa* evades the host defenses by various mechanisms initiating the destruction of periodontal tissues. After this initial attack, adequate immune defenses are stimulated to produce opsonic antibodies that enhance the clearance of invading bacteria. This way, colonization of other site may be prevented.
2. Bacteria antagonistic to *Aa* may colonize the periodontal tissues and inhibit it from further colonization.
3. For unknown reasons, *Aa* may lose its leucotoxin-producing ability.
4. A defect in the cementum formation may be responsible for the localization of the lesions.

It is characterized by more pronounced systemic antibody titers against periodontal pathogens than are found in patients with GAP. This could indicate that, in individuals who are susceptible to disease but who also have the ability to enact a robust response against

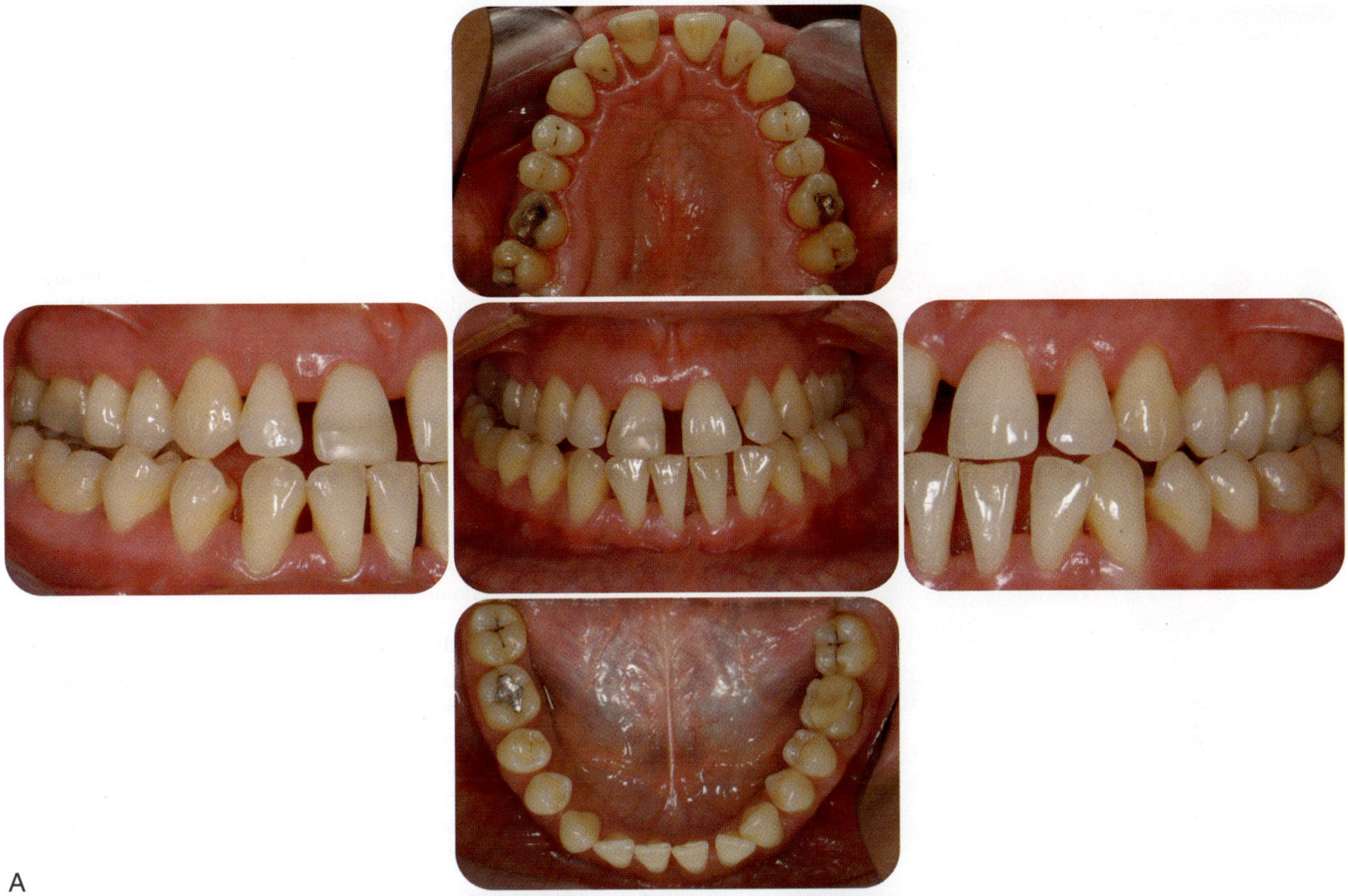

A

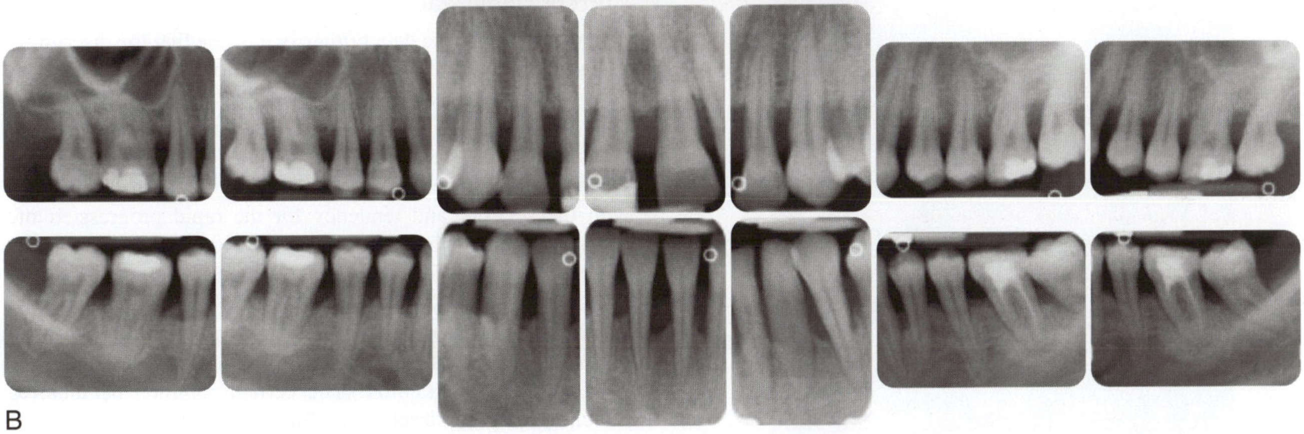

B

Fig. 21.7 Generalized aggressive periodontitis. Generalized aggressive periodontitis in a 28-year-old Caucasian, female, nonsmoking patient. A, Clinical views with minimal amounts of calculus and plaque. B, Radiographically, bone loss of 50% or more was present at all teeth.

pathogens, the disease might be limited in extent (i.e., LAP). Alternatively, in individuals with a lesser humoral response, the disease would not be limited to the first permanent teeth, and the patient would develop GAP. This would mean that LAP and GAP would merely be phenotypic variations of the same underlying disease. This assumption is backed by several reports that show a sequence of LAP and GAP in the same individuals over time.

At the same time, there exist several lines of evidence that support the claim that LAP constitutes a disease on its own, with dissimilar underlying molecular and cellular mechanisms.

Prevalence and Distribution by Age and Gender

The prevalence of LAP in an Israeli army population between the ages of 18 and 30 years old was 4.3%. In this cohort, the presence of LAP was highly correlated with North African origin and current smoking.

In addition to these recent data, there exist several studies on the prevalence of localized juvenile periodontitis (LJP) among diverse populations. LJP is the predecessor of LAP although the two conditions are not exactly interchangeable. The prevalence of this disease in geographically diverse adolescent populations was estimated to

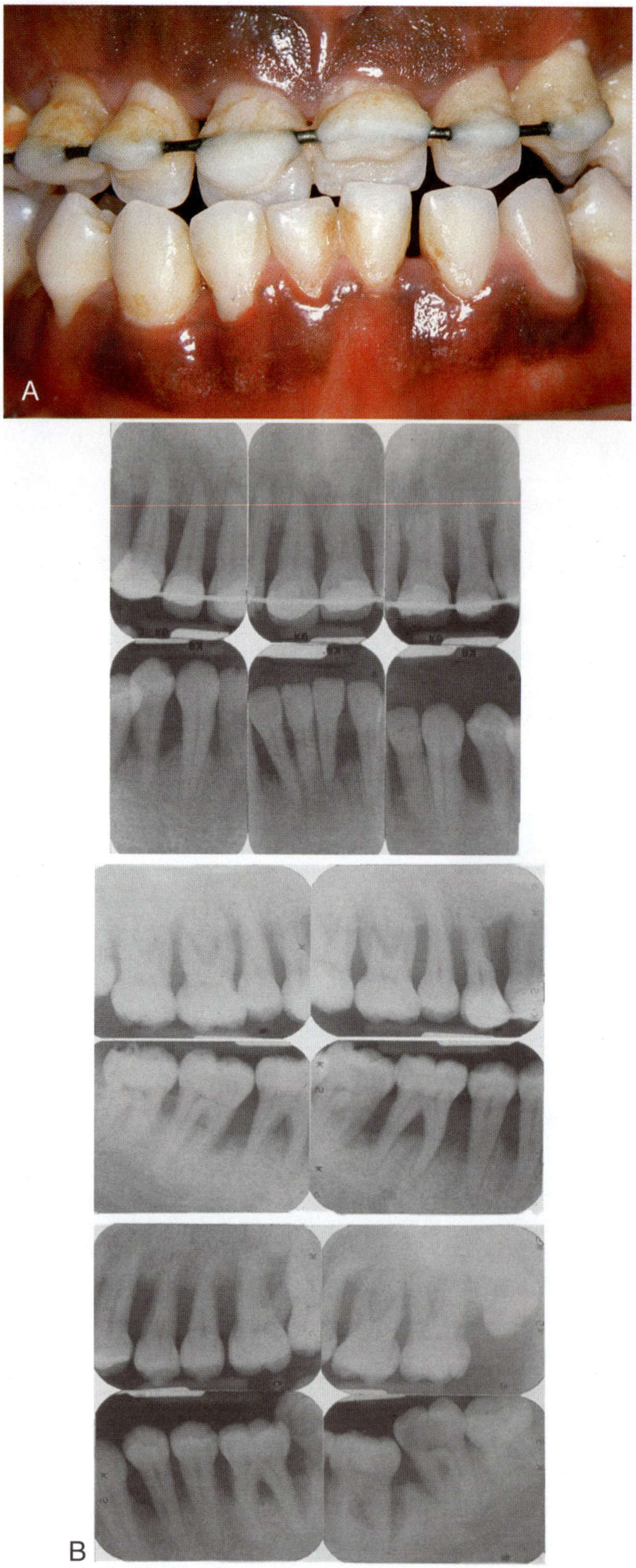

Fig. 21.8 Generalized aggressive periodontitis. Severe generalized aggressive periodontitis in a 22-year-old black, male patient with a family history of early tooth loss through periodontal disease. A, Clinical view showing minimal plaque and inflammation. A provisional wire-and-resin splint had been placed by the general practice dentist to stabilize the teeth. B, Radiographs showing the severe and generalized nature of the disease, with all erupted teeth affected.

be less than 1%. Most reports suggested a low prevalence of about 0.2%. Two independent radiographic studies of 16-year-old adolescents (one in Finland and the other in Switzerland) followed the strict diagnostic criteria, delineated by Baer, and reported a prevalence rate of 0.1%. A clinical and radiographic study of 7266 English adolescents who were 15–19 years old also showed a prevalence rate of 0.1%. In the United States, a national survey of adolescents between the ages of 14 and 17 years reported that 0.53% had LJP. Blacks were at a much higher risk for LJP, and black male teenagers were 2.9 times more likely to have the disease than black female adolescents. By contrast, white female teenagers were more likely to have LJP than white male adolescents. Several other studies have found the highest prevalence of LJP among black males, who are followed in descending order by black females, white females, and white males.

LJP was reported to affect both males and females and it is seen most frequently in the period between puberty and 20 years of age. Some studies have suggested a predilection for female patients, particularly in the youngest age groups, whereas others reported no male or female differences in incidence when studies are designed to correct for ascertainment bias.

Radiographic Findings

Vertical loss of alveolar bone noted around the first molars and incisors begin around puberty in otherwise healthy teenagers. Classical arc-shaped loss of alveolar bone extending from the distal surface of second premolar to the mesial surface of second molar is appreciated in LAP.

Bone defects are usually wider than those that are usually seen with chronic periodontitis.

Current Understanding

Taken together, these data primarily indicate that the discrimination of aggressive periodontitis from other forms of periodontitis is not always easy, especially when seeing the patient only for a single examination as it is the case in most epidemiological studies. The prevalence of aggressive periodontitis of approximately 1%–15% among subjects, who are 35 years old or younger, in combination with the severity and tendency for the rapid progression of this disease, strongly suggest that all patients in this age group should be screened regularly for the presence of periodontal disease.

Pathobiology and Risk Factors

All forms of periodontitis share certain common pathobiological principles as polymicrobial, biofilm-mediated, and chronic inflammatory diseases at the biofilm–gingival interface. For now, we will focus on the biological reasons for the rapid course of destruction in patients with aggressive periodontitis, including looking at research that has investigated the specific properties of aggressive periodontitis in periodontal microbiology, immunology, and genetics.

Microbiology

Periodontitis is caused by specific microorganisms in a susceptible host. In the subgingival biofilm, up to 700 bacterial species have been identified, some of which have been identified as being causative.

The observed higher rate of disease progression in aggressive versus chronic periodontitis could possibly be explained by the presence of specific microorganisms that cause and perpetuate tissue destruction. In addition, the reported familiar aggregation of aggressive periodontitis cases could be also, to a certain point,

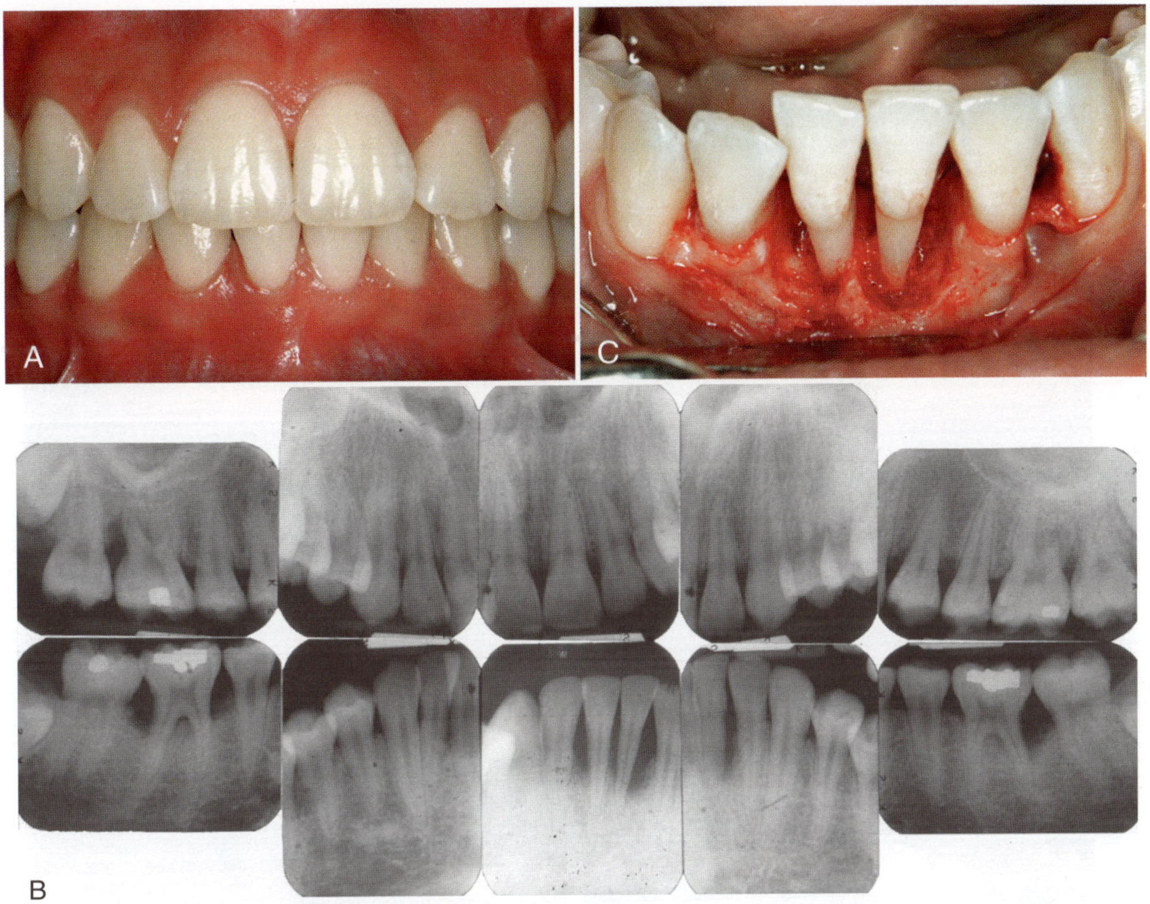

Fig. 21.9 Localized aggressive periodontitis. Localized aggressive periodontitis in a 15-year-old black, female patient who had a twin with similar disease. A, Clinical view showing minimal plaque and inflammation, except for localized inflammation on the distal side of the maxillary left central incisor and the mandibular right central incisor. B, Radiographs showing localized, vertical, angular bone loss associated with the maxillary and mandibular first molars and the mandibular central incisors. The maxillary incisors show no apparent involvement. C, Surgical appearance of the localized, vertical, angular bony defects affecting the mandibular incisors. Note the wide circumferential nature of the defects and the lack of calculus on the root surfaces.

explained by an infection or the within-family transmission of specific microorganisms.

Therefore, several studies have sought to identify the specific microbial properties of aggressive periodontitis cases. However, when evaluating GAP and LAP as a single entity and solely focusing on a small number of "classic" pathogens, it has been concluded that microbiological infection patterns could not reliably distinguish between this entity and chronic periodontitis cases.

However, data from a limited number of studies, involving both classic microbiological tools and more recent molecular techniques, suggest that differences exist in microbiological composition between (1) LAP and both GAP and chronic periodontitis and (2) CAP and chronic periodontitis.

Specific Bacteria in Localized Aggressive Periodontitis

In patients with LAP, the situation seems to be different. In these cases, several lines of evidence point to a strong role of specific microorganisms, most notably *A. actinomycetemcomitans*. For decades, this bacterial species has been associated with LAP, and its presence predicted the development of LAP in two longitudinal studies. Longitudinal studies are of critical importance for the demonstration of a causal relationship, whereas cross-sectional studies can by definition only show correlations that cannot be used to infer causality.

In the first longitudinal study, age-, gender-, and race-matched juvenile carriers and noncarriers of *A. actinomycetemcomitans* (serotypes a, b, and c were equally distributed, with no presence of *A. actinomycetemcomitans* strain JP2) were followed longitudinally. After 1 year of follow-up, 80% of the carriers and only 10% of the noncarriers had developed periodontitis.

In the second and larger longitudinal study, the highly leukotoxic *A. actinomycetemcomitans* (serotype b) strain JP2, which has a 530-bp deletion in its leukotoxin gene operon that leads to a 10- to 20-fold higher production of leukotoxin, was found to be directly related to the occurrence of LAP in children in Northern Africa. Specifically, the odds ratio for future attachment loss among carriers of the JP2 strain was 18.0 as compared to 3.0 for carriers of other, non-JP2 strains of *A. actinomycetemcomitans*. Similar findings can also be found in West African countries, such as Ghana. This is in contrast with the eastern parts of Africa where no studies have reported the presence of JP2 clone strains in patients with periodontitis.

A recent study of the occurrence of JP2 clone strains in patients with aggressive periodontitis demonstrated a high incidence of both LAP and GAP, which suggests that both subclasses could be more related than initially thought.

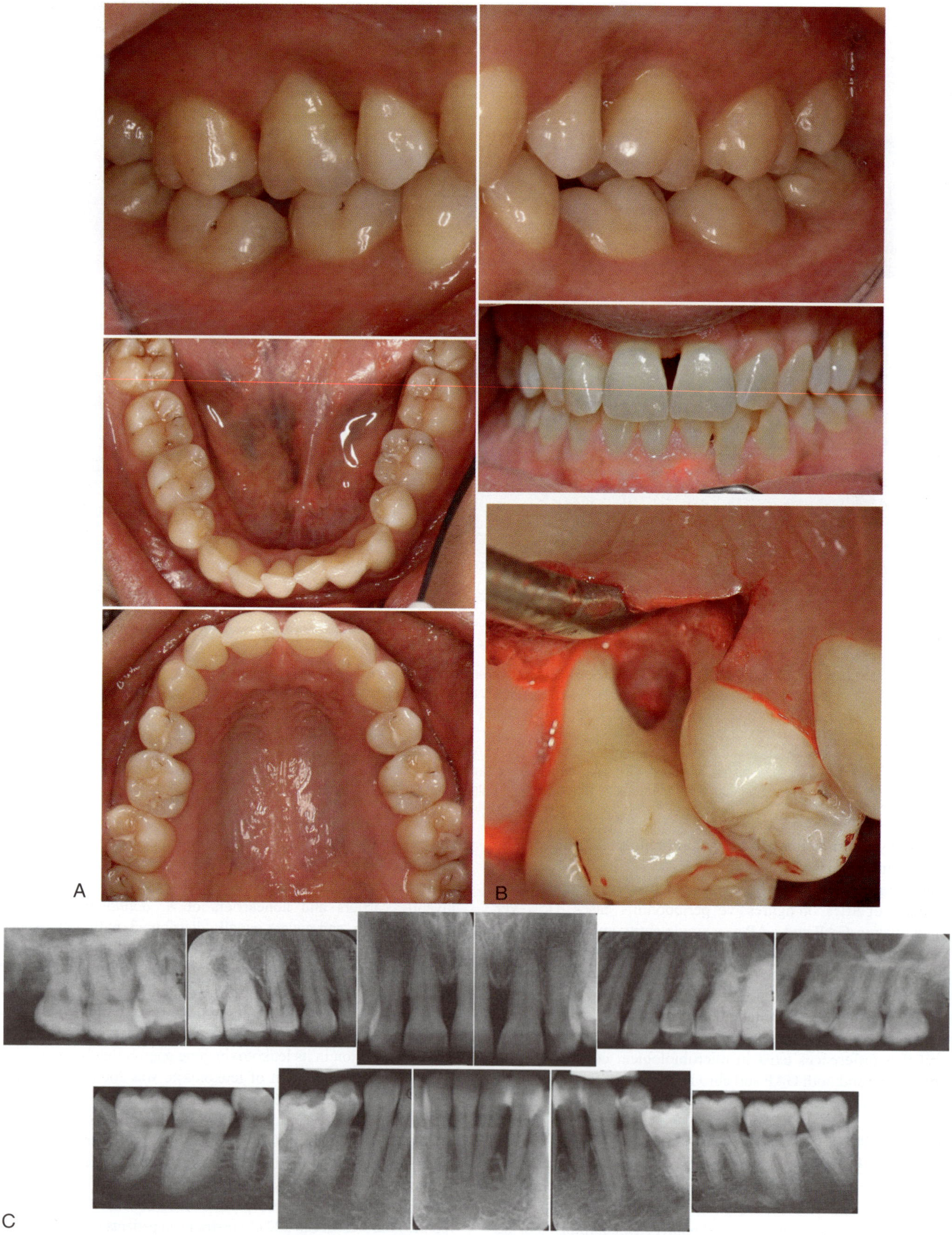

Fig. 21.10 Localized aggressive periodontitis. Localized aggressive periodontitis in an 18-year-old Caucasian, female, nonsmoking patient. Familiar aggregation was reported. A, Clinical view showing recessions at the incisors and first molars. B, Intraoperative view showing advanced, localized, angular bony defect associated with a first molar. C, Radiographs showing pronounced localized, angular bone loss. *(Courtesy: Dr Hendrik Schulze, Bonn, Germany.)*

In addition, it needs to be noted that LAP is clearly not a monoinfection with *A. actinomycetemcomitans*; as with all entities involving periodontitis, LAP features a polymicrobial biofilm. In support of this notion is the fact that there are also reports of confirmed cases of LAP that did not involve *A. actinomycetemcomitans*.

Host Response to Bacterial Challenge

The inflammatory host response toward pathogens is generally attributed to be responsible for a larger proportion of the tissue destruction in periodontitis than the invading periodontal pathogens themselves. The rapid progression of aggressive periodontitis implies that—in addition to the aforementioned composition of the subgingival microbiological flora—specific properties of this inflammatory response render the individuals with aggressive periodontitis, both more susceptible to disease and to the loss of more attachment in a shorter amount of time.

Host Response Specific to Aggressive Periodontitis

With regard to GAP, a recent review concluded that "there appears to be no difference between aggressive and chronic periodontitis in terms of their histopathology and immunopathology." Still, it has to be acknowledged that this could mean that there exist no differences or, rather, that "the differences between both disease entities only reflect variations in the degree of severity of susceptibility rather than actual different immunopathologies."

Most recently, the stronger activation of natural killer cells and natural killer T cells in patients with aggressive periodontitis was suggested to be causative for the enhanced tissue destruction that has been observed in these patients.

Abnormalities in Localized Aggressive Periodontitis

Earlier work suggested that individuals with LAP were characterized by an inherited defect of neutrophil function that led to a dampened immune response against the microflora inhabiting the periodontal pocket. Specifically, when challenged with periodontal pathogens, the LAP neutrophils were reported to show impaired chemotaxis, phagocytosis, and killing of bacteria. Alternatively, it was also hypothesized that these impaired defense properties were in fact acquired defects caused by prolonged exposure to an inflammatory microenvironment.

Today, the understanding of neutrophil biology is that neutrophils arriving at a site with uncontrolled periodontal inflammation are primed to attack the invading pathogens by releasing lytic enzymes. These enzymes may, on the other hand, accelerate tissue destruction. It is hypothesized that the observed dampened neutrophil function in deep aggressive periodontitis lesions is due to the heavy commitment of primed neutrophils to debridement and decreased potency for chemotaxis and defense.

Genetics: Family Studies

A familial aggregation of aggressive periodontitis cases is a secondary feature of the disease entity; it is often (but not always) found with aggressive periodontitis. To assess the familial component of the disease, twin studies were performed, and these demonstrated a strong genetic component with a likely autosomal-dominant inheritance pattern and a 70% (African-Americans) to 73% (Caucasians) penetrance.

Genetics: Polymorphisms

Accordingly, extensive work has been carried out to determine the inherent genetic traits that underlie this familiar aggregation.

First, it was suspected that an inherent susceptibility to periodontitis would be likely the result of mutations in the DNA encoding for proteins of inflammatory mediators; this is the candidate gene approach. DNA regions that were selected on the basis of a priori knowledge of the disease pathobiology were assessed for sequence variations, and these were most often SNPs. On the basis of small sample sizes and often suboptimal study designs that conceivably led to false-positive results, SNPs within genes that encoded for cytokines, such as interleukins-1α, -1β, -6, and so on, were reported to be associated with aggressive periodontitis. However, with current knowledge, it has to be realized that these findings were possibly spurious or the result of confounding: all of the "classical" candidate gene associations could not be replicated in today's larger and better-controlled cohorts. Note that, in the case of genetic association studies, metaanalyses are not generally suitable tools to overcome the problems of small, heterogeneous cohorts.

Use of the genome-wide association study (GWAS) has been made possible by technologic advances in the field of high-throughput analysis. Using a GWAS of a large number of aggressive periodontitis cases and controls identified a common susceptibility locus for aggressive periodontitis and myocardial infarction, and these findings were replicated in independent cohorts.

Taken together, these data indicate that there is evidence for a strong genetic component in aggressive periodontitis. It is very likely that the low number of identified and replicated susceptibility loci for aggressive periodontitis are the result of extremely low sample numbers and issues in study design than the lack of biological association.

Environmental Factors That Affect Susceptibility

The amount and duration of smoking are important variables that can influence the extent of destruction seen in young adults. Patients with GAP who smoke have more affected teeth and a greater loss of clinical attachment than nonsmoking patients with GAP. However, smoking may not have the same impact on the attachment levels in younger patients with LAP.

Diagnosis

Assessment of Clinical Presentation

The most reliable diagnostic marker for periodontitis is periodontal probing. However, this technique merely assesses a loss of attachment; it does not classify subcategories of periodontal disease.

The diagnosis of aggressive periodontitis in the clinic is therefore made by jointly assessing the primary and secondary features of aggressive periodontitis, as described previously.

As a result of the small but significant prevalence of this severe category of periodontal disease, it is also recommended to routinely screen for the presence of attachment loss in younger patients with the use of Periodontal Screening and Recording or the PSI every year. In patients with significant findings, a more thorough clinical assessment that includes the evaluation of periodontal probing depth and attachment loss at six sites per tooth should be performed.

In addition, patients who are at risk for developing aggressive periodontitis should be more closely monitored. These are primarily subjects with a known familiar aggregation of aggressive periodontitis (e.g., the child of a patient with aggressive periodontitis who is already being treated in the practice).

The diagnosis of systemic health is made by assessing the medical history of the patient, usually with the use of a questionnaire and a short interview; this process is repeated every other year. In subjects with suspected aggressive periodontitis, the primary-care physician can be consulted to rule out any underlying systemic illnesses or conditions. Radiographs will help in confirming the diagnosis based on clinical findings.

Current Developments

Based on the aforementioned still incomplete current understanding of the specific microbiologic, immunologic, and genetic properties of the clinical symptom-based periodontitis entities aggressive and chronic periodontitis, research now focuses on the assessment of whether these entities are in fact sufficiently distinct with respect to their underlying pathobiology to form etiology-based clinical classes. For these analyses, novel unbiased high-throughput methodology such as microarrays and next-generation sequencing are employed.

Therapeutic Considerations in Aggressive Periodontitis Patients

Clinician's Corner

Aggressive periodontitis is defined by rapid attachment loss in clinically healthy individuals. There is considerable familiar aggregation. Aggressive periodontitis is most often found in younger individuals but can occur at any age. The entity is subdivided into two categories, localized and generalized aggressive periodontitis.

LAP primarily affects first molars and incisor teeth in adolescents with deep pockets and advanced bone loss. It occurs in less than 1% of adolescents. There is a strong, hitherto only partially understood genetic component. In addition, the anaerobic gram-negative bacterium *A. actinomycetemcomitans* in the subgingival plaque biofilm was causally linked to LAP development in adolescents.

GAP usually occurs first in young adults and may be present in some populations in up to 15% of the age group. Smoking may play a role because smokers with GAP have more teeth involved and more advanced pockets than nonsmokers.

Considerations for Antiinfective Therapy of Aggressive Periodontitis

Antiinfective therapy in patients with aggressive periodontitis seems to benefit strongly from the adjunctive use of systemic antibiotics (see Chapter 52).

Considerations for Surgical Therapy of Aggressive Periodontitis

In general, individuals with aggressive periodontitis, especially LAP, have to undergo surgical therapy more often than the average periodontitis patient. This is due to (1) the often much more pronounced loss of attachment with deep periodontal pockets that are challenging to instrument and (2) the high prevalence of vertical defects, notably in LAP, that need to be resolved.

Considerations for Supportive Periodontal Therapy of Aggressive Periodontitis Patients

Aggressive periodontitis patients are understood to suffer from an especially virulent microbiologic burden in combination with alterations in their host defense that render them more prone to rapid attachment loss, even in the absence of seemingly adequate numbers of etiologic factors. This suggests that during the maintenance phase, utmost care needs to be taken to optimize the self-performed oral hygiene in order to minimize the amount of plaque that could eventually lead to a new, rapid loss of attachment. Therefore, many clinicians recommend performing supportive periodontal therapy, including regular assessments of periodontal parameters, at least every 3 months—even in subjects who show particularly high levels of oral hygiene proficiency and independent of the periodontal risk assessment tool that seems to be of limited use in aggressive periodontitis.

Considerations for Oral Rehabilitation and Implant Therapy in Aggressive Periodontitis Patients

Dental implants today allow for the routine, predictable, functional, and esthetic replacement of lost teeth. Still, there are concerns about the incidence of peri-implantitis, an inflammatory condition of dental implants with parallels to periodontal disease for which no defined, predictable treatment protocols exist to date. Peri-implantitis risk is linked to a history of periodontal disease in the individual treated with dental implants. Limited data exist that show an even stronger risk for developing the disease in patients suffering from aggressive periodontitis, as compared to chronic periodontitis patients or periodontally healthy controls.

Why Chronic and Aggressive Periodontitis Were Included in a Single Category as Periodontitis in 2017 World Workshop Classification?

In the 1999 classification, periodontitis was further classified as chronic and aggressive periodontitis which were subclassified into localized and generalized and based on severity into mild, moderate, and severe. Distinguishing between different types of periodontitis relies on understanding their underlying causes and physiological processes rather than solely relying on variations in clinical presentation such as extent and severity. While localized early-onset periodontitis demonstrates recognizable clinical features like early onset, a preference for molar and incisor involvement, and the progression of attachment loss, the precise etiological and pathological factors contributing to this distinct presentation remain inadequately elucidated. Similarly, the mechanisms driving the onset of generalized periodontitis in young individuals are not thoroughly understood. In essence, while clinical manifestations serve as indicators, the true differentiation among periodontitis entities necessitates a deeper comprehension of their respective etiologies and pathophysiologies.

Current evidence, that is, according to the 2017 World Workshop Classification, does not support the distinction between chronic and aggressive periodontitis, as defined by the 1999 Classification Workshop, as two separate diseases; however, a substantial variation in clinical presentation exists concerning extent and severity throughout the age spectrum, suggesting that there are population subsets with distinct disease trajectories due to differences in exposure and/or susceptibility.

Key points

- Formerly known as "adult periodontitis" or chronic adult periodontitis" is the most prevalent form of periodontitis.
- It is generally a slowly progressing disease. However, in the presence of systemic or environmental factors that may modify the host response to plaque accumulation such as diabetes, smoking, or stress, disease progression may become aggressive.
- Chronic periodontitis has recently been defined as "an infectious disease resulting in inflammation within the supporting tissues of the teeth, progressive attachment loss, and bone loss."
- Clinical features include supragingival and subgingival plaque accumulation frequently associated with calculus formation, gingival inflammation, pocket formation, loss of periodontal attachment, and loss of alveolar bone. Tooth mobility often appears in advanced cases when bone loss has been considerable.
- A differential diagnosis is based on the age of the patient, rate of disease progression over time, familial nature of the aggressive disease, and a relative absence of local factors in aggressive disease compared to the presence of abundant plaque and calculus in chronic periodontitis.

- Chronic periodontitis is considered a site-specific disease. It is classified as localized periodontitis when <30% of sites assessed in the mouth demonstrate attachment loss and bone loss. It is termed as generalized periodontitis when >30% of the sites assessed in the mouth demonstrate attachment loss and bone loss.
- Based on the severity, chronic periodontitis is classified as slight (mild) when periodontal destruction is generally considered slight when no more than 1–2 mm of clinical attachment loss has occurred. Moderate periodontitis is when periodontal destruction is generally considered moderate when 3–4 mm of clinical attachment loss has occurred. Severe periodontitis is when periodontal destruction is considered severe when 5 mm or more of clinical attachment loss has occurred.
- Symptoms include gingival tenderness or itchiness, root exposure may lead to pain and sensitivity to heat, cold, or both. The presence of areas of food impactions may add to the patient's discomfort.
- Chronic periodontitis disease progression model includes the continuous model, the random or episodic burst model, and the asynchronous multiple burst model.
- The risk factors for chronic periodontitis include—prior history of periodontitis, local factors, systemic factors, environmental or behavioral factors, and genetic factors.
- Necrotizing ulcerative periodontitis (NUP) is an extension of necrotizing ulcerative gingivitis into the periodontal structures, leading to attachment and bone loss.
- Two types of NUP have been described according to their relationship with acquired immunodeficiency syndrome (AIDS)—non-AIDS type necrotizing ulcerative periodontitis and AIDs-associated necrotizing ulcerative periodontitis.
- Pseudomembrane—a whitish yellowish soft material covering the necrosed gingival margin. This inflammatory infiltrate in lesions of NUG, especially in long-standing cases can extend to the underlying bone, resulting in deep, crater-like osseous lesions, most often located in the interdental areas.
- NUP is characterized by deep interdental osseous craters, but deep conventional pockets are not found because the ulcerative and necrotizing character of the gingival lesion destroys the marginal epithelium, resulting in recession. Lesions of NUP can lead to advanced bone loss, tooth mobility, and tooth loss.
- The HIV-associated periodontal diseases include linear gingival erythema (LGE), NUG, and NUP. In these patients, complications include large areas of soft tissue necrosis with exposure of bone and sequestration of bone fragments, which sometimes extend to the vestibular area, palate, and become necrotizing stomatitis.
- Refractory periodontitis has been defined by the AAP as those patients who are unresponsive to any treatment provided, whatever the thoroughness or frequency. The etiology may be abnormal host response, an unusually pathogenic and virulent microflora, failure to eliminate plaque retentive factors, or combination of any of these factors.
- Periodontitis can be a manifestation of systemic diseases like Papillon–Lefèvre syndrome, Down syndrome, neutropenia, Chédiak–Higashi Syndrome, hypophosphatasia, and leukocyte adhesion deficiency.
- Aggressive periodontitis generally affects systemically healthy individuals less than 30 years old or older.
- It is universally distinguished from chronic periodontitis by the age of onset, the rapid rate of progression, nature and composition of microflora, alteration in the host's immune response, and familial aggregation of the diseased individuals.
- Aggressive periodontitis is classified as localized aggressive periodontitis (LAgP) and generalized aggressive periodontitis (GAaP).
- Localized aggressive periodontitis is usually characterized as having "localized first molar/incisor presentation with interproximal attachment loss on at least two permanent teeth, one of which is a first molar, and involving no more than two teeth other than first molars and incisors."
- *A. actinomycetemcomitans* is the major organism seen in aggressive periodontitis.
- Arc-shaped bone loss extending from the distal surface of the second premolar to the mesial surface of the second molar.
- Generalized aggressive periodontitis usually affects individuals under the age of 30, but older patients also may be affected.
- Generalized aggressive periodontitis is characterized by generalized interproximal attachment loss affecting at least three permanent teeth other than first molars and incisors.
- Radiographic picture in generalized aggressive periodontitis can range from severe bone loss associated with minimal number of teeth to majority of teeth.
- Risk factors for aggressive periodontitis include microbiologic factors, immunologic factor, genetic factors, and environmental factors.

Suggested Readings

Chronic Periodontitis

Chung WO, Dommisch H, Yin L, et al: Expression of defensins in gingiva and their role in periodontal health and disease, *Curr Pharm Des* 13:3073–3083, 2007.

Eke PI, Dye BA, Wei L, et al: Prevalence of periodontitis in adults in the United States: 2009 and 2010, *J Dent Res* 91:914–920, 2012.

Flemmig TF: Periodontitis, *Ann Periodontol* 4:32–38, 1999.

Kebschull M, Demmer RT, Papapanou PN: "Gum bug, leave my heart alone!"—epidemiologic and mechanistic evidence linking periodontal infections and atherosclerosis, *J Dent Res* 89:879–902, 2010.

Lang NP, Schatzle MA, Loe H: Gingivitis as a risk factor in periodontal disease, *J Clin Periodontol* 36(Suppl 10):3–8, 2009.

Lindhe J, Okamoto H, Yoneyama T, et al: Longitudinal changes in periodontal disease in untreated subjects, *J Clin Periodontol* 16:662–670, 1989.

Pihlstrom BL, Michalowicz BS, Johnson NW: Periodontal diseases, *Lancet* 366:1809–1820, 2005.

Preshaw PM, Alba AL, Herrera D, et al: Periodontitis and diabetes: a two-way relationship, *Diabetologia* 55:21–31, 2012.

Schaefer AS, Richter GM, Nothnagel M, et al: A 3' UTR transition within DEFB1 is associated with chronic and aggressive periodontitis, *Genes Immun* 11:45–54, 2010.

Tonetti MS: Cigarette smoking and periodontal diseases: etiology and management of disease, *Ann Periodontol* 3:88–101, 1998.

Necrotizing Ulcerative Periodontitis

Cobb CM, Ferguson BL, Keselyak NT, et al: A TEM/SEM study of the microbial plaque overlying the necrotic gingival papillae of HIV-seropositive, necrotizing ulcerative periodontitis, *J Periodontal Res* 38(2):147–155, 2003.

Feller L, Lemmer J: Necrotizing periodontal diseases in HIV-seropositive subjects: pathogenic mechanisms, *J Int Acad Periodontol* 10(1):10–15, 2008.

Glick M, Muzyka BC, Salkin LM, et al: Necrotizing ulcerative periodontitis: a marker for immune deterioration and a predictor for the diagnosis of AIDS, *J Periodontol* 65 (5):393–397, 1994.

Jimenez LM, Duque FL, Baer PN, et al: Necrotizing ulcerative periodontal diseases in children and young adults in Medellin, Colombia, 1965–2000, *J Int Acad Periodontol* 7(2):55–63, 2005.

Novak MJ: Necrotizing ulcerative periodontitis, *Ann Periodontol* 4(1): 74–78, 1999.

Winkler JR, Grassi M, Murray PA: *Clinical description and etiology of HIV-associated periodontal diseases*, Littleton, MA, 1988, PSG Publishing.

Aggressive Periodontitis

Armitage GC: Comparison of the microbiological features of chronic and aggressive periodontitis, *Periodontol 2000* (53):70–88, 2010.

Armitage GC, Cullinan MP: Comparison of the clinical features of chronic and aggressive periodontitis, *Periodontol 2000* (53):12–27, 2010.

Demmer RT, Papapanou PN: Epidemiologic patterns of chronic and aggressive periodontitis, *Periodontol 2000* (53):28–44, 2010.

Fine DH, Markowitz K, Furgang D, et al: *Aggregatibacter actinomycetemcomitans* and its relationship to initiation of localized aggressive periodontitis: longitudinal cohort study of initially healthy adolescents, *J Clin Microbiol* 45(12):3859–3869, 2007.

Haubek D, Ennibi OK, Poulsen K, et al: Risk of aggressive periodontitis in adolescent carriers of the JP2 clone of *Aggregatibacter (Actinobacillus) actinomycetemcomitans* in Morocco: a prospective longitudinal cohort study, *Lancet* 371(9608):237–242, 2008.

Kebschull M, Guarnieri P, Demmer RT, et al: Molecular differences between chronic and aggressive periodontitis, *J Dent Res* 92(12):1081–1088, 2013.

Laine ML, Crielaard W, Loos BG: Genetic susceptibility to periodontitis, *Periodontol* 58(1):37–68, 2012, 2000.

Nowak M, Kramer B, Haupt M, et al: Activation of invariant NK T cells in periodontitis lesions, *J Immunol* 190(5):2282–2291, 2013.

Schaefer AS, Richter GM, Dommisch H, et al: CDKN2BAS is associated with periodontitis in different European populations and is activated by bacterial infection, *J Med Genet* 48(1):38–47, 2011.

Smith M, Seymour GJ, Cullinan MP: Histopathological features of chronic and aggressive periodontitis, *Periodontol 2000* (53):45–54, 2010.

References

References and MCQs with answers for the chapter are available on www.medenact.com.

CHAPTER 22

Pathology and Management of Periodontal Problems Associated With Viral Infection, Including HIV, COVID, and Others

AG Martinezi | PS Kumar | YL Hernandez-Kapila | N Ambalavanan

CHAPTER OUTLINE

The human oral microbiome consists of a complex community that spans all three domains of life (Archaea, Bacteria, Eukarya), including eukaryotic RNA and deoxyribonucleic acid (DNA) viruses and prokaryotic viruses. Viruses can cause acute, persistent, or latent infections as they have the capacity to integrate into the human genome as seen with endogenous retroviruses. Conversely, viruses also play a role in the formation of our commensal microbiome which begins shortly after birth and continuously develops throughout our lifetime. Due to early life variables, antibiotic use, host genetics, and the distinct selective pressures present between body sites, there are compositional variations of the human microbiome within this holobiont complex.

It has been postulated that enhanced bacterial pathogenicity may result from the reactivation of common herpes viruses and their intimate topographic relationship with putative periodontopathogens within diseased periodontal pockets. Viruses may compound the destructive inflammatory process by modulation of the host immune response which affects a similar cytokine and chemokine profile found in patients with periodontitis.

Oral Viral Ecology

Some viruses that reproduce in the lungs, nasal mucosa, or salivary glands are shed into the oral cavity. Transmission may occur through aerosols, contaminated hands, kissing, or spitting. Saliva that forms aerosol also contains both pathogenic bacteria (Staphylococcus species, *Porphymonas gingivalis*) and viruses (HIV, HSV, Epstein-Barr virus [EBV], hepatitis B virus) which are involved in the development of caries and periodontitis. Both the direct exchange and aerosolized particles can carry virus-like particles per milliliter of saliva, which is mainly composed of bacteriophages of the taxon Caudovirales with limited homologs of herpesviruses and circoviruses. Perhaps the best-known eukaryotic virus that is transmitted via saliva is EBV which results in mononucleosis or "kissing disease."

Viruses

Papilloma Viruses

Human papilloma viruses (HPVs) are a family of small, nonenveloped, double-stranded DNA viruses with cutaneous and mucosal tropism, causing the most common sexually transmitted disease. HPV has been isolated from inflamed periodontal tissues as HPV persists within the basal layer of stratified epithelium, which is found in ulcerated gingival sulcular epithelium. Indicators of microabrasions associated with oral inflammation, such as high interproximal plaque index and gingival bleeding index, are significantly correlated with the detection of oral HPV of any type. An association between HPV and periodontitis is biologically plausible due to the synergistic effects of extensive exposure of damaged crevicular epithelium and the ecological proximity to periodontopathogens. However, there is very little evidence to show a positive relationship between oral HPV infection and periodontitis.

Herpes Viruses

Herpes viruses are typically spread by close contact between infectious and susceptible hosts as they are fragile viruses that cannot survive independently for much time in the external environment. Human herpes viruses can spread in a variety of ways: transmitted directly from mother to child in breast milk (CMV) and spread among family members and close contact via saliva (HSV-1, CMV, EBV, HHV-6, -7, and -8). Of these viruses, HHV-6 and -7 are the most successful, infecting almost everyone worldwide. The prevalence of asymptomatic infections of EBV, CMV, and HSV-1 lies between 50% and 90% of the population, whereas the prevalence of herpesvirus-associated malignancies continues to rise (Table 22.1).

TABLE 22.1 Herpesvirus

Virus	Characteristics	Disease Association	Oral Pathos
Herpes simplex virus-1	Latency in sensory ganglia Causes orolabial disease	Herpetic gingivostomatitis Recurrent orolabial lesions Herpetic whitlow Keratoconjunctivitis Eczema herpeticum Pharyngitis Mononucleosis-like syndrome Encephalitis Neonatal infection	Adult herpetic gingivostomatitis HIV-/AIDS-related oral ulcers Recurrent oral aphthous stomatitis Behçet syndrome Oral pemphigus vulgaris Erythema multiforme Dry socket after tooth extraction
Herpes simplex virus-2	Latency in sensory ganglia Causes genital and newborn infections	Genital infection Aseptic meningitis Sacral autonomic nervous system dysfunction	—
Varicella-Zoster virus	Latency in sensory ganglia Only three major genotypes of the wild-type virus are known More than 90% are infected before adolescence in an unvaccinated population	Varicella (chickenpox) Herpes zoster (shingles) Central nervous system involvement pneumonia Secondary bacterial infections Death Available varicella vaccines include a single-antigen vaccine and a combination vaccine against measles-mumps-rubella-varicella	Recurrent oral aphthous stomatitis Osteomyelitis herpes zoster (Ramsay Hunt Syndrome)
Epstein-Barr virus	Identified initially in 1964 from African Burkitt lymphoma Infects epithelial cells with a cytolytic infection and B lymphocytes with a latent infection	Infectious mononucleosis Hairy leukoplakia of the tongue Burkitt lymphoma B lymphoproliferative disease Hodgkin lymphoma X-linked lymphoproliferative disease Nasal T-cell lymphoma Nasopharyngeal carcinoma Gastric carcinoma Parotid carcinoma Leiomyosarcoma	Recurrent oral aphthous stomatitis Erythema multiforme Various epithelial type tumors, such as lymphoepithelioma-like carcinoma, salivary gland lymphoepithelial carcinoma, Warthin tumor (cystadenolymphoma) of the parotid gland, oral squamous cell carcinoma, tonsillar carcinoma, oral undifferentiated carcinomas, and oral hairy leukoplakia Various lymphoid type tumors, such as Hodgkin lymphoma, T-cell/natural killer cell lymphoma, Burkitt lymphoma, cyclosporine-related posttransplant lymphoproliferative disorder, oral posttransplant lymphoproliferative disorder/ B-cell lymphoma, follicular lymphoid hyperplasia, and plasmablastic lymphoma Infectious mononucleosis
Human cytomegalovirus	Infects mainly T lymphocytes and macrophages The gB protein in the virion envelope participates in the virus-cell interaction and is a major target of the immune response	Preterm birth Preeclampsia Transplant rejection Immunosenescence Hemorrhagic retinal necrosis (patients with HIV) Encephalitis Infectious mononucleosis Atherosclerosis Gastrointestinal disease Pneumonia	HIV-/AIDS-related oral ulcers Recurrent oral aphthous stomatitis Behçet syndrome Oral pemphigus vulgaris Erythema multiforme Cyclosporine-steroid associated lymphoproliferative disorder Benign infantile hemangioendothelioma Kaposi sarcoma Occasionally infectious mononucleosis Sialadenitis Osteomyelitis
Human herpesvirus-6	Cell tropism for T lymphocytes and the neural cells Frequently shed in the saliva of healthy donors	Roseola infantum (sixth disease) Meningitis Encephalitis Possibly multiple sclerosis	Uvulopalatoglossal junctional ulcers Oral squamous cell carcinoma Oral leukoplakia Oral lichen planus
Human herpesvirus-7	Latency in macrophages and T lymphocytes Frequently shed in the saliva of healthy donors	Exanthema subitem Macular–papular rashes Transplant–recipient pathogens	—

TABLE 22.1 Herpesvirus—cont'd

Virus	Characteristics	Disease Association	Oral Pathos
Human herpesvirus-8	Six genetic subtypes with marked clustering to geographic area B lymphocytes and monocytes serve as reservoirs	Kaposi sarcoma Multicentric Castleman disease Primary effusion lymphoma Mononucleosis-like illness Aplastic anemia (unlike Epstein-Barr virus, herpesvirus-8 is not involved in epithelial tumors)	Recurrent oral aphthous stomatitis Kaposi sarcoma

AIDS, Acquired immunodeficiency syndrome; *HIV*, human immunodeficiency virus

Latency and active replication have been demonstrated to occur within various microenvironments of the oral cavity and the different cell types that comprise the periodontium. This state of dormancy can be disturbed by a number of environmental stresses that lead to the reactivation of viral replication, cellular lysis, viral transmission, and eventually clinical symptoms. In the oral cavity, an infection with herpesviruses can present itself as a primary herpetic stomatitis, herpes labialis (cold sores), chickenpox (varicella), or shingles (zoster). Herpes virus active infections can remain asymptomatic but still give rise to viral shedding, or they can cause illness that ranges from classic infectious diseases to benign and malignant tumors, especially in immunocompromised hosts (e.g., patients with acquired immunodeficiency syndrome [AIDS], organ transplant recipients).

Epstein-Barr Virus

EBV is classified into the γ-herpesviruses subfamily due to its very restrictive host range. Along with HHV-8, γ-herpesviruses are oncogenic viruses associated with Burkitt and Hodgkin lymphoma. Persistent infection and latency of EBV occur in epithelial cells of the oropharynx and in B-cells. It is estimated that more than 90% of adult humans present with a latent infection of EBV and are subject to EBV reactivation causing classic mononucleosis and several life-threatening diseases. The mechanisms which promote and regulate the reactivation of EBV are still being uncovered and are critical for potential prophylactic treatment. Close contact behaviors like kissing or sharing personal objects such as eating utensils, toothbrushes, food, and drinks with an infected individual can lead to the spread of EBV. EBV generally infects silently during childhood but may manifest as infectious mononucleosis in adolescents or young adults.

Periodontal epithelium, specifically the junctional epithelium, is commonly infected with EBV where one in vivo study found 13.2% of healthy and 30% of inflamed epithelium expressing elevated latent transcripts. Along with the presence in the periodontal epithelium, oral fluid samples further implicate EBV in the development or progression of periodontitis. Viral load within salivary samples may reflect the status of periodontal inflammation as there is a significant elevated difference of EBV in patients with periodontitis compared to healthy patients. A similar association of EBV levels in gingival crevicular fluid to the severity of periodontitis has been documented. However, an established association using these samples has not been achieved as several studies report a lack of association between EBV and periodontitis.

The high prevalence of EBV seen in ulcerated periodontal pockets demonstrates the potential contributions that the virus has on the multifactorial pathogenesis of periodontitis. Disruption of the innate immune response to bacterial challenges occurs during coinfection with herpesviruses. Architectural and functional changes occur within key periodontal inflammatory cells as herpesvirus-like viral bodies are identified within these cells in early-onset periodontitis.

Cytomegalovirus

Cytomegalovirus is classified into the β-herpesviruses subfamily due to its long replicative cycle and restricted host range. Cytomegalovirus is transmitted via close interpersonal contact with body fluids, including blood, semen, breast milk, urine, and saliva. The ubiquity of cytomegalovirus infection is reflected in an 80% worldwide seroprevalence in immunocompetent adults that increases with age. Primary infection, re-infection, or reactivation of cytomegalovirus typically manifests as asymptomatic in immunocompetent hosts. However, with an immature or compromised immune system, such as in neonates, transplant recipients, or HIV-infected individuals, the true pathogenic potential of cytomegalovirus may be realized.

Persistent cytomegalovirus replication occurs in oral structures, such as the salivary glands and oral manifestations may present. Approximately 30% of HIV-infected individuals with an asymptomatic infection shed cytomegalovirus through salivary secretions compared to only 1%–2% of immunocompetent individuals. Oral manifestations of cytomegalovirus infections are a rare occurrence but are characterized as painful necrotic oral mucosal ulcerations with a punched-out appearance and nonindurated borders that affect the lips, gingiva, tongue, or buccal mucosa.

Isolation of cytomegalovirus within advanced or necrotic periodontal lesions is often accompanied by gram-negative periodontopathogens. A significant association was noted for *Aggregatibacter actinomycetemcomitans*, *P. gingivalis* and cytomegalovirus, and aggressive periodontitis; however, the strongest dual infection association belonged to *A. actinomycetemcomitans* and cytomegalovirus. Thus, dual infection with cytomegalovirus may allude to additive or synergistic effects of herpesviruses in aggressive periodontitis-diseased sites. Modulation of the immune host response by cytomegalovirus may influence *A. actinomycetemcomitans* and *P. gingivalis* in ulcerated periodontal pockets. All of these pathogens invade and disrupt epithelial cells and potentially benefit from chemotaxis upregulation and inhibition of apoptosis in neutrophils modulated by cytomegalovirus.

Severe Acute Respiratory Syndrome Coronavirus

An outbreak of a viral respiratory illness originating from Wuhan, China, in late 2019 had its causative agent identified as a novel species from the genus beta coronavirus. In March 2020, the crisis was declared a pandemic as the RNA virus is responsible for more than 250 million cases worldwide that can result in diffuse alveolar damage, thromboembolism, and nonspecific shock injury in multiple organs. Transmission occurs mainly by exposure to infected aerosolized particles, droplet inhalation, and contact with infected individuals. Transmission by close contact is defined as being within 1 m of a known SARS-CoV-2 infected individual for over 15 min over a 24-h period. The incubation period for SARS-CoV-2 ranges from 2 to 14 days and transmission of the virus may occur during or after this period. A large proportion of transmission of SARS-CoV-2 appears to be through exposure to infected aerosols produced by presymptomatic and asymptomatic individuals during breathing or speaking. Infected tissues of the oral cavity may play a role in presymptomatic and asymptomatic spread as sources of cellular and acellular SARS-CoV-2 are commonly isolated in saliva.

The high percentage of asymptomatic carriers and unequivocal presence of SARS-CoV-2 in saliva evokes the risk of SARSCoV-2 infection during dental clinical treatments that generate aerosols. Limitations on various dental instruments such as high- or low-speed handpieces, ultrasonic scalers, and air-water sprays had been recommended at the early stages of the COVID-19 pandemic to diminish possible airborne transmission. Persistence of SARSCoV-2 within the oral cavity has been identified as oral tissues are enriched with ACE2 receptors and pose a risk for prolonged virus shedding even after respiratory symptoms. Despite the high viral loads in saliva, these viral particles may not be infectious as intraoral innate immune mechanisms such as oral epithelial cells produced β-defensins provide antiviral protection.

Mouth-SARS-CoV-2 Connection

A high density of ACE2 receptors and a high frequency of oral symptoms associated with COVID-19 suggest a greater role of the oral cavity in the pathogenesis of SARS-CoV-2 infection. The palate, tongue, gingiva, and lips represent the most frequent locations for oral COVID-19 symptoms that were present in 25% of mild to moderate cases. These oral lesions healed within 3–21 days, either spontaneously or through topical treatment and oral hygiene. Studies that have documented the onset of these oral mucosal lesions associate mild COVID-19 cases to oral symptoms that develop before or at the same time as initial respiratory symptoms, whereas lesions developed 7–24 days after respiratory symptoms were associated with COVID-19 hospitalizations. One hallmark prodromal symptom that is present in over half (54%) of patients presenting with mild to moderate SARS-CoV-2 infections as the sudden loss of taste (dysgeusia/ageusia) occurs prior to the onset of general COVID-19 symptoms. Characterizing oral prodromal symptoms of COVID-19 can alert individuals and dental practitioners of a progressing infection for which treatment in a timely manner is crucial.

Etiological agents and risk factors associated with COVID-19 indicate a potential relationship to periodontitis. The exact shared mechanisms between these two conditions are still sought after as COVID-19 patients with periodontitis are at a higher risk for complications (and ICU admission). Respiratory symptoms are exacerbated as SARS-CoV-2 interacts with both the lung and oral microbiome that modulates cytokine and immune cell regulation. Aspiration of *P. gingivalis* and *Fusobacterium nucleatum* have previously been implicated in the pathogenesis of respiratory illness and may stimulate ACE2 expression in the lungs during a SARS-CoV-2 infection due to cellular recognition of bacterial adhesion molecules and endotoxins.

Dysregulation in the functions of periodontal structures occurs during infection of SARS-CoV-2 which may further aggravate the bacterial dysbiosis that is essential in the development of periodontitis. Inflamed periodontal states in COVID-19 patients would subside as symptoms of COVID-19 resolved. The most apparent connection between COVID-19 and periodontitis is the hyperinflammatory response that may result in adverse outcomes. Chronic inflammatory conditions commonly associated with periodontitis such as diabetes, obesity, and cardiovascular disease also constitute high-risk factors for severe forms of COVID-19. In these conditions, the low- to moderate-grade inflammation and bacterial dysbiosis can create an environment for heightened SARS-CoV-2 virulence. More specifically, the keystone cytokines (IL-6, IL-1β, IL-8, TNF-α, INF-γ) released by immune cells in periodontitis stimulated by periodontopathogens overlap with the cytokines involved in the cytokine storm described in severe forms of COVID-19 manifestations. Although there is no established mechanism on how periodontitis directly affects systemic inflammation, these cytokines can enter the systemic circulation when transferred from the gingival crevicular fluid to saliva.

Preventative Measures

Dental practitioners should understand the fundamental characteristics of COVID-19 and implement protective measures that reduce the risk of cross-infection during dental procedures. Patient screening prior to scheduled dental appointments should be performed in order to identify symptomatic or asymptomatic SARS-CoV-2 infected individuals. At the appointment, the patient's temperature should be taken, and any signs of fever, coughing, or shortness of breath should be assessed.

In preparation to treat patients during viral outbreaks, the execution of universal infection control protocols by all dental personnel is imperative. Infectious droplets from saliva or blood during dental procedures may be inhaled by the dental staff or come in contact with dental instruments that should be sterilized after every patient encounter. Reduction of aerosol production can be achieved by switching to hand instruments, use of rubber dams, and performing four-handed dentistry. A preprocedural therapeutic mouthrinse with chlorhexidine may be helpful in significantly reducing the microbial and SARS-CoV-2 load transiently in dental aerosols. Increasing the ventilation in health care facilities during and after dental procedures has the potential to reduce the circulating concentration of infectious viral particles as aerosolized SAR-CoV-2 can remain in the air for up to 3–12 h. Inactivation of SARS-CoV-2 can be achieved by aerosolized hydrogen peroxide, hydrogen peroxide vapor, hydrogen ultraviolet C light, and gaseous ozone.

Human Immunodeficiency Virus

Acquired immunodeficiency syndrome (AIDS) is characterized by profound impairment of the immune system. The condition was first reported in 1981, and a viral pathogen, the *human immunodeficiency virus (HIV)*, was identified in 1984. The condition was originally thought to be restricted to male homosexuals. Subsequently, it was also identified in male and female heterosexuals and bisexuals who participated in unprotected sexual activities or who abused injected drugs. Currently, sexual activity and drug abuse remain the primary means of transmission.

HIV has a strong affinity for cells of the immune system, most specifically those that carry the CD4 cell surface receptor molecule. Thus, helper T lymphocytes (T4 cells) are most profoundly affected, but monocytes, macrophages, Langerhans cells, and some neuronal and glial brain cells may also be involved. Viral replication occurs continuously in the lymphoreticular tissues of the lymph nodes, the spleen, the gut-associated lymphoid cells, and the macrophages.

Pathogenesis

In patients with untreated or inadequately treated HIV infection, the overall effect is the gradual impairment of the immune system via interference with T4 (CD4) lymphocytes and other immune cell functions. Evidence indicates that innate immune response may play a role in controlling HIV replication. Chemokine receptor type 5 (CCR5) is found on the surface of CD4 cells, and it often serves as a point of entry for HIV into the cell.

B lymphocytes are not infected, but the altered function of infected T4 lymphocytes secondarily results in B-cell dysregulation and altered neutrophil function. This may place HIV-positive individuals at increased risk for malignancy and disseminated infections with microorganisms such as viruses, mycobacterioses, and mycoses. HIV-positive individuals are also at increased risk for adverse drug reactions as a result of altered antigenic regulation. Epithelial cells of the mucosa may become infected, and they may allow the virus to access the bloodstream. Some evidence suggests that oral epithelial cells may harbor HIV virions and infect CD4+ cells by direct cell-to-cell transfer or by transporting and releasing low levels of infectious virions. Most evidence, however, indicates that oral transmucosal viral transmission occurs after mild or severe traumatic injury or puncture of the mucous membranes. This allows for the infection of circulating host defense cells such as lymphocytes, macrophages, and dendritic cells. HIV has been detected in most body fluids, although it is found in high quantities only in blood, semen, and cerebrospinal fluid. Transmission occurs almost exclusively by sexual contact, illicit use of injection drugs, or exposure to blood or blood products. Transmission after human bites has been reported, although the risk is extremely low.

The high-risk population includes homosexual and bisexual men, users of illegal injection drugs, persons with hemophilia or other coagulation disorders, recipients of blood transfusions before April 1985, infants of HIV-infected mothers (in whom transmission occurs by fetal transmission, at delivery, or by breastfeeding), promiscuous heterosexuals, and individuals who engage in unprotected sex with HIV-positive cohorts.

Highly Active Antiretroviral Therapy

With highly active antiretroviral therapy (HAART), combinations of three or more antiretroviral drugs are administered simultaneously for long periods of time in an effort to block HIV replication and plasma viral load and to restore immune function while minimizing antiretroviral drug resistance and adverse drug effects. The goals are to improve the patient's quality of life and reduce HIV-related morbidity and mortality. Three commonly used combinations are one nonnucleoside reverse transcriptase inhibitor plus two nucleoside reverse transcriptase inhibitors (NRTIs), one or two protease inhibitors plus two NRTIs, or three NRTIs. One NRTI three-drug combination is available in a single tablet, but this antiretroviral therapy does not necessarily qualify as HAART. It has now been many years since the advent of HAART, and some authorities propose that drug combinations be personalized for each HIV-positive individual on the basis of the specific characteristics of the drugs (e.g., toxicity, potency, central nervous system/sanctuary site penetration), the virus (e.g., resistance pattern, history of antiretroviral use, CCR5 tropism), and the host (e.g., lifestyle, compliance, drug interactions, non-AIDS comorbidities, organ dysfunction, pregnancy). In addition, evidence has indicated that early treatment is far more successful than delayed treatment. Before the advent of antiretroviral therapy, opportunistic infections were the principal cause of morbidity and mortality among HIV-infected persons. Opportunistic infections continue to occur among those who are unaware of their HIV infection, those who do not take recommended medications, and those who are resistant or react adversely to recommended medications. In some instances, HAART has not altered the rate of occurrence or severity of certain opportunistic infections, whereas it is associated with the increased occurrence of others. Commonly described systemic conditions that may be found more often after HAART are lipodystrophy, increased insulin resistance, gynecomastia, blood dyscrasias, and dermatologic disorders. In the oral cavity, candidal infections are markedly reduced among individuals who are responsive to antiretroviral therapy; hairy leukoplakia, Kaposi sarcoma (KS), deep mycoses, necrotizing ulcerative gingivitis (NUG), and necrotizing ulcerative periodontitis (NUP) are reduced in these patients as well. Conversely, the incidence and severity of oral condylomata and HSV infection appear unchanged, whereas neutropenia-associated oral aphthous-like ulcers; lichenoid reactions; and oral melanotic macules of the lip, gingiva, palate, or buccal mucosa may increase. On the basis of these observations, the presence or absence of oral opportunistic infections associated with HIV infection or its treatment may serve as markers for the success or failure of antiretroviral therapy.

Oral and Periodontal Manifestations of Human Immunodeficiency Virus Infection

Oral lesions are common in HIV-infected patients, although geographic and environmental variables may exist. Previous reports have indicated that most patients with AIDS have head and neck lesions, whereas oral lesions are common among HIV-positive individuals who do not yet have AIDS. Several reports have identified a strong correlation between HIV infection and oral candidiasis, oral hairy leukoplakia, atypical periodontal diseases, oral KS, and oral non-Hodgkin lymphoma (NHL).

Oral lesions less strongly associated with HIV infection include melanotic hyperpigmentation, mycobacterial infections, necrotizing ulcerative stomatitis (NUS), miscellaneous oral ulcerations, and viral infections (e.g., herpes simplex virus [HSV], herpes zoster, and condyloma acuminatum). Lesions that are seen in HIV-infected individuals with undetermined frequency include less common viral infections (e.g., CMV, molluscum contagiosum), recurrent aphthous stomatitis, and bacillary angiomatosis (epithelioid angiomatosis) (Box 22.1).

The advent of HAART has resulted in a greatly diminished frequency of oral lesions associated with HIV infection and AIDS.

However, some medical protocols delay the use of HAART drugs until immune suppression is relatively severe. These protocols also discontinue HAART if immune stability has been achieved or if the targeted virus becomes drug resistant. In theory, these protocols suggest that patients with HIV and AIDS may experience a greater number of oral manifestations than patients who start HAART therapy earlier. The dental practitioner must continue to be prepared to diagnose and manage these conditions in coordination with the patient's physician. However, HIV resistance to antiretroviral drug therapy is an ongoing problem, and this resistance may even be transmitted to newly infected sexual partners or newborns of infected mothers.

Oral Candidiasis

Candidiasis is the most common oral lesion associated with HIV disease, and it has been found in approximately 90% of patients with AIDS. It usually has one of four clinical presentations: pseudomembranous, erythematous, or hyperplastic candidiasis or angular cheilitis.

Pseudomembranous candidiasis (thrush) presents as painless or slightly sensitive, yellow-white, curd-like lesions that can be readily scraped and separated from the surface of the oral mucosa. This type is most common on the hard and soft palate and the buccal or labial mucosa, but it can occur anywhere in the oral cavity.

BOX 22.1 Oral Manifestations of HIV Infection

Oral candidiasis	Non-Hodgkin lymphoma
Oral hairy leukoplakia	Bacillary (epithelioid) angiomatosis
Kaposi sarcoma	Oral hyperpigmentation

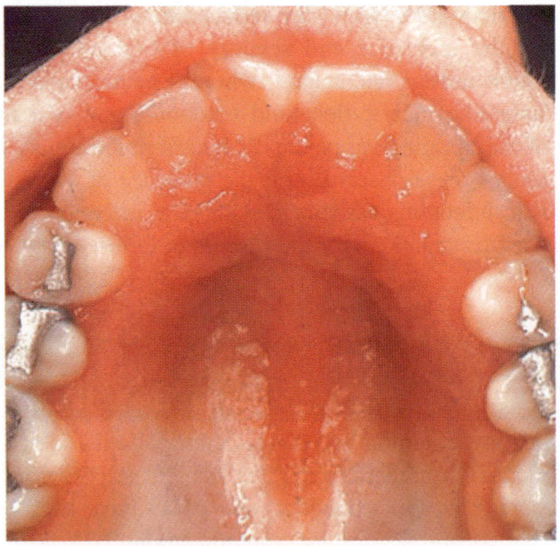

Fig. 22.1 Palatal erythematous candidiasis.

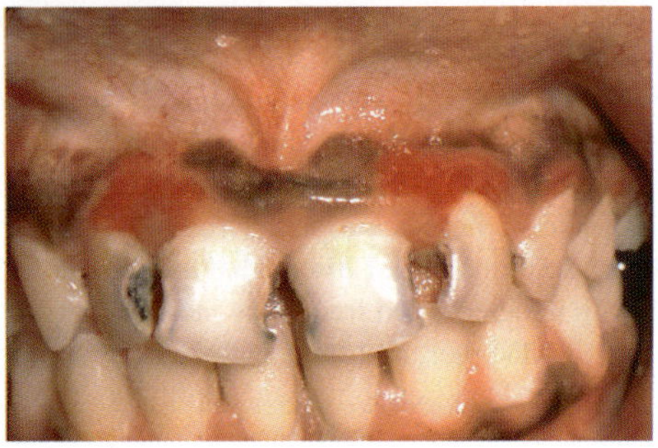

Fig. 22.2 Gingival erythematous candidiasis that is suggestive of desquamative gingivitis.

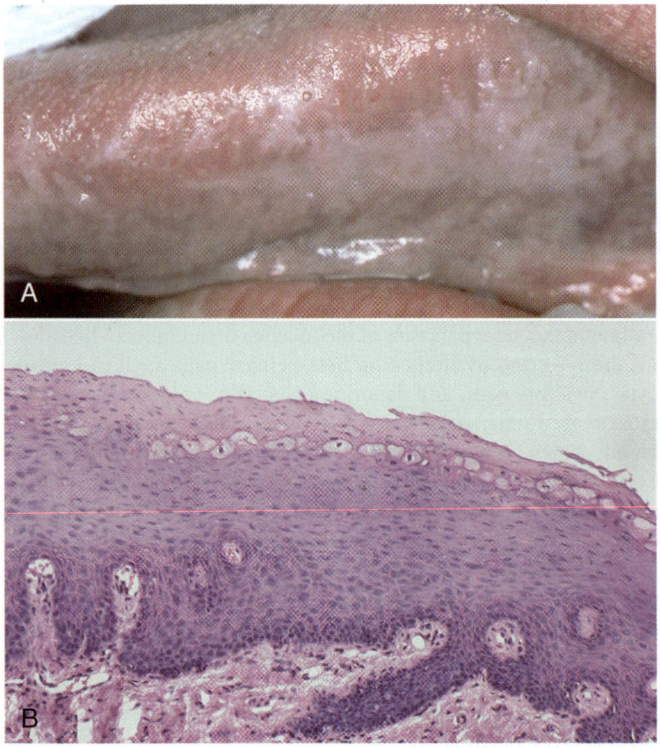

Fig. 22.3 Oral hairy leukoplakia on the left lateral border of the tongue. A, Clinical view. B, Biopsy confirmation of oral hairy leukoplakia. Note the ballooned epithelial cells near the surface of the epithelium.

Erythematous candidiasis may be present as a component of the pseudomembranous type, appearing as red patches on the buccal or palatal mucosa, or it may be associated with depapillation of the tongue. If the gingiva is affected, it may be misdiagnosed as desquamative gingivitis (Figs. 22.1 and 22.2). Some evidence suggests that erythematous candidiasis is more common among HIV-positive individuals with CD4+ counts between 200 and 500 cells/μL, whereas the pseudomembranous form occurs in patient with less than 200 CD4+ cells/μL. Viral load is most often elevated to more than 100,000 copies/mL. However, it should be emphasized that any form of candidiasis can be found in individuals who are only minimally immunocompromised.

Hyperplastic candidiasis is the least common form, and it may be seen in the buccal mucosa and the tongue. It is more resistant to removal than the other types.

In *Candida*-related *angular cheilitis*, the commissures of the lips appear erythematous, with surface crusting and fissuring.

The diagnosis of candidiasis is made by clinical evaluation, culture analysis, or microscopic examination of a tissue sample or smear of material scraped from the lesion (oral cytology), which shows hyphae and yeast forms of the organisms. When oral candidiasis appears in patients with no apparent predisposing cause, the clinician should be alerted to the possibility of HIV infection. Many patients who are at risk for HIV infection who present with oral candidiasis also have esophageal candidiasis, which is a diagnostic sign of AIDS.

Oral Hairy Leukoplakia

Oral hairy leukoplakia (OHL) primarily occurs in persons with HIV infection. It is found on the lateral borders of the tongue, it frequently has a bilateral distribution, and it may extend to the ventrum. OHL is caused by the EBV, and it is the only EBV lesion with which viral shedding in saliva is common. The lesion is characterized by an asymptomatic, poorly demarcated, keratotic area that ranges in size from a few millimeters to several centimeters (Fig. 22.3A). Often, characteristic vertical striations are present, and these impart a corrugated appearance; the surface may also be shaggy and appear hairy when dried. The lesion does not rub off, and it may resemble other keratotic oral lesions.

Microscopically, the OHL lesion shows a hyperparakeratotic surface with projections that often resemble hairs. Beneath the parakeratotic surface, acanthosis and some characteristic "balloon cells" that resemble koilocytes are seen (Fig. 22.3B). It has been demonstrated that these cells contain viral particles of the human herpesvirus group; these particles have been interpreted as EBV.

Epithelial dysplasia is not a feature, and, in most OHL lesions, little or no inflammatory infiltrate in the underlying connective tissue is present.

OHL is found almost exclusively on the lateral borders of the tongue, although it has been reported on the dorsum of the tongue, the buccal mucosa, the floor of the mouth, the retromolar area, and the soft palate. In addition, most of these lesions reveal surface colonization by *Candida* organisms, which are secondary invaders and not the cause of the lesion.

OHL was originally thought to be caused by the human papillomavirus, but subsequent evidence has indicated an association with EBV. Regardless of the cause, biopsy identification of a lesion that is suggestive of OHL should dictate that HIV testing be performed. It should be emphasized that the severity of the lesion is not correlated with the likelihood of developing AIDS; thus small lesions are as diagnostically significant as extensive lesions.

The differential diagnosis of OHL includes several white lesions of the mucosa, such as dysplasia, carcinoma, frictional and idiopathic

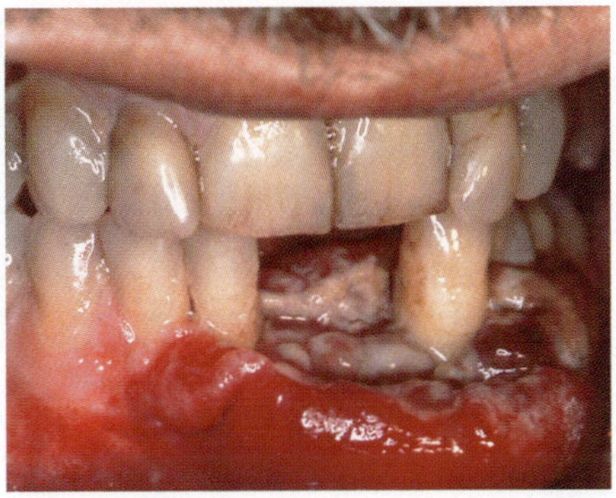

Fig. 22.4 Non-Hodgkin lymphoma of the anterior mandibular gingiva.

keratosis, lichen planus, tobacco-related leukoplakia, secondary syphilis, psoriasiform lesions (e.g., geographic tongue), and hyperplastic candidiasis. The microscopic confirmation of OHL of the tongue in a high-risk patient is considered to be a specific early sign of HIV infection and an indication that the patient will develop AIDS. Before the advent of effective therapy for HIV, survival analysis indicated that 83% of HIV-infected patients with hairy leukoplakia would develop AIDS within 31 months, and the number of patients with hairy leukoplakia who eventually developed AIDS approached 100%. The use of HAART, however, has resulted in a greatly diminished incidence of OHL.

Kaposi Sarcoma and Other Malignancies

Oral malignancies occur more frequently in severely immunocompromised individuals than in the general population. An HIV-positive individual with NHL or KS is categorized as having AIDS. Oral lesions are reported in approximately 4% of individuals with NHL, and the gingiva and palate are common sites. The incidence of oral squamous cell carcinoma may also increase among HIV-infected individuals. KS was a rare disease until the early 1980s. In its classic form, it is found in older men and occasionally in patients after organ transplants, and it is endemic in parts of Africa. An epidemic form has subsequently been described in HIV-positive individuals, and it is an AIDS-defining condition.

KS is the most common oral malignancy associated with AIDS. This angioproliferative tumor is a rare, multifocal, vascular neoplasm; it was originally described in 1872 as occurring in the skin of the lower extremities of older men of Mediterranean origin. Today, it is closely associated with homosexual and heterosexual transmission, but it occurs 5–10 times more often among male homosexuals than in other groups at high risk for HIV. The causative agent has been identified as human herpesvirus-8 (HHV-8).

Lymphedema of the neck and face has been reported in association with oral lesions. The cause of lymphedema has not been determined, but it may result from the compression of lymphatics by expanding lesions. The presence of facial lymphedema is considered to be an ominous sign that is associated with a fatal outcome.

During the early stages, the oral lesions are painless, reddish-purple macules of the mucosa. As they progress, the lesions frequently become nodular, and they can easily be confused with other oral vascular entities, such as hemangiomas, hematomas, varicosities, or pyogenic granulomas (when occurring in the gingiva).

Lesions may manifest as nodules, papules, or nonelevated macules that are usually brown, blue, or purple, although occasionally they may display normal pigmentation. The lesions may become painful if they become ulcerated or traumatized by opposing teeth as they enlarge. Diagnosis is based on histologic findings.

Gingival KS lesions may be exacerbated by existing periodontal lesions, or necrotizing periodontal diseases may be superimposed on existing gingival KS. On occasion, the expansion of gingival lesions may result in bone resorption, and increased tooth mobility and loss has been reported.

The advent of HAART has resulted in a marked reduction in the incidence of KS. However, the lesions may still be found in severely immunocompromised individuals who are unaware of their HIV-positive status or who are untreated or unresponsive to therapy. HHV-8 may be found more frequently in the saliva of HIV-positive individuals with higher CD4 cell counts, which suggests that viral shedding may occur relatively early during the disease process. Treatment of oral KS includes antiretroviral agents, laser excision, cryotherapy, radiation therapy, and intralesional injection with vinblastine, interferon-γ, sclerosing agents, or other chemotherapeutic drugs. Nichols and colleagues described the successful use of intralesional vinblastine injections at a dose of 0.1 mg/cm^2 with the use of a 0.2 mg/mL solution of vinblastine sulfate in saline. However, comparable results may be obtained with injections of 3% sodium tetradecyl sulfate, a sclerosing agent that was previously used for the treatment of varicose veins. The sclerosing agent offers the advantage of being relatively inexpensive and easy to use. Destructive periodontitis has also been reported in conjunction with gingival KS. In such patients, scaling and root planing as well as other periodontal therapy may be indicated in addition to intralesional or systemic chemotherapy.

Today, some authorities recommend treating oral KS with a combination of HAART and systemic cytotoxic therapy.

Non-Hodgkin Lymphoma

Lymphoma represents a heterogeneous malignancy that is characterized by the proliferation of lymphoid cells. It is broadly classified as Hodgkin disease (14%) or NHL. NHL in individuals with HIV infection is an AIDS-defining condition, and elevated cumulative viremia may be a strong predictor of AIDS-related lymphoma.

The risk of NHL is associated with a number of infections; EBV-associated lesions may include Burkitt lymphoma and HIV-associated lymphoma. NHL is characterized by malignancy of B or T lymphocytes, and tumors are typed by the WHO classification system as indolent, aggressive, or highly aggressive. NHL is treated by chemotherapy, and HAART does not appear to significantly reduce the incidence or prognosis of the malignancies, although HIV-associated NHL may be less common.

Oral lesions usually appear as erythematous, painless enlargements that may become ulcerated as a result of traumatic injury. In some cases, bone involvement occurs. Lesions commonly affect the gingival, palatal, and alveolar mucosa, and they may mimic dental infections (Fig. 22.4). Diagnosis is based on physical examination, complete blood count with differential, imaging studies, and lymph node and tissue biopsy.

Patients with AIDS and NHL may require management of HIV-related opportunistic infections, chemotherapy-induced mucositis and thrombocytopenia, and possibly graft-versus-host disease, if hematopoietic cell transplantation is performed.

Bacillary (Epithelioid) Angiomatosis

Bacillary (epithelioid) angiomatosis (BA) is an infectious vascular proliferative disease with clinical and histologic features similar to those of KS. BA is caused by facultative intracellular gram-negative mobile bacilli of the genus *Bartonella* and the order Rickettsia (e.g., *Bartonella henselae, Bartonella quintana*). Cats are the primary host of *B. henselae*, and the infection is usually transmitted to

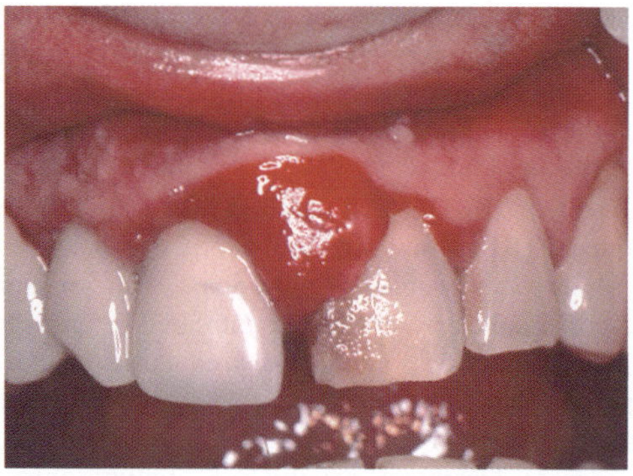

Fig. 22.5 Bacillary angiomatosis mimicking Kaposi sarcoma.

humans by bites, scratches, or fleas (i.e., cat-scratch fever). Humans are the primary reservoir for *B. quintana*, and it is usually transmitted by human lice. BA can occur in immunocompetent persons, but it is most commonly associated with AIDS. Skin lesions are similar to those associated with KS or cat-scratch disease. Gingival BA manifests as red, purple, or blue edematous soft-tissue lesions that may cause the destruction of periodontal ligament and bone (see Fig. 22.5).

The condition is more prevalent in HIV-positive individuals with low CD4 levels.

The diagnosis of BA is based on biopsy, which reveals an "epithelioid" proliferation of angiogenic cells accompanied by an acute inflammatory cell infiltrate. The causative organism in the biopsy specimen may be identified with the use of Warthin–Starry silver staining or electron microscopy.

The differential diagnosis of BA includes KS, angiosarcoma, hemangioma, pyogenic granuloma, and nonspecific vascular proliferation. BA is usually treated with broad-spectrum antibiotics such as erythromycin or doxycycline. Gingival lesions may be managed by using the antibiotic in conjunction with conservative periodontal therapy and possibly excision of the lesion. To date, no reports have been found regarding the effect of HAART on BA incidence among HIV-positive individuals. However, one case report described a fatal outcome of *B. quintana*-derived BA during HAART-induced immunity restoration.

Oral Hyperpigmentation

An increased incidence of *oral hyperpigmentation* has been described in HIV-infected individuals. Oral pigmented areas often appear as spots or striations on the buccal mucosa, the palate, the gingiva, or the tongue (Fig. 22.6B & C). At present, most reports describing the oral features of HIV/AIDS or post-HAART HIV/AIDS come from areas of the world where racial pigmentation may be common. In these areas, oral evaluation may often be accomplished by nondental health care workers. Consequently, it is not possible to accurately assess the degree of HIV-related oral hyperpigmentation before or after ART.

In some cases, the pigmentation may relate to the prolonged use of drugs such as zidovudine, ketoconazole, or clofazimine. Zidovudine is also associated with excessive pigmentation of the skin and nails, although similar hyperpigmentation has been reported in some individuals who have never taken zidovudine. On occasion, oral pigmentation may be the result of adrenocorticoid insufficiency that has been induced in an HIV-positive individual via the prolonged use of ketoconazole or by *Pneumocystis jiroveci*, CMV, or other viral infections (see Fig. 22.6A).

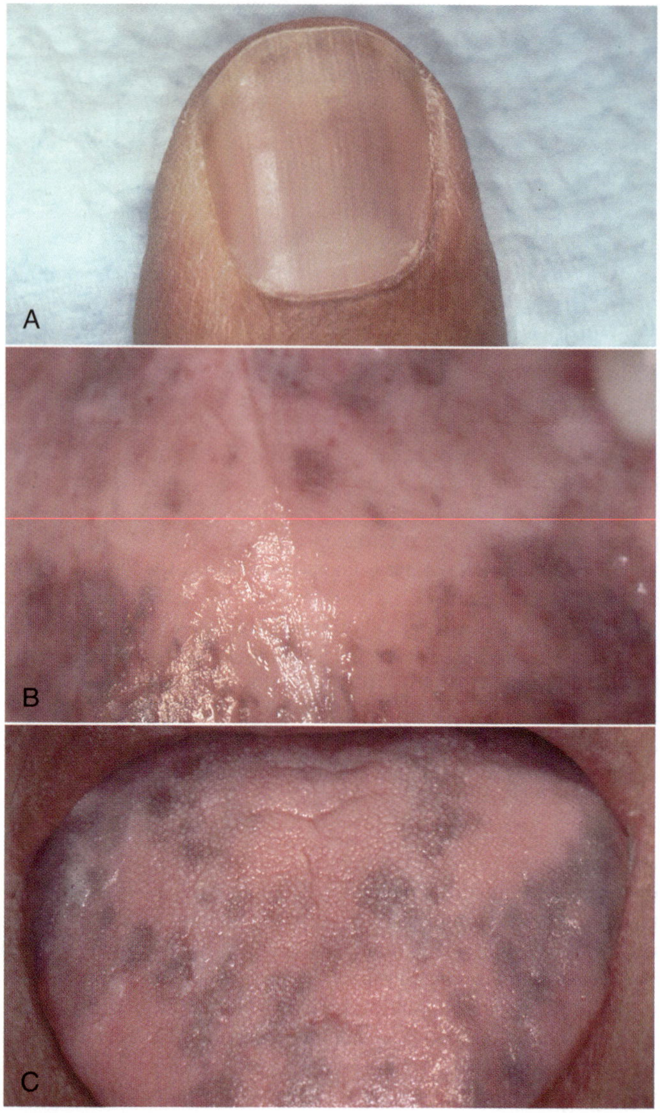

Fig. 22.6 Drug-induced hyperpigmentation as a result of zidovudine use. A, Palatal hyperpigmentation in the same patient. B, Tongue hyperpigmentation in the same patient.

Dental Treatment Complications

Concerns have been expressed regarding the potential for postoperative complications (e.g., hemorrhage, infection, delayed wound healing) in individuals with HIV or AIDS. Medically compromised patients must be carefully managed in the dental office to avoid undue treatment complications. On occasion, the poor overall health status of an individual with AIDS may limit periodontal therapy to conservative, minimally invasive procedures, and antibiotic therapy may be required. When possible, antibiotics should be avoided in significantly immunocompromised individuals to minimize the risk of opportunistic infections (e.g., candidiasis), superinfection, and microorganism drug resistance.

Gingival and Periodontal Diseases (Box 22.2)

Considerable research has focused on the nature and incidence of periodontal diseases in HIV-infected individuals. Some studies suggest that chronic periodontitis is more common in this patient population, but others do not. Periodontal diseases are more common

BOX 22.2 Periodontal Manifestations of HIV Infection

Linear gingival erythema	Necrotizing ulcerative stomatitis
Necrotizing ulcerative gingivitis	Chronic periodontitis
Necrotizing ulcerative periodontitis	

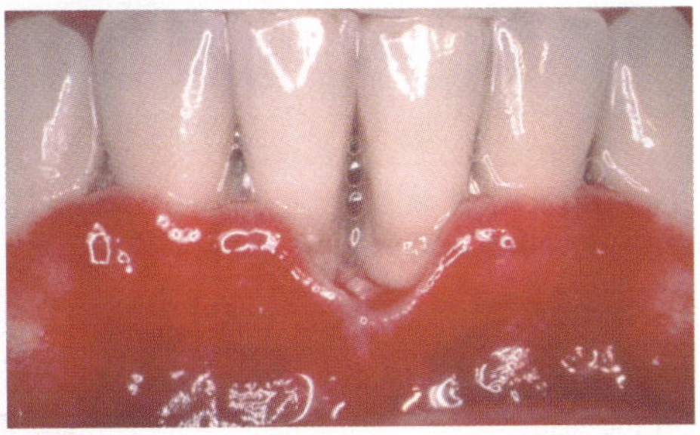

Fig. 22.7 Linear gingival erythema and necrotizing ulcerative gingivitis in a patient with acquired immunodeficiency syndrome.

among HIV-infected users of injection drugs, but this may relate to poor oral hygiene and a lack of dental care rather than decreased CD4 cell counts. However, some unusual types of periodontal diseases do seem to occur with greater frequency among HIV-positive individuals.

Linear Gingival Erythema

A persistent, linear, easily bleeding, erythematous gingivitis has been described in some HIV-positive patients. The intensity of the erythema is disproportionate to the amount of plaque present. There is no ulceration, pocketing, or attachment loss, and the condition does not respond predictably to conventional periodontal therapy. Lesions that are clinically identical to linear gingival erythema (LGE) were observed before the advent of HIV in association with severely immunocompromised individuals or in those with NUG.

LGE may or may not serve as a precursor to rapidly progressive NUP (Fig. 22.7). The microflora of LGE may closely mimic that of periodontitis rather than gingivitis. However, *Candida* infection has been implicated as a major etiologic factor, and human herpesviruses have been proposed as possible triggers or cofactors. Linear gingivitis lesions may be localized or generalized in nature. The erythematous gingivitis may be limited to marginal tissue, extend into attached gingiva in a punctate or diffuse erythema, or extend into the alveolar mucosa.

Although LGE may sometimes be unresponsive to corrective therapy, such lesions may undergo spontaneous remission. Concomitant oral candidiasis and LGE lesions have been identified, which suggests a possible etiologic role for candidal species in LGE. In one study, direct microscopic cultures from LGE lesions implicated *Candida dubliniensis* in four patients, all of whom experienced complete or partial remission after systemic antifungal therapy. It is not yet known whether candidal infection is an etiologic factor in all LGE cases. A systematic review indicates that LGE is more common among HIV-infected populations but that most individuals who are HIV positive do not experience LGE.

Others have reported that LGE is most often found in HIV-positive individuals whose CD4+ counts are depressed (200–500 cells/mm^3 or <200 cells/mm^3) or whose viral loads are elevated, suggesting that it may represent an early marker of progressive immunodeficiency or even the transition to outright AIDS.

LGE-like lesions can sometimes be adequately managed by following the therapeutic principles associated with marginal gingivitis. However, as mentioned previously, it has been suggested that gingivitis lesions that respond to conventional therapy do not represent LGE. The affected sites should be scaled and polished. Subgingival irrigation with chlorhexidine or 10% povidone–iodine may be beneficial. The patient should be carefully instructed regarding the performance of meticulous oral hygiene procedures. The condition should be reevaluated 2–3 weeks after initial therapy. If the patient is compliant with home care procedures and the lesions persist, the possibility of a candidal infection should be considered. It is doubtful that topical antifungal rinses will reach the base of the gingival crevices. Consequently, the treatment of choice may be the empiric administration of a systemic antifungal agent, such as fluconazole, for 7–10 days.

It is important to remember that LGE is often refractory to treatment. If so, the patient should be carefully monitored for developing signs of more severe periodontal conditions (e.g., NUG, NUP, NUS). The patient should be placed on a 2- to 3-month recall maintenance interval and re-treated as necessary. As mentioned previously, despite the occasional resistance of LGE to conventional periodontal therapy, spontaneous remission may occur for reasons that are not yet known.

Necrotizing Ulcerative Gingivitis

Some reports have described an increased incidence of NUG among HIV-infected individuals, although this has not been substantiated by other studies.

There is no consensus regarding whether the incidence of NUG increases in HIV-positive patients. However, one study evaluated the HIV status of individuals who presented with necrotizing periodontal diseases, and 69% were found to be HIV seropositive. The treatment of NUG in these patients does not differ from that in HIV-negative individuals.

The affected gingiva may be exquisitely painful, and caution must be taken to avoid undue patient discomfort. Basic treatment may consist of the cleaning and debriding affected areas with a cotton pellet soaked in peroxide after applying a topical anesthetic. Escharotic oral rinses such as hydrogen peroxide should be used only rarely for any patient, and they are especially contraindicated in immunocompromised individuals. The patient should be seen daily or every other day for the first week, and debridement of affected areas is repeated at each visit. Plaque-control methods are gradually introduced. A meticulous plaque-control program should be taught and started as soon as the sensitivity of the area allows it. After initial healing has occurred, the patient should be able to tolerate scaling and root planing, if needed.

The patient should avoid tobacco, alcohol, and condiments. An antimicrobial oral rinse such as chlorhexidine gluconate 0.12% should be prescribed.

Systemic antibiotics such as metronidazole or amoxicillin may be prescribed for patients with moderate to severe tissue destruction, localized lymphadenopathy, or systemic symptoms. Metronidazole may be the antibiotic of choice, because it has been demonstrated to be effective for the treatment of NUG, and its narrow bactericidal spectrum may minimize the risk of secondary opportunistic infections such as candidiasis. The use of prophylactic antifungal medication should be considered if antibiotics are prescribed.

The periodontium should be reevaluated 1 month after the resolution of acute symptoms to assess the results of treatment and to determine whether further therapy will be necessary.

Necrotizing Ulcerative Periodontitis

A necrotizing, ulcerative, rapidly progressive form of periodontitis occurs more frequently among HIV-positive individuals, although

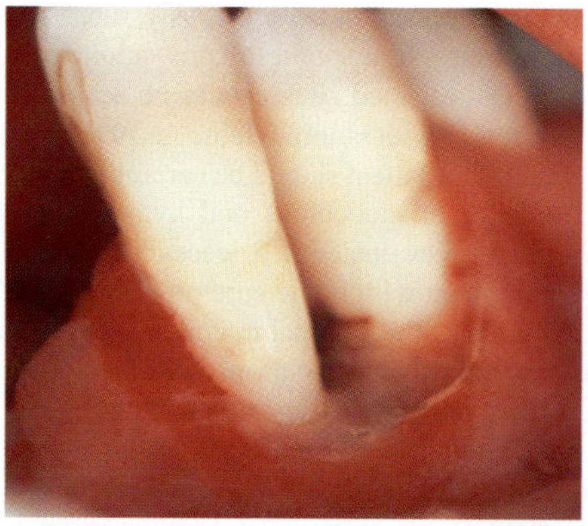

Fig. 22.8 Necrotizing ulcerative periodontitis. Note the adjacent linear gingival erythema.

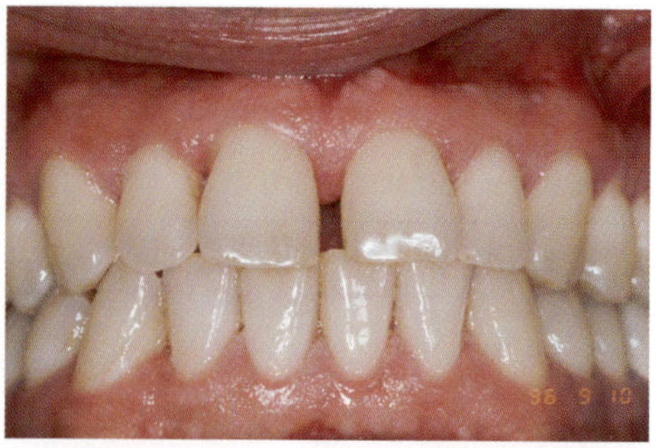

Fig. 22.9 Periodontal health in an individual with advanced acquired immunodeficiency syndrome.

such lesions were described long before the onset of the AIDS epidemic. NUP appears to represent an extension of NUG in which bone loss and periodontal attachment loss occur.

NUP is characterized by soft-tissue necrosis, rapid periodontal destruction, and interproximal bone loss (Fig. 22.8). Lesions may occur anywhere in the dental arches; they are usually localized to a few teeth, although generalized NUP is sometimes present after marked CD4+ cell depletion. Bone is often exposed, which results in necrosis and subsequent sequestration. NUP is severely painful at onset, and immediate treatment is necessary. Occasionally, however, patients undergo spontaneous resolution of the necrotizing lesions, which leave painless, deep, interproximal craters that are difficult to clean and that may lead to conventional periodontitis.

Some evidence suggests slight differences between the microbial flora found in NUP lesions and that found in chronic periodontitis, but most data implicate a similar microbial component in both diseases. An increasing number of studies, however, have identified the presence of candidal organisms and human herpesviruses of various types in individuals with necrotizing ulcerative periodontal diseases. The exact role of these organisms is not yet fully understood. As discussed previously, the reported periodontal health of HIV-infected individuals is subject to wide variations. Therapy for NUP includes local debridement; scaling and root planing; in-office irrigation with an effective antimicrobial agent such as chlorhexidine gluconate or povidone–iodine (Betadine); and the establishment of meticulous oral hygiene, including the home use of antimicrobial rinses or irrigation. This therapeutic approach is based on reports that involved only a small number of patients.

In patients with severe NUP, antibiotic therapy may be necessary, but it should be used with caution in HIV-infected patients to avoid an opportunistic and potentially serious localized candidiasis or even candidal septicemia. If an antibiotic is necessary, metronidazole (250 mg, with two tablets taken immediately and then two tablets taken four times daily for 5–7 days) is the drug of choice. The prophylactic prescription of a topical or systemic antifungal agent is prudent if an antibiotic is used.

Chronic Periodontitis

A number of longitudinal studies and prevalence studies have suggested that HIV-positive individuals are more likely to experience chronic periodontitis than the general population. Most studies, however, do not take into account the level of oral hygiene, the presence of preexisting gingivitis, poor diet, the age of the patient, smoking, other periodontal disease risk factors, the degree of immunodeficiency in the population studied, or whether the individuals in the study are injection drug users; these confounding factors cloud the issue.

With proper home care and appropriate periodontal treatment and maintenance, HIV-positive individuals can anticipate reasonably good periodontal health throughout the course of their disease. The median period between initial HIV infection and outright AIDS is approximately 15 years, and the life expectancy of persons living with AIDS has been significantly prolonged with current anti-HIV drug therapy.

This indicates that HIV-infected patients are potential candidates for conventional periodontal treatment procedures, including surgery and implant placement. Treatment decisions should be based on the overall health status of the patient, the degree of periodontal involvement, and the motivation and ability of the patient to perform effective oral hygiene (Fig. 22.9).

Periodontal Treatment Protocol

It is imperative that medically compromised patients, including those with HIV or AIDS, be safely and effectively managed in dental practice. Several universal treatment considerations are important to ensure that this goal is achieved.

Health Status

The patient's health status should be determined from the health history, the physical evaluation, and consultation with the patient's physician. Treatment decisions will vary, depending on the patient's state of health. For example, delayed wound healing and an increased risk of postoperative infection are possible complicating factors in patients with AIDS, but neither concern should significantly alter treatment planning for an otherwise healthy, asymptomatic, HIV-infected patient with a normal or near-normal CD4 count and a low viral bioload.

Infection Control Measures

The clinical management of HIV-infected periodontal patients requires strict adherence to established methods of infection control, which should be based on guidance from the American Dental Association and the CDC. Compliance, especially with universal precautions, will eliminate or minimize risks to both patients and the dental staff. Immunocompromised patients are potentially at risk for acquiring as well as transmitting infections in the dental office and other health care facilities.

Goals of Therapy

A thorough oral examination will determine the patient's dental treatment needs. The primary goal of dental therapy should be the restoration and maintenance of oral health, comfort, and function.

At the very least, periodontal treatment goals should be directed toward the control of HIV-associated mucosal diseases, such as chronic candidiasis and recurrent oral ulcerations. Acute periodontal and dental infections should be managed, and the patient should receive detailed instructions regarding the performance of effective oral hygiene procedures.

Conservative nonsurgical periodontal therapy should be a treatment option for virtually all HIV-positive patients, and the performance of elective surgical periodontal procedures, including implant placement, has been reported. NUP or NUS can be severely destructive to periodontal structures, but a history of these conditions does not automatically dictate the extraction of involved teeth, unless the patient is unable to maintain effective oral hygiene in the affected areas. Decisions regarding elective periodontal procedures should be made with the informed consent of the patient and after medical consultation, when possible.

Maintenance Therapy

It is imperative for the patient to maintain meticulous personal oral hygiene. In addition, periodontal maintenance recall visits should be conducted at short intervals (i.e., every 2–3 months), and any progressive periodontal disease should be treated vigorously.

As mentioned previously, systemic antibiotic therapy should be administered with caution. Blood and other medical laboratory tests may be required to monitor the patient's overall health status, and close consultation and coordination with the patient's physician are necessary.

Key points

- Viruses can cause acute, persistent, or latent infections as they have the capacity to integrate into the human genome.
- Viruses may compound the destructive inflammatory process of periodontitis by modulation of the host immune response.
- Altered functions of T4 lymphocytes secondarily result in B-cell dysregulation and altered neutrophil function, which places the HIV-positive individuals at greater risk for malignancy and disseminated infections.
- A CD4 count of less than 350/mm^3 is considered diagnostic for AIDS in adults and in children who are 5 years old or older.
- With HAART (highly active antiretroviral therapy), combinations of three or more antiretroviral drugs are administered simultaneously for long periods of time in an effort to block HIV replication and plasma viral load and to restore immune function while minimizing antiretroviral drug resistance and adverse drug effects.
- Oral lesions more strongly associated with HIV infection are oral candidiasis, oral hairy leukoplakia, atypical periodontal diseases, oral Kaposi sarcoma, and oral non-Hodgkin lymphoma.
- Kaposi sarcoma, an angioproliferative tumor is a multifocal, vascular neoplasm and is the most common oral malignancy associated with AIDS.
- Gingival bacillary angiomatosis manifests as red, purple, or blue edematous soft-tissue lesions that lead to the destruction of periodontal ligament and bone.
- Salivary gland hypofunction and xerostomia are most common among HIV-infected men during both the early and advanced stages of HIV infection and immunosuppression.
- Linear gingival erythema is most often found in HIV-positive individuals whose CD4+ counts are depressed (200–500 cells/mm^3 or $<$200 cells/mm^3) or whose viral loads are elevated.
- Linear gingival erythema may represent an early marker of progressive immunodeficiency or even the transition to outright AIDS.
- A necrotizing, ulcerative, rapidly progressive form of periodontitis occurs more frequently among HIV-positive individuals, which is characterized by soft tissue necrosis, rapid periodontal destruction, and interproximal bone loss.
- The clinical management of HIV-infected periodontal patients requires strict adherence to established methods of infection control.
- Periodontal treatment goals should be directed toward the control of HIV-associated mucosal diseases, such as chronic candidiasis and recurrent oral ulcerations. Acute periodontal and dental infections should be managed, and the patient should receive detailed instructions regarding the performance of effective oral hygiene procedures.

Suggested Readings

AIDS Education and Training Centers: HIV classification: CDC and WHO staging systems, 2006.

González OA, Ebersole JL, Huang CB: Oral infectious diseases: a potential risk factor for HIV virus recrudescence? *Oral Dis* 15:313–332, 2009.

Kaplan JE, Benson C, Holmes KK, Centers for Disease Control and Prevention (CDC), National Institutes of Health, HIV Medicine Association of the Infectious Diseases Society of America, et al: Guidelines for prevention and treatment of opportunistic infections in HIV-infected adults and adolescents: recommendations from CDC, the National Institutes of Health and the HIV Medicine Association of the Infectious Diseases Society of America, *MMWR* 58(RR-4):1–207, 2009.

Matafsi M, Skoura L, Sakellari D: HIV infection and periodontal diseases: an overview of the post-HAART era, *Oral Dis* 17:13–25, 2011.

Mosca NG, Hathorn AR: HIV-positive patients: dental management considerations, *Dent Clin North Am* 50:635–657, 2006.

Pantanowitz L, Khammissa RAG, Lemmer J, et al: Oral HIV-associated Kaposi sarcoma, *J Oral Pathol Med* 42:201–207, 2013.

Toppuni AR: Immune reconstitution inflammatory syndrome, *Adv Dent Res* 23:90–96, 2011.

Umadevi M, Adeyemi O, Patel M, et al: Periodontal diseases and other bacterial infections, *Adv Dent Res* 19:139–145, 2006.

Vacharajsa A, Asrani AC, Gebhard KH, et al: Oral keratinocytes support nonreplicative infection and transfer or harbored HIV-1 to permissive cells, *Retrovirology* 5:66, 2008.

References

References and MCQs with answers for the chapter are available on www.medenact.com.

CHAPTER 23

Impact of Periodontal Infection on Systemic Health

BL Mealey | PR Klokkevold | YL Hernandez-Kapila | N Ambalavanan

CHAPTER OUTLINE

Pathobiology of Periodontitis

Our understanding of the pathogenesis of periodontitis has changed remarkably over the last 40 years. The nonspecific accumulation of bacterial plaque was once thought to be the cause of periodontal destruction, but it is now recognized that periodontitis is an infectious disease associated with a relatively small number of predominantly gram-negative microorganisms that exist in a subgingival biofilm. Furthermore, the importance of the host in disease initiation and progression is clearly recognized. Although pathogenic bacteria are necessary for periodontal disease, they are not sufficient alone to cause the disease. A susceptible host is also imperative. In a host who has relatively low susceptibility to disease, bacterial pathogens may have minimal clinical effect. This may be due to a particularly effective host immunoinflammatory response that eliminates pathogenic organisms while minimizing destruction of native tissues. Conversely, in a host with relatively high disease susceptibility, marked destruction of periodontal tissues may result.

Because of differences in host susceptibility, not all individuals are equally vulnerable to the destructive effects of periodontal pathogens and the immunoinflammatory response to those organisms. Thus, patients may not necessarily have similar disease expression despite the presence of similar bacteria. Likewise, the response to periodontal treatment may vary depending on the wound-healing capacity and susceptibility of the host to further disease progression.

Although the potential impact of many systemic disorders on the periodontium is well documented, evidence suggests that periodontal infection may significantly enhance the risk for certain systemic diseases or alter the natural course of systemic condition,

Although more than 50 different systemic conditions have been associated with periodontal diseases, the evidence base is quite large for many of these conditions and small for others. For example, conditions in which the influences of periodontal infection are well documented include coronary heart disease (CHD) and CHD-related events such as angina, infarction, atherosclerosis, and other vascular conditions; stroke; diabetes mellitus; preterm labor, low-birth-weight delivery, and preeclampsia; and respiratory conditions such as chronic obstructive pulmonary disease (Box 23.1). A smaller but growing evidence base supports an association between poor oral health, tooth loss, or periodontitis and conditions such as chronic kidney disease and renal insufficiency; certain forms of cancer affecting the liver, pancreas, and colorectal region; rheumatoid arthritis; and altered cognitive function, dementia, and Alzheimer disease. This chapter focuses on those conditions with the strongest evidence base, recognizing that ongoing research will further elucidate relationships between inflammatory periodontal diseases and systemic health.

Focal Infection Theory Revisited

Research in the area of periodontal medicine marks resurgence in the concept of focal infection. In 1900, British physician William Hunter first developed the idea that oral microorganisms were responsible for a wide range of systemic conditions that were not easily recognized as being infectious in nature. He claimed that restoration of carious teeth, instead of extraction, resulted in the trapping of infectious agents under restorations. In addition to caries, pulpal necrosis, and periapical abscesses, Hunter identified gingivitis and periodontitis as foci of infection. He advocated the extraction of teeth with these conditions to eliminate the source of sepsis. Hunter thought that teeth were prone to septic infection primarily because of their structure and their relationship to alveolar bone. He stated that the degree of systemic effect produced by oral sepsis depended on the virulence of the oral infection and the individual's degree of resistance. He also thought that oral organisms had specific actions on different tissues and that these organisms acted by producing toxins, thereby resulting in low-grade "subinfections" that produced systemic effects over prolonged periods. Finally, Hunter thought that the connection between oral sepsis and resulting systemic conditions could be shown via removal of the

BOX 23.1 Organ Systems and Conditions Possibly Influenced by Periodontal Infection

Cardiovascular and Cerebrovascular Systems
Atherosclerosis
Coronary heart disease
Angina
Myocardial infarction
Cerebrovascular accident (stroke)
Erectile dysfunction
Anemia

Endocrine System
Metabolic syndrome
Diabetes mellitus

Reproductive System
Preterm and low-birth-weight infants
Preeclampsia

Respiratory System
Chronic obstructive pulmonary disease
Acute bacterial pneumonia

Kidney Diseases
Renal insufficiency
Chronic kidney disease
End-stage kidney disease

Autoimmune Diseases
Rheumatoid arthritis
Ankylosing spondylitis

Cognitive Function
Dementia
Alzheimer disease

Cancers
Colorectal
Pancreatic
Hepatocellular
Others

causative sepsis through tooth extraction and observation of the improvement in systemic health. Because it explained a wide range of disorders for which there was no known explanation at the time, Hunter's theory became widely accepted in Britain and eventually in the United States, leading to the wholesale extraction of teeth.

The focal infection theory fell into disrepute during the 1940s and 1950s, when widespread extraction—often of the entire dentition—failed to reduce or eliminate the systemic conditions to which the supposedly infected dentition had been linked. The theory, while offering a possible explanation for perplexing systemic disorders, had been based on very little (if any) scientific evidence. Hunter and other advocates of the theory were unable to explain how focal oral sepsis produced these systemic maladies. They were also unable to elucidate possible interactive mechanisms between oral and systemic health. Furthermore, the suggested intervention of tooth extraction often had no effect on the systemic conditions for which patients sought relief. However, Hunter's ideas did encourage extensive research in the areas of microbiology and immunology.

Evidence-Based Clinical Practice

Many of the precepts of the focal infection theory are being revived today in light of recent research demonstrating links between oral and systemic health. However, as expressed by Newman, for the "hypothesis not to fall into disrepute for a second time, there must be no unsubstantiated attributions, no theories without evidence." Today's era of evidence-based medicine and dentistry provides an excellent environment in which to examine the possible relationships between oral infection and systemic disorders. To establish a relationship between conditions A and B, different levels of evidence must be examined. All scientific evidence is not given the same weight. The stronger the evidence, the more likely it is that a true relationship exists between the conditions. Table 23.1 describes these various levels of evidence.

Subgingival Environment as a Reservoir for Bacteria

The subgingival microbiota in patients with periodontitis provides a significant and persistent gram-negative bacterial challenge to the host that is met with a potent immunoinflammatory response. These organisms and their products, such as *lipopolysaccharides* (LPSs), have ready access to the periodontal tissues and to the circulation via the sulcular epithelium, which is frequently ulcerated and discontinuous. Even with treatment, complete eradication of these organisms is difficult, and their reemergence is often rapid. The total surface area of pocket epithelium in contact with subgingival bacteria and their products in a patient with generalized moderate periodontitis has been estimated to be approximately the size of the palm of an adult hand, with even larger areas of exposure in cases

TABLE 23.1 Evaluation of Evidence

Type of Evidence	Strength of Evidence	Description
Case report	+/–	• Provides relatively weak retrospective anecdotal evidence • May suggest that further study is needed
Cross-sectional study	+	• Compares groups of subjects at a single point in time • Stronger than a case report • Fairly easy to conduct • Relatively inexpensive to conduct
Longitudinal study	++	• Follows groups of subjects over time • Stronger than a cross-sectional study • Studies with a control group much stronger than studies without controls • More difficult and expensive to conduct
Intervention trial	+++	• Examines the effects of some intervention • Studies with a control group (i.e., placebo) much stronger than studies without controls • Strongest form of evidence is the randomized controlled intervention trial • Difficult and expensive to conduct
Systematic review	++++	• Systematically evaluates evidence from multiple studies, especially randomized controlled trials • Uses clearly defined guidelines for the selection of evidence to be included or excluded from the review • Examines for heterogeneity in the overall data to indicate variations in study design, sample populations, and assessment methodologies

of more advanced periodontal destruction. Bacteremias are common after mechanical periodontal therapy, and they also occur frequently during normal daily function and oral hygiene procedures. Just as the periodontal tissues mount an immunoinflammatory response to bacteria and their products, systemic challenge with these agents also induces a major vascular response. This host response may offer explanatory mechanisms for the interactions between periodontal infection and a variety of systemic disorders.

Periodontal Disease and Mortality

The ultimate medical outcome measure is mortality. A number of studies suggest that an increased mortality rate from various causes is associated with inflammatory periodontal diseases. Periodontal status at the baseline examination was a significant predictor of mortality independent of other factors such as smoking, alcohol use, cholesterol levels, blood pressure, family history of heart disease, education level, and body mass. For those subjects with the most alveolar bone loss (>21% alveolar bone loss at baseline), the risk of dying during the follow-up period was 70% higher than for all other subjects. Interestingly, alveolar bone loss increased the risk of mortality more than smoking (52% increased risk), which is a well-known risk factor for mortality. A later evaluation of these same subjects confirmed a higher incidence of CHD-related events such as myocardial infarction (MI) and unstable angina among men younger than 60 years of age with alveolar bone loss compared to those without bone loss.

Those with the highest levels of periodontal attachment loss have a significantly higher risk of death compared to those with the least attachment loss. The mortality rate over a 9-year period was 15.7% in those with the greatest attachment loss and 7.9% in those with the lowest level of periodontal attachment loss. When examining research that suggests oral health status is a possible risk factor for systemic conditions, it is important to recognize when other known risk factors for those systemic conditions have been accounted for in the analysis. Host susceptibility factors that place individuals at risk for periodontitis may also place them at risk for systemic diseases such as cardiovascular disease. In these patients, the association may actually be among the risk factors rather than among the diseases. For example, periodontitis and cardiovascular disease share risk factors such as smoking, age, race, male gender, and stress. Genetic risk factors may also be shared. However, studies do support an association between poor oral health and an increased risk of mortality. In a prospective longitudinal study of subjects with type 2 diabetes, those with severe periodontitis had 3.2 times the risk of death from ischemic heart disease or kidney disease as subjects without periodontitis or with only slight periodontitis, after adjusting for other risk factors, including age, sex, duration of diabetes, glycemic control, macroalbuminuria, body mass index, serum cholesterol concentration, hypertension, and current smoking.

Periodontal Disease and Oncogenesis

Periodontal disease is associated with an increased risk for oral cancer. Bacterial pathogens in the oral cavity responsible for chronic inflammation and chronic immune cell infiltration are an accompanying feature of oral and head and neck cancer. The leading bacteria at sites with periodontal destruction include members of the red complex, namely *Porphyromonas gingivalis*, *Tannerella forsythia*, and *Treponema denticola*. Also, *Fusobacterium nucleatum* is one of the most abundant oral bacteria present in periodontal disease biofilms. *F. nucleatum* has strong intermicrobial binding properties with most oral biofilm colonizers, and it can help other bacteria cross host-epithelial and -endothelial barriers. *P. gingivalis* and *F. nucleatum* have been implicated in the pathogenesis of several chronic diseases and cancer. Indeed, although the relationship between these bacteria and cancer has been reported in colon and pancreatic cancer, involvement of these oral pathogens in the etiology and progression of oral cancer and in potential mechanistic contributions to oral cancer is emerging.

Epidemiological data suggest that there is an association between tooth loss, periodontal disease, or periodontal microbial pathogens and cancer. For example, risk of pancreatic cancer is increased in people with tooth loss or periodontal disease. In addition, in a large European cohort study, participants with elevated antibody titers to the periodontal pathogen, *P. gingivalis*, had a 2.14 times greater risk for pancreatic cancer compared to those with undetectable or low antibody levels. Tooth loss and periodontal disease have also been associated with oral or head and neck cancer. However, knowledge about the direct link between periodontal pathogens and oral cancer and the mechanisms involved are limited.

Several mechanisms and processes have been postulated for the causal role of pathogenic bacteria and microbial dysbiosis in cancer and the host, including modulation of the host-immune response, heightened inflammation, altered metabolism, and altered host-cell signaling. A direct relationship between *F. nucleatum* and colorectal cancer was demonstrated. Other studies found that *P. gingivalis* and *F. nucleatum* seem to promote migration and invasion of oral cancer cells by triggering an epithelial to mesenchymal transition, acquisition of stemness properties, and cytokine signaling *P. gingivalis* can also promote invasion in oral squamous cell carcinoma and esophageal cancer. The specific carcinogenic mechanisms induced or potentiated by pathogenic oral bacteria on the host or cancer are also emerging.

Periodontal Disease, Coronary Heart Disease, and Atherosclerosis

CHD-related events are a major cause of death. MI has been associated with acute systemic bacterial and viral infections and is sometimes preceded by influenza-like symptoms. Traditional risk factors such as smoking, dyslipidemia, hypertension, and diabetes mellitus do not explain the presence of coronary atherosclerosis in a large number of patients. Localized infection that results in a chronic inflammatory reaction has been suggested as a mechanism underlying CHD in these individuals.

In cross-sectional studies of patients with acute MI or confirmed CHD who were compared with age- and gender-matched control patients, patients with MI had significantly worse dental health (e.g., periodontitis, periapical lesions, caries, pericoronitis) than controls. This association between poor dental health and MI was independent of known risk factors for heart disease, such as age, cholesterol levels, hypertension, diabetes, and smoking. Because atherosclerosis is a major determinant of CHD-related events, dental health has also been related to coronary atheromatosis. There is evidence that the extent of periodontal disease may be associated with CHD. For example, there may be a greater risk for CHD-related events, such as MI, in subjects who have periodontitis affecting a greater number of teeth in the mouth compared to those who have periodontitis involving fewer teeth.

Longitudinal studies provide compelling data regarding this relationship. In a 7-year follow-up study of the patients, dental disease was significantly related to the incidence of new fatal and nonfatal coronary events as well as overall mortality. In a prospective study, subjects with periodontitis had a 25% increased risk for

CHD compared to those with no or minimal periodontal disease, after adjusting for other known risk factors. Among males between the ages of 25 and 49 years, periodontitis increased the risk of CHD by 70%. The level of oral hygiene was also associated with heart disease. Patients with poor oral hygiene, as indicated by higher debris and calculus scores, had a twofold increased risk for CHD.

Perhaps the best evidence available comes from systematic reviews of studies examining the relationship between periodontal infection and cardiovascular disease. A systematic review and meta-analysis of data from 15 studies showed a significant 14%–222% increase in the risk of CHD-related events in patients with periodontal disease as compared to those without periodontal disease. A similar systematic review of longitudinal cohort and case–control studies showed a significant increase in the risk of incident MI, angina, or CHD-related death in subjects with periodontitis in five of the six studies reported. This increased risk was noted mainly in younger subjects (i.e., <65 years old). Extensive systematic reviews by Scannapieco and colleagues and by an American Heart Association working group concluded that a moderate degree of evidence exists to support an association between periodontal disease and atherosclerosis, MI, and cardiovascular disease independent of known confounders; however, causality is unclear. The results of the 2013 AAP/EFP Workshop on Periodontitis and Systemic Diseases concluded that "there is consistent and strong epidemiologic evidence that periodontitis imparts increased risk for future cardiovascular disease," but whereas many studies support multiple biologic mechanisms to explain this relationship, "intervention trials to date are not adequate to draw further conclusions." That is, insufficient evidence exists to show that the treatment of periodontal disease has any impact on the risk of heart disease.

Effects of Periodontal Infection

There are numerous mechanisms—both direct and indirect—through which periodontal infection may affect the onset or progression of atherosclerosis and CHD. Periodontitis and atherosclerosis both have complex etiologic factors that combine genetic and environmental influences. In addition to smoking, the diseases share many risk factors and have distinct similarities with regard to their basic pathogenic mechanisms.

Ischemic Heart Disease

Ischemic heart disease is associated with the processes of atherogenesis and thrombogenesis. Damage to the vascular endothelium, with a subsequent inflammatory reaction, plays a major role in atherosclerosis and ischemic organ damage. Increased viscosity of blood may promote major ischemic heart disease and cerebrovascular accident (stroke) by increasing the risk of thrombus formation. Fibrinogen is a major factor in the promotion of this hypercoagulable state. *Fibrinogen* is the precursor to fibrin, and increased fibrinogen levels increase blood viscosity. Increased plasma fibrinogen is a recognized risk factor for cardiovascular events and peripheral vascular disease. An elevated white blood cell count is also a predictor of heart disease and stroke, and circulating leukocytes may promote the occlusion of blood vessels. Coagulation factor VIII (von Willebrand factor) has likewise been associated with a risk of ischemic heart disease.

Systemic Infections

Systemic infections are known to induce a hypercoagulable state and increase blood viscosity (Fig. 23.1). Fibrinogen levels and white blood cell counts are often increased in patients with periodontal disease. Individuals with poor oral health may also have significant elevations in coagulation factor VIII/von Willebrand factor antigen, thereby increasing the risk of thrombus formation. Thus, periodontal infection may also promote increased blood viscosity and thrombogenesis, which leads to an increased risk for central and peripheral vascular disease.

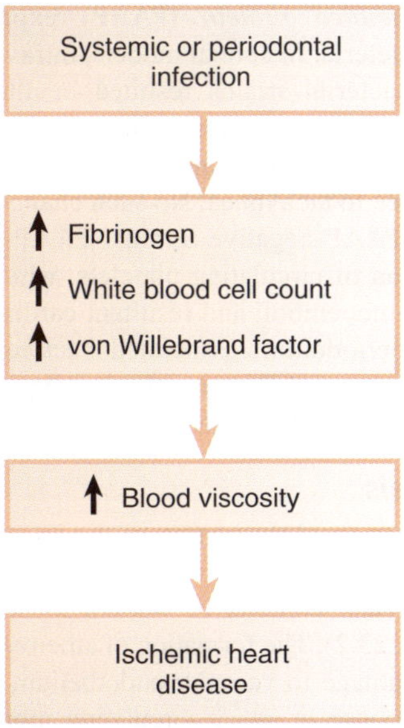

Fig. 23.1 The effect of infection on blood viscosity. Increased plasma fibrinogen and von Willebrand factor cause hypercoagulability. When they are combined with an increased white blood cell count, the blood viscosity increases, thereby increasing the risk of coronary ischemia.

Daily Activity

Routine daily activities such as mastication and oral hygiene procedures result in frequent bacteremia with oral organisms. Periodontal disease may predispose the patient to an increased incidence of bacteremia, including the presence of virulent gram-negative organisms associated with periodontitis. There is a greater risk of bacteremia after toothbrushing in patients with higher levels of plaque, calculus, and gingivitis as compared to those with minimal plaque and gingival inflammation. In fact, subjects with generalized gingival bleeding after brushing showed an almost eightfold increase in their incidence of bacteremia as compared to those with minimal gingival bleeding. An estimated 8% of all cases of infective endocarditis are associated with periodontal or dental disease without a preceding dental procedure. The periodontium, when affected by periodontitis, also acts as a reservoir of *endotoxins* (LPSs) from gram-negative organisms. Endotoxins can pass readily into the systemic circulation during normal daily function, thereby inducing damage to the vascular endothelium and precipitating many negative cardiovascular effects. In a study of the incidence of endotoxemia after simple chewing, subjects with periodontitis were four times more likely to have endotoxin present in the bloodstream than subjects without periodontitis. Furthermore, the concentration of endotoxin in the bloodstream was more than fourfold greater in those with periodontitis as compared to healthy subjects.

Thrombogenesis

Platelet aggregation plays a major role in thrombogenesis, and most cases of acute MI are precipitated by thromboembolism. Oral organisms may be involved in coronary thrombogenesis. Platelets selectively bind some strains of *Streptococcus sanguinis*, which is a common component of supragingival plaque, and *P. gingivalis*, which is a pathogen closely associated with periodontitis. The aggregation of platelets is induced by the *platelet aggregation–associated protein* (PAAP) expressed on some strains of these bacteria. In animal models, intravenous infusion of PAAP-positive bacterial strains resulted in alterations of heart rate, blood pressure, cardiac contractility, and electrocardiogram readings consistent with MI. Platelet accumulation also occurred in the lungs and led to tachypnea. No such changes were seen with the infusion of PAAP-negative strains. PAAP-positive bacteria caused aggregation of circulating platelets, which resulted in the formation of thromboemboli and resultant cardiac and pulmonary changes. Thus, periodontitis-associated bacteremia with certain strains of *S. sanguinis* and *P. gingivalis* may promote acute thromboembolic events via interaction with circulating platelets.

Atherosclerosis

Atherosclerosis is a focal thickening of the arterial *intima*, the innermost layer lining the vessel lumen, and the *media*, the thick layer under the intima that consists of smooth muscle, collagen, and elastic fibers (Fig. 23.2). The formation of atherosclerotic plaques is precipitated by damage to vascular endothelium that results in an inflammatory response in which circulating monocytes adhere to the vascular endothelium. Damage to vascular endothelium can occur because of the presence of intravascular microorganisms and their products; chemical damage, often resulting from elements of tobacco and other exogenous toxins; and increased shear force along the vascular lining, such as that occurring in hypertension. The adherence of monocytes to the damaged vascular endothelium is mediated by several adhesion molecules on the endothelial cell surface, including intercellular adhesion molecule-1 (ICAM-1), endothelial leukocyte adhesion molecule-1 (ELAM-1), and vascular cell adhesion molecule-1 (VCAM-1). These adhesion molecules are upregulated by a number of factors, including bacterial LPSs, prostaglandins, and proinflammatory cytokines. After binding to the endothelial cell lining, monocytes penetrate the endothelium and migrate under the arterial intima. The monocytes ingest circulating low-density lipoprotein in its oxidized state and become engorged, thereby forming the foam cells that are characteristic of atheromatous plaque.

Atheromatous plaque formation and thickening of the vessel wall narrow the lumen and dramatically decrease blood flow through the vessel. Arterial thrombosis often occurs after an atheromatous plaque ruptures. Plaque rupture exposes circulating blood to arterial collagen and tissue factor from monocytes and macrophages that activate platelets and the coagulation pathway. Platelet and fibrin accumulation forms a thrombus that may occlude the vessel and result in an ischemic event such as angina or MI. The thrombus may separate from the vessel wall and form an embolus, which may also occlude vessels, again leading to an acute event such as MI or cerebral infarction (stroke).

Role of Periodontal Disease in Atherosclerotic Myocardial or Cerebral Ischemia

Patients with periodontitis are at increased risk for thickening of the walls of the major coronary arteries. In several studies of atheromas obtained from humans during endarterectomy, more than half of the lesions contained periodontal pathogens, and many atheromas contained multiple different periodontal species. Periodontal diseases result in chronic systemic exposure to products of these organisms. Low-level bacteremia may initiate host responses that alter coagulability, endothelial and vessel wall integrity, and platelet function, thereby resulting in atherogenic changes and possible thromboembolic events (Fig. 23.3).

Research has clearly shown a wide variation in host response to bacterial challenge. Some individuals with heavy plaque accumulation

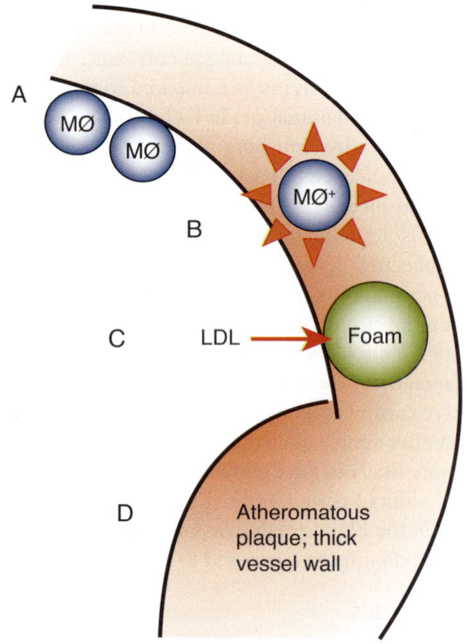

Fig. 23.2 Pathogenesis of atherosclerosis. A, Monocytes and macrophages *(MØ)* adhere to the vascular endothelium. B, Monocytes and macrophages penetrate into the arterial media and produce proinflammatory cytokines and growth factors. C, The ingestion of oxidized low-density lipoprotein *(LDL)* enlarges monocytes to form foam cells. D, Smooth muscle proliferation and plaque formation thicken vessel walls and narrow the lumen. *MØ+*, Hyperinflammatory monocyte/macrophage phenotype.

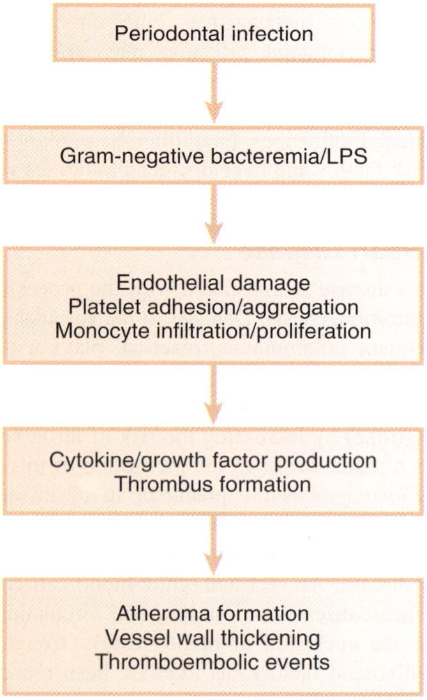

Fig. 23.3 The influence of periodontal infection on atherosclerosis. Periodontal pathogens and their products result in damage to the vascular endothelium. Monocytes and macrophages enter the vessel wall and produce cytokines that further increase the inflammatory response and propagate the atheromatous lesion. Growth factor production leads to smooth muscle proliferation in the vessel wall. Damaged endothelium also activates platelets, thereby resulting in platelet aggregation and potentiating thromboembolic events. *LPS*, Lipopolysaccharide.

and high proportions of pathogenic organisms appear relatively resistant to bone and attachment loss. Others develop extensive periodontal destruction in the presence of small amounts of plaque and low proportions of putative pathogens. Patients with an abnormally exuberant inflammatory response often have a hyperinflammatory monocyte and macrophage phenotype (MØ$^+$). Monocytes and macrophages from these individuals secrete significantly increased levels of proinflammatory mediators (e.g., IL-1, TNF-α, PGE_2) in response to bacterial LPSs compared to patients with a normal monocyte and macrophage phenotype. Patients with aggressive periodontitis, refractory periodontitis, and type 1 diabetes mellitus often possess the MØ$^+$ phenotype, which appears to be under both genetic and environmental control.

The monocyte and macrophage cell line is intimately involved in the pathogenesis of both periodontal disease and atherosclerosis. Diet-induced elevations in serum low-density lipoprotein levels upregulate monocyte and macrophage responsiveness to bacterial LPSs. Thus, elevated low-density lipoprotein levels, which is a known risk factor for atherosclerosis and CHD, may increase the secretion of destructive and inflammatory cytokines by monocytes and macrophages. This may result not only in the propagation of atheromatous lesions but also in enhanced periodontal destruction in the presence of pathogenic organisms. This is one example of a potential shared mechanism in the pathogenesis of cardiovascular and periodontal diseases. The presence of an MØ$^+$ phenotype may place patients at risk for both CHD and periodontitis (Fig. 23.4). Periodontal infections may contribute to atherosclerosis and thromboembolic events by repeatedly challenging the vascular endothelium and arterial wall with bacterial LPSs and proinflammatory cytokines. Vascular monocytes and macrophages in patients with an MØ$^+$ phenotype meet this challenge with an abnormally elevated inflammatory response that may directly contribute to atherosclerosis and may precipitate thromboembolic events.

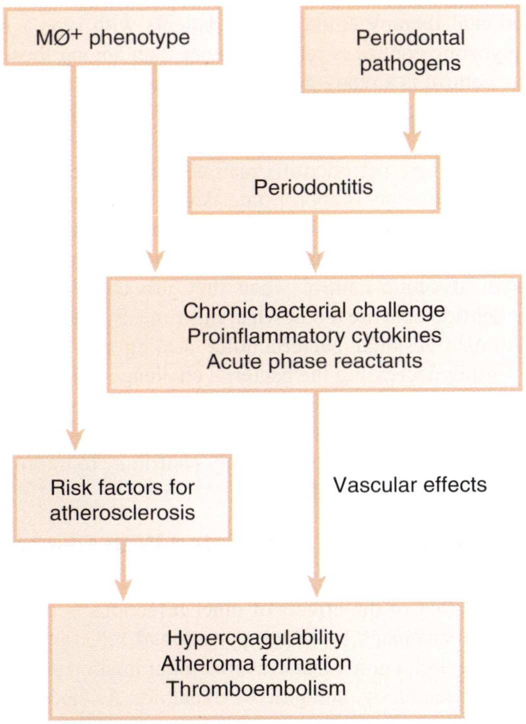

Fig. 23.4 The cardiovascular and periodontal consequences of the hyperresponsive monocyte/macrophage phenotype *(MØ$^+$)*. In combination with other risk factors, the MØ$^+$ phenotype predisposes individuals to both atherosclerosis and periodontitis. Bacterial products and inflammatory mediators associated with periodontitis affect vascular endothelium, monocytes and macrophages, platelets, and smooth muscle and may increase blood coagulability. This may further increase atherosclerosis and may result in thromboembolism and ischemic events.

Acute-phase proteins such as *C-reactive protein* (CRP) and fibrinogen are produced in the liver in response to inflammatory or infectious stimuli and act as inflammatory markers. CRP induces monocytes and macrophages to produce tissue factor, which stimulates the coagulation pathway and increases blood coagulability. Increased fibrinogen levels may contribute to this process. CRP also stimulates the complement cascade, further exacerbating inflammation.

Elevations in serum CRP and fibrinogen levels are well-accepted risk factors for cardiovascular disease. Research has focused on periodontitis as a potential trigger for systemic inflammation. Serum CRP and fibrinogen levels are often elevated in subjects with periodontitis as compared to subjects without periodontitis. These acute-phase proteins may act as intermediary steps in the pathway from periodontal infection to cardiovascular disease (see Figs. 23.3 and 23.4). Thus, periodontal diseases may have both direct effects on the major blood vessels (e.g., atheroma formation) and indirect effects that stimulate changes in the cardiovascular system (e.g., elevation of systemic inflammatory responses).

In subjects with chronic periodontitis, serum levels of IL-6 and CRP are reduced after scaling and root planing. Inflammatory periodontal disease (compared to periodontal health) is also associated with altered vascular endothelial function. Altered vascular endothelial function is a major risk factor for acute thrombotic events. After scaling and root planing with a resultant decrease in periodontal inflammation, markers of vascular health improve significantly over time. The functional assessment of vascular endothelial function also returns to normal after scaling and root planing. These results suggest that periodontal inflammation adversely affects the health of the vascular endothelium, whereas a reduction in inflammation improves endothelial health. Whether these changes directly impact the risk of acute cardiovascular events remains to be determined.

Role of Periodontal Disease in Erectile Dysfunction

Erectile dysfunction (ED) is associated with endothelial dysfunction, and elevated levels of oxidative stress and systemic inflammation are common to both periodontal disease and ED. Studies have shown a relationship between ED and periodontitis, but more research is needed to understand the mechanisms of interaction.

Periodontal Disease and Stroke

Ischemic cerebral infarction, or stroke, is often preceded by systemic bacterial or viral infection. In one study, patients with cerebral ischemia were five times more likely to have had a systemic infection within 1 week before the ischemic event than nonischemic control subjects. Recent infection was a significant risk factor for cerebral ischemia; it was independent of other known risk factors such as hypertension, history of a previous stroke, diabetes, smoking, and CHD. Interestingly, the presence of systemic infection before the stroke resulted in significantly greater ischemia and a more severe postischemic neurologic defect than stroke not preceded by infection. Stroke patients with a preceding infection had slightly higher levels of plasma fibrinogen and significantly higher levels of CRP compared to those without infection.

Stroke is classified as either hemorrhagic or nonhemorrhagic. Nonhemorrhagic stroke, or ischemic stroke, is usually caused by thromboembolic events and cerebrovascular atherosclerosis, whereas hemorrhagic stroke often results from a vascular bleed such as an aneurysm. Periodontal disease has been associated primarily with an increased risk of nonhemorrhagic stroke. Numerous studies have shown that periodontal disease is associated with an increased risk of stroke.

Periodontal infection may contribute directly to the pathogenesis of atherosclerosis by providing a persistent bacterial challenge to the arterial endothelium, thereby contributing to the monocyte- and macrophage-driven inflammatory process that results in atheromatosis and narrowing of the vessel lumen. Furthermore, periodontal infection may stimulate a series of indirect systemic effects, such as elevated production of fibrinogen and CRP, which increases the risk of stroke (see Figs. 23.3 and 23.4). Finally, bacteremia with PAAP-positive bacterial strains from supragingival and subgingival plaque can increase platelet aggregation, thereby contributing to thrombus formation and subsequent thromboembolism, which is the leading cause of stroke.

Periodontal Disease and Diabetes Mellitus

It is clear from epidemiologic research that diabetes increases the risk for and severity of periodontal diseases. The increased prevalence and severity of periodontitis typically seen in patients with diabetes—especially those with poor metabolic control—has led to the designation of periodontal disease as the "sixth complication" of diabetes. In addition to the five "classic" complications of diabetes (Box 23.2), the American Diabetes Association has officially recognized that periodontal disease is common among patients with diabetes, and its Standards of Care include taking a history of current or past dental infections as part of the physician's examination. Since 2009, the American Diabetes Association's Standards of Medical Care in Diabetes has specifically recommended that physicians refer patients with diabetes to a dentist for a comprehensive dental and periodontal examination.

Periodontitis has also been associated with the classic complications of diabetes. Diabetic adults with severe periodontitis at baseline had a significantly greater incidence of kidney and macrovascular complications over the subsequent 1–11 years than did diabetic adults with only gingivitis or mild periodontitis. This was true despite both groups' having similar glycemic control. One or more cardiovascular complications occurred in 82% of patients with severe periodontitis versus 21% of patients without severe periodontitis. Again, severe periodontitis preceded the onset of clinical diabetic complications in these subjects.

Among diabetic patients with periodontitis, periodontal therapy may have beneficial effects on glycemic control. This may be especially true for patients with relatively poor glycemic control and more advanced periodontal destruction before treatment. A large number of studies, starting as far back as 1960, have examined the impact of periodontal therapy on glycemic control in patients with diabetes. Most of these studies compared scaling and root planing (with or without adjunctive systemic antibiotics) with no periodontal therapy and followed patients for several months to assess changes in glycemic control measured by glycated hemoglobin (HbA1c) values. Others included in the treatment regimen not only scaling and root planing but also extraction of periodontally hopeless teeth and even periodontal surgery. Many of these studies showed a significant improvement in glycemic control, as determined by reductions in HbA1c values, in the periodontal treatment group compared to the nontreatment group. Other studies showed minimal change in glycemic control in periodontally treated patients.

BOX 23.2 Complications of Diabetes Mellitus

1. Retinopathy
2. Nephropathy
3. Neuropathy
4. Macrovascular disease
5. Altered wound healing
6. Periodontal disease

(From Löe H: Periodontal disease: the sixth complication of diabetes mellitus. *Diabetes Care* 16(Suppl 1):329, 1993.)

Numerous systematic reviews and meta-analyses have consistently shown that periodontal therapy is associated with a statistically significant and clinically relevant improvement in glycemic control in patients with diabetes and periodontitis. However, clinicians must understand that individual patients may or may not have outcomes similar to the average outcome in any given study or systematic review. That is, treatment results vary from patient to patient, and clinicians should not expect the same result in all patients. These studies suggest that periodontal therapy is most likely to result in short-term improvement in glycemia in those diabetic patients with severe periodontitis and poor metabolic control who demonstrate marked reduction in periodontal inflammation after treatment.

Research suggests that periodontal therapy may have a smaller impact on glycemic control in patients with type 1 diabetes than in those with type 2 disease. In a study of subjects with type 1 and type 2 diabetes with periodontitis, periodontal therapy was associated with a significant improvement in glycemic control overall in those with type 2 diabetes but not in those with type 1 disease, despite improvement in the periodontal condition of both groups.

However, clinician may anticipate a greater glycemic response to periodontal therapy among those patients with type 1 diabetes whose glycemic control is relatively poor than among those whose glycemic control is already good before periodontal treatment.

Although the routine use of systemic antibiotics for treatment of chronic periodontitis is not justified, patients with poorly controlled diabetes and severe periodontitis may constitute one patient group for whom such therapy is appropriate. Antibiotics remain an adjunct to the necessary mechanical removal of plaque and calculus. The mechanisms by which adjunctive antibiotics may induce positive changes in glycemic control when they are combined with mechanical debridement are unknown at this time. Systemic antibiotics may eliminate residual bacteria after scaling and root planing, thereby further decreasing the bacterial challenge to the host. Tetracyclines are also known to suppress the glycation of proteins and decrease the activity of tissue-degrading enzymes such as matrix metalloproteinases. These changes may contribute to improvements in the metabolic control of diabetes.

Periodontal Infection Associated With Glycemic Control in Diabetes

An understanding of the effects of other infections is useful to delineate the mechanisms by which periodontal infection influences glycemia. It is well known that systemic inflammation plays a major role in insulin sensitivity and glucose dynamics. As discussed previously, periodontal diseases can induce or perpetuate an elevated systemic chronic inflammatory state, which is reflected in increased serum CRP, IL-6, and fibrinogen levels seen in many people with periodontitis.

It is possible that chronic gram-negative periodontal infections may also result in increased insulin resistance and poor glycemic control. In patients with periodontitis, persistent systemic challenge with periodontopathic bacteria and their products results in an

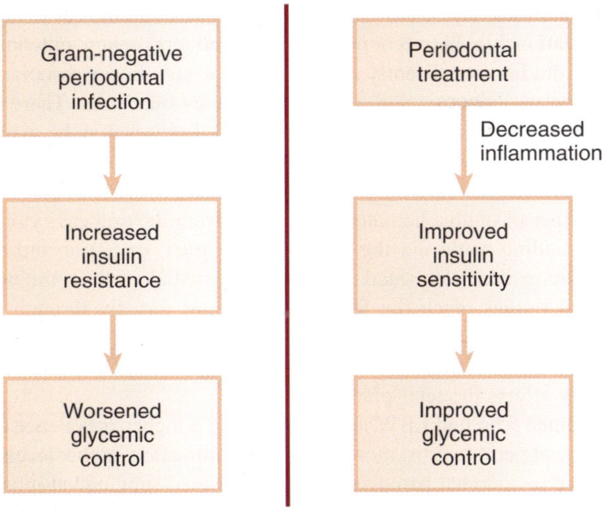

Fig. 23.5 Potential effects of periodontal infection and periodontal therapy on glycemia in patients with diabetes.

upregulation of the immunoinflammatory response, with elevation in serum levels of proinflammatory mediators such as IL-1β, TNF-α, and IL-6, similar to well-recognized systemic infections but on a more persistent, chronic basis (Fig. 23.5). Increased serum levels of several cytokines, including TNF-α and IL-6, are associated with increased insulin resistance. This mechanism would explain the worsening of glycemic control associated with severe periodontitis. Periodontal treatment designed to decrease the bacterial insult and reduce inflammation may result in decreased systemic inflammation, restoring insulin sensitivity over time and thereby resulting in improved metabolic control. The improved glycemic control seen in many studies of periodontal therapy would support such a hypothesis. This mechanism may also explain differences in the glycemic response to periodontal therapy between individuals with type 1 and type 2 diabetes. Because type 2 diabetes is strongly associated with insulin resistance, periodontal therapy that reduces systemic inflammation may improve insulin sensitivity and result in improved glycemic control. Conversely, type 1 diabetes is not strongly associated with insulin resistance, so reduced inflammation after periodontal therapy may not have a major effect on insulin sensitivity in patients with type 1 disease, which would minimize the impact of periodontal treatment in these patients.

Periodontal Disease and Asthma

Evidence evaluating the relationship between periodontal disease and asthma is now emerging. A systematic review evaluating the association between asthma and periodontal diseases found significantly less gingival inflammation in patients without asthma compared to those with asthma. However, the relationship between asthma and parameters of periodontitis, such as probing depth and clinical attachment levels, was unclear, with conflicting results between studies. More research is needed to clarify the relation.

Periodontal Disease and Rheumatoid Arthritis

An association between periodontitis and rheumatoid arthritis (RA) has been a topic of research for decades. Both are chronic destructive conditions in which inflammation plays the primary role. Studies consistently show a strong and statistically significant association between the prevalence of RA and periodontitis. Proinflammatory cytokine profiles are similar in RA and periodontitis, and matrix metalloproteinase enzymes play a major role in tissue destruction found in both conditions. Altered proteins called "citrullinated proteins" are commonly found in inflamed tissues, and they can elicit a profound autoimmune response resulting in production of anticitrullinated protein antibodies. Anticitrullinated protein antibodies play a predominant role in RA and higher antibody levels are associated with more severe RA over time.

P. gingivalis in strongly implicated in periodontal inflammation. *P. gingivalis* is also unique in its ability to produce citrullination of proteins. This may then prime the immune response to respond rapidly and robustly to the presence of citrullinated proteins present in other tissues, such as the synovium, by producing high levels of anticitrullinated protein antibodies. Translocation of *P. gingivalis* from the oral cavity to the joint space via the bloodstream may result in production of citrullinated proteins, such as fibrinogen and fibrin, in the joint synovium. This then stimulates rapid local production of anticitrullinated protein antibodies in the synovium, leading to complement activation, stimulation of proinflammatory cytokine production, and activation of osteoclasts. While these mechanisms may provide a possible link between periodontal diseases and RA, a causal relationship cannot be established without extensive confirmatory research.

Periodontal Disease and Pregnancy Outcome

Low-birth-weight (LBW) infants (i.e., those weighing <2500 g at birth) are 40 times more likely to die during the neonatal period than normal-birth-weight (NBW) infants. LBW infants who survive the neonatal period are at increased risk for congenital anomalies, respiratory disorders, and neurodevelopmental disabilities.

The primary cause of LBW deliveries is *preterm labor* or *premature rupture of membranes* (PROM). Factors such as smoking, alcohol, or drug use during pregnancy; inadequate prenatal care; race; low socioeconomic status; hypertension; old or young maternal age; diabetes; and genitourinary tract infections increase the risk of preterm LBW delivery. However, these risk factors are not present in approximately one-fourth of preterm LBW cases, which results in a continued search for other causes.

Research has examined the relationship between maternal infection and preterm labor, PROM, and LBW delivery. The true extent of this relationship is difficult to determine because the majority of maternal infections may be subclinical. Genitourinary tract infections have been associated with adverse pregnancy outcomes. Women with bacteriuria have increased rates of preterm delivery, and the antibiotic treatment of bacteriuria has resulted in a significant decrease in preterm delivery rates as compared to placebo treatment. Vaginal colonization with group B streptococci or *Bacteroides* species increases the risk of PROM, preterm delivery, and LBW infants.

Although the direct effects of microorganisms may play an important role in many cases of preterm labor, PROM, and LBW delivery, indirect mechanisms may also be operative. Bacterial infection of the chorioamnion, or extraplacental membrane, may lead to chorioamnionitis, a condition that is strongly associated with PROM and preterm delivery. However, many cases of histologic chorioamnionitis demonstrate negative bacterial cultures, indicating that infection is not the sole cause of this condition. It is likely that an indirect mechanism may be active in which the cascade of host products produced in response to infection is often responsible for preterm labor. Maternal infection may lead to the presence of amniotic bacterial products, such as LPSs from gram-negative

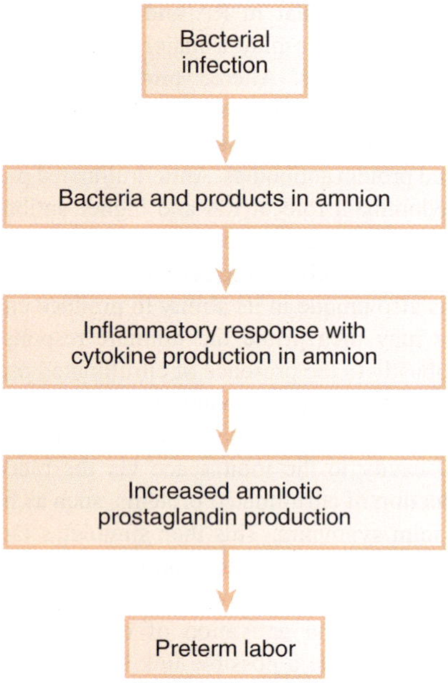

Fig. 23.6 Mechanisms by which infection may induce preterm labor.

organisms, which stimulate the production of host-derived cytokines in the amnion and the decidua (Fig. 23.6). These cytokines, including IL-1, TNF-α, and IL-6, stimulate increased prostaglandin production from the amnion and the decidua, which leads to the onset of preterm labor. A premature rise in PGE_2 and $PGF_2\alpha$ is characteristic of preterm labor, regardless of whether clinical or subclinical maternal genitourinary tract infection is detected.

The question then arises as to what stimulates the increased cytokine levels and the resultant increased prostaglandin levels seen during preterm delivery in patients with no evidence of genitourinary infection. Many cases of preterm LBW could result from infections of unknown origin, such as those that originate in areas other than the genitourinary tract.

Role of Periodontitis

Periodontitis is a remote gram-negative infection that may play a role in LBW infants. As discussed previously, periodontopathic organisms and their products may have wide-ranging effects that are most likely mediated through the stimulation of host cytokine production in target tissues. A remote nondisseminated infection with *P. gingivalis* may result in abnormal pregnancy outcomes

P. gingivalis-induced experimental periodontitis in animal models resulted in decreased fetal birth weight and increased amniotic fluid levels of TNF-α and PGE_2. This provides direct evidence that periodontal infection can affect the fetal environment and pregnancy outcomes.

These animal studies have led to an examination of the potential effects of periodontitis on pregnancy outcomes in humans. It was found that women who had LBW infants also had significantly greater clinical attachment loss than women who had NBW infants. After adjusting for known risk factors for LBW delivery, women with periodontitis that resulted in more than 3 mm of attachment loss in at least 60% of sites had a 7.5-fold increased risk of having an LBW infant. In a large prospective study of more than 1300 pregnant women, those with generalized periodontitis had a fivefold increased risk of preterm birth before 35 weeks' gestation and a sevenfold increased risk of delivery before 32 weeks' gestation as compared to women without periodontitis. These studies and others indicate a strong association between periodontal infection and adverse pregnancy outcomes. Excellent systematic reviews with meta-analyses have examined the wide range of studies evaluating the relationship between periodontitis and pregnancy outcomes. These studies consistently demonstrated a significant association between periodontitis and adverse pregnancy outcomes. There are two major pathways by which periodontal diseases may be associated with increased adverse pregnancy outcomes: (1) a direct pathway in which oral microorganisms disseminate to the fetal-placental unit either through a hematogenous route from the oral cavity or by an ascending route via the genitourinary tract, or (2) an indirect pathway in which elevated inflammatory mediators from the periodontal tissues reach the fetal-placental unit directly through the systemic vasculature or reach the liver and stimulate hepatic production of even more proinflammatory cytokines, which subsequently affects the fetal-placental unit.

Women who had LBW infants often had a higher prevalence and severity of periodontitis, more gingival inflammation, higher levels of putative periodontal pathogens, and an elevated subgingival inflammatory response than women who had NBW infants; furthermore, the increased bacterial challenge may have broader systemic effects, thereby resulting in an elevated challenge to the fetal immune system.

Periodontal disease may also increase the risk for preeclampsia. This hypertensive disorder affects about 5%–10% of pregnancies, and it is a major cause of perinatal and maternal morbidity and mortality. Preeclampsia has multiple potential etiologies, several of which involve vascular changes in the placenta that are similar to those seen with atherosclerosis. The presence of periodontitis during pregnancy or a worsening of periodontal disease during pregnancy is associated with a 2-fold to 2.5-fold increased risk for preeclampsia.

Systematic reviews with meta-analyses have produced conflicting results regarding the impact of periodontal therapy on pregnancy outcome. They have also emphasized the difficulty inherent in analyzing such studies due to the variability among studies with regard to the definitions of periodontal disease used and the types of periodontal treatment provided to patients. Given the conflicting evidence, it is currently unclear whether periodontal therapy provided during gestation has a beneficial effect on pregnancy outcome. What is clear is that scaling and root planing provided during the second and third trimesters of gestation are safe procedures. Every intervention trial published to date has shown that scaling and root planing during pregnancy are associated with either a decrease or no change in adverse pregnancy outcome rates. Not a single study has shown an increase in adverse outcome rates. In addition, the children of women who received scaling and root planing during gestation had similar cognitive, motor, and language development during the first 2 years of life when compared to the children of women who did not receive periodontal therapy until the postpartum period. Thus, the clinician should feel comfortable providing scaling and root planing during the second and third trimesters of pregnancy.

Periodontal Disease and Chronic Obstructive Pulmonary Disease

Chronic obstructive pulmonary disease (COPD) is characterized by airflow obstruction that results from chronic bronchitis or emphysema. Bronchial mucous glands enlarge, and an inflammatory process occurs during which neutrophils and mononuclear inflammatory cells accumulate within the lung tissue.

COPD shares similar pathogenic mechanisms with periodontal disease. With both diseases, a host inflammatory response is mounted in response to chronic challenge by bacteria in periodontal disease and by factors such as cigarette smoking in COPD. The resulting neutrophil influx leads to the release of oxidative and hydrolytic enzymes that cause tissue destruction directly. The recruitment of monocytes and macrophages leads to further release of proinflammatory mediators.

Less is known about the clinical relationship between periodontal disease and COPD as compared to CHD and other systemic conditions. A case–control study showed significantly deeper probing depth and more clinical attachment loss in patients with COPD than in controls without COPD. Individuals with poor oral hygiene have also been found to be at increased risk for chronic respiratory diseases such as bronchitis and emphysema. Conversely, a large epidemiologic study revealed no significant overall association between periodontal disease and COPD. Among nonsmokers and former smokers, even severe periodontitis did not increase the risk for COPD. In current smokers, however, the presence of severe periodontitis was associated with an increased risk of COPD. These results suggest that smoking may act as a major effect modifier in the relationship between COPD and periodontal disease and that this modifier's presence may be required to generate an effect. Conversely, tooth loss may modify the effect of smoking on COPD. In a large epidemiologic study of more than 400,000 people, both smoking and tooth loss were associated with an increased likelihood of COPD. Compared to nonsmokers with no tooth loss, smokers with tooth loss were at much higher risk for COPD, and the risk of COPD increased as the number of missing teeth increased. In COPD patients with periodontitis, periodontal therapy may impact respiratory health. COPD exacerbation is an acute event in which respiratory symptoms are worsened, usually to the point where a change in medication is needed. Most COPD exacerbations are caused by infections. In controlled clinical trials, scaling and root planing were associated with a decrease in the frequency of COPD exacerbations compared to nontreatment.

Periodontal Disease and Acute Respiratory Infections

The upper respiratory passages are often contaminated with organisms derived from the oral, nasal, and pharyngeal regions. Conversely, the lower airways, in which gas exchange occurs, are generally maintained free of microorganisms by a combination of host immune factors and mechanical clearance through the cough reflex, the ciliary transport of aspirated contaminants, and the movement of secretions from the lower airways into the trachea. Pneumonia is an infection of the lungs that is caused by bacteria, viruses, fungi, or mycoplasma and is broadly categorized as either community-acquired or hospital-acquired. A wide variety of bacteria can cause pneumonia, and the spectrum of offending organisms differs greatly between community-acquired and hospital-acquired infections.

Community-acquired bacterial pneumonia is caused primarily by the inhalation of infectious aerosols or the aspiration of oropharyngeal organisms. *Streptococcus pneumoniae* and *Haemophilus influenzae* are the most common, although numerous other species may be found, including anaerobic bacteria. Antibiotic therapy is highly successful for the resolution of most cases of community-acquired bacterial pneumonia. To date, no associations have been found between oral hygiene or periodontal disease and the risk for acute respiratory conditions such as pneumonia in community-dwelling individuals.

The same cannot be said for individuals in the hospital setting. *Hospital-acquired (nosocomial) bacterial pneumonia* has a very high morbidity and mortality rate. The incidence of nosocomial pneumonia is highest among severely ill patients, such as those in intensive care units or on ventilatory support. Although nosocomial pneumonia is most often caused by gram-negative aerobic organisms, many cases are the result of infection by anaerobic bacteria, including those that are typically found in the subgingival environment.

Hospital-acquired pneumonia is usually caused by the aspiration of oropharyngeal contents. Oropharyngeal colonization with *potential respiratory pathogens* (PRPs) is generally a transient phenomenon; however, such colonization increases during hospitalization. The longer the hospital stay, the greater the prevalence of PRPs. PRPs are found predominantly in the gastrointestinal tract, and they may be passed via esophageal reflux into the oropharynx, where they colonize. Subsequent aspiration may lead to pneumonia. Patients whose posterior oropharynx becomes colonized with PRPs have a significantly increased risk of developing nosocomial pneumonia as compared to those without oropharyngeal colonization by PRPs. Dental plaque has been shown to serve as a reservoir of PRPs; such colonization in plaque results in a persistent source of potential aspiration.

Selective decontamination is a technique that combines systemic antibiotics with orally administered nonabsorbable antibiotics in an attempt to eradicate PRPs from the digestive tract and the oropharynx and thereby minimize the risk of nosocomial respiratory infections. The technique is used primarily for patients who are intubated and on mechanical ventilators. Selective decontamination significantly decreases the incidence of nosocomial pneumonia. Decontamination of only the digestive tract does not reduce the incidence of pneumonia, but decontamination of the oropharynx alone does. This provides further evidence that the oropharynx is the primary site of PRP colonization, with the subsequent aspiration of causative organisms leading to pneumonia.

PRPs may also originate in the oral cavity, with dental plaque serving as a reservoir of these organisms. Poor oral hygiene is common in hospital and nursing home settings, especially among severely ill patients. PRPs are more often isolated from the supragingival plaque and buccal mucosa of patients in intensive care units than from those in outpatient settings. Organisms that are not routinely found in dental plaque become plaque colonizers after prolonged hospitalization. Subgingival plaque may also harbor PRPs, and putative periodontal pathogens have been associated with nosocomial pneumonia. Furthermore, anaerobic organisms from periodontal pockets may serve as the primary inoculum for suppurative respiratory diseases (e.g., pulmonary abscesses) that involve significant morbidity and mortality.

Systematic reviews of the evidence have determined that interventions used to improve oral hygiene, such as mechanical toothbrushing and chemical antimicrobial rinses, have the potential to decrease the risk of nosocomial pneumonia in high-risk patients, such as those in intensive care units or those on ventilators. Improved oral hygiene by the patient in combination with frequent professional oral health care reduces both the incidence and progression of respiratory diseases in older patients living in nursing homes, and these practices have a major impact on individuals in intensive care units, for whom the risk for nosocomial pneumonia is markedly elevated. One systematic review showed that mechanical oral hygiene performed in nursing homes and hospitals significantly decreased the occurrence and progression of respiratory tract infections and pneumonia; and that "one in 10 cases of death from pneumonia in elderly nursing home residents may be prevented by improving oral hygiene."

Periodontal Medicine in Clinical Practice

The concept of periodontal diseases as localized entities that affect only the teeth and the supporting apparatus is oversimplified. Rather than being confined to the periodontium, inflammatory periodontal diseases may have wide-ranging systemic effects. In most people, these effects are relatively inconsequential, or at least not clinically evident. In susceptible individuals, however, periodontal infection may act as an independent risk factor for systemic disease, and it may be involved in the basic pathogenic mechanisms of these conditions. Furthermore, periodontal infection may exacerbate existing systemic disorders.

Periodontal Disease and Systemic Health

Proper use of the knowledge of potential relationships between periodontal disease and systemic health requires the dental professional to recognize the oral cavity as one of many interrelated organ systems. A palm-sized infection on the leg of a pregnant woman would be of major concern to the patient and her health care provider, given the potential negative consequences of this localized infection on fetal and maternal health. Similarly, a suppurating infection on the foot of a person with diabetes would be cause for immediate evaluation and aggressive treatment, considering the effects of such infections on the metabolic control of diabetes.

Periodontal infection must be viewed in a similar manner. Periodontitis is a gram-negative infection that often results in severe inflammation, and it potentially involves the intravascular dissemination of microorganisms and their products throughout the body. However, periodontitis tends to be a "silent" disease until destruction results in acute oral symptoms. Most patients—and many medical professionals—do not recognize the potential infection that may exist within the oral cavity.

Patient Education

Patient education is a priority. Only 30 years ago, the factors involved in CHD were unclear. At present, however, it would be difficult to find an individual who was unfamiliar with the link between cholesterol and heart disease. This change was precipitated by research that clearly demonstrated the increased risk for heart disease among individuals with high cholesterol levels, followed by intensive education efforts to spread the message from the scientific community to the public at large. It is important to recognize that high cholesterol levels have not been shown to *cause* heart disease in all individuals; rather, they significantly *increase the risk* of disease. Cholesterol has also been demonstrated to have a biologically plausible role in the pathogenesis of CHD.

Similarly, patient education efforts in the realm of periodontal medicine must emphasize the inflammatory nature of periodontal infections, the increased risk for systemic disease associated with the infection, and the biologically plausible role that periodontal infection may play in systemic disease. Few individuals had their cholesterol levels evaluated until knowledge of the link between cholesterol and heart disease became widespread. Likewise, an increased appreciation of the potential effects of periodontal infection on systemic health may result in increased patient demand for periodontal evaluation.

Enhanced community awareness may be derived from newspapers, magazines, and other lay sources. However, the most reliable origin of information should be dental and medical professionals, through daily contact with patients. A pregnant woman usually knows that infections may adversely affect her pregnancy. Individuals with diabetes generally know that infections impair glycemic control. However, many of these patients do not know that occult periodontal infections can have the same effect as more clinically evident infections. The dentist is responsible for diagnosing periodontal infections, providing appropriate treatment, and preventing disease recurrence or progression. Because many medical professionals are unfamiliar with the oral cavity and oral health research, dentists must reach out to the medical community to improve patient care through education and communication. Likewise, patients must be educated about disease prevention. Just as patients know that lowering their cholesterol levels may decrease their risk for heart disease, similar knowledge regarding the prevention of periodontal infection should be emphasized. A physician would be remiss if he or she did not provide education about decreasing cholesterol level, losing weight, and ceasing a smoking habit to a patient at risk for CHD. Likewise, controlling the risk factor of periodontal infection requires the dentist to emphasize personal and professional preventive measures that are focused on oral hygiene and regular recall.

Key points

- There is consistent and strong epidemiologic evidence that periodontitis imparts increased risk for future cardiovascular disease.
- Periodontal infection may also promote increased blood viscosity and thrombogenesis, which leads to an increased risk for central and peripheral vascular disease.
- Periodontal diseases may have both direct effects on the major blood vessels (e.g., atheroma formation) and indirect effects that stimulate changes in the cardiovascular system (e.g., elevation of systemic inflammatory responses).
- Bacteremia with PAAP-positive bacterial strains from supragingival and subgingival plaque can increase platelet aggregation, thereby contributing to thrombus formation and subsequent thromboembolism, which is the leading cause of stroke.
- Among diabetic patients with periodontitis, periodontal therapy may have beneficial effects on glycemic control.
- There is a significant association between periodontitis and adverse pregnancy outcomes (delivery of preterm and low birth weight infants).
- The presence of periodontitis during pregnancy or a worsening of periodontal disease during pregnancy is associated with a 2-fold to 2.5-fold increased risk for preeclampsia.
- Patient education efforts in the realm of periodontal medicine must emphasize the inflammatory nature of periodontal infections, the increased risk for systemic disease associated with the infection, and the biologically plausible role that periodontal infection may play in systemic disease.

Suggested Readings

Beck JD, Offenbacher S: The association between periodontal diseases and cardiovascular diseases: a state-of-the-art review, *Ann Periodontol* 6:9–15, 2001.

D'Aiuto F, Parkar M, Andreou G: Periodontitis and systemic inflammation: control of the local infection is associated with a reduction in serum inflammatory markers, *J Dent Res* 83:156–160, 2004.

Kebschull M, Demmer RT, Papapanou PN: Gum bug, leave my heart alone"—epidemiologic and mechanistic evidence linking periodontal infections and atherosclerosis, *J Dent Res* 89:879–902, 2010.

Lockhart PB, Bolger AF, Papapanou PN, American Heart Association Rheumatic Fever, Endocarditis, and Kawasaki Disease Committee of the Council on Cardiovascular Disease in the Young, Council on Epidemiology and Prevention, Council on Peripheral Vascular Disease, and Council on Clinical Cardiology: et al: Periodontal disease and atherosclerotic vascular disease: does the evidence support an independent association? A scientific statement from the American Heart Association, *Circulation* 125:2520–2544, 2012.

Mealey BL, Oates TW: Diabetes mellitus and periodontal diseases, *J Periodontol* 77:1289–1303, 2006.

Ross RL: Atherosclerosis—an inflammatory disease, *N Engl J Med* 342: 115–126, 1999.

Scannapieco FA, Bush RB, Paju S: Associations between periodontal disease and risk for nosocomial bacterial pneumonia and chronic obstructive pulmonary disease: a systematic review, *Ann Periodontol* 8:54–69, 2003.

Tonetti MS, D'Aiuto F, Nibali L: Treatment of periodontitis and endothelial function, *New Engl J Med* 356:911–920, 2007.

Williams RC: Understanding and managing periodontal diseases: a notable past, a promising future, *J Periodontol* 79:1552–1559, 2008.

Xiong X, Beukens P, Fraser WD, et al: Periodontal disease and adverse pregnancy outcomes: a systematic review, *BJOG* 113:135–143, 2006.

References

References and MCQs with answers for the chapter are available on www.medenact.com.

CHAPTER 24

Periodontal Examination and Diagnosis

S Elangovan | JH Do | HH Takei | FA Carranza | G Avila-Ortiz | CD Dwarakanath

CHAPTER OUTLINE

Diagnosis can be defined as the art of identifying a condition or disease and differentiating it from other entities.

Proper diagnosis is essential for effective treatment. **Periodontal** diagnosis is primarily aimed at determining whether the disease is present, as well as its severity and extent. An accurate diagnosis can also provide valuable information pertaining to the underlying pathologic processes and their causes, which is fundamental to formulating a personalized **treatment plan**. In other chapters of this book, detailed descriptions of the different diseases that can affect the **periodontium** and associated treatment modalities are provided.

The periodontal diagnosis is determined after careful analysis of the case history and evaluation of the clinical signs and symptoms, as well as the results of various diagnostic procedures (e.g., probing, mobility assessment, radiographs, blood tests, and biopsies).

The oral cavity mirrors the general health of an individual; and the oral health can affect the general health. Hence, arriving at a diagnosis, determining the prognosis, establishing a treatment plan, and the treatment outcomes are all affected by the systemic health of an individual. Diagnosis must therefore include a general evaluation of the patient and an overall consideration of the oral cavity. For example, the 2017 **periodontal disease** classification system endorses this view and utilizes a holistic approach to arrive at the diagnosis of **periodontitis**, one of the most prevalent human diseases.

Diagnostic procedures must be systematic and organized for specific purposes. It is not enough to assemble facts. Findings must be pieced together so that they provide a meaningful explanation of the patient's periodontal status. The following is a recommended sequence of procedures for the diagnosis of periodontal diseases and conditions.

Overall Appraisal of the Patient

From the first interaction, the clinician should attempt to make an overall appraisal of the patient. This includes consideration of the patient's mental and emotional status, temperament, attitude, and physiologic age. An example is the observation of a patient's gait when walking in the clinic. This observation could provide valuable information on the patient's neurological status and the existence of physical challenges that could potentially affect the patient's oral hygiene practices.

Demographics like name, age, gender, educational status, occupation, income, and address are also recorded not only for medicolegal reasons but for many other purposes. They help in establishing a rapport with the patient which helps in confidence and trust building. Certain conditions are age and gender (hormones) related; the educational and socioeconomic status of the patient could affect the treatment plan; the occupation could have a bearing on the periodontal condition and treatment plan (stress, wasting diseases, esthetics, etc.); the area of residence could help in diagnosis of certain conditions as well as in treatment schedules; and, the prognosis could also be affected by age.

Health History

A thorough health/medical history should be obtained at the first visit. This information can be supplemented and updated by pertinent questioning on subsequent visits. The health history can be obtained verbally by questioning the patient and recording his or her responses in the patient's health record or by means of a questionnaire that the patient completes prior to the appointment. Fig. 24.1 shows the health history form recommended by the American Dental Association.

The importance of the health history should be clearly explained because patients often omit relevant information that they cannot relate to their dental problems or that they are not willing to share. In some situations, it is prudent to communicate with the patient's medical provider to obtain a complete history prior to treatment. The patient should be made aware of the following: (1) the possible impact of certain systemic diseases, conditions, behavioral factors, and medications on periodontal diseases and conditions, their treatment, and treatment outcomes; (2) certain conditions may require special precautions or modifications of the treatment procedure; and (3) the impact that oral **infections** may have on systemic health.

Health History Form

ADA. American Dental Association www.ada.org

E-mail: Today's Date:

As required by law, our office adheres to written policies and procedures to protect the privacy of information about you that we create, receive or maintain. Your answers are for our records only and will be kept confidential subject to applicable laws. Please note that you will be asked some questions about your responses to this questionnaire and there may be additional questions concerning your health. This information is vital to allow us to provide appropriate care for you. This office does not use this information to discriminate.

Name: (Last / First / Middle) Home Phone: *Include area code* ( ) Business/Cell Phone: *Include area code* ( )

Address: (Mailing address) City: State: Zip:

Occupation: Height: Weight: Date of birth: Sex: M F

SS# or Patient ID: Emergency Contact: Relationship: Home Phone: ( ) Cell Phone: ( ) *Include area codes*

If you are completing this form for another person, what is your relationship to that person?

Your Name Relationship

Do you have any of the following diseases or problems: ***(Check DK if you Don't Know the answer to the question)***

	Yes	No	DK
Active tuberculosis	☐	☐	☐
Persistent cough greater than a 3 week duration	☐	☐	☐
Cough that produces blood	☐	☐	☐
Been exposed to anyone with tuberculosis	☐	☐	☐

If you answer yes to any of the 4 items above, please stop and return this form to the receptionist.

Dental Information *For the following questions, please mark (X) your responses to the following questions.*

	Yes	No	DK
Do your gums bleed when you brush or floss?	☐	☐	☐
Are your teeth sensitive to cold, hot, sweets or pressure?	☐	☐	☐
Does food or floss catch between your teeth?	☐	☐	☐
Is your mouth dry?	☐	☐	☐
Have you had any periodontal (gum) treatments?	☐	☐	☐
Have you ever had orthodontic (braces) treatment?	☐	☐	☐
Have you had any problems associated with previous dental treatment?	☐	☐	☐
Is your home water supply fluoridated?	☐	☐	☐
Do you drink bottled or filtered water?	☐	☐	☐
If yes, how often? Circle one: DAILY / WEEKLY / OCCASIONALLY			
Are you currently experiencing dental pain or discomfort?	☐	☐	☐

	Yes	No	DK
Do you have earaches or neck pains?	☐	☐	☐
Do you have any clicking, popping or discomfort in the jaw?	☐	☐	☐
Do you brux or grind your teeth?	☐	☐	☐
Do you have sores or ulcers in your mouth?	☐	☐	☐
Do you wear dentures or partials?	☐	☐	☐
Do you participate in active recreational activities?	☐	☐	☐
Have you ever had a serious injury to your head or mouth?	☐	☐	☐

Date of your last dental exam:
What was done at that time?

Date of last dental x-rays:

What is the reason for your dental visit today?

How do you feel about your smile?

Medical Information *Please mark (X) your response to indicate if you have or have not had any of the following diseases or problems.*

	Yes	No	DK
Are you now under the care of a physician?	☐	☐	☐

Physician Name: Phone: *Include area code* ( )

Address/City/State/Zip:

	Yes	No	DK
Are you in good health?	☐	☐	☐
Has there been any change in your general health within the past year?	☐	☐	☐

If yes, what condition is being treated?

Date of last physical exam:

	Yes	No	DK
Have you had a serious illness, operation or been hospitalized in the past 5 years?	☐	☐	☐

If yes, what was the illness or problem?

	Yes	No	DK
Are you taking or have you recently taken any prescription or over the counter medicine(s)?	☐	☐	☐

If so, please list all, including vitamins, natural or herbal preparations and/or diet supplements:

Fig. 24.1 Medical history form from the American Dental Association. *(From ©American Dental Association. Reprinted with permission.)*

Medical Information

Please mark (X) your response to indicate if you have or have not had any of the following diseases or problems.

(Check DK if you Don't Know the answer to the question)

	Yes	No	DK
Do you wear contact lenses?	☐	☐	☐
Joint Replacement. Have you had an orthopedic total joint (hip, knee, elbow, finger) replacement?	☐	☐	☐
Date: ______ If yes, have you had any complications? ______			
Are you taking or scheduled to begin taking either of the medications, alendronate (Fosamax®) or risedronate (Actonel®) for osteoporosis or Paget's disease?	☐	☐	☐
Since 2001, were you treated or are you presently scheduled to begin treatment with the intravenous bisphosphonates (Aredia® or Zometa®) for bone pain, hypercalcemia or skeletal complications resulting from Paget's disease, multiple myeloma or metastatic cancer?	☐	☐	☐
Date Treatment began: ______			
Do you use controlled substances (drugs)?	☐	☐	☐
Do you use tobacco (smoking, snuff, chew, bidis)?	☐	☐	☐
If so, how interested are you in stopping? (Circle one) VERY / SOMEWHAT / NOT INTERESTED			
Do you drink alcoholic beverages?	☐	☐	☐
If yes, how much alcohol did you drink in the last 24 hours? ______			
If yes, how much do you typically drink In a week? ______			
WOMEN ONLY Are you:			
Pregnant?	☐	☐	☐
Number of weeks: ______			
Taking birth control pills or hormonal replacement?	☐	☐	☐
Nursing?	☐	☐	☐

Allergies - Are you allergic to or have you had a reaction to:
To all **yes** responses, specify type of reaction.

	Yes	No	DK
Local anesthetics ______	☐	☐	☐
Aspirin ______	☐	☐	☐
Penicillin or other antibiotics ______	☐	☐	☐
Barbiturates, sedatives, or sleeping pills ______	☐	☐	☐
Sulfa drugs ______	☐	☐	☐
Codeine or other narcotics ______	☐	☐	☐
Metals ______	☐	☐	☐
Latex (rubber) ______	☐	☐	☐
Iodine ______	☐	☐	☐
Hay fever/seasonal ______	☐	☐	☐
Animals ______	☐	☐	☐
Food ______	☐	☐	☐
Other ______	☐	☐	☐

Please mark (X) your response to indicate if you have or have not had any of the following diseases or problems.

	Yes	No	DK
Artificial (prosthetic) heart valve	☐	☐	☐
Previous infective endocarditis	☐	☐	☐
Damaged valves in transplanted heart	☐	☐	☐
Congenital heart disease (CHD)			
Unrepaired, cyanotic CHD	☐	☐	☐
Repaired (completely) in last 6 months	☐	☐	☐
Repaired CHD with residual defects	☐	☐	☐

Except for the conditions listed above, antibiotic prophylaxis is no longer recommended for any other form of CHD.

	Yes	No	DK
Cardiovascular disease.	☐	☐	☐
Angina	☐	☐	☐
Arteriosclerosis	☐	☐	☐
Congestive heart failure	☐	☐	☐
Damaged heart valves	☐	☐	☐
Heart attack	☐	☐	☐
Heart murmur	☐	☐	☐
Low blood pressure	☐	☐	☐
High blood pressure	☐	☐	☐
Other congenital heart defects	☐	☐	☐
Mitral valve prolapse	☐	☐	☐
Pacemaker	☐	☐	☐
Rheumatic fever	☐	☐	☐
Rheumatic heart disease	☐	☐	☐
Abnormal bleeding	☐	☐	☐
Anemia	☐	☐	☐
Blood transfusion	☐	☐	☐
If yes, date: ______			
Hemophilia	☐	☐	☐
AIDS or HIV infection	☐	☐	☐
Arthritis	☐	☐	☐
Autoimmune disease	☐	☐	☐
Rheumatoid arthritis	☐	☐	☐
Systemic lupus erythematosus.	☐	☐	☐
Asthma	☐	☐	☐
Bronchitis	☐	☐	☐
Emphysema	☐	☐	☐
Sinus trouble	☐	☐	☐
Tuberculosis	☐	☐	☐
Cancer/Chemotherapy/Radiation Treatment	☐	☐	☐
Chest pain upon exertion	☐	☐	☐
Chronic pain	☐	☐	☐
Diabetes Type I or II	☐	☐	☐
Eating disorder	☐	☐	☐
Malnutrition	☐	☐	☐
Gastrointestinal disease	☐	☐	☐
G.E. Reflux/persistent heartburn	☐	☐	☐
Ulcers	☐	☐	☐
Thyroid problems	☐	☐	☐
Stroke	☐	☐	☐
Glaucoma	☐	☐	☐
Hepatitis, jaundice or liver disease	☐	☐	☐
Epilepsy	☐	☐	☐
Fainting spells or seizures	☐	☐	☐
Neurological disorders	☐	☐	☐
If yes, specify: ______			
Sleep disorder	☐	☐	☐
Mental health disorders	☐	☐	☐
Specify: ______			
Recurrent infections	☐	☐	☐
Type of infection: ______			
Kidney problems	☐	☐	☐
Night sweats	☐	☐	☐
Osteoporosis	☐	☐	☐
Persistent swollen glands in neck	☐	☐	☐
Severe headaches/migraines	☐	☐	☐
Severe or rapid weight loss	☐	☐	☐
Sexually transmitted disease	☐	☐	☐
Excessive urination	☐	☐	☐

	Yes	No	DK
Has a physician or previous dentist recommended that you take antibiotics prior to your dental treatment?	☐	☐	☐

Name of physician or dentist making recommendation: ______ Phone: ______

	Yes	No	DK
Do you have any disease, condition, or problem not listed above that you think I should know about?	☐	☐	☐

Please explain:

NOTE: Both doctor and patient are encouraged to discuss any and all relevant patient health issues prior to treatment.
I certify that I have read and understand the above and that the information given on this form is accurate. I understand the importance of a truthful health history and that my dentist and his/her staff will rely on this information for treating me. I acknowledge that my questions, if any, about inquiries set forth above have been answered to my satisfaction. I will not hold my dentist, or any other member of his/her staff, responsible for any action they take or do not take because of errors or omissions that I may have made in the completion of this form.

Signature of Patient/Legal Guardian: ______ Date: ______

FOR COMPLETION BY DENTIST

Comments: ______

Fig. 24.1, cont'd

The health history should include the following information:

1. Vital signs and other morphometric assessments, including blood pressure readings, heart rate, and temperature, as well as height and weight measures to determine the patient's body mass index.
2. The date of the last physical exam and the frequency of physical exams and physician visits. If the patient is under current medical care, the nature and duration of the problem(s) and associated therapy should be discussed. The name, address, and telephone number of the physician's practice should be recorded, because direct communication may be necessary.
3. Details regarding previous hospitalizations and surgical operations, including the diagnosis, the type of operation, and any untoward events (e.g., anesthetic, hemorrhagic, or **infectious** complications), should be obtained.
4. All medical problems, including cardiovascular, hematologic, and endocrine conditions, infectious diseases, high-risk behavior for **human immunodeficiency virus** infection, and possible occupational disease, should be identified and recorded.
5. Abnormal bleeding, such as nosebleeds, prolonged bleeding time after minor skin cuts, spontaneous ecchymosis, a tendency toward excessive bruising, and profuse menstrual bleeding, should be noted. These symptoms should be cross-checked with the medications that the patient takes on a regular basis.
6. Specifically for females, information regarding the onset of puberty, menopause, menstrual disorders, hysterectomy, pregnancies, and miscarriages should be recorded.
7. Need for **antibiotic** prophylaxis should be assessed.
8. A list of all medications being currently taken and whether they were prescribed or obtained over-the-counter should be included. All possible effects and drug interactions of these medications should be carefully analyzed to determine their effect, if any, on the oral tissues. It is of paramount importance to avoid administering other medications that would interact adversely with them. A special inquiry should be made regarding the dosage and duration of therapy with anticoagulants and corticosteroids. Patients who are taking any medications in the family of drugs called bisphosphonates (e.g., alendronate, zoledronic acid), which are often prescribed for osteoporosis, should be cautioned about possible complications related to osteonecrosis of the jaw prior to undergoing any intervention involving trauma to bone tissue.
9. The patient's history of allergies should be recorded, including hay fever, asthma, sensitivity to foods, drugs (e.g., aspirin, codeine, barbiturates, sulfonamides, antibiotics, procaine, laxatives), and dental materials (e.g., latex, eugenol, acrylic resins).
10. Pertinent information regarding family history should be gathered, including bleeding disorders, cardiovascular disease, diabetes, and periodontal diseases.
11. Detailed information on current and history of alcohol, recreational drugs, and tobacco use and the desire to quit should be obtained.

For patients who are on medications (e.g., bisphosphonates and anticoagulants); patients who do not know the current status of their systemic disease, such as diabetes, hypertension, or immunodeficiency; or patients who elicit signs and symptoms of systemic diseases but have not as yet been diagnosed, a medical consultation is often required before any periodontal treatment can be rendered.

Dental History

Chief Complaint and Current Illness

Some patients may be unaware of existing periodontal diseases and conditions. However, many patients presenting with severe diseases usually report profuse **gingival** bleeding, tooth mobility, spreading of the teeth with the appearance of spaces where none existed before, "longer" teeth, a foul taste in the mouth, bad breath, or an itchy feeling in the gums that is relieved by digging with a toothpick. Some patients may also present with pain of varied types and duration, including constant, dull, gnawing pain; sensitivity when chewing; dull pain after eating; burning sensation in the gums; deep radiating pain in the jaws; spontaneous **acute** throbbing pain; sensitivity to hot and cold foods and beverages; or extreme sensitivity to inhaled air.

The chief complaint is recorded in the patient's own words. This is for medicolegal purposes and this also gives us an idea of the patient's concerns and expectations. When the patient has multiple complaints, they are recorded in a chronological order. The onset, duration, progress, aggravating factors, and relieving factors of the chief complaint are then noted. Any treatment that has been sought and rendered for the same complaint and its outcome are also noted.

The dental history should include reference to the following:

1. The frequency of past visits to the dentist, the date of the most recent visit, and the nature of the treatment, including whether it was a dental prophylaxis, **periodontal maintenance**, or root **debridement** (**scaling** and **root planing**) by a dentist or hygienist.
2. The patient's oral hygiene habits, including toothbrushing frequency, time of day, method, type of toothbrush and dentifrice, and interval when brushes are replaced. Other methods for oral care, such as mouthwashes, interdental brushes, dental floss, water irrigation, and other devices.
3. Any previous or current orthodontic treatment, including its duration and the approximate date of completion.
4. Presence of deleterious and parafunctional habits, such as grinding or clenching of the teeth during the day or at night (Some leading questions to ascertain this information are: Do the teeth or jaw muscles feel "sore" in the morning?), tobacco smoking or chewing (duration of the habit, frequency of usage, etc.), nail biting, or biting on objects.
5. The patient's history of previous dental and periodontal problems, including the nature of the condition and, if previously treated, the type of treatment received (surgical and/or nonsurgical) and the approximate period of disease resolution.
6. Note whether the patient wears any tooth-, mucosa-, or implant-supported prostheses for tooth replacement and the patient's satisfaction with it.
7. History of tooth extractions and the reason for extraction (mobility or caries).
8. History of any alarming events or any complications during or due to dental or periodontal treatment in the past like an adverse or allergic reaction to local anesthesia or any dental materials or drugs, syncopal episodes, or other medical complications or emergencies in the dental chair or operatory. (Such an event can impart anxiety and fear in patients, which could negatively impact future treatment and management. This history can aid the clinician to better prepare and effectively manage the patient in future appointments while minimizing risks.)

Photographic Documentation and Study Models

An important element of the periodontal examination is the documentation of clinical findings. Digital photographic documentation is useful for record-keeping, education of both the clinician and the patient, communication with referrals and colleagues, and planning and treatment of patients with high esthetic demands. Photographs can provide details that a clinician may not otherwise remember, or even perceive while performing an intraoral exam, and allow the clinician to evaluate extra- and intraoral structures after the patient leaves and to monitor tissue changes over time. If possible, prior to initiating the clinical examination, a set of intraoral photos should be taken before the tissue is probed and manipulated to obtain an undisturbed baseline of the patient's mouth with intact **gingiva** and **biofilm** (Fig. 24.2). These initial photos, when presented to the patient on a large-screen monitor, can be extremely powerful in educating and helping the patient to understand the conditions of his or her mouth; the presence and location of biofilm, **inflammation**, and any tissue abnormality; and the need for improvement of oral hygiene habits (Fig. 24.3).

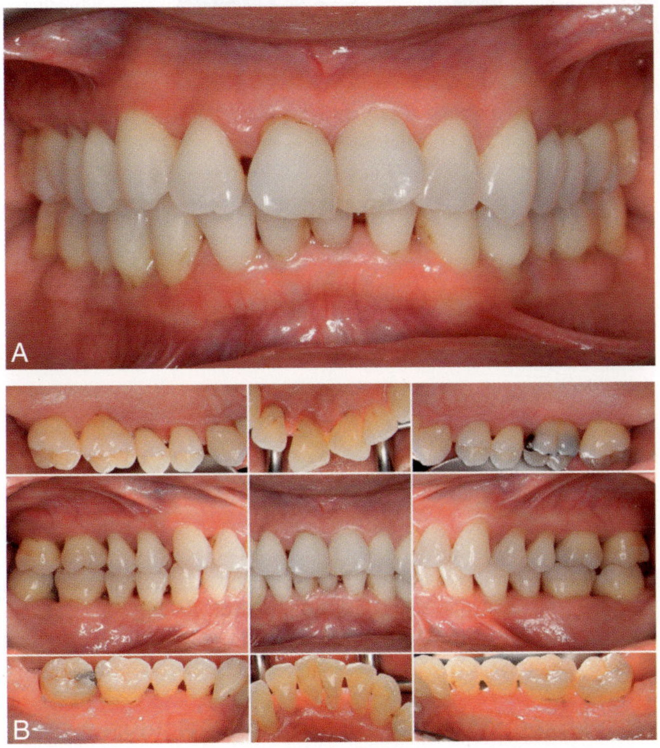

Fig. 24.2 At a minimum, an initial set of intraoral photographs contains nine images: A, The retracted frontal image is a direct shot. B, The two buccal shots are flipped horizontally and compiled with the remaining seven images to create a composite of the whole dentition. *(Copyright Jonathan H. Do, DDS. All rights reserved.)*

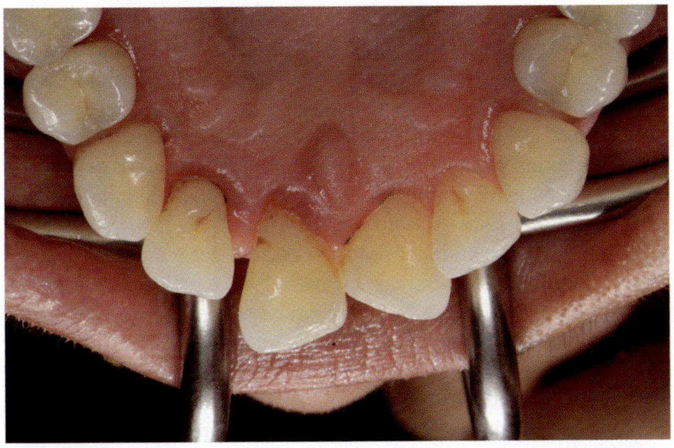

Fig. 24.3 An image capturing the palatal surfaces of the anterior maxilla is presented on a 27-inch computer screen to help a patient understand her periodontal status. *(Copyright Jonathan H. Do, DDS. All rights reserved.)*

Similar to photographic documentation, a set of dental models can be a valuable diagnostic and patient-education tool. Models may be obtained with a conventional physical impression or through digital scanning and subsequent 3D printing. The three-dimensional nature of dental models may allow the clinician to not only study the case more precisely but also explain dynamic concepts, such as occlusion, to patients, as a complement to radiographs and photographs. Models may also be used to fabricate appliances like night guard, a protective palatal stent for **autogenous** soft tissue graft donor sites, or a surgical guide for implant placement.

Clinical Examination

Examination of Extraoral Structures

Clinical examination should begin with an evaluation of the extraoral structures for abnormalities. The temporomandibular joints should be assessed for pain, crepitus, clicking, popping, and their range of motions. Masticatory muscles and salivary glands should be palpated for pain and tenderness.

Because periodontal and periapical pathosis and other oral diseases may result in lymph node changes, the clinician should routinely examine and evaluate the lymph nodes of the head and neck. Lymph nodes can become palpable, enlarged, or indurated as a result of an acute infectious episode, malignant metastases, or residual fibrotic changes. Inflamed nodes typically become enlarged, palpable, tender, and fairly immobile. The overlying skin may be red and warm. **Primary herpetic gingivostomatitis, necrotizing ulcerative gingivitis**, and acute **periodontal abscesses** may produce lymph node enlargement. After successful therapy, lymph nodes typically return to normal in a matter of days to weeks.

Examination of the Oral Cavity

The entire oral cavity, including the lips, the vestibule, the buccal mucosa, the floor of the mouth, the tongue, the palate, and the oropharyngeal region should be examined in a sequence, to detect any abnormalities or pathological changes. The oral mucosa in the apical region of the alveolar ridge may be palpated for tenderness to detect periapical and periodontal abscesses.

The oral cavity should be assessed for oral hygiene efficiency. The cleanliness of the oral cavity may be visually appraised in terms of the extent of accumulated food debris, biofilm, **calculus**, and tooth surface stains, as well as biofilm coating of the dorsum of the tongue (Fig. 24.4). The oral cavity is also assessed for the presence of oral malodor. Oral malodor, also termed *fetor ex ore, fetor oris,* or *halitosis,* is a foul or offensive odor that emanates from the oral cavity. When present, mouth odors may be of diagnostic significance, and their origin may be either oral or extraoral (such as the gastrointestinal tract).

Assessment of Oral Hygiene Performance

Prior to initiating the periodontal examination *per se*, it is important to assess the patient's oral hygiene performance. This can be done in a simple and unbiased manner by giving the patient a toothbrush and a piece of floss and asking the patient to perform **plaque** removal as they would normally do on a day-to-day basis. This exercise can provide very valuable information regarding technical efficiency, dexterity and time spent, which can be further utilized for patient education purposes.

Examination of the Periodontium

The periodontal examination should be systematic and not immediately begin with the insertion of the periodontal probe into the

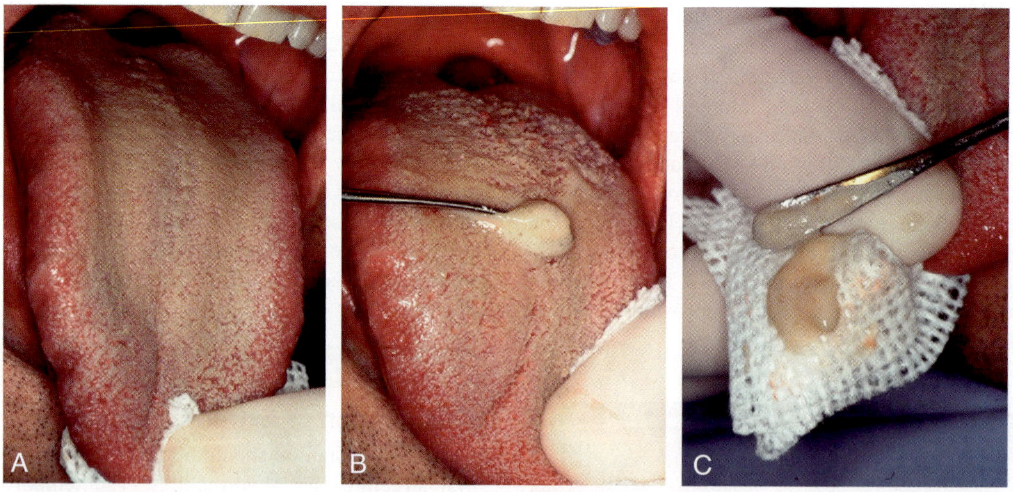

Fig. 24.4 Biofilm coating of the dorsum surface of the tongue (A) can be a source of oral malodor. When the tongue is heavily coated, the biofilm may need to be scraped off with a spatula or a tongue scraper (B and C).

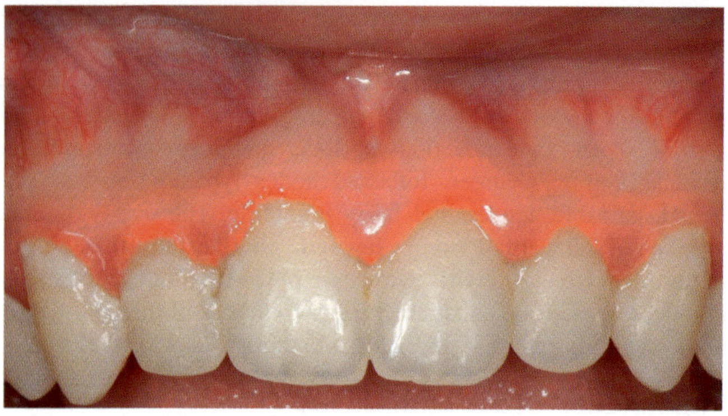

Fig. 24.5 The inflammatory response in the marginal gingiva is typically the result of biofilm accumulation on the tooth surface along the gingival margin. *(Copyright Jonathan H. Do, DDS. All rights reserved.)*

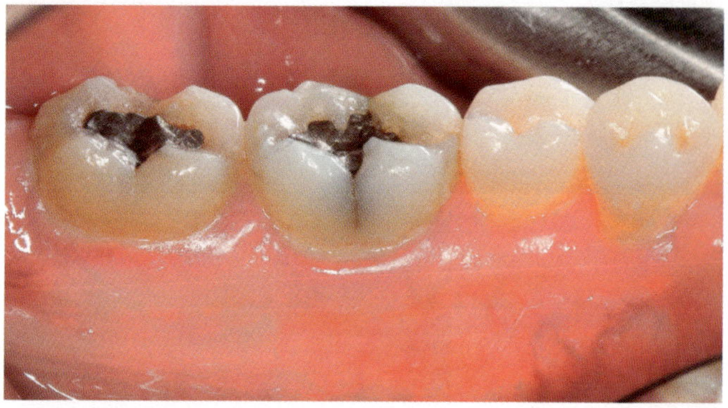

Fig. 24.6 Biofilm frequently accumulates on tooth surfaces in concavities along the gingival margin and interproximal spaces. *(Copyright Jonathan H. Do, DDS. All rights reserved.)*

gingival crevice, which can be uncomfortable and traumatic for a patient and may induce bleeding that could make visualization of inflammatory changes in the soft tissue challenging. Therefore, the periodontal examination should begin with a thorough and careful visual evaluation of the gingival margin to assess biofilm and calculus **accumulation**, inflammatory changes in the soft tissue (Fig. 24.5), as well as alterations of the normal soft tissue contours and position, such as gingival recession defects and tooth mobility. Once a thorough visual periodontal assessment has been completed, the gingiva, the gingival crevice, and the subgingival tooth surface are carefully probed (tactile periodontal examination). Thorough probing of the gingival crevice and tactile assessment of the surrounding tissues provides a wealth of valuable information, such as **probing depth** measures, **bleeding on probing**, and the position of the gingival margin with respect to the CEJ and clinical attachment loss, which are essential parameters for the diagnosis and treatment of periodontal diseases and conditions (e.g., periodontitis).

Visual Periodontal Examination

Visual examination begins with taking a survey of biofilm and calculus accumulation to assess oral hygiene. This can be facilitated by the use of disclosing agents. The gingiva is then examined for clinical signs of inflammation (e.g., erythema and edema) and apical migration of the gingival margin to assess the presence, extent, and severity of disease.

Visual Examination of Biofilm and Calculus

There are many methods available for assessing biofilm and calculus accumulation. The presence of biofilm and supragingival calculus can be observed directly. Biofilm frequently accumulates in concavities along the gingival margins and in embrasure spaces, especially in difficult-to-reach areas, such as the distal surface of the distal-most tooth in the quadrant and the lingual surfaces of mandibular posterior teeth (Fig. 24.6). Supragingival calculus tends to accumulate on the lingual surfaces of the mandibular anterior teeth and the buccal surfaces of the maxillary molars, mainly due to the presence of the Wharton and Stensen salivary ducts, respectively, and ineffective biofilm removal. The amount and location of biofilm and supragingival calculus may provide insights into the effectiveness of the patient's biofilm control as well as possible inflammatory changes in the tissue. Biofilm on the buccal and facial surfaces of teeth closest to the midline is most accessible for removal. The presence of biofilm in these areas is generally suggestive of inadequate oral hygiene (see Fig. 24.5). The absence of biofilm may not necessarily indicate that the patient practices good oral hygiene or that the disease is absent, as many patients thoroughly brush their teeth before seeing a dentist. The presence or absence of biofilm should be correlated with the presence and severity or absence of gingival inflammation, as well as the presence of subgingival deposits.

The presence of subgingival calculus may not be easily detected. Sometimes, subgingival calculus may be identified along the gingival

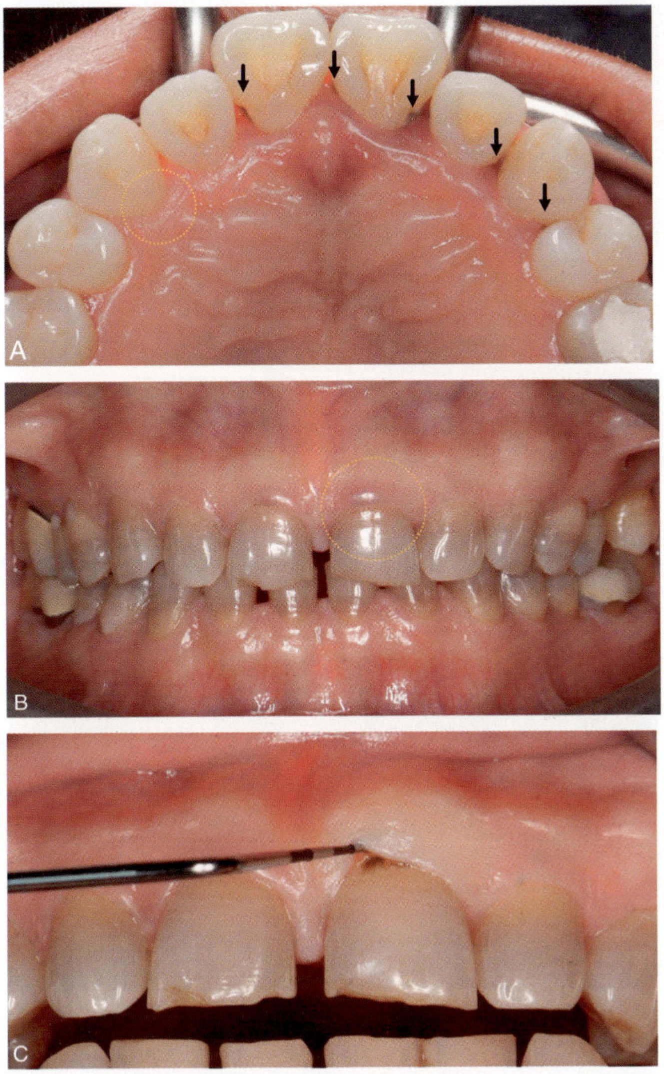

Fig. 24.7 A, Subgingival calculus can be visible on the tooth surface *(arrows)* along the gingival margin. Its presence is associated with inflammatory changes in the tissue. In places where biofilm and calculus are absent, the gingiva is usually pink, firm, and stippled *(circle)*. B, Subgingival calculus may be visible through the marginal gingiva. C, Retraction of the gingiva confirms its presence. *(Copyright Jonathan H. Do, DDS. All rights reserved.)*

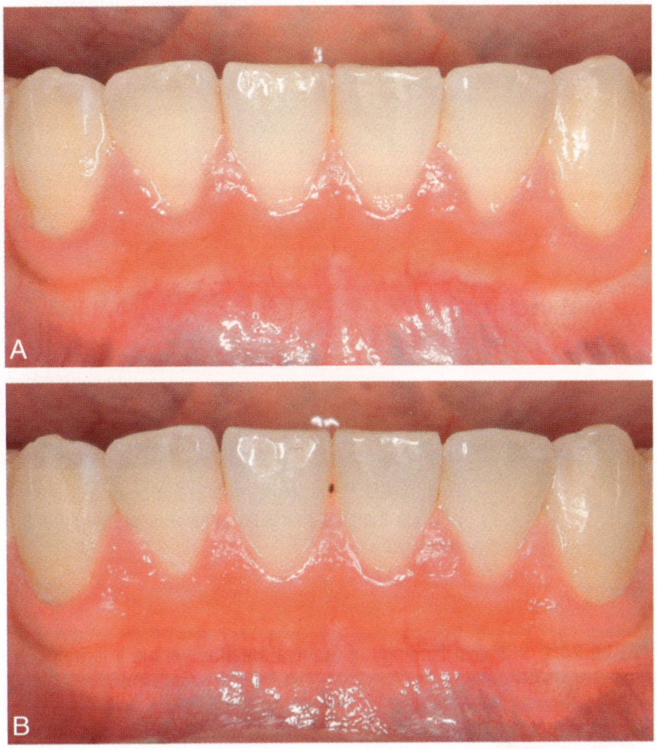

Fig. 24.8 Saliva obscures details. A, The gingiva appears smooth when covered in saliva. B, Once dried, stippling is visible, and erythema and edema become more obvious. *(Copyright Jonathan H. Do, DDS. All rights reserved.)*

margin with gentle separation of the marginal gingiva or periodontal pocket wall with a periodontal probe or may even be visible through the soft tissue in sites exhibiting a thin gingival **phenotype** (Fig. 24.7). However, subgingival calculus is usually detected by careful tactile examination of the root surface using an instrument (e.g., periodontal probe or explorer). The presence of signs of gingival inflammation (e.g., discoloration and swelling) may provide clues to the location of subgingival calculus deposits.

Although radiographs may sometimes reveal heavy calculus deposits interproximally and even on the facial and lingual surfaces, they cannot be relied on for thorough calculus detection.

Visual Examination of the Gingiva

The gingiva is the collar of soft tissue that invests the cervical region of a tooth and is contiguous with its periodontal ligament and the alveolar mucosa. It extends from the gingival margin to the mucogingival junction. On the palate, where the mucogingival junction is absent, the gingiva extends apically and merges seamlessly with the masticatory mucosa that invests the hard palate.

Gingival width is the distance from the gingival margin to the mucogingival junction. The mucogingival junction, which demarcates the immobile attached gingiva from the mobile alveolar mucosa, can be determined by stretching the lip and cheek outwards and away from the vestibule or by placing a probe **horizontally** in the vestibule and rolling it from the alveolar mucosa toward the gingiva coronally. The mucogingival junction is where the mucosa stops moving or rolling, respectively. All teeth are surrounded by a variable amount of gingiva. However, there may be sites where the keratinized tissue is minimal and cannot be clinically appreciated, giving the impression that the tooth is surrounded by nonkeratinized mucosa (Fig. 24.8). The gingiva is then dried and evaluated for inflammatory changes. Although not always the case, when there is adequate gingival width, subtle inflammatory changes in the marginal gingiva may be best detected by comparing the marginal gingiva to the gingival tissue 2 or 3 mm apical to the gingival margin, where the tissue is likely to be healthier (Fig. 24.9). Local inflammatory changes tend to be correlated with the presence and severity of biofilm and calculus. If supragingival biofilm and calculus deposits are insignificant in sites exhibiting signs of inflammation, the presence of subgingival calculus or other contributing factors should be carefully investigated.

The appearance of the soft tissues investing a tooth and the underlying alveolar bone may vary from site to site and from individual to individual, depending on the location and the specific anatomical features of the area, as well as genetic and environmental determinants. Generally, healthy gingiva is pink in color. The color depends on the vascularity, thickness of the gingiva, and the degree of keratinization. The color could vary due to pigmentation. The physiologic cause of pigmentation is the presence of melanin in the epithelium and the amount of pigmentation varies in different races. The gingival contour consists of sharp, thin, knife-edge

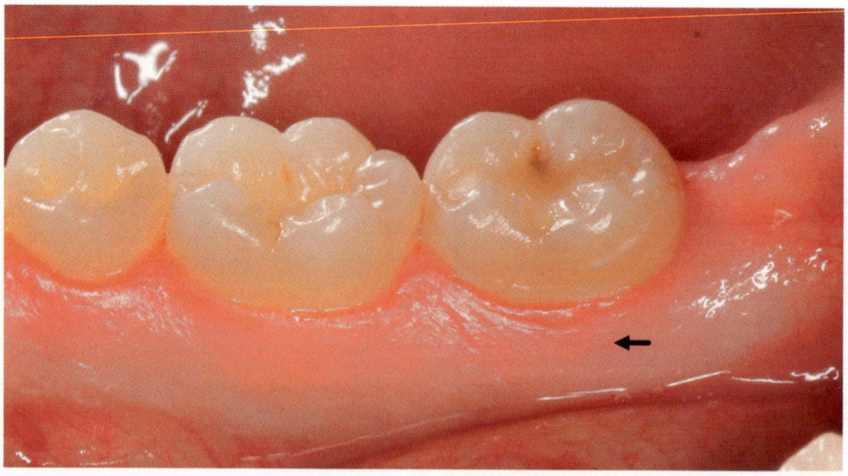

Fig. 24.9 When compared to the gingival tissue located at 2–3 mm apical to the gingival margin *(arrow)*, it is obvious that the marginal gingiva is erythematous and edematous. *(Copyright Jonathan H. Do, DDS. All rights reserved.)*

TABLE 24.1 Clinical Findings of Gingiva: Healthy Versus Inflamed

Gingiva: Healthy	Gingiva: Inflammation
• Color: pink, pigmentation could be present	• Color: erythematous or cyanotic
• Consistency: firm, tight, resilient, well adapted	• Consistency: edematous, spongy, loosely adapted, or fibrotic
• Contour: scalloped, sharp papillae, knife-edge margin	• Contour: blunt, bulbous, swollen papillae, rolled margin
• Surface texture: stippled, matte	• Surface texture: smooth, shiny
• Marginal bleeding: absent or slight	• Marginal bleeding: moderate or severe
• Probing depth: 1–3 mm	• Probing depth: >3 mm
• Noticeable tissue resistance to probe penetration	• Minimal tissue resistance to probe penetration
• Bleeding on probing: absent or slight	• Bleeding on probing: moderate to severe
• Discomfort on probing: absent or slight	• Could present with moderate to severe pain

margins with scalloped gingival architecture and sharp pointed papillae. The surface texture of healthy gingiva is matte and may be stippled in the attached gingiva and the central portion of the interdental papillae. The presence of stippling can vary across individuals and also in different sites within the same individual. Stippling is absent in very young children and also reduces with aging. Hence the absence of stippling does not necessarily imply inflammatory changes in the tissue.

In the presence of inflammatory disease, the color of the gingiva may be erythematous (reddish) or cyanotic (bluish). Instead of having knife-edge margins and sharp interdental papillary gingival contours, inflamed gingival tissue typically has rolled margins and blunt or bulbous papillae. The surface of the gingiva in the presence of inflammation tends to be smooth and shiny, mainly due to tissue edema. Table 24.1 summarizes clinical findings of healthy and inflamed gingiva.

Pigmented gingiva exhibits similar characteristics of gingival inflammation as the nonpigmented gingiva. However, the color changes which could be masked or altered due to the presence of pigmentation (Fig. 24.10).

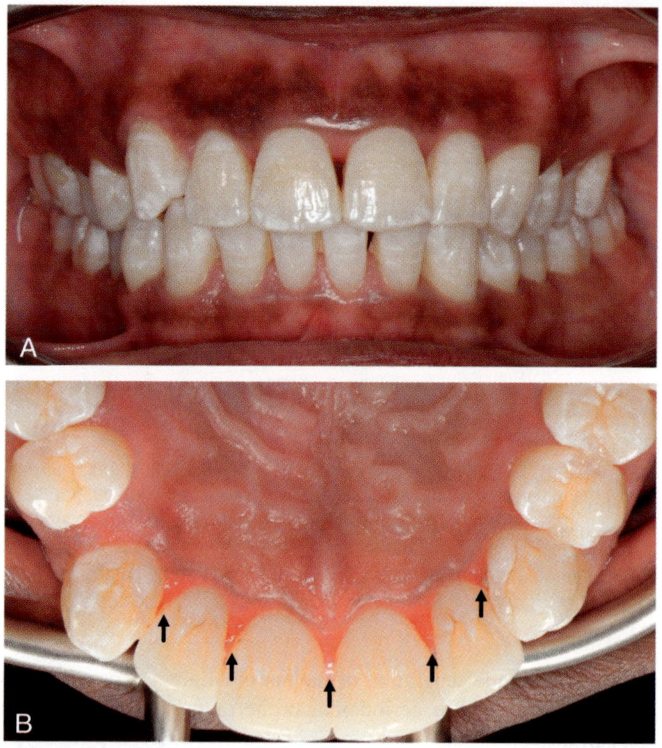

Fig. 24.10 Edema, papillary *(arrows)*, and marginal erythema in a patient with physiologic pigmentation. Frontal view (A) and palatal view (B). *(Copyright Jonathan H. Do, DDS. All rights reserved.)*

Gingival Recession

The location of the gingival margin around teeth should be evaluated and recorded. In the absence of attachment loss, the gingival margin is normally located coronal to the cementoenamel junction. In these instances, measuring the exact distance between the gingival margin and the cementoenamel junction can be challenging as it is a purely tactile, blinded assessment. Gingival recession is defined as the apical migration of the gingival margin. The presence of recession indicates that attachment loss has occurred but not necessarily that inflammation is present. Depending on the extent of attachment loss and the anatomical features of the teeth and the periodontium

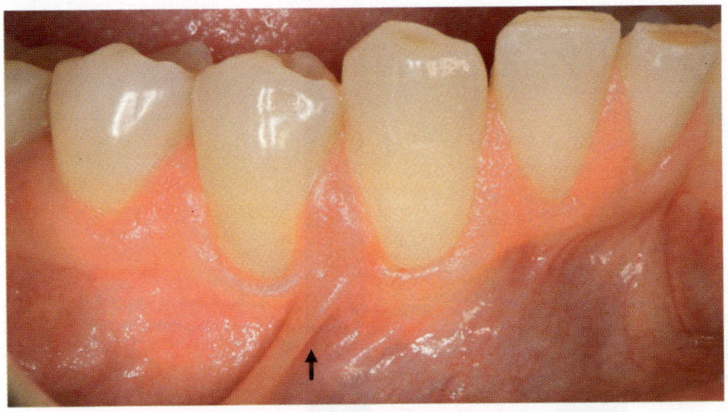

Fig. 24.11 The canine and first premolar exhibit gingival recession defects and minimal keratinized tissue. Both teeth are at risk of further recession depth increase due to the presence of gingival inflammation and a frenum pull *(arrow)*. *(Copyright Jonathan H. Do, DDS. All rights reserved.)*

at a specific site, the gingival margin may remain in a supragingival location, which is not common but certainly possible, or have shifted apically into a juxta- or subgingival location. When the cementoenamel junction is supragingival, recession depth can be measured using a standardized periodontal probe as the distance from the cementoenamel junction to the gingival margin. At sites exhibiting gingival recession defects, the amount of recession should be recorded. Additionally, the presence of biofilm and calculus, inflammatory changes in the gingiva, width of the keratinized tissue, and gingival thickness (phenotype) should be carefully evaluated and accounted for to establish a proper diagnosis and treatment plan (Fig. 24.11).

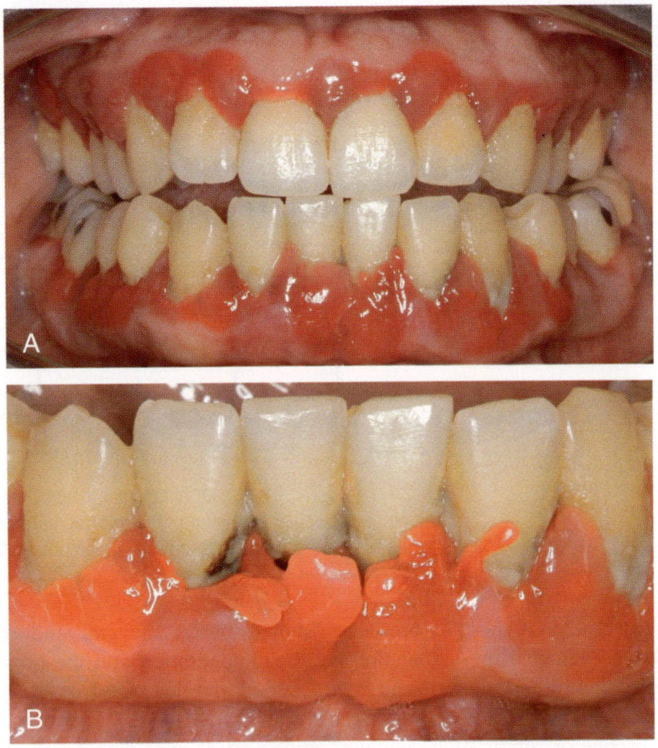

Fig. 24.12 The severely inflamed gingiva is loosely adapted to the tooth. The marginal gingiva is easily retracted to reveal heavy subgingival biofilm and calculus. Maxillary and mandibular frontal view (A) and mandibular frontal view (B). *(Copyright Jonathan H. Do, DDS. All rights reserved.)*

Tactile Periodontal Examination

Tactile periodontal examination begins with the evaluation of the consistency of the gingiva and its adaptation to the tooth, as well as the presence of marginal bleeding and **suppuration**. The gingival crevice is probed to evaluate the **subgingival** environment. The tooth surface should be carefully probed for aberrations, concavities, furcation defects, and subgingival calculus. The response of the gingival tissue to probing is measured in terms of resistance to and depth of probe penetration, as well as bleeding, suppuration, and pain upon probing.

Tactile Examination of the Marginal Gingiva

The marginal gingiva is palpated with a periodontal probe to assess its consistency and adaptation to the tooth. Healthy gingiva is typically firm, resilient, and well-adapted to the tooth due to the presence of dense, well-organized **collagen** fiber bundles in the lamina propria of the gingiva. When inflamed, the gingiva normally appears edematous, spongy, and loosely adapted to the tooth surface due to the degradation of collagen and the influx of inflammatory cells and fluid into the lamina propria (Fig. 24.12). In cases of **chronic** inflammation and in smokers, the gingival tissue may clinically appear fibrotic yet inflamed at the microscopic level.

Marginal Bleeding

Marginal bleeding is normally associated with inflammatory changes in the coronal aspect of the gingiva. Marginal bleeding can be evaluated by running an instrument, such as a periodontal probe or rubber tip, along the gingival margin. Under pressure, healthy gingival tissue normally blanches and does not bleed, whereas in the presence of gingival inflammation, marginal bleeding is triggered. The ease and severity of marginal bleeding are usually correlated with the actual severity of gingival inflammation, although bleeding can be masked in some instances (e.g., smokers).

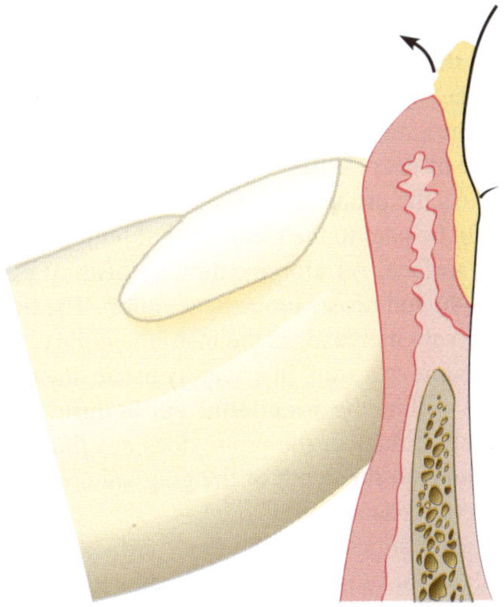

Fig. 24.13 Purulent exudate expressed from a periodontal pocket by digital pressure.

Suppuration

The palpation of the marginal gingiva with a probe or digitally, by placing the ball of the index finger on the gingiva apical to the margin and pushing coronally toward the gingival margin (Fig. 24.13), may trigger the release of a white-yellowish **exudate** from the gingival crevice. The presence of an abundance of **neutrophils** in the gingival fluid transforms it into a purulent exudate. Suppuration does not occur in all **periodontal pockets**, but pressure may reveal

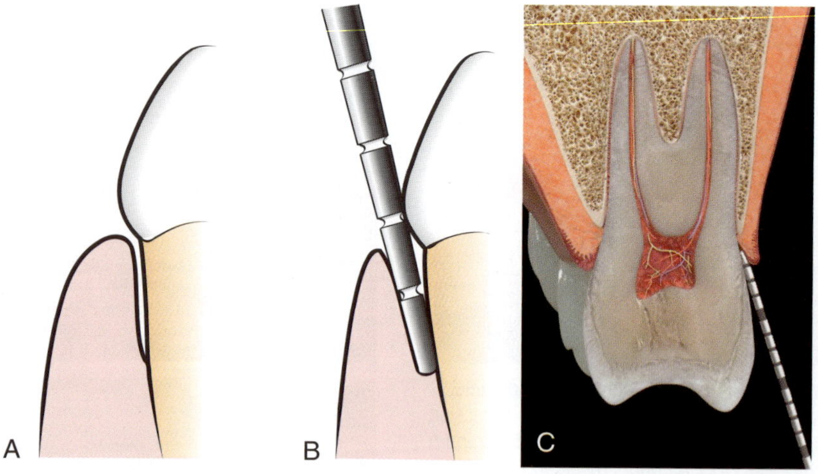

Fig. 24.14 A, The biologic or histologic pocket depth is the distance between the gingival margin and the base of the gingival sulcular epithelium. B, The probing or clinical pocket depth is the distance from the gingival margin to the bottom of the probeable crevice. C, Graphical illustration showing periodontal probing. *(© Periopixel.)*

it in **pockets** where its presence is not suspected. Several studies have evaluated the association between suppuration and the progression of periodontitis and have reported that this sign is present in a very low percentage of diseased sites (i.e., 3%–5%). Therefore, absence of suppuration does not indicate absence of disease. Suppuration is also not associated with the severity of disease or depth of the pocket. Suppuration only indicates that the disease is in an active phase.

Tactile Examination of the Gingival Crevice

The periodontal probe should be inserted into the gingival sulcus vertically with the tip of the probe touching and sliding down along the tooth surface to the bottom of the crevice. The probe should be "walked" circumferentially around each surface of each tooth to detect the areas of deepest penetration, instead of making "pinpoint assessments." As the probe tip slides down along the tooth surface, attention should be paid to the tactile feel of both the gingival tissue and the tooth surface. As aforementioned, healthy gingival tissue usually feels tight and resists probe penetration. The tightness of the tissue progressively increases as the instrument moves apically, and the probe will come to a stop. In a healthy tissue, the tip of the probe typically stops within the **junctional epithelium**. If the gingival tissue is severely inflamed, the probe does not find as much resistance and it "falls" to the depth of the gingival crevice, penetrating into the connective tissue region.

As the probe tip slides along the tooth surface, if there is no anatomical irregularity or subgingival calculus, the tooth surface will feel smooth. On the contrary, if the tooth surface feels rough and/or if the advancement of the probe tip is impeded, the presence of subgingival calculus should be suspected. The probe may need to be moved axially away from the tooth to navigate around the calculus in order for it to penetrate to depth. As previously mentioned in this chapter, the presence of subgingival calculus is usually associated with inflammatory changes in the gingival tissue (see Fig. 24.7), the absence of gingival tightness, and the presence of bleeding on probing. For a thorough assessment of the extent and location of subgingival calculus around the dentition, tactile examination using specific instruments (e.g., Old Dominion 11/12 explorer) is recommended.

Additionally, attention should be directed to the detection of periodontal bone defects (e.g., interdental craters and furcation defects) and root surface abnormalities (e.g., developmental grooves, cemental tears, and **enamel** pearls). Periodontal defects tend to be associated with deep probing depths and gingival inflammation. To detect an *interdental crater*, the probe should be placed obliquely from both the facial and lingual surfaces to explore the deepest point of the pocket located beneath the contact point. Regarding furcation defects, the use of specially designed probes (e.g., Nabers probe) allows for an easier and more accurate exploration of the horizontal component of lesions affecting the furcation of multirooted teeth.

Probing Depth

There are two different pocket depths: (1) the biologic or histologic depth and (2) the clinical or probing depth (Fig. 24.14).

Biologic depth is the distance between the gingival margin and the base of the **gingival sulcular epithelium** (i.e., the coronal boundary of the junctional epithelium). This can be measured only in carefully prepared and adequately oriented histologic sections.

Probing depth is the distance from the gingival margin to the bottom of the probable crevice (i.e., where the probe tip stops).

Probing depth is generally ≤3 mm in gingival health and greater than 3 mm in the presence of gingival inflammation. Several studies have been conducted to determine the depth of penetration of a probe in a sulcus or pocket. Armitage and colleagues used beagle dogs to evaluate the penetration of a probe with the use of a standardized force of 25 g. They reported that in healthy gingiva, the probe penetrated the junctional epithelium to about two-thirds of its length; in **gingivitis** cases, it stopped 0.1 mm short of its apical end; and in cases of periodontitis, the probe tip consistently went past the most apical cells of the junctional epithelium and into the connective tissue compartment (Fig. 24.15). In human periodontal pockets, it has been demonstrated that the probe tip penetrates until it finds the most coronal intact fibers of the connective tissue attachment.

Probing depth is a dynamic parameter that may naturally change over time, even in healthy patients with no history of periodontitis, as a result of changes in the position of the gingival margin. Therefore, probing depth changes may be unrelated to attachment loss. This is important to consider when evaluating differences in probing depth before and after treatment, because the reduction in probe penetration may be primarily related to a reduction in gingival inflammation and shrinkage of tissues, rather than a gain in attachment.

Periodontal Probing

The use of a manual, nonautomated periodontal probe is the classic method to detect probing depth and attachment loss. However, it

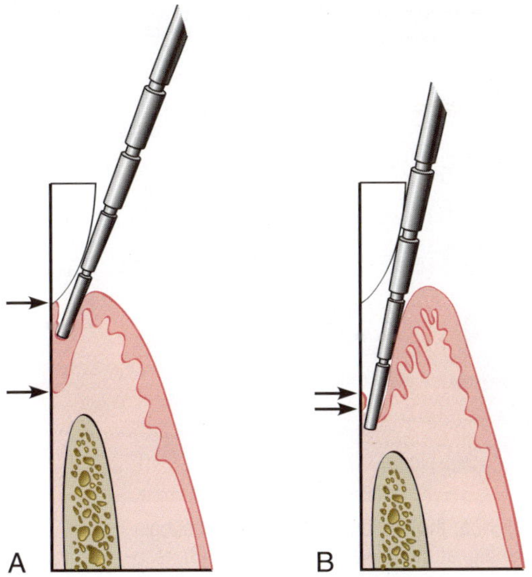

Fig. 24.15 A, In a normal sulcus, the probe penetrates about one-third to half the length of the junctional epithelium *(between arrows)*. B, In an inflamed periodontal pocket, the probe penetrates beyond the apical end of the junctional epithelium *(between arrows)*.

presents some limitations in terms of the reproducibility of the measurements.

Factors that affect probing:

1. Size of the probe
2. Direction of probing
3. Probing pressure
4. Convexity of the crown, restorations, subgingical calculus, etc.
5. Condition of the gingival tissues (edematous or fibrotic)
6. Landmarks to be considered while probing
7. Crest of the gingival margin
8. Cemento-enamel junction
9. Base of the probable sulcus
10. Crest of the alveolar bone
11. Mucogingival junction

Standardized probes such as William's periodontal probe should be used. It is a common mistake to use explorers to probe gingival sulcus. Probe penetration can vary depending on the probing force applied, the shape and size of the probe tip, the direction or angulation of penetration, tooth contours, root morphology, the presence of subgingival calculus, and the resistance of the tissues, which is typically related to the degree of tissue inflammation. Accuracy and reproducibility also depend on the precision of the probe's calibration.

Probing Force

One of the main factors affecting reproducibility is the variation of probing force, which several investigators have explored. A maximum force of 0.75 N (1 N is approximately 102 g) has been found to be generally well tolerated and accurate. With forces up to 30 g, the tip of the probe remains within the junctional epithelium, whereas forces over 50 g are necessary to go through the connective tissue and reach the bone level. The development of pressure-sensitive probes has helped to provide a consistent probing force.

Probe Angulation

Standardization of the probe tip (i.e., <1 mm) and the addition of registration stents to maintain a reproducible probe angulation have been used to overcome this error. This is particularly relevant in the context of clinical research.

Interexaminer Probing Errors

Interexaminer error (i.e., depth discrepancies between examiners) has been reported to be as much as 2.1 mm (with an average of 1.5 mm). This variability should be taken into account when more than one examiner is involved in the periodontal examination of a patient that is being monitored over a period of time. Interexaminer standardization depends on the factors affecting periodontal probing discussed earlier. In fact, intraexaminer standardization is also difficult for the same reasons. For measurements of clinical attachment loss, it is necessary to identify the location of the cementoenamel junction, which adds another hurdle for the standardization of measurements.

Automated Probing

Computer-assisted technology has been used to improve inter- and intraexaminer probing accuracy and reproducibility. In addition to being more accurate, the data derived from automated probing can be directly added to an electronic record, which can facilitate monitoring of clinical changes and patterns of disease progression. These records can also be used to provide feedback to patients. An example of automated probing is the Florida Probe System, which consists of a probe handpiece, a digital readout, a foot switch, a computer interface, and a computer. The end of the probe has a width of 0.4 mm, and it reciprocates through a sleeve that provides a reference by which measurements are made. These measurements are made electronically and transferred automatically when the foot switch is pressed or when a voice command is given. Constant probing force is provided by coil springs inside the probe handpiece and a digital readout. This method combines the advantages of a constant probing force with precise electronic measurement and computer storage of data, thereby minimizing potential errors associated with visual reading and eliminating the need for an assistant to record the measurements.

Several studies have been made comparing the Florida Probe with conventional probing. The automated probe appears to underestimate deep probing depths but shows less variability than conventional probing. The automated probe also presents the problem of providing little tactile sensitivity, thereby making it more difficult to "walk" the probe within the sulcus.

Other electronic systems, such as the Interprobe and the Periprobe, provide constant probing force and computer storage of data, but their reproducibility is only slightly better than that of conventional methods.

Bleeding on Probing

If the gingiva is inflamed, the insertion of a probe into the bottom of the sulcus or pocket typically elicits a bleeding response. Noninflamed sites rarely bleed, and if they do, it is often the result of an inadequate probing technique (e.g., excessive probing force). In most cases, bleeding on probing is an earlier sign of inflammation than gingival color changes. However, gingival color changes may be identified without concomitant bleeding on probing. Depending on the severity of inflammation, bleeding can vary from a tenuous red line along the gingival margin to profuse bleeding. If periodontal treatment is successful and biofilm control is optimal, bleeding on probing will cease.

To test for bleeding after probing, the probe is carefully introduced to the bottom of the sulcus or pocket and gently moved laterally along the sulcus or pocket wall. Sometimes bleeding appears immediately after the removal of the probe; other times it may be delayed. Therefore, it is generally recommended that the examiner recheck for bleeding 30–60 s after probing.

As a single test, bleeding on probing is not a reliable predictor of progression of attachment loss; however, its absence is an excellent

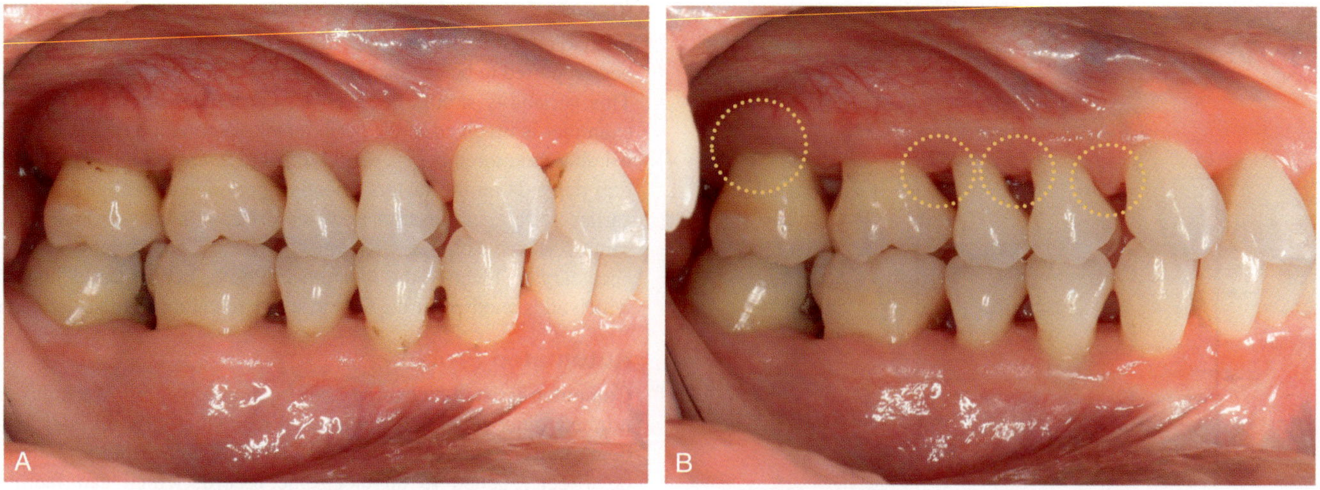

Fig. 24.16 Clinical presentation prior to scaling and root planing (A). Note the presence of supra- and subgingival calculus along the gingival margin. Following scaling and root planing, at the 6-week reevaluation (B), resolution of gingival inflammation resulted in dramatic gingival shrinkage or apical migration of the gingival margin *(circles). (Copyright Jonathan H. Do, DDS. All rights reserved.)*

indicator of periodontal stability. When bleeding is present in multiple sites that exhibit other signs of advanced periodontitis (e.g., probing depth >5 mm), bleeding on probing is a good indicator of attachment loss progression.

Pain on Probing

Pain is a cardinal sign of inflammation. However, gingival inflammation in gingivitis and periodontitis is generally not associated with pain. Probing of healthy sites does not typically induce pain, as long as the probing technique is adequate, while probing of sites presenting inflammation is more likely to produce pain. The level of pain is usually related to the severity and extent of gingival inflammation. Unless gingival inflammation is generalized and severe, patients do not normally report the same level of pain upon probing at every site. Although the clinician cannot directly measure pain on probing, for education purposes, it is useful to make the patient aware that pain usually indicates the presence of inflammation.

Probing Around Implants

Similar to the periodontium, the peri-implant tissues are susceptible to biofilm-induced inflammatory diseases. Hence, probing around implants is an integral component of the periodontal examination. It has been demonstrated that a conventional periodontal probe may be used under light force (e.g., 0.25 N) without damaging the peri-implant mucosal seal. Although conventional probes can be used for probing around implants, a flexible probe like PP12 Periodontal Probe, made of Polyether Ether Ketone thermoplastic, is preferred as it can be safely used on titanium surface; and its flexible, thin, and solid tip adapts easily to the implant anatomy.

Probing in the Presence of Severe Disease

Recording probing depth measurements before, during, and after treatment is essential for effective diagnosis and monitoring of periodontal diseases and conditions, such as periodontitis. In the presence of severe gingival inflammation (see Figs. 24.5 and 24.12), accurate probing depth measurement may be difficult to obtain without anesthesia due to the pain and discomfort associated with the insertion of the periodontal probe into the inflamed periodontal pocket. Therefore, when periodontal disease is overt and obvious clinically and radiographically, local anesthesia may facilitate the conduction of a thorough clinical periodontal examination, including probing depth assessments. Additionally, in cases presenting heavy **subgingival calculus** deposits, probing depth measurements may not be accurate until after completion of subgingival debridement. Clinicians should keep in mind that, in moderate and advanced periodontitis cases, a dramatic change in probing depths is normally observed after improvements in biofilm control and following scaling and root planing (Fig. 24.16). Obtaining accurate probing depths at the reevaluation following nonsurgical therapy holds more clinical relevance than obtaining accurate probing depths at the pretreatment periodontal examination, as the post-therapy measurements have more value in the context of clinical decision-making processes pertaining to recommendations for further treatment, be it corrective or supportive therapy.

Attachment Loss

Attachment loss is the apical migration of the dentogingival junction. Attachment loss may be induced by a variety of etiologies, such as inflammatory disease (e.g., periodontitis) or sustained trauma. The dentogingival junction is constituted by the junctional epithelium and the connective tissue attachment. The classic term to refer to the apicocoronal dimension of the dentogingival junction is the biologic width, which has been recently replaced with the term "**supracrestal tissue attachment**" (Fig. 24.17).

The supracrestal tissue attachment averages 2.04 mm in humans. In healthy conditions, without attachment loss, the connective tissue attachment of the dentogingival junction inserts into the root surface immediately apical to the cementoenamel junction. *Clinical attachment loss* refers to the *amount* of apical migration of the dentogingival junction that has occurred, using the cementoenamel junction as the reference point. If the cementoenamel junction is absent, another fiduciary mark can be used (e.g., restorative margin). Clinical attachment loss is typically measured using a calibrated probe as the distance from the cementoenamel junction to the bottom of the probeable crevice (i.e., attachment level). When the gingival margin is located coronal to the cementoenamel junction (on the anatomic crown), the clinical parameter "*clinical attachment loss*" is determined by subtracting the distance from the gingival margin to the cementoenamel junction from the probing depth. If both are the same, the actual clinical attachment loss is zero. When the gingival margin coincides with the cementoenamel junction, clinical attachment loss is equal to the probing depth. When

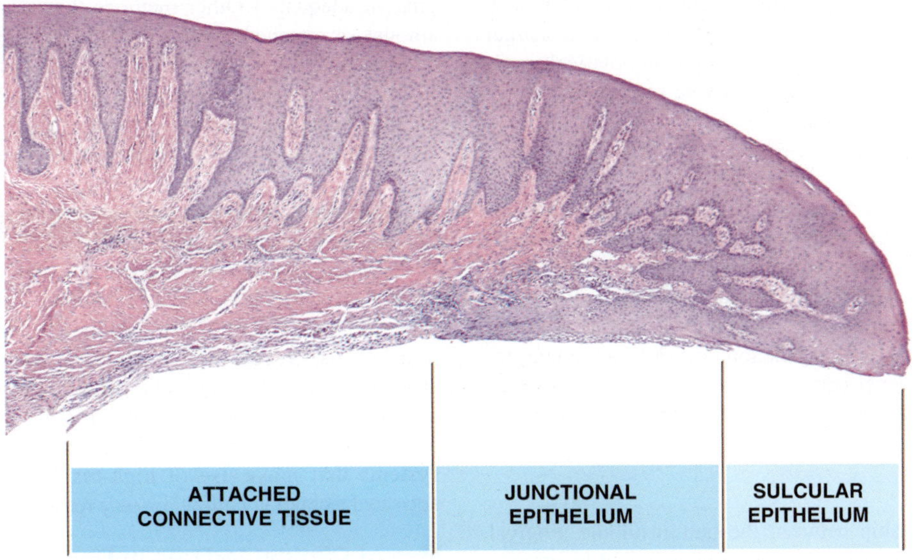

Fig 24.17 Histologic image of a human gingival sample depicting the apicocoronal dimension of the dentogingival junction showing the sulcular epithelium, the junctional epithelium, and the attached connective tissue. *(Copyright Gustavo Avila-Ortiz, DDS, MS, PhD. All rights reserved.)*

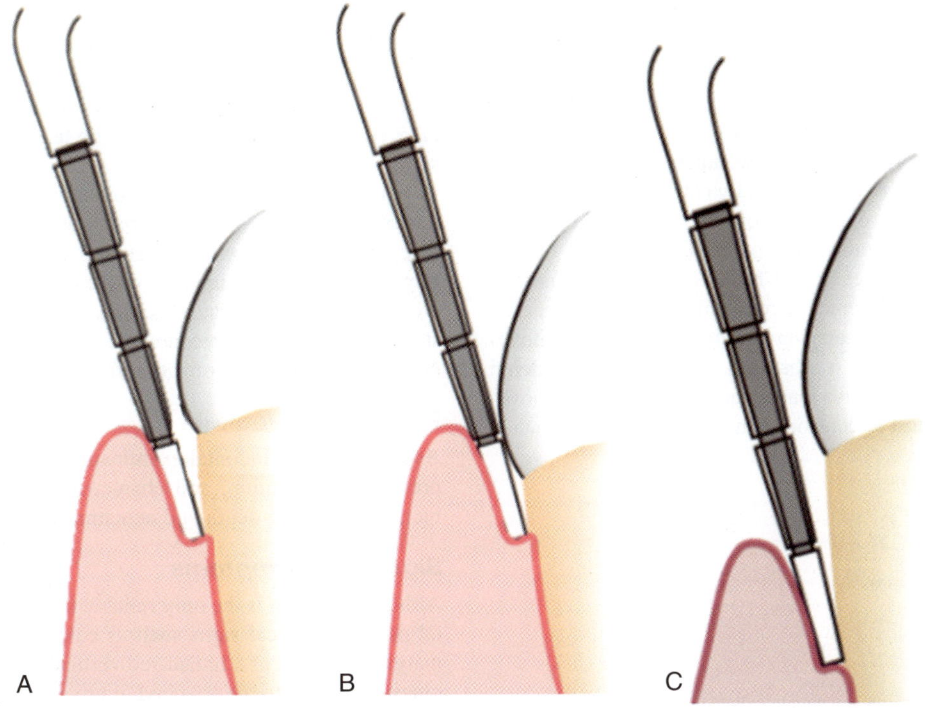

Fig. 24.18 Schematic illustration of three clinical scenarios where the probing depth is the same but with differing gingival margin locations with respect to the cementoenamel junction (CEJ), which result in different clinical attachment loss (CAL) measures. In scenario A, the gingival margin is at the level of the CEJ and, hence, the probing depth equals the CAL. In scenario B, the gingival margin is coronal to the CEJ, therefore CAL is calculated by subtracting the distance from the gingival margin to the CEJ from the probing depth. Scenario C presents a gingival recession defect. In this case, CAL is determined by adding the gingival recession measure (distance from the CEJ to the gingival margin) and the probing depth.

the gingival margin is located apical to the cementoenamel junction, clinical attachment loss is greater than the probing depth. Therefore, clinical attachment loss is the sum of gingival recession depth and probing depth. Refer to Fig. 24.18 to see how clinical attachment loss is determined in different clinical scenarios. Entering the probing depths and drawing the gingival margin on the periodontogram allows one to determine this important clinical landmark.

Clinical attachment loss is automatically calculated in many dental practice management software programs as the sum of probing depth and recession depth. This calculation is accurate only when both the probing and the recession depth are entered into the software correctly. However, when recession depth is not entered, many software programs assume the cementoenamel junction is at the level of the gingival margin and equate clinical attachment loss to probing depth. This is not necessarily correct, as many clinicians do not enter a value for recession depth when the cementoenamel junction is subgingival and not visible. As such, automatically calculated clinical attachment loss values must be scrutinized before they are used to establish a diagnosis.

Attachment Level

Attachment level refers to the most coronal location of the dentogingival junction on the tooth surface. For example, the attachment level of a tooth can be on the coronal third of the root or the apical third of the root. As aforementioned, **clinical attachment loss** measures the distance between the attachment level and a reference point, such as the cementoenamel junction or a restorative margin. Changes in attachment level can be the result of gain or loss of attachment, and they can provide valuable information to make clinical decisions.

Attached Gingiva

Establishing the relationship between the bottom of the gingival sulcus (or the periodontal pocket) and the mucogingival junction is a critical component of the periodontal examination, especially at sites presenting gingival recession defects and narrow gingival width (see Fig. 24.11). The width of the attached gingiva is the distance between the mucogingival junction and the bottom of the gingival sulcus (or the periodontal pocket). Attached gingiva width should not be confused with the gingival width, a dimension that also includes the marginal gingiva (Fig. 24.19).

The width of the attached gingiva is determined by subtracting the sulcus or pocket depth from the total gingival width (i.e., the distance from the gingival margin to the mucogingival junction). The amount of attached gingiva is generally considered to be insufficient when it presents a dimension of less than 1 mm, which sometimes correlates with movement of the free gingival margin when the lip or cheek are stretched. (Checking for the adequacy of the attached gingiva by stretching or retracting the lips and cheeks is called the Tension test. On carrying out this test, if visible movement of the gingival margin is observed, the test is considered positive, and the attached gingiva inadequate. However, if no movement is observed, the test is considered negative, and the attached gingiva adequate.) Other methods that are used to determine the amount of attached gingiva include pushing or rolling the apical alveolar mucosa coronally with a dull instrument, or swabbing Schiller's potassium iodine solution or Lugol's iodine solution over the mucosa, which stains the nonkeratinized alveolar mucosa due to its glycogen content, thus demarcating the mucogingival junction.

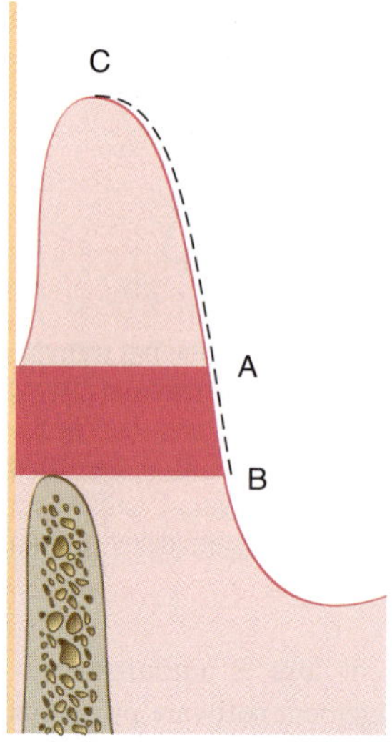

Fig. 24.19 The *shaded area* shows the attached gingiva, which extends between the projection on the external surface of the bottom of the gingival sulcus or periodontal pocket (A) and the mucogingival junction (B). The keratinized tissue (gingiva) extends from the mucogingival junction (B) to the gingival margin (C).

Periodontal Charting

Periodontograms provide a record of a comprehensive examination of the patient's periodontal condition and associated findings (Fig. 24.20A and B). These records are necessary to evaluate the initial status, the response to treatment, and for further comparison at recall visits. Electronic clinical records provide rapid and easy access to information and allow for the incorporation of digital clinical and radiographic images. Computerized dental examination systems that make use of high-resolution graphics and voice-activated technology allow for easy retrieval and comparison of data.

Use of Clinical Indices in Dental Practice

In recent decades, there has been a tendency to extend the use of indices that were originally designed for **epidemiologic studies** into dental practice. Of all of the available indices, the gingival index and the sulcus bleeding index appear to be the most useful and most easily transferrable to clinical practice.

The *gingival index* is based on a visual assessment of the gingival inflammatory status. This index can be used in practice to compare gingival health before and after phase 1 therapy or before and after surgical therapy. It can also be used to compare the gingival status at recall visits.

The **sulcus bleeding index** provides an objective and easily reproducible assessment of the gingival status. It is extremely useful for detecting early inflammatory changes and the presence of inflammatory lesions located at the base of the periodontal pocket, which is an area inaccessible to visual examination. Patients can easily understand this index; therefore, it can be used for educational purposes to enhance the patient's motivation for effective plaque control.

Periodontal Pockets

As part of the periodontal examination, it is important to record the presence, distribution, and characteristics of periodontal pockets, including probing depth and attachment level.

Signs and Symptoms

Although probing is the only reliable method of detecting periodontal pockets, clinical signs such as color changes (i.e., a bluish-red marginal gingiva or a bluish-red vertical zone that extends from the gingival margin to the attached gingiva); a "rolled" edge separating the gingival margin from the tooth surface; or an enlarged, edematous gingiva may suggest their presence. Gingival bleeding and/or suppuration, and loose, extruded teeth may also denote the presence of a pocket.

Periodontal pockets are generally painless, but they may give rise to symptoms such as localized or sometimes radiating pain, or gnawing pain with an urge to "dig" which is relieved on "digging" with a pin or toothpick, or the sensation of pressure after eating that gradually diminishes. A foul taste, sensitivity to hot and cold, and toothache in the absence of **caries** are also sometimes reported by periodontitis patients.

Detection of Periodontal Pockets

As previously mentioned, the only accurate method of detecting and measuring periodontal pockets is careful exploration with

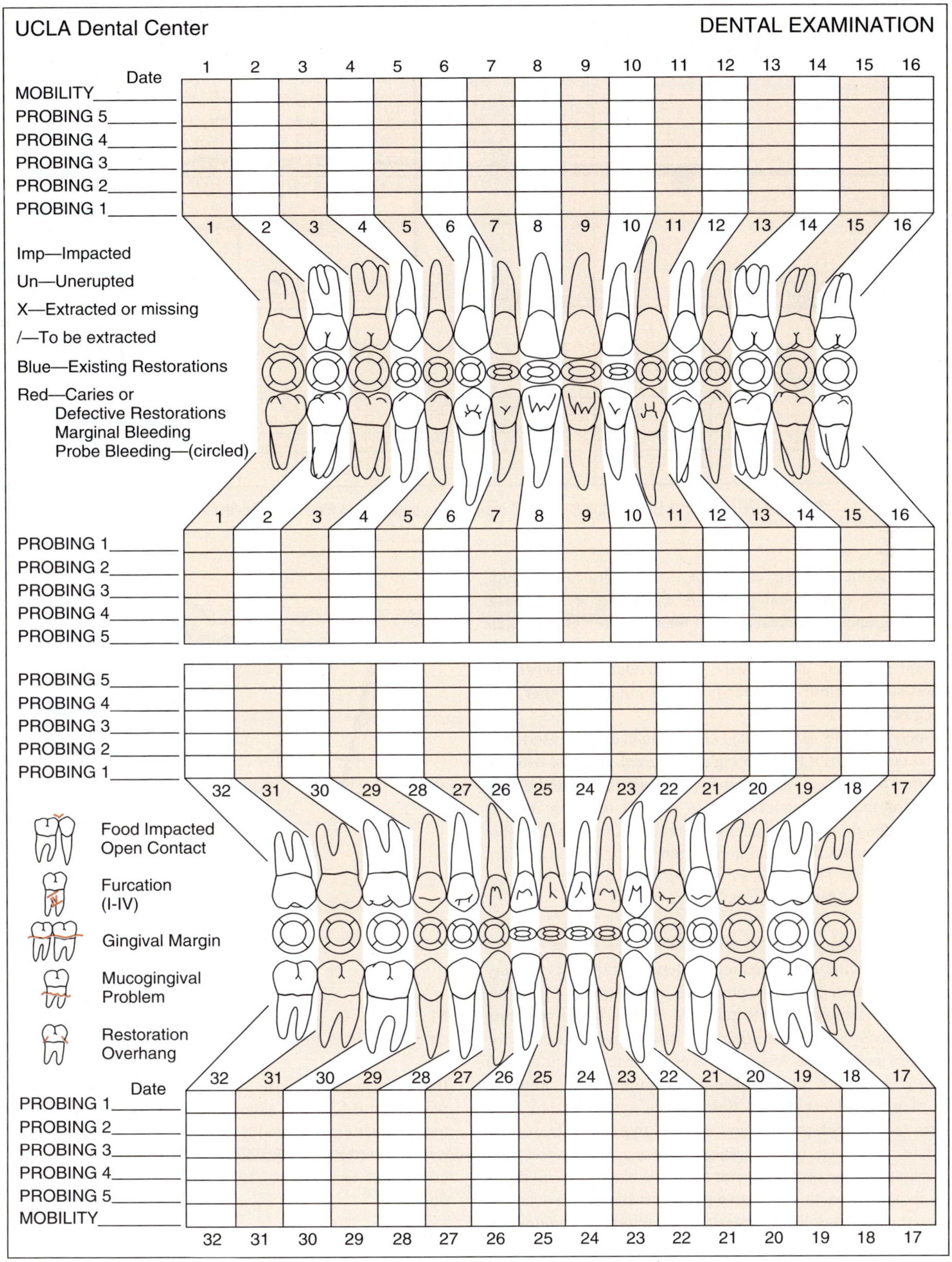

A

Fig. 24.20 A, Periodontal chart (periodontogram) used at the University of California, Los Angeles.

Continued

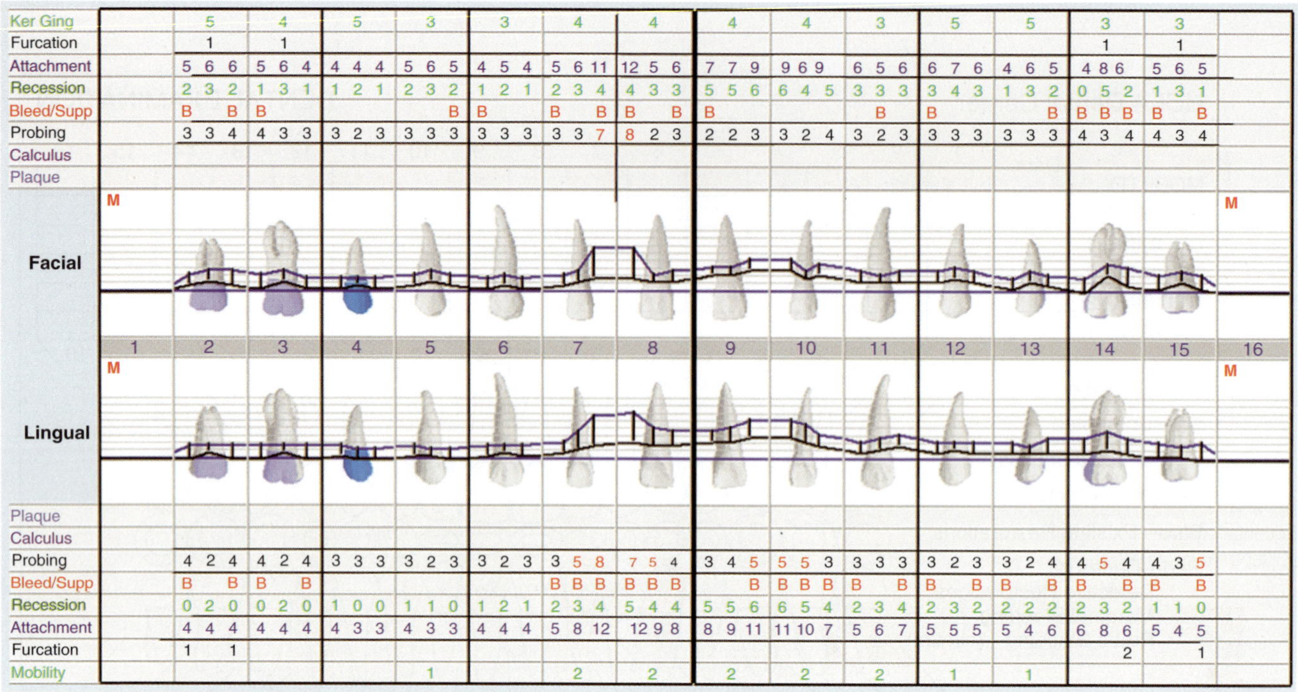

Fig. 24.20, cont'd B, Periodontal chart of maxillary teeth within an Electronic Health Record System.

a periodontal probe. Pockets cannot be detected by radiographic examination. The periodontal pocket is essentially a soft tissue change. Radiographs can reveal areas of bone loss in which pockets may be suspected, but they do not show pocket presence or depth, and consequently, they are not valid to differentiate between the periodontal status before and after pocket elimination, other than monitoring bone levels.

Gutta-percha points or calibrated silver points can be inserted in periodontal pockets prior to obtaining a radiograph to assist with the determination of the level of attachment. This approach can be used effectively for individual pockets or in clinical research, but its routine use throughout the mouth is impractical and unacceptable from a radiation protection standpoint. Again, clinical examination, including meticulous probing, is a direct and efficient way to assess the presence of periodontal pockets.

Determination of Disease Activity

A precise, site-specific determination of periodontitis activity may have a direct effect on diagnosis, prognosis, and therapy (e.g., treatment goals and strategy). Unfortunately, there are no accurate chairside methods currently available to determine the activity or inactivity of a periodontal lesion. In general, inactive (quiescent) lesions may show little or no bleeding on probing and minimal amounts of **gingival crevicular fluid**, while active lesions may bleed more readily with probing and exhibit large amounts of fluid and exudate. However, no differences between both active and nonactive sites may be observed with regard to bleeding with probing, even in patients with **aggressive periodontitis** (i.e., a separate category in the previous disease classification to group periodontitis patients presenting a rapid progression pattern with a tendency to occur in relatively young patients).

Assessment and comparison of clinical attachment level at different time points allows the examiner to determine whether attachment loss has occurred over time, which can be used as an indicator of disease progression. The automated Florida Probe provides a means of recording relative clinical attachment level changes over time. A later model of the probe has a modified sleeve with a prominent 0.125-mm edge to facilitate a "catch" of the cementoenamel junction. The width of this edge is considered small enough not to interfere with probing-depth measurements, thus providing concurrent assessments of clinical attachment level and pocket depth.

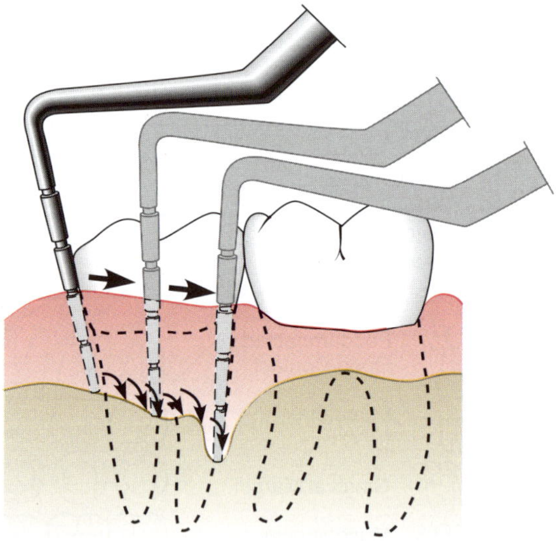

Fig. 24.21 Bone sounding: under local anesthesia, the probe is inserted down to the bone crest to explore the bone architecture.

Alveolar Bone Loss

Interproximal alveolar bone levels are primarily evaluated via radiographic examination. Probing can be helpful for estimating the following: (1) the approximate height and contour of the facial and lingual bone, which are obscured by the roots on conventional 2D radiographs, and (2) the architecture of the interdental bone. Transgingival probing, also known as Bone Sounding (Figs. 24.21 and 24.22),

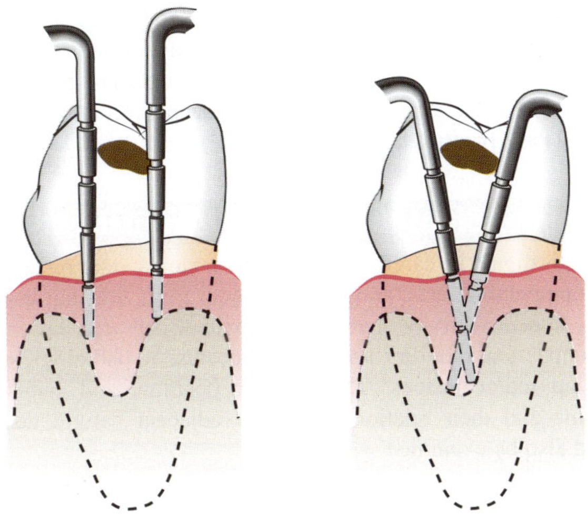

Fig. 24.22 A straight vertical insertion of the probe *(left)* may not detect interdental craters; oblique positioning of the probe *(right)* helps to reach the true depth of the crater.

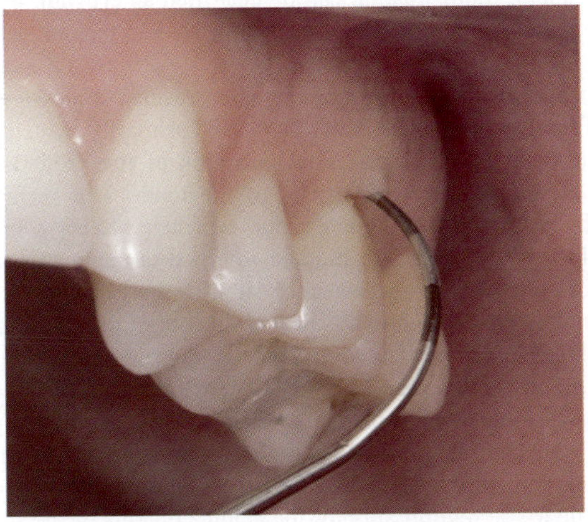

Fig. 24.23 Assessment of furcation involvement on the buccal aspect of the maxillary left first molar using a Nabers probe. Note the alternating colored bands in the probe, which are 3 mm in length.

which should be performed after anesthesia is achieved, can be used as a method of evaluation of the crestal bone architecture.

Furcation Invasion

Attachment loss can result in *furcation invasion*, which is the pathologic resorption of interradicular bone within the furca of a multirooted tooth. Furcation invasion is detected by carefully probing the root surface for horizontal concavities where the roots start to diverge. As previously mentioned, specialized probes, such as the Nabers probe (Fig. 24.23), may facilitate detection of furcation invasion. Knowledge of the morphology of the teeth is important for detecting furcation invasion. (For example, Maxillary first premolar furcation invasion is assessed from the mesial and distal aspects; maxillary first molar is assessed from buccal aspect for buccal furcation invasion, from buccal or palatal aspect for distal furcation invasion, and from palatal aspect for mesial furcation invasion; mandibular molars are assessed for furcation invasion from buccal and lingual aspects.) Several classifications of furcation invasion exist. The Glickman Classification of furcation invasion is one of the most commonly used, and it is as follows:

- Grade I: pocket formation into the flute but intact interradicular bone.
- Grade II: loss of interradicular bone and pocket formation of varying depths into the furcation but not completely through to the opposite side of the tooth.
- Grade III: through-and-through lesion.
- Grade IV: same as grade III with gingival recession, rendering the furcation clinically visible.

Another popular classification scheme is the one proposed by Hamp, Nyman, and Lindhe in 1975 that categorizes furcation invasion into three degrees:

- Degree I: horizontal loss of periodontal tissue supports less than 3 mm.
- Degree II: horizontal loss of periodontal tissue support exceeding 3 mm but not encompassing the total width of the furcation area.
- Degree III: horizontal "through and through" destruction of the periodontal tissue in the furcation.

Periodontal Abscess

A periodontal abscess is a localized accumulation of exudate within the gingival wall of a periodontal pocket. Periodontal abscesses may be acute or chronic.

The *acute periodontal abscess* appears as an ovoid elevation of the gingiva along the surface of the root. The gingiva usually appears edematous and red, with a smooth, shiny surface. The shape and consistency of the elevated area may vary; it may be domelike and relatively firm, or pointed and soft. In most cases, gentle digital pressure elicits exudate discharge through the gingival margin. An acute periodontal abscess is typically accompanied by symptoms such as throbbing, radiating pain, and tenderness to gingival palpation. Other symptoms may include sensitivity to tooth palpation or percussion; tooth mobility and lymphadenitis; and, less frequently, systemic effects such as fever, leukocytosis, and malaise. Occasionally, a patient may refer symptoms of an acute periodontal abscess without any notable clinical lesion or radiographic changes.

A *chronic periodontal abscess* usually presents a sinus tract that opens onto the gingival mucosa. There may be a history of intermittent exudation. The orifice of the sinus tract may appear as a difficult-to-detect pinpoint opening, which, when probed, reveals a sinus tract that leads deep into the periodontium. The sinus tract orifice may be covered by a small, pink, beadlike mass of granulomatous tissue. A chronic periodontal abscess is usually asymptomatic. However, the patient may report episodes of dull, gnawing pain; a slight elevation of the tooth; and a desire to bite down and grind the tooth. A chronic periodontal abscess may undergo acute exacerbation with all or some of the associated symptoms described previously. Fig. 24.24 is a clinical image that shows periodontal abscess on a mandibular molar tooth with **furcation involvement**.

Diagnosis of a periodontal abscess requires the correlation of the patient's medical and dental history with the clinical and radiographic findings. The suspected area should be probed carefully along the gingival margin in relation to each tooth surface to detect a channel from the marginal area to the deeper periodontal tissues. Continuity of the lesion with the gingival margin is clinical evidence that the abscess is periodontal.

An abscess is not necessarily located on the same surface of the root as the pocket from which it is formed. For example, a pocket on an interproximal surface may give rise to a periodontal abscess on the facial aspect of the tooth.

In children, a sinus orifice along the lateral aspect of a root is usually the result of a periapical infection of a **deciduous tooth**. In the permanent dentition, such an orifice may be caused by a periodontal abscess or by apical involvement of endodontic origin and, therefore, a thorough examination is required to establish whether it is a purely periodontal, endodontic, or a combined lesion.

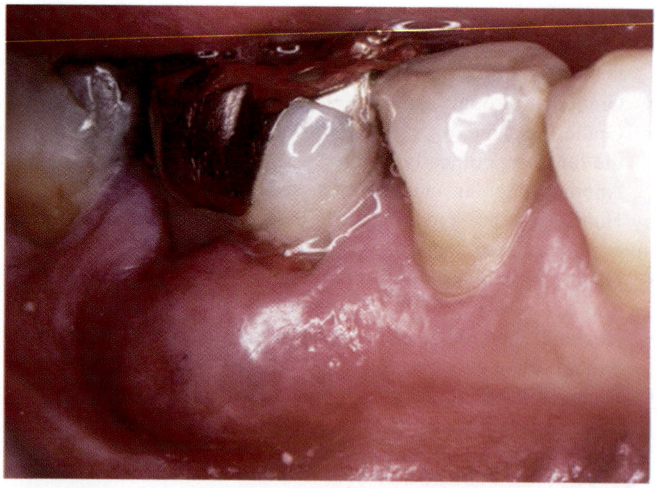

Fig. 24.24 Periodontal abscess associated with a furcation-involved mandibular molar.

Periodontal Abscess and Gingival Abscess

The principal differences between the periodontal abscess and the gingival abscess are location and history. The gingival abscess is confined to the marginal gingiva, and it often occurs in previously disease-free areas. It is usually an acute inflammatory response to the presence of foreign material introduced into the gingiva. On the contrary, periodontal abscess involves supporting periodontal structures beyond the gingiva, and it generally occurs during the course of periodontitis or for other reasons (e.g., endodontic involvement, root fracture).

Periodontal Abscess and Periapical Abscess

Several characteristics can be used as guidelines when differentiating a periodontal abscess from a periapical abscess. If the tooth is nonvital, the lesion most likely has a periapical/endodontic origin. However, a previously nonvital tooth can have a deep periodontal pocket that may lead to the formation of a true periodontal abscess. Moreover, a deep periodontal pocket can extend to the apex and cause pulpal involvement and secondary **necrosis**.

A periapical abscess may spread along the root surface to the gingival margin. However, when the root apex and surface are involved with a single lesion that can be probed directly from the gingival margin, the lesion is more likely to have originated as a periodontal abscess.

Radiographic imaging can be helpful in differentiating between a periodontal and a periapical lesion. Early acute periodontal and periapical abscesses typically present with no radiographic changes. Ordinarily, a radiolucent area along the surface of the root suggests the presence of a periodontal abscess, whereas apical rarefaction suggests a periapical abscess. However, acute periodontal abscesses that show no radiographic changes may cause symptoms in teeth with long-standing, radiographically detectable periapical lesions that are not contributing to the patient's complaint. Clinical findings such as the presence of extensive caries, pocket formation, lack of tooth vitality, the existence of continuity between the gingival margin, and the abscess area often prove to be of greater diagnostic value than the radiographic appearance.

A draining sinus tract in the proximity of the gingival margin is suggestive of periodontal rather than periapical involvement, while a sinus tract from a periapical lesion is more likely to be located further apically. However, sinus location is not conclusive. In many instances, particularly in children, the sinus from a periapical lesion tends to drain coronally rather than at the apex. Radiographs can be taken after inserting Gutta-percha points or silver points in the sinus tracts to help track its origin. It is also important to note that abscesses are also associated with other dental conditions, such as **vertical root fractures** or cracked teeth.

Examination of the Teeth and Implants

The teeth should be carefully examined for caries, poor restorations, developmental defects, anomalies of tooth form, wasting diseases, stains, hypersensitivity, inadequate proximal contact relationships, food impaction, mobility, trauma from occlusion, pathologic migration and malocclusions. The number, position, and stability of implants and their relationship to the adjacent natural dentition should also be examined.

Wasting Disease of the Teeth

Wasting is a generic term that refers to any gradual loss of tooth substance, which is characterized by the formation of smooth, polished surfaces. Depending on etiological factors and the process of development, tooth wasting can be classified as **erosion**, abrasion, attrition, and abfraction. For more details, refer to the online version of this chapter.

Erosion, also known as *biocorrosion*, results in an irreversible loss of hard tissues of the dentition caused primarily by acids without microbial involvement. The long axis of the eroded area is perpendicular to the vertical axis of the tooth. The surfaces are smooth, hard, and polished. Erosion typically affects a group of teeth. In the early stages, it may be confined to the enamel and, in cases of concomitant gingival recession, to the **cementum**, but in most situations, it eventually extends into the underlying **dentin**. The etiology of erosion is multifactorial. Decalcification by acidic beverages in combination with the effect of acidic salivary secretion is a possible cause. Erosion is also seen in patients with eating disorders like Bulimia nervosa, which is characterized by induced vomiting and in patients with GERD (gastroesophageal reflux disease) due to the regurgitation of the acidic contents of the stomach. Another cause of erosion is occupational, where the acid fumes generated in factories like battery factory affects the teeth of the workers. Sognnaes referred to these lesions as *dentoalveolar ablations* and attributed them to forceful frictional action between the oral soft tissues and the adjacent hard tissues. Interestingly, in patients with erosion, the salivary pH, the buffering capacity, and the calcium and phosphorus content have been reported as normal, while the mucin level is elevated.

Abrasion refers to the loss of tooth substance that is induced by mechanical wear other than that of mastication. Abrasion results in saucer-shaped or wedge-shaped indentations with a smooth, shiny surface. Abrasion may start on enamel or, mainly, on exposed cementum surfaces, and it may extend into the dentin. A sharp "ditching" around the cementoenamel junction appears to be the result of the softer cemental surface as compared to the much harder enamel surface. A variety of factors, such as the action of prosthetic clasps, have been pointed to as etiological factors, but aggressive toothbrushing with an abrasive dentifrice is the most common cause of abrasion. Tooth malposition (e.g., too facial) can also be a major factor in the abrasive loss of tooth structure. The degree of tooth wear from toothbrushing depends on the abrasive effect of the dentifrice and the angle of brushing. Horizontal brushing at right angles respective to the vertical axis of the teeth typically results in the most extreme loss of tooth substance. Occasionally, abrasion of the incisal edges occurs as a result of habits such as holding objects (e.g., bobby pins, tacks, toothpicks) between the teeth.

Attrition is occlusal wear that typically results from sustained parafunctional contact with opposing teeth. Wear facets may result from functional or parafunctional wear as well as dental treatment, sometimes iatrogenic, through coronoplasty (i.e., **occlusal adjustment**). However, coronoplasty does not appear to contribute to higher ratings of wear. Functional wear patterns may occur on incisal, occlusal, or approximal tooth surfaces. A certain amount of tooth wear occurs physiologically with aging, but accelerated wear may be caused by abnormal anatomic or unusual functional factors. Excessive wear may result in the obliteration of the cusps and the formation of either a flat or cuneiform (cupped-out) occlusal surface. These affected regions are usually not sensitive to thermal or tactile stimulation. Occlusal or incisal surfaces worn by attrition are called *wear facets*. When active tooth grinding occurs, the enamel rods are fractured and become highly reflective to light. Thus, shiny, smooth, and curvilinear facets are usually reliable indicators of ongoing frictional activity. If dentin is exposed, a yellowish-brown discoloration is frequently present in the central aspect of the lesion. Facets vary with regard to size and location, depending on whether they are produced by physiologic or abnormal wear. Attrition has been correlated with age when older adults are considered. It has been reported that at least one significant wear facet can be observed in 92% of adults, while other authors have indicated that facet **prevalence** approaches universality. Contrary to earlier thought, attrition in young adults from modern societies is not age related. This suggests that a significant amount of attrition when present in young adults is unlikely to occur as a result of functional wear, and it is probably the result of bruxing activity.

Another mechanism of tooth wear that has been studied is called *abfraction*, which results from occlusal loading that causes tooth flexure and mechanical microfractures in the cervical area. Mechanical microfractures from abfraction weaken the cervical tooth structure and make it susceptible to loss of tooth structure via abrasion.

The four mechanisms of tooth wear, namely erosion, abrasion, attrition, and abfraction, can combine to increase the degree of loss of tooth substance.

Dental Stains

Dental stains are pigmented deposits on teeth that are not to be mistaken with calculus deposits. They could be extrinsic (due to food or beverages, chromogenic bacteria, habits like tobacco chewing or smoking, etc.) or intrinsic (due to fluorosis, tetracycline administration during tooth development, etc.). They should be carefully examined to determine their origin.

Hypersensitivity

Exposed root surfaces and sites presenting tooth wear may be hypersensitive to thermal changes or tactile stimulation due to exposure of the dentinal tubules. Patients often direct the clinician to the sensitive areas. These may be located by gentle exploration with an instrument (e.g., probe or explorer) or the direct application of cold air.

Proximal Contact Relations

Open contacts allow for food impaction, which can contribute to attachment loss. Open contacts may also be a result of inflammatory changes associated with periodontal diseases and conditions. The tightness of contacts should be checked by means of clinical observation and with dental floss. Abnormal contact relationships may also trigger occlusal changes, such as a shift in the median line between the central incisors with labial flaring of the maxillary canine, buccal or lingual displacement of the posterior teeth, and an uneven relationship of the marginal ridges. Teeth opposing an **edentulous** site may supraerupt, thereby altering their proximal contacts.

Tooth Mobility

All teeth have a slight degree of physiologic mobility, which varies for different teeth and at different times of the day. Tooth mobility is usually greatest when arising in the morning, and it progressively decreases through the day. The increased mobility in the morning is attributed to slight extrusion of the tooth as a result of limited occlusal contact during sleep. During the waking hours, mobility is reduced by chewing and swallowing forces, which "re-intrude" the teeth into the sockets. These 24-h variations (diurnal variation) are less marked in persons with a healthy periodontium than in those with a history of attachment loss due to periodontitis or occlusal habits such as bruxism and clenching.

Single-rooted teeth typically exhibit greater mobility than multirooted teeth, with incisors having the most mobility. Mobility occurs primarily in a horizontal direction, although some axial mobility can also be detected to a lesser degree.

Tooth mobility occurs in the following two stages:

1. The initial or intrasocket stage: It occurs when the tooth moves within the confines of the periodontal ligament. This is associated with viscoelastic distortion of the principal fibers of the periodontal ligament and the redistribution of the periodontal fluids, interbundle content, and other interstitial fibers. This initial movement occurs with forces exceeding about 100 lbs., and it is in the order of 0.05–0.10 mm (50–100 μm).
2. The secondary stage: This is a gradual process that entails elastic deformation of the alveolar bone in response to increased horizontal forces. When a force of 500 g is applied to the crown, the resulting displacement is about 100–200 μm for incisors, 50–90 μm for canines, 8–10 μm for premolars, and 40–80 μm for molars.

When a force such as that applied to teeth in occlusion is discontinued, the teeth return to their original position in two stages: the first is an immediate, spring-like elastic recoil; the second is a slow, asymptomatic recovery movement. Interestingly, the recovery movement is pulsating, and it is apparently associated with the normal pulsation of the periodontal vessels, which occurs in synchrony with the cardiac cycle (this is called the periodontal pulse).

Many attempts have been made to develop mechanical or electronic devices for the precise measurement of tooth mobility. Although standardization of grading mobility would be helpful for the diagnosis of some periodontal diseases and conditions and for the evaluation of treatment outcomes, these devices are not widely used. As a general rule, mobility is graded clinically by holding the tooth firmly between the handles of two rigid instruments (Fig. 24.25) or with one rigid instrument and one finger. An effort is then made to move the tooth in all directions. Abnormal mobility most often exhibits a faciolingual pattern. Tooth mobility is generally scored in daily practice according to the ease and extent of tooth movement according to the Miller Index, as follows:

- Class 0: Normal (physiologic) movement when force is applied.
- Class1: First distinguishable sign of movement in horizontal direction greater than physiologic.
- Class 2: Movement in a lateral direction (buccolingual or mesiodistal) of 1 mm or more but inability to depress the tooth in a vertical direction (apicocoronal).
- Class 3: Movement in a lateral direction (buccolingual or mesiodistal) of 1 mm or more with ability to depress the tooth in a vertical direction (apicocoronal).

Physiologic mobility is generally defined as tooth movement up to 0.2 mm horizontally and 0.02 mm vertically. Mobility beyond the physiologic range is termed *abnormal* or *pathologic*. However, the periodontium is not *necessarily* diseased at the time of examination.

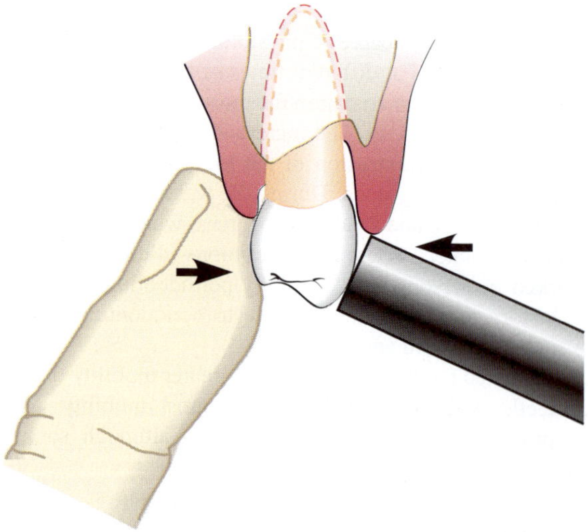

Fig. 24.25 Assessment of tooth mobility using two flat ends of rigid instruments (in this case mouth mirrors).

Increased mobility can be caused by one or more of the following factors:

1. The amount of mobility is related to the severity and distribution of bone loss around individual root surfaces; and the shape and length of the roots as compared to that of the crown. For the same amount of bone loss, a tooth with short, tapered roots is more likely to exhibit mobility than one with normal-sized or bulbous roots. Postorthodontic cases should be carefully evaluated for possible apical shortening of the root, which may lead to supraphysiologic mobility.
2. *Trauma from occlusion* (i.e., injury produced by excessive occlusal forces as a result of parafunctional habits, such as bruxism and clenching; or due to diminished withstanding capacity of the periodontium to normal occlusal forces, due to reduced periodontal support) is a common cause of tooth mobility. Mobility produced by trauma from occlusion occurs initially as a result of resorption of the inner cortical layer of bone (i.e., alveolar bone proper), which leads to reduced fiber support, and later, as an adaptation phenomenon that results in a widened periodontal ligament space. Notably, mobility may also be increased in response to hypofunction.
3. *Spread of inflammation* from the gingiva or the periapex into the periodontal ligament results in tissue changes that may increase tooth mobility. A good example of this is the spread of inflammation from an acute periapical abscess that increases tooth mobility in the absence of periodontitis.
4. *Periodontal surgery* causes transient tooth mobility immediately after the intervention, due to postoperative inflammation. This is especially so, if a **resective** intervention to correct osseous deformities is performed.
5. Tooth mobility can increase during *pregnancy*, and it is sometimes associated with the *menstrual cycle* or the use of *hormonal contraceptives*. This is unrelated to periodontitis, and it occurs presumably because of physicochemical changes in the periodontal tissues in response to fluctuations in **hormone** levels.
6. *Pathologic processes of the jaws* that destroy the alveolar bone or the roots of the teeth can also result in mobility. **Osteomyelitis** and tumors of the jaws belong in this category.

Trauma From Occlusion

Trauma from occlusion refers to *tissue injury* produced by supraphysiologic occlusal forces. The threshold that defines a "supraphysiologic" force is different depending on multiple local and functional factors inherent to the site and the patient, respectively. The criterion that determines whether an occlusion is traumatic is whether it causes damage to the periodontal tissues. Therefore, the diagnosis of trauma from occlusion is made considering the condition of the periodontal tissues, not the magnitude of the force *per se*. The periodontal findings are used as a guide to identify etiological occlusal relationships.

Periodontal findings that suggest the presence of trauma from occlusion include abnormal tooth mobility, particularly in teeth that show radiographic evidence of a widened periodontal space; vertical or **angular** bone destruction; and pathologic migration, especially of the anterior teeth. The teeth could exhibit attrition and have wear facets. Trauma from occlusion can be detected by the Fremitus test (functional mobility test) and using articulating papers or occlusion registration strips.

Fremitus test checks for vibrations in the teeth in contacting position and movements. It is carried out by placing a dampened, ungloved, index finger along the buccal and labial surfaces of the maxillary teeth, taking care to place the finger partly on the gingiva as well. The patient is then asked to tap the teeth together in the maximum intercuspal position, as well as grind them systematically in the lateral, protrusive, and latero-protrusive contacting movements and positions. The vibrations and displacement are then observed and grading is done as follows:

- Class 0: Normal, no vibrations or movement.
- Class 1: Only mild vibrations or movements palpable.
- Class 2: Easily palpable vibrations and no/barely visible movements.
- Class 3: Movements visible clearly to naked eyes.

Articulating papers or occlusion registration strips can also be used to detect "High pressure points" by the pattern of impression made by them in contacting positions and movements.

Pathologic Tooth Migration

Alterations in tooth position should be carefully noted as part of the periodontal examination, particularly with a view toward identifying abnormal forces, a tongue-thrusting habit, or other habits that may be contributing etiologic factors (Fig. 24.26). Premature tooth contacts in the posterior region that deflect the mandible anteriorly contribute to the destruction of the periodontium of the maxillary anterior teeth and, secondarily, to pathologic migration. The loss of posterior teeth can also lead to facial "flaring" of the anterior dentition. This is due to the increased trauma that the mandibular anterior dentition places against the palatal surface of the maxillary anterior dentition. Pathologic migration (distolabial) of the anterior teeth in young individuals may be a sign of periodontitis with a molar-incisor pattern (previously termed "**localized aggressive** or **juvenile periodontitis**").

Sensitivity to Percussion

Sensitivity to percussion may be indicative of acute inflammation of the periodontal ligament. Gentle tooth percussion at different angles with respect to the long axis often helps to localize the inflamed site.

Dentition With the Jaws Closed

Examination of the dentition with the jaws closed should be performed to detect conditions, such as irregularly aligned teeth, supraerupted teeth, improper proximal contacts, and areas of food impaction, all of which may favor microbial biofilm accumulation.

Excessive *overbite*, which is seen most often in the anterior region, may cause impingement of the teeth on the gingiva and food impaction, which may subsequently lead to gingival inflammation and periodontal pocket formation. The real significance of the

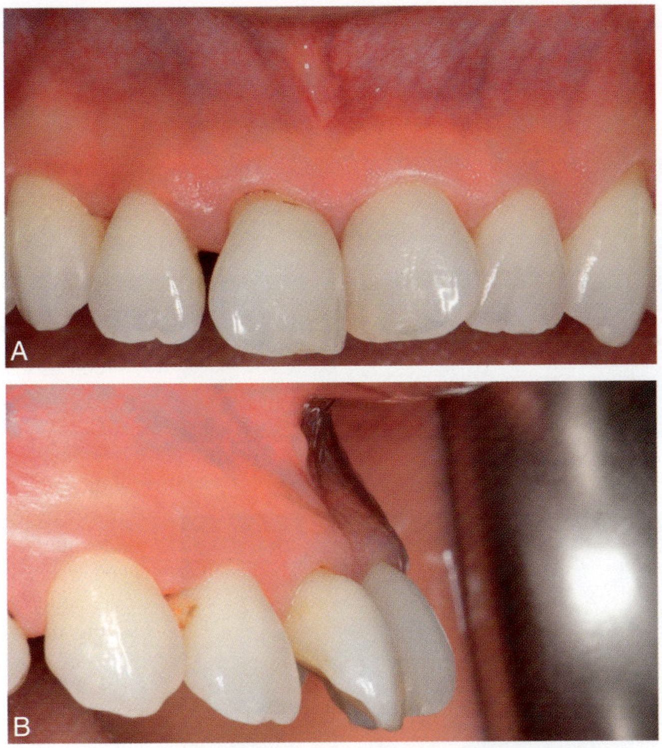

Fig. 24.26 Facial flaring and supraeruption of the right central incisor and spacing between the lateral and central incisors result from pathologic migration due to chronic periodontitis. Facial view (A) and side view (B). *(Copyright Jonathan H. Do, DDS. All rights reserved.)*

detrimental effect of an excessive anterior overbite on gingival health is still controversial.

In *open-bite* relationships, abnormal spacing exists between the maxillary and mandibular teeth. This condition is more common in the anterior region, although posterior open bite can be occasionally seen. Reduced mechanical cleansing by the passage of food may lead to the accumulation of plaque and debris, calculus formation, and tooth extrusion.

Crossbite is an inversion of the normal transversal relationship of the mandibular teeth with the maxillary teeth in which the maxillary teeth are lingual to the mandibular teeth. Crossbite may be anterior or posterior, and if posterior, it may be bilateral or unilateral. It may also affect multiple teeth or only a pair of antagonists. Crossbite may lead to food impaction, tooth migration, trauma from occlusion, and other periodontal disturbances.

Functional Occlusal Relationships

A meticulous examination of functional occlusal relationships is an important part of the diagnostic procedure. Dentitions that appear to be normal when the jaws are closed may actually present marked functional abnormalities.

Radiographic Examination

The standard radiographic survey in a complete dentition normally consists of a minimum of 14 periapical and 4 posterior bitewing radiographs (Fig. 24.27). Panoramic radiographs are a simple and convenient method of obtaining a survey view of the dental arch and the surrounding structures (Fig. 24.28). They are helpful for the detection of developmental anomalies, pathologic lesions of the teeth and jaws, and fractures. Panoramic radiographs provide an overall radiographic picture of the distribution and severity of bone destruction in periodontitis cases, but *a complete intraoral series consisting of periapical and bitewing radiographs is required for a proper periodontal diagnosis and treatment planning.* In patients with severe bone loss, vertical rather than horizontal bitewings are the preferred radiographs to adequately capture the location of the crestal bone.

Laboratory Tests to Aid Clinical Diagnosis

When unusual gingival or periodontal findings that cannot be explained by local causes are detected, the possible contribution of systemic factors must be explored. The signs and symptoms of oral manifestations of systemic disease have to be clearly understood and analyzed, and their presence discussed with the patient's physician.

Laboratory tests may aid in the diagnosis of systemic diseases that contribute to periodontitis and other oral diseases; these tests may also be needed to make treatment decisions when dealing with medically compromised patients. Analyses of blood smears, blood cell counts, white blood cell differential counts, and erythrocyte **sedimentation** rates are used to evaluate the presence of blood dyscrasias and generalized infections. Determinations of platelet counts, coagulation time, bleeding time, clot retraction time, prothrombin time, and capillary fragility, as well as bone marrow studies, may be required to determine the presence of coagulation disorders. In a patient presenting with a suspicious oral lesion, biopsy of the abnormal tissue followed by histopathological evaluation is warranted.

Diagnosis and Classification of Periodontitis

Once the patient's medical and dental history have been obtained; clinical, radiographic, and other necessary examinations have been performed; and a diagnosis of periodontitis has been confirmed, the information acquired can be synthesized and utilized in a multidimensional staging and grading system to classify the periodontitis case. This system, which was devised in the context of the 2017 World Workshop on the Classification of Periodontal and Peri-Implant Diseases and Conditions, takes the following factors into consideration: severity, treatment complexity, tooth loss due to periodontitis, rate of disease progression, and the presence of **risk factors**. The process of classifying a case of periodontitis is carried out according to the following key steps:

Step 1: Confirm the Case of Periodontitis

A patient is considered to have periodontitis if one of the following two criteria is satisfied: Interdental clinical attachment loss is detectable at ≥2 nonadjacent teeth or buccal or oral clinical attachment loss ≥3 mm with pocketing greater than 3 mm is detectable at ≥2 teeth and the observed clinical attachment loss cannot be attributed to the following clinical scenarios: (1) trauma-induced gingival recession, (2) dental caries extending subgingivally, (3) clinical attachment loss on the distal aspect of second molar (associated with malposition or extraction of third molar), (4) endodontic pathology draining through periodontium, and (5) vertical root fracture.

Step 2: Establish the Stage and Extent

There are four **stages** (I through IV). Stage is determined based on the site with the most severe disease (attachment loss) and tooth loss. Stages I and II represent mild to moderate periodontitis without any tooth loss due to periodontitis. Stages III and IV represent

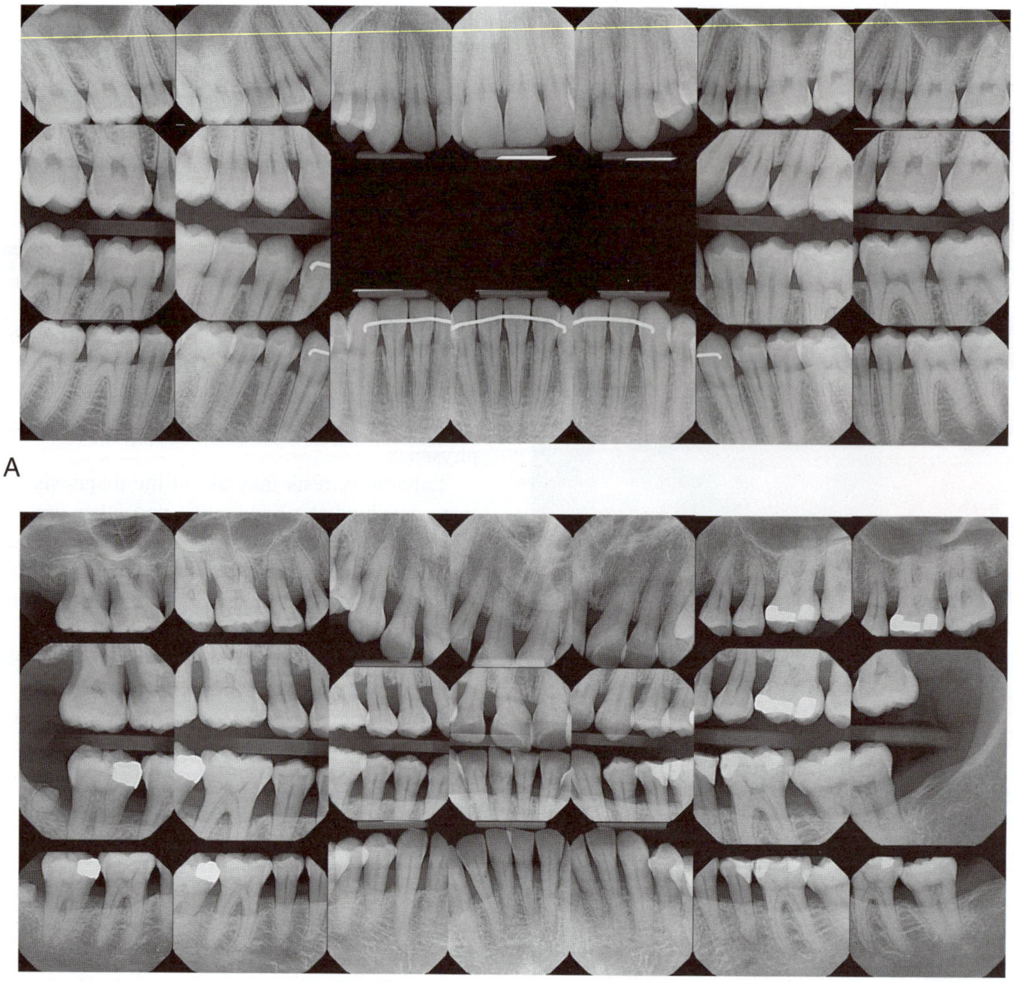

A

B

Fig. 24.27 A complete intraoral radiographic set is an essential adjunct to periodontal diagnosis component of the periodontal examination. A, Intraoral radiographs of a patient with gingivitis. Note the radiopaque fixed lingual orthodontic retainer. B, Intraoral radiographs of a patient with generalized moderate to severe chronic periodontitis. Vertical bitewing radiographs are useful to evaluate crestal bone loss. *(Copyright Jonathan H. Do, DDS. All rights reserved.)*

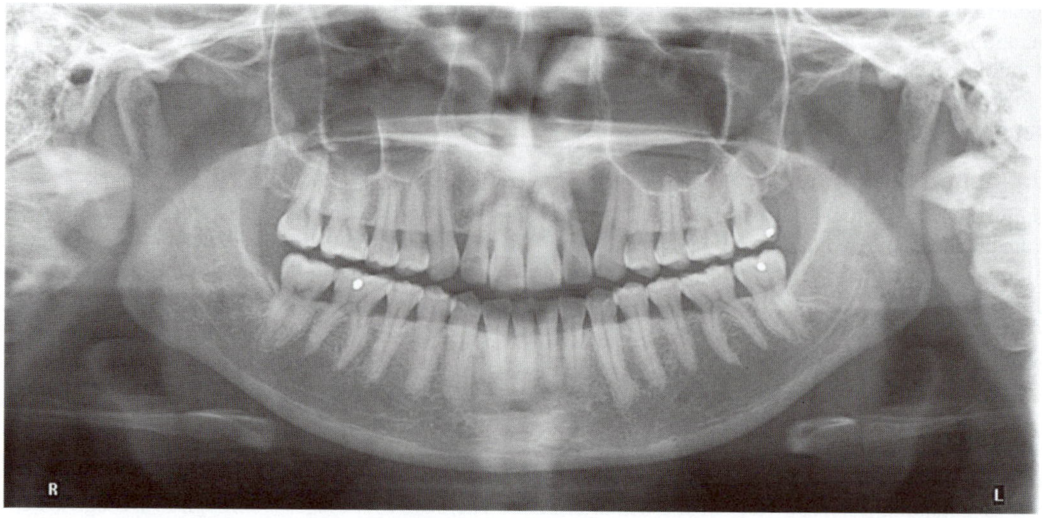

Fig. 24.28 Panoramic radiographs provide an overview of the dental arch and the surrounding structures.

TABLE 24.2 Salient Clinical and Radiographic Features of the Four Different Stages of Periodontitis According to the Classification Released in 2018

Stage I	Stage II	Stages III and IV
• Incipient periodontitis 1–2 mm interdental CAL • Probing depths ≤4 mm • No tooth loss or planned for extraction due to periodontitis	• Progression beyond incipient periodontitis • 3–4 mm interdental CAL • Probing depths ≤5 mm • No tooth loss or planned to be removed due to periodontitis	• Tooth loss or planned for extraction due to periodontitis • ≥5 mm interdental CAL and probing depths ≥6 mm • Deep vertical bony defects • Deep furcation involvements • Extent of tooth loss and complexity of management distinguishes stage III from stage IV disease.
Radiographic Findings		
• Bone loss in the coronal third (<15% of the root)	• Bone loss in the coronal third (15%–33% of the root)	• Bone loss extending to middle third of root and beyond

CAL, Clinical attachment loss.

severe periodontitis associated with (or potential for) tooth loss (≤4 in stage III and ≥5 teeth in stage IV). Table 24.2 presents the key features of each of the stages of periodontitis.

The extent should be described after the determination of the stage. Assessment of extent describes the percentage of teeth at the stage-defining severity level based on a 30% threshold. Localized periodontitis is defined as periodontitis affecting ≤30% of teeth, while periodontitis affecting greater than 30% of teeth is considered generalized. If the periodontal attachment loss is completely or mostly confined to the first molars and incisors, the term molar-incisor pattern is used for the disease extent.

Step 3: Establish the Grade

There are three grades (A, B, and C). Grade A denotes a slow rate of disease progression, while grades B and C denote a moderate and severe rate of disease progression, respectively. When direct evidence of radiographic or clinical disease progression over time is not available, indirect evidence in the form of % bone loss/age is used as the primary method to assign a grade. For grades A, B, and C, the corresponding % bone loss age measures are less than 0.25, 0.25–1.0. and greater than 1.0, respectively. Established periodontal risk factors such as smoking and its frequency and glycemic control status are both used as grade modifiers.

Assessment of Biofilm Control and Patient Education

Patients presenting for periodontal consultations typically expect to find out the problems they have and the treatments they need. By the end of the periodontal consultation, it may not be possible to determine a detailed prognosis and formulate a complete treatment plan, as a careful analysis of the information obtained, the acquisition of more diagnostic information, or consultation with other dental and medical professionals may be required. However, the patient can be educated on the problems identified in his or her mouth upon initial examination, the need for further diagnostics, and the etiologies and prevention of these problems. Clinical photographs, radiographs, and models may be useful to help the patient understand their current status of oral health. Upon completion of the periodontal examination, the patient may be presented with a preliminary treatment plan that may include emergency and palliative treatments as well as nonsurgical periodontal therapy as part of infection control therapy.

Although patient education and biofilm control are not the focus of this chapter, a preventive approach to oral health care demands behavior modification through effective patient education, which requires time, effort, and repetition. As such, every opportunity to educate and motivate patients should be seized in order to implement positive behavioral changes. Patients should be given personalized, site-specific oral hygiene instructions for biofilm control and to improve their oral health, including periodontal health. It is not uncommon for patients presenting with poor plaque control and the presence of disease to report brushing and flossing multiple times daily. For that reason, the effectiveness of the patient's biofilm control must be evaluated and monitored over time. If suboptimal plaque control is evident, the patient should be asked to demonstrate biofilm control (toothbrushing, flossing, etc.) in front of a mirror so that both the patient and the clinician can see their oral hygiene techniques. The patient should then be taught proper biofilm control techniques with a demonstration in their own mouth in front of a mirror.

Ideally, unless emergency treatment is required, patients should be given at least 1 or 2 weeks to improve their oral hygiene, to control biofilm and reduce periodontal inflammation, and to appreciate how meticulous biofilm control can positively impact their oral health before any periodontal treatment is rendered.

Conclusion

Periodontal examination begins with the acquisition of a thorough medical and dental history. Although, for didactic purposes, the sequence of periodontal examination presented in this chapter is divided into two parts (visual and tactile examination), in practice, both visual and tactile assessments overlap and occur simultaneously, as do the evaluations of the teeth and the periodontium. A proper periodontal examination should include an overall survey of biofilm and calculus, clinical signs of inflammation, and other obvious signs of disease to obtain insights into the patient's oral hygiene performance and disease status.

Once a detailed patient history has been obtained and a thorough clinical examination has been completed, the information collected is analyzed and synthesized to arrive at a diagnosis or a list of diagnoses. The periodontal examination is the basis from which the diagnosis, prognosis, and treatment plan are derived. Therefore, a thorough and accurate periodontal examination is of the utmost importance to render optimal periodontal therapy.

Key points

- To arrive at an accurate diagnosis an orderly and comprehensive clinical examination is mandatory. It includes a thorough history, medical background of the patient and a phased step-by-step identification of all the presenting features.
- Detailed history includes the patient chief complaint, past dental and periodontal visits, family history, habits such as smoking and oral hygiene practices.
- Oral cavity is examined for any changes in the mucosa and teeth are examined for caries, occlusion and wasting diseases.
- A thorough evaluation of periodontium includes examination of gingiva, periodontal pockets, clinical attachment level, mobility, migration, furcation involvement and presence of any mucogingival problems.

SUGGESTED READING

Salvi GE, Roccuzzo A, Imber JC, Stähli A, Klinge B, Lang NP. Clinical periodontal diagnosis. Periodontology 2000. Published online July 14, 2023. doi:10.1111/prd.12487.

CHAPTER 25

Radiographic Aids in the Diagnosis of Periodontal Disease

SM Mallya | S Tetradis | CD Dwarakanath

CHAPTER OUTLINE

Radiologic imaging provides essential information that contributes to diagnosis and management of patients with periodontal disease. Objectives of imaging include assessment of the extent and pattern of osseous changes, identification of local causative factors, and an assessment of local anatomy. Radiographs illustrate the current status of calcified tissues—these imaging findings reflect the cumulative effects of inflammation on bone and teeth and do not always reflect current cellular activity in the periodontium. *Thus, radiographs must be used as an adjunct to and not as a substitute for a clinical examination.* Radiologic evaluation provides information on the morphology of intrabony defects, the extent of furcation bone loss, and anatomic restrictions to root instrumentation—factors that contribute to treatment planning and outcome. In addition, radiographs provide longitudinal assessment of bone loss.

Imaging Modalities for Periodontal Assessment

Intraoral Imaging

Intraoral radiologic imaging with periapical and bite-wing projections serves as the primary imaging examination to assess periodontal disease. Radiologic assessments include evaluation of the bone level, the **destruction pattern**, periodontal ligament (PDL) space width, and the radiodensity, trabecular pattern, and marginal contour of the interdental bone. Depiction of these details requires optimization of technique for radiographic projection and exposure. Standardized, reproducible techniques are important to obtain reliable radiographs for pretreatment and posttreatment comparisons.

Prichard established the following four criteria to determine adequate angulation of periapical radiographs (Fig. 25.1):

1. The radiograph should show the tips of molar cusps with little or none of the occlusal surface showing.
2. Enamel caps and pulp chambers should be distinct.
3. Interproximal spaces should be open.
4. Proximal contacts should not overlap unless teeth are anatomically misaligned.

For periapical radiographs, the long-cone paralleling technique accurately projects the alveolar bone level (Fig. 25.2). The bisecting angle technique typically elongates the projected image, making the bone margin appear closer to the crown; the facial bone level is distorted more than the lingual alveolar crest. Inappropriate horizontal angulation results in tooth overlap, changes the shape of the interdental bone image, alters the radiographic width of the PDL space and the appearance of the **lamina dura**, and may distort the extent of **furcation involvement** (see Fig. 25.2). Periapical radiographs frequently do not reveal the correct relationship between the alveolar bone and the cementoenamel junction (CEJ). This is particularly true when a shallow palate or high floor of the mouth does not allow ideal placement of the receptor parallel to the tooth.

Bite-wing radiographs are a better approach to evaluate periodontal bone levels. For a bite-wing projection, the image receptor is placed lingual to the crowns of the upper and lower teeth and parallel to the long axis of the crowns. The X-ray beam is directed through the contact areas of the teeth and perpendicular to the image receptor. Thus, the bite-wing projection geometry permits evaluation of the relationship between the interproximal alveolar crest and the CEJ without distortion (Figs. 25.3 and 25.4). When the periodontal bone loss is severe and the bone level cannot be visualized on horizontally positioned bite-wing radiographs, receptors may be placed vertically to encompass more root length (Fig. 25.5). More than two vertical bite-wing images may be necessary to cover all of the interproximal spaces in the area of interest.

A full mouth radiologic examination with periapical and bite-wing radiographs provides detailed evaluation of the periodontal bone and is the preferred examination to assess the osseous impact of periodontal disease (Fig. 25.6).

Panoramic Imaging

Panoramic imaging (Fig. 25.7) encompasses regions of the jaw beyond the dentoalveolar region, including the basal body and rami of the mandible, the temporomandibular joints, the maxillary sinuses, and nasal cavity. Panoramic imaging is a low-radiation-dose procedure, is relatively quicker and easier than a full mouth intraoral survey, and is more comfortable for the patient. However, panoramic image resolution is lower than that of intraoral radiographs, and assessments of root shape and resorption are more accurate on intraoral radiographs.

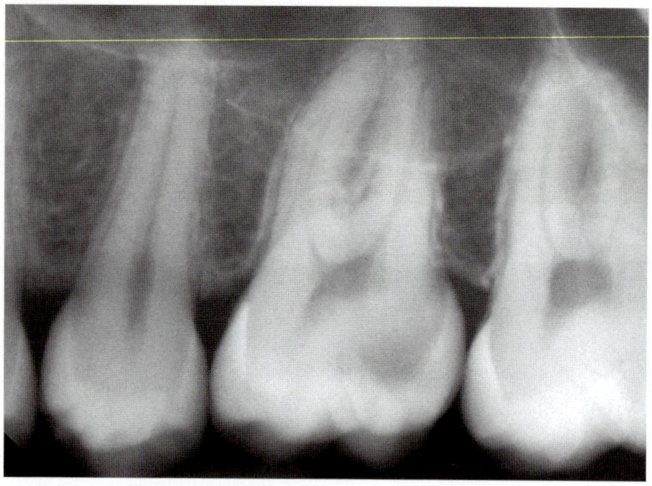

Fig. 25.1 Periapical radiograph of the posterior maxilla. Note that the cusps are superimposed and the enamel appears as a distinct cap separated from the pulp space. The approximal surfaces are separated, and the interdental bone is distinct.

For periodontal purpose, the role of conventional radiographs may be summarized as under:

Features recognizable:

1. Height of the remaining bone.
2. Location of cementoenamel junction.
3. Type of bone loss viz. horizontal/vertical.
4. Trabecular pattern of bone.
5. Width of periodontal ligament space.
6. Integrity of lamina dura.
7. Root resorption.
8. Dental caries, periapical pathology.
9. Impacted, unerupted teeth.
10. Advanced stages of furcation involvement.
11. Other bone pathologies such as osteoporosis and cyst.

Features nonrecognizable:

1. Periodontal pocket—They are soft tissue lesions and can only be ascertained by accurate probing.
2. Current cellular activity.
3. Number of walls involved in an osseous defect.
4. Osseous defects on the facial or lingual surface of the teeth such as fenestration and dehiscence.
5. Early stage of furcation involvement.
6. Early stage of abscesses.
7. Accurate determination of proximity of maxillary sinus.
8. Location of mandibular canal and mental foramen.

Digital Radiologic Imaging

Globally, the use of digital technologies for intraoral and extraoral imaging has grown rapidly over the past two decades. Digital imaging provides several advantages over film-based imaging and, importantly, also decreases patient radiation dose. In the United States, more than 80% of intraoral imaging is done using digital receptors. Two technologies are used for digital intraoral imaging—solid-state detectors and photostimulable phosphors (PSPs). Solid-state sensor-based systems use complementary metal oxide semiconductor (CMOS) or charge-coupled device (CCD) chips to detect X-ray photons and record an image. These systems provide immediate image display after acquisition. PSP technology uses rare earth crystals to store energy and record a latent radiographic image. The stored energy is then released by stimulating the plate with an appropriate wavelength of light causing the crystal to emit light photons. Unlike CCD/CMOS receptors, PSP plates do not provide an instantaneous display of the radiographic image. Irrespective of acquisition method, digital images can be modulated, and most vendors provide software tools to adjust density and contrast, magnify images, and enhance edges to sharpen the image. Some software vendors have incorporated preprogrammed algorithms that can be applied to enhance digital images for specific diagnostic tasks (e.g., to enhance visualization of interproximal caries, periodontal bone [Fig. 25.8], and pulp canals). However, it is important

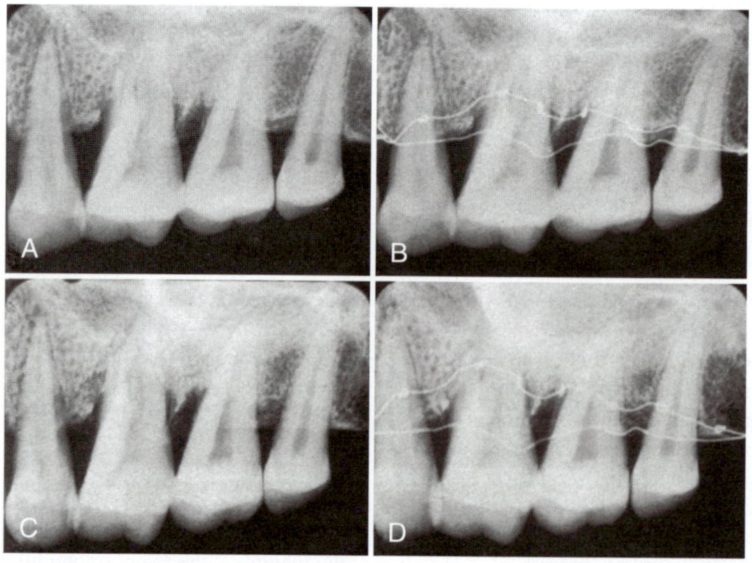

Fig. 25.2 Comparison of long-cone paralleling and bisection-of-the-angle techniques. A, Long-cone paralleling technique, radiograph of dried specimen. B, Long-cone paralleling technique, same specimen as shown in part A. Smooth wire is on the margin of the facial plate and knotted wire is on the lingual plate to show their relative positions. C, Bisecting angle technique, same specimen as in parts A and B. D, Bisecting angle technique, same specimen. Both bone margins are shifted toward the crown, the facial margin (smooth wire) more than the lingual margin (knotted wire), creating the illusion that the lingual bone margin has shifted apically. *(Courtesy Dr. Benjamin Patur, Hartford, Connecticut.)*

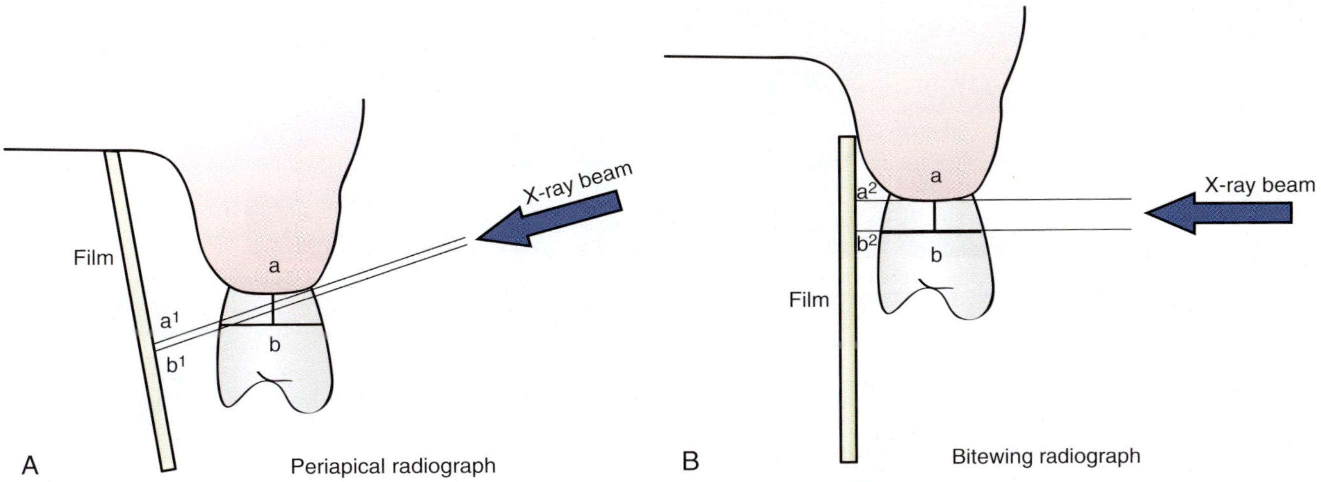

Fig. 25.3 Schematic diagram of periapical (A) and bite-wing (B) radiographs. Angulation of the X-ray beam and the receptor on the periapical radiograph distort the distance between the alveolar crest and the cementoenamel junction (CEJ) (compare a–b vs a^1–b^1). In contrast, the projection geometry of the bitewing radiograph allows a more accurate depiction (a^2–b^2) of the distance between the alveolar crest and the CEJ (a–b).

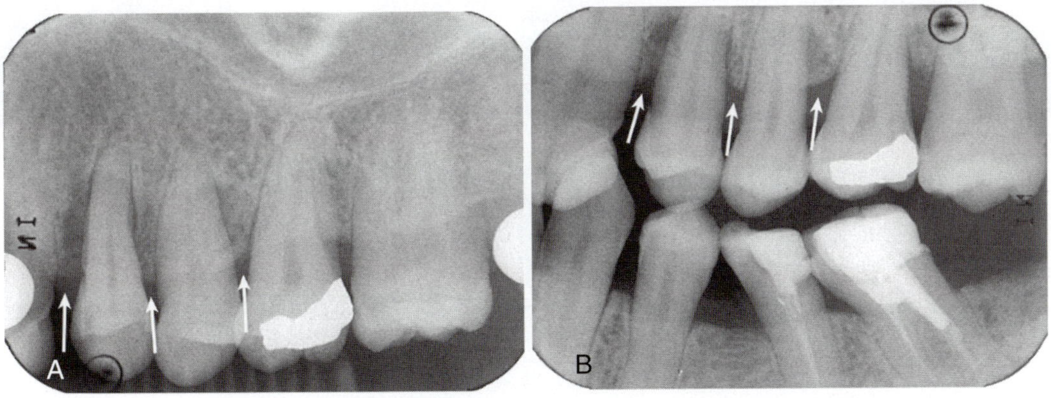

Fig. 25.4 Periapical (A) and bitewing (B) radiographs from a full-mouth series of a patient with periodontitis. The periapical film clearly underestimates the amount of bone loss *(white arrows)*. Because of appropriate projection geometry, the alveolar crest height is accurately depicted on the bite-wing radiograph *(white arrows)*.

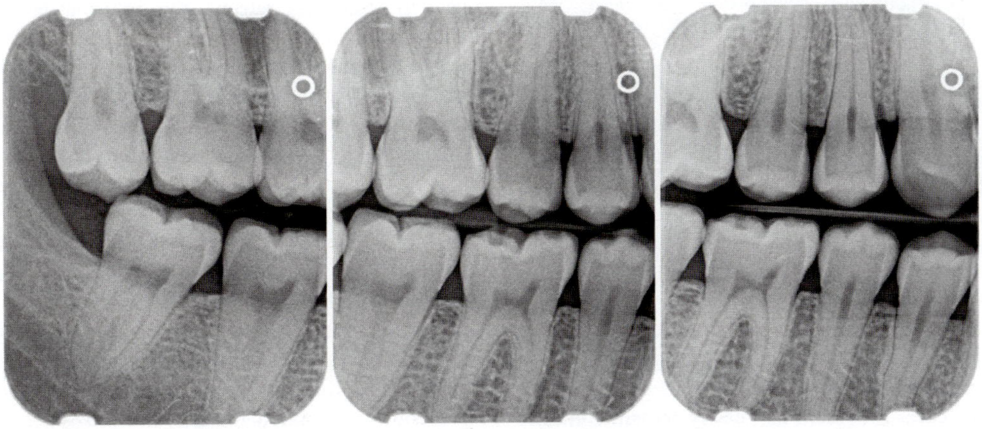

Fig. 25.5 Vertical bite-wing radiographs can be used to encompass a longer length of root and alveolar bone.

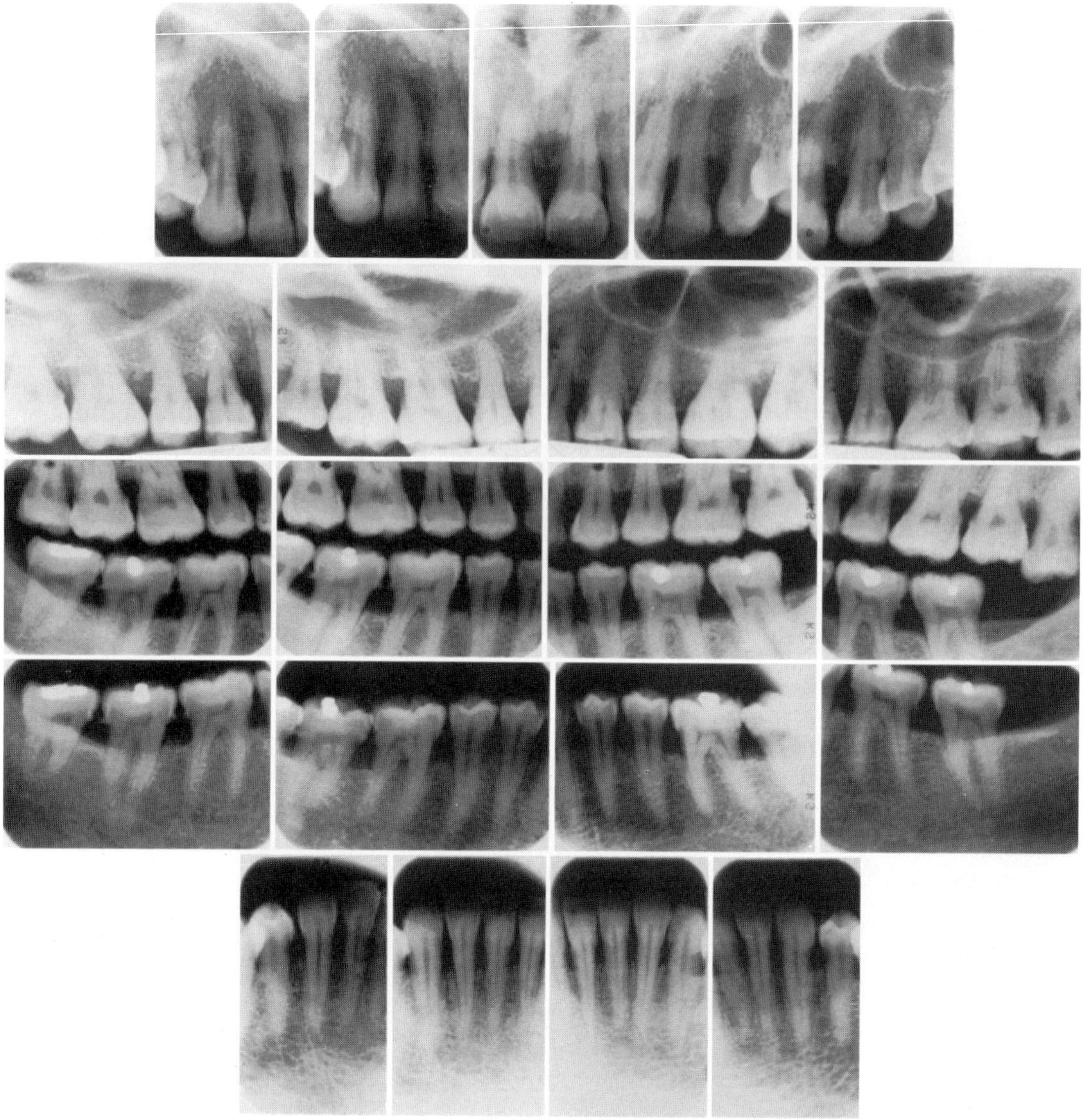

Fig. 25.6 Image display of a full-mouth radiographic series acquired using digital receptors. Specific features of the software program allow for image manipulation, measurements, and annotations.

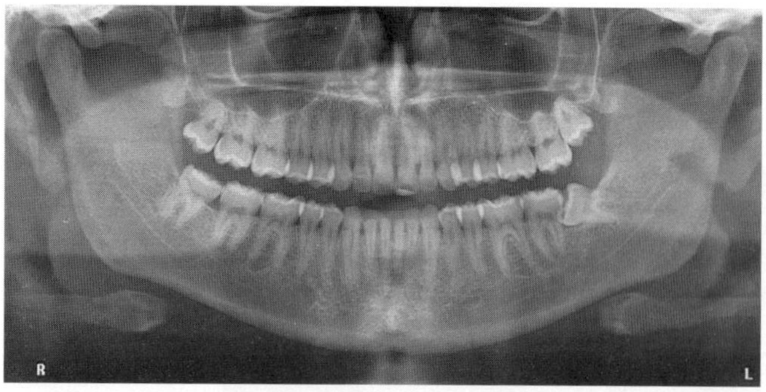

Fig. 25.7 Panoramic radiograph. Note the extended anatomic coverage relative to a full-mouth radiographic series.

to recognize that such image manipulations produce artifacts that may be misinterpreted as disease (see Fig. 25.8).

Digital radiologic imaging offers additional conveniences for documentation of care. Providers can easily transmit images to other providers for consultation or transfer of care and to insurance companies and other payors. Digital radiologic images are typically stored with metadata that identifies the patient, exam date, and other information regarding the acquisition. Coupling this information along with the image pixel data allows an end user to accurately retrieve this information. The digital imaging and communication in medicine (DICOM) standard is an international standard that allows interoperability of this information, irrespective of the patient management software used by individual offices. This standard specifies how clinical and radiologic images are to be transmitted, stored, retrieved, archived, and displayed, allowing vendors to develop interoperable products for image display and archival.

More recently, **artificial intelligence** (AI) algorithms have been applied for image-based pattern recognition to highlight unusual patterns or areas of altered radiodensity. In dentomaxillofacial imaging, AI-based approaches have been developed to aid caries detection, score periodontal bone loss, and identify periapical lesions. Such products may facilitate radiologic review by presenting annotated images that are subsequently validated by the clinician (Fig. 25.9).

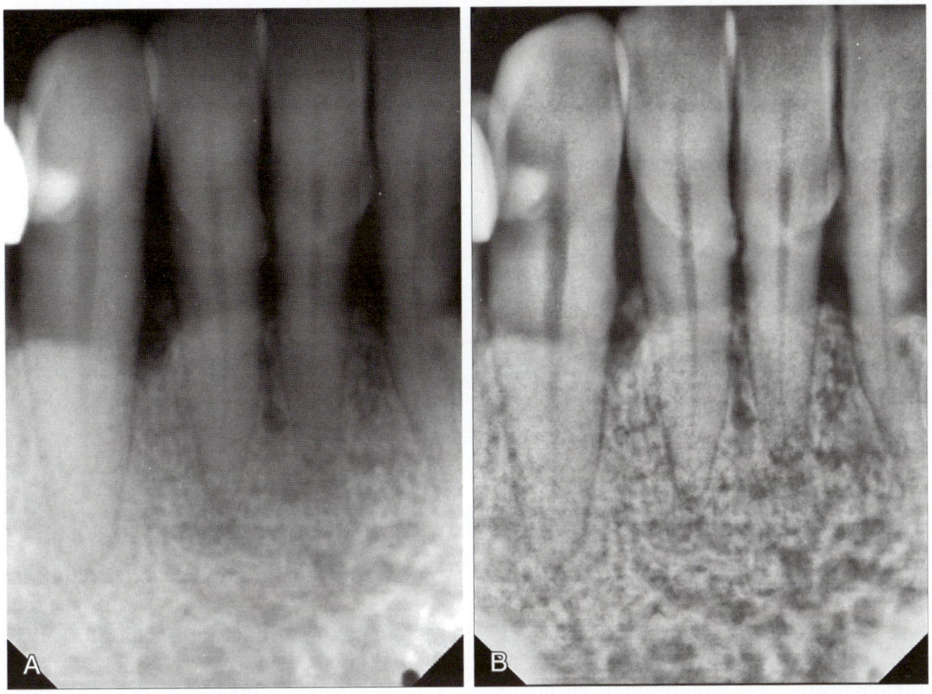

Fig. 25.8 A, Periapical radiograph acquired with a digital complementary metal oxide semiconductor sensor. B, Radiograph with a "perio" image enhancement filter applied to highlight the contrast of alveolar bone. Note the enhanced image highlights the contrast of calculus and the alveolar crest. Note artifactual radiolucent area adjacent to the restoration on the mandibular canine, which may be mistaken for caries.

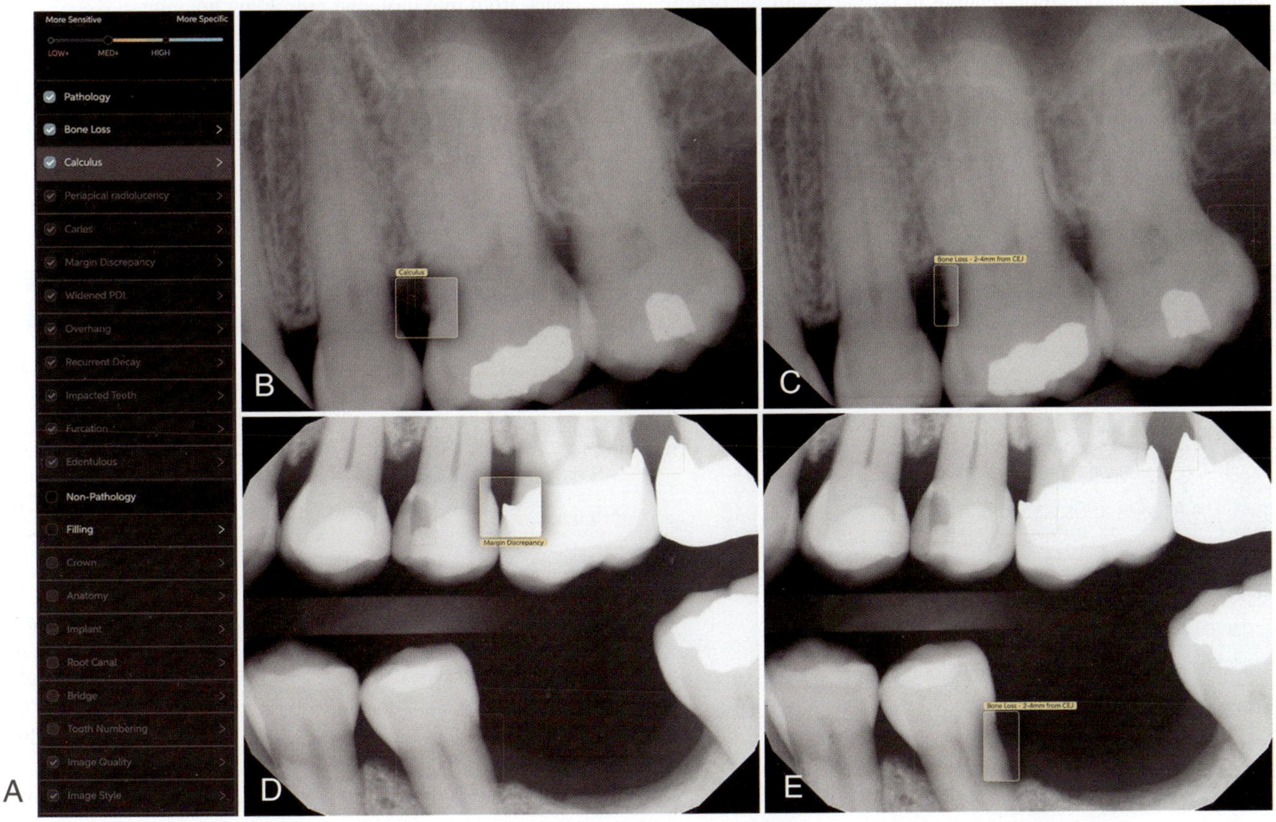

Fig. 25.9 Example of artificial intelligence-based assessments of relevance to periodontal evaluation. A, Tool panel to select specific assessments. Note that the assessments parallel the assessments of morphology and disease that are performed during a systematic human radiologic evaluation of an intraoral radiograph. B and C, Periapical radiograph with calculus deposits and bone loss highlighted by the program. D and E, Bite-wing radiograph with an overhanging margin and periodontal bone loss highlighted by the program. *(Radiographs evaluated using "Second Opinion" [Pearl, West Hollywood, CA, United States], a computer vision platform for intraoral radiographic analysis. Images courtesy of Dr. Kyle Stanley.)*

Cone-Beam Computed Tomography

Computed tomography (CT) is an advanced imaging technique that provides three-dimensional evaluation of the anatomy examined. In CT imaging, the X-ray source and detector revolve around the patient, acquiring projection images at hundreds of angles. Attenuation data from these projections are spatially reconstructed to provide a three-dimensional volumetric dataset that can be evaluated in multiple planes. CT imaging is dimensionally accurate and overcomes the limitations of image superimposition that are inherent to two-dimensional projection radiography. Maxillofacial cone-beam CT (CBCT) is a type of CT that uses an X-ray beam with a cone-shaped geometry to image the dentomaxillofacial hard tissues, including teeth and bones. Depending on the extent of anatomy imaged, referred to as field of view (FOV), CBCT imaging protocols are categorized as:

- **Limited** FOV: Typically 3–5 cm and encompasses a dentoalveolar region with two to four teeth.
- **Single arch** FOV: Encompasses *one* dentoalveolar arch.
- **Dentoalveolar** FOV: Encompasses *both* dentoalveolar arches.
- **Maxillofacial** FOV: Encompasses the entire mandible and maxilla and part of the craniofacial skeleton extending cranially to the nasion.

In general, images acquired at a smaller FOV have a higher resolution. Imaging periodontal structures requires high resolution to detect the PDL space and the lamina dura, and thus limited and single arch protocols are preferred to evaluate the teeth and periodontium in three dimensions.

Due to its inherent three-dimensional nature, CBCT provides significantly more information relative to intraoral and panoramic imaging. For example, interdental craters, an early sign of periodontal bone loss, is often masked on intraoral images but will be evident with multiplanar imaging. Specifically for periodontal management, two-dimensional imaging does not accurately depict the morphology of the periodontal defect—information that is important to determine disease severity and access to periodontal instrumentation, both important prognostic factors. Indeed, CBCT imaging is superior to intraoral imaging for identification of interdental craters, furcation involvement, and dehiscence and fenestration defects (see example in Fig. 25.17). Despite these demonstrated advantages, an American Academy of Periodontology Best Evidence Review found limited evidence to justify CBCT imaging for routine diagnosis and treatment planning of moderate-to-severe (**stage II, III, or IV**) periodontitis. Nevertheless, the review identified specific situations where CBCT imaging provides value beyond intraoral imaging. These include periodontal bone loss that has extended to the maxillary sinus or inferior alveolar canal, suspected endodontic and periodontal-endodontic lesions with equivocal findings on intraoral radiographs, to assess the periodontal impact of orthodontic tooth movement, and periodontal retreatment cases that fail to respond to localized therapy.

Selection of Appropriate Imaging

The decision to prescribe radiologic imaging is based on:

- The *diagnostic objectives* to be accomplished by imaging—the minimum essential information that is needed to diagnose and manage the patient.
- The *diagnostic efficacy* of the radiologic procedure—the ability of the radiologic technique to provide the required information.
- The *radiation-associated risks* of the procedure—to ensure that the benefits from the radiologic procedure far exceed the associated risk of radiation-induced cancer, the only risk of significance from maxillofacial radiologic imaging.
- The *cost of imaging*—to ensure that the added benefits from imaging are provided at an appropriate cost.

Table 25.1 provides information on the radiation doses and associated risks from select radiologic examinations. Relative to

TABLE 25.1 Radiation Doses and Risks From Dentomaxillofacial Radiologic Imaging

Examination	Effective Dose (mSv)[a]	Equivalent Background Radiation[b]	Estimated Cancer Risk[c]	Relative Radiation Level[d]
Four bite-wing radiographs	0.005	<1 day	1 in 4 million	●●
Air travel, Los Angeles to New York, 5 h	0.015	~1.5 days		
Panoramic, direct digital	0.02	~2 days	1 in a million	●●
Full mouth, digital sensor, rectangular collimation	0.03	~3 days	1 in 600,000	●
Air travel, Los Angeles to Osaka, 15 h	0.045	~5 days		
CBCT, limited FOV	0.05	~6 days	1 in 400,000	●
Full mouth, digital sensor, round collimation	0.1	~12 days	1 in 200,000	●●
CBCT, dentoalveolar				●●
Air travel, Los Angeles to Singapore, round trip, 33 h	0.1	~12 days		
CBCT, maxillofacial with cranium	0.15	~2 weeks	1 in 130,000	●●
Mammogram	0.4	~7 weeks	1 in 50,000	●●
MDCT, maxillofacial	0.8	~14 weeks	1 in 25,000	●●
MDCT, chest	7.0	~2 years	1 in 3000	●●●

CBCT, Cone-beam computed tomography; *FOV*, field of view; *MDCT*, multidetector computed tomography.
[a]Median effective doses of typical imaging protocols collated from multiple published studies.
[b]Equivalent background radiation is based on the average annual US background exposure of 3.1 mSv.
[c]Cancer risk estimated at 5.5%/Sv as per ICRP publication no. 103.
[d]Relative radiation levels. From American College of Radiology. *ACR Appropriateness Criteria*.
(Adapted from Table 2 in Mallya SM. Effective and safe use of x-rays: understanding the risks for decision-making. *J Calif Dent Assoc*. 2021;49:301–309.)

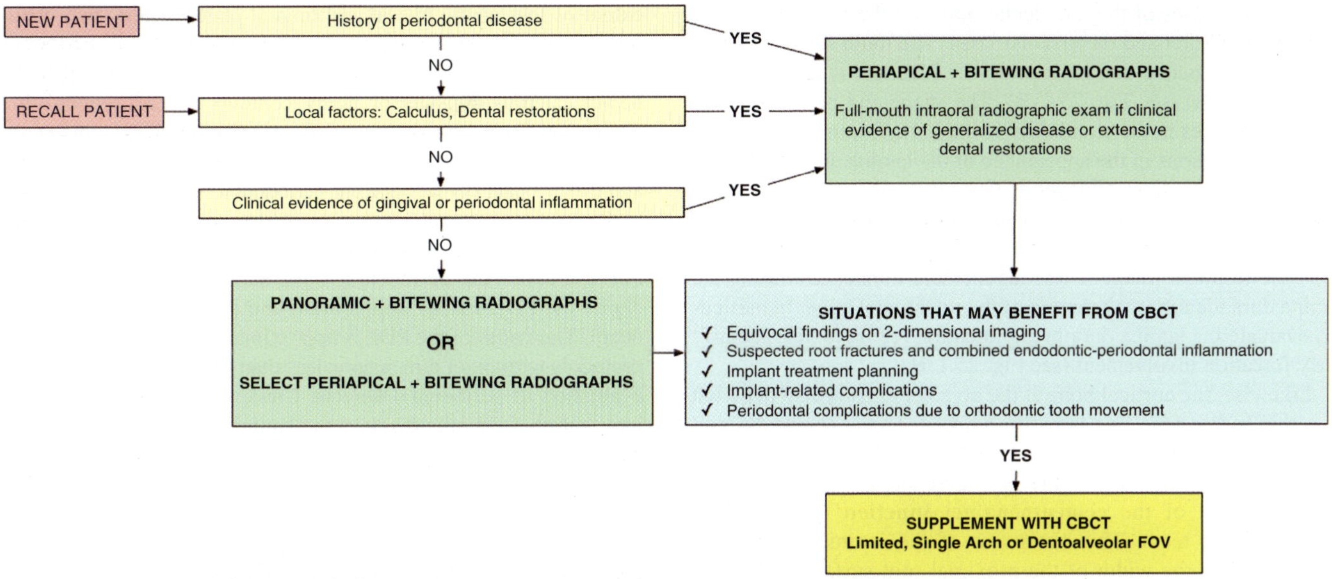

Fig. 25.10 Flowchart to guide imaging evaluation of teeth and periodontal structures. The goal of this flowchart is to provide a broad guideline with respect to selection of radiographs in the management of periodontal conditions. The need and selection must be assessed on a case-by-case basis. Information collated from the recommendations, position statements, and best evidence reviews from the American Association of Endodontists, the American Association of Oral and Maxillofacial Radiology, the American Academy of Periodontology Best Evidence Reviews, and the American Dental Association.

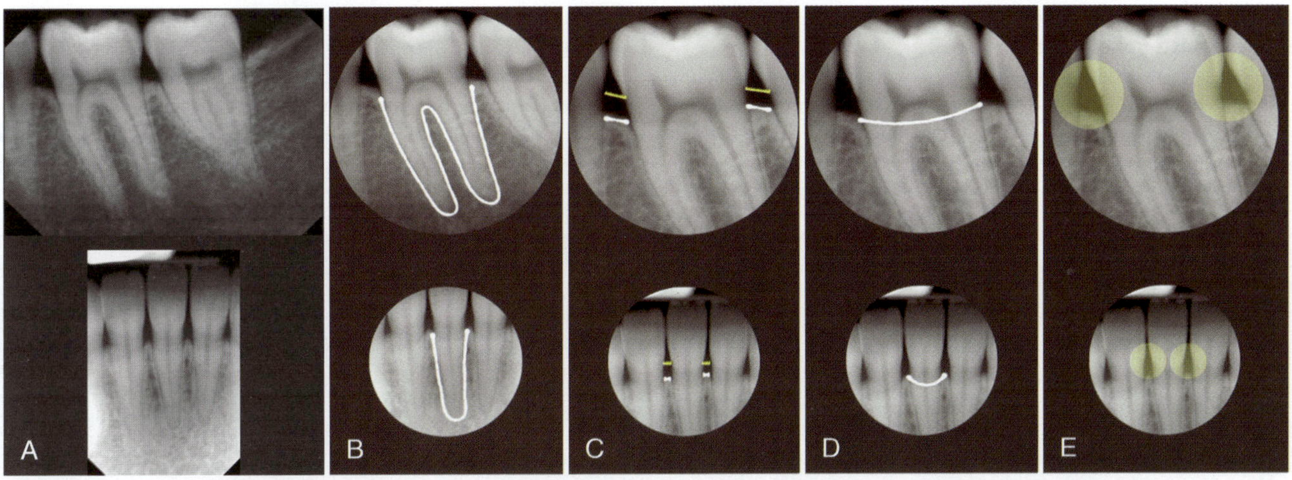

Fig. 25.11 Systematic approach to evaluate periodontal bone. A, Periapical radiographs of the mandibular posterior region *(top)* and mandibular anterior region *(bottom)*. B, Evaluate the lamina dura *(white lines)* for continuity, in particular, in the furcation region. C, Identify the line joining the adjacent cementoenamel junctions *(yellow line)*. The interdental bone level (*white* line) is normally 1–2 mm below this line. D, Trace the contour of the facial and lingual alveolar crest over the roots and examine their relation to the furcation. E, Examine the embrasure spaces *(yellow highlight)* for evidence of calculus or overhanging restoration margins.

most radiologic procedures used in health care, doses from dental radiologic examinations are low and are considered low risk. Thus, the decisions to select an imaging technique are driven predominantly by its efficacy and cost. Fig. 25.10 provides guidance for imaging of the teeth and periodontal structures based on current evidence and recommended best practices. This imaging algorithm considers benefits, costs, and risks and is based on current evidence and follows the recommendations of the American Association of Endodontists, the American Association of Oral and Maxillofacial Radiology, the American Academy of Periodontology, and the American Dental Association.

Normal Interdental Bone

Standard radiologic assessments for periodontal disease use intraoral radiographs. On these projections, the facial and lingual bony plates are obscured by the relatively dense root structure (Fig. 25.11D). Thus, evaluation of bone changes in periodontal disease is based predominantly on the appearance of the interdental bone. It is important to recognize normal appearances of the interdental bone—periodontal bone loss is categorized based on the extent and the pattern of resorption relative to this normal interdental bone level. Fig. 25.11 outlines a systematic approach to periodontal bone evaluation on intraoral radiographs.

The boundaries of the interdental bone are the cortical outlines of the tooth socket and the alveolar crest. The tooth socket appears as a thin, radiopaque line adjacent to the PDL and is referred to as the *lamina dura* (see Fig. 25.11B). The shape and position of the root and changes in the angulation of the X-ray beam produce considerable variations in the appearance of the lamina dura. When the X-ray photons traverse a longer distance through the cortical bone, the lamina dura appears as a well-demarcated radiopaque line. When the X-ray photons intersect a shorter segment of the lamina dura, the resultant image is less distinct and thinner. Outlining the lamina dura identifies the margin of the interdental bone. In particular, evaluate the lamina dura in the furcation region to help identify early furcation involvement (see Fig. 25.11B).

Likewise, the cortical bone at the alveolar crest is also depicted as a thin radiopaque line between adjacent teeth. The width and shape of the interdental bone and the angle of the crest normally vary with the convexity of the proximal tooth surfaces and the relative levels of the **cementoenamel junction** (CEJ) of the approximating teeth. The dimension of the interdental bone is determined by the width of the proximal root surface and space between approximal teeth. In the posterior dentition, the crestal table of the interdental bone appears as a corticated line parallel to a line between the CEJs of the approximating teeth and approximately 1–2 mm below this line (see Fig. 25.11C, top panel). When there is a difference in the level of the CEJs, as with tooth migration or tipping, the crest of the interdental bone appears inclined, relative to the crowns. In the anterior dentition, the interproximal spaces are narrower, and the interdental bone is triangular in shape (see Fig. 25.11C, bottom panel).

The dense root structure superimposes over and masks the facial and lingual plates of the tooth socket. On close examination, the crest of the facial and lingual plates can be identified as a faint radiopaque line across the root surface (see Fig. 25.11D). When the extent of loss of the buccal and lingual plates differs, two distinct bone levels may be apparent over the root surface.

In addition to evaluation of periodontal bone, radiographs also depict calculus deposits or faulty contours of restorations—local factors that increase risk for periodontal disease. Radiologic evaluation must include an assessment for the presence of these risk factors and their impact on the adjacent periodontal bone (see Fig. 25.11D).

The same systematic approach is also applied to the evaluation of periodontal bone support on CBCT examinations (Fig. 25.12). For evaluation of periodontal bone support, limited FOV scans depict the PDL space, lamina dura, and trabecular bone with high detail. The width of the PDL is approximately 0.2 mm, and imaging protocols with pixel dimensions less than 0.15 mm provide optimal evaluation of periodontal defects. Unlike with conventional imaging, sectional imaging displays the lamina dura and PDL spaces on all the root surfaces, and these structures must be evaluated in the sagittal, coronal, and axial planes (see Fig. 25.12).

Radiographic Appearance of Periodontal Disease

Early destructive changes of bone that do not remove sufficient mineralized tissue cannot be captured on radiographs. Therefore, radiographic manifestations suggest that the disease has progressed beyond its initial stages. The earliest signs of periodontal disease must be detected clinically. Radiographic changes of periodontal inflammation follow the pathophysiology of periodontal tissue destruction and include the following:

1. *Fuzziness and disruption of lamina dura and crestal cortication* are the earliest radiographic changes of periodontitis (Fig. 25.13A and B) and results from bone resorption activated by extension of gingival inflammation into the periodontal bone. Depicting these early changes depends greatly on the radiographic technique

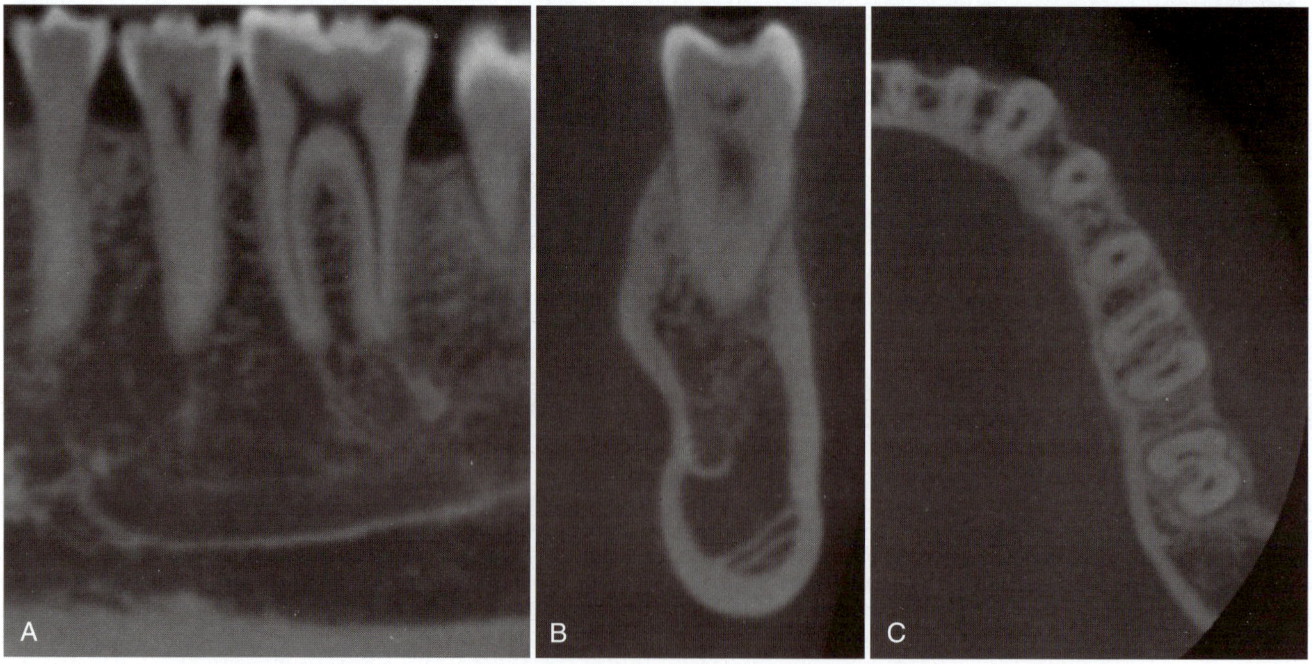

Fig. 25.12 Evaluation of periodontal bone on cone-beam computed tomography (CBCT) examinations. A, Sagittal plane sections resemble the projection of a periapical radiograph and the lamina dura and periodontal ligament (PDL) space should be examined along the root length and in the furcation. B, Coronal plane section shows the facial and lingual plates and the crest height on the root surface. C, Axial section shows the PDL circumferentially around the root and continuity of the facial and lingual bone adjacent to the roots. Videos corresponding the CBCT sections presented in this figure are available on the Expert Consult version of the book.

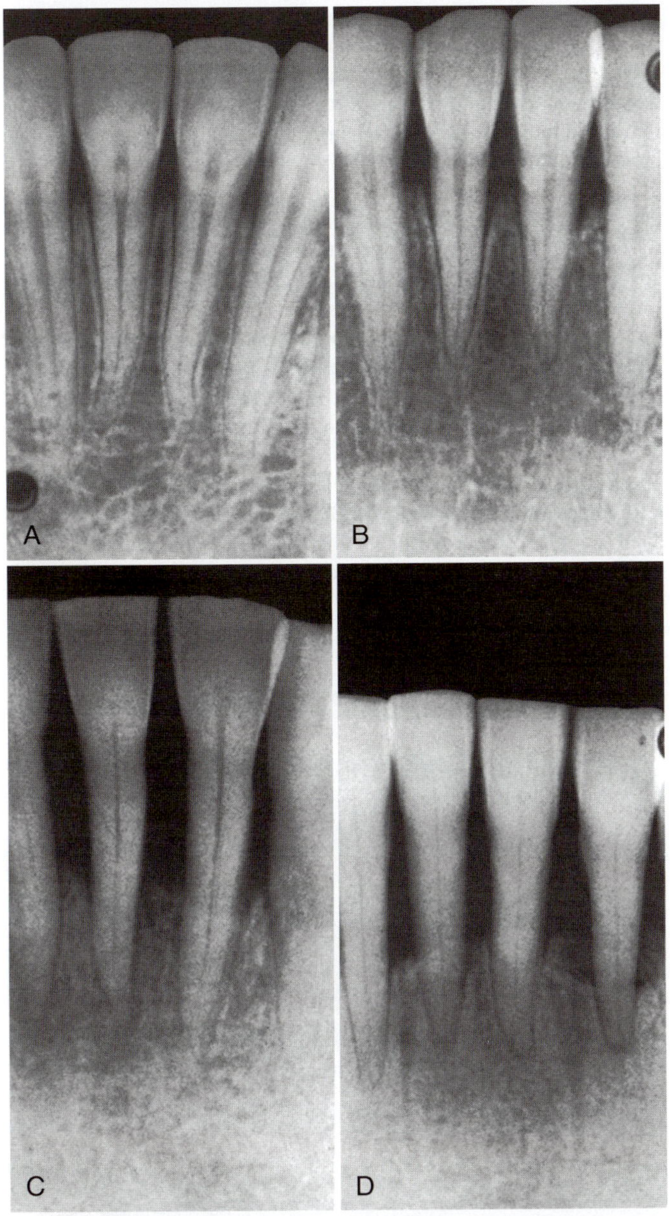

Fig. 25.13 Radiographic changes in periodontitis. A, Normal appearance of interdental bone. B, Fuzziness and a break in the continuity of the lamina dura at the crest of the bone distal to the central incisor *(left)*. There are wedge-shaped radiolucent areas at the crest of the other interdental bone. C, Radiolucent projections from the crest into the interdental bone indicate extension of destructive processes. D, Severe bone loss.

and on anatomic variations (thickness and density of interdental bone, position of adjoining teeth). The presence of crestal lamina dura on radiographs is associated with periodontal stability, but its absence is not associated with clinical inflammation, bleeding on probing, periodontal pockets, or loss of attachment. Therefore, the presence of an intact crestal lamina dura is considered an indicator of periodontal health, whereas its absence does not always imply periodontal disease.

2. Continued periodontal bone loss and widening of the periodontal space results in a *wedge-shaped radiolucency* at the mesial or distal aspect of the crest (see Fig. 25.13A and B). The apex of the area is pointed in the direction of the root.
3. Subsequently, the destructive process extends across the alveolar crest, reducing the height of the interdental bone. As increased osteoclastic activity results in increased bone resorption along the endosteal margins of the medullary spaces, the remaining interdental bone may appear partially eroded (see Fig. 25.13C).
4. The height of the interdental septum is progressively reduced by the extension of inflammation and the resorption of bone (see Fig. 25.13D).
5. Frequently a radiopaque horizontal line can be observed across the roots of a tooth. This opaque line demarcates the portion of the root where the labial or lingual bony plate has been partially or completely destroyed from the remaining bone-supported portion (Fig. 25.14 and see Fig. 25.11D).

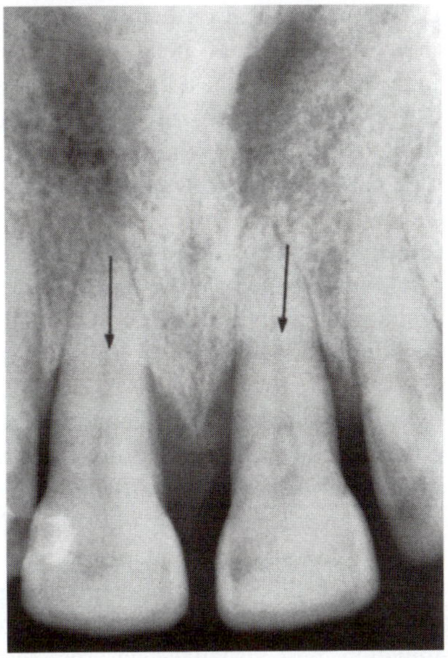

Fig. 25.14 Horizontal lines across the roots of the central incisors *(arrows)*. The area of the roots below the horizontal lines is partially or completely denuded of the facial and lingual bony plates.

Radiographic Bone Loss

Bone loss is the final manifestation of the periodontal inflammatory process. The radiographic image tends to underestimate the severity of bone loss. The difference between the alveolar crest height and the radiographic appearance ranges from 0 to 1.6 mm, mostly accounted for by X-ray angulation. Radiologic assessment of bone loss must include both the amount of bone loss and the distribution and pattern of bone destruction.

Radiographs are an indirect method for determining the amount of bone loss in periodontal disease; they show the amount of remaining bone rather than the amount lost. The amount of bone lost is estimated to be the difference between the physiologic bone level and the height of the remaining bone. Several investigators have analyzed the distance from the CEJ to the alveolar crest—it is generally accepted that the alveolar crest is less than 2 mm from this reference line. Current periodontal disease staging and grading relies on radiographic bone loss (RBL) at the site of greatest loss. RBL is categorized based on the extent of bone loss along the root length (Fig. 25.15), with increasing bone loss associated with later stage disease. The distribution of bone loss is an important assessment. It identifies the locations of destructive local factors in different areas of the mouth and in relation to different surfaces of the same tooth.

Patterns of Bone Destruction

Periodontal bone loss changes the height and contour of the bone. The patterns of bone destruction are broadly categorized as horizontal bone loss and vertical or angular defects. In horizontal bone loss, the height of interdental bone is reduced with the crest perpendicular to the long axis of the adjacent teeth (Fig. 25.16A). In contrast, vertical or angular defects are oblique trough-like bone loss adjacent to the root surface, with base of the defect located apically (see Fig. 25.16B). The defects are classified as *one-*, *two-*, or *three-*wall defects, depending on the number of bony walls that surround the defect. Contiguous defects that form a trough along more than one surface are called *circumferential* defects.

The internal morphology and depth of vertical defects are not apparent on two-dimensional radiographs. Furthermore, radiographs do not reveal the extent of involvement on the facial and lingual surfaces. Bone destruction of facial and lingual surfaces is masked by the dense root structure, and bone destruction on the mesial and distal root surfaces may be partially hidden by superimposed anatomy, such as a dense mylohyoid ridge (Fig. 25.17). In most cases, it can be assumed that bone loss seen interdentally continues in either the facial or lingual aspect, creating a trough-like lesion. Bone loss along the facial and lingual alveolar crest is apparent on CBCT examination, best visualized on cross-sectional images (Fig. 25.18).

Dense cortical facial and lingual plates of interdental bone obscure destruction of the intervening cancellous bone. Thus a deep, crater-like defect between the facial and lingual plates might not be depicted on conventional radiographs. To record destruction of the interproximal cancellous bone radiographically, the cortical bone must be involved. A reduction of only 0.5–1 mm in the thickness of the cortical plate is sufficient to permit radiographic visualization of the destruction of the inner cancellous trabeculae.

Interdental craters are a specific type of two-wall defect—they are concavities in the interdental bone between the facial and lingual plates. Interdental craters are common manifestations of periodontal destruction and constitute a third of osseous defects. They are more common in the mandible, especially in the posterior regions. Radiographically, interdental craters are recognized as irregular areas of reduced density on the alveolar bone crests. Craters are generally not sharply demarcated but gradually blend with the rest of the bone. Conventional radiographs do not accurately depict the morphology or depth of interdental craters, which sometimes appear as vertical defects. CBCT imaging allows for better evaluation of the three-dimensional morphology of the defect (Fig. 25.19).

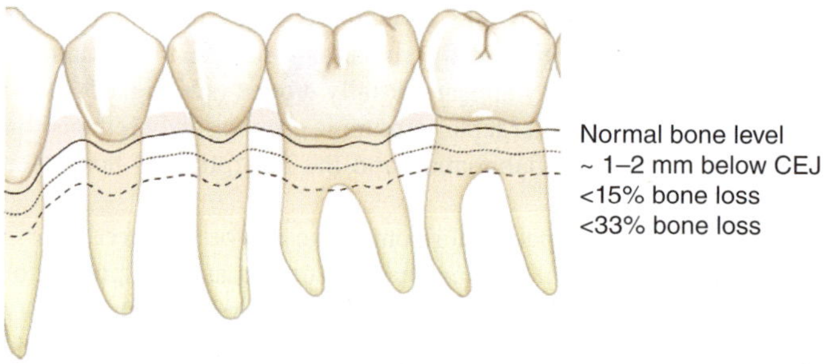

Fig. 25.15 Scoring radiographic bone loss for periodontal disease staging. Note that bone loss extending to and beyond the middle third of the root may involve the furcation of molar teeth. *(Modified from Mallya S, Lam E.* White and Pharoah's Oral Radiology. *8th ed. Mosby.)*

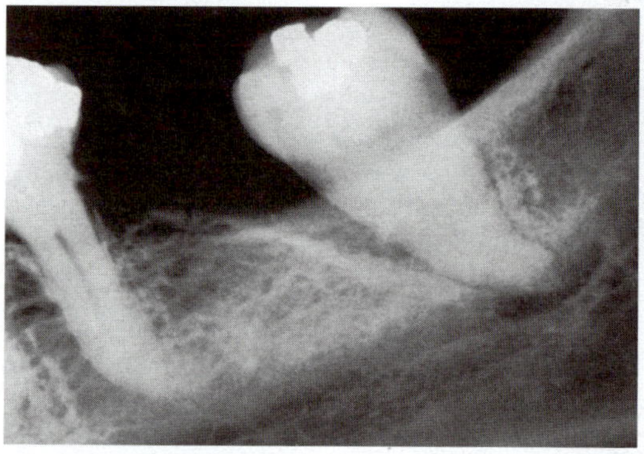

Fig. 25.17 Angular bone loss on mandibular molar partially obscured by a dense mylohyoid ridge.

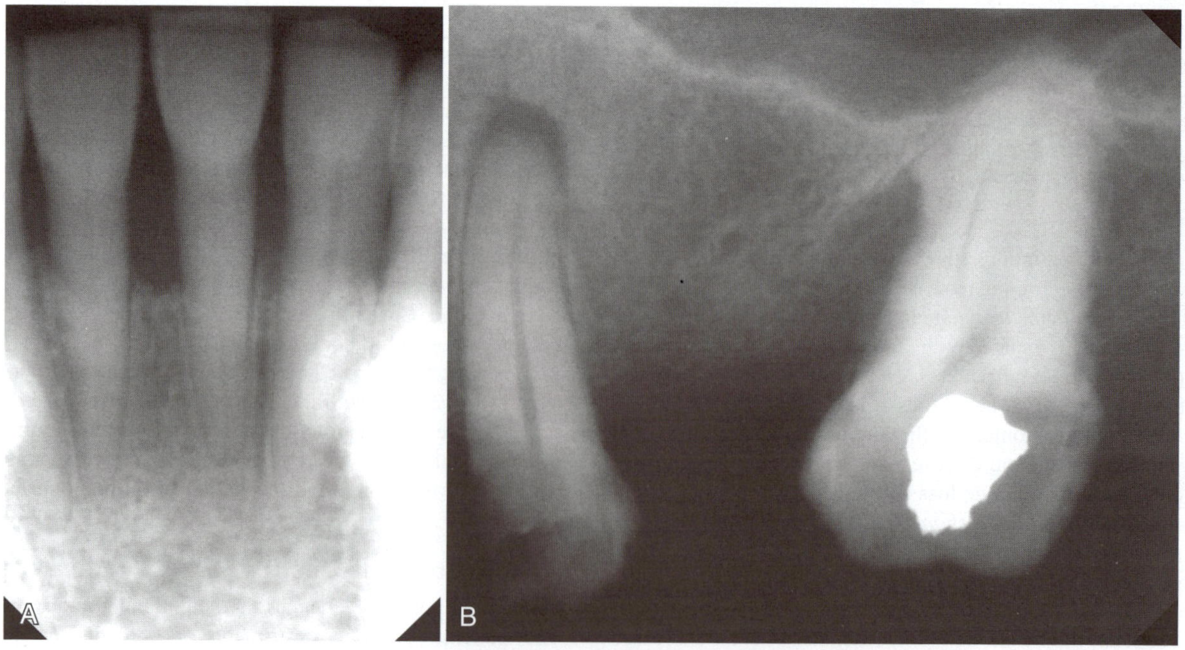

Fig. 25.16 A, Horizontal bone loss. B, Vertical or angular defect.

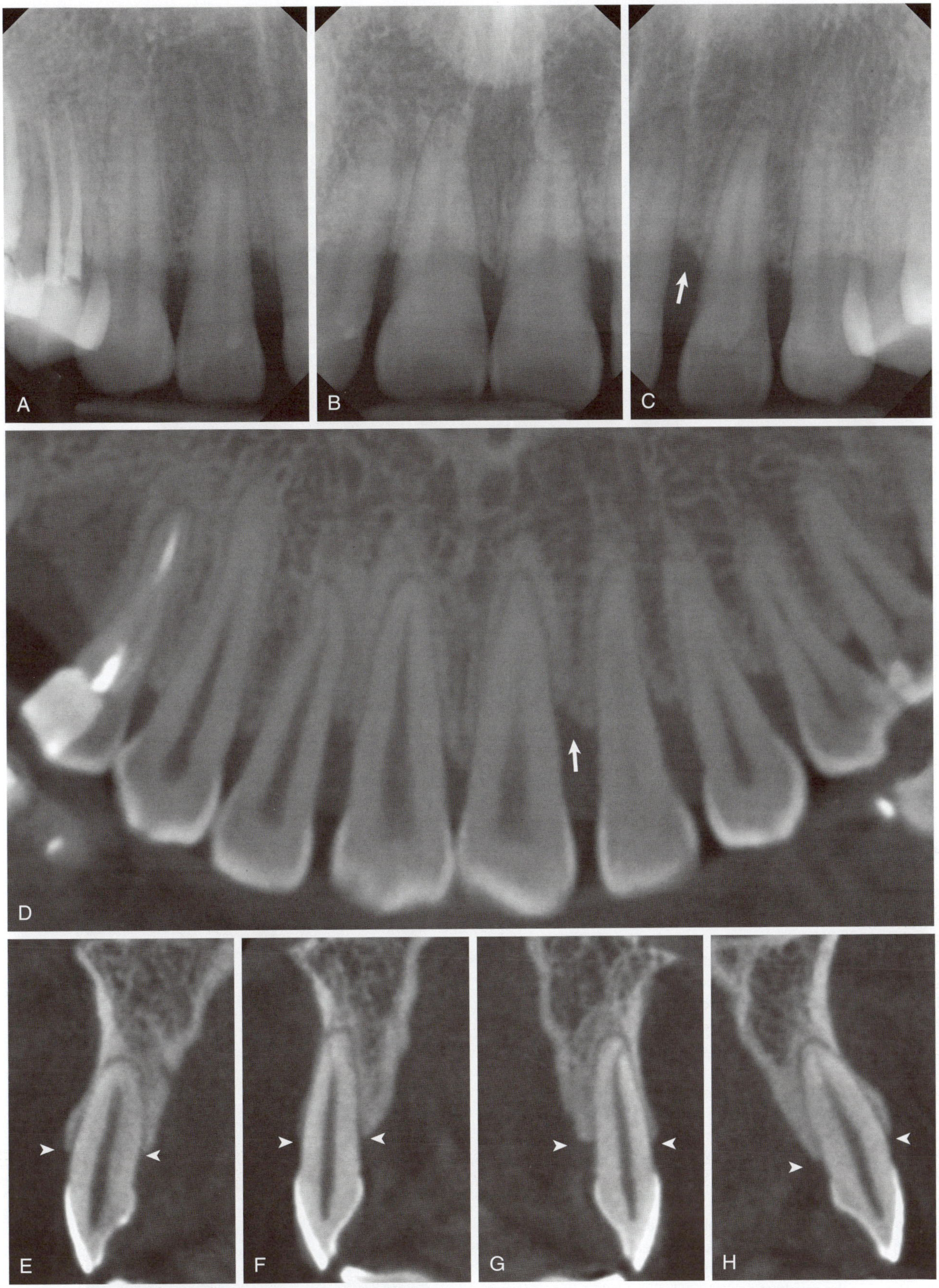

Fig. 25.18 Cone-beam computed tomography (CBCT) examination of the anterior maxilla. A–C, Periapical radiographs show horizontal bone loss and a vertical defect between the left maxillary central incisor and the maxillary left lateral incisor *(arrow).* D, Panoramic reconstruction of a CBCT examination depicting the vertical periodontal defect noted in panel A *(arrow).* E–H, Cross-sections through the long axes of the maxillary incisors. The height of the crestal bone is evident *(arrow heads).* Note that the facial bone adjacent to the maxillary right central incisor (panel F) is markedly thin.

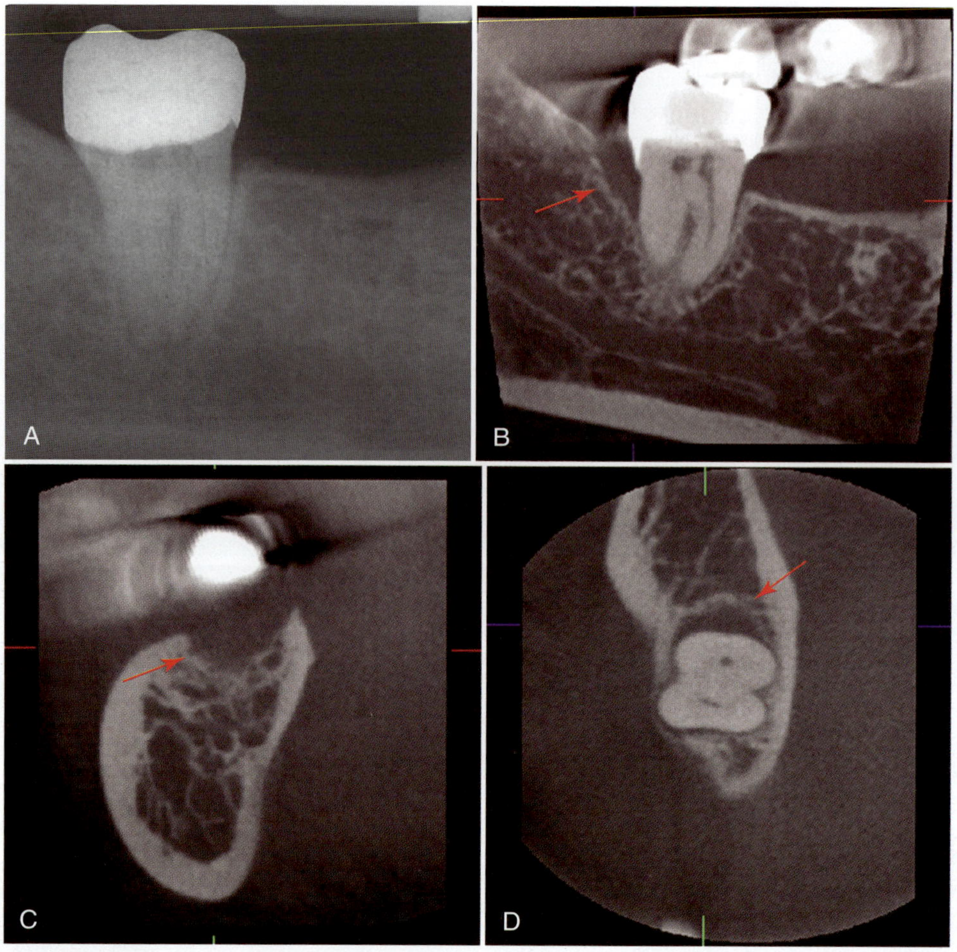

Fig. 25.19 Periapical radiograph (A) and sagittal (B), cross-sectional (C), and axial (D) cone-beam computed tomography (CBCT) sections of the mandibular right second molar. No periodontal defect is apparent on the periapical radiograph. However, CBCT images clearly illustrate a deep, vertical, three-wall defect on the distal surface of the mandibular right second molar *(red arrow)*.

Interdental bone loss may continue facially or lingually to form a trough-like defect that could be difficult to interpret on radiographs. These lesions may terminate on the radicular surface or may communicate with the adjacent interdental area to form one continuous lesion (Fig. 25.20).

Fig. 25.21 shows two adjacent interdental lesions connecting on the radicular surface to form one interconnecting osseous lesion. In addition to clinical probing to identify pocket depth, imaging with a radiopaque pointer, such as a gutta-percha point, placed into the defect will demonstrate the extent of the bone loss.

Periodontal bone loss should be differentiated from normal anatomy or anatomic variants that can resemble disease. For example, nutrient canals in the alveolar bone can appear as linear and circular radiolucent areas (Fig. 25.22). These canals can be seen more frequently in the anterior mandible, although they can be present throughout the alveolar ridge.

Finally, as emphasized earlier, radiographs can assess only the amount of existing periodontal bone to deduce the extent of prior bone loss. However, it is sometimes necessary to determine whether the reduced bone level is the result of periodontal disease that is no longer destructive (usually after treatment and proper maintenance) or whether active periodontal disease is present. Differentiation between treated versus active periodontal disease can only be achieved by clinical assessment.

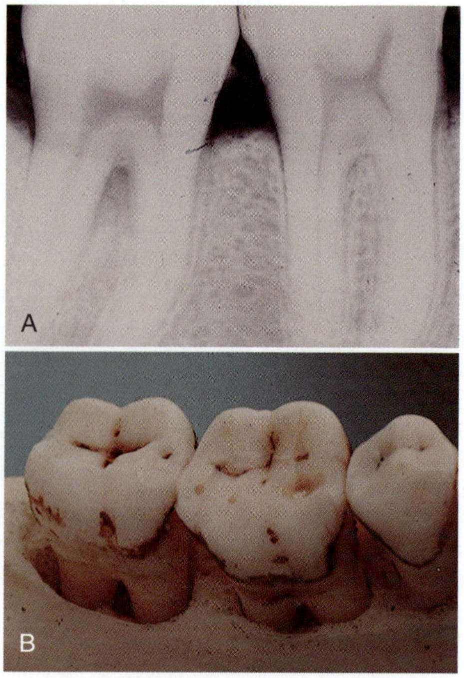

Fig. 25.20 (A & B) Interdental lesion that extends to the facial or lingual surfaces in a trough-like manner.

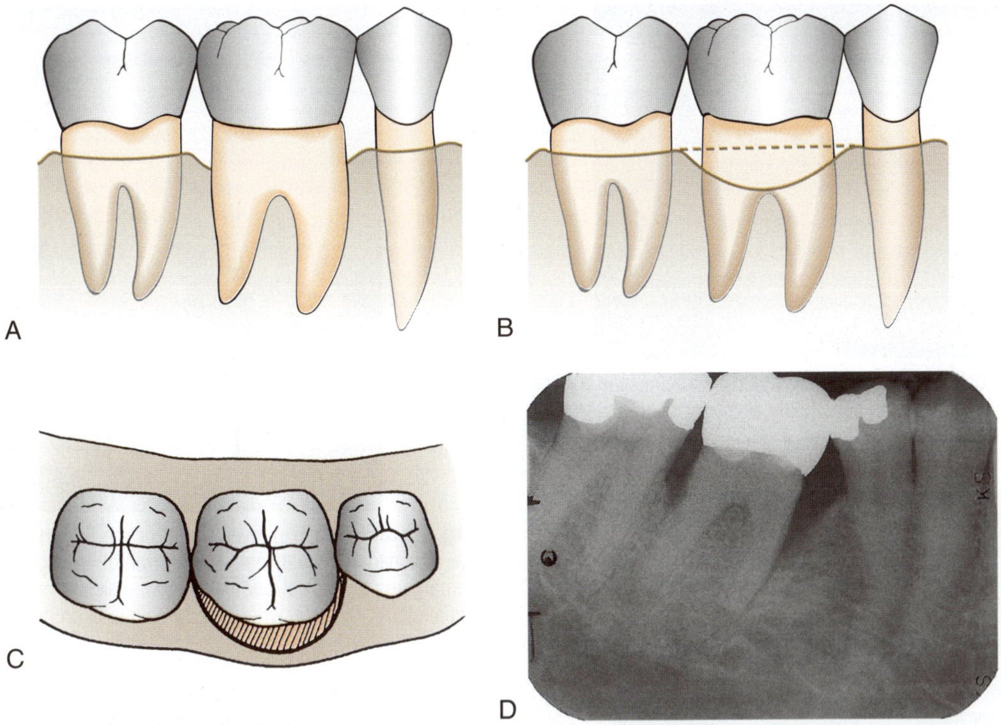

Fig. 25.21 A, Interdental mesial and distal lesions. B, Facial or lingual outlines of the actual lesion. C, Occlusal view of the lesion. D, Radiograph of mesial and facial lesions.

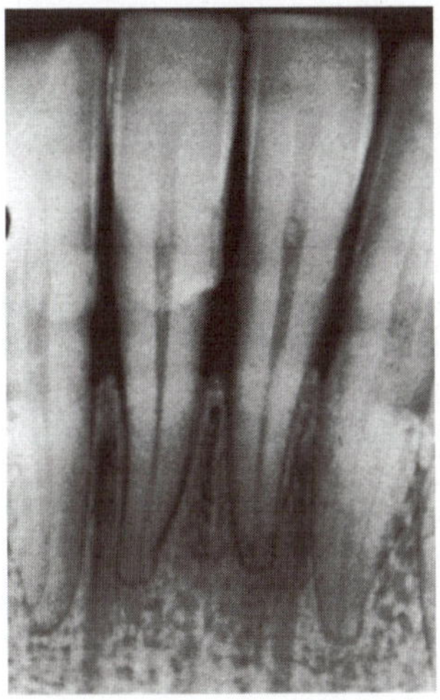

Fig. 25.22 Prominent nutrient canals in the mandible.

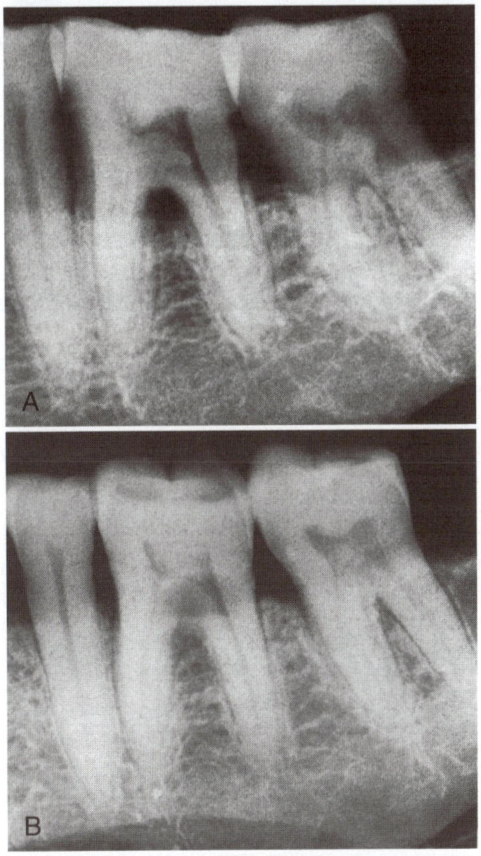

Fig. 25.23 A, Furcation involvement indicated by triangular radiolucency in the bifurcation area of mandibular first molar. The second molar presents only a slight thickening of the periodontal space in the bifurcation area. B, Radiograph of the same region as in A with different angulation. The triangular radiolucency in the bifurcation of the first molar is obliterated, and furcation involvement of the second molar is apparent.

Furcation Involvement

Definitive diagnosis of furcation involvement is made by clinical examination, which includes careful probing with a specially designed probe (e.g., Nabers). Radiographs are helpful, but root superimposition, caused by anatomic variations or improper technique, can obscure bone loss in the furcation. As a general rule, bone loss is greater than it appears in the radiograph. A tooth may present marked furcation involvement in one image (Fig. 25.23A) but appear to be uninvolved in another (see Fig. 25.23B). Radiographs should be taken at different angles to reduce the risk of missing furcation involvement.

A large, clearly defined radiolucency in the furcation area is easy to identify (see Fig. 25.23A), but less clearly defined radiographic changes are often overlooked. To assist in the radiographic

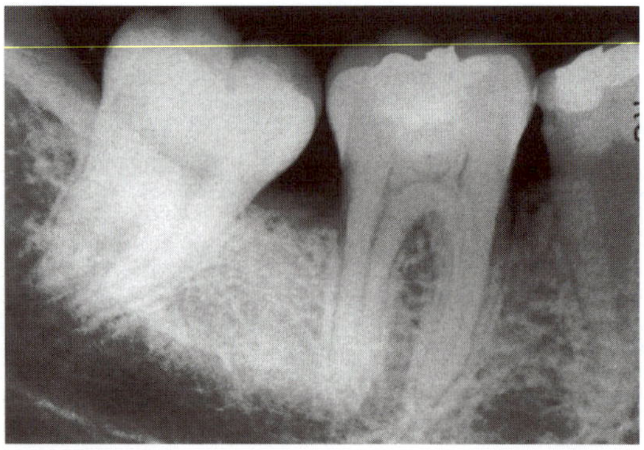

Fig. 25.24 Early furcation involvement suggested by fuzziness in the furcation of the mandibular first molar, particularly when associated with bone loss on the roots.

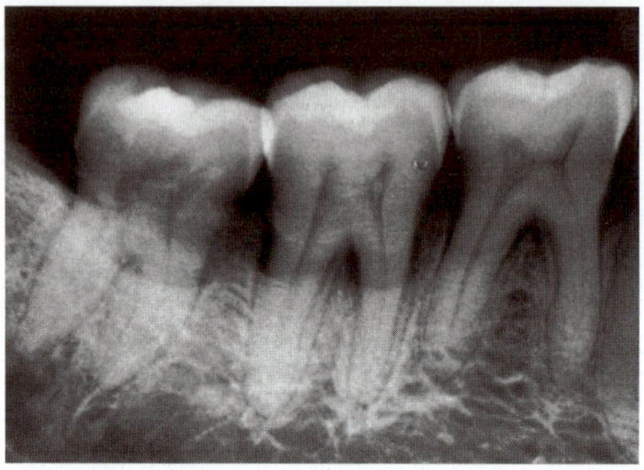

Fig. 25.25 Furcation involvement of mandibular first and second molars indicated by thickening of the periodontal space in the furcation area. The furcation of the third molar is also involved, but the thickening of the periodontal space is partially obscured by the external oblique line.

detection of furcation involvement, the following evaluation scheme is suggested:

1. The slightest radiographic change in the furcation area should be investigated clinically, especially if there is bone loss on adjacent roots (Figs. 25.24 and 25.27A).
2. Diminished radiodensity in the furcation area in which outlines of bony trabeculae are visible suggests furcation involvement (Figs. 25.25 and 25.27A).
3. Whenever there is marked bone loss in relation to a single molar root, it may be assumed that furcation is also involved (Figs. 25.26 and 25.27A).

Bone loss patterns and furcation involvement is often masked by superimposition of teeth and osseous structures on intraoral radiographs. The complexity of the bone loss extent and pattern is better depicted on CBCT images, especially for multirooted teeth (see Fig. 25.27).

Periodontal Abscess

The typical radiographic appearance of a periodontal abscess is a discrete area of radiolucency along the lateral aspect of the root (Figs. 25.28 and 25.29). However, the radiographic manifestation is often not characteristic (Fig. 25.30). This can be due to the following:

1. *The stage of the lesion.* The early stages of an acute periodontal abscess are extremely painful but present no radiographic changes.
2. *The extent of bone destruction and the morphologic changes of the bone.*
3. *The location of the* **abscess**. Lesions in the soft tissue wall of a periodontal pocket are less likely to produce radiographic changes than those deep in the supporting tissues. Abscesses on the facial or lingual surface are obscured by the radiopacity of the root; interproximal lesions are more likely to be visualized radiographically.

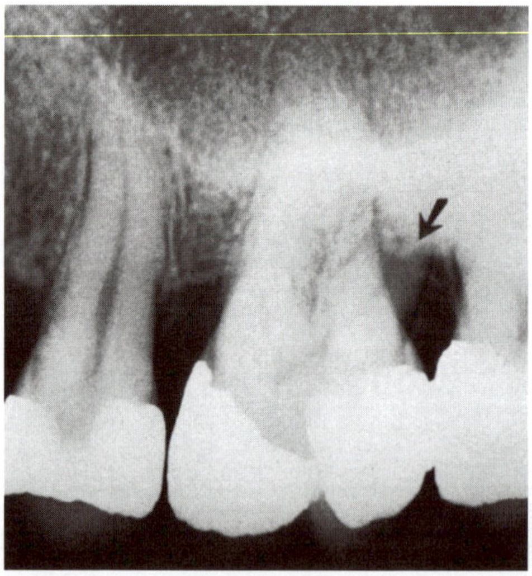

Fig. 25.26 Furcation involvement of the first molar partially obscured by the radiopaque lingual root. The horizontal line across the distobuccal root demarcates the apical portion *(arrow)*, which is covered by bone, from the remainder of the root, where the bone has been destroyed.

Therefore, radiographs alone cannot provide a final diagnosis of a periodontal abscess but need to be accompanied by careful clinical examination.

Clinical Probing

Regenerative and resective flap designs and incisions require prior knowledge of the underlying osseous topography. Careful probing of these pocket areas ("bone sounding") after scaling and root instrumentation often requires local anesthesia and definitive radiographic evaluation of the osseous lesions. Radiographs taken with periodontal probes, gutta-percha points, or other indicators (e.g., Hirschfeld pointers) placed into the anesthetized pocket show the true extent of the bone lesion. As indicated previously, the attachment level on the radicular surface or interdental lesions with thick facial or lingual bone cannot be visualized in the radiograph. The use of radiopaque indicators is an efficient and necessary diagnostic aid (Fig. 25.31).

Localized Aggressive Periodontitis

Prior classifications of periodontal disease considered "aggressive periodontitis" as a separate entity distinct from other forms of periodontal inflammation. However, the distinction between these two entities has not been consistently applied. Currently, there is no evidence that these disease patterns are due to distinct pathophysiologic pathways, and the evidence to consider them as separate diseases is inconsistent. In the 2018 disease classification, in addition to localized and generalized extent categories, "molar-incisor pattern" was added, which is now used to describe the previous disease category "localized aggressive periodontitis." As the name suggests, in this condition, the radiographic bone loss (mostly vertical) typically occurs in younger individuals and is restricted primarily to first molars and incisors.

Trauma From Occlusion

Trauma from occlusion can produce radiographically detectable changes in the thickness of the lamina dura, morphology of the alveolar crest, width of the PDL space, and density of the surrounding cancellous bone.

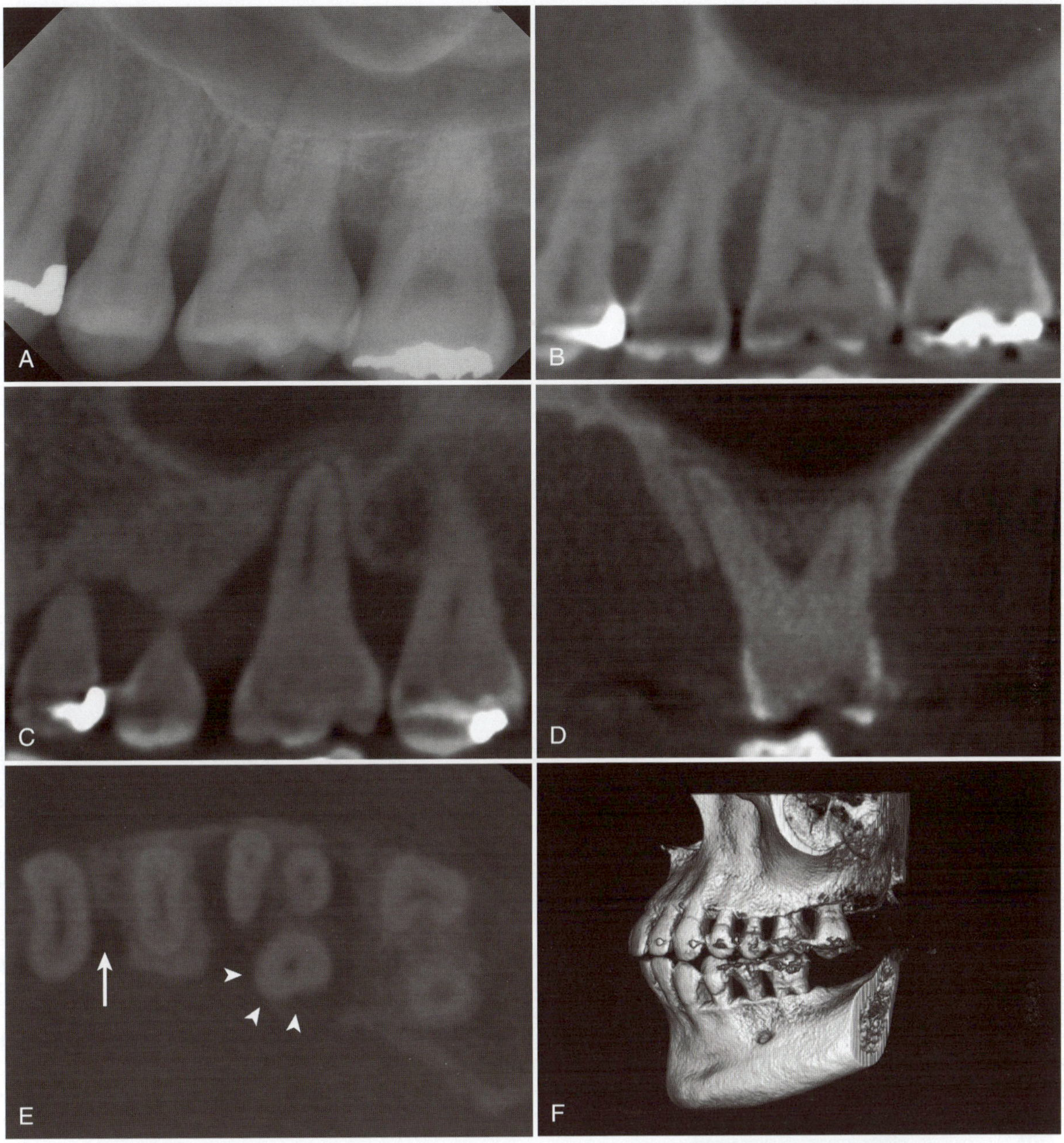

Fig. 25.27 A, Periapical radiograph showing a vertical defect on the mesial and distal aspects of the maxillary first molar. The palatal root is superimposed over the furcation. B, Sagittal section through the maxillary first molar buccal roots. Note clear depiction of extent of bone loss along the root length. C, Sagittal section through the palatal root. Note that bone loss along this root is underestimated on the periapical radiograph. D, Coronal section through the furcation of the maxillary first molar. Note bone loss between the palatal and mesiobuccal root that is not evident of the periapical radiograph in panel A. E, Axial section at a level immediately apical to the furcation. Note bone loss along the mesiobuccal root extending to cause palatal dehiscence and merging with the circumferential bone loss around the palatal root *(arrow heads)*. Note palatal bone loss between the premolars *(arrows)* that is obscured on the periapical radiograph in panel A by the remnant interdental bone. F, Volume-rendered cone-beam computed tomography (CBCT) image.

Traumatic lesions manifest more clearly in faciolingual aspects because mesiodistally, the tooth has added stability provided by the contact areas with adjacent teeth. Therefore, slight variations in the proximal surfaces may indicate greater changes in the facial and lingual aspects. *The radiographic changes listed next are not pathognomonic for trauma from occlusion and must be interpreted in combination with clinical findings*, particularly tooth mobility, presence of wear facets, pocket depth, and analysis of occlusal contacts and habits.

The *injury phase* of trauma from occlusion produces a loss of the lamina dura that may be noted in apices, furcations, and marginal areas. This loss of lamina dura results in widening of the PDL space (Fig. 25.32). The *repair phase* of trauma from occlusion results in an attempt to strengthen the periodontal structures to better support the increased loads. Radiographically, this is manifested by a widening of the PDL space, which may be generalized or localized.

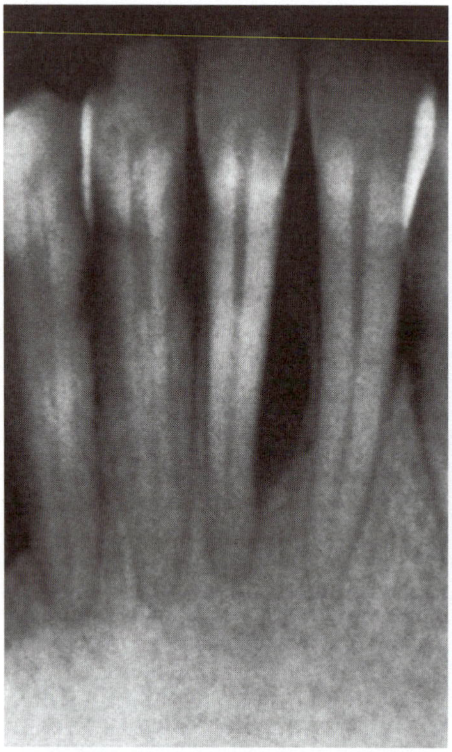

Fig. 25.28 Radiolucent area on lateral aspect of root with chronic periodontal abscess.

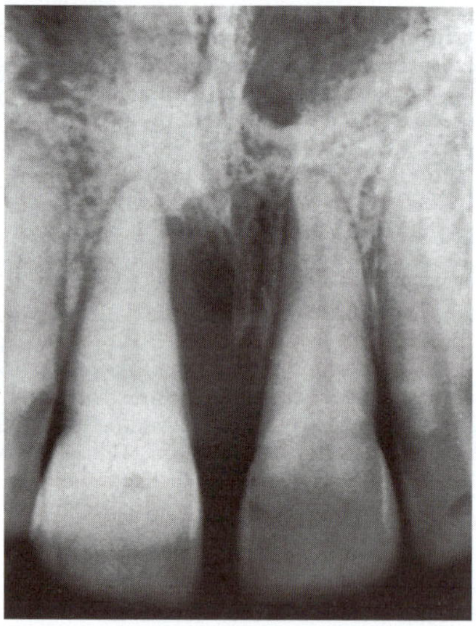

Fig. 25.29 Typical radiographic appearance of periodontal abscess on right central incisor.

Although microscopic measurements have determined normal variations in the PDL space width along the root surface, these are generally not detected radiographically. Thus, when seen on radiographs, variations in PDL space width suggest that the tooth is being subjected to increased forces. Successful attempts to reinforce the periodontal structures by widening the PDL space can be accompanied by increased width of the lamina dura and sometimes by condensation of the perialveolar cancellous bone.

More advanced traumatic lesions may result in deep angular bone loss, which, when combined with marginal inflammation, may lead to intrabony pocket formation. In terminal stages, these lesions extend around the root apex, producing a wide, radiolucent periapical image (cavernous lesions).

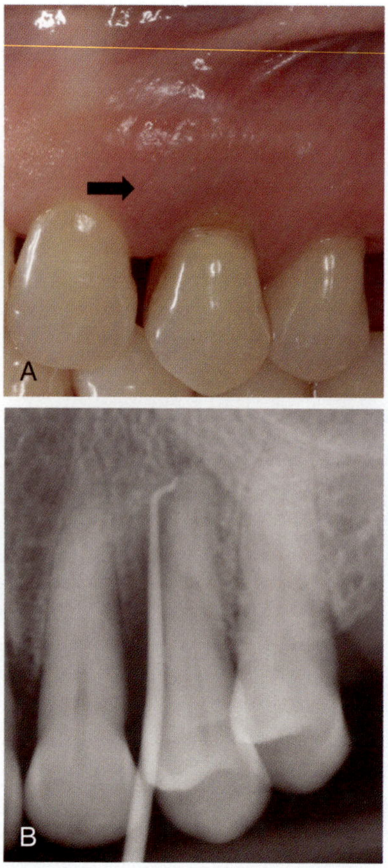

Fig. 25.30 Chronic periodontal abscess. A, Periodontal abscess in the left maxillary first premolar area. B, Extensive bone destruction on the mesial surface of the first premolar. Gutta-percha point traces to the root apex.

Root resorption may also result from excessive forces on the periodontium, particularly those caused by orthodontic appliances. Although trauma from occlusion produces many areas of root resorption, these areas are usually of a magnitude insufficient to be detected radiographically.

Conclusion

Intraoral radiographic examination with periapical and bite-wing radiographs should supplement a thorough history and clinical evaluation of manifestations of gingival and periodontal inflammation, including a detailed recording of probing depths and clinical attachment loss. Radiographic evaluation should be updated based on clinical need. Periapical radiographs often underestimate the amount of periodontal bone loss, and early periodontal disease is usually not apparent on radiographs. Significant interdental bone loss can occur and on periapical radiographs may be masked by the radiodensity of the intact buccal and lingual or palatal bone plates. Despite these limitations, intraoral radiographs taken with a reproducible technique provide adequate information to diagnose and treat periodontal disease and periodically monitor outcomes. Three-dimensional imaging with CBCT provides additional value in select cases, either by providing better diagnostic accuracy or by providing morphological information of relevance to treatment planning.

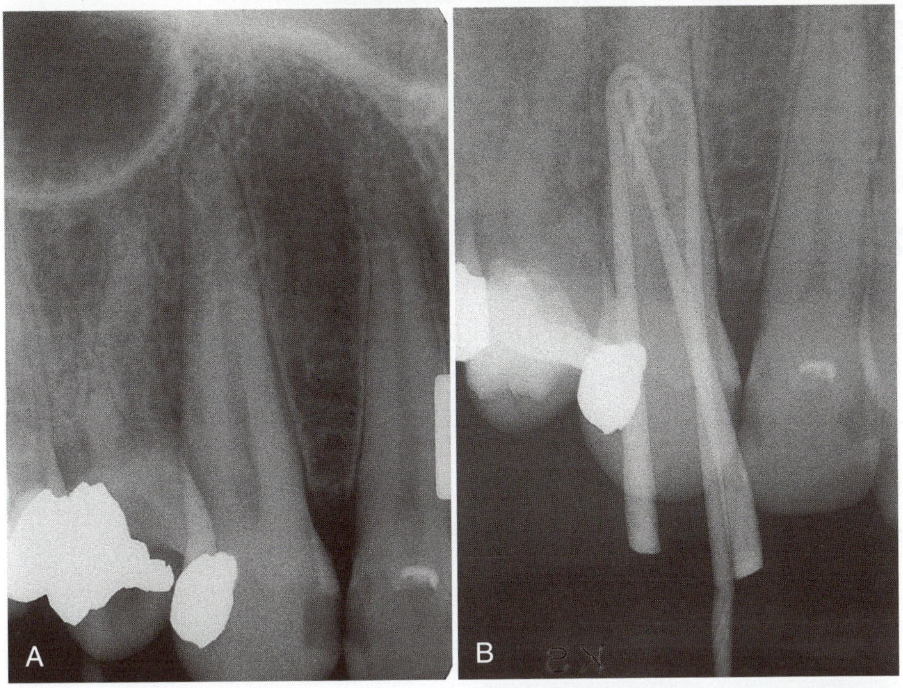

Fig. 25.31 A, Radiograph of maxillary cuspid. This view does not show facial bone loss. B, Radiograph of same maxillary cuspid as in part A, with gutta-percha points placed in the facial pocket to indicate bone loss.

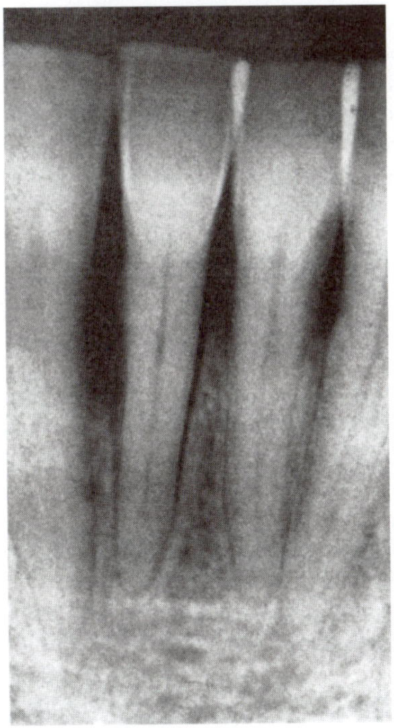

Fig. 25.32 Widened periodontal space caused by trauma from occlusion. Note the increased density of the surrounding bone caused by new bone formation in response to increased occlusal forces.

Key points

- Accurate radiographs are valuable in the diagnosis of periodontal disease and to formulate treatment. They are adjuncts to some clinical examination, not a substitute to it.
- Conventional radiographs are helpful to evaluate the height and form of interdental bone, width of PDL, continuity of lamina dura, trabecular pattern of bone, root resorption, caries and periapical pathology, etc. However they may not depict bony changes in the facial and lingual surfaces such as fenestration and dehiscences, early stages of furcation involvement, osseous defects like craters. Moreover they do not inform about current disease activity.
- Advanced imaging techniques such as digital radiography and CBCT provide more accurate details.

SUGGESTED READINGS

Lang NP, Hill RW. Radiographs in periodonties. Journal of clinical periodontology. 1977;4(1):16–28.

Brägger I. Radiographic diagnosis of periodontal disease progression. Current Opinion in Periodontology. 1996;3:59–67.

Corbet EF, Ho DK, Lai SM. Radiographs in periodontal disease diagnosis and management. Aust Dent J. 2009;54 Suppl 1:S27–S43.

CHAPTER 26

Clinical Risk Assessment

JM White | S Elangovan | C-T Lee | CD Dwarakanath

CHAPTER OUTLINE

Definitions

Risk assessment is defined by numerous components. Disease risk is the probability that an individual will develop a specific disease in a given period. The risk of developing the disease will vary from individual to individual.

Risk factors may be environmental, behavioral, or biologic factors that, when present, increase the likelihood that an individual will develop the disease. Risk factors are identified through longitudinal studies of patients with the disease of interest. Exposure to a risk factor or factors may occur at a single point in time, over multiple separate points in time, or continuously. However, to be identified as a risk factor, the exposure must occur before disease onset. Interventions often can be identified and, when implemented, can help modify risk factors.

The term *risk determinant/background characteristic*, which is sometimes substituted for the term *risk factor*, should be reserved only for factors that cannot be modified. *Risk indicators* are *probable* or *putative* risk factors that have been identified in cross-sectional studies but not confirmed through longitudinal studies. *Risk predictors/markers*, although associated with increased risk for disease, do not cause the disease. These factors also are identified in cross-sectional and longitudinal studies. Box 26.1 lists elements of these categories of risk for periodontal disease.

Clinical Correlation

Lack of bleeding on probing does appear to serve as an excellent indicator of periodontal health, but the presence of bleeding on probing alone is not a good predictor of future attachment loss.

Risk Factors for Periodontal Disease

Tobacco Smoking

Tobacco smoking is a well-established risk factor for **periodontitis**. A direct relationship exists between smoking and the **prevalence** of periodontal disease. This association is independent of other factors such as oral hygiene or age. Studies comparing the response to periodontal therapy in smokers, previous smokers, and nonsmokers have shown that smoking has a negative impact on the response to therapy. However, former smokers respond similarly to nonsmokers. These studies demonstrate the therapeutic impact of smoking cessation on patients who smoke

Diabetes

Diabetes is a clear risk factor for periodontitis. Epidemiologic data demonstrate that the prevalence and severity of periodontitis are significantly higher in patients with type 1 or type 2 diabetes mellitus than in those without diabetes and that the level of diabetic control is an important variable in this relationship.

Pathogenic Bacteria and Biofilm Deposit

It is well documented that the accumulation of bacterial **plaque** at the gingival margin results in the development of gingivitis and that the gingivitis can be reversed with the implementation of oral hygiene measures. These studies demonstrate a causal relationship between the accumulation of bacterial plaque and gingival inflammation. However, a causal relationship between *plaque accumulation* and *periodontitis* has been more difficult to establish. We come across clinical scenarios in which patients with severe loss of attachment have minimal levels of bacterial plaque on the affected teeth, indicating that the *quantity* of plaque is not of major importance in the disease process. However, although quantity may not indicate risk, there is evidence that the composition, or *quality*, of the complex plaque biofilm is important.

In terms of the quality of plaque, three specific bacteria have been identified as etiologic agents for periodontitis: *Aggregatibacter actinomycetemcomitans* (formerly *Actinobacillus actinomycetemcomitans*), *Porphyromonas gingivalis*, and *Tannerella forsythia* (formerly *Bacteroides forsythus*). To be considered periodontal **pathogens**, these bacteria have to fulfill a set of criteria (in relation to the disease in question): association, elimination, host response, **virulence** factor, animal studies, and risk assessment. *P. gingivalis* and *T. forsythia* are often found in periodontitis, whereas *A. actinomycetemcomitans* is often associated with aggressive periodontitis (a separate disease category in the previous disease classification to group periodontitis patients with rapid progression pattern occurring in relatively younger patients). Additional evidence that these organisms are causal agents includes the following:

1. Their elimination or suppression impacts the success of periodontal therapy (elimination).

BOX 26.1 Categories of Risk Elements for Periodontal Disease

Risk Factors
Tobacco smoking
Diabetes
Pathogenic bacteria in dental biofilm deposit

Risk Determinants/Background Characteristics
Genetic factors
Age
Gender
Socioeconomic status
Stress

Risk Indicators
Human immunodeficiency virus (HIV)/acquired immunodeficiency syndrome (AIDS)
Osteoporosis
Infrequent dental visits

Risk Markers/Predictors
Previous history of periodontal disease
Bleeding on probing

2. There is elevated antibody in serum, **saliva**, or in periodontal tissue to these pathogens (host response).
3. Virulence factors (e.g., leukotoxin, endotoxin) are associated with these pathogens (virulence factor).
4. Inoculation of these bacteria into animal models induces periodontal disease (animal studies).
5. Cross-sectional and longitudinal studies support the delineation of these three bacteria as risk factors for periodontal disease (risk assessment).

Although not completely supported by these criteria for causation, moderate evidence also suggests that *Campylobacter rectus, Eubacterium nodatum, Fusobacterium nucleatum, Prevotella intermedia, Prevotella nigrescens, Peptostreptococcus micros, Streptococcus intermedius,* and *Treponema denticola* are etiologic factors in periodontitis.

It is becoming clear from recent investigations that the plaque composition shifts from a more symbiotic **microbial** community to one that is more dysbiotic (an imbalance in the relative abundance of microbes leading to disease), composed primarily of anaerobes, as we go from periodontal health to periodontal disease. Certain pathogens (termed *keystone pathogens*) such as *P. gingivalis* play a major role in inducing such a shift, converting commensals into disease-provoking microbes (termed *pathobionts*). Therefore, the quantity of plaque present may not be as important as the quality of the plaque in determining the risk for periodontitis.

Anatomic factors, such as furcations, root concavities, developmental grooves, cervical enamel projections, enamel pearls, and bifurcation ridges, may predispose the **periodontium** to disease as a result of their potential to harbor bacterial plaque and present a challenge to the clinician during instrumentation. Similarly, the presence of **subgingival** and overhanging margins in restorations can result in increased plaque accumulation, increased inflammation, and increased bone loss. Although not clearly defined as risk factors for periodontitis, anatomic factors and restorative factors that influence plaque accumulation may play a role in disease susceptibility for specific teeth.

The presence of calculus, which serves as a reservoir of bacterial plaque, has been suggested as a risk factor for periodontitis. Although the presence of some calculus in healthy individuals receiving routine dental care does not result in a significant loss of attachment, the presence of calculus in other groups of patients, such as those not receiving regular care and those with poorly controlled diabetes, can have a negative impact on periodontal health.

Risk Determinants/Background Characteristics for Periodontal Disease

Genetic Factors

Evidence indicates that genetic differences between individuals may explain why some patients develop periodontal disease and others do not. Studies conducted on twins have shown that genetic factors influence clinical measures of gingivitis, probing **pocket** depth, attachment loss, and interproximal bone height. The familial aggregation seen in localized and generalized aggressive periodontitis (periodontitis with rapid progression in relatively younger patients) also indicates genetic involvement in these diseases.

Kornman and colleagues demonstrated that alterations (**polymorphisms**) in specific genes encoding inflammatory cytokines such as interleukin-1α (IL-1α) and interleukin-1β (IL-1β) were associated with severe periodontitis in nonsmoking subjects. However, the results of other studies have shown a limited association between these altered genes and the presence of periodontitis. Overall, it appears that changes in the IL-1 genes may be only one of several genetic changes involved in the risk for periodontitis. Therefore, although an alteration in the IL-1 genes may be a valid marker for periodontitis in defined populations, its usefulness as a genetic marker in the general population may be limited.

Immunologic alterations, such as neutrophil abnormalities, monocytic hyperresponsiveness to lipopolysaccharide stimulation in patients with a molar-incisor pattern of periodontitis (formerly called localized aggressive periodontitis), and alterations in the **monocyte**/macrophage **receptors** for the Fc portion of an antibody, also appear to be under genetic control. In addition, genetics plays a role in regulating the titer of the protective immunoglobulin G2 (IgG2) antibody response to *A. actinomycetemcomitans* in patients with aggressive periodontitis.

Age

Both the prevalence and severity of periodontal disease increase with age. It is possible that degenerative changes related to aging may increase susceptibility to periodontitis. However, it is also possible that the attachment loss and bone loss seen in older individuals are the result of prolonged exposure to other risk factors over a person's life, creating a cumulative effect over time. In support of this theory, studies have shown minimal loss of attachment in aging subjects enrolled in preventive programs throughout their lives. Therefore, it is suggested that periodontal disease is not an inevitable consequence of the aging process and that aging alone does not increase disease susceptibility. However, it remains to be determined whether changes related to the aging process, such as medication intake, decreased immune function, and altered nutritional status, interact with other well-defined risk factors to increase susceptibility to periodontitis.

Evidence of loss of attachment may have more consequences in younger patients. The younger the patient, the longer the time for continuous exposure to causative factors since the disease starts early. In addition, aggressive periodontitis (periodontitis with rapid progression in relatively younger patients) in young individuals is often associated with unmodifiable risk factors, such as a genetic predisposition to disease. Therefore, young individuals with periodontal disease may be at greater risk for continued disease as they age.

Gender

Gender plays a role in periodontal disease. Surveys conducted in the United States since 1960 demonstrate that men have more loss of attachment than women. In addition, men have poorer oral hygiene than women, as evidenced by higher levels of plaque and calculus. Therefore, gender differences in the prevalence and severity of periodontitis appear to be related to preventive practices rather than any genetic factor.

Socioeconomic Status

Gingivitis and poor oral hygiene can be related to lower socioeconomic status (SES). This most likely can be attributed to decreased dental awareness and decreased frequency of dental visits compared to more educated individuals with higher SES. Emerging evidence suggests low education attainment to be an important factor associated with periodontitis.

Stress

The incidence of **necrotizing ulcerative gingivitis** increases during periods of emotional and physiologic stress, suggesting a link between the two. Emotional stress may interfere with normal immune function and may result in increased levels of circulating hormones, which can affect the periodontium. Specifically, it is known that stress deregulates the immune system via the hypothalamic-pituitary-adrenal cortex axis or via the sympathetic-adrenal medullary axis. The resulting increase in cortisol and epinephrine/norepinephrine, respectively, are shown to cause hyperglycemia, affect the immune system, and also affect the wound healing process.

Stressful life events, such as bereavement and divorce, appear to lead to a greater prevalence of periodontal disease, and an apparent association exists between psychosocial factors and risk behaviors such as smoking, poor oral hygiene, and periodontitis. Adult patients with periodontitis who are resistant to therapy are more stressed than those who respond to therapy. Individuals with financial strain, distress, depression, or inadequate coping mechanisms have a more severe loss of attachment. Although epidemiologic data on the relationship between stress and periodontal disease are limited, stress can be a putative risk factor for periodontitis. Stress is listed as a risk determinant, but it is important to know that unlike other risk determinants listed above, it can be alleviated and hence its negative effect on periodontium can be minimized or negated.

Clinical Correlation

The ultimate goal of performing a periodontal risk assessment is to develop a more personalized treatment plan for a specific patient, taking into account the periodontal risk profile of that patient. Once an at-risk patient is identified and a diagnosis is made, the treatment plan may be modified accordingly.

Risk Indicators for Periodontal Disease

Human Immunodeficiency Virus/Acquired Immunodeficiency Syndrome

It has been hypothesized that the immune dysfunction associated with human immunodeficiency **virus** (HIV) infection and acquired immunodeficiency syndrome (AIDS) increases susceptibility to periodontal disease. Early reports on the periodontal status of patients with AIDS or those who are HIV seropositive revealed that these patients often had severe periodontal destruction characteristic of **necrotizing periodontitis**. More recent reports, however, have failed to demonstrate significant differences in the periodontal status of individuals with HIV infection and healthy controls. The apparent discrepancy in these reports may have been caused by the inclusion of patients with AIDS (vs patients who were exclusively HIV seropositive) in some studies.

Conflicting results also exist in studies examining the level of immunosuppression and severity of periodontal destruction. Some studies support the observation that as the degree of immunosuppression increases in adults with AIDS, **periodontal pocket** formation and loss of clinical attachment also increase. Results of other studies have found no relationship between periodontal diseases and HIV/AIDS status. Evidence also suggests that AIDS-affected individuals who practice good preventive oral health measures, including effective home care and seeking appropriate professional therapy, can maintain periodontal health. Therefore, although it seems reasonable to hypothesize that HIV infection and immunosuppression are risk factors for periodontal disease, the evidence is not conclusive.

Osteoporosis

Osteoporosis has been suggested as another risk factor for periodontitis. Although studies in animal models indicate that osteoporosis does not initiate periodontitis, evidence indicates that the reduced bone mass seen in osteoporosis may aggravate periodontal disease progression. However, reports on humans are conflicting. In a study of 12 women with osteoporosis and 14 healthy women, von Wowern and coworkers reported that the women with osteoporosis had greater loss of attachment than the control subjects. In contrast, Kribbs examined pocket depth, bleeding on probing, and gingival recession in women with and without osteoporosis. Although the two groups had significant differences in bone mass, no differences in periodontal status were noted. However, it appears that a link may exist between osteoporosis and periodontitis, and additional studies may need to be conducted to determine whether osteoporosis is a true risk factor for periodontal disease.

Infrequent Dental Visits

Identifying failure to visit the dentist regularly as a risk factor for periodontitis is controversial. One study demonstrated an increased risk for severe periodontitis in patients who had not visited the dentist for 3 or more years, whereas another demonstrated that there was no more loss of attachment or bone loss in individuals who did not seek dental care compared to those who did over a 6-year period. However, differences in the ages of the subjects in these two studies may explain the different results. Additional longitudinal and intervention studies are necessary to determine whether the infrequency of dental visits is a risk factor for periodontal disease.

Risk Markers/Predictors for Periodontal Disease

Previous History of Periodontal Disease

A history of previous periodontal disease is a good clinical predictor of risk for future disease progression. Patients with the most severe existing loss of attachment are at the greatest risk for future loss of attachment. Conversely, patients currently free of periodontitis have a decreased risk of developing loss of attachment compared to those who currently have periodontitis.

Bleeding on Probing

Bleeding on probing is the best clinical indicator of gingival inflammation. Although this indicator alone does not serve as a predictor for loss of attachment, bleeding on probing coupled with increasing pocket depth may serve as an excellent predictor for future loss of attachment. Lack of bleeding on probing does appear to serve as an excellent indicator of periodontal health.

Clinical Risk Assessment for Periodontal Disease

Information concerning individual risk for developing periodontal disease is obtained through careful evaluation of the patient's demographic data, medical history, dental history, and clinical examination.

The elements that contribute to increased risk can be identified through the collection of demographic data, including the patient's age, gender, and SES. The medical history may reveal elements such as a history of diabetes, smoking, HIV/AIDS, or osteoporosis, as well as a perceived level of stress. The dental history can reveal a family history of early tooth loss (suggestive of a genetic predisposition to an aggressive form of periodontitis), a previous history of periodontal disease, and information concerning the frequency of oral health care in the past. Important elements identified during the clinical examination can include the location and extent of bacterial plaque accumulation, presence of plaque-retentive factors (e.g., overhanging restorations, subgingival margins), presence of anatomic plaque-retentive areas (e.g., grooves, furcation involvement), presence of calculus, the extent of attachment loss, and presence or absence of bleeding on probing.

- Demographic Data
  - Age
  - Duration of exposure to risk elements
  - Postmenopausal
  - Male sex
  - Socioeconomic status
  - Education attainment
- Medical and Behavioral History
  - Preventive practices (regular medical exams)
  - Diabetes
  - Tobacco smoking
  - Human immunodeficiency virus (HIV)/acquired immunodeficiency syndrome (AIDS)
  - Osteoporosis
  - Stress
  - Genetic disorders and other systemic conditions that influence the pathogenesis of periodontal diseases
  - Dental History
  - Dental awareness
  - Family history of early tooth loss
  - Previous history of periodontal disease
  - Evidence of aggressive destruction of periodontal tissues
  - Frequency of personal and professional oral care
  - History and compliance with past dental visits
  - Clinical examination
  - Plaque accumulation
  - Microbial sampling for putative periodontal pathogens
  - Calculus deposition
  - Bleeding on probing
  - Extent and severity (stage of disease) of loss of attachment and alveolar bone
  - Rate of disease progression (grade of disease)
  - Tooth examination
  - Plaque retentive areas
  - Anatomic factors
  - Restorative factors

Once the social, demographic, medical history, dental history, and clinical presentation data are collected, they must be analyzed to identify whether the patient is at risk for developing **periodontal disease** or for periodontal disease progression. Over the years, several periodontal risk assessment systems were developed in order to stratify patients based on the risk for disease progression (attachment loss) or tooth loss. Periodontal risk assessment (PRA) and periodontal risk calculator (PRC) are the more frequently used and validated ones, compared to others. PRA is a multifactorial risk assessment tool used to evaluate the risk for recurrence or progression of periodontitis in patients who are in **supportive periodontal therapy** (SPT). PRA has six clinical parameters: (1) full-mouth bleeding on probing percentage, (2) the number of sites with **probing depth** of ≥5 mm, (3) the number of teeth lost (wisdom teeth are excluded), (4) the percentage of loss of periodontal support (bone) in the worst posterior sites in relation to patient's age (bone loss (%)/age), (5) systemic and/or genetic conditions, and (6) environmental factors (e.g., smoking status). The result of each clinical parameter can be categorized into low, moderate, or high-risk levels. Then the SPT patients can be assigned to one of the three risk profiles: low, moderate, or high, based on the risk level of each of the above-mentioned parameters. In spite of being in SPT, patients with a high-risk profile were shown to experience higher periodontitis recurrence and tooth loss than patients with a low-risk profile.

PRC is a computer-based risk assessment tool designed to assess the risk of developing periodontitis in those patients who do not have the disease and to assess the risk for disease progression in periodontitis patients. The calculation of risk is a multistep process involving mathematical algorithms that use nine risk factors: age, smoking history, diabetes, history of periodontal surgery, pocket depth, furcation involvements, restorations or calculus below the gingival margin, radiographic bone height, and vertical bone defects. Information from baseline examination can be analyzed by the risk calculator, and a risk score on a scale of 1–5 for periodontal deterioration will be calculated for each patient. The risk score was shown to have a direct correlation with tooth loss in nonperiodontitis and periodontitis patients. This tool can provide a more objective, quantitative way to assess risk for periodontitis than clinical opinion.

Once an at-risk patient is identified and a diagnosis is made, the treatment plan may be modified accordingly. For example, patients with a history of cigarette smoking should be informed of the relationship between smoking and periodontitis. They should also be informed of the impact of smoking on their prognosis and the likelihood of success of periodontal therapy if they continue to smoke. Part of their recommended treatment plan for initial therapy may include referral to a smoking cessation program or the use of self-administered smoking cessation aids. As another example, a patient diagnosed with severe periodontitis may be encouraged to be examined and tested for systemic disorders, such as diabetes. If the diagnosis is confirmed, control of the systemic disorder is important for periodontal health, and periodontal treatment may involve the administration of systemic antimicrobial or other adjunctive agents. Previously identified risk elements may also need to be reassessed at the re-evaluation stage of treatment. This is especially important for patients who do not respond favorably to periodontal therapy.

Electronic Health Records and Periodontal Risk Assessment

Periodontal disease risk assessments and calculations are paper-based, available on the Internet (https://www.perio-tools.com/), commercially available cloud-based (https://www.previser.com/), or integrated within the electronic health record (EHR). Risk assessments and calculations provide useful clinic decision support for the provider and the patient. The challenge in clinic decision support is providing the right information, to the right person, in the right intervention format, through the right channel at the right time in the workflow. Although all methods—paper, Internet, cloud-based, and within the EHR—provide a risk assessment, risk assessments within the EHR are well accepted and preferred.

Risk assessment integrated within the EHR draws on data and condenses it into a useable format providing clinic decision support for the provider. This information in its simplest form summarizes data within the EHR, such as providing a summary of periodontal clinical findings. More complex clinic decision support can utilize the data within the EHR to provide a calculated periodontal risk assessment and calculate a periodontal diagnosis. Within the EHR assessment, management and re-evaluation are all captured and depicts a model periodontal assessment including information that summarizes a number of factors which includes most recent periodontal charting, most recent radiographs, number of natural teeth, number of teeth lost to periodontal disease, risk assessment factors (smoking status, diabetes/HbA1c, plaque index), pocket depth distribution, clinical attachment level distribution, bleeding on probing, most severe bone loss percent, and **subgingival calculus**. The assessment summary calculates a periodontal risk score that is determined by an algorithm. The provider uses this information and then selects a periodontal risk assessment. The assessment form also provides clinic decision support and suggests a periodontal diagnosis that the provider then selects. It depicts the periodontal management plan selected by the provider, including the treatment procedures, general prevention therapy, and expected outcomes.

Risk assessment enabled by clinic decision support is likely to expand in dentistry as machine learning and artificial intelligence are developed and applied to **periodontology**. As this technology expands, it will need to be fully validated for clinical use in periodontology. We envision artificial intelligence to be used in many aspects of dentistry and it is likely to be integrated within the EHR providing clinical decision support for providers.

Conclusion

Risk assessment involves identifying elements that either may predispose patients to develop periodontal disease or may influence the progression of disease that already exists. In either case, these patients may require modification of their prognosis and treatment plan. In addition to an evaluation of the factors contributing to their risk, these patients should be educated concerning their risk, and, when appropriate, suitable intervention strategies should be implemented.

Key points

- Risk factors are those, when present increase the chances of development of a disease. They are not etiological factors. They can be environmental, behavioral or biologic factors. Some of them are modifiable whereas others such as genetic factors cannot be modified. Such unmodifiable factors are called risk determinants.
- Risk assessment should not be confused with determining the prognosis. The latter is determined when disease is already present and its response to therapy needs to be evaluated.
- Common risk factors of periodontal disease include tobacco smoking, diabetes mellitus, and presence of pathogenic bacteria. These can be controlled. Whereas other factors such as genetic, age, and gender cannot be controlled.
- A computer-based risk assessment tool called the periodontal assessment tool (PAT) which utilizes input from 23 items helps in quantification of the current disease and a risk score for the future.

Suggested Reading

Lang NP, Tonetti MS. Periodontal risk assessment (PRA) for patients in supportive periodontal therapy (SPT). Oral Health Prev Dent. 2003;1(1):7–16.

Philstrom BL. Periodontal risk assessment, diagnosis and treatment planning. Periodontology 2000. 2001;25:37–58.

CHAPTER 27

Determination of Prognosis

C-T Lee | JH Do | HH Takei | KF Novak | S Elangovan | CD Dwarakanath

CHAPTER OUTLINE

Prognosis is a forecast. It is a prediction of the probable course, duration, and outcome of a disease and the likelihood of its response to treatment, based on a general knowledge of the pathogenesis of the disease and the presence of risk factors. It is established after the diagnosis is made and before the treatment plan is established. The prognosis is based on specific information about the disease and the manner in which it can be treated, but it can also be influenced by the clinician's previous experience with treatment outcomes (successes and failures) as they relate to the particular case. It is important to note that determination of prognosis is a dynamic process. As such, the prognosis initially assigned should be reevaluated after completion of all phases of therapy, including periodontal maintenance.

Prognosis is often confused with the term risk. Risk generally deals with the likelihood that an individual will develop a disease in a specified period. *Risk factors* are those characteristics of an individual that put the person at increased risk for developing a disease. In contrast, *prognosis* is the prediction of the course or outcome of a disease. *Prognostic factors* are characteristics that predict the outcome of disease once the disease is present. In some cases, risk factors and prognostic factors are the same. For example, patients with diabetes or patients who smoke are more at risk for acquiring periodontal disease, and once they have it, they generally have a worse prognosis.

Determination of prognosis is mostly based upon the past events and may not depict accurately what is going to happen in the future as the actual outcome may vary. The reader can refer to excellent reports of McGuire and Nunn in their study "Prognosis versus Actual outcome."

For descriptive purposes and better understanding, prognosis is classified as follows:

1. *Overall prognosis*: which is concerned with the patient and dentition as a whole and determined by several factors including the type of disease, age of the patient, and systemic background.
2. *Individual tooth prognosis*: The *individual tooth prognosis* is determined after the overall prognosis and is affected by it. For example, in a patient with a poor overall prognosis, the dentist in all likelihood would not attempt to retain a tooth that has a questionable prognosis because of local conditions (see Box 27.1). Many of the factors listed under local, prosthetic, and restorative factors have a direct effect on the prognosis of individual teeth, in addition to any overall systemic or environmental factors that may be present.

Prognosis is also classified as:

1. *Therapeutic prognosis*: It deals with the response of the tissues to treatment and successful arrest of disease process.
2. *Prosthetic prognosis*: which indicates the ability of the remaining teeth to support a prosthesis.

Further, prognosis can be divided as:

1. *Short-term prognosis*: where estimation is made for the next 3–5 years.
2. *Long-term prognosis*: where the teeth are expected to remain in health and function beyond 5 years.

Types of Prognosis

Although some factors may be more important than others when assigning a prognosis, consideration of each factor may be beneficial to the clinician.

Historically, prognosis classification schemes have been designed based on studies evaluating tooth mortality. One scheme follows the below-mentioned classification:

Good prognosis: Control of etiologic factors and adequate periodontal support ensure the tooth will be easy to maintain by the patient and clinician.

Fair prognosis: Approximately 25% attachment loss and/or Class I furcation involvement (location and depth allow proper maintenance with good patient compliance).

Poor prognosis: 50% attachment loss, Class II furcation involvement (location and depth make maintenance possible but difficult).

Questionable prognosis: >50% attachment loss, poor crown-to-root ratio, poor root form, Class II furcations (location and depth make access difficult), or Class III furcation involvements; >2+ mobility; root proximity.

Hopeless prognosis: Inadequate attachment to maintain health, comfort, and function.

It should be recognized that good, fair, and hopeless prognoses in this classification system could be established with a reasonable degree of accuracy. However, poor and questionable prognoses are likely to change to other categories because they depend on a large number of factors that can interact in unpredictable number of ways.

BOX 27.1 Factors to Consider When Determining a Prognosis

Overall Clinical Factors
Patient age
Disease severity
Biofilm control
Patient compliance

Systemic and Environmental Factors
Smoking
Systemic disease or condition
Genetic factors
Stress

Local Factors
Biofilm and calculus
Anatomic factors
- Short, tapered roots
- Cervical enamel projections
- Enamel pearls
- Bifurcation ridges
- Root concavities
- Developmental grooves
- Root proximity
- Furcation invasion

Tooth mobility
Caries
Tooth vitality
Root resorption

Prosthetic and Restorative Factors
Subgingival restorations
Tooth-supported prosthesis
Abutment selection

In contrast to schemes based on tooth mortality, Kwok and Caton have proposed a scheme based on "the probability of obtaining stability of the periodontal supporting apparatus." This scheme is based on the probability of disease progression as related to local and systemic factors (see Box 27.1). Although some of these factors may affect disease progression more than others, consideration of each factor is important in assigning a prognosis. It is as follows:

Favorable prognosis: Comprehensive periodontal treatment and maintenance will stabilize the status of the tooth. Future loss of periodontal support is unlikely.

Questionable prognosis: Local and/or systemic factors influencing the periodontal status of the tooth may or may not be controllable. If controlled, the periodontal status can be stabilized with comprehensive periodontal treatment. If not, future periodontal breakdown may occur.

Unfavorable prognosis: Local and/or systemic factors influencing the periodontal status cannot be controlled. Comprehensive periodontal treatment and maintenance are unlikely to prevent future periodontal breakdown.

Hopeless prognosis: The tooth must be extracted.

Since periodontal stability is assessed on a regular basis using clinical measures, it may be more useful in making treatment decisions and prognosis predictions than trying to determine the likelihood of the tooth being lost.

In many of these cases, it may be advisable to establish a *provisional prognosis* until phase I therapy is completed and evaluated. The provisional prognosis allows the clinician to initiate treatment of teeth that have a doubtful outlook in the hope that a favorable response may tip the balance and allow the teeth to be retained. The reevaluation phase in the treatment sequence allows the clinician to examine the tissue response to scaling, oral hygiene, and root planing, as well as to the possible use of chemotherapeutic agents where indicated. The patient's compliance with the proposed treatment plan also can be determined.

Factors in Determination of Prognosis

Overall Clinical Factors

Patient Age

For two patients with comparable levels of remaining connective tissue attachment and alveolar bone, the prognosis is generally better for the older of the two. For the younger patient, the prognosis is not as good because of the shorter time frame in which the periodontal destruction has occurred; the younger patient may also have an aggressive pattern of disease progression because of systemic disease, smoking, or other factors. In addition, although the younger patient would ordinarily be expected to have a greater reparative capacity, the occurrence of so much destruction in a relatively short period would exceed any naturally occurring periodontal repair.

Disease Severity

Studies have demonstrated that a patient's history of previous periodontal disease may be indicative of their susceptibility to future periodontal breakdown. Therefore, the following variables should be carefully recorded because they are important in determining the patient's past history of periodontal disease: probing **pocket** depth, **clinical attachment level**, amount of bone loss, and type of bony defect. These factors are determined by clinical and radiographic evaluation.

Determining clinical attachment loss reveals the approximate extent of root surface that is devoid of periodontal ligament; the radiographic examination shows the amount of root surface still invested in bone. Probing pocket depth is less important than the level of attachment in determining the severity of tissue destruction because sometimes the pocket depth is not necessarily related to bone loss. In general, it is necessary to consider clinical attachment level, radiographic bone level, and probing pocket depth together to assess disease severity, which in turn affects prognosis. Lower attachment level, less remaining bone, and deeper pocket depth are associated with a worse prognosis.

Prognosis is adversely affected if the probing pocket depth is deep ($\geq$5 mm). Compared to a site with a shallower probing pocket depth, it will be challenging to remove biofilm and calculus from a deeper pocket site. When the base of the pocket (level of attachment) is too deep and close to the root apex, the presence of apical disease as a result of endodontic involvement also worsens the prognosis. However, surprisingly, optimal repair of the attachment apparatus can sometimes be achieved by combining endodontic and periodontal therapy.

The prognosis also can be related to the height of remaining bone. Assuming bone destruction can be arrested, is there enough bone remaining to support the teeth? The answer is readily apparent in extreme cases—that is, when there is so little bone loss that tooth support is not in jeopardy (Fig. 27.1) or when bone loss is so severe that the remaining bone is obviously insufficient for proper tooth support (Fig. 27.2). Most patients, however, do not fit into these extreme categories. The height of remaining bone is usually somewhere in between, making bone level assessment alone insufficient for determining the overall prognosis.

The type of defect also must be determined. The prognosis for **horizontal** bone loss depends on the height of the existing bone because it is unlikely that clinically significant bone height regeneration will be induced by therapy. In the case of **angular**, intrabony defects, if the contour of the existing bone and the number of osseous walls are favorable (e.g., a narrow three-wall defect), there is an excellent chance that therapy could regenerate bone to approximately the level of the existing alveolar crest. The extent of bone loss around a tooth will also affect the prognosis. For example, a tooth with a circumferential bone loss may have worse prognosis than a tooth with bone loss limited to a localized area.

When greater bone loss has occurred on one surface of a tooth, the bone height on the less involved surfaces should be taken into consideration when determining the prognosis. Because of the greater height of bone in relation to other surfaces, the center of rotation of the tooth will be nearer the crown (Fig. 27.3). This

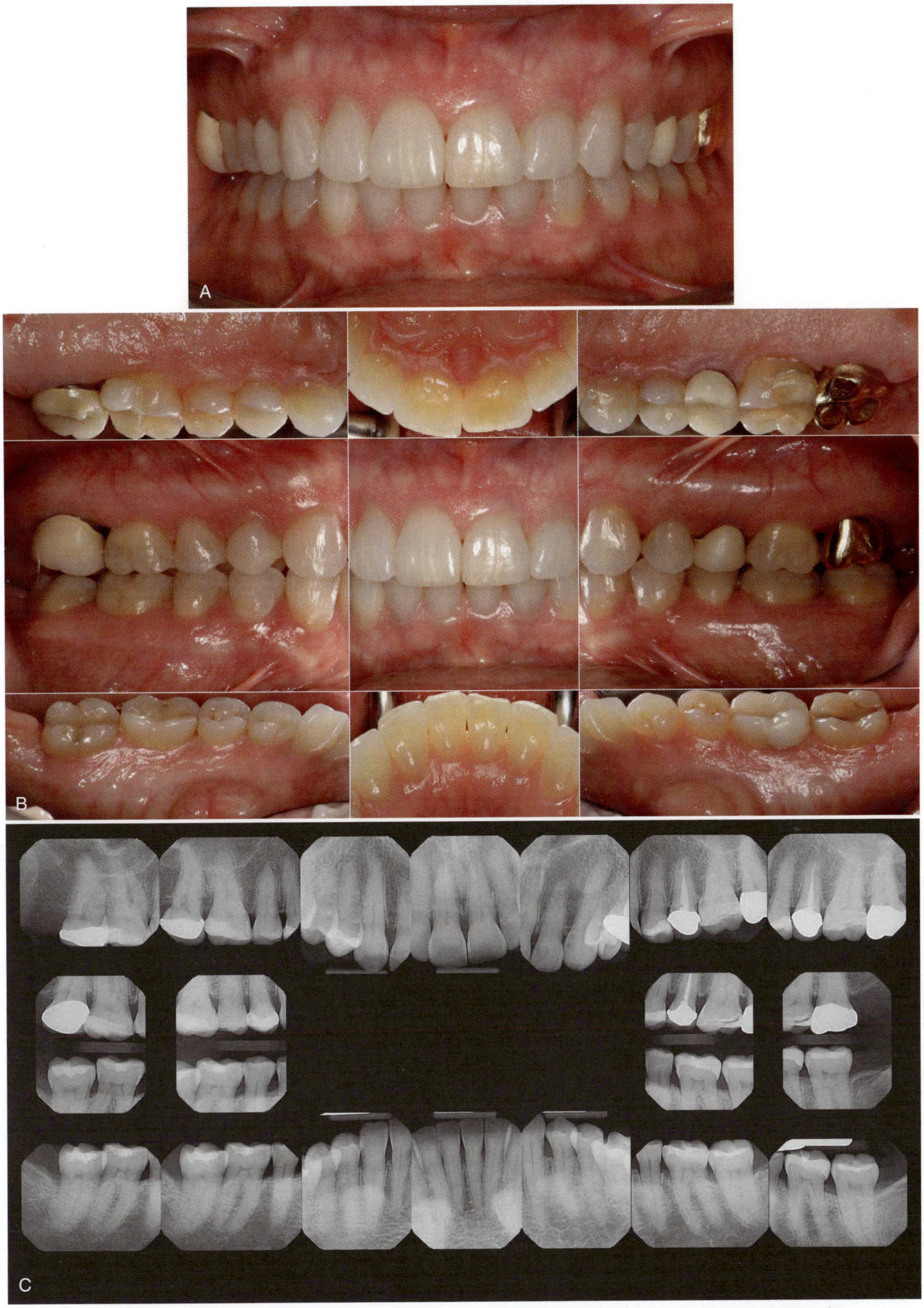

Fig. 27.1 Generalized stage I, grade B periodontitis in a healthy, nonsmoking 67-year-old female. Minimal clinical biofilm and gingival inflammation (A and B) and radiographic bone loss (C). Overall prognosis is favorable. *(Copyright Jonathan H. Do, DDS. All rights reserved.)*

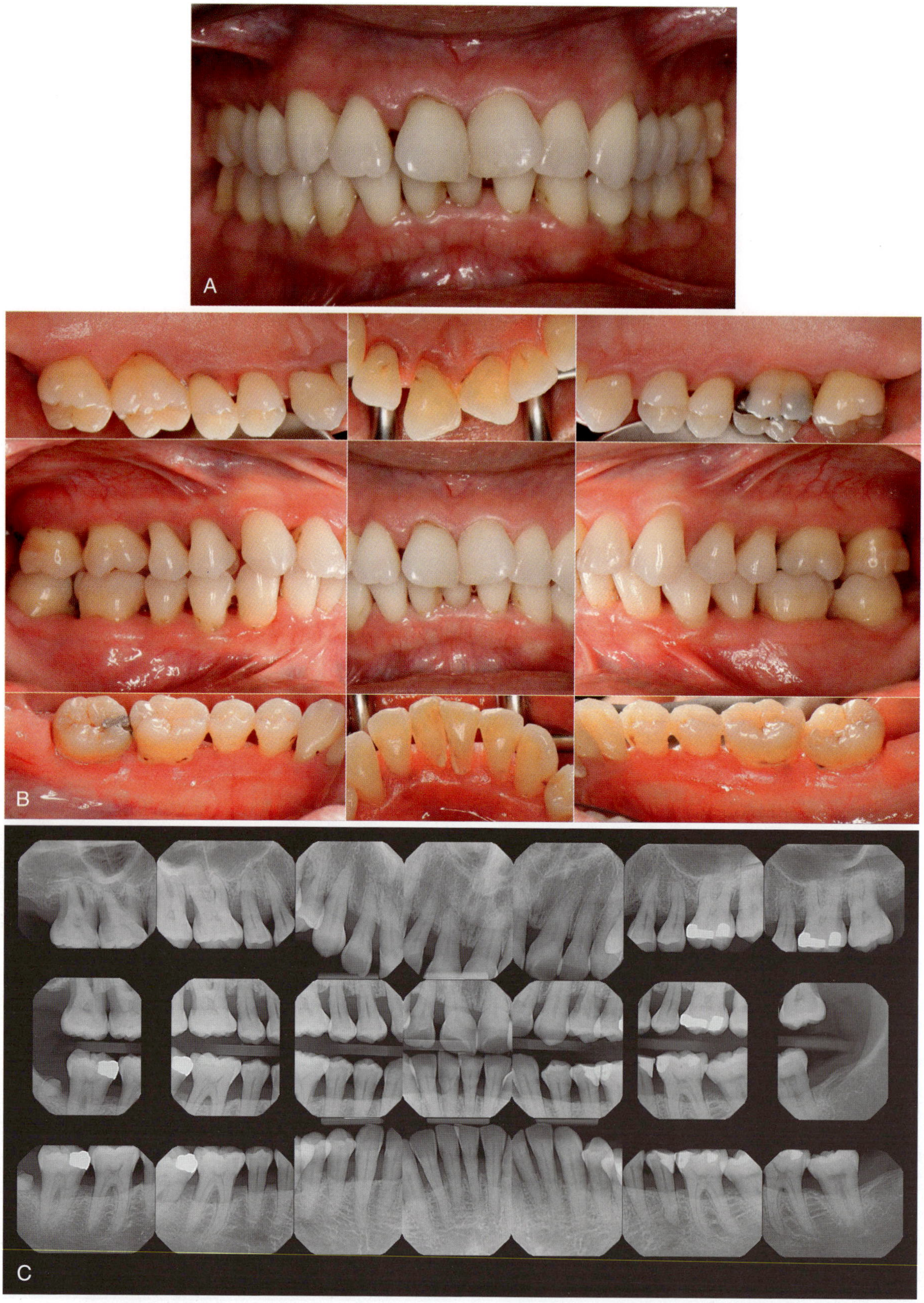

Fig. 27.2 Generalized, stage III, grade C periodontitis in a healthy, nonsmoking 49-year-old female. A and B, Moderate clinical biofilm, calculus, and gingival inflammation. C, Moderate to severe radiographic bone loss. Overall prognosis is questionable/unfavorable. *(Copyright Jonathan H. Do, DDS. All rights reserved.)*

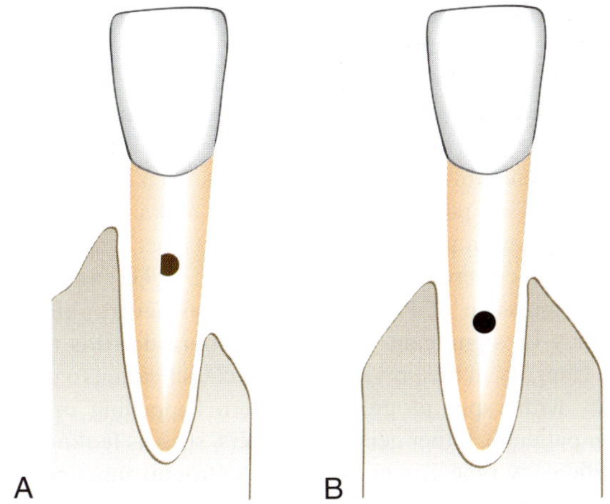

Fig. 27.3 Prognosis for tooth A is better than for tooth B, despite less bone on one of the surfaces of A. Because the center of rotation of tooth A is closer to the crown, the distribution of occlusal forces to the periodontium is more favorable than in B.

results in a more favorable distribution of forces to the **periodontium** and less tooth mobility.

In dealing with a tooth that has an unfavorable prognosis, the chances of successful treatment should be weighed against any benefits that would accrue to the adjacent teeth if the tooth under consideration was extracted. Strategic extraction of teeth was first proposed as a means of improving the overall prognosis of adjacent teeth or enhancing the prosthetic treatment plan. It has now been expanded to include the extraction of teeth with an unfavorable prognosis to enhance the likelihood of partial restoration of the bone support of the adjacent teeth (Fig. 27.4A–D) or **successful implant** placement. With the growing evidence of the long-term success of dental implants, it is proposed that a "watch and wait" approach may allow an area to deteriorate to the point that placing an implant is no longer a viable option. This means that the practitioner should carefully weigh the potential success of one treatment option (extraction and implant placement) versus the other (periodontal therapy and maintenance) when dealing with a tooth with unfavorable prognosis. Having said that, a patient's needs and expectations should be taken into account prior to performing any irreversible treatment such as tooth extraction.

Biofilm Control

Bacterial biofilm is the primary etiologic factor associated with periodontal disease. Therefore, effective removal of biofilm on a daily basis by the patient is critical to the success of periodontal therapy and the overall prognosis.

Patient Compliance

The prognosis for patients with **gingival** and periodontal disease is critically dependent on the patient's attitude, desire to retain the natural teeth, and willingness and ability to effectively control biofilm. Without these, treatment cannot succeed. Patients should be educated on the etiology and prevention of dental **caries** and periodontal diseases, and they should be clearly informed of the important role they must play for treatment to succeed. Additionally, it is well known that patients' noncompliance with supportive periodontal therapy (periodontal maintenance) is significantly associated with periodontal disease progression and tooth loss. Maintaining good oral hygiene and being compliant with the recommended professional periodontal maintenance visits are critical

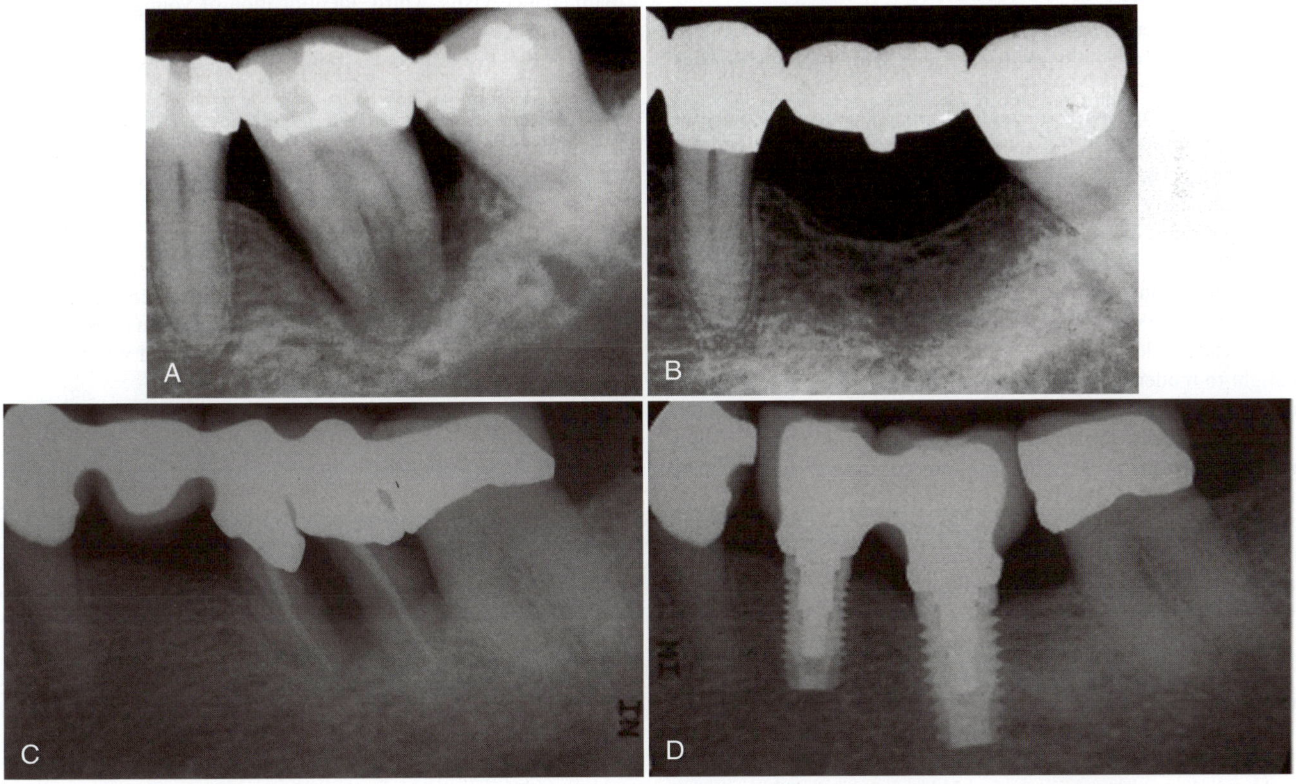

Fig. 27.4 Extraction of severely involved tooth to preserve bone on adjacent teeth. A, Extensive bone destruction around the mandibular first molar. B, Radiograph made years after extraction of the first molar and replacement by a prosthesis. Note the excellent bone support. C, Extraction of periodontally involved bicuspid and molar. D, Implant replacement of both teeth. *(Courtesy Dr. S. Angha, University of California, Los Angeles.)*

to maintaining better prognosis. If a patient is unwilling to perform adequate biofilm control and receive the timely periodic maintenance checkups and treatments that the dentist deems necessary, the dentist can refuse to accept the patient for treatment. The dentist should make it clear to the patient and in the patient record that further treatment is needed but will not be performed because of a lack of patient cooperation.

Systemic and Environmental Factors

Smoking

Epidemiologic evidence suggests that smoking may be the most important environmental risk factor impacting the development and progression of periodontal disease. Therefore, it should be made clear to patients that a direct relationship exists between smoking and the **prevalence** and **incidence** of **periodontitis**. In addition, patients should be informed that smoking affects not only the severity of periodontal destruction but also the healing potential of the periodontal tissues. As a result, patients who smoke do not respond as well to conventional periodontal therapy as patients who have never smoked. There is a dose-response effect with the more the patient smokes, the more severe the tissue destruction and the poorer the treatment outcome. Therefore, the prognosis in patients who smoke and have slight to moderate (**stage** I or stage II) periodontitis is generally questionable. In smokers with severe periodontitis (stage III or stage IV), the prognosis may be unfavorable or hopeless.

However, it should be emphasized that smoking cessation can affect the treatment outcome and therefore the prognosis. As such, for patients who stop smoking, the prognosis can improve to favorable in those with slight to moderate periodontitis and questionable in those with severe periodontitis.

Systemic Disease or Condition

The patient's systemic background affects the overall prognosis in several ways. For example, evidence from **epidemiologic studies** clearly demonstrates that the prevalence and severity of periodontitis are significantly higher in patients with poorly controlled diabetes than in those whose diabetes is well controlled or those who do not have diabetes. Therefore, patients at risk for diabetes should be identified as early as possible and informed of the relationship between periodontitis and diabetes. Similarly, patients diagnosed with diabetes must be informed of the impact of diabetic control on the development and progression of periodontitis. It follows that the prognosis in these cases depends on patient compliance relative to both medical and dental status. Patients with well-controlled diabetes and slight to moderate periodontitis who comply with their recommended periodontal treatment should generally have a favorable prognosis. Similarly, in patients with other systemic disorders that could affect disease progression, prognosis improves with correction of the systemic problem.

The prognosis is questionable when surgical periodontal treatment is required but cannot be provided because of the patient's systemic health. Incapacitating conditions that limit the patient's performance of oral procedures (e.g., Parkinson disease) also adversely affect the prognosis. Newer "automated" oral hygiene devices, such as electric toothbrushes, may be helpful for these patients and may improve their prognosis.

Genetic Factors

Periodontal diseases represent a complex interaction between a microbial challenge and the host's response to that challenge, both of which may be influenced by environmental factors such as smoking. In addition to these external factors, evidence also indicates that genetic factors may play an important role in determining the nature of the host response. Evidence for this type of genetic influence exists for patients with periodontitis. Genetic **polymorphisms** in the **interleukin**-1 (IL-1) genes, resulting in increased production of IL-1β, have been associated with a significant increase in risk for severe and generalized periodontitis. It has been demonstrated that knowledge of the patient's IL-1 **genotype** and smoking status can aid the clinician in assigning a prognosis. Genetic factors also appear to influence serum immunoglobulin G2 (IgG2) **antibody** titers and the expression of FcγRII **receptors** on **neutrophils**, both of which may be significant in **aggressive periodontitis** (a separate disease category in the previous disease classification to group periodontitis with rapid progression pattern happening in relatively younger patients). Other genetic disorders, such as **leukocyte adhesion** deficiency type 1, can influence neutrophil function, creating an additional risk factor for this aggressive pattern of periodontitis. Finally, the familial aggregation that is characteristic of this periodontitis with rapid progression pattern (previously termed aggressive periodontitis) indicates that additional, as yet unidentified, genetic factors may be important in one's susceptibility to this form of disease.

The influence of genetic factors on prognosis is not simple. Although microbial and environmental factors can be altered through conventional periodontal therapy and patient education, genetic factors currently cannot be altered. However, detection of genetic variations linked to periodontal disease can potentially influence the prognosis in several ways. First, early detection of patients at risk because of genetic factors can lead to early implementation of preventive and treatment measures for these patients. Second, identification of genetic risk factors later in the disease or during the course of treatment can influence treatment recommendations, such as the use of adjunctive **antibiotic** therapy or increased frequency of maintenance visits. Third, identification of young individuals who have not been evaluated for periodontitis but who are recognized as being at risk because of the familial aggregation seen in periodontitis with rapid progression (previously termed aggressive periodontitis) pattern can lead to the development of early intervention strategies. In each of these cases, early diagnosis, intervention, and alterations in the treatment regimen may lead to an improved prognosis for the patient.

Stress

Physical and emotional **stress**, as well as substance abuse, may alter the patient's ability to respond to the periodontal treatment performed. These factors must be realistically faced when attempting to establish a prognosis.

Local Factors

Biofilm and Calculus

The microbial challenge presented by bacterial biofilm and calculus is the most important local factor in periodontal diseases. Therefore, in most cases, having a favorable prognosis depends on the ability of the patient and the clinician to remove these etiologic factors.

Anatomic Factors

Anatomic factors that may predispose the periodontium to disease and therefore affect the prognosis include short, tapered roots with large crowns, cervical **enamel** projections and enamel pearls, intermediate bifurcation ridges, root concavities, and developmental grooves. The clinician must also consider root proximity and the location and anatomy of furcations when assigning a prognosis.

Prognosis is less favorable for teeth with short, tapered roots and relatively large crowns. Because of the disproportionate crown-to-root ratio and the reduced root surface available for periodontal support, the periodontium may be more susceptible to injury by occlusal forces.

Cervical enamel projections (CEPs) are flat, ectopic extensions of enamel that extend beyond the normal contours of the cementoenamel junction. CEPs extend into the furcation of 28.6% of mandibular molars and 17% of maxillary molars. CEPs are most likely to be found on buccal surfaces of mandibular second molars. Enamel pearls are larger, round deposits of enamel that can be located in furcations or other areas on the root surface. Enamel pearls are seen less frequently (1.1%–5.7% of permanent molars; most prevalent in maxillary third molars) than CEPs. An intermediate bifurcation ridge has been described in 73% of mandibular first molars, crossing from the mesial to the distal root at the midpoint of the furcation. The presence of these enamel projections on the root surface interferes with the attachment apparatus and may prevent **regenerative** procedures from achieving their maximum potential. Therefore, their presence may have a negative effect on the prognosis for an individual tooth.

Subgingival root instrumentation ("scaling and root planing") is a fundamental procedure in periodontal therapy. Anatomic factors that decrease the efficiency of this procedure can have a negative impact on the prognosis. Therefore, the morphology of the tooth root is an important consideration when discussing prognosis. *Root concavities* exposed through loss of attachment can vary from shallow flutings to deep depressions. They appear more marked on maxillary first premolars, the mesiobuccal root of the maxillary first molar, both roots of mandibular first molars, and the mandibular incisors (Fig. 27.5 and Fig. 27.6). Any tooth, however, can have a proximal concavity. Although these concavities increase the attachment area and produce a root shape that may be more resistant to torquing forces, they also create areas that can be difficult for both the clinician and the patient to clean.

Other anatomic considerations that present accessibility problems are developmental grooves, root proximity, and furcation involvement. The presence of any of these can worsen the prognosis.

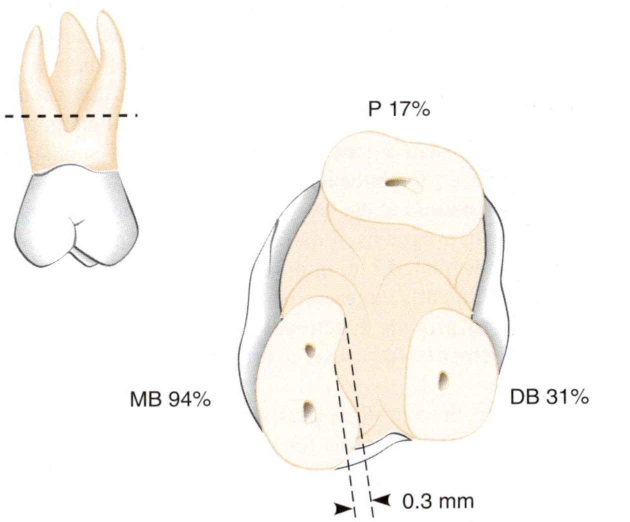

Fig. 27.5 Root concavities in maxillary first molars sectioned 2 mm apical to the furca. The furcal aspect of the root is concave in 94% of the mesiobuccal *(MB)* roots, 31% of the distobuccal *(DB)* roots, and 17% of the palatal *(P)* roots. The deepest concavity is found in the furcal aspects of the mesiobuccal roots (mean concavity, 0.3 mm). The furcal aspect of the buccal roots diverges toward the palate in 97% of teeth (mean divergence, 22 degrees). *(Redrawn from Bower RC. Furcation morphology relative to periodontal treatment. Furcation root surface anatomy.* J Periodontol. *1979;50:366.)*

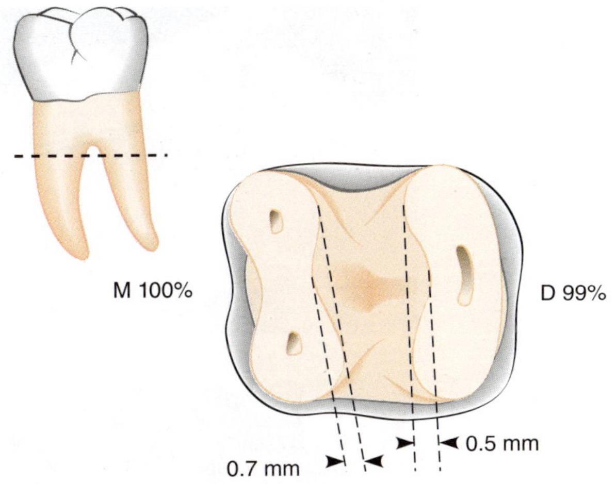

Fig. 27.6 Root concavities in mandibular first molars sectioned 2 mm apical to the furca. Concavity of the furcal aspect was found in 100% of mesial *(M)* roots and 99% of distal *(D)* roots. Deeper concavity was found in the mesial roots (mean concavity, 0.7 mm). *(Redrawn from Bower RC. Furcation morphology relative to periodontal treatment. Furcation root surface anatomy.* J Periodontol. *1979;50:366.)*

Developmental grooves, which sometimes appear in the maxillary lateral incisors (palatogingival groove; Fig. 27.7) or in the lower incisors, create an accessibility problem. They initiate on enamel and can extend a significant distance on the root surface, providing a plaque-retentive area that is difficult to instrument. These palatogingival grooves are found on 5.6% of maxillary lateral incisors and 3.4% of maxillary central incisors. Similarly, *root proximity* can result in interproximal areas that are difficult for the clinician and patient to access. Also, when periodontally involved, the narrow interproximal bone associated with the root proximity is susceptible to rapid bone loss. Finally, *access to the furcation area* is usually difficult to obtain. In 58% of maxillary and mandibular first molars, the furcation entrance diameter is narrower than the width of conventional periodontal curettes (Fig. 27.8). Maxillary first premolars present the greatest difficulty, and therefore their prognosis is usually unfavorable when the lesion reaches the mesiodistal furcation which is averaged at 7–8 mm below the cementoenamel junction. Maxillary molars also present some difficulty in access when interproximal furcation defects are present. The root trunk length of maxillary and mandibular molars is approximately 2.5–5 mm. Therefore, attachment loss over 3 mm at these areas can be a sign of furcation involvement in molars and should be carefully assessed. Generally, furcation involvement is associated with a poorer prognosis due to difficult access for both the clinician and the patient to clean these sites. When buccal and lingual furcations of mandibular molars or buccal furcations of maxillary molars offer good access for oral hygiene measures, the prognosis is usually better.

Tooth Mobility

The principal causes of tooth mobility are loss of alveolar bone, inflammatory changes in the periodontium, and trauma from occlusion. Tooth mobility caused by inflammation and trauma from occlusion may be correctable. However, tooth mobility resulting from loss of alveolar bone is not likely to be corrected. The likelihood of restoring tooth stability is inversely proportional to the extent to which mobility is caused by the loss of supporting alveolar bone. A longitudinal study of the response to treatment of teeth with different degrees of mobility revealed that pockets on clinically mobile teeth do not respond as well to periodontal therapy as pockets

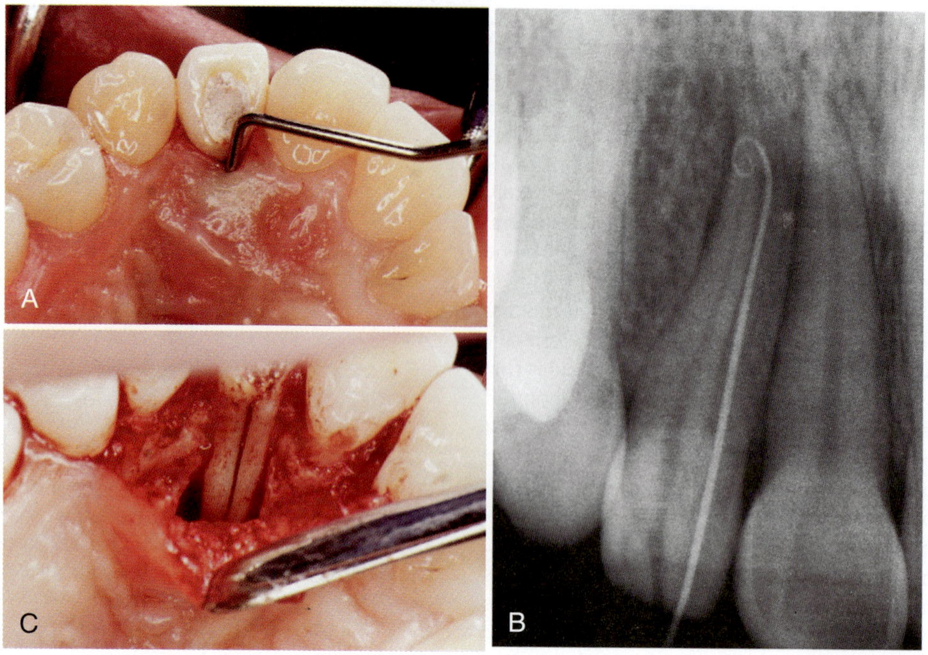

Fig. 27.7 Palatogingival groove. A, Probe in place to indicate a deep pocket along the palatogingival groove. B, Radiograph with a gutta-percha point placed in the pocket. C, The area is surgically opened. Note the palatogingival groove along the entire palatal portion of the root. *(Courtesy Dr. Nadia Chugal, University of California, Los Angeles.)*

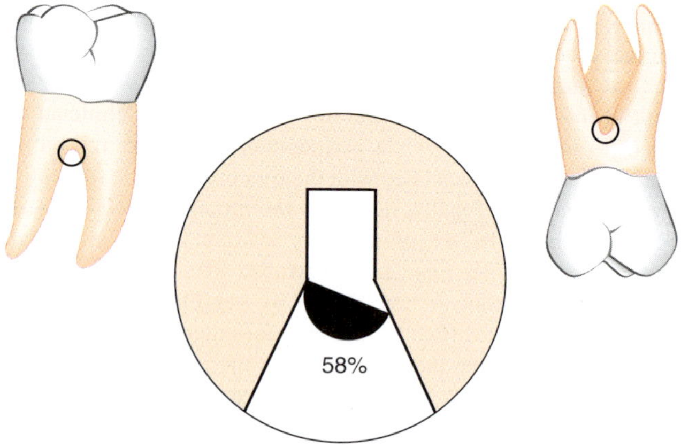

Fig. 27.8 The furcation entrance is narrower than a standard curette in 58% of first molars. *(Redrawn from Bower RC. Furcation morphology relative to periodontal treatment. Furcation root surface anatomy.* J Periodontol. *1979;50:366.)*

on nonmobile teeth exhibiting the same initial disease severity. Another study, however, in which ideal **plaque** control was attained, found similar healing in both hypermobile and firm teeth. The stabilization of tooth mobility through the use of splinting may have a beneficial impact on the overall and individual tooth prognosis during treatment. However, it should be noted that splinting may potentially increase biofilm **accumulation**, resulting in inflammation. It is important to identify the cause of mobility, and assess patient's oral hygiene and compliance before splinting is considered.

Caries, Tooth Vitality, and Root Resorption

For teeth mutilated by extensive caries, the feasibility of adequate restoration and endodontic therapy should be considered before undertaking periodontal treatment. Extensive idiopathic root resorption or root resorption resulting from orthodontic therapy or endodontic **infection** jeopardizes the stability of teeth and adversely affects the response to periodontal treatment. The periodontal prognosis of treated nonvital teeth does not differ from that of vital teeth. New attachment can occur to the **cementum** of both nonvital and vital teeth.

Restorative and Prosthetic Factors

Subgingival margins may contribute to increased biofilm accumulation, increased inflammation, and increased bone loss when compared to **supragingival** margins. Furthermore, discrepancies in these margins (e.g., overhangs) can negatively impact the periodontium. The size of these discrepancies and duration of their presence are important factors in the amount of destruction that occurs. In general, a tooth with a discrepancy in its subgingival margins has a worse prognosis than a tooth with well-contoured supragingival margins. However, for esthetic reasons, it is common to keep the anterior crown margin at the level or below the gingival margin.

The overall prognosis requires a general consideration of bone levels (evaluated radiographically) and attachment levels (determined clinically) to establish whether enough teeth can be saved either to provide functional and esthetic dentition or to serve as **abutments** for a useful prosthetic replacement of the missing teeth.

At this point, the overall prognosis and individual tooth prognosis overlap because the prognosis for key individual teeth may affect the overall prognosis for prosthetic rehabilitation. For example, saving or losing a key tooth may determine whether other teeth are saved or extracted or whether the prosthesis is fixed or removable (see Fig. 27.4). When few teeth remain, the prosthodontic needs become more important, and sometimes periodontally treatable teeth may have to be extracted if they are not compatible with the design of the prosthesis.

Teeth that serve as abutments are subjected to increased functional demands. Therefore, more rigid standards are required when evaluating the prognosis of teeth adjacent to **edentulous** areas. A tooth with a post that has undergone endodontic treatment is more likely to fracture when serving as a distal abutment supporting a distal removable partial **denture**. Additionally, special oral hygiene measures must be instituted in these areas.

In general, prognostication systems in periodontics were proposed to assign prognosis of a tooth based on its periodontal condition. However, clinically, it is important to consider restorability and the overall prosthetic plan when assigning individual or overall prognosis.

Prognosis of Specific Periodontal Diseases

Many of the criteria used in the diagnosis of periodontal diseases and conditions are also used in assigning prognosis (see Box 27.1). Factors such as patient age, severity of disease, genetic susceptibility, and presence of systemic disease are important criteria in the diagnosis of the condition and in developing a prognosis.

Prognosis for Patients With Gingival Disease

Dental Plaque-induced Gingivitis Associated With Biofilm Alone

Dental plaque-induced **gingivitis** is a reversible disease that occurs when bacterial biofilm accumulates at the gingival margin. This disease can occur on a periodontium that has experienced no attachment loss or on a periodontium with nonprogressing attachment loss. In either case, the prognosis is good for patients with gingivitis associated with bacterial biofilm only, provided that all local irritants are removed, other local factors contributing to biofilm retention are eliminated, gingival contours conducive to the preservation of health are attained, and the patient cooperates by maintaining good oral hygiene.

Dental Plaque-Induced Gingivitis Mediated by Systemic or Local Risk Factors

Gingivitis is primarily induced by dental plaque but the inflammatory response to bacterial biofilm at the gingival margin can be influenced by systemic and local factors. Systemic factors include endocrine-related changes associated with puberty, menstruation, pregnancy, and diabetes; the presence of blood dyscrasias; smoking; and malnutrition. Local factors include dental plaque retention factors (e.g., prominent subgingival restoration margins) and hyposalivation.

In many cases, the frank signs of gingival inflammation that occur in these patients are seen in the presence of relatively small amounts of bacterial biofilm. Therefore, the long-term prognosis for these patients depends not only on control of bacterial biofilm but also on control or correction of these systemic and local factors.

Dental Plaque-Induced Gingivitis—Drug-Influenced Gingival Enlargement

The third group of conditions under dental plaque-induced gingivitis is drug-influenced gingival enlargement. This is often seen in patients taking antiepileptic medication such as phenytoin, immunosuppressants like cyclosporine, or calcium channel blockers like nifedipine. In drug-influenced gingival enlargement, the severity of the lesions is associated with inflammation, which is usually induced by bacterial biofilm. Inflammation may also be induced by repeated trauma (Fig. 27.9). Eliminating the source of inflammation, either biofilm or trauma, can limit the severity of the gingival overgrowth. However, surgical intervention is usually necessary to correct the alterations in gingival contour. Continued use of the drug and persistence of inflammation usually result in recurrence of the enlargement, even after surgical intervention. Therefore, the long-term prognosis depends on whether the etiology of the inflammation

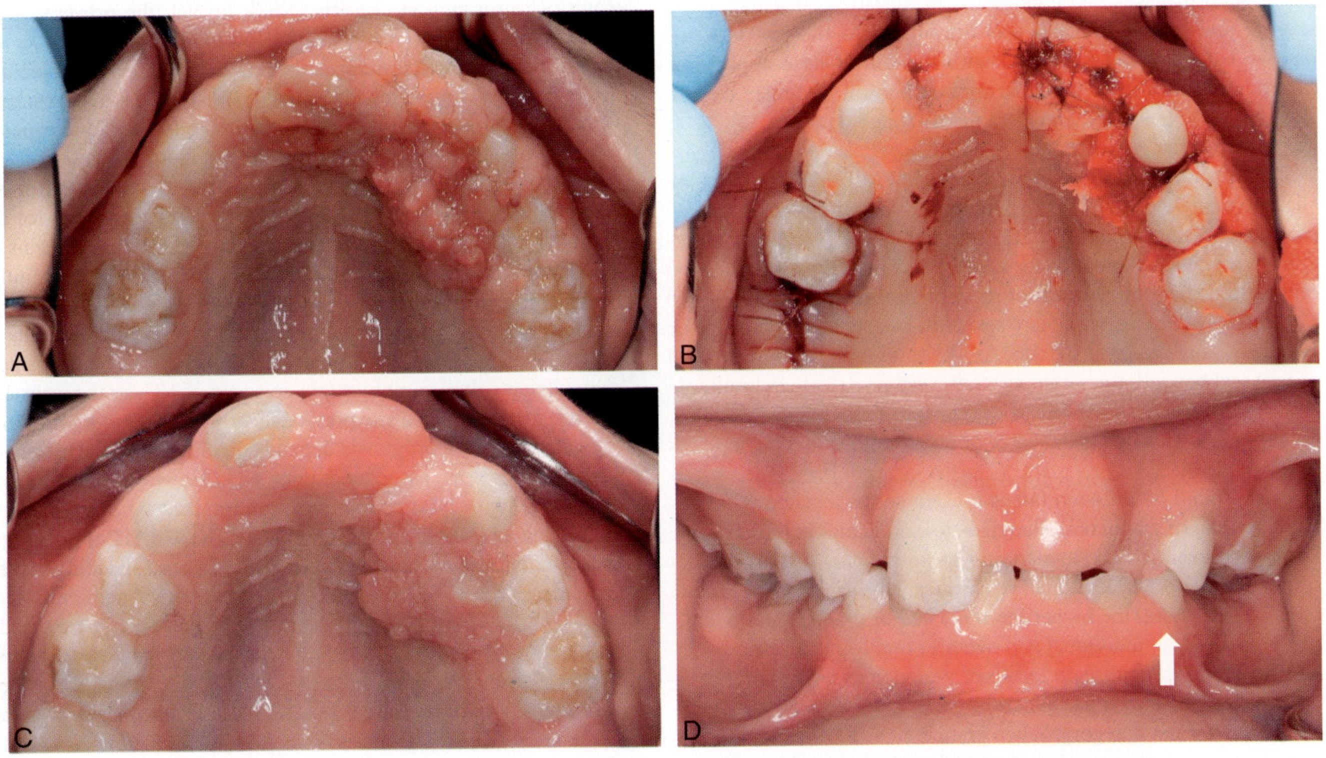

Fig. 27.9 A, Gingival overgrowth in a 5-year-old male patient who was taking cyclosporine for the management of aplastic anemia. B, The gingival overgrowth was resected surgically. C, Recurrence of gingival overgrowth on the maxillary left quadrant at 1-year postop due to trauma from the opposing mandibular teeth occluding on the maxillary left palatal tissue (D). *(Copyright Jonathan H. Do, DDS. All rights reserved.)*

can be completely eliminated, or the patient's systemic problem can be treated with an alternative medication that does not have gingival enlargement as a side effect.

Nondental Plaque-Induced Gingival Diseases

Some gingival diseases are primarily induced genetic/developmental disorders (hereditary gingival fibromatosis), specific infections (bacterial, viral, or fungal origin), inflammatory and immune conditions (hypersensitivity reactions, **autoimmune diseases** of skin and mucous membranes, granulomatous inflammatory lesions), reactive processes (epulides), neoplasms, endocrine disorders, nutritional deficiency (vitamin C deficiency), metabolic diseases, or trauma. These gingival conditions will not be fully resolved by removal of dental plaque alone. However, uncontrolled plaque accumulation can worsen these conditions. Therefore, the long-term prognosis in these patients depends on the control of these contributing factors along with dental plaque control.

Prognosis for Patients With Periodontitis

Periodontitis

In general, there is a significant overlap in the prognostic factors for gingivitis and periodontitis. However, with the same prognostic factor(s), the prognosis for a periodontally affected tooth is worse than a tooth with gingival inflammation only.

Previously, periodontitis was further categorized into **chronic periodontitis** and aggressive periodontitis. Chronic periodontitis is a slowly progressive disease associated with well-known risk factors, such as biofilm and calculus. Aggressive periodontitis is a rapidly progressive disease associated with abnormal host responses and featured bacterial species. However, since there is no strong evidence supporting the differences in etiology and pathophysiology between these two types of diseases, they are both categorized as periodontitis in the 2018 classification of periodontal diseases and conditions. In the 2018 classification, a staging and grading system was introduced to the periodontitis disease category and presented with the following components: generalized, localized, or molar-incisor pattern (extent); stage I, II, III, or IV (severity and complexity); and grade A, B, or C (progression rate).

In cases in which the clinical attachment loss and bone loss are slight to moderate (stage I or II periodontitis) with slow or moderate progression rate (grade A or B), the prognosis is generally favorable, provided the inflammation can be controlled through good oral hygiene and the removal of local biofilm-retentive factors (see Fig. 27.1). In patients with more severe disease (stage III or IV) (see Fig. 27.2), as evidenced by bone loss extending to the middle third of root and beyond, furcation invasion, vertical defect, and multiple tooth loss due to periodontitis, with rapid progression rate (grade C), the prognosis may be questionable or unfavorable, or even hopeless for some teeth.

When rapid progression rate is present and associated with systemic factors (e.g., uncontrolled diabetes) and smoking history, the host response might be altered and these patients usually do not respond well to conventional nonsurgical or surgical periodontal therapy. Therefore, the higher the stage and/or grade of periodontitis, the poorer the individual and overall prognoses will be.

The overall prognosis in localized periodontitis is generally better than in generalized periodontitis since the disease is less extensive in the former category. When compared to localized periodontitis, the molar/incisor pattern of periodontitis that tends to occur in younger patients (previously known as **localized aggressive periodontitis**) is associated with rapid disease progression and therefore has worse overall prognosis (Fig. 27.10).

Periodontitis as a Manifestation of Systemic Diseases

Although the primary etiologic factor in periodontal diseases is bacterial plaque, systemic diseases that alter the ability of the host to respond to the microbial challenge may affect the progression of disease and therefore the prognosis for the case. For example, decreased numbers of circulating neutrophils (as in acquired neutropenia) may contribute to widespread destruction of the periodontium. Unless the neutropenia can be corrected, these patients can present with a questionable to unfavorable prognosis. Similarly, genetic disorders that alter the way the host responds to bacterial plaque (as in leukocyte adhesion deficiency syndrome) also can contribute to the development of periodontitis. Because these disorders generally manifest early in life, the destruction of periodontium can be severe and aggressive. The prognosis in these cases will be questionable or unfavorable.

Other systemic disorders do not affect the host's ability to combat infections but still affect the development of periodontitis. Examples include (1) hypophosphatasia, in which patients have decreased levels of circulating alkaline phosphatase, severe alveolar bone loss, and premature loss of **deciduous** and permanent teeth, and (2) Ehlers–Danlos syndrome, a connective tissue disorder in which patients may present with clinical characteristics of severe periodontitis. In both examples, the prognosis can be questionable or unfavorable.

Necrotizing Periodontal Disease

Necrotizing periodontal disease can be divided into necrotic diseases that affect the gingival tissues exclusively (necrotizing gingivitis [NG]); necrotic diseases that affect deeper tissues of the periodontium, resulting in a loss of connective tissue attachment and alveolar bone (necrotizing periodontitis [NP]); and necrotic diseases that affect **gingiva**, periodontium and mucosa in the oral cavity (necrotizing **stomatitis** [NS]). In NG, the primary **predisposing factor** is bacterial plaque. However, this disease is usually complicated by the presence of secondary factors such as **acute** psychological stress, tobacco smoking, and poor nutrition, all of which can contribute to immunosuppression. The superimposition of these secondary factors on preexisting gingivitis can result in the painful, necrotic lesions characteristic of NG. With control of the bacterial plaque and the secondary factors, the prognosis for a patient with NG is favorable. Uncontrolled and repeated NG may progress to NP, negatively affecting the prognosis.

The clinical presentation of NP is similar to that of NG, except the **necrosis** extends from the gingiva into the periodontal ligament and alveolar bone. In systemically healthy patients, this progression may have resulted from multiple episodes of NG, or the necrotizing disease may occur at a site previously affected with periodontitis. In these patients, the prognosis depends on alleviating the biofilm and secondary factors associated with NG. However, many patients presenting with NP are immunocompromised by systemic conditions such as **human immunodeficiency virus (HIV)** infection. In these patients, the prognosis depends not only on reducing local and secondary factors but also on dealing with the systemic problem.

Determination and Reassessment of Prognosis

Determination of prognosis of a tooth or teeth requires a careful and thorough assessment of the presence of disease and its severity, extent, and progression rate. An accurate prognosis cannot be made without an accurate diagnosis. Once disease has been properly and accurately diagnosed, determining the prognosis can still be

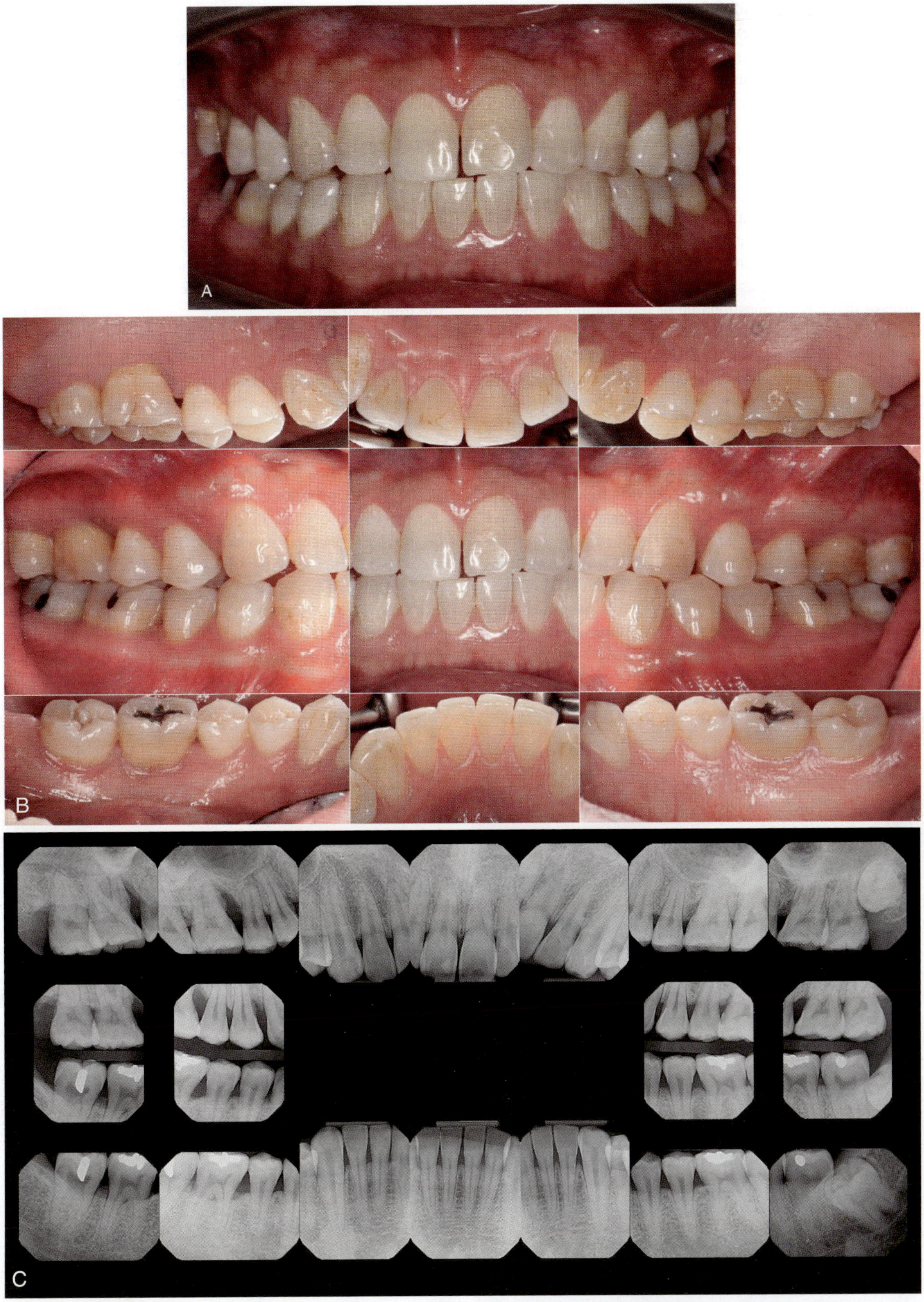

Fig. 27.10 Clinical photos (A and B) and full mouth radiographic series (C) of a patient who had molar-incisor pattern of periodontitis (used to be called "localized aggressive periodontitis"). The overall prognosis is favorable except for the maxillary right first molar (unfavorable), maxillary left first molar (questionable), and mandibular right first molar (questionable).

difficult, particularly for teeth with disease. Many factors can influence disease progression and the response to therapy, and the specific influence of any factor is unknown and likely different from one patient to another. In addition, each patient can respond differently at different times. Moreover, the outcome of therapy significantly depends on the treatment to be rendered, the quality of the treatment, the skills and knowledge of the treating clinician, and patient home care. For these reasons, determining an accurate prognosis can be challenging.

Prognosis of teeth with minimal disease is favorable and by far the easiest to assign with accuracy and precision. As disease develops and severity increases, prognosis becomes progressively harder to assign correctly and accurately, especially for teeth with moderate to advanced disease that have a questionable or unfavorable prognosis. Once disease progresses to a point that teeth are no longer functional or treatable, the prognosis is again easy to determine. These teeth are assigned a hopeless prognosis and the treatment is extraction. However, the treatability of a tooth can be easily skewed by the skills and expertise of the treating clinician, or lack thereof. It is also easier for a clinician to make a diagnosis, determine a prognosis, and create a treatment plan that aligns with his or her expertise. For example, a prosthodontist may assign mandibular incisors with moderate attachment loss and grade 2 mobility a hopeless prognosis and develop a treatment plan that involves replacement of these teeth with a removable partial denture or dental implants. However, a periodontist may assign these teeth a questionable prognosis if the patient is compliant. With the proper periodontal treatment and effective patient biofilm control, the health and function of these mandibular anterior teeth may be restored and maintained for many years.

It is not always possible to accurately determine the prognosis prior to initiating periodontal treatment. During the periodontal examination, due to the lack of anesthesia, it may not be possible to accurately and carefully probe a tooth to determine the true extent of bone loss and severity of disease. During subgingival root instrumentation ("scaling and root planing") under anesthesia, it is possible to probe to the depth of the **periodontal pocket**. However, the anatomy of the osseous defect may not be determined until a periodontal flap has been elevated and all the granulation tissue removed. Additionally, heavy **subgingival calculus** deposits before treatment may affect the accuracy of the examination, resulting in an imprecise diagnosis and prognosis. As such, the prognosis may change as more specific diagnostic information is discovered during the treatment phase.

Prognosis may also change with periodontal treatment or disease progression. During therapy, the patient's motivation and commitment, acknowledged as critical in all forms of periodontal therapy, can be determined, as well as the host response and the healing capacity of the patient.

A frank reduction in **probing depth** and inflammation after therapy indicates a favorable response to treatment and may suggest a better prognosis than previously assumed (Fig. 27.11). If the inflammatory changes cannot be controlled or reduced by therapy, the overall prognosis would be poorer. Adverse treatment outcomes usually indicate existence of uncontrolled or unidentified local and/or systemic factors. Therapy allows the clinician an opportunity to work with the patient and the patient's other care providers to control local, systemic, and environmental factors such as overhanging restorations, diabetes, and smoking,

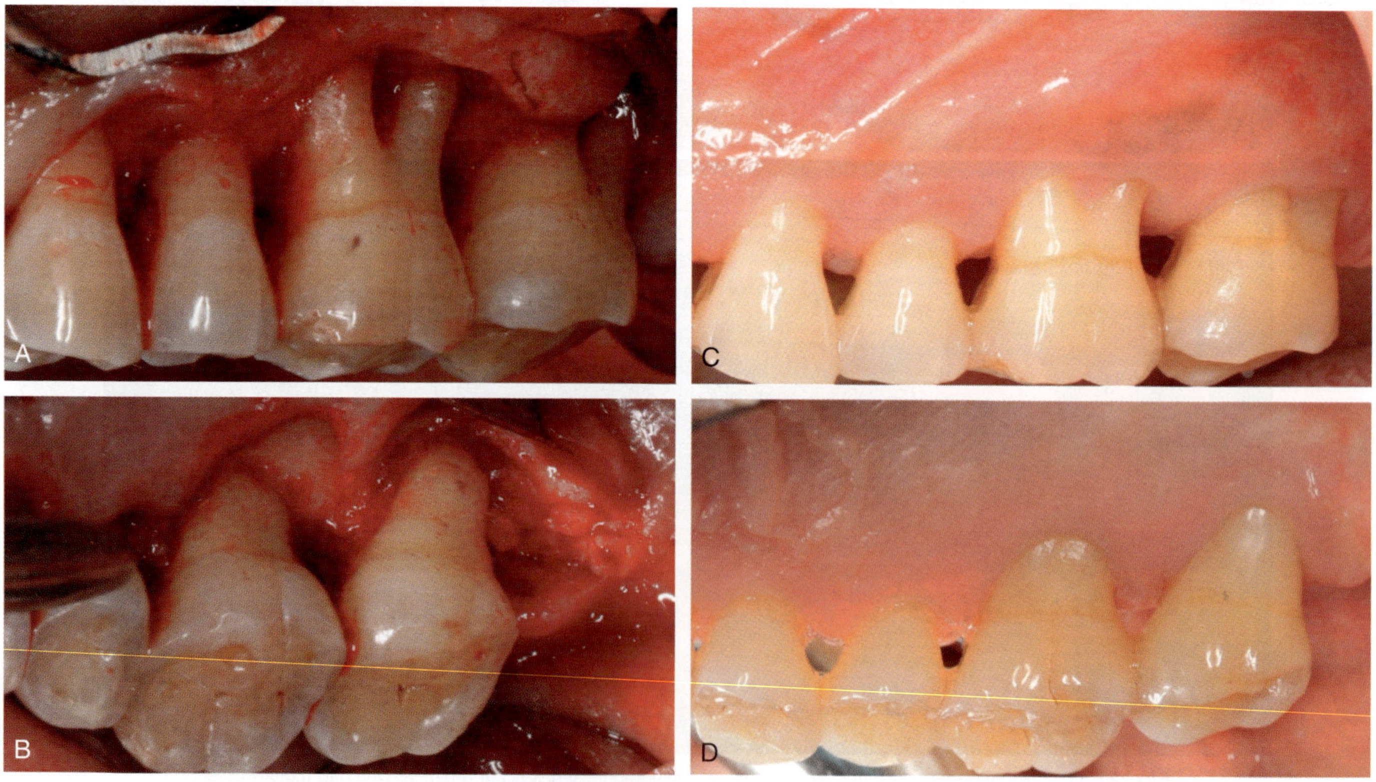

Fig. 27.11 Prognosis changes with treatment. The maxillary left first and second molars were initially assigned an unfavorable prognosis due to advanced bone loss and deep grade II furcation invasion (A and B). The clinician contemplated extraction of both teeth. However, both teeth were vital, stable, and did not require any restorative treatment, and the patient wanted to keep them and was willing to effectively control biofilm. Both teeth were treated with periodontal surgery. After 5 years, they remain healthy, functional with shallow probing pocket depths, and the prognosis improved to favorable (C and D). *(Copyright Jonathan H. Do, DDS. All rights reserved.)*

respectively, which may have a positive effect on prognosis, if adequately controlled.

The progression of periodontitis generally occurs in an episodic manner, with alternating periods of quiescence and shorter destructive stages. No methods are available at present to accurately determine whether a given lesion is in a stage of remission or exacerbation. Advanced lesions, if active, may progress rapidly to a hopeless stage, whereas similar lesions in a quiescent stage may be maintainable for long periods. Stable lesions in a patient in periodontal maintenance may also break down and advance due to changes in biofilm control, systemic health, or stress level. For these reasons, prognosis along with diagnosis must be carefully evaluated and reassessed throughout the course of treatment and over time during supportive maintenance therapy.

Conclusion

The periodontal prognosis plays a pivotal role in therapy, as treatment decisions are made based on prognosis and to improve prognosis. Teeth with a hopeless prognosis are extracted, whereas teeth with more favorable prognoses are treated, with the intent of restoring health and stability and ultimately improving the prognosis. A hopeless prognosis is perhaps the easiest prognosis to assign because hopeless teeth usually have overt and severe disease. The hopeless prognosis is also perhaps the easiest to be erroneously assigned, due to clinical bias or lack of training and expertise. Therefore, the hopeless prognosis must be assigned with caution, as the consequences are irreversible. It must also be recognized that patients and diseases are dynamic. As such, a prognosis will change and must be reevaluated over time. Depending on the controllability of local and systemic factors that affect the prognosis, the questionable or unfavorable prognostic categories can change and could go in either direction and therefore should be continually monitored.

Key points

- Prognosis is essentially a prediction of the course of disease and its response to treatment. It is determined after diagnosis and based upon it the treatment plan is worked out. Prognosis is made both at the level of overall dentition and individual tooth
- The factors that determine the overall prognosis of the dentition include the type of disease, patient's age, systemic background, habits such as smoking, height of the remaining bone, genetic background and the attitude and compliance of the patient.
- Factors that determine the individual tooth prognosis include caries, endodontic status, mobility, furcation involvement, anatomical factors and prosthetic and restorative considerations.
- Often prognosis at the initial visit cannot be made accurately and needs to be reassessed at subsequent visits based upon the response of the patients to phase I therapy.
- No methods are available at present to determine whether the disease is in a state of remission or exacerbation.

Suggested Readings

Kwok V, Caton JG: Commentary: prognosis revisited: a system for assigning periodontal prognosis. *J Periodontol* 78(11):2063–2071, 2007.

McGuire MK: Prognosis versus actual outcome: a long-term survey of 100 treated periodontal patients under maintenance care. *J Periodontol* 62(1):51–58, 1991.

McGuire MK, Nunn ME: Prognosis versus actual outcome. II. The effectiveness of clinical parameters in developing an accurate prognosis. *J Periodontol* 67(7):658–665, 1996.

McGuire MK, Nunn ME: Prognosis versus actual outcome. III. The effectiveness of clinical parameters in accurately predicting tooth survival. *J Periodontol* 67(7):666–674, 1996.

McGuire MK, Nunn ME: Prognosis versus actual outcome. IV. The effectiveness of clinical parameters and IL-1 genotype in accurately predicting prognoses and tooth survival. *J Periodontol* 70(1):49–56, 1999.

CHAPTER 28

Rationale for Periodontal Treatment and Treatment Plan

S Elangovan | JH Do | HH Takei | FA Carranza | MG Newman | CD Dwarakanath

CHAPTER OUTLINE

What Does Periodontal Therapy Accomplish?

The effectiveness of periodontal therapy is made possible by the remarkable healing capacity of the periodontal tissues. Periodontal therapy can restore chronically inflamed gingiva so that, from a clinical and structural point of view, it is almost identical with gingiva that has never been exposed to excessive plaque accumulation.

Properly performed, periodontal treatment can eliminate pain, exudate, gingival inflammation, and bleeding. It can also reduce periodontal pockets, eliminate infection, arrest the destruction of soft tissue and bone, and reduce abnormal tooth mobility. Other benefits are to establish optimal occlusal function, restore tissue destroyed by disease, reestablish physiologic gingival contour, and prevent the recurrence of disease, which will all help to maintain the natural dentition (Fig. 28.1).

Local Therapy

The cause of periodontitis and gingivitis is bacterial plaque accumulation on the tooth surface close to the gingival tissue. The accumulation of plaque can be favored by a variety of local factors, such as calculus, overhanging margins of restorations, and food impaction. *The removal of plaque and all of the factors that favor its accumulation is the primary goal in local therapy.*

Abnormal forces on the tooth can increase tooth mobility. The thorough elimination of plaque and the prevention of its formation can help maintain periodontal health, even if traumatic forces are allowed to persist. However, the elimination of trauma may increase the chances for bone regeneration and the gain of attachment. Although this point is not widely accepted, it appears that creating occlusal relationships that are more tolerable to the periodontal tissues increases the margin of safety of the periodontium to the buildup of plaque, in addition to reducing tooth mobility. It should be remembered that total plaque elimination as obtained in experimental studies may not be possible in human subjects.

Systemic Therapy

Systemic therapy may be employed as an adjunct to local measures for specific purposes such as controlling systemic complications from acute infections or chemotherapy and preventing harmful effects of posttreatment bacteremia. The control of systemic diseases that aggravate the patient's periodontal condition is always a consideration so proper precautions can be instituted during therapy.

Systemic therapy for treatment of the periodontal condition in conjunction with local therapy is indicated in patients with aggressive periodontitis. In these diseases, systemic antibiotics are used to eliminate the bacteria that invade the gingival tissues and can repopulate the pocket after scaling and root planing.

In addition, periodontal manifestations of systemic diseases are treated primarily by other local measures.

In the late 20th century, the concept of *host modulation* was introduced as a medical approach to periodontal treatment. The classic 1979 paper by Nyman, Schroeder, and Lindhe reported that it was possible to block periodontal bone loss in animals with the aspirin-like drug indomethacin. Evidence was then presented that some *nonsteroidal antiinflammatory drugs* (NSAIDs), such as flurbiprofen and ibuprofen, can reduce the development of experimental gingivitis as well as the loss of alveolar bone in periodontitis. These drugs are propionic acid derivatives and act by inhibiting the cyclooxygenase pathway of arachidonic acid metabolism, thereby reducing prostaglandin formation. These NSAIDs can be administered by mouth or applied topically.

Another drug that has a strong inhibitory effect on bone resorption is alendronate, a *bisphosphonate*, which is currently used to treat metabolic diseases in humans, such as Paget disease or hypercalcemia of malignancy, which result in bone resorption. Experimental studies in monkeys have shown that alendronate reduced the bone loss associated with periodontitis.

Host modulation is still in its experimental stages, and protocols for its clinical use have not been established. However, current studies indicate that future treatment modalities may attempt not only to control the bacterial cause of the disease but also to suppress the self-destructive components of the host inflammatory response.

Factors That Affect Healing

In the periodontium, as elsewhere in the body, healing is affected by local and systemic factors.

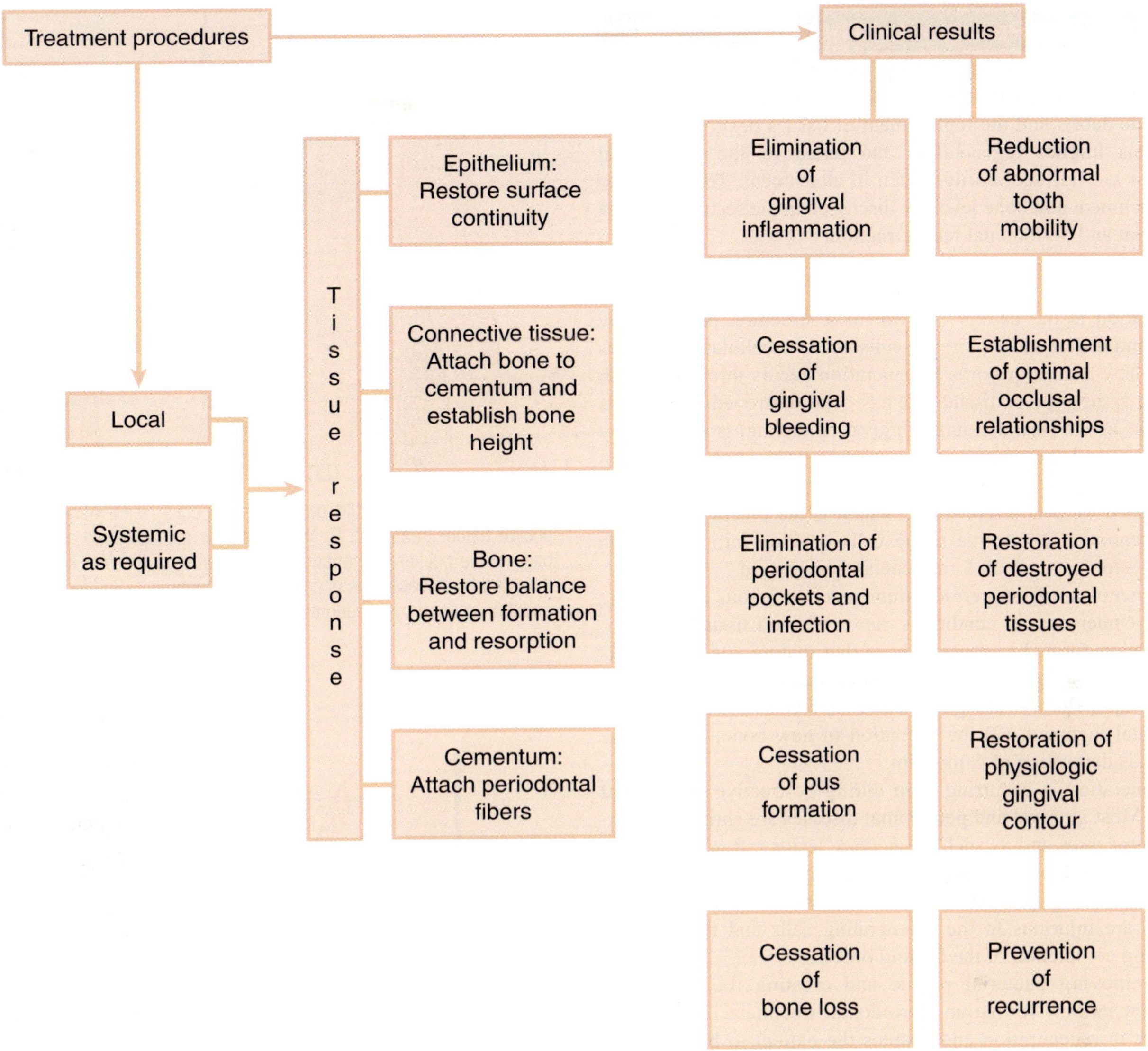

Fig. 28.1 Tissue response and clinical results after periodontal treatment.

Local Factors

Systemic conditions that impair healing may reduce the effectiveness of local periodontal treatment and should be corrected before or during local procedures. However, local factors, particularly plaque microorganisms are the most common deterrents to healing after periodontal treatment.

Healing is also delayed by (1) excessive tissue manipulation during treatment, (2) trauma to the tissues, (3) the presence of foreign bodies, and (4) repetitive treatment procedures that disrupt the orderly cellular activity in the healing process. An adequate blood supply is needed for the increased cellular activity during healing. If the blood supply is impaired or insufficient, areas of necrosis will develop and delay the healing process.

Healing is improved by debridement (removal of degenerated and necrotic tissue), immobilization of the healing area, and pressure on the wound. The cellular activity in healing entails an increase in oxygen consumption, but healing of the gingiva is not accelerated by artificially increasing the oxygen supply beyond the normal requirements.

Systemic Factors

The effects of systemic conditions on healing have been extensively documented in animal experiments but are less clearly defined in humans. Healing capacity diminishes with age, probably because of the atherosclerotic vascular changes common in aging and the resulting reduction in blood circulation. Healing is delayed in patients with generalized infections and in those with diabetes and other debilitating diseases.

Healing is impaired by insufficient food intake; bodily conditions that interfere with the use of nutrients; and deficiencies in vitamin C, proteins, and other nutrients. However, the nutrient requirements of the healing tissues in minor wounds, such as those created by periodontal surgical procedures, are usually satisfied by a well-balanced diet.

Healing is also affected by hormones. Systemically administered glucocorticoids such as cortisone hinder repair by depressing the inflammatory reaction or by inhibiting the growth of fibroblasts, the production of collagen, and the formation of endothelial cells. Systemic stress, thyroidectomy, testosterone, adrenocorticotropic hormone (ACTH), and large doses of estrogen suppress the formation of granulation tissue and impair healing. Progesterone increases and accelerates the vascularization of immature granulation tissue and appears to increase the susceptibility of the gingiva to mechanical injury by causing dilation of the marginal vessels.

Healing After Periodontal Therapy

The basic healing processes are the same after all forms of periodontal therapy. These processes consist of the removal of degenerated tissue debris and the replacement of tissues destroyed by disease. This implies regeneration and repair of the periodontal structures but not necessarily a gain in attachment. Techniques to gain attachment and bone level are discussed in the sections on new attachment and periodontal reconstruction.

Regeneration

Regeneration is the natural renewal of a structure, produced by growth and differentiation of new cells and intercellular substances to form new tissues or parts. Regeneration occurs through growth from the same type of tissue that has been destroyed or from its precursor. In the periodontium, gingival epithelium is replaced by epithelium, and the underlying connective tissue and periodontal ligament are derived from connective tissue. Bone and cementum are replaced by connective tissue, which is the precursor of both. Undifferentiated connective tissue cells develop into osteoblasts and cementoblasts, which form bone and cementum.

Regeneration of the periodontium is a continuous physiologic process. Under normal conditions, new cells and tissues are constantly being formed to replace those that mature and die; this is termed a *wear and tear repair*. It is manifested by (1) mitotic activity in the epithelium of the gingiva and the connective tissue of the periodontal ligament, (2) the formation of new bone, and (3) the continuous deposition of cementum.

Regeneration is occurring even during destructive periodontal disease. Most gingival and periodontal diseases are chronic inflammatory processes and as such are *healing* lesions. Regeneration is part of healing. However, bacteria and bacterial products that perpetuate the disease process, along with the resulting inflammatory exudate, are injurious to the regenerating cells and tissues, thus preventing completion of the healing process.

By removing bacterial plaque and creating the conditions to prevent its new formation, periodontal treatment removes the obstacles to regeneration and enables the patient to benefit from the inherent regenerative capacity of the tissues. A brief "spurt" in regenerative activity occurs immediately after periodontal treatment, but no local treatment procedures promote or accelerate regeneration.

Repair

Repair simply restores the continuity of the diseased marginal gingiva and reestablishes a normal gingival sulcus at the same level on the root as the base of the preexisting periodontal pocket (Fig. 28.2). This process, called *healing by scar*, arrests bone destruction but does not result in gain of gingival attachment or bone height. This return of the destroyed periodontium to health involves regeneration and mobilization of epithelial and connective tissue cells into the damaged area and increased local mitotic divisions to provide sufficient numbers of cells (Fig. 28.3).

For the diseased gingiva and attachment apparatus to regain (totally or partially) their level on the root (Fig. 28.2C), therapy must include special materials and techniques. If these are not used or are not successful, tissues undergo repair only, which involves regeneration of tissue to remodel the attachment apparatus but does not include regaining attachment level or new bone height. For this reason, we prefer to use the term *reconstruction of the periodontium* to refer to the crucial therapeutic techniques that seek to rebuild the periodontium and result in a significant gain of attachment and bone height.

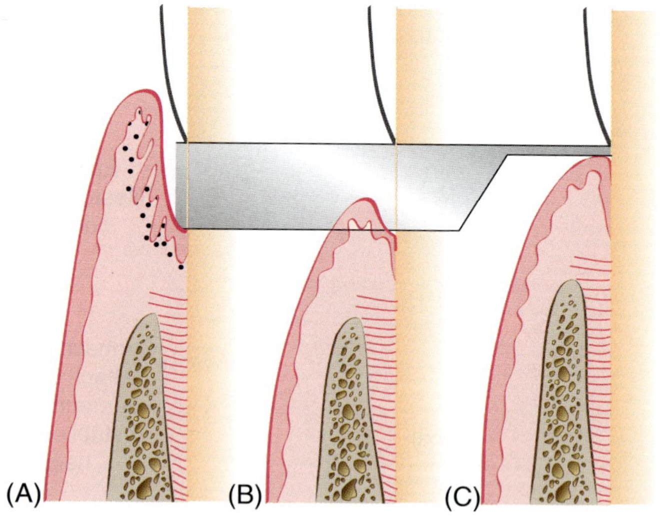

Fig. 28.2 Two possible outcomes of pocket elimination. A, Periodontal pocket before treatment. B, Normal sulcus reestablished at the level of the base of the pocket. C, Periodontium restored on the root surface previously denuded by disease; this is called new attachment. Shaded areas show denudation caused by periodontal disease.

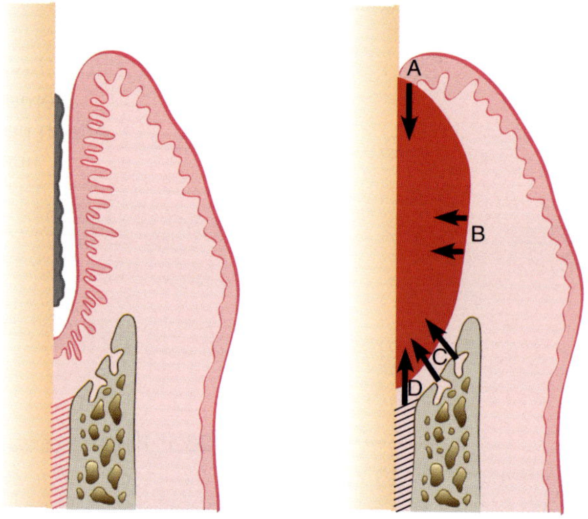

Fig. 28.3 Sources of regenerating cells in the healing stages of a periodontal pocket. Left, Intrabony pocket. Right, After therapy the clot formed is invaded by cells from, A, the marginal epithelium; B, the gingival connective tissue; C, the bone marrow; and D, the periodontal ligament.

New Attachment

New attachment is the embedding of new periodontal ligament fibers into new cementum and the attachment of the gingival epithelium to a tooth surface previously denuded by disease.

The critical phrase in this definition is "tooth surface previously denuded by disease" (Fig. 28.4, area B). The attachment of the gingiva or the periodontal ligament to areas of the tooth from which they have been removed in the course of treatment (or during preparation of teeth for restorations) represents simple healing or reattachment of the periodontium, not new attachment. The term *reattachment* refers to repair in areas of the root not previously exposed to the pocket, such as after surgical detachment of the tissues or following traumatic tears in the cementum, tooth fractures, or the treatment of periapical lesions (Fig. 28.4, area D).

Epithelial adaptation differs from new attachment in that it is the close apposition of the gingival epithelium to the tooth surface,

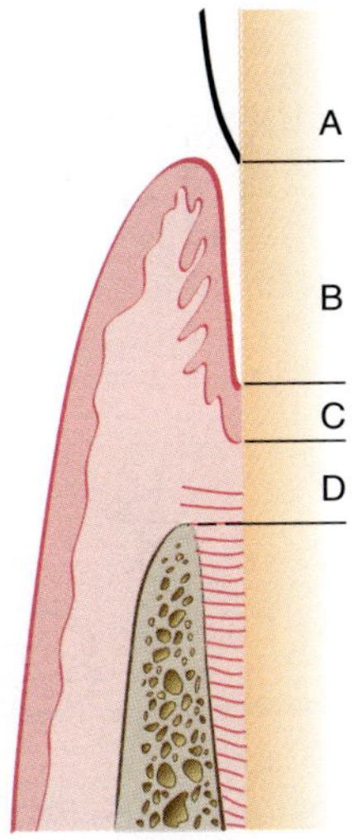

Fig. 28.4 Enamel surface (A). Area of cementum denuded by pocket formation (B). Area of cementum covered by junctional epithelium (C). Area of cementum apical to junctional epithelium (D). The term new attachment refers to a new junctional epithelium and attached connective tissue fibers formed on area B.

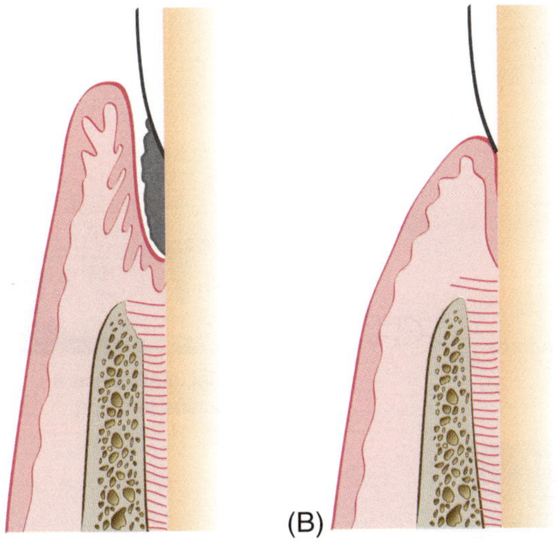

Fig. 28.5 Epithelial adaptation after periodontal treatment. A, Periodontal pocket. B, After treatment. The pocket epithelium is closely adapted to but not attached to the root.

with no gain in height of gingival fiber attachment. The pocket is not completely obliterated, although it may not permit passage of a probe (Fig. 28.5).

However, studies have shown that these deep sulci lined by long, thin epithelium may be as resistant to disease as true connective tissue attachments. The absence of bleeding or secretion on probing, the absence of clinically visible inflammation, and the absence of stainable plaque on the root surface when the pocket wall is deflected from the tooth may indicate that the "deep sulcus" persists in an inactive state, causing no further loss of attachment. A post therapies depth of 4 mm or even 5 mm may, therefore, be acceptable in these cases.

Periodontal Reconstruction

As previously discussed, the term *periodontal reconstruction* refers to the process of regeneration of cells and fibers and remodeling of the lost periodontal structures that results in (1) gain of attachment level, (2) formation of new periodontal ligament fibers, and (3) a level of alveolar bone significantly coronal to that present before treatment.

A technique to attain these ideal results has been a constant but elusive goal of periodontal therapy for centuries. Since the 1970s, renewed laboratory and clinical research efforts have resulted in new concepts and techniques that have moved us much closer to attaining this ideal result of therapy. Melcher pointed out that the regeneration of the periodontal ligament is the key to periodontal reconstruction because it "provides continuity between the alveolar bone and the cementum and also because it contains cells that can synthesize and remodel the three connective tissues of the alveolar part of the periodontium."

During the healing stages of a periodontal pocket, the area is invaded by cells from four different sources (Fig. 28.3): oral epithelium, gingival connective tissue, bone, and periodontal ligament.

The final outcome of periodontal pocket healing depends on the sequence of events during the healing stages. If the epithelium proliferates along the tooth surface before the other tissues reach the area, the result will be a long junctional epithelium. If the cells from the gingival connective tissue are the first to populate the area, the result will be fibers parallel to the tooth surface and remodeling of the alveolar bone with no attachment to the cementum. If bone cells arrive first, root resorption and ankylosis may occur. Finally, only when cells from the periodontal ligament proliferate coronally is there a new formation of cementum and periodontal ligament.

Several methods, based on different concepts and resulting in various techniques, have been recommended to improve the likelihood of gaining new attachment and increased bone levels.

Treatment Plan

A thorough and diligent "information gathering" process is an absolute prerequisite for the clinician to formulate a comprehensive **treatment plan** that takes into account not just local factors in the oral cavity but also the systemic health status of the patient and other critical treatment modifiers like psychosocial and behavioral factors. With the growing body of scientific evidence and validation of molecular markers of health and disease, the information-gathering process now expands to these domains as well in order to render preventive and/or therapeutic precision health care. In addition, digitalization of diagnostic information—be it **periodontal** charting, radiographs, or intraoral scans—allows for the effective integration of artificial intelligence and machine-learning capabilities that can aid the clinician in the decision-making process. In addition, three-dimensional imaging like cone-beam computed tomography (CBCT), with its seamless capability to connect to third-party software programs and the ability to link intraoral scanning images to CBCT images, has greatly expanded the diagnostic and treatment planning possibilities. The previous chapters in this section provide a more detailed information on the process of information gathering and how that information is utilized to diagnose **periodontal diseases** and conditions and to generate a personalized treatment plan for a patient. Fig. 28.6 provides a broad overview of this process and how and where "arriving at diagnosis," "prognostication," and "formulating a treatment plan" fit in the broader scheme of things.

A proper treatment plan is a blueprint for case management. An ideal treatment plan should be based on the following factors.

1. Should be comprehensive. The well-being of the entire oral health which includes structural integrity, functional balance, and esthetic harmony must be planned.
2. Should be long term.

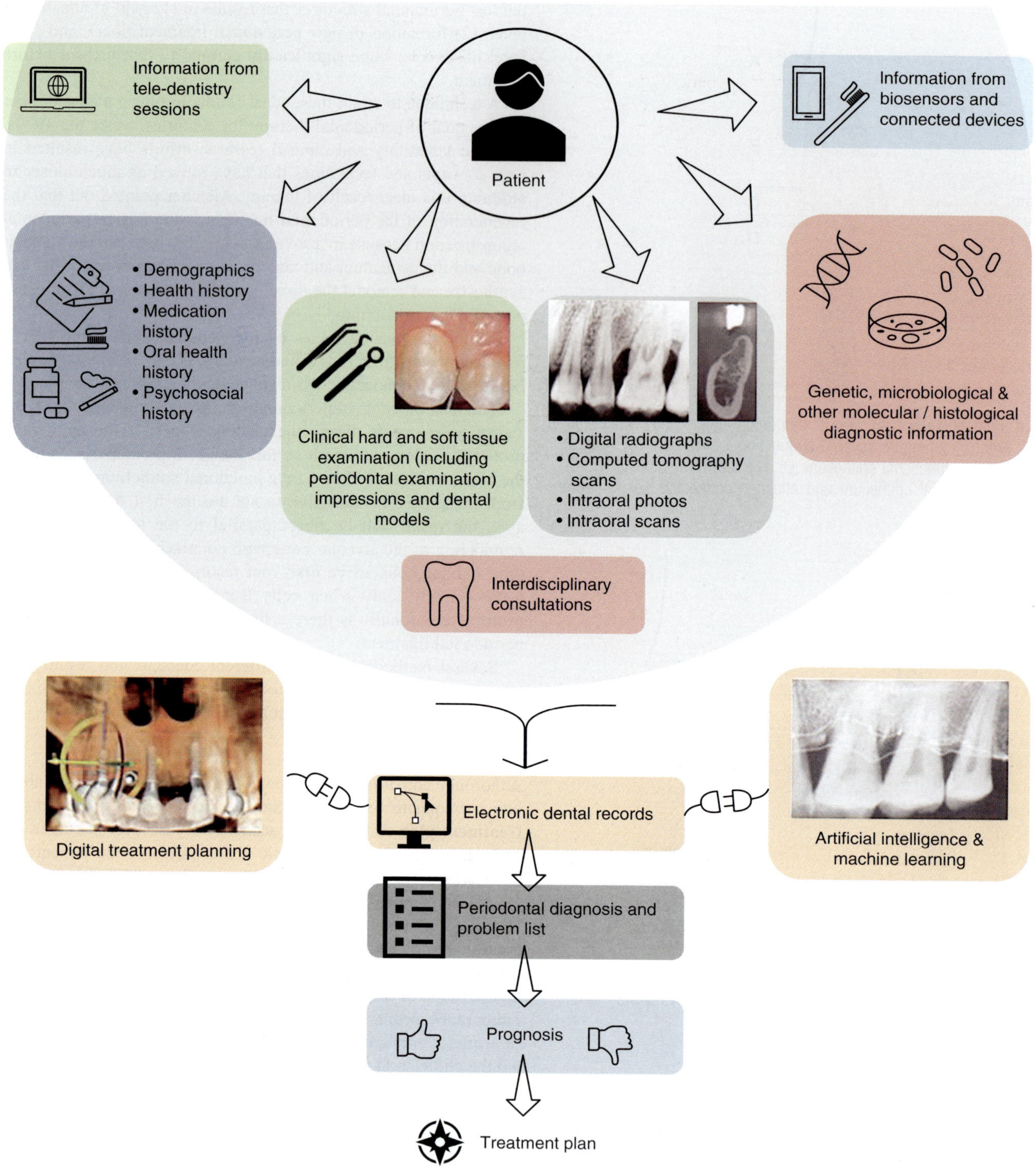

Fig. 28.6 Schematic diagram illustrating the information-gathering process and how it leads to the formulation of a periodontal treatment plan in the era of precision dentistry.

3. Should not be rigid. For example, the success of the treatment should not depend on maintenance of a single tooth or a group of teeth. Often the periodontal status changes midway during the treatment necessitating modifications.

As shown in Fig. 28.6, after the periodontal diagnosis and prognosis have been established, the treatment is planned. The plan should encompass immediate, intermediate, and long-term goals.

The *immediate goals* are the elimination and resolution of **infectious** and inflammatory processes, respectively, that cause periodontal and other oral problems that may hinder the patient's general health. Basically, the immediate goals are to bring the oral cavity to a state of health. This may require patient education on infectious oral diseases and disease prevention, periodontal procedures, endodontics, **caries** control, extractions, and treatment of oral mucous membrane pathologies. Referral to other dental and medical specialties may be necessary at this stage of therapy.

From a periodontal viewpoint, the immediate goals are important because they consist of the resolution of **gingival inflammation** and the correction of conditions that cause and perpetuate it. These include not only elimination of root surface accretions but also **pocket** reduction and the establishment of good gingival contours and mucogingival relationships conducive to periodontal health. Extraction of hopeless teeth, restoration of carious lesions, and correction of defective existing restorations may be necessary.

The *intermediate goals* are the reconstruction of a healthy dentition that not only fulfills all functional and esthetic requirements but lasts many years. Restoration of health, function, esthetics, and longevity involves endodontic, orthodontic, periodontal, and prosthodontic considerations as well as the age, health, and desires of the patient. The financial impact of restoring the dentition to health, function, esthetics, and longevity requires careful consideration and understanding by the patient. The intermediate goals may be quickly achieved or require treatments over months or even years depending on the complexity of the case, the therapy involved, and the financial/compliance status of the patient.

The *long-term goal* is maintenance of health through prevention and professional supportive periodontal therapy. The long-term goal is set, and both the patient and the clinician work toward it from the very first visit. Once active disease has been controlled, all infectious and inflammatory processes have been addressed, and health has been attained, health should be maintainable for the rest of the patient's life. Maintenance of health requires patient education on disease prevention and oral hygiene at the onset of treatment and at repeated intervals, meticulous daily home care by the patient, and patient adherence to professional recall maintenance.

The treatment plan is the blueprint for case management. It includes all procedures required for the establishment and maintenance of oral health and involves decisions regarding the following:

- Emergency treatment (pain, **acute infections**).
- Removal of nonfunctional and diseased teeth and possibly strategic extraction of healthy teeth to facilitate the prosthetic reconstruction of the patient.
- Treatment of periodontal diseases (nonsurgical or surgical).
- Endodontic therapy (necessary and intentional).
- Caries removal and placement of temporary and final restorations.
- **Occlusal adjustment** and orthodontic therapy.
- Replacement of missing teeth with removable or tooth/implant-supported fixed **dental prostheses.**
- Esthetic demands.
- Sequence of therapy.

Treatment decisions are made with the diagnosis and prognosis of the individual teeth and the overall dentition in mind. The prognosis is usually established based on the diagnosis. Treatment decisions are made based on the prognosis and to improve the prognosis, and therefore prognosis will change with treatment. In the 2017 World Workshop, it was determined that once a stage of **periodontitis** is established, it cannot regress even with successful treatment outcomes—with the exception of successful regeneration of vertical defects and furcation with regenerative approaches changing the stage from III to possibly II.

Unforeseen developments during treatment may necessitate modification of the initial treatment plan. However, except for emergencies, no therapy should be initiated until a treatment plan has been established.

Overall Treatment Plan

The aim of the treatment plan is to render comprehensive care—that is, the coordination of all the immediate, intermediate, and long-term goals for the purpose of creating a well-functioning dentition in a healthy periodontal environment. The periodontal treatment encompasses different areas of therapeutic objectives for each patient according to his or her needs. It is based on the diagnosis, prognosis, disease severity, risk factors, and other factors outlined in previous chapters.

Extracting or Preserving a Tooth

Periodontal treatment requires long-range planning. Its value to the patient is measured in years of healthy functioning of the entire dentition and not by the number of teeth retained at the time of treatment. Treatment is directed to establishing and maintaining the health of the **periodontium** throughout the mouth rather than attempting spectacular efforts to "tighten loose teeth."

Implant replacement of missing teeth has become a predictable course of therapy. Therefore, attempts to save questionable teeth may jeopardize adjacent teeth and may lead to the loss of bone needed for implant therapy. Teeth on the borderline of a hopeless prognosis do not contribute to the overall usefulness of the dentition. Such teeth become sources of recurrent problems for the patient and detract from the value of the greater service rendered by the establishment of periodontal health in the remainder of the oral cavity.

Removal, retention, or temporary (interim) retention of one or more teeth is an important part of the overall treatment plan. A tooth should be extracted under the following conditions:

- Grade III mobility as a result of advanced bone loss.
- Advanced stages of furcation involvement.
- Advanced stages of endodontics—periodontal lesions.
- Circumferential bone loss extending to the apical third of root.
- Strategically unimportant tooth in the dentition.

It should be borne in the mind that since the advent of dental implants as a highly predictable and effective method of replacement of lost teeth, heroic periodontal therapeutic measures to salvage teeth with questionable and hopeless prognosis are not recommended.

In some cases, a tooth can be retained temporarily, postponing the decision to extract until after treatment is completed. A tooth in this category can be retained under the following conditions:

- It maintains posterior stops; the tooth can be removed after treatment when it can be replaced by an implant or another type of prosthesis.
- It maintains posterior stops and may be functional after implant placement in adjacent areas. When the implant is restored, these teeth can be extracted.
- In the anterior esthetic zone, a tooth can be retained during periodontal therapy and removed when treatment is completed and a permanent restorative procedure can be performed. The retention of this tooth should not jeopardize the adjacent teeth. This approach avoids the need for temporary appliances in the esthetic zone during therapy.
- Extraction of hopeless teeth can be delayed during the nonsurgical periodontal therapy and can be performed during periodontal surgery of the adjacent teeth. This approach reduces the number of appointments needed for surgery in the same area.

In addition to the proper function of the dentition, esthetic considerations play an important role in the formulation of the treatment plan. Different patients value esthetics differently according to their age, gender, profession, social status, and life experiences. The clinician should carefully evaluate and consider a final esthetic outcome of treatment that will be acceptable to the patient without jeopardizing the basic need of attaining health.

With the predictable use of implants, questionable teeth should be carefully evaluated as to whether their removal and replacement with an implant may be a better and more satisfactory course of therapy.

In complex cases, interdisciplinary consultation with other specialty areas is necessary before a final plan can be made. The opinions of orthodontists and prosthodontists are especially important for the final decision in these patients.

Occlusal evaluation and therapy may be necessary during treatment, which may necessitate planning for occlusal adjustment, orthodontics, and splinting. The correction of bruxism and other occlusal habits may also be necessary.

Systemic conditions should be carefully evaluated because they may require special precautions during the course of periodontal treatment. The tissue response to treatment procedures may be affected, or the preservation of periodontal health may be threatened after treatment is completed. The patient's physician should always be consulted when the patient presents with medical and systemic problems that may affect the periodontal therapy.

Supportive periodontal therapy is also of paramount importance for maintenance of treatment outcomes. Such care entails all procedures for maintaining periodontal health after it has been attained. It consists of instruction in oral hygiene and recall therapy at regular intervals, according to the patient's needs. Please refer to Chapter 70 for detailed information on supportive periodontal therapy.

Sequence of Therapy

The periodontal treatment sequence is presented in Box 28.1, and a nonsurgical periodontal treatment decision tree is presented in Fig. 28.7. Periodontal therapy is an inseparable part of dental therapy, and all treatments must be well coordinated.

Although the phases of treatment are numbered, the recommended sequence does not follow the numbers (Fig. 28.8). Phase I, or the *nonsurgical phase*, is directed to the elimination of the etiologic factors of dental, gingival, and periodontal diseases. When successfully performed, this phase controls and stops the progression of dental and periodontal disease.

Immediately after completion of phase I therapy, the patient should be placed on the *maintenance phase* (phase IV) to preserve the results obtained and prevent any further deterioration and recurrence of disease. While on the maintenance phase with its periodic evaluation based on need, the patient enters into the *surgical phase* (phase II) and the *restorative phase* (phase III) of treatment (Fig. 28.9). These phases include periodontal surgery to treat and improve the condition of the periodontal and surrounding tissues. This may include reconstruction of gingival and bone defects for function and esthetics, placement of implants, and restorative therapy.

Explaining the Treatment Plan to the Patient

The following discussion includes suggestions for explaining the treatment plan to the patient.

Be specific. Tell your patient, "You have **gingivitis**" or "You have periodontitis," then explain exactly what the condition is.

BOX 28.1 Periodontal Treatment Sequence

Periodontal Evaluation

Comprehensive periodontal examination
Diagnosis, prognosis, and risk assessment
Patient education
- Clinical findings and disease status
- Disease **pathogenesis** and prevention
- Personalized oral hygiene instruction

Reduction of systemic and environmental risk factors
- Physician consultation
- Smoking cessation

Periodontal treatment plan
- Oral hygiene assessment and education

Nonsurgical Therapy

Oral hygiene assessment and education[a]
Infection control
- Nonsurgical periodontal therapy
- Supragingival **scaling** and subgingival **root instrumentation** ("**scaling** and **root planing**")
- Extraction of hopeless teeth

Reduction of local risk factors
- Removal or reshaping of overhangs and overcontoured restorations
- Restoration of carious lesions
- Restoration of open contacts

Periodontal Reevaluation

Inquiry of new concerns or problems
Inquiry of changes in patient's medical and oral health status
Oral hygiene assessment and education[a]
Comprehensive periodontal examination
Assessment of outcome of nonsurgical therapy
Determination of required additional nonsurgical and adjunctive therapy

Surgical Therapy

Adjunct to nonsurgical therapy
Should only occur once patient demonstrates proficient **biofilm** control
Objectives:
- Primary: Access for root instrumentation
- Secondary: Pocket reduction through soft tissue resection, osseous resection, or periodontal regeneration

Periodontal pocket reduction surgery
- Resective
- Regenerative

Extraction of hopeless teeth
Periodontal plastic surgery
- Mucogingival surgery
- Esthetic crown lengthening

Preprosthetic surgery
- Prosthetic crown lengthening
- Implant site preparation and implant placement

Periodontal Maintenance Therapy

Inquiry of new concerns or problems
Inquiry of changes in patient's medical and oral health status
Oral hygiene assessment and education[a]
Comprehensive periodontal examination
Professional maintenance care
- **Supragingival** and **subgingival biofilm and calculus** removal
- Selective subgingival **root instrumentation** ("**scaling** and **root planing**")

Assessment of recall interval and plan for next visit

[a]Patient oral hygiene is critical to the overall short-term and long-term treatment outcome. Therefore, oral hygiene must be repeatedly assessed and reinforced.

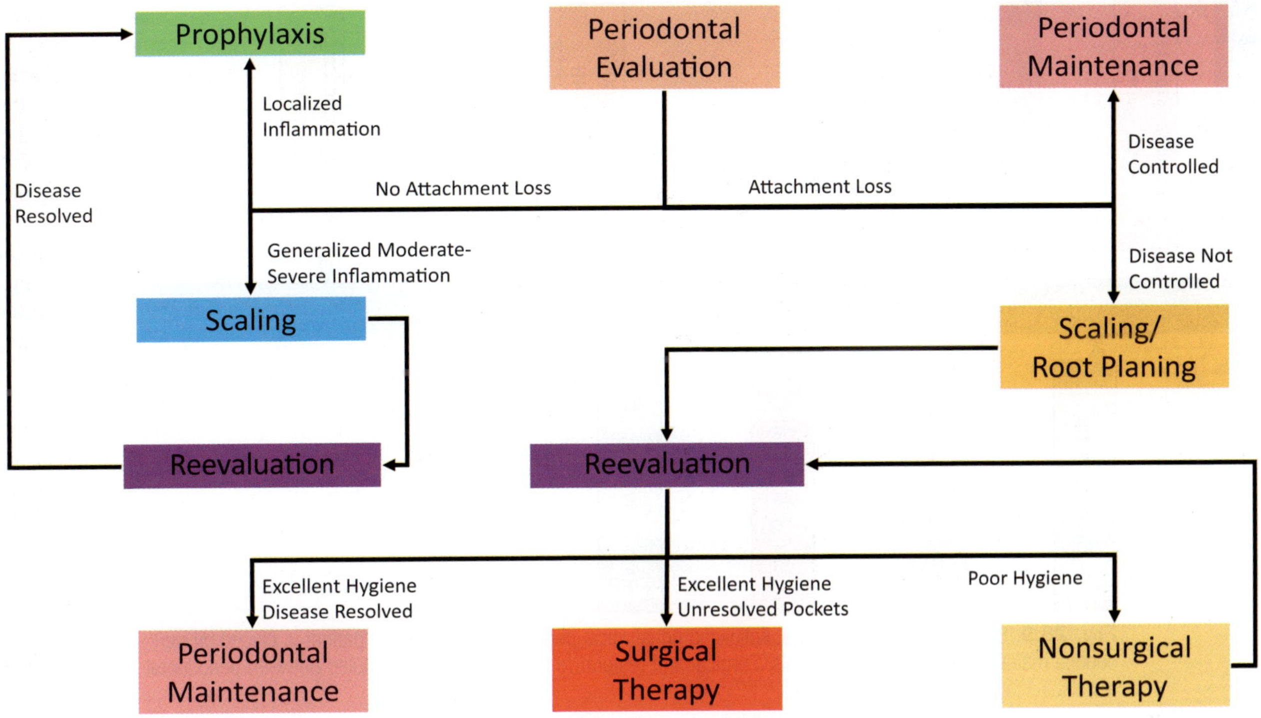

Fig. 28.7 Periodontal treatment decision tree.

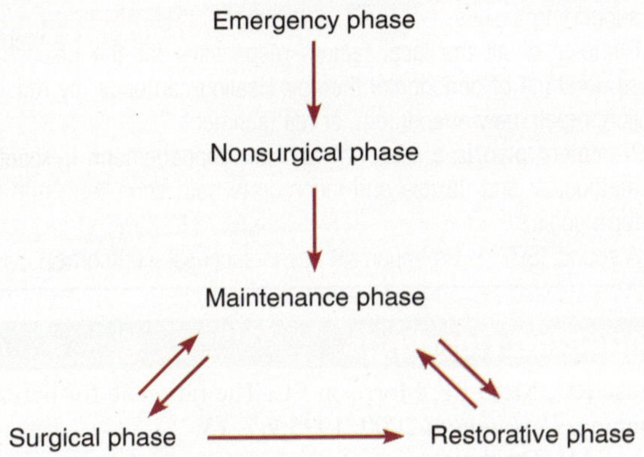

Fig. 28.8 Preferred sequence of therapy.

Avoid vague statements. Do not use statements such as, "You have trouble with your gums" or "Something should be done about your gums." The patient may not understand the significance of such statements and may disregard them.

Begin your discussion on a positive note. Talk about the teeth that can be retained and the long-term service they can be expected to render. Do not begin your discussion with the statement "The following teeth have to be extracted." This creates a negative impression, which adds to the erroneous attitude of hopelessness the patient may already have regarding his or her mouth. Make it clear that every effort will be made to retain as many teeth as possible, but do not dwell on the patient's loose teeth. Emphasize that the important purpose of the treatment is to prevent the other teeth from becoming as severely diseased as the loose teeth.

Present the entire treatment plan as one unit. Avoid creating the impression that treatment consists of separate procedures, some—or all—of which may be selected by the patient. Make it clear that dental restorations and prostheses contribute as much to the health of the gingiva as the elimination of inflammation and **periodontal pockets**. Do not speak in terms of "having the gums treated and then taking care of the necessary restorations later" as if these were unrelated treatments.

Patients often seek guidance from the dentist with questions such as the following:

- "Are my teeth worth treating?"
- "Would you have them treated if you had my problem?"
- "Why don't I just go along the way I am until the teeth really bother me and then have them all extracted?"

Explain that "doing nothing" or holding on to hopelessly diseased teeth as long as possible is inadvisable for the following reasons:

1. Periodontal disease with inflammation as a bridge is associated with several medical conditions such as stroke, cardiovascular disease, pulmonary disease, and diabetes, as well as the possibility for premature, low-birth-weight babies in women of child-bearing age.
2. It is not feasible to place restorations or fixed bridges on teeth with untreated periodontal disease, because the usefulness of the restoration would be limited by the uncertain condition of the supporting structures.
3. Failure to eliminate periodontal disease not only results in the loss of teeth already severely involved but also shortens the life span of other teeth. With proper treatment, these teeth can serve as the foundation for a healthy and functioning dentition.

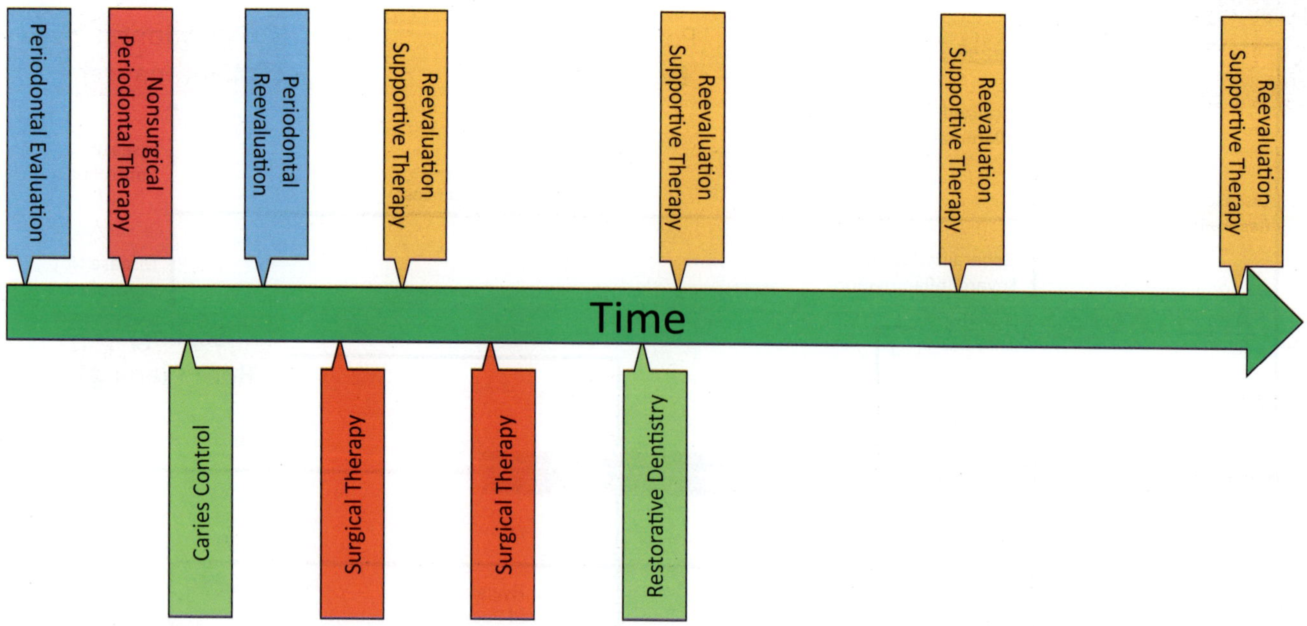

Fig. 28.9 Sample treatment timeline. Following nonsurgical periodontal therapy, the patient is placed on periodontal maintenance at regular intervals. Surgical and restorative treatments are scheduled between periodontal recalls.

Therefore, the dentist should make it clear to the patient that if the periodontal condition is treatable, the best results are obtained by prompt treatment. If the condition is not treatable, the teeth should be extracted.

It is the dentist's responsibility to advise the patient of the importance of periodontal treatment. However, if treatment is to be successful, the patient must be sufficiently interested in retaining his or her natural teeth and to maintain the necessary oral hygiene. Individuals who are not particularly perturbed by the thought of losing their teeth are generally not good candidates for periodontal treatment.

Conclusion

The ultimate goal for every patient is to bring his or her mouth to a state of health and maintain it long term. This begins with educating the patient on the problems in his or her mouth and the etiologies, treatment, and prevention of these problems. A properly formulated treatment plan is paramount to achieving this goal. A treatment plan is a plan for therapy formulated only after a thorough examination has been completed, the diagnosis and prognosis have been determined, and the needs and desires of the patient have been taken into consideration. It must be recognized that as the diagnosis (in select cases) and prognosis will change with treatment, therapeutic needs may also change. As such, the treatment plan must be changed accordingly.

Key points

- Properly performed periodontal treatment can eliminate pain, exudate, gingival inflammation, and bleeding. It also reduces periodontal pockets, eliminates infection, and arrests further destruction of supporting tissues.
- Removal of all the local factors responsible for the disease is a cornerstone of periodontal therapy. Healing can occur by regeneration, repair, new attachment, or reattachment.
- Treatment plan is a blueprint for case management. It should be methodical and flexible and incorporate both short-term and long-term goals.
- A sound "SPT" is an important key to successful outcome.

Suggested Readings

Caffesse RG, Mota LF, Morrison EC. The rationale for periodontal therapy. *Periodontol* 2000. 1995;9:7–13.

Melcher AH. On the repair potential of periodontal tissues. *J Periodontol*. 1976;47(5):256–260.

References

References and MCQs with answers for the chapter are available on www.medenact.com.

CHAPTER 29

Periodontal Treatment of Medically Compromised Patients and Patients With Special Needs

PR Klokkevold | BL Mealey | J Otomo-Corgel | CD Dwarakanath

CHAPTER OUTLINE

Many patients seeking dental care have significant medical conditions that can alter the course of their oral disease and the therapy provided. This is especially true for older patients who are more likely to have underlying disease(s). The therapeutic responsibility of the clinician includes identification of the patient's medical problems to formulate a proper **treatment plan**. A thorough medical history is paramount. If significant findings are unveiled, consultation with or referral of the patient to an appropriate physician is indicated. This ensures correct management and provides medicolegal coverage for the clinician.

This chapter covers common medical conditions that clinicians will encounter when managing patients with **periodontal disease**. The review of each topic area can be supplemented by consulting other references for more detailed coverage of specific disorders. Understanding these conditions enables the clinician to appropriately treat the total patient, rather than focusing solely on their **periodontal** needs.

Cardiovascular Diseases

Cardiovascular diseases are the most prevalent category of systemic disease in the United States and many other countries, and they are more common with increasing age. Health histories should be closely scrutinized for cardiovascular problems, including hypertension, angina pectoris, atrial fibrillation, myocardial infarction (MI), cardiac bypass surgery, cerebrovascular accident (CVA), congestive heart failure (CHF), infective endocarditis (IE), and implanted cardiac pacemakers or automatic cardioverter-defibrillators.

In most cases, the patient's physician should be consulted, especially if stressful or prolonged treatment is anticipated. Short appointments and a calm, relaxing environment help minimize **stress** and maintain hemodynamic stability.

Hypertension

Hypertension, the most common cardiovascular disease, affects more than 100 million American adults, many of whom are undiagnosed. In 2017, the American Heart Association, the American College of Cardiology, and nine other health professional organizations revised the 2003 high blood pressure guidelines, lowering the definition of high blood pressure from 140/90 to 130/80 mm Hg. Nearly half (46%) of the US adult population has high blood pressure based on the new definitions (Table 29.1).

The new guidelines were developed following the Systolic Blood Pressure Intervention Trial, which included more than 9000 adults aged 50 years old and older with at least one risk factor and a systolic blood pressure of 130 mm Hg or higher. The results demonstrated that a systolic blood pressure of 120 mm Hg or less reduced the chances of heart attack, heart failure, or stroke over a 3-year period. The new guidelines eliminate the category of prehypertension, categorizing these patients as elevated (systolic 120–129 and diastolic <80) or stage 1 hypertension (systolic 130–139 or diastolic 80–89).

Hypertension is not diagnosed from a single elevated blood pressure (BP) recording. Rather, the diagnosis is based on the average value of two or more BP readings taken at two or more appointments. Both the systolic and diastolic pressure readings are considered in the diagnosis.

Hypertension is divided into primary and secondary types. *Primary* (i.e., essential) *hypertension* occurs when no underlying pathologic abnormality can be found to explain the disease. Approximately 90%–95% of hypertensive patients have primary hypertension. The remaining 5%–10% have *secondary hypertension*, in which an underlying cause can be found and is often treated. Conditions responsible for secondary hypertension include renal disease, endocrinologic changes, and neurogenic disorders.

In early hypertension, the patient may be asymptomatic. If not identified, diagnosed, and treated, hypertension can persist and increase in severity, leading eventually to coronary artery disease, angina, MI, CHF, CVA, or kidney failure. Patients with hypertension enter dental practices every day. Hypertension is more common among the older populations who are frequently seen in

TABLE 29.1 Blood Pressure Categories

Category	Systolic (mm Hg)		Diastolic (mm Hg)
Normal	<120	and	<80
Elevated	120–129	and	<80
Stage 1 hypertension	130–139	or	80–89
Stage 2 hypertension	≥140	or	≥90
Hypertensive crisis	>180	and/or	>120

periodontal practices, and the **prevalence** of patients with hypertension will certainly increase with the new, lower threshold guidelines. Prior evidence from the Framingham Heart Study revealed that people with normal BP at age 55 still have a 90% risk of becoming hypertensive later in life.

The dental office can play a vital role in the detection of hypertension and maintenance care of the patient with hypertensive disease. The first dental office visit should include two BP readings spaced at least 10 min apart, which are averaged and used as a baseline. Before the clinician refers a patient to a physician because of elevated BP, readings should be taken at a minimum of two appointments, unless the measurements are extremely high (i.e., systolic pressure > 180 mm Hg or diastolic pressure > 120 mm Hg).

The periodontal recall maintenance visit is an ideal time for hypertension detection and monitoring. Only about one in four (24%) adults with hypertension in the United States have their condition under control. Lack of compliance with antihypertensive therapy is the primary reason for this failure. Dentists can help patients achieve greater success in managing hypertension by taking BP readings at each periodontal recall maintenance visit and informing them about the readings.

Periodontal or other dental procedures should not be performed until accurate BP measurements and a thorough medical history have been taken to identify patients with significant hypertensive disease. The time of day should be recorded because BP varies significantly throughout the day. Patient position and arm used to record blood pressure should also be recorded (e.g., right arm, seated).

Dental treatment for hypertensive patients is safe as long as stress is minimized. If a patient is receiving antihypertensive therapy, consultation with the physician may be warranted regarding the current medical status, medications, periodontal treatment plan, and patient care. Many physicians are not knowledgeable about the details of dental or periodontal procedures. It is important for the dentist to inform the physician regarding the estimated degree of stress, length of the procedures, and complexity of the individualized treatment plan. Morning dental appointments were once suggested for hypertensive patients, but evidence indicates that BP usually increases around awakening and peaks at midmorning. Because lower BP levels occur in the afternoon, afternoon dental appointments may be preferable.

No routine periodontal treatment should be given to a patient who is hypertensive and not under medical management. For patients with systolic BP greater than 180 mm Hg or diastolic BP greater than 120 mm Hg, treatment should be limited to emergency care only until hypertension is controlled. Immediate referral to manage hypertension should be considered. Analgesics are prescribed for pain and **antibiotics** for infection. **Acute** infections may require surgical incision and drainage, but the surgical field should be limited because excessive bleeding can occur with elevated BP.

When treating hypertensive patients, the clinician should not use a local anesthetic containing an epinephrine concentration greater than 1:100,000 or a vasopressor to control local bleeding. Local anesthesia without epinephrine can be used for short procedures (<30 min). In a patient with hypertensive disease, however, it is important to minimize pain by providing profound local anesthesia to avoid an increase in **endogenous** epinephrine secretion.

The benefits of the small doses of epinephrine used in dentistry far outweigh the potential for hemodynamic compromise. The smallest possible dose of epinephrine should be used, and aspiration before injection of local anesthetics is critical. Intraligamentary (i.e., periodontal ligament) injection is usually contraindicated because hemodynamic changes are similar to an intravascular injection. If the hypertensive patient exhibits anxiety, the use of **conscious sedation** in conjunction with periodontal procedures may be warranted.

Although there is success with nonpharmacologic methods to control hypertension including diet, exercise, weight control, and limiting alcohol, most people require one or more medications to achieve blood pressure control. There are several categories of antihypertensive medications (Table 29.2). See online material for a brief description of the various classes of medications used to control hypertension.

Alpha-adrenergic blockers work by reducing arterial **resistance**, relaxing muscle tone of the vascular walls. Some possible side effects include rapid heart rate, dizziness, and orthostatic hypotension.

Alpha-2 **receptor** agonists reduce blood pressure by decreasing the sympathetic activity of the nervous system. These medications may cause drowsiness or dizziness.

Direct vasodilators relax the muscle in vessel walls, allowing the vessel to dilate. Possible side effects include headaches, fluid retention, heart palpitations, and joint pain.

Peripheral adrenergic inhibitors reduce blood pressure by blocking neurotransmitters, which blocks smooth muscle constriction. Side effects include stuffy nose, diarrhea, insomnia, depression, dizziness, orthostatic hypotension, and more. These drugs are rarely used unless other medications are not effective.

Beta-adrenergic blockers reduce heart rate, workload, and output, which lowers blood pressure. Side effects include insomnia, tiredness, depression, slow heart rate, asthma symptoms, and more.

The β-adrenergic receptor antagonists (i.e., β-blockers) are used to treat hypertension. They are either *cardioselective*, blocking only β1 cardiac receptors (i.e., β1 receptors), or *nonselective*, blocking both β1 cardiac receptors and β2 peripheral receptors (i.e., β2 receptors). Epinephrine, an α-adrenergic and β-adrenergic agonist, increases heart rate through direct stimulation of cardiac β1 receptors. Epinephrine also stimulates α-adrenergic receptors, producing **vasoconstriction** of arteries, and β2 receptors, causing vasodilation of skeletal muscle arterioles.

Administration of local anesthetics containing epinephrine to patients taking nonselective β-blockers (e.g., propranolol) can elevate BP. Epinephrine-induced α-adrenergic stimulation results in vasoconstriction and increased BP. Because the patient's nonselective medication has blocked the β2 receptors, epinephrine cannot stimulate the normal compensatory β2 receptor-induced vasodilation. This can result in dramatically increased BP, followed by reflex bradycardia mediated by the vagus nerve and carotid baroreceptors. The end result is a patient with severe hypertension and bradycardia, producing a dangerous decrease in vascular perfusion and possibly causing death. Because of this potential complication, epinephrine-containing local anesthetics should be used cautiously and only in very small amounts in patients taking nonselective β-blockers, with careful monitoring of vital signs.

TABLE 29.2 Classes of Medication Available in the United States to Treat Hypertension

Medication Categories	Common Examples
Alpha-adrenergic blockers	Doxazosin (Cardura) Prazosin (Minipress) Terazosin (Hytrin)
Central alpha-adrenergic (alpha 2) agonists	Clonidine (Catapres) Guanfacine (Tenex) Methyldopa (Aldomet)
Direct vasodilators	Hydralazine (Apresoline) Minoxidil (Loniten)
Peripheral adrenergic inhibitors	Guanadrel (Hylorel) Reserpine (Serpasil)
Beta-adrenergic blockers	Atenolol (Tenormin) Bisoprolol (Zebeta) Metoprolol (Toprol XL) Propranolol (Inderal) Timolol (Blocadren)
Beta-adrenergic blockers with intrinsic sympathomimetic activity	Acebutolol (Sectral) Pindolol (Visken)
Beta-adrenergic blockers with alpha-blocking properties	Carvedilol (Coreg) Labetalol (Normodyne, Trandate)
Beta-adrenergic blockers with nitric-oxide mediated vasodilating activity	Nebivolol (Bystolic)
Calcium-channel blockers—dihydropyridines	Amlodipine (Norvasc, Lotrel) Isradipine (DynaCirc) Nicardipine (Cardene SR) Nifedipine (Adalat CC, Procardia XL)
Calcium-channel blockers—nondihydropyridines	Diltiazem (Cardizem CD, Cardizem SR, Dilacor XR, Tiazac) Verapamil (Calan SR, Covera HS, Isoptin SR, Verelan)
Diuretics—thiazide/thiazide-like	Chlorthalidone (Hygroton, Thalitone, Chlorthalidone) Chlorothiazide (Diuril) Hydrochlorothiazide (Dyazide, Maxzide)
Diuretics—loop	Bumetanide (Bumex) Ethacrynic acid (Edecrin) Furosemide (Lasix) Torsemide (Demadex)
Diuretics—potassium-sparing	Amiloride (Midamor) Triamterene (Dyrenium)
Diuretics—aldosterone antagonists	Eplerenone (Inspra) Spironolactone (Aldactone)
Renin-angiotensin system inhibitors angiotensin-converting enzyme (ACE) inhibitors	Enalapril (Vasotec) Captopril (Capoten) Fosinopril (Monopril) Lisinopril (Prinivil, Zestril)
Renin-angiotensin system inhibitors angiotensin II receptor blockers (ARB)	Candesartan (Atacand) Irbesartan (Avapro) Losartan (Cozaar) Valsartan (Diovan)
Renin-angiotensin system inhibitors direct renin inhibitor	Aliskiren (Tekturna)

Calcium channel blockers prevent calcium from entering smooth muscle cells in the heart and vessel walls, which reduces cardiac contraction and vessel constriction thereby reducing blood pressure. Some possible side effects include palpitations, peripheral edema, constipation, headache, and dizziness.

Diuretics control blood pressure by excreting sodium and water. These medications are often used in combination with other antihypertensive medications. The mechanism of action for diuretics can result in depletion of potassium. As a result, side effects include weakness, muscle cramps, and tiredness. Dietary potassium or supplements may be helpful. Some diuretics are potassium sparing. Patients who are diagnosed with diabetes may need to adjust diet and medication because diuretics can increase blood glucose levels.

Angiotensin-converting **enzyme** (ACE) inhibitors reduce production of angiotensin, which facilitates vasodilation resulting in lower blood pressure. Angiotensin causes vasoconstriction. Side effects include skin rash, loss of taste, **chronic** dry cough, and rarely kidney damage.

Angiotensin II receptor blockers (ARB), as the name implies, block the receptor and the effects of angiotensin, thereby reducing vasoconstriction and blood pressure. Side effects include dizziness. ARBs should not be used during pregnancy.

Clinicians need to be familiar with antihypertensive medications and recognize their side effects and potential drug interactions. *Postural hypotension* is common and can be minimized by slow positional changes of the dental chair. *Depression* is a side effect of some antihypertensive medications that many patients are unaware of. Nausea, sedation, oral dryness, lichenoid drug reactions, and **gingival** enlargement are associated with certain classes of antihypertensive agents.

Clinical Correlation

Hypertension, the most common cardiovascular disease, affects more than 100 million American adults, many of whom are undiagnosed. Three of every four (76%) adults with hypertension do not control their blood pressure well enough. The dental office can play a vital role in the detection of undiagnosed hypertension and the compliance of patients being treated for hypertension. Blood pressure should be taken at the initial visit and at each periodontal recall maintenance visit.

Ischemic Heart Diseases

Ischemic heart disease (Fig. 29.1) includes disorders such as angina pectoris and MI. Angina pectoris occurs when myocardial oxygen demand exceeds supply, resulting in temporary myocardial ischemia. Patients with a history of unstable angina pectoris (i.e., angina that occurs irregularly or on multiple occasions without **predisposing factors**) should be treated only for emergencies and then in consultation with their physician. Patients with stable angina (i.e., angina that occurs infrequently is associated with exertion or stress and is easily controlled with medication and rest) can undergo elective dental procedures. Because stress can induce an acute anginal attack, stress reduction is important. Profound local anesthesia is vital, and conscious sedation may be indicated for anxious patients. Supplemental oxygen delivered by nasal cannula can also help prevent intraoperative anginal attacks.

Patients who manage acute anginal attacks with nitroglycerin should be instructed to bring their medication to dental appointments. Nitroglycerin should also be kept in the office medical emergency kit. For particularly stressful procedures, the patient may take a nitroglycerin tablet preoperatively to prevent angina, although this usually is not necessary. The patient's nitroglycerin should be readily accessible on the dental tray in case it is needed

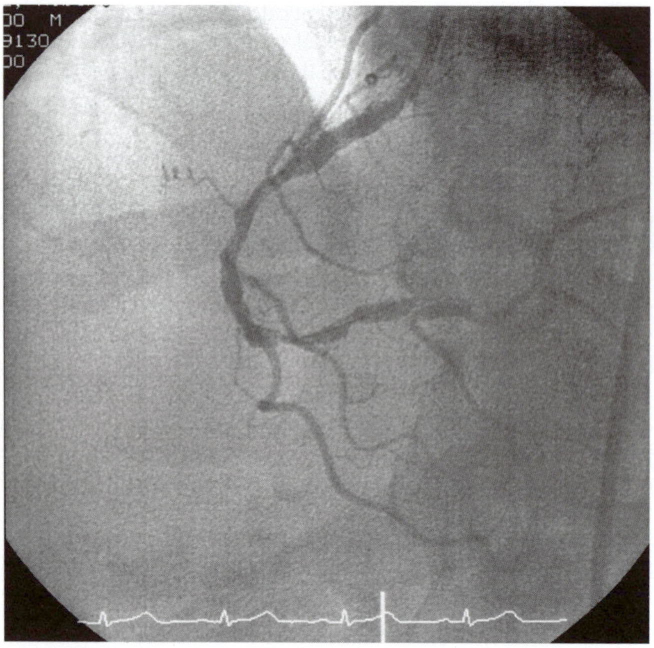

Fig. 29.1 As seen on a coronary angiogram, atherosclerosis can result in narrowing of the coronary arteries, producing signs and symptoms of ischemic heart disease.

BOX 29.1 Emergency Treatment Protocol for Patients Who Experience Angina in the Dental Chair

1. Discontinue the periodontal procedure.
2. Administer one tablet (0.3–0.6 mg) of nitroglycerin sublingually.
3. Reassure the patient and loosen restrictive garments.
4. Administer oxygen with the patient in a reclined position.
5. If the signs and symptoms cease within 3 min, complete the periodontal procedure if possible, making sure that the patient is comfortable. Terminate the procedure at the earliest convenient time.
6. If the anginal signs and symptoms do not resolve with this treatment within 5 min, administer another dose of nitroglycerin, monitor the patient's vital signs, call the patient's physician, and be ready to accompany the patient to the emergency department.
7. A third nitroglycerin tablet can be given 5 min after the second. Chest pain that is not relieved by three tablets of nitroglycerin indicates likely MI. The patient should be transported to the nearest emergency medical facility immediately.

during treatment. Because the shelf life of nitroglycerin is relatively short, the expiration date of the patient's nitroglycerin and that of the nitroglycerin in the office's medical emergency kit should be regularly checked and updated.

Patients with angina may be taking longer-acting forms of nitroglycerin (e.g., tablet, patch), β-blockers, or calcium channel blockers (also used for treating hypertension) for prevention of angina. Restrictions on the use of local anesthetics containing epinephrine are similar to those for the patient with hypertension. Intraosseous injection with epinephrine-containing local anesthetics using special systems (e.g., Stabident, Fairfax Dental) should be done cautiously in patients with ischemic heart disease because it results in transient increases in heart rate and myocardial oxygen demand.

If the patient becomes fatigued or uncomfortable or has a sudden change in heart rhythm or rate during a periodontal procedure, the procedure should be discontinued as soon as possible. Box 29.1 outlines the emergency medical treatment protocol for a patient who has an anginal episode in the dental chair.

Nitroglycerin lingual spray formulations have been popular in hospital pharmacies because of the increased shelf life compared to nitroglycerin tablets. The lingual spray can provide greater and more rapid vasodilation with a longer duration of action. The convenience and advantages of a nitroglycerin lingual spray are appealing, but the accuracy of dose delivery has been questioned and warrants additional studies before the spray can be recommended to replace the known tablet regimen.

MI is the other category of ischemic heart disease encountered with patients in dental practice. Dental treatment is usually deferred for at least 6 months after MI because the peak mortality rate occurs during this time. After 6 months, MI patients can usually be treated using techniques similar to those for stable angina patients.

Cardiac (aortocoronary) bypass, femoral artery bypass, angioplasty, arterial stent insertion, and endarterectomy have become common surgical procedures in patients with ischemic heart disease. If one of these procedures was recently performed, the physician should be consulted before elective dental therapy to determine the degree of heart damage or arterial occlusive disease, the stability of the patient's condition, and the potential for infective endocarditis or graft rejection. Prophylactic antibiotics are not usually necessary for cardiac bypass patients unless recommended by the cardiologist.

Congestive Heart Failure

CHF is a condition in which the pump function of the heart is unable to supply sufficient amounts of oxygenated blood to meet the body's needs. CHF usually begins with left ventricular failure caused by a disproportion between the hemodynamic load and the capacity to handle that load. CHF can be caused by a chronic increase in workload (as in hypertension or aortic, mitral, pulmonary, or tricuspid valvular disease), direct damage to the myocardium (as in MI or rheumatic fever), or an increase in the body's oxygen requirements (as in anemia, thyrotoxicosis, or pregnancy).

Patients with poorly controlled or untreated CHF are not candidates for elective dental procedures. These individuals are at risk for sudden death, usually from ventricular arrhythmias. For patients with treated CHF, the clinician should consult with the physician regarding the severity of CHF, underlying cause, and current medical management. Medical management of CHF can include the use of calcium channel blockers, direct vasodilators, diuretics, ACE inhibitors, α-receptor blockers, or cardiotonic agents such as digoxin. Each medication has potential side effects that can affect periodontal therapy. Because of orthopnea (i.e., inability to breathe unless in an upright position) in some CHF patients, the dental chair should be adjusted to a comfortable level for the patient rather than placed in a supine position. Short appointments, stress reduction, profound local anesthesia, possibly conscious sedation, and use of supplemental oxygen should be considered.

Cardiac Pacemakers and Implantable Cardioverter-Defibrillators

Cardiac arrhythmias are most often treated with medications, but some are also treated with implantable pacemakers or automatic cardioverter-defibrillators. Pacemakers are usually implanted in the chest wall and enter the heart via transvenous catheter. Automatic cardioverter-defibrillators are more often implanted subcutaneously near the umbilicus and have electrodes passing into the heart via transvenous catheter or directly attached to the epicardium. Consultation with the patient's physician allows determination of the underlying cardiac status, the type of pacemaker or automatic cardioverter-defibrillator, and any precautionary measures to be taken.

Older pacemakers were unipolar and could be disrupted by dental equipment that generated electromagnetic fields, such as ultrasonic and electrocautery units. Newer units are bipolar and are usually not affected by dental equipment. Automatic cardioverter-defibrillators activate without warning when certain arrhythmias occur. This can endanger the patient during dental treatment because activation often causes sudden patient movement. Stabilization of the operating field during periodontal treatment with bite blocks or other devices can prevent trauma or injury from unexpected movements.

Infective Endocarditis

Infective endocarditis (IE) is a disease in which **microorganisms** colonize damaged endocardium or heart valves. Although the incidence of IE is low, it is a serious disease with a poor prognosis despite modern therapy. The term *infective endocarditis* is preferred to the previous term *bacterial endocarditis* because the disease can also be caused by **fungi** or **viruses**. The organisms most often encountered in IE are α-hemolytic streptococci (e.g., *Streptococcus viridans*). However, nonstreptococcal organisms, often found in the **periodontal pocket**, have been increasingly implicated, including *Eikenella corrodens, Aggregatibacter actinomycetemcomitans, Capnocytophaga*, and *Lactobacillus* species.

IE has been divided into acute and subacute forms. The acute form involves virulent organisms, usually nonhemolytic streptococci and strains of staphylococci, which invade normal cardiac tissue, produce septic emboli, and cause infections that run a rapid, usually fatal course. The subacute form results from colony formation on damaged endocardium or heart valves by low-grade pathogenic organisms. The classic example is rheumatic carditis from rheumatic fever.

Following the earlier American Heart Association (AHA) publication on prevention of IE in 1997, many questioned the efficacy of antimicrobial prophylaxis to prevent IE in patients who undergo dental or other procedures. Members of the Rheumatic Fever, Endocarditis, and Kawasaki Disease Committee of the AHA Council on Cardiovascular Disease in the Young and a national and international group of experts on IE extensively reviewed data published on the prevention of IE. The committee concluded that only an extremely small number of IE cases might be prevented by antibiotic prophylaxis for dental procedures (even if such therapy was 100% effective). Consequently, the guidelines were changed and published in a 2007 report. The new guidelines advise that IE prophylaxis should be recommended only for cardiac conditions with the highest risk of adverse outcome from IE (Box 29.2). For these patients, antibiotic prophylaxis continues to be recommended for all dental procedures that involve manipulation of the gingival or periapical tissues, or perforation of the oral mucosa. Antibiotic prophylaxis is *not* indicated for individuals on the basis of an increased lifetime risk of contracting IE. A recent (2021) scientific statement from the American Heart Association, following review of currently available evidence, confirmed there are no changes to the 2007 viridans group streptococcal (VGS) IE prevention guidelines.

The practice of periodontics is intimately concerned with the prevention of IE. However, bacteremia may occur even in the absence of dental procedures, especially in individuals with poor oral hygiene and significant periodontal **inflammation**. IE is much more likely to result from frequent **exposure** to random bacteremias associated with daily activities than to be caused by bacteremia associated with a dental procedure. Prevention of periodontal inflammation is paramount. The AHA states that patients who are at risk for IE should "establish and maintain the best possible oral health to reduce potential sources of bacterial seeding." To provide adequate preventive measures for IE, the clinician's major concern should be to reduce the microbial **biofilm** in the oral cavity to minimize soft tissue inflammation and bacteremia.

BOX 29.2 Cardiac Conditions Associated With the Highest Risk of Adverse Outcome From Infective Endocarditis for Which Prophylaxis With Dental Procedures Is Recommended[a]

Previous history of infective endocarditis
Prosthetic cardiac valves or prosthetic material used for cardiac valve repair
Congenital heart disease (CHD), with the following conditions:

- Unrepaired cyanotic CHD, including palliative shunts and conduits
- Completely repaired congenital heart defect with prosthetic material or device, whether placed by surgery or catheter intervention, during the first 6 months after the procedure
- Repaired CHD with residual defects at or adjacent to the site of a prosthetic patch or prosthetic device (which inhibits endothelialization)

Cardiac transplantation recipients who develop cardiac valvulopathy.

[a]American Heart Association recommendations.
(From Wilson W, Taubert KA, Gewitz M, et al. Prevention of infective endocarditis: guidelines from the American Heart Association Rheumatic Fever, Endocarditis, and Kawasaki Disease Committee, Council on Cardiovascular Disease in the Young, and the Council on Clinical Cardiology, Council on Cardiovascular Surgery and Anesthesia, and the Quality of Care and Outcomes Research Interdisciplinary Working Group. *Circulation.* 2007;116:1736–1754.)

Preventive measures to reduce the risk of IE (for those with cardiac conditions with the highest risk of adverse outcomes) consist of the following:

1. *Define the susceptible patient.* A careful medical history can disclose a susceptible patient. Health questioning should cover the history in all categories of risk. If any doubt exists, the patient's physician should be consulted.
2. *Provide oral hygiene instruction.* Oral hygiene should be practiced with methods that improve gingival health. In patients with significant gingival inflammation, oral hygiene should initially be limited to gentle procedures (i.e., oral rinses and gentle toothbrushing with a soft brush) to minimize bleeding. As gingival health improves, more definitive oral hygiene procedures can be initiated. Oral irrigators are usually not recommended because their use can induce bacteremia. Susceptible patients should be encouraged to maintain the highest level of oral hygiene to control soft tissue inflammation.
3. *Recommended antibiotic prophylactic regimens should be practiced with all high-risk patients during periodontal treatment* (Table 29.3). If any doubt regarding susceptibility exists, the patient's physician should be consulted. In patients who have been receiving continuous oral penicillin for secondary prevention of rheumatic fever, penicillin-resistant α-hemolytic streptococci are occasionally found in the oral cavity. An alternate regimen is recommended instead. If the patient is taking a systemic antibiotic, changes in the IE prophylaxis regimen may be indicated. For example, a patient taking a penicillin agent after regenerative therapy can be placed on azithromycin before the next periodontal procedure. Patients with **periodontitis grade C** (**aggressive periodontitis**) often have high levels of *A. actinomycetemcomitans* in the **subgingival plaque** (biofilm). This organism has been associated with IE and is often resistant to penicillins. In patients with periodontitis grade C (aggressive periodontitis) who warrant antibiotic prophylaxis, Slots and colleagues suggested using tetracycline (250 mg four times daily for 14 days) to eliminate or reduce *A. actinomycetemcomitans*, followed by the conventional prophylaxis protocol at the time of dental treatment.

TABLE 29.3 Recommended Antibiotic Prophylaxis Regimens for Periodontal/Dental Procedures in Patients at Risk for Infective Endocarditis (Single Dose 30–60 Minutes Prior to Procedure)

Regimen	Antibiotic	Adult Dosage	Child Dosage
Standard oral regimen	Amoxicillin	2.0 g	50 mg/kg
Regimen for patients unable to take oral medications	Ampicillin or	2.0 g IM or IV	50 mg/kg IM or IV
	Cefazolin or ceftriaxone	1.0 g IM or IV	50 mg/kg IM or IV
Alternate regimen[a] for patients allergic to penicillin or ampicillin (oral)	Cephalexin[b] or	2.0 g	50 mg/kg
	Azithromycin or clarithromycin or	500 mg	15 mg/kg
	Doxycycline	100 mg	2.2 mg/kg (<45 kg) 100 mg (>45 kg)
Regimen for patients unable to take oral medications and allergic to penicillin or ampicillin	Cefazolin or Ceftriaxone[a]	1.0 g IM or IV	

(Table updated according to Wilson WR, Gewitz M, Lockhart PB, et al. Prevention of viridans group streptococcal infective endocarditis: a scientific statement from the American Heart Association. *Circulation.* 2021;143(20):e963-e978.)

[a]Clindamycin is no longer recommended for antibiotic prophylaxis due to frequent and severe reactions compared to other antibiotics.

[b]Cephalosporins should not be used in patients with immediate-type hypersensitivity reactions (e.g., urticaria, angioedema, anaphylaxis) to penicillin or ampicillin.

4. *Periodontal treatment should be designed for susceptible patients to accommodate their degree of periodontal involvement.* The nature of periodontal therapy enhances the problems related to the prophylaxis of subacute IE. Patients are faced with long-term therapy, healing periods that extend beyond a 1-day antibiotic regimen, multiple visits, and procedures that easily elicit gingival bleeding.

The following guidelines can aid in the development of periodontal treatment plans for patients who are highly susceptible to IE:

- Periodontal disease is an **infection** with potentially wide-ranging systemic effects. For patients at risk for IE, every effort should be made to eliminate this infection. Teeth with severe periodontitis and a poor prognosis may require extraction. Teeth with less severe involvement in a motivated patient should be retained, treated, and monitored closely.
- All periodontal treatment procedures (including probing) require antibiotic prophylaxis; gentle oral hygiene methods are excluded. Pretreatment **chlorhexidine** rinses are recommended before all procedures, including periodontal probing, because these oral rinses significantly reduce the **bacteria** on mucosal surfaces.
- To reduce the number of visits required and thereby minimize the risk of developing resistant bacteria, numerous procedures can be accomplished at each appointment, depending on the patient's needs and ability to tolerate dental treatment.
- When possible, allow at least 7 days between appointments (preferably 10–14 days). If this is not possible, select an alternative antibiotic regimen for appointments within a 7-day period.
- Evidence does not support or refute a need to place patients at risk for IE on extended antibiotic regimens after treatment. Patients who have had periodontal surgery are not usually placed on antibiotics for the first week of healing unless there are specific indications to do so. If patients are placed on these regimens, the dosages are inadequate to prevent endocarditis during ensuing appointments. The standard prophylactic antibiotic dose is still needed. For example, if a patient was placed on 250 mg of amoxicillin three times a day for 10 days after periodontal surgery and was to return to the office for more treatment on the seventh day, the patient would require a full 2.0-g dose of amoxicillin before that treatment. Alternatively, clindamycin or azithromycin could be used at the second appointment.
- Regular recall appointments, with an emphasis on oral hygiene reinforcement and maintenance of periodontal health, are extremely important for patients susceptible to IE.

There may be instances when health care providers and patients do not agree with the stated guidelines. In these cases, clinicians must be familiar with and understand the guidelines in order to inform patients about risks and benefits of antibiotic prophylaxis. The decision to premedicate is made by the treating clinician in consultation with the patient's physician and based on the specific assessment and needs of the individual patient at the time.

Cerebrovascular Accident

A CVA or stroke is caused by ischemic changes such as a cerebral thrombosis from an embolus or a hemorrhagic phenomenon. Hypertension and **atherosclerosis** are predisposing factors for CVA and should alert the clinician to evaluate the patient's medical history carefully for the possibility of early cerebrovascular insufficiency and to be aware of symptoms of the disease. A physician's referral should precede periodontal therapy if the signs and symptoms of early cerebrovascular insufficiency are evident.

To prevent a repeat stroke, active infections should be treated aggressively because even a minor infection can alter blood coagulation and trigger thrombus formation and ensuing cerebral infarction. The clinician should counsel the patient about maintaining periodontal health and the importance of thorough oral hygiene (biofilm control). Poststroke weakness of the facial area or paralysis of extremities can make oral hygiene procedures extremely difficult. The clinician may need to modify oral hygiene instruments for ease of use, perhaps in consultation with an occupational therapist. Long-term chlorhexidine rinses greatly aid in biofilm control.

Dental clinicians should treat post-CVA patients with the following guidelines:

1. No periodontal therapy (except for an emergency) should be performed for 6 months after CVA because of the high risk of recurrence during this period.
2. After 6 months, periodontal therapy can be performed during short appointments with an emphasis on minimizing stress. Profound local anesthesia should be obtained, using the minimal effective dose of local anesthetic agents. Concentrations of epinephrine greater than 1:100,000 are contraindicated.
3. Light conscious sedation (i.e., inhalation, oral, or **parenteral**) can be used for anxious patients. Supplemental oxygen is indicated to maintain thorough cerebral oxygenation.
4. Stroke patients are frequently placed on oral anticoagulants. Previously, it was thought that for procedures entailing significant bleeding, such as periodontal surgery or tooth extraction, the anticoagulant regimen might need adjustment to lower the risk of bleeding. However, evidence regarding the risks of altering anticoagulation therapy suggests that it is safer and more prudent to provide treatment without changing it (see Antiplatelet and Anticoagulant Therapies under Medications below). Any changes in anticoagulant therapy regimens for a stroke patient should only be done in consultation with the patient's physician.

5. Blood pressure should be monitored regularly. Recurrence rates for CVAs are high, as are the rates of associated functional deficits.
6. Dental clinicians are advised to locate and access the nearest stroke center that can screen patients for embolic versus hemorrhagic diagnosis. If screened early and diagnosed with a thromboembolic stroke, treatment with tissue plasminogen activator within 3 h can be lifesaving and decrease morbidity.

Endocrine Disorders

The endocrine system comprises a network of glands that produce and release **hormones** that regulate and control numerous physiologic functions from energy storage and consumption to tissue repair and maintenance and controlling responses. Alterations or disruptions in the normal functioning of the endocrine system can lead to various diseases and disorders, including diabetes mellitus, thyroid or parathyroid disorders, and adrenal insufficiency.

Diabetes

The patient with diabetes requires special precautions before periodontal therapy. Type 1 diabetes was formerly known as insulin-dependent diabetes, and type 2 diabetes was referred to as noninsulin-dependent diabetes. During the past decade, the medical management of diabetes has changed significantly in an effort to minimize the debilitating complications associated with this disease.

Blood glucose (i.e., glycemia) levels are more tightly managed through diet, oral agents, and insulin therapy.

If the clinician detects intraoral signs of undiagnosed or poorly controlled diabetes, a thorough history is indicated. The classic signs of diabetes include **polydipsia** (i.e., excessive thirst), **polyuria** (i.e., excessive urination), and **polyphagia** (i.e., excessive hunger, often with unexplained concurrent weight loss). If the patient has any of these signs or symptoms or the clinician suspects diabetes, further investigation with laboratory studies and physician consultation is indicated. Periodontal therapy has limited success in the setting of undiagnosed or poorly controlled diabetes.

If a patient is suspected of having undiagnosed diabetes, the following procedures should be performed:

1. Consult the patient's physician.
2. Analyze laboratory tests (Box 29.3), including fasting blood glucose and casual glucose test results.
3. Rule out acute orofacial infection or severe dental infection; if present, provide emergency care immediately.
4. Establish the best possible oral health through nonsurgical **debridement** of plaque (biofilm) and **calculus**. Institute oral hygiene instruction. Limit more advanced care until the diagnosis has been established and good glycemic control obtained.

If a patient is known to have diabetes, it is critical that the level of glycemic control be established before initiating periodontal treatment. The fasting glucose and casual glucose tests provide snapshots of the blood glucose concentration at the time the blood was drawn; these tests reveal nothing about long-term glycemic control. The primary test used to assess glycemic control is the glycated hemoglobin (Hb) assay, also called the HbA1c test (Box 29.4). This assay has been shown by a large international study to provide an accurate measure of the average blood glucose concentrations over the preceding 2–3 months. Fig. 29.2 is a simplified graphic representation of the data from that study depicting the average blood glucose concentrations for HbA1c values.

The therapeutic goal for many patients with diabetes is to achieve and maintain an HbA1c below 7%. Patients with well-controlled diabetes (HbA1c < 7%) usually respond to therapy in

BOX 29.3 Diagnostic Criteria for Diabetes Mellitus

Diabetes mellitus can be diagnosed by any one of the following laboratory methods. Initial results using any method must be confirmed on a subsequent day.

1. Fasting plasma glucose level ≥126 mg/dL (≥7.0 mmol/L). *Fasting* is defined as no caloric intake for at least 8 h. The normal fasting glucose level is 70–100 mg/dL.
2. Two-hour postprandial glucose level ≥200 mg/dL (≥11.1 mmol/L) during an oral glucose tolerance test. The test should be performed using a glucose load containing the equivalent of 75 g anhydrous glucose dissolved in water. The normal 2-h postprandial glucose level is <140 mg/dL.
3. Glycated hemoglobin (HbA1c) value ≥6.5% (≥48 mmol/L). The test should be performed in a laboratory using a method that is certified by the National Glycohemoglobin Standardization Program (NGSP) and standardized according to the Diabetes Control and Complications Trial (DCCT) assay.[a]
4. Random plasma glucose level ≥200 mg/dL (≥11.1 mmol/L) for a patient with classic symptoms of hyperglycemia or hyperglycemic crisis, which include polyuria, polydipsia, and unexplained weight loss. Blood for casual glucose testing can be drawn without regard to the time since the last meal.

[a]In the absence of unequivocal hyperglycemia, results should be confirmed by repeat testing.

(Data from American Diabetes Association. Classification and diagnosis of diabetes. *Diabetes Care.* 2021;44(suppl. 1):S15–S33.)

BOX 29.4 Laboratory Evaluation of Diabetes Control by Glycated Hemoglobin (HbA1c) Assay Values

Normal	4%–6%
Good diabetes control	<7%
Moderate diabetes control	7%–8%
Action suggested to improve diabetes control	>8%

(Data from American Diabetes Association. Classification and diagnosis of diabetes. *Diabetes Care.* 2021;44(suppl. 1):S15–S33.)

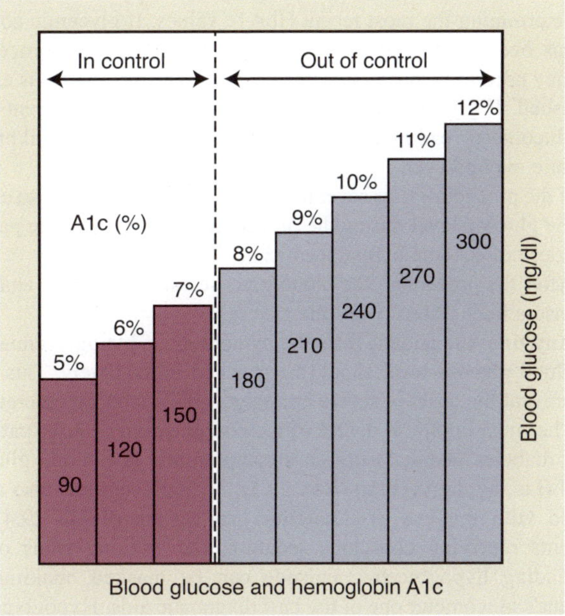

Fig. 29.2 Graphic representation of glycated hemoglobin (HbA1c) values that correspond to estimated average blood glucose levels.

a manner similar to nondiabetic individuals. Poorly controlled patients often have a poor response to treatment, with more postoperative complications and less favorable long-term results. Improvements in HBA1c values after periodontal therapy may provide an indication of the potential response.

Periodontal infection can worsen glycemic control and should be managed aggressively. Patients with diabetes and periodontitis should receive oral hygiene instructions, mechanical debridement to remove local factors, and regular maintenance. Periodontally hopeless teeth should also be extracted. When possible, HbA1c of less than 8% should be established before elective surgical treatment is performed. Systemic antibiotics are not needed routinely, although evidence indicates that tetracycline antibiotics in combination with **scaling** and **root planing** (root debridement) may positively influence glycemic control. If the patient has poor glycemic control and surgery is absolutely needed, prophylactic antibiotics can be given; penicillins are most often used for this purpose. Frequent reevaluation after active therapy is needed to assess treatment response and prevent recurrence of periodontitis.

Almost all patients with diabetes use a glucometer for blood glucose self-monitoring. These devices use capillary blood from a fingerstick to provide blood glucose readings in seconds. Patients with diabetes should be asked whether they have a glucometer and how often they use it. Because these devices provide instantaneous assessment of blood glucose, they are highly beneficial in the dental office environment. The following guidelines should be observed:

1. Patients should be asked to bring their glucometer to the dental office at each appointment.
2. Patients should check their blood glucose before any long procedure to obtain a baseline level. Patients with a blood glucose level at or below the lower end of normal before the procedure may become hypoglycemic intraoperatively. It is advisable to have the patient consume some carbohydrate before starting treatment. For example, if a 2-h procedure is planned and the pretreatment glucose level is 70 mg/dL (i.e., lower end of normal range), providing 4 ounces of juice preoperatively may help prevent hypoglycemia during treatment. If the pretreatment glucose level is excessively high, the clinician should determine whether the patient's glycemic control has been poor recently. This can be done with thorough patient questioning and by determining the most recent HbA1c values. If glycemic control has been poor over the preceding few months, the procedure may need to be postponed until better glycemic control is established. If glycemic control has been good and the current high glucometer reading is a fairly isolated event, the surgical procedure may proceed.
3. If the procedure lasts several hours, it is often beneficial to check the glucose level during the procedure to ensure that the patient does not become hypoglycemic.
4. After the procedure, the blood glucose can be checked again to assess fluctuations over time.
5. Any time the patient feels the symptoms of hypoglycemia, the blood glucose level should be checked immediately. This may prevent the onset of severe hypoglycemia, a medical emergency.

The most common dental office complication seen in patients with diabetes taking insulin is a symptomatic low blood glucose level (i.e., hypoglycemia) (Box 29.5). Hypoglycemia is also associated with the use of numerous oral agents (Table 29.4). In patients receiving conscious sedation, the warning signs of an impending hypoglycemic episode can be masked, making the patient's glucometer one of the best diagnostic aids. Hypoglycemia does not usually occur until the blood glucose level falls below 60 mg/dL. However, in patients with poor glycemic control who have prolonged hyperglycemia (i.e., high blood glucose levels), a rapid drop in glucose can precipitate signs and symptoms of hypoglycemia at levels well above 60 mg/dL.

As medical management of diabetes has intensified, the incidence of severe hypoglycemia has risen. The clinician should question

BOX 29.5 Signs and Symptoms of Hypoglycemia

Shakiness or tremors	Dizziness
Confusion	Feeling of impending doom
Agitation and anxiety	Unconsciousness
Sweating	Seizures
Tachycardia	

TABLE 29.4 Oral Agents Used for the Management of Diabetes

Agent	Action	Risk of Hypoglycemia[a]
Sulfonylureas (1st gen): Chlorpropae, Tolbutamide, Tolazamide	Stimulate pancreatic insulin secretion	++
Sulfonylureas (2nd gen): Glyburide, Glipizide	Stimulate pancreatic insulin secretion	+++
Sulfonylureas (3rd gen): Glimepiride	Stimulate pancreatic insulin secretion	+
Meglitinides: Repaglinide, Nateglinide	Stimulate rapid pancreatic insulin secretion (different mechanism from sulfonylureas)	+
Biguanides: Metformin	Block production of glucose by liver; improve tissue sensitivity to insulin	–
Thiazolidinedione: Rosiglitazone, Pioglitazone	Improve tissue sensitivity to insulin	–
α-Glucosidase inhibitors: Acarbose, Miglitol	Slow absorption of some carbohydrates from gut, decreasing postprandial peaks in glycemia	–
Dipeptidyl peptidase-4 (DPP-4) inhibitors: Sitagliptin, Saxagliptin, Alogliptin, Linagliptin	Inhibit the enzyme DPP-4; enable the pancreas to produce more insulin but only after food ingestion	–
Sodium-glucose co-transporter 2 (SGLT-2) inhibitors: Canagliflozin, Dapagliflozin, Empagliflozin	Inhibit reabsorption of glucose in the kidney	–
Combination agents	Combine two different oral agents into single drug	Risk depends on which drugs are combined

[a]Hypoglycemia risk: +++, high; ++, moderate; +, low; –, none.

TABLE 29.5 Types of Insulin

Type	Classification	ACTIVITY Onset	Peak	Duration
Lispro (Humalog), aspart (Novolog), glulisine (Apidra)	Rapid-acting	15 min	30–90 min	<5 h
Regular R or Novolin R, Velosulin (used in insulin pump)	Short-acting	30–60 min	2–3 h	3–6 h
			1–2 h	2–3 h
NPH (N), Humulin N, Novolin N	Intermediate-acting	2–4 h	4–12 h	14–18 h
Insulin detemir (Levemir)	Long-acting	1–2 h	Relatively flat (fairly even over 24 h)	Up to 24 h
Glargine (Lantus, Basaglar); Glargine U-300 (Toujeo)	Long-acting	6–8 h	There is no peak	20–24+ h
Degludec (Tresiba U-100 or U-200)	Long-acting	4–6 h	There is no peak	24 h

patients about past episodes of hypoglycemia. Hypoglycemia is more common in patients with better glycemic control. When planning dental treatment, it is best to schedule appointments before or after periods of peak insulin activity. This requires knowledge of the pharmacodynamics of the drugs. Patients taking insulin are at greatest risk, followed by those taking sulfonylurea agents. Oral agents such as metformin, thiazolidinediones, α-glucosidase inhibitors, dipeptidyl peptidase 4 (DPP-4) inhibitors, and sodium-glucose cotransporter-2 (SGLT-2) inhibitors usually do not cause hypoglycemia (see Table 29.4). Likewise, injectable agents known as incretin mimetics (exenatide; liraglutide; albiglutide) generally do not cause hypoglycemia.

Insulins are classified as rapid-acting, short-acting, intermediate-acting, or long-acting agents (Table 29.5). The categories vary in onset, peak, and duration of activity. It is important that the clinician establish exactly which insulin the patient takes, the amount, the number of times per day, and the time of the last dose. Periodontal treatment often can be timed to avoid peak insulin activity. Many patients with diabetes take multiple injections each day, in which case it is difficult, if not impossible, to avoid peak insulin activity. Checking the pretreatment glucose with the patient's glucometer, checking again during a long procedure, and checking again at the end of the procedure provides a better understanding of the patient's insulin pharmacodynamics and can help prevent hypoglycemia.

If hypoglycemia occurs during dental treatment, therapy should be immediately terminated. If a glucometer is available, the blood glucose level should be checked. Treatment guidelines include the following:

1. Provide approximately 15 g of oral carbohydrate to the patient:
   - 4–6 ounces of juice or soda
   - 3–4 teaspoons of table sugar
   - Hard candy with 15 g of sugar
2. If the patient is unable to take food or drink by mouth or if the patient is sedated:
   - Give 25–30 mL of 50% dextrose intravenously, which provides 12.5–15.0 g of dextrose, or
   - Give 1 mg of glucagon intravenously (i.e., glucagon results in rapid release of stored glucose from the liver), or
   - Give 1 mg of glucagon intramuscularly or subcutaneously (if no intravenous access).

Emergencies resulting from hyperglycemia are rare in the dental office. They usually take days to weeks to develop. However, the glucometer may be used to rule out hyperglycemic emergencies such as diabetic ketoacidosis, a life-threatening event.

Because periodontal therapy can render the patient unable to eat for some time, adjustment in insulin or oral agent dosages may be required. It is critical that patients eat a normal meal before dental treatment. Taking insulin without eating is the primary cause of hypoglycemia. If the patient is restricted from eating before treatment (e.g., for conscious sedation), normal insulin doses need to be reduced. As a general guideline, *well-controlled patients with diabetes undergoing routine periodontal treatment may take their normal insulin doses as long as they also eat their normal meal.* If the procedure is going to be particularly long, the insulin dose before treatment may need to be reduced. Likewise, if the patient will have dietary restrictions after treatment, insulin or sulfonylurea dosages may need to be reduced.

Consultation with the patient's physician is prudent and allows both practitioners to review the proposed treatment plan and determine whether modifications are needed. When periodontal surgery is indicated, it is usually best to limit the size of the surgical field so that the patient will be comfortable enough to resume a normal diet immediately.

Thyroid and Parathyroid Disorders

Periodontal therapy requires minimal alterations for the patient with adequately managed thyroid disease. Patients with *thyrotoxicosis* and those with inadequate medical management should not receive periodontal therapy until their condition is stabilized. Patients with a history of *hyperthyroidism* should be carefully evaluated to determine the level of medical management, and they should be treated in a way that limits stress and infection. Hyperthyroidism can cause tachycardia and other arrhythmias, increased cardiac output, and myocardial ischemia. Medications such as epinephrine and other vasopressor amines should be given with caution to patients with treated hyperthyroidism, although the small amounts used in dental anesthetics rarely cause problems. These drugs should not be given to patients with thyrotoxicosis or poorly controlled thyroid disorders. Patients with *hypothyroidism* require careful administration of sedatives and narcotics because of the potential for excessive sedation.

Routine periodontal therapy can be provided to patients with parathyroid disease after the disorder has been identified and the proper medical treatment given. However, patients who have not received medical care may have significant renal disease, uremia, and hypertension. If hypercalcemia or hypocalcemia exists, the patient may be more prone to cardiac arrhythmias.

Adrenal Insufficiency

Acute adrenal insufficiency is associated with significant morbidity and mortality rates as a result of peripheral vascular collapse and cardiac arrest. The periodontist should be aware of the clinical manifestations and ways of preventing acute adrenal insufficiency in patients with a history of *primary* adrenal insufficiency (i.e., Addison disease) or *secondary* adrenal insufficiency (i.e., most often caused by use of exogenous glucocorticosteroids).

The use of systemic corticosteroids is common in patients with allergic, endocrine, respiratory, joint, intestinal, neurologic, renal, liver, skin, or connective tissue disorders. Significant complications associated with corticosteroid use include alterations in glucose metabolism (i.e., steroid-induced diabetes), increased risk of infection, altered wound healing, osteoporosis, skin disorders, cataracts, glaucoma, and suppression of the hypothalamic-pituitary-adrenal (HPA) axis. In the normal healthy patient, stress activates the HPA axis, stimulating increased endogenous cortisol production by the adrenal glands. **Exogenous** steroids may suppress the HPA axis and impair the patient's ability to respond to stress with increased endogenous cortisol production, leading to the potential for acute adrenal crisis. The degree of adrenal suppression depends on the drugs used, dose, duration of administration, time elapsed since steroid therapy was terminated, and route of administration.

It was common practice in the past to administer prophylactic systemic steroids before dental treatment for patients who were taking or had recently taken exogenous steroids. However, steroid supplementation may not be required for many periodontal procedures. *Adrenal crisis* is rare in dentistry, especially when associated with secondary adrenal suppression caused by steroid use. Shapiro and associates found that patients taking 5–20 mg/day of prednisone maintained at least some adrenal reserve after immediate termination of steroid therapy. Higher doses can suppress the adrenal glands to a greater degree. Although exogenous steroids can suppress normal adrenal cortisol secretion for an extended period, the ability of the adrenal gland to respond to stress can return quickly after termination of steroid therapy.

Despite its rarity, the severe consequences of adrenal crisis suggest caution in patient care. Before providing extensive dental treatment to a patient with a history of recent or current steroid use, physician consultation is indicated to determine whether the patient's treatment needs warrant supplemental steroids. Use of a stress-reduction protocol and profound local anesthesia helps minimize the physical and psychologic stress associated with therapy and reduce the risk of acute adrenal crisis.

Most individuals with adrenal insufficiency can receive routine dental treatment without the need for supplemental glucocorticosteroids. Patients currently taking corticosteroids usually have enough exogenous and endogenous cortisol to handle routine dental procedures if their usual dose is taken within 2 h of the planned procedure. For most patients, supplemental corticosteroid administration is not required when uncomplicated minor surgical procedures, including periodontal surgery, are performed with local anesthesia with or without sedation.

Individuals at risk for adrenal crisis requiring supplementation include those who are undergoing lengthy major surgical procedures, those expected to have significant blood loss, and those who have extremely low adrenal function. For these individuals, consultation with their physician and steroid supplementation is indicated. Low adrenal function can be identified with an adrenocorticotropic hormone (ACTH) stimulation test. A rapid assay is also available to determine the degree of adrenal reserve by measurement of serum cortisol levels 30 and 60 min after intravenous administration of synthetic corticotropin.

For the patient who is identified as being at risk, the need for corticosteroid prophylaxis depends on the drug used because of the variance in equivalent therapeutic doses.

Glucocorticosteroid coverage regimens vary, but most provide a twofold to fourfold increase in coverage, depending on the stress produced by the procedure. In an emergency situation, when testing is not possible, increasing the steroid dose before the procedure can decrease the chances of acute adrenal crisis.

Management of the patient in an acute adrenal insufficiency crisis is as follows:

1. Terminate periodontal treatment.
2. Summon medical assistance.
3. Give oxygen.
4. Monitor vital signs.
5. Place the patient in a supine position.
6. Administer 100 mg of hydrocortisone sodium succinate (Solu-Cortef) intravenously over 30 s or intramuscularly.

Hemorrhagic Disorders

Patients with a history of bleeding problems caused by disease or drugs should be managed to minimize the risks of hemorrhage. Identification of these patients through the health history, clinical examination, and clinical laboratory tests is paramount. Health questioning should cover (1) the history of bleeding after previous surgery or trauma, (2) past and current drug history, (3) history of bleeding problems among relatives, and (4) illnesses associated with potential bleeding problems.

Clinical examination can detect jaundice, ecchymosis, spider telangiectasia, hemarthrosis, petechiae, hemorrhagic vesicles, spontaneous gingival bleeding, and gingival enlargement. Laboratory tests include methods to measure the hemostatic, coagulation, or lytic phase of the clotting mechanism, depending on clues regarding which phase is involved (Table 29.6). These tests include bleeding time, tourniquet test, complete blood cell count, prothrombin time (PT), partial thromboplastin time (PTT), and coagulation time. Bleeding disorders are classified as coagulation disorders, thrombocytopenic purpuras, or nonthrombocytopenic purpuras.

Coagulation Disorders

The main inherited coagulation disorders include hemophilia A, hemophilia B, and von Willebrand disease (Table 29.7). *Hemophilia A* results in a deficiency of coagulation factor VIII, and the clinical severity of the disorder depends on the level of factor VIII remaining. Patients with severe hemophilia who have less than 1% of normal factor VIII levels can have severe bleeding on the slightest provocation, whereas those with more moderate hemophilia (i.e., 1%–5% of factor VIII) have less frequent spontaneous hemorrhage but still bleed with minimal trauma. Patients with mild hemophilia (i.e., 6%–30% of factor VIII) rarely bleed spontaneously but may still hemorrhage after severe trauma or during surgical procedures.

The clinician should consult the patient's physician before dental treatment to determine the risk of bleeding and treatment modifications required. To prevent surgical hemorrhage, a factor VIII level of at least 30% is needed. Parenteral 1-deamino-8-D-arginine vasopressin (DDAVP; desmopressin) can be used to raise factor VIII levels twofold to threefold in patients with mild or moderate hemophilia. DDAVP has the significant advantage of avoiding the risk of viral disease transmission from factor VIII infusion and is considered the drug of choice in responsive patients. Most patients with moderate or severe hemophilia require infusion of factor VIII concentrate before surgical procedures. Before 15, the risk of viral disease transmission from these infusions was high. Since then, virally safe, highly purified monoclonal **antibody** or recombinant **deoxyribonucleic acid (DNA)** factor VIII products have come into widespread use.

Hemophilia B (i.e., Christmas disease) results in a deficiency of factor IX. The severity of the disorder depends on the relative

TABLE 29.6 Laboratory Tests for Bleeding Disorders

HEMOSTATIC TESTS			
Vascular	**Platelet**	**Coagulation**	**Lysis**
1. Tourniquet test *N:* 10 petechiae *Abn:* >10 petechiae	1. Platelet count *N:* 150,000–300,000/mm^3 *Abn:* Thrombocytopenia occurs at <100,000/mm^3; clinical bleeding occurs at <80,000/mm^3; spontaneous bleeding occurs at <20,000/mm^3	1. PT measures extrinsic and common pathways: factors I, II, V, VII, and X. *N:* 11–14 s (depending on laboratory) measured against control PT reported as international normalized ratio (INR): *N:* INR = 1.0 *Abn:* INR > 1.5	1. Euglobulin clot lysis time *N:* <90 min *Abn:* >90 min
2. Bleeding time *N:* 1–6 min *Abn:* >6 min	2. Bleeding time 3. Clot retraction 4. Complete blood cell count	2. PTT measures intrinsic and common pathways: factors III, IX, XI, and low levels of factors I, II, V, X, and XII. *N:* 25–40 s (depending on laboratory) measured against control *Abn:* >1.5 times normal 3. Clotting (coagulation) time *N:* 30–40 min *Abn:* >1 h	
CLINICAL DISEASE ASSOCIATIONS			
Vascular (Capillary) Wall Defect	**Thrombocytopenia**		**Increase in Fibrinolytic Activity**
Rule out:	*Rule out:*	*All three tests:*	
Thrombocytopenia purpuras Telangiectasia Aspirin or NSAID therapy Leukemia Renal dialysis	Vascular wall defect Acute or chronic leukemia Aplastic anemia Liver disease Renal dialysis	Liver disease Warfarin therapy Aspirin or NSAID therapy Malabsorption syndrome or long-term antibiotic therapy (lack of vitamin K metabolism) PT: factor VII deficiency PTT: hemophilia Renal dialysis	

Abn, Abnormal; *N*, normal; *NSAID*, nonsteroidal antiinflammatory drug; *PT*, prothrombin time; *PTT*, partial thromboplastin time.

TABLE 29.7 Inherited Coagulation Disorders

Type	Prolonged	Normal	Treatment
Hemophilia A	PTT	PT Bleeding time	DDAVP factor VIII concentrate or cryoprecipitate Fresh frozen plasma Fresh whole blood ϵ-Aminocaproic acid (Amicar) Tranexamic acid
Hemophilia B	PTT	PT Bleeding time	Purified prothrombin complex concentrate Factor IX concentrates Fresh-frozen plasma
Von Willebrand disease	Bleeding time PTT Variable factor VIII deficiency	PT Platelet count	DDAVP factor VIII concentrate or cryoprecipitate

DDAVP, 1-Deamino-8-d-arginine vasopressin (desmopressin); *PT*, prothrombin time; *PTT*, partial thromboplastin time.

amount of existing factor IX. Surgical therapy requires a factor IX level of 30%–50%, which is usually achieved by administration of purified prothrombin complex concentrate or factor IX concentrate.

Von Willebrand disease results from a deficiency of von Willebrand factor, which mediates **adhesion** of platelets to the injured vessel walls and is required for primary hemostasis. Von Willebrand factor also carries the coagulant portion of factor VIII in the plasma. The disorder has three major subtypes, with a wide range of clinical severity. Many cases of von Willebrand disease go undiagnosed, and bleeding during dental treatment may be the first sign of the underlying disease. More severe forms require preoperative factor VIII concentrate or cryoprecipitate infusion. Patients with milder forms respond favorably to administration of DDAVP before periodontal surgery or tooth extraction.

Periodontal treatment can be performed in patients with these coagulation disorders, provided that sufficient precautions are taken. Probing, scaling, and prophylaxis can usually be done without medical modification. More invasive treatment, such as local block anesthesia, root planing (root debridement), or surgery, dictates prior physician consultation.

During treatment, local measures to ensure clot formation and stability are of major importance. Complete wound closure and application of pressure can reduce hemorrhage. Antihemostatic agents, such as oxidized cellulose or purified bovine **collagen**, can be placed over surgical sites or into extraction sockets. The antifibrinolytic agent *ϵ-aminocaproic acid* (Amicar), given orally or intravenously, is a potent inhibitor of initial clot dissolution. *Tranexamic acid* is a more potent antifibrinolytic agent than Amicar and can prevent excessive oral hemorrhage after periodontal surgery and tooth extraction. It is available as an oral rinse and may be used alone or in combination with systemic tranexamic acid for several days after surgery.

Not all coagulation disorders are hereditary. Liver disease affects all phases of blood clotting because most coagulation factors are synthesized and removed by the liver. Long-term alcohol abusers or chronic hepatitis patients often demonstrate inadequate coagulation. Coagulation can be impaired by vitamin K deficiency, often caused by malabsorption syndromes, or by prolonged antibiotic administration, which alters the intestinal microflora that produces vitamin K. Dental treatment planning for patients with liver disease should include the following:

1. Physician consultation
2. Laboratory evaluations: PT, bleeding time, platelet count, and PTT (for patients in later stages of liver disease)
3. Conservative, nonsurgical periodontal therapy whenever possible
4. When surgery is required (may require hospitalization)
   - International normalized ratio (INR; PT) in the range of 2.0–3.0 is manageable.
   - Platelet count should be more than 80,000/mm^3.

Thrombocytopenic Purpuras

Thrombocytopenia is defined as a platelet count of less than 100,000/mm^3. Bleeding caused by thrombocytopenia can be seen with idiopathic thrombocytopenic purpuras, radiation therapy, myelosuppressive drug therapy (e.g., chemotherapy), leukemia, or infections. Purpuras are hemorrhagic diseases characterized by extravasation of blood into the tissues under the skin or mucosa, producing spontaneous petechiae (i.e., small red patches) or ecchymoses (i.e., bruises).

Periodontal therapy for patients with thrombocytopenia should be directed toward reducing inflammation by removing local irritants to avoid the need for more aggressive therapy. Oral hygiene instructions and frequent maintenance visits are paramount. Physician referral is indicated for a definitive diagnosis and to determine alterations in planned therapy. Scaling and root planing (root debridement) is usually safe unless the platelet count is less than 60,000/mm^3. No surgical procedure should be performed unless the platelet count is greater than 80,000/mm^3. Platelet transfusion may be required before surgery. Surgical technique should be as minimally invasive as possible, and local hemostatic measures should be applied.

Nonthrombocytopenic Purpuras

Nonthrombocytopenic purpuras result from vascular wall fragility or thrombasthenia (i.e., impaired platelet aggregation). Vascular wall fragility can result from hypersensitivity reactions, scurvy, infections, chemicals (e.g., phenacetin, aspirin), dysproteinemia, and other causes. Thrombasthenia occurs in uremia, Glanzmann disease, aspirin ingestion, and von Willebrand disease. Both types of nonthrombocytopenic purpura can cause immediate bleeding after gingival injury. Treatment consists primarily of direct pressure applied for at least 15 min. This initial pressure should control the bleeding unless coagulation times are abnormal or reinjury occurs. Surgical therapy should be avoided until the qualitative and quantitative platelet problems are resolved.

Blood Dyscrasias

Numerous disorders of red and white blood cells can affect the course of periodontal therapy. Alterations in wound healing, bleeding, tissue appearance, and susceptibility to infection can occur. Clinicians should be aware of the clinical signs and symptoms of blood dyscrasias, availability of screening laboratory tests, and need for physician referral.

Leukemia

Altered periodontal treatment for patients with leukemia is based on their enhanced susceptibility to infections, bleeding tendency, and effects of chemotherapy. The treatment plan for leukemia patients is as follows:

1. Refer the patient for medical evaluation and treatment. Close coordination with the physician is required.
2. Before chemotherapy, a complete periodontal treatment plan should be developed with a physician.
   - Monitor hematologic laboratory values daily: bleeding time, coagulation time, PT, and platelet count.
   - Administer antibiotic coverage before periodontal treatment because infection is a major concern.
   - If systemic conditions allow, extract all hopeless, nonmaintainable, or potentially **infectious** teeth at least 10 days before the initiation of chemotherapy.
   - Root debridement (i.e., scaling and root planing) should be performed and thorough oral hygiene instructions given if the patient's condition allows.
   - Twice-daily rinsing with 0.12% chlorhexidine gluconate is recommended after oral hygiene procedures.
   - Recognize the potential for bleeding caused by thrombocytopenia. Use pressure and topical hemostatic agents as indicated.
3. During the acute phases of leukemia, patients should receive only emergency periodontal care. Any source of potential infection must be eliminated to prevent systemic dissemination. Antibiotic therapy is frequently the treatment of choice, combined with nonsurgical or surgical debridement as indicated.
4. Oral ulcerations and mucositis are treated palliatively with agents such as viscous lidocaine. Systemic antibiotics may be indicated to prevent secondary infection.
5. Oral **candidiasis** is common in patients with leukemia and can be treated with nystatin suspension (400,000–600,000 U/mL four times daily) or clotrimazole vaginal suppositories (10 mg four or five times daily).
6. For patients with chronic leukemia and those in remission, scaling and root planing (root debridement) can be performed without complication, but periodontal surgery should be avoided if possible. Platelet count and bleeding time should be measured on the day of the procedure. If either is low, postpone the appointment and refer the patient to a physician.

Agranulocytosis

Patients with agranulocytosis (i.e., cyclic neutropenia and granulocytopenia) have an increased susceptibility to infection. The total white blood cell count is reduced, and granular **leukocytes** (i.e., **neutrophils**, eosinophils, and basophils) are reduced in number or disappear. These disorders are often marked by early, severe periodontal destruction. When possible, periodontal treatment should be done during periods of disease remission. At such times, treatment should be as conservative as possible while reducing potential sources of systemic infection. After physician consultation, severely affected teeth should be extracted. Oral hygiene instruction should include chlorhexidine rinses twice daily. Scaling and root planing (root debridement) should be performed carefully under antibiotic protection.

Renal Diseases

The most common causes of renal failure are glomerulonephritis, pyelonephritis, kidney cystic disease, renovascular disease, drug **nephropathy**, obstructive uropathy, and hypertension. Renal failure can result in severe electrolyte imbalance, cardiac arrhythmias, pulmonary congestion, CHF, and prolonged bleeding. Because the dental management of patients with renal disease may need to be drastically altered, physician consultation is necessary to determine the stage of renal disease, regimen for medical management, and alterations in periodontal therapy. The patient in chronic renal failure has a progressive disease that ultimately may require kidney transplantation or dialysis. It is preferable to treat the patient before transplantation or dialysis.

The following treatment modifications should be made:

1. Consult the patient's physician.
2. Monitor BP; patients in end-stage renal failure are usually hypertensive.
3. Check laboratory values: PTT, PT, bleeding time, and platelet count; hematocrit; blood urea nitrogen (do not treat if >60 mg/dL); and serum creatinine (do not treat if >1.5 mg/dL).
4. Eliminate areas of oral infection to prevent systemic infection.
   - Good oral hygiene should be established.
   - Periodontal treatment should aim at eliminating inflammation or infection and providing easy maintenance. Questionable teeth should be extracted if medical parameters permit.
   - Frequent recall appointments should be scheduled.
5. Drugs that are nephrotoxic or metabolized by the kidney should not be given (e.g., phenacetin, tetracycline, aminoglycoside antibiotics, nonsteroidal antiinflammatory drugs [NSAIDs]). Acetaminophen may be used for **analgesia** and diazepam for sedation. Local anesthetics such as lidocaine are usually safe.

The patient who is receiving dialysis requires modifications in treatment planning. The three modes of dialysis are intermittent peritoneal dialysis (IPD), chronic ambulatory peritoneal dialysis (CAPD), and hemodialysis. Only hemodialysis patients require special precautions. They have a high incidence of viral hepatitis, anemia, and prolonged hemorrhage. The risk of hemorrhage is related to anticoagulation during dialysis, platelet trauma from dialysis, and the uremia that develops with renal failure. Hemodialysis patients have an internal arteriovenous fistula or an external arteriovenous shunt. The shunt is often located in the arm and must be protected from trauma. In addition to guidelines for patients with chronic renal disease, the following recommendations are made for those receiving hemodialysis:

1. Screen for hepatitis B and hepatitis C **antigens** and antibodies before any treatment.
2. Provide antibiotic prophylaxis to prevent endarteritis of the arteriovenous fistula or shunt. IPD and CAPD patients do not usually require prophylactic antibiotics.
3. Patients receive heparin anticoagulation on the day of hemodialysis. Periodontal treatment should be provided on the day *after* dialysis, when the effects of heparinization have subsided. Hemodialysis treatments are usually performed three or four times per week. (IPD and CAPD patients are not systemically heparinized; they usually do not have the potential bleeding problems associated with hemodialysis.)
4. The hemodialysis shunt or fistula must be protected when the patient is in the dental chair. If the shunt or fistula is placed in the arm, do not cramp the limb; *blood pressure readings should be taken from the other arm.* Do not use the limb for the injection of medication. Patients with leg shunts should avoid sitting with the leg dependent for longer than 1 h. If the appointment lasts longer, allow the patient to walk about for a few minutes, then resume therapy.
5. Refer the patient to the physician if uremic problems develop, such as uremic **stomatitis**. To prevent systemic dissemination, refer to the physician if oral infections do not resolve promptly.

The renal transplant patient's greatest foe is infection. Transplant recipients take immunosuppressive drugs that greatly reduce resistance to infection. Excessive bleeding can occur during or after periodontal treatment because of drug-induced thrombocytopenia or anticoagulation, or both. A **periodontal abscess** is a potentially life-threatening situation, and a dental team approach should be used *before* transplantation to determine which teeth can be easily maintained. Many organ transplantation centers include dental examination in their standard protocols. Teeth with severe bone and attachment loss, **furcation** invasion, periodontal abscesses, or extensive surgical requirements should be extracted, leaving an easily maintainable dentition. In addition to the recommendations for patients with chronic renal failure, the following should be considered for the renal transplant recipient:

1. Hepatitis B and C screening.
2. Determination of the level of immune system compromise resulting from antirejection drug therapy.
3. Prophylactic antibiotics using AHA recommendations or a specific regimen based on physician consultation; not all transplant recipients require antibiotic coverage, and physician consultation is warranted before prescribing.

Liver Diseases

Liver diseases range from mild conditions to complete liver failure. Major causes of liver disease include drug toxicity, cirrhosis, viral infections (e.g., hepatitis B, hepatitis C), neoplasms, and biliary tract disorders. Because the liver is the site of production of most clotting factors, excessive bleeding during or after periodontal treatment can occur in patients with severe liver disease. Many drugs are metabolized in the liver, and liver disease alters normal drug metabolism. Treatment recommendations for patients with liver disease include the following:

1. Consultation with the physician concerning the current stage of disease, risk of bleeding, potential drugs to be prescribed during treatment, and required alterations to periodontal therapy.
2. Screening for hepatitis B and C.
3. Laboratory values for PT and PTT.
4. Laboratory values for INR.

For the liver transplant recipient, as with kidney and other organ transplantation, infection is a major concern. Patients take immunosuppressive drugs that greatly reduce resistance to infection. Excessive bleeding can occur during or after periodontal treatment because of drug-induced thrombocytopenia, anticoagulation, or both. Dental or periodontal infections are potentially life-threatening. A pretransplantation evaluation is recommended to determine which teeth can be maintained without risk of infection. Teeth with severe bone and attachment loss, furcation invasion, periodontal abscesses, or extensive surgical requirements should be extracted.

Pulmonary Diseases

The periodontal treatment of a patient with pulmonary disease may require alteration, depending on the nature and severity of the respiratory problem. Pulmonary diseases range from obstructive lung diseases (e.g., asthma, emphysema, bronchitis, acute obstruction) to restrictive ventilatory disorders caused by muscle weakness, scarring, obesity, or any condition that can interfere with effective lung ventilation. Combined restrictive-obstructive lung disease may also develop.

The clinician should be aware of the signs and symptoms of pulmonary disease, such as increased respiratory rate, cyanosis, clubbing of the fingers, chronic cough, chest pain, hemoptysis, dyspnea or orthopnea, and wheezing. Patients with any of these problems should be referred for medical evaluation and treatment. Most patients with chronic lung disease can undergo routine periodontal therapy if they are receiving adequate medical management. Caution should be practiced in relation to any treatment that may depress respiratory function.

Acute respiratory distress can be caused by slight airway obstruction or depression of respiratory function. Because of limited vital lung capacity, patients also have decreased cough effectiveness. They must continually deal with the mental anxiety caused by air hunger and alter their position in attempts to improve their ventilatory efficiency.

The following guidelines should be used during periodontal therapy:

1. Identify and refer patients with signs and symptoms of pulmonary disease to their physician.
2. For patients with known pulmonary disease, consult with their physician regarding medications (e.g., antibiotics, steroids, chemotherapeutic agents) and the degree and severity of pulmonary disease.
3. Avoid elicitation of respiratory depression or distress:
   - Minimize the stress of a periodontal appointment. The patient with emphysema should be treated in the afternoon, several hours after sleep, to allow for airway clearance.
   - Avoid medications that could cause respiratory depression (e.g., narcotics, sedatives, general anesthetics).
   - Avoid bilateral mandibular block anesthesia, which could cause increased airway obstruction.
   - Position the patient to allow maximal ventilatory efficiency, be careful to prevent physical airway obstruction, keep the patient's throat clear, and avoid excess periodontal packing.
4. For a person with a history of asthma, especially if asthma attacks are frequent, make sure the patient's medication (inhaler) is available. The inhaler should be readily accessible on the countertop in the dental treatment room.
5. Patients with active fungal or bacterial respiratory diseases should not be treated unless the periodontal procedure is an emergency.

Medications

Some medications that are prescribed to cure, manage, or prevent diseases may have effects on periodontal tissues, wound healing, or the host immune response that need to be recognized, considered, and possibly modified for treatment. The following medication categories are briefly addressed: bisphosphonates and antiresorptive agents, antiplatelet and anticoagulation therapies, and corticosteroids. Additional information and advice can be found in other sources.

Bisphosphonates and Antiresorptive Agents

Bisphosphonate medications are used to treat metastatic cancer or multiple myeloma via intravenous (IV) administration. They are commonly used to treat osteoporosis via oral and IV administration, albeit with less frequency and lower doses. They act by inhibiting osteoclastic activity, which leads to less bone resorption, **remodeling**, and turnover. Bisphosphonates are used in cancer treatment to prevent the often-lethal imbalance of osteoclastic activity. In the treatment of osteoporosis, the goal is to harness osteoclastic activity to minimize or prevent bone loss. The major difference between these applications is the potency and route of administration. Potency is influenced by the chemical properties and pharmacokinetics of these agents in bone. Other nonbisphosphonate antiresorptive agents such as denosumab are also associated with osteonecrosis of the jaw.

Denosumab (Prolia, Xgeva) is an antiresorptive agent used to treat osteoporosis. It is a fully human monoclonal antibody that binds the **cytokine RANKL (receptor activator of NFκβ** ligand), which is an essential factor that initiates bone turnover. RANKL blocks **osteoclast** maturation and activity-reducing bone resorption. Thus, denosumab reduces bone resorption.

Although other terms have been suggested and used, the term antiresorptive agent-induced osteonecrosis of the jaw (ARONJ) is currently adopted and is now used to describe the nonhealing exposure of bone induced by bisphosphonates or other antiresorptive agents.

Romosozumab (Evenity) is an antiresorptive agent used to treat osteoporosis. It is a humanized monoclonal antibody that targets sclerostin, an osteocyte-derived **glycoprotein** that inhibits the Wnt signaling cascade and activation of **osteoblast** function, leading to inhibition of bone formation. Thus, romosozumab increases bone formation and reduces bone resorption. Initial animal studies suggest that the osteoporosis dose of romosozumab inhibits bone resorption without inducing ONJ-like lesions.

Clinically, ARONJ manifests as exposed **alveolar** bone occurring spontaneously or after a dental procedure. Individuals treated with high-potency, nitrogen-containing bisphosphonates, especially those administered intravenously for cancer treatment (e.g., zoledronate), appear to be at greater risk for ARONJ than individuals taking oral bisphosphonates or other antiresorptive agents for prevention and treatment of osteoporosis. In patients treated for cancer, the incidence ranges from 1% to 15%. Estimating the incidence for patients taking oral bisphosphonates for osteoporosis is more difficult but appears to range from 0.001% to 0.01%. Other reports suggest a slightly higher incidence that ranges from 0.004% to 0.11%. Even if this is an underestimation of the actual risk for individuals taking oral bisphosphonates, the incidence appears to be low. The risk for individuals treated with oral bisphosphonates for a period of less than 3 years appears to be minimal or very near zero. Regular use of oral bisphosphonates for a period greater than 3 years suggests a risk profile that increases with time and length of use.

As with many multifactorial diseases and conditions, it is likely that factors in addition to bisphosphonate therapy contribute to the individual risk of ARONJ. Potential comorbidity **risk factors** include systemic corticosteroid therapy, smoking, alcohol, poor oral hygiene, periodontal disease, chemotherapy, radiotherapy, diabetes, hematologic disease, and the concomitant use of antiresorptive agents with agents that inhibit angiogenesis. Reported treatment-related factors for ARONJ include extractions, root canal treatment, periodontal surgery, and dental **implant** surgery. Periodontal disease and treatment (especially surgery) poses a risk for patients treated with bisphosphonates or other antiresorptive medications. The bacteria-induced inflammatory process of periodontitis that causes bone resorption can lead to bone **necrosis**. Likewise, periodontal treatment can cause bone necrosis in the setting of bisphosphonates.

Caution is warranted for all patients treated with bisphosphonates or other antiresorptive agents.

Health care providers need to evaluate patients carefully, communicate with other medical health care providers, inform patients, and consider treatment options and risks carefully. A careful intraoral examination is prudent for all patients treated with intravenous or oral bisphosphonate therapy (or other antiresorptive agents) to determine whether bone exposure exists and to assess local conditions that may predispose them to ARONJ. A thorough medical history should be reviewed, evaluated, and annotated with details about bisphosphonate or other antiresorptive agent, including medication type, dose, route of administration, and duration. Comorbidities, such as previous and current medications, treatments, and existing disease or pathology, should be considered as well. Radiographs should be carefully evaluated for signs of ARONJ.

Marx suggested that a laboratory blood test for the serum C-terminal telopeptide fragment of type I collagen (CTX) could be used to assess an individual's risk of developing antiresorptive agent-induced ONJ. Marx reported that lower CTX values were associated with greater risk. It is important to recognize that these values are based on retrospective evaluation of patients with osteonecrosis of the jaws and that prospective studies to validate these findings have not been done. The CTX laboratory test is a measure of the specific C-terminal fragment of type I collagen cleaved by osteoclasts and indicates bone resorption activity. However, its use as a measure of the risk for ARONJ is controversial and not confirmed by prospective studies.

Optimal periodontal and oral health should be achieved and maintained for all patients. A thorough inspection of all intraoral tissues should be completed at each periodontal recall maintenance visit. For individuals treated with intravenous bisphosphonates, invasive surgical treatment should be avoided. Risks must be considered before treatment of individuals with a history of taking oral bisphosphonates or antiresorptive agents for longer than 3 years. This area of research will continue to evolve as the pathophysiology becomes better understood. Providers are encouraged to consult other sources for updates on this important topic.

Antiplatelet and Anticoagulant Therapies

Many patients with a variety of conditions are placed on antiplatelet or anticoagulant medications to prevent thrombosis (i.e., blood clotting) or thromboembolism (Table 29.8). Some patients are treated with a combination of these medications. Patients at risk who may be on antiplatelet or anticoagulant therapy include those with heart valve replacements, heart rhythm disorders, congenital heart defects, or those with a history or risk of myocardial infarction, stroke, or deep vein thrombosis. These patients are frequently placed on oral anticoagulants such as the vitamin K antagonists (VKAs) using coumarin derivatives such as dicumarol and warfarin. Over the past decade, there has been increased use of a new class of novel oral anticoagulants (NOACs) or direct oral anticoagulants (DOACs) that have some advantages over VKAs. While antiplatelet and anticoagulant therapies are effective in reducing the risk of

TABLE 29.8 Antiplatelet and Anticoagulation Medications

Medication	Class	Mode of Action	Onset/Offset	Reversal
Aspirin	Antiplatelet	Impairs platelet aggregation via inhibition of thromboxane A_2 synthesis. Blocks production of prostaglandins via irreversibly inhibiting cyclooxygenase (COX)	Peak plasma concentration (uncoated 30–40 min; enteric coated 3–4 h)/half-life effect ~7–10 days	None
Clopidogrel (Plavix)	Antiplatelet	Active metabolite irreversibly blocks ADP $P2Y_{12}$ receptor preventing platelet activation	Peak plasma concentration (2 h)/half-life effect ~7 days	None
Prasugrel (Effient)	Antiplatelet	Active metabolite irreversibly blocks ADP $P2Y_{12}$ receptor preventing platelet activation	Peak plasma concentration (30 min)/half-life effect ~7 days	None
Ticagrelor (Brilinta)	Antiplatelet	Active metabolite reversibly binds to ADP $P2Y_{12}$ receptor preventing platelet activation	Peak plasma concentration (2–3 h)/half-life effect ~12–48 h	PB2452 potential reversal agent under investigation
Dabigatran (Pradaxa)	Direct oral anticoagulant	Direct thrombin inhibitor	Peak plasma concentration (0.5–2 h)/~24 h	Idarucizumab (Praxbind)
Apixaban (Eliquis)	Direct oral anticoagulant	Activated factor Xa inhibitor	Peak plasma concentration (1–2 h)/~24 h	Andexanet alfa (Andexxa)
Edoxaban (Savaysa)	Direct oral anticoagulant	Activated factor Xa inhibitor	Peak plasma concentration (1–2 h)/~24 h	Andexanet alfa (Andexxa)
Rivaroxaban (Xarelto)	Direct oral anticoagulant	Activated factor Xa inhibitor	Peak plasma concentration (2–4 h)/~24 h	Andexanet alfa (Andexxa)
Heparin (various)	Anticoagulant	Binds to enzyme inhibitor antithrombin III, which inactivates thrombin, Xa and other proteases	Onset of action (IV immediate; subcutaneous [SQ] 2–4 h)/duration of action ~2–6 h (IV) ~8–12 h (SQ)	Protamine
Warfarin (Coumadin)	Anticoagulant	Competitively inhibits the vitamin K epoxide reductase complex 1 (VKORC1), which depletes functional vitamin K reserves and reduces synthesis of active clotting factors II, VII, IX, and X	Onset of action (24–72 h)/duration of action ~2–5 days	Oral or IV vitamin K; fresh frozen plasma

thrombosis, they may increase the risk for bleeding complications in patients undergoing surgical procedures.

The traditional approach to managing surgery for patients on antiplatelet or anticoagulant therapy *was* to discontinue therapy about 3–5 days (antiplatelet therapy) or 7–10 days (anticoagulant therapy) before a planned surgical procedure, in consultation with the patient's physician. However, evidence regarding the care of patients on antiplatelet or anticoagulant therapy suggest that treating them (e.g., with periodontal surgery or extractions) without altering their antiplatelet or anticoagulant medications may be safer and does not lead to greater intraoperative or postoperative bleeding complications. The increased risk of morbidity and mortality for those discontinuing the antiplatelet or anticoagulant therapy may be significant.

Antiplatelet Medications

Many patients are taking oral antiplatelet medications to prevent vascular thrombosis. Aspirin is the most common of these and well known for its antiplatelet activity. It interferes with normal platelet aggregation by irreversibly acetylating cyclooxygenase-1, which inhibits thromboxane-A2 production and reduces platelet aggregation. The effects of aspirin last at least 4–7 days. The normal half-life for platelets is 7–10 days. Aspirin is typically used in small doses ≤325 mg per day, which can increase bleeding time.

Controlled clinical studies have demonstrated that intraoperative bleeding is not likely to be a problem with simple extractions or periodontal surgery if low-dose aspirin antiplatelet therapy is continued. In these studies, there were no episodes of uncontrolled bleeding, all bleeding was controlled with local measures, and there were no cases of postoperative bleeding problems. Conversely, the risk of stopping antiplatelet therapy may be serious.

Recent evidence suggests that discontinuing antiplatelet therapy may pose a risk of thrombus formation. A **metaanalysis** of 474 studies, including 49,590 patients evaluating the thromboembolic risk of discontinuing low-dose aspirin compared to the hemorrhagic risks of continuation for a variety of surgical procedures, including dental, found that discontinuing aspirin therapy resulted in thromboembolic complications, including death. The surgeons who were blinded to the aspirin status were unable to detect a difference in intraoperative bleeding and postoperative bleeding management was identical for both groups. A metaanalysis including 14,981 patients who either continued or discontinued low-dose aspirin in preparation for various surgical procedures revealed that 95 (0.6%) patients who discontinued aspirin experienced an acute vascular event. Fourteen (15.1%) of these were associated with dental surgery. Yet, another review and metaanalysis including 50,279 patients revealed that discontinuing aspirin had a detrimental effect. Thus, it is not advised to discontinue low-dose aspirin therapy prior to oral surgical procedures.

Clopidogrel (Plavix) is an oral antiplatelet medication that reduces platelet aggregation by irreversibly binding and inhibiting adenosine diphosphate (ADP) receptors on platelet **membranes**. In a prospective study of 192 patients, 5 of 91 patients (5.5%) who had antiplatelet therapy discontinued for surgery experienced an adverse cardiac event. None of the patients who continued antiplatelet therapy experienced an adverse event. The authors suggest that clopidogrel should not be stopped or altered prior to oral surgical procedures.

In a retrospective study of 222 patients receiving one or more extractions (75.7%) or other minor oral surgery (24.3%) with a history of taking antiplatelet medications including aspirin (n = 123; 55.4%), clopidogrel (n = 22; 9.9%), ticagrelor (n = 17; 7.7%), or dual antiplatelet therapy (n = 60; 27%), the overall frequency of bleeding was 4.9% (11 of 222). Postoperative bleeding frequency for aspirin, clopidogrel, ticagrelor, and dual antiplatelet therapy was 3.2%, 4.5%, 5.9%, and 8.3%, respectively, with no statistically significant difference between groups. None of the patients experienced prolonged bleeding. The practical implication of this review, according to published studies and guidelines, is that antiplatelet therapy should not be interrupted for extractions or minor oral surgery.

NSAIDs such as ibuprofen also inhibit platelet function. Because NSAIDs bind reversibly, the effect is transitory, lasting only a short time after the last drug dose. However, due to the antiplatelet effect, these medications should not be prescribed for patients who are receiving antiplatelet or anticoagulation therapy or who have an illness with bleeding tendencies.

Anticoagulant Medications

Oral anticoagulants are prescribed for a variety of conditions to prevent thromboembolic events. The most common oral anticoagulants are the VKAs, such as warfarin, that decrease production of vitamin K-dependent coagulation factors II, VII, IX, and X. The effectiveness of anticoagulation therapy is monitored by a PT laboratory test (PT/INR). The recommended level of therapeutic anticoagulation for most patients is an INR of 2.0–3.0, with prosthetic heart valve patients usually in the range of 2.5–3.5.

The traditional recommendations for surgical management of patients taking anticoagulants *was*:

1. Consult the patient's physician to understand medical problem and degree of anticoagulation.
2. Assess the risk of bleeding for the planned procedure and determine an acceptable INR level.
3. The dentist informs physician about anticipated risk of intraoperative and postoperative bleeding.
4. The physician must be consulted about any changes (i.e., discontinuing or reducing) in anticoagulant dosage.
5. The INR was checked on the day of surgery. If the INR was within the acceptable target range, the procedure was done and the anticoagulant resumed immediately after treatment.
6. Meticulous technique and complete wound closure were paramount. Application of cold pressure and other local measures were used to establish hemostasis (e.g., use of oxidized cellulose, microfibrillar collagen, topical thrombin, and tranexamic acid).

Discontinuing anticoagulant therapy before dental surgery *was* common in the past. However, it is no longer recommended because it poses significant risks for the patient. Evidence related to the risks of altering anticoagulant therapy and the lack of evidence for bleeding complications suggest that treating patients without reducing or discontinuing medications is safe. Specifically, international guidelines, clinical trials, and reviews suggest that **dentoalveolar** surgical procedures can be safely completed for patients with an INR ≤ 3.5.

Clinical studies of patients on anticoagulant therapy undergoing extractions and other oral surgical procedures have demonstrated minimal bleeding problems when anticoagulant therapy is continued. In a review of the literature, Wahl and colleagues reported that only 12 of 950 patients (<1.3%) receiving continuous anticoagulant therapy required more than local measures to control hemorrhage after 2400 minor oral surgical procedures. Most of the 950 patients had anticoagulation levels that were well above currently recommended therapeutic levels. Only three patients (<0.31%) had anticoagulation levels within or below currently recommended therapeutic levels. In contrast, 5 of 526 patients (0.95%) who experienced 575 interruptions of continuous anticoagulant therapy suffered serious embolic complications; four patients died.

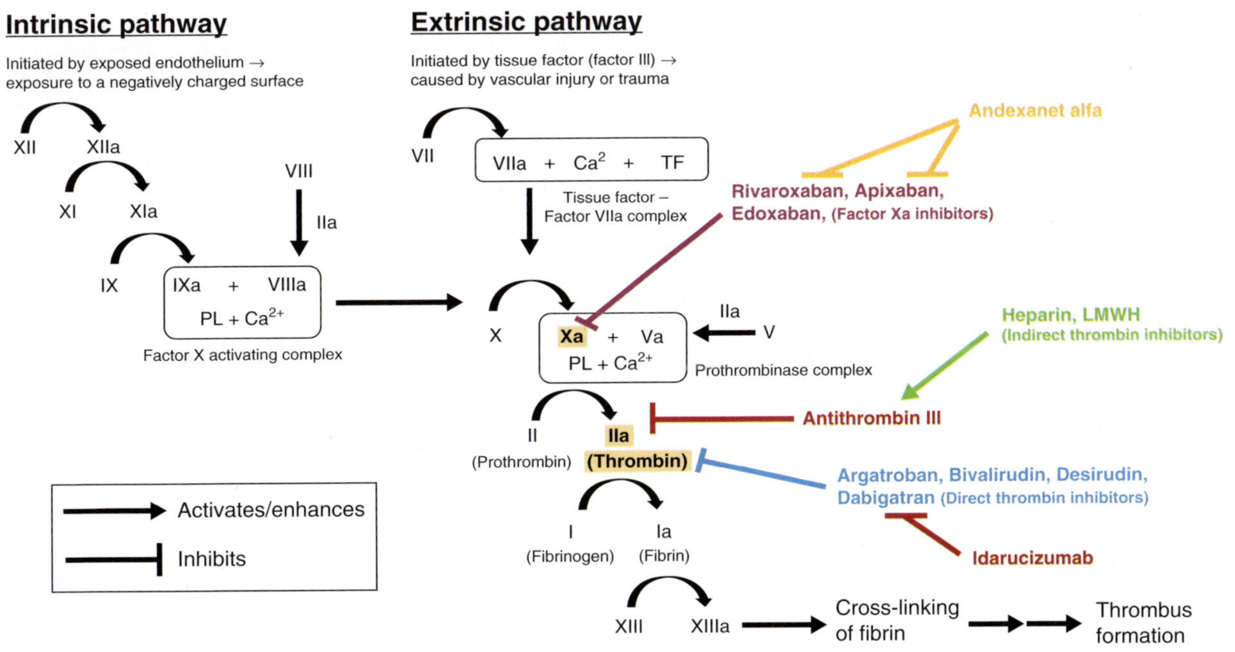

Fig. 29.3 Diagram of the intrinsic and extrinsic coagulation pathways showing factors that are inhibited by various anticoagulation medications.

In a prospective study of 131 patients undergoing 511 extractions, those patients whose oral anticoagulant therapy was reduced 72 h before surgery to achieve an INR of 1.5–2.0 (target INR, 1.8) had postoperative bleeding that warranted subsequent local intervention in 10 of 66 patients (15.1%). Postoperative bleeding occurred in only 6 of 65 patients (9.2%) in the group that continued the regular dosage of oral anticoagulant therapy (mean INR, 2.9).

DOACs are medications that inhibit specific activated clotting factors IIa and Xa (Fig. 29.3). They are also known as NOACs or target-specific oral anticoagulants (TSOACs). However, according to the International Society of Thrombosis and Haemostasis, the preferred nomenclature for these medications is DOACs.

This relatively new class of oral anticoagulants includes dabigatran (Pradaxa), rivaroxaban (Xarelto), apixaban (Eliquis), and edoxaban (Savaysa) (see Table 29.8). They act by directly inhibiting an activated clotting factor, either IIa or Xa. Since being approved, physicians are prescribing them more and more as alternatives to the VKA anticoagulant medications. The most significant advantages of these DOACs over VKAs are their predictable pharmacology, limited interaction with other drugs, and rapid onset and offset of activity. The pharmacokinetic and pharmacodynamic properties are more predictable so routine PT testing is not required. Reversal agents are now available for DOACs. Idarucizumab (Praxbind) is the reversal agent for dabigatran (Pradaxa). Andexanet alfa (Andexxa) is the reversal agent for apixaban (Eliquis), edoxaban (Savaysa), and rivaroxaban (Xarelto).

There are a limited number of studies reporting the risks of bleeding associated with continuing DOAC therapy versus the risks of thromboembolic complications associated with discontinuing them. In a prospective clinical comparative study aimed to analyze postoperative bleeding risk in patients continuing their anticoagulation therapy while undergoing dental implant surgery and bone grafting procedures, there were no postoperative bleeding problems reported for patients taking DOACs. A retrospective study including 100 patients (64 with comorbidities; 50% with diabetes) undergoing tooth extraction according to the European Heart Rhythm Association protocol (i.e., continuation of DOAC therapy for up to three extractions at the presumed time of DOAC trough concentration) reported only 4 of 64 patients (6.25%) with bleeding episodes in the comorbidity group (one moderate episode at 1 h after extraction and three mild episodes the day after extraction) and no bleeding episodes (0 of 36 patients) in the group without comorbidities. Another retrospective study including 120 patients who received 153 dental procedures while continuing or discontinuing NOACs reported 9 postoperative bleeding episodes in 153 treatments (5.88%). There was no difference in bleeding episodes between groups and all were managed with local measures.

A literature review, including nine studies evaluating bleeding risk in patients undergoing dental implant surgery while taking antiplatelet drugs, oral anticoagulants, or direct oral anticoagulants, found that postoperative bleeding occurred in 10 of 456 cases (2.2%). The bleeding incidence for those on antiplatelet therapy was 1 of 253 (0.4%). For those taking oral anticoagulants, the bleeding incidence was 6 of 105 (5.7%). The incidence of postoperative bleeding for patients taking direct oral anticoagulants was 3 of 90 (3.3%). The authors concluded that the evidence supports continuing antiplatelet, oral anticoagulant, or direct oral anticoagulant therapy during implant surgery.

These studies suggest that the risk of serious morbidity associated with discontinuing antiplatelet or anticoagulant therapy should be avoided and that the risk of bleeding while maintaining antiplatelet or anticoagulant therapy is minimal.

Patients on anticoagulation therapy should be treated while in the therapeutic range and clinicians must be knowledgeable about and prepared to use local hemostasis procedures. Oral anticoagulant therapy should be continued for periodontal/oral surgical procedures to avoid the risk of thromboembolic complications. It is advisable to request a preoperative PT test to assess the INR level close to the day of surgery (ideally, same day). Clinicians should plan surgical procedures with a minimally invasive approach and attention to local hemostatic measures in these patients to minimize bleeding complications.

Corticosteroids

Approximately 5% of adults in the United States habitually take corticosteroids for the treatment of various conditions, potentially putting them at risk for secondary adrenal insufficiency. Patients who habitually use corticosteroids have an increased likelihood of developing hypertension, osteoporosis, and peptic **ulcer** disease. Care should be taken to minimize the risk of adverse outcomes in these patients. Blood pressure should be monitored, and medications that may exacerbate peptic ulceration (e.g., aspirin, NSAIDs) should be avoided.

Stressful events, such as trauma, illness, surgery, emotional upset, or athletic events, normally increase circulating endogenous cortisol levels through stimulation of the HPA axis. Pain appears to increase the requirement for cortisol release. There is concern that the normal release of cortisol in response to a stressful event, such as a dental procedure, may be impaired in patients exposed to habitual corticosteroid use. The concern is about whether these patients require perioperative supplementation for dental procedures. Historically, recommendations were based on the type, amount, and duration of corticosteroid use. However, current thinking about the need for perioperative corticosteroid supplementation has been adjusted.

Studies investigating the stress response to minor general and oral surgical procedures concluded that significant increases in cortisol were usually not seen until 1–5 h after surgery and appeared to be associated more with postoperative pain and the loss of local anesthesia than with the preoperative and intraoperative stress of the procedure. Administration of adequate analgesics in the postoperative period can diminish the release (requirement) of cortisol.

Most individuals with adrenal insufficiency can receive routine dental treatment without the need for supplemental glucocorticosteroids. Patients taking corticosteroids usually have enough exogenous and endogenous cortisol to handle routine dental procedures if the usual dose is taken within 2 h of the planned procedure. For most patients, supplemental corticosteroid administration is not required when uncomplicated minor surgical procedures, including periodontal surgery, are performed with local anesthesia with or without sedation. Topical corticosteroids usually have minimal HPA effect, and steroid supplementation is not required for these patients.

Individuals at risk for adrenal crisis who require supplementation include those undergoing lengthy major surgical procedures, those expected to have significant blood loss, and those who have extremely low adrenal function. Low adrenal function can be identified with an ACTH stimulation test. For these individuals, consultation with the physician and steroid supplementation are indicated.

Cancer Therapies

Many patients are treated for various cancers. These treatments may involve surgery, chemotherapy, or radiation as stand-alone therapies or in combination. Cancer therapy can have adverse effects on the patient and may need special consideration or modifications for periodontal treatment. Chemotherapy and radiation therapy are briefly addressed in this section. Additional information and advice can be found in other sources.

Immunosuppression and Chemotherapy

Immunosuppressed patients have an impaired host defense as a result of an underlying immunodeficiency or use of drugs (primarily related to organ transplantation or cancer chemotherapy). Because chemotherapy is often cytotoxic to bone marrow, destruction of platelets and red and white blood cells results in thrombocytopenia, anemia, and leukopenia. Immunosuppressed individuals are at greatly increased risk for infection, and even minor periodontal infections can become life-threatening if immunosuppression is severe. Bacterial, viral, and fungal infections can manifest intraorally. Patients undergoing bone marrow transplantation require special attention because they receive extremely high-dose chemotherapy and are particularly susceptible to dissemination of oral infections.

Treatment should be directed toward prevention of oral complications that can be life-threatening. The greatest potential for infection occurs during periods of extreme immunosuppression; treatment should be conservative and palliative. It is always preferable to evaluate the patient before initiation of chemotherapy. Teeth with a poor prognosis should be extracted, with thorough debridement of remaining teeth to minimize the microbial load. The clinician must teach and emphasize the importance of good oral hygiene. Antimicrobial rinses, such as chlorhexidine, are recommended, especially for patients with chemotherapy-induced mucositis, to prevent secondary infection.

Chemotherapy is usually performed in cycles, with each cycle lasting several days, followed by intervening periods of myelosuppression and recovery. If periodontal therapy is needed during chemotherapy, it is best done the day *before* chemotherapy is given, when white blood cell counts are relatively high. Coordination with the oncologist is critical. Dental treatment should be done when the white blood cell count is above 2000/mm^3, with an absolute granulocyte count of 1000–1500/mm^3.

In consultation with the patient's physician, antibiotic premedication should be considered for any patient who is immunocompromised, including those who are undergoing chemotherapy.

Radiation Therapy

The use of radiotherapy, alone or in conjunction with surgical resection, is common in the treatment of head and neck tumors. The side effects of ionizing radiation include dramatic perioral changes of significant concern to dental health personnel. The extent and severity of mucositis, dermatitis, **xerostomia**, dysphagia, gustatory alteration, radiation **caries** (Fig. 29.4), vascular changes, trismus, **temporomandibular** joint degeneration, and periodontal changes depend on the type of radiation used, field of irradiation, number of ports, type of tissue in the field, and dosage.

Patients scheduled to receive head and neck radiation therapy require dental consultation *at the earliest possible time* to reduce the morbidity of known perioral side effects. Preirradiation treatment depends on the patient's prognosis, compliance, and residual dentition in addition to the field, ports, dose, and immediacy of radiotherapy. The initial visit should include panoramic and intraoral radiographs, a clinical dental examination, a periodontal evaluation, and a physician consultation. The physician should be asked about the type and amount of radiation to be administered, extent and location of the lesion, nature of surgical procedures already performed or to be performed, number of radiation ports, exact fields to be irradiated, mode of radiation therapy, and patient's prognosis (i.e., likelihood of metastasis). Preirradiation treatment should commence immediately after the physician consultation. The first decision should involve possible extractions because radiation can cause side effects that interfere with healing.

For head and neck **squamous cell carcinomas**, the radiation dose is usually 5000–7000 cGy (1 cGy = 1 rad) delivered in a fractionated method (150–200 cGy/day over a 6- to 7-week course). This is considered full-course radiation treatment, and the degree of perioral side effects depends on which tissues are irradiated (i.e., radiation fields). If the radiation is administered to the salivary gland tissues, xerostomia will ensue. The parotid is the most radiosensitive of the salivary glands; **saliva** may become extremely viscous or nonexistent, depending on the dose delivered to the

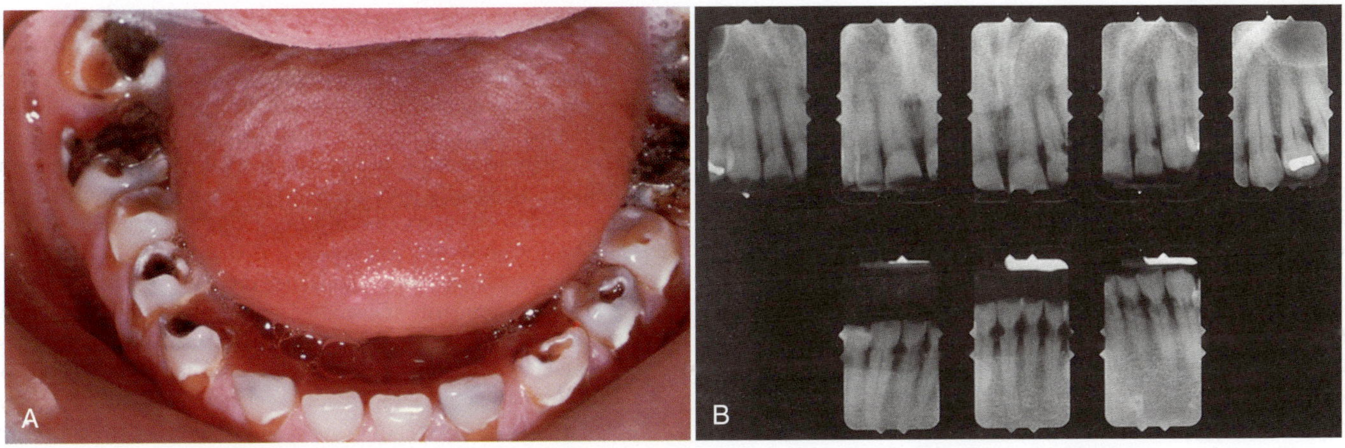

Fig. 29.4 A, In a clinical view of a patient with radiation caries, notice how the caries primarily affected the smooth tooth surfaces, especially cervical areas and cusp tips. B, Radiographs of anterior teeth of 52-year-old man with postradiation caries. The patient received a dose of 6000 cGy for radiation treatment of the posterior mandible and base of the tongue for squamous cell carcinoma. Radiation caries developed within 1 year after radiation treatment, affecting the cervical areas and incisal edges of the anterior teeth. *(A, Courtesy Dr. Eric Sung, Hospital Dentistry, University of California, Los Angeles.)*

particular gland. Xerostomia causes a decrease in the normal salivary cleansing mechanisms, buffering capacity of saliva, and pH of oral fluids. Oral bacterial populations shift to a preponderance of cariogenic forms (e.g., *Streptococcus mutans*, *Actinomyces* spp., *Lactobacillus* spp.). Radiation-induced caries may progress rapidly, and they primarily affect smooth tooth surfaces (see Fig. 29.4).

High-dose radiation therapy results in hypovascularity of irradiated tissues, with a reduction in wound-healing capacity. Most severe among the resulting oral complications is osteoradionecrosis (ORN). Decreased vascularity renders the bone less capable of resolving trauma or infection. These events can cause severe destruction of bone. The risk of ORN continues for the remainder of the patient's life and does not decrease with time.

Periodontal disease can be a precipitating factor in ORN. Tooth extraction after radiation treatment involves a high risk of developing ORN, and surgical flap procedures are usually discouraged after radiation therapy. For these reasons, it is important that the clinician address the patient's periodontal disease *before* radiation begins, when possible. Teeth that are nonrestorable or severely periodontally diseased should be extracted, ideally at least 2 weeks before radiation therapy. Extractions should be performed in a manner that allows primary closure. Mucoperiosteal flaps should be gently elevated; teeth should be extracted in segments; alveolectomy should be performed, allowing no rough bony spicules to remain; and primary closure should be provided without tension. It is not necessary to extract teeth that can be retained with conservative restorative, endodontic, or periodontal therapy. However, prudence dictates extraction of questionable teeth because periodontal treatment after irradiation may be limited to nonsurgical forms of therapy. Flap surgery or extraction of teeth after radiation can lead to ORN. Management of ORN is often difficult and costly, involving progressively more aggressive treatment if bone does not respond to conservative therapy. Costly hyperbaric oxygen therapy is frequently required for complete resolution.

During radiation therapy, patients should receive weekly prophylaxis, oral hygiene instruction, and professionally applied fluoride treatments, unless mucositis prevents treatment. Patients should be instructed to brush daily with a 0.4% stannous or 1.0% sodium fluoride gel. Custom gel trays allow optimal fluoride application. All remaining teeth should receive thorough root debridement (i.e., scaling and root planing).

Postirradiation follow-up consists of palliative treatment provided as needed. Viscous lidocaine can be prescribed for painful mucositis, and salivary substitutes can be given for xerostomia. Daily topical fluoride application and oral hygiene are the best means of preventing radiation caries over time. A long-term, 3-month recall interval is ideal.

Prosthetic Joint Replacement

The main treatment consideration for patients with **prosthetic** joint replacement *was* the potential need for antibiotic prophylaxis before periodontal therapy. No scientific evidence indicates that prophylactic antibiotics prevent late prosthetic joint infections, which can occur from transient bacteremia induced by dental treatment. Although dental-induced bacteremia can theoretically cause prosthetic joint infection, scan reports demonstrate dental treatment as a source of joint infection, and none actually documents a cause-and-effect relationship.

Reports of the American Dental Association (ADA), American Academy of Orthopedic Surgeons (AAOS), American Academy of Oral Medicine (AAOM), and British Society for Antimicrobial Chemotherapy (BSAC) agree that routine antibiotic prophylaxis before dental treatment is not indicated for most patients with prosthetic joint replacement.

Between 2009 and 2014, there was controversy and debate among experts, with a complete shift toward recommending prophylactic antibiotics before dental treatment for all patients with prosthetic joint replacement for life. After further review of the evidence and consensus among experts, new recommendations were published that did not recommend prophylactic antibiotics for dental procedures in patients with prosthetic joint replacement to prevent prosthetic joint infection.

Current advice for patients with orthopedic joint replacement stresses the importance of maintaining good dental health and hygiene and seeking prompt attention and treatment for oral infections when they occur. Dental procedures have not been associated with an increased risk of prosthetic joint infection, and the use of prophylactic antibiotics before dental procedures does not reduce the risk of infection. Given the lack of evidence to support the need for prophylactic antibiotics, the AAOM, ADA, AAOS, and BSAC advise against the universal use of antibiotic prophylaxis before dental procedures for the prevention of prosthetic joint infections.

In 2013, the ADA in conjunction with the AAOS published a joint guideline on the prevention of orthopedic implant infections in patients undergoing dental procedures. The publication stated that there was no convincing evidence to support the routine use of prophylactic antibiotics for patients with prosthetic joints. In 2015, the ADA Council on Scientific Affairs published a clinical practice guideline to clearly state the findings of the 2013 ADA/AAOS joint guideline. The clinical practice guideline states that prophylactic antibiotics are *not* recommended before dental procedures for patients with prosthetic joint implants to prevent prosthetic joint infections.

Pregnancy

The aim of periodontal therapy for the pregnant patient is to minimize the exaggerated inflammatory response related to pregnancy-associated hormonal alterations. Meticulous plaque control, scaling, root planing, and polishing should be the only nonemergency periodontal procedures performed.

The second trimester is the safest time to perform treatment. However, long, stressful appointments and periodontal surgical procedures should be delayed until the postpartum period. As the **uterus** increases in size during the second and third trimesters, obstruction of the vena cava and aorta can occur if the patient is placed in a supine position. The reduction in return cardiac blood supply can cause *supine hypotensive syndrome*, with decreased placental perfusion. Decreasing blood pressure, syncope, and loss of consciousness can occur. This can be prevented by placing the patient on her left side or by elevating the right hip 5–6 inches during treatment. Appointments should be short, and the patient should be allowed to change positions frequently. A fully reclined position should be avoided if possible.

Other precautions during pregnancy relate to the potential toxic or teratogenic effects of therapy on the fetus. Ideally, no medications should be prescribed. However, analgesics, antibiotics, local anesthetics, and other drugs may be required during pregnancy, depending on the patient's needs. Before being prescribed, all drugs should be reviewed for potential adverse effects on the fetus.

As for any patients, use of dental radiographs during pregnancy should be kept to a minimum. The small amount of radiation exposure during diagnostic dental radiography poses little or no risk to the fetus as long as the mother is properly shielded. The ADA has stated that "normal radiographic guidelines do not need to be altered because of pregnancy." Use of a properly positioned lead apron is an absolute requirement.

Infectious Diseases

Because many infectious diseases are occult in nature and medical histories are often inaccurate or incomplete, all periodontal patients should be treated as though they have an infectious disease. Protection of patients, clinicians, and office staff requires the use of universal (standard) precautions for all patients, maximizing prevention of infection and cross-contamination. This section provides a brief discussion of hepatitis, **human immunodeficiency virus (HIV)** and **acquired immunodeficiency syndrome (AIDS)**, and **tuberculosis** in relation to the precautions required in periodontal therapy.

Hepatitis

Six distinct viruses that cause viral hepatitis have been identified: hepatitis A, B, C, D, E, and G viruses. A single-stranded DNA virus known as *transfusion-transmitted virus* has been identified in cases of acute and chronic hepatitis; its role as an etiologic agent is undetermined. These forms of hepatitis differ in their virology, epidemiology, and prophylaxis. Because most hepatitis infections are undiagnosed, the clinician must be aware of high-risk groups such as renal dialysis patients, health care workers, immunosuppressed patients, patients who have received multiple blood transfusions, homosexuals, drug users, and institutionalized patients.

Hepatitis A virus (HAV) and *hepatitis E virus* (HEV) produce self-limited infections with no associated chronic liver disease. These viruses are primarily transmitted by the fecal-oral route. HAV transmission in the United States usually results from close personal household, sexual, or day care center contact. HEV is transmitted mainly through feces-contaminated drinking water and is relatively uncommon in the United States. A vaccination is available to protect against HAV infection but not HEV infection.

Hepatitis B virus (HBV) infection can result in chronic liver disease and a chronic carrier state. Chronic HBV infection develops in about 5%–10% of infected individuals, with much higher rates among infants and children. Because it is transmitted primarily through a hematogenous route, HBV is a major concern for health care workers; the highest rates of HBV infection are found among dentists and oral surgeons. Percutaneous or permucosal injury with contaminated instruments or needles is the most common route of infection in the dental office. The HBV vaccine is recommended for all health care workers.

Hepatitis D virus (HDV) is a defective virus that requires the presence of HBV for its survival, replication, and infectivity. The HDV genetic material is packaged in the HBV surface-antigen coating. Prevention of HDV infection is similar to prevention of HBV and relies strongly on HBV vaccination. After antibody titers to HBV are elevated to a protective level, the patient is also protected against HDV infection.

Hepatitis C virus (HCV) is probably the most serious of all viral hepatitis infections because of its high chronic infection rate. Only 15% of patients infected with HCV recover completely; 85% develop chronic HCV infection, which dramatically increases the risk of cirrhosis, hepatocellular carcinoma, and liver failure. HCV infection is the leading cause of liver transplantation in the United States. Unfortunately, no vaccine is available for HCV. Because HCV is transmitted primarily through a percutaneous or permucosal route, health care workers are at risk from injury with contaminated instruments.

Hepatitis G virus (HGV) is a **ribonucleic acid (RNA)** virus, and its epidemiology and virology are not fully understood. HGV rarely occurs as a solitary infection, instead usually appearing as a coinfection with hepatitis A, B, or C. HGV is transmitted through the blood and has frequently been associated with transfusions.

Transfusion-transmitted virus (TTV) was first identified in 1997 and is common in the general population. The virus is often present in patients with hepatitis and chronic liver disease. Similar to HGV, TTV may not cause a specific form of hepatitis. Patients infected with TTV can develop a chronic carrier state without having clinically evident disease, or they can develop frank disease. Evidence indicates that TTV can be transmitted through the blood (e.g., transfusions), by a fecal-oral route, and from mother to child. As with HGV, TTV is often associated with HCV.

The following guidelines are offered for treating hepatitis patients:

1. If the disease, regardless of type, is active, do not provide periodontal therapy unless the situation is an emergency. In an

emergency case, follow the protocol for patients testing positive for hepatitis B surface antigen (HBsAg).

2. For patients with a history of hepatitis, consult the physician to determine the type of hepatitis, course and length of the disease, mode of transmission, and any chronic liver disease or viral carrier state.
3. For recovered HAV and HEV patients, perform routine periodontal care.
4. For recovered HBV and HDV patients, consult with the physician and order HBsAg and anti-HBs (i.e., antibody to HBV surface antigen) laboratory tests.
   - If HBsAg and anti-HBs test results are negative but HBV is suspected, order another HBs determination.
   - Patients who are HBsAg positive are probably infective (i.e., chronic carriers); the degree of infectivity is measured by an HBsAg determination.
   - Patients who are anti-HBs positive may be treated routinely because they have antibody to HBsAg.
   - Patients who are HBsAg negative may be treated routinely.
5. For HCV patients, consult with the physician to determine the patient's risk for transmissibility and current status of chronic liver disease.
6. If a patient with active hepatitis, positive-HBsAg (i.e., HBV carrier) status, or positive-HCV carrier status requires emergency treatment, use the following precautions:
   - Consult the patient's physician regarding status.
   - If bleeding is likely during or after treatment, measure the PT and bleeding time. Hepatitis can alter coagulation; change the treatment accordingly.
   - All personnel in clinical contact with the patient should use full barrier techniques, including masks, gloves, glasses or eye shields, and disposable gowns.
   - Use as many disposable covers as possible, covering light handles, drawer handles, and bracket trays. Headrest covers should also be used.
   - All disposable items (e.g., gauze, floss, saliva ejectors, masks, gowns, gloves) should be placed in one lined wastebasket. After treatment, these items and all disposable covers should be bagged, labeled, and disposed of following proper guidelines for biohazardous waste.
   - **Aseptic** technique should be followed at all times. Minimize aerosol production by not using ultrasonic instrumentation, air syringe, or high-speed handpieces; remember that saliva contains a distillate of the virus. Prerinsing with chlorhexidine gluconate for 30 s is highly recommended.
   - When the procedure is completed, all equipment should be scrubbed and sterilized. If an item cannot be sterilized or disposed of, it should not be used.

If a percutaneous or permucosal injury occurs during dental treatment of an HBV carrier, Centers for Disease Control and Prevention (CDC) guidelines recommend administration of *hepatitis B immune globulin* (HBIG). The HBV vaccine should also be administered if the injured individual has not previously received it. Unfortunately, postexposure prophylaxis with immune globulin or antiviral agents is usually ineffective if a percutaneous injury occurs during treatment of a hepatitis C carrier.

Human Immunodeficiency Virus and Acquired Immunodeficiency Syndrome

Since the beginning of the AIDS epidemic, a wide range of oral lesions has been associated with HIV infection. As with hepatitis, not all HIV-infected patients know that they are infected when they present for dental treatment. Individuals with known HIV infection may not admit their status on the medical history. Every patient receiving dental treatment should be managed as a potentially infected person, using universal precautions for all therapy.

Extensive periodontal treatment plans must be considered in regard to the patient's systemic health, prognosis, and survival time. Large variations in progression of HIV disease exist among individuals, and selecting an appropriate treatment plan depends on the state of the patient's overall health. Although there appear to be few contraindications to routine dental treatment for many HIV-infected patients, the periodontal treatment plan is influenced by the patient's overall systemic health and coincident oral infections or diseases. An awareness of oral disorders associated with HIV infection may allow the clinician to recognize previously undiagnosed disease or modify treatment protocols appropriately.

COVID-19

The COVID-19 pandemic is a serious worldwide infectious disease problem that was recognized in early 2020, but likely began in late 2019. The novel virus was first identified in the Chinese city of Wuhan and quickly spread throughout the world. The virus is highly **contagious**, and although vaccines have been developed, the pandemic continues due to the highly infective nature and the ongoing variety of emerging mutations. The coronavirus pandemic is caused by the severe acute respiratory syndrome coronavirus 2 (SARS-CoV-2). As with many infectious diseases, infected individuals may not know that they are infected when they present for dental treatment, especially in the early stage before the onset of symptoms, yet these individuals can transmit the virus. Thus, COVID-19 symptom screening and universal precautions are imperative for all patients. Every patient receiving dental treatment should be managed as a potentially infected person.

Tuberculosis

The patient with tuberculosis should receive only emergency care, following the guidelines listed in the section on hepatitis. If the patient has completed chemotherapy, the patient's physician should be consulted regarding infectivity and the results of sputum **cultures** for *Mycobacterium tuberculosis*. When medical clearance has been given and sputum culture results are negative, the patient can be treated normally. Any patient who gives a history of poor medical follow-up (e.g., lack of yearly chest radiographs) or shows signs or symptoms indicative of tuberculosis should be referred for evaluation. Adequate treatment of tuberculosis requires a minimum of 18 months, and thorough posttreatment follow-up should include chest radiographs, sputum cultures, and a review of the patient's symptoms by the physician at least every 12 months.

Management of Patients With Special Needs

Conscious Sedation and General Anesthesia

Periodontal and implant surgery should be performed painlessly and with minimal or no apprehension. The patient should be assured at the initial consultation. The most reliable means of providing painless surgery is effective administration of local anesthesia. However, patients who are apprehensive may require treatment under mild or moderate sedation. The use of sedation can help make patients more comfortable during periodontal and implant surgery, especially when the procedure is expected to continue for 2 h or more. Routes of administration for sedation agents include inhalation, oral, intramuscular, and intravenous. The specific agents and modality of administration are based on the desired level of sedation, anticipated length of the procedure, overall condition of the patient, and training of the clinician and staff.

Rationale for Sedation During Periodontal and Implant Surgical Procedures

Many patients delay or avoid having needed dental treatment because of fear and anxiety. This avoidance behavior often results in compromised health and quality of life. In a study of 174 patients referred for dental implant therapy, only 40.8% proceeded with therapy, and 24% listed dental fear as the reason for refusing to accept treatment. Those who proceeded with therapy had low anxiety ratings as measured by the Modified Dental Anxiety Scale. Anxiety about dental therapy has not changed significantly during the past 50 years; publications report that about 30%–50% of patients are at least somewhat fearful of dental procedures. Evidence suggests that genetic variations are associated with anxiety related to dental care, which could help to explain the consistent avoidance patterns despite improved treatment methods. Anxiety reduction that includes moderate sedation is an important part of delivering advanced periodontal services. Because dental anxiety results in avoidance behavior and is associated with more dental and periodontal problems, it is likely that disproportionate numbers of patients referred to periodontal specialists have dental anxiety. There appears to be a close relationship between anxiety and postoperative pain, and preoperative anxiety can be a predictor of postoperative pain. High levels of anxiety (i.e., stress) can affect wound healing after periodontal treatment. Sedation techniques have been effective in reducing physiologic markers of stress. For these reasons, it is important for clinicians who provide advanced periodontal and implant therapy to be knowledgeable and skilled in providing sedation to reduce anxiety in their patients.

Periodontal Treatment for Older Adults

Older adults are expected to comprise a larger proportion of the population than in the past. Population growth among long-lived older adults contributes to this increase worldwide. For dentistry, this means that older adults are retaining more of their natural dentition. Almost 70% of older adults in the United States have natural teeth. However, retention of teeth may result in more teeth at risk for periodontal disease, and the prevalence of periodontal disease can be associated with aging.

Periodontal disease in older adults usually is not a rapidly progressive disease but often manifests as a long-standing chronic disease. The goal of clinically managing periodontal disease in older adults is based on specific, individualized care. The major consideration is improving or maintaining function, with an emphasis on quality-of-life issues. Emphasizing care over cure is the cornerstone of any proposed treatment plan. Prevention, comfort, function, esthetics, and ease of maintenance are the criteria for successful care of an older adult, particularly a frail or functionally dependent older patient.

Several factors must be considered during treatment planning for older individuals. It is important first to remember that periodontal healing and recurrence of disease are not influenced by age. Factors to consider in the older patient are medical and mental health status, medications, functional status, and lifestyle behaviors that influence periodontal treatment, outcome, or progression of disease. Periodontal disease severity, ability to perform oral hygiene procedures, and ability to tolerate treatment should be evaluated during treatment planning. The risks and benefits of surgical and nonsurgical therapy should be considered. The amount of remaining periodontal support or past periodontal destruction, tooth type, number of occlusal contacts, and individual patient preferences are also important.

Dental implants are reliable replacements for missing teeth in older adults; age alone is not a contraindication for implant placement. Risk factors for the success of implants have been investigated. Although aging is a factor in decision making, most failures are associated with smoking, diabetes, head and neck irradiation, and postmenopausal estrogen therapy. For older adults, a nonsurgical approach is often the first treatment choice. Depending on the nature and extent of periodontal disease, surgical therapy may be indicated. Surgical technique should minimize the amount of additional root exposure. Individuals who respond best to surgical therapy are those who are able to maintain the surgical result. Age alone is not a contraindication to surgery. For individuals who are unable to comply with treatment, have poor oral hygiene, or are medically or mentally compromised or functionally impaired, palliative supportive periodontal care instead of surgical periodontal treatment is often the optimal approach.

A common goal for all older adults is to decrease bacteria through oral hygiene and mechanical debridement. Clinical trials enrolling older adults showed that the development or progression of periodontal disease could be prevented or arrested by controlling plaque. For certain patients, topical antibiotic therapy may complement repeated subgingival instrumentation during supportive care. Oral hygiene maintenance should also focus on root surfaces susceptible to caries. Decision making for frail and functionally dependent older adults may be challenging for the general dentist. For this reason, dentists, other health care professionals, and other scientists are creating high-quality office-based methods to access evidence-based decision-making programs and accommodating websites to help with complicated oral health care issues.

Sleep-Related Breathing Disorders and the Periodontium

The **prevalence** of impaired breathing in patients may be as high as four times more likely among those who are experiencing **periodontitis** or have shown to be susceptible to **periodontal disease**, while periodontitis occurs twice as frequently among patients affected by sleep-related breathing disorders and the periodontium (SRBD). Periodontitis is best understood as an inflammatory bone disease most similar to rheumatoid arthritis. Sleep disturbances, especially when occurring in stressed individuals, are associated with elevated systemic **inflammation** as does periodontitis. The occurrence of periodontitis among individuals with an SRBD is significant, and the severity of both conditions run parallel. As essential members of the health care team, dentists must determine if both conditions are being experienced by any patient presenting with either.

Whereas a qualified physician is responsible for diagnosing obstructive sleep apnea (OSA), the dentist can identify and differentiate between clinical signs of possible airway issues, often before the patient becomes suspicious of the health risk. Information shared by the patient regarding his or her overall health status should be reviewed and correlated with clinical observations of oral indicators of attempted compensation by the patient for a significant degree of airway obstruction or resistance.

The value of early recognition and intervention cannot be overstated. The deleterious effects of SRBD and resultant periods of asphyxia on cardiovascular health, endocrine function, neurologic function, and masticatory system integrity add to the urgency for dentists to include recognition protocols during initial and recurring evaluations of their patients. A multidisciplinary team approach that incorporates respect for each team member's professional role is essential to make an accurate diagnosis and facilitate provision of the most appropriate treatment.

Conclusion

Patients with periodontal treatment needs often present with medical diseases or conditions that need to be understood by dentists and dental hygienists. Although some diseases/conditions are mild and may not have an impact on periodontal treatment, others may pose a serious risk of an adverse outcome or complication. Patients also take a variety of medications. It is imperative to review a patient's medical history and to assess the stability of their condition, and the possible need to modify treatment. Whenever a patient's health status is complex, it is prudent to consult with their physician to better understand their condition and to ascertain appropriate modifications for safe periodontal treatment. This chapter reviewed common diseases, conditions, and medications that can have an impact on oral health and patient care.

Key points

- A detailed medical history should be taken for every patient. Coordination with the patient's physician or referring to a medical consultant is mandatory.
- Approximately 95% of all hypertensive patients have primary (external) hypertension.
- No treatment should be provided if systolic pressure is above 180 mm Hg or diastolic pressure is above 110 mm Hg.
- Use local anesthesia of adrenaline concentration of 1:100,000 or less.
- Make sure bleeding has stopped completely before discharging the patient.
- Keep nitroglycerin tablets (0.3–0.6 mg) readily available for patients with ischaemic heart disease (IHD).
- Follow AHA guidelines for prophylaxis against infective endocarditis.
- Standard oral regimen of prophylactic antibiotics in 2 g amoxicillin 30–40 min before procedure.
- In a controlled diabetes for nonsurgical therapy, antibiotics are not needed.
- Prophylactic antibiotics are administered prior to surgical procedures.
- Always be on guard against symptoms of hypoglycemia.
- Short mid-morning appointments are ideal.
- Limit the size of surgical fields.
- Anticoagulant and antiplatelet medication like aspirin (less than 325 mg/day) should not be stopped.
- Check the INR. Preferable for most patients is 2.0–3.0. Consult the patient's physician.
- Periodontal therapy in patients with renal transplantation require prophylactic antibiotics similar to AHA guidelines.
- Follow standard barrier techniques while treating hepatitis patients.
- Avoid unnecessary medication for a pregnant patient.
- Avoid ultrasonic scalers in patients treated by radiotherapy and with infective diseases.
- Avoid dental treatment in patients who have undergone chemotherapy if white cell counts are less than 2500/mm^3.

Suggested Reading

Malamed SF: *Medical emergencies in the dental office*, ed 7, London, 2014, Elsevier Health Sciences.

Rose LF, Steinberg BJ, Atlas SL. Periodontal management of the medically compromised patient. *Periodontol* 2000. 1995;9:165-175.

CHAPTER 30

Treatment of Aggressive and Atypical Forms of Periodontitis

PR Klokkevold | A Uppoor

CHAPTER OUTLINE

The majority of patients with common forms of periodontal disease respond predictably well to conventional therapy, including oral hygiene instruction, nonsurgical debridement, surgery, and supportive periodontal maintenance. However, patients diagnosed with aggressive and some atypical forms of periodontal disease often do not respond as predictably or as favorably to conventional therapy. Fortunately, only a small percentage of patients with periodontal disease are diagnosed with aggressive periodontitis. Patients who are diagnosed with periodontal disease (any type) that is refractory to treatment present in small numbers as well. Even fewer patients are diagnosed with necrotizing ulcerative periodontitis. Each of these atypical disease entities poses significant challenges for the clinician not only because they are infrequently encountered but also because they may not respond favorably to conventional periodontal therapy. Furthermore, the severe loss of periodontal support associated with these cases leaves the clinician faced with uncertainty about treatment outcomes and difficulty in making decisions about whether to save compromised teeth or to extract them.

Aggressive Periodontitis

Aggressive periodontitis, by definition, causes rapid destruction of the periodontal attachment apparatus and the supporting alveolar bone. The responsiveness of aggressive periodontitis to conventional periodontal treatment is unpredictable, and the overall prognosis for these patients is poorer than for patients with chronic periodontitis. Because these patients do not respond "normally" to conventional methods and their disease progresses unusually fast, the logical question is whether there are problems associated with an impaired host immune response that may contribute to such a *different* disease and result in a *limited* response to the usual therapeutic measures. Indeed, defects in polymorphonuclear leukocyte (PMN, neutrophil) function have been identified in some patients with aggressive periodontitis. Also, in a small number of cases, a systemic disease, such as neutropenia, can be identified that clearly explains the unusual severity of the periodontal disease for that individual. In most patients with aggressive periodontitis, however, systemic diseases or disorders cannot be identified. In fact, the irony is that these patients are typically quite healthy. Numerous attempts to examine immunologic profiles in patients with aggressive periodontitis have failed to identify any specific etiologic factors common to all patients.

The prognosis for patients with aggressive periodontitis depends on (1) whether the disease is generalized or localized, (2) the degree of destruction present at the time of diagnosis, and (3) the ability to control future progression. *Generalized* aggressive periodontitis rarely undergoes spontaneous remission, whereas *localized* forms of the disease have been known to arrest spontaneously. This unexplained curtailment of disease progression has sometimes been referred to as a "burnout" of the disease. It appears that cases of localized aggressive periodontitis often have a limited period of rapid periodontal attachment and alveolar bone loss, followed by a slower, more chronic phase of disease progression. Overall, patients with generalized aggressive periodontitis tend to have a poorer prognosis because they typically have more teeth affected by the disease and because the disease is less likely to go spontaneously into remission compared to patients with localized forms of aggressive periodontitis.

Therapeutic Modalities

Early detection is critically important in the treatment of aggressive periodontitis (generalized or localized) because preventing further destruction is often more predictable than attempting to regenerate lost supporting tissues. Therefore, at the initial diagnosis, it is helpful to obtain any previously taken radiographs to assess the rate of progression of the disease. Together with future radiographs, this documentation will also facilitate the clinician's assessment of treatment success and control of the disease.

Treatment of aggressive periodontitis must be pursued with a logical and regimented approach. Several aspects of treatment must be particularly considered when managing a patient with aggressive periodontitis. One of the most important aspects of treatment success is to educate the patient about the disease, including the causes and the risk factors for disease, and to stress the importance of the patient's role in the success of treatment. Essential therapeutic considerations for the clinician are to control the infection, arrest disease progression, correct anatomic defects, replace missing teeth, and ultimately help the patient maintain periodontal health with frequent periodontal maintenance care. Educating family members is another important factor because aggressive periodontitis is known to have familial aggregation. Thus family members, especially younger siblings, of the patient diagnosed with aggressive periodontitis should be examined for signs of disease, educated about preventive measures, and monitored closely. It cannot be stressed enough that early diagnosis, intervention, and if possible, prevention of disease is more desirable than attempting to reverse the destruction that results from aggressive periodontitis.

Conventional Periodontal Therapy

Because aggressive periodontitis is primarily a bacterial infection, initial treatment is comparable to treatment rendered for chronic periodontitis. Conventional periodontal therapy for aggressive periodontitis consists of patient education, oral hygiene improvement, scaling and root planing, and regular (frequent) recall maintenance. It may or may not include periodontal flap surgery. Unfortunately, the response of aggressive periodontitis to conventional therapy alone has been limited and unpredictable. Patients who are diagnosed with aggressive periodontitis at an early stage and who are able to enter therapy may have a better outcome than those who are diagnosed at an advanced stage of destruction. In general, the earlier the disease is diagnosed, the more conservative the therapy and the more predictable the outcome.

Teeth with moderate to advanced periodontal attachment loss and bone loss often have a poor prognosis and pose the most difficult challenge. Depending on the condition of the remaining dentition, treatment of these teeth may have a limited prospect for improvement and may even diminish the overall treatment success for the patient. Clearly, some of these teeth should be extracted; however, other teeth may be pivotal to the stability of that individual's dentition, and thus it may be desirable to attempt treatment to maintain them. Treatment options for teeth with deep periodontal pockets and bone loss may be nonsurgical or surgical. Surgery may be purely resective, regenerative, or a combination of these approaches.

KEY FACT

Patients who are diagnosed with aggressive periodontitis at an early stage and who are able to enter therapy may have a better outcome than those who are diagnosed at an advanced stage of destruction. In general, the earlier the disease is diagnosed, the more conservative the therapy and the more predictable the outcome. Teeth with advanced periodontal attachment loss and bone destruction often have a poor prognosis and pose the biggest challenge for treatment.

Surgical Resective Therapy

Resective periodontal surgery can be effective to reduce or eliminate pocket depth in patients with aggressive periodontitis. However, it may be difficult to accomplish if adjacent teeth are unaffected, as often seen in cases of localized aggressive periodontitis. If a significant height discrepancy exists between the periodontal support of the affected tooth and the adjacent unaffected tooth, the gingival transition (following the bone) will often result in deep probing pocket depth around the affected tooth despite surgical efforts. A less-than-ideal outcome must be taken into consideration before deciding to treat increased pocket depth surgically.

It is important to realize the limitations of surgical therapy and to appreciate the possible risk that surgical therapy may further compromise teeth that are mobile because of extensive loss of periodontal support. For example, in a patient with severe horizontal bone loss, surgical resective therapy may result in increased tooth mobility that is difficult to manage, and a nonsurgical approach may be indicated. Therefore, careful evaluation of the risks versus the benefits of surgery must be considered on a case-by-case basis.

Regenerative Therapy

The concept and application of periodontal regeneration has been established in patients with chronic forms of periodontal disease. The use of regenerative materials, including bone grafts, barrier membranes, and wound-healing agents, are well documented and often used. Intrabony defects, particularly vertical defects with multiple osseous walls, are often amenable to regeneration with these techniques. Most of the success and predictability of periodontal regeneration have been achieved in patients with chronic periodontitis; much less evidence is available about the use of periodontal regeneration for patients with aggressive periodontitis.

Periodontal regenerative procedures have been successfully demonstrated in patients with localized aggressive periodontitis in some clinical case reports. Dodson et al. demonstrated the regenerative potential of a severe, localized osseous defect around a mandibular incisor in a healthy, 19-year-old black man diagnosed with localized aggressive periodontitis. The patient presented with severe bone loss localized around one of the mandibular incisors. Using open-flap surgical debridement, root surface conditioning (tetracycline solution), and an allogenic bone graft reconstituted with sterile saline and tetracycline powder, the surgeons reduced the probing pocket depth from 9 to 12 mm down to 1 to 3 mm (3 mm of recession was noted), and significant bone fill of the defect (about 80%) was reported (Fig. 30.1). This case illustrates the potential for healing severe defects in patients with localized aggressive periodontitis, especially when local factors are controlled and sound surgical principles are followed. The authors cited several factors that likely contributed to the success of this case, including a probable transition of disease activity from aggressive to chronic, tooth stabilization before surgery, sound surgical management of hard and soft tissues, and good postoperative care.

It is important to note that although the potential for regeneration in patients with aggressive periodontitis appears to be good, expectations are limited for patients with severe bone loss. This is especially true if the bone loss is horizontal and if it has progressed to involve furcations.

KEY FACT

Periodontal regeneration has been successfully demonstrated in patients with localized aggressive periodontitis, illustrating the potential for healing severe defects in these patients. As with periodontal regeneration in nonaggressive forms of periodontitis, it is important to control local factors and follow sound surgical principles.

Antimicrobial Therapy

The presence of periodontal pathogens, specifically *Aggregatibacter actinomycetemcomitans*, has been implicated as the reason that aggressive periodontitis does not respond to conventional therapy alone. These pathogens are known to remain in the tissues after therapy to reinfect the pocket. In the late 1970s and early 1980s, the identification of *A. actinomycetemcomitans* as a major culprit and the discovery that this organism penetrates the tissues offered another perspective to the pathogenesis of aggressive periodontitis and offered new hope for therapeutic success, namely, antibiotics. The use of systemic antibiotics was thought to be necessary to eliminate pathogenic bacteria (especially *A. actinomycetemcomitans*)

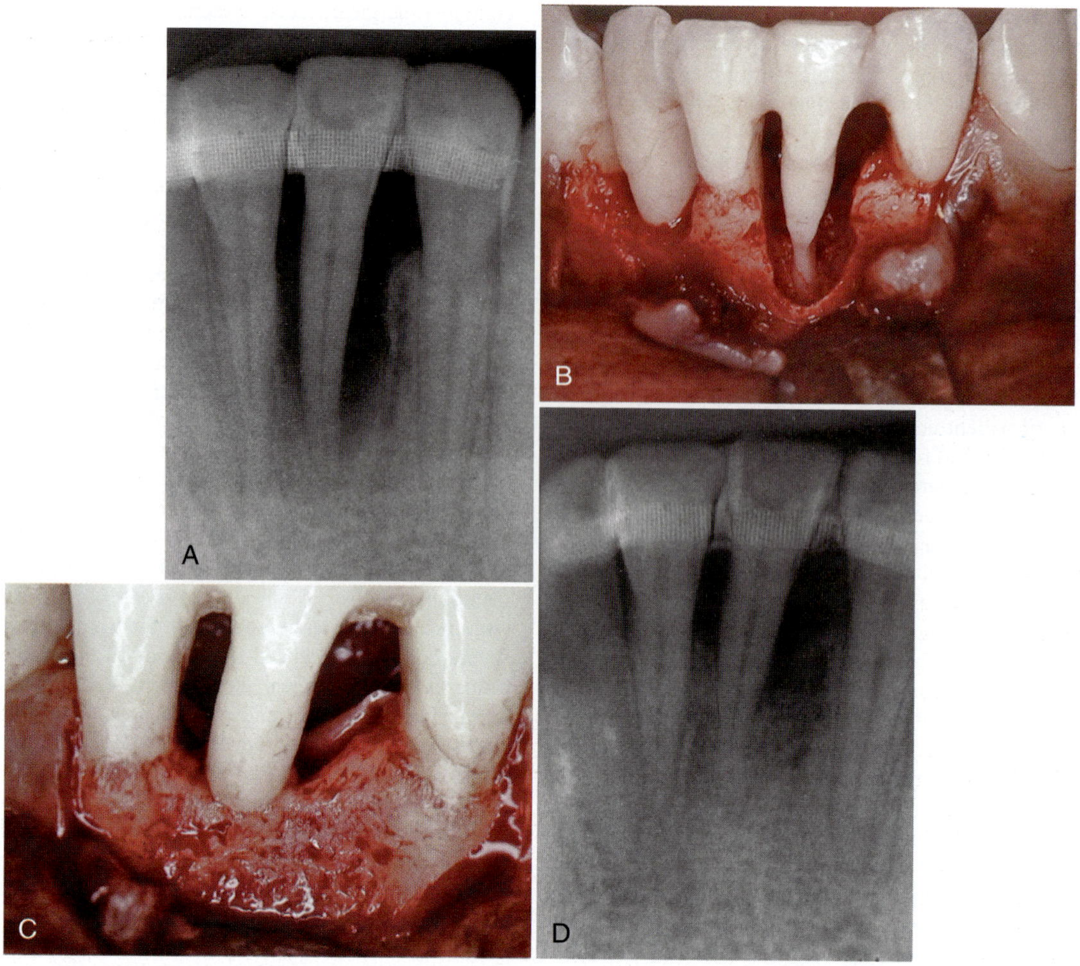

Fig. 30.1 Clinical photographs and periapical radiographs demonstrating regenerative success in patient with localized aggressive periodontitis. A, Periapical radiograph of the right lateral incisor at the initial diagnosis. Notice the severe, vertical bone loss associated with the right lateral incisor. Tooth has been splinted to adjacent teeth for stability. B, Facial view of the circumferential osseous defect around the lower right lateral incisor during open flap surgery. There is complete loss of buccal, lingual, mesial, and distal bone around the lateral incisor, with minimal bone support limited to the apical few millimeters. C, Facial view of reentered surgical site 1 year after treatment. Bone fill around all surfaces demonstrates remarkable potential for regeneration of a large osseous defect in a young patient with localized aggressive periodontitis. D, Periapical radiograph taken 1 year after regenerative therapy. Note the increased radiopacity and bone fill. *(From Dodson SA, Takei HH, Carranza FA Jr:* Int J Periodont Restor Dent *16:455, 1996.)*

from the tissues. Indeed, several authors have reported success in the treatment of aggressive periodontitis using antibiotics as adjuncts to standard therapy.

There is compelling evidence that adjunctive antibiotic treatment frequently results in a more favorable clinical response than mechanical therapy alone. Systemic antimicrobials in conjunction with scaling and root planing offer benefits over scaling and planing alone in terms of clinical attachment level, probing pocket depth, and reduced risk of additional attachment loss. Patients with deeper, progressive pockets seem to benefit the most from systemic administration of adjunctive antibiotics. Many different antibiotic types and regimens were reviewed, but because of limitations in comparing data from different studies, definitive recommendations were not possible. In a metaanalysis of the literature (including six randomized clinical trials), Sgolastra and associates found that the systemic use of combined amoxicillin and metronidazole as an adjunct to scaling and root planing for the treatment of generalized aggressive periodontitis resulted in significant clinical attachment gain ($P < 0.05$) and pocket reduction ($P < 0.05$) compared to scaling and root planing alone.

Fig. 30.2 shows the before and after results of an aggressive periodontitis case treated nonsurgically with scaling and root planing and adjunctive antibiotic therapy. The patient, a 34-year-old Asian male, presented with a complaint of loose teeth and bleeding gums. He requested treatment to save his teeth. Treatment consisted of patient education including oral hygiene instructions and nonsurgical therapy with adjunctive antibiotics. All teeth were thoroughly scaled and root planed under local anesthesia over two treatment appointments, and the patient was treated with systemic amoxicillin (500 mg, 3 times a day for 2 weeks) during the period of treatment. All areas responded favorably with probing pocket depths decreasing from 3 to 13 mm down to 2 to 5 mm. Bleeding on probing diminished from generalized to very few isolated areas. He has been on periodontal maintenance with good results for more than 5 years.

Genco and coworkers treated localized aggressive periodontitis with scaling and root planing plus systemic administration of tetracycline (250 mg, four times daily for 14 days every 8 weeks). Measurements of vertical defects were made at intervals of up to 18 months after the initiation of therapy. Bone loss stopped, and

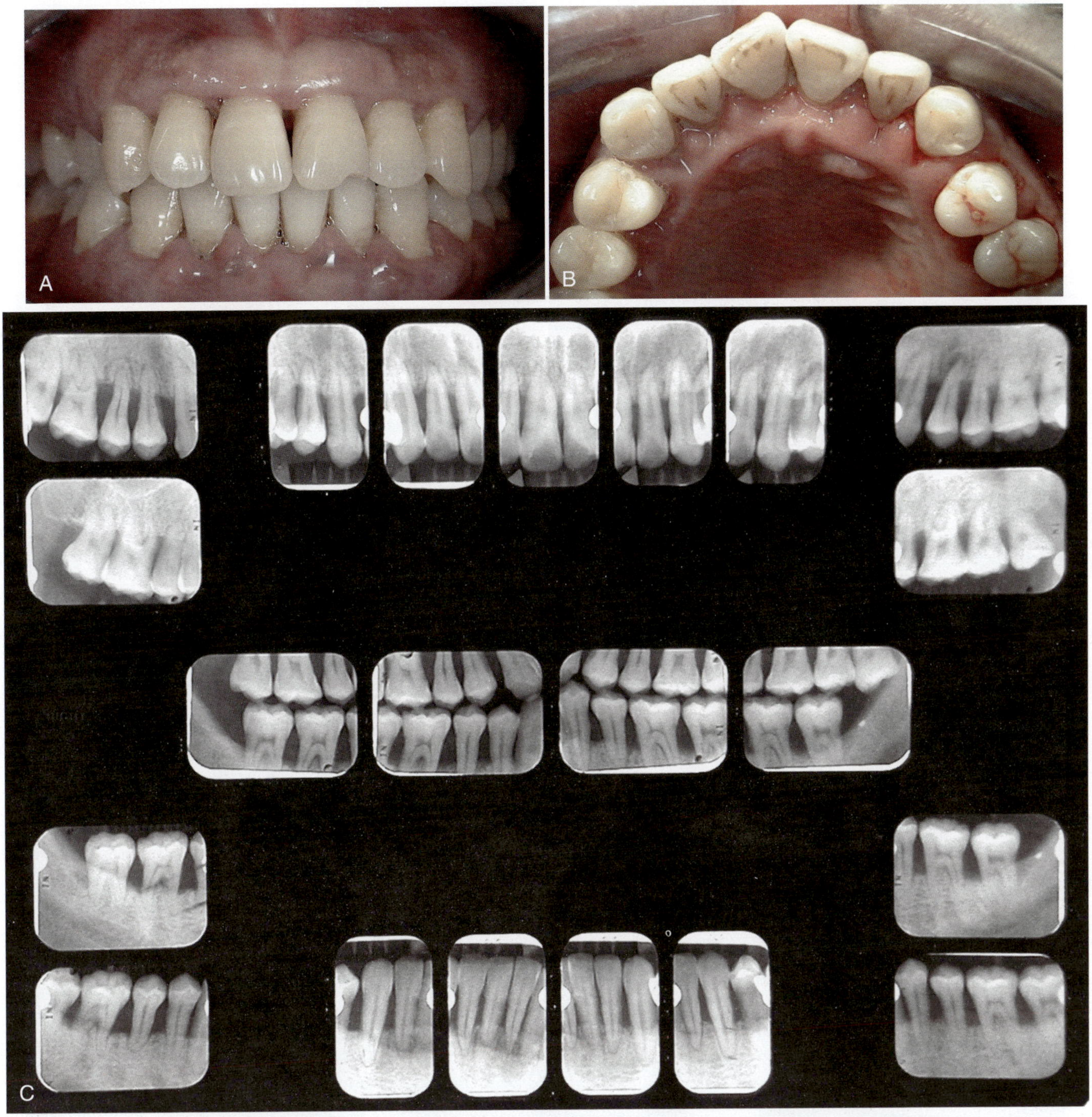

Fig. 30.2 Intraoral clinical photographs and full-mouth radiographs (before and after treatment) of a 34-year-old Asian male with aggressive periodontitis. A and B, Intraoral clinical photographs of pretreatment periodontal condition. Note the gingival edema, inflammation, and bleeding. Probing pocket depths ranged from 3 to 13 mm with generalized bleeding on probing and purulent exudate. C, Pretreatment full-mouth radiographs demonstrating generalized severe horizontal bone loss. Note the periapical radiolucency at the apex of the upper left premolar indicating pulpal disease.

Continued

one-third of the defects demonstrated an increase in bone level, whereas in the control group, bone loss continued.

Liljenberg and Lindhe treated localized aggressive periodontitis with systemic administration of tetracycline (250 mg, four times daily for 2 weeks), modified Widman flaps, and periodic recall visits (one visit every month for 6 months, then one visit every 3 months). The lesions healed more rapidly and more completely than similar lesions in control patients. These investigators reevaluated their results after 5 years and found that the treatment group continued to demonstrate resolution of gingival inflammation, gain of clinical attachment, and refill of bone in angular defects.

Clearly, numerous studies support the use of adjunctive tetracycline along with mechanical debridement for the treatment of *A. actinomycetemcomitans*-associated aggressive periodontitis (Box 30.1). Given the possible emergence of tetracycline-resistant *A. actinomycetemcomitans*, there is concern that tetracycline may

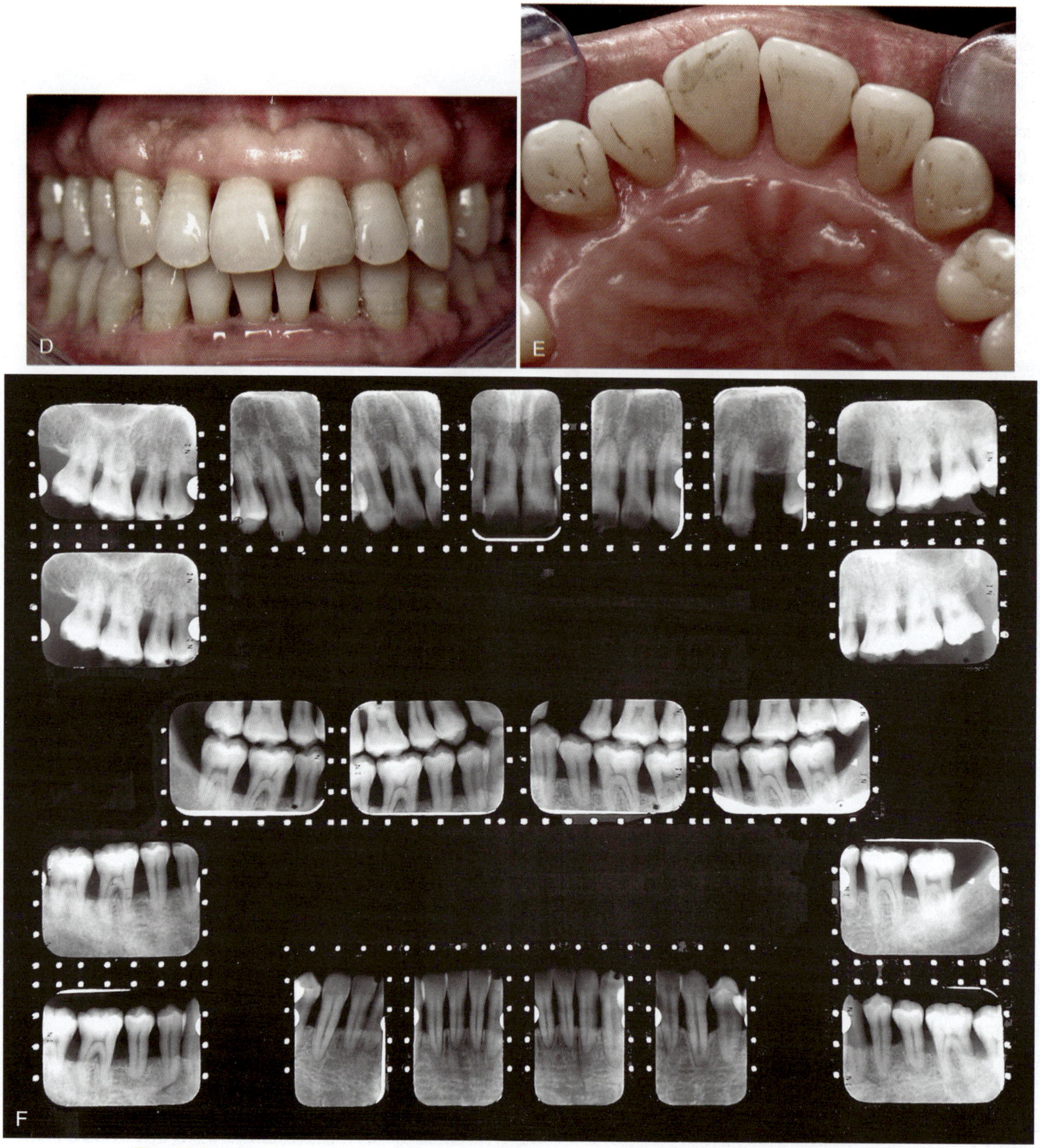

Fig. 30.2, cont'd D and E, Intraoral clinical photographs of posttreatment (5 years) results. Treatment included nonsurgical scaling and root planing along with adjunctive systemic antibiotics (amoxicillin). Patient improved oral hygiene and continued to be seen for professional maintenance every 3 months. Probing pocket depths have been maintained in the range of 2–5 mm with only a few localized areas of bleeding on probing. F, Posttreatment (5 years) full-mouth radiographs demonstrating no additional bone loss. Endodontically involved maxillary premolar was extracted and replaced with a removable partial denture.

not be effective. In these cases, the combination of metronidazole and amoxicillin may be advantageous. The combination of these two antibiotics with conventional periodontal therapy provides better disease control and better clinical improvement in attachment levels in difficult-to-manage periodontitis cases than similar periodontal therapy without antibiotics. Similar effects were seen for a variety of antibiotic types. However, a lack of sufficient sample sizes among studies makes it difficult to offer specific recommendations about which antibiotics were most effective.

The criteria for selection of antibiotics are not clear. Good clinical and microbiologic responses have been reported with several individual antibiotics and antibiotic combinations (Table 30.1). The

BOX 30.1 Systemic Tetracycline in Treatment of Aggressive Periodontitis

Systemic tetracycline (250 mg of tetracycline hydrochloride four times daily for at least 1 week) should be given in conjunction with local mechanical therapy. If surgery is indicated, systemic tetracycline should be prescribed and the patient instructed to begin taking the antibiotic approximately 1 h before surgery. Doxycycline, 100 mg/day, may be used instead of tetracycline. Chlorhexidine rinses should be prescribed and continued for several weeks to enhance plaque control and facilitate healing.

TABLE 30.1 Antibiotic Therapy for Aggressive Periodontitis

Associated Microflora	Antibiotic of Choice
Gram-positive organisms	Amoxicillin–clavulanate potassium (Augmentin)
Gram-negative organisms	Clindamycin
Nonoral gram-negative, facultative rods *Pseudomonads, Staphylococci*	Ciprofloxacin
Black-pigmented bacteria and Spirochetes	Metronidazole
Prevotella intermedia, Porphyromonas gingivalis	Tetracycline
Aggregatibacter actinomycetemcomitans	Metronidazole–amoxicillin Metronidazole–ciprofloxacin Tetracycline
P. gingivalis	Azithromycin

optimal antibiotic or combination for any particular infection probably depends on the case. Choices must be made based on patient-related and disease-related factors.

Microbial Testing

Some investigators and clinicians advocate microbial testing to identify the specific periodontal pathogens responsible for disease and to select an appropriate antibiotic based on sensitivity and resistance. There may be specific cases in which bacterial identification and antibiotic-sensitivity testing is invaluable. For example, in localized aggressive periodontitis cases, tetracycline-resistant *Actinobacillus* species have been suspected. If antibiotic susceptibility tests determine that tetracycline-resistant species exist in the lesion, the clinician may be advised to consider another antibiotic or an antibiotic combination, such as amoxicillin and metronidazole.

In practice, antibiotics are often used empirically without microbial testing. One study evaluated and compared the results of microbial testing offered by two independent laboratories. Two microbiologic cultures, sampled simultaneously from the same sites in 20 patients, were submitted separately to each of the two laboratories for bacterial identification and antibiotic-sensitivity testing. The reported presence of bacterial species varied between the two laboratories, as did their antimicrobial recommendations. The combination of amoxicillin and metronidazole yielded the highest level of agreement (80%), likely because of the effectiveness of this combination and a clinical predisposition to favor a known regimen. These findings suggested that the usefulness of microbial testing may be limited and led the authors to conclude that the empiric use of antibiotics, such as a combination of amoxicillin and metronidazole, may be more clinically sound and cost-effective than bacterial identification and antibiotic-sensitivity testing.

Nonetheless, the use of microbial testing should be considered whenever a case of aggressive periodontitis is not responding or if the destruction continues despite good therapeutic efforts.

Local Delivery

The use of local delivery to administer antibiotics offers a novel approach to the management of periodontal "localized" infections. The primary advantage of local therapy is that smaller total dosages of topical agents can be delivered inside the pocket, avoiding the side effects of systemic antibacterial agents while increasing the exposure of the target microorganisms to higher concentrations, and therefore more therapeutic levels, of the medication. Local delivery agents have been formulated in many different forms, including solutions, gels, fibers, and chips.

Full-Mouth Disinfection

Another approach to antimicrobial therapy in the control of infection associated with periodontitis is the concept of full-mouth disinfection. The concept, described by Quirynen et al., consists of full-mouth debridement (removal of all plaque and calculus) completed in two appointments within a 24-h period. In addition to scaling and root planing, the tongue is brushed with a chlorhexidine gel (1%) for 1 min, the mouth is rinsed with a chlorhexidine solution (0.2%) for 2 min, and periodontal pockets are irrigated with a chlorhexidine solution (1%).

In a clinical and microbiologic study, 10 patients with advanced chronic periodontitis were randomly assigned to a test or control group. Test patients were treated as just described, whereas control patients received scaling and root planing by quadrant at 2-week intervals along with oral hygiene instructions. At 1 and 2 months after treatment, the test group showed significantly higher reduction in probing pocket depth, especially for deeper pockets (7–8 mm). Patients in the test group also had significantly lower concentrations of pathogenic microorganisms after treatment compared to controls. Several follow-up studies by the same center demonstrated similar results for up to 6 months after therapy. In another study, the same researchers included a test group who did *not* use chlorhexidine as part of the one-stage, full-mouth disinfection. The results for both test groups (i.e., with and without chlorhexidine) were similar and were significantly better than for controls. The authors concluded that the beneficial effects of one-stage, full-mouth disinfection probably result from the full-mouth debridement within 24 h rather than the adjunctive chlorhexidine treatment.

A few reports have included patients with aggressive (early-onset) periodontitis in their evaluation of the one-stage, full-mouth disinfection protocol. As with the advanced chronic periodontitis group, De Soete et al. found a significant reduction in probing pocket depth and gain in clinical attachment in patients with aggressive periodontitis up to 8 months after treatment compared to controls (scaling and root planing by quadrant at 2-week intervals). They also found significant reductions in periodontal pathogens up to 8 months after therapy. *Porphyromonas gingivalis* and *Tannerella forsythia* were reduced to levels below detection.

Host Modulation

A novel approach in the treatment of aggressive periodontitis and difficult-to-control forms of periodontal disease is the administration of agents that modulate the host response. Several agents have been used or evaluated to modify the host response to disease.

Treatment Planning and Restorative Considerations

Successful management of patients with aggressive periodontitis must include tooth replacement as part of the treatment plan. In some advanced cases of aggressive periodontitis, the overall treatment success for the patient may be enhanced if severely compromised teeth are extracted. The outcome of treatment for these teeth is limited, and more importantly, the retention of severely diseased teeth over time may result in additional bone loss and teeth that are further compromised. The risk of further bone loss is even a greater concern now with the current success and predictability of dental implants and the desire to preserve bone for implant placement. Any additional alveolar bone loss in an area that has already undergone severe bone loss may further compromise residual anatomy and impair the opportunity for tooth replacement with a dental implant. This is especially true for certain areas with poor bone quality or limited bone volume, such as the posterior maxilla. Fortunately, healing of extraction sites is typically uneventful in patients with aggressive periodontitis, and bone augmentation of defect sites is predictable.

In the patient with aggressive periodontitis, the approach to restorative treatment should be chosen based on a single premise: Extract severely compromised teeth early, and plan treatment to accommodate future tooth loss. The teeth with the best prognosis should be identified and considered when planning the restorative treatment. The lower cuspids and first premolars are typically more resistant to loss, probably because of the favorable anatomy (i.e., single roots, no furcations) and easier access for patient oral hygiene. As a rule, an extensive fixed prosthesis should be avoided, and removable partial dentures should be planned in such a way as to allow for the addition of teeth.

When hopeless teeth are extracted, they need to be replaced. The desire to replace missing teeth in a permanent manner without preparation of adjacent teeth for a fixed partial denture motivated clinicians to attempt transplantation of teeth from one site to another. Transplantation of developing third molars to the sockets of hopeless first molars has been attempted with limited success. Clearly, the success and predictability of dental implants have obviated the need for attempting to transplant teeth to edentulous sites.

Use of Dental Implants

Initially, the use of dental implants was suggested and implemented with much caution in patients with aggressive periodontitis because of an unfounded fear of bone and implant loss. However, evidence to the contrary appears to support the use of dental implants in patients treated for aggressive periodontal disease. Thus, it is possible to consider the use of dental implants in the overall treatment plan for patients with aggressive periodontitis.

There is scant evidence to support the use of bone augmentation procedures in preparation for or in combination with implant placement in patients being treated for aggressive periodontitis. One case report with short-term follow-up suggested that it was successful. A prospective study of 10 patients treated for generalized aggressive periodontitis who underwent guided bone regeneration followed by implant placement found that the implant survival rate was 100% after 3 years. However, slightly greater attachment loss (0.65 mm) and bone loss (1.78 mm) were observed in the aggressive periodontitis group compared to 10 periodontally healthy controls who received implants without bone augmentation.

Clinical Consideration

It is important to recognize that special consideration must be given to the risk of occlusal overload of implants placed in a periodontally compromised dentition. This is especially true when only one or a few implants are used to replace a limited number of teeth with an implant-supported fixed crown or bridge in a patient with a majority of the remaining dentition being mobile. The immobility of implants in a dentition that does not have a stable vertical occlusal stop may lead to implant overload.

Periodontal Maintenance

When patients with aggressive periodontitis are transferred to maintenance care, their periodontal condition must be stable (i.e., no clinical signs of disease and no periodontal pathogens). Each maintenance visit should consist of a medical history review, an inquiry about any recent periodontal problems, assessment risk of factors, a comprehensive periodontal and oral examination, thorough root debridement, and prophylaxis, followed by a review of oral hygiene instructions. If oral hygiene is not good, patients may benefit most from a review of oral hygiene instructions and visualization of plaque in their own mouth before debridement and prophylaxis.

Frequent maintenance visits appear to be one of the most important factors in the control of disease and the success of treatment in patients with aggressive periodontitis. In a study of 25 individuals with aggressive (early-onset) periodontitis followed with maintenance every 3–6 months for 5 years, it was concluded that these patients can be effectively maintained with clinical and microbiologic improvements after active periodontal therapy. High bacterial counts (particularly *P. gingivalis* and *Treponema denticola*), number of acute episodes, number of teeth lost, smoking, and stress appeared to be significant factors in the small percentage of sites that showed progressive bone loss. In a 5-year follow-up study of 13 patients with aggressive periodontitis treated with comprehensive mechanical, surgical, and antimicrobial therapy and supportive periodontal maintenance every 3–4 months, periodontal disease progression was arrested in 95% of the initially affected lesions. Only 2%–5% experienced discrete episodes of loss of periodontal support.

A supportive periodontal maintenance program aimed at early detection and treatment of sites that begin to lose attachment should be established. The duration between these recall visits is usually short during the first period after the patient's completion of therapy, generally no longer than 3-month intervals. Acute episodes of gingival inflammation can be detected and managed earlier when the patient is on a frequent monitoring cycle. Monitoring as frequently as every 3–4 weeks may be necessary when the disease is thought to be active. If signs of disease activity and progression persist despite therapeutic efforts, frequent visits, and good patient compliance, microbial testing may be indicated. The rate of disease progression may be faster in younger individuals, and therefore the clinician should monitor such patients more frequently. Over time, the recall maintenance interval can be adjusted (more or less often) to suit the patient's level of oral hygiene and control of disease, as determined by each examination.

Close collaboration among members of the treatment team, including the periodontist, general dentist, dental hygienist, and patient's physician, is required for continuity of care and for patient motivation and encouragement. It is important to monitor and observe the patient's overall physical status as well because weight loss, depression, and malaise have been reported in patients with generalized aggressive periodontitis. Finally, there is a constant need to reinforce patient education about disease etiology and preventive practices (i.e., oral hygiene and control of risk factors).

Periodontitis Refractory to Treatment

Although refractory periodontitis is not currently considered a separate disease entity, patients who fail to respond to conventional therapy are considered to have periodontitis that is "refractory" to treatment. It is possible to characterize any form of periodontal disease (e.g., chronic periodontitis, aggressive periodontitis) as refractory to treatment.

These cases are difficult to manage because the etiology behind their lack of response to therapy is unknown. Initially, because contributing factors may have been overlooked, it is important to evaluate the adequacy of treatment attempts thoroughly and to consider other possible etiologies before concluding that a case truly is refractory. A patient with periodontitis that is refractory to treatment often does not have any distinguishing clinical characteristics on initial examination compared to cases of periodontitis that respond normally. Therefore, the initial treatment would follow conventional therapeutic modalities for periodontitis. After treatment, if the patient has not responded as expected, the clinician should rule out the following conditions:

1. *Inadequately treated periodontitis.* Most forms of periodontitis can be treated effectively with currently available modalities if they are performed properly. After treatment, if it is determined that the patient has not responded, the clinician must evaluate whether the therapy was adequately performed. Undetected or inaccessible subgingival calculus may be present in one or more areas. Retreatment may be the best way to ensure that therapy was adequately performed. All root surfaces must be meticulously inspected.
2. *Poor plaque control.* Plaque control is essential to the success of periodontal therapy. Patients must understand the role of bacterial plaque in their disease process, and they must comply with daily oral hygiene instructions. Thus, patient compliance and the adequacy of their daily plaque control should be assessed before concluding that a case of periodontitis is refractory to treatment.
3. *Endodontic infection.* The presence of nonperiodontal infections in the area can perpetuate periodontal disease activity and prevent a normal healing response to conventional periodontal therapy. Endodontic infection of teeth in the area should be suspected and ruled out before concluding that a case is refractory to treatment. The clinician should suspect an endodontic etiology especially in those patients with localized recurrent disease.

A case may be considered *refractory* to treatment only when loss of periodontal attachment and bone continues after well-executed treatment in a patient with good oral hygiene and no other infections or etiologic factors.

Clinicians are in a quandary when presented with a patient who is not responding to periodontal therapy. Therapeutic means must be broad in scope and thorough to ensure that all aspects of the host response are addressed. At a minimum, a frequent and intensive recall maintenance and home care program is necessary. Mechanical debridement with scaling and root planing can reduce total supragingival and subgingival bacterial masses, but major periodontal pathogens may persist. Surgical treatment may aid in providing access for debridement and in elimination of bacterial pathogens. In addition, the morphology of the gingival tissues should be modified to facilitate daily plaque removal by the patient.

Systemic antibiotic therapy is administered to reinforce mechanical periodontal treatment and support the host defense system in overcoming the infection by killing subgingival pathogens that remain after conventional mechanical periodontal therapy. Many antibiotics have been used according to the target microflora with various degrees of success (Table 30.1). For patients with refractory disease who fail to respond to initial antibiotic therapy, subsequent treatment should include microbial testing with bacterial identification and antimicrobial susceptibility.

Antibiotic resistance is a potential problem. Patients with periodontitis that is refractory to treatment often present with a history of previous tetracycline therapy, and thus they may have a microflora that is resistant to this drug. Tetracycline-resistant bacteria have been isolated from patients with periodontitis refractory to treatment. However, some patients with refractory disease may still benefit from the use of tetracycline or one of its derivatives.

Cases of periodontitis (refractory), in which the associated microflora consists primarily of Gram-positive microorganisms, have been successfully treated with *amoxicillin–clavulanate potassium.* Many efforts have been made to establish the most appropriate regimen of antibiotic therapy for these patients. Similar antimicrobial regimens, consisting of 250 mg of amoxicillin and 125 mg of clavulanate potassium, have been administered three times daily for 14 days, with scaling and root planing, and produced a reduction in attachment loss for at least 12 months. A regimen of one capsule containing the same amount of drug every 6 h for 2 weeks, with intrasulcular full-mouth lavage using a 10% povidone-iodine solution and chlorhexidine oral rinses twice daily, resulted in a reduction in attachment loss that persisted at approximately 34 months. A regimen of 500 mg of metronidazole three times daily for 7 days was shown to be effective in treating periodontitis (refractory) in patients who were culture positive for *T. forsythia* in the absence of *A. actinomycetemcomitans.*

Clindamycin is a potent antibiotic that penetrates well into gingival fluid, although it is not usually effective against *A. actinomycetemcomitans* and *Eikenella corrodens.* However, clindamycin has been effective in controlling the extent and rate of disease progression in refractory cases in patients who have a microflora susceptible to this antibiotic. A regimen of clindamycin hydrochloride, 150 mg, four times daily for 7 days, combined with scaling and root planing produced a decrease in the incidence of disease activity from an annual rate of 8% to an annual rate of 0.5% of sites per patient. Clindamycin should be prescribed with caution because of the potential for pseudomembranous colitis from superinfections with *Clostridium difficile.* Patients should be warned and advised to discontinue the antibiotic if symptoms of diarrhea develop.

Azithromycin may be effective in periodontitis that is refractory to treatment, especially in patients infected with *P. gingivalis.*

Combinations of antibiotic therapy may offer greater promise as adjunctive treatment for the management of refractory periodontitis. The rationale is based on the diversity of putative pathogens and no single antibiotic being bactericidal for all known pathogens. Combination antibiotic therapy may help broaden the antimicrobial range of the therapeutic regimen beyond that attained by any single antibiotic. Other advantages include lowering the dose of individual antibiotics by exploiting possible synergy between two drugs against targeted organisms. In addition, combination therapy may prevent or forestall the emergence of bacterial resistance. Many combinations of antibiotics have demonstrated significant improvement in the clinical aspects of the disease. Examples of combinations include amoxicillin–clavulanate or metronidazole–amoxicillin for the treatment of *A. actinomycetemcomitans*-associated periodontitis; metronidazole-doxycycline for the prevention of recurrent periodontitis; metronidazole-ciprofloxacin for the treatment of recurrent cases containing a microflora associated with enteric rods and pseudomonads; and amoxicillin-doxycycline in the treatment of periodontitis associated with *A. actinomycetemcomitans* and *P. gingivalis.*

Some cases of periodontitis that are refractory to treatment may not respond to a given antibiotic regimen. When this occurs, the clinician should consider a different antimicrobial therapy based on microbial susceptibility analysis. At this point in the therapy, strong consideration should be given to consulting with the patient's physician for an evaluation of a possible host immune system deficiency or a metabolic problem such as diabetes.

Necrotizing Ulcerative Periodontitis

Necrotizing ulcerative periodontitis (NUP) is a rare disease, especially in developed countries. Often, NUP is diagnosed in individuals with a compromised host immune response. The incidence of NUP in specific populations, such as patients who are positive for human immunodeficiency virus (HIV) infection or have acquired immunodeficiency syndrome (AIDS), has been reported to be between 0% and 6%. These patients often have an underlying predisposing systemic factor that renders them susceptible to necrotizing ulcerative periodontal disease. For this reason, patients presenting with NUP should be treated in consultation with their physician.

A comprehensive medical evaluation and diagnosis of any condition that may be contributing to an altered host immune response should be completed. It is also important to rule out any hematologic disease (e.g., leukemia) before initiating treatment of a case that has a similar presentation to NUP.

Treatment can be initiated only after a thorough medical history and examination to identify the existence of any systemic diseases. Treatment for NUP includes local debridement of lesions with scaling and root planing, lavage, and instructions for good oral hygiene. It may be necessary to use local anesthesia during the debridement because lesions are frequently painful. The use of ultrasonic instrumentation with profuse irrigation may enhance debridement and flushing of the deep lesions. Achieving good oral hygiene may be challenging as well until the lesions and associated pain resolve.

Antimicrobial adjuncts, such as chlorhexidine, added to the oral hygiene regimen may be effective in contributing to the daily reduction of bacterial loads. Patients frequently complain of pain. The use of locally applied topical antimicrobials and systemic antibiotics, as well as systemic analgesics, should be used as indicated by signs and symptoms.

Patients with NUP often harbor bacteria, fungi, viruses, and other nonoral microorganisms, complicating the selection of antimicrobial therapy. Superinfection or overgrowth of fungi and viruses may be propagated by antibiotic therapy. Antifungal and/or antiviral agents can be considered prophylactically against these infections or after they are diagnosed. Since oral hygiene for these patients is complicated by the painful lesions, alternative methods should be encouraged. In such patients, irrigation with diluted cleansing and antibacterial agents can be of some benefit.

Ultimately, the successful treatment of NUP may depend on the resolution or treatment of the systemic condition (e.g., immune compromise) that predisposed the individual to the disease. Evaluation and treatment of patients with known systemic conditions, such as HIV infection, should be coordinated with the patient's physician.

Conclusion

Treatment of aggressive and atypical forms of periodontal disease is challenging for clinicians because these forms are infrequently encountered, can manifest with more severe bone loss, and do not respond as predictably or as favorably to conventional therapy. Fortunately, only a small percentage of patients are diagnosed with these forms of periodontitis. This chapter discussed therapies and rationales for management of these challenging cases.

Key points

- Patients diagnosed with aggressive and some atypical forms of periodontal disease often do not respond as predictably or as favorably to conventional therapy.
- The prognosis for patients with aggressive periodontitis depends on (1) whether the disease is generalized or localized, (2) the degree of destruction present at the time of diagnosis, and (3) the ability to control future progression.
- One of the most important aspects of treatment success in aggressive periodontitis is to educate the patient about the disease, including the causes and the risk factors for disease, and to stress the importance of the patient's role in the success of treatment. Essential therapeutic considerations for the clinician are to control the infection, arrest disease progression, correct anatomic defects, replace missing teeth, and ultimately help the patient maintain periodontal health with frequent periodontal maintenance care. Patients who are diagnosed with aggressive periodontitis at an early stage and who are able to enter therapy may have a better outcome than those who are diagnosed at an advanced stage of destruction. Treatment options for teeth with deep periodontal pockets and bone loss may be nonsurgical or surgical. Surgery may be purely resective, regenerative, or a combination of these approaches.
- The presence of periodontal pathogens, specifically *Aggregatibacter actinomycetemcomitans*, has been implicated as the reason that aggressive periodontitis does not respond to conventional therapy alone. These pathogens are known to remain in the tissues after therapy to reinfect the pocket.
- The antimicrobial therapy includes antibiotic susceptibility test, systemic and local antibiotic therapy, full mouth disinfection, and use of host modulating agents.
- Each maintenance visit should consist of a medical history review, an inquiry about any recent periodontal problems, assessment risk of factors, a comprehensive periodontal and oral examination, thorough root debridement, and prophylaxis, followed by a review of oral hygiene instructions.
- Although refractory periodontitis is not currently considered a separate disease entity, patients who fail to respond to conventional therapy are considered to have periodontitis that is "refractory" to treatment. It is possible to characterize any form of periodontal disease (e.g., chronic periodontitis, aggressive periodontitis) as refractory to treatment.
- A case may be considered *refractory* to treatment only when loss of periodontal attachment and bone continues after well-executed treatment in a patient with good oral hygiene and no other infections or etiologic factors.
- Various antibiotic regimens have been tried in treatment of refractory periodontitis but development of antibiotic resistance is the common problem associated with it.
- Necrotizing ulcerative periodontitis (NUP) is a rare disease, especially in developed countries. These patients often have an underlying predisposing systemic factor that renders them susceptible to necrotizing ulcerative periodontal disease. For this reason, patients presenting with NUP should be treated in consultation with their physician.
- Treatment for NUP includes local debridement of lesions with scaling and root planing, lavage, and instructions for good oral hygiene. It may be necessary to use local anesthesia during the debridement because lesions are frequently painful. The use of ultrasonic instrumentation with profuse irrigation may enhance debridement and flushing of the deep lesions.

Suggested Readings

Al-Zahrani MS: Implant therapy in aggressive periodontitis patients: a systematic review and clinical implications, *Quintessence Int* 39:211–215, 2008.

Bollen CM, Mongardini C, Papaioannou W, et al: The effect of a one-stage full-mouth disinfection on different intra-oral niches. Clinical and microbiological observations, *J Clin Periodontol* 25:56–66, 1998.

Buchmann R, Nunn ME, Van Dyke TE, et al: Aggressive periodontitis: 5-year follow-up of treatment, *J Periodontol* 73:675–683, 2002.

Haffajee AD, Uzel NG, Arguello EI, et al: Clinical and microbiological changes associated with the use of combined antimicrobial therapies to treat "refractory" periodontitis, *J Clin Periodontol* 31:869–877, 2004.

Herrera D, Sanz M, Jepsen S, et al: A systematic review on the effect of systemic antimicrobials as an adjunct to scaling and root planing in periodontitis patients, *J Clin Periodontol* 29(Suppl 3):136–159, 2002.

Lang N, Bartold PM, Cullinan M, et al: Consensus report: aggressive periodontitis, *Ann Periodontol* 4, 1999.

Lindhe J, Liljenberg B: Treatment of localized juvenile periodontitis. Results after 5 years, *J Clin Periodontol* 11:399–410, 1984.

Nevins M, Langer B: The successful use of osseointegrated implants for the treatment of the recalcitrant periodontal patient, *J Periodontol* 66: 150–157, 1995.

Quirynen M, Mongardini C, de Soete M, et al: The role of chlorhexidine in the one-stage full-mouth disinfection treatment of patients with advanced adult periodontitis. Long-term clinical and microbiological observations, *J Clin Periodontol* 27:578–589, 2000.

Waerhaug J: Subgingival plaque and loss of attachment in periodontosis as evaluated on extracted teeth, *J Periodontol* 48:125–130, 1977.

References

References and MCQs with answers for the chapter are available on www.medenact.com.

CHAPTER 31

Treatment of Acute Gingival Disease

PR Klokkevold | FA Carranza | DG Naik | A Uppoor

CHAPTER OUTLINE

The treatment of acute gingival disease entails the alleviation of the acute symptoms and elimination of all other periodontal diseases, both chronic and acute, throughout the oral cavity. Treatment is not complete if periodontal pathologic changes or factors capable of causing them are still present. Systemic risk factors that increase susceptibility to these acute gingival diseases also need to be assessed and eliminated or modified if possible.

Necrotizing Ulcerative Gingivitis

Necrotizing ulcerative gingivitis (NUG) results from an impaired host response to a potentially pathogenic microflora. Depending on the degree of immunosuppression, NUG may occur in a mouth essentially free of other gingival involvement or may be superimposed on underlying chronic gingival disease. Treatment should include the alleviation of the acute symptoms and the correction of the underlying chronic gingival disease. The former is the simpler part of the treatment, whereas the latter requires more comprehensive procedures.

The treatment of NUG consists of (1) alleviation of the acute inflammation by reducing the microbial load and removal of necrotic tissue, (2) treatment of chronic disease either underlying the acute involvement or elsewhere in the oral cavity, (3) alleviation of generalized symptoms such as fever and malaise, and (4) correction of systemic conditions or factors that contribute to the initiation or progression of the gingival changes. Chapter 24 provides further information on the management and treatment of NUG in patients with acquired immunodeficiency syndrome (AIDS).

Treatment of NUG should follow an orderly sequence according to specific steps at three clinical visits.

First Visit

At the first visit, the clinician should do a complete evaluation of the patient, including a comprehensive medical history with special attention to recent illness, living conditions, dietary background, cigarette smoking, type of employment, hours of rest, risk factors for HIV, and psychosocial parameters (e.g., stress, depression). The patient is questioned regarding the history of the acute disease and its onset and duration, as follows:

- Is the disease recurrent?
- Are the recurrences associated with specific factors such as menstruation, particular foods, exhaustion, or mental stress?
- Has there been any previous treatment? When and for how long?

The clinician should also inquire as to the type of treatment received and the patient's impression regarding its effect.

The examination of the patient should include general appearance, presence of halitosis, presence of skin lesions, vital signs including temperature, and palpation for the presence of enlarged lymph nodes, especially submaxillary and submental nodes.

The oral cavity is examined for the characteristic lesion of NUG (see Chapters 15 and 21) distribution and the possible involvement of the oropharyngeal region. Oral hygiene is evaluated, with special attention to the presence of pericoronal flaps, periodontal pockets, and local factors (e.g., poor restorations, distribution of calculus). Periodontal probing of NUG lesions is likely to be very painful and may need to be deferred until after the acute lesions are resolved.

KEY FACT

The goals of initial therapy for NUG are reduction of the microbial load and removal of necrotic tissue to facilitate the healing process of repair and regeneration so that normal tissue barriers can be reestablished.

The goals of initial therapy are to reduce the microbial load and remove necrotic tissue to the degree that repair and regeneration of normal tissue barriers are reestablished. Treatment during this initial visit is confined to the acutely involved areas, which are isolated with cotton rolls and dried. A topical anesthetic is applied, and after 2 or 3 min, the areas are gently swabbed with a moistened cotton pellet to remove the pseudomembrane and nonattached surface debris. Bleeding may be profuse. Each cotton pellet is used in a small area, then discarded; sweeping motions over large areas with a single pellet are not recommended. After the area is cleansed with warm water, the superficial calculus is removed. Ultrasonic scalers are very useful for this purpose because they do not elicit pain, and the water jet and cavitation aid in lavage of the area.

Subgingival scaling and curettage are contraindicated at this time because these procedures may extend the infection into the deeper tissues and may also cause bacteremia. Unless an emergency exists, procedures, such as extractions or periodontal surgery, are postponed until the patient has been symptom free for 4 weeks to minimize the likelihood of exacerbating the acute symptoms.

Patients with moderate or severe NUG and local lymphadenopathy or other systemic signs or symptoms are placed on an antibiotic regimen of amoxicillin, 500 mg orally every 6 h for 10 days. For amoxicillin-sensitive patients, other antibiotics are prescribed, such as erythromycin (500 mg every 6 h) or metronidazole (500 mg twice daily for 7 days). Systemic complications should subside in 1–3 days. Antibiotics are not recommended in NUG patients who do not have systemic complications.

Instructions to the Patient

The patient is discharged with the following instructions:

1. Avoid tobacco, alcohol, and condiments.
2. Rinse with a glassful of an equal mixture of 3% hydrogen peroxide and warm water every 2 h and/or twice daily with 0.12% chlorhexidine solution.
3. Get adequate rest. Pursue usual activities, but avoid excessive physical exertion or prolonged exposure to the sun, as in golf, tennis, swimming, or sunbathing.
4. Confine toothbrushing to the removal of surface debris with a bland dentifrice and an ultrasoft brush; overzealous brushing and the use of dental floss or interdental cleaners will be painful. Chlorhexidine mouth rinses are also helpful in controlling plaque throughout the mouth.
5. An analgesic, such as a nonsteroidal antiinflammatory drug (NSAID; e.g., ibuprofen), is appropriate for pain relief.
6. Patients who have systemic complications, such as high fever, malaise, anorexia, and general debility and who have been put on an antibiotic treatment are told that bed rest is necessary, as well as copious fluid consumption and administration of analgesics for relief of pain.

Patients are asked to report back to the clinician in 1–2 days. The patient should be advised of the extent of total treatment that the condition requires and warned that treatment is not complete when pain stops. The patient should be informed of the presence of chronic gingival or periodontal disease, which must be eliminated to reduce the likelihood of recurrence of the acute symptoms.

A large variety of drugs have been used in the treatment of NUG. Topical drug therapy, however, is only an adjunctive measure; no drug, when used alone, can be considered complete therapy. Systemic antibiotics, when used, also reduce the oral bacterial flora and alleviate the oral symptoms, but they are only an adjunct to the complete local treatment that the disease requires. In patients treated by drugs alone or by systemic antibiotics alone, the acute painful symptoms often recur after treatment is discontinued.

Second Visit

At the second visit, 1 or 2 days after the first visit, the patient is evaluated for amelioration of signs and symptoms. The patient's condition is usually improved; the pain is diminished or no longer present. The gingival margins of the involved areas are erythematous but without a superficial pseudomembrane.

Scaling is performed if necessary and sensitivity permits. Shrinkage of the gingiva may expose previously covered calculus, which is gently removed. The instructions to the patient are the same as those given previously.

Third Visit

At the next visit, approximately 5 days after the second visit, the patient is evaluated for resolution of symptoms, and a comprehensive plan for the management of the patient's periodontal conditions is formulated. The patient should be essentially symptom free. Some erythema may still be present in the involved areas, and the gingiva may be slightly painful on tactile stimulation (Fig. 31.1A and B). The patient is instructed in plaque control procedures which are essential for the success of the treatment and the maintenance of periodontal health. The patient is further counseled on nutrition, smoking cessation, and other conditions or habits associated with a potential recurrence. The hydrogen peroxide rinses are discontinued, but chlorhexidine rinses can be maintained for 2 or 3 weeks. Scaling and root planing are repeated if necessary. Unfortunately, the patient often discontinues treatment because the acute condition has subsided; however, this is when comprehensive treatment of the patient's chronic periodontal problem should start.

Appointments should be scheduled for the treatment of chronic gingivitis, periodontal pockets, and pericoronal flaps, as well as for the elimination of all forms of local irritation. The patient should be reevaluated at 1 month to determine compliance with oral hygiene, health habits, psychosocial factors, the potential need for

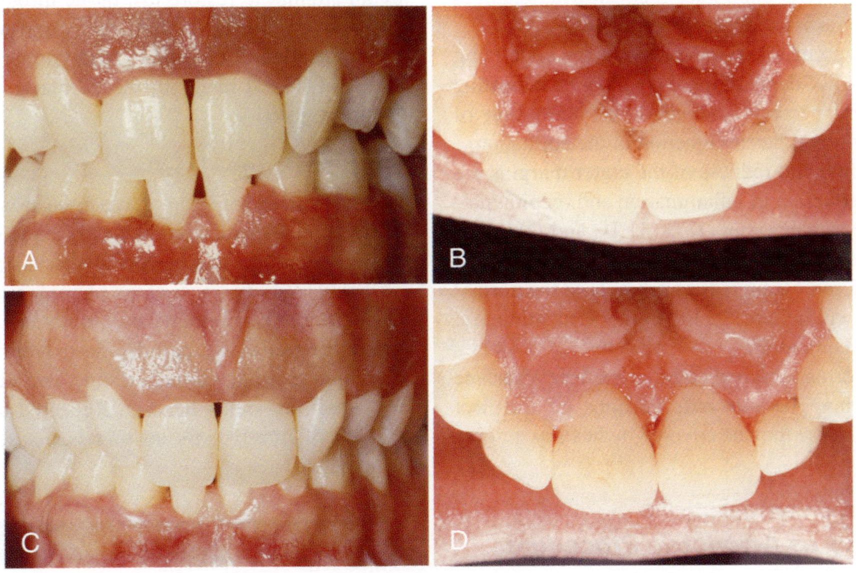

Fig. 31.1 A, Initial view of the anterior gingival tissues in a 22-year-old white female smoker with acute NUG. B, Palatal view of the same patient. C, Facial view of the same patient, 2 days after initial scaling and cessation of smoking. D, Palatal view of the same patient, 2 days after initial scaling and cessation of smoking. *(From Rose LF, Mealey BL, Genco RJ, Cohen DW: Periodontics: medicine, surgery, and implants, Mosby, St. Louis, 2005.)*

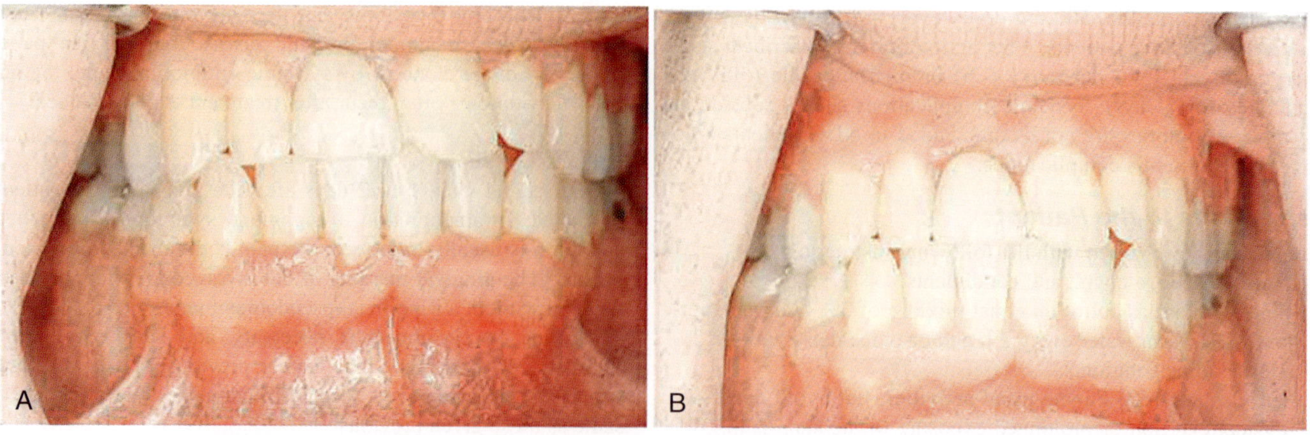

Fig. 31.2 Treatment of acute NUG. A, Before treatment. Note the characteristic interdental lesions. B, After treatment, showing restoration of healthy gingival contour.

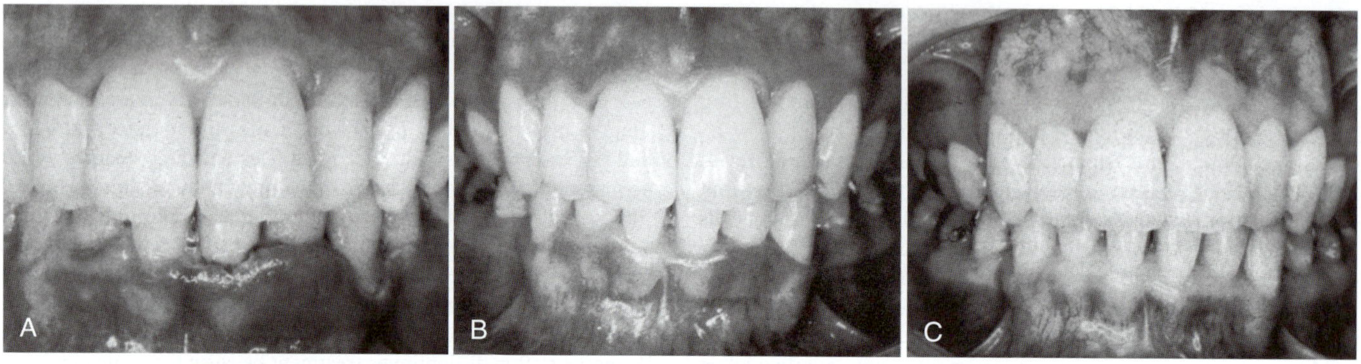

Fig. 31.3 Reshaping the gingiva in the treatment of acute NUG. A, Before treatment, showing bulbous gingiva and interdental necrosis in the mandibular anterior area. B, After treatment. Gingival contours still undesirable. C, Final result. Physiologic contours obtained by reshaping the gingiva.

reconstructive or esthetic surgery, and the interval of subsequent recall visits.

Gingival Changes With Healing

The characteristic lesion of NUG undergoes the following changes in the course of healing in response to treatment:

1. Removal of the surface pseudomembrane exposes the underlying red, hemorrhagic, crater-like depressions in the gingiva, indicating inflammation caused by necrosis and microbial infiltration of tissue that has lost the normal barrier function of the epithelium.
2. In the next stage, the bulk and redness of the crater margins are reduced, indicating a reduction in inflammation and reepithelialization, but the surface remains shiny (Fig. 31.1C and D).
3. This is followed by the early signs of restoration of normal gingival contour and color, indicating reestablishment of the normal barrier function of the epithelium, including keratinization and further reduction of inflammation.
4. In the final stage, the normal gingival color, consistency, surface texture, and contour may be restored. Portions of the root exposed by the acute disease may be covered by healthy gingiva (Fig. 31.2).

Additional Treatment Considerations

Contouring of Gingiva as Adjunctive Procedure

Even in cases of severe gingival necrosis, healing often leads to restoration of the normal gingival contour although normal architecture of the gingiva may be achieved only after several weeks or months. However, if there has been loss of interdental bone, if the teeth are irregularly aligned, or if the entire papilla is lost, healing sometimes results in the formation of a shelf-like gingival margin, which favors retention of plaque and recurrence of gingival inflammation as well as being an esthetic problem. This can be corrected by an attempt to restore lost tissue through periodontal plastic procedures or by reshaping the gingiva surgically (Fig. 31.3). Effective plaque control by the patient is particularly important to establish and maintain the normal gingival contour in areas of tooth irregularity.

Role of Drugs

A large variety of drugs have been used for topical treatment of NUG. Topical drug therapy is only an adjunctive measure. No drug, when used alone, can be considered complete treatment.

Escharotic drugs, such as phenol, silver nitrate, chromic acid, or potassium bichromate, should not be used. They are necrotizing agents that alleviate pain by destroying the nerve endings of the ulcerated gingiva. However, they also destroy young cells needed for repair and delay healing. Repeated use of these agents results in loss of gingival tissue that is not restored when the disease subsides.

KEY FACT

No drug, when used alone, can be considered complete treatment for the resolution of acute gingival disease (e.g., NUG). Local therapy and elimination of risk factors are essential for complete resolution.

Persistent or Recurrent Cases

Adequate local therapy with optimal home care will resolve most cases of NUG. If a case of NUG persists despite therapy or if it recurs, the patient should be reevaluated, with a focus on the following factors:

1. Reassessment of differential diagnosis to rule out diseases that resemble NUG. Several diseases and conditions may initially present with a similar appearance as NUG, such as desquamative gingivitis. A renewed search for skin lesions and other signs or symptoms should be undertaken, with a biopsy if warranted.
2. Underlying systemic disease causing immunosuppression. In particular, HIV infection may frequently present with symptoms of NUG or necrotizing ulcerative periodontitis (NUP). The patient should be reassessed for risk factors and may need counseling about testing for HIV or other suspected underlying systemic diseases (e.g., lymphoproliferative disease). The patient will likely need referral to his or her physician for further evaluation.
3. Inadequate local therapy. Too often, treatment is discontinued when the symptoms have subsided, without eliminating the chronic gingival disease and periodontal pockets that remain after the superficial acute condition is relieved. Remaining calculus and other local factors that predispose to gingival inflammation may permit recurrence. Recurrent acute involvement in the mandibular anterior area can be associated with persistent pericoronal inflammation arising from partial eruption and pericoronal inflammation of third molars. The anterior involvement is less likely to recur after the third molar situation is corrected.
4. Inadequate compliance. Poor plaque control, heavy use of tobacco, ineffective stress management, and continued malnutrition can also contribute to persistence or recurrence of NUG.

The clinician should evaluate the quality and consistency of plaque control. Further assessment and counseling on tobacco use will also determine the role of tobacco in this patient. If the clinician perceives that psychosocial factors are unresolved and are complicating health behaviors and contributing to immunosuppression, the patient should be referred to the appropriate professional. A reassessment of the patient's nutritional state, with potential dietary analysis or nutritional testing, may be required.

CLINICAL CORRELATION

Acute gingival disease may be a sign of a more serious systemic condition, such as acquired immunodeficiency disease or another condition that renders the host immunocompromised.

Acute Pericoronitis

The treatment of pericoronitis depends on the severity of the inflammation, the systemic complications, and the advisability of retaining the involved tooth. All pericoronal flaps should be viewed with suspicion. Persistent symptom-free pericoronal flaps should be removed as a preventive measure against subsequent acute involvement.

The treatment of acute pericoronitis consists of (1) gently flushing the area with warm water to remove debris and exudate and (2) swabbing with antiseptic after elevating the flap gently from the tooth with a scaler. The underlying debris is removed, and the area is flushed with warm water (Fig. 31.4). The occlusion is evaluated to determine if an opposing tooth is occluding with the pericoronal flap. It may be necessary to reduce soft tissue surgically and/or to adjust the opposing tooth to alleviate pain. Antibiotics can be prescribed in severe cases and for patients who may have clinical evidence of diffuse microbial infiltration of the tissue. If the gingival flap is swollen and fluctuant, an incision may be necessary to establish drainage and relieve pressure.

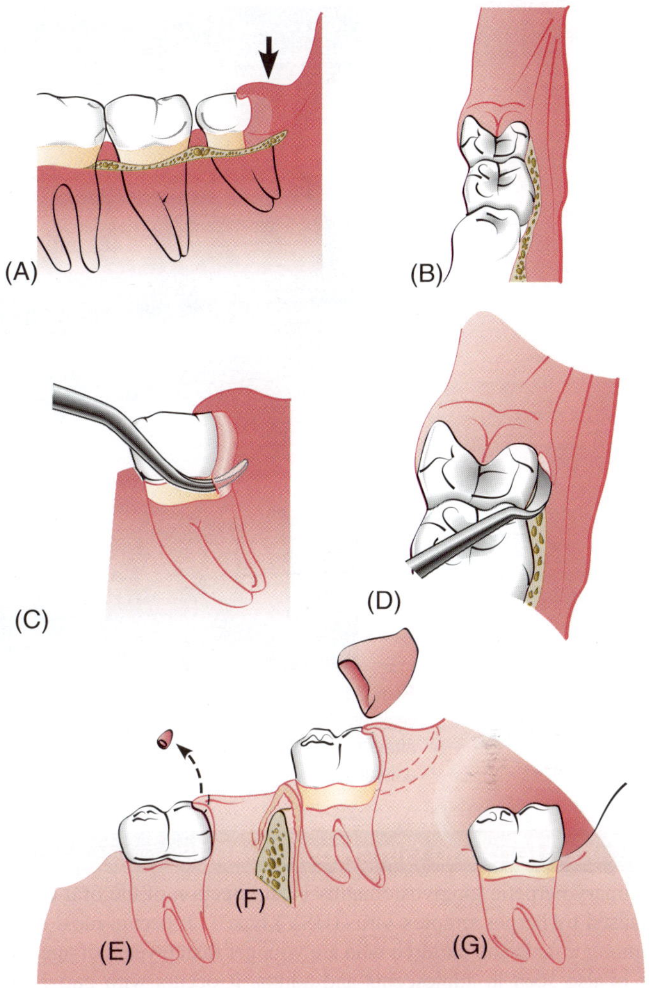

Fig. 31.4 Treatment of acute pericoronitis. Osseous surgery may be necessary in some cases. A, Inflamed pericoronal flap (arrow) in relation to the mandibular third molar. B, Anterior view of third molar and flap. C, Lateral view with scaler in position to gently remove debris under flap. D, Anterior view of scaler in position. E, Incorrect removal of the tip of the flap, permitting the deep pocket to remain distal to the molar. F, Removal of section of the gingiva distal to the third molar after the acute symptoms subsided. The line of incision is indicated by the broken line. G, Appearance of the healed area.

Once the acute symptoms have subsided, the prognosis of the tooth can be evaluated. The decision will be governed by the likelihood of whether the tooth will continue eruption into a functional position or if impaction and the factors predisposing to pericoronitis will persist. Bone loss on the distal surface of the second molar is a concern when third molars are impacted along the distal surface. The problem is significantly greater if the third molars are extracted after the roots are formed or when patients are older (i.e., mid-20s or later). To reduce the risk of bone loss around second molars, partially or completely impacted third molars should be extracted early in their development.

If the decision is made to retain the tooth, the pericoronal flap is surgically reduced (see Fig. 31.4). It is necessary to remove the tissue distal to the tooth, as well as the flap on the occlusal surface. Incising only the occlusal portion of the flap leaves a deep distal pocket, which invites recurrence of acute pericoronal involvement. It is critical to leave the patient with a cleansable site. On healing, the patient needs appropriate instruction in long-term maintenance.

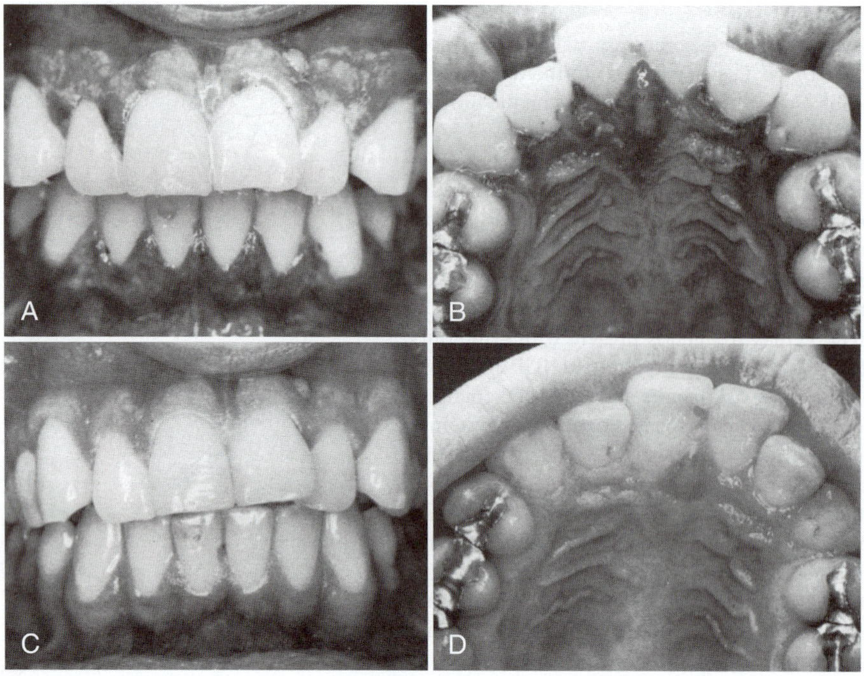

Fig. 31.5 Treatment of acute herpetic gingivostomatitis. A, Before treatment. Note diffuse erythema and surface vesicles. B, Before treatment, palatal view, showing gingival edema and ruptured vesicle on palate. C, One month after treatment, showing restoration of normal gingival contour and stippling. D, One month after treatment, palatal view.

Acute Herpetic Gingivostomatitis

Primary herpetic gingivostomatitis is an infection of the oral cavity caused by herpes simplex virus (HSV) type 1. It occurs most often among infants and children who are younger than 6 years of age, but it is also seen in adolescents and adults. It occurs with equal frequency in male and female patients. In most individuals, however, the primary infection is asymptomatic. It runs a 7 to 10-day course and usually heals without scarring. A recurrent herpetic episode may be precipitated in individuals with a history of herpesvirus infections by dental treatment, respiratory infections, sunlight exposure, fever, trauma, exposure to chemicals, and emotional stress.

Treatment consists of early diagnosis and immediate initiation of antiviral therapy. Until recently, therapy for primary herpetic gingivostomatitis consisted of palliative care. With the development of antiviral therapy, however, the standard of care has changed. In a randomized double-blind placebo-controlled study, Amir et al. demonstrated that antiviral therapy with 15 mg/kg of an acyclovir suspension given five times daily for 7 days substantially changes the course of the disease without significant side effects. Acyclovir reduced symptoms, including fever, from 3 days to 1 day; decreased new extraoral lesions from 5.5 to 0 days; and reduced difficulty with eating from 7 to 4 days. Furthermore, viral shedding stopped at 1 day for the acyclovir group compared to 5 days for the control group. Overall, oral lesions were present for only 4 days in the acyclovir group but for 10 days in the control group. Although no clear clinical evidence indicates that this regimen will reduce recurrences, research data suggest that a greater number of latent virus copies incorporated into ganglia will increase the severity of recurrences.

In summary, if primary herpetic gingivostomatitis is diagnosed within 3 days of onset, acyclovir suspension should be prescribed: 15 mg/kg five times daily for 7 days. If diagnosis occurs after 3 days in an immunocompetent patient, acyclovir therapy may have limited value. All patients, including those presenting more than 3 days after disease onset, may receive palliative care, including removal of plaque and food debris. An NSAID (e.g., ibuprofen) can be given systemically to reduce fever and pain. Patients may use either nutritional supplements or topical anesthetics (e.g., viscous lidocaine) before eating to aid in proper nutrition during the early phases in acute herpetic gingivostomatitis. Periodontal therapy should be postponed until the acute symptoms subside to avoid the possibility of exacerbation (Fig. 31.5).

Local or systemic application of antibiotics is sometimes advised to prevent opportunistic infection of ulcerations, especially in the immunocompromised patient. If the condition does not resolve within 2 weeks, the patient should be referred to a physician for medical consultation. The patient should be informed that herpetic gingivostomatitis is contagious at certain stages such as when vesicles are present (highest viral titer). All individuals exposed to an infected patient should take precautions. Herpetic infection of a clinician's finger, referred to as herpetic whitlow, can occur if a seronegative clinician becomes infected with a patient's herpetic lesions.

Key points

- The treatment of acute gingival disease entails the alleviation of the acute symptoms and elimination of all other periodontal diseases, both chronic and acute, throughout the oral cavity.
- The treatment of NUG consists of (1) alleviation of the acute inflammation by reducing the microbial load and removal of necrotic tissue, (2) treatment of chronic disease either underlying the acute involvement or elsewhere in the oral cavity, (3) alleviation of generalized symptoms such as fever and malaise, and (4) correction of systemic conditions or factors that contribute to the initiation or progression of the gingival changes.
- The treatment of NUG includes three visit pattern. The entire treatment is provided under first, second, and third visit.

- Treatment during this initial visit is confined to the acutely involved areas, which are isolated with cotton rolls and dried. A topical anesthetic is applied, and after 2 or 3 min, the areas are gently swabbed with a moistened cotton pellet to remove the pseudomembrane and nonattached surface debris.
- During first visit, subgingival scaling and curettage are contraindicated at this time because these procedures may extend the infection into the deeper tissues and may also cause bacteremia.
- Second visit is usually 1–2 days after the first visit. Usually the superficial area will be free of pesudomembrane.
- Adequate local therapy with optimal home care will resolve most cases of NUG. If a case of NUG persists despite therapy or if it recurs, the patient should be reevaluated, with a focus on factors such as reassessment of differential diagnosis to rule out diseases that resemble underlying systemic disease causing immunosuppression, inadequate local therapy, and inadequate patient's compliance.
- The treatment of pericoronitis depends on the severity of the inflammation, the systemic complications, and the advisability of retaining the involved tooth. Persistent symptom-free pericoronal flaps should be removed as a preventive measure against subsequent acute involvement.
- Primary infection with herpes simplex virus in the oral cavity results in a condition known as acute herpetic gingivostomatitis, which is an oral infection often accompanied by systemic signs and symptoms. Usually occurs in children and duration of 7–10 days.
- Early diagnosis and prompt antiviral therapy will give better prognosis.

Suggested Readings

Amir J, Harel L, Smetana Z, et al: Treatment of herpes simplex gingivostomatitis with acyclovir in children: a randomised double-blind placebo-controlled study, *BMJ* 314:1800, 1997.

Ash MM Jr, Costich ER, Hayward JR: A study of periodontal hazards of third molars, *J Periodontol* 33:209, 1962.

Corbet EF: Diagnosis of acute periodontal lesions, *Periodontol* 2000 34:204–216, 2004.

Johnson BD, Engel D: Acute necrotizing ulcerative gingivitis: a review of diagnosis, etiology and treatment, *J Periodontol* 57(3):141–150, 1986.

Kureishi A, Chow AW: The tender tooth. Dentoalveolar, pericoronal, and periodontal infections, *Infect Dis Clin North Am* 2(1):163–182, 1988.

Langlais RP, Miller CS: *Color atlas of common oral diseases*, ed 2, New York, 1998, Williams & Wilkins.

Matusow RJ: Acute primary herpetic gingivostomatitis in non-immunocompromised adults and an HSV-1 isolation technique, *Compendium* 13(8):662–666, 1992.

Regezi JA, Sciubba JJ: *Oral pathology: clinical-pathologic correlations*, Philadelphia, 1989, Saunders.

Wade DN, Kerns DG: Acute necrotizing ulcerative gingivitis-periodontitis: a literature review, *Mil Med* 163(5):337–342, 1998.

Williamson RT: Diagnosis and management of recurrent herpes simplex induced by fixed prosthodontic tissue management: a clinical report, *J Prosthet Dent* 82:1, 1999.

References

References and MCQs with answers for the chapter are available on www.medenact.com.

CHAPTER 32

Treatment of Periodontal Abscess

PR Melnick | HH Takei | A Uppoor | DG Naik

CHAPTER OUTLINE

Specific Treatment Approaches

Treatment of the periodontal abscess includes two phases: resolving the acute lesion, followed by the management of the resulting chronic condition (Box 32.1).

Acute Abscess

The acute abscess is treated to alleviate symptoms, control the spread of infection, and establish drainage. Before treatment, the patient's medical history, dental history, and systemic condition are reviewed and evaluated to assist in the diagnosis and to determine the need for systemic antibiotics (Boxes 32.2 and 32.3).

Drainage Through Periodontal Pocket

The peripheral area around the abscess is anesthetized with sufficient topical and local anesthetic to ensure comfort. The pocket wall is gently retracted with a periodontal probe or curette in an attempt to initiate drainage through the pocket entrance (see Fig. 32.1). Gentle digital pressure and irrigation may be used to express exudates and clear the pocket (Fig. 32.2). If the lesion is small and access uncomplicated, debridement in the form of scaling and root planing may be undertaken.

If the lesion is large and drainage cannot be established, root debridement by scaling and root planing or surgical access should be delayed until the major clinical signs have abated. In these patients, use of adjunctive systemic antibiotics with short-term high-dose regimens is recommended (Box 32.3). Antibiotic therapy alone without subsequent drainage and subgingival scaling is contraindicated.

Drainage Through External Incision

The abscess is dried and isolated with gauze sponges. Topical anesthetic is applied, followed by local anesthetic injected peripheral to the lesion. A vertical incision through the most fluctuant center of the abscess is made with a no. 15 surgical blade. The tissue lateral to the incision can be separated with a curette or periosteal elevator. Fluctuant matter is expressed, and the wound edges approximated under light digital pressure with a moist gauze pad.

In abscesses presenting with severe swelling and inflammation, aggressive mechanical instrumentation should be delayed in favor of antibiotic therapy so as to avoid damage to healthy contiguous periodontal tissues.

Once bleeding and suppuration have ceased, the patient may be dismissed. For those who do not need systemic antibiotics, posttreatment instructions include frequent rinsing with warm salt water (1 tbsp/8-oz glass) and periodic application of chlorhexidine gluconate either by rinsing or locally with a cotton-tipped applicator. Reduced exertion and increased fluid intake are often recommended for patients showing systemic involvement. Analgesics may be prescribed for comfort. By the following day, the signs and symptoms have usually subsided. If not, the patient is instructed to continue the previously recommended regimen for an additional 24 h. This often results in satisfactory healing and the lesion can be treated as a chronic abscess.

Chronic Abscess

As with a periodontal pocket, the chronic abscess is usually treated with scaling and root planing or surgical therapy. Surgical treatment is suggested when deep vertical or furcation defects are encountered that are beyond the therapeutic capabilities of nonsurgical instrumentation (Fig. 32.3). The patient should be advised of the possible postoperative sequelae usually associated with periodontal nonsurgical and surgical procedures. As with the acute abscess, antibiotic therapy may be indicated.

KEY FACT

Periodontal abscess due to a deep periodontal pocket often requires a surgical flap to access the subgingival calculus. This also allows the clinician to reduce the pocket at the same surgical appointment.

Gingival Abscess

Treatment of the gingival abscess is aimed at reversal of the acute phase and when applicable, immediate removal of the cause. To ensure procedural comfort, topical, or local anesthesia by infiltration is administered. When possible, scaling and root planing are completed to establish drainage and remove microbial deposits.

BOX 32.1 Treatment Options for Periodontal Abscess

1. Drainage through pocket retraction or incision
2. Scaling and root planing
3. Periodontal surgery
4. Systemic antibiotics
5. Tooth removal

(Modified from Sanz M, Herrera D, van Winkelhoff AJ: The periodontal abscess. In Lindhe, J: Clinical periodontology, Copenhagen, 2000, Munksgaard.)

BOX 32.2 Indications for Antibiotic Therapy in Patients With Acute Abscess

1. Cellulitis (nonlocalized, spreading infection)
2. Deep, inaccessible pocket
3. Fever
4. Regional lymphadenopathy
5. Immunocompromised patient

BOX 32.3 Antibiotic Options for Periodontal Infections

Antibiotic of Choice

Amoxicillin, 500 mg

- 1.0-g loading dose, then 500 mg 3 times a day for 3 days.
- Reevaluation after 3 days to determine the need for continued or adjusted antibiotic therapy.

Penicillin Allergy

Clindamycin

- 600-mg loading dose, then 300 mg four times a day for 3 days.

Azithromycin (or Clarithromycin) (To be used with caution in patients with high baseline cardiovascular risk.)

- 1.0-g loading dose, then 500 mg 4 times a day for 3 days.

(Data from American Academy of Periodontology: *J Periodontol* 67:1553, 2004.)

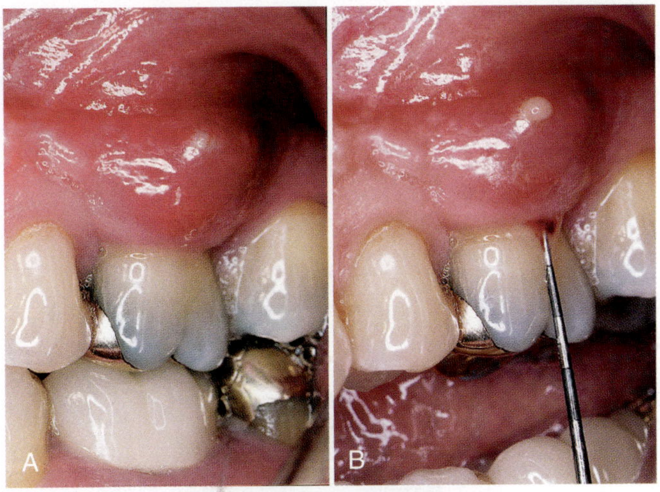

Fig. 32.1 Diagnosis of periodontal abscess.

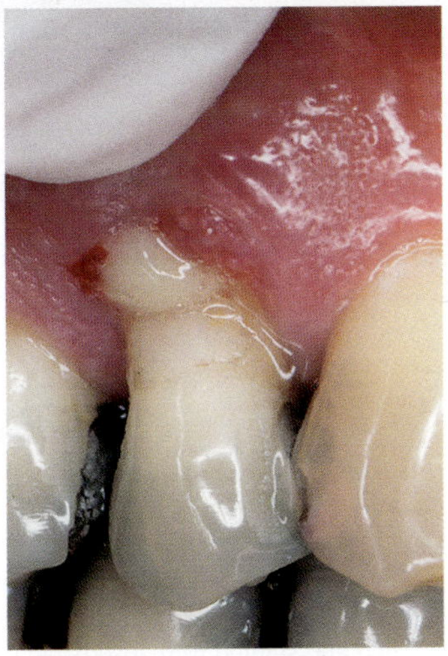

Fig. 32.2 Gentle digital pressure may be sufficient to express purulent discharge.

In more acute situations, the fluctuant area is incised with a no. 15 scalpel blade, and exudate may be expressed by gentle digital pressure. Any foreign material (e.g., dental floss, impression material) is removed. The area is irrigated with warm water and covered with moist gauze under light pressure.

Once bleeding has stopped, the patient is dismissed with instructions to rinse with warm salt water every 2 h for the remainder of the day. After 24 h, the area is reassessed, and if resolution is sufficient, scaling not previously completed is undertaken. If the residual lesion is large or poorly accessible, surgical access may be required.

Pericoronal Abscess

As with the other abscesses of the periodontium, the treatment of the pericoronal abscess is aimed at management of the acute phase, followed by resolution of the chronic condition. The acute pericoronal abscess is properly anesthetized for comfort, and drainage is established by gently lifting the soft tissue operculum with a periodontal probe or curette. If the underlying debris is easily accessible, it may be removed, followed by gentle irrigation with sterile saline. If there is regional swelling, lymphadenopathy, or systemic signs, systemic antibiotics may be prescribed.

The patient is dismissed with instructions to rinse with warm salt water every 2 h, and the area is reassessed after 24 h. If discomfort was one of the original complaints, appropriate analgesics should be employed. Once the acute phase has been controlled, the partially erupted tooth may be definitively treated with either surgical excision of the overlying tissue or removal of the offending tooth.

Key points

- Treatment of the periodontal abscess includes two phases: resolving the acute lesion, followed by the management of the resulting chronic condition.
- Before treatment, the patient's medical history, dental history, and systemic condition are reviewed and evaluated to assist in the diagnosis and to determine the need for systemic antibiotics.
- Abscess drainage can be done through periodontal pocket, through external incision.
- If there is regional swelling, lymphadenopathy, or systemic signs, systemic antibiotics may be prescribed.
- Once the acute phase has been controlled, the partially erupted tooth may be definitively treated with either surgical excision of the overlying tissue or removal of the offending tooth.

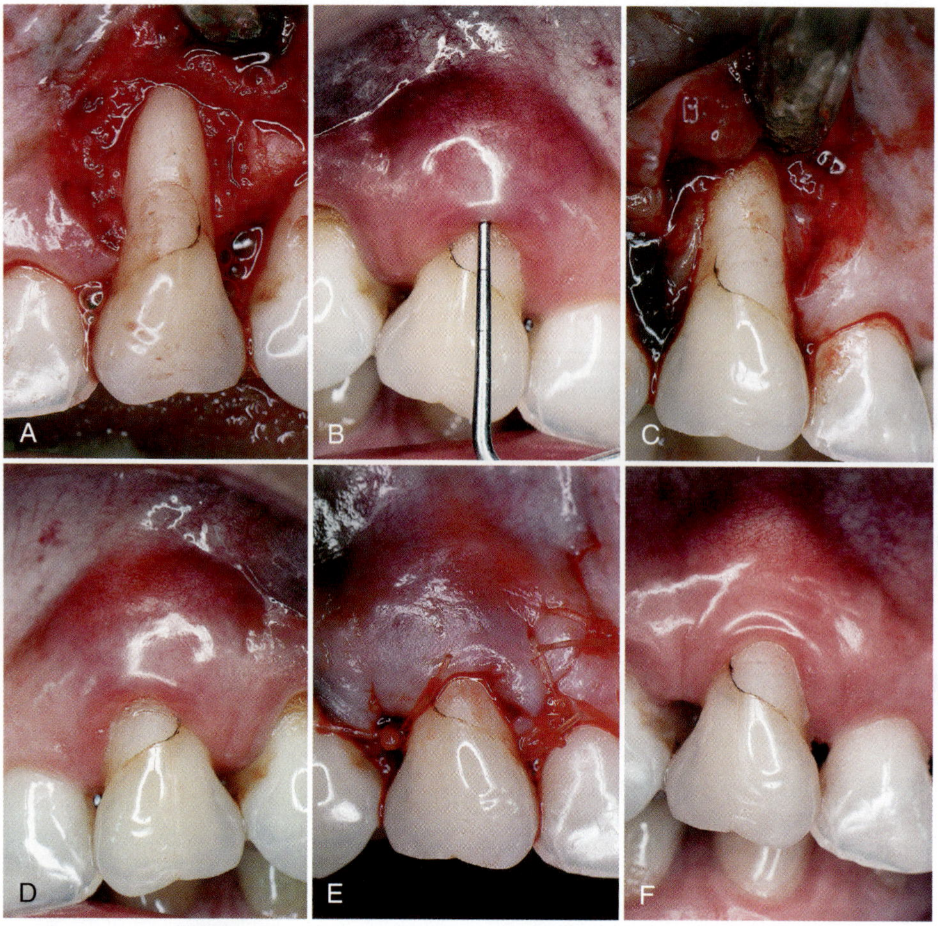

Fig. 32.3 A, Chronic periodontal abscess of maxillary right canine. B, Using local anesthesia, periodontal probe is inserted to determine severity of the lesion. C, Using mesial and distal vertical incisions, a full-thickness flap is elevated, exposing severe bone dehiscence, a subgingival restoration, and root calculus. D, Root surface has been planed free of calculus and the restoration smoothed. E, Full-thickness flap has been replaced to its original position and sutured with absorbable sutures. F, At 3 months, gingival tissues are pink, firm, and well adapted to the tooth, with minimal periodontal probing depth.

Suggested Readings

American Academy of Periodontology: parameter on acute periodontal diseases, *J Periodontol* 71 (5 Suppl):863–866, 2000.

Corbet EF: Diagnosis of acute periodontal lesions, *Periodontol 2000* 34:204, 2004.

Dahlen G: Microbiology and treatment of dental abscesses and periodontal-endodontic lesions, *Periodontol 2000* 28:206, 2002.

Herrera D, Roldan S, Gonzalez I, et al: The periodontal abscess. I. Clinical and microbiology findings, *J Clin Periodontol* 27:287, 2000a.

Herrera D, Roldan S, Sanz M: The periodontal abscess: a review, *J Clin Periodontol* 27:377, 2000b.

Lang N, Soskolne WA, Greenstein G, et al: Consensus report: abscesses of the periodontium, *Ann Periodontol* 4 (1):83, 1999.

Meng HX: Periodontal abscess, *Ann Periodontol* 4:79, 1999.

Minsk L: Diagnosis and treatment of acute periodontal conditions, *Compend Contin Educ Dent* 27 (1):8–11, 2006.

Sanz M, Herrera D, van Winkelhoff AJ: The periodontal abscess. In Lindhe J, editor: *Clinical periodontology*, Copenhagen, 2000, Munksgaard.

References

References and MCQs with answers for the chapter are available on www.medenact.com.

CHAPTER 33

Phase I Periodontal Therapy

DA Perry | HH Takei | A Jain

CHAPTER OUTLINE

Phase I therapy or cause-related therapy is the first step in the chronologic sequence of procedures that constitute periodontal treatment. The objective of phase I therapy is to alter or eliminate the microbial etiology and factors that contribute to gingival and periodontal diseases to the greatest extent possible, therefore halting the progression of disease and returning the dentition to a state of health and comfort. Phase I therapy is referred to by a number of names, including initial therapy, nonsurgical periodontal therapy, and cause-related therapy. All terms refer to the procedures performed to treat gingival and periodontal infections, up to and including tissue reevaluation, which is the point at which the course of ongoing care is determined.

Rationale

Phase I therapy is defined by the evidence-based American Association of Periodontology practice guidelines as the initiation of a comprehensive daily plaque-control regimen, management of periodontal-systemic interrelationships as needed, thorough removal of supra- and subgingival bacterial plaque biofilm and calculus, chemotherapeutic agents as necessary, and elimination of local factors, such as defective restorations and treatment of carious lesions. These procedures are a required part of periodontal therapy, regardless of the extent of disease present. In many cases, only phase I therapy will be required to restore periodontal health, or it will constitute the preparatory phase for surgical therapy. Figs. 33.1 and 33.2 show the results of phase I therapy in two patients with chronic periodontitis. The goal of cause-related phase I periodontal therapy has been succinctly stated as the approach *aimed at removal of pathogenic biofilms, toxins and calculus, and the reestablishment of a biologically acceptable root surface*.

Phase I therapy is a critical aspect of periodontal treatment. Data from clinical research indicate that the long-term success of periodontal surgical treatment is dependent upon maintaining the plaque-biofilm control results achieved with phase I therapy. In fact, patients who do not have an adequate plaque-biofilm control will continue to lose attachment regardless of the surgical procedures performed. In addition, phase I therapy provides an opportunity for the dentist to evaluate tissue response and provide reinforcement about homecare, both of which are crucial elements to the overall success of treatment.

Based on the knowledge that microbial plaque biofilm is the major etiologic agent in gingival inflammation, one specific aim of phase I therapy for every patient is *effective daily plaque-biofilm removal* at home. These homecare procedures can be complex, time-consuming, and often require changing long-standing habits. Good oral hygiene is more easily accomplished if the tooth surfaces are free of calculus deposits and other irregularities so that surfaces are easily accessible. Management of contributing all local factors is required in phase I therapy. The following list of elements makes up phase I therapy:

1. Patient education and oral hygiene instruction;
2. Complete removal of calculus (see Chapter 36);
3. Correction or replacement of poorly fitting restorations and prosthetic devices (see Chapter 53);
4. Restoration or temporization of carious lesions;
5. Orthodontic tooth movement (see Chapter 55);
6. Treatment of food impaction areas;
7. Treatment of occlusal trauma;
8. Extraction of hopeless teeth; and
9. Possible use of antimicrobial agents including necessary plaque sampling and sensitivity testing (see Chapters 8 and 37).

Treatment Sessions

After careful analysis and diagnosis of the specific periodontal condition present, the dentist must develop a treatment plan that includes all required procedures and estimates the number of appointments necessary to complete phase I therapy. In most cases, patients require several treatment sessions for the complete debridement of tooth surfaces. All of the following conditions must be considered when determining the phase I treatment plan:

- General health and tolerance of treatment;
- Number of teeth present;
- Amount of subgingival calculus;
- Probing pocket depths;
- Attachment loss;
- Furcation involvements;
- Alignment of teeth;
- Margins of restorations;
- Developmental anomalies;
- Physical barriers to access (i.e., limited opening or tendency to gag); and

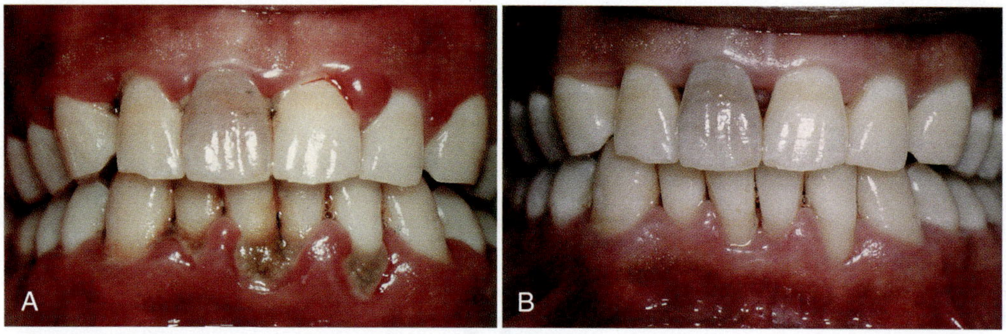

Fig. 33.1 Results of phase I therapy, severe chronic periodontitis. A, A 45-year-old patient with deep-probe depths, bone loss, severe swelling, and redness of the gingival tissues. B, Results 3 weeks after the completion of phase I therapy. Note that the gingival tissue has returned to a normal contour, with redness and swelling dramatically reduced.

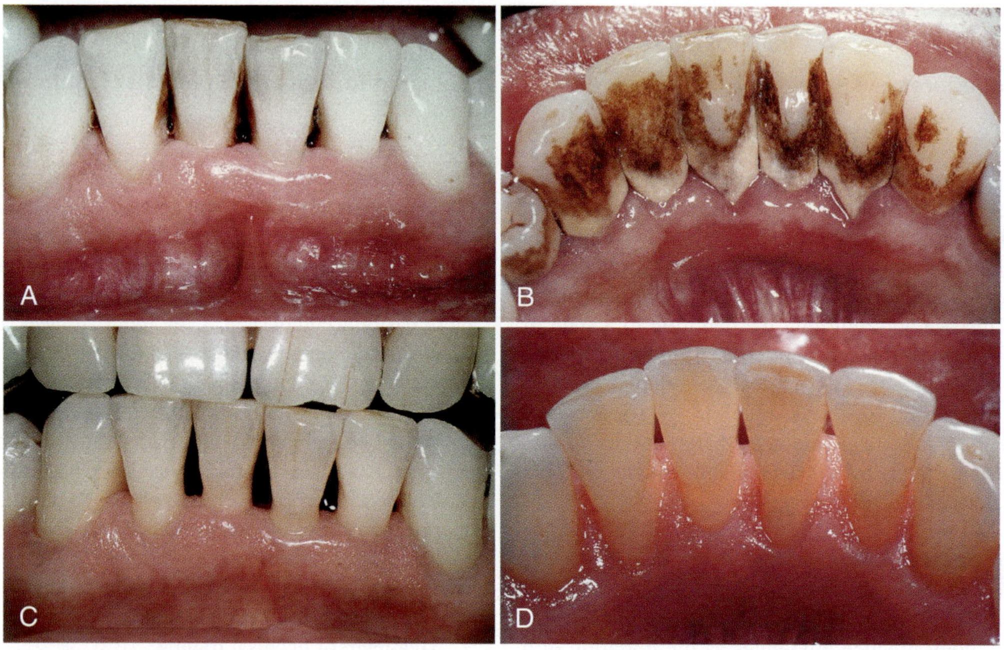

Fig. 33.2 Results of phase I therapy, moderate chronic periodontitis. A, A 52-year-old patient with moderate attachment loss and probe depths in the 4–6 mm range. Note that the gingiva appears pink because it is fibrotic. Inflammation is present in the periodontal pockets but disguised by the fibrotic tissue. Bleeding occurs on probing. B, Lingual view of the patient with more visible inflammation and heavy calculus deposits. C and D, 18 months after phase I therapy, the same areas show significant improvement in gingival health. The patient returned for regular maintenance visits at 4-month intervals.

- Patient cooperation and sensitivity (requiring use of anesthesia or analgesia).

Sequence of Procedures

Step 1. Plaque-Biofilm Control Instruction

Plaque-biofilm control is an essential component to the successful periodontal therapy and instruction should begin at the first treatment appointment. The patient must learn to correctly brush the teeth, focusing on applying the bristles at the gingival third of the clinical crowns of the teeth and begin using floss or other aids for interdental cleaning. This is sometimes referred to as *targeted oral hygiene* and emphasizes thorough biofilm removal around the periodontal tissues. The multiple appointment approach to phase I therapy permits the dentist to evaluate, reinforce, and improve the patient's oral-hygiene skills (Chapter 34 details plaque-control options).

Step 2. Removal of Supragingival and Subgingival Plaque Biofilm and Calculus

Removal of calculus is accomplished using scalers, curettes, ultrasonic instrumentation, or combinations of these devices during one or more appointments. Evidence suggests that the treatment results for chronic periodontitis are similar for all instruments which could be hand instrumentation or other mechanical instruments, such as ultrasonic scalers. In addition to calculus removal, bacterial plaque biofilm and some cementum are removed by instrumentation procedures as a matter of course. At one time it was thought that all cementum had to be systematically planed off of root surfaces in order to leave a glassy hard surface free of accumulated bacterial toxins. The rationale was that cementum became necrotic from penetration of lipopolysaccharide endotoxins from the microbial biofilm and would interfere with healing. However, it is now well known that lipopolysaccharides are only loosely attached and easily removed from cementum, so the instrumentation beyond the thorough removal of calculus and plaque biofilm will not improve treatment outcomes. As a consequence, the term *debridement* is now used as commonly than root planing.

Laser treatment has also been advocated for periodontal therapy by and some dentists. However, recent reviews suggest that further well-designed studies are needed to confirm improved outcomes. In addition, gingival curettage, the systematic removal of the soft-tissue lining of the pockets, has not been shown to improve results of treatment and there is, little if any, change in outcomes from performing irrigation or lavage of periodontal pockets during phase I-treatment appointments.

Photodynamic therapy has also been posited as an adjunct to scaling and root planing. This therapy uses lasers at specific wavelengths to "target microorganisms treated with a photosensitizer." Studies have not found this intervention to be useful as an alternative to scaling and root planing, or to improve treatment outcomes, and further research needs to be conducted to ascertain the efficacy of this treatment.

One other interesting approach to calculus removal and debridement is full-mouth disinfection. The technique is to perform the full-mouth treatment at one session, or multiple sessions within a day or so, and using disinfectants with the intention to prevent reinfection of treated sites from untreated sites. This treatment approach may also be used for phase I therapy, but it has not been shown to be superior to any other phase I-therapy treatment plan.

There are multiple approaches to planning and performing nonsurgical phase I therapy. Decisions as to how to proceed should be discussed and agreed upon by the patient and the dentist based on the amount of disease present and patient comfort. Staged therapy permits the advantage of evaluating and reinforcing oral-hygiene care and the one or two appointment therapies can be more efficient in reducing the number of office visits the patient is required to attend.

Step 3. Recontouring Defective Restorations and Crowns

Corrections for restorative defects, which are plaque traps, may be made by smoothing surfaces and overhangs with burs or hand instruments or by replacing restorations. These procedures can be completed concurrently with other phase I procedures.

Step 4. Management of Carious Lesions

Removal of the carious tooth structure and placement of either temporary or permanent restorations is indicated in phase I therapy because of the infectious nature of dental caries. Healing of the periodontal tissues will be maximized by removing the reservoir of bacteria in these lesions so that they cannot repopulate the microbial plaque.

Step 5. Tissue Reevaluation

After scaling, root planing, and other phase I procedures, the periodontal tissues require approximately 4 weeks to heal so that the connective tissues heal well and accurate probe depths can be measured for assessing the treatment outcomes. Patients also need the opportunity to improve their homecare skills required to reduce inflammation and adopt new habits that ensure the success of treatment. At the reevaluation appointment, periodontal tissues are probed, and all related anatomic conditions are carefully evaluated to determine if further treatment, including periodontal surgery, is indicated. Additional improvement from periodontal surgical procedures can be expected only if phase I therapy resulted in the gingiva being free of overt inflammation and the patient has adopted effective daily plaque-biofilm control procedures.

Results

Scaling and root planing therapy has been studied extensively to evaluate its effects on periodontal disease. Many studies indicated that this treatment is both effective and reliable. Studies ranging from 1 month to 2 years in length demonstrated up to 80% reduction in bleeding on probing and mean probing-depth reductions of 2–3 mm. Others demonstrated that the percentage of periodontal pockets of 4-mm or greater depth was reduced more than 50% and up to 80%. Figs. 33.1 and 33.2 show examples of the effectiveness of phase I therapy.

It is also important to recognize that deeper probing depths present the dentist with greatly increased instrumentation challenges due to the complexity of root anatomy and difficulty of access. Badersten et al. showed in 1980s that more residual calculus remained in deeper pockets on up to 44% of the surfaces. Other studies have confirmed these findings, including those comparing the use of hand instruments to powered scaling instruments.

Additional individual treatments, such as caries control and correction of poorly fitting restorations, clearly augment the healing gained through good plaque-biofilm control and debridement by making tooth surfaces accessible to cleaning procedures. Fig. 33.3 demonstrates the effects of an overhanging amalgam restoration on gingival inflammation in an otherwise healthy periodontium. Maximal healing from phase I treatment is not possible when local conditions retain biofilm and provide reservoirs for repopulation of periodontal pathogens.

Healing

Healing of the gingival epithelium consists of the formation of a long junctional epithelium rather than new connective tissue attachment to the root surfaces. The attachment epithelium reappears about 1 week after therapy. Gradual reductions in inflammatory cell population, crevicular fluid flow, and repair of connective tissue result in decreased clinical signs of inflammation, including less redness and swelling. One or two millimeters of recession are often apparent as the result of tissue shrinkage. Connective tissue fibers are disrupted and lysed by the disease process and also by the inflammatory reaction to treatment. These tissues require 4 or more weeks to reorganize and heal, and complete healing can take months.

Transient root sensitivity frequently accompanies the healing process. Although evidence suggests that relatively few teeth in a few patients become highly sensitive, this development is common and can be disconcerting to patients. The extent of the sensitivity can be diminished through good plaque-biofilm removal. Warning patients about the potential outcomes of the teeth appearing longer because of shrinkage of periodontal tissues and tooth root sensitivity at the beginning of the treatment sequence will avoid surprise if these changes occur. Unexpected and possibly uncomfortable consequences to treatment may result in distrust and loss of motivation to continue therapy.

Decision to Refer for Specialist Treatment

Often, periodontal conditions heal sufficiently well after phase I therapy and no further treatment is required beyond routine maintenance, making the treatment of most periodontal patients the responsibility of the general dentist. However, advanced or complicated cases benefit from specialist care. It has been demonstrated by Heitz-Mayfield and Lang that surgical treatment in deep pockets, those >6 mm, gained 0.6 mm more probing depth reduction and 0.2 mm more clinical attachment gain than did deep pockets treated with

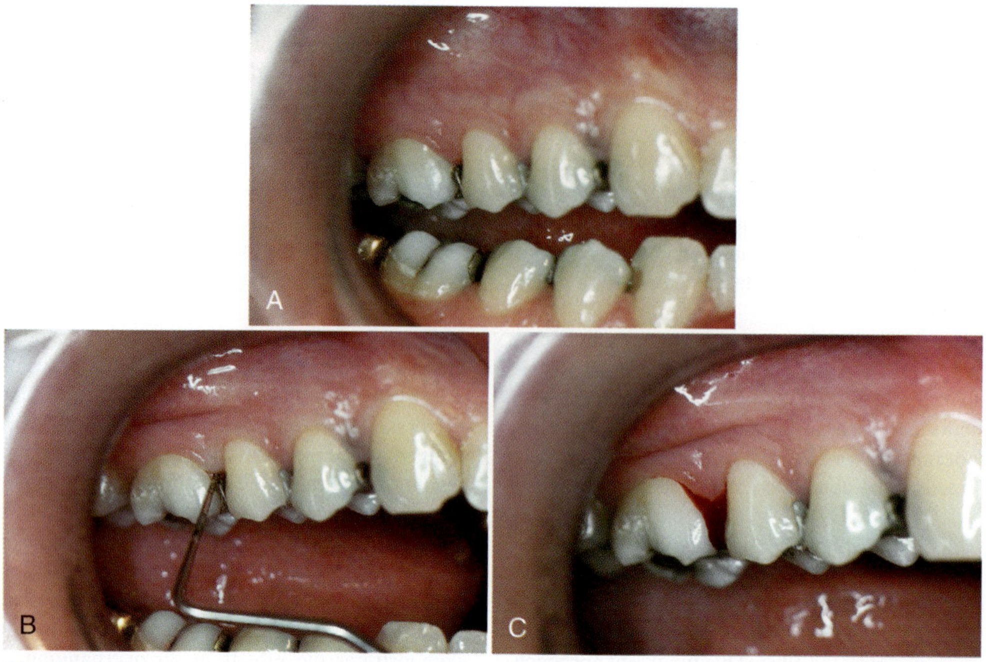

Fig. 33.3 Effects of overhanging amalgam margin on interproximal gingiva of maxillary first molar in otherwise healthy mouth. A, Clinical appearance of rough, irregular, and overcontoured amalgam. B, Gentle probing of interproximal pocket. C, Extensive bleeding elicited by gentle probing indicating severe inflammation in the area.

scaling and root planing alone. That group also confirmed that in pockets of 4–6 mm probing depth, scaling and root planing resulted in 0.4 mm more attachment gain than surgical procedures, and shallow pockets of 1–3 mm had 0.5 mm less attachment loss compared to surgical results. It is critical to be skilled in determining which patients would benefit from specialist care and should be referred.

The concept of the *critical probing depth* of 5.4 mm has been advanced to assist in making the determination to proceed to surgical intervention. This is the measurement above which therapy will result in clinical attachment gain and below it will result in clinical attachment loss. This determination was made based on statistical analysis of surgical outcomes data. A similar *5-mm standard* has been commonly used as a guideline for identifying candidates for surgical referral based on the understanding that the typical root length is about 13 mm and the crest of the alveolar bone is at a level approximately 2 mm apical to the bottom of the pocket. When there is 5 mm of clinical attachment loss, the crest of bone is about 7 mm apical to the cementoenamel junction, therefore only about half the bony support for the tooth remains. Periodontal surgery can help improve support for teeth in these cases through pocket reduction, bone augmentation, and regeneration procedures. Fig. 33.4 depicts the relationship of clinical attachment loss to tooth support.

In addition to consideration of 5-mm probing depths, other factors must also be factored into the decision to refer are listed.

1. *Extent of disease and generalized or localized deep involvement.* Extensive bone loss, even in localized areas, suggests the need for specialized surgical techniques.
2. *Root length.* Short roots are more seriously jeopardized by 5 mm of clinical attachment loss than long roots.
3. *Hypermobility.* Excessive tooth mobility suggests contributing factors and a more guarded prognosis.
4. *Difficulty of scaling and root planing.* The presence of deep pockets and furcations makes instrumentation much more difficult and results can often be improved with surgical access.
5. *Restorability and importance of particular teeth for reconstruction.* Long-term prognosis of each tooth is important when considering extensive restorative work.
6. *Age of the patient.* Younger patients with extensive attachment loss are more likely to have aggressive forms of disease that require extensive therapy.

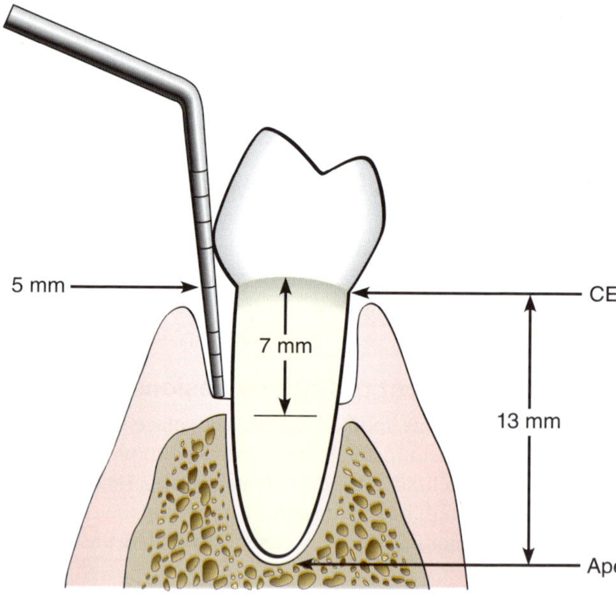

Fig. 33.4 The 5-mm standard for referral to a periodontist is based on root length, probing depth, and clinical attachment loss. The standard serves as a reasonable guideline to analyze the case for referral for specialist care. *CEJ,* Cementoenamel junction. *(Redrawn with permission from Armitage G, editor: Periodontal maintenance therapy, Berkeley, California, 1974, Praxis.)*

7. *Lack of resolution of inflammation after scaling and planing.* If inflammation persists, further therapy is often necessary to gain the most positive results.

Every patient is unique, and the decision process for each patient is complex. The considerations presented in this chapter should provide guidance in understanding the significance of phase I therapy and making referral decisions.

Conclusion

The major goal of phase I therapy is to control the factors responsible for the periodontal inflammation; the removal of subgingival bacterial biofilms and the subsequent control of plaque biofilm levels by patients are particularly significant. Phase I therapy should be comprehensive and include scaling, root planing, and oral hygiene instructions and other therapies, such as caries control, replacement of defective restorations, occlusal therapy, orthodontic tooth movement, and cessation of confounding habits, such as tobacco use. Comprehensive reevaluation after phase I therapy is essential to determine treatment options and to estimate prognosis. Many patients can have their periodontal disease controlled with phase I therapy alone and may not require further surgical intervention. For patients who do need surgical intervention, phase I therapy is an advantageous element of treatment in that it permits tissue healing, thus improving the surgical management and healing response of the tissues.

Periodontal surgical intervention should be considered for patients with critically deep pocket depths and those with 5 mm or more of attachment loss still present after phase I therapy. Periodontal specialists can best provide treatment to preserve the teeth for these patients with advanced disease. It is also important to note that patients who do not demonstrate the ability to successfully control plaque biofilm at home, on a daily basis, are poor candidates for successful surgical outcomes and should be closely monitored on a recall maintenance program unless conditions change.

Key points

- Phase I therapy is also known as initial therapy, nonsurgical periodontal therapy, and cause-related therapy.
- Phase I therapy is aimed at removal of pathogenic biofilms, toxins and calculus, and the reestablishment of a biologically acceptable root surface.
- The elements which make up phase I therapy are complete removal of calculus; correction or replacement of poorly fitting restorations and prosthetic devices; restoration or temporization of carious lesions; orthodontic tooth movement; treatment of food impaction areas; treatment of occlusal trauma; extraction of hopeless teeth; and possible use of antimicrobial agents including necessary plaque sampling and sensitivity testing.
- Critical probing depth of 5.4 mm assists in making the decision regarding surgical intervention. Surgery in cases with probing depth above this will result in clinical attachment gain, and in cases with probing depth below this will result in clinical attachment loss.

Suggested Readings

American Academy of Periodontology, Ad Hoc Committee on the Parameters of Care: Phase I therapy, *J Periodontol* 71 (Suppl 5):856, 2000.

American Academy of Periodontology, Task Force to Update the Guidelines for Periodontal Therapy: Comprehensive periodontal therapy: a statement by the American Academy of Periodontology, *J Periodontol* 82:943, 2011.

Dentino A, Lee S, Mailhot J, et al: Principles of periodontology, *Periodontol 2000* 61:16, 2013.

Heitz-Mayfield LJA, Lang NP: Surgical and nonsurgical periodontal therapy. Learned and unlearned concepts, *Periodontol 2000* 62:218, 2013.

References

References and MCQs with answers for the chapter are available on www.medenact.com.

CHAPTER 34

Plaque Biofilm Control

DA Perry | A Jain | V Grover

CHAPTER OUTLINE

Microbial plaque biofilm control is an effective way of treating and preventing gingivitis and is an essential part of all the procedures involved in the treatment and prevention of periodontal diseases. It is critical to the long-term success of all periodontal and dental treatment. In 1965, Löe et al. conducted the classic study demonstrating the relationship between microbial plaque biofilm accumulation and the development of experimental gingivitis in humans. Subjects in the study stopped brushing and other plaque biofilm control procedures, resulting in the development of gingivitis in every person within 7–21 days. The composition of the biofilm bacteria also shifted so that more virulent Gram-negative organisms predominated, and these changes were shown to be reversible within 7 days. Good supragingival biofilm control has also been shown to affect the growth and composition of subgingival plaque so that it favors a healthier microflora and reduces calculus formation. Carefully performed daily home plaque biofilm control, combined with frequent professionally delivered plaque biofilm and calculus removal, reduces the amount of supragingival biofilm; decreases the total number of microorganisms in moderately deep pockets, including furcation areas; and greatly reduces the quantity of periodontal pathogens. Reviews of home care procedures in 2011 and 2013 confirm the positive effects of daily plaque biofilm removal but cautions that these gains appear to be small and best results also require professional maintenance care.

Microbial biofilm growth occurs within hours, and it must be completely removed at least once every 48 h in the experimental setting with periodontally healthy subjects to prevent inflammation. The American Dental Association (ADA) recommends that individuals brush twice per day and use floss or other interdental cleaners once per day to effectively remove microbial plaque biofilms and prevent gingivitis. They recommend twice daily brushing because most individuals do not adequately remove microbial biofilms at one brushing and doing it a second time improves the results.

Periodontal lesions are predominantly found in interdental locations, so toothbrushing alone is not sufficient to control gingival and periodontal diseases. It has been demonstrated in healthy subjects that plaque biofilm formation begins on the interproximal surfaces where the toothbrush does not reach. Masses of biofilm first develop in the molar and premolar areas, followed by the proximal surfaces of the anterior teeth and the facial surfaces of the molars and premolars. Lingual surfaces accumulate the least amount of biofilm. Patients consistently leave more plaque biofilm on the posterior teeth than the anterior teeth, with interproximal surfaces retaining the highest amounts of biofilm, exactly the places in which periodontal infections begin. In addition, periodontal patients have increased susceptibility to disease, complex defects in gingival architecture, and long exposed root surfaces to clean, compounding the difficulty of doing a thorough job of cleaning.

Chemical inhibitors of plaque biofilm and calculus that are incorporated in mouthwashes or dentifrices also play important roles in controlling microbial biofilms. Fluorides delivered through toothpastes and mouthrinses are essential for caries control. Many products are available as adjunctive agents to mechanical techniques. These medicaments, as with any drug, should be recommended and prescribed according to the needs of individual patients. Also note that the interest in supplementing oral hygiene procedures with natural products has increased in our society. However, the evidence base supporting the use of these products is currently lacking valid studies to determine their efficacy.

Daily plaque biofilm control permits each patient to assume responsibility for oral health every day. Without it, optimal oral health through periodontal treatment cannot be attained or preserved. Elements of biofilm control include mechanical cleaning and chemical adjuncts.

The Toothbrush

Toothbrushes vary in size and design as well as in length, hardness, and arrangement of the bristles (Fig. 34.1A–D). The ADA has described the range of dimensions of acceptable brushes: as having a brushing surface 1–1.25 in. long and 5/16–3/8 in. wide, 2–4 rows of bristles, and 5–12 tufts per row. A study compared four commercially

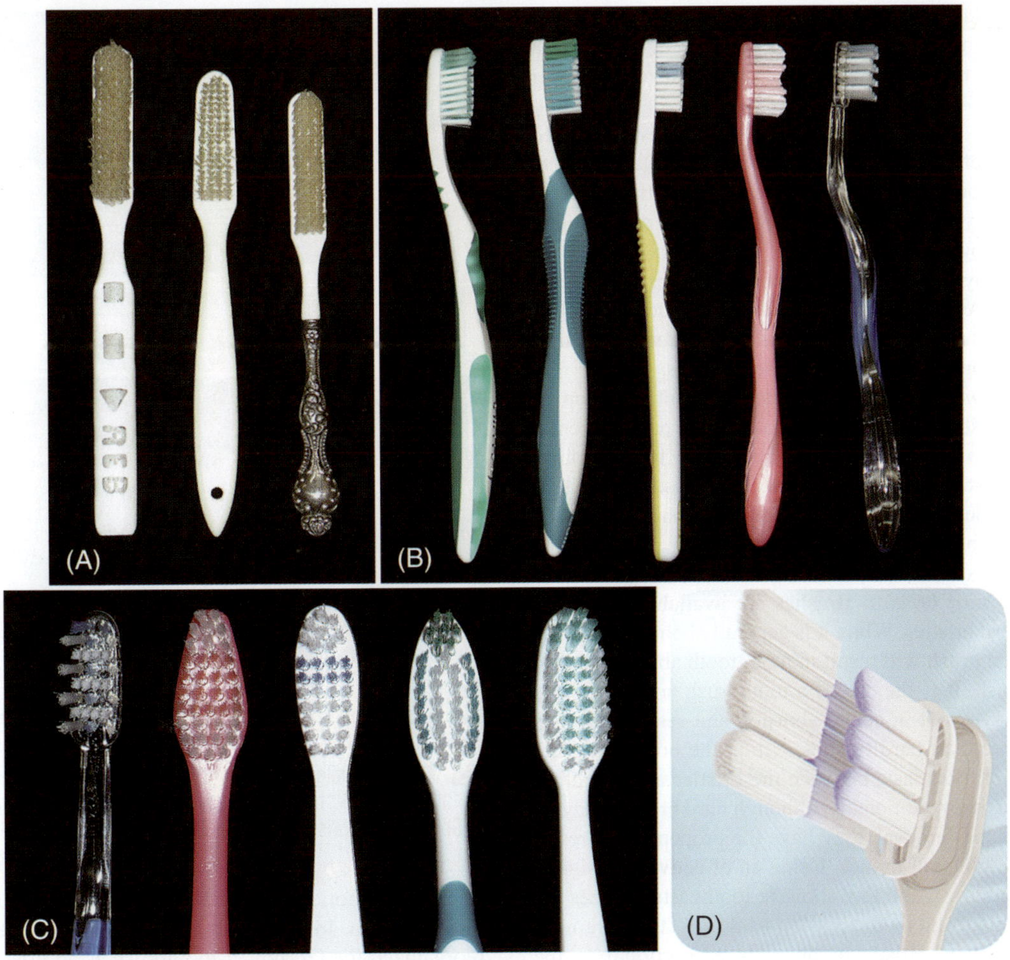

Fig. 34.1 **Manual toothbrushes.** A, Toothbrushes from the 19th and 20th centuries, one with an ivory handle from about 1890 *(left)*, one with a composition handle from the 1950s *(center)*, and one with a sterling silver handle from the early 20th century *(right)*. The ivory-handled brush belonged to a dental student who used the handle to practice cutting preparations and filling the "preps" with amalgam or gold foil. B, Various types of toothbrushes are available; note the variation in brush head and handle design. C, Brush heads, showing various bristle configurations. *(Antique brushes courtesy: Dean John D.B. Featherstone, University of California, San Francisco School of Dentistry Historical Collection, San Francisco.)* D, Anchor free tufting technology (AFT) utilized in Gum expert toothbrush design. (*Courtesy: Colgate-Palmolive, India)*

available toothbrushes for total plaque biofilm removal at a single brushing; all four toothbrushes removed biofilms equally, and the authors concluded that no one design was superior to others.

When recommending a particular toothbrush, ease of use by the patient and the perception that the brush works well are the important considerations. The effectiveness of and potential injury from different types of brushes depend to a great degree on how the brushes are used. Data from in vitro studies of abrasion by different manual toothbrushes suggest that brush designs permitting the bristles to carry more toothpaste while brushing contribute to abrasion more than brush bristles themselves. However, it has been shown that use of hard toothbrushes, vigorous horizontal brushing, and use of extremely abrasive dentifrices may lead to cervical abrasions of teeth and recession of gingiva.

Toothbrush Design

Toothbrush bristles are grouped in tufts that are usually arranged in three or four rows (Fig. 34.1). Two types of bristle material are used in toothbrushes: natural bristles from hogs and artificial filaments made of nylon. Both remove microbial plaque biofilms, but nylon bristle brushes vastly predominate the market.

The amount of force used to brush is not critical for effective plaque biofilm removal. Vigorous brushing is not necessary and can lead to gingival recession, wedge-shaped defects in the cervical area of root surfaces, and painful ulceration of the gingiva.

Toothbrushes must also be replaced periodically although the amount of visible bristle wear does not appear to affect plaque biofilm removal for up to 9 weeks. Most clinicians recommend that toothbrushes be replaced every 3–4 months.

Introduction of modern bristle designs provided for safer and more effective brushing and laid the foundation for the further development of brush heads, bristle designs, and ergonomic handles. Successive innovations addressing clinical/patient needs have included the introduction of end-rounded filaments, indicator filaments, multilevel filaments, polishing cup filaments, toe tufts, bristles of varying density, and tapered filaments. Some of the advantages of such innovations are

End rounding: End-rounded bristles are less likely to result in gingival trauma and are gentler and safer than stiff, sharp-edged filament.

The indicator bristles: They are created by infusing a blue food-grade dye into the outer layer of the bristles. As the brush is used, the color gradually dissipates. Since worn filaments are more likely to damage the gingivae and are less effective at removing plaque, they inform the users when to replace their toothbrush.

Trim: Research has consistently shown that multilevel-trimmed brushes are more effective for plaque removal than flat trimmed, especially at interproximal sites. Brushes incorporating rows of tall, thin, elliptically shaped tufts, together with rows consisting of shorter tufts in a row along both sides of the brush head, enhance cleaning efficacy by improving reach into interproximal areas and gingival margins. As a result, major manufactures such as Oral-B, Colgate, GSK, and so on introduced brushes with multilevel trim to improve brushing efficacy in hard-to-reach areas.

Polishing cup filaments: Another innovation was introduction of polishing cup bristles. These consist of tightly packed center bristles that help to keep the dentifrice against the tooth surface, thereby aiding extrinsic stain removal. The bristles feel stiff because they are densely packed and short. They are surrounded by taller, angled bristle tufts that hug the tooth and help the dentifrice polish extrinsic stain off the tooth surfaces.

Soft, medium, and hard bristles: Brushes are available with soft, medium, and hard bristles. While it is generally believed that use of a hard-bristled brush will result in more tooth abrasion than a soft-bristled brush, it is the use of a toothbrush and toothpaste together that may result in dental abrasion and sensitivity. Soft bristles flex more than hard bristles, letting the brush head accommodate more toothpaste between the bristles and therefore more of the abrasive. Additionally, although hard bristles may be effective for plaque removal, they have the propensity to result in trauma to the gingival tissues. Using an effectively designed soft-bristled toothbrush and low abrasive toothpaste reduces the risk of both gingival and tooth abrasion while effectively removing plaque and stain. Bristle hardness is proportional to the square of the diameter and inversely proportional to the square of bristle length. Diameters of common bristles range from 0.007 in. (0.2 mm) for soft brushes to 0.012 in. (0.3 mm) for medium brushes and 0.014 in. (0.4 mm) for hard brushes.

Angled bristles: Brushes with cross-action bristles have been demonstrated to be superior to numerous manual toothbrush designs in short- and long-term clinical trials, for example, Oral-B Cross Action Power Toothbrush (Fig. 34.2). The angled, multilevel bristles and tufts of just the right stiffness together ensure the most effective brushing under normal home care conditions.

The introduction of "Anchor Free Tufting Technology (AFT)" marks a recent advancement in toothbrush design, offering increased versatility in hole size, density, shape variety, and trimming profile of the bristles which has been incorporated in Colgate PerioGard Gum Expert toothbrush by Colgate, with multiheight bristles, slender tufts on both sides, and high-density ultraslim bristles. These enhancements facilitate improved adaptation and access of the toothbrush at the tooth-gingival junction, leading to enhanced cleaning efficacy.

Clinical investigations have demonstrated significant improvements in plaque and gingivitis reduction after 1, 6, and 12 weeks of product use compared to baseline examinations before brushing and in comparison to contemporary available alternatives.

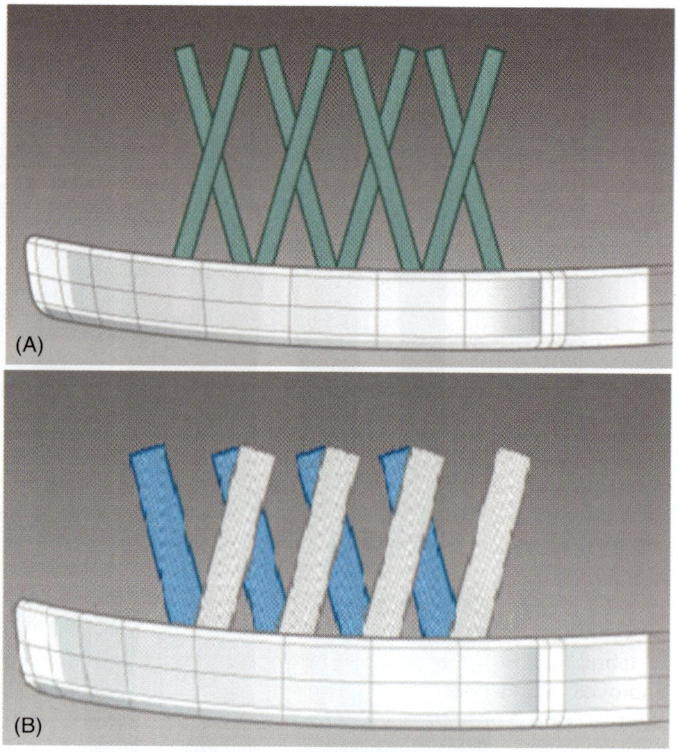

Fig. 34.2 Multilevel bristles for effective plaque disruption and removal. A, Tall thin bristle tufts that crisscross that optimize interproximal cleaning. B, Short, dense bristle tufts that crisscross effectively clean smooth surfaces.

Powered Toothbrushes

By 1937, the first powered toothbrush had been created in Switzerland. In the same year, Motodent Inc. of Los Angeles launched a powered toothbrush that had individual arms designated for each family member. The movement of the early brush heads used side-to-side or elliptical motions aimed to mimic the motion of a person using a manual brush. In 1964, the ADA Council on Dental Therapeutics reorganized the GE power toothbrush as an effective cleansing device. At this time, powered toothbrushes were only recommended for people with limited physical and mental capacities. However, by the 1980s–1990s, a new generation of power brushes had arrived. This period witnessed innovative brush designs and modes of action that improved the effectiveness of this toothbrush category and allowed people to remove plaque more effectively. Numerous clinical studies confirmed that power toothbrushes were more effective than manual. Improved tooth surface cleaning, as well as a reducing and controlling gingivitis, were shown to be the greatest benefits of power toothbrushes. In long-term studies, power toothbrushes provided better plaque reduction and protection against gingivitis than manual toothbrushes. Nevertheless, within the power toothbrush category, there are significant differences in efficacy between toothbrushes with different modes of action [e.g., oscillating/rotating, side-to-side (sonic), and counter-oscillation].

Currently, powered toothbrushes have oscillating and rotating motions in which the brush head rotates in one direction and then the other (Fig. 34.3). Other types of motion can be oscillating-rotating pulsating, in which the entire brush head oscillates, rotates, and pulsates; side-to-side (sonic), in which the brush head moves laterally in a side-to-side motion; multidirectional, in which the brush sweeps from side-to-side and pulsates; counter-oscillation, in which the adjacent tufts rotate in opposite directions to each other or circular/rotary, in which the entire brush head rotates in a full circle moving in one.

The frequency at which the brush head oscillates should be in the range of 8500–9000 oscillations per minute. In addition, the brush head should be angled 3–5 degrees from the handle to help users reach posterior regions and allow effortless progression from tooth to tooth.

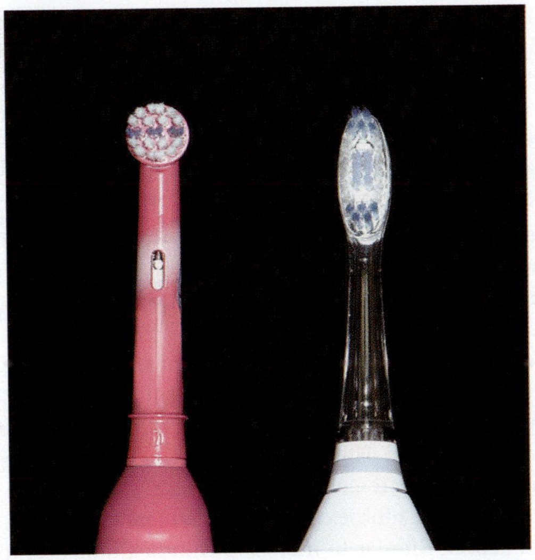

Fig. 34.3 Powered toothbrush designs offer options in head shape and size.

Typically, comparison studies of powered toothbrushes, manual toothbrushes, or other powered devices demonstrate slightly improved plaque biofilm removal by powered toothbrushes in short-term clinical trials. A recent Cochrane review reported that mechanical brushes with oscillating and rotating motions reduced microbial plaque biofilm 11% and demonstrated 6% greater reduction in gingival bleeding than manual brushing. These improvements were maintained over 3 months. Although long-term benefits have not been established, this particular style of mechanical brush resulted in better microbial plaque biofilm and gingivitis reduction in a number of well-controlled studies.

Patient acceptance of powered toothbrushes is good. One study reported that 88.9% of patients introduced to a powered toothbrush would continue to use it. However, patients have also been reported to quit using powered toothbrushes after 5 or 6 months, presumably when the novelty is gone. Powered toothbrushes have been shown to improve oral health for (1) children and adolescents, (2) children with physical or mental disabilities, (3) hospitalized patients, including older adults who need to have their teeth cleaned by caregivers, and (4) patients with fixed orthodontic appliances. Patients who want to use powered toothbrush should be encouraged to do so.

Dentifrices

People have used various compounds (e.g., pumice, oyster shells, and chalk) to clean their teeth since around 5000 BC. However, only since the 1950s have dentifrices been used to prevent and treat specific diseases and conditions. The most recent advances in dentifrices have been in the area of delivering multiple benefits in one dentifrice and in the introduction of new products to treat dentinal hypersensitivity. Dentifrice's ingredients help reduce caries, plaque, gingivitis, calculus, stain, halitosis, and hypersensitivity. Some ingredients provide a therapeutic benefit while other ingredients or additives contribute to the cosmetic benefits or physical properties of the dentifrice. This section describes the most common dentifrice ingredients used to provide anticaries, antibacterial, anticalculus, whitening, and antihypersensitivity benefits.

Anticaries agents

Caries is simply the result of a series of demineralization/remineralization cycles where, over time, demineralization conditions prevail. One of the most effective methods to prevent caries is by promoting remineralization and slowing down demineralization. This can be accomplished with fluoride therapy. Fluoride's presence in low concentration and high frequency is more effective at preventing caries than high levels of fluoride used in low frequency. Fluoridated dentifrice is the best method for delivering fluoride to the tooth surface.

Fluoride can be delivered in several different chemical forms:

- Stannous fluoride (SnF_2)
- Sodium fluoride (NaF)
- Sodium monofluorophosphate
- Amine fluoride
- Aluminium fluoride (AlF_3)

a. *Stannous fluoride*. Stannous fluoride (SnF_2; also called tin fluoride) was first formulated successfully into a dentifrice to deliver an anticaries benefit by Proctor and Gamble. Its CREST formulation included 0.454% stannous fluoride and the abrasive calcium pyrophosphate.

b. *Sodium fluoride*. Sodium fluoride (NaF) has greater stability than stannous fluoride and thus is easier to formulate. Sodium fluoride delivers a highly reactive fluoride ion (Crest with Fluoristat).

c. *Sodium monofluorophosphate*. Sodium monofluorophosphate (MFP) is a fluoridated compound that requires enzymatic activation by a salivary enzyme (alkaline phosphatase) to release bioavailable fluoride. Omnident toothpaste from Group pharmaceuticals provides the additional benefit of fluoride and xylitol which prevent the formation of plaque and helps remineralize the teeth while strengthening the gums.

d. *Arginine*. Arginine, an amino acid, has been studied as a potential preventive measure against dental caries. Clinical trials in both adults and children have confirmed its effectiveness at a concentration of 1.5% in preventing dental cavities. By incorporating arginine into oral products containing fluoride (Colgate Total Whole Mouth health), it is possible to augment the remineralization process, thereby enhancing their overall effectiveness. Furthermore, arginine serves as a regulator of plaque metabolism and has the capability to elevate the pH of plaque by generating ammonia and other natural arginolytic substances within the oral biofilm. This aids in sustaining a pH-neutral environment, a crucial factor in combating dental caries, as demineralization occurs when the pH decreases due to acid production by cariogenic bacteria.

Anticalculus Agents

By 1980s, agents were discovered that could provide better calculus and stain control. The chemical agents used for calculus control in dentifrice are:

a. *Pyrophosphate*. Pyrophosphate occurs naturally in saliva and plays a role in inhibiting calculus formation. These molecules chelate calcium, slowing the rate of nucleation (crystal formation) and calcification of plaque. The pyrophosphate binds to calcium in a growing crystal, essentially blunting further crystal growth at that site and effectively decreasing calculus buildup. Crest Tartar Control contains 3.3% pyrophosphate. It was the first tartar control dentifrice introduced to the market and the first dentifrice to receive the ADA seal for tartar control.

b. *Sodium hexametaphosphate (HMP)*. Sodium HMP is a large polyphosphate molecule and has multiple calcium binding sites in one molecule. It is a very effective calculus inhibitor. Sodium HMP is too large of a molecule to enter into tooth enamel, so there is no danger of it entering between enamel rods and sequestering calcium from sound enamel. Since it works only on the surface, it is sometimes called a calcium surface-active builder.

c. *Zinc*. Zinc salts (e.g., zinc citrate, zinc chloride, zinc lactate, zinc sulphate) are used in some tartar control dentifrices and oral rinses and have been shown to be moderately effective at controlling calculus. Positively charged zinc ion (Zn^{2+}) inhibits crystal growth by substituting for calcium in the crystal lattice of calcium phosphate. This corrupts the crystal formation and slows crystal growth. In addition, Zn ion, in the form of zinc sulphate, as present in Omnident toothpaste, also helps maintain the integrity of the tooth enamel surface

Whitening Agents

Stain control and whitening are key benefits of modern dentifrices. These are accomplished via ingredients that target specific types of tooth stain. Dentifrices primarily work against extrinsic stains. Bleaching products that contain hydrogen peroxide or carbamide peroxide (i.e., dental office bleaching trays) address intrinsic stains as well as extrinsic stains.

a. *Extrinsic stain*. Extrinsic (surface) stains can be relatively easily removed on a daily basis by proper toothbrushing with a dentifrice.
   Physical action. Most dentifrices contain mild abrasives that help clean precipitated stain particles from the tooth surface; controlling surface stains with home care. The abrasivity of dentifrice is measured in terms of Relative Dentin Abrasivity, or RDA. The lower the RDA, the less abrasive the dentifrice. This means less potential to wear tooth structure through toothbrushing. Since dentifrices with lower RDA values are less abrasive, they also tend to have less potential to remove surface stain. The International Standards Organization (ISO) specification states that a dentifrice should not exceed an RDA of 250, which is considered safe for hard tissues.
   Chemical action. Polyphosphates, which are dentifrice ingredients used to control calculus, also target extrinsic stain. One of the most effective ingredients with this dual action is sodium HMP, which is used in several dentifrices. Stain molecules, or *chromogens*, are usually negatively charged molecules and have an affinity for positively charged ions like calcium (Ca^{2+}) in the tooth enamel and cross-link pellicle proteins. HMP is also negatively charged with a strong affinity for calcium. HMP can displace stain molecules from calcium binding sites. It binds to the tooth surface and integrates into the pellicle to prevent additional stain molecules from binding.
b. *Intrinsic stain*. Intrinsic stains are stains and discolorations that are located below the enamel surface. Due to their diverse etiology, intrinsic stain treatment varies with the cause. Bleaching is usually used to remove or minimize intrinsic discolorations.

Antibacterial and Antibiofilm Agents

Adding antibacterial action to dentifrice was another major therapeutic breakthrough. Several modern dentifrice ingredients have the potential to kill or inhibit bacteria that cause plaque, gingivitis, and oral malodor.

a. *Zinc*. Zinc ion (Zn^{2+}), in addition to having anticalculus benefits, has an effective antibacterial action also, by virtue of its binding ability to the membranes of microorganisms, inhibiting cell division and slowing the cell growth cycle. Zinc citrate 2% (Periogard from Colgate) provides an antiplaque and antimicrobial action to combat bacteria and inhibits the volatilization of compounds that causes bad breath or halitosis. Clinical studies have observed 70.7% and 68.5% reduction in plaque and gingival index scores over 6 months of duration.
b. *Stannous*. Stannous ion (Sn^{2+}) is an effective antibacterial agent. In early formulations of stannous fluoride dentifrices, stannous was not stable or bioavailable. Current stannous-containing dentifrices have been formulated to circumvent stannous instability and bioavailability challenges. Crest Gum Care, introduced in 1995, contained stabilized stannous and delivered antibacterial benefits. Stannous exerts antibacterial effects by two actions. One is by being bactericidal and its nonspecific interaction with the bacterial membrane that causes membrane disruption. The second mode of antibacterial activity is through stannous ion's inhibition of metabolic enzymes, which further lead to reduction of bacterial growth, prevention of bacterial adhesion to oral surfaces (e.g., enamel), and reduction in bacterial byproducts. Stannous can also have an astringent taste and cause extrinsic staining of teeth and fillings.
c. *Triclosan*. Triclosan is a broad-spectrum antibacterial agent that inserts into and disrupts the bacterial membrane. Being a nonpolar molecule, it has an affinity for the hydrophobic environment of the lipid bilayer. This causes leakage of cellular components, ultimately leading to cell death.
d. *Chlorhexidine*. Chlorhexidine is a chemical agent with a bactericidal action. Similar to triclosan, chlorhexidine acts to disrupt bacterial membranes, resulting in bacterial death. Chlorhexidine is primarily used as a therapeutic ingredient in mouthwash and some dentifrices; however, it has some side effects such as poor taste and staining.
e. *Sodium bicarbonate*. Newly developed dentifrices with sodium bicarbonate formulation like Parodontax from Haleon provides a strong antiplaque advantage by interrupting the sticky polysaccharide matrix when it penetrates the plaque layer, loosening the biofilm, and facilitating the physical removal of plaque. Clinical studies showed statistically significant improvements for gingival inflammation, gingival bleeding, and supra-gingival plaque in participants using sodium bicarbonate-containing toothpaste as opposed to regular fluoride toothpaste, over six week period of observation .Gingival health and plaque control in individuals with mild to moderate gingivitis were shown to be significantly improved after a professional dental cleaning and twice-daily brushing with a 67% sodium bicarbonate toothpaste compared with a regular (non-sodium bicarbonate) toothpaste, according to a pooled analysis of patient-level data from six similarly designed studies.
f. *Arginine*. It been demonstrated to directly impact oral health by modifying plaque metabolism and composition. The Dual Zinc plus Arginine (DZA) technology not only harnesses the benefits of arginine but also incorporates the mineral zinc. The "dual zinc" component in DZA technology as in Colgate total toothpaste includes both zinc citrate and zinc oxide. Zinc, known for its antimicrobial properties, has been utilized in toothpaste formulations for many years, such as in the form of zinc citrate, to reduce the presence of bacteria responsible for dental plaque. In a randomized double-blind clinical trial, a toothpaste containing DZA technology (consisting of 0.96% dual zinc and 1.5% arginine along with 1450 ppm fluoride as sodium fluoride) exhibited significantly greater reductions in plaque and gingivitis at 3 and 6 months compared to a standard sodium fluoride toothpaste with the same fluoride concentration.

Antihypersensitivity agents

It has been reported that up to 57% of the adult population suffers from dentinal hypersensitivity. Dentinal hypersensitivity is generally treated in one of the two ways:

- Chemical desensitization of the tooth nerve endings.
- Tubule occluding agents or barriers to reduce dentin permeability.
   a. *Nerve depolarization agents*. Potassium ion (K^+), sodium ion (Na^+), and chloride ion (Cl^-) are important ions involved in the electrical activity of nerve cells. When the nerve cell is at rest, the potassium ion concentration is higher on the

inside of the cell than on the outside, while the sodium ion concentration is higher on the outside of the cell than on the inside. When the nerve cell is stimulated, these ions cross the nerve cell membrane through channels and move from an area of high concentration to an area of lower concentration (referred to as the concentration gradient). Thus, potassium ions flow from the inside to the outside of the cell and the sensation of pain is transmitted. Potassium ion is a desensitization agent because it diffuses through dentin tubules and increases the extracellular potassium concentration at the nerve ending, eliminating the potassium ion concentration gradient across the nerve cell membrane. Without this concentration gradient, the nerve cell becomes depolarized and will not respond to stimuli, thus the sensation of pain will not be transmitted. Potassium ion can be delivered in a variety of salt forms (e.g., potassium nitrate, potassium citrate). The most common potassium salt used in sensitivity dentifrice is potassium nitrate (KNO_3).

Most of the toothpastes contain potassium salts, strontium salts, and fluorides. Potassium salts are now most commonly used agents incorporated in toothpastes for the treatment of DH. Most of the studies have shown that potassium-containing toothpastes demonstrated improvement in patients' perceived symptoms of DH and the effectiveness increased with time. Toothpastes containing potassium salts penetrate into dentinal tubules and depolarize the nerve synapse, thereby reducing sensitivity by preventing conduction of pain impulses.

b. *Tubule blocking or occluding agents*. Another strategy to treat/prevent dentinal hypersensitivity is to reduce the permeability of the dentin by occluding or blocking the exposed dentin tubules. This prevents stimuli from causing fluid flow in the tubules, thereby preventing the nerve endings inside the tooth from being stimulated. Strontium chloride was one such desensitizing ingredient which worked via formation of strontium salt precipitates.

c. *Newer tubule-occluding agents*. Other tubule-occluding agents are new to the market, including arginine with calcium carbonate (Pro-Argin), strontium acetate, calcium sodium phosphosilicate (Novamin), and fluoro calcium phosphosilicate.

Arginine, found naturally in saliva, when combined with calcium carbonate and phosphate, creates a positively charged glycoprotein which is deposited on exposed dentin surfaces that are negatively charged and aids in closing open tubules and enhances the natural mechanism of sealing dentin tubules. The distinct Pro-Argin formula containing 8% arginine, adheres to the dentin surface, forming a physical seal by incorporating arginine, calcium carbonate, and phosphate into a "plug" structure. This seal diminishes fluid flow within the tubules and shields against painful external stimuli. Additionally, it establishes an acid-resistant barrier over the dentin surface, safeguarding it from acids.

Strontium (Sr^{2+}) is a metal ion, and in the oral cavity, it can form insoluble metal salts that can plug dentin tubules.

Stannous ion is also a tubule-occluding agent that treats dentinal hypersensitivity through hydrolysis and oxidation reactions, which form many insoluble metal salts that can precipitate in dentinal tubules and on the dentin surface. A study utilizing synchrotron-based imaging revealed that the updated formulation of 0.454% stannous fluoride (Sensodyne Deep Repair) penetrates deeply into the microstructure of tubules and constructs a robust repair layer fortified with fluoride across the dentin surface, ensuring longer lasting protection against sensitivity.

Calcium sodium phosphosilicate—Formulations containing calcium sodium phosphosilicate (NovaMin) create a shielding layer over exposed dentine, providing enduring defense against dentine hypersensitivity. Sensodyne Repair and Protect incorporates NovaMin specifically to mend exposed dentine. Upon contact with saliva, NovaMin triggers a series of ionic exchanges, leading to an elevation in pH levels in the immediate area. This facilitates its bonding to collagen fibers in exposed dentine. Once attached to the dentine, these particles serve as reservoirs for calcium and phosphate, forming a resilient and reparative hydroxyapatite-like layer over exposed dentine tubules, aiding in the prevention of dentine hypersensitivity discomfort. The protective hydroxyapatite layer forms immediately, with the first brushing after application which keeps on maturing to a complete layer within 3–4 days . With regular use , this structural layer formed is maintained, protecting vital pulp tissues by occluding dentin tubules, and preventing fluid movement that results in transmission of painful stimuli.

An in-vitro study using serial block-face SEM technology, demonstrated 100% tubular occlusion in dentine samples treated with NovaMin®, reduction in tubular diameter (0.79 ± 0.05 to $0.66 \pm 0.21\mu m$), and a superior occlusive layer at surface and at 30μm depth. Clinical trial data from United States, India, China, Thailand, and Ireland shows significant reduction in pain of tooth sensitivity, reduction upto 50% in two weeks, 70% in 6–8 weeks and 91% over a period of 12 weeks of continued twice daily use.

Clinical studies have reported 53% reduction in the proportion of teeth qualifying as sensitive in response to an evaporative air test (Schiff Sensitivity Scale) and 2.2% improvement in dentine hypersensitivity in response to tactile pressure after 24 weeks of twice-daily brushing with 5% NovaMin containing toothpaste. In in-vitro tests Vs marketed products in India, NovaMin® demonstrated superior hardness score of 0.34 GPa, highest among all compared dental desensitize molecules.

Fluoro calcium phosphosilicate—The bioactive glass utilized in BioMin technology facilitates a unique and continuous release of low-level fluoride for up to 12 h following each brushing session, ensuring optimal protection. Fluoro calcium phosphosilicate, an active ingredient of Elsenz toothpaste by Group Pharmaceuticals Ltd., helps in enhanced occlusion of dentinal tubules, resulting in a more significant reduction in hydraulic conductance. It mitigates the demineralization of enamel and dentin by reducing bacterial plaque's acid production and decreasing apatite crystal solubility. Furthermore, it readily integrates as a fluorapatite layer, reducing apatite dissolution during acid attacks and progressively fortifying protection against tooth sensitivity to cold, heat, acids, sweets, or contact.

Other Dentifrice Ingredients

Nontherapeutic dentifrice components include binders, surfactants, buffering agents, humectants, preservatives, sweeteners, flavorings, and dyes. These components are essential to keep the dentifrice properly mixed with a smooth consistency, and they make the product palatable to the consumer. Three dentifrice ingredients (abrasive, humectants, and solvent) typically represent about 95% of the dentifrice ingredients.

Humectants

Humectants retain moisture so that the dentifrice does not dry out. Humectants, such as glycerin and sorbitol, also inhibit bacterial growth and provide flowability to the dentifrice.

Binders

Binders, also referred to as thickeners, provide texture and determine how "thick" or "runny" the dentifrice is. Binders are used for cohesiveness, to provide body, and to prevent ingredients from separating. Xanthan gum, carboxymethyl cellulose carbomers, carrageenan, and synthetic cellulose are all commonly used dentifrice binders.

Buffers

Manufacturers use buffers as part of their dentifrice formulation to keep the pH constant. Trisodium phosphate, pyrophosphates, and sodium citrate are examples of dentifrice buffers.

Flavors/Sweeteners

Flavoring agents and sweeteners are added to improve the dentifrice taste. Common flavoring agents and sweeteners include peppermint, saccharin, and xylitol. Toothpaste like Omnident, with artificial sweeteners like xylitol shall prove more suitable as a regular toothpaste and safe in diabetic patients.

Surfactants

Surfactants (detergents) create the foaming and aid in the cleaning process by helping to loosen plaque and debris. Sodium lauryl sulfate (SLS) is the surfactant most commonly used.

Colors/Visuals

Finally, coloring agents are added to provide dentifrice with pleasing colors. The opacity of a paste dentifrice comes from the addition of titanium dioxide. Mica is used to provide a sparkly appearance in some dentifrices, such as those marketed to children.

Toothbrushing Methods

Many methods for brushing the teeth have been described and promoted as being efficient and effective. These methods can be categorized primarily according to the pattern of motion when brushing and are primarily of historic interest, as follows:

Roll: Roll or modified Stillman technique
Vibratory: Stillman, Charters, and Bass techniques
Circular: Fones technique
Vertical: Leonard technique
Horizontal: Scrub technique

Patients with periodontal disease are most frequently taught a sulcular brushing technique using a vibratory motion to improve access to the gingival margin areas. It is important for patients to understand that the plaque biofilm removal at the dento-gingival junction is necessary to prevent caries as well as periodontal disease. This is referred to as "target hygiene." The method most often recommended is the *Bass technique* because it emphasizes the placement of the bristles at this most important area. This sulcular placement of the bristle and adapting the bristle tips to the gingival margin to reach the supragingival plaque biofilm and accessing some of the subgingival biofilm may be the most important aspect of "target hygiene." A controlled vibrating motion is used to dislodge microbial plaque biofilm and avoid trauma. The brush is systematically placed on all the teeth in both arches. Figs. 34.4 and 34.5 illustrate this brushing technique.

Bass Technique

1. Place the head of a soft brush parallel with the occlusal plane, with the brush head covering three to four teeth, beginning at the most distal tooth in the arch.
2. Place the bristles at the gingival margin, pointing at a 45-degree angle to the long axis of the teeth.
3. Exert gentle vibratory pressure, using short, back-and-forth motions without dislodging the tips of the bristles. This motion forces the bristle ends into the gingival sulcus area (Fig. 34.4), as well as partly into the interproximal embrasures. The pressure should be firm enough to blanch the gingiva.

The Bass method has certain advantages over other techniques, such as: (1) The short back-and-forth motion is easy to master because it is a simple movement familiar to most patients who brush using a scrub technique. (2) It concentrates the cleaning action on the cervical and interproximal portions of the teeth, where microbial plaque is most likely to have accumulated. The Bass technique is efficient and can be recommended for any patient with or without periodontal involvement.

Modified Stillman Method

The modified Stillman method requires that the brush be placed with the bristle ends resting partly on the cervical portion of the teeth and partly on the adjacent gingiva, pointing in an apical direction and at an oblique angle to the long axis of the

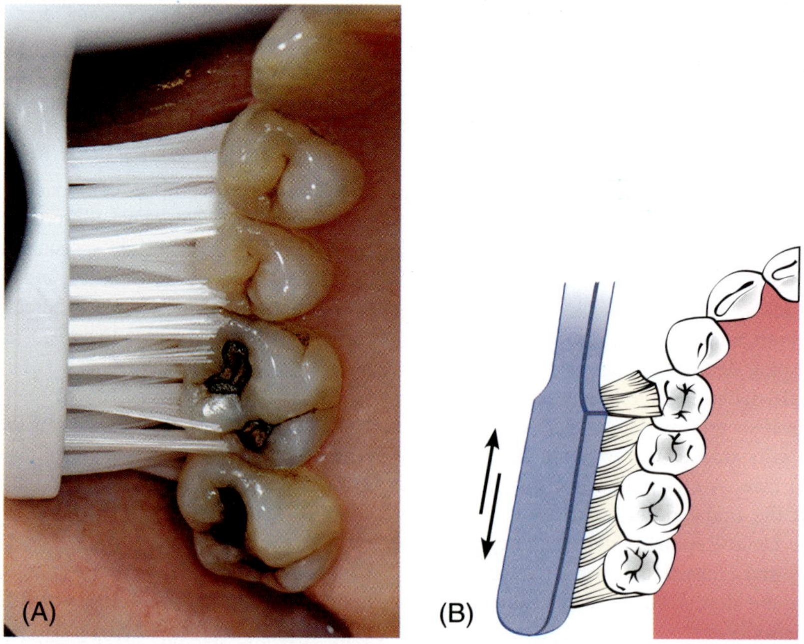

Fig. 34.4 Bass method. A, Place the toothbrush so that the bristles are angled approximately 45 degree from the tooth surfaces. B, Start at the most distal tooth in the arch and use a vibrating, back-and-forth motion to brush.

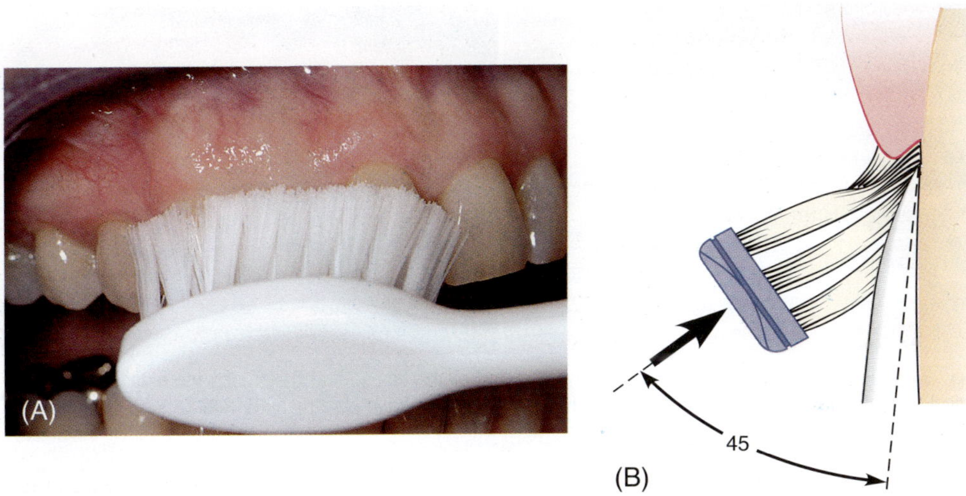

Fig. 34.5 Bass method. A, Proper position of the brush in the mouth aims the bristle tips toward the gingival margin. B, Diagram shows the ideal placement, which permits slight subgingival penetration of the bristle tips.

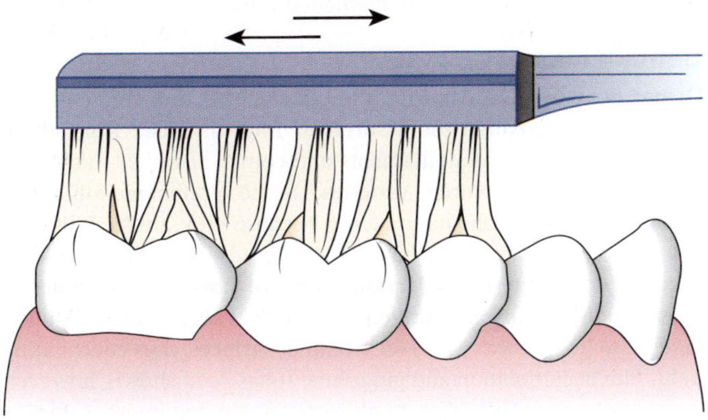

Fig. 34.6 Modified Stillman method. This method requires placement of the sides of the bristles against the teeth and gingival while moving the brush with short, back-and-forth strokes in a coronal direction.

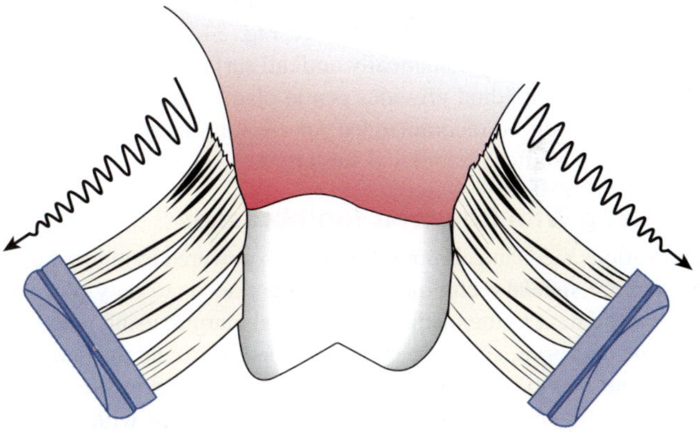

Fig. 34.7 This brush position on occlusal surfaces of the teeth is used with any technique, including the Bass, Stillman, or Charters method.

teeth (Fig. 34.6). Apply pressure against the gingival margin to produce a perceptible blanching. Then move the brush about 20 short back-and-forth strokes while simultaneously moving it coronally along the attached gingiva, the gingival margin, and the tooth surface. A soft or medium multitufted brush should be used with this technique to minimize trauma to the gingiva. This process must be repeated on all tooth surfaces, proceeding systematically around the mouth. To reach the lingual surfaces of the maxillary and mandibular incisors, the handle of the brush can be held in a vertical position, engaging the end of the brush. With this technique, the sides rather than the ends of the bristles do the work. The bristles tend not to penetrate into the gingival sulcus. The occlusal surfaces of molars and premolars are cleaned with the bristles placed perpendicular to the occlusal plane and penetrating into the grooves and interproximal embrasures (see Fig. 34.7). The modified Stillman method may be recommended for cleaning in areas with progressing gingival recession and root exposure to minimize abrasive tissue destruction.

Charters Method

The Charters method requires placement of a soft or medium multitufted brush on the teeth with the bristles pointed toward the crown at a 45-degree angle to the long axis of the teeth (Fig. 34.8). The sides of the bristles should be flexed

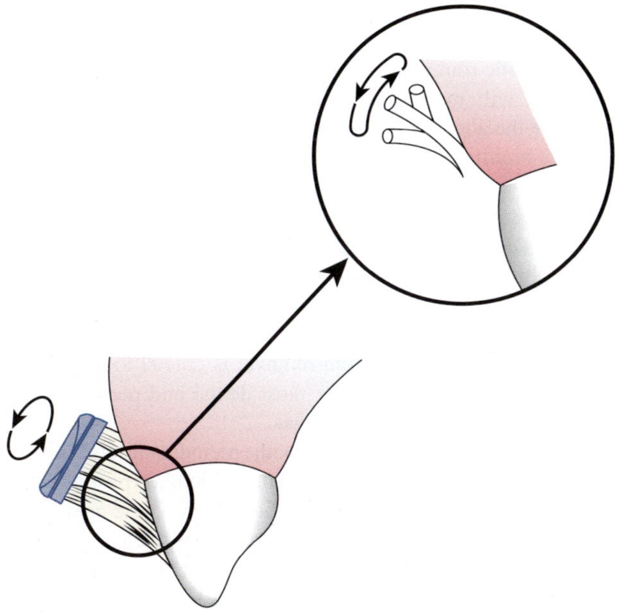

Fig. 34.8 Charters method. The Charters method requires that the bristles be pressed against the sides of the teeth and gingiva. The brush is moved with short circular or back-and-forth strokes.

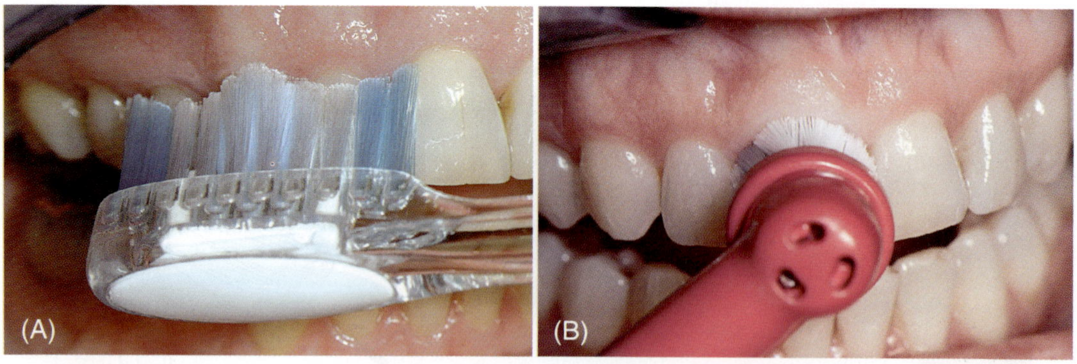

Fig. 34.9 Positioning the powered toothbrush head and bristle tips so that they reach the gingival margin is critical to achieving the most effective cleaning results. A, Straight-head placement. B, Round-head placement.

against the gingiva, and a back-and forth vibratory motion used to brush. The technique was designed to gently massage the gingiva, so the bristle tips should not drag across the gingiva. The bristle tips should be placed in the pits and fissures, and short back-and-forth strokes should be used to clean the occlusal surfaces (see Fig. 34.7). The procedures are repeated systematically until all surfaces are cleaned. The Charters method provides gentle plaque removal. This technique can be recommended for cleaning in areas of healing wounds after periodontal surgery.

Brushing With Powered Toothbrushes

The various mechanical motions built into powered toothbrushes do not require special techniques. The patient needs to only place the brush head next to the teeth at the gingival margin, using a targeted hygiene approach, and proceed systematically around the dentition. A routine method of brushing all the teeth, similar to the method described for manual brushing, should also be used with powered toothbrushes (Fig. 34.9).

Recommendations

- Targeted hygiene focuses brushing efforts on the cervical and interproximal portions of the teeth where microbial plaque biofilm accumulates first.
- Brushing with either a manual or a powered toothbrush requires a systematic routine to clean all the accessible areas.
- Patients will modify any technique to their needs but must achieve the goal of brushing effectively until the teeth are free of plaque biofilm on all accessible surfaces.

Interdental Cleaning Aids

Any toothbrush, regardless of the brushing method used, does not completely remove interdental plaque biofilms. This is true for all brushers, even periodontal patients with wide-open embrasures. Daily interdental plaque biofilm removal is crucial to augment the effects of toothbrushing because most dental and periodontal diseases originate in interproximal areas.

Tissue destruction associated with periodontal disease often leaves large, open spaces between teeth and long, exposed root surfaces with anatomic concavities and furcations. These areas shelter plaque biofilms and are both difficult for patients to clean and poorly accessible to the toothbrush. In addition, dental floss does not reach these concave surfaces. Patients need to understand that the purpose of interdental cleaning is to remove microbial plaque biofilms, not just dislodge food wedged between teeth. Many tools are available for interproximal cleaning and they should be recommended based on the size of interdental spaces, presence of furcations, tooth alignment, and presence of orthodontic appliances or fixed prostheses. Also, ease of use and patient cooperation are important considerations. Common aids are dental floss and interdental cleaners such as wooden or plastic tips and interdental brushes.

Dental Floss

Dental floss is the most widely recommended tool for removing biofilm from proximal tooth surfaces. Floss is made from nylon filaments or plastic monofilaments and comes in waxed, unwaxed, thick, thin, and flavored varieties. Some prefer monofilament flosses made of a nonstick material because they are slick and do not fray. Clinical research has demonstrated no significant differences in the ability of the various types of floss to remove dental plaque biofilm; they all work equally well. Waxed dental floss was thought to leave a waxy film on proximal surfaces, thus contributing to biofilm accumulation and gingivitis. It has been shown, however, that wax is not deposited on tooth surfaces and that improvement in gingival health is unrelated to the type of floss used. Factors influencing the choice of dental floss include the tightness of tooth contacts, roughness of proximal surfaces, and the patient's manual dexterity, not the superiority of any one product. Therefore, recommendations about type of floss should be based on ease of use and personal preference. As indicated previously, the limitations of dental floss must also be explained to the patient, and alternative methods must be demonstrated.

Technique

The floss must contact the proximal surface from line angle to line angle to clean effectively. It must also clean the entire proximal surface, including accessible subgingival areas, not just be slipped apical into the contact area. Flossing technique requires the following:

1. Start with a piece of floss long enough to grasp securely; 12–18 in. is usually sufficient. It may be wrapped around the fingers, or the ends may be tied together in a loop.
2. Stretch the floss tightly between the thumb and forefinger (Fig. 34.10), or between both forefingers, and pass it gently through each contact area with a firm back-and-forth motion. Do not snap the floss past the contact area because this may injure the interdental gingiva. In fact, zealous snapping of floss through contact areas creates proximal grooves in the gingiva.
3. Once the floss is apical to the contact area between the teeth, wrap the floss around the proximal surface of one tooth and slip it under the marginal gingiva. Move the floss firmly along the tooth up to the contact area and gently down into the sulcus again, repeating this up-and-down stroke two or three times (Fig. 34.11). Then, move the floss across the interdental gingiva,

and repeat the procedure on the proximal surface of the adjacent tooth.

4. Continue through the whole dentition, including the distal surface of the last tooth in each quadrant. When the working portion of the floss shreds or becomes dirty, move to a fresh portion of floss.

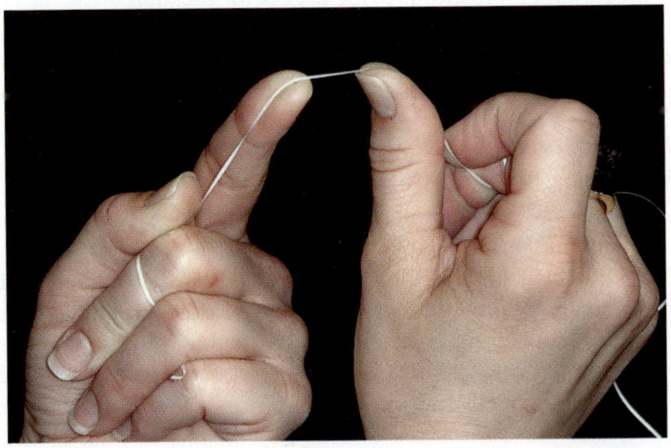

Fig. 34.10 Dental floss should be held securely in the fingers or tied in a loop.

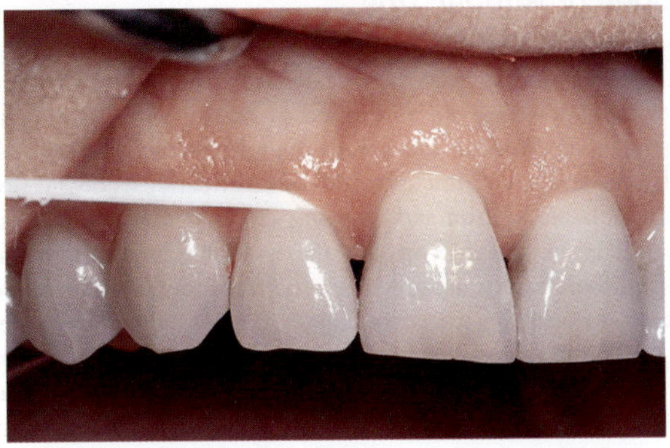

Fig. 34.11 Dental floss technique. The floss is slipped between the contact area of the teeth (in this case, teeth #7 and #8), is wrapped around the proximal surface, and removes plaque by using several up-and-down strokes. The process must be repeated for the distal surface of tooth #8.

Flossing can be facilitated by using a *floss holder* (Fig. 34.12A). Floss holders are helpful for patients lacking manual dexterity and for caregivers assisting patients in cleaning their teeth. A floss holder should be rigid enough to keep the floss taut when penetrating into tight contact areas, and it should be simple to string with floss. The disadvantage is that floss tools are time-consuming because they must be rethreaded frequently when the floss shreds.

Disposable, single-use floss holders with prethreaded floss are also available. Short-term clinical studies suggest that plaque biofilm reduction and improvement in gingivitis scores are similar for patients using disposable floss devices as for patients who hold the floss with their fingers (Fig. 34.12B).

Powered flossing devices are also available (Fig. 34.13). The devices have been shown to be safe and effective but no better at plaque biofilm removal than holding the floss in the fingers.

Establishing a lifelong habit of flossing the teeth is difficult to achieve for both patients and dentists, regardless of whether one uses a tool or flosses with the fingers. In fact, the daily use of floss is universally low. It has been reported that only about 8% of young teenagers in Great Britain flossed daily, with similar percentages reported for other countries. No information is available about the establishment of long-term flossing habits comparing the various tools to finger flossing. However, the tools may be useful to help some individuals begin flossing or to make flossing possible if patients have limited dexterity.

Recommendations

- The benefits of interproximal cleaning using dental floss are undisputed.
- Flossing tools work as well as flossing with the traditional method.
- The flossing habit is difficult to establish.

Interdental Brushes

Probably the most effective plaque biofilm removal method for interdental areas, where the papilla does not completely fill the space, is the use of interdental brushes. As indicated earlier, concave root surfaces such as the mesial aspect of the maxillary first bicuspid and furcations areas are usually not cleaned efficiently with dental floss. A comparison study of dental floss and interdental brushes used by patients with moderate to severe periodontal disease showed that the interproximal brushes removed slightly more interproximal

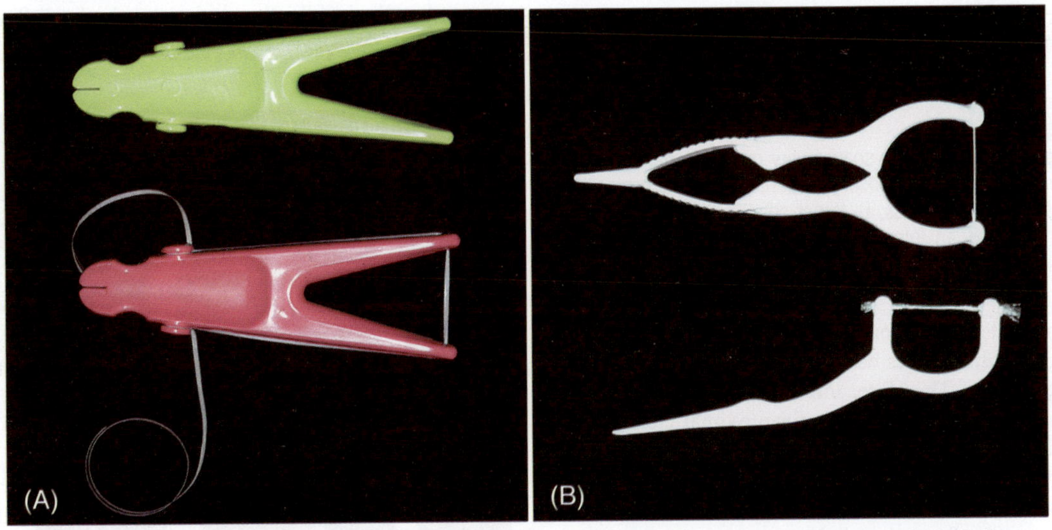

Fig. 34.12 Floss holders can simplify the manipulation of dental floss. A, Reusable floss tools require stringing the floss around a series of knobs and grooves to secure it. B, Disposable floss tools have prestrung floss and are easy to use, but the floss may shred and break, requiring several tools to complete flossing the teeth.

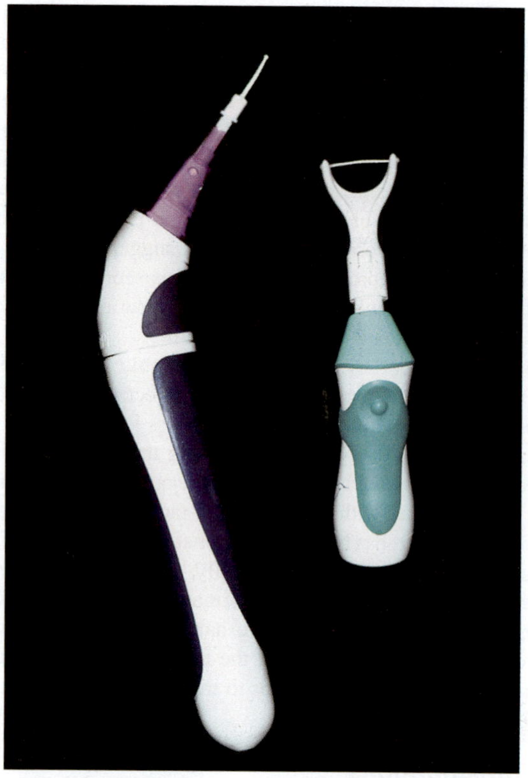

Fig. 34.13 Powered flossing devices can be easier for some patients to use than handheld floss. The tip is inserted into the proximal space, and a bristle or wand comes out of the tip and moves in a circular motion when the device is turned on *(left)*. Alternately, the device moves the prestrung floss in short motions to provide interproximal cleaning *(right)*.

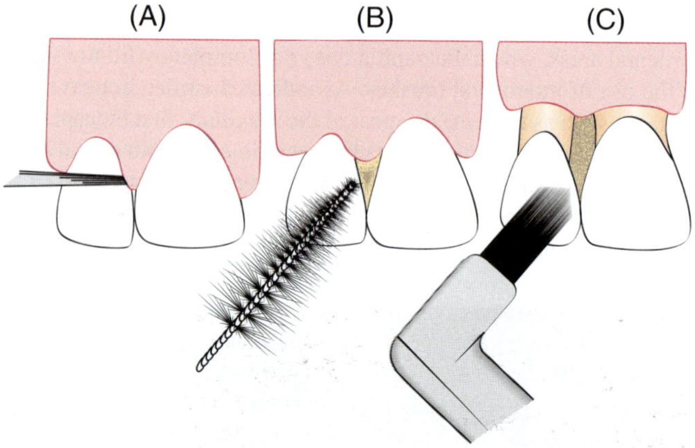

Fig. 34.14 Interproximal embrasure spaces vary greatly in patients with periodontal disease. In general, A, embrasures with no gingival recession are adequately cleaned using dental floss; B, larger spaces with exposed root surfaces require the use of an interproximal brush; and C, single-tufted brushes clean efficiently in interproximal spaces with no papillae.

plaque biofilm and that subjects found them easier to use than dental floss. However, no differences were seen in probe depth reductions or bleeding indices. Therefore, interproximal cleaning aids, such as interdental brushes, are adequate for proximal cleaning of teeth when interdental spaces permit access.

Embrasure spaces vary greatly in size and shape. Fig. 34.14 provides a representation of the size and anatomy of three types of embrasures and the type of interdental cleaner often recommended for each. As a general rule, the larger the space, the larger the device needed to clean it.

Technique

Interdental brushes of any style are inserted through interproximal spaces and moved back and forth between the teeth with short strokes. The diameter of brush should be slightly larger than the gingival embrasures to be cleaned. This size permits bristles to exert pressure on both proximal tooth surfaces, working their way into concavities on the roots.

Single-tufted brushes provide access to furcation areas, or isolated areas of deep recession, and work well on the lingual surfaces of mandibular molars and premolars. These areas are often missed when using a toothbrush and floss.

Other Interdental Cleaning Devices: Rubber Tips, Wooden Toothpicks, and Tufted Brushes

A wide variety of other interdental cleaning devices are available for removing microbial plaque biofilm from between the teeth (Fig. 34.15). Rubber tips with angled shanks, tapered wooden toothpicks that are round or triangular in cross-section, and single-tufted brushes are all helpful in attaining interdental hygiene.

Many interdental devices have handles for convenient manipulation around the teeth and in posterior areas. Clinical research has shown that the devices are effective on lingual and facial tooth surfaces as well as on proximal surfaces.

Wooden or Rubber Tips

Wooden toothpicks are used either with or without a handle (Fig. 34.15A and B). Access is easier from the buccal surfaces for tips without handles but is limited primarily to the anterior and bicuspid areas. Wooden toothpicks used on handles improve access to all areas and have been shown to be as effective as dental floss in reducing plaque biofilm and bleeding scores in subjects with gingivitis. Triangular wooden tips are also available; this design is most useful in the anterior areas when used from the buccal surfaces of the teeth. Rubber tips are conical and are mounted on handles or the ends of toothbrushes; they are reusable and can be easily adapted to all proximal surfaces in the mouth. Plastic tips that resemble wooden or rubber tips are also available and are used in the same way.

Technique

Toothpicks are common devices and readily available in most homes. They can be used around all surfaces of the teeth when attached to commercially available handles (Fig. 34.15B). Once mounted on the handle, the toothpick is broken off so that it is only

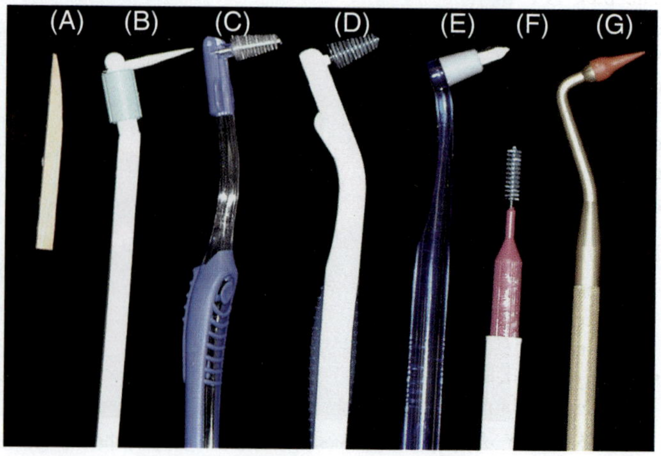

Fig. 34.15 Interproximal cleaning devices include wooden tips (A and B), interproximal brushes (C–F), and rubber tip stimulators (G).

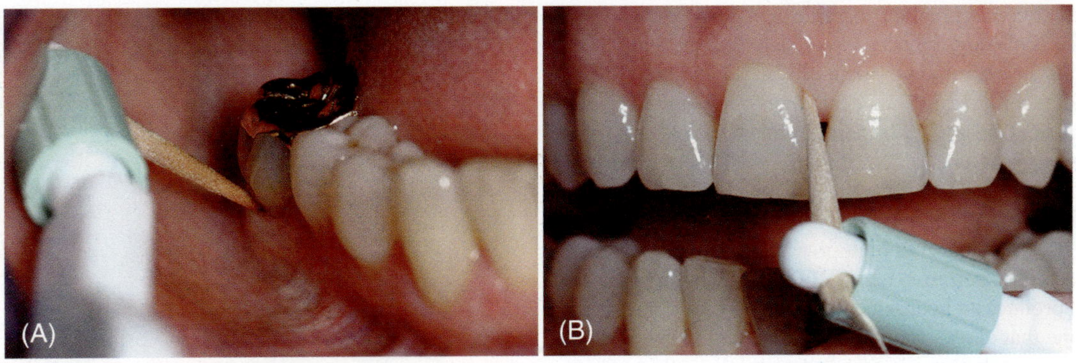

Fig. 34.16 Wooden toothpick. A, The tip is a common wooden toothpick held in a handle and broken off. It is used to clean subgingivally and reach into periodontal pockets. B, The tip can also be used to clean along the gingival margins of the teeth and reach under the gingiva.

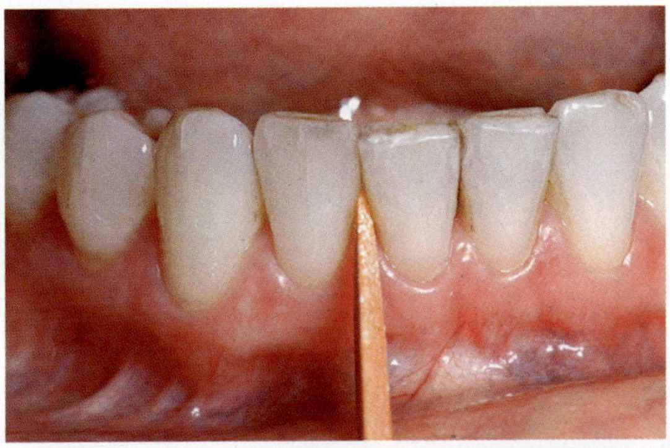

Fig. 34.17 Triangular wooden tips are also popular with patients. The tip is inserted between the teeth, with the triangular portion resting on the gingival papilla. The tip is moved in and out to remove plaque; however, it is very difficult to use on posterior teeth and from the lingual aspect of all teeth.

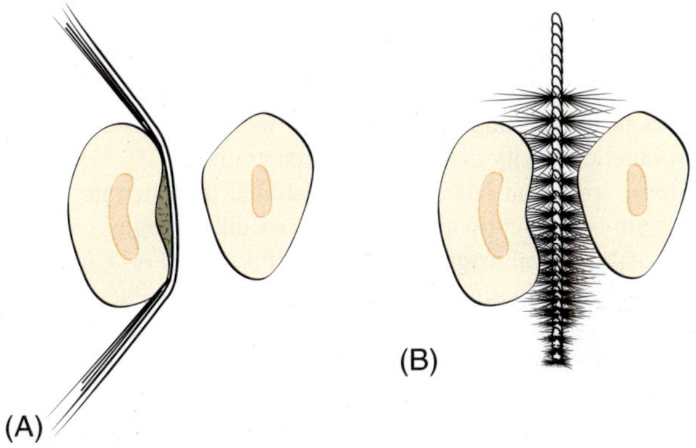

Fig. 34.18 Cleaning of concave or irregular proximal tooth surfaces. Dental floss (A) may be less effective than an interdental brush (B) on long root surfaces with concavities.

5- or 6-mm long. The tip of the toothpick is used to trace along the gingival margin and into the proximal areas from both the facial and the lingual surface of each tooth (Fig. 34.16). Toothpicks mounted on handles are efficient for cleaning along the gingival margin, can penetrate into periodontal pockets and furcations, and permit patients to target their hygiene efforts at the gingival margin.

Soft, triangular wooden picks or plastic picks are placed in the interdental space with the base of the triangle resting on the gingiva and the sides in contact with the proximal tooth surfaces (Fig. 34.17). The pick is then repeatedly moved in and out of the embrasure several times to remove the biofilm. The disadvantage of triangular wooden or plastic tips is that they do not reach well into the posterior areas or on the lingual surfaces.

Rubber tips should be placed into the embrasure space, resting on the gingiva, and used in a circular motion. They can be applied to interproximal spaces and other defects throughout the mouth and are easily adaptable to lingual surfaces.

Recommendations

- Often a toothbrush and dental floss are not sufficient to clean interdental spaces adequately, so it is extremely important to find an interdental device that the patient likes and will use.
- Many interdental cleaning aids are available for patients. The patient might need to try several devices before finding one that is acceptable and cleans adequately.
- In general, the largest brush or device that fits into a space will clean most efficiently (Fig. 34.18).

Gingival Massage

Massaging the gingiva with a toothbrush or an interdental cleaning devices produces epithelial thickening, increased keratinization, and increased mitotic activity in the epithelium and connective tissue. The increased keratinization occurs only on the gingiva facing the oral cavity and not on the areas more vulnerable to microbial attack, which are the sulcular epithelium and the interdental areas where the gingival col is present. Epithelial thickening, increased keratinization, and increased blood circulation have not been shown to be beneficial for restoring gingival health. Improved gingival health associated with interdental stimulation is much more likely the result of microbial plaque biofilm removal than gingival massage.

Oral Irrigation

Home/Self-Applied Irrigation

The body of evidence on the oral irrigators (also called water flosser and dental water jet) consistently has been shown to significantly reduce gingivitis, bleeding on probing, and periodontal pathogens. These oral health improvements have been demonstrated with the use of either water or an antimicrobial agent. The evidence indicates that the oral irrigators effectively remove biofilm and are more effective than dental floss when added to toothbrushing.

Mechanism of Action of Irrigation

The mechanism of action of irrigation occurs through the direct application of a pulsed stream of water or other solution. Studies have found pulsation and pressure to be critical components of an irrigation device. Pulsating devices have been shown to be three times as effective as a continuous-stream irrigating syringe. Pulsation provides for a compression and decompression phase that may account for expedient clearing of bacteria from the pocket. A pulsating device allows for control of the pressure rate. The majority of studies on home irrigation that have demonstrated clinical efficacy have been done using a water flosser with 1200–1400 pulsations per minute set on a medium to a high pressure setting (50–90 psi) (Fig. 34.19A). A higher pulsation rate of 1600/min in newer systems (Colgate Blast) produces a hydrokinetic activity creating an impact and flushing zone that allows for debris and bacteria to be expelled from the sulcus or pocket and is reported to be three times more effective than a continuous-stream device. This cordless, portable, and rechargeable water flosser system works at three pressure settings, that is, gentle (37–68 PSI), regular (42–92 PSI), and pulse (27–60 PSI), to meet the variable individual needs of the patients (Fig. 34.19B). A pulsation device has been shown to create two zones of hydrokinetic energy: the impact zone, in which the solution initially contacts, and the flushing zone, in which the solution reaches in to the subgingival sulcus (Fig. 34.20). The outcome of hydrokinetic activity is subgingival penetration.

Home irrigation has been demonstrated to penetrate subgingivally with both a jet tip and a soft, site-specific, subgingival tip (Pik Pocket subgingival irrigation tip, Water Pik, Inc., Fort Collins, CO). Supragingival irrigation is irrigation with a jet tip placed above the gingival margin resulting in penetration of a solution into the subgingival sulcus to approximately 50%. The jet tip is generally used for full-mouth irrigation. Recently, other types of supragingival tips enhanced with soft, tapered bristles have been introduced and shown to be effective in increasing the removal of plaque. Irrigation with the soft, site-specific tip is called *subgingival irrigation.* This refers to the placement of the tip, which is placed slightly below the gingival margin (Fig. 34.21). The subgingival tip is used for the localized irrigation of a specific site such as a deep pocket, furcation, implant, or crown and bridge. Studies with this site-specific, subgingival tip show that it can deliver a solution into a pocket of 6 mm or less up to 90% of its depth. In pockets deeper than 6 mm, the depth of penetration has been shown to be 64%. Numerous novel tip designs utilizing innovative nozzles have emerged to meet the varied requirements of individual patients and enhance clinical benefits of subgingival irrigation systems (Fig. 34.22).

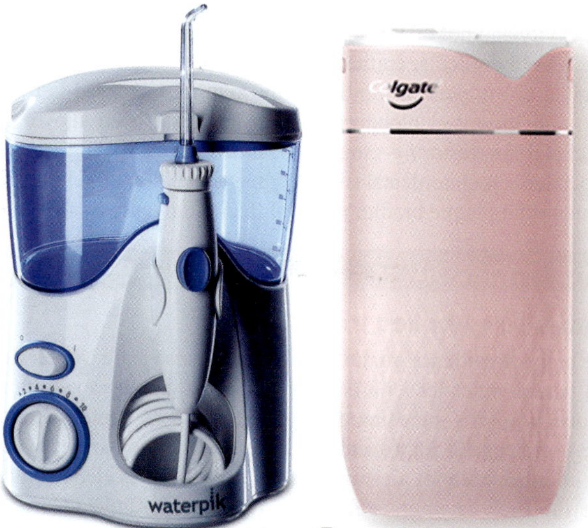

A B

Fig. 34.19 A, Water flosser with 1400 ppm and a pressure setting that ranges from 20 to 90 psi. B, A portable water flosser with 1600 ppm and three pressure setting modes, that is, gentle (37–68 psi), regular (42–92 psi), and pulse (27–60 psi). (*A, Courtesy: Water Pik, Inc., Fort Collins, CO; B, Courtesy: Colgate-Palmolive, India.*)

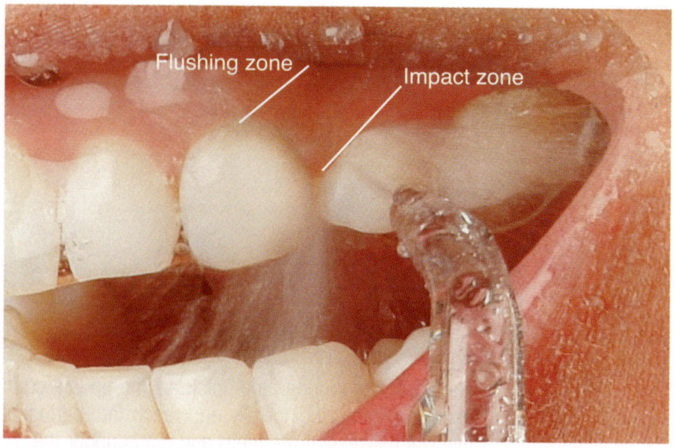

Fig. 34.20 Pulsation creates two zones of hydrokinetic activity: the impact zone and the flushing zone. (*Courtesy: Water Pik, Inc., Fort Collins, CO.*)

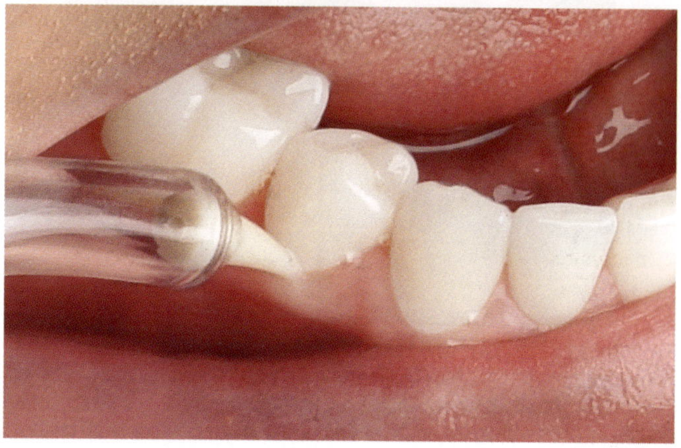

Fig. 34.21 The Pik Pocket tip is gently placed slightly subgingivally. (*Courtesy: Water Pik, Inc., Fort Collins, CO.*)

Technique of Supragingival Irrigation

1. The common home-use irrigator tip is a plastic nozzle with a 90-degree bend at the tip attached to a pump providing pulsating beads of water at speeds regulated by a dial. Patients should be instructed to aim the pulsating jet across the proximal papilla, hold it there for 10–15 s, trace along the gingival margin to the next proximal space, and repeat the procedure.
2. The irrigator should be used for both the buccal and lingual surface.
3. Patients with gingival inflammation should start at low pressure, and they can increase the pressure comfortably to about medium as tissue health improves. Some individuals like to use the device on the highest pressure setting, with no reported harm. Patient comfort should be the guide for pressure setting.

Technique of Subgingival Irrigation

The soft rubber irrigator tip reduces the pressure and flow of the pulsating jet of water when it is inserted subgingivally, and it permits penetration of irrigant to up to 70% of pocket depth in laboratory simulations. The subgingival irrigation tip should be

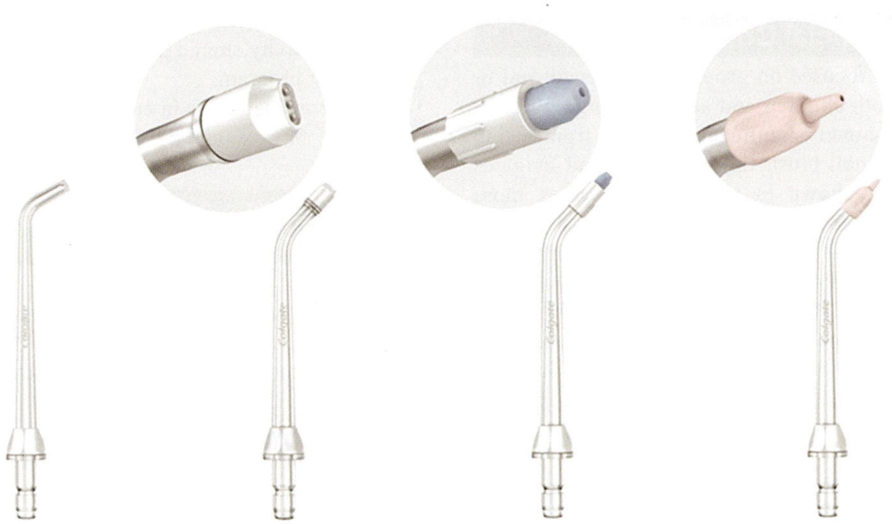

Fig. 34.22 Innovative nozzle designs of water flosser tips. (*Courtesy: Colgate-Palmolive, India.*)

gently inserted into pockets or furcation areas, 3 mm if possible, and each pocket should be flushed for a few seconds.

Safety

Concerns regarding the safety of oral irrigation with regard to soft tissue damage and penetration of bacteria into the pocket have been voiced although no scientific evidence exists to support these assumptions. The published research shows a different profile starting with early studies that showed a histological reduction of inflammation. Subsequent studies showed the reduction of subgingival pathogens even in pockets up to 6 mm and an ultrastructural study found no differences in the epithelial lining of the pocket compared to the nonirrigated sites. Studies that have measured the clinical attachment level and probing pocket depth have reported either no change or a significant improvement supporting no detrimental effects on the attachment or junctional epithelium. Manipulation of tissue in any level of periodontal disease will cause a bacteremia. The incidence of bacteremia using a pulsating oral irrigator ranges from 7% in people with gingivitis to 50% in people with periodontitis. These findings are in line with other self-care techniques such as toothbrushing and flossing (20%–68%), wooden toothpicks or sticks (20%–40%), and mastication (7%–51%).

Clinical Outcomes of Irrigation

Evaluated outcomes include removal of plaque biofilm and reductions in calculus, gingivitis, bleeding on probing, probing depth, periodontal pathogens, and inflammatory mediators. Home irrigation has been studied and found safe and effective for those with gingivitis, implants, crown and bridge, orthodontics, intermaxillary fixation, and diabetes; patients who are noncompliant with dental floss; and in periodontal maintenance.

Early studies found that irrigation with water leads to a reduction in calculus: up to as much as 50% over brushing alone. A study conducted with the scanning electron microscope found that a 3-s pulsating lavage at a 60 psi with either a jet tip or small brush tip removed 99% of plaque biofilm (Fig. 34.23). A single-use study that compared irrigation to string floss, each in addition to manual brushing found irrigation to be 29% more effective at whole mouth plaque removal.

As early as the 1960s, it was shown that oral irrigation with water added to toothbrushing reduced gingivitis by 52% compared to a 30% reduction for toothbrushing alone. Throughout the years, other researchers have found concurring results with the use of plain water. The use of an antimicrobial agent, such as diluted chlorhexidine (Table 34.1), or an essential oil, generally enhances reductions in gingivitis and bleeding.

Emerging evidence indicates that home irrigation may play a role in modulating the host response, particularly the inflammatory mediators associated with clinical attachment loss and alveolar bone loss. This evidence lends support to the safety of irrigation, as well as its potential for helping periodontal maintenance patients maintain stability.

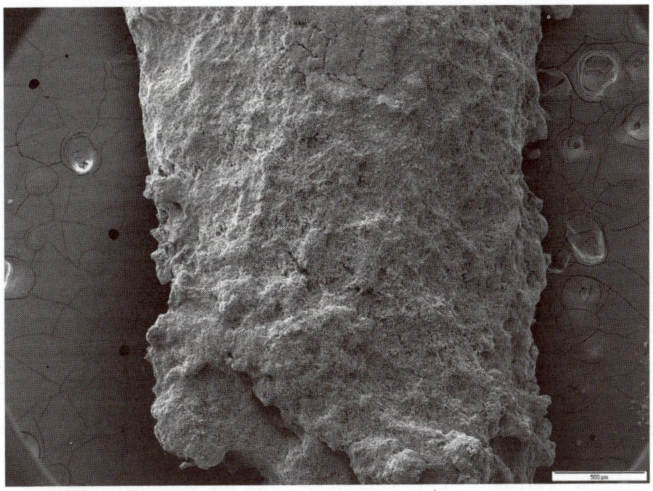
Fig. 34.23 Control tooth with no irrigation. (*Courtesy: Water Pik, Inc., Fort Collins, CO.*)

TABLE 34.1 Chlorhexidine Dilutions (Based on 0.12% Concentration) Shown Effective in Clinical Trials

Concentrations	Amount of Water	Amount of Chlorhexidine
0.02%	5 parts	1 part
0.04%	3 parts	1 part
0.06%	1 part	1 part

Individuals With Special Considerations

Some clinical trials have focused on groups with special oral or medical health needs. Both children and adults undergoing orthodontic therapy have shown significant benefits from using a water flosser. A new, small brush tip that cleans and irrigates simultaneously has been shown to remove 3.76 times more plaque than brushing and flossing with a floss threader. For individuals with implants, manual brushing and irrigating with water over 4 weeks showed an 81.8% reduction in bleeding which was 2.45 times better than using string floss. For those with special medical considerations, home irrigation has been studied and shown safe and effective in a group of individuals with either type 1 or type 2 diabetes.

Conclusion

Home irrigation is safe and effective for a wide variety of patients, including those in periodontal maintenance; those with calculus buildup, gingivitis, orthodontic appliances, maxillary fixation, crown and bridge, implants, and diabetes; and those who are noncompliant with floss. Clinical outcomes include the reduction of plaque, calculus, gingivitis, bleeding on probing, probing depth, periodontal pathogens, and inflammatory mediators.

The recommendations for caries prevention are discussed online.

Caries Control

Dental caries, particularly root caries, is a problem for periodontal patients because of attachment loss and exposed root surfaces associated with the disease process and periodontal therapeutic procedures. *Root caries* develops through a process similar to coronal caries, in the alternating cycle of demineralization and remineralization of the surfaces and other risk factors associated with diet and salivary flow. The demineralization process requires the fermentation of carbohydrates in the plaque biofilm by oral bacteria, resulting in loss of mineral from the root surface. *Lactobacillus* and *Streptococcus* species are involved in the root caries process, as with coronal caries. The major difference is that the amount of organic material in the root surfaces is greater than in enamel, so once the demineralization has occurred, the organic matrix—mostly collagen—is exposed. Organic material is then further broken down by bacterial enzymes, resulting in rapid destruction of the root surface.

Fluoride works primarily by topical effects to prevent and reverse the caries process, whether in enamel, cementum, or dentin. Low concentrations of topical fluoride inhibit demineralization, enhance remineralization, and inhibit the enzyme activity in bacteria by acidifying the cells. Adult patients benefit from the prevention and reversal of root caries provided by low concentration topical fluoride delivered by toothpastes or other topical applications. It also has been demonstrated that the use of fluoride dentifrice containing 5000 ppm of fluoride was more effective in reversing active root caries lesions than the fluoride level of 1100 ppm found in conventional toothpastes.

Recommendations

- All periodontal patients should be encouraged to use a fluoride-containing toothpaste daily, 1000–1100 ppm, to reduce demineralization and enhance remineralization of tooth surfaces.
- Patients at high risk for caries, including those with a history of root lesions or who have active lesions, should use higher-concentration fluoride toothpaste or gels, 5000 ppm, daily until the risk for caries is controlled, then maintain with the lower concentration toothpastes and mouthrinses.
- Periodic chlorhexidine rinsing to control cariogenic bacteria in the oral cavity should also be used as part of a caries risk management program.
- Other considerations in caries control, such as diet and reduced salivary flow, should be evaluated as with all dental patients.

Chemical Plaque Biofilm Control With Oral Rinses

Plaque control is the key to prevention of periodontal diseases. It can be achieved mechanically (as discussed earlier) or chemically. Chemical plaque control, however, should be regarded as an adjunct to and not a substitute for mechanical plaque control.

Mouthwash, mouthrinse, oral rinse, or mouth bath is a liquid which is held in the mouth passively or swirled around the mouth by contraction of the perioral muscles and/or movement of the head and gargled.

An ideal chemical plaque control agent should possess the properties of *Substantivity* (ability of agent to bind to tissue surfaces and be released over time); *Penetrability* (ability to penetrate deeply into the biofilm); and *Selectivity* (ability to affect specific bacteria in a mixed population).

The extent of *stability* of the active agent in the presence of salivary and/or bacterial enzymes, its *solubility* into the oral environment, its adequate *bioavailability*, its *accessibility* to the site of action, and the *ionic interactions* between agent and receptor sites are other important factors which affect delivery to and clearance of the plaque control agents from the oral cavity.

Chemical plaque control agents may be grouped into first-, second-, and third-generation antimicrobial agents (Table 34.2).

Some of the antimicrobial agents are discussed here:

Chlorhexidine rinse: The agent that has shown the most positive antibacterial results to date is chlorhexidine, a diguanidohexane with pronounced antiseptic properties. Several other clinical investigations confirmed the initial finding that two daily rinses with 10 mL of a 0.2% aqueous solution of chlorhexidine digluconate almost completely inhibited the development of dental plaque, calculus, and gingivitis in the human model for experimental gingivitis. Clinical studies of several months' duration have reported plaque reductions of 45%–61% and, more importantly, gingivitis reductions of 27%–67%. A randomized, cross-over, double blind clinical trial proved the equal efficacy of the lower concentrations of CHX 0.12% solutions, yet some inadvertent side effects, such as variable dental staining, was observed with both concentrations. The novel formula of Periogard Low Stain containing 0.12% chlorhexidine gluconate combines sodium tripolyphosphate as a stain prevention technology and SLS+Poloxamer, a surfactant complex and provides effective chlorhexidine action to minimize the staining effect during long-term usage. The low-stain chlorhexidine mouthwash clinically demonstrated significantly less stain than the standard chlorhexidine formula, while maintaining its efficacy against plaque and gingivitis over 6 months. It has a broad antimicrobial spectrum. At low concentrations, it causes leakage of intracellular potassium and reduction in bacterial acid production. At higher concentrations, it is able to induce bacterial cell wall disruption and coagulation of the cytoplasmic constituents. It also inhibits enzymes involved in bacterial adhesion, bacterial growth, and metabolism. Approximately 30% of the chlorhexidine applied is retained in the oral soft tissues, which serve as a reservoir for slow release of the agent over extended periods of time. Localized, reversible side effects to chlorhexidine use may occur, primarily brown staining of the teeth, tongue, and silicate and

TABLE 34.2 Classification of Chemical Plaque Control Agents

First-Generation Chemical Plaque Control Agents	Second-Generation Chemical Plaque Control Agents	Third-Generation Chemical Plaque Control Agents
Phenolic compounds Phenol Thymol Triclosan Listerine (menthol, thymol, eucalyptol) Hexylresorcinol	*Bisbiguanides* Chlorhexidine Alexidine	Delmopinol
Quaternary ammonium compounds Cetylpyridinium chloride Benzethonium chloride	*Bispyridinamines* Octenidine dihydrochloride	
Antibiotics		
Vancomycin, niddamycin, kanamycin		
Halogens		
Iodine, fluorides		
Metallic ions		
Zinc, copper, tin, silver, mercury ions		
Herbal extracts		
Sanguinaria extract		
Antiplaque enzymes		
Mucinase, mutanase, dextranase, amyloglucosidase		
Oxygenating/Oxidizing agents		
Peroxides		

resin restorations and transient impairment of taste perception. Chlorhexidine has very low systemic toxic activity in humans, has not produced any appreciable resistance of oral microorganisms, and has not been associated with teratogenic alterations.

Nonprescription essential oil rinse: One of the most extensively used and researched mouthrinse, Listerine (named after Lister), is a combination of phenol-related essential ions, thymol, and eucalyptol, mixed with menthol and methyl salicylate in a hydroalcoholic base. It is antiinflammatory and has the ability to suppress odorigenic bacteria. The nonionized molecules cause inactivation of essential enzymes at low concentrations and disruption of cell proteins at high concentrations.

Heavy metal ions: Divalent metal ions possess antiplaque potential as a result of their ability to bind plaque components via electrostatic forces, thereby altering the surface charge and adherence potential of bacteria. They are able to displace calcium ions from the pellicle and bacterial surfaces, have antiglycolytic effect, and reduce pathogenecity of established plaque by suppressing plaque acidogenecity.

Quaternary ammonium compounds: These cationic antiseptics interact with plaque in a manner similar to that of chlorhexidine but are less effective because of their rapid clearance from the oral cavity.

Sanguinarine: A mixture of bezophenanthridine alkaloids, this extract of the bloodroot plant *Sanguinaria canadensis* is effective against both gram-positive and gram-negative bacteria. Its ability to interfere with the steps in bacterial cell wall synthesis may be responsible for its antimicrobial activities.

Hexetidine: A synthetic hexahydropyridine with mechanism of action similar to chlorhexidine. However, it has little antiplaque effect at clinically acceptable concentrations. Higher concentrations are associated with corresponding increase in frequency of desquamative lesions.

Enzymes: Peroxidases have been added to mouthrinses and dentifrices to ensure presence of sufficient hydrogen peroxide to control proliferation of plaque bacteria.

Triclosan: This is a nonionic, broad spectrum antimicrobial agent, currently being incorporated into dentifrices and mouthrinses because of its high retentivity in the oral cavity and hence a positive, linear dose-response antiplaque and antigingivitis efect. Its antiinflammatory effect can be attributed to its ability to inhibit both cyclooxygenase and lipooxygenase, thereby retarding prostaglandin and leukotriene production. Total (Colgate Oral Pharmaceuticals Inc. Canton, Mass.) contains triclosan and Gantrez (a copolymer of polyvinyl methyl and maleic acid) and is the first dentifrice sold in the United States to receive the ADA's Seal of Acceptance for the reduction of plaque and gingivitis.

Octenidine dihydrochloride: It has high antimicrobial activity together with good tolerability. It provides antibacterial and antifungal activity during oral rinsing which is maintained between rinsing. It is a positively charged compound that exerts its bactericidal action by binding to the negatively charged bacterial cell membranes as well as to the soft and hard tissue surfaces of the oral cavity. It has both lipophilic and hydrophilic properties, allowing it to embed in the phospholipid bilayer, disrupting the regular distribution of phospholipids, and attacking the enzyme systems. This causes the cell wall to lose integrity and leak cytoplasmic contents. It also has a high affinity for cardiolipin, which is a lipid only present in bacterial cell membranes, and is therefore lethal only to bacterial cells, leaving human tissue and epithelium unaffected. Octenidine dihydrochloride is a potential alternative to chlorhexidine.

Delmopinol: This is a substituted amino-alcohol, which disrupts the bacterial matrix formation, thereby interfering with bacterial attachment. This surface-modifying agent is less effective than chlorhexidine on established gingivitis patients. Transient anesthesia of the dorsum of the tongue, mucosal soreness, taste disturbances, and erosions are the various side effects attributed to this compound.

Disclosing Agents

Removal of plaque at regular intervals is critical for oral health maintenance. However, plaque is relatively invisible to the naked eye. Therein comes the role of plaque disclosing agents, which are agents capable of staining bacterial biofilms on the surfaces of teeth, tongue, and gingiva, making it visible for easy detection and removal (Fig. 34.24). They play a vital role in patient motivation and education; help the clinicians in determining the plaque indices; and also help the researcher in evaluating the effectiveness of plaque control devices.

Various dyes that have been utilized to detect plaque are erythrosine (most widely used, stains the plaque area red, but may also stain the soft tissues), Skinners Iodine solution (formerly widely used, unacceptable taste, high incidence of allergic reactions), Fast green, Mercurochrome preparations, Bismark Brown, Merbromin, Basic Fuchsin, Phloxine B plus Patent Blue (two-tone dye, stains older/mature plaque blue and newer/immature plaque pink/red, does not stain the soft tissues), and Fluorescein (fluoresces yellow–green under UV light, expensive, does not stain the soft tissues, but a special light is required to visualize the stained plaque).

Disclosing agents are available as solutions or wafers commercially. Solutions are applied to the teeth as concentrates on cotton swabs or diluted as rinses. Wafers are crushed between the teeth and swished around the mouth for a few seconds and then spit out. Either form can be used for plaque biofilm control instruction in the office and dispensed for home use to aid periodontal patients in evaluating the effectiveness of their oral hygiene routines.

Frequency of Plaque Biofilm Removal

In the controlled and supervised environment of clinical research, where well-trained individuals remove all visible plaque biofilm, gingival health can be maintained by one thorough cleaning with brush, floss, and toothpicks every 24–48 h. However, this is not true with most patients. The average daily home care routine lasts less than 2 min and removes only 40% of plaque biofilm. It has been reported that improved plaque biofilm removal and therefore improved periodontal health are associated with increasing the frequency of brushing to twice per day. Cleaning three or more times per day does not appear to improve periodontal conditions further. Clinical experience has also indicated that more important than the number of times the patient practices oral hygiene during a given day is effective to target hygiene, meaning thorough plaque biofilm removal at the proper location. One could be cleaning several times a day, but if the target areas are missed, plaque biofilm will persist in these critical areas.

Patient Motivation and Education

In periodontal therapy, plaque biofilm control has two important purposes: to minimize gingival inflammation and to prevent the recurrence or progression of periodontal diseases and caries. Daily mechanical removal of plaque biofilm by the patient, including the use of appropriate antimicrobial agents, is the only practical means for improving oral health on a long-term basis. The process requires interest on the part of the patient and education and instruction from the dentist, followed by encouragement and reinforcement. Keeping records of patient performance facilitates this process. Fig. 34.25 provides an example of a plaque biofilm control record that permits repeated measures and comparison over time.

Motivation for Effective Plaque Biofilm Control

Motivating patients to perform effective plaque biofilm control is one of the most critical and difficult elements of long-term success in periodontal therapy. It requires both commitment by the patient to change daily habits and regular return visits for maintenance and reinforcement. The scope of this compliance problem is immense. It has been shown that patients stop using interproximal cleaning aids after a very short time. Heasman et al. followed 100 patients treated for moderate to severe periodontal disease and taught to use one or more interdental cleaning aids. It was found that only 20% used the aids after 6 months. Of those who had started using three devices, one-third had stopped all interdental cleaning at 6 months; the others used one or two of the aids. The situation is no better when looking at patient willingness to return for office visits. In one study of 1280 patients, most of whom had periodontal surgery in multiple sites after intensive scaling, root planing, and home care instruction,

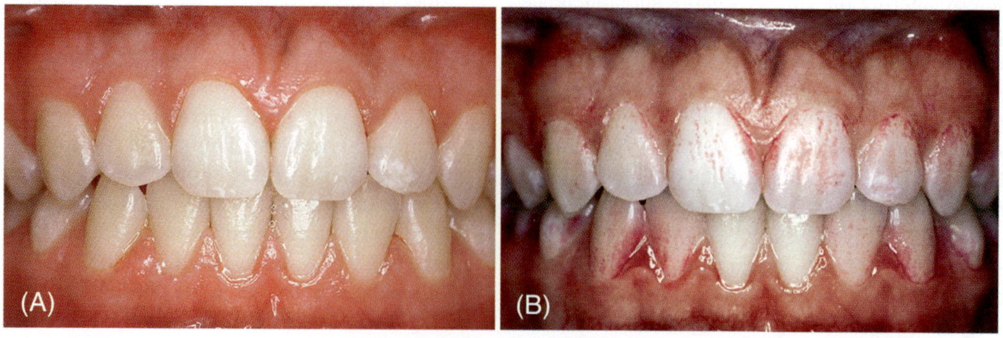

Fig. 34.24 Effect of a disclosing agent. A, Unstained, the teeth look clean, but close inspection shows subtle signs of gingivitis. B, Plaque shows as dark-red particulate matter when stained with a disclosing dye. It is useful to demonstrate toothbrushing in the patient's mouth with the teeth disclosed and plaque visible.

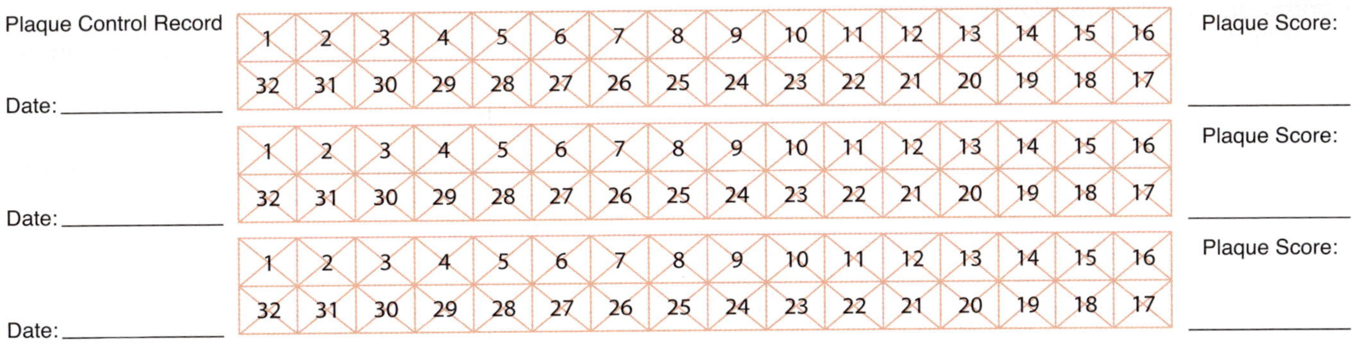

Fig. 34.25 The plaque control record can be an effective motivator for patients. This form permits easy comparison of scores over time. (*Courtesy: Dean John D.B. Featherstone, University of California, San Francisco School of Dentistry, San Francisco.*)

25% never returned for a follow-up visit; only 40% returned regularly. Wilson et al. reported that 67% of periodontal patients were noncompliant with return visits in a 20-year retrospective of a private periodontal practice.

Adopting new habits and returning for office visits is not an impossible task. To be successful, the patient (1) must be receptive and understand the concepts of pathogenesis, treatment, and prevention of periodontal disease; (2) must be willing to change the habits of a lifetime; and (3) must be able to adjust personal beliefs, practices, and values to accommodate new regimens. Manual skills must be developed to establish an effective plaque biofilm control regimen. In addition, the patient must understand the dentist's critical role in treating and maintaining periodontal health. If not, long-term success of treatment is much less likely.

Education and Scoring Systems

Many patients prefer to believe that treatment is a passive process, so it is incumbent on the dentist to educate and reinforce to each patient their personal role in long-term success of therapy. Our health-conscious society is an advantage with regard to patient education. Most patients know what gingivitis is because they have heard about it on television or read about it in magazines or on the web. They are willing to spend time and money to try new products such as toothbrushes and mouthrinses.

Patients must also be informed that periodic assessment and debridement of the teeth in the dental office are required to prevent recurrence of periodontal diseases and identify problems that may arise. These procedures work best when combined with an individualized oral hygiene regimen practiced daily at home. Therefore, time spent in the dental office teaching the patient how to perform microbial plaque biofilm control procedures is central to care. Patients sometimes have the concept that "cleanings" every few months are sufficient for calculus and biofilm removal and disease control. Only the combination of regular office visits with conscientious home care has been shown to significantly reduce gingivitis and loss of supporting periodontal tissues over the long term.

Periodontal patients should be shown how periodontal disease has manifested in their own mouth. Stained plaque biofilm, the bleeding of inflamed gingiva, and demonstrations of the periodontal probe inserted into pockets are impressive demonstrations of the presence of pathogens and symptoms of disease. It also is of educational value to patients to have their oral cleanliness and periodontal condition recorded periodically so that improvements in performance can be used for positive reinforcement. The plaque biofilm control record index, bleeding points index, and their significance in patient education and motivation are discussed in detail online.

Plaque Biofilm Control Record (O'Leary Index)

Have the patient use a disclosing solution or tablet and examine each tooth surface (except occlusal surfaces) for the presence or absence of stained biofilm at the dento-gingival junction. Plaque biofilm is recorded on the appropriate box in a diagram for four surfaces on each tooth. After all teeth have been scored, the index number is calculated for the percentage of surfaces with biofilm by dividing the number of surfaces with microbial plaque biofilm by the total number of surfaces scored and then multiplying by 100. A reasonable goal for patients is 10% or fewer surfaces with plaque biofilm. If biofilm is always present in the same areas, provide instructions to improve cleaning procedures in those areas. It is extremely difficult to achieve a perfect score of 0, so patients should be rewarded for approaching it.

Some frequently used plaque biofilm indices do not require staining the teeth including the Plaque Index of Silness and Löe. These are more convenient to use and often more acceptable to patients, but they are not as dramatic for patient education.

Bleeding Points Index

The bleeding points index provides an evaluation of gingival inflammation around each tooth in the patient's mouth. Retract the cheek and place the periodontal probe 1 mm into the sulcus or pocket at the distal aspect of the most posterior tooth in the quadrant on the buccal surface. Carry the probe lightly across the length of the sulcus to the mesial interproximal area on the facial aspect. Continue along all the teeth in the quadrant from the facial aspect. Wait 30 s and record the presence of bleeding on the distal, facial, and mesial surfaces on the chart. Repeat on the lingual-palatal aspect, recording bleeding only for the direct lingual surface, not for the mesial or distal surfaces. This results in four separate scores for each tooth and does not score the mesial and distal surfaces twice. Repeat the steps for each quadrant. The percentage of the number of bleeding surfaces is calculated by dividing the number of surfaces that bled by the total number of tooth surfaces (four per tooth) and by multiplying by 100 to convert the score to a percentage. This index is designed to demonstrate gingival inflammation characterized by bleeding rather than presence of microbial plaque biofilm. Again, a goal of 10% or fewer bleeding points is good, but 0 is ideal. If a few bleeding points repeatedly occur in the same areas, cleaning procedures for those areas should be reinforced or modified.

Significance of Plaque Biofilm Scores and Bleeding Scores

Plaque biofilm scores are helpful as indicators of patient compliance and success with daily home care procedures. However, biofilm levels themselves do not necessarily reflect gingival health or risk of disease progression, even though the location of the plaque biofilm is highly correlated with the presence of gingivitis. Bleeding is a much better indicator of predicting success in controlling inflammation and reducing the chance of disease progression. Although bleeding on probing is not the most specific or sensitive measures of health, it has a strong negative correlation to disease progression. If bleeding is absent at any given site in the mouth, reflecting good plaque biofilm control and disease management, it is unlikely that periodontal disease will progress.

Instruction and Demonstration

Patients can reduce the incidence of plaque biofilm and gingivitis with repeated instruction and encouragement much more effectively than with self-acquired oral hygiene habits. However, instruction in how to clean teeth must be more than a cursory chairside demonstration on the use of a toothbrush. It is a painstaking procedure that requires patient participation, careful supervision with correction of mistakes, and reinforcement during return visits, until the patient achieves the necessary proficiency. Any strategy for introducing plaque biofilm control to the periodontal patient includes several elements. At the first instruction visit, the patient should be given a new toothbrush, an interdental cleaner, and a disclosing agent. The patient's plaque biofilm should be disclosed otherwise it is difficult for the patient to see (Fig. 34.24). Polished dental restorations do not take up the stain, but the oral mucosa and the lips may retain it for up to several hours. Use petroleum jelly to keep the dye off the patient's lips. For these patients, the location and true color of the plaque biofilm can be demonstrated with the rubber tip. Once the plaque biofilm is demonstrated, the clinician can proceed with the hygiene instruction in the patient's mouth.

The rubber tip is used to demonstrate the plaque biofilm located at the gingival margin, which is the target area. The nondisclosed plaque biofilm is almost the same color as the teeth, which impresses and educates the patient about the reason for not recognizing biofilm in the past. Toothbrushing should also be demonstrated in the patient's mouth while he or she observes with a hand mirror. The patient then repeats the procedure with the clinician giving assistance, correction, and positive reinforcement. Repeat the demonstration and instruction with dental floss and other interdental cleaning aids according to the patient's needs. Depending on the patient's skill and understanding of the technique, instruction on interdental hygiene may be postponed until the patient is able to manipulate the toothbrush properly. The rubber tip is an excellent instrument to demonstrate plaque biofilm, but it is also used to clean the interdental area. The rubber tip is placed interdentally, and the plaque biofilm is removed with a scooping motion.

Encourage patients to clean the teeth thoroughly at least once a day. Be sure to inform them that home care procedures on a full dentition take 5–10 min, and for complex periodontal cases, home care procedures may take 30 min. The patient should set aside a convenient time and place in the daily schedule to perform the procedures reliably every day. Subsequent instruction visits should be used to reinforce or modify previous instructions, periodically recording the state of gingival health and amount of plaque biofilm.

Some strategies simply do not work. Waiting until the end of the appointment, for example, when the patient is sore, exhausted, and possibly anesthetized is not conducive to learning. Failing to provide positive reinforcement, handing the patient too many tools, and relying only on pamphlets and printed material to provide education are likely to result in an insufficient or ineffective instruction process.

Recommendations

The following list provides some strategies that will assist you in educating and motivating your patients:

- Provide encouragement.
- Demonstrate how devices work, and allow the patient to practice with them.
- Provide samples so that the patient does not have to stop and buy products on the way home; the patient may not follow through with the purchase.
- Show improvements at subsequent appointments, even if they are modest.
- Use positive reinforcement; threats are not effective.

Conclusion

All patients require the regular use of a toothbrush, either manual or electric, at least once per day. The brushing method should emphasize access to the gingival margins (dento-gingival junction) of all accessible tooth surfaces, referred to as targeted hygiene,and extension as far onto the proximal surfaces as possible. Dental floss should be used in all interdental spaces that are filled with gingiva. Interdental aids such as interproximal brushes, wooden tips, rubber tips, or toothpicks should be used in all areas where the toothbrush and floss techniques cannot adequately remove the plaque biofilm. This includes large embrasure spaces and furcation areas as well as the mesial surface of the maxillary first bicuspid, which presents a concavity on the root surface near the cementoenamel junction. Daily at-home subgingival irrigation is useful for reduction of inflammation and maintenance for patients with residual deep pockets and those who struggle with mechanical interproximal cleaning devices. The effectiveness of irrigation is enhanced by the addition of a chlorhexidine or essential oil rinse as an irrigant. Caries control requires the daily use of a dentifrice with lowconcentration fluoride. Topical oral rinses and gels with higher concentrations of fluoride should be used if the patient demonstrates caries risk, and chlorhexidine rinses should be used in a caries risk management program for patients at high risk for caries. Chemical antimicrobial agents, such as chlorhexidine and essential oils, can be used to disinfect the patient's mouth and control infection. These oral rinses may be continued indefinitely. Staining of teeth and taste alteration are side effects that may limit the use of these products. Reinforcement of daily plaque biofilm control practices and routine visits to the dental office for maintenance care are essential to successful microbial plaque biofilm control and the long-term success of therapy.

Key points

- ADA specifications for acceptable brushes: brushing surface 1–1.25 in. long and 5/16–3/8 in. wide, 2–4 rows of bristles, and 5–12 tufts per row.
- Bristles diameters are 0.2 mm for soft brushes, 0.3 mm for medium brushes and 0.4 mm for hard brushes.
- Sodium hexametaphosphate (HMP) works only on the surface and, hence, is sometimes called a calcium surface-active builder.
- The abrasivity of a dentifrice is measured in terms of Relative Dentin Abrasivity, or RDA. The lower the RDA, the less abrasive the dentifrice.
- As per ISO, a dentifrice should not exceed an RDA of 250.

- Dentinal hypersensitivity is generally treated by chemical desensitization of the tooth nerve endings or by tubule occluding agents or barriers to reduce dentin permeability.
- Oral irrigators create two zones of hydrokinetic activity: the impact zone and the flushing zone. The outcome of hydrokinetic activity is subgingival penetration.
- Irrigation with the soft, site-specific tip is called "subgingival irrigation."
- An ideal chemical plaque control agent should possess the substantivity (ability of agent to bind to tissue surfaces and be released over time); penetrability (ability to penetrate deeply into the biofilm); and selectivity (ability to affect specific bacteria in a mixed population).
- The 0.12% chlorhexidine digluconate preparation has been shown to be equally effective as the higher-concentration product (0.2%) is for reducing plaque and gingivitis.

Suggested Readings

Arabaci T, Cicek Y, Canakci CF: Sonic and ultrasonic scalers in periodontal treatment: a review, *Int J Dent Hygiene* 5:2, 2007.

Axelsson P: *Preventive materials, methods and programs* vol 4, Chicago, 2004, Quintessence Publishing, 155.

Axelsson P: *Preventive materials, methods and programs* vol 4, Chicago, 2004a, Quintessence Publishing, 159.

Axelsson P: *Preventive materials, methods and programs* vol 4, Chicago, 2004b, Quintessence Publishing, 163.

Axelsson P: *Preventive materials, methods and programs* vol 4, Chicago, 2004c, Quintessence Publishing, p. 153.

Canter MT, Stahl SS: Interdental col tissue responses to the use of a water pressure cleansing device, *J Periodontol* 40:292, 1969.

Ciancio SG: The dental water jet: a product ahead of its time, *Compend Contin Educ Dent* 30 (special 1):7, 2009.

Cobb CM, Rodgers RL, Killoy WJ: Ultrastructural examination of human periodontal pockets following the use of an oral irrigation device in vivo, *J Periodontol 59*:155, 1988.

Conforti NJ, Cordero RE, Liebman J, et al: A clinical comparison of the efficacy of a new and a worn manual toothbrush, *J Dent Res* 81, 2002 (special issue): Abstract 2863.

Conforti NJ, Cordero RE, Liebman J, et al: An investigation into the effect of three months' clinical wear on toothbrush efficacy: results from two independent studies, *J Clin Dent* 14 (2):29–33, 2003.

Dils ES: Toothbrushes and toothbrushing methods. In Harris NO, Garcia-Godoy F, Nathe CN, editors: *Primary preventive dentistry*, ed 7, Upper Saddle River, NJ, 2009, Pearson Education, pp 121–140.

Drisko C: Academy report: sonic and ultrasonic scalers in periodontics, *J Periodontol* 71:1792, 2000.

Drisko CL: Periodontal self-care: evidence-based support, *Periodontol 2000* (62):243, 2013.

Drisko C, Henderson R, Yancy J: A review of current toothbrush bristle end-rounding studies, *Compend Contin Educ Dent* 7:694–698, 1995.

Dyer D, Addy M, Newcombe RG: Studies in vitro of abrasion by different manual toothbrush heads and a standard toothpaste, *J Clin Periodontol* 27 (2):99–103, 2000.

Featherstone JD: Prevention and reversal of dental caries: role of low level fluoride, *Community Dent Oral Epidemiol* 27:31, 1999.

Flex JE, Rosen S, App GR: Detection of bacteremia after the use of an oral irrigation device in subjects with periodontitis, *J Periodontol* 42:785, 1971.

Genovesi AM, Lorenzi C, Lyle DM, et al: Periodontal maintenance following scaling and root planing. A randomized single-center study comparing minocycline treatment and daily oral irrigation with water, *Minerva Stomatol* 62:1, 2013.

Gorur A, Lyle DM, Schaudinn C: Biofilm removal with a dental water jet, *Compend Contin Educ Dent* 30 (Special Issue 1):1–6, 2009.

Goyal CR, Lyle DM, Qaqish JG, Schuller R: The addition of a water flosser to power tooth brushing: Effect on bleeding, gingivitis and plaque, *J Clin Dent* 23:57, 2012.

Grover V, Kumar A, Jain A, Chatterjee A, Grover HS, Pandit N, et al.: ISP good clinical practice recommendations for the management of dentin hypersensitivity. *J Indian Soc Periodontol* 26:307–333, 2022.

Harrel SK, Barnes JB, Rivera-Hidalgo F: Reduction of aerosols produced by ultrasonic scalers, *J Periodontol* 67:28, 1996.

Jolkovsky DL, Lyle DM: Safety of a water flosser: a literature review, *Compend Contin Dent Ed* 36:146, 2015.

Khambay BS, Walmsley AD: Acoustic microstreaming: detection and measurement around ultrasonic scalers, *J Periodontol* 70:626, 1999.

Kumar A, Grover V, Satpathy A, Jain A, Grover HS, Khatri M, et al: ISP good clinical practice recommendations for gum care. *J Indian Soc Periodontol* 27:4–30, 2023.

Lindhe J, Nyman S: The effect of plaque control and surgical pocket elimination on the establishment and maintenance of periodontal health: a longitudinal study of periodontal therapy in cases of advanced disease, *J Clin Periodontol* 2:67, 1975.

Lockhart PB, Brennan MT, Sasser HC, et al: Bacteremia associated with tooth brushing and dental extraction, *Circulation* 117:3118, 2008.

Matthews RW: Hot salt water mouth baths, *Br Dent J* 195:3, 2003.

Newman MG, Flemmig TF, Nachnani S, et al: Irrigation with 0.06% chlorhexidine in naturally occurring gingivitis. II. 6 months microbiological observations, *J Periodontol* 61:427, 1990.

Newman MG, Cattabriga M, Etienne D, et al: Effectiveness of adjunctive irrigation in early periodontitis: multi-center evaluation, *J Periodontol* 65:224, 1994.

Obeid PR, D'Hoore W, Bercy P: Comparative clinical responses related to the use of various periodontal instrumentation, *J Clin Periodontol* 31:193, 2004.

Robinson P, Deacon SA, Deery C, et al: Manual versus powered toothbrushing for oral health, *Cochrane Database Syst Rev* (2): CD002281, 2005.

Romans AR, App GR: Bacteremia, a result from oral irrigation in subjects with gingivitis, *J Periodontol* 43:757, 1971.

Rosema NAM, Hennequin Hoenderdos NL, Berchier CE, et al: The effect of different interdental cleaning devices on gingival bleeding, *J Int Acad Periodontol* 13:2–10, 2011.

Sambunjak D, Nickerson JW, Poklepovic T, et al: Flossing for the management of periodontal diseases and dental caries in adults, *Cochrane Database Syst Rev* (12): CD008829, 2011.

Sanders PC, Linden GJ, Newman HN: The effects of a simplified mechanical oral hygiene regimen plus supragingival irrigation with chlorhexidine or metronidazole on subgingival plaque, *J Clin Periodontol* 13:237, 1986.

Segrave K: *America brushes up: the use and marketing of toothpaste and toothbrushes in the twentieth century*, Jefferson, North Carolina, 2010, McFarland & Company, Inc.

Warren PR, Jacobs D, Low MA, et al: A clinical investigation into the effect of toothbrush wear on efficacy, *J Clin Dent* 13:119–124, 2002.

Wilson TG Jr, Glover ME, Schoen J, et al: Compliance with maintenance therapy in a private dental practice, *J Periodontol* 55:468, 1984.

Wilson W, Taubert KA, Gewitz M, et al: Prevention of infective endocarditis: guidelines from the American Heart Association: a guideline from the American Heart Association Rheumatic Fever, Endocarditis, and Kawasaki Disease Committee, Council on Cardiovascular Disease in the Young, and the Council on Clinical Cardiology, Council on Cardiovascular Surgery and Anesthesia, and the Quality of Care and Outcomes Research Interdisciplinary Working Group, *Circulation* 116:1736, 2007.

Zimmer S, Öztürk M, Barthel CR, et al: Cleaning efficacy and soft tissue trauma after use of manual toothbrushes with different bristle stiffness, *J Periodontol* 82 (2):267–271, 2011.

References

References and MCQs with answers for the chapter are available on www.medenact.com.

CHAPTER 35

Periodontal Instruments and Instrumentation

AM Pattison | GL Pattison | PR Klokkevold | HH Takei | FA Carranza | A Jain

CHAPTER OUTLINE

Periodontal instruments are designed for specific purposes such as removing calculus, planing root surfaces, curetting the gingiva, and removing diseased tissue. On first investigation, the variety of instruments available for similar purposes appears confusing. With experience, however, clinicians select a relatively small set that fulfills all requirements.

Classification of Periodontal Instruments

Periodontal instruments are classified according to the purposes they serve, as follows:

1. *Periodontal probes* are used to locate, measure, and mark pockets, as well as determine their course on individual tooth surfaces.
2. *Explorers* are used to locate calculus deposits and caries.
3. *Scaling, root-planing, and curettage instruments* are used for removal of biofilm and calcified deposits from the crown and root of a tooth, removal of altered cementum from the subgingival root surface, and debridement of the soft tissue lining the pocket. Scaling and curettage instruments are classified as follows:
   - *Sickle scalers* are heavy instruments used to remove supragingival calculus.
   - *Curettes* are fine instruments used for subgingival scaling, root planing, and removal of the soft tissue lining the pocket.
   - *Hoe, chisel, and file scalers* are used to remove tenacious subgingival calculus and altered cementum. Their use is limited compared to that of curettes.
   - *Implant instruments* are plastic or titanium scalers and curettes designed for use on implants and implant restorations.
   - *Ultrasonic and sonic instruments* are used for scaling and cleansing tooth surfaces and curetting the soft tissue wall of the periodontal pocket.
4. *Periodontal endoscopes* are used to visualize deeply into subgingival pockets and furcations, allowing the detection of deposits.
5. *Cleansing and polishing instruments*, such as rubber cups, brushes, and dental tape, are used to clean and polish tooth surfaces. Also available are air-powder abrasive systems for tooth, root, and implant polishing.

The wearing and cutting qualities of some types of steel used in periodontal instruments have been tested, but specifications vary among manufacturers. Stainless steel is used most often in instrument manufacture. High-carbon-content steel instruments are also available and are considered by some clinicians to be superior.

Each group of instruments has characteristic features; individual therapists often develop variations with which they operate most effectively. Small instruments are recommended to fit into periodontal pockets without injuring the soft tissues.

The parts of each instrument are referred to as the working end, shank, and handle (Fig. 35.1).

Periodontal Probes

Periodontal probes are used to measure the depth of pockets and to determine their configuration. The typical probe is a tapered, rodlike instrument calibrated in millimeters, with a blunt, rounded tip (Fig. 35.2). There are several other designs with various millimeter calibrations (Fig. 35.3). The World Health Organization probe (WHO) probe has millimeter markings and a small, round ball at the tip (Fig. 35.3E). Ideally, these probes are thin, and the shank is angled to allow easy insertion into the pocket. Furcation areas can best be evaluated with the curved, blunt Naber's probe (Fig. 35.4).

When measuring a pocket, the probe is inserted with a firm, gentle pressure to the bottom of the pocket. The shank should be aligned with the long axis of the tooth surface to be probed. Several measurements are made to determine the level of attachment along the surface of the tooth.

Explorers

Explorers are used to locate subgingival deposits and carious areas and to check the smoothness of the root surfaces after root planing. Explorers are designed with different shapes and angles, with various uses (Fig. 35.5), as well as limitations (Fig. 35.6). The periodontal probe can also be useful in the detection of subgingival deposits (Fig. 35.6D).

Scaling and Curettage Instruments

Scaling and curettage instruments are illustrated in Fig. 35.7.

Sickle Scalers

Sickle scalers have a flat surface and two cutting edges that converge in a sharply pointed tip. The shape of the instrument makes the tip strong so that it will not break off during use (Fig. 35.8). The

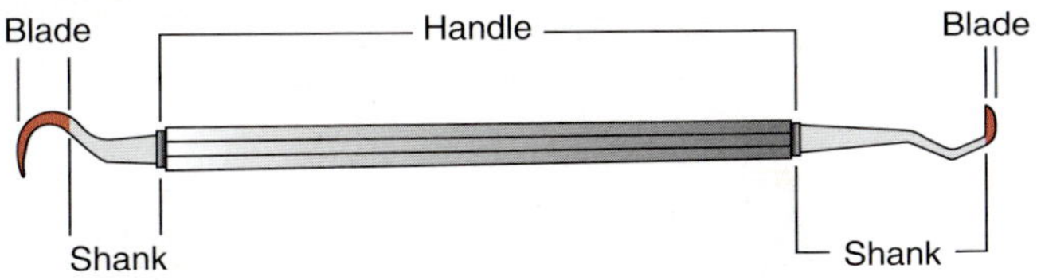

Fig. 35.1 Parts of a typical periodontal instrument.

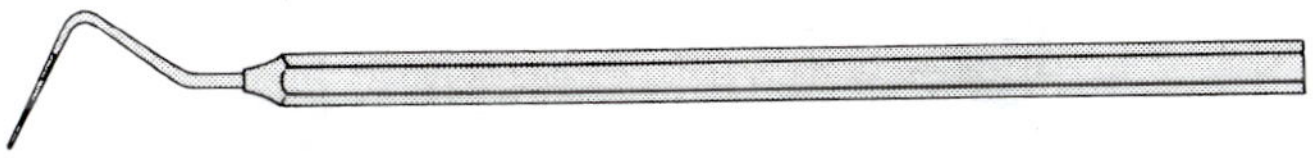

Fig. 35.2 Periodontal probe is composed of the handle, shank, and calibrated working end.

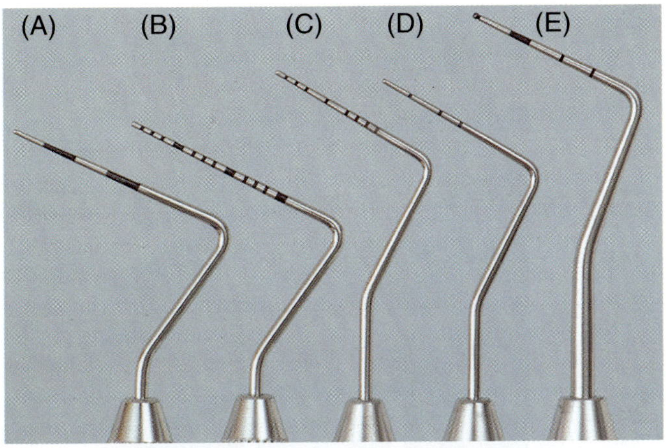

Fig. 35.3 Types of periodontal probes. A, Marquis color-coded probe. Calibrations are in 3-mm sections. B, University of North Carolina-15 probe, a 15-mm long probe with millimeter markings at each millimeter and color coding at the 5, 10, and 15 mm. C, University of Michigan "O" probe, with Williams markings (at 1, 2, 3, 5, 7, 8, 9, and 10 mm). D, Michigan "O" probe with markings at 3, 6, and 8 mm. E, WHO probe, which has a 0.5-mm ball at the tip and millimeter markings at 3.5, 8.5, and 11.5 mm and color coding from 3.5 to 5.5 mm.

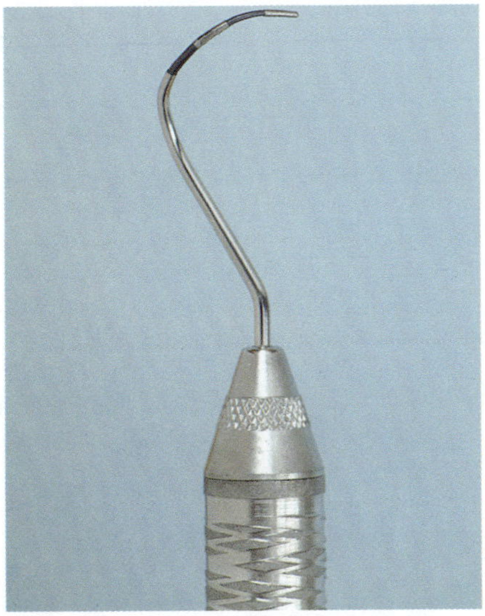

Fig. 35.4 Curved #2 Naber's probe for detection of furcation areas, with color-coded markings at 3, 6, 9, and 12 mm.

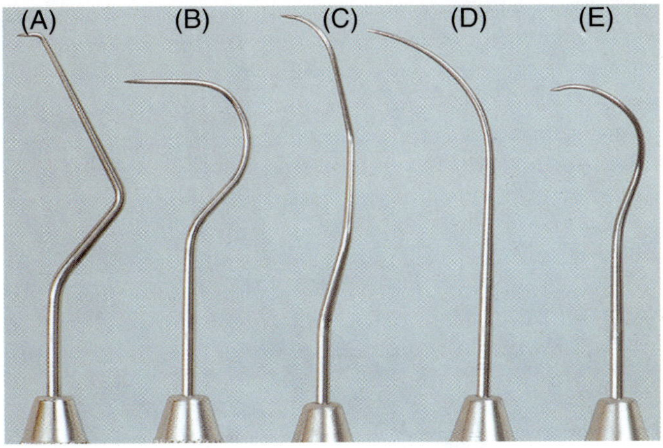

Fig. 35.5 Five typical explorers. A, #17; B, #23; C, EXD 11-12; D, #3; E, #3CH Pigtail.

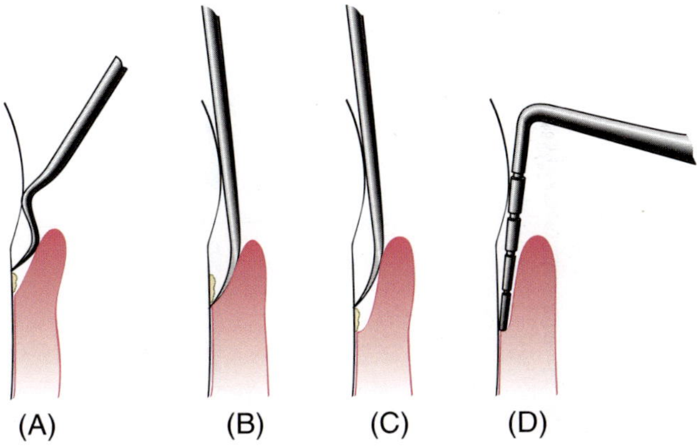

Fig. 35.6 Insertion of two types of explorers and a periodontal probe in a pocket for calculus detection. A, The limitations of the pigtail explorer in a deep pocket. B, Insertion of the #3 explorer. C, Limitations of the #3 explorer. D, Insertion of the periodontal probe.

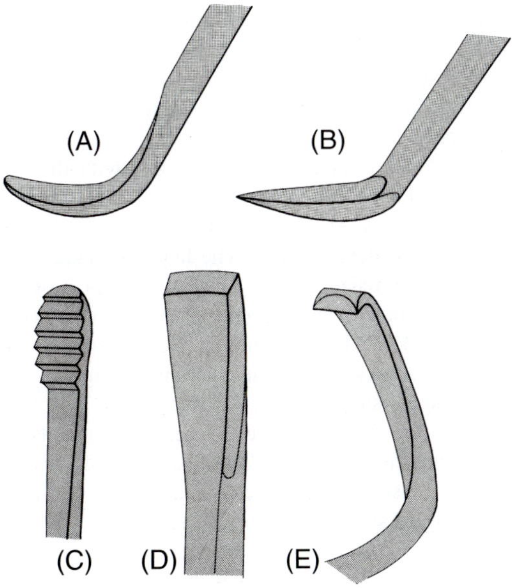

Fig. 35.7 The five basic scaling instruments. A, Curette; B, sickle; C, file; D, chisel; E, hoe.

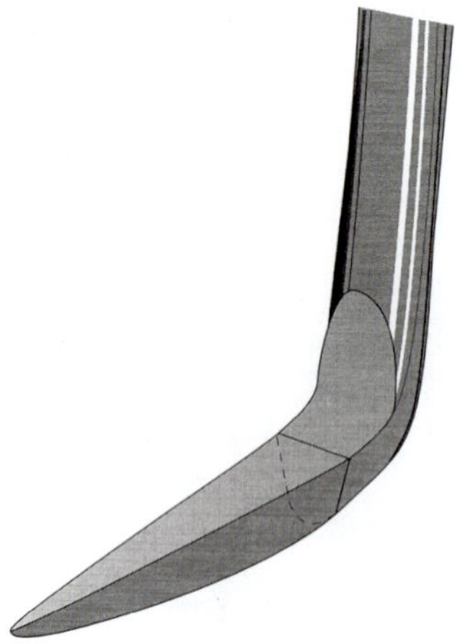

Fig. 35.8 Basic characteristics of a sickle scaler: triangular shape, double-cutting edge, and pointed tip.

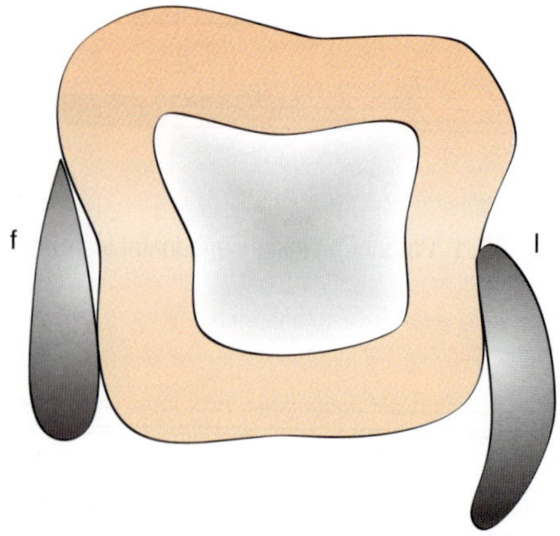

Fig. 35.10 Subgingival adaptation around the root is better with the curette than with the sickle; *f*, facial; *l*, lingual.

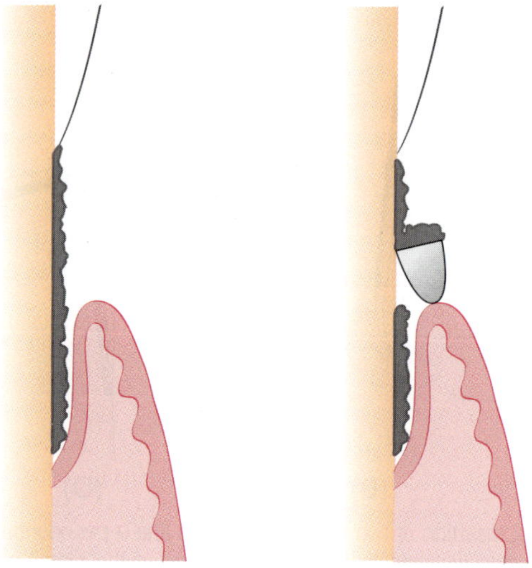

Fig. 35.9 Use of a sickle scaler for removal of supragingival calculus.

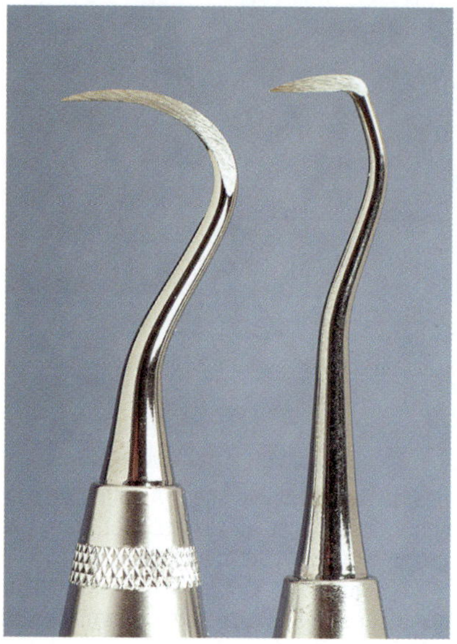

Fig. 35.11 Both ends of a U15/30 scaler.

sickle scaler is used primarily to remove supragingival calculus (Fig. 35.9). Due to the design of this instrument, it is difficult to insert a large sickle blade under the gingiva without damaging the surrounding gingival tissues (Fig. 35.10). Small, curved sickle scaler blades such as the 204SD can be inserted under the ledges of calculus several millimeters below the gingiva. Sickle scalers are used with a pull stroke.

It is important to note that sickle scalers with the same basic design can be obtained with different blade sizes and shank types to adapt to specific uses. The U15/30 (Fig. 35.11), Ball, and Indiana University sickle scalers are large. The Jaquette sickle scalers #1, 2, and 3 have medium-size blades. The curved 204 posterior sickle scalers are available with large, medium, or small blades (Fig. 35.12). The Montana Jack sickle scaler and the Nevi 2, Nevi 3, and Nevi 4 curved posterior sickle scalers are all thin enough to be inserted several millimeters subgingivally for removal of light to moderate ledges of calculus. The selection of these instruments should be based on the area to be scaled. Sickle scalers with straight shanks are designed for use on anterior teeth and premolars. Sickle scalers with contra-angled shanks adapt to posterior teeth.

Curettes

The curette is the instrument of choice for removing deep subgingival calculus, root planing altered cementum, and removing the soft

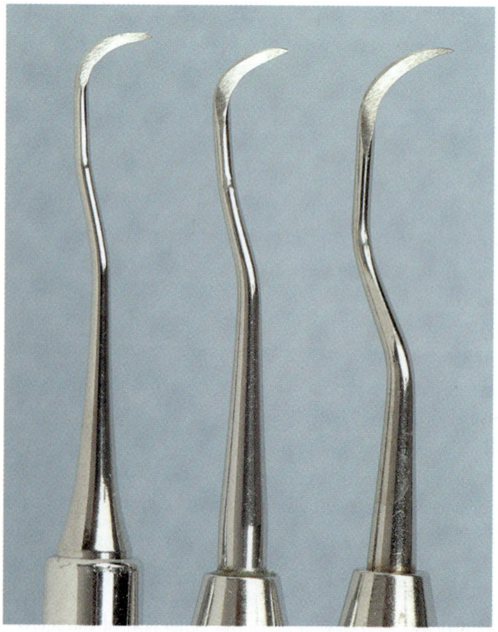

Fig. 35.12 Three different sizes of 204 sickle scalers.

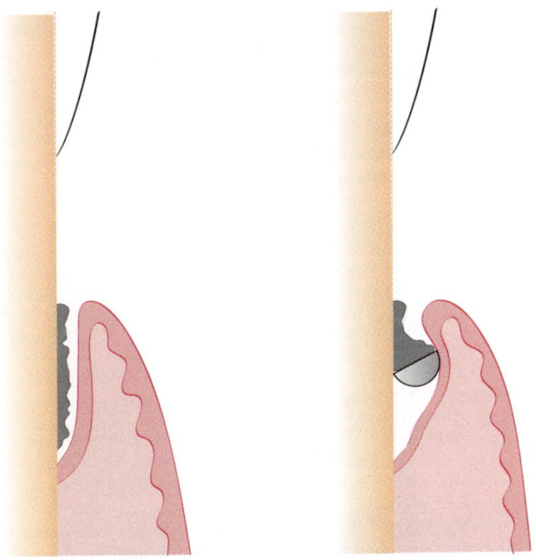

Fig. 35.13 The curette is the instrument of choice for subgingival scaling and root planing.

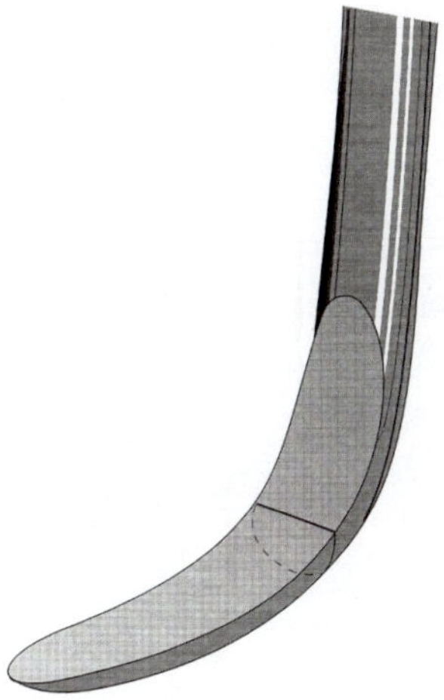

Fig. 35.14 Basic characteristics of a curette: spoon-shaped blade and rounded tip.

tissue lining the periodontal pocket (Fig. 35.13). Each working end has a cutting edge on both sides of the blade and a rounded toe. The curette is finer than the sickle scalers and does not have any sharp points or corners other than the cutting edges of the blade (Fig. 35.14). Therefore, curettes can be adapted and provide good access to deep pockets, with minimal soft tissue trauma (Fig. 35.10). In cross-section, the blade appears semicircular with a convex base. The lateral border of the convex base forms a cutting edge with the face of the semicircular blade. There are cutting edges on both sides of the blade. Both single- and double-end curettes may be obtained, depending on the preference of the operator.

As shown in Fig. 35.10, the curved blade and rounded toe of the curette allow the blade to adapt better to the root surface, unlike the straight design and pointed end of a sickle scaler, which can cause tissue laceration and trauma. There are two basic types of curettes: universal and area specific.

Universal Curettes

Universal curettes have cutting edges that may be inserted in most areas of the dentition by altering and adapting the finger rest, fulcrum, and hand position of the operator. The blade size and the angle and length of the shank may vary, but the face of the blade of every universal curette is at a 90-degree angle (perpendicular) to the lower shank when seen in cross-section from the tip (Fig. 35.15A). The blade of the universal curette is curved in one direction from the head of the blade to the toe. The Barnhart curettes #1–2 and 5–6 and the Columbia curettes #13–14, 2R–2L, and 4R–4L (Figs. 35.16 and 35.17A) are examples of universal curettes. Other popular universal curettes are the Younger-Good #7–8, McCall's #17–18, and the Indiana University #17–18 (Fig. 35.17B).

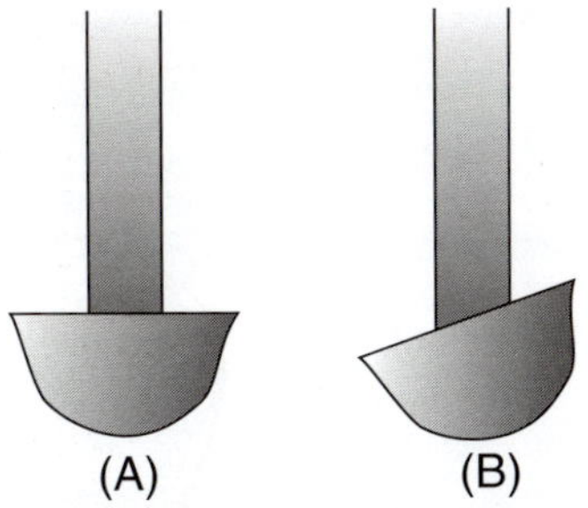

Fig. 35.15 Principal types of curettes as seen from the toe of the instrument. A, Universal curette. B, Gracey curette. Note the offset blade angulation of the Gracey curette.

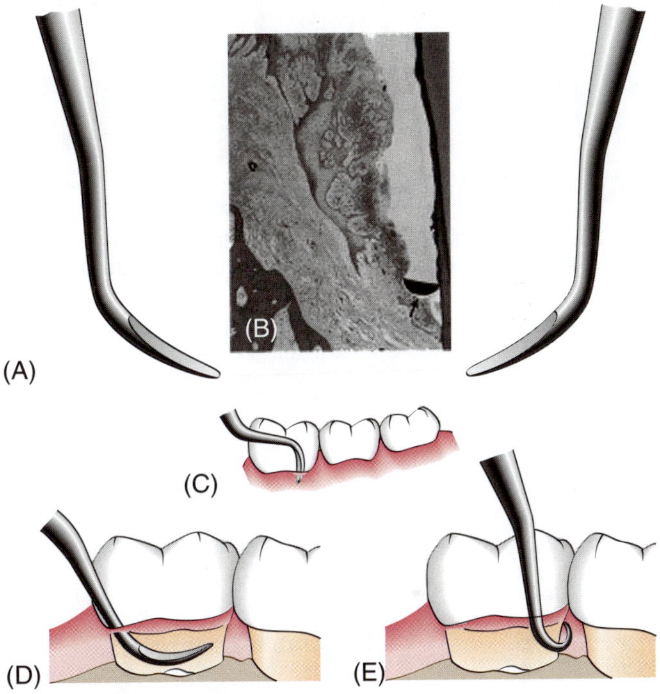

Fig. 35.16 A, Double-ended curette for the removal of subgingival calculus. B, Cross-section of the curette blade *(arrow)* against the cemental wall of a deep periodontal pocket. C, Curette in position at the base of a periodontal pocket on the facial surface of a mandibular molar. D, Curette inserted in a pocket with the tip directed apically. E, Curette in position at the base of a pocket on the distal surface of the mandibular molar.

Area-Specific Curettes

Gracey Curettes. Gracey curettes are representative of the area-specific curettes, a set of several instruments designed and angled to adapt to specific anatomic areas of the dentition (Fig. 35.18). These curettes and their modifications are probably the best instruments

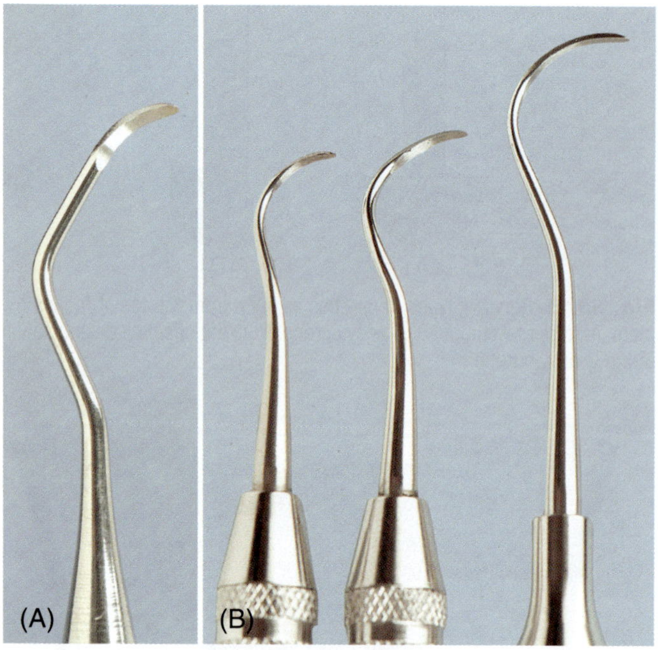

Fig. 35.17 A, Columbia #4R-4L universal curette. B, Younger-Good #7–8, McCall's #17–18, and Indiana University #17–18 universal curettes.

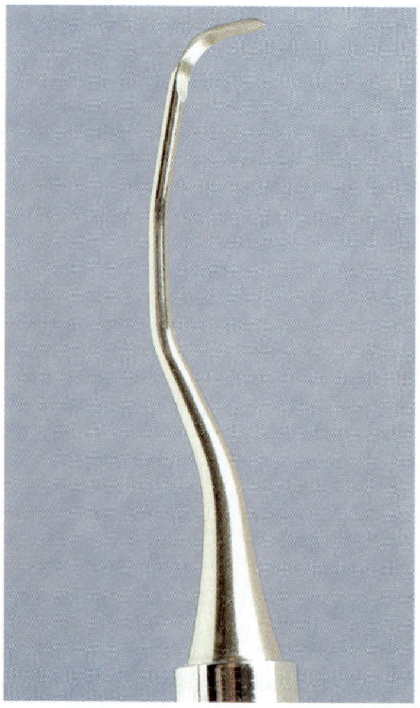

Fig. 35.19 Gracey #11–12 curette. For mesial surfaces.

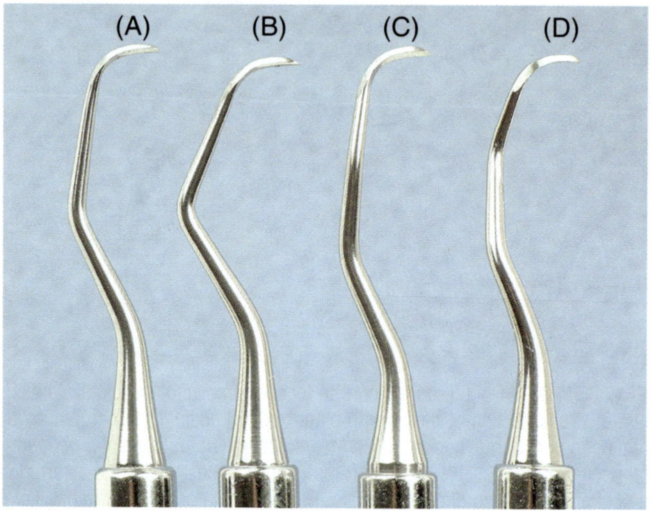

Fig. 35.18 Reduced set of Gracey curettes. A, #5–6; B, #7–8; C, #11–12; and D, #13–14.

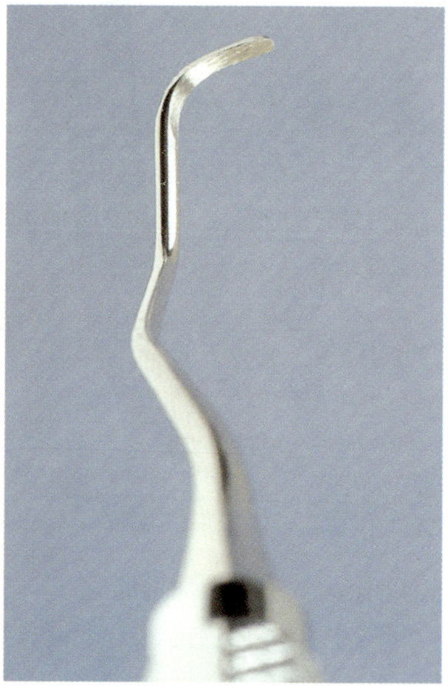

Fig. 35.20 Gracey #13–14 curette. For distal surfaces.

for subgingival scaling and root planing because they provide the best adaptation to complex root anatomy.

Double-ended Gracey curettes are paired in the following manner:
Gracey #1–2 and #3–4: Anterior teeth
Gracey #5–6: Anterior teeth and premolars
Gracey #7–8 and #9–10: Posterior teeth: facial and lingual
Gracey #11–12: Posterior teeth: mesial (Fig. 35.19)
Gracey #13–14: Posterior teeth: distal (Fig. 35.20)

Single-ended Gracey curettes can also be obtained; a set of these curettes comprises 14 instruments. Although these curettes are designed to be used in specific areas, an experienced operator can adapt each instrument for use in several different areas by altering the position of his or her hand and the position of the patient.

The Gracey curettes also differ from the universal curettes in that the blade is not at a 90-degree angle to the lower shank. The term *offset blade* is used to describe Gracey curettes because they are angled approximately 60–70 degrees from the lower shank (Fig. 35.15B). This unique angulation allows the blade to be inserted in the precise position necessary for subgingival scaling and root planing, provided that the lower shank is parallel with the long axis of the tooth surface being scaled.

Area-specific curettes also have a curved blade. Whereas the blade of the universal curette is curved in one direction (Fig. 35.21A), the Gracey blade is curved from head to toe and also along the side of the cutting edge (Fig. 35.21B). Thus, only a pull stroke can be used. Table 35.1 lists some of the major differences between Gracey (area-specific) curettes and universal curettes.

Gracey curettes are available with either a "rigid" or a "finishing" type of shank. The rigid Gracey has a larger, stronger, and less flexible shank and blade than the standard finishing Gracey. The rigid shank allows the removal of moderate to heavy calculus without using a separate set of heavy scalers, such as sickles and hoes.

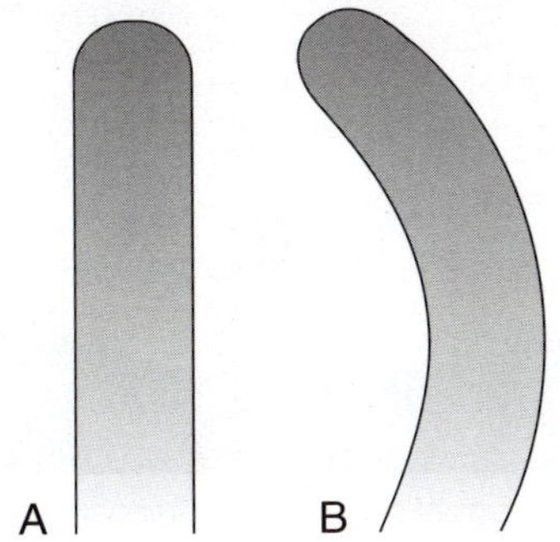

Fig. 35.21 A, Universal curette as seen with the face of the blade parallel to the floor. Note that the blade is straight. B, Gracey curette as seen with the face of the blade parallel to the floor. Only the outer convex cutting edge is used.

TABLE 35.1 Comparison of Area-Specific (Gracey) and Universal Curettes

	Gracey Curette	Universal Curette
Area of use	Set of many curettes designed for specific areas and surfaces.	One curette designed for all areas and surfaces.
Cutting Edge		
Use	One cutting edge used; work with outer edge only.	Both cutting edges used; work with either outer or inner edge.
Curvature	Curved in two planes; blade curves up and to the side.	Curved in one plane; blade curves up, not to the side.
Blade angle	Offset blade; face of blade beveled at 60 degrees to shank.	Blade not offset; face of blade beveled at 90 degrees to shank.

(Modified from Pattison G, Pattison A: *Periodontal instrumentation*, ed 2, Norwalk, CT, 1992, Appleton & Lange.)

Although some clinicians prefer the enhanced tactile sensitivity that the flexible shank of the finishing Gracey provides, both types of Gracey curettes are suitable for root planing.

Recent additions to the Gracey curette set have been the Gracey #15–16 and #17–18. The Gracey #15–16 is a modification of the standard #11–12 and is designed for the mesial surfaces of posterior teeth (Fig. 35.22). It consists of a Gracey #11–12 blade combined with the more acutely angled #13–14 shank. When the clinician is using an intraoral finger rest, it is often difficult to position the lower shank of the Gracey #11–12 so that it is parallel with the mesial surfaces of the posterior teeth, especially on the mandibular molars. The new shank angulation of the Gracey #15–16 allows better adaptation to posterior mesial surfaces from a front position with intraoral rests. If alternative fulcrums, such as extraoral or opposite-arch rests, are used, the Gracey #11–12 works well and the new #15–16 is not essential. The Gracey #17–18 is a modification of the #13–14. It has a terminal shank elongated by 3 mm and a more accentuated angulation of the shank to provide complete occlusal clearance and better access to all posterior distal surfaces. The horizontal handle position minimizes interference from opposing arches and allows a more relaxed hand position when scaling distal surfaces. In addition, the blade is 1-mm shorter to allow better adaptation of the blade to distal tooth surfaces.

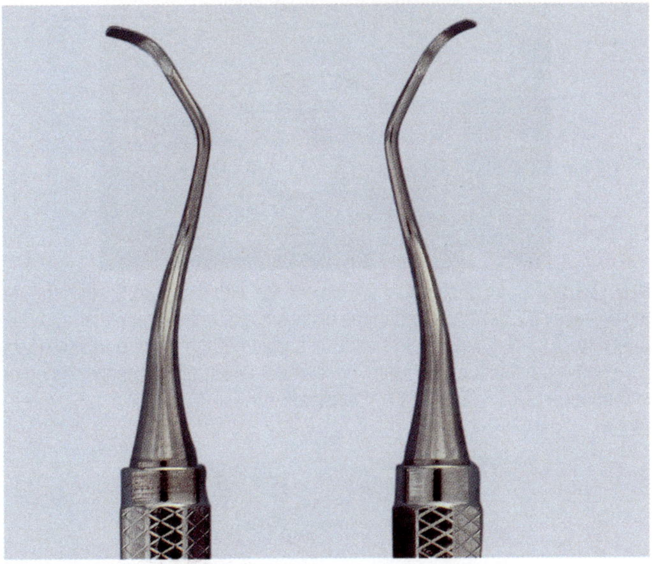

Fig. 35.22 Gracey #15–16. New Gracey curette, designed for mesioposterior surfaces, combines a Gracey #11–12 blade with a Gracey #13–14 shank. *(Copyright A. Pattison.)*

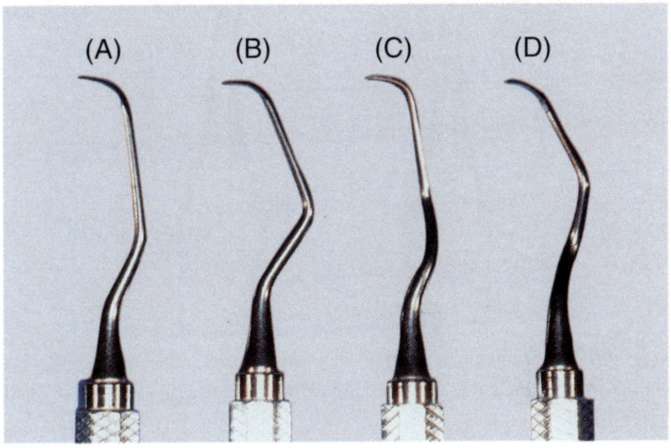

Fig. 35.23 After Five curette. Note the extra 3 mm in the terminal shank of the After Five curette compared to the standard Gracey curette. A, #5–6; B, #7–8; C, #11–12; D, #13–14. *(Copyright A. Pattison.)*

Extended-Shank Curettes. Extended-shank curettes, such as the *After Five* curettes (Hu-Friedy, Chicago), are modifications of the standard Gracey curette design. The terminal shank is 3-mm longer, allowing extension into deeper periodontal pockets of 5 mm or more (Figs. 35.23 and 35.24). Other features of the After Five curette include a thinned blade for smoother subgingival insertion and reduced tissue distention and a large-diameter, tapered shank. All standard Gracey numbers except for the #9–10 (i.e., #1–2, #3–4, #5–6, #7–8, #11–12, or #13–14) are available in the After Five series. The After Five curettes are available in finishing or rigid designs. For heavy or tenacious calculus removal, rigid After Five curettes should be used. For light scaling or deplaquing in a periodontal maintenance patient, the thinner, finishing After Five curettes will insert subgingivally more easily.

Mini-Bladed Curettes. Mini-bladed curettes, such as the Hu-Friedy *Mini Five* curettes, are modifications of the After Five curettes. The Mini Five curettes feature blades that are half the length of the After Five or standard Gracey curettes (Fig. 35.25).

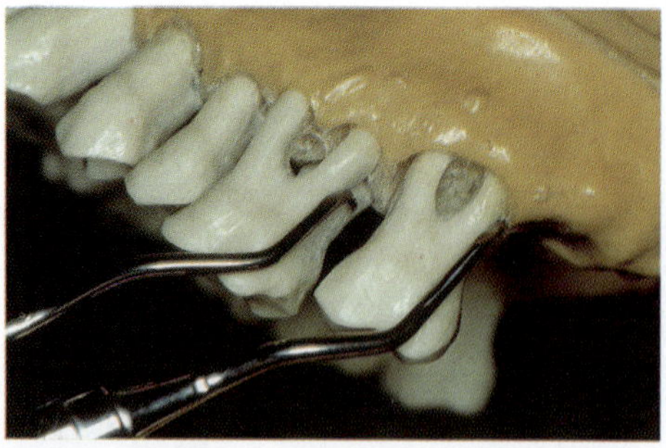

Fig. 35.24 Comparison of After Five curette with standard Gracey curette. Rigid Gracey #13–14 adapted to the distal surface of the first molar and rigid After Five #13–14 adapted to the distal surface of the second molar. Notice the extra-long shank of the After Five curette, which allows deeper insertion and better access. *(Copyright A. Pattison.)*

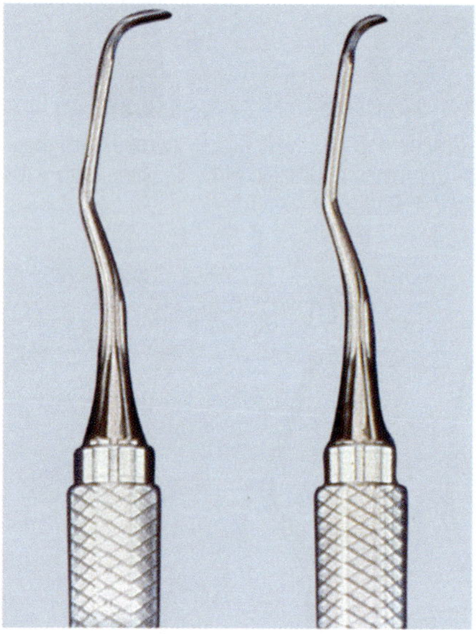

Fig. 35.25 Comparison of After Five curette and Mini Five curette. The shorter Mini Five blade (half the length) allows increased access and reduced tissue trauma.

The shorter blade allows easier insertion and adaptation in deep, narrow pockets; furcations; developmental grooves; line angles; and deep, tight, facial, lingual, or palatal pockets. In any area in which root morphology or tight tissue prevents full insertion of the standard Gracey or After Five blade, the Mini Five curettes can be used with vertical strokes, with reduced tissue distention, and without tissue trauma (Fig. 35.26).

In the past, the only solution in most of these areas of difficult access was to use the Gracey curettes with a toe-down horizontal stroke. Mini Five curettes, along with other short-bladed instruments relatively recently introduced, opened a new chapter in the history of root instrumentation by allowing access to areas that previously were extremely difficult or impossible to reach with standard instruments. Mini Five curettes are available in both finishing and rigid designs. Rigid Mini Five curettes are recommended for calculus removal. The more flexible shanked, finishing Mini Five curettes are appropriate for light scaling and deplaquing in periodontal maintenance patients with tight pockets. As with the After Five series, the Mini Five curettes are available in all standard Gracey numbers, except the #9–10.

The recently introduced *Micro Mini Five* Gracey curettes (Hu-Friedy, Chicago) have blades that are 20% thinner and smaller

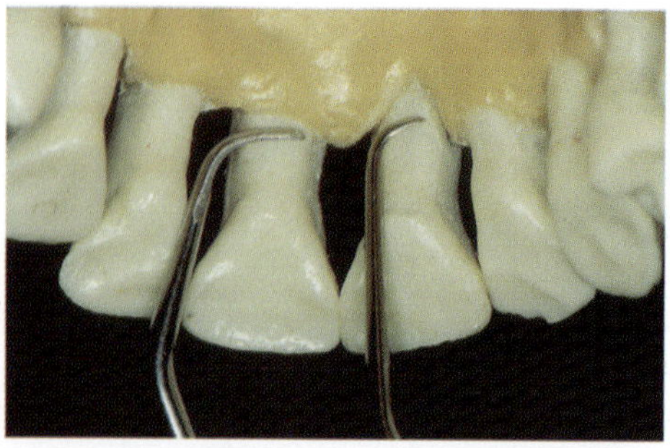

Fig. 35.26 Comparison of standard rigid Gracey #5–6 with rigid Mini Five #5–6 on the palatal surfaces of the maxillary central incisors. Mini Five curette can be inserted to the base of these tight anterior pockets and used with a straight vertical stroke. Standard Gracey or After Five curette usually cannot be inserted vertically in this area because the blade is too long. *(Copyright A. Pattison.)*

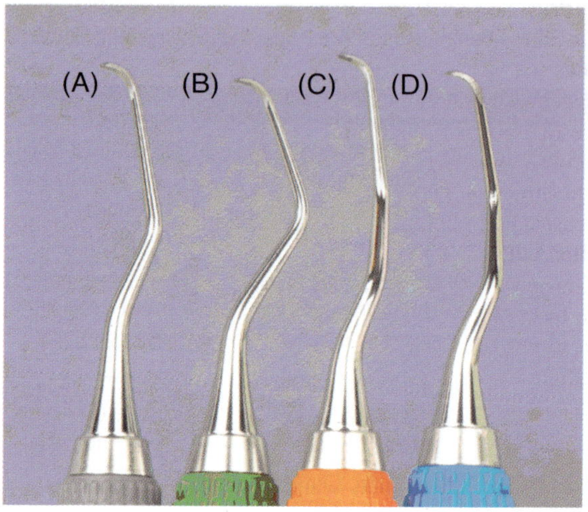

Fig. 35.27 Micro Mini Five Gracey curettes. A, #1–2; B, #7–8; C, #11–12; D, #13–14. *(Copyright A. Pattison.)*

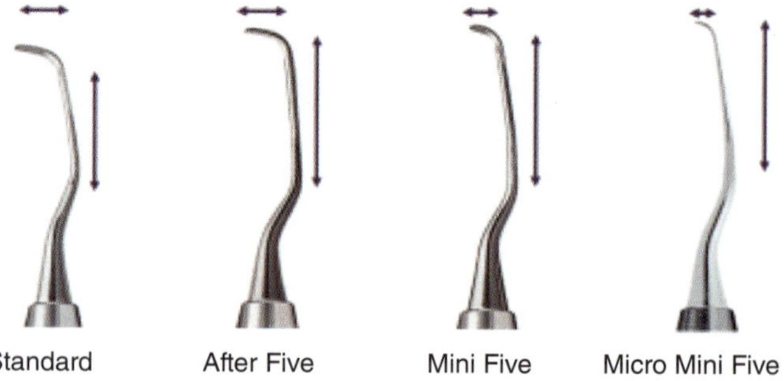

Fig. 35.28 Comparison of Gracey curette designs. *Left to right,* Standard #1–2, After Five #1–2, Mini Five #1–2, Micro Mini Five #1–2. *(Courtesy: Hu-Friedy, Chicago, IL.)*

than the Mini Five curettes (Figs. 35.27 and 35.28). These are the smallest of all curettes, and they provide exceptional access and adaptation to tight, deep, or narrow pockets; narrow furcations; developmental depressions; line angles; and deep pockets on facial, lingual, or palatal surfaces. In areas in which root morphology or tight, thin tissue prevents easy insertion of other mini-bladed curettes, the Micro Mini Five curettes can be used with vertical strokes without causing tissue distension or tissue trauma.

The *Gracey Curvettes* are another set of four mini-bladed curettes; the Sub-0 and the #1–2 are used for anterior teeth and premolars, the

#11–12 is used for posterior mesial surfaces, and the #13–14 for posterior distal surfaces. The blade length of these instruments is 50% shorter than that of the conventional Gracey curette and the blade has been curved slightly upward (Fig. 35.29). This curvature allows the Gracey curettes to adapt more closely to the tooth surface than any other curettes, especially on the anterior teeth and on line angles (Fig. 35.30). However, this curvature also carries the risk of gouging or "grooving" into the root surfaces on the proximal surfaces of the posterior teeth when the Gracey Curvette #11–12 or 13–14 is used. Additional features that represent improvements on the standard Gracey curettes are a precision-balanced blade tip in direct alignment with the handle, a blade tip perpendicular to the handle, and a shank closer to parallel with the handle.

For many years, the *Morse scaler*, a miniature sickle, was the only mini-bladed instrument available. However, the mini-bladed curettes have largely replaced this instrument (Fig. 35.31).

Periodontal Maintenance Curettes. The most recent Gracey curette innovation is a category called periodontal maintenance Gracey curettes, introduced in November 2015. These instruments are specifically designed for patients with tight tissue, recession, and residual pocket depth following initial periodontal therapy or periodontal surgery. They can also be used on maintenance patients with healthier tight tissue without attachment loss or recession. In both cases, patients require a small, thin blade to allow subgingival insertion with ease (Fig. 35.32).

This newer blade is 1 mm shorter and 20% thinner, and the face of the blade is offset from the terminal shank at 60 degrees as opposed to all other Gracey designs, which are offset at 70 degrees. This slight modification to the blade-to-shank angle and the thinner, narrow blade allow easier insertion and better access to root surfaces with tight tissue and loss of attachment. Working angulation can be achieved without as much tissue distention, thus increasing patient comfort. The three-quarter blade length of this new type of Gracey curette is between the blade lengths of the standard and mini-bladed Gracey curettes. The shorter blade adapts more easily to root anatomy and furcation areas and helps to prevent spanning across root depressions.

The shank length is 2 mm longer than that of the standard Gracey curette, but 1 mm shorter than that of the extended shank Gracey curette. This length enables better access to molar areas with attachment loss but still allows ease of use in the anterior areas where a very long shank is not necessary. The shank angle of the new Gracey #11–12 is between the regular Gracey #11–12 and the Gracey #15–16, and the shank angle of the new Gracey #13–14 is between the regular Gracey #13–14 and the Gracey #17–18. These shank angle modifications were developed to enhance access to the mesial and distal surfaces of the posterior teeth.

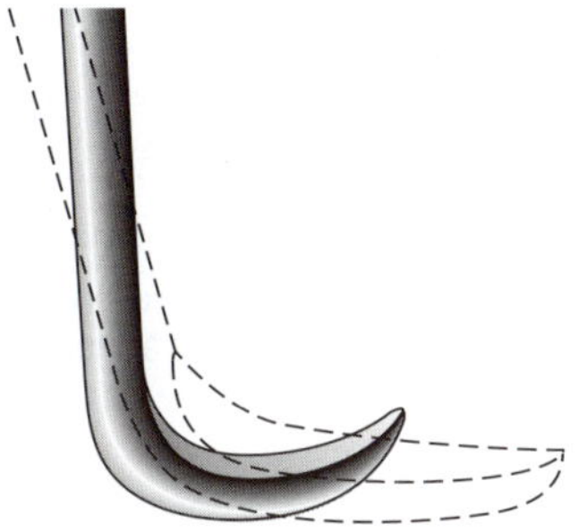

Fig. 35.29 Gracey Curvette blade. This diagram shows the 50% shorter blade of the Gracey Curvette superimposed on the standard Gracey curette blade *(dotted lines)*. Notice the upward curvature of the Curvette blade and blade tip. *(Redrawn from Pattison G, Pattison A: Periodontal instrumentation, ed 2, Norwalk, Conn, 1992, Appleton & Lange.)*

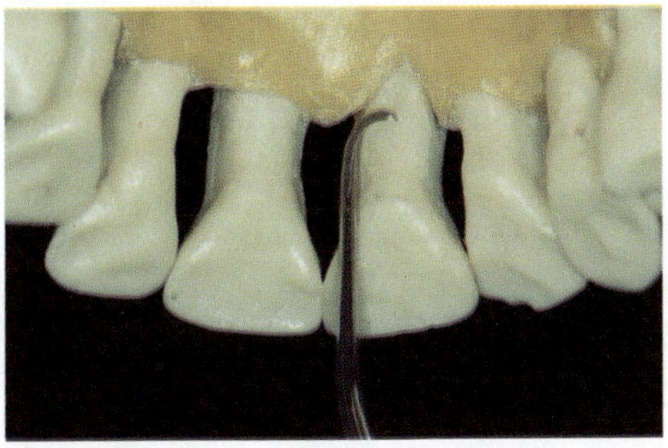

Fig. 35.30 Gracey Curvette Sub-0 on the palatal surface of a maxillary central incisor. The long shank and short, curved, and blunted tip make this a superior instrument for deep anterior pockets. This curette provides excellent blade adaptation to the narrow root curvatures of the maxillary and mandibular anterior teeth. *(Copyright A. Pattison.)*

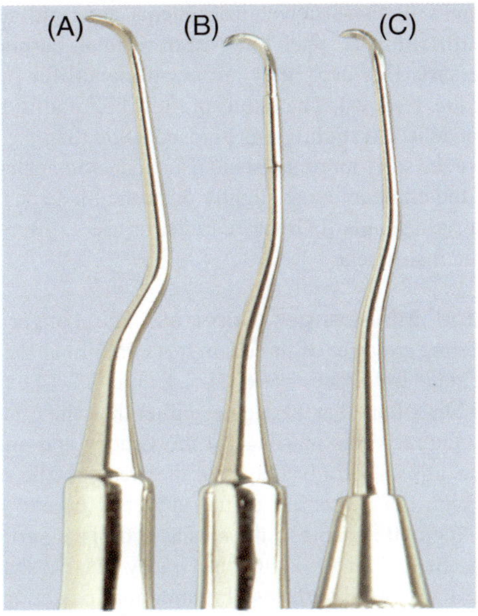

Fig. 35.31 Comparison of three different mini-bladed instruments designed for use on the maxillary and mandibular anterior teeth. A, Hu-Friedy Mini Five #5–6; B, Hu-Friedy Curvette Sub-0; C, Hartzell Sub-0. *(Copyright A. Pattison.)*

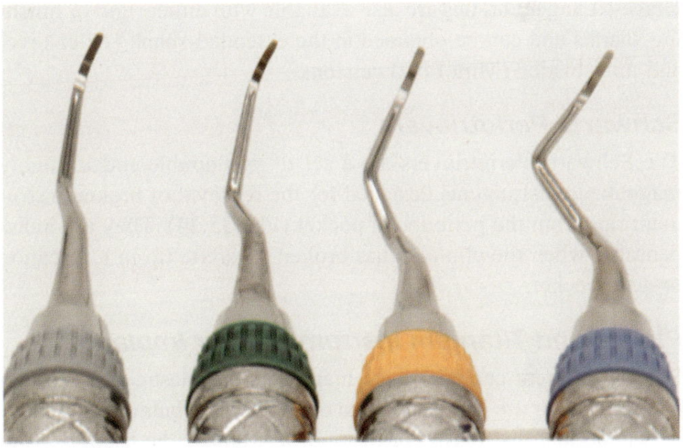

Fig. 35.32 Periodontal maintenance Gracey curettes (Hu-Friedy). Shorter, thinner three-quarter–sized Gracey curettes with modified rigid shanks. *Left to right,* Pattison Gracey Lite #1–2, Pattison Gracey Lite #7–8, Pattison Gracey Lite #11–12, Pattison Gracey Lite #13–14. *(Copyright A. Pattison.)*

The shanks of these newer instruments are rigid so they can withstand firm pressure when removal of residual burnished calculus is necessary. However, they are not designed for moderate or heavy calculus removal. The clinician must be mindful that the instrument blade is at a slightly more closed angle than the traditional Gracey curette, so if more substantial or tenacious calculus is encountered, the clinician must slightly open the blade angulation, or switch to a rigid standard Gracey curette, or use a different manual or ultrasonic instrument.

Langer and Mini-Langer Curettes. The Langer and Mini Langer curettes are a set of three curettes combining the shank design of the standard Gracey #5–6, 11–12, and #13–14 curettes with a universal blade honed at 90 degrees rather than the offset blade of the Gracey curette. This marriage of the Gracey and universal curette designs allows the advantages of the area-specific shank to be combined with the versatility of the universal curette blade. The Langer #5–6 curette adapts to the mesial and distal surfaces of anterior teeth; the Langer #1–2 curette (Gracey #11–12 shank) adapts to the mesial and distal surfaces of mandibular posterior teeth; and the Langer #3–4 curette (Gracey #13–14 shank) adapts to the mesial and distal surfaces of maxillary posterior teeth (Fig. 35.33). These instruments can be adapted to both mesial and distal tooth surfaces without changing instruments. The standard Langer curette shanks are heavier than a finishing Gracey but less rigid than the rigid Gracey. Langer curettes are also available with either rigid or finishing shanks and can be obtained in the extended-shank (After Five) and mini-bladed (Mini Five) versions.

Schwartz Periotrievers

The Schwartz Periotrievers are a set of two double-ended, highly magnetized instruments designed for the retrieval of broken instrument tips from the periodontal pocket (Fig. 35.34). They are indispensable when the clinician has broken a curette tip in a furcation or deep pocket.

Plastic and Titanium Instruments for Implants

Several different companies are manufacturing plastic and titanium instruments for use on titanium and other implant abutment materials. It is important that plastic or titanium instruments be used to avoid scarring and permanent damage to the implants (Figs. 35.35–35.37).

Mini-bladed titanium implant instruments are now available in both universal and Gracey curette designs (Fig. 35.37B). Although most standard titanium implant instrument blades are large, the newer mini-bladed titanium curettes insert more easily under tight tissue and

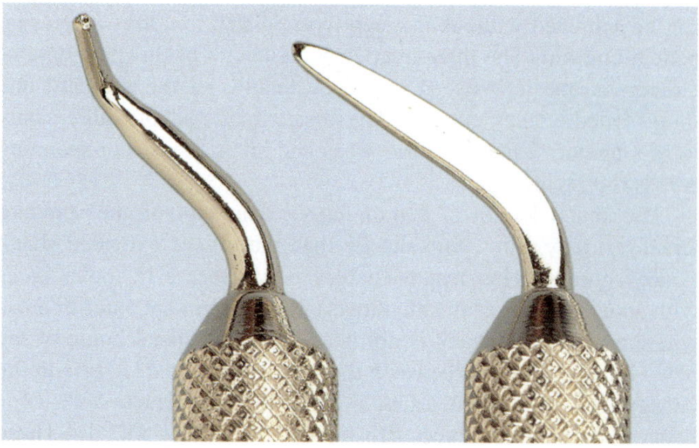

Fig. 35.33 Langer curettes combine Gracey-type shanks with universal curette blades. A, #5–6; B, #1–2; and C, #3–4. (*Copyright A. Pattison.*)

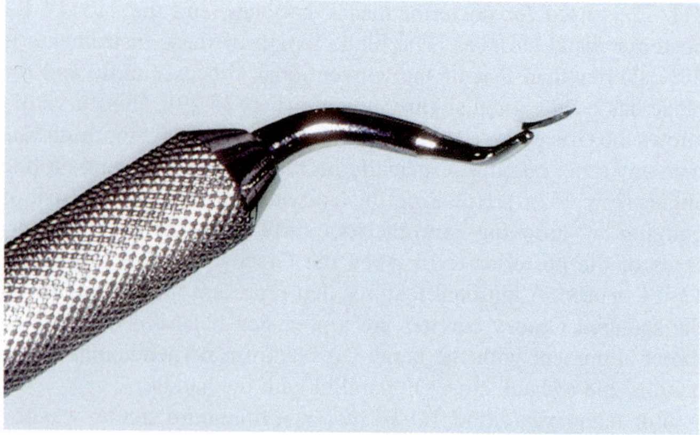

Fig. 35.34 Broken instrument tip attached to the magnetic tip of the Schwartz Periotriever (Daness Dental Distributors, Nyack, N.Y). (*From Pattison G, Pattison A: Periodontal instrumentation, ed 2, Norwalk, CT, 1992, Appleton & Lange.*)

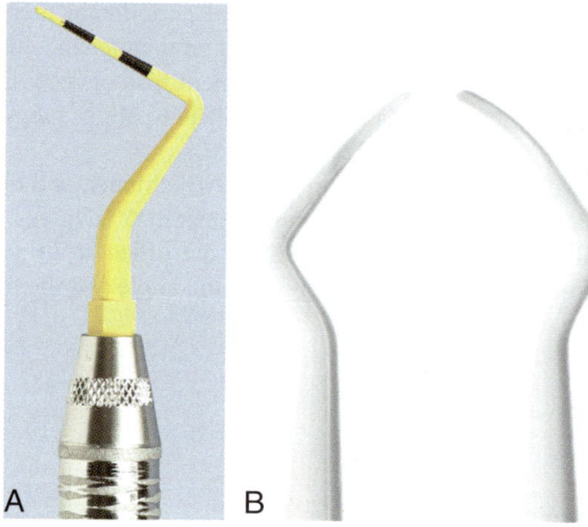

Fig. 35.35 A, Plastic probe: Colorvue. B, New Implacare II Barnhart #5–6 cone socket plastic curette tips that screw into an autoclavable stainless steel handle. (*Courtesy: Hu-Friedy, Chicago, IL.*)

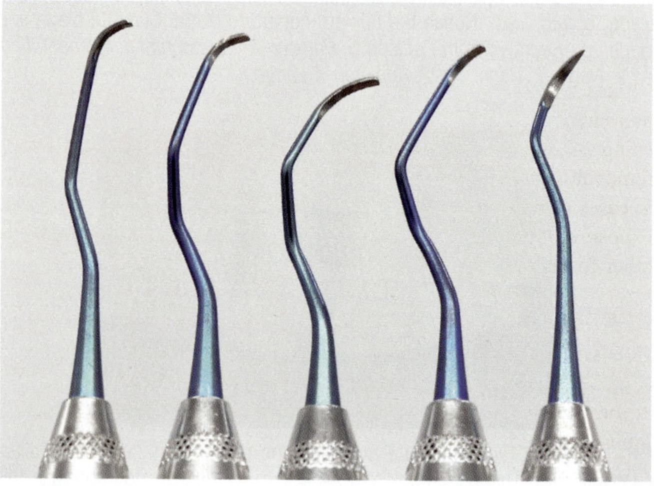

Fig. 35.36 New mini titanium implant scalers (Hu-Friedy, Chicago). *Left to right*, Mini Five Gracey #1–2, Mini Five Gracey #11–12, Langer #1–2, Mini Five Gracey #13–14, 204SD Sickle Scaler.

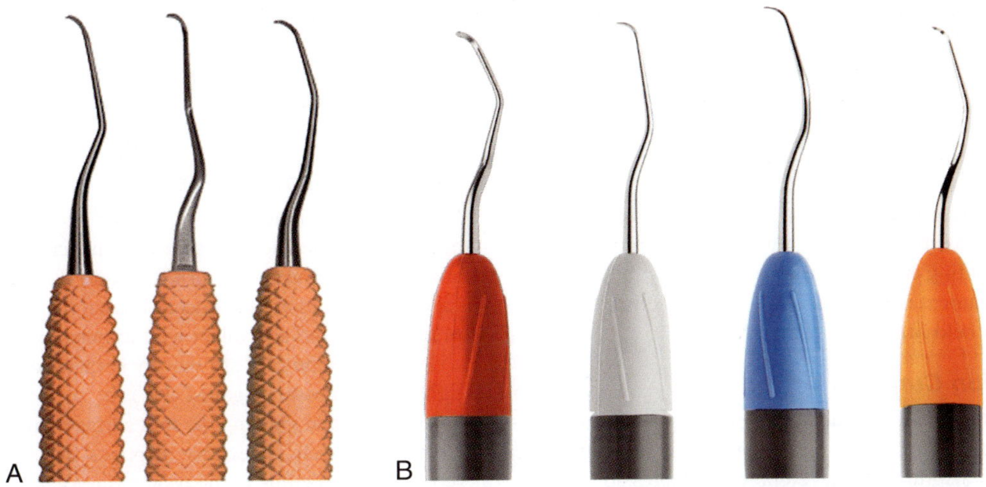

Fig. 35.37 A, Micro Mini titanium implant curettes (Paradise Dental Technologies, Missoula, MT). *Left to right*, Gracey #1–2 Micro Mini, Gracey #11–12 Micro Mini, Gracey #13–14 Micro Mini. B, Mini-bladed titanium implant curettes (LM Instruments, Parainen, Finland): Mini universal curette, Mini Gracey #1–2, Mini Gracey #13–14, Mini Gracey #11–12.

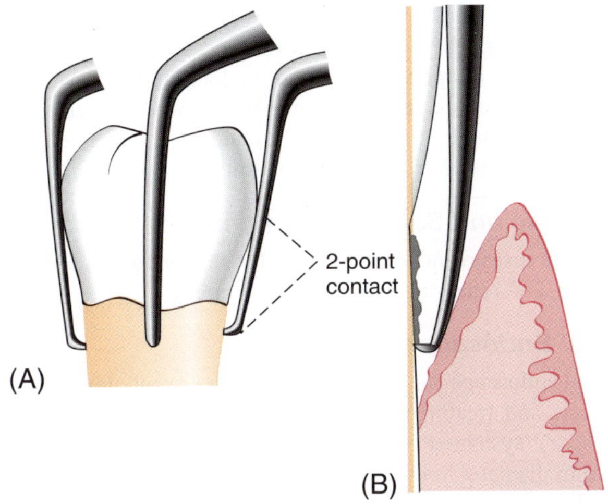

Fig. 35.38 A, Hoe scalers designed for different tooth surfaces, showing "two-point" contact. B, Hoe scaler in a periodontal pocket. The back of the blade is rounded for easier access. The instrument contacts the tooth at two points for stability.

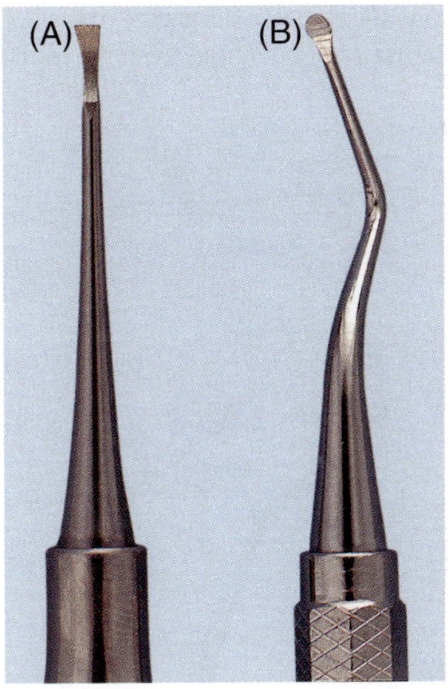

Fig. 35.39 A, Chisel scaler and B, file scaler.

adapt more easily around implants and implant restorations. They may be used for implant maintenance with careful, light-pressured strokes for biofilm and light calculus removal. Moderate- or heavy-pressured strokes should be avoided to prevent scratching or roughening of implant surfaces. These instruments are not intended for removal of heavy calculus or cement. Such deposits are often found in cases of peri-implantitis with moderate to advanced bone loss and exposure of implant threads. Removal of tenacious deposits requires other forms of instrumentation and surgical treatment of the implant.

Hoe Scalers

Hoe scalers are used for scaling of ledges or rings of calculus (Fig. 35.38). The blade is bent at a 99-degree angle; the cutting edge is formed by the junction of the flattened terminal surface with the inner aspect of the blade. The cutting edge is beveled at 45 degrees. The blade is slightly bowed so that it can maintain contact at two points on a convex surface. The back of the blade is rounded, and the blade has been reduced to minimal thickness to permit access to the roots without interference from the adjacent tissues.

Hoe scalers are used in the following manner:

1. The blade is inserted to the base of the periodontal pocket so that it makes two-point contact with the tooth (Fig. 35.38). This stabilizes the instrument and prevents nicking of the root.
2. The instrument is activated with a firm pull stroke toward the crown, with every effort being made to preserve the two-point contact with the tooth.

McCall's #3, #4, #5, #6, #7, and #8 are a set of six hoe scalers designed to provide access to all tooth surfaces. Each instrument has a different angle between the shank and handle.

Files

Files have a series of blades on a base (Fig. 35.39). Their primary function is to fracture or crush large deposits of tenacious calculus or burnished sheets of calculus. Files can easily gouge and roughen root surfaces when used improperly. Therefore, they are not suitable for fine scaling and root planing. Mini-bladed curettes are currently preferred for fine scaling in areas where files were once used. Files are sometimes used for removing overhanging margins of dental restorations.

Chisel Scalers

The chisel scaler, designed for the proximal surfaces of teeth too closely spaced to permit the use of other scalers, is usually used in the anterior part of the mouth. It is a double-ended instrument with a curved shank at one end and a straight shank at the other (Fig. 35.39); the blades are slightly curved and have a straight cutting edge beveled at 45 degrees.

The chisel is inserted from the facial surface. The slight curve of the blade makes it possible to stabilize it against the proximal surface, whereas the cutting edge engages the calculus without nicking the tooth. The instrument is activated with a push motion while the side of the blade is held firmly against the root.

Quétin Furcation Curettes

The Quétin furcation curettes are actually hoes with a shallow, half-moon radius that fits into the roof or floor of the furcation. The curvature of the tip also fits into developmental depressions on the inner aspects of the roots. The shanks are slightly curved for better access, and the tips are available in two widths (Fig. 35.40). The BL1 *(buccal-lingual)* and MD1 *(mesial-distal)* instruments are small and fine, with a 0.9-mm blade width. The BL2 and MD2 instruments are larger and wider, with a 1.3-mm blade width.

These instruments remove burnished calculus from recessed areas of the furcation where curettes, even the mini-bladed curettes, are often too large to gain access. Using mini-bladed Gracey curettes and Gracey Curvettes in the roof or floor of the furcation may unintentionally create gouges and grooves. The Quétin instruments, however, are well suited for this area and lessen the likelihood of root damage.

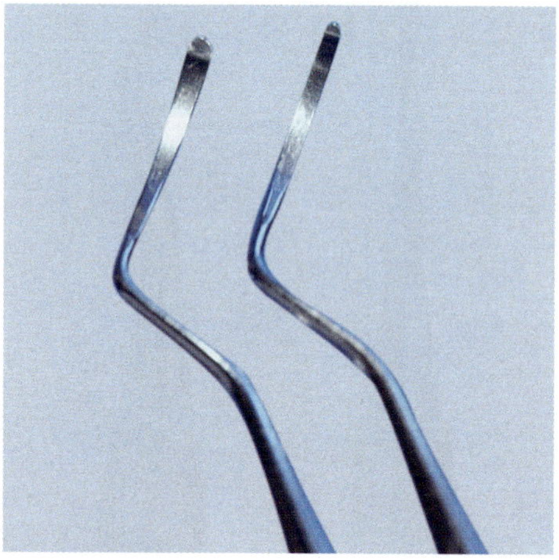

Fig. 35.40 Quétin furcation curettes: BL2 (larger) and BL1 (smaller). *(Copyright A. Pattison.)*

Diamond-Coated Files

Diamond-coated files are unique instruments used for final finishing of root surfaces. These files do not have cutting edges; instead, they are coated with very-fine-grit diamond (Fig. 35.41). The most useful diamond files are the buccal-lingual instruments, which are used in furcations and also adapt well to many other root surfaces.

New diamond files are sharply abrasive and should be used with light, even pressure against the root surface to avoid gouging or grooving. When viewing the root surface with the dental endoscope after all tactilely detectable deposits are gone, small embedded remnants of calculus in the root surface can be observed. Diamond files are used similar to an emery board to remove these minute remnants of calculus from the root, creating a surface that is free of all visible accretions. Diamond files can produce a smooth, even, clean, and highly polished root surface.

Diamond files must be used carefully because they can cause overinstrumentation of the root surface. They will remove too much root structure if they are used with excessive force, are poorly adapted to root morphology, or used too long in one place.

Diamond files are particularly effective when used with the dental endoscope, which reveals residual deposits and directs the clinician to the exact area for instrumentation.

Ultrasonic and Sonic Instruments

Ultrasonic instruments may be used for removing plaque, scaling, curetting, and removing stain (see Chapter 36).

Dental Endoscope

A dental endoscope has been introduced for use subgingivally in the diagnosis and treatment of periodontal disease (Fig. 35.42). The *Perioscopy* system (Perioscopy, Inc., Oakland, CA) consists of a 0.99-mm diameter, reusable fiberoptic endoscope over which is fitted a disposable, sterile sheath. The fiberoptic endoscope fits onto periodontal probes and ultrasonic instruments that have been designed to accept it (Fig. 35.43). The sheath delivers water irrigation that flushes the pocket while the endoscope is being used, keeping the field clear. The fiberoptic endoscope attaches to a medical-grade

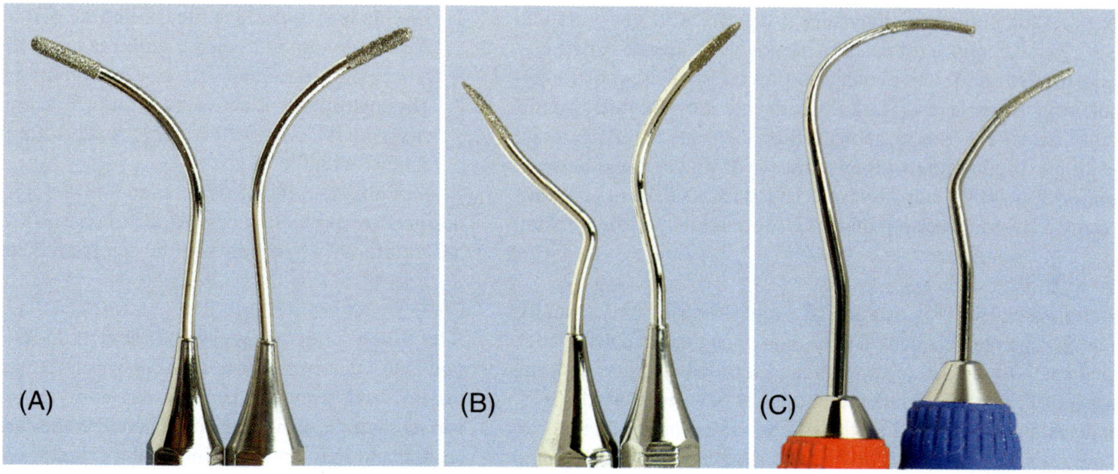

Fig. 35.41 Diamond files. A, #1,2 (Brasseler, Savannah, GA); B, #3,4 (Brasseler); C, SDCN 7, SDCM/D 7. (Hu-Friedy, Chicago.) *(Copyright A. Pattison.)*

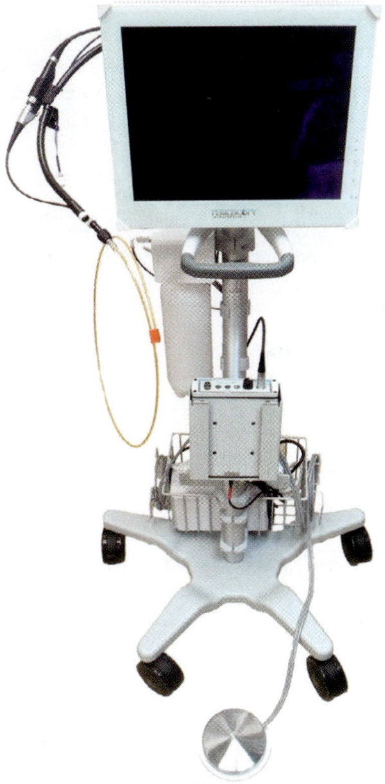

Fig. 35.42 Perioscopysystem, dental endoscope. (*Courtesy: Perioscopy Incorporated, Oakland, CA.)*

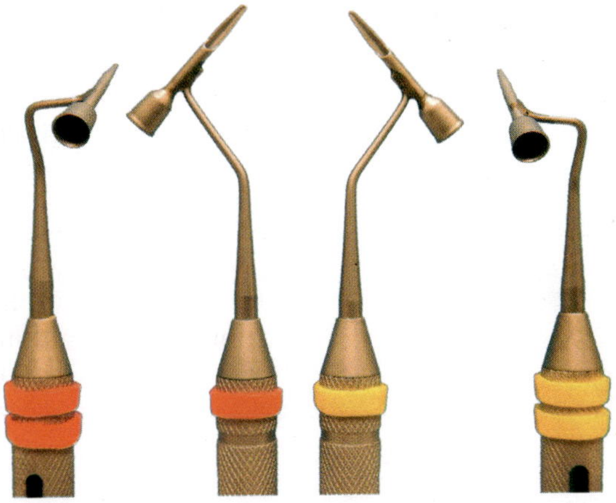

Fig. 35.43 Viewing periodontal explorers (left/right/full viewing) for the Perioscopy system. (*Courtesy: Perioscopy Incorporated, Oakland, CA.)*

charged-coupled device video camera and light source that produces an image on a flat-panel monitor for viewing during subgingival exploration and instrumentation. This device allows clear visualization deeply into subgingival pockets and furcations (Fig. 35.44). It permits operators to detect the presence and location of subgingival deposits and guides them in the thorough removal of these deposits. Magnification ranges from 24 to 48 times, enabling visualization of even minute deposits of plaque and calculus. Using this device, operators can achieve levels of root debridement and cleanliness that are much more difficult or impossible to produce without it. The perioscopy system can also be used to evaluate subgingival areas for caries, defective restorations, root fractures, and resorption.

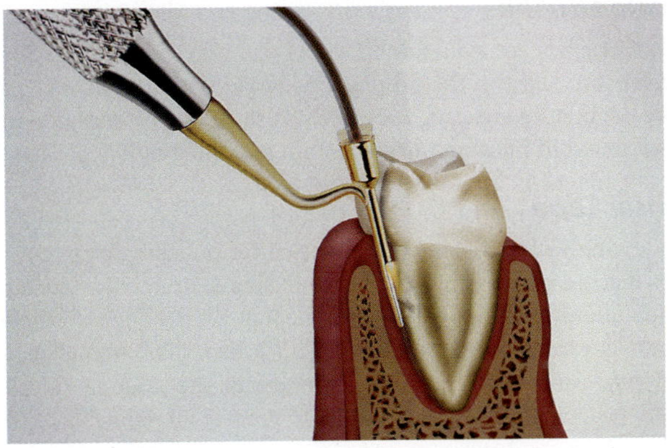

Fig. 35.44 Perioscopic instrumentation permits deep subgingival visualization in pockets and furcations. (*Courtesy: Perioscopy Incorporated, Oakland, CA.)*

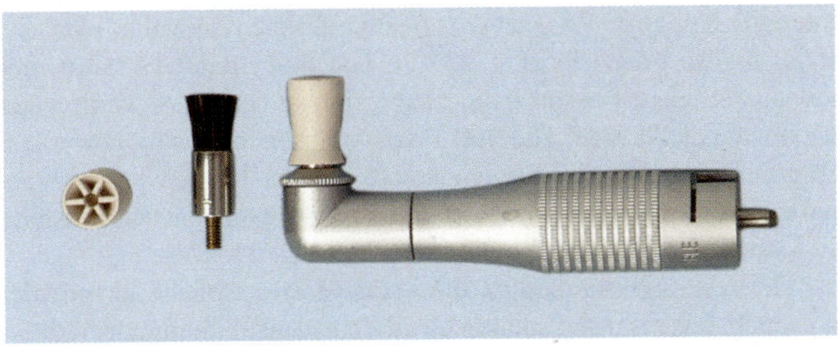

Fig. 35.45 Metal prophylaxis angle with rubber cup and brush.

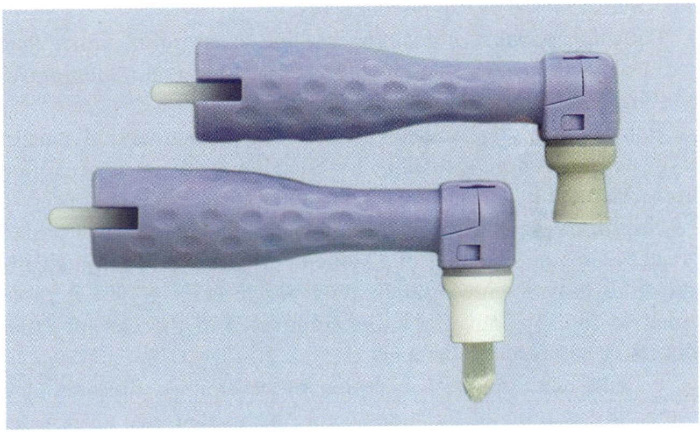

Fig. 35.46 Disposable plastic prophylaxis angle with rubber cup and with brush.

Cleansing and Polishing Instruments

Rubber Cups

Rubber cups consist of a rubber shell with or without webbed configurations in the hollow interior (Fig. 35.45). They are used in the handpiece with a special prophylaxis angle. The handpiece, prophylaxis angle, and rubber cup must be sterilized after each patient use, or a disposable plastic prophylaxis angle and rubber cup may be used and then discarded (Fig. 35.46). A good cleansing and polishing paste that contains fluoride should be used and kept moist to minimize frictional heat as the cup revolves. Polishing pastes are available in fine, medium, or coarse grits and are packaged in small, convenient, single-use containers. Aggressive use of the rubber cup with any abrasive may remove the layer of cementum, which is thin in the cervical area.

Bristle Brushes

Bristle brushes are available in wheel and cup shapes (Fig. 35.45). The brush is used in the prophylaxis angle with a polishing paste. Since the bristles are stiff, use of the brush should be confined to the crown to avoid injuring the cementum and the gingiva.

Dental Tape

Dental tape with polishing paste is used for polishing proximal surfaces that are inaccessible to other polishing instruments. The tape is passed interproximally while being kept at a right angle to the long axis of the tooth and is activated with a firm labiolingual motion. Particular care is taken to avoid injury to the gingiva. The area should be cleansed with warm water to remove all remnants of paste.

Air-Powder Polishing

The first specially designed handpiece to deliver an air-powered slurry of warm water and sodium bicarbonate for polishing was introduced in the early 1980s. This device, called the *Prophy-Jet* (Dentsply International, York, PA), is very effective for the removal of extrinsic stains and soft deposits (Fig. 35.47). The slurry removes stains rapidly and efficiently by mechanical abrasion and provides warm water for rinsing and lavage. The flow rate of abrasive cleansing power can be adjusted to increase the amount of powder for heavier stain removal. Currently, many manufacturers produce air-powder polishing systems that use various powder formulas Fig. 35.48.

The results of studies on the abrasive effect of the air-powder polishing devices using sodium bicarbonate and aluminum trihydroxide on cementum and dentin show that significant tooth substance can be lost. Damage to gingival tissue is transient and insignificant clinically, but amalgam restorations, composite resins, cements, and other nonmetallic materials can be roughened.

Polishing powders containing glycine or erythritol rather than sodium bicarbonate are commonly used in Europe for subgingival biofilm removal from root surfaces.

Both supragingival and subgingival air polishing with glycine or erythritol powder are safe and very effective for removal of biofilm from titanium implant surfaces and restorative materials (Fig. 35.49).

No soft tissue abrasion occurs, and at probing depths of 1 mm to greater than 5 mm, the use of glycine or erythritol powder in an air-polishing device with a subgingival nozzle (Fig. 35.50) is more effective for subgingival biofilm removal than the use of either manual or ultrasonic instruments.

Patients with medical histories of respiratory illnesses and hemodialysis are not candidates for the use of the air-powder

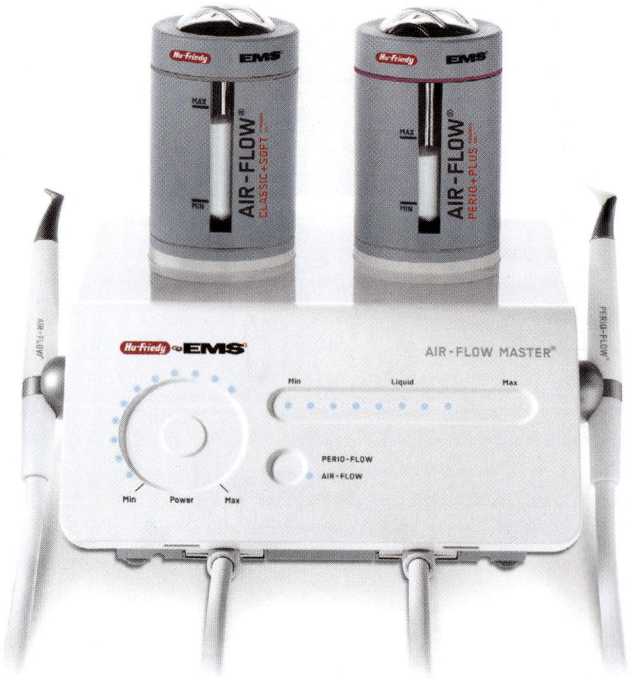

Fig. 35.48 Hu-Friedy EMS Air Flow Master air polishing device with perio and standard handpieces and tips for both supragingival and subgingival air polishing. (*Courtesy: Hu-Friedy, Chicago, IL.*)

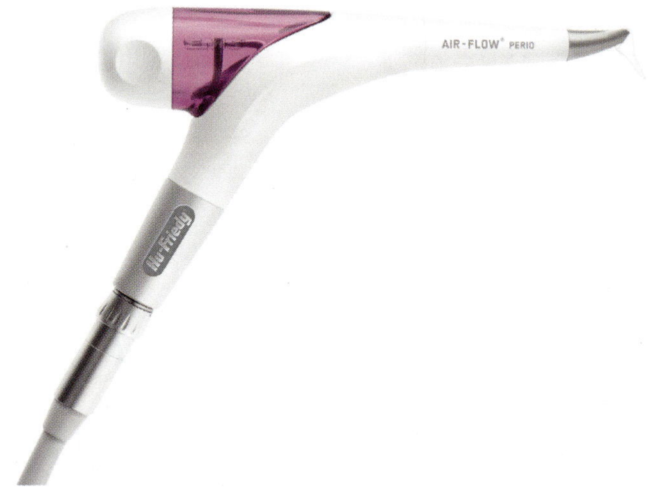

Fig. 35.49 Hu-Friedy EMS Air Flow Perio Handy smaller air polishing device with subgingival air polishing tip for glycine or erythritol powder polishing. (*Courtesy: Hu-Friedy, Chicago, IL.*)

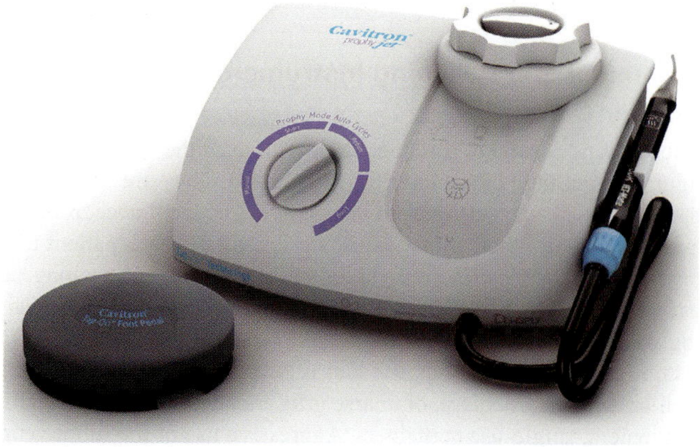

Fig. 35.47 Cavitron Prophy Jet air-powder polishing device. (*Courtesy: Dentsply International, York, PA.*)

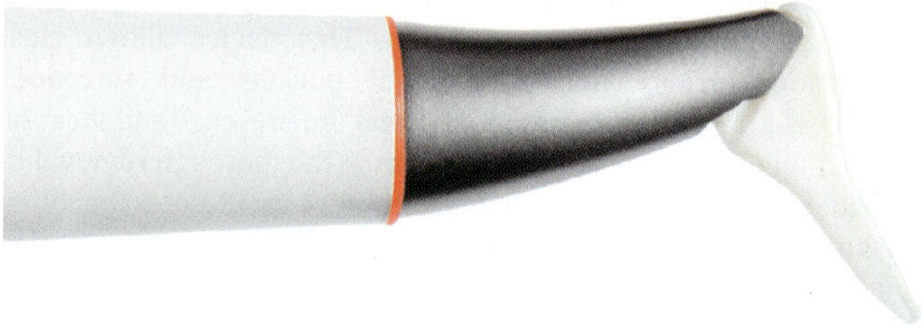

Fig. 35.50 Hu-Friedy EMS Perio Flow Tip disposable plastic tip with millimeter markings for subgingival air polishing of implants or deep pockets with glycine or erythritol powder. (*Courtesy: Hu-Friedy, Chicago IL.*)

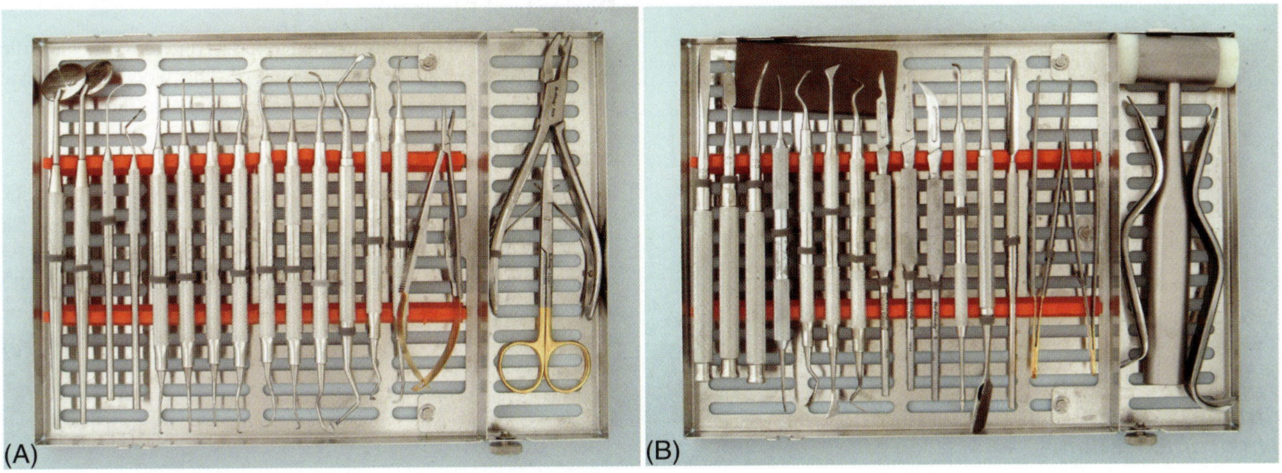

Fig. 35.51 A typical series of periodontal surgical instruments divided into two cassettes. A, From left, Mirrors, explorer, probe, series of curettes, needleholder, rongeurs, and scissors. B, From left, Series of chisels, Kirkland knife, Orban knife, scalpel handles with surgical blades (nos. 15C, 15, and 12D), periosteal elevators, spatula, tissue forceps, cheek retractors, mallet, and sharpening stone. *(Courtesy: A, Hu-Friedy, Chicago, IL; Courtesy: B, G. Hartzell & Son, Concord, CA.)*

polishing device. Powders containing sodium bicarbonate should not be used on patients with histories of hypertension, sodium-restricted diets, or medications affecting the electrolyte balance. Patients with infectious diseases should not be treated with this device because of the large quantity of aerosol created. A preprocedural rinse with 0.12% chlorhexidine gluconate should be used to minimize the microbial content of the aerosol. High-speed evacuation should also be used to eliminate as much of the aerosol as possible.

Aerosol-Generating Devices and Communicable Diseases

Aerosol-generating devices such as air polishers and ultrasonic scalers create a large amount of contaminated aerosol. Patients with diseases that can be transmitted by aerosols should not be treated in the dental office or clinic. However, since any patient could be an asymptomatic or prodromal carrier of coronavirus disease 2019 (COVID-19), tuberculosis, or other communicable blood-borne or airborne disease, air polishers should only be used with proper aerosol control measures. Aerosols linger in the air for 30 min up to several hours in the entire operatory and in areas of the dental office outside the operatory. Unprotected patients are more susceptible to infection by aerosols than dental personnel who wear protective barriers such as face shields, respirators, masks, gloves, eyewear, and disposable clinical clothing. High volume evacuation, preprocedural rinsing with antimicrobial mouth wash, flushing of the handpiece and water lines or a self-contained sterile water source, disinfection of environmental surfaces, adequate ventilation and air filtration units with high-efficiency particulate air (HEPA) filters are all important measures to minimize the hazards of microbial aerosols.

Surgical Instruments

Periodontal surgery is accomplished with numerous instruments; Fig. 35.51 shows a typical surgical cassette. Periodontal surgical instruments are classified as follows:

1. Excisional and incisional instruments
2. Surgical curettes and sickles
3. Periosteal elevators
4. Surgical chisels
5. Surgical files

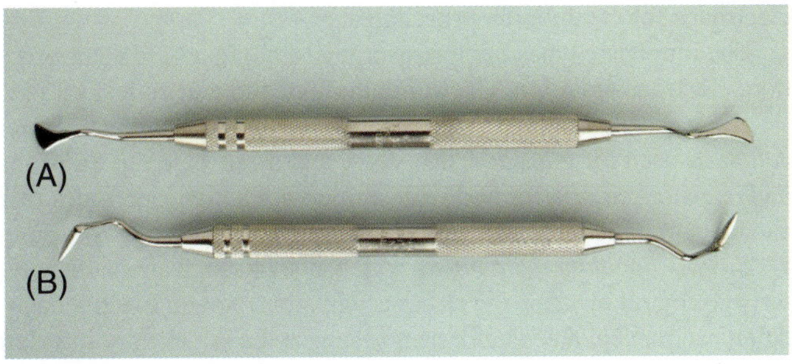

Fig. 35.52 Gingivectomy knives. A, Kirkland knife; B, Orban interdental knife.

6. Scissors
7. Hemostats and tissue forceps

Excisional and Incisional Instruments

Periodontal Knives (Gingivectomy Knives)

The Kirkland knife is representative of the knives that are typically used for gingivectomy. These knives can be obtained as either double-ended or single-ended instruments. The entire periphery of these kidney-shaped knives is the cutting edge (Fig. 35.52A).

Interdental Knives

The Orban knife (nos. 1 and 2; Fig. 35.52B) and the Merrifield knife (nos. 1 through 4) are examples of knives that can be used for interdental areas. These spear-shaped knives have cutting edges on both sides of the blade, and they are designed with either double-ended or single-ended blades.

Surgical Blades

Scalpel blades of different shapes and sizes are used in periodontal surgery. The most common blades are nos. 12D, 15, and 15C (Fig. 35.53). The no. 12D blade is a beak-shaped blade with cutting edges on both sides, which allow the operator to engage narrow, restricted areas with both pushing and pulling cutting motions. The no. 15 blade is used for thinning flaps and general purposes. The no. 15C blade, which is a narrower version of the no. 15 blade, is useful for making the initial, scalloping-type incision. The slim design of this blade allows for incising into the narrow interdental portion of the flap. All of these blades are discarded after one use.

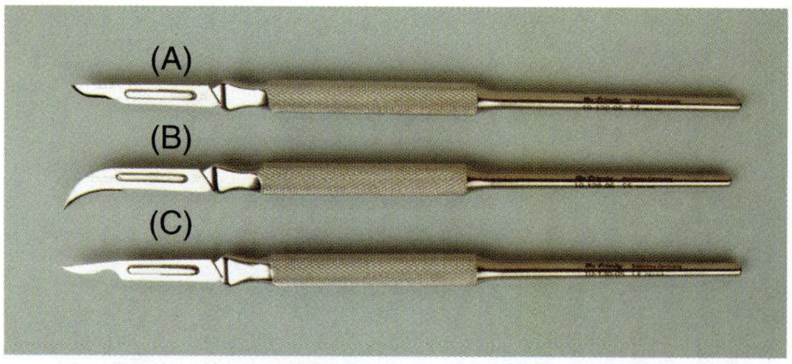

Fig. 35.53 Surgical blades. A–C, Nos. 15, 12D, and 15C. These blades are disposable.

Electrosurgery (Radiosurgery) Techniques and Instrumentation

The terms *electrosurgery* and *radiosurgery* are currently used to identify surgical techniques performed on soft tissue with the use of controlled, high-frequency electrical (radio) currents in the range of 1.5–7.5 million cycles per second (megahertz). There are three classes of active electrodes: single-wire electrodes for incising or excising; loop electrodes for planing tissue; and heavier, bulkier electrodes for coagulation procedures.

The four basic types of electrosurgical techniques are electrosection, electrocoagulation, electrofulguration, and electrodesiccation.

Electrosection, which is also referred to as *electrotomy* or *acusection*, is used for incisions, excisions, and tissue planing. Incisions and excisions are performed with single-wire active electrodes that can be bent or adapted to accomplish any type of cutting procedure.

Electrocoagulation provides a wide range of coagulation and hemorrhage control by using the electrocoagulation current. Electrocoagulation can prevent bleeding or hemorrhage at the initial entry into soft tissue, but it cannot stop bleeding after blood is present. All forms of hemorrhage must be stopped first by some form of direct pressure (e.g., air, compress, hemostat). After bleeding has momentarily stopped, the final sealing of the capillaries or large vessels can be accomplished with a short application of the electrocoagulation current. The active electrodes that are used for coagulation are much bulkier than the fine tungsten wire used for electrosection. Electrosection and electrocoagulation are the procedures that are most often used in all areas of dentistry. The two monoterminal techniques, electrofulguration and electrodesiccation, are not in general use in dentistry.

The most important basic rule of electrosurgery is this: *always keep the tip moving*. The prolonged or repeated application of current to tissue induces heat accumulation and undesired tissue destruction, whereas interrupted application at intervals adequate for tissue cooling (5–10 s) reduces or eliminates heat buildup. Electrosurgery is not intended to destroy tissue; it is a controllable means of sculpturing or modifying oral soft tissue with little discomfort and hemorrhage for the patient.

The indications for electrosurgery in periodontal therapy and a description of wound healing after electrosurgery are presented in Chapter 44. Electrosurgery is contraindicated for patients who have incompatible or poorly shielded cardiac pacemakers.

Surgical Curettes and Sickles

Larger and heavier curettes and sickles are often needed during surgery for the removal of granulation tissue, fibrous interdental tissues, and tenacious subgingival deposits. The Prichard curette (Fig. 35.54) and the Kirkland surgical instruments are heavy curettes, whereas the Ball scaler (nos. B2 and B3) is a popular heavy sickle. The wider, heavier blades of these instruments make them suitable for surgical procedures.

Periosteal Elevators

The periosteal elevators are needed to reflect and move the flap after the incision has been made for flap surgery. The Woodson and Prichard elevators are well-designed periosteal instruments (Fig. 35.55).

Surgical Chisels

The back-action chisel is used with a pull motion (Fig. 35.56), whereas the straight chisel [e.g., Wedelstaedt, Ochsenbein (nos. 1 and 2)] is used with a push motion (Fig. 35.57). The Ochsenbein chisel is a useful chisel with a semicircular indentation on both sides of the shank that allows the instrument to engage around the tooth and into the interdental area. The Rhodes chisel is another popular back-action chisel.

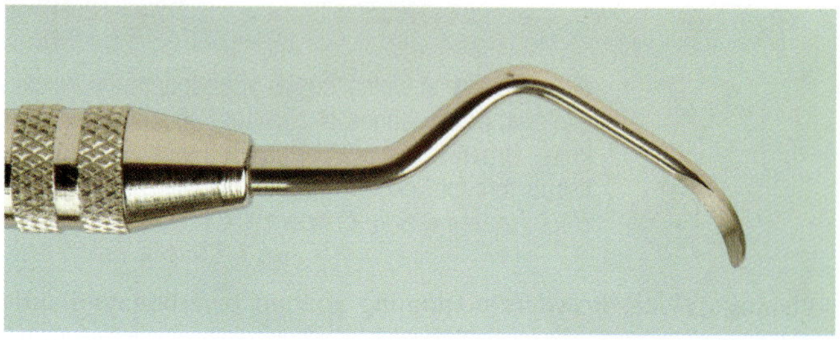

Fig. 35.54 A Prichard surgical curette. The curettes that are used in surgery have wider blades than those that are used for conventional scaling and root planing.

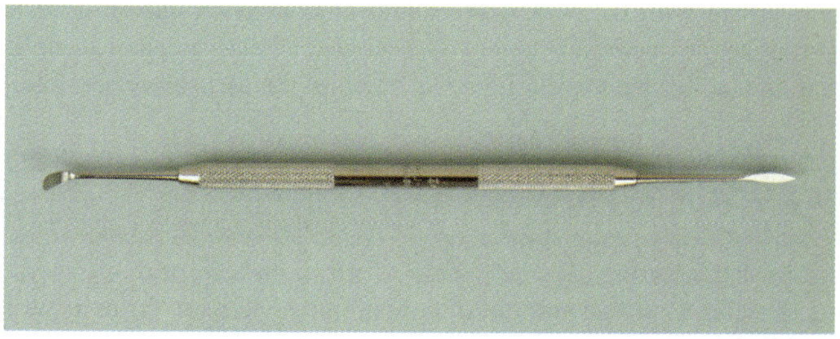

Fig. 35.55 Woodson periosteal elevator.

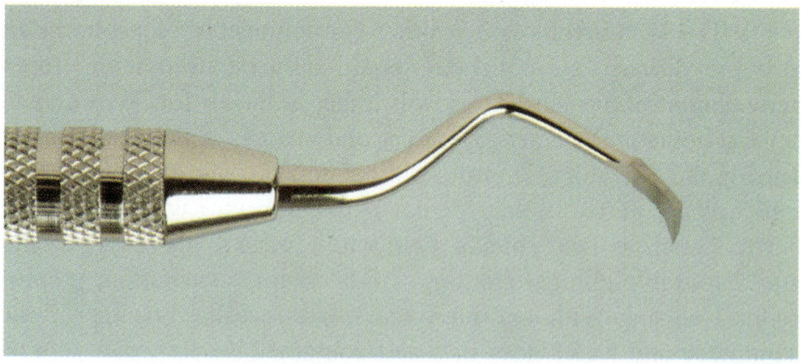

Fig. 35.56 Back-action chisel.

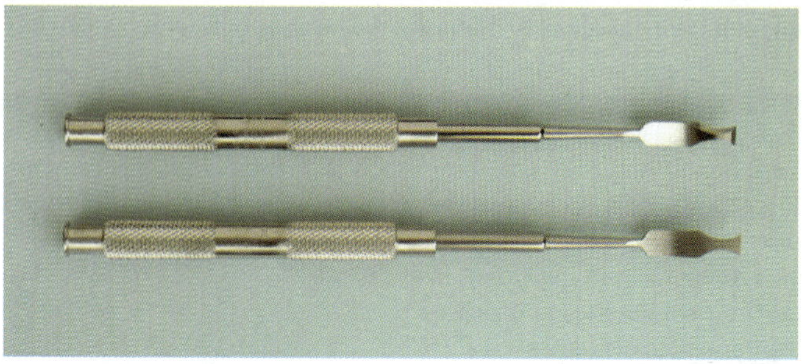

Fig. 35.57 Ochsenbein chisels are paired, with their cutting edges in opposite directions.

Tissue Forceps

The tissue forceps is used to hold the flap during suturing. It is also used to position and displace the flap after the flap has been reflected. The DeBakey forceps is an extremely efficient instrument (Fig. 35.58).

Scissors and Nippers

Scissors and nippers are used in periodontal surgery to remove tabs of tissue during gingivectomy, to trim the margins of flaps, to enlarge incisions in periodontal abscesses, and to remove muscle attachments in mucogingival surgery. Many types are available, and individual preference determines the choice. The Goldman–Fox no. 16 scissors has a curved, beveled blade with serrations (Fig. 35.59).

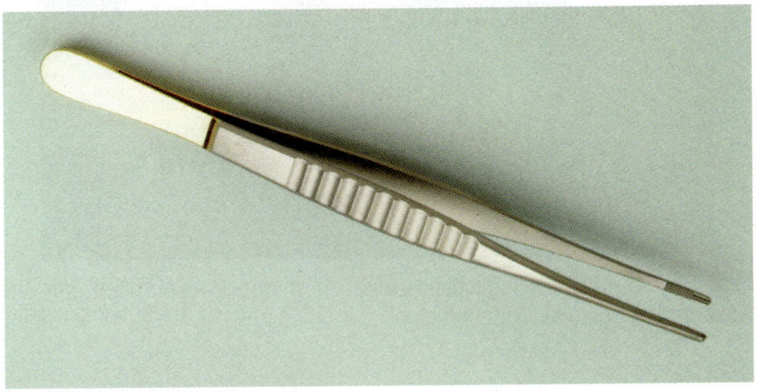

Fig. 35.58 DeBakey tissue forceps.

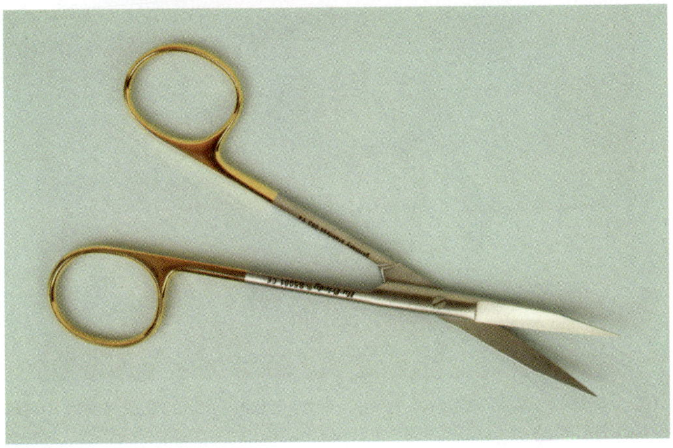

Fig. 35.59 Goldman–Fox scissors.

Needleholders

Needleholders are used to suture the flap at the desired position after the surgical procedure has been completed. In addition to the regular types of needleholders (Fig. 35.60A), the Castroviejo needleholder is used for delicate, precise techniques that require the quick and easy grasp and release of the suture (Fig. 35.60B).

General Principles of Instrumentation

Effective instrumentation is governed by a number of general principles that are common to all periodontal instruments. Proper position of the patient and the operator, illumination and retraction for optimal visibility, and sharp instruments are fundamental prerequisites. A constant awareness of tooth and root morphologic features and of the condition of the periodontal tissues is also essential. Knowledge of instrument design enables the clinician to select the proper instrument for the procedure and the correct area in which it will be performed. In addition to these principles, the basic concepts of grasp, finger rest, adaptation, angulation, and stroke must be understood before clinical instrument-handling skills can be mastered.

Accessibility: Positioning of Patient and Operator

Accessibility facilitates thoroughness of instrumentation. The position of the patient and operator should provide maximal accessibility to the area of operation. Inadequate accessibility impedes thorough instrumentation, prematurely tires the operator, and diminishes his or her effectiveness.

The clinician should be seated on a comfortable operating stool that has been positioned so that the clinician's feet are flat on the floor with the thighs parallel to the floor. The clinician should be able to observe the field of operation while keeping the back straight and the head erect.

The patient should be in a supine position and placed so that the mouth is close to the resting elbow of the clinician. For instrumentation of the maxillary arch, the patient should be asked to raise the chin slightly to provide optimal visibility and accessibility. For instrumentation on the mandibular arch, it may be necessary to raise the back of the chair slightly and request that the patient lower the chin until the mandible is parallel to the floor. This will especially facilitate work on the lingual surfaces of the mandibular anterior teeth.

Visibility, Illumination, and Retraction

Whenever possible, *direct vision* with *direct illumination* from the dental light is most desirable (Fig. 35.61). If this is not possible, *indirect vision* may be obtained by using the mouth mirror (Fig. 35.62) and *indirect illumination* may be obtained by using the mirror to

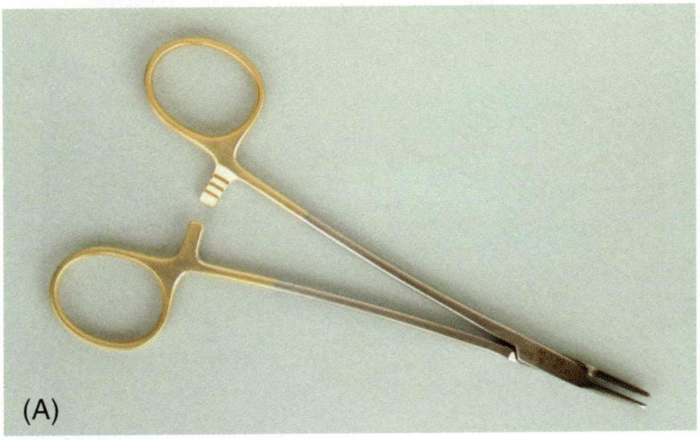
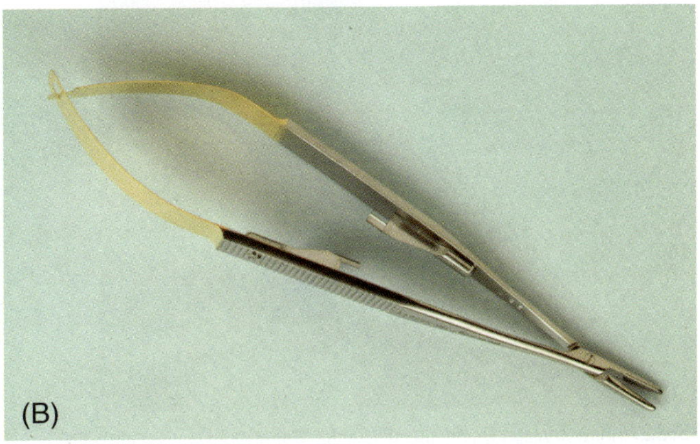

Fig. 35.60 A, Conventional needleholder; B, Castroviejo needleholder.

reflect light to where it is needed (Fig. 35.63). Indirect vision and indirect illumination are often used simultaneously (Fig. 35.64).

Retraction provides visibility, accessibility, and illumination. Depending on the location of the area of operation, the fingers and/or the mirror are used for retraction. The *mirror* may be used for retraction of the cheeks or the tongue; the *index finger* is used for retraction of the lips or cheeks. The following methods are effective for retraction:

1. Use of the mirror to deflect the cheek while the fingers of the nonoperating hand retract the lips and protect the angle of the mouth from irritation by the mirror handle.
2. Use of the mirror alone to retract the lips and cheek (Fig. 35.65).
3. Use of the fingers of the nonoperating hand to retract the lips (Fig. 35.66).
4. Use of the mirror to retract the tongue (Fig. 35.67).
5. Combinations of the preceding methods.

When retracting, care should be taken to avoid irritation to the angles of the mouth. If the lips and skin are dry, softening the lips with petroleum jelly before instrumentation is a helpful precaution against cracking and bleeding. Careful retraction is especially important for patients with a history of recurrent *herpes labialis* because these patients may easily develop herpetic lesions after instrumentation.

Condition and Sharpness of Instruments

Before any instrumentation, all instruments should be inspected to make sure that they are clean, sterile, and in good condition. The working ends of pointed or bladed instruments must be sharp to be effective. Sharp instruments enhance tactile sensitivity and allow the clinician to work more precisely and efficiently (see later discussion). Dull instruments may lead to incomplete calculus removal and unnecessary trauma because of the excess force usually applied to compensate for their ineffectiveness.

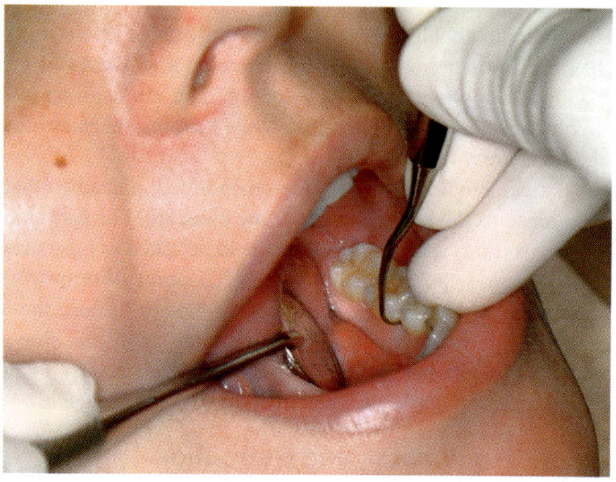

Fig. 35.61 Direct vision and direct illumination in the mandibular left premolar area.

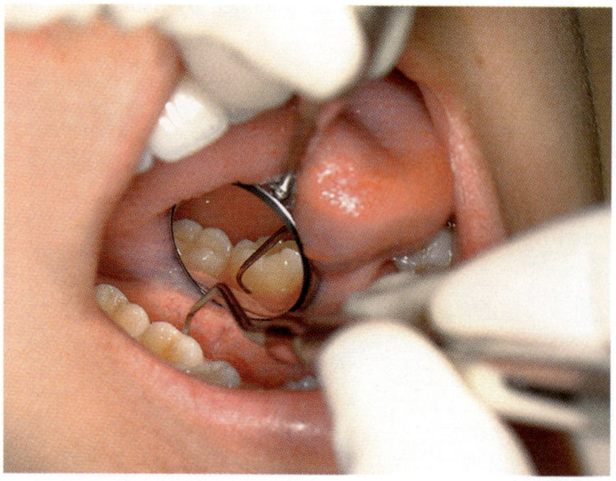

Fig. 35.62 Indirect vision using the mirror for the lingual surfaces of the mandibular anterior teeth.

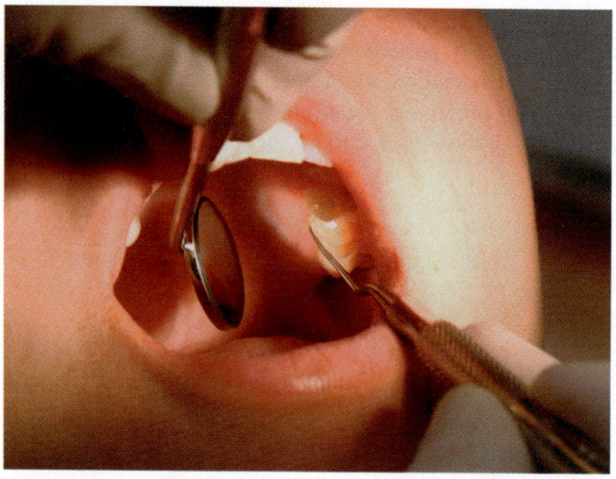

Fig. 35.63 Indirect illumination using the mirror to reflect light onto the maxillary left posterior lingual region.

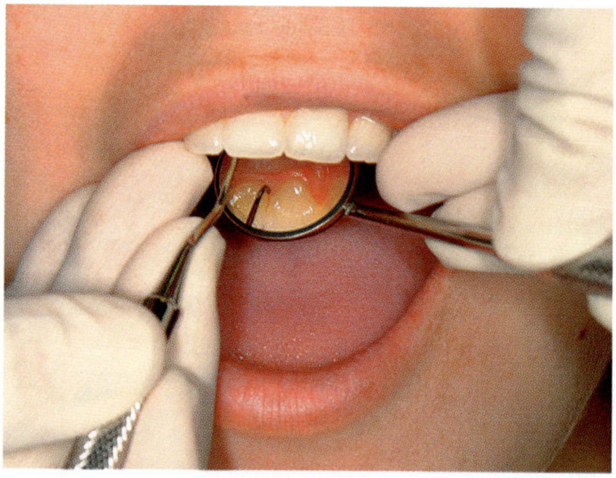

Fig. 35.64 Combination of indirect illumination and indirect vision for the lingual surfaces of the maxillary anterior teeth.

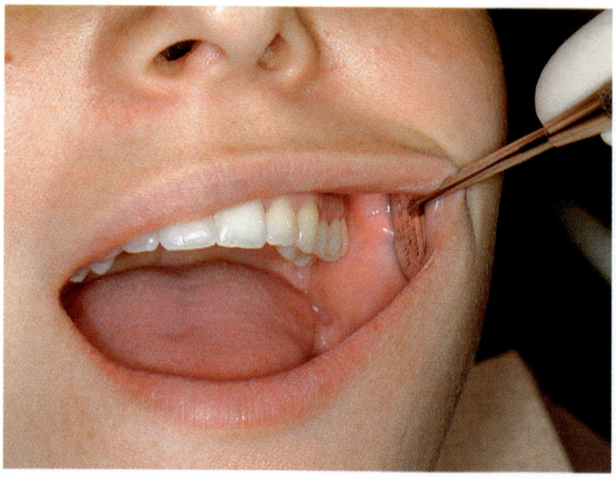

Fig. 35.65 Retracting the cheek with the mirror.

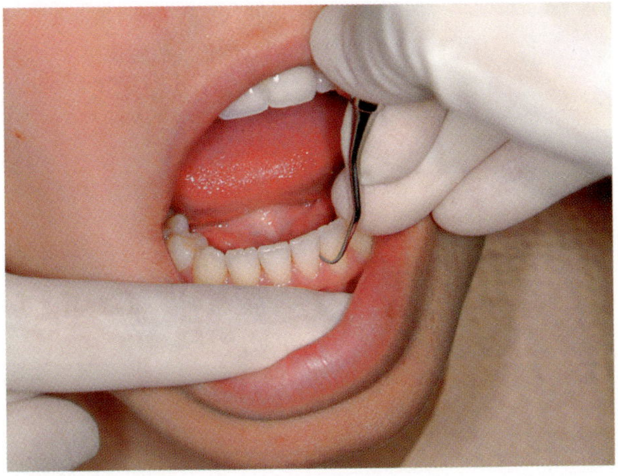

Fig. 35.66 Retracting the lip with the index finger of the nonoperating hand.

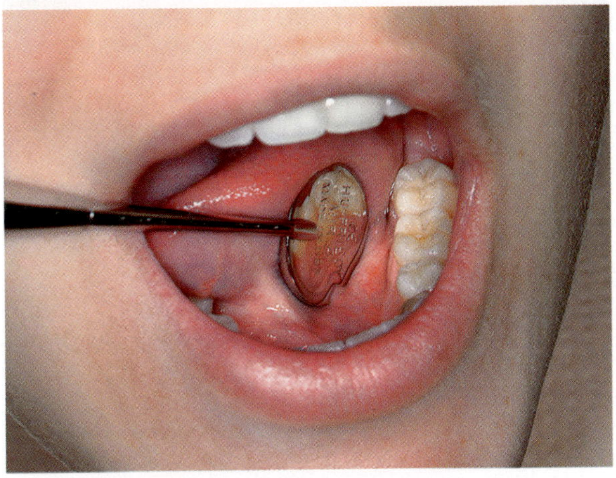

Fig. 35.67 Retracting the tongue with the mirror.

Maintaining a Clean Field

Despite good visibility, illumination, and retraction, instrumentation can be hampered if the operative field is obscured by saliva, blood, and debris. The pooling of saliva interferes with visibility during instrumentation and impedes control because a firm finger rest cannot be established on wet, slippery tooth surfaces. Adequate suction is essential and can be achieved with a saliva ejector or, if working with an assistant, an aspirator.

Gingival bleeding is an unavoidable consequence of subgingival instrumentation. In areas of inflammation, bleeding is not necessarily an indication of trauma from incorrect technique but rather may indicate ulceration of the pocket epithelium. Blood and debris can be removed from the operative field with suction and by wiping or blotting with gauze squares. The operative field should also be flushed occasionally with water.

Compressed air and gauze squares can be used to facilitate visual inspection of tooth surfaces just below the gingival margin during instrumentation. A jet of air directed into the pocket deflects a retractable gingival margin. Retractable tissue can also be deflected away from the tooth by gently packing the edge of gauze square into the pocket with the back of a curette. Immediately after the gauze is removed, the subgingival area should be clean, dry, and clearly visible for a brief interval.

Instrument Stabilization

Stability of the instrument and the hand is the primary requisite for controlled instrumentation. Stability and control are essential for effective instrumentation and avoidance of injury to the patient or clinician. The two factors of major importance in providing stability are the instrument grasp and the finger rest.

Instrument Grasp

A proper grasp is essential for precise control of movements made during periodontal instrumentation. The most effective and stable grasp for all periodontal instruments is the *modified pen grasp* (Fig. 35.68). Although other grasps are possible, this modification of the *standard pen grasp* (Fig. 35.69) ensures the greatest control in performing intraoral procedures.

The thumb, index finger, and middle finger are used to hold the instrument as a pen is held, but the middle finger is positioned so that the side of the pad next to the fingernail is resting on the instrument shank. The index finger is bent at the second joint from the fingertip and is positioned well above the middle finger on the same side of the handle.

The pad of the thumb is placed midway between the middle and index fingers on the opposite side of the handle. This creates a triangle of forces, or *tripod effect*, that enhances control because it counteracts the tendency of the instrument to turn uncontrollably

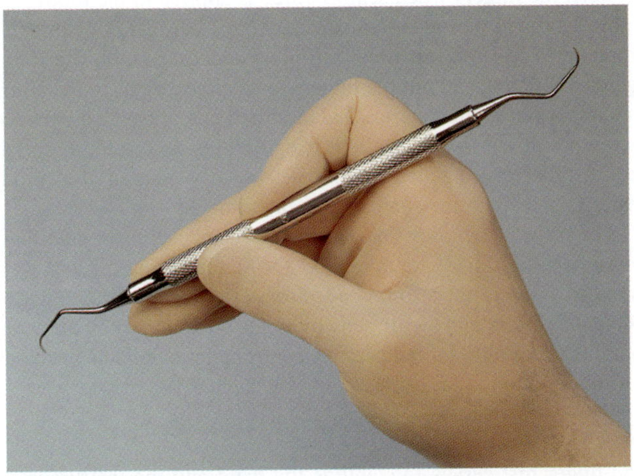

Fig. 35.68 Modified pen grasp. The pad of the middle finger rests on the shank. *(Copyright A. Pattison.)*

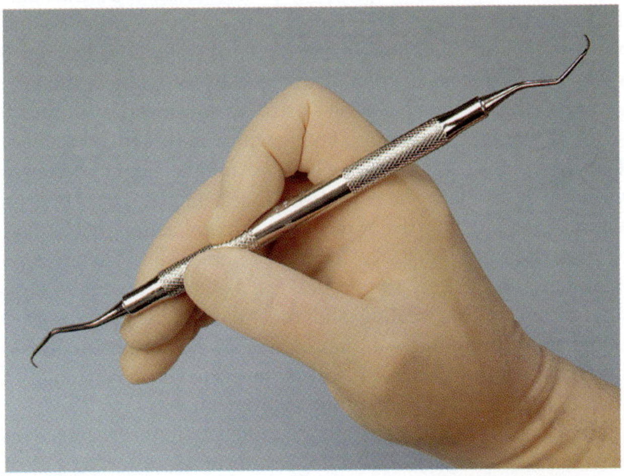

Fig. 35.69 Standard pen grasp. The side of the middle finger rests on the shank. *(Copyright A. Pattison.)*

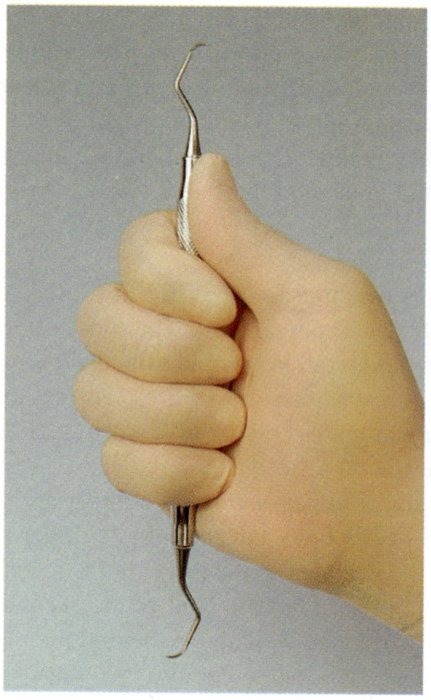

Fig. 35.70 Palm and thumb grasp, used for stabilizing instruments during sharpening. The fourth finger rests on the occlusal surfaces of adjacent teeth. (*Copyright A. Pattison.*)

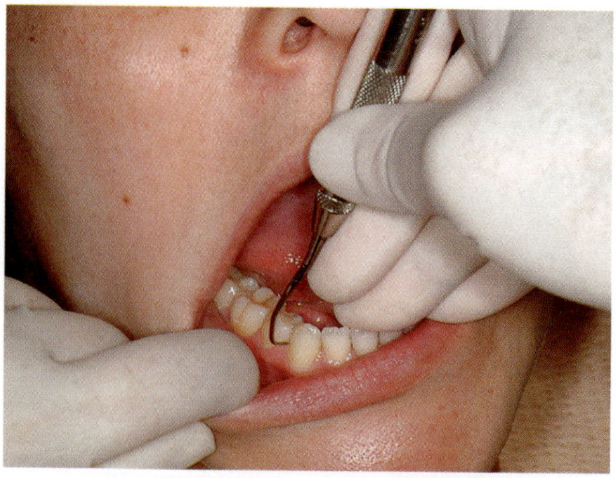

Fig. 35.71 Intraoral conventional finger rest.

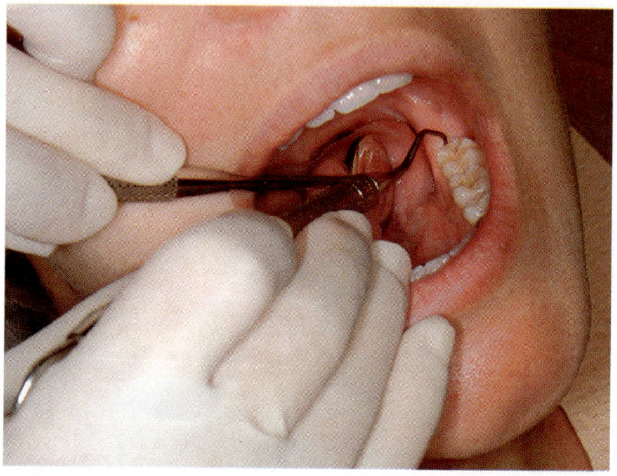

Fig. 35.72 Intraoral cross-arch finger rest. The fourth finger rests on the incisal surfaces of teeth on the opposite side of the same arch.

between the fingers when scaling force is applied to the tooth. This stable modified pen grasp enhances control because it enables the clinician to roll the instrument in precise degrees with the thumb against the index and middle fingers to adapt the blade to the slightest changes in tooth contour. The modified pen grasp also enhances tactile sensitivity because slight irregularities on the tooth surface are best perceived when the tactile-sensitive pad of the middle finger is placed on the shank of the instrument.

The *palm and thumb grasp* (Fig. 35.70) is useful for stabilizing instruments during sharpening and for manipulating air and water syringes, but it is not recommended for periodontal instrumentation. Maneuverability and tactile sensitivity are so inhibited by this grasp that it is unsuitable for the precise, controlled movements necessary during periodontal procedures.

Finger Rest

The finger rest serves to stabilize the hand and the instrument by providing a firm fulcrum as movements are made to activate the instrument. A good finger rest prevents injury and laceration of the gingiva and surrounding tissues by poorly controlled instruments. The fourth (ring) finger is preferred by most clinicians for the finger rest. Although it is possible to use the third (middle) finger for the finger rest, this is not recommended because it restricts the arc of movement during the activation of strokes and severely curtails the use of the middle finger for both control and tactile sensitivity. Maximal control is achieved when the middle finger is kept between the instrument shank and the fourth finger. This "built-up" fulcrum is an integral part of the wrist-forearm action that activates the powerful working stroke for calculus removal. Whenever possible, these two fingers should be kept together to work as a one-unit fulcrum during scaling and root planing. Separation of the middle and fourth fingers during scaling strokes results in a loss of power and control because it forces the clinician to rely solely on finger flexing for activation of the instrument.

Finger rests may be generally classified as intraoral finger rests or extraoral fulcrums. Intraoral finger rests on tooth surfaces ideally are established close to the working area. Variations of intraoral finger rests and extraoral fulcrums are used whenever good angulation and a sufficient arc of movement cannot be achieved by a finger rest close to the working area. The following examples illustrate the different variations of the intraoral finger rest:

1. *Conventional:* The finger rest is established on tooth surfaces immediately adjacent to the working area (Fig. 35.71).
2. *Cross-arch:* The finger rest is established on tooth surfaces on the other side of the same arch (Fig. 35.72).
3. *Opposite arch:* The finger rest is established on tooth surfaces on the opposite arch (e.g., mandibular arch finger rest for instrumentation on the maxillary arch) (Fig. 35.73).
4. *Finger on finger:* The finger rest is established on the index finger or thumb of the nonoperating hand (Fig. 35.74).

Extraoral fulcrums are essential for effective instrumentation of some aspects of the maxillary posterior teeth. When properly established, they allow optimal access and angulation while providing adequate stabilization. Extraoral fulcrums are not "finger rests" in the literal sense because the tips or pads of the fingers are not used for extraoral fulcrums as they are for intraoral finger rests. Instead, as much of the front or back surface of the fingers as possible is placed on the patient's face to provide the greatest degree of stability. The two most common extraoral fulcrums are used as follows:

1. *Palm up:* The palm-up fulcrum is established by resting the backs of the middle and fourth fingers on the skin overlying the lateral aspect of the mandible on the right side of the face (Fig. 35.75).

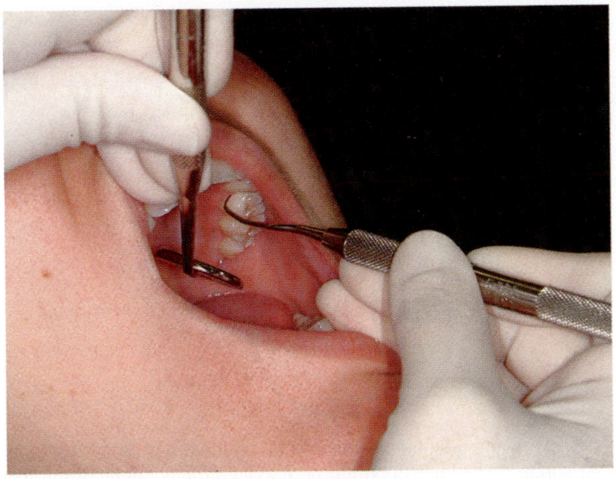

Fig. 35.73 Intraoral opposite-arch finger rest. The fourth finger rests on the mandibular teeth while the maxillary posterior teeth are instrumented.

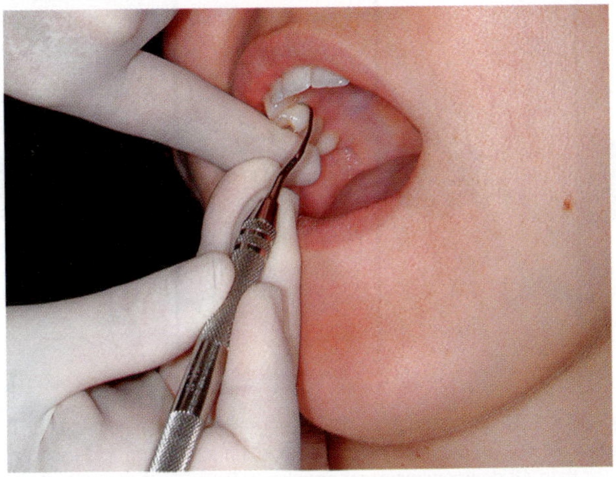

Fig. 35.74 Intraoral finger-on-finger rest. The fourth finger rests on the index finger of the nonoperating hand.

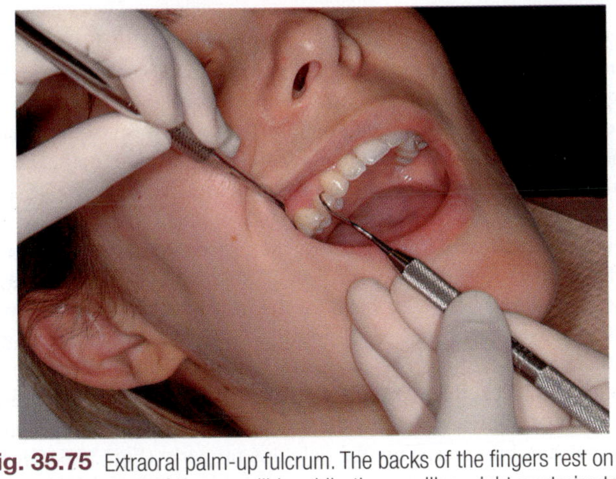

Fig. 35.75 Extraoral palm-up fulcrum. The backs of the fingers rest on the right lateral aspect of the mandible while the maxillary right posterior teeth are instrumented.

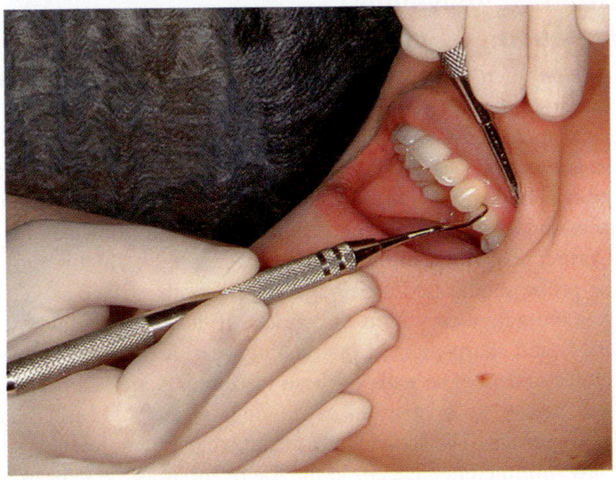

Fig. 35.76 Extraoral palm-down fulcrum. The front surfaces of the fingers rest on the left lateral aspect of the mandible while the maxillary left posterior teeth are instrumented.

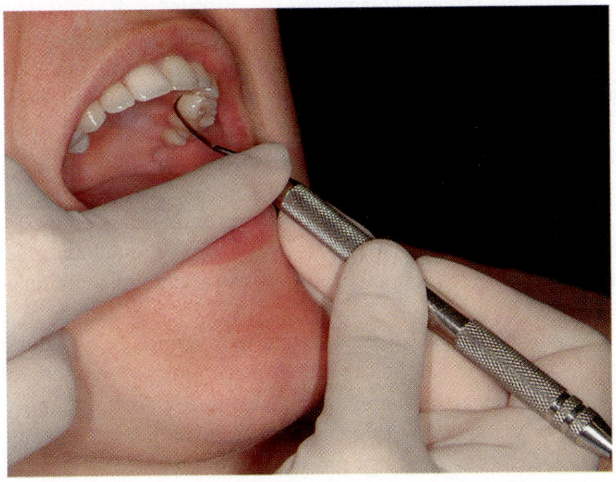

Fig. 35.77 Index finger-reinforced rest. The index finger is placed on the shank for pressure and control in the maxillary left posterior lingual region.

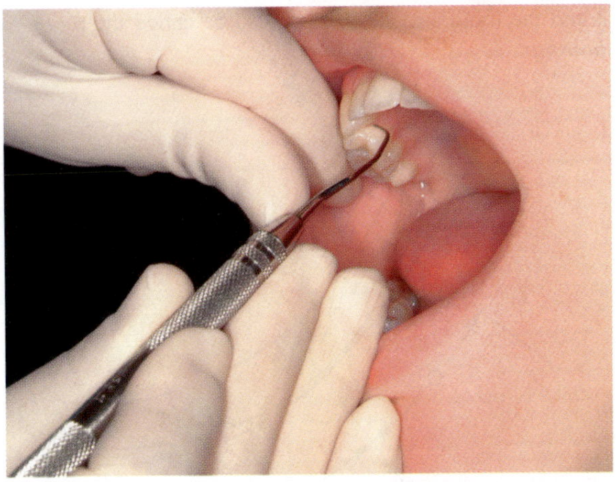

Fig. 35.78 Thumb-reinforced rest. The thumb is placed on the handle for control in the maxillary right posterior lingual region.

2. *Palm down:* The palm-down fulcrum is established by resting the front surfaces of the middle and fourth fingers on the skin overlying the lateral aspect of the mandible on the left side of the face (Fig. 35.76).

Both intraoral finger rests and extraoral fulcrums may be reinforced by applying the index finger or thumb of the nonoperating hand to the handle or shank of the instrument for added control and pressure against the tooth. The reinforcing finger is usually employed for opposite-arch or extraoral fulcrums when precise control and pressure are compromised by the longer distance between the fulcrum and the working end of the instrument. Fig. 35.77 shows the index finger-reinforced rest, and Fig. 35.78 shows the thumb-reinforced rest.

Instrument Activation

Adaptation

Adaptation refers to the manner in which the working end of a periodontal instrument is placed against the surface of a tooth. The objective of adaptation is to make the working end of the instrument conform to the contour of the tooth surface. Precise adaptation must be maintained with all instruments to avoid trauma to the soft tissues and root surfaces and to ensure maximum effectiveness of instrumentation.

Correct adaptation of the probe is quite simple. The tip and side of the probe should be flushed against the tooth surface as vertical strokes are activated within the crevice. Bladed instruments (e.g., curettes) and sharp-pointed instruments (e.g., explorers) are more difficult to adapt. The ends of these instruments are sharp and can lacerate tissue, so adaptation in subgingival areas becomes especially important. The lower third of the working end, which is the last few millimeters adjacent to the toe or tip, must be kept in constant contact with the tooth while it is moving over varying tooth contours (Fig. 35.79). Precise adaptation is maintained by carefully rolling the handle of the instrument against the index and middle fingers with the thumb. This rotates the instrument in slight degrees so that the toe or tip leads into concavities and around convexities. On convex surfaces such as line angles, it is not possible to adapt more than 1 or 2 mm of the working end against the tooth. Even on what appear to be broader, flatter surfaces, no more than 1 or 2 mm of the working end can be adapted because the tooth surface, although it may seem flat, is actually slightly curved.

If only the middle third of the working end is adapted on a convex surface so that the blade contacts the tooth at a tangent, the toe or sharp tip will jut out into soft tissue, causing trauma and discomfort (Fig. 35.80).

If the instrument is adapted so that only the toe or tip is in contact, the soft tissue can be distended or compressed by the back of the working end, also causing trauma and discomfort. A curette that is improperly adapted in this manner can be particularly damaging because the toe can gouge or groove the root surface.

Angulation

Angulation refers to the angle between the face of a bladed instrument and the tooth surface. It may also be called the *tooth–blade relationship*.

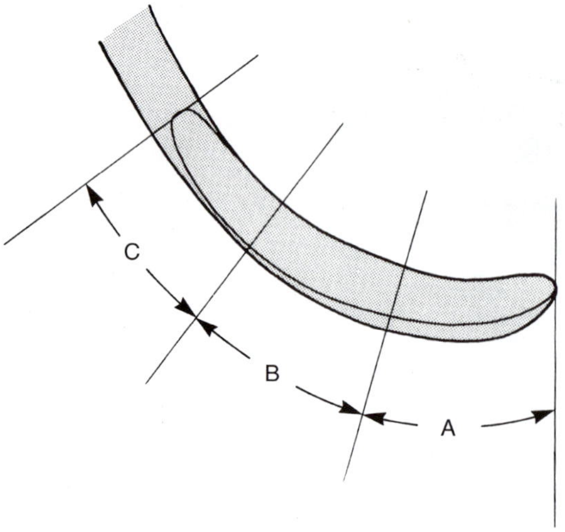

Fig. 35.79 Gracey curette blade divided into three segments. A, The lower one-third of the blade, consisting of the terminal few millimeters adjacent to the toe; B, the middle one-third; and, C, the upper one-third, which is adjacent to the shank.

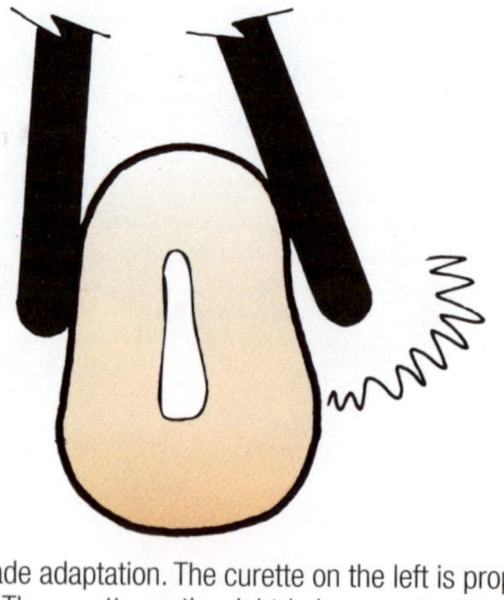

Fig. 35.80 Blade adaptation. The curette on the left is properly adapted to the root surface. The curette on the right is incorrectly adapted; the toe juts out, lacerating the soft tissues.

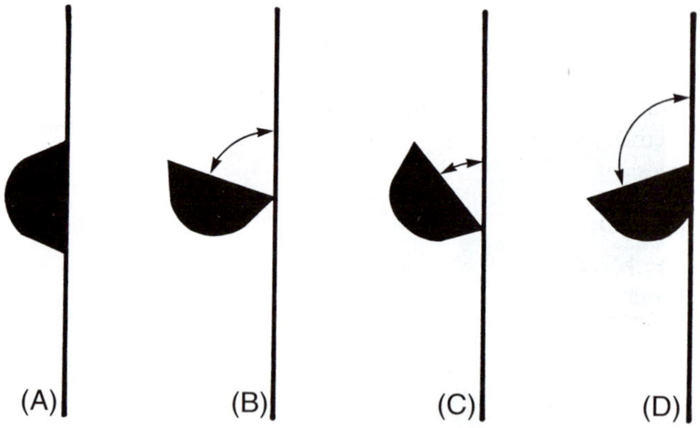

Fig. 35.81 Blade angulation. A, 0 degree: correct angulation for blade insertion. B, 45–90 degrees: correct angulation for scaling and root planing. C, Less than 45 degrees: incorrect angulation for scaling and root planing. D, More than 90 degrees: incorrect angulation for scaling and root planing, correct angulation for gingival curettage.

Correct angulation is essential for effective calculus removal. For subgingival insertion of a bladed instrument such as a curette, angulation should be as close to 0 degree as possible (Fig. 35.81A). The end of the instrument can be inserted to the base of the pocket more easily with the face of the blade flush against the tooth. During scaling and root planing, optimal angulation is between 45 and 90 degrees (Fig. 35.81B). The exact blade angulation depends on the amount and nature of the calculus, the procedure being performed, and the condition of the tissue. Blade angulation is diminished or closed by tilting the lower shank of the instrument toward the tooth. It is increased or opened by tilting the lower shank away from the tooth. During scaling strokes on heavy, tenacious calculus, angulation should be just less than 90 degrees so that the cutting edge "bites" into the calculus. With angulation of less than 45 degrees, the cutting edge will not bite into or engage the calculus properly (Fig. 35.81C). Instead, it will slide over the calculus, smoothing or "burnishing" it. If angulation is more than 90 degrees, the lateral surface of the blade, rather than the cutting edge, will be against the tooth, and the calculus will not be removed and may become burnished (Fig. 35.81D). After the calculus has been removed, angulation of just less than 90 degrees may be maintained, or the angle may be slightly closed as the root surface is smoothed with light, root-planing strokes.

When gingival curettage is indicated, angulation greater than 90 degrees is deliberately established so that the cutting edge will engage and remove the pocket lining (Fig. 35.81D).

Lateral Pressure

Lateral pressure refers to the pressure created when force is applied against the surface of a tooth with the cutting edge of a bladed instrument. The exact amount of pressure applied must be varied according to the nature of the calculus and according to whether the stroke is intended for initial scaling to remove calculus or for root planing to smooth the root surface.

Lateral pressure may be firm, moderate, or light. When removing calculus, lateral pressure is initially applied firmly or moderately and is progressively diminished until light lateral pressure is applied for the final root-planing strokes. When insufficient lateral pressure is applied for the removal of heavy calculus, rough ledges or lumps may be shaved to thin, smooth sheets of burnished calculus that are difficult to detect and remove. This burnishing effect often occurs in areas of developmental depressions and along the cementoenamel junction.

Although firm lateral pressure is necessary for the thorough removal of calculus, indiscriminate, unwarranted, or uncontrolled application of heavy forces during instrumentation should be avoided. Repeated application of excessively heavy strokes often nicks or gouges the root surface.

The careful application of varied and controlled amounts of lateral pressure during instrumentation is an integral part of effective scaling and root-planing techniques and is critical to the success of both these procedures.

Strokes

Three basic types of strokes are used during instrumentation: the exploratory stroke, the scaling stroke, and the root-planing stroke. Any of these basic strokes may be activated by a pull or a push motion in a vertical, oblique, or horizontal direction (Fig. 35.82). *Vertical* and *oblique* strokes are used most frequently. *Horizontal* strokes are used selectively on line angles or deep pockets that cannot be negotiated with vertical or oblique strokes. The direction, length, pressure, and number of strokes necessary for either scaling or root planing are determined by four major factors: (1) gingival position and tone, (2) pocket depth and shape, (3) tooth contour, and (4) the amount and nature of the calculus or roughness.

The *exploratory stroke* is a light, "feeling" stroke that is used with probes and explorers to evaluate the dimensions of the pocket and to detect calculus and irregularities of the tooth surface. With bladed instruments such as the curette, the exploratory stroke is alternated with scaling and root-planing strokes for these same purposes of evaluation and detection. The instrument is grasped lightly and adapted with light pressure against the tooth to achieve maximal tactile sensitivity.

The *scaling stroke* is a short, powerful pull stroke that is used with bladed instruments for the removal of both supragingival and subgingival calculus. The muscles of the fingers and hands are tensed to establish a secure grasp, and lateral pressure is firmly applied against the tooth surface. The cutting edge engages the apical border of the calculus and dislodges it with a firm movement in a coronal direction. The scaling motion should be initiated in the forearm and transmitted from the wrist to the hand with a slight flexing of the fingers. Rotation of the wrist is synchronized with movement of the forearm. The scaling stroke is neither initiated in the wrist or fingers nor is it carried out independently without the use of the forearm.

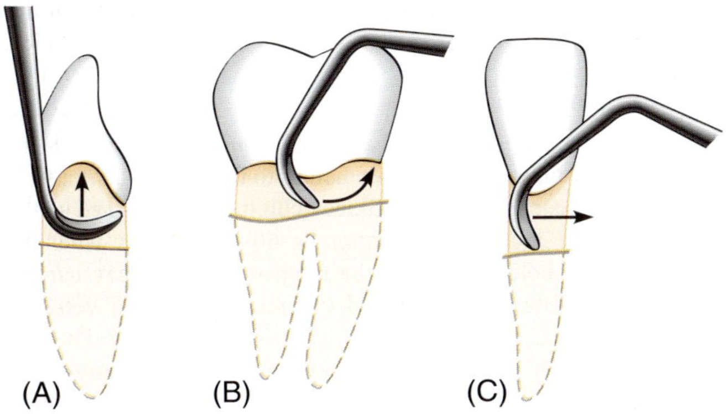

Fig. 35.82 Three basic stroke directions. A, Vertical; B, oblique; C, horizontal.

It is possible to initiate the scaling motion by rotating the wrist and forearm or by flexing the fingers. The use of wrist and forearm action versus finger motion has long been debated among clinicians. Perhaps the strong opinions on both sides should be the most valid indication that there is a time and a place for each. Neither method can be advocated exclusively because a careful analysis of effective scaling and root-planing technique reveals that both types of stroke activation are necessary for complete instrumentation. The wrist and forearm motion, pivoting in an arc on the finger rest, produces a more powerful stroke and is therefore preferred for scaling. *Finger flexing* is indicated for precise control over stroke length in areas such as line angles and when horizontal strokes are used on the lingual or facial aspects of narrow-rooted teeth.

The *push scaling* motion has been advocated by some clinicians. In the push stroke, the instrument engages the lateral or coronal border of the calculus, and the fingers provide a thrust motion that dislodges the deposit. Since the push stroke may force calculus into the supporting tissues, its use, especially in an apical direction, is not recommended.

The *root-planing stroke* is a moderate to light pull stroke that is used for final smoothing and planing of the root surface. Although hoes, files, and ultrasonic instruments have been used for root planing, curettes are widely acknowledged to be the most effective and versatile instruments for this procedure. The design of the curette, which allows it to be more easily adapted to subgingival tooth contours, makes curettes particularly suitable for root planing in periodontal patients. With a moderately firm grasp, the curette is kept adapted to the tooth with even, lateral pressure. A continuous series of long, overlapping shaving strokes is activated. As the surface becomes smoother and resistance diminishes, lateral pressure is progressively reduced.

Instruments for Scaling and Root Planing

Universal Curettes

The working ends of the universal curette are designed in pairs so that all surfaces of the teeth can be treated with one double-ended instrument or a matched pair of single-ended instruments (Fig. 35.16).

In any given quadrant, when approaching the tooth from the facial aspect, one end of the universal curette adapts to the mesial surfaces and the other end adapts to the distal surfaces. When approaching from the lingual aspect in the same quadrant, the double-ended universal curette must be turned end for end because the blades are mirror images. This means that the end that adapts to the mesial surfaces on the facial aspect also adapts to the distal surfaces on the lingual aspect, and vice versa. Both ends of the universal curette are used for instrumentation of the anterior teeth. On posterior teeth, however, because of the limited access to distal surfaces, a single working end can be used to treat both mesial and distal surfaces by using both its cutting edges. To do this, the instrument is first adapted to the mesial surface with the handle nearly parallel to the mesial surface. Since the face of the universal curette blade is honed at 90 degrees to the lower shank, if the lower shank is positioned so that it is absolutely parallel to the surface being

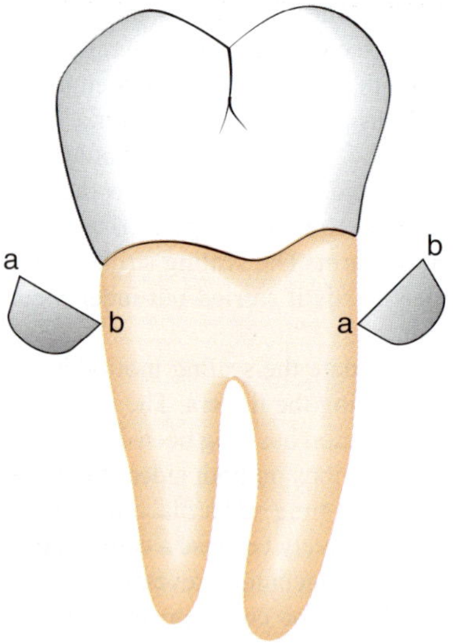

Fig. 35.83 Adaptation of the universal curette on a posterior tooth. Cross-sectional representations of the same universal curette blade as its cutting edges (A and B) are adapted to the mesial and distal surfaces of a posterior tooth.

instrumented, the tooth-blade angulation is 90 degrees. To close this angle and thus obtain proper working angulation, the lower shank must be tilted slightly toward the tooth. The distal surface of the same posterior tooth can be instrumented with the opposite cutting edge of the same blade. This cutting edge can be adapted at proper working angulation by positioning the handle so that it is *perpendicular* to the distal surface (Fig. 35.83).

When adapting the universal curette blade, as much of the cutting edge as possible, should be in contact with the tooth surface, except on narrow convex surfaces such as line angles. Although the entire cutting edge should contact the tooth, pressure should be concentrated on the lower third of the blade during scaling strokes. During root-planing strokes, however, lateral pressure should be distributed evenly along the cutting edge.

The primary advantage of these curettes is that they are designed to be used universally on all tooth surfaces in all regions of the mouth. However, universal curettes have limited adaptability for the treatment of deep pockets in which apical migration of the attachment has exposed furcations, root convexities, and developmental depressions. For this reason, many clinicians prefer the Gracey curettes and the new modifications of Gracey curettes, which are area specific and specially designed for subgingival scaling and root planing in periodontal patients.

Gracey Curettes

As discussed earlier, Gracey curettes are a set of area-specific instruments that were designed by Dr Clayton H. Gracey of Michigan in the mid-1930s (Fig. 35.18). Four design features make the Gracey curettes unique: (1) they are area specific, (2) only one cutting edge on each blade is used, (3) the blade is curved in two planes, and (4) the blade is "offset" (Table 35.1) Each of these features directly influences the manner in which the Gracey curettes are used, as discussed next.

Area Specificity

There are seven pairs of curettes in the set. The Gracey curettes #1–2 and # 3–4 are used on anterior teeth. The Gracey #5–6 may be used on both anterior and premolar teeth. The facial and lingual surfaces of posterior teeth are instrumented with Gracey curettes #7–8 and #9–10. The Gracey #11–12 is designed for mesial surfaces of posterior teeth, and the #13–14 adapts to the distal surfaces of posterior teeth. Although these guidelines for areas of use were originally established by Dr Gracey, it is possible to use a Gracey curette in an area of the mouth other than the one for which it was specifically designed if the general principles regarding these curettes are understood and applied. Gracey curettes need not be reserved exclusively for periodontal patients. In fact, many clinicians prefer Gracey curettes for general scaling because of their excellent adaptability.

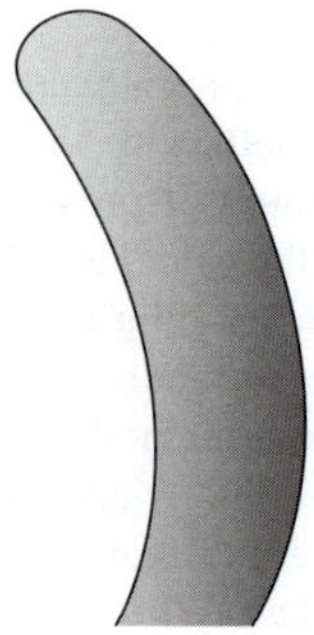

Fig. 35.84 Determining the correct cutting edge of a Gracey curette. When viewed from directly above the face of the blade, the correct cutting edge is the one forming the larger, outer curve on the right.

Single Cutting Edge Used

As with a universal curette, the Gracey curette has a blade with two cutting edges. Unlike the universal curette, however, the Gracey instrument is designed so that only one cutting edge is used. To determine which of the two is the correct cutting edge to adapt to the tooth, the blade should be held face up and parallel to the floor. When viewed from this angle, the blade can be seen to curve to the side. One cutting edge forms a larger outer curve, and the other forms a shorter, small inner curve. The larger outer curve, which has also been described as the "inferior cutting edge" or as the cutting edge farther away from the handle, is the correct cutting edge (Fig. 35.84).

Blade Curves in Two Planes

As with the toe of the universal curette, the toe of the Gracey curette curves upward. However, the toe of the Gracey curette also curves to the side, as previously mentioned. This unique curvature enhances the blade's adaptation to convexities and concavities as the working end is advanced around the tooth. Only the lower third or half of the Gracey blade is in contact with the tooth during instrumentation. The cutting edge of a universal curette blade, however, is straight and does not curve to the side, making it less adaptable to root concavities.

Offset Blade

Gracey curette blades are honed at an *offset angle*, which means that the face of the blade is not perpendicular to the lower shank as it is on a universal curette. Instead, Gracey curettes are designed so that the tooth-blade working angulation is 60–70 degrees when the lower shank is held parallel to the tooth surface. Gracey curettes were originally designed to be used with *push strokes* and were beveled to provide a tooth-blade angulation of 40 degrees when the lower shank was parallel to the tooth surface; for many years, Gracey curettes were available only in this form. Currently, Gracey curettes are available not only in the original push design but also in a modified version to be used with pull strokes. It is important to understand this when purchasing Gracey curettes to avoid obtaining instruments that are not properly designed for *pull strokes*. If Gracey curettes that are designed to be used with push strokes are used with pull strokes instead, they are likely to burnish calculus rather than completely remove it. The design of the Gracey curette was modified in response to requests from clinicians who liked the shank design and adaptability of the original Gracey instruments but were opposed to the use of push strokes for scaling and root planing. The push stroke is not recommended, especially for the novice clinician, because it is likely to cause undue trauma to the junctional epithelium and to embed fragments of dislodged calculus in the soft tissues.

Principles of Use

The following general principles of use of the Gracey curettes are essentially the same as those for the universal curette; italicized principles apply only to Gracey curettes:

1. *Determine the correct cutting edge.* The correct cutting edge should be determined by visually inspecting the blade and confirmed by lightly adapting the chosen cutting edge to the tooth with the lower shank parallel to the surface of the tooth. With the toe pointed in the direction to be scaled (e.g., mesially with a #7–8 curette), only the back of the blade can be seen if the correct cutting edge has been selected (Fig. 35.85). If the wrong cutting edge has been adopted, the flat, shiny face of the blade will be seen instead (Fig. 35.86).
2. *Make sure the lower shank is parallel to the surface to be instrumented.* The lower shank of a Gracey curette is that portion of the shank between the blade and the first bend in the shank. Parallelism of the handle or upper shank is not an acceptable guide with Gracey curettes because the angulations of the shanks vary. On anterior teeth, the lower shank of the Gracey #1–2, 3–4, or # 5–6 should be parallel to the mesial, distal, facial, or lingual surfaces of the teeth (Fig. 35.87). On posterior teeth the lower shank of the #7–8 or # 9–10 should be parallel to the facial or lingual surfaces of the teeth (Fig. 35.88); the lower shank of the #11–12 should be parallel to the mesial surfaces of the teeth (Fig. 35.89); and the lower shank of the #13–14 should be parallel to the distal surfaces of the teeth (Fig. 35.90).
3. When using intraoral finger rests, keep the fourth and middle fingers together in a built-up fulcrum for maximum control and wrist-arm action.
4. Use extraoral fulcrums or mandibular finger rests for optimal angulation when working on the maxillary posterior teeth.

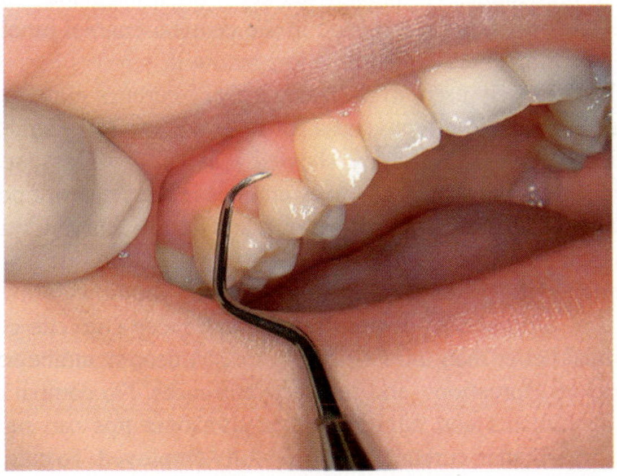

Fig. 35.85 Correct cutting edge of a Gracey curette adapted to the tooth.

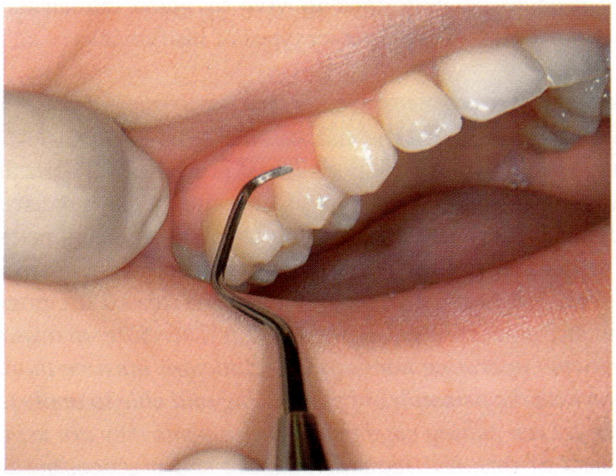

Fig. 35.86 Incorrect cutting edge of a Gracey curette adapted to the tooth.

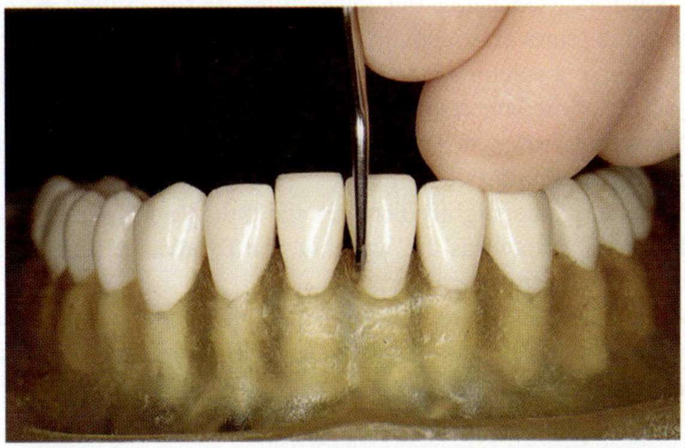

Fig. 35.87 Gracey #5–6 curette adapted to an anterior tooth. *(Copyright A. Pattison.)*

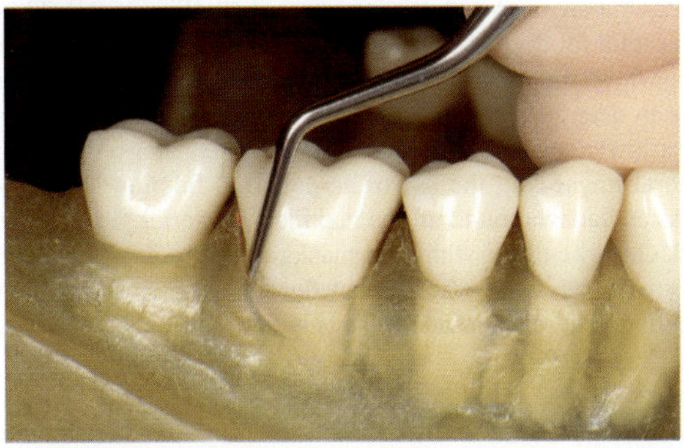

Fig. 35.88 Gracey #7–8 curette adapted to the facial surface of a posterior tooth. *(Copyright A. Pattison.)*

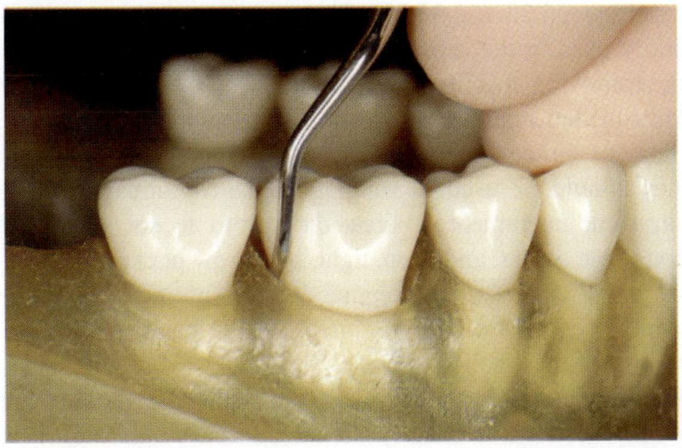

Fig. 35.89 Gracey #11–12 curette adapted to the mesial surface of a posterior tooth. *(Copyright A. Pattison.)*

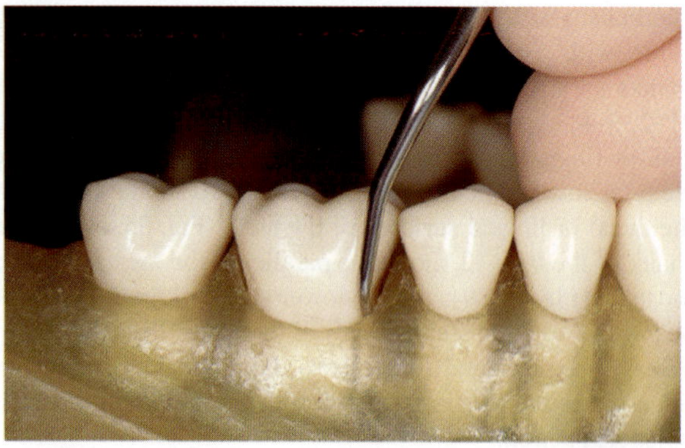

Fig. 35.90 Gracey #13–14 curette adapted to the distal surface of a posterior tooth. *(Copyright A. Pattison.)*

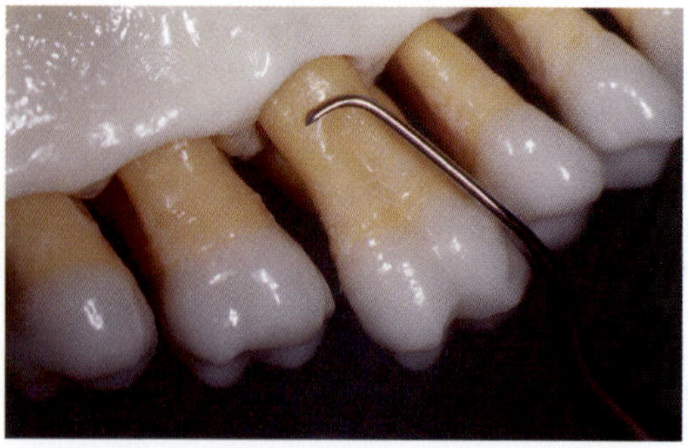

Fig. 35.91 Mini Five #13–14 curette adapted to the palatal surface of a maxillary molar with the toe directed distally. *(Copyright A. Pattison.)*

5. Concentrate on using the lower third of the cutting edge for calculus removal, especially on line angles or when attempting to remove a calculus ledge by breaking it away in sections, beginning at the lateral edge.
6. Allow the wrist and forearm to carry the burden of the stroke rather than flexing the fingers.
7. Roll the handle slightly between the thumb and fingers to keep the blade adapted as the working end is advanced around line angles and into concavities.
8. Modulate lateral pressure from firm to moderate to light depending on the nature of the calculus and reduce pressure as the transition is made from scaling to root-planing strokes.

Extended-Shank Gracey Curettes

Extended-shank Gracey curettes, such as the After Five curettes, are 3-mm longer in the terminal shank than the standard Gracey curettes but are used with the same technique (Fig. 35.23). They are most useful for deep pockets on maxillary and mandibular posterior teeth, where the longer terminal shank allows better access, especially to deep mesial and distal pockets (Fig. 35.24). Although the longer lower shank makes access easier while using a conventional intraoral finger rest, the use of an extraoral fulcrum allows better access and adaptation to all the maxillary posterior teeth. Extended shank Gracey curettes with rigid shanks should be used for scaling of heavy calculus; those with regular, finishing shanks should be used for periodontal maintenance patients with deep residual pockets.

Mini-Bladed Gracey Curettes

Mini-bladed Gracey curettes, such as the Mini Five curettes and the Gracey Curvettes, have a terminal shank that is 3-mm longer than the standard Gracey curettes and a blade that is 50% shorter. Micro Mini Five curette blades are 20% smaller than Mini Five curette blades (Figs. 35.28 and 35.29). These mini-bladed instruments are generally used in the same manner as the Gracey curettes, except for the following specific differences:

1. Mini-bladed curettes should not be used routinely in place of standard Gracey or extended shank Gracey curettes. Instead, they should be used to supplement conventional curettes and ultrasonic instruments in areas difficult to access, such as furcations, line angles, and deep, tight, or narrow pockets (Fig. 35.30).
2. Large #4 handles are recommended for any mini-bladed instruments because the larger diameter of the handles allows better control of the small blades.
3. Mini-bladed curettes can be used to scale with the toe directed either mesially or distally. In fact, these curettes often adapt more effectively to the root curvatures of many posterior teeth when the blade is inserted with the toe pointed distally and when strokes are activated from the mesial toward the distal line angle (Fig. 35.91).
4. Use rigid-shank mini-bladed curettes for calculus removal. Use the thinner, standard-shank mini-bladed curettes for deplaquing during maintenance.
5. When using mini-bladed curettes for calculus removal, use intraoral finger rests close to the working area. When performing light root planing or deplaquing, either intraoral rests or extraoral fulcrums may be used. Extraoral fulcrums are usually necessary to gain access to deep pockets on maxillary second and third molars.
6. Mini-bladed curettes are generally used with straight, vertical strokes. They may also be used with oblique or horizontal strokes, but because of the shortness of the blade, these strokes might not extend far enough subgingivally unless the tissue is very retractable. Horizontal strokes with mini-bladed curettes are most effective when used in the cementoenamel junction or in developmental depressions just below it.

When properly used, mini-bladed Gracey curettes allow unprecedented access and effectiveness for both nonsurgical and surgical root debridement. One study showed that Gracey Curvettes performed better than standard Gracey curettes in deep anterior pockets. In areas such as line angles, furcations, and narrow, curved, facial, or palatal root surfaces, these miniature curettes provide excellent adaptation with better tactile sensitivity than modified, slim ultrasonic tips. Studies also demonstrated that Gracey Curvette curettes performed better than ultrasonic slim tips on deep mandibular anterior pockets, furcations, and furcation entrances. No comparison of hand instruments and modified, slim ultrasonic tips can be made unless mini-bladed curettes have been fully employed. To date, some research has been done to compare the effectiveness of mini-bladed instruments with the modified, slim ultrasonic tips. More of these studies need to be performed in vivo to guide clinicians in the optimal utilization of these newer types of instruments.

Instrument Sharpening

It is impossible to carry out periodontal procedures efficiently with dull instruments. A sharp instrument cuts more precisely and quickly than a dull instrument. To do its job at all, a dull instrument must be held more firmly and pressed harder than a sharp instrument. This reduces tactile sensitivity and increases the possibility that the instrument will inadvertently slip. *Therefore, to avoid wasting time and operating haphazardly, clinicians must be thoroughly familiar with the principles of sharpening and able to apply them to produce a keen cutting edge on the instruments they are using.* Development of this skill requires patience and practice, but clinical excellence cannot be attained without it.

Evaluation of Sharpness

The *cutting edge* of an instrument is formed by the angular junction of two surfaces of its blade. The cutting edges of a curette, for example, are formed where the face of the blade meets the lateral surfaces (Fig. 35.92).

When the instrument is sharp, this junction is a fine line running the length of the cutting edge. As the instrument is used, metal is worn away at the cutting edge, and the junction of the face and lateral surface becomes rounded or dulled (Fig. 35.93). Thus, the cutting edge becomes a rounded surface rather than an acute angle, which is why a dull instrument cuts less efficiently and requires more pressure to do its job.

Sharpness can be evaluated by sight and touch in one of the following ways:

1. When a dull instrument is held under a light, the rounded surface of its cutting edge reflects light back to the observer. It appears as a bright line running the length of the cutting edge (Fig. 35.94). The acutely angled cutting edge of a sharp instrument, conversely, has no surface area to reflect light. When a sharp instrument is held under a light, no bright line can be observed (Fig. 35.92).
2. Tactile evaluation of sharpness is performed by drawing the instrument lightly across an acrylic rod known as a "sharpening test stick." A dull instrument will slide smoothly without "biting" into the surface and raising a light shaving as a sharp instrument would.

Objective of Sharpening

The objective of sharpening is to restore the fine, thin, linear cutting edge of the instrument. This is done by grinding the surfaces of the blade until their junction is once again sharply angular rather than rounded. For any given instrument, several sharpening techniques may produce this result. A technique is acceptable if it produces a sharp cutting edge without unduly wearing the instrument or altering its original design. To maintain the original design, the operator must understand the location and course of the cutting edges and the angles between the surfaces that form them. It is important to restore the cutting edge without distorting the original angles of the instrument. When these angles have been altered, the instrument does not function as it was designed to function, which limits its effectiveness.

Sharpening Stones

Sharpening stones may be quarried from natural mineral deposits or produced artificially. In either case, the surface of the stone is made up of abrasive crystals that are harder than the metal of the instrument to be sharpened. Coarse stones have larger particles and cut more rapidly; they are used on instruments that are dull. Finer stones with smaller crystals cut more slowly and are reserved for final sharpening to produce a finer edge and for sharpening instruments that are only slightly dull. India and Arkansas oilstones are examples of natural abrasive stones. Carborundum, ruby, and ceramic stones are synthetically produced (Fig. 35.95).

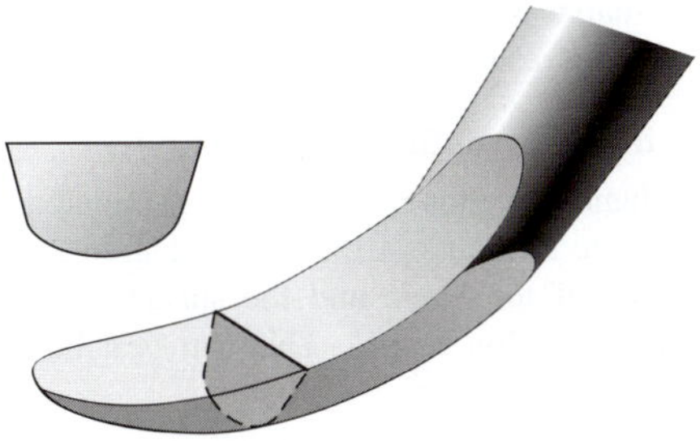

Fig. 35.92 The cutting edge of a curette is formed by the angular junction of the face and the lateral surfaces of the instrument. When the instrument is sharp, the cutting edge is a fine line.

Fig. 35.93 The cutting edge of a dull curette is rounded.

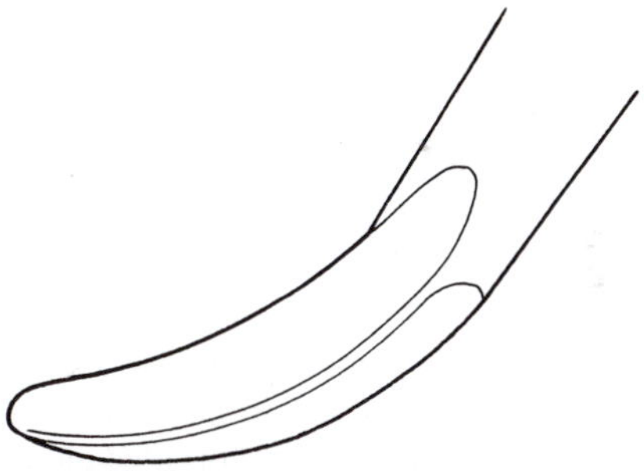

Fig. 35.94 Light reflected from the rounded cutting edge of a dull instrument appears as a bright line.

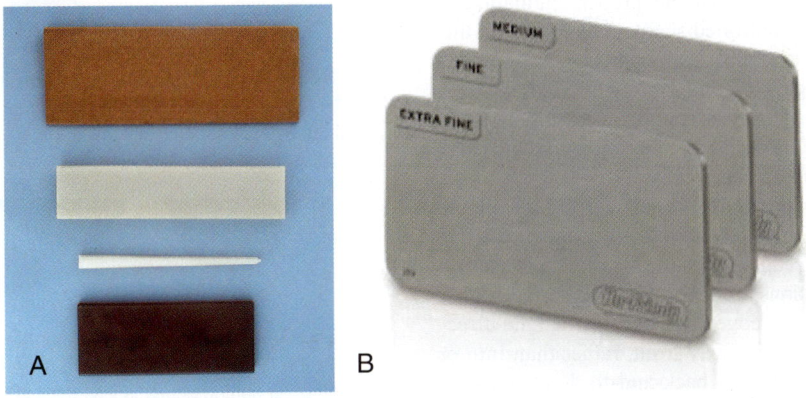

Fig. 35.95 A, Sharpening stones. *Top* to *bottom*, a flat India stone, a flat Arkansas stone, a cone-shaped Arkansas stone, and a ceramic stone. B, Diamond sharpening cards. *Left to right*, extra fine grit, fine grit and medium grit one-sided diamond sharpening cards. (*Courtesy: Hu-Friedy, Chicago, IL.*)

Sharpening stones can also be categorized by their method of use.

Mounted Rotary Stones

These stones are mounted on a metal mandrel and used in a motor-driven handpiece. They may be cylindrical, conical, or disk shaped. These stones are generally not recommended for routine use because they (1) are difficult to control precisely and can ruin the shape of the instrument, (2) tend to wear down the instrument quickly, and (3) can generate considerable frictional heat, which may affect the temper of the instrument.

Unmounted Stones

Unmounted stones come in a variety of sizes and shapes. Some are rectangular with flat or grooved surfaces, whereas others are cylindrical or cone shaped. Unmounted stones may be used in two ways: the instrument may be stabilized and held stationary while the stone is drawn across it, or the stone may be stabilized and held stationary while the instrument is drawn across it.

Diamond Sharpening Cards

The abrasive surface of the diamond sharpening card is made up of small, industrial-grade diamonds coated onto one or both sides of a stainless steel card. Three grits are available: extra fine, fine, and medium (Fig. 35.95B). The medium card has somewhat larger diamond crystals. These sharpen faster and are used to recondition instruments that are very dull. Fine-grit cards are used for routine sharpening, and extra fine is used to further refine an already sharp instrument. One advantage of diamond sharpening cards is that the surface does not wear away with use the way conventional stones do. The durable surface remains flat even after repeated use. Another advantage is that these cards do not require lubrication. They can be used dry or moistened with water. Oil is not required. Diamond sharpening cards can be cleaned in an ultrasonic instrument cleaner or scrubbed and rinsed with water to remove metal filings. They are sterilized in a steam autoclave between uses.

Principles of Sharpening

1. Choose a stone suitable for the instrument to be sharpened—one that is of an appropriate shape and abrasiveness.
2. Use a sterilized sharpening stone if the instrument to be sharpened will not be resterilized before it is used on a patient.
3. Establish the proper angle between the sharpening stone and the surface of the instrument on the basis of an understanding of its design.
4. Maintain a stable, firm grasp of both the instrument and the sharpening stone. This ensures that the proper angulation is maintained throughout the controlled sharpening stroke. In this manner, the entire surface of the instrument can be reduced evenly, and the cutting edge is not improperly beveled.
5. Avoid excessive pressure. Heavy pressure causes the stone to grind the surface of the instrument more quickly and may shorten the instrument's life unnecessarily.
6. Avoid the formation of a "wire edge," characterized by minute filamentous projections of metal extending as a roughened ledge from the sharpened cutting edge. When the instrument is used on root surfaces, these projections produce a grooved surface rather than a smooth surface. A wire edge is produced when the direction of the sharpening stroke is away from, rather than into or toward, the cutting edge. When back-and-forth or up-and-down sharpening strokes are used, formation of a wire edge can be avoided by finishing with a down stroke toward the cutting edge.
7. Lubricate the stone during sharpening. This minimizes clogging of the abrasive surface of the sharpening stone with metal particles removed from the instrument. It also reduces heat produced by friction. Oil should be used for natural stones and water for synthetic stones.
8. Sharpen instruments at the first sign of dullness. A grossly dull instrument is inefficient and requires more pressure when used, which hinders control. Furthermore, sharpening such an instrument requires the removal of a great deal of metal to produce a sharp cutting edge. This shortens the effective life of the instrument.

Sharpening Individual Instruments

Universal Curettes

Several techniques will produce a properly sharpened curette. Regardless of the technique used, the clinician must keep in mind that the angle between the face of the blade and the lateral surface of any curette is 70–80 degrees (Fig. 35.96). This is the most effective design for removing calculus and root planing (Fig. 35.97A). Changing this angle distorts the design of the instrument and makes it less effective. A cutting edge of less than 70 degrees is quite sharp but also thin (Fig. 35.97B). It wears down quickly and becomes dull. A cutting edge of 90 degrees or more requires heavy lateral pressure to remove deposits (Fig. 35.97C). Calculus removal with such an instrument is often incomplete, and root planing cannot be done effectively.

The following technique is recommended because it enables the clinician to visualize the critical 70–80 degree angle easily and thereby consistently restores an effective cutting edge:

Sharpening the Lateral Surface

When a flat, handheld stone is correctly applied to the lateral surface of a curette to maintain the 70–80 degree angle, the angle between the face of the blade and the surface of the stone will be 100–110 degrees (Fig. 35.96). This can best be visualized by

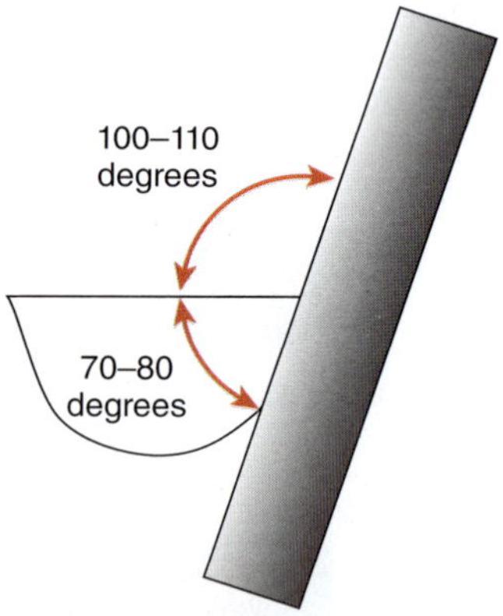

Fig. 35.96 When the sharpening stone forms a 100–110-degree angle with the face of the blade, the 70–80-degree angle between the face and the lateral surface is automatically preserved.

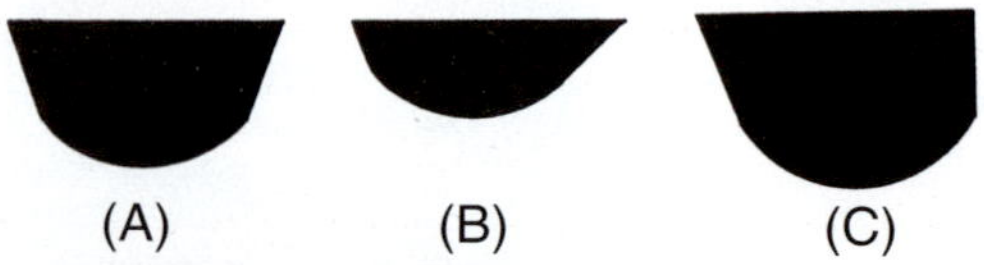

Fig. 35.97 A, Properly sharpened curette maintains a 70–80-degree angle between its face and lateral surface. B, Curette has been sharpened so that one of its cutting edges is less than 70 degrees. This fine edge is quite sharp but dulls easily. C, One of the cutting edges of the curette has been sharpened to 90 degrees. Heavy lateral pressure must be applied to the tooth to remove deposits with such an instrument.

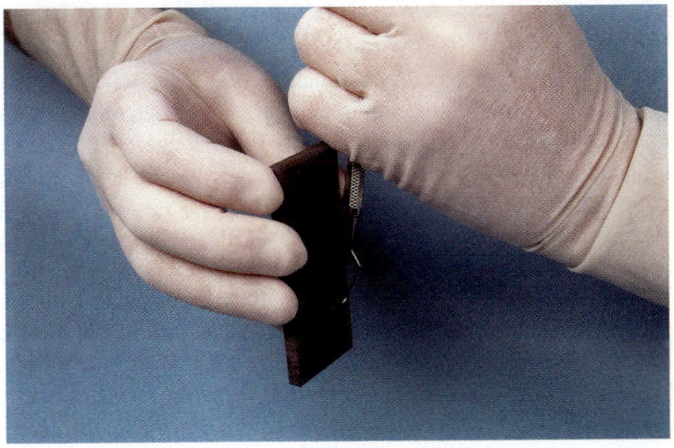

Fig. 35.98 Using a palm grasp, operator holds the universal curette so that the face of the blade is parallel to the floor. The stone makes a 100–110-degree angle with the face of the blade.

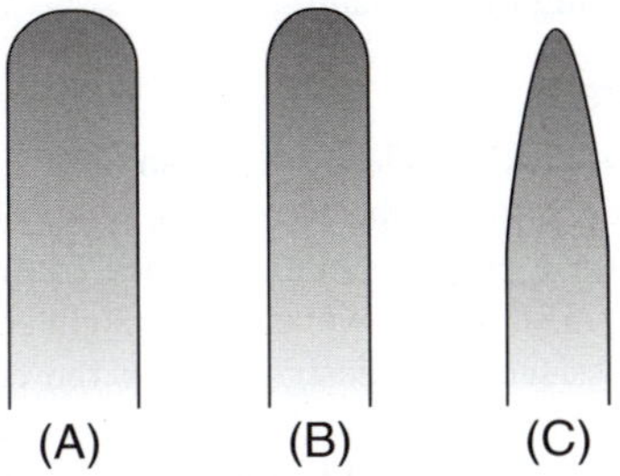

Fig. 35.99 A, New, unsharpened curette viewed from directly above the face of the blade. B, curette has been correctly sharpened to maintain the rounded toe. C, curette has been incorrectly sharpened, producing a pointed toe.

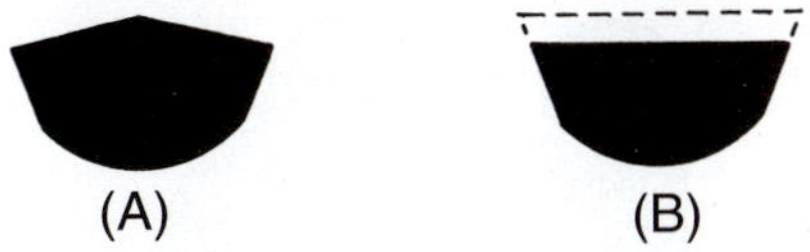

Fig. 35.100 A, Angulation is difficult to control when sharpening the face of the blade and often results in unwanted beveling. B, Sharpening the face also weakens the blade by narrowing it from face to back.

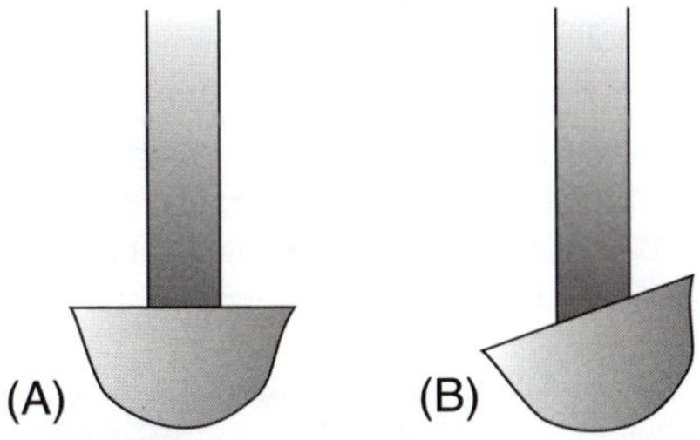

Fig. 35.101 A, Face of a universal curette is at 90 degrees to its shank. B, Face of a Gracey curette is offset, forming a 70-degree angle with its shank.

holding the curette so that the face of the blade is parallel with the floor. A palm grasp should be used and the upper arm braced against the body for support.

1. Apply the sharpening stone to the lateral surface of the curette so that the angle between the face of the blade and the stone is 100–110 degrees (Fig. 35.98; see also Fig. 35.96).
2. Beginning at the shank end of the cutting edge and working toward the toe, activate the stone with short, up-and-down strokes. Use consistent, light pressure and keep the stone continuously in contact with the blade. Make sure that the 100–110-degree angle is constantly maintained (Fig. 35.98).
3. Check for sharpness as previously described and continue sharpening as necessary. To prevent the toe of the curette from becoming pointed, sharpen the entire blade from shank end to toe. When approaching the toe, be sure to sharpen around it to preserve its rounded form (Fig. 35.99).
4. As the stone is moved along the cutting edge, finish each section with a down stroke into or toward the cutting edge; this will minimize the formation of a wire edge. Check the cutting edge under a light.
5. Sharpening the curette in this manner tends to flatten the lateral surface. This can be corrected by lightly grinding the lateral surface and the back of the instrument, away from the cutting edge, each time the instrument is sharpened.
6. When one edge has been properly sharpened, the opposite cutting edge can be sharpened in the same manner.

Sharpening the Face of the Blade

This may be done by moving a handheld cylindrical or cone-shaped stone back and forth across the face of the blade. A similar stone mounted in a handpiece may also be used by applying it to the face of the blade with the stone rotating toward the toe. These methods are not recommended for routine use for the following reasons:

1. The angulation between the instrument and the stone is difficult to maintain, and therefore the blade may be improperly beveled (Fig. 35.100A).
2. Sharpening the face of the blade narrows the working end from face to back. This weakens the blade and makes it likely to bend or break while in use (Fig. 35.100B).
3. Sharpening the face of the blade with a handheld stone using a back-and-forth motion produces a wire edge that interferes with the sharpness of the blade.

Area-Specific (Gracey) Curettes

As with a universal curette, a Gracey curette has an angle of 70–80 degrees between the face and lateral surface of its blade. Therefore, the technique described for sharpening a universal curette can be used to sharpen a Gracey curette. However, several unique design features that distinguish a Gracey from a universal curette must be understood to avoid distorting the design of the instrument while sharpening (see earlier discussion).

As previously noted, Gracey curettes have an offset blade; that is, the face of the blade is not perpendicular to the shank of the instrument as it is on a universal curette but is offset at a 70-degree angle (Fig. 35.101). A Gracey curette is further distinguished by the curvature of its cutting edges. When viewed from directly above the face of the blade, the cutting edges of a universal curette extend in straight lines from shank to toe; both cutting edges can be used for scaling and root planing. The cutting edges of a Gracey curette, conversely, curve gently from shank to toe, and only the larger, outer cutting edge is used for scaling and root planing (Fig. 35.102).

With these points in mind, a Gracey curette is sharpened in the following manner:

1. Hold the curette so that the face of the blade is parallel with the floor. Since the blade is offset, the shank of the instrument will not be perpendicular to the floor as it is with universal curettes (Fig. 35.103).
2. Identify the edge to be sharpened. Remember that only one cutting edge is used, so only that edge must be sharpened (Fig. 35.104, left). Apply the stone to the lateral surface so that

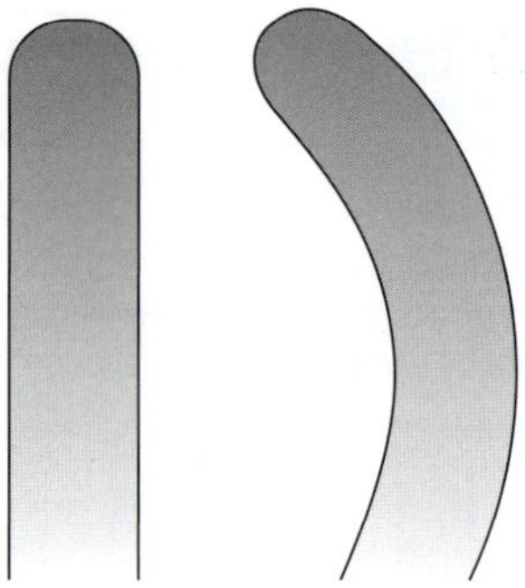

Fig. 35.102 Cutting edges of a universal curette extend straight from shank to toe. The cutting edges of a Gracey curette gently curve from shank to toe. Only the larger, outer cutting edge at the right is used for scaling and needs to be sharpened.

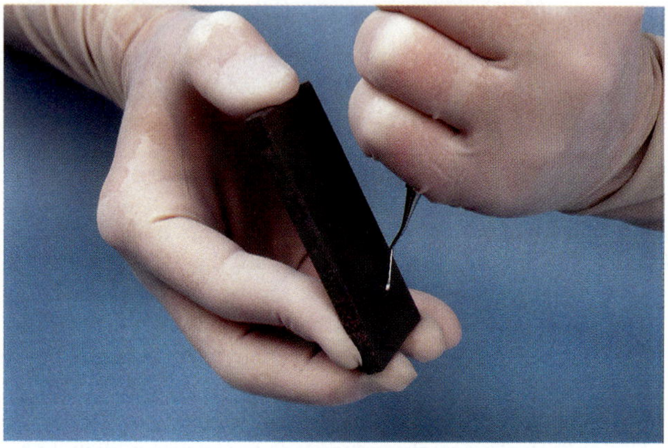

Fig. 35.103 Note that when a Gracey curette is held in proper sharpening position, its shank is not perpendicular to the floor because of its offset blade angle. The stone meets the blade at an angle of 100–110 degrees.

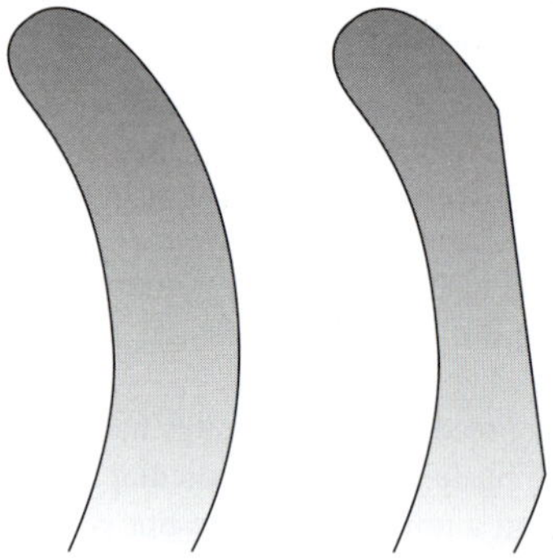

Fig. 35.104 Gracey curette on the left has been properly sharpened to maintain a symmetric curve on its outer cutting edge. For the curette on the right, the sharpening stone was activated too long in one place, thereby flattening the blade.

the angle between the face of the blade and the stone is 100–110 degrees.

3. Activate short, up-and-down strokes, working from the shank end of the blade to the curved toe. Finish with a down stroke.
4. Remember that the cutting edge is curved. Preserve the curve by turning the stone while sharpening from shank to toe. If the stone is kept in one place for too many strokes, the blade will be flattened (Fig. 35.104, right).
5. Evaluate sharpness as previously described. Continue sharpening as necessary.

Extended-Shank, Mini-Bladed, and Periodontal Maintenance Gracey Curettes

Extended-shank Gracey curettes, such as the After Five curettes, are sharpened in exactly the same manner as the standard Gracey curettes. Although the terminal shank is 3-mm longer, the blade size and shape are very similar, and thus there is no difference in the sharpening technique.

Mini-bladed Gracey curettes, such as the Mini Five curettes, Micro Mini curettes, or Gracey Curvettes, are also sharpened with the same technique. These blades are only half the length of a standard Gracey blade, but the angle between the face and the lateral surface of the blade is still 70–80 degrees. Similarly, Periodontal Maintenance Gracey curettes have the same 70–80 degree angle between the face of the blade and the lateral surface and are therefore sharpened with the same technique. They also have a shorter blade, being only three-fourths the length of a standard Gracey curette. With any of these modified Gracey curettes, sharpening too heavily or too often around the toe should be avoided to prevent excessive shortening of the blade.

Sickle Scalers

The two types of sickle scalers are the straight sickle and curved sickle. On a straight sickle, the face of the blade is flat from shank to tip, whereas on a curved sickle, the face of the blade forms a gentle curve (Fig. 35.105). However, the straight and curved sickles have similar cross-sectional designs. As in the curette, the angle between the face of the blade and the lateral surface of a sickle is 70–80 degrees (Fig. 35.106). When a sharpening stone is correctly applied to the lateral surface to preserve this angle, the angle between the face of the blade and the surface of the stone is 100–110 degrees. With this in mind, the sickle scaler can be sharpened in a manner similar to that described for the curette, except that the sickle has a sharp, pointed toe that must not be rounded.

A large, flat stone may also be used to sharpen sickles (Fig. 35.107). The stone is stabilized on a table or cabinet with the left hand. The

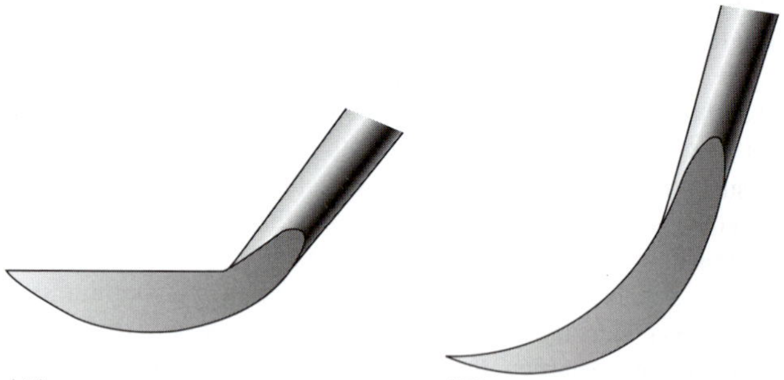

Fig. 35.105 Face of the blade on a straight sickle is flat from shank to tip, A, whereas on the curved sickle the blade face forms a gentle arc, B.

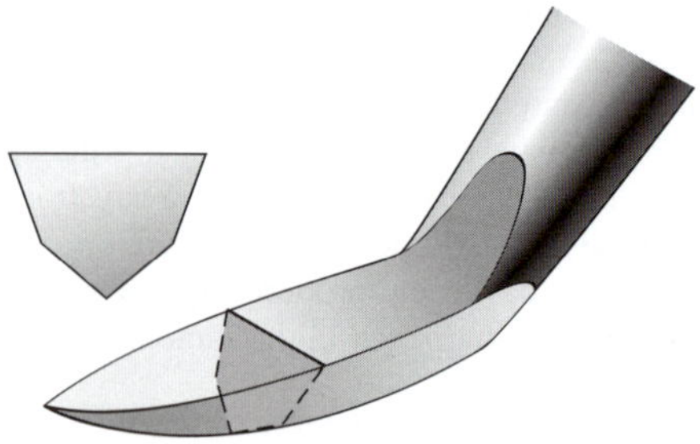

Fig. 35.106 As with the curette, the sickle has an angle of 70–80 degrees between the face of the blade and the lateral surface.

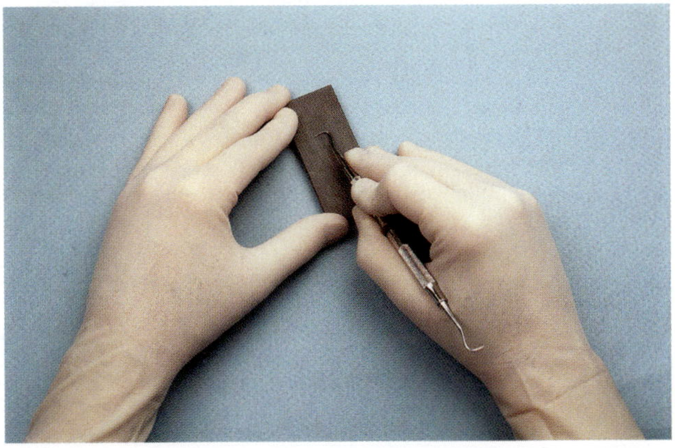

Fig. 35.107 Large, flat stone may also be used to sharpen the sickle. The stone is stabilized on a flat surface. The fourth finger of the right hand guides the sharpening stroke as the instrument is pulled across the face of the stone toward the operator.

sickle is held in the right hand with a modified pen grasp and applied to the stone so that the angle between the face of the blade and the stone is 100–110 degrees. The fourth finger is placed on the right-hand edge of the stone to stabilize and guide the sharpening movement. The right hand then pushes and pulls the sickle across the surface of the stone.

To avoid a wire edge, the operator finishes with a pull stroke, being sure that the proper angulation is always maintained.

Chisels and Hoes

Chisels have a single, straight cutting edge that is perpendicular to the shank. The face of the blade is continuous with the shank of the instrument, which may be directly in line with the handle or slightly curved. The end of the blade is beveled at 45 degrees to form the cutting edge.

To sharpen a chisel, stabilize a flat sharpening stone on a flat surface. Grasp the instrument with a modified pen grasp. Establish a finger rest with the pads of the third and fourth fingers against the straight edge of the sharpening stone. Apply the flat beveled surface of the chisel to the surface of the stone. If the entire surface of the bevel is contacting the stone, the 45-degree angle between the beveled surface and the face of the blade will be maintained, and the design of the instrument will not be altered (Figs. 35.108 and 35.109).

Using moderate, steady pressure, with the hand and arm acting as a unit and the finger resting on the edge of the stone as a guide, push the instrument across the surface of the sharpening stone. Release pressure slightly and draw the instrument back to its starting point. Repeat the sharpening stroke until a sharp edge has been obtained. Remember to finish with a push stroke to prevent the formation of a wire edge. Check for sharpness as previously described. Examine the instrument carefully to be sure that its design has not been inadvertently altered.

Back-action surgical chisels and hoe scalers are sharpened with exactly the same technique described for chisels except that a pull stroke is used rather than a push stroke (Fig. 35.110).

Periodontal Knives

There are two general types of periodontal knives. The first type includes the disposable scalpel blades that come prepackaged and are presharpened and sterilized by the manufacturer. These knives are not resharpened when they become dull but are discarded and replaced.

The second type of periodontal knife is reusable and must be sharpened when it becomes dull. The most common knives in this group are the flat-bladed gingivectomy knives (e.g., Kirkland knives #15K and 16K) and the narrow, pointed interproximal knives.

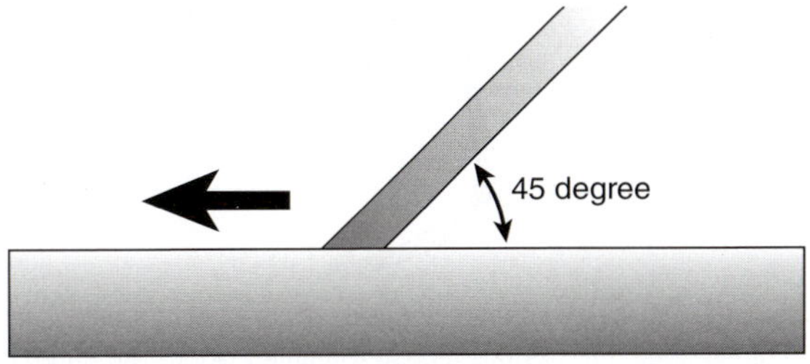

Fig. 35.108 When the entire bevel on a chisel contacts the sharpening stone, the angle between the instrument and the stone is 45 degrees. The cutting edge will be properly sharpened if this angle is maintained as the instrument is pushed across the stone.

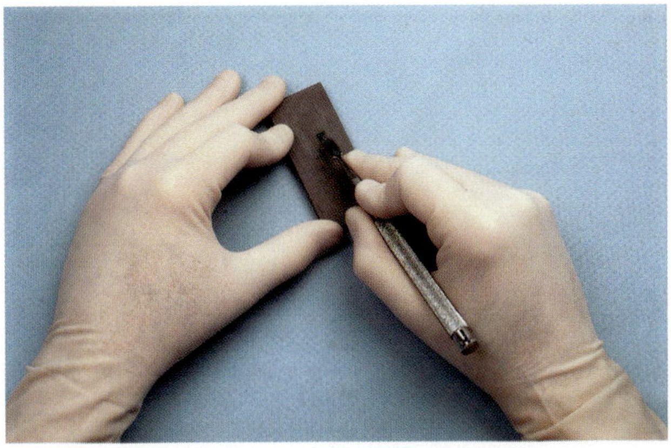

Fig. 35.109 Chisel can also be sharpened on a stationary, flat sharpening stone.

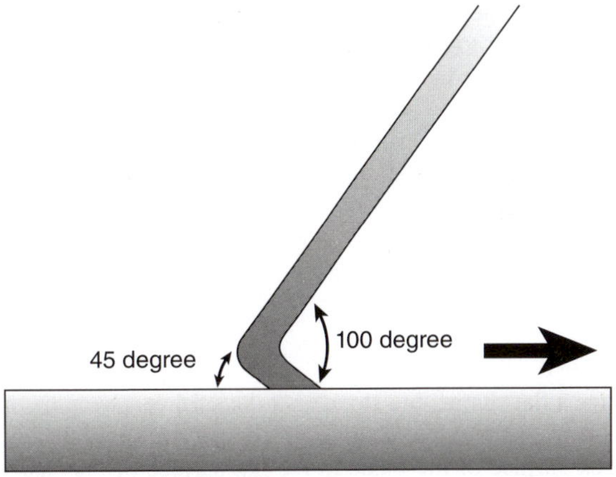

Fig. 35.110 Back-action chisels and hoes are sharpened with a pull stroke.

Flat-Bladed Gingivectomy Knives

These knives have broad, flat blades that are nearly perpendicular to the lower shank of the instrument. The curved cutting edge extends around the entire outer edge of the blade and is formed by bevels on both the front and the back surface of the blade (Fig. 35.111).

When sharpening these instruments, only the bevel on the back surface of the instrument needs to be ground. This can be done by drawing the blade across a stationary, flat sharpening stone or by holding the instrument stationary and drawing the stone across its blade.

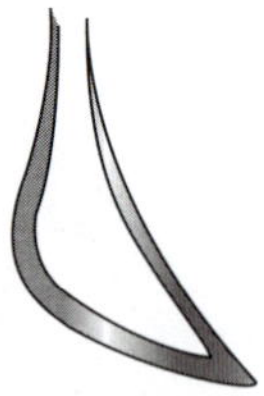

Fig. 35.111 Flat-bladed gingivectomy knives, such as this Kirkland knife, have a cutting edge that extends around the entire blade. The entire cutting edge must be sharpened.

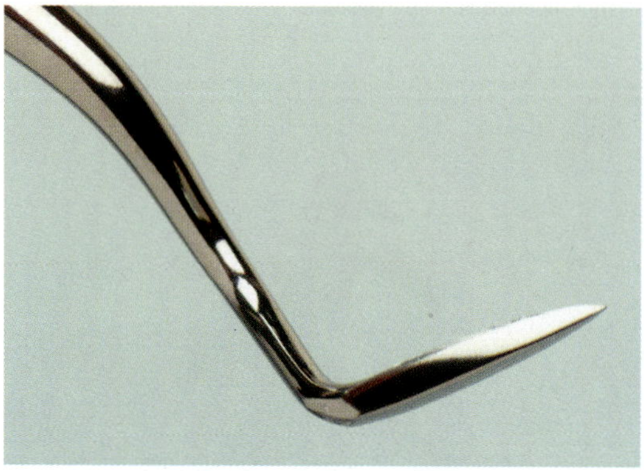

Fig. 35.112 The two cutting edges of an interproximal knife are formed by bevels on the front and back surfaces of the blade.

Interproximal Knives

The blades of interproximal knives have two long, straight cutting edges that come together at the sharply pointed tip of the instrument. The cutting edges are formed by bevels on the front and back surfaces of the blade. The entire blade is roughly perpendicular to the lower shank of the instrument (Fig. 35.112).

As with the flat-bladed gingivectomy knives, only the bevels on the back surface of the interproximal knives need to be sharpened. Again, this can be accomplished by drawing the instrument across a stationary stone or by holding the instrument stationary and moving the stone across it.

Stationary Stone Technique

Stabilize a flat sharpening stone on a flat surface. Grasp the handle of the instrument with a modified pen grasp, and apply the bevel on the back surface of the blade to the flat surface of the sharpening stone. With moderate pressure, pull the instrument toward you (Figs. 35.113 and 35.114). Release pressure slightly, and return to the starting point. Begin at one end of the cutting edge, and continue around the blade by rolling the handle of the instrument slightly between the thumb and the first and second fingers. Finish each section of the blade with a pull stroke to prevent formation of a wire edge. Check for sharpness as described previously.

Stationary Instrument Technique

Grasp the instrument with the palm. Apply the flat surface of a handheld sharpening stone to the bevel on the back surface of the blade (Fig. 35.115). Begin at one end of the cutting edge, and with moderate pressure, draw the stone back and forth across the instrument. To prevent the formation of a wire edge, finish each section with a stroke into or toward the cutting edge. Proceed around the entire length of the cutting edge by gradually rotating the instrument and the stone in relation to one another.

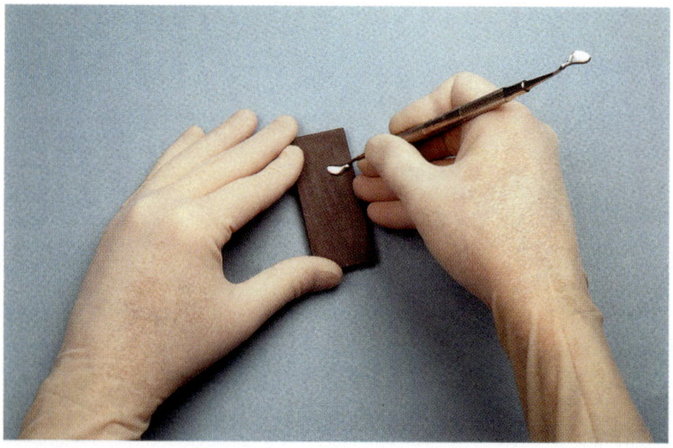

Fig. 35.113 Gingivectomy knife may be sharpened on a stationary flat stone. The instrument is held with a modified pen grasp. The fourth finger guides the sharpening stroke as the instrument is rolled between the fingers so that all sections of the blade are sharpened.

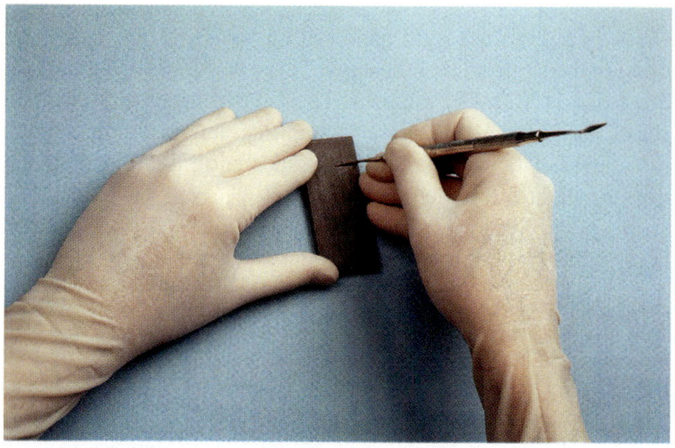

Fig. 35.114 Interproximal knife may be sharpened on a flat stationary stone. The blade is drawn toward the operator.

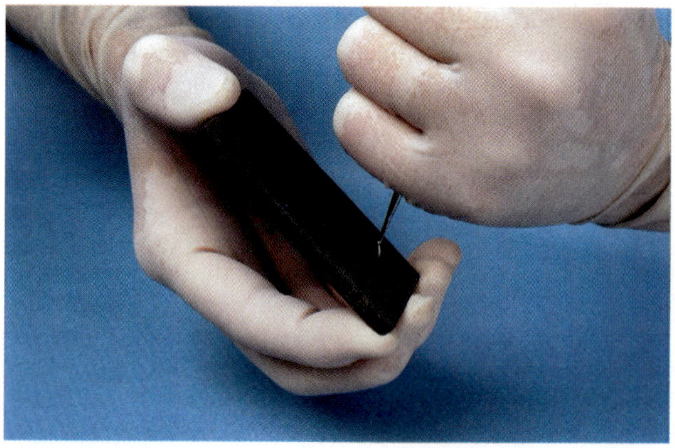

Fig. 35.115 Interproximal knife may also be sharpened with a handheld stone. The instrument is held with a palm grasp, and the stone is applied to the entire cutting edge.

Key points

- Periodontal instruments are classified into periodontal probes, explorers, scaling, root-planing, and curettage instruments, periodontal endoscopes and cleansing and polishing instruments.
- The term offset blade is used to describe Gracey curettes because they are angled approximately 60–70 degrees from the lower shank.

- The Gracey #15–16 is a modification of the standard #11–12 and is designed for the mesial surfaces of posterior teeth. It consists of a Gracey #11–12 blade combined with the more acutely angled #13–14 shank.
- The Gracey #17–18 is a modification of the #13–14. It has a terminal shank elongated by 3 mm and a more accentuated angulation of the shank to provide complete occlusal clearance and better access to all posterior distal surfaces.
- Extended-shank curettes, such as the After Five curettes, are modifications of the standard Gracey curette design. The terminal shank is 3-mm longer, blade is thinner, and the shank is tapered, with a large diameter.
- After Five series are available in all standard Gracey numbers except for the #9–10.
- Mini Five curettes feature blades that are half the length of the After Five or standard Gracey curettes. Mini Five curettes are available in all standard Gracey numbers, except the #9–10.
- Micro Mini Five Gracey curettes have blades that are 20% thinner and smaller than the Mini Five curettes. They are the smallest of all curettes.
- The Gracey Curvettes have blade length 50% shorter than that of the conventional Gracey curette, and the blade is curved slightly upward.
- The Langer and Mini Langer curettes combine the shank design of the standard Gracey #5–6, 11–12, and 13–14 curettes with a universal blade honed at 90 degrees rather than the offset blade of the Gracey curette.
- Chisel scalers are activated with a push motion.
- The most effective and stable grasp for all periodontal instruments is the modified pen grasp. Finger rests may be generally classified as intraoral finger rests (conventional, cross-arch, opposite arch, and finger on finger) or extraoral fulcrums (palm-up and palm-down).
- Angulation refers to the angle between the face of a bladed instrument and the tooth surface. It may also be called the tooth–blade relationship.
- During scaling and root planing, optimal angulation is between 45 and 90 degrees.
- For gingival curettage, angulation greater than 90 degrees is deliberately established so that the cutting edge will engage and remove the pocket lining.
- Lateral pressure refers to the pressure created when force is applied against the surface of a tooth with the cutting edge of a bladed instrument.
- The exploratory stroke is a light, "feeling" stroke.
- Scaling stroke is a short, powerful pull stroke.
- Root-planing stroke is a moderate to light pull stroke.
- Oil should be used to lubricate a natural sharpening stone and water to lubricate synthetic sharpening stones.

Suggested Readings

Cadosch J, Zimmermann U, Ruppert M, et al: Root surface debridement and endotoxin removal, *J Periodontal Res* 38:229, 2003.

Claffey N: Decision making in periodontal therapy: the reevaluation, *J Clin Periodontol* 18:364, 1991.

Drisko CL, Cochran DL, Blieden T, et al: Position paper: sonic and ultrasonic scalers in periodontics. Research, Science and Therapy Committee of the American Academy of Periodontology, *J Periodontol* 71:1792, 2000.

Greenstein G: Nonsurgical periodontal therapy in 2000: a literature review, *J Am Dent Assoc* 131:1580, 2000.

Kaldahl WB, Kalkwarf KL, Patil KD, et al: Long-term evaluation of periodontal therapy. I. Response to 4 therapeutic modalities, *J Periodontol* 67:93, 1996.

Lindhe J, Nyman S: Long-term maintenance of patients treated for advanced periodontal disease, *J Clin Periodontol* 11:504, 1984.

Lindhe J, Nyman S, Karring T: Scaling and root planing in shallow pockets, *J Clin Periodontol* 9:415, 1982.

Magnusson I, Lindhe J, Yoneyama T, et al: Recolonization of a subgingivalmicrobiota following scaling in deep pockets, *J Clin Periodontol* 11:193, 1984.

Pattison AM: The use of hand instruments in supportive periodontal treatment, *Periodontol 2000* 12:71, 1996.

Quirynen M, Mongardini C, Pauwels M, et al: One stage full-versus partial-mouth disinfection in the treatment of chronic adult or generalized early-onset periodontitis. II. Long-term impact on microbial load, *J Periodontol* 70:646, 1999.

References

References and MCQs with answers for the chapter are available on www.medenact.com.

CHAPTER 36

Scaling and Root Planing

AM Pattison | GL Pattison | CA Jahn | A Jain

CHAPTER OUTLINE

Principles of Scaling and Root Planing

Definitions and Rationale

Scaling is the process by which biofilm and calculus are removed from both supragingival and subgingival tooth surfaces. No deliberate attempt is made to remove tooth substance along with the calculus. *Root planing* is the process by which residual embedded calculus and portions of cementum are removed from the roots to produce a smooth, hard, and clean surface.

The primary objective of scaling and root planing is to restore gingival health by completely removing elements that provoke gingival inflammation (i.e., biofilm, calculus, and endotoxin) from the tooth surface (Fig. 36.1). Instrumentation has been shown to reduce dramatically the numbers of subgingival microorganisms and produce a shift in the composition of subgingival biofilm from one with high numbers of gram-negative anaerobes to one dominated by gram-positive facultative bacteria compatible with health. After thorough scaling and root planing, a profound reduction in spirochetes, motile rods, and putative pathogens, such as *Actinobacillus actinomycetemcomitans, Porphyromonas gingivalis,* and *Prevotella intermedia*, and an increase in coccoid cells occur. These changes in the microbiota are accompanied by a reduction or elimination of inflammation clinically. This positive microbial change must be sustained by the periodic scaling and root planing performed during supportive periodontal therapy.

Scaling and root planing are not separate procedures; all the principles of scaling apply equally to root planing. The difference between scaling and root planing is only a matter of degree. The nature of the tooth surface determines the degree to which the surface must be scaled or planed.

Biofilm and calculus on enamel surfaces provoke gingival inflammation. Unless they are grooved or pitted, enamel surfaces are relatively smooth and uniform. When biofilm and calculus form on enamel, the deposits are usually superficially attached to the surface and are not locked into irregularities. Scaling alone is sufficient to remove biofilm and calculus completely from enamel, leaving a smooth, clean surface.

Root surfaces exposed to biofilm and calculus pose a different problem. *Deposits of calculus on root surfaces are frequently embedded in cemental irregularities*. Subgingival calculus is porous and harbors bacteria and endotoxin and therefore should be removed completely. When dentin is exposed, biofilm bacteria may invade dentinal tubules. Therefore, scaling alone is insufficient to remove them, and a portion of the root surface must be removed to eliminate these deposits. Furthermore, when the root surface is exposed to biofilm and the pocket environment, its surface is contaminated by toxic substances, notably endotoxins. Evidence suggests that these toxic substances are only superficially attached to the root and do not permeate it deeply. Removal of extensive amounts of dentin and cementum is not necessary to render the roots free of toxins and should be avoided. In areas where cementum is thin, however, instrumentation may expose dentin. Although this is not the aim of treatment, such exposure may be unavoidable.

Scaling and root planing should not be viewed as separate procedures unrelated to the rest of the treatment plan. These procedures belong to the initial phase of an orderly sequence of treatment. After careful analysis of a case, the number of appointments needed to complete this phase of treatment is estimated. Patients with small amounts of calculus and relatively healthy tissues can be treated in one appointment. Most other patients require several treatment sessions. The dentist should estimate the number of appointments needed on the basis of the number of teeth in the mouth, severity of inflammation, amount and location of calculus, depth and activity of pockets, presence of furcation invasions, patient's comprehension of and compliance with oral hygiene instructions, and need for local anesthesia.

When the rationale for scaling and root planing is thoroughly understood, it becomes apparent that mastery of these skills is essential to the ultimate success of any course of periodontal therapy. Of all clinical dental procedures, subgingival scaling and root planing in deep pockets are the most difficult and exacting skills to master. It has been argued that such proficiency in instrumentation cannot be attained, and therefore periodontal surgery is necessary to gain access to root surfaces. Others have argued that although proficiency is possible, it need not be developed because access to the roots can be gained more easily with surgery. However, without mastering subgingival scaling and root-planing skills, the clinician will be severely hampered and unable to treat adequately those patients for whom surgery is contraindicated.

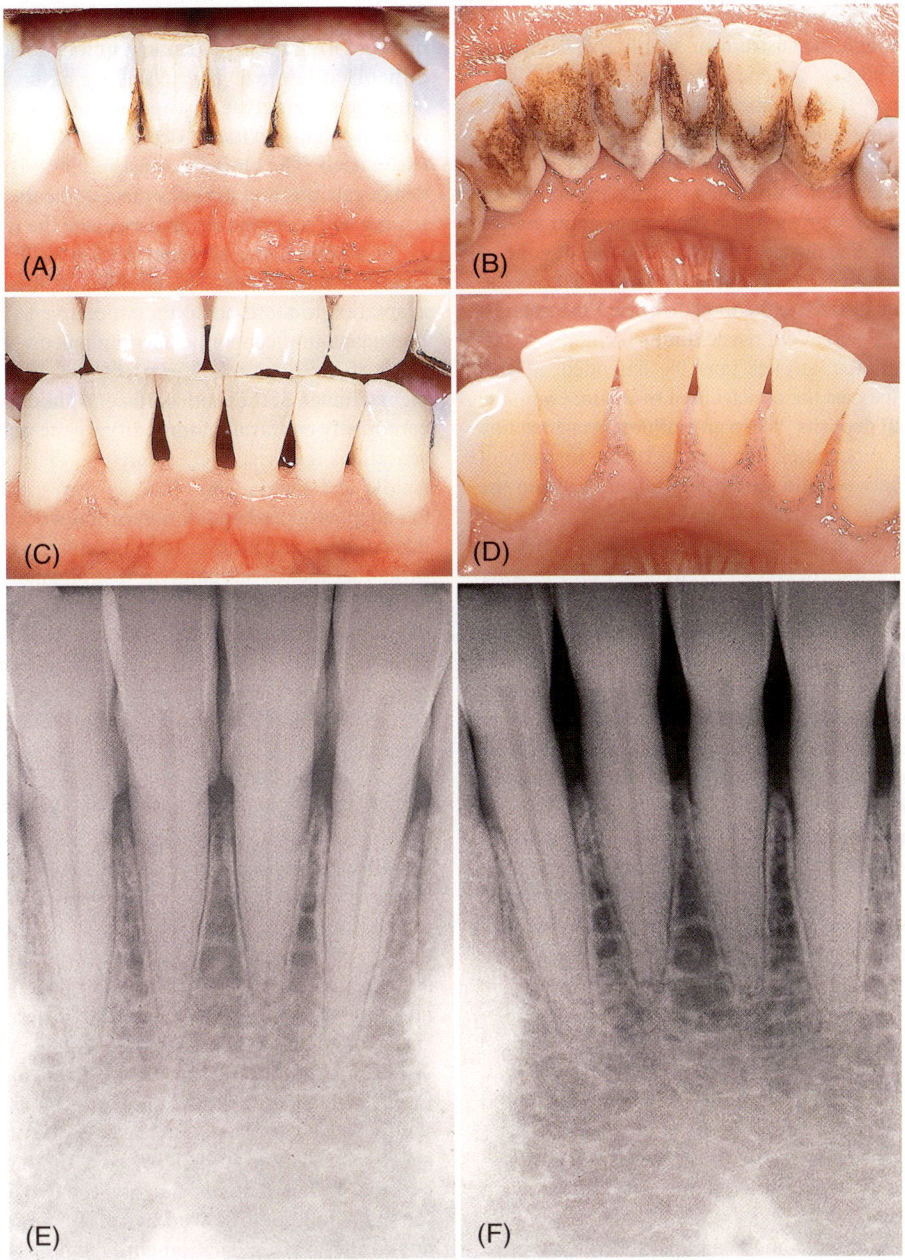

Fig. 36.1 Results of Phase I therapy. A–F, Moderate chronic periodontitis. A, Patient presenting with moderate attachment loss and probe depths in the 4–6-mm range. Note the gingiva appears pink because it is fibrotic and the inflammation is deep in the periodontal pockets. B, Lingual view before treatment, with more visible inflammation and heavy deposits of calculus. C and D, The same areas with significant improvement in gingival health 18 months after scaling, root planing, and plaque control therapy were provided; the patient returned for regular maintenance visits. E and F, Presenting radiographs of the lower anterior teeth. Radiograph taken 18 months after Phase I therapy and maintenance shows no increase in bone loss.

Detection Skills

Good visual and tactile detection skills are required for the accurate initial assessment of the extent and nature of deposits and root irregularities before scaling and root planing. Valid evaluation of results of instrumentation depends on these detection skills.

Visual examination of supragingival and subgingival calculus just below the gingival margin is not difficult with good lighting and a clean field. Light deposits of supragingival calculus are often difficult to see when they are wet with saliva. Compressed air may be used to dry supragingival calculus until it is chalky white and readily visible. Air also may be directed into the pocket in a steady stream to deflect the marginal gingiva away from the tooth so that subgingival deposits near the surface can be seen.

Tactile exploration of the tooth surfaces in subgingival areas of pocket depth, furcations, and developmental depressions is much more difficult than visual examination of supragingival areas and requires the skilled use of a fine-pointed explorer or probe. The explorer or probe is held with a light but stable modified pen grasp. This provides maximal tactile sensitivity for detection of subgingival calculus and other irregularities. The pads of the thumb and fingers, especially the middle finger, should perceive the slight vibrations conducted through the instrument shank and handle as irregularities in the tooth surface are encountered.

After a stable finger rest is established, the tip of the instrument is carefully inserted subgingivally to the base of the pocket. Light exploratory strokes are activated vertically on the root surface. When calculus is encountered, the tip of the instrument should be advanced apically over the deposit until the termination of the calculus on the root is felt. The distance between the apical edge of the calculus and the bottom of the pocket usually ranges from 0.2 to 1.0 mm. The tip is adapted closely to the tooth to ensure the greatest degree of tactile sensitivity and avoid tissue trauma. When a proximal surface is being explored, strokes must be extended at least halfway across that surface past the contact area to ensure complete detection of interproximal deposits. When an explorer is used at line angles, convexities, and concavities, the handle of the instrument must be rolled slightly between the thumb and fingers to keep the tip constantly adapted to the changes in tooth contour.

Although exploration technique and good tactile sensitivity are important, *interpreting various degrees of roughness and making clinical judgments based on these interpretations* also require much expertise. The beginning student usually has difficulty detecting fine calculus and altered cementum. Such detection must begin with the recognition of ledges, lumps, or spurs of calculus, then smaller spicules, then slight roughness, and finally a slight graininess that feels like a sticky coating or film covering the tooth surface. Overhanging or deficient margins of dental restorations, caries, decalcification, and root roughness caused by previous instrumentation are all typically found during exploration. These and other irregularities must be recognized and differentiated from subgingival calculus. Because this requires a great deal of experience and a high degree of tactile sensitivity, many clinicians agree that the development of detection skills is as important as the mastery of scaling and root-planing technique.

Supragingival Scaling Technique

Supragingival calculus is generally less tenacious and less calcified than subgingival calculus. Because instrumentation is performed coronal to the gingival margin, scaling strokes are not confined by the surrounding tissues. This makes adaptation and angulation easier. It also allows direct visibility, as well as a freedom of movement not possible during subgingival scaling.

Sickles, curettes, and ultrasonic and sonic instruments are most often used for the removal of supragingival calculus; hoes and chisels are less frequently used. To perform supragingival scaling, the sickle or curette is held with a modified pen grasp, and a firm finger rest is established on the teeth adjacent to the working area. The blade is adapted with an angulation of slightly less than 90 degrees to the surface being scaled. The cutting edge should engage the apical margin of the supragingival calculus while short, powerful, overlapping scaling strokes are activated coronally in a vertical or an oblique direction. The sharply pointed tip of the sickle can easily lacerate marginal tissue or gouge exposed root surfaces, so careful adaptation is especially important when this instrument is being used. The tooth surface is instrumented until it is visually and tactilely free of all supragingival deposits. If the tissue is retractable enough to allow easy insertion of the bulky blade, the sickle may be used slightly below the free gingival margin. If the sickle is used in this manner, final scaling and root planing with the curette should always follow.

Subgingival Scaling and Root-Planing Technique

Subgingival scaling and root planing are much more complex and difficult to perform than supragingival scaling. *Subgingival calculus* is usually harder than supragingival calculus and is often locked into root irregularities, making it more tenacious and therefore more difficult to remove. The overlying tissue creates significant problems in subgingival instrumentation. Vision is obscured by the bleeding that inevitably occurs during instrumentation and by the tissue itself. The clinician must rely heavily on tactile sensitivity to detect calculus and irregularities, guide the instrument blade during scaling and root planing, and evaluate the results of instrumentation.

In addition, the adjacent pocket wall limits the direction and length of the strokes. The confines of the soft tissue make careful adaptation to tooth contours imperative to avoid trauma. Such precise adaptation cannot be accomplished without a thorough knowledge of tooth morphologic features. The clinician must form a mental image of the tooth surface to anticipate variations in contour, continually confirming or modifying the image in response to tactile sensations and visual cues, such as the position of the instrument handle and shank. The clinician then must instantaneously adjust the adaptation and angulation of the working end to the tooth. It is this complex and precise coordination of visual, mental, and manual skills that makes subgingival instrumentation one of the most difficult of all dental skills. *The curette is preferred by most clinicians for subgingival scaling and root planing because of the advantages afforded by its design.* Its curved blade, rounded toe, and curved back allow the curette to be inserted to the base of the pocket and adapted to variations in tooth contour with minimal tissue displacement and trauma.

Sickles, hoes, files, and ultrasonic instruments also are used for subgingival scaling of heavy calculus. Some small files (e.g., Hirschfeld file) may be inserted to the base of the pocket to crush or initially fracture tenacious deposits. Larger files, hoes, sickles, and standard ultrasonic tips for supragingival use are too bulky and cannot be inserted easily into deep pockets or areas where tissue is firm and fibrotic. Hoes and files cannot be used to produce as smooth a surface as curettes. Hoes, files, and standard large ultrasonic tips are all more hazardous than the curette in terms of trauma to the root surface and surrounding tissues. Although thin ultrasonic tips designed for scaling of deep pockets and furcations can be inserted more easily subgingivally, they must be used on low power. When low-power scaling is performed on heavy calculus or tenacious sheets of calculus, thin ultrasonic tips are likely to burnish the calculus rather than thoroughly remove it. Therefore, ultrasonic scaling should be followed by careful assessment with an explorer and further instrumentation with curettes when necessary.

Subgingival scaling and root planing are accomplished with either universal or area-specific (Gracey) curettes using the following basic procedure. The curette is held with a modified pen grasp, and a stable finger rest is established. The correct cutting edge is slightly adapted to the tooth, with the lower shank kept parallel to the tooth surface. The lower shank is moved toward the tooth so that the face of the blade is nearly flush with the tooth surface. The blade is then inserted under the gingiva and advanced to the base of the pocket by a light exploratory stroke. When the cutting edge reaches the base of the pocket, a working angulation of between 45 and 90 degrees is established, and pressure is applied laterally against the tooth surface. Calculus is removed by a series of controlled, overlapping, short, powerful strokes primarily using wrist-arm motion (Fig. 36.2). As calculus is removed, resistance to the passage of the cutting edge diminishes until only a slight roughness remains. Longer, lighter root-planing strokes are then activated with less lateral pressure until the root surface is completely smooth and hard. The instrument handle must be rolled carefully between the thumb and fingers to keep the blade adapted closely to the tooth surface as line angles, developmental depressions, and other changes in tooth

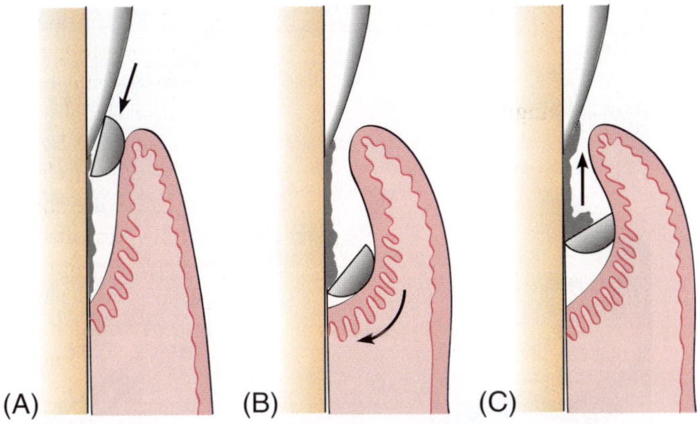

Fig. 36.2 Subgingival scaling procedure. A, Curette inserted with the face of the blade flush against the tooth. B, Working angulation (45–90 degrees) is established at the base of the pocket. C, Lateral pressure is applied, and the scaling stroke is activated in the coronal direction.

contour are followed. Scaling and root-planing strokes should be confined to the portion of the tooth where calculus or altered cementum is found; this area is known as the *instrumentation zone*. Sweeping the instrument over the crown where it is not needed wastes operating time, dulls the instrument, and causes loss of control.

The amount of lateral pressure applied to the tooth surface depends on the nature of the calculus and whether the strokes are for initial calculus removal or final root planing. If heavy lateral pressure is continued after the bulk of calculus has been removed and the blade is repeatedly readapted with short, choppy strokes, the result will be a root surface roughened by numerous nicks and gouges, resembling the rippled surface of a washboard. If heavy lateral pressure is continued with long, even strokes, the result will be excessive removal of root structure, producing a smooth but "ditched" or "riffled" root surface. To avoid these hazards of overinstrumentation, a deliberate transition from short, powerful scaling strokes to longer, lighter root-planing strokes must be made as soon as the calculus and initial roughness have been eliminated.

When scaling strokes are used to remove calculus, force can be maximized by concentrating lateral pressure onto the lower third of the blade. This small section, the terminal few millimeters of the blade, is positioned slightly apical to the lateral edge of the deposit, and a short vertical or oblique stroke is used to split the calculus from the tooth surface. Without withdrawing the instrument from the pocket, the lower third of the blade is advanced laterally and repositioned to engage the next portion of the remaining deposit. Another vertical or oblique stroke is made slightly overlapping the previous stroke. This process is repeated in a series of powerful scaling strokes until the entire deposit has been removed. The overlapping of these pathways or "channels" of instrumentation ensures that the entire instrumentation zone is covered (Fig. 36.3).

Engaging a large, tenacious ledge or piece of calculus with the entire length of the cutting edge is not recommended because the force is distributed through a longer section of the cutting edge rather than concentrated. Much more lateral pressure is required to dislodge the entire deposit in one stroke. Although some clinicians may possess the strength to remove calculus completely in this manner, the heavier forces required diminish tactile sensitivity and contribute to a loss of control that results in tissue trauma. A single heavy stroke usually is not sufficient to remove calculus entirely. Instead, the blade skips over or skims the surface of the deposit. Subsequent strokes made with the entire cutting edge tend to shave the deposit down layer by layer. When a series of these repeated whittling strokes is applied, the calculus may be reduced to a thin, smooth, burnished sheet that is difficult to distinguish from the surrounding root surface.

A common error in instrumenting proximal surfaces is failing to reach the midproximal region apical to the contact. This area is relatively inaccessible, and the technique requires more skill than instrumentation of buccal or lingual surfaces. It is extremely important to extend strokes at least halfway across the proximal surface so that no calculus or roughness remains in the interproximal area. With properly designed curettes, this can be accomplished by keeping the lower shank of the curette parallel with the long axis of the tooth (Fig. 36.4A). With the lower shank parallel to the long axis, the blade of the curette will reach the base of the pocket and the toe will extend beyond the midline as strokes are advanced across the proximal surface. This extension of strokes beyond the midline ensures thorough exploration and instrumentation of these surfaces. If the lower shank is angled or tilted away from the tooth, the toe will move toward the contact area. Because this prevents the blade from reaching the base of the pocket, calculus apical to the contact will not be detected or removed. Strokes will be hampered because the toe tends to become lodged in the contact. If the instrument is angled or tilted too far toward the tooth, the lower shank will hit the

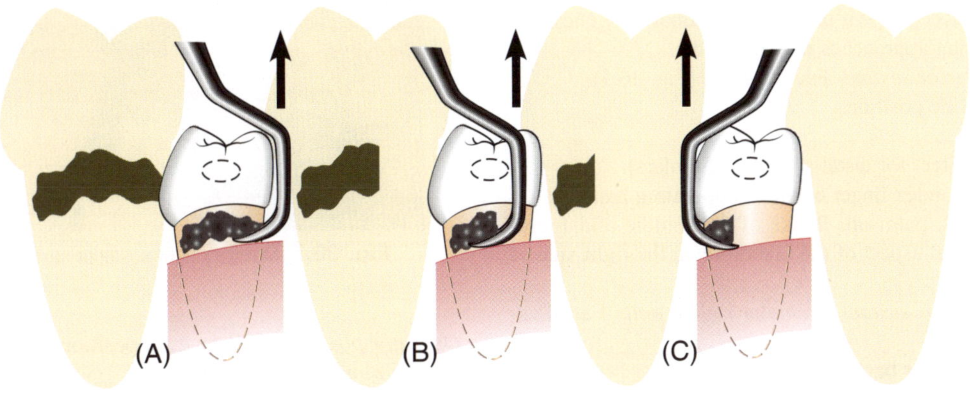

Fig. 36.3 Instrumentation for calculus removal. A, Calculus is removed by engaging the apical or lateral edge of the deposit with the cutting edge of a scaler; vertical movement of the instrument will remove the fragment of calculus engaged by the instrument, as seen in the shaded drawing. B, The instrument is moved laterally and again engages the edge of the calculus, overlapping the previous stroke to some extent; the shaded drawing shows further removal. C, The final portion of the deposit is engaged and removed. Note how the procedure is performed in an interdental space by entering facially and lingually.

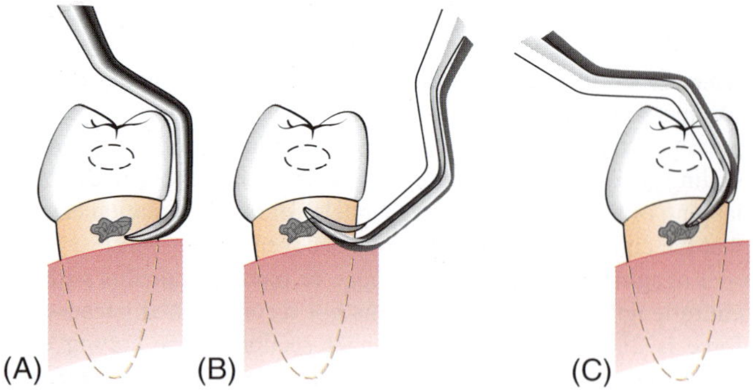

Fig. 36.4 Shank position for scaling proximal surfaces. A, Correct shank position, parallel with the long axis of the tooth. B, Incorrect shank position, tilted away from the tooth. C, Incorrect shank position, tilted too far toward the tooth. Sextant: lingual aspect.

tooth or the contact area, preventing extension of strokes to the midproximal region (Fig. 36.4B and C).

The relationship between the location of the finger rest and the working area is important for two reasons. First, the finger rest or fulcrum must be positioned to allow the lower shank of the instrument to be parallel or nearly parallel to the tooth surface being treated. This parallelism is a fundamental requirement for optimal working angulation. Second, the finger rest must be positioned to enable the operator to use wrist-arm motion to activate strokes. On some aspects of the maxillary posterior teeth, these requirements can be met only with the use of extraoral or opposite-arch fulcrums. When intraoral finger rests are used in other regions of the mouth, the finger rest must be close enough to the working area to fulfill these two requirements. A finger rest that is established too far from the working area forces the clinician to separate the middle finger from the fourth finger in an effort to obtain parallelism and proper angulation. Effective wrist-arm motion is possible only when these two fingers are kept together in a built-up fulcrum. Separation of the fingers commits the clinician to the exclusive use of finger flexing for the activation of strokes.

As instrumentation proceeds from one tooth to the next, the body position of the operator and the location of the finger rest must be frequently adjusted or changed to allow parallelism and wrist-arm motion. Various approaches to instrumentation in different areas of the mouth are illustrated here. The examples shown provide maximal efficiency for the clinician and comfort for the patient. For most areas, more than one approach is presented. Other approaches are possible and are acceptable if they provide equal efficiency and comfort. The following approaches may be used:

Maxillary right posterior sextant: Facial aspect (Fig. 36.5).
Operator position: Side position.
Illumination: Direct.
Visibility: Direct (indirect for distal surfaces of molars).
Retraction: Mirror or index finger of the nonoperating hand.
Finger rest: Extraoral, palm up. Backs of the middle and fourth fingers on the lateral aspect of the mandible on the right side of the face.

Maxillary right posterior sextant, premolar region only: Facial aspect (Fig. 36.6).
Operator position: Side or back position.
Illumination: Direct.
Visibility: Direct.
Retraction: Mirror or index finger of the nonoperating hand.
Finger rest: Intraoral, palm up. Fourth finger on the occlusal surfaces of the adjacent maxillary posterior teeth.

Maxillary right posterior sextant: Lingual aspect (Fig. 36.7).

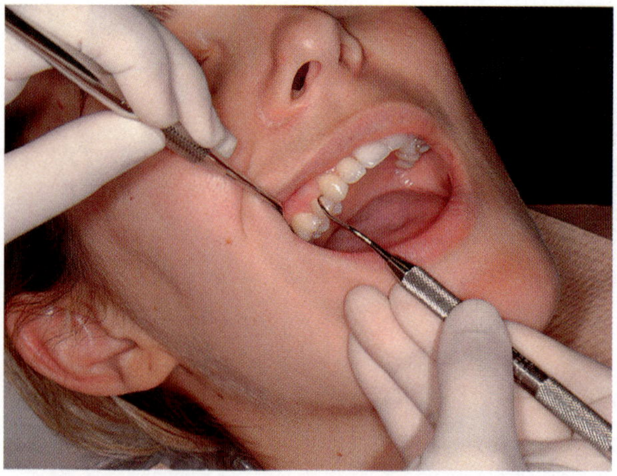

Fig. 36.5 Maxillary right posterior sextant: facial aspect.

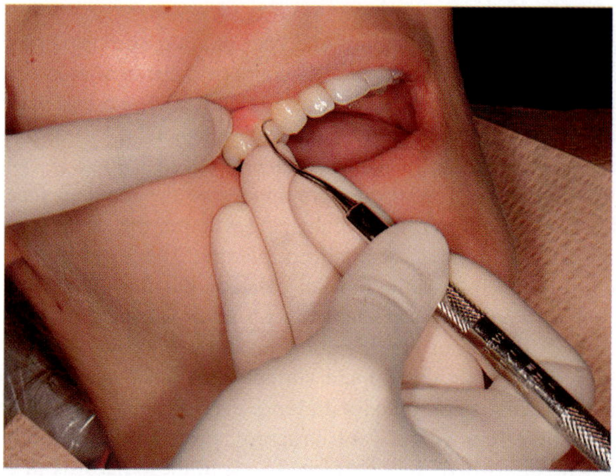

Fig. 36.6 Maxillary right posterior sextant, premolar region only: facial aspect.

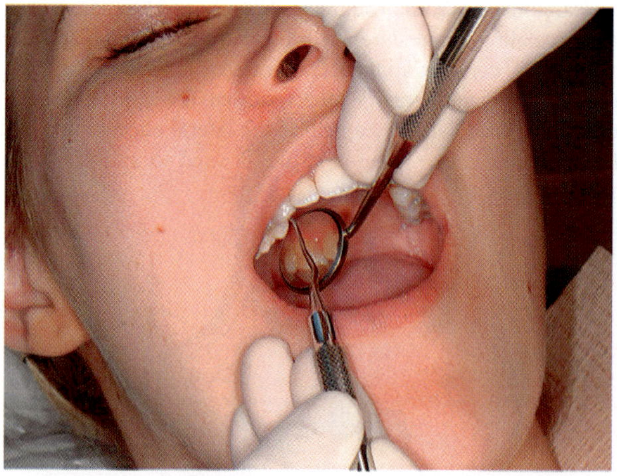

Fig. 36.7 Maxillary right posterior sextant: lingual aspect.

Operator position: Side or front position.
Illumination: Direct and indirect.
Visibility: Direct or indirect.
Retraction: None.
Finger rest: Extraoral, palm up. Backs of the middle and fourth fingers on the lateral aspect of the mandible on the right side of the face.

Maxillary right posterior sextant: Lingual aspect (Fig. 36.8).

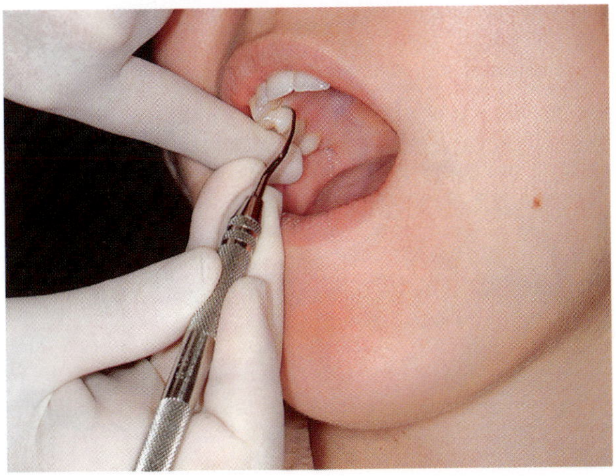

Fig. 36.8 Maxillary right posterior sextant: lingual aspect.

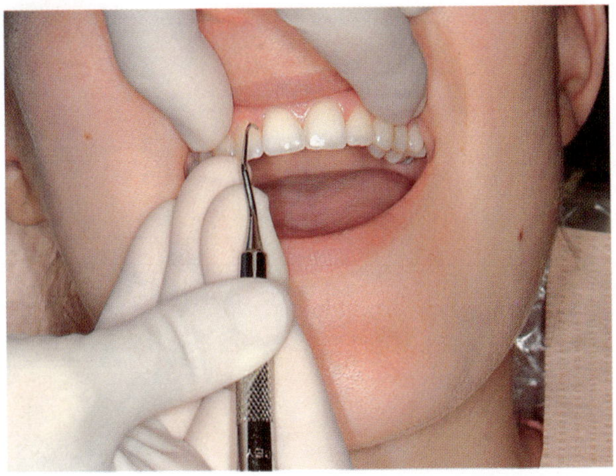

Fig. 36.9 Maxillary anterior sextant: facial aspect, surfaces away from the operator.

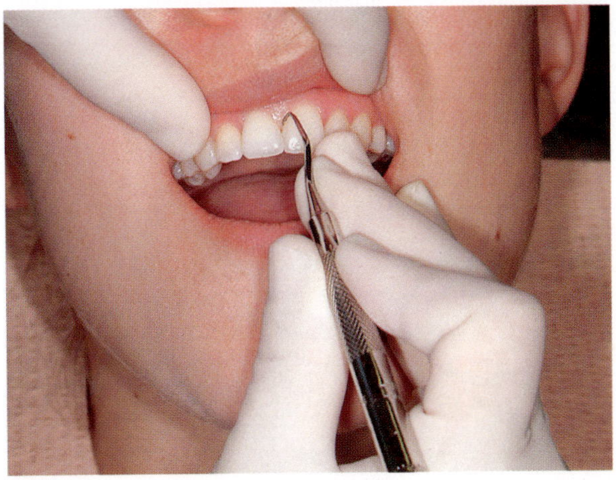

Fig. 36.10 Maxillary anterior sextant: facial aspect, surfaces toward the operator.

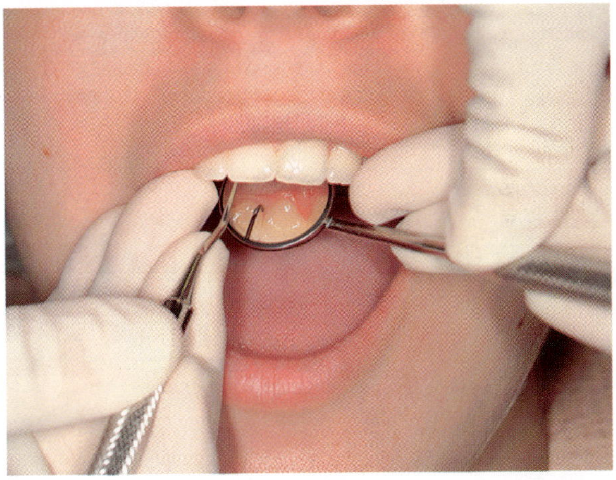

Fig. 36.11 Maxillary anterior sextant: lingual aspect, surfaces away from the operator (surfaces toward the operator are scaled from a front position).

Operator position: Front position.
Illumination: Direct.
Visibility: Direct.
Retraction: None.
Finger rest: Intraoral, palm up, finger on finger. Index finger of the nonoperating hand on the occlusal surfaces of the maxillary right posterior teeth; fourth finger of the operating hand or the index finger of the nonoperating hand.

Maxillary anterior sextant: Facial aspect, surfaces away from the operator (Fig. 36.9).
Operator position: Back position.
Illumination: Direct.
Visibility: Direct.
Retraction: Index finger of the nonoperating hand.
Finger rest: Intraoral, palm up. Fourth finger on the incisal edges or occlusal surfaces of adjacent maxillary teeth.

Maxillary anterior sextant: Facial aspect, surfaces toward the operator (Fig. 36.10).
Operator position: Front position.
Illumination: Direct.
Visibility: Direct.
Retraction: Index finger of the nonoperating hand.
Finger rest: Intraoral, palm down. Fourth finger on the incisal edges or the occlusal or facial surfaces of adjacent maxillary teeth.

Maxillary anterior sextant: Lingual aspect, surfaces away from the operator (surfaces toward the operator are scaled from a front position) (Fig. 36.11).
Operator position: Back position.
Illumination: Indirect.
Visibility: Indirect.
Retraction: None.
Finger rest: Intraoral, palm up. Fourth finger on the incisal edges or the occlusal surfaces of adjacent maxillary teeth.

Maxillary left posterior sextant: Facial aspect (Fig. 36.12).
Operator position: Side or back position.
Illumination: Direct or indirect.
Visibility: Direct or indirect.
Retraction: Mirror.
Finger rest: Extraoral, palm down. Front surfaces of the middle and fourth fingers on the lateral aspect of the mandible on the left side of the face.

Maxillary left posterior sextant: Facial aspect (Fig. 36.13).
Operator position: Back or side position.
Illumination: Direct or indirect.
Visibility: Direct or indirect.
Retraction: Mirror.
Finger rest: Intraoral, palm up. Fourth finger on the incisal edges or the occlusal surfaces of adjacent maxillary teeth.

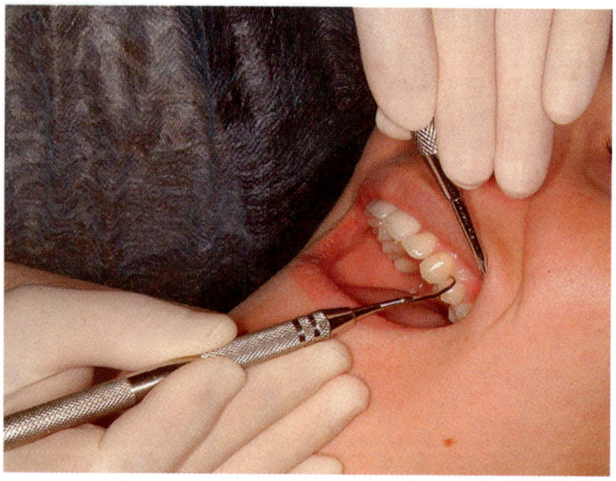

Fig. 36.12 Maxillary left posterior sextant: facial aspect.

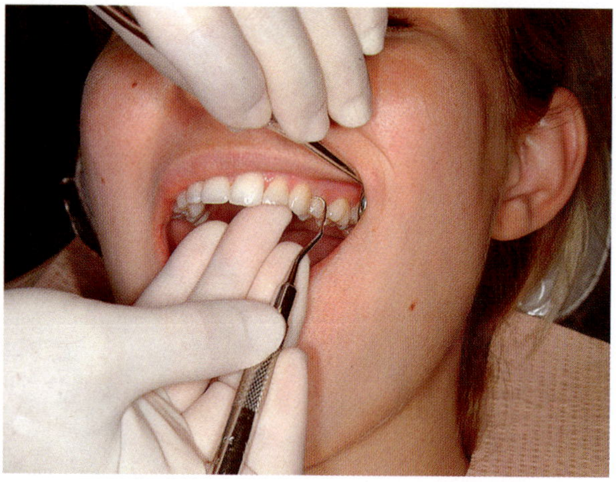

Fig. 36.13 Maxillary left posterior sextant: facial aspect.

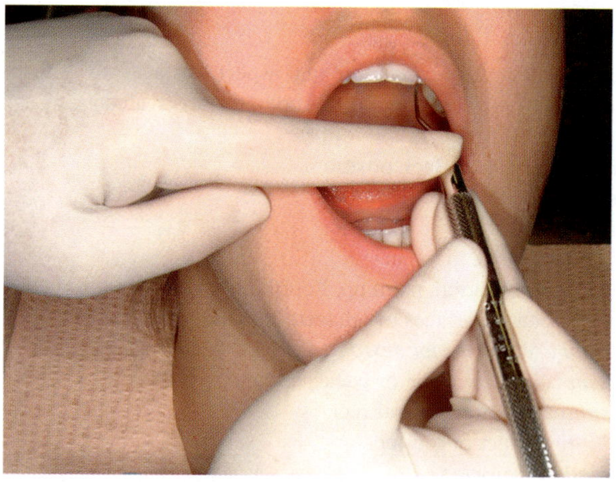

Fig. 36.14 Maxillary left posterior sextant: lingual aspect.

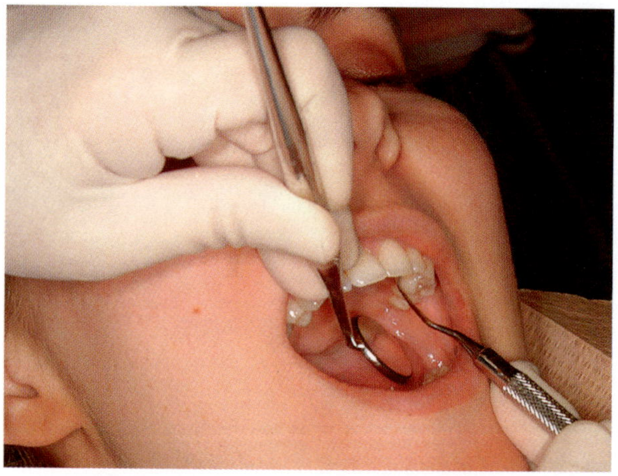

Fig. 36.15 Maxillary left posterior sextant: lingual aspect.

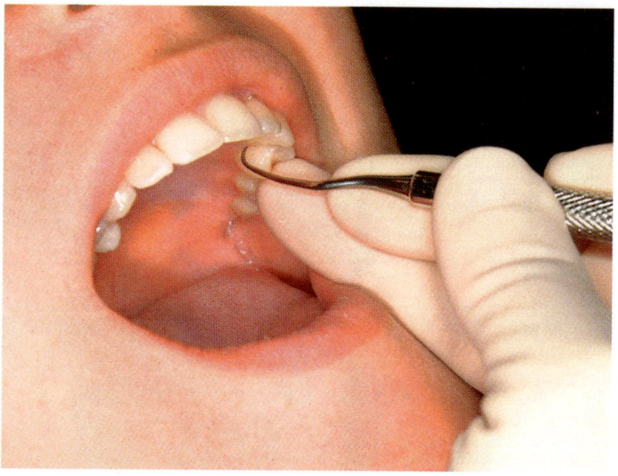

Fig. 36.16 Maxillary left posterior sextant: lingual aspect.

Maxillary left posterior sextant: Lingual aspect (Fig. 36.14).
Operator position: Front position.
Illumination: Direct.
Visibility: Direct.
Retraction: None.
Finger rest: Intraoral, palm down, opposite arch, reinforced. Fourth finger on the incisal edges of the mandibular anterior teeth or the facial surfaces of the mandibular premolars, reinforced with the index finger of the nonoperating hand.

Maxillary left posterior sextant: Lingual aspect (Fig. 36.15).
Operator position: Front position.
Illumination: Direct and indirect.
Visibility: Direct and indirect.
Retraction: None.
Finger rest: Extraoral, palm down. Front surfaces of the middle and fourth fingers on the lateral aspect of the mandible on the left side of the face. The nonoperating hand holds the mirror for indirect illumination.

Maxillary left posterior sextant: Lingual aspect (Fig. 36.16).
Operator position: Side or front position.
Illumination: Direct.
Visibility: Direct.
Retraction: None.
Finger rest: Intraoral, palm up. Fourth finger on the occlusal surfaces of adjacent maxillary teeth.

Mandibular left posterior sextant: Facial aspect (Fig. 36.17).
Operator position: Side or back position.
Illumination: Direct.
Visibility: Direct or indirect.
Retraction: Index finger or mirror of the nonoperating hand.
Finger rest: Intraoral, palm down. Fourth finger on the incisal edges or the occlusal or facial surfaces of adjacent mandibular teeth.

Mandibular left posterior sextant: Lingual aspect (Fig. 36.18).

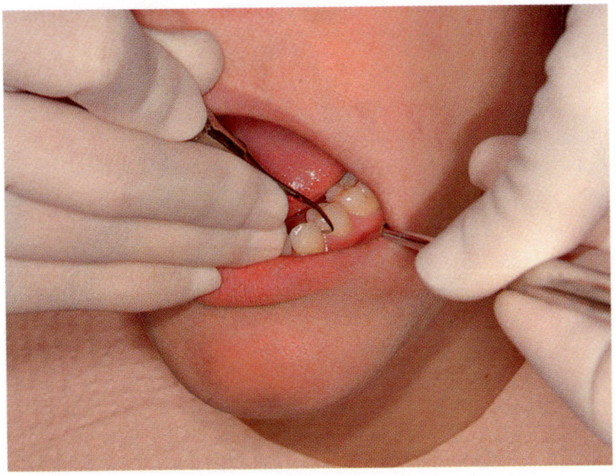

Fig. 36.17 Mandibular left posterior sextant: facial aspect.

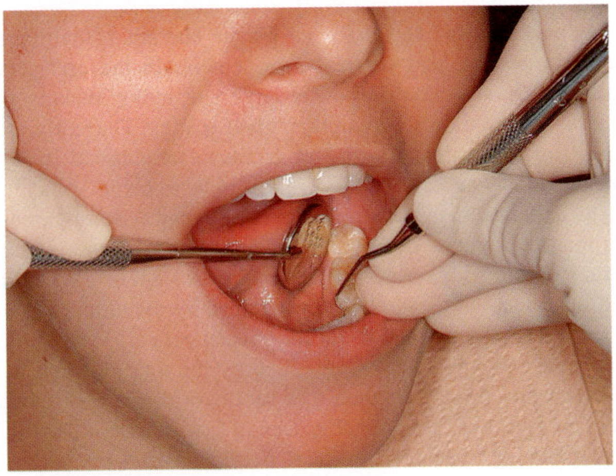

Fig. 36.18 Mandibular left posterior sextant: lingual aspect.

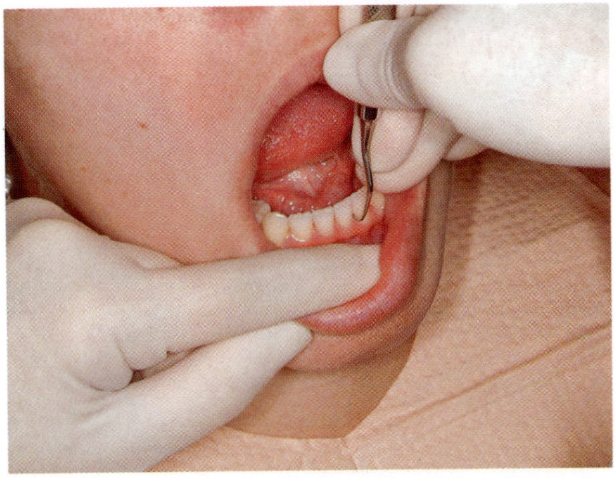

Fig. 36.19 Mandibular anterior sextant: facial aspect, surfaces toward the operator.

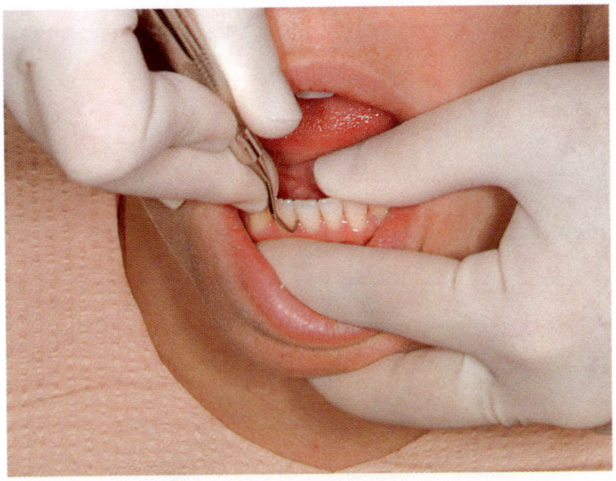

Fig. 36.20 Mandibular anterior sextant: facial aspect, surfaces away from the operator.

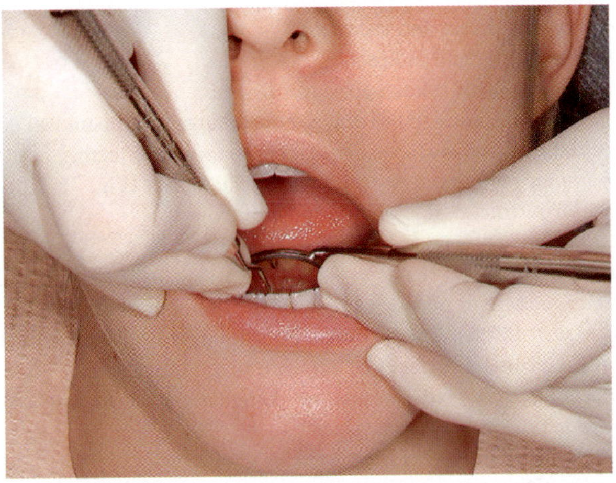

Fig. 36.21 Mandibular anterior sextant: lingual aspect, surfaces away from the operator.

Operator position: Front or side position.
Illumination: Direct and indirect.
Visibility: Direct.
Retraction: Mirror retracts tongue.
Finger rest: Intraoral, palm down. Fourth finger on the incisal edges or the occlusal surfaces of adjacent mandibular teeth.
Mandibular anterior sextant: Facial aspect, surfaces toward the operator (Fig. 36.19).
Operator position: Front position.
Illumination: Direct.
Visibility: Direct.
Retraction: Index finger of the nonoperating hand.
Finger rest: Intraoral, palm down. Fourth finger on the incisal edges or the occlusal surfaces of adjacent mandibular teeth.
Mandibular anterior sextant: Facial aspect, surfaces away from the operator (Fig. 36.20).
Operator position: Back position.
Illumination: Direct.
Visibility: Direct.
Retraction: Index finger or thumb of the nonoperating hand.
Finger rest: Intraoral, palm down. Fourth finger on the incisal edges or the occlusal surfaces of adjacent mandibular teeth.
Mandibular anterior sextant: Lingual aspect, surfaces away from the operator (Fig. 36.21).
Operator position: Back position.
Illumination: Direct and indirect.
Visibility: Direct and indirect.
Retraction: Mirror retracts tongue.
Finger rest: Intraoral, palm down. Fourth finger on the incisal edges or the occlusal surfaces of adjacent mandibular teeth.
Mandibular anterior sextant: Lingual aspect, surfaces toward the operator (Fig. 36.22).
Operator position: Front position.

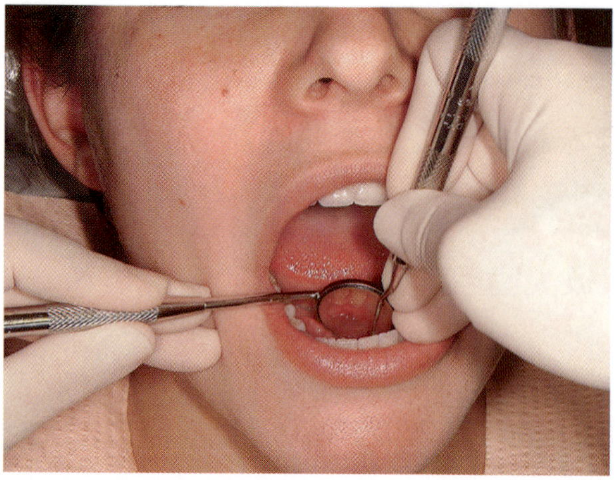

Fig. 36.22 Mandibular anterior sextant: lingual aspect, surfaces toward the operator.

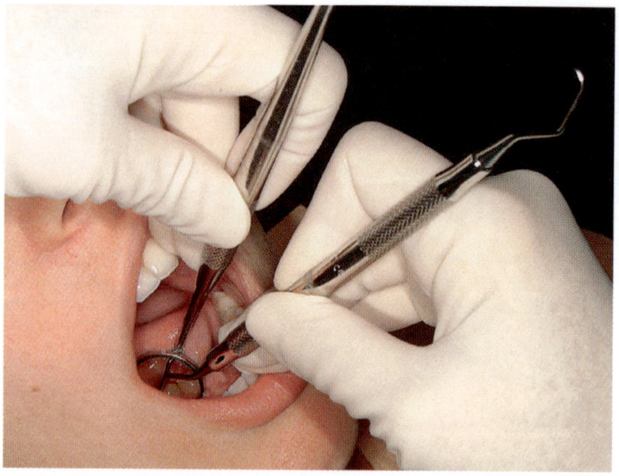

Fig. 36.24 Mandibular right posterior sextant: lingual aspect.

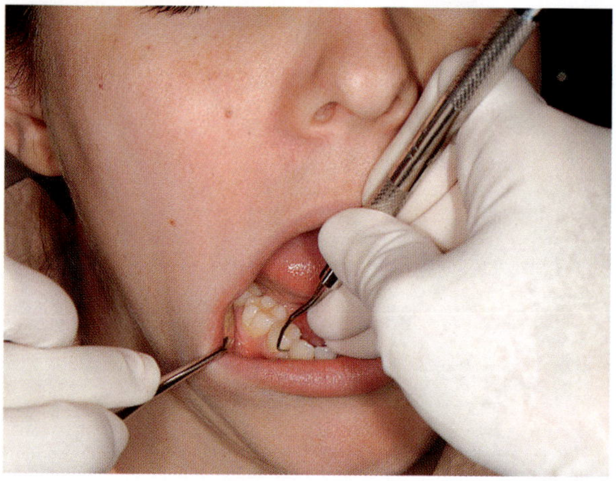

Fig. 36.23 Mandibular right posterior sextant: facial aspect.

Illumination: Direct and indirect.
Visibility: Direct and indirect.
Retraction: Mirror retracts tongue.
Finger rest: Intraoral, palm down. Fourth finger on the incisal edges or the occlusal surfaces of adjacent mandibular teeth.
Mandibular right posterior sextant: Facial aspect (Fig. 36.23).
Operator position: Side or front position.
Illumination: Direct.
Visibility: Direct.
Retraction: Mirror or index finger of the nonoperating hand.
Finger rest: Intraoral, palm down. Fourth finger on the incisal edges or the occlusal surfaces of adjacent mandibular teeth.
Mandibular right posterior sextant: Lingual aspect (Fig. 36.24).
Operator position: Front position.
Illumination: Direct and indirect.
Visibility: Direct and indirect.
Retraction: Mirror retracts tongue.
Finger rest: Intraoral, palm down. Fourth finger on the incisal edges or the occlusal surfaces of adjacent mandibular teeth.

Ultrasonic and Sonic Scaling

For many years, practitioners have sought ways to enhance and prolong the outcomes from scaling and root planing. In the office setting, technologic advances and new designs of ultrasonic and sonic power scalers have transformed the role of power-driven oscillating instruments in periodontal therapy. Ultrasonic and sonic scalers may be used for removing plaque and stain, scaling, root planing, curetting, and surgical debridement. In the early era of ultrasonic scaling, most tips were large and bulky, making them generally suitable only for supragingival scaling. Currently, many thinner ultrasonic tips allow better access to subgingival areas that were previously accessible only with hand instruments. It is important to understand this historical perspective when attempting to interpret the literature comparing the effects of hand and ultrasonic instruments on root surfaces. The selection of either ultrasonic or hand instrumentation should be determined by the clinician's preference and experience and the needs of each patient. The success of either treatment method is determined by the time devoted to the procedure and the thoroughness of root debridement. In practice, clinicians typically use a combination of both ultrasonic and hand instrumentation to achieve thorough debridement.

Mechanism of Action of Power Scalers

Various physical factors play a role in the mechanism of action of power scalers. These factors include frequency, stroke, and water flow. In addition to rate of flow, the physiologic effects of water may play a role in the efficacy of power instrument.

Frequency: Frequency is defined as the number of times per second an insert tip moves back and forth during one cycle in an orbital, elliptic, or linear stroke path. For example, a frequency of 25,000 (25K) equates to the tip moving 25,000 times per second, and a 30,000 (30K) frequency equates to the tip moving 30,000 times per second. Frequency is important because it determines the area of the insert tip that is considered active. Only the active portion of the insert can remove hard and soft debris. A higher frequency results in a smaller active area of an insert tip. An insert working in the frequency of 30K would have an active tip area of 4.2 mm, and a 25K tip has a working area of 4.3 mm. The working area of a sonic scaler tip has not been determined.

Stroke: Stroke is the maximum distance the insert tip travels during one cycle or stoke path. Amplitude is equal to one-half the distance of the stroke. The power knob on an ultrasonic unit controls the stroke length of the insert during one cycle. Increasing the power knob increases the distance the tip travels while the frequency remains constant. High power settings produce a longer stroke pattern, and lower power settings provide a shorter stroke pattern.

Water flow: Ultrasonic scalers may be designed as manually or automatically tuned devices (Fig. 36.25). Both types of technology

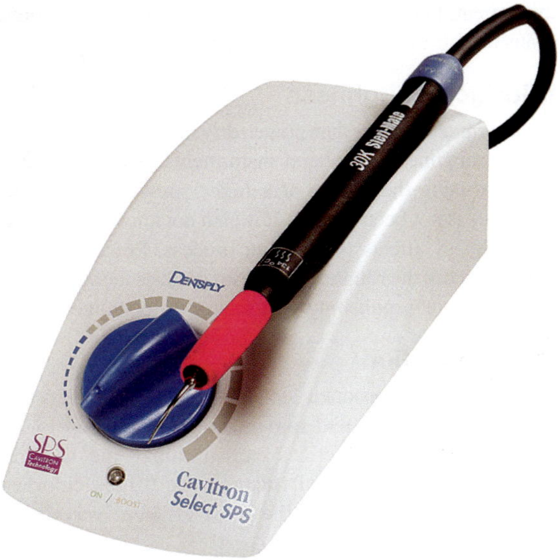

Fig. 36.25 Magnetostrictive ultrasonic device with turning knob for power and water.

contain a water knob; this controls the volume of water being delivered to the insert tip. Manual-tuned units have three control knobs on the front panel labeled water, tuning, and power. Manual technology allows the clinician to control the frequency of the unit by adjusting the tuning knob. Auto-tuned units have two control knobs, water and power, and maintain a stable frequency. These units work through feedback that constantly adjusts the insert to ensure it is vibrating at the predetermined frequency level.

Water contributes to three physiologic effects that enhance the efficacy of power scalers: acoustic streaming, acoustic turbulence, and cavitation. Acoustic streaming is the unidirectional fluid flow caused by ultrasound waves. Acoustic turbulence is created when the movement of the tip causes the coolant to accelerate, producing an intensified swirling effect. This turbulence continues until cavitation occurs. Cavitation is the formation of bubbles in water caused by the high turbulence. The bubbles implode and produce shock waves in the liquid, creating further shock waves throughout the water. In vitro, the combination of acoustic streaming, acoustic turbulence, and cavitation has been shown to disrupt microflora.

Type and Benefit of Power Instruments

Sonic units work at a frequency of 2000–6500 cycles per second and use a high- or low-speed air source from the dental unit. Water is delivered via same tubing used to deliver water to a dental handpiece. Sonic scaler tips are large in diameter and universal in design. A sonic scaler tip travels in an elliptical or orbital stroke pattern. This stroke pattern allows the instrument to be adapted to all tooth surfaces. Box 36.1 outlines the advantages and disadvantages of mechanized instruments as compared to manual instruments.

Magnetostrictive ultrasonic devices work in a frequency range of 18,000–50,000 cycles per second. Metal stacks that change dimension when electrical energy is applied to power magnetostrictive technology. Vibrations travel from the metal stack to a connecting body that causes the vibration of the working tip. Tips move in an elliptical or orbital stroke pattern. This allows the tip four active working surfaces.

Piezoelectric ultrasonic units work in a frequency range of 18,000–50,000 cycles per second (Fig. 36.26). They have ceramic disks that are located in the handpiece power piezoelectric technology. They change in dimension as electrical energy is applied to the tip. Piezoelectric tips move in a linear pattern, giving the tip two active surfaces (Fig. 36.27). A variety of insert tip designs and shapes are available for use.

BOX 36.1 Advantages and Disadvantages of Mechanized Instruments as Compared to Manual Instruments

Advantages

Increased efficiency
Multiple surfaces of tip are capable of removing deposits
No need to sharpen
Less chance for repetitive stress injuries
Handpiece size large
Reduced lateral pressure
Less tissue distention
Water
Lavage
Irrigation
Acoustic microstreaming

Disadvantages

More precautions and limitations
Client comfort (water spraying)
Aerosol production
Temporary hearing shifts
Noise
Less tactile sensation
Reduced visibility

(From Darby ML, Walsh MM: *Dental hygiene*, ed 3, Saunders, St Louis, 2010.)

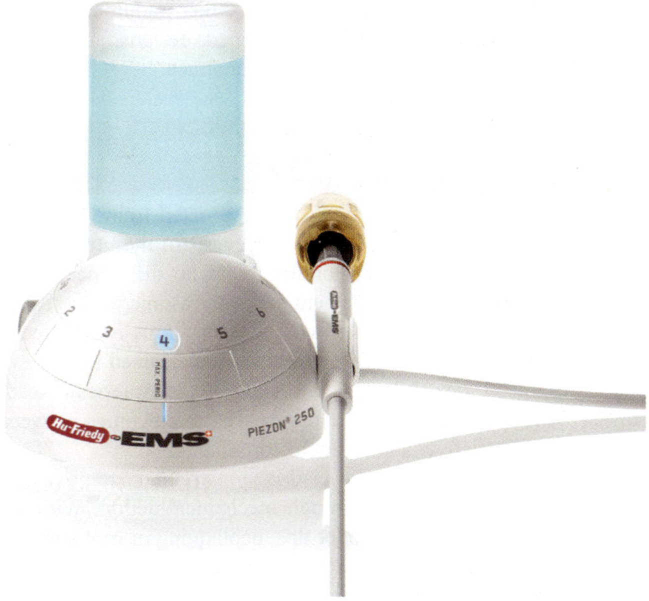

Fig. 36.26 A piezoelectric ultrasonic device. *(Courtesy: Hu-Friedy, Chicago.)*

Efficiency

Power instrumentation has the potential to make scaling less demanding, more time efficient, and more ergonomically friendly. Modified tip designs allow for improved access in many areas, including furcations. Newer, slimmer designs operate effectively at lower power settings, thus improving patient comfort. Sonic and ultrasonic tips can reduce the time needed for scaling.

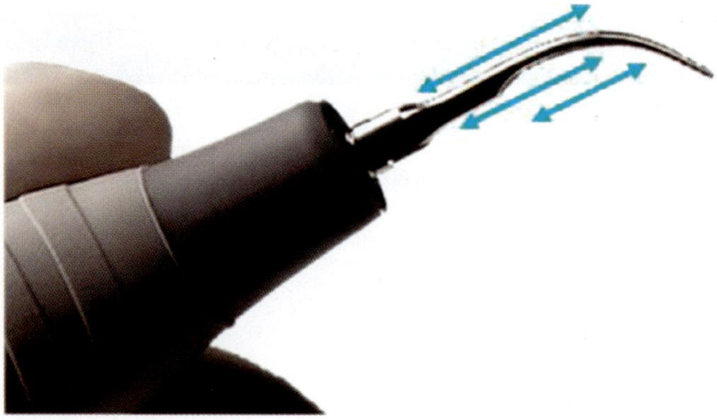

Fig. 36.27 Working sides of a piezoelectric tip. *(Courtesy: Hu-Friedy, Chicago.)*

Tip Designs

There are tips designed to remove heavy supragingival calculus or to definitively debride periodontal pockets. Large diameter tips are created in a universal design and are indicated for the removal of large, tenacious deposits. A high power setting is generally recommended. Thinner diameter tips may be site specific in design. The straight tip design is ideal for use in treating patients with gingivitis and deplaquing maintenance patients. The right and left contra-angled instruments allow for greater access and adaptation to root morphology. These inserts are designed to work in a low power setting. They can be used for exploration. The amount of water delivered for lavage can be controlled through the selection of either traditional flow or a focused tip delivery flow. Contra-angled designs and larger, ergonomic grips enhance comfort and ergonomics.

Clinical Outcomes of Power-Driven Instruments

Numerous clinical outcomes have been evaluated from the use of power-driven instruments. A systematic review of the literature on the treatment of chronic periodontitis found no difference in the efficacy of subgingival debridement using ultrasonic/sonic scalers versus hand instruments in the treatment of single-rooted teeth. A benefit for multirooted teeth could not be determined because of a lack of clinical data. Likewise, a review by the American Academy of Periodontology found no differences in outcomes between sonic, magnetostrictive, and piezoelectric scalers.

It is well established that power-driven instruments remove biofilms, bacteria, and calculus through mechanical action. With the advent of new designs and thinner tips, deplaquing of root surfaces may be effectively accomplished by power scalers. Both sonic and ultrasonic instruments have been shown to be effective in removing calculus similar to hand instrumentation. Ultrasonic instruments through high-speed action produce a cavitational activity and acoustic microstreaming that some believe may help enhance the disruption of the bacteria in subgingival biofilms.

The primary expected clinical outcomes from scaling and root planing are a reduction in bleeding and probing depth and a gain in clinical attachment. In comparing power scalers to hand instruments, both types demonstrate similar outcomes for reductions in bleeding on probing and probing depth and gains in clinical attachment.

Special Considerations

Furcations present one of the greatest scaling challenges. In many instances, the opening of the furcation is narrower than the conventional hand instrument. For this reason, power scalers may be recommended as a means to improve access when scaling furcations.

Root Surface Roughness

The data are mixed on whether power-driven instruments cause more root surface roughness than hand instruments. Although it could be assumed that using the device at a higher power may cause more roughness, this is not been proven. It is also not known how much root surface roughness affects the healing process. Power-driven instruments may increase the roughness of resin or glass ionomer restorative materials; therefore, repolishing post scaling is recommended.

Aerosol Production

Power-driven devices produce bioaerosols and splatter, which can contaminate the operator and remain in the air for up to 30 min. Good infection control practices can minimize the hazard. Data have shown that preprocedural rinsing with 0.12% chlorhexidine and high-speed evacuation are the most efficient ways to reduce bioaerosols.

Cardiac Pacemakers

The use of ultrasonics on patients with cardiac pacemakers is somewhat controversial. Newer models of pacemakers often have bipolar titanium insulation that is believed to make ultrasonic and sonic instruments generally safe for use. An in vivo study supports this; 12 patients underwent continuous electrocardiogram monitoring during piezoelectric ultrasonic scaling and had no abnormal pacemaker functions. Conversely, an in vitro study found that ultrasonic scalers interfered with the activity of dual-system pacemakers. If in doubt, consult with the physician regarding any precautions or warnings from the manufacturer of the product. Box 36.2 outlines

BOX 36.2 Indications, Precautions, and Contraindications for Use of Mechanized Instruments

Indications
- Supragingival debridement of dental calculus and extrinsic stain
- Subgingival debridement of calculus, oral biofilm, root surface constituents, and periodontal pathogens
- Removal of orthodontic cement
- Gingival and periodontal conditions and diseases
- Surgical interventions
- Margination (reduces amalgam overhangs)

Precautions
- Unshielded pacemakers
- Infectious diseases: human immunodeficiency virus, hepatitis, tuberculosis (active stages)
- Demineralized tooth surface
- Exposed dentin (especially associated with sensitivity)
- Restorative materials (porcelain, amalgam, gold, composite)
- Titanium implant abutments unless using special insert, for example, Quixonic Sonic scaler with SofTip Prophy Tips
- Children (primary teeth)
- Immunosuppression from disease or chemotherapy
- Uncontrolled diabetes mellitus

Contraindications
- Chronic pulmonary disease: asthma, emphysema, cystic fibrosis, pneumonia
- Cardiovascular disease with secondary pulmonary disease
- Swallowing difficulty (dysphagia)

(From Darby ML, Walsh MM: *Dental hygiene*, ed 3, Saunders, St Louis, 2010.)

the indications, precautions, and contraindications of using mechanized instrumentation.

Principles and Technique of Powered Instrumentation

Ultrasonic technique is different from instrumentation with hand scalers. A modified pen grasp is used with an ultrasonic scaler along with an extraoral fulcrum. The purpose of the extraoral fulcrum is that it allows the operator to maintain a light grasp and easier access physically and visually to the oral cavity. Alternate fulcrums of cross arch or opposite arch fulcrums are acceptable alternatives.

Light pressure is needed with a power instrument. The tip is traveling at a set frequency in a set stroke pattern. Increased clinician pressure on the tip causes decreased clinical efficacy.

Sonic/ultrasonic instrumentation requires removal from the coronal to the apical portion of the deposit. This stroke pattern allows the insert to work at its optimal stroke pattern and frequency for quick effective deposit removal. A deplaquing stroke should be used when the focus is removal of biofilm and soft debris for the resolution of gingival inflammation. This stroke entails accessing every square millimeter of the tooth surface during ultrasonic deplaquing as a result of the limited lateral dispersion of the lavage subgingivally.

Technique

Ultrasonic instrumentation is accomplished with a light-to-moderate grasp and varying pressure depending on the amount and tenacity of the deposit. Excessive pressure is not recommended because it can cause dampening of the vibration of the tip. The tip should be kept in constant motion and parallel to the tooth surface. Leaving the tip in one place for too long or using the point of the tip against the tooth can produce gouging and roughening of the root surface or overheating of the tooth. Using a lower-power setting and applying only slight pressure reduces the volume and depth of tooth structure removal.

The ultrasonic tip must come in direct physical contact with calculus to fracture and remove it. The tip must also contact all aspects of the root surface to remove biofilm and toxins thoroughly. Although as much as 10 mm or more of the length of the ultrasonic tip vibrates, only the terminal few millimeters of the tip produce maximum vibration. At any point in time, it is only possible for this terminal 1- to 2-mm portion of the tip to be in contact with the tooth because of the curved anatomy of teeth. On convex surfaces such as depressions or line angles, it is not possible to adapt more than 1 or 2 mm of the tip against the tooth. Even on what appear to be broader, flatter surfaces, no more than this small terminal portion of the tip can be adapted because the tooth surface, although it may seem flat, is actually slightly curved.

If a longer portion of the tip is adapted to a convex surface so that it contacts the tooth at a tangent, this less effective part of the tip is likely to burnish calculus or miss it altogether. Additionally, the tip will jut out into the soft tissue, thus possibly causing trauma and discomfort.

A series of focused, overlapping strokes must be activated to keep this small active portion of the tip adapted to the root surface at all times. The handpiece and the blunt working end of the ultrasonic tip impair tactile sensitivity, and the constant water spray hampers visibility. For these reasons, during ultrasonic instrumentation, the tooth surface should be frequently examined with an explorer to evaluate the completeness of debridement.

With these points in mind, the ultrasonic device is used in the following manner:

1. Thoroughly wipe the ultrasonic unit with a disinfectant. Use a sterile, autoclavable ultrasonic handpiece, or wipe the handpiece with disinfectant. Cover the ultrasonic unit or control knobs and the handpiece with plastic or latex barriers. Flush the water lines and handpiece for 2 min to decrease the number of microorganisms in the lines. Use water line filters or sterile water whenever possible.
2. Direct the patient to rinse for 1 min with an antimicrobial oral rinse such as 0.12% chlorhexidine to reduce the contaminated aerosol.
3. The clinician and the assistant should wear protective eyewear or face shields and masks. Use high-speed evacuation to minimize contaminated aerosol produced during instrumentation.
4. Turn on the unit, select an insert, place it into the handpiece, and then adjust the water control knob to produce a light mist of water at the working tip. Adequate aspiration is necessary to remove the water as it accumulates in the mouth. The power setting should begin on low and be adjusted no higher than necessary to remove calculus. Medium- to high-power settings have been shown to cause damage to roots when the tip is not parallel to the root surface.
5. The instrument is grasped with a light to moderate pen or modified pen grasp, and a finger rest or extraoral fulcrum should be established to allow a light touch. Extraoral hand rests should be used for the maxillary teeth. For the mandibular teeth, either intraoral or extraoral fulcrums may be used.
6. Use short, light, vertical, horizontal, or oblique overlapping strokes. Keep the working tip adapted to the tooth surface as it passes over the deposit. Heavy lateral pressure is unnecessary because the vibrational energy of the instrument dislodges the calculus. However, the working end must touch the deposit for this to occur.
7. The working end should be kept in constant motion, and the tip should be kept parallel to the tooth surface or at no more than a 15-degree angle to avoid etching or grooving the tooth surface.
8. The instrument should be switched off periodically to allow for aspiration of water, and the tooth surface should be examined frequently with an explorer.
9. Any remaining irregularities of the root surface may be removed with sharp standard or mini-bladed curettes if necessary.

Evaluation of Adequacy of Scaling and Root Planing

The adequacy of scaling and root planing is evaluated when the procedure is performed and again later, after a period of soft tissue healing.

Immediately after instrumentation, the tooth surfaces should be carefully inspected visually with optimal lighting and the aid of a mouth mirror and compressed air; surfaces also should be examined with a fine explorer or probe. Subgingival surfaces should be hard and smooth. Although complete removal of calculus is definitely necessary for the health of the adjacent soft tissue, little documented evidence of the necessity for root smoothness is available. Nevertheless, relative smoothness is still the best immediate clinical indication that calculus has been completely removed.

Although smoothness is the criterion by which scaling and root planing are immediately evaluated, the ultimate evaluation is based on *tissue response*. Clinical evaluation of the soft tissue response to scaling and root planing, including probing, should not be conducted earlier than 2 weeks postoperatively. Reepithelialization of the wounds created during instrumentation takes 1–2 weeks. Until then, gingival bleeding on probing can be expected even when calculus has been completely removed because the soft tissue wound is not epithelialized. Any gingival bleeding on probing noted after this interval is more likely the result of persistent inflammation produced by residual deposits not removed during the initial procedure or inadequate plaque control. Positive clinical changes after instrumentation often continue for weeks or months. Therefore, a longer period of evaluation may be indicated before deciding whether to intervene with further instrumentation or surgery.

Occasionally, the clinician may find that some slight root roughness remains after scaling and root planing. If sound principles of instrumentation have been followed, the roughness may not be calculus. Because calculus removal, not root smoothness, has been shown to be necessary for tissue health, it might be more prudent in such a case to stop short of perfect smoothness and reevaluate the patient's tissue response after 2–4 weeks or longer. This avoids overinstrumentation and removal of excessive root structure in the pursuit of smoothness for its own sake. If the tissue is healthy after an interval of 2–4 weeks or longer, no further root planing is necessary. If the tissue is inflamed, the clinician must determine to what extent this is caused by biofilm accumulation or the presence of residual calculus and to what degree further root planing is necessary.

Key points

- Scaling is the process by which biofilm and calculus are removed from both supragingival and subgingival tooth surfaces.
- Root planing is the process by which residual embedded calculus and portions of cementum are removed from the roots to produce a smooth, hard, and clean surface.
- The distance between the apical edge of the calculus and the bottom of the pocket usually ranges from 0.2 to 1.0 mm.
- Scaling and root-planing strokes should be confined to the portion of the tooth where calculus or altered cementum is found which is also known as instrumentation zone.
- The finger rest or fulcrum must be positioned to allow the lower shank of the instrument to be parallel or nearly parallel to the tooth surface being treated. Also, the finger rest must be positioned to enable the operator to use wrist-arm motion to activate strokes.
- Acoustic streaming is the unidirectional fluid flow caused by ultrasound waves.
- Acoustic turbulence is created when the movement of the tip of the power scaler causes the coolant to accelerate, producing an intensified swirling effect.
- Cavitation is the formation of bubbles in water caused by the high turbulence.
- Sonic units work at a frequency of 2000–6500 cycles per second, whereas ultrasonic devices work at a frequency range of 18,000–50,000 cycles per second.
- Tips of magnetostrictive ultrasonic devices move in an elliptical or orbital stroke pattern and have four active working surfaces.
- Tips of piezoelectric ultrasonic units move in a linear pattern and have two active working surfaces.

Suggested Readings

Arabaci T, Cicek Y, Canakci CF: Sonic and ultrasonic scalers in periodontal treatment: a review, *Int J Dent Hygiene* 5:2, 2007.Cadosch J, Zimmermann U, Ruppert M, et al: Root surface debridement and endotoxin removal, *J Periodontal Res* 38:229, 2003.

Claffey N: Decision making in periodontal therapy: the reevaluation, *J Clin Periodontol* 18:364, 1991.

Drisko C: Academy report: sonic and ultrasonic scalers in periodontics, *J Periodontol* 71:1792, 2000.

Drisko CL, Cochran DL, Blieden T, et al: Position paper: sonic and ultrasonic scalers in periodontics. Research, Science and Therapy Committee of the American Academy of Periodontology, *J Periodontol* 71:1792, 2000.

Greenstein G: Nonsurgical periodontal therapy in 2000: a literature review, *J Am Dent Assoc* 131:1580, 2000.

Harrel SK, Barnes JB, Rivera-Hidalgo F: Reduction of aerosols produced by ultrasonic scalers, *J Periodontol* 67:28, 1996.

Kaldahl WB, Kalkwarf KL, Patil KD, et al: Long-term evaluation of periodontal therapy. I. Response to 4 therapeutic modalities, *J Periodontol* 67:93, 1996.

Khambay BS, Walmsley AD: Acoustic microstreaming: detection and measurement around ultrasonic scalers, *J Periodontol* 70:626, 1999.

Lindhe J, Nyman S: Long-term maintenance of patients treated for advanced periodontal disease, *J Clin Periodontol* 11:504, 1984.

Lindhe J, Nyman S, Karring T: Scaling and root planing in shallow pockets, *J Clin Periodontol* 9:415, 1982.

Magnusson I, Lindhe J, Yoneyama T, et al: Recolonization of a subgingivalmicrobiota following scaling in deep pockets, *J Clin Periodontol* 11:193, 1984.

Obeid PR, D'Hoore W, Bercy P: Comparative clinical responses related to the use of various periodontal instrumentation, *J Clin Periodontol* 31:193, 2004.

Pattison AM: The use of hand instruments in supportive periodontal treatment, *Periodontol* 2000 12:71, 1996.

Quirynen M, Mongardini C, Pauwels M, et al: One stage full- versus partial-mouth disinfection in the treatment of chronic adult or generalized early-onset periodontitis. II. Long-term impact on microbial load, *J Periodontol* 70:646, 1999.

References

References and MCQs with answers for the chapter are available on www.medenact.com.

CHAPTER 37

Antiinfective Therapy

SG Ciancio | A Mariotti | RD Finkelman | HL Sarmiento | AM Polson | A Jain

CHAPTER OUTLINE

It is well established that the various periodontal diseases are caused by bacterial infection. Bacteria begin reattaching to the crowns of teeth soon after the teeth have been cleaned and begin to form a *biofilm*. Over time, this supragingival plaque biofilm becomes more complex, which leads to a succession of bacteria that are more pathogenic. Bacteria grow in an apical direction and become subgingival. Eventually, as bone is destroyed, a periodontal pocket is formed. In a periodontal pocket, the bacteria form a highly structured and complex biofilm. As this process continues, the bacterial biofilm extends so far subgingivally that the patient cannot reach it during oral hygiene efforts. In addition, this complex biofilm may now offer some protection from the host's immunologic mechanisms in the periodontal pocket as well as from antibiotics used for treatment. It has been suggested that an antibiotic strength that is 500 times greater than the usual therapeutic dose may be needed to be effective against bacteria that have become arranged in biofilms.

It is, therefore, logical to treat periodontal pockets via the mechanical removal of local factors (including the calculus that harbors bacteria) and also by the disruption of the subgingival plaque biofilm itself. Mechanical removal includes manual instrumentation (e.g., scaling and root planing) and machine-driven instrumentation (e.g., ultrasonic scalers), and these procedures can be considered "antiinfective therapy." Many chemotherapeutic agents are now available to clinicians who treat periodontal diseases. *Systemic* antiinfective therapy (oral antibiotics) and *local* antiinfective therapy (placing antiinfective agents directly into the periodontal pocket) can reduce the bacterial challenge to the periodontium. It is also possible that systemically administered nonsteroidal antiinflammatory agents may play a role in future adjunctive therapy.

Bacteria and their toxic products cause a loss of attachment and a loss of bone. Ultimately, however, the host's own immunologic response to this bacterial infection can cause even more bone destruction (i.e., indirect bone loss) than that caused by pathogenic bacteria and their by-products. This immunologic response can be influenced by environmental (e.g., tobacco use), acquired (e.g., systemic disease), and genetic risk factors. Chemotherapeutic agents can modulate the host's immune response to bacteria and reduce the host's self-destructive immunologic response to bacterial pathogens, thereby reducing bone loss. It is also incumbent on health care providers to counsel patients about the detrimental effects of systemic factors, including medications, stress, and tobacco use.

This chapter reviews the indications and protocols for optimizing the use of antiinfective agents during the treatment of periodontal diseases. It is important to note that significant work has been performed with the use of a systematic *evidence-based approach* to evaluate the various antiinfective and host modulation therapies. The metaanalysis of similar research studies has given power to statistical analysis to evaluate antiinfective chemotherapeutic agents for the treatment of periodontal diseases. Unfortunately, a standardized research protocol has not yet been implemented. As a result, some studies—although relevant—have not been used in the evidence-based approach because of their study design. Further evidence-based and similar research is needed to define protocols more precisely for the use of antiinfective agents to treat periodontal diseases.

An antiinfective agent is a *chemotherapeutic agent* that acts by reducing the number of bacteria present. An antibiotic is a naturally occurring, semisynthetic, or synthetic type of antiinfective agent that destroys or inhibits the growth of selective microorganisms, generally at low concentrations. An antiseptic is a chemical antimicrobial agent that can be applied topically or subgingivally to mucous membranes, wounds, or intact dermal surfaces to destroy microorganisms and to inhibit their reproduction or metabolism. In dentistry, antiseptics are widely used as the active ingredient in antiplaque and antigingivitis oral rinses and dentifrices. Disinfectants (a subcategory of antiseptics) are antimicrobial agents that are generally applied to inanimate surfaces to destroy microorganisms.

Antiinfective agents can be administered *locally* or *orally*. When administered orally, many of these agents can be found in gingival crevicular fluid (GCF). With either approach, their purpose is to reduce the number of bacteria present in the diseased periodontal pocket. The *systemic administration* of antibiotics may be a necessary adjunct for the controlling of bacterial infection because bacteria can invade periodontal tissues, thereby making mechanical therapy alone sometimes ineffective. The *local administration* of antiinfective agents, generally directly to the pocket, has the potential to provide greater concentrations directly to the infected area and thus reduce possible systemic side effects.

A single chemotherapeutic agent can also have a dual mechanism of action. For example, tetracyclines (especially doxycycline)

TABLE 37.1 Antibiotics Used to Treat Periodontal Diseases

Category	Agent	Major Features
Penicillin[a]	Amoxicillin Augmentin[b]	Extended spectrum of antimicrobial activity; excellent oral absorption; used systemically Effective against penicillinase-producing microorganisms; used systemically
Tetracyclines	Minocycline Doxycycline	Effective against a broad spectrum of microorganisms; used systemically and applied locally (subgingivally)
	Tetracycline	Effective against a broad spectrum of microorganisms; used systemically and applied locally (subgingivally) Chemotherapeutically used in subantimicrobial doses for host modulation (Periostat) Effective against a broad spectrum of microorganisms
Quinolone	Ciprofloxacin	Effective against gram-negative rods; promotes health-associated microflora
Macrolide	Azithromycin	Concentrates at sites of inflammation; used systemically
Lincomycin derivative	Clindamycin	Used in penicillin-allergic patients; effective against anaerobic bacteria; used systemically
Nitroimidazole[c]	Metronidazole	Effective against anaerobic bacteria; used systemically and applied locally (subgingivally) as gel

[a]Indications: localized aggressive periodontitis, generalized aggressive periodontitis, medically related periodontitis, and refractory periodontitis.
[b]Amoxicillin and clavulanate potassium.
[c]Indications: localized aggressive periodontitis, generalized aggressive periodontitis, medically related periodontitis, refractory periodontitis, and necrotizing ulcerative periodontitis.

are chemotherapeutic agents that can reduce collagen and bone destruction via their ability to inhibit the enzyme collagenase. As antibiotic agents, they can also reduce periodontal pathogens in periodontal tissues.

Systemic Administration of Antibiotics

Background and Rationale

The treatment of periodontal diseases is based on the infectious nature of these diseases (Table 37.1). Ideally, the causative microorganisms should be identified, and the most effective agent should be selected with the use of antibiotic-sensitivity testing. Although this appears simple, the difficulty lies primarily in identifying the specific etiologic microorganisms rather than the microorganisms that are simply associated with various periodontal disorders.

An ideal antibiotic for use in the prevention and treatment of periodontal diseases should be specific for periodontal pathogens, allogenic, nontoxic, substantive, not in general use for the treatment of other diseases, and inexpensive. Currently, however, an ideal antibiotic for the treatment of periodontal diseases does not exist. Although oral bacteria are susceptible to many antibiotics, no single antibiotic at the concentrations achieved in body fluids inhibits all putative periodontal pathogens. Indeed, a combination of antibiotics may be necessary to eliminate all putative pathogens from some periodontal pockets (Table 37.2).

As always, the clinician—in concert with the patient—must make the final decision regarding any treatment. Thus, the treatment of the individual patient must be based on the patient's clinical status, the nature of the colonizing bacteria, the ability of the agent to reach the site of infection, and the risks and benefits associated with the proposed treatment plan. The clinician is responsible for choosing the correct antimicrobial agent. Some adverse reactions include allergic or anaphylactic reactions, superinfections of opportunistic bacteria, the development of resistant bacteria, interactions with other medications, upset stomach, nausea, and vomiting. Most adverse reactions take the form of gastrointestinal upset. Other concerns include the cost of the medication and the patient's willingness and ability to comply with the proposed therapy.

No consensus exists regarding the magnitude of the risk for the development of bacterial resistance. The common and indiscriminate use of antibiotics worldwide has contributed to increasing numbers of resistant bacterial strains over the last 15–20 years, and this trend is likely to continue given the widespread use of antibiotics. The overuse, misuse, and widespread prophylactic application of antiinfective drugs are some of the factors that have led to the emergence of resistant microorganisms. Increasing levels of resistance of subgingivalmicroflora to antibiotics has been correlated with the increased use of antibiotics in individual countries. However, researchers have noted that the subgingivalmicroflora tends to revert to similar proportions of antibiotic-resistant isolates 3 months after therapy.

TABLE 37.2 Common Antibiotic Regimens Used to Treat Periodontal Diseases[a]

	Regimen	Dosage/Duration
Single Agent		
Amoxicillin	500 mg	Three times daily for 8 days
Azithromycin	500 mg	Once daily for 4–7 days
Ciprofloxacin	500 mg	Twice daily for 8 days
Clindamycin	300 mg	Three times daily for 10 days
Doxycycline or minocycline	100–200 mg	Once daily for 21 days
Metronidazole	500 mg	Three times daily for 8 days
Combination Therapy		
Metronidazole + amoxicillin	250 mg of each	Three times daily for 8 days
Metronidazole + ciprofloxacin	500 mg of each	Twice daily for 8 days

(Data from Jorgensen MG, Slots J: *Compend Contin Educ Dent* 21:111, 2000.)
[a]These regimens are prescribed after a review of the patient's medical history, periodontal diagnosis, and antimicrobial testing. Clinicians must consult pharmacology references such as *Mosby's GenRx* or the manufacturer's guidelines for warnings, contraindications, and precautions.

Tetracyclines

Tetracyclines have been widely used for the treatment of periodontal diseases. They have been frequently used to treat refractory periodontitis, including *localized aggressive periodontitis* (LAP) (Table 37.1). Tetracyclines have the ability to concentrate in the periodontal tissues and to inhibit the growth of *Aggregatibacter actinomycetemcomitans*. In addition, tetracyclines exert an anticollagenase effect that can inhibit tissue destruction and that may help with bone regeneration.

Pharmacology

The tetracyclines are a group of antibiotics that are produced naturally from certain species of *Streptomyces* or that are derived semisynthetically. These antibiotics are bacteriostatic, and they are effective against rapidly multiplying bacteria. They generally are more effective against gram-positive bacteria than gram-negative bacteria. Tetracyclines are effective for the treatment of periodontal diseases in part because their concentration in the gingival crevice is 2–10 times that found in serum. This allows a high drug concentration to be delivered into the periodontal pockets. In addition, several studies have demonstrated that tetracyclines at a low GCF concentration (i.e., 2–4 μg/mL) are very effective against many periodontal pathogens.

Clinical Use

Tetracyclines have been investigated as adjuncts for the treatment of LAP. *A. actinomycetemcomitans* is a frequent microorganism that is associated with LAP, and it invades tissue. Therefore, the mechanical removal of calculus and plaque from root surfaces may not eliminate this bacterium from the periodontal tissues. Systemic tetracycline can eliminate tissue bacteria, and it has been shown to arrest bone loss and to suppress *A. actinomycetemcomitans* levels in conjunction with scaling and root planing. This combination therapy allows for the mechanical removal of root surface deposits and for the elimination of pathogenic bacteria from within the tissues. Increased posttreatment bone levels have been noted with the use of this method. Due to increased resistance to tetracyclines, metronidazole, or amoxicillin with metronidazole has been found to be more effective for the treatment of aggressive periodontitis in children. Some investigators think that metronidazole in combination with amoxicillin–clavulanic acid is the preferable antibiotic.

The long-term use of low antibacterial doses of tetracyclines has been advocated in the past. One long-term study of patients taking low doses of tetracycline (i.e., 250 mg/day for 2–7 years) demonstrated the persistence of deep pockets that did not bleed after probing. These sites contained high proportions of tetracycline-resistant, gram-negative rods *(Fusobacterium nucleatum)*. After the antibiotic was discontinued, the flora was characteristic of sites with disease. Therefore, it is not advisable to prescribe long-term regimens of tetracyclines because of the possible development of resistant bacterial strains. Although tetracyclines were often used in the past as antiinfective agents, especially for LAP and other types of aggressive periodontitis, they are now frequently replaced by more effective combination antibiotics.

Specific Agents

Tetracycline, minocycline, and doxycycline are semisynthetic members of the tetracycline group that have been used in periodontal therapy.

Tetracycline

Treatment with tetracycline hydrochloride requires the administration of 250 mg 4 times daily. It is inexpensive, but compliance may be reduced by the need to take the medication so frequently. Side effects include gastrointestinal disturbances, photosensitivity, hypersensitivity, increased blood urea nitrogen levels, blood dyscrasias, dizziness, and headache. In addition, tooth discoloration occurs when this drug is administered to children who are 12 years old or younger.

Minocycline

Minocycline is effective against a broad spectrum of microorganisms. In patients with adult periodontitis, it suppresses spirochetes and motile rods as effectively as scaling and root planing, with suppression evident up to 3 months after therapy. Minocycline can be given twice daily, thereby facilitating compliance as compared to tetracycline. Although it is associated with less phototoxicity and renal toxicity than tetracycline, minocycline may cause reversible vertigo. Minocycline administered at a dose of 200 mg/day for 1 week results in a reduction in total bacterial counts, the complete elimination of spirochetes for up to 2 months, and the improvement of all clinical parameters.

Side effects are similar to those of tetracycline; however, there is an increased incidence of vertigo. It is the only tetracycline that can discolor permanently erupted teeth and gingival tissue when administered orally.

Doxycycline

Doxycycline has the same spectrum of activity as minocycline, and it may be equally effective. Since doxycycline can be given only once daily, patients may be more compliant. Compliance is also favored because its absorption from the gastrointestinal tract is only slightly altered by calcium, metal ions, or antacids, as is the absorption of other tetracyclines. Side effects are similar to those of tetracycline hydrochloride; however, it is the most photosensitizing agent in the tetracycline category.

The recommended dosage when doxycycline is used as an antiinfective agent is 100 mg twice daily the first day, which is then reduced to 100 mg daily. To reduce gastrointestinal upset, 50 mg can be taken twice daily after the initial dose. When given as a subantimicrobial dose (to inhibit collagenase), 20 mg of doxycycline twice daily is recommended. Periostat (CollaGenex Pharmaceuticals Inc, Newtown, PA) and generic forms are currently available in a dose of 20 mg of doxycycline.

Metronidazole

Pharmacology

Metronidazole is a nitroimidazole compound that was developed in France to treat protozoal infections. It is bactericidal to anaerobic organisms, and it is thought to disrupt bacterial DNA synthesis in conditions with a low reduction potential. Metronidazole is not the drug of choice for treating *A. actinomycetemcomitans* infections. However, metronidazole is effective against *A. actinomycetemcomitans* when it is used in combination with other antibiotics. Metronidazole is also effective against anaerobes such as *Porphyromonas gingivalis* and *Prevotella intermedia*.

Clinical Use

Metronidazole (MTX) has been used clinically to treat gingivitis, acute necrotizing ulcerative gingivitis, chronic periodontitis, and aggressive periodontitis. It has been used as monotherapy and also in combination with both root planing and surgery or with other antibiotics. Metronidazole has been used successfully to treat necrotizing ulcerative gingivitis.

Studies in humans have demonstrated the efficacy of metronidazole for the treatment of gingivitis and periodontitis. A single dose of metronidazole (250 mg orally) appears in both serum and GCF in sufficient quantities to inhibit a wide range of suspected periodontal pathogens. When it is administered systemically (i.e., 750–1000 mg/day for 2 weeks), metronidazole reduces the growth of anaerobic flora, including spirochetes, and it decreases the clinical and histopathologic signs of periodontitis. The most common regimen is 250 mg 3 times daily for 7 days. Currently, the critical level of spirochetes that is needed to diagnose an anaerobic infection, the appropriate time to give metronidazole, and the ideal dosage or duration of therapy are unknown. As monotherapy (i.e., with no concurrent root planing), metronidazole is inferior and at best only equivalent to root planing. Therefore, if it is used, metronidazole should not be administered as monotherapy.

Soder and colleagues demonstrated that metronidazole was more effective than placebo for the management of sites that were unresponsive to root planing. Nevertheless, many patients still had sites that bled with probing, despite metronidazole therapy. The existence of refractory periodontitis as a diagnostic consideration indicates that some patients do not respond to conventional therapy, which may include root planing, surgery, or both.

Studies have suggested that, when it is combined with amoxicillin or amoxicillin–clavulanate potassium (Augmentin), metronidazole may be of value for the management of patients with LAP or refractory periodontitis. This is discussed in more detail later in this chapter.

Side Effects

Metronidazole has an Antabuse effect when alcohol is ingested. The response is generally proportional to the amount ingested, and it can result in severe cramps, nausea, and vomiting. Products that contain alcohol should be avoided during therapy and for at least 1 day after therapy is discontinued. Metronidazole also inhibits warfarin metabolism. Patients who are undergoing anticoagulant therapy should avoid metronidazole because it prolongs prothrombin time. It also should be avoided in patients who are taking lithium. This drug produces a metallic taste in the mouth, which may affect compliance.

Penicillins

Pharmacology

Penicillins are the drugs of choice for the treatment of many serious infections in humans, and they are the most widely used antibiotics. Penicillins are natural and semisynthetic derivatives of broth cultures of the *Penicillium* mold. They inhibit bacterial cell wall production and therefore are bactericidal.

Clinical Use

Penicillins other than amoxicillin and amoxicillin–clavulanate potassium (Augmentin) have not been shown to increase periodontal attachment levels, and their use in periodontal therapy does not appear to be justified.

Side Effects

Penicillins may induce allergic reactions and bacterial resistance; up to 10% of patients may be allergic to penicillin.

Amoxicillin

Amoxicillin (AMX) is a semisynthetic penicillin with an extended antiinfective spectrum that includes gram-positive and gram-negative bacteria. It demonstrates excellent absorption after oral administration. Amoxicillin is susceptible to penicillinase, which is a β-lactamase produced by certain bacteria that breaks the penicillin ring structure and thus renders penicillins ineffective.

Amoxicillin may be useful for the management of patients with aggressive periodontitis in both localized and generalized forms. The recommended dosage is 500 mg 3 times daily for 8 days.

Amoxicillin–Clavulanate Potassium

The combination of amoxicillin with clavulanate potassium makes this antiinfective agent resistant to penicillinase enzymes produced by some bacteria. Amoxicillin with clavulanate (Augmentin) may be useful for the management of patients with LAP or refractory periodontitis. Bueno and colleagues reported that Augmentin arrested alveolar bone loss in patients with periodontal disease that was refractory to treatment with other antibiotics, including tetracycline, metronidazole, and clindamycin.

Cephalosporins

Pharmacology

The family of β-lactams known as cephalosporins is similar in action and structure to the penicillins. These drugs are frequently used in medicine, and they are resistant to a number of β-lactamases that are normally active against penicillin.

Clinical Use

Cephalosporins are generally not used to treat dental-related infections. The penicillins are superior to cephalosporins with regard to their range of action against periodontal pathogenic bacteria.

Side Effects

Patients who are allergic to penicillins must be considered to be allergic to all β-lactam products. Rashes, urticaria, fever, and gastrointestinal upset have all been associated with cephalosporins.

Clindamycin

Pharmacology

Clindamycin is effective against anaerobic bacteria, and it has a strong affinity for osseous tissue. It is effective for situations in which the patient is allergic to penicillin.

Clinical Use

Clindamycin has demonstrated efficacy in patients with periodontitis that is refractory to tetracycline therapy. Walker and colleagues showed that clindamycin assisted with the stabilization of refractory patients; the dosage used was 150 mg 4 times daily for 10 days. Jorgensen and Slots recommend a regimen of 300 mg twice daily for 8 days.

Side Effects

Clindamycin has been associated with pseudomembranous colitis, but the incidence is higher with cephalosporins and ampicillin. When needed, however, clindamycin can be used with caution, but it is not indicated for patients with a history of colitis. Diarrhea or cramping that develops during clindamycin therapy may be indicative of colitis, and clindamycin should be discontinued. If symptoms persist, the patient should be referred to an internist.

Ciprofloxacin

Pharmacology

Ciprofloxacin is a quinolone that is active against gram-negative rods, including all facultative and some anaerobic putative periodontal pathogens.

Clinical Use

Since it demonstrates a minimal effect on *Streptococcus* species, which are associated with periodontal health, ciprofloxacin therapy may facilitate the establishment of a microflora that is associated with periodontal health. At present, ciprofloxacin is the only antibiotic in periodontal therapy to which all strains of *A. actinomycetemcomitans* are susceptible. It has also been used in combination with metronidazole.

Side Effects

Nausea, headache, metallic taste in the mouth, and abdominal discomfort have been associated with ciprofloxacin. Quinolones inhibit the metabolism of theophylline, and caffeine and concurrent administration can produce toxicity. Quinolones have also been reported to enhance the effect of warfarin and other anticoagulants.

Macrolides

Pharmacology

Macrolide antibiotics contain a many-membered lactone ring to which one or more deoxy sugars are attached. They inhibit protein synthesis by binding to the 50S ribosomal subunits of sensitive microorganisms. Macrolides can be bacteriostatic or bactericidal, depending on the concentration of the drug and the nature of the microorganism. The macrolide antibiotics used for periodontal treatment include erythromycin, spiramycin, and azithromycin.

Clinical Use

Erythromycin does not concentrate in GCF, and it is not effective against most putative periodontal pathogens. For these reasons, erythromycin is not recommended as an adjunct to periodontal therapy.

Spiramycin is active against gram-positive organisms; it is excreted in high concentrations in saliva. It is used as an adjunct to periodontal treatment in Canada and Europe, but it is not available in the United States. Spiramycin has a minimal effect on increasing attachment levels.

Azithromycin is a member of the azalide class of macrolides. It is effective against anaerobes and gram-negative bacilli. After an oral dosage of 500 mg 4 times daily for 3 days, significant levels of azithromycin can be detected in most tissues for 7–10 days. The concentration of azithromycin in tissue specimens from periodontal lesions is significantly higher than that of normal gingiva. It has been proposed that azithromycin penetrates fibroblasts and phagocytes in concentrations that are 100–200 times greater than that of the extracellular compartment. The azithromycin is actively transported to sites of inflammation by phagocytes, where it is then released directly into the sites of inflammation as the phagocytes rupture during phagocytosis. Therapeutic use requires a single dose of 250 mg/day for 5 days after an initial loading dose of 500 mg.

Data have suggested that azithromycin may be an effective adjunctive therapy for increasing attachment levels in patients with aggressive periodontitis as well as for reducing the degree of gingival enlargement. At this time, these data must be carefully considered because the data were derived from small subject populations. Currently, the literature presents conflicting reports regarding the efficacy of this antibiotic as an adjunct to periodontal therapy. A recent study concluded that adjunctive azithromycin provides no additional benefit over nonsurgical periodontal treatment for the parameters investigated in patients with severe generalized chronic periodontitis. Furthermore, a study in the *New England Journal of Medicine* in 2012 reported that there was an increase in cardiovascular deaths among patients who were receiving azithromycin; this increase was most pronounced among patients with a high baseline risk of cardiovascular disease. As a result of this study, the US Food and Drug Administration issued a warning that the drug can alter the electrical activity of the heart, which may lead to a potentially fatal heart rhythm known as *prolonged QT interval.* This rhythm causes the timing of the heart's contractions to become irregular. The warning stated that physicians should use caution when giving the antibiotic to patients who are known to have this condition or who are at risk for cardiovascular problems.

To ascertain the efficacy of azithromycin for the management of periodontal diseases, future studies will need to increase the number of subjects, improve diagnostic methods and tools, and determine the appropriate dose, duration, and frequency of azithromycin therapy.

Serial and Combination Antibiotic Therapy

Rationale

Since periodontal infections may contain a wide diversity of bacteria, no single antibiotic is effective against all putative pathogens. Indeed, differences exist in the microbial flora associated with the various periodontal disease syndromes. These "mixed" infections can include a variety of aerobic, microaerophilic, and anaerobic bacteria, which may be both gram-negative and gram-positive. In these cases, it may be necessary to use more than one antibiotic, either serially or in combination. Before combinations of antibiotics are used, however, the periodontal pathogens being treated must be identified and antibiotic-susceptibility testing performed.

Clinical Use

Antibiotics that are bacteriostatic (e.g., tetracycline) generally require rapidly dividing microorganisms to be effective. They do not function well if a bactericidal antibiotic (e.g., amoxicillin) is given concurrently. *When both types of drugs are required, they are best given serially rather than in combination.*

Rams and Slots reviewed combination therapy involving the use of systemic metronidazole along with amoxicillin, amoxicillin–clavulanate (Augmentin), or ciprofloxacin. The metronidazole–amoxicillin and metronidazole–Augmentin combinations provided excellent elimination of many organisms in adults with LAP who had been treated unsuccessfully with tetracyclines and mechanical debridement. These drugs have an additive effect that involves the suppression of *A. actinomycetemcomitans*. Tinoco and colleagues found metronidazole and amoxicillin to be clinically effective for the treatment of LAP, although 50% of patients who were treated with this regimen harbored *A. actinomycetemcomitans* 1 year later. The metronidazole–ciprofloxacin combination is effective against *A. actinomycetemcomitans;* metronidazole targets obligate anaerobes, and ciprofloxacin targets facultative anaerobes. This is a powerful combination against mixed infections. Studies of this drug combination for the treatment of refractory periodontitis have documented marked clinical improvement. This combination may provide a therapeutic benefit by reducing or eliminating pathogenic organisms and a prophylactic benefit by giving rise to a predominantly streptococcal microflora.

Systemic antibiotic therapy in combination with mechanical therapy appears to be valuable for the treatment of recalcitrant periodontal infections and LAP infections that involve *A. actinomycetemcomitans*. Antibiotic treatment should be reserved for specific subsets of periodontal patients who do not respond to conventional therapy. The selection of specific agents should be guided by the results of cultures and sensitivity tests for subgingival plaque microorganisms.

Pharmacologic Implications

Principles of antibiotic therapy for the proper selection of an antibiotic minimally require the identification of the causative organism, the determination of the antibiotic sensitivity, and an effective method of administration. The use of antibiotics to treat gingival diseases is contraindicated because this is a local infection that can be easily treated with scaling and appropriate home care by the patient. With regard to destructive periodontal diseases, there are limited data to support the use of systemic antibiotic treatment. Although bacterial infections of the periodontium are considered to

TABLE 37.3 Therapeutic Uses of Systemic Antimicrobial Agents for Various Periodontal Diseases

Disease	Systemic Antimicrobial Agents	Adjunct or Stand-Alone Therapy
Gingival diseases	Antibiotic use not recommended	Not applicable
Necrotizing ulcerative gingivitis	Antibiotics use not recommended unless accompanied by systemic complications (e.g., fever, swollen lymph nodes)	As an adjunct when necessary
Chronic periodontitis	Limited benefit; antibiotic use not recommended	Not applicable
Aggressive periodontitis	Antibiotic use recommended; for greatest benefit, therapeutic levels of antibiotics should be achieved by the time scaling and root planing are completed (all debridement should be completed within a week); the optimal antibiotic type, dose, frequency, and duration have not been identified	As an adjunct
Necrotizing ulcerative periodontitis	Antibiotic use dependent on the systemic condition of the patient	As an adjunct when necessary
Periodontitis as a manifestation of systemic diseases	Antibiotic use dependent on the systemic condition of the patient	As an adjunct when necessary
Periodontal abscess	Antibiotic use not recommended	Not applicable

be important for the initiation of the disease, currently there is no one microbe or group of microbes that has been demonstrated to be the cause of these diseases. It is therefore not surprising that systemic antibiotics have had only a modest effect on the management of periodontal diseases. At this time, systemic antibiotics for the treatment of periodontal diseases have been indicated primarily for adjunctive use in the treatment of aggressive periodontal diseases (Table 37.3).

Guidelines for the use of antibiotics in periodontal therapy include the following:

1. The clinical diagnosis and situation dictate the need for possible antibiotic therapy as an adjunct for controlling active periodontal disease (Fig. 37.1). The patient's diagnosis can change over time. For example, a patient who presents with generalized, mild chronic periodontitis can return to a diagnosis of periodontal health after initial therapy. However, if this patient has been treated and continues to have active disease, the diagnosis may change to generalized severe chronic periodontitis.
2. Disease activity as measured by continuing attachment loss, purulent exudate, and bleeding on probing may be an indication for periodontal intervention and possible microbial analysis through plaque sampling.
3. When they are used to treat periodontal disease, antibiotics are selected on the basis of the patient's medical and dental status, his or her current medications, and the results of microbial analysis, if it is performed.
4. Microbiologic plaque sampling may be performed according to the instructions of the reference laboratory. The samples are usually taken at the beginning of an appointment before instrumentation of the pocket. Supragingival plaque is removed, and an endodontic paper point is inserted subgingivally into the deepest pockets present to absorb bacteria in the loosely associated plaque. This endodontic point is placed in reduced transfer fluid or a sterile transfer tube and sent overnight to the laboratory. The laboratory will then send the referring dentist a report that includes the pathogens that are present and any appropriate antibiotic regimen. At this time, there are scant data to suggest that microbial identification from a plaque sample can be used to clinically improve the periodontal condition of the patient.
5. Meta-analyses of randomized clinical trials and quasi-experimental studies have shown that systemic antibiotics can improve attachment levels when they are used as adjuncts to scaling and root planing. The same benefits could not be demonstrated when antibiotics were used as a stand-alone therapy.
6. When systemic antibiotics were used as adjuncts to scaling and root planing, improvements were observed in the attachment levels of patients with chronic and aggressive periodontitis, although patients with aggressive periodontitis experienced greater benefits. The mean attachment level change depended on the antibiotic used; it ranged from 0.09 to 1.10 mm.
7. The identification of which antibiotics were most effective for the treatment of destructive periodontal diseases was limited by the insufficient sizes of the samples found in the randomized clinical trials used as part of a systematic review. With the use of a metaanalysis to evaluate eight different antibiotics or antibiotic combinations, only tetracycline and metronidazole were shown to significantly improve attachment levels when they were used as adjuncts to scaling and root planing for patients with destructive periodontal diseases.
8. Debridement of root surfaces, optimal oral hygiene, and frequent periodontal maintenance therapy are important parts of comprehensive periodontal therapy. As mentioned previously, an antibiotic strength that is 500 times greater than the systemic therapeutic dose may be required to be effective against bacteria that has been arranged into biofilms. It is therefore important to disrupt this biofilm physically so that the antibiotic agents can have access to the periodontal pathogens.
9. Although there are adequate data to suggest that systemic antibiotics can be of benefit for the treatment of destructive periodontal diseases, there are limited data available to identify which antibiotics are suitable for which infection; the optimum dosage, frequency, and duration of antibiotic therapy; when the regimen with antibiotics should be introduced during the treatment schedule; the long-term outcomes of antibiotic use; the potential hazards of these agents (e.g., antibiotic resistance, changes in oral microflora); and the economic ramifications of this type of pharmacologic intervention.

The selection of an antibiotic must be made on the basis of factors other than the empirical decisions made by the clinician. Unfortunately, there is no one best choice of antibiotic at present (i.e., there is no "silver bullet"). Therefore, the clinician must integrate the history of the patient's disease, the clinical signs and symptoms, and the results of radiographic examinations and possibly of microbiologic sampling to determine the course of periodontal

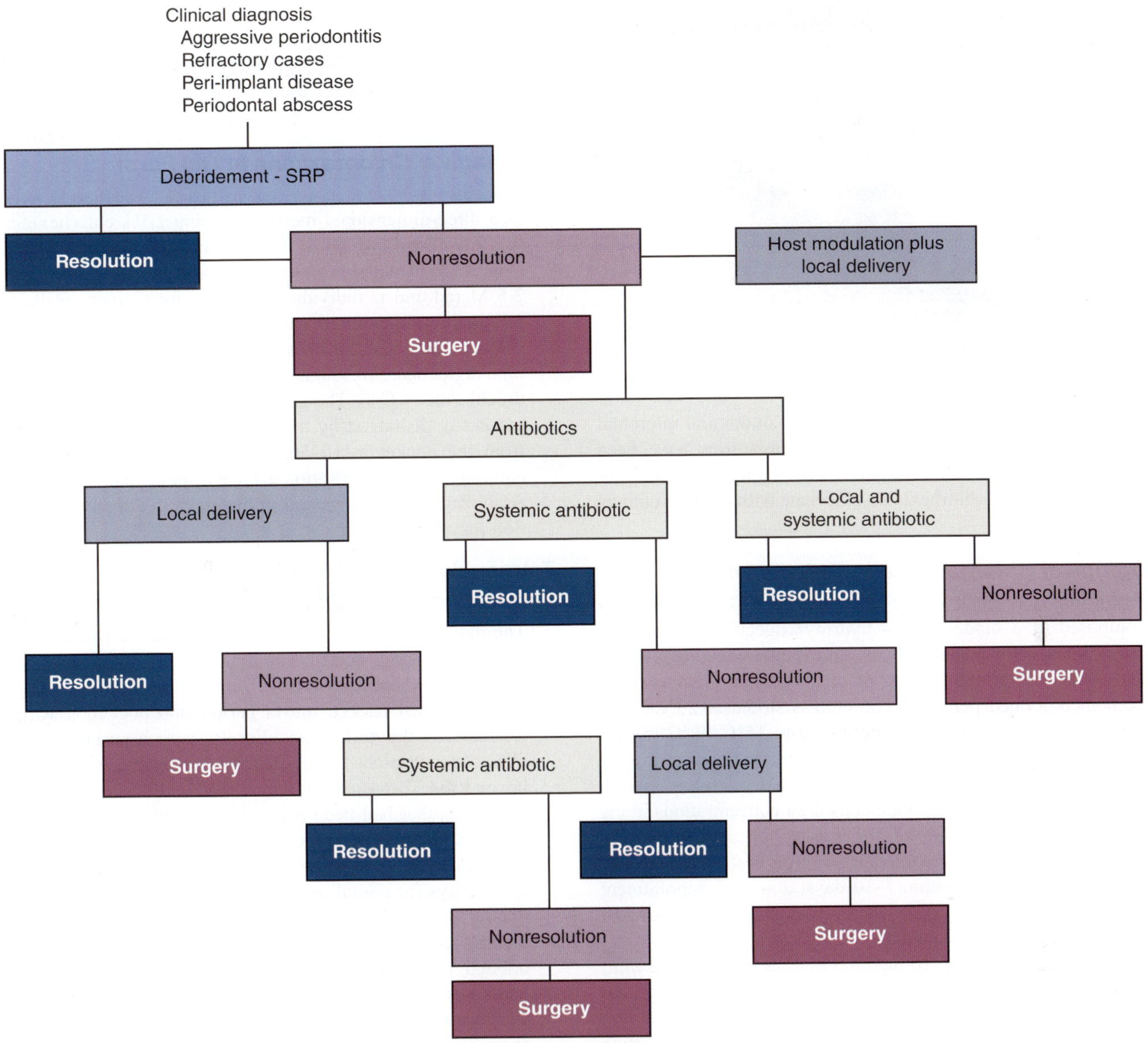

Fig. 37.1 A decision tree for the selection of antibiotic therapy.

therapy. The clinician must obtain a thorough medical history, including current medications and the possible adverse effects of combining these medicines, before prescribing any antibiotic therapy. The clinician must make the final decision with the patient. Risks and benefits concerning antibiotics as adjuncts to periodontal therapy should be discussed with the patient before antibiotics are used.

Locally Delivered, Controlled-Release Antimicrobials

Rationale for Local Delivery and Controlled Release

Locally delivered antimicrobial agents are available as adjuncts to scaling and root planing and as aids for the control of growth of bacteria on barrier membranes. When they are placed into periodontal pockets, they reduce the subgingival microflora, the probing depths, and the clinical signs of inflammation. In some cases, they are used as monotherapy, and in other cases, they are administered adjunctively with SRP, which is generally considered by the professional community to be the best approach.

A systematic review concluded that "adjunctive local therapy generally reduced probing depth levels. Differences between treatment and SRP-only groups in the baseline to follow-up period typically favored treatment groups but usually only modestly (e.g., from about 0.1 to nearly 0.5 mm). Effects for clinical attachment level gains were smaller and statistical significance less common." A report about locally delivered agents that was prepared by the American Academy of Periodontology stated that "the clinician's decision to use locally delivered agents should be based upon a consideration of clinical findings, the patient's dental and medical history, scientific evidence, patient preferences and advantages and disadvantages of alternative therapies." The report also stated that use of locally delivered agents may be of value when probing depths of more than 5 mm with inflammation are still present after conventional therapy. However, if multiple sites are present in the same quadrant, therapy other than locally delivered agents should be considered.

Chlorhexidine-Based Products

Chlorhexidine is active against a broad range of microbes. It disrupts the cell membrane and causes precipitation of the cytoplasm,

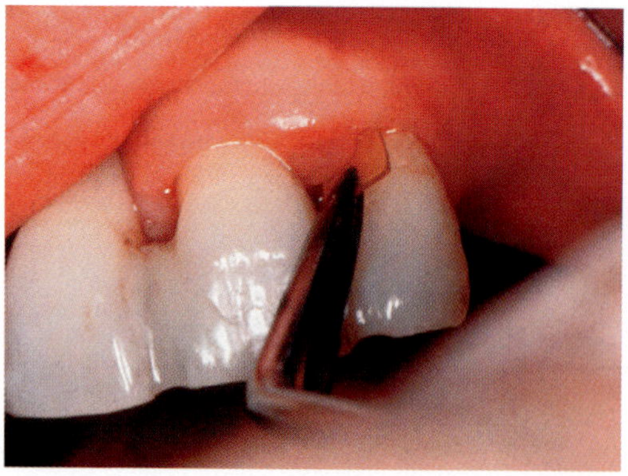

Fig. 37.2 Placement of a chlorhexidine gluconate chip (PerioChip).

resulting in cell death. No adverse alterations in the oral microbial flora or overgrowth of opportunistic microorganisms have been observed. A resorbable delivery system has been tested for the subgingival placement of chlorhexidine gluconate with positive clinical results (Fig. 37.2).

Subgingival Chlorhexidine in Chip Form

a. PerioChip is a small chip (4.0 × 5.0 × 0.35 mm) that is composed of a biodegradable hydrolyzedgelatin matrix. It is cross-linked with glutaraldehyde, and it also contains glycerin and water into which 2.5 mg of chlorhexidine gluconate has been incorporated per chip. The chip is stored at 20°C–25°C (68°F–77°F), with excursions permitted to 15°C–30°C (59°F–86°F). The chlorhexidine chip is placed into the pocket directly from the foil container using a forceps. This delivery system releases chlorhexidine and maintains drug concentrations in the GCF of more than 100 μg/mL for at least 7 days; these concentrations are well above the tolerance of most oral bacteria. Since the chip biodegrades within 7–10 days, a second appointment for removal is not needed. However, dental floss should be avoided for 10 days to avoid dislodging it.

b. PerioCol-CG is a small, 10-mg chip (4 × 5 × 0.25–0.32 mm) designed as a collagen matrix into which chlorhexidine gluconate (2.5 mg) is incorporated from a 20% chlorhexidine solution that is its active ingredient. The chip is designed for insertion into the periodontal pocket and resorbs after 30 days, but its coronal edge degrades within 10 days. It releases chlorhexidine in vitro at a rate of approximately 40%–45% in the first 24 h, followed by a linear release for 7–8 days, and it has a shelf-life of 2 years.

Subgingival Chlorhexidine in Gel Form

c. Chlo-Site is a xanthan gel, consisting of a saccharide polymer as a three-dimensional mesh containing 1.5% chlorhexidine in 0.5 mL of gel, which is injected into the periodontal pocket (Fig. 37.3). The gel product is sterilized by gamma radiation at 2.5 M rad and is individually packed for delivery in 0.25-mL prefilled syringes fitted with a blunt side-exit needle. The gel contains two types of chlorhexidine: a slow-release chlorhexidine digluconate (0.5%) and a rapid-release chlorhexidine dihydrochloride (1.0%). The gel is retained within the pocket and is not easily dislodged by the GCF or saliva. The gel disappears from the pocket in 10–30 days and is reported to achieve a chlorhexidine concentration in GCF of more than 100 μg/mL for an average of 6–9 days and to maintain an effective concentration for at least 15 days.

Tetracycline-Based Products

Tetracycline-Containing Fibers

a. The first local delivery product available in the United States—an ethylene/vinyl acetate copolymer fiber (diameter, 0.5 mm) that contained tetracycline (12.7 mg per 9 in.)—was extensively studied. When packed into a periodontal pocket, it was well tolerated by the oral tissues. For 10 days, it sustained tetracycline concentrations that exceeded 1300 μg/mL, which was well beyond the 32–64 μg/mL required to inhibit the growth of the pathogens that had been isolated from periodontal pockets. By contrast, GCF concentrations of only 4–8 μg/mL were reported after systemic tetracycline administration (250 mg 4 times daily for 10 days for a total oral dose of 10 g). Studies demonstrated that tetracycline fibers applied with or without scaling and root planing reduced probing depth, bleeding with probing, and periodontal pathogens and provided gains in clinical attachment level. Such effects were significantly better than those attained with scaling and root planing alone or with placebo fibers. No change in antibiotic resistance to tetracycline was found after

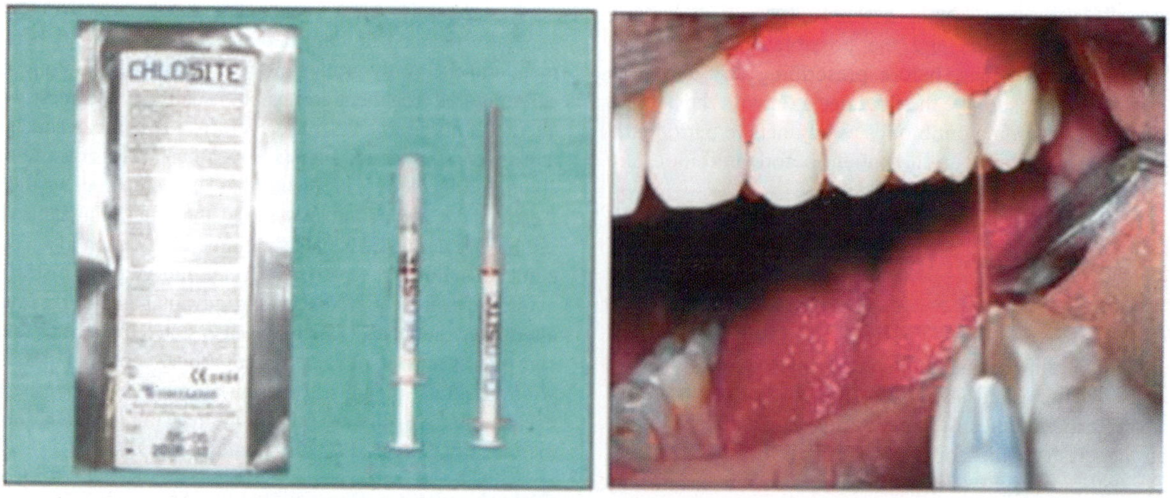

Fig. 37.3 Chlo-Site gel packaging is shown *(left)*. The xanthan gel with chlorhexidine is inserted into the periodontal pocket *(right)*. *(Reprinted from Gill, et al: Nonsurgical management of chronic periodontitis with two local drug delivery agents—a comparative study.* J Clin Exp Dent *3:e424–e429, 2011.)*

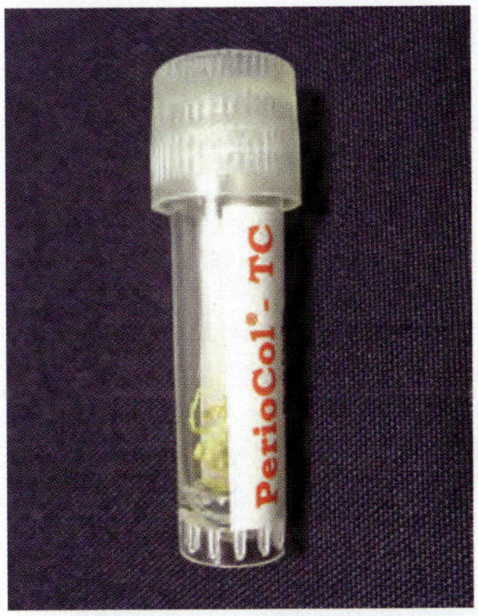

Fig. 37.4 PerioCol-TC fibers are packaged in an individual vial. *(Courtesy: Eucare Pharmaceuticals, Ltd., Chennai, India. http://www.eucare.in/dental-regeneration-concepts.html.)*

tetracycline fiber therapy among the tested putative periodontal pathogens. However, these fibers are no longer commercially available.

b. As reported by the manufacturer, each PerioCol-TC vial contains fish type I collagen (approximately 25 mg) impregnated with approximately 2.0 mg of tetracycline hydrochloride, which is sterilized by gamma radiation (Fig. 37.4). PerioCol-TC releases tetracycline in vitro for 8–10 days. A periodontal dressing should be placed to avoid dislodging the fibers. PerioCol-TC is indicated for the treatment of adult periodontitis as an adjunct to SRP for pockets more than 5 mm deep, and it can be administered every 3 months. The fibers are moistened with saline and placed into the periodontal pocket to the depth of the pocket base; they are biodegradable and do not have to be removed. PerioCol-TC is stored in a dry place between 5°C (41° F) and 25°C (77°F) and has a shelf life of 2 years with proper storage.
c. Periodontal Plus AB is a bioresorbable tetracycline fiber. It is 25 mg of pure fibrillar collagen evenly impregnated with approximately 2 mg of tetracycline hydrochloride (Fig. 37.5). The fibers are packaged as a strip containing four individually packed and separable sterile product packs. The fiber biodegrades in the periodontal pocket within 7 days. The fiber should be retained with a periodontal dressing or covered with a dental adhesive for 10 days.

Doxycycline-Based products

Doxycycline in Gel Form

a. A gel system involving the use of a syringe with 10% doxycycline (Atridox) is available. It was the only local delivery system accepted by the American Dental Association when the association had an acceptance program for professional products, although that program was terminated in 2008. This product is available in the United States and in a number of other countries. Doxycycline gel is a subgingival, controlled-release delivery product composed of a two-syringe mixing system (Fig. 37.6A). Syringe A contains 450 mg of a bioabsorbable polymeric formulation of 36.7% poly (D,L,-lactide) dissolved in 63.3% *N*-methyl-2-pyrrolidone. Syringe B contains 50 mg of doxycycline hyclate, equivalent to 42.5 mg of doxycycline. The two syringes are stored at 2°C–30°C (36°F to 86°F). When mixed, the product is a viscous liquid of 500 mg, which contains 50 mg (10%) of doxycycline hyclate. Doxycycline gel is indicated for the treatment of chronic adult periodontitis for a gain in clinical attachment, reduction in probing depth, and reduction of bleeding on probing. Doxycycline, a broad-spectrum semisynthetic tetracycline, is bacteriostatic, inhibiting bacterial protein biosynthesis by interfering with transfer RNA (tRNA) and messenger RNA (mRNA) at the ribosome. No overgrowth of opportunistic organisms was observed after use of the doxycycline gel. The gel has been reported to release doxycycline in the GCF over 7 days. The doxycycline gel is biodegradable and does not require removal. If not used immediately, the mixed contents in syringe A can be stored in an airtight container at room temperature for a maximum of 3 days. The doxycycline gel is used by injecting the mixed contents of the two syringes directly into the pocket (see Fig. 37.6B). The pocket contents are then covered with a periodontal dressing or a cyanoacrylate dental adhesive.
b. Ligosan Slow Release is a 14% (w/w), resorbable doxycycline gel for periodontal application provided in a laminate pouch and stored under refrigeration. It contains 1, 2, 4, 8, 10, or 16 single-application cylinder cartridges, each containing 260 mg of Ligosan Slow Release (Fig. 37.7). The product is used by inserting the cartridge into the caulking gun, opening the spray nozzle,

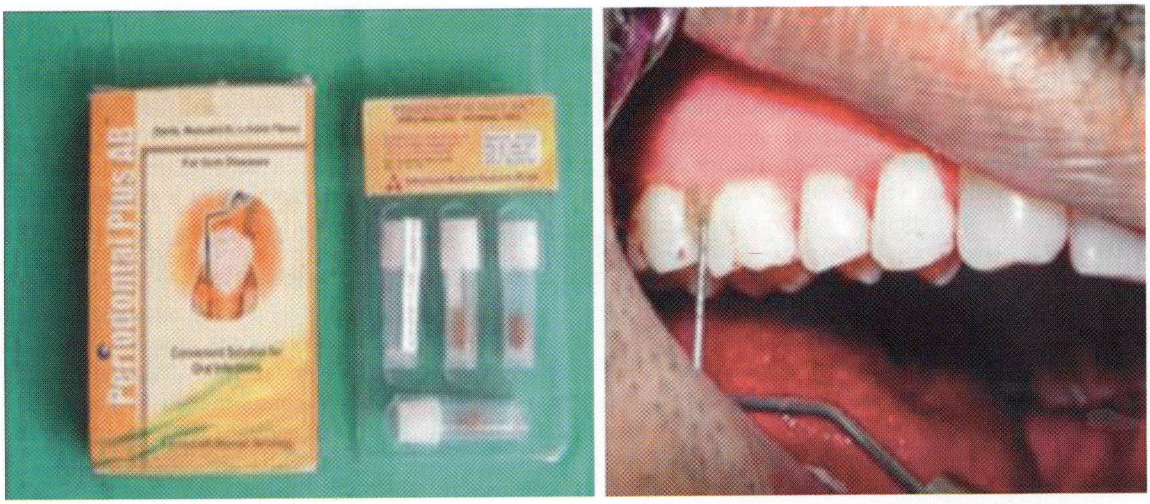

Fig. 37.5 Periodontal Plus AB packaging *(left)*. Fibers are Inserted into the periodontal pocket *(right)*. *(Reprinted from Gill, et al:* J Clin Exp Dent *3:e424–e429, 2011.)*

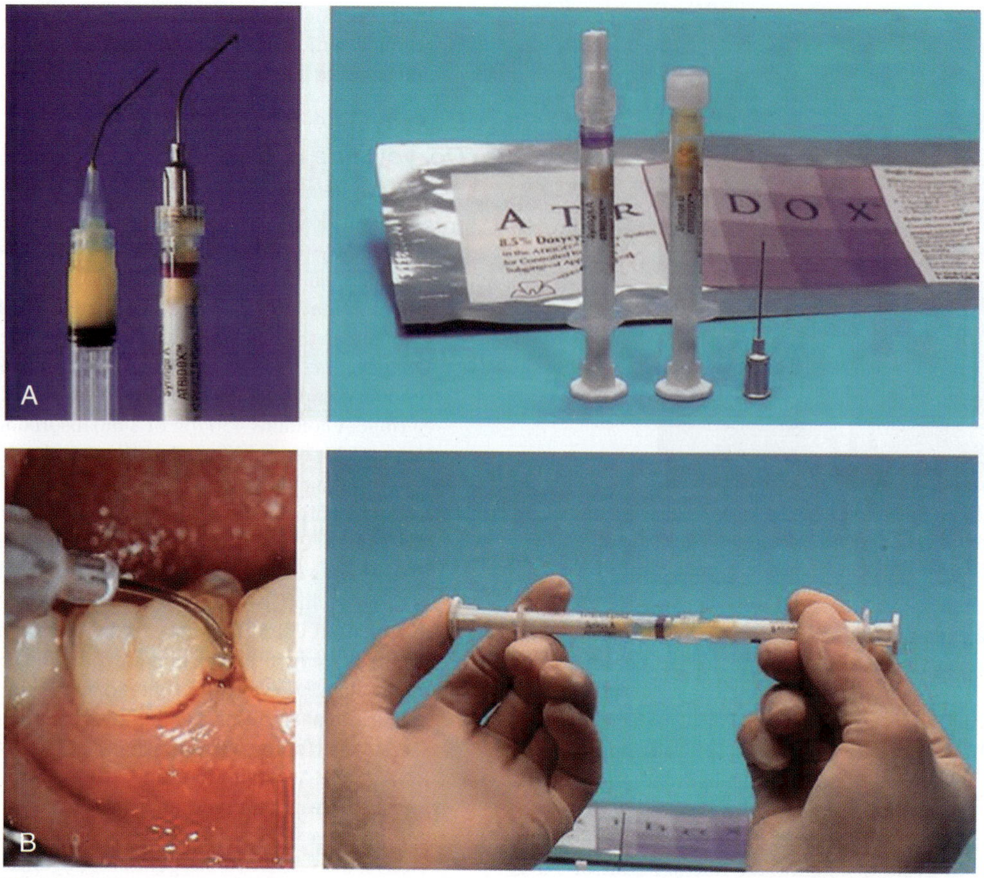

Fig. 37.6 Doxycycline hyclate gel (Atridox). A, Doxycycline gel is packaged as a two-syringe mixing system *(right)*. After mixing the gel, a cannula is attached for injection *(left)*. B, The two syringes are coupled, and the liquid contents of syringe A are injected into the powder within syringe B; the contents are mixed within the two syringes for 100 cycles (1 cycle/s) and then left within syringe A *(right)*. The mixed solution is injected into the pocket through the cannula attached to syringe A until the pocket is completely filled *(left)*. The pocket contents are covered with a periodontal dressing or a cyanoacrylate dental adhesive. *(Reprinted from Wolf HF, Hassell TM: Color atlas of dental hygiene: periodontology, ed 1, Stuttgart, Germany, 2006, Thieme, with permission.)*

and then discharging the gel to the bottom of the pocket. The doxycycline release profile was studied in 20 patients. The maximal value in the GCF within the first 5 h (i.e., at 15 min) was 19.97 ± 5.58 mg/mL; after 3 days, the concentration was 577.1 ± 127.3 μg/mL. Concentrations in the GCF remained above 16 μg/mL for at least 12 days. Mechanical hygiene in the area should be avoided for 7 days.

Subgingival Minocycline

A locally delivered, sustained-release form of minocycline microspheres (Arestin) is available for subgingival placement as an adjunct to scaling and root planing (Fig. 37.8). The minocycline microspheres product is a subgingival, controlled-release delivery system containing the antibiotic minocycline hydrochloride incorporated into a bioresorbable poly (glycolide-co-D,L-lactide) polymer in unit-dose cartridges. Each cartridge delivers minocycline hydrochloride equivalent to 1 mg of minocycline free base. Minocycline microspheres are indicated as an adjunct to SRP for the reduction of pocket depth in patients with adult periodontitis and as part of a periodontal maintenance program, which includes good oral hygiene and SRP.

Minocycline belongs to the tetracycline class of antibiotics and has a broad spectrum of activity. Its bacteriostatic, antimicrobial activity results from the inhibition of protein biosynthesis. No overgrowth of opportunistic microorganisms was reported from clinical studies. No changes in the number of minocycline-resistant bacteria, *Candida albicans* or *Staphylococcus aureus*, in the gastrointestinal tract were detected at the end of a 56-day study, although there was a slight increase in the numbers of minocycline-resistant bacteria in periodontal pocket plaque samples after 9 months. The clinical significance of the changes is unknown.

Patients should avoid hard or sticky foods at the treated teeth for 1 week and interproximal cleaning devices for about 10 days. The minocycline microspheres formulation is biodegradable and does not require removal. The cartridges are stored at 20°C–25°C (68°F–77°F), with excursions permitted to 15°C–30°C (59°F–86°F). Excessive heat should be avoided. The minocycline microspheres are used by injecting the contents of a unit-dose cartridge into the pocket. Neither a periodontal dressing nor an adhesive is needed.

Subgingival Metronidazole

A topical medication that contains an oil-based metronidazole 25% dental gel (glycerylmonooleate and sesame oil) has been tested in a number of studies. This product is not available in the United States. It is applied in a viscous consistency to the pocket, where it is liquidized by the body heat and then hardens again, forming crystals when it comes in contact with water. As a precursor, the preparation contains metronidazole–benzoate, which is converted into the active substance by esterases in GCF. Two 25% gel applications at a 1-week interval have been used.

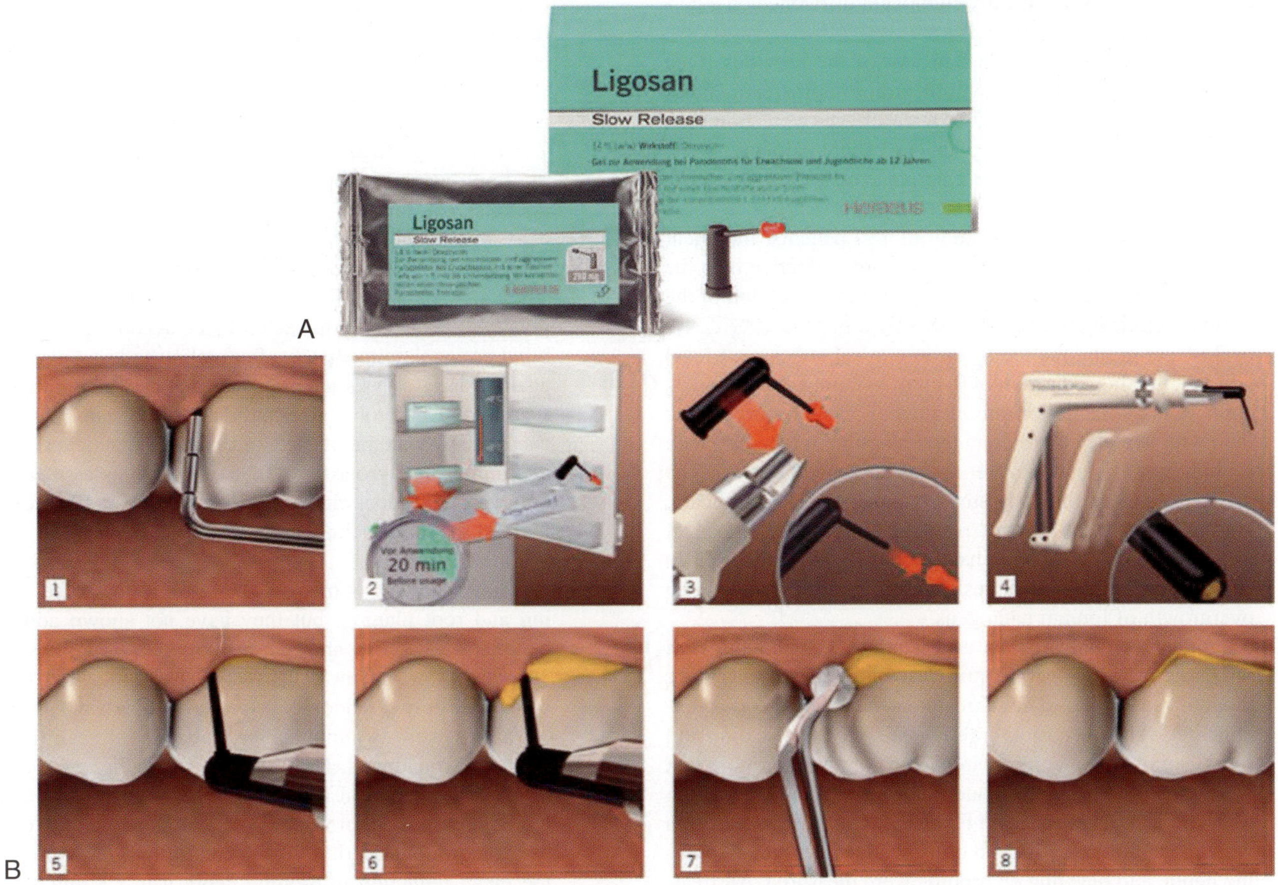

Fig. 37.7 A, Ligosan Slow Release; box, laminate pouch and caulking gun tip. B, Steps 1 through 8 in the placement procedure. *(A) (From http://www.zm-online.de/markt/heraeus-kulzer/produkte/Ligosan-Slow-Release-in-Einer-Packung_69583.html). (B) (From http://heraeus-kulzer.de/media/webmedia_local/downloads_new/ligosan_4/Ligosan_Produktinformation_DE.pdf.)*

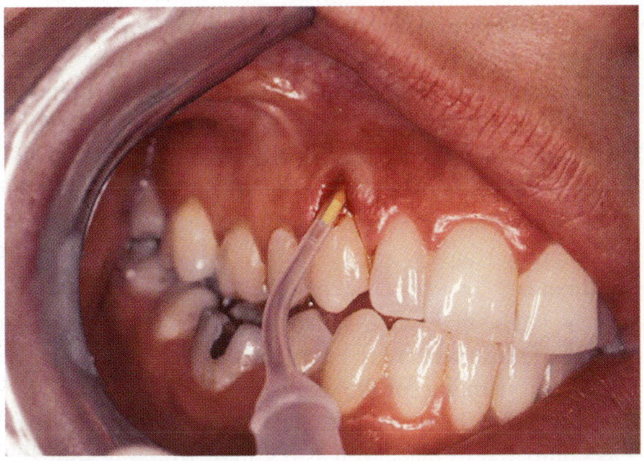

Fig. 37.8 Placement of minocycline microspheres (Arestin).

Subgingival Moxifloxacin

Moxifloxacin is a fourth-generation synthetic fluoroquinolone with broad-spectrum antibacterial activity. This antibiotic inhibits cell replication by modifying the actions of DNA gyrase and topoisomerase IV. Since moxifloxacin has been shown to have antimicrobial activity against aerobic and anaerobic bacteria, including a number of periodontal pathogens, it has been introduced as a local delivery agent for the treatment of destructive periodontal diseases.

Related Studies

1. PerioChip

   Two multicenter, randomized, double-blind, parallel-group, controlled clinical trials of this chip were conducted in the United States and included a total of 447 patients from 10 centers. In these studies, patients received supragingival prophylaxis for up to 1 h, which was followed by scaling and root planing for 1 h. Chips were placed in target sites with probing depths of 5–8 mm at baseline that bled with probing and again at 3 and 6 months if the probing depth remained at 5 mm or more. Sites in control subjects received either a placebo chip (inactive) with scaling and root planing or scaling and root planing alone. Sites in test subjects received either a chlorhexidine chip (active) with scaling and root planing or scaling and root planing alone. Examinations were performed at baseline and again at 3, 6, and 9 months. At 9 months, significant decreases in probing depth from baseline that favored the active chip as compared to controls were observed: chlorhexidine chip with scaling and root planing, -0.95 ± 0.05 mm; placebo chip with scaling and root planing, -0.69 ± 0.05 mm ($P = 0.001$); and scaling and root planing alone, -0.65 ± 0.05 mm ($P = 0.00001$). Although statistically significant, the net clinical changes were limited. The proportion of pocket sites with a probing depth reduction of 2 mm or more was increased in the chlorhexidine chip group (30%) as compared to scaling and root planing alone

(16%); this was a statistically significant difference on a per-patient basis ($P < 0.0001$).

No signs of staining were noted in any of the previous three studies as a result of the chlorhexidine chip treatment as measured by a stain index. Adverse effects were minimal, although a few patients complained of slight pain and swelling during the first 24 h after chip placement.

2. Atridox

During a 9-month multicenter study of 180 patients, treatment with 10% doxycycline gel alone was more effective than the other treatments at all time periods, with the exception of the 3-month clinical attachment level value. For the 10% doxycycline gel group, the reduction in clinical attachment level at 9 months showed a gain of 0.4 mm as compared to vehicle control; the reduction in probing depth was 0.6 mm greater than with vehicle control; and the reduction of bleeding with probing was 0.2 units greater than with vehicle control. The differences were clinically small but statistically significant. Although resistance was not evaluated in this study, the local application of doxycycline has previously been reported to show transient increases in resistance in oral microbes and no overgrowth of foreign pathogens.

Two multicenter clinical trials each studied 411 patients with moderate to severe periodontitis. At baseline, patients were randomized to one of four treatment groups: 10% doxycycline gel, vehicle control, oral hygiene only, and scaling and root planing. Sites with probing depths of 5 mm or more that bled with probing were treated at baseline and then again with the same treatment at 4 months. Clinical assessments were made for 9 months, and clinical attachment level, probing depth, and bleeding on probing were measured. All treatment groups in both studies showed clinical improvements as compared to baseline over the 9-month period. The results for all parameters measured were significantly better in the 10% doxycycline gel group as compared to vehicle control and oral hygiene only. As compared to scaling and root planing, the effects of 10% doxycycline gel as monotherapy on clinical attachment level gain and probing depth reduction were equivalent. Most recently, a 6-month, randomized, multicenter, placebo-controlled, examiner-masked study of 171 subjects evaluated the combined use of systemically delivered doxycycline hyclate (20 mg twice daily) plus locally delivered doxycycline hyclate gel (10%) in combination with scaling and root planing versus scaling and root planing plus placebo. The results of the study showed that the combination therapy provided statistically significantly greater clinical benefits than control therapy for all clinical measures at both 3 and 6 months. The clinical parameters measured were probing depth, clinical attachment level, bleeding with probing, and gingival health.

3. Minocycline

In a four-center, double-blind, randomized trial, patients with periodontal pockets at least 5 mm deep were selected, and either 2% minocycline gel or vehicle was applied once every 2 weeks for four applications after initial scaling and root planing. A total of 343 teeth (976 sites) were included in the minocycline group, with 299 teeth (810 sites) being included in the control group. Reductions in *P. gingivalis* and *P. intermedia* at weeks 2, 4, 6, and 12 and at weeks 6 and 12 for *A. actinomycetemcomitans* were statistically significant. These results demonstrated the advantages of supplementing standard subgingival debridement with the application of minocycline gel. The three primary clinical efficacy variables in this study were probing depth, clinical attachment level, and bleeding index. There was a trend toward clinical improvement in both treatment groups for all three measures, and the reduction in probing depth was significantly greater with minocycline gel. When sites with probing depth of at least 7 mm and significant bleeding at baseline were considered, the improvements were greater than those seen with 5-mm pockets. The improvements with minocycline were statistically significantly better than those seen in the control group.

Applications of 2% minocycline were also evaluated in a 3-month study in 30 patients. Active or placebo gel was placed subgingivally at planed sites in each subject, according to a double-blind protocol, immediately after scaling and root planing and again 2 and 4 weeks later. Differences between groups with regard to mean probing depth did not reach statistical significance at any visit, but mean clinical attachment levels favored the minocycline group ($P < 0.05$) at both reassessments. The number of sites that bled after deep probing at 12 weeks also favored the minocycline group ($P < 0.05$).

4. Metronidazole gel

Studies have shown that metronidazole gel is equivalent to scaling and root planing, but they have not shown adjunctive benefits with scaling and root planing. In a 6-month study of 30 patients, treatment consisted of two applications of the dental gel in two randomly selected quadrants at 1-week intervals as well as simultaneous subgingival scaling of the remaining quadrants. Oral hygiene instructions were given on day 21. Statistical analyses showed that both treatments effectively reduced probing depth and bleeding with probing over the 6-month period. At the end of the follow-up period, the mean reduction in probing depth was 1.3 mm after gel treatment and 1.5 mm after subgingival scaling. Bleeding with probing was reduced by 35% and 42%, respectively. No significant differences between the two treatments were detected. Dark-field microscopy showed a shift toward a seemingly healthier microflora for both treatment modalities; this effect persisted throughout the 6-month period.

A large, multicenter study of 206 subjects investigated two applications of metronidazole gel in two randomly selected quadrants versus two quadrants of scaling. Probing depths were reduced by 1.2 mm in the gel and by 1.5 mm in the scaling group. At 6 months, the differences between treatments were statistically but not clinically significant. In addition, bleeding on probing was reduced by 88% for both treatment groups.

5. Moxifloxacin

A recent study in Europe suggested that the local delivery of 0.4% moxifloxacin may be of benefit as an adjunct to scaling and root planning for the treatment of periodontitis. It should be noted that the mean incremental reduction in probing depth as compared to placebo was 0.4 mm, which is similar to the reduction found with other commercially available local delivery agents. As of this writing, this drug is not available in the United States, but it is available in other parts of the world.

Comparative Studies

Few researchers have attempted to compare these devices side by side. However, in one study, doxycycline polymer, metronidazole gel, and PerioChip were compared in 47 periodontal patients. The study found that all controlled-release polymer devices increased gingival attachment levels but that there was a slightly greater improvement among patients who were treated with the doxycycline polymer.

Overview of Local Delivery of Antimicrobial Agents and Peri-implant Mucositis/Implantitis

Since there are a number of similarities between the pathogens involved in periodontitis peri-implant mucositis and peri-implantitis, it is logical that similar clinical approaches should be implemented for these two conditions. An early study by Mombelli and colleagues that made use of tetracycline-containing fibers that are no longer available demonstrated in 25 patients with peri-implant mucositis that there was a significant reduction of four periopathogenic species; however, other species (e.g., *P. gingivalis, A. actinomycetemcomitans*) had very low baseline levels and were not significantly affected. There was a slight but not significant improvement in the probing depth at 12 months. The study showed that the local delivery of tetracycline from polymeric fibers may be used to improve the clinical and microbiologic parameters around infected implants as compared to scaling and root planing alone.

In another study, investigators applied controlled-release doxycycline (Atridox) into peri-implant pockets and noted differences as compared to scaling and root planing alone. This study also showed the efficacy of such devices for the treatment of peri-implant mucositis. Patients who received the doxycycline treatment showed significantly greater probing attachment levels and lesser pocket probing depths and bleeding indexes ($P < 0.05$) as compared with those who received scaling and root planing alone.

A study by Persson and colleagues evaluated 31 implants with peri-implantitis in 25 patients and monitored clinical and radiographic changes over 12 months after the adjunctive placement of minocycline microspheres (Arestin). Minocycline microspheres (Arestin) were locally delivered to each implant site with bone loss and with a probing pocket depth (PPD) of 5 mm or more. Rescue therapy with Arestin was allowed at days 180 and 270 at any site exhibiting an increase in PPD of 2 mm or more as compared to the previous visit. Six implants in six subjects were either rescued or exited as a result of persisting active peri-implantitis. Successful implants showed a statistically significant reduction in both PPD and the percentage of sites with bleeding with probing between baseline and day 360 ($P < 0.05$). At mesial implant sites, the mean PPD reduction amounted to 1.6 mm (95% confidence interval, 0.9–2.2 mm; $P < 0.001$), and this was accompanied by a statistically significant reduction of the bleeding with probing value ($P < 0.001$).

Although studies evaluating the use of the PerioChip (chlorhexidine) for periimplantmucositis were not identified, one 12-month study compared the clinical and microbiologic results after the application of minocycline microspheres as an adjunct to the mechanical treatment of incipient peri-implant infections as compared to an adjunctive treatment involving the application of 1 mL of a 1% chlorhexidine gel. Sixteen patients in the minocycline group and fourteen patients in the chlorhexidine group completed the study. The findings of the study were that the adjunctive use of minocycline microspheres resulted in improvements of probing depths and bleeding scores, whereas the adjunctive use of chlorhexidine only resulted in the limited reduction of bleeding scores. For the deepest sites of the treated implants in the minocycline group, the mean probing depth was reduced from 5.0 to 4.4 mm at 12 months. This study did not demonstrate any significant difference in the levels of bacterial species or groups at any time point between the two antimicrobial agents tested.

Pharmacokinetics

The pharmacokinetic principles of controlled-release local delivery are illustrated in Fig. 38.9. Drug delivered locally to the periodontal pocket but not in a controlled-release formulation (e.g., by irrigation) is washed out of the pocket by the GCF flow, quickly reducing the concentration of drug in the GCF. Locally delivered, controlled-release antimicrobials have been designed to maintain high and clinically relevant concentrations of drug in the GCF for extended periods. The pharmacokinetics of the chlorhexidine chip, doxycycline gel, and minocycline microspheres have been studied in clinical trials and are dicussed in detail online.

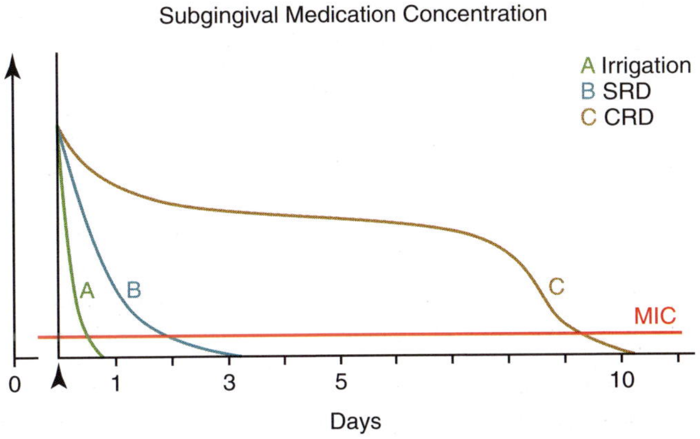

Fig. 37.9 Graph shows the release profile of locally delivered, sustained-release or controlled-release antimicrobials by irrigation. Drug concentration in the gingival crevicular fluid (GCF) is diminished rapidly after irrigation (A). Drug concentration can be extended for several days with drug administered in a modified, sustained-release formulation (B). Drug concentration in the GCF can be maintained at therapeutically relevant concentrations for up to 10 days with controlled-release formulations (C). Area under the curve but above the minimal inhibitory concentration *(MIC)* line represents drug concentration in the gingival crevicular fluid greater than MIC values. The MIC for subgingival plaque bacteria may be substantially greater than typically reported bacterial MIC values because of the potentially protective effect of a subgingival biofilm formation. *CRD*, Controlled-release delivery; *SRD*, sustained-release delivery; *arrowhead*, administration of locally delivered agent. *(Adapted from Wolf HF, Hassell TM:* Color atlas of dental hygiene: periodontology, *ed 1, Stuttgart, Germany, 2006, Thieme, with permission.)*

Chlorhexidine Chip

The release profile of the chlorhexidine chip was evaluated in a single-center, 10-day clinical trial in 19 patients with chronic adult periodontitis. Each patient received a single chip administered into each of four pocket sites, and concentrations of chlorhexidine were determined in GCF, plasma, and urine at various times after dosing. Peak GCF concentrations were achieved 2 h after dosing (2007 ± 422 μg/mL), with GCF concentrations maintained between approximately 1300 and 1900 μg/mL to 4 days after dosing. Mean chlorhexidine concentrations then steadily decreased to 57 ± 13 μg/mL at 9 days. Chlorhexidine was below detectable limits in plasma and urine at all time points. For perspective, Wilson and colleagues reported that chlorhexidine (125 μg/mL) killed 99.9% of cultivable bacteria from plaque samples from patients with chronic periodontitis within 15 min.

Doxycycline Gel

The release profile of the doxycycline gel was evaluated in a single-center, 28-day clinical trial in 32 patients with adult periodontitis and compared with oral doxycycline. All patients assigned to receive local delivery had doxycycline gel administered to all pocket sites with probing depths of 5 mm or more that bled on probing. Drug was retained after placement with a noneugenol (NE) periodontal dressing ($n = 13$) or 2-octyl cyanoacrylate (2-O) ($n = 13$). Mean GCF concentrations peaked 2 h after dosing (1473 ± 328 μg/mL for NE; 1986 ± 445 μg/mL for 2-O). At day 7, mean concentrations were 309 ± 127 μg/mL (NE) and 148 ± 49 μg/mL (2-O). Mean salivary concentrations peaked at 2 h (4.05 ± 1.24 μg/mL for NE; 8.78 ± 1.48 μg/mL for 2-O) and were 2 μg/mL or less at 24 h. Serum concentrations after local administration remained at 0.1 μg/mL or less.

For oral doxycycline (200 mg on day 0 and then 100 mg/day for 7 days; $n = 6$), GCF concentrations peaked at 12 h after dosing (2.53 ± 1.56 μg/mL), and serum concentrations ranged from 0.91 to 2.26 μg/mL for the 8 days of data collection. Salivary concentrations never exceeded 0.11 μg/mL.

Minocycline Microspheres

The release profile of minocycline microspheres was studied in 18 patients with moderate to advanced chronic periodontitis. Minocycline microspheres (mean dose, 46.2 mg; 25–112 unit doses) were administered to eligible periodontal pocket sites with a 5 mm or more probing depth (i.e., minimum of 30 sites on at least eight teeth; 1 mg/treatment site) after SRP. Serum and saliva samples were collected before dosing and at various times after dosing to 14 days. The mean dose-normalized saliva area under the curve and maximal concentration (C_{max}) were approximately 125 and 1000 times that of serum parameters, respectively. In saliva, the minocycline C_{max} was 254.0 ± 139.3 mg/mL at 0.75 ± 0.56 h after dosing, with a half-life of 44.7 ± 19.2 h. In serum, the mean minocycline concentrations peaked at 4.8 ± 1.8 h after dosing (C_{max}: 216.4 ± 122.9 μg/mL) and were undetectable by 7 days. Minocycline concentrations in saliva and GCF were sufficient (>1 μg/mL) to kill bacteria associated with periodontal disease in vitro. These concentrations were evident for up to 14 days without significant systemic exposure.

Phases of Drug Development

The typical investigational drug is studied in many clinical trials before an application [i.e., new drug application (NDA)] and can be submitted to the US Food and Drug Administration (FDA) for clearance for commercial marketing in the United States. Clinical trials before registration are often conducted in three phases. Phase I trials usually enroll small numbers of healthy volunteers to determine preliminary safety and dosing. Phase II trials typically enroll larger numbers of patients to characterize preliminary safety in patients and to determine dosing that is evaluated in later trials. Large phase III trials often are called pivotal or registration trials and usually are multicenter, blinded, and randomized studies that enroll sufficiently large numbers of patients to provide conclusive evidence of safety and efficacy to support the submission of an NDA to the FDA for registration for marketed use.

After FDA registration, phase IV trials may be performed to provide additional information about drug products, including longer-term safety and efficacy in a broader number of patients or in alternative practice settings. The objectives of the phases of clinical research as described by the National Institutes of Health are given in Table 37.4. The typical phases of drug development seem less distinct when trials are considered in exploratory or confirmatory stages. Specialized clinical pharmacology trials may be conducted at any phase to provide specific information such as pharmacokinetics or to address treatment conditions such as specific patient populations (e.g., geriatric or pediatric patients, patients with hepatic or renal impairment) or the effect of the drug on cardiac electrophysiology (e.g., QT prolongation). The drug development process has been reviewed by Tonkens and by Mathieu and Milne. The FDA offers an overview of the drug review process to ensure that drugs are safe and effective

TABLE 37.4 Phases of Clinical Research

Phase	Description
I	Researchers test a new drug or treatment in a small group of people for the first time to evaluate its safety, determine a safe dosage range, and identify side effects.
II	The drug or treatment is given to a larger group of people to see if it is effective and to further evaluate its safety.
III	The drug or treatment is given to large groups of people to confirm its effectiveness, monitor side effects, compare it with commonly used treatments, and collect information that will allow the drug or treatment to be used safely.
IV	Studies are done after the drug or treatment has been marketed to gather information on the drug's effect in various populations and side effects associated with long-term use.

(From U.S. National Library of Medicine, National Institutes of Health: FAQ Clinicaltrials.gov—clinical trial phases. https://www.nih.gov/health-information/nih-clinical-research-trials-you/basics.)

TABLE 37.5 Characteristics of Adequate and Well-Controlled (Phase III) Clinical Trial Designs

1. Type I error rate control
2. Clear statement of the proposed and actual objectives
3. Methods of analysis in the protocol, statistical analysis plan, and reports
4. Methods of adequate assurance of patient selections
5. Patient assignments that minimize bias and group comparability
6. Methods to minimize bias for all parties: patients, investigators, and data analysts
7. Well-defined endpoints that address the primary hypothesis
8. Analysis of results that allows for interpretation of the effects of the study drug

(Modified from U.S. Food and Drug Administration: Electronic Code of Federal Regulations. §314.126 https://www.ecfr.gov/cgi-bin/text-idx?SID=6d23d836424edd2eeb76d932e75aca7b&mc=true&node=se21.5.314_1126&rgn=div8.)

Trial Design Considerations

Regulatory decisions depend on the data produced by adequate and well-controlled Phase III clinical trials providing evidence that a drug is safe and effective when used as intended. These trials are usually large and conducted in many investigational centers to enroll a sufficient number of patients to give the proper statistical power and to complete the trial within a reasonable length of time. Multicenter trials are enormously expensive and difficult to perform. Clinical trials must be designed appropriately to test the hypotheses. Some important design features of trials that are considered adequate and well controlled are listed in Table 37.5 and discussed in the following sections.

Type I Error Rate Control

A type I error occurs when the investigator rejects the null hypothesis when it is true (i.e., rejecting the null hypothesis that there is no effect of the treatment or drug in question and concluding that there is an effect). The probability of a type I error is the level of significance of the statistical test of the hypothesis and is denoted by *alpha*. This error contrasts with a type II error, when the alternative hypothesis (i.e., fails to reject the null hypothesis) is rejected although the alternative hypothesis is actually true. A clinical trial should be adequately designed so that the *alpha* level is set at $P \leq 0.05$, the value that is most commonly used as the cutoff for statistical significance.

Statement of the Proposed and Actual Objectives

The primary and secondary objectives of the trial must be clearly defined in the protocol at the start of the study. The stated objectives should adequately address the study hypotheses. Exploratory objectives may also be included in the trial protocol, but they are typically considered as hypothesis-generating rather than hypothesis-testing objectives. Analyses not predefined and generated during the course of the study or assessed at the end of the study are typically denoted as post hoc analyses and are usually not appropriate for regulatory evaluation or decision.

Analysis in the Protocol, Statistical Plan, and Reports

The statistical methods planned for the analysis of trial data should be prespecified in the protocol and perhaps expanded in a statistical analysis plan, ideally before the start of the trial but at least before locking of the study data. In this fashion, all methods are predefined and not subject to bias as a result of the trial outcomes. Manuscripts or reports arising from the trial should adequately describe the analytic methods so that readers can appropriately consider and interpret the results of the trial.

Patient Selection and Assignment

The protocol should include methods for appropriately enrolling patients to ensure the study population represents the broader population and that study outcomes can be generalized to a broader population of similar patients. Multicenter trials (vs a single center or a few centers) increase the heterogeneity of the study population and make the study results more generalizable. There must be adequate procedures in place to ensure that patients are randomly included and not specifically selected, which can skew study results.

Patients should be randomly assigned to treatment groups to minimize the chances for systematic differences between groups. Treatment groups should be as comparable as possible so that any differences in study outcomes between groups can confidently be ascribed to the study treatment. Treatment assignments should be sequential and generated by appropriate randomization schemes (usually computer generated) to eliminate the potential for bias in treatment selection by investigators or sponsors. For particular characteristics of interest (e.g., smoking status for periodontal trials), treatment assignments can be stratified to ensure an equal distribution of the characteristics among all treatment groups.

Dental studies often use teeth randomized to different treatment assignments in the same patient (i.e., split-mouth designs), using patients to serve as their own controls. This type of assignment should be discouraged because the units of statistical analysis are no longer independent. With this intrapatient design, there are considerable concerns that treatment for one or more teeth (i.e., periodontal pockets) in one treatment group could affect the other treatment sites in the same patient or that all treatment groups could be affected by host factors equally or differentially. The parallel-group design is preferable because the statistical unit is the patient, ensuring that sites in a treatment group are completely independent and not subject to confounding by the other treatment groups.

Minimizing Bias for Patients, Investigators, and Data Analysts

Pivotal trials are typically double blinded or triple blinded to prevent patients, investigators, and statistical analysts from being aware of treatment assignments. In this fashion, no patients, investigators, study staff, or those who analyze the data can consciously or inadvertently influence the study outcome.

Well-Defined Endpoints That Address the Primary Hypothesis

The study protocol should clearly describe all endpoints that will be assessed and the methods of assessment. Pivotal trials can include many dozens of study sites, and there is considerable risk of systematic differences among different investigators. Protocols must standardize study methods as much as possible among study sites so that all treatments and study procedures are performed and all endpoints are assessed in the same manner at all study centers. The endpoints chosen should be relevant to the study objectives.

Current designs of clinical trials to assess periodontal outcomes usually are limited to the evaluation of surrogate endpoints (e.g., probing depth, attachment level) rather than direct and more clinically relevant endpoints such as tooth survival. An endpoint of tooth survival, although arguably better, is not practical for a clinical trial conducted within a reasonable period or with a reasonable number of patients. Surrogate variables are considered acceptable endpoints in periodontal clinical trials and relevant to tooth retention, although surrogate outcomes have inherent weaknesses. Discordance among surrogate periodontal endpoints further highlights the need for long-term data from clinical trials with tooth survival as the primary objective.

Analysis of the Study Drug's Effects

Statistical analysis of the results allows differentiation of the effects of the study drug or treatment from those caused by systematic differences between treatment groups or biases of the participants in any aspect of the trial. The objective of a clinical trial is to answer a particular research question. The worst result possible is trial completion without being able to interpret the outcome of the trial with confidence, a nonresult that would require repeating the trial. The many elements of study design contribute to the degree of confidence with which investigators can consider the outcome of the trial and the interpretation of results.

The pivotal trials for the chlorhexidine chip and the minocycline microspheres are examples of phase III designs for the study of adjunctive, locally delivered, controlled-release antimicrobials for the treatment of periodontitis. Representative populations of patients with chronic adult periodontitis were enrolled in multicenter, double-blind clinical trials and were randomly assigned to treatment groups. Target pocket sites received SRP at baseline with or without adjunctive drug according to the randomization protocol. At 3 and 6 months, sites randomized to drug received additional drug only if probing depth remained 5 mm or more. Final results showed a reduction of probing depth from baseline at 9 months as expected in all groups, but the treatment group (i.e., SRP plus adjunctive therapy) showed a significantly greater reduction from baseline compared to the control group (i.e., SRP alone or SRP plus placebo).

If the adjunctive therapy had no effect, probing depth at these sites would have trended toward baseline as in the SRP alone (or SRP plus placebo) sites. The observation that probing depth remained reduced demonstrated that the drug was efficacious. For the chlorhexidine chip trials, baseline measurements were obtained after supragingival scaling. Because a supragingival scaling can result in a mean probing depth reduction of approximately 0.3–0.4 mm, interpretation of the absolute changes in probing depth as a result of treatment should consider this potential prebaseline change.

It has been hypothesized that these trial results might have been different had control groups also received repeated treatment (i.e., repeated SRP). However, if the control group had received repeated SRP, the adjunctively treated group also would have had to receive repeated instrumentation to maintain design balance. It cannot be assumed that results might have been different only for the control group. Locally delivered, controlled-release antimicrobials also can be effective in the setting of calculus or with reduced amounts of instrumentation. Additional instrumentation would have made data interpretation more difficult, and multiple treatments at multiple times make it more difficult to separate treatment effects meaningfully. In further support of the lack of an impact of additional instrumentation on the outcome, a similarly significant difference was reported when both treatment arms received SRP at baseline and a supragingival prophylaxis at 3 months.

When considering locally delivered, controlled-release antimicrobials as adjunctive therapy or monotherapy, the general consensus of the professional community seems to be that the best use for these products is in the adjunctive setting. Considerable data, however, support efficacy in the monotherapy setting, and Garrett and colleagues suggested that monotherapy was equally as effective as mechanical instrumentation for supportive periodontal maintenance. The investigators cautioned, however, that further studies are needed to validate this treatment regimen, and they emphasized the importance of compliance, including frequent visits for professional supportive maintenance.

Evaluating Safety and Efficacy

To approve a drug for market in the United States, the FDA requires conclusive evidence that it is safe and effective for its intended use. Data from at least two pivotal phase III trials usually are required for regulatory decisions, although in some circumstances (e.g., life-threatening disease such as cancer), only one trial may be required, such as when it would be unethical to withhold an effective treatment from patients and conduct a second trial. The concern is that results of one trial may represent a chance occurrence and should be confirmed by a second trial. Earlier trials (i.e., phase I and II) cannot provide data on which to base regulatory or clinical decisions. The FDA states that each of these pivotal trials must be "adequate and well controlled" and describes common characteristics of designs that are considered adequate and well-controlled studies (see Table 37.5). Comments about trial design, especially phase III trials, and these characteristics were provided earlier in this chapter.

Informed Consent and Legal Considerations

Concerns about malpractice litigation and the legal aspects of dentistry are realities of dental practice. Often at the core of malpractice issues is the concept of informed consent, and adjunctive therapy may have a place in this legal framework.

Informed consent is the standard for dental practice. Clinicians must treat all patients under the principles of informed consent, and all patients must provide their consent for treatment. For clinical research, the FDA [adapted from 21CFR 50.25(a)] describes eight elements of informed consent (Table 37.6). These elements also apply to clinical practice. Appropriate treatment that satisfies the principles of informed consent includes treatment that is evidence based; it is supported by appropriate research data. Because locally delivered, controlled-release antimicrobials as adjuncts have been consistently shown in adequate and well-controlled clinical trials to enhance the efficacy of SRP and provide an additional incremental benefit, performing SRP but not at least offering an adjunctive agent seems to violate the principles of informed consent.

Undiagnosed or undertreated periodontitis is a major source of dental malpractice litigation. Because SRP procedures are commonly considered the standard of care for nonsurgical periodontal therapy and available data confirm that adjunctive locally delivered, controlled-release antimicrobials enhance the efficacy of SRP, SRP plus adjunctive therapy could potentially be considered a new standard. Other investigators have supported the clinical relevance of locally delivered, controlled-release antimicrobials, and SRP without adjunctive therapy could be considered less than maximally effective. In a malpractice litigation of alleged improperly managed periodontitis, it could be claimed that the patient had not been offered maximally effective therapy (i.e., SRP with an adjunctive agent).

TABLE 37.6 Elements of Informed Consent

1. Description of planned treatment
2. Description of reasonably foreseeable risks or discomforts
3. Description of any reasonably expected benefits
4. Disclosure of appropriate alternative treatment
5. Description of procedures to maintain confidentiality
6. Disclosure of associated costs or payments
7. Answering all patient questions
8. Disclosure that all treatment or study participation is voluntary

(Modified from U.S. Food and Drug Administration: 21CFR50.25, revised April 1, 2017. https://www.accessdata.fda.gov/scripts/cdrh/cfdocs/cfcfr/cfrsearch.cfm?=50.25.)

Clinical Use

Potential Indications

Additional dental indications for locally delivered, controlled-release antimicrobials have not been evaluated by the FDA. Examples include combination adjunctive therapy and adjuncts for surgical therapy or peri-implantitis. Preliminary data for these indications are available and discussed in the following sections.

Combination Adjunctive Therapy

Many local and systemic adjunctive therapies are available with supportive data on their use in patients. None is labeled for use in combination therapy. It seems likely, however, that some practitioners may already be providing off-label combination adjunctive therapy for their patients, even though appropriate data do not exist.

Locally delivered, controlled-release antimicrobials enhance the clinical efficacy of SRP. Similarly, adjunctive systemic therapy with low-dose (20 mg) doxycycline, given orally twice daily as a host-modulating agent (later reported as a once-daily, modified-release formulation) also can enhance the clinical efficacy of SRP. Reddy and colleague and Ryan and Golub have reviewed matrix metalloproteinase modulation as a treatment strategy. The question is whether a combination of local antimicrobial and host-modulating adjunctive therapies can provide greater clinical benefit than either adjunctive agent used alone.

In a 6-month clinical trial, combination adjunctive therapies resulted in significantly greater improvements in probing depth and clinical attachment compared to SRP alone. More sites showed a probing depth reduction of 2.0 mm or more, and fewer sites had a residual probing depth 5.0 mm or more. A single case report from this trial was published. Because the appropriate control groups (i.e., SRP plus single adjunctive therapy) were not included in the trial, definitive conclusions regarding increased benefit from combination versus single adjunctive therapy cannot be made. The potential for combined adjunctive therapy to enhance clinical benefit is promising and warrants additional research.

The focus of this chapter is locally delivered, controlled-release antimicrobials. Data support the efficacy of locally delivered, controlled-release antimicrobials, supporting the conclusion that SRP plus adjunctive therapy could be considered a new standard for nonsurgical periodontal therapy. Available data also support the adjunctive efficacy of systemic, low-dose oral doxycycline to an extent that is numerically similar to that reported for locally delivered, controlled-release antimicrobials. Because appropriate comparative data are not available, comparisons of these therapies is not appropriate, and no conclusion can be reached regarding the most efficacious approach for adjunctive therapy, local or systemic adjunctive therapy, or with single or combined agents.

In addition to the possibility of combination adjunctive therapy with a locally delivered agent and host modulatory therapy with low-dose oral doxycycline, Goodson and coworkers reported outcomes from a randomized trial enrolling 231 patients that considered SRP alone and various combinations of SRP, systemic antimicrobials, and surgery using a $2 \times 2 \times 2$ factorial design. Patients were followed for 24 months. Maximal reductions in probing depth and gains in attachment level were observed at 6 months, which were maintained at 24 months in all treatment groups. At 24 months, gains in attachment were increased by systemic antimicrobials (0.50 mm), and probing depth reductions were further augmented by systemic antimicrobials (0.51 mm) and surgical treatment (0.36 mm). Both types of improvements were reduced by smoking.

Surgical Therapy

Pocket sites that do not seem to respond adequately to nonsurgical therapy and evidence residual probing depth with inflammation are often treated with follow-up surgical therapy. A question is whether locally delivered, controlled-release antimicrobials could augment surgical results. This hypothesis was tested in a pilot study by Hellström and coworkers with minocycline microspheres at all pocket sites of 5 mm or more. Sixty patients with at least one nonmolar pocket site with a probing depth of 6 mm or more in each of two quadrants were treated with (1) microspheres at baseline and immediately after each of two surgical procedures at weeks 2 and 3 and again at week 5 or (2) standard surgical therapy. The mean probing depth was reduced in both treatment groups, but the reduction was significantly greater in the test group than in controls at 25 weeks (2.51 ± 0.10 mm vs 2.18 ± 0.10 mm, $P = 0.027$). In contrast, the probing depth reduction after SRP with a limited surgical approach using adjunctive minocycline microspheres was not significantly different compared to SRP in a smaller pilot trial.

A specialized periodontal surgical procedure, regenerative surgery, has become a standard procedure in periodontal practice. It had been suggested verbally as early as 1993 (Killoy WJ, personal communication, 2002) and in print in 1998 that adjunctive locally delivered, controlled-release antimicrobials might improve outcomes after regenerative periodontal surgery. In a pilot trial, the adjunctive use of the chlorhexidine chip with regenerative surgery resulted in more than a 100% greater mean improvement from baseline in bone height and mass 9 months after surgical treatment compared to SRP alone and surgery. Both groups had also received prophylactic systemic antimicrobial treatment before surgery, but the addition of a locally administered antimicrobial resulted in a significant benefit compared to the control arm.

Other reports support the lack of efficacy of systemic antimicrobials and the benefit of locally delivered antimicrobials as adjunctive treatments in the regenerative setting. A microbiologic rationale for the use of locally delivered antimicrobials (i.e., tetracycline fiber) in the regenerative setting was also supported by Sbordone and colleagues. Aichelmann-Reidy and coworkers suggested that regenerative surgical procedures should include an adjunctive, locally delivered, controlled-release antimicrobial agent to provide a more consistent clinical benefit.

These preliminary reports suggested that the adjunctive use of locally delivered, controlled-release antimicrobials can improve clinical outcomes after periodontal surgery in regenerative and nonregenerative settings. These hypotheses require testing in prospective, adequate, and well-controlled trials. None of the three available agents is approved as an adjunct to surgery.

Peri-Implantitis

Similar to periodontitis, peri-implantitis is an inflammatory disease process that is initiated by local microorganisms and that affects the tissues surrounding an implant. An opportunity exists to treat diseased implant sites chemically by targeting the local microflora. There is a potential rationale for the use of locally delivered, controlled-release antimicrobials for the treatment of peri-implantitis. Although the treatment of peri-implantitis is an off-label use, it seems likely that some clinicians have tried local delivery in this setting.

Renvert and coworkers studied 32 patients with at least one implant site with a probing depth of 4 mm or more plus bleeding or exudate on probing. Patients were treated with debridement followed by minocycline microspheres (17 patients, 57 implants) or a chlorhexidine gel formulation (15 patients, 38 implants). Treatments were repeated at 30 and 90 days. Follow-up examinations were performed at 10 days and 1, 3, 6, 9, and 12 months. There were significant reductions in probing depth compared to chlorhexidine at 1, 3, and 6 months and marked reductions in indicator microorganisms in both treatment groups. The study authors concluded that adjunctive minocycline microspheres could be of value in treating peri-implant lesions.

Buchter and colleagues studied 28 patients with a total of 48 peri-implant defects. Two to 18 weeks before baseline measurements, patients had been treated for peri-implantitis (including scaling with a plastic instrument). Patients then continued to receive this treatment alone or with the additional adjunctive use of the doxycycline gel. At 18 weeks, the test group evidenced a significant reduction in mean probing depth and a significant gain in mean attachment levels compared to controls.

Schar and associates and Bassetti coworkers studied 40 patients with peri-implantitis who had probing depths of 4–6 mm and less than 2 mm of radiographic bone loss that was treated with mechanical debridement and air polishing and adjunctively with local minocycline microspheres or photodynamic therapy for 12 months. A significant decrease in probing depth from baseline values was observed in photodynamic sites up 9 months and in minocycline sites up to 12 months. Decreases in *P. gingivalis* and *Tannerella forsythia* concentrations and in GCF levels of IL-1β were seen in both groups. There were no significant differences between groups, and no conclusions can be drawn about either therapy compared to mechanical therapy alone because an appropriate control group was not included.

Labels for the available locally delivered, controlled-release antimicrobials do not include an indication for peri-implantitis. Their potential treating peri-implantitis, however, is an exciting possibility, and one that warrants additional research. Phase III trials are needed to test the hypothesis that locally delivered, controlled-release antimicrobials offer clinical benefit as part of a treatment regimen to manage peri-implantitis.

Tobacco Smoking

Smoking is a well-known risk factor for the development or progression of periodontitis, and it can limit the effectiveness of periodontal therapy. The adjunctive use of locally delivered, controlled-release antimicrobials can enhance the efficacy of SRP in smokers. In a 3-month trial, SRP plus adjunctive doxycycline gel resulted in significantly greater probing depth reduction and clinical attachment gain compared to SRP alone about equally in smokers and nonsmokers. This result was consistent with subset analyses of current smokers, former smokers, and nonsmokers from two 9-month, multicenter trials of doxycycline gel and of microspheres smokers versus nonsmokers in studies of minocycline microsphers. Subset analyses of therapy with minocycline microspheres showed that results for smokers were consistent with overall trial results.

Consistent results also were seen in a later clinical trial of minocycline microspheres. Beneficial periodontal microbiologic alterations in adjunctively treated sites compared to SRP alone were reported for doxycycline gel and minocycline microspheres. A 2-year trial of doxycycline gel with a small number of patients provided further evidence of clinical efficacy.

In a pilot trial to test the use of adjunctive minocycline microspheres in a surgical setting, clinical improvement was seen similarly in smokers and nonsmokers. Adjunctive therapy may lessen the adverse impact of smoking on the periodontium and improve treatment outcomes for patients who smoke. A systematic review of the doxycycline gel and minocycline microspheres found that available data are insufficient to conclude that adjunctive therapy significantly enhances SRP specifically in smokers, and it recommended additional clinical trials (i.e., adequate and well-controlled trials) to assess outcomes for smokers.

Adverse Effects and Cautions for Use

A complete listing of cautions for use and possible adverse effects as listed on the FDA labels for these locally delivered, controlled-release antimicrobials is beyond the scope of this chapter, but complete details about the use of these products and their safety profiles are available in the full prescribing information.

Clinicians are cautioned about adverse effects of this class of drugs:

- Potential for hypersensitivity reactions (i.e., not to be used in patients with a known sensitivity to any ingredient).
- Potential for the overgrowth of nonsusceptible microorganisms, including fungi.
- Use in pregnancy.
- Potential for discoloration during tooth development (i.e., tetracyclines only).
- Use in an acutely abscessed periodontal pocket or in extremely severe periodontal defects with little remaining periodontium.
- Use of local mechanical oral hygiene procedures (e.g., toothbrushing, interdental cleaning devices) for approximately 7–10 days after administration.

The most frequently reported adverse reactions reported in the clinical trials without mention of causality include headache, infection (including upper respiratory tract infection), flu syndrome, pain, tooth disorder and toothache, and various oral signs or symptoms. Toothache was the only adverse reaction that was significantly higher ($P = 0.042$) in the chlorhexidine chip group compared to placebo.

Costs and Outcomes

Locally delivered, controlled-release antimicrobials entail costs. Adjunctive therapy with these products adds cost for the patient in addition to that of SRP, depending on fees charged by the practice. Concerns about the costs and the cost-effectiveness of these agents have proved to be a deterrent to routine clinical use. Although a thorough cost-effectiveness analysis is beyond the scope of this chapter, incorporation of adjunctive therapy into clinical practice warrants some assessment of costs and outcomes.

In an economic evaluation of adjunctive therapy, the relevant issues are the additional costs associated with treatment compared to the additional benefits obtained. Because all therapies entail costs, and very few result in a cost savings, the issue is the value of the incremental benefit obtained. An analysis of the additional benefit obtained by adjunctive periodontal therapy in relation to the additional costs is challenging.

In a clinical trial enrolling more than 450 patients to study the costs associated with the chlorhexidine chip, adjunctive therapy increased total treatment costs by approximately 50% but reduced the likelihood for surgical treatment by about 50% compared to patients treated with standard care. There was a sufficient reduction in other dental treatment to offset about one-half of the acquisition costs of the chip. The result was consistent with a previously published modeled assessment. After 12 months, the examining periodontists recommended similar further degrees of surgery for both groups. No information was available, however, regarding any further disease progression or tooth mortality or whether patients received further surgical care. No information was available for these patients about differential outcomes with follow-up surgical care or continued nonsurgical maintenance with SRP and adjunctive therapy.

A cost-effectiveness comparison of three locally delivered, controlled-release antimicrobial agents was performed by Niederman and colleagues based on a review of published data. The measures used in the analysis included the number needed to treat (i.e., number of teeth or sites treated to produce one site with a probing depth reduction of $\geq$2 mm) and the total cost of treatment. The analysis concluded with a cost-effectiveness ranking of tetracycline fibers > chlorhexidine chips > minocycline microspheres. Use of the number needed to treat analysis has been reviewed; the key message is the inappropriateness of this method for a comparison of different therapies assessed in dissimilar populations at different times and perhaps with different baselines of disease or with different comparators.

What might be the outcomes if locally delivered, controlled-release antimicrobials were included in a long-term periodontal maintenance program? Phase III pivotal trials have provided evidence for the safety and efficacy of these agents to improve clinical signs of periodontitis (e.g., probing depth, attachment level) over the length of the trials (i.e., 6–9 months). Longer-term clinical trials, including studies of minocycline microspheres, doxycycline gel, and the chlorhexidine chip, have provided evidence for the safety and efficacy of locally delivered, controlled-release antimicrobials for periodontal maintenance. The data suggest a benefit in improving tooth retention, but long-term adequate and well-controlled clinical trials are needed to provide conclusive data that adjunctive therapy reduces tooth mortality. Other potential outcomes may include an increase in nonsurgical periodontal therapy, with a corresponding reduction in surgical therapy.

In a meta-analysis of the effects of adjunctive therapy of chlorhexidine, metronidazole, minocycline, and tetracycline with SRP, Bonito and coworkers concluded that the benefit in favor of adjunctive therapy with respect to changes in clinical attachment was significant for all antimicrobials assessed. Little information is available regarding the effect of adjunctive therapy on alveolar bone levels. In a subset of patients from the chlorhexidine chip phase III clinical trials, some patients receiving SRP alone had reduced alveolar bone over 9 months as measured by subtraction radiography, but no patient treated adjunctively showed radiographic evidence of bone loss. In another small study of periodontitis patients treated adjunctively with another formulation of a chlorhexidine chip (i.e., PerioCol-CG), Grover and associates reported that although most sites showed no changes in alveolar bone height, 5% of SRP-alone sites showed bone loss, and 21% of sites showed a bone gain. In contrast, 47% of SRP plus chlorhexidine chip sites showed bone gain, and no site lost alveolar bone.

Treatment with SRP plus adjunctive minocycline microspheres resulted in a significant reduction of markers associated with bone resorption [i.e., pyridinoline cross-linked carboxy terminal telopeptide of type I collagen (ICTP) and interleukin 1-beta (IL-1β)] in the GCF of sites with probing depths of 5 mm or more compared to SRP alone at 1 month. GCF levels of ICTP and IL-1β were significantly increased in periodontitis patients compared to healthy controls. SRP plus chlorhexidine chip reduced levels of matrix metalloproteinase-8 activity and prostaglandin E_2 (PGE_2) in GCF compared to SRP alone. Adequate and well-controlled clinical trials are needed to test the hypothesis that adjunctive, locally delivered controlled-release antimicrobials can reduce alveolar bone loss.

Consideration of the incremental costs of adjunctive therapy requires estimation of the cost-effectiveness of SRP alone compared to no treatment. The data reported by Antczak-Bouckoms and Weinstein, perhaps the first cost-effectiveness analysis of periodontal therapy, support the idea that all treatment entails cost but that addition of antimicrobials can provide an incremental benefit with an additional incremental cost. Just as the benefit of SRP is derived from continued maintenance treatment and repeated instrumentation for life, it seems likely that the benefits of locally delivered, controlled-release antimicrobials are derived from their routine incorporation as adjuncts to SRP procedures and as part of a periodontal maintenance program as indicated.

A detailed review of the cost-effectiveness of locally delivered, controlled-release antimicrobials in periodontal therapy has been provided by Heasman and coworkers. The authors also emphasized the need for long-term studies to assess effects on tooth mortality and other patient-reported outcomes.

Considerations for Future Research

Additional research is warranted for locally delivered, controlled-release antimicrobials for periodontal therapy. For example, research could include large, open-label extension trials or registries to assess outcomes with long-term maintenance therapy. Research is needed to explore new indications or cost-effectiveness issues, along with the suggestions made throughout this chapter for current agents. Other research regarding locally delivered treatment strategies for periodontitis (e.g., targeting the periodontal pocket) could include different treatment regimens using currently available agents. For example, a Phase III clinical trial (ClinicalTrials.gov NCT01249846) to study more frequent administration of a chlorhexidine chip has been completed.

Other classes of agents such as growth factors or antiinflammatory agents could be developed for local delivery into periodontal pockets. A multicenter, randomized clinical trial provided evidence that the delivery of recombinant human platelet-derived growth factor BB in combination with a beta-tricalcium phosphate (β-TCP) resulted in greater bone fill and attachment gain after treatment of advanced periodontal osseous defects compared to β-TCP as an active control; gains were continued in a 36-month extension study. This combination product has been approved for marketed use.

A Phase II trial of fibroblast growth factor 2 (FGF2) in a hydroxypropylcellulose vehicle has been published. Phase II and III trials (NCT00199290, NCT00734708, NCT00514657, NCT01015404) of recombinant human basic FGF (i.e., trafermin) have been completed. Another growth factor, granulocyte-macrophage colony-stimulating factor (sargramostim), has been studied in a Phase I trial (NCT00689143).

An example of the local delivery of antiinflammatory agents is NSAID flurbiprofen. A Phase II trial (NCT00425451) of a combination chip of chlorhexidine and flurbiprofen was completed, and a flurbiprofen chip was compared to a chlorhexidine chip in another completed Phase II trial (NCT01040286). Other NSAIDs (e.g., ketoprofin, meloxicam) have been studied.

A controlled-release system for the steady delivery of a chemoattractant for regulatory lymphocytes offers an exciting alternative. Local administration in preclinical canine and murine models led to reduced alveolar bone resorption and a reduction in clinical measures of inflammation. Gamal and Kumper reported the use of a doxycycline-loaded, biodegradable membrane in a randomized trial of regenerative surgical procedures with or without EDTA root surface etching.

Antimicrobial Photodynamic Therapy (aPDT)

Need for aPDT

Periodontal disease is a polymicrobial infection and involves an immune-inflammatory response to the biofilm. Hence eliminating the infection remains the mainstay of periodontal therapy. Mechanical therapy in the form of SRP is technique sensitive, difficult and time-consuming especially in root concavities, furcations, and areas with deep pockets. *T. forsythia* and *A. actinomycetemcomitans* have been shown to persist in periodontal pockets after routine SRP. Supporting therapy with antibiotics is believed to further suppress the periodontal pathogens, increasing the benefits of conventional mechanical therapy. However, unwanted side effects such as allergies or gastrointestinal complaints, and emergence of antibiotic resistant strains is a major cause of concern.

Biofilms further increase the resistance of bacteria to antibiotics by reducing the penetration of antimicrobials through its matrix and by allowing transfer of potential resistances among various bacterial species by horizontal gene transer. Herein comes the role of aPDT as an alternate approach with a different modus operandi than the key-lock mechanism of action of conventional antimicrobials.

Historical Background

The history of PDT dates back to the ancient Egyptians who used the staining properties of dyes to treat skin diseases. Oxygen-dependent photodynamic reactions were accidently discovered by a medical student in Munich, Oscar Raab in 1900, who was involved in a study on the toxicity of the dye acridine red on *Paramecium* sp. as part of his doctoral thesis. Raab and his supervisor Hermann von Tappeiner recognized that the observed toxicity of acridine was dependent on the time of the day and the amount of daylight. The term "photodynamic phenomenon" was coined by von Tappeiner, who went on to further utilize this knowledge for the treatment of skin cancers. The concept of photodynamic inactivation of bacteria was first described by Jodlbauer and von Tappeiner in 1904 and Huber in 1905.

Mechanism of Action

The three prerequisites of aPDT are (1) the presence of a nontoxic, photoactivatable substance, the photosensitizer, which is capable of binding to the targeted cell; (2) light of an appropriate wavelength for exciting the photosensitizer (preferably in the visible to near infra red spectrum); (3) Molecular oxygen. Photosensitizer in ground state, on excitation with light of a specific wavelength, gets excited into either a doublet or triplet state, which then reacts with the biomolecules by either of the two mechanisms as described in Fig. 37.10, damaging the target cells via highly reactive oxygen species, particularly singlet oxygen. In type I mechanism, charge (i.e., electrons) is transferred to surrounding substrates leading to formation of superoxide ions, hydrogen peroxide, and free hydroxyl radicals. In type II mechanism, energy (but no charge) is transferred directly to the ground state molecular oxygen, leading to emergence

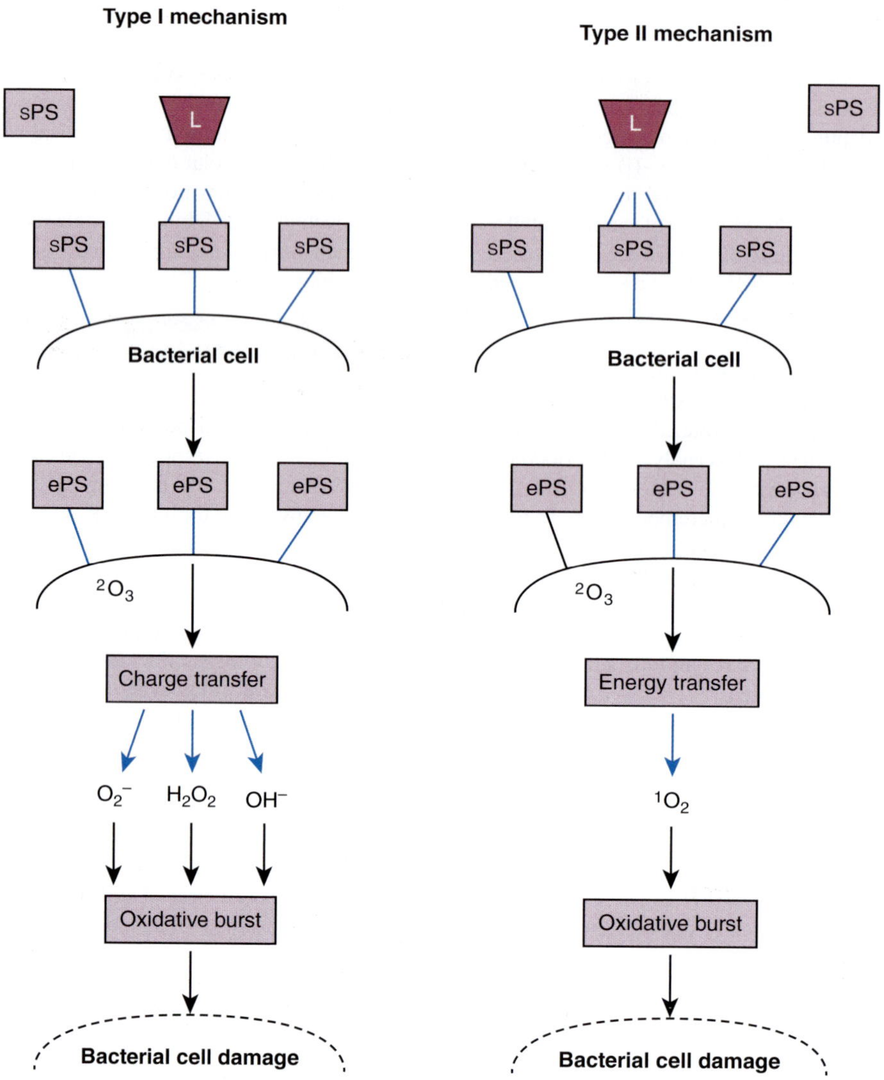

Fig. 37.10 Adapted Jablonski diagram depicting the mechanism of action of antimicrobial photodynamic therapy. *L*, Light of appropriate wavelength; *sPS*, singlet state photosensitizer; *ePS*, excited state photosensitizer; ($^2O_3$), molecular oxygen; (O_2^-), superoxide radical; (H_2O_2), hydrogen peroxide; (OH^-), free hydroxyl radical; ($^1O_2$), singlet oxygen.

of singlet oxygen. These ions further go on to cause bacterial cell damage via oxidative burst. aPDT causes nonselective oxidative damage of bacterial proteins, lipids, and nucleic acids, targeting primarily cytoplasmic membranes and DNA.

Photosensitizers

Since the discovery of photodynamic process, many dyes have been tried as photosensitizers. An ideal photosensitizer must be nontoxic, soluble in water, and have high quantum yield of singlet oxygen in vivo. It should bind to bacteria in plaque without staining gingiva and be acceptable to patients. The major classes of photosensitizers with their salient properties are presented in Table 37.7.

Light Source

The spectral emission, intensity of light source, and the mode of light delivery are more important characteristics than the type of the light source, which can be either:

1. LASERS (e.g., argon, diode, Nd:YAG lasers): monochromatic, can be easily coupled into a single optical fiber and mounted on different light delivery devices.
2. Light-emitting diodes (LEDs): inexpensive compared to lasers, wider spectrum of emission, highly flexible, small, lightweight.
3. Gas-discharge lamps (e.g., quartz-tungsten-halogen or xenon-discharge lamps): cannot be efficiently coupled into optical fiber bundles; cause more heating as compared to lasers and LEDs.

aPDT in Periodontitis

aPDT treatment may augment periodontal treatment by increasing bacterial killing, inactivating bacterial virulence factors, and inactivating host cytokines that impair periodontal restoration. Periopathogens, such as *P. gingivalis*, are commonly found in diseased sites, and this bacterium is believed to contribute to the destruction of the host tissue by expression of proteases. *P. gingivalis* proteases have been shown to be virulent factors, in that they can degrade host connective tissue, disarm the innate host response, and are required for virulence in animal models of disease. In vivo and in vitro studies done to evaluate the bactericidal and protease inactivation effect of photosensitizers reported that protease inactivation requires lower concentrations of photosensitizer and less time of light exposure than that needed for bacterial killing. Crevicular IL-1beta, IL-6, and

TABLE 37.7 Major Classes of Photosensitizers Used in PDT

Photosensitizer	Salient Properties
Phenothiazinium derivatives	Three-ring p-system with auxochromic side groups Singlet oxygen quantum yield below 0.5 Work by type I mechanism Show absorption in (600–680 nm) For example, methylene blue, toluidine blue, new methylene blue, di-methyl-methylene blue First clinically approved photosensitizers for use in dentistry Used as a standard for in vitro studies
Xanthene derivatives	Singlet oxygen quantum yield 0.6–0.8 Show absorption in green spectrum (480–550 nm) Work by type II mechanism Eosin Y, Erythrosine, Rose Bengal
Fullerene derivatives	Soccer-ball shaped cage molecules Show strong absorption in UV and visible range Work by both type I and type II mechanisms
Porphyrin, chlorin and phthalocyanine derivatives	Singlet oxygen quantum yield 0.5 and 0.8 Work by type II mechanism Intense absorption at 405 nm, with smaller peaks at wavelength longer than 500 nm For example, TMPyP [5,10,15,20-tetrakis (1-methyl-4-pyridinium)-porphyrin tetra-(p-toluenesulfonate], XF-73 [5,15-bis-[4–(3-trimethylammoniopropyloxy)-phenyl]-porphyrin chloride], photodithazine VR [a commercially available chlorin-e6 derivative]
Phenalenone derivatives	Singlet oxygen quantum yield above 0.9 Work by type II mechanism Show absorption in UV/blue spectrum (320–430 nm) SAPYR is the first water-soluble exclusive type II photosensitizer
Curcumin derivatives	Work by type I mechanism Show absorption in UV/blue spectrum (300–500 nm) Approved as a food additive
Riboflavin derivatives	Singlet quantum yield 0.7 and 0.8 Show absorption in UV/blue spectrum (350–470 nm) Safe for humans

TNF-alpha are inactivated during aPDT, thereby promoting tissue healing. aPDT increases the expression of bFGF gene, an important factor in periodontal tissue regeneration. aPDT is also beneficial in the treatment of halitosis. Immediate results have been reported following a single session of PDT. As adjunct to SRP in patients of chronic periodontitis, modest gains in CAL (0.36 mm) and reductions in probing depth (0.21 mm) have been reported. aPDT has an additional positive effect on reduction of gingival bleeding in generalized aggressive periodontitis patients when used as an adjunct to nonsurgical periodontal treatment. PDT has no negative side effects on gingival fibroblasts and osteoblasts in vitro, suggesting that it can be safely used in periodontal conditions.

aPDT in Peri-Implantitis Management

Implant decontamination remains the primary objective in peri-implantitis treatment. However, the disinfection of implant surfaces and peri-implant tissues by mechanical debridement alone remains difficult due to the complexity of the design and topography of the implant surface. Following aPDT, several studies have reported a reduction in *T. denticola, T. forsythia, Fusobacterium* sp., and *S. beta-hemolytic* counts. Renato Silva Fraga et al. in their systematic review and metaanalysis also reported a significant reduction in *A. actinomycetemcomitans, P. gingivalis*, and *P. intermedia* CFU counts after aPDT therapy in peri-implantitis cases. They summarized that aPDT has positive potential to act as an alternative therapy for peri-implantitis. Better bone gain and reduction in probing depth following adjunctive use of PDT has been reported by Shibli et al. and Romeo et al., respectively. aPDT in conjunction with mechanical debridement is also more beneficial in treating peri-mucositis in individuals vaping e-cigarettes than mechanical debridement alone. Although Best Evidence Review 2018 of AAP indicates that evidence is lacking supporting the benefit of aPDT as an adjunct in treatment of peri-implantitis, it agrees that PDT therapy is safe and no adverse events have been reported till date.

aPDT in Smokers

Smokers have an unfavorable response to periodontal treatment compared to nonsmokers. Systemic antibiotics are often prescribed to augment healing in such situations. There is no universally accepted antibiotic regime to be followed for periodontal therapy in smokers, although several studies advocate the use of MTX-AMX combination for a period of 7–14 days. Keeping in mind the emergence of resistance against antibiotics, aPDT could be a promising adjunct to mechanical debridement in the presence of such systemic modifying factors like smoking, which have the potential to alter the healing response of tissues.

Though some studies do not report any clinical advantage in terms of probing depth reduction after a single session, there are others who have reported multiple sessions (preferably three sessions conducted at 48 h interval) to be equally beneficial as MTX-AMX combination in reducing probing depth, bleeding on probing, and the levels of *Prevotella intermedia* and *Prevotella nigrescens* in deep pockets. Some studies have also reported a reduction in IL-1 beta and MMP-8 levels after a single session of aPDT in smokers.

Conclusion

Scaling and root planing alone are effective for reducing pocket depths, gaining increases in periodontal attachment levels, and decreasing inflammation levels (i.e., bleeding with probing). When systemic antibiotics are used as adjuncts to scaling and root planing, the evidence indicates that some systemic antibiotics (e.g., metronidazole, tetracycline) provide additional improvements in attachment levels (0.35 mm for metronidazole; 0.40 mm for tetracycline) when used as adjuncts to scaling and root planing. When scaling and root planing are combined with the subgingival placement of sustained-release vehicles, additional clinical benefits are possible, including the further reduction of pocket depths, additional gains in clinical attachment levels (e.g., 0.39 mm with minocycline gel), and further decreases in inflammation. Improvements in clinical attachment levels also occur with the chlorhexidine chip (0.16 mm) and doxycycline gel (0.34 mm). The use of antiinfective chemotherapeutic treatment adjuncts does not result in significant patient-centered adverse effects.

The decision regarding when to use local or systemic antimicrobials should be made on the basis of the clinician's consideration of the clinical findings, the patient's medical and dental history, the patient's preferences, and the potential benefits of adjunctive therapy with these agents.

The benefits of aPDT therapy include reduce treatment time, no reported adverse effects, no need for anesthesia, destruction of bacteria in a very short period of time (less than 1 min), and avoidance of damage to adjoining tissues. Also, it is unlikely that target bacteria will develop resistance to PDT.

On the other hand, aPDT has few limitations. Firstly, it is a nonspecific process. Secondly, majority of the in vitro studies conducted so far have essentially been performed on pure cultures of bacteria, not taking into account the fact that oral microbes essentially occur as mixed species, that too in the form of biofilms. Hence, the results of the in vitro studies may not hold true for in vivo situations, where presence of blood in the periodontal pockets could decrease the effectiveness of aPDT.

Key points

- An antiinfective agent is a chemotherapeutic agent that acts by reducing the number of bacteria present.
- An antibiotic is a naturally occurring, semisynthetic, or synthetic type of antiinfective agent that destroys or inhibits the growth of selective microorganisms, generally at low concentrations.
- Disinfectants are antimicrobial agents that are generally applied to inanimate surfaces to destroy microorganisms.
- Tetracyclines have the ability to concentrate in the periodontal tissues and to inhibit the growth of *Aggregatibacter actinomycetemcomitans*. In addition, tetracyclines exert an anticollagenase effect that can inhibit tissue destruction and that may help with bone regeneration.
- Metronidazole has an Antabuse effect when alcohol is ingested.
- Metronidazole inhibits warfarin metabolism.
- The combination of amoxicillin with clavulanate potassium makes amoxicillin resistant to penicillinase enzymes produced by some bacteria.
- At present, ciprofloxacin is the only antibiotic in periodontal therapy to which all strains of *A. actinomycetemcomitans* are susceptible.
- Azithromycin can alter the electrical activity of the heart, which may lead to a potentially fatal heart rhythm known as prolonged QT interval. This rhythm causes the timing of the heart's contractions to become irregular.
- When both bacteriostatic and bactericidal antibiotics are required, they are best given serially rather than in combination.
- Controlled-release agents maintain clinically effective intrapocket concentrations of antimicrobial for an extended period of time.
- The three prerequisites of aPDT: (1) the presence of a nontoxic, photoactivatable substance, the photosensitizer, which is capable of binding to the targeted cell; (2) light of an appropriate wavelength for exciting the photosensitizer (preferably in the visible to near infrared spectrum); and (3) molecular oxygen.

References

References and MCQs with answers for the chapter are available on www.medenact.com.

CHAPTER 38

Host Modulation

ME Ryan | Y Gu | A Jain

CHAPTER OUTLINE

Host modulation is a relatively new term that has been incorporated into our dental jargon, but it has not been well defined. *Host* can be defined as "the organism from which a parasite obtains its nourishment," or in the transplantation of tissue, "the individual who receives the graft." *Modulation* is defined as "the alteration of function or status of something in response to a stimulus or an altered chemical or physical environment" (*Taber's Medical Dictionary*, 2004). In diseases of the periodontium that are initiated by bacteria, the "host" clearly is the individual who harbors these pathogens; however, it was not clear for many years whether it was possible to modulate the host response to these pathogens and other stimuli leading to the breakdown of the attachment apparatus. Host modulation with chemotherapeutic agents or drugs is the latest adjunctive therapeutic option for the management of periodontal diseases. The concept of host modulation is fairly new to the field of dentistry but is universally understood by most physicians who routinely apply the principles of host modulation to the management of a number of chronic progressive disorders such as arthritis and osteoporosis. The concept of host modulation was first introduced to dentistry by Williams and Golub et al. and then expanded on by many other scholars in the dental profession. In 1990, Williams concluded "there are compelling data from studies in animals and human trials indicating that pharmacologic agents, that modulate the host responses believed to be involved in the pathogenesis of periodontal destruction, may be efficacious in slowing the progression of periodontitis." In 1992, Golub and colleagues discussed "host modulation with tetracyclines and their chemically modified analogs."

To better understand the host factors that clinicians are attempting to modulate, a more detailed assessment of the role of the host response in periodontal pathogenesis is needed (Fig. 38.1). Elevations in the proinflammatory or destructive mediators in response to bacterial challenge are counterbalanced by elevations in antiinflammatory or protective mediators such as the cytokines IL-4 and IL-10, other mediators such as IL-1ra (receptor antagonist), and tissue inhibitors of metalloproteinases (TIMPs) (Fig. 38.2). Under conditions of health, the antiinflammatory or protective mediators control tissue destruction. If there are adequate levels of these antiinflammatory or protective mediators to keep the host response to the bacterial challenge in check, the individual will be disease resistant. If an imbalance occurs, with excessive levels of the proinflammatory or destructive mediators present in the host tissues, tissue destruction will ensue in the susceptible host. Host modulatory therapy (HMT) is a *means of treating the host side of the host–bacteria interaction*. The host response is responsible for most of the tissue breakdown that occurs, leading to the clinical signs of periodontitis (i.e., loss of connective tissue attachment and bone). HMTs offer the opportunity for modulating or reducing this destruction by treating aspects of the chronic inflammatory response. HMTs do not "switch off" normal defense mechanisms or inflammation; instead, they ameliorate excessive or pathologically elevated inflammatory processes to enhance the opportunities for wound healing and periodontal stability.

HMT can be used to reduce excessive levels of enzymes, cytokines, and prostanoids and should not reduce levels below constitutive levels. HMTs can also modulate osteoclast and osteoblast function (Fig. 38.3) but should not impact normal tissue turnover. HMT is key to addressing many of the risk factors that have adverse effects on the host response, which are either not easily managed (e.g., smoking, diabetes) or cannot be changed (e.g., genetic susceptibility). In addition, host modulatory agents might be used to increase the levels of a person's own protective or antiinflammatory mediators. Use of systemic HMTs for treatment of a patient's periodontal condition may also provide benefits for other inflammatory disorders such as arthritis, cardiovascular disease, dermatologic conditions, diabetes, rheumatoid arthritis, and osteoporosis. Also, patients who are currently taking host modulatory agents, such as nonsteroidal antiinflammatory drugs (NSAIDs), bisphosphonates, or tetracyclines, as well as newer agents targeting specific cytokines for the management of medical conditions, may be experiencing periodontal benefits from these systemic medications prescribed for the management of other chronic inflammatory conditions.

A variety of different drug classes have been evaluated as host modulation agents, including the NSAIDs, bisphosphonates, tetracyclines, enamel matrix proteins, growth factors, and bone morphogenetic proteins. This section discusses chemotherapeutics developed as HMTs researched as adjuncts to treat periodontitis to date, use of HMTs in clinical practice, and what the future might hold for HMTs.

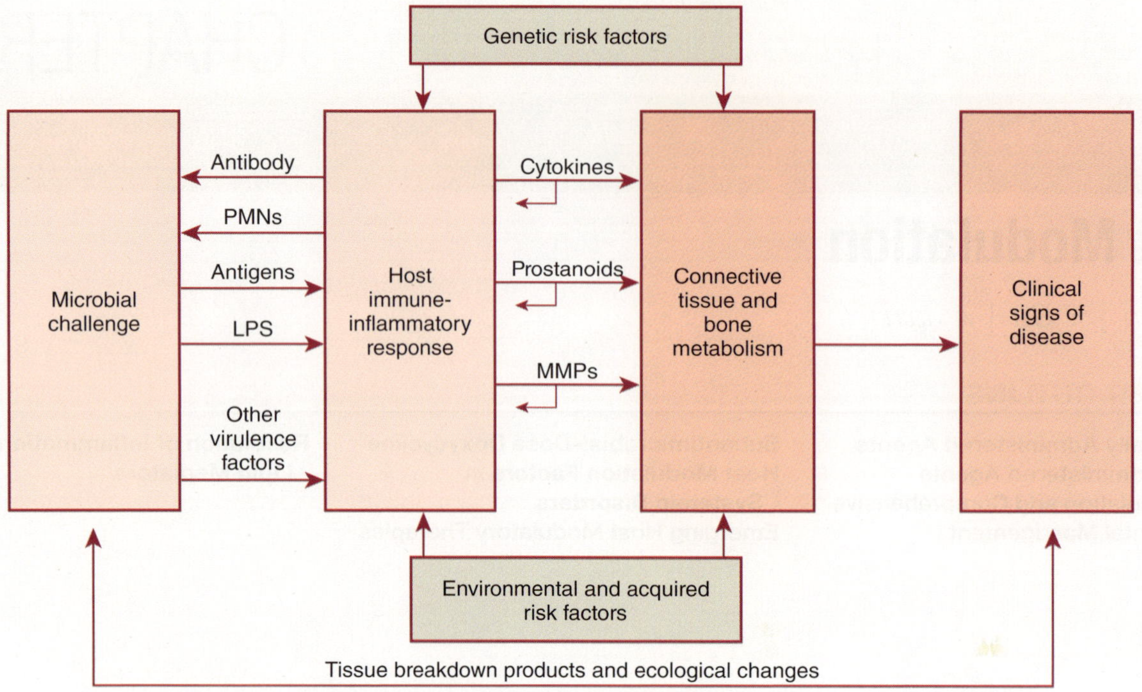

Fig. 38.1 Schematic illustration of the pathogenesis of periodontitis. The microbial challenge presented by subgingival plaque bacteria results in an upregulated host immune-inflammatory response in the periodontal tissues that is characterized by the excessive production of inflammatory cytokines (e.g., interleukins, tumor necrosis factor), prostanoids (e.g., prostaglandin E_2), and enzymes, including the matrix metalloproteinases *(MMPs).* These proinflammatory mediators are responsible for the majority of periodontal breakdown that occurs, leading to the clinical signs and symptoms of periodontitis. The process is modified by environmental (e.g., tobacco use) and acquired risk factors (e.g., systemic diseases) and genetic susceptibility. *PMNs*, Polymorphonuclear leukocytes; *LPS*, lipopolysaccharide. (*Modified from Page RC, Kornman KS: The pathogenesis of human periodontitis: an introduction*, Periodontology *20:127, 2009.)*

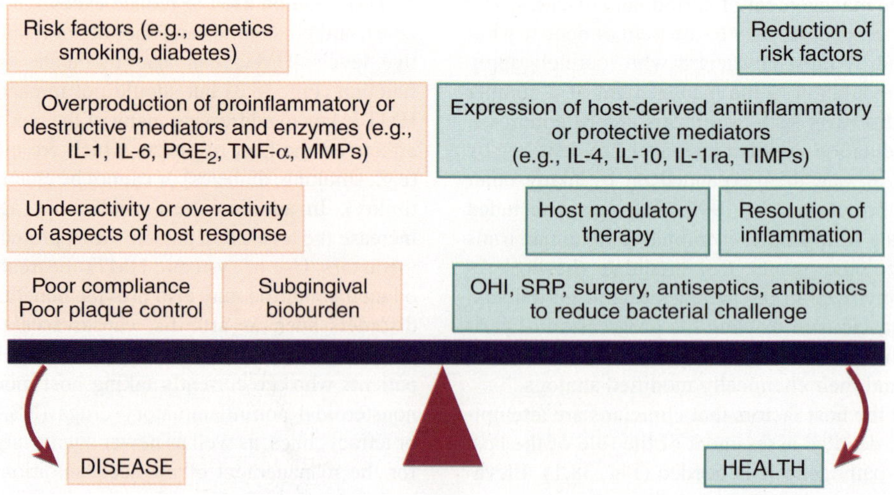

Fig. 38.2 The periodontal balance. The balance between periodontal breakdown (disease) and periodontal stability (health) is tipped toward disease by risk factors, excessive production of inflammatory cytokines and enzymes (e.g., *IL-1* and *IL-6*, interleukin-1 and -6; PGE_2, prostaglandin E_2; *TNF-α*, tumor necrosis factor alpha; *MMPs*, matrix metalloproteinases), underactivity or overactivity of aspects of the immune-inflammatory host response, poor compliance, and a pathogenic microflora. The balance can be tipped toward health by risk factor modification, upregulation, and restoration of balance between naturally occurring inhibitors of inflammation (e.g., *IL-4* and *IL-10*, interleukins-4 and -10; *IL-1ra*, interleukin-1 receptor antagonist; *TIMPs*, tissue inhibitors of metalloproteinases); *HMT*, host modulatory therapy and antibacterial treatments such as *OHI* (oral hygiene instructions); *SRP*, scaling and root planing, surgery, antiseptics, and antibiotics.

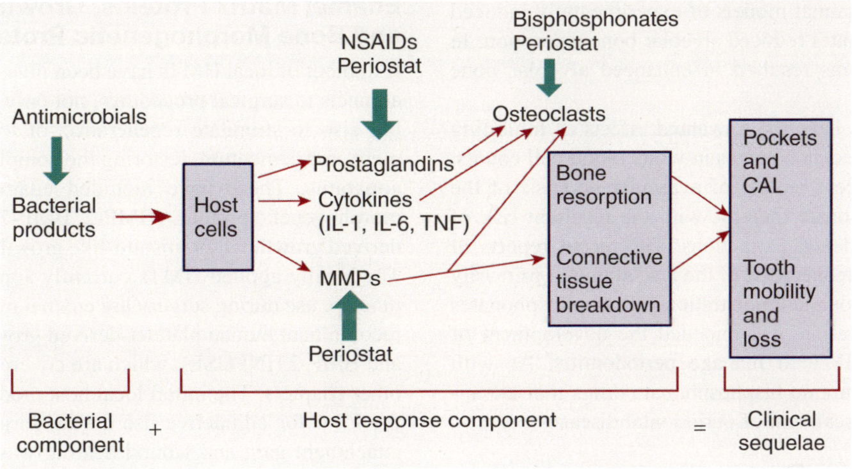

Fig. 38.3 Potential adjunctive therapeutic approaches. Possible adjunctive therapies and points of intervention in the treatment of periodontitis are presented related to the pathologic cascade of events. *CAL*, Clinical attachment loss.

Systemically Administered Agents

A variety of drug classes have been evaluated as host modulation agents, including NSAIDs, bisphosphonates, tetracyclines, enamel matrix proteins, growth factors, and bone morphogenetic proteins. Chemotherapeutic agents have been researched as adjunct treatments for periodontitis in clinical practice, and HMTs are still evolving.

Nonsteroidal Antiinflammatory Drugs

NSAIDs inhibit the formation of prostaglandins, including PGE_2, which is produced by neutrophils, macrophages, fibroblasts, and gingival epithelial cells in response to the presence of LPS, a component of the cell wall of gram-negative bacteria. PGE_2 has been extensively studied in periodontal disease because it upregulates bone resorption by osteoclasts. Levels of PGE_2 have been shown to be elevated in patients with periodontal disease compared to healthy patients. PGE_2 also inhibits fibroblast function and has inhibitory and modulatory effects on the immune response.

NSAIDs inhibit prostaglandins and therefore reduce tissue inflammation. They are used to treat pain, acute inflammation, and a variety of chronic inflammatory conditions. NSAIDs include the salicylates (e.g., aspirin), indomethacin, and the propionic acid derivatives (e.g., ibuprofen, flurbiprofen, and naproxen). The ability of NSAIDs to block PGE_2 production, thereby reducing inflammation and inhibiting osteoclast activity in the periodontal tissues, has been investigated in patients with periodontitis. Short-term administration of NSAIDs reduced gingival crevicular fluid (GCF) MMP-8 levels, but no statistically significant differences were observed in clinical attachment levels (CALs). Studies also suggested that low-dose aspirin as an adjunct periodontal therapy was beneficial in reducing periodontal attachment loss. Studies have shown that systemic NSAIDs, such as indomethacin, flurbiprofen, and naproxen administered daily for up to 3 years, significantly slowed the rate of alveolar bone loss compared to placebo. However, NSAIDs have some serious disadvantages when considered for use as a HMT for periodontitis. Daily administration for extended periods is necessary for periodontal benefits to become apparent, and NSAIDs are associated with significant side effects, including gastrointestinal problems, hemorrhage (from decreased platelet aggregation), and renal and hepatic impairment. Furthermore, research shows that the periodontal benefits of taking long-term NSAIDs are lost when patients stop taking the drugs, with a return to or even an acceleration of the rate of bone loss seen before NSAID therapy, often referred to as a "rebound effect." For these reasons, the long-term use of NSAIDs as an adjunctive treatment for periodontitis has never really developed beyond research studies.

It was previously anticipated that the selective cyclooxygenase-2 (COX-2) inhibitors may offer promise as adjunctive treatments in the management of periodontitis. The enzyme cyclooxygenase, which converts arachidonic acid to prostaglandins, exists in two functionally distinct isoforms, COX-1 and COX-2. COX-1 is constitutively expressed and has antithrombogenic and cytoprotective functions. Therefore, inhibition of COX-1 by nonselective NSAIDs causes side effects such as gastrointestinal ulceration and impaired hemostasis. COX-2 is induced after stimulation by various cytokines, growth factors, and LPS and results in the production of elevated quantities of prostaglandins. Inhibition of COX-2 by selective COX-2 inhibitors results in reduction of inflammation. Researchers considered that the use of selective COX-2 inhibitors offered the prospect for reducing periodontal inflammation without the side effects typically observed after long-term (nonselective) NSAID therapy, and preliminary studies identified that selective COX-2 inhibitors slowed alveolar bone loss in animal models and modified prostaglandin production in human periodontal tissues. However, the selective COX-2 inhibitors were later identified to be associated with significant and life-threatening adverse effects (i.e., myocardial infarction), resulting in some drugs being withdrawn from the market. In summary, NSAIDs (including the selective COX-2 specific inhibitors) are presently not indicated as adjunctive HMTs in the treatment of periodontal disease.

Bisphosphonates

The bisphosphonates are bone-seeking agents that inhibit bone resorption by disrupting osteoclast activity. Their precise mechanism of action is unclear, but research has shown that bisphosphonates interfere with osteoblast metabolism and secretion of lysosomal enzymes. More recent evidence has suggested that bisphosphonates also possess anticollagenase properties. The ability of bisphosphonates to modulate osteoclast activity clearly may be useful in the treatment of periodontitis. Research has demonstrated that in naturally occurring periodontitis in beagle dogs, treatment with the bisphosphonate, alendronate, significantly increased bone density compared to placebo. In animal models of experimentally induced periodontitis, bisphosphonates reduced alveolar bone resorption. In human studies, these agents resulted in enhanced alveolar bone status and density.

Some bisphosphonates have the unwanted effects of inhibiting bone calcification and inducing changes in white blood cell counts. Also, there have been recent reports of avascular necrosis of the jaws following bisphosphonate therapy, with the resultant risk of bone necrosis following dental extractions. The recent reports of bisphosphonate-related osteonecrosis of the jaw, although primarily associated with intravenous administration of bisphosphonates rather than oral administration, has impeded the development of bisphosphonates as an HMT to manage periodontitis. As with NSAIDs, at present there are no bisphosphonate drugs that are approved and indicated for treatment of periodontal diseases.

Subantimicrobial-Dose Doxycycline

Subantimicrobial-dose doxycycline (SDD) is a 20-mg dose of doxycycline (Periostat) that is approved and indicated as an adjunct to scaling and root planing (SRP) in the treatment of chronic periodontitis. It is taken twice daily for 3 months, up to a maximum of 9 months of continuous dosing. The 20-mg dose exerts its therapeutic effect by enzyme, cytokine, and osteoclast inhibition rather than by any antibiotic effect. Research studies have found no detectable antimicrobial effect on the oral flora or the bacterial flora in other regions of the body and have identified clinical benefit when used as an adjunct to SRP.

At present, SDD (Periostat) is the only systemically administered HMT specifically indicated for the treatment of chronic periodontitis that is approved by the US Food and Drug Administration (FDA) and accepted by the American Dental Association (ADA). Studies conducted by Preshaw et al., using this same modified-release SDD versus placebo in 266 subjects with periodontitis as an adjunct to SRP, resulted in significantly greater clinical benefits than SRP alone.

A review paper on the nonsurgical treatment of chronic periodontitis by means of SRP with or without adjuncts showed that clinical improvements with SRP alone resulted in a mean gain of 0.5 mm in CALs, whereas adjunctive therapy with SDD resulted in an additional 0.35 mm gain in CALs beyond that seen with mechanical therapy alone, representing a 70% improvement in CALs.

A modified-release SDD (i.e., Oracea) was approved by the FDA for the treatment of the common skin disorder rosacea, and it is routinely prescribed within the dermatology community. It will be interesting to see what the long-term benefits to oral health will be in rosacea patients prescribed the time-release formulation of SDD. There has been considerable off-label use of this drug for the treatment of periodontal disease based on the understanding that once-daily administration can increase the level of compliance compared to twice-daily oral administration. Preshaw and coworkers demonstrated that this modified-release SDD resulted in significantly improved clinical benefits in the treatment of periodontitis.

Locally Administered Agents

Nonsteroidal Antiinflammatory Drugs

Topical NSAIDs have shown benefit in the treatment of periodontitis. One study of 55 patients with chronic periodontitis who received topical ketorolac mouth rinse reported that GCF levels of PGE_2 were reduced by approximately half over 6 months and that bone loss was halted. In addition, locally administered ketoprofen has been investigated. To date, topically administered NSAIDs have not been approved as local HMTs for the management of periodontitis.

Enamel Matrix Proteins, Growth Factors, and Bone Morphogenetic Proteins

A number of local HMTs have been investigated for potential use as adjuncts to surgical procedures, not only to improve wound healing but also to stimulate regeneration of lost bone, periodontal ligament, and cementum, restoring the complete periodontal attachment apparatus. These have included enamel matrix proteins, bone morphogenetic proteins (BMP-2, BMP-7), growth factors (platelet-derived growth factor, insulin-like growth factor), and tetracyclines. The locally applied HMTs currently approved by the FDA for adjunctive use during surgery are enamel matrix proteins (Emdogain), recombinant human platelet-derived growth factor-BB (GEM 21S), and BMP-2 (INFUSE), which are covered in much greater detail in other chapters. The initial local host modulatory agent approved by the FDA for adjunctive use during surgery to assist with clinical attachment gain and wound healing was Emdogain; this has been followed by platelet-derived growth factor combined with a resorbable synthetic bone matrix (GEM 21S) to assist in regenerative procedures approved recently by the FDA, as well as rhBMP-2 (INFUSE) soaked onto an absorbable collagen sponge to assist with ridge and sinus augmentation. The technology behind GEM 21 has also been approved and marketed for use in wound healing, particularly in patients with diabetes, and INFUSE has been used for quite some time for the healing of fractures by the orthopedic community. However, adverse events associated with the administration of BMPs have been reported, including osteolysis, seroma or hematoma, infection, arachnoiditis, dysphagia, increased neurologic deficits, and cancer.

The remainder of this chapter focuses on the clinical utility of host modulation for nonsurgical procedures in clinical practice and the use of SDD (Periostat) in clinical practice.

Host Modulation and Comprehensive Periodontal Management

The term *periodontal management* suggests a much broader concept of periodontal care than the term *periodontal treatment.* This concept is extremely important considering the chronic nature of the disease. Management includes thorough medical and dental history and examination (clinical charting and radiographs), assessment of risk factors, diagnosis, development of a treatment strategy, initial and definitive treatment planning, review of treatment outcomes and reevaluation, long-term supportive periodontal therapy (maintenance care), and assessment of prognosis. In addition, as new data continue to emerge regarding biochemical assessments of disease activity (measuring levels of proinflammatory mediators, bone and connective tissue breakdown products in the GCF, saliva, and tissues of the oral cavity), new diagnostic and prognostic tests may become part of our established protocols for comprehensive periodontal disease management in the future. However, controlling the bacteria that cause periodontal infections remains a central focus of effective periodontal treatment. Understanding the importance of the host response and the impact of risk factors now allows clinicians to provide complementary treatment strategies simultaneously for their patients (Fig. 38.4).

The patients most likely requiring the use of HMT include those with risk factors that are either nonmodifiable or not easily modified. If the decision is made to use HMT, this must be discussed with the patient and the rationale for treatment thoroughly explained. This takes time at the chair side, but it is time well spent; patients become increasingly interested in their periodontal status and are more likely to develop ownership of their management, thereby enhancing compliance with all aspects of care, including

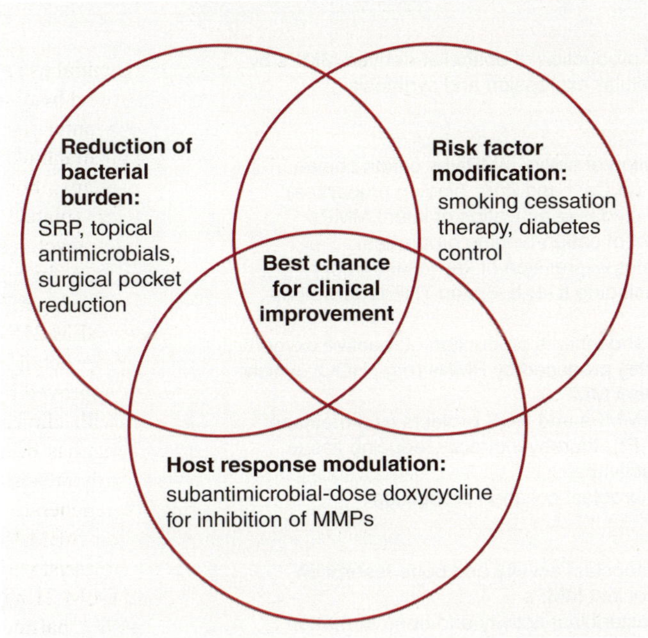

Fig. 38.4 Complementary treatment strategies in periodontitis. The best chance for clinical improvement may come from implementing complementary treatment strategies that target different aspects of the periodontal balance. Reduction of the bacterial burden by scaling and root planing *(SRP)* is the cornerstone of treatment and can be augmented by the use of topical antimicrobials and surgical pocket therapy. In addition to this antibacterial treatment approach, the host response can be treated by the use of host modulatory therapy, such as subantimicrobial-dose doxycycline, for the inhibition of matrix metalloproteinases *(MMPs)*. Risk factor assessment and modification must form a key part of any periodontal treatment strategy, including smoking cessation counseling. These different but complementary treatment strategies can be used together as part of a comprehensive management approach.

plaque control, risk reduction, and treatment protocols. Compliance with HMT is greatly facilitated if the rationale for prescribing is clearly explained. The need for compliance with the prescribed drug regimen is important because with SDD, for example, a tablet must be taken twice daily (once in the morning and once in the evening) and should not be taken with calcium supplements. Compliance may be improved by administration of a modified-release SDD capsule taken only once a day. It should be emphasized to the patient that the use of HMT is not a substitute for excellent plaque control (just as it is not a substitute for excellent debridement and root surface instrumentation by the treating clinician). To achieve the best results, patients must be interested and well informed about their condition so that compliance is maximized. Furthermore, patients must also be convinced that comprehensive and frequent recall appointments are absolutely necessary in the maintenance phase of this chronic and often progressive disease, which can be very well controlled with adequate follow-up.

In addition to patient motivation, oral hygiene instruction, and SRP to reduce the bacterial challenge, a key treatment strategy when managing periodontitis patients is *risk factor modification.* The harmful effects of smoking on the periodontal tissues are well documented, and successful smoking cessation therapy will likely be a major benefit to patients with periodontitis. Smoking cessation counseling can be undertaken in the dental office (if staff are appropriately trained) or through collaboration with the patient's physician or specialized clinics. Given the evidence that smokers have worse periodontal disease than nonsmokers and that the magnitude and predictability of clinical improvements after treatment are significantly reduced in smokers, smoking cessation counseling should form a major part of treatment for smokers with periodontitis. Patients with poorly controlled diabetes are also at increased risk for periodontitis, and periodontal therapy may have an impact on diabetic control. Collaboration with medical colleagues when treating diabetic patients with periodontitis is warranted to ascertain the degree of diabetic control. Other possible risks for periodontitis include nonmodifiable factors such as genetics, gender, and race. As the relevance of different risk factors is established through epidemiologic research, clinicians must remain aware of their responsibilities for informing and attempting to change patients' behaviors in relation to modifiable risks.

The management of patients with periodontitis can, therefore, involve the following complementary treatment strategies:

- Patient education and motivation, including oral hygiene instruction; use of powered toothbrushes, antiseptics in rinses, toothpastes, and irrigation; and explanation of the rationale for any adjunctive treatments.
- Reduction of the bacterial burden by high-quality SRP.
- Site-specific antibacterial treatment with local delivery systems or systemic antimicrobial therapy in select cases.
- Host response modulation by HMT.
- Risk factor modification and risk reduction strategies.
- Periodontal surgery with or without HMT.

It is the responsibility of the dentist to customize the treatment plan for each individual patient by selecting and providing appropriate treatments, following discussion and informed decision making by the patient. Good communication and showing an interest in the patient's condition are essential to maximize compliance and modify risk factors. The best chance for clinical improvement may come from a combination of targeted treatment approaches for each patient (Fig. 38.4). In fact, Novak et al. published very striking improvements in probing depth reductions and CAL gains in a 6-month, randomized, multicenter, examiner-blinded, placebo-controlled study, which showed that combination therapy of HMT (SDD) plus a locally delivered antimicrobial (doxycycline hyclate gel) and SRP provided optimal improvements in clinical parameters when compared to SRP alone in the treatment of moderate-to-severe periodontitis.

Subantimicrobial-Dose Doxycycline

As previously discussed, SDD is currently the only FDA-approved, systemically administered HMT indicated specifically in the treatment of periodontitis. SDD is used as an adjunct to SRP and must not be used as a stand-alone therapy (monotherapy). Because SDD, previously called "low-dose doxycycline" (LDD) and currently marketed as Periostat, is based on SDD, a member of the tetracycline family of compounds, the use of tetracyclines for the management of periodontal diseases must be put in perspective.

In regard to incorporation of a medical pharmacologic approach into the management of a disease in the dental practice setting, no class of drugs has made more of an impact on periodontal therapy than the tetracyclines. They have been used in conjunction with SRP, the "gold standard" of nonsurgical therapy, as well as with both resective and regenerative surgical procedures. The tetracyclines have been used locally and systemically as antimicrobial agents and more recently, systemically as a host modulation agent (SDD). The tetracyclines have been prescribed not only to address chronic periodontitis but also to manage specific and often more aggressive types of periodontitis. Most recently, the tetracyclines have been advocated for the management of patients with systemic

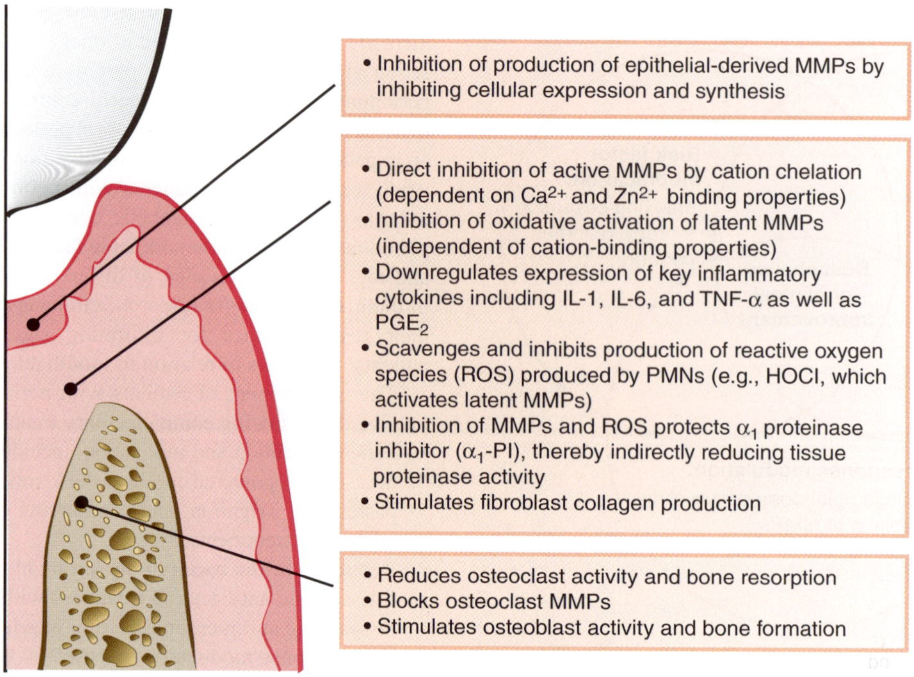

Fig. 38.5 Schematic of periodontal pocket indicating the pleiotropic mechanisms by which doxycycline inhibits connective tissue breakdown. Downregulation of destructive events occurring in the periodontal tissues by doxycycline results from modulation of a variety of different proinflammatory pathways. (*From Golub LM, Lee HM, Ryan ME, et al:* Adv Dent Res *12:12, 1998.*)

diseases such as diabetes, rheumatoid arthritis, and rosacea [doxycycline (Oracea)]; doxycycline has led to improvements in both the periodontal health of compromised diabetic patients and long-term markers of glycemic control (e.g., glycated hemoglobin). As an adjunct to mechanical therapies, the goal of tetracycline therapy has been to enhance reattachment or even to stimulate new attachment of the supporting apparatus and osseous formation.

This section concentrates on the use of these pleiotropic compounds for modulation of the host response in the treatment of periodontitis under the following subheads:

E only: Clinical Research Data on Distinct Patient Population, General Patient Populations, High Risk Patients: Smokers, Special Patient Populations, Suggested Uses and Other Considerations, Candidate Patients, Treatable Periodontal Conditions, Side Effects, Sequencing Prescription With Periodontal Treatment, Combining With Periodontal Surgery or Local Delivery Systems, Monitoring Benefits of Therapy, Host Modulation Factors in Systemic disorders.

Mechanisms of Action

In addition to its antibiotic properties, doxycycline (as well as the other members of the tetracycline family) has the ability to downregulate MMPs, a family of zinc-dependent enzymes that are capable of degrading extracellular matrix molecules, including collagen. MMPs are secreted by the major cell types in the periodontal tissues (fibroblasts, keratinocytes, macrophages, PMNs, endothelial cells) and play a key role in periodontitis. Excessive quantities of MMPs are released in inflamed periodontal tissues, resulting in breakdown of the connective tissue matrix. The predominant MMPs in periodontitis, particularly MMP-8 and MMP-9, derive from PMNs and are extremely effective in degrading type I collagen, the most abundant collagen type in gingiva and periodontal ligament. Levels of PMN-type MMPs have been shown to increase with severity of periodontal disease and decrease after therapy. The release of large quantities of MMPs in the periodontium leads to significant anatomic disruption and breakdown of the connective tissues, contributing to the clinical signs of periodontitis.

The rationale for using SDD as a HMT in the treatment of periodontitis is that doxycycline downregulates the activity of MMPs by a variety of synergistic mechanisms, including reductions in cytokine levels, and stimulates osteoblastic activity and new bone formation by upregulating collagen production (Fig. 38.5).

Clinical Research Data on Distinct Patient Populations

Tetracyclines work well as host modulation agents because of their pleiotropic effects on multiple components of the host response (Fig. 38.3). The only enzyme (MMP) inhibitors that have been approved for clinical use and tested for the treatment of periodontitis are members of the tetracycline family of compounds. In early studies investigating the use of different commercially available tetracyclines, Golub et al. reported that the semisynthetic compound (e.g., doxycycline) was more effective than the parent compound tetracycline in reducing excessive collagenase activity in the GCF of chronic periodontitis patients. Because doxycycline was found to be a more effective inhibitor of collagenase than either minocycline or tetracycline and because of its safety profile, pharmacokinetic properties, and ready systemic absorption, recent clinical trials have focused on this compound. In an effort to eliminate the side effects of long-term tetracycline therapy, especially the emergence of tetracycline-resistant organisms, SDD capsules were prepared and tested. Each capsule contained 20 mg of doxycycline versus the commercially available 50 mg and 100 mg, antimicrobially effective, capsules or tablets. Multiple clinical studies using SDD have shown no difference in the composition or resistance level of the oral flora. More recent studies also demonstrate no appreciable differences in either fecal or vaginal microflora samples. In addition, these studies have shown no overgrowth of opportunistic pathogens, such as *Candida*, in the oral cavity, gastrointestinal system, or genitourinary system.

With regard to MMP inhibition, Golub et al. reported that a 2-week regimen of SDD reduced collagenase in GCF and in the adjacent gingival tissues surgically excised for therapeutic purposes. Subsequent studies using SDD therapy adjunctive to routine scaling and prophylaxis indicated continued reductions in the excessive levels of collagenase in the GCF after 1 month of treatment. After cessation of SDD administration, however, there was a rapid rebound of collagenase activity to placebo levels, suggesting that a 1-month treatment regimen with this host modulation agent was insufficient to produce a long-term benefit. In contrast, during the same study, a 3-month regimen produced a prolonged drug effect without a rebound in collagenase levels to baseline during the no-treatment phase of the study. The mean levels of GCF collagenase were significantly reduced (47.3% from baseline levels) in the SDD group versus the placebo group, who received scaling and prophylaxis alone (29.1% reduction from baseline levels). Accompanying these reductions in collagenase levels were gains in the relative attachment levels in the SDD group. Continuous drug therapy over several months appears to be necessary for maintaining collagenase levels near normal over prolonged periods. However, it is reasonable to speculate that levels of these MMPs will eventually increase again in the more susceptible patients, and those individuals having the most risk factors and the greatest microbial challenge will require more frequent HMT than other patients.

General Patient Populations

Data from clinical trials of SDD are summarized in Table 38.1. In addition, a series of double-blind, placebo-controlled studies of 3, 6, and 9 months' duration all showed clinical efficacy based on reductions in probing depth and gains in clinical attachment as well as biochemical efficacy, based on the inhibition of collagenase activity and protection of serum α_1-antitrypsin (a naturally occurring protective mediator) from collagenase attack in the periodontal pocket. Golub et al. showed that a 2-month regimen of SDD significantly decreased both the level of bone-type collagen breakdown products (carboxy terminal telopeptide of type 1 collagen [ICTP]; carboxy terminal peptide, a pyridinoline-containing cross-linked peptide of type 1 collagen) and MMP-8 and MMP-13 enzyme levels (neutrophil and bone-type collagenase) in chronic periodontitis subjects (Fig. 38.6).

The Phase III, 9-month, randomized, double-blind, placebo-controlled trial conducted at five dental centers demonstrated clinical efficacy and safety of SDD versus placebo as an adjunct to SRP. The benefits of HMT as an adjunct to mechanical therapy were again seen, with statistically significant reductions in probing depths and gains in CALs, as well as the prevention of disease progression. When SDD administration was discontinued after 9 months of continuous therapy, the incremental improvements demonstrated in the SDD group were maintained for at least 3 months. There was no rebound effect in either the pocket depth reductions or the CAL gains; in fact, there appeared to be slight continued improvement in both these clinical parameters, presumably because of the enhanced clinical status of the patients who had benefited from adjunctive SDD, and possibly also because of the known persistence or substantivity of doxycycline in the bone and soft tissue of the periodontium. The clinical relevance of such findings confirms the utility of an MMP inhibitor in the management of chronic periodontitis.

High-Risk Patients: Smokers

The harmful effects of cigarette smoking and the reduced response to periodontal treatment in smokers compared to nonsmokers are well established. A recent meta-analysis of randomized clinical trials of SDD used as an adjunct to SRP revealed a benefit when using SDD in smokers with periodontitis (Table 39.1). A hierarchic treatment response was observed such that nonsmokers who received SDD demonstrated the best clinical improvements and smokers who received placebo had the poorest treatment response. The responses of the smokers who received SDD and the nonsmokers who received placebo were intermediate to the two extremes and were broadly identical. This suggests that even patients traditionally considered resistant to periodontal treatment (i.e., smokers) can benefit from SDD, with a treatment response similar to that expected when treating a nonsmoker by SRP alone.

Special Patient Populations

More recent Phase IV (i.e., postlicensing) clinical studies have revealed success using SDD in particular populations of susceptible individuals. Much interest has focused on genetic susceptibility to periodontal disease, particularly whether a specific variation in the genes that regulate the cytokine IL-1 confers increased susceptibility to disease. This polymorphism is known as the *periodontitis-associated genotype* (PAG), the presence of which can be characterized using a commercially available screening test, the Periodontal Susceptibility Test (PST) genetic susceptibility test. Investigation of patients who possess this gene polymorphism has been driven by the assumption that local phenotypic differences exist in chronic periodontitis associated with this genotype (e.g., that PAG-positive patients produce more IL-1 cytokines for a given bacterial challenge, resulting in increased tissue damage and more extensive periodontal disease). However, few studies exist of the impact of cytokine gene polymorphism on tissue IL-1 cytokine levels in periodontal disease to support this, although IL-1β levels in shallow periodontal pockets have been reported to be higher in patients with the genotype than those without. The studies that have investigated associations between PAG and periodontal disease status have thus far generated conflicting data (as reviewed by Taylor et al.). A reasonable assumption currently is that there are genetic associations between polymorphisms in the IL-1 gene cluster and periodontal disease but that unambiguous results are not yet apparent because of the heterogeneity of the disease and/or the variable design of the reported studies. Cullinan et al. concluded that IL-1 genotype is a contributory but nonessential risk factor for periodontal disease progression.

A 5-month preliminary investigation by Ryan et al. was designed to evaluate the impact of treatment on IL-1β and MMP levels in PST-positive (PAG) patients who presented with elevated levels of these biochemical markers in their GCF. These patients were initially treated with SRP, resulting in no change in the levels of these biochemical markers after 1 month. Al-Shammari et al. reported similar findings, with no changes in GCF levels of IL-1β and ICTP before and after SRP in patients who had not been genotyped. When the genotype-positive patients received SDD and these biochemical markers were monitored at 2 and 4 months, a significant decrease (50%–61%) in the IL-1β and MMP-9 levels was noted after treatment with SDD. Correspondingly, gains in clinical attachment and reduced probing depths were also observed. The study concluded that SDD may provide PST-positive patients with a therapeutic strategy that specifically addresses their exaggerated host response.

Another recent study was conducted in susceptible patients with severe generalized periodontitis using host modulation (SDD) as an adjunct to repeated subgingival debridement. Seventy percent of the patients who completed this 9-month double-blind, placebo-controlled study were smokers. SDD as an adjunct to mechanical

TABLE 38.1 Summary of Data Reported in Clinical Trials of Subantimicrobial-Dose Doxycycline (SDD)

			Mean Cal Change (mm)		Mean PD Reduction (mm)		% Sites with Cal Gain[c]		% Sites with PD Reduction[b]	
Study (Year)	Duration	Study groups (*N*)	4–6 mm Pockets	7+ mm Pockets	4–6 mm Pockets	7+ mm Pockets	≥2 mm	≥3 mm	≥2 mm	≥3 mm
Caton et al. (2000)	Study: 9 months (drug: 9 months)	SRP + SDD (90)	1.03[a]	1.55[a]	0.95[b]	1.68[b]	46	22	47[a]	22[a]
		SRP + placebo (93)	0.86	1.17	0.69	1.20	38	16	35	13
Novak et al. (2002)	Study: 9 months (drug: 6 months)	SRP + SDD (10)	1.00	1.78	1.20	3.02	29	15	48	26
		SRP + placebo (10)	0.56	1.24	0.97	1.42	21	11	21	6
Emingil et al. (2004)	Study: 12 months (drug: 3 months)	SRP + SDD (10)	0.21 (all sites)	1.59[a] (all sites)						
		SRP + placebo (10)	0.05 (all sites)	1.32 (all sites)						
Preshaw et al. (2004)	Study: 9 months (drug: 9 months)	SRP + SDD (107)	1.27[b]	2.09[a]	1.29[b]	2.31[b]	58[a]	33[b]	62[b]	37[b]
		SRP + placebo (102)	0.94	1.60	0.96	1.77	44	20	45	21
Lee et al. (2004)	Study: 9 months (drug: 9 months)	SRP + SDD (240)	1.56[a] (all sites)	1.63[a] (all sites)						
		SRP + placebo (17)	0.80 (all sites)	1.19 (all sites)						
Choi et al. (2004)	Study: 4 months (drug: 4 months)	SRP + SDD (15)	2.2[a] (test sites)	1.6[a] (test sites)						
		SRP + placebo (17)	0.6 (test sites)	1.1 (test sites)						
Gurkan et al. (2005)	Study: 6 months (drug: 3 months)	SRP + SDD (13)	1.12	2.15	1.80	3.38				
		SRP + placebo (13)	0.78	1.76	1.46	2.57				
Preshaw et al. (2005)[e]	Study: 9 months (drug: 9 months)	SRP + SDD# (116)	1.23[a]	1.89[b]	1.22[b]	2.16[a]	59[b]	33[b]	63[d]	37
		SRP + placebo# (135)	0.96	1.43	0.88	1.53	43	19	44	18
		SRP + SDD## (81)	1.03	1.71	1.01	1.80	44	21	45[b]	20
		SRP + placebo## (60)	0.85	1.58	0.80	1.62	37	15	31	13
Mohammad et al (2005)	Study: 9 months (drug: 9 months)	SRP + SDD (12)	2.14[d]	3.18[a]	1.57[d]	3.22[d]				
		SRP + placebo (12)	0.02	0.25	0.63	0.98				
Górska and Nedzi-Góra (2006)	Study: 3 months (drug: 3 months)	SRP + SDD (33)	0.33[a] (all sites)	0.29[a] (all sites)						
		SRP + placebo (33)	0.04 (all sites)	0.08 (all sites)						
Needleman et al. (2007)	Study: 6 months (drug: 3 months)	SRP + SDD## (18)	0.65 (all sites)	1.40 (all sites)						
		SRP + placebo## (16)	0.40 (all sites)	0.98 (all sites)						

N, Number of subjects; *SRP*, scaling and root planing; *CAL*, clinical attachment level, *CAL* change can be positive (CAL gain) or negative (CAL loss); *PD*, probing depth.

[a]$P < 0.05$ compared to placebo.

[b]$P < 0.01$ compared to placebo.

[c]Percentage of sites with CAL gain and PD reduction ≥2 mm and ≥3 mm calculated for all sites that had 6+ mm probing depths at baseline.

[d]$P < 0.001$ compared to placebo.

[e]Same study population as Preshaw et al. (2004), stratified by smoking status: #, nonsmokers, ##, smokers.

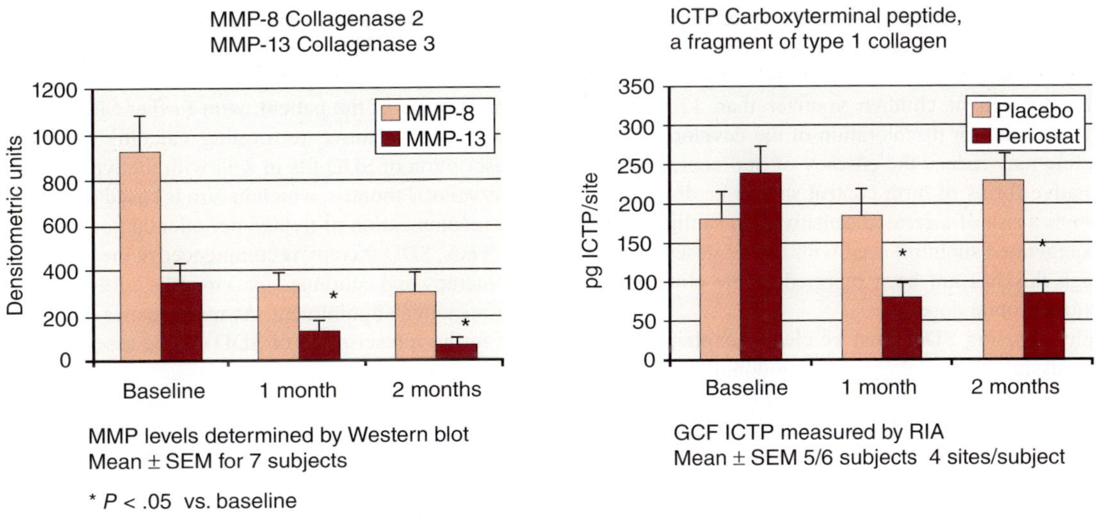

Fig. 38.6 Effect of subantimicrobial-dose doxycycline (SDD) on gingival crevicular fluid (GCF) collagenase (MMP-8, MMP-13) and ICTP. A 2-month regimen of SDD significantly decreased levels of matrix metalloproteinases (MMP-8 and MMP-13, neutrophil, and bone-type collagenases, respectively) and ICTP compared to placebo in GCF samples of adult periodontitis patients. Decreased levels of GCF bone-type collagen breakdown products (ICTP, pyridinoline-containing cross-linked peptide of type 1 collagen) in the SDD group versus the placebo group provides biochemical evidence of a reduction in bone resorption. *RIA*, Radioimmunoassay. (*From Golub LM, Lee HM, Greenwald RA, et al:* Inflamm Res *46:310, 1997.)*

therapy versus mechanical therapy alone resulted in significantly greater mean probing depth reductions in pockets of 7 mm or greater at baseline as early as 1 month after therapy (2.52 vs 1.25 mm, respectively). These improvements in the SDD group compared to the group receiving mechanical therapy only were maintained during the 5.25 months of therapy (2.85 vs 1.48 mm, respectively) and even at 3 months after stopping drug therapy (3.02 vs 1.41 mm), demonstrating that no rebound effect occurred. Because of the beneficial effects of HMT in susceptible patients, multicenter studies are using SDD in other susceptible populations, including diabetic, osteoporotic, and institutionalized geriatric patients, as well as smokers.

Since periodontitis is associated with many systemic diseases [e.g., osteoporosis, diabetes, and cardiovascular disease (CVD)], researchers have investigated the effect of SDD on these systemic conditions. Payne et al. conducted a 2-year randomized, double-blind, placebo-controlled trial in osteopenic women at two dental centers demonstrating that SDD can effectively reduce the levels of localized and systemic inflammatory mediators in osteopenic patients in addition to improving on the clinical measurements of periodontitis; SDD significantly reduced the progression of periodontal attachment loss and the severity of gingival inflammation and alveolar bone loss in postmenopausal osteopenic women. Golub et al. reported that collagenase activity in the GCF of these osteopenic women was significantly reduced by SDD treatment. ICTP showed a similar pattern of change during SDD treatment with GCF collagenase activity and ICTP levels positively correlated at all time periods ($P < 0.001$). MMP-8 accounted for approximately 80% of total collagenase in the GCF, with much lower levels of MMP-1 and -13. SDD dramatically reduced the elevated MMP-8 levels by 60%. This 2-year study also demonstrated that long-term continuous use of SDD did not produce antibiotic side effects, confirming what had been reported previously in studies of continuous use of up to 12 months. Previously reported studies had demonstrated a relationship between serum high-sensitivity C-reactive protein (hsCRP) concentration and biochemical bone turnover markers in healthy pre- and postmenopausal women. These findings suggested that low-grade systemic inflammation may be a common linking factor between the development of atherosclerosis and an increased bone turnover rate. A recently published study by Payne et al. demonstrated that the 2-year SDD regimen described above in postmenopausal women significantly reduced serum inflammatory biomarkers (hs-CRP and MMP-9) and, among women more than 5 years postmenopausal, increased the high-density lipoprotein (HDL) cholesterol level. These preliminary findings suggest that SDD may play a role in managing the care of patients at risk for developing coronary artery disease. Other studies have shown that SDD reduces systemic inflammatory biomarkers in CVD patients and SDD decreases glycosylated hemoglobin (HbA_{1c}) assay in patients who are taking normally prescribed hypoglycemic agents. The impact of SDD therapy on periodontitis may be amplified by the concurrent use of other HMTS used to manage other inflammatory diseases. Additional studies are being conducted to investigate the impact of combined HMT use not only on periodontal disease but on other chronic inflammatory conditions.

Suggested Uses and Other Considerations

Earlier, treatment options for periodontal disease have focused solely on reducing the bacterial challenge by nonsurgical therapy, surgery, and systemic or local antimicrobial therapy. The development of SDD as an HMT, driven by research into the pathogenesis of periodontal disease, is a great example of how translational research can lead to new treatments. By better understanding the biochemical processes that are important in periodontal disease, a pharmacologic principle (doxycycline downregulates MMP activity) has been used in the development of a new drug treatment. Data presented from research studies show the clinical benefits of adjunctive SDD, and the science behind SDD has been transferred into clinical practice. In other words, dentists now have the opportunity to use SDD for patient care, with the aim being to enhance the treatment response to conventional therapy.

Candidate Patients

When deciding whether to use SDD as an adjunct to SRP, first consider the patient's motivation toward periodontal care, the medical history, and the patient's willingness to take a systemic drug treatment. SDD is contraindicated in any patient with a history of allergy or hypersensitivity to tetracyclines. It should not be given to pregnant or lactating women or children younger than 12 years old (because of the potential for discoloration of the developing dentition). Doxycycline may reduce the efficacy of oral contraceptives; therefore alternative forms of birth control should be discussed, if necessary. There is a risk of increased sensitivity to sunlight (manifested by an exaggerated sunburn) seen with higher doses of doxycycline, although this has not been reported in the clinical trials using the subantimicrobial dose.

The rationale for using SDD must be clearly explained to the patient. By discussing the etiology of periodontal disease, the available treatment options, and the anticipated outcomes, patients become more interested in their periodontal management, are more likely to comply with treatment, and take more responsibility for managing their disease. Therefore, the anticipated compliance and likely commitment to treatment must also be gaged when considering SDD therapy. Patients who show little enthusiasm for complying with the treatment plan or with oral hygiene practices are less likely to be good candidates for systemic drug therapy.

Treatable Periodontal Conditions

SDD is indicated in the management of chronic periodontitis, and studies to date have focused on chronic and aggressive forms of periodontitis. SDD should not be used in conditions such as gingivitis and periodontal abscess or when an antibiotic is indicated. SDD can be used in patients with aggressive periodontitis who are being treated nonsurgically. Furthermore, emerging studies have supported efficacy of SDD as an adjunct to periodontal surgery. SDD may also be of benefit in cases that are refractory to treatment, as well as in patients with risk factors such as smoking, diabetes, osteoporosis/osteopenia, genetic susceptibility, and in whom the treatment response might be limited.

Side Effects

Doxycycline at antibiotic doses (≥100 mg) is associated with adverse effects, including photosensitivity, hypersensitivity reactions, nausea, vomiting, and esophageal irritation. However, in the clinical trials of SDD (20-mg dose), it was reported that the drug was well tolerated, and the profile of unwanted effects was virtually identical in the SDD and placebo groups. The types of adverse events did not differ significantly between treatment groups, and the typical side effects of the tetracycline class were not observed indicating that the appearance of adverse events is dose related. Furthermore, there was no evidence of adverse events that could be attributed to antimicrobial effects of treatment and no evidence of developing antibiotic resistance of the microflora after 2 years of continuous use. Therefore, the drug appears to be well tolerated, with a very low incidence of adverse effects.

Sequencing Prescription With Periodontal Treatment

SDD is indicated as an adjunct to mechanical periodontal therapy and should not be used as a stand-alone or monotherapy. SDD should be prescribed to coincide with the first round of SRP and is prescribed for 3 months, up to a maximum of 9–24 months of continuous dosing depending on the patient risk. Modification of any risk factors, such as smoking, nutrition, stress, contributing medications, faulty restorations, poor oral hygiene, and poor diabetic control, should also be addressed at this time. A patient's refusal or inability to modify contributing risk factors is an important consideration for treatment planning and evaluation of therapeutic responses.

After initial periodontal treatment, the patient is enrolled into an intensive periodontal maintenance program. This involves regular monitoring of probing depths, reinforcement of oral hygiene, and remotivation of the patient, with further SRP to disrupt the plaque biofilm and remove re-forming calculus deposits. The 3-month prescription of SDD fits in well with the typical maintenance recall interval of 3 months, which in turn is based on the duration reported for recolonization of treated periodontal pockets.

Thus, SDD therapy is commenced at the start of initial periodontal therapy and continues for 3 months until the first reevaluation or maintenance appointment. At maintenance appointments, the need for further prescription of SDD can be assessed. For patients demonstrating a good treatment response with significant reductions in probing depths, further SDD may not be necessary. Periodontal maintenance care must continue, with an emphasis on plaque control, monitoring, and prophylaxis. In other patients, the treatment response after completion of initial therapy may be less favorable. Sites with persisting or progressing pockets may require additional instrumentation, and the prescription of SDD may be extended for an additional 3 months. SDD may be combined with the use of locally applied antimicrobials and surgical procedures. Remember that periodontitis is a chronic disease, and the treatment (whether SDD is used or not) is long term. The patient must be regularly reevaluated to determine disease stability or progression and the need for additional active therapy.

Therefore, patients may cycle between phases of "active" treatment (SRP + SDD) and long-term periodontal maintenance. The success of the maintenance phase of treatment will be affected by many factors, including the following:

- Compliance with the maintenance regimen.
- Compliance with oral hygiene instruction.
- Presence of risk factors, such as smoking, poorly controlled diabetes, or stress.
- Extent (i.e., number) and severity (i.e., depth) of residual deep pockets.

Maintenance therapy is more likely to be successful in patients with good compliance, good oral hygiene, minimal or no systemic risk factors, and minimal residual deep pocketing. The patient who enters the maintenance program may have periodontal stability for months or years. However, plaque control may deteriorate, the patient may develop or acquire new risk factors, and disease progression (i.e., further loss of attachment) may become apparent, indicating that a further course of treatment is required. A further course of SRP will then be undertaken together with adjunctive SDD to restore periodontal stability.

Combining With Periodontal Surgery or Local Delivery Systems

Most clinical research to date has focused on using SDD as an adjunct to nonsurgical periodontal treatment. However, emerging data in which SDD was used as an adjunct to access flap surgery in 24 patients revealed better probing depth reductions in surgically treated sites greater than 6 mm compared to surgically treated sites in patients given placebo. Furthermore, the SDD group demonstrated greater reductions in ICTP (carboxy-terminal peptide, a breakdown product of collagen) than the placebo group, indicating that collagenolytic activity was reduced in the patients taking SDD.

SDD treatment can also be combined with the local delivery of antibiotics into the periodontal pocket through sustained-delivery systems. The two treatment approaches target different aspects of the pathogenic process: Local delivery systems deliver antimicrobial concentrations of an antibacterial agent directly into the site of the pocket, whereas SDD is a systemic host response modulator.

Thus, combining these two complementary treatment strategies is another example of how antibacterial therapy (SRP + local antibiotics) can be combined with HMT (SDD) to maximize the clinical benefit for patients. Preliminary results from a 6-month, 180-patient clinical trial designed to evaluate the safety and efficacy of SDD combined with a locally applied antimicrobial [doxycycline hyclate (Atridox)] and SRP versus SRP alone demonstrated that patients receiving the combination of treatments experienced more than a 2-mm improvement in mean attachment gains and probing depth reductions ($P < 0.0001$) compared to SRP alone.

Monitoring Benefits of Therapy

To improve the ability of dentists to make appropriate treatment decisions for patients undergoing periodontal therapy, it would be extremely useful if they had access to the types of diagnostic tests available to their medical colleagues. Such tests might be used, for example, to distinguish between active and inactive lesions. Studies have shown that SRP alone, although effective for improving clinical parameters such as probing depths, may not be sufficient to reduce excessive levels of many underlying destructive mediators, particularly in more susceptible patients. It would be valuable, therefore, if it is possible to monitor the levels of such inflammatory mediators as treatment progresses. SDD results in downregulation of MMP activity in inflamed periodontal tissues. Therefore, in theory, MMP levels could be monitored before, during, and after SRP plus SDD treatment. Published data support a concomitant reduction in MMP levels in GCF and improvements in clinical parameters when combining SDD and SRP. Although chair-side tests for MMPs have been developed, they are not in widespread use because of concerns about their specificity or sensitivity.

In the absence of new chair-side tests or a centralized diagnostic facility for monitoring the inflammatory status of the tissues, dentists must rely on clinical periodontal monitoring to assess the outcomes of treatment. In addition to the reductions in probing depths and gains in attachment that may be observed after SRP plus SDD, the quality of the periodontal tissues also tends to improve after treatment with SDD. More sensitive radiographic techniques, assessments of bone density, and bone height changes used solely in clinical trials in the past may be possible in clinical practice in the future. Until such diagnostic techniques are made widely available, however, clinicians must rely on clinical judgment to determine the most appropriate course of therapy.

Host Modulation Factors in Systemic Disorders

In susceptible patients demonstrating an excessive local inflammatory response to the bacterial stimuli leading to periodontal disease, another consideration involves the loss of epithelial integrity in the periodontal pocket. This tissue response allows for bacterial penetration into the inflamed tissues and eventual entry of the bacteria into the systemic circulation. Patients with untreated periodontitis have an increased risk for transient bacteremias. Bacteremia and associated endotoxemia may incite the overproduction of destructive proinflammatory mediators at distant sites in the periodontitis patient. Therefore, patients with periodontitis may be at greater risk for developing a number of systemic conditions associated with a similar overactive host response to external stimuli such as cardiovascular disease and diabetic complications. Elevated levels of cytokines, prostanoids, and enzymes are evident in all these conditions.

In the era of periodontal medicine, systemic host modulatory approaches need to be considered. As mentioned, host modulators used to manage periodontal disease, such as an MMP, cytokine, and prostanoid inhibitors, may have additional beneficial effects on systemic diseases that have been linked to periodontal disease, such as CVD and diabetes. In CVD, preliminary studies have indicated that individuals with periodontal disease are almost twice as likely to have a fatal heart attack and three times as likely to have a stroke. MMPs and cytokines have been found to play a major role in weakening the plaques formed with CVD, leading to rupture and eventual thrombosis and infarction. In fact, Golub et al. suggested that tetracyclines could reduce the incidence of acute myocardial infarction by blocking collagenase and stabilizing the collagen cap on the atheroscleromatous arterial plaques. In diabetes, the same MMPs and cytokines involved in the development of periodontitis as the sixth long-term complication of diabetes also play a role in the development of other well-known complications of diabetes such as nephropathy, angiopathy, retinopathy, and wound-healing problems. Modulation of these proinflammatory mediators in patients with diabetes may impede the development of multiple long-term complications. An inhibitor of MMPs, cytokines, and prostanoids used in the treatment of periodontitis may have an indirect effect on these disease processes if a patient's risk for developing these disorders is increased by the presence of untreated periodontitis. HMT may also directly aid in the treatment and prevention of CVD and diabetic complications.

Emerging Host Modulatory Therapies

In the future, a variety of HMTs will likely be developed as adjunctive treatments for periodontitis. One of the most promising groups of potential HMTs is the *chemically modified tetracyclines* (CMTs). These nonantibiotic tetracycline analogs are tetracycline molecules that have been modified to remove all antibiotic properties, but which retain host modulatory, anticollagenolytic effects. The CMTs are also designed to be more potent inhibitors of proinflammatory mediators and can increase levels of antiinflammatory mediators such as IL-10. Because they have no antimicrobial properties, the clinician would be able to increase the dose for more susceptible patients with more risk factors and who might be more difficult to manage without getting side effects seen with antibiotics. CMTs, such as CMT-3 and CMT-8 (both of which lack antibiotic activity but retain anti-MMP activity), have been shown to inhibit osteoclastic bone resorption and promote bone formation, enhance wound healing, and inhibit proteinases produced by periodontal pathogens. CMTs also are being studied for other effects, such as inhibition of tumor cell invasion and attenuation of intimal thickening after arterial injury. CMTs will likely emerge as drugs that have beneficial effects in a variety of disease states because of their host modulation capabilities.

Other potential HMTs include the novel *anticytokine drugs* developed for the management of rheumatoid arthritis, a disease with a pathobiology similar to that of periodontitis. Cytokines such as TNF-α have been targeted by TNF-α antagonists (e.g., infliximab, etanercept), which have been shown to be effective in treating rheumatoid arthritis. As yet, such drugs have not been evaluated in the treatment of periodontal disease, but they could offer potential benefits given the importance of inflammatory cytokines, such as TNF-α, in periodontal pathogenesis. In addition, drugs designed to increase the levels of antiinflammatory or protective mediators, such as IL-1ra, can perform similar functions. In addition, evidence is emerging to support the benefits of combining HMTs that target different aspects of the disease processes. For example, the combination of SDD with bisphosphonates has also showed synergy in animal models of bone loss.

As the concept of host modulation has become more widely accepted, we have seen much research looking toward the development of new HMTs. Studies have revealed that *probiotics* can be beneficial in the management of periodontitis. From animal studies to human clinical trials, Lactobacillus-based probiotics demonstrated potential therapeutic effects on reduction of gingival index (GI) and PD, with gains in CAL compared to a placebo control when administered as an adjunctive treatment to SRP. The underlying mechanisms are not completely understood, as probiotics seem to modulate both the periodontal pathogens and host inflammatory responses. Probiotics have been used to reduce the levels of gram-negative bacteria, temporarily shifting the oral microbial environment to a more healthy microbiome. With regard to host modulation, it is proposed that probiotics can modulate T-regulatory cell activity to inhibit inflammation and periodontal bone loss and may play a role in the inhibition of nitric oxide synthesis. It is clear that more extensive studies of probiotics demonstrating safety and efficacy are needed before this approach can be available clinically. Some have focused in the efficacy of available nutritional supplements such as fish oils. Studies have indicated that n-3 polyunsaturated fatty acid (n-3 PUFA; fish oil), as an adjunct to oral hygiene instructions, can significantly lower GCF, IL-8, IL-6, and PGE_2 levels compared to placebo controls. Other studies have found that a combination therapy with n-3 PUFA and low-dose aspirin as an adjunct to regenerative procedures using decalcified freeze-dried bone allografts result in greater mean probing depth reductions ($P < 0.001$) and gains in clinical attachment ($P < 0.05$) accompanied by a trend for modulation of the cytokine profile of IL-1β and IL-10 in GCF compared to placebo controlled regenerative therapy.

Collagenase (i.e., MMP) inhibitors known as *polyenolic zinc-binding compounds* (PEZBINs) for periodontitis have been investigated. These new inhibitors are based on the natural product curcumin, which contains a calcium- and zinc-binding β-diketone moiety that is similar to that found in tetracyclines. The antiinflammatory properties of curcumin have been demonstrated in periodontal disease, cardiovascular diseases, cancer, arthritis, and diabetes. A novel group of chemically modified curcumins with increased bioavailability and improved antiinflammatory activity have been tested. In vitro and in vivo findings demonstrate that these potential host modulatory agents can decrease pathologically elevated MMP levels in the plasma and gingiva of animal models of periodontitis. One of the lead compounds demonstrated a significant effect on reducing alveolar bone loss in experimental periodontitis models.

More research is being conducted to evaluate this new group of compounds as an HMT in periodontal diseases and in other systemic chronic inflammatory conditions such as arthritis and diabetes. Reports indicate the therapeutic potential of a novel semisynthetic glycosaminoglycan ether (SAGE) or sulfated polysaccharide to suppress inflammatory mediators in high-risk individuals, such as smokers and those with diabetes, based on the ability to reduce the impact of advanced glycation end products (AGEs) reducing the proinflammatory mediators of disease. In vitro and in vivo studies found that systemic administration of SAGE significantly reduced local and systemic inflammation by modulating the production of cytokines and MMPs. Periodontal bone loss was significantly attenuated in the diabetic rats with infection.

Research may enable the application of *stem cells* in HMT, offering interesting alternatives to existing therapies. Human periodontal stem cells can modulate neutrophil function and reduce excessive inflammation. Bone marrow-derived mesenchymal stem cells have shown great potential for periodontal regeneration in animal models. Additional studies are needed to characterize dental stem cells and evaluate the therapeutic efficacy of stem cell-based periodontal therapy. Enhanced stem cell approaches may result in innovative HMT strategies to achieve desired periodontal outcomes.

Resolution of Inflammation and Lipid Mediators

Periodontal disease is a polymicrobial infection and involves an immune-inflammatory response to the biofilm. Inflammation is defined as "a complex reaction to injurious agents such as microbes and damaged, usually necrotic, cells that consists of vascular responses, migration and activation of leukocytes, and systemic reactions." Recent research has indicated that there is an active biochemical resolution phase involved in inflammation. Failure of this resolution pathway may play a role in the pathogenesis of periodontal diseases. Restoration of the resolution pathway by the introduction of resolving molecules may provide new potential therapeutic methods for the management of inflammatory periodontitis.

An acute-inflammatory response that is resolved in a timely manner prevents tissue injury. However, an inadequate resolution and failure to tissue homeostasis results in neutrophil- mediated destruction. A greater understanding of the pathways and processes underlying resolution of inflammation has led to increased interest in pro-resolving lipid mediators that contribute to the restoration of tissue homeostasis. As novel lipid mediators are small molecules (<500 MW), amenable to total organic synthesis and manufacturable with currently available pharmaceutical facilities, they are very attractive for new therapeutic interventions. Examples of such mediators are: Resolvins (the first "pro-resolution" pathway—novel lipid mediators); lipoxins; aspirin triggered lipoxins (ATLs); docosahexaenoic acid (DHA) derivatives; an abundant omega-3 fatty acid in neural tissues, now coined as docosatrienes; and protections.

The use of pro-resolution agents has already been tested in animal models where it has been shown to markedly reduce periodontal inflammation, with regeneration of bone to preligature height and regeneration of cementum and an organized periodontal ligament. PGs and leukotrienes (LTs) mediate cardinal signs of inflammation; hence, their enzymes are targets of current antiinflammatory therapies. Products of arachidonate 15-lipoxygenases (LO) types I and II display both beneficial roles, such as lipoxins (LXs) that stereoselectively signal counterregulation, as well as potential deleterious actions (i.e., nonspecific phospholipid degradation). Serhan and Jain et al. examined transgenic (TG) rabbits overexpressing 15-LO type I and their response to inflammatory challenge. Microbe-associated inflammation and leukocyte-mediated bone destruction were assessed initiating acute periodontitis. 15-LO TG rabbits exhibited markedly reduced bone loss and local inflammation. The authors hence concluded that enhanced LX production was associated with an increased antiinflammatory status of 15-LO TG rabbits.

The endogenous lipid mediator Resolvin E1 (RvE1) counter regulates leukocyte-mediated tissue injury and pro-inflammatory gene expression as was noticed in a mouse peritonitis model. Promotion of resolution of inflammation as a therapeutic target with RvE1 resulted in complete restoration of the *P. gingivalis*-induced local periodontal lesion and reduction in the systemic inflammatory markers C-reactive protein and IL-1β in rabbits. This report was the first to show that resolution of inflammation by a naturally occurring endogenous lipid mediator resulted in complete regeneration of pathologically lost tissues, including bone. In the future, a combination of antiinflammatory drugs with resolving agents tested in human clinical trials may provide evidence to support a brand new host modulation therapy for the management of periodontal diseases.

Conclusion

Periodontal pathogens and destructive host responses are involved in the initiation and progression of periodontitis. Therefore, the successful long-term management of this disease may require a treatment strategy that integrates therapies that address both etiologic components. Evidence for the role of MMPs, cytokines, and other mediators in the pathogenesis of periodontal disease distinguishes them as viable targets for a chemotherapeutic approach. The introduction of novel, adjunctive therapies such as host modulation to enhance the efficacy of existing mechanical procedures can contribute favorably to an integrated approach for the long-term, clinical management of periodontitis.

HMTs are an emerging treatment concept in the management of periodontitis. The use of HMT as an adjunct may be particularly useful in susceptible, high-risk patients in whom a prolonged and excessive host response to the presence of bacteria promotes the activity of MMPs and osteoclasts. SDD is the only systemically administered HMT currently approved and indicated as an adjunct to SRP for treating periodontitis. Clinical trials have demonstrated a clear treatment benefit when using SDD versus SRP alone. SDD should be used as part of a comprehensive treatment strategy that includes antibacterial treatments (SRP, plaque control, oral hygiene instruction, local antimicrobials, and periodontal surgery), host response modulation (SDD), and assessment and management of periodontal risk factors. In the future, a range of HMTs targeting different aspects of the destructive cascade of breakdown events in the periodontal tissues are likely to be developed as adjunctive treatments for periodontitis. The further development of these agents will permit dentists to treat specific aspects of the underlying biochemical basis for periodontal disease. The goal is to maximize and make more predictable the treatment response by reducing inflammation and inhibiting destructive processes in the tissues, which will result in enhanced periodontal stability after conventional periodontal treatments such as SRP and surgery. The dentist is now in the exciting position to be able to combine established treatment strategies with new systemic and local drug treatments for this common, chronic disease.

The findings discussed with regard to the use of HMT to better manage chronic periodontal disease may have applications to other chronic systemic diseases such as arthritis, diabetes, osteoporosis, and cardiovascular disease. In addition, studies using locally applied antimicrobials as part of an intensive periodontal therapy (IPT) regimen have shown very promising results. Future studies may demonstrate that in addition to our current standard therapies, IPT with adjunctive antibiotics and/or host modulation for the management of periodontal disease may have profound positive effects on the overall health status of high-risk patients. The proper management of local infection and inflammation (periodontitis) will have a significant impact on the general overall health of the population.

Key points

- The concept of host modulation was first introduced to dentistry by Williams and Golub et al.
- HMT is a means of treating the host side of the host–bacteria interaction.
- HMTs ameliorates excessive or pathologically elevated inflammatory processes to enhance the opportunities for wound healing and periodontal stability.
- Bisphosphonate therapy can lead to avascular necrosis of the jaws, with resultant risk of bone necrosis following dental extractions.
- Chemically modified tetracyclines (CMTs) are nonantibiotic tetracycline analogs that have been modified to remove all antibiotic properties, but retain host modulatory, anticollagenolytic effects.
- An FDA-approved agent for host modulation treatment of periodontal disease is subantimicrobial-dose doxycycline (SDD) at 20 mg, taken twice daily.
- SDD is the only systemically administered HMT approved, and it is indicated as an adjunct to scaling and root planing (SRP) for treating periodontitis.
- Clinical trials have demonstrated a clear benefit for SDD compared to SRP alone.

Suggested Readings

Caton JG, Ciancio SG, Blieden TM, et al: Treatment with subantimicrobial dose doxycycline improves the efficacy of scaling and root planing in patients with adult periodontitis, *J Periodontol* 71:521, 2000.

Genco RJ: Current view of risk factors for periodontal diseases, *J Periodontol* 67:1041, 1996.

Golub LM, Ciancio S, Ramamurthy NS, et al: Low-dose doxycycline therapy: effect on gingival and crevicular fluid collagenase activity in humans, *J Periodontal Res* 25:321, 1990.

Mariotti A: The extracellular matrix of the periodontium: dynamic and interactive tissues, *Periodontol 2000* 3:39, 1993.

Novak MJ, Dawson DR III, Magnusson I, et al: Combining host modulation and topical antimicrobial therapy in the management of moderate to severe periodontitis: a randomized multicenter trial, *J Periodontol* 79(1):33, 2008.

Payne JB, Golub LM, Stoner JA, et al: The effect of subantimicrobial-dose-doxycycline periodontal therapy on serum biomarkers of systemic inflammation: a randomized, double-masked, placebo-controlled clinical trial, *J Am Dent Assoc* 142(3):262, 2011.

Preshaw PM: Host response modulation in periodontics, *Periodontol 2000* 48:92, 2008.

Ryan ME, Ramamurthy NS, Golub LM: Matrix metalloproteinases and their inhibition in periodontal treatment, *Curr Opin Periodontol* 3:85, 1996.

Walker C, Preshaw PM, Novak J, et al: Long-term treatment with subantimicrobial dose doxycycline has no antibacterial effect on intestinal flora, *J Clin Periodontol* 32:1163, 2005.

Williams RC: Periodontal disease, *N Engl J Med* 322(6):373, 1990.

References

References and MCQs with answers for the chapter are available on www.medenact.com.

CHAPTER 39

Occlusal Therapy and Splinting

MJ McDevitt | A Jain

CHAPTER OUTLINE

Among the numerous local and systemic factors with the potential to influence the progression of periodontitis, the patient's occlusion remains a variable that requires an exact diagnosis. All of the disciplines of dentistry include the comprehensive analysis of occlusal relationships for determination of appropriate care.

The functional demands of the occlusion may fall within or substantially exceed the tolerances and the adaptability of the patient's periodontium and masticatory system. The full range of knowledge and skill needed to analyze all aspects of occlusal anatomy and function is beyond the scope of this chapter, which does present practical guidelines for the assessment and management of the occlusion specific to a patient's unique susceptibility to periodontitis.

Pathogenesis

The host-driven inflammatory response of each patient to a pathogenic bacterial biofilm is so specific that the patient is his or her only reference for the interpretation of possible contributing factors to the progressive loss of supporting bone. Destructive events can be episodic and are site specific.

A dentist's diagnostic responsibility includes careful measurement of periodontal structures in the entire circumference of each tooth, accurate documentation, and timely reassessment. Periodontal deterioration that occurs rapidly or that is excessive for a person's age should prompt the clinician to investigate all variables that can amplify his or her periodontitis. If a local factor such as an occlusal relationship can influence the course of the disease, its analysis must be as precise as any other aspect of the periodontal examination.

Evidence-Based Decision Making

In a perfect world, all diagnostic and therapeutic decisions would reflect evidence from multiple prospective clinical trials that have been subject to systematic review. Prospective human investigations of occlusal trauma are considered unethical, and periodontics has conscientiously struggled to reach discipline-wide consensus regarding the interaction of a patient's occlusion with his or her periodontal status. To be clinically applicable, the investigation's methodology must parallel the clinical diagnosis and treatment of an individual with periodontitis.

Historically, data management and statistical credibility and methodology within retrospective studies limited the ability of dedicated researchers to interpret the role of occlusion in an individual's periodontitis experience. The grouping of data points, especially for large study populations, departs from the site specificity that periodontal diagnosis requires. If occlusal trauma is affecting a tooth, the effect on the periodontium is site specific for only that tooth. Treatment for a patient with periodontitis would never be based on an average of diagnostic references, but rather on his or her unique susceptibility, anatomy, occlusion, and history.

> In 2001, Nunn and Harrell reported the retrospective findings for a group of patients with periodontitis. The analysis was based on measurement of the loss of attachment of each tooth and the presence or absence of occlusal interferences. This study and a similar investigation confirmed that trauma from occlusion amplified the loss of attachment. Harrell and Nunn also reported that eliminating occlusal interferences had a positive influence on the outcome of treatment when trauma from occlusion was found to be a contributing local factor. The positive influence of occlusal adjustment on the outcome of surgical and non-surgical periodontal therapies was also reported by Burgett. Evidence supports the possibility that trauma from occlusion can amplify damage to an inflamed periodontium.

Although animal studies do not carry the evidence-based hierarchic weight of ideally structured clinical trials, several newer studies seem to support the potential for excessive occlusal forces to amplify damage from inflammatory periodontitis. In two studies using a periodontitis-induced rat model, occlusal trauma resulted in readily identifiable changes in the periodontal ligament of the experimental group compared to the controls. Greater numbers of osteoclasts, perhaps related to increased receptor activator of nuclear factor kappa-B ligand (RANKL) expression, supported the observation of greater alveolar bone loss in the inflammation plus trauma group. That group also demonstrated increased numbers of immune complexes, which may be a product of the damaged periodontal ligament collagen fibers' greater permeability. An in vitro study of human periodontal ligament fibroblasts from healthy individuals and chronic periodontitis patients also supported the observation of

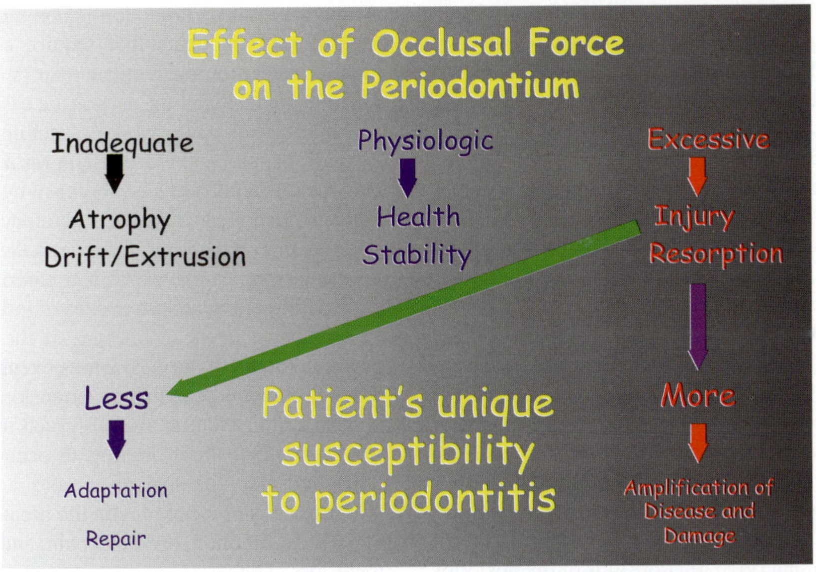

Fig. 39.1 The degree of occlusal force is depicted as a spectrum of white to black, representing none to excessive force.

significant differences in healthy and diseased periodontal ligament fibroblasts when subjected to compression. Several matrix metalloproteins, interleukin-l6 and -21, and other inflammation-associated proteins were expressed by the diseased, compressed fibroblasts compared to healthy fibroblasts, suggesting the diseased fibroblasts could produce additional damage to the periodontium of patients with chronic periodontitis.

Interest in occlusion in the discipline of periodontics appears to be increasing, especially with the rapid growth of the replacement of missing teeth with implants. Despite some conflicting reports in the literature, common ground for consensus exists, as shown in Fig. 39.1.

Occlusal force has an effect on the periodontium and that susceptibility to periodontitis is unique to each patient. Occlusal forces occur across a broad spectrum. No or minimal occlusal contact on a tooth results in disuse atrophy of the periodontium, which can result in instability of that tooth. Harmonious occlusal force on a tooth stimulates the physiologic arrangement of the periodontal attachment fibers and osseous architecture and encourages stability. Forces that exceed the tolerance of the periodontium result in resorption of the bone and disruption of the attachment. In the healthy person, the periodontium around teeth that are subject to excessive occlusal force experiences adaptation and repair or remodeling with no loss of attachment, which often occurs with orthodontics.

For the patient who is losing bone as a result of periodontitis, coupling the ongoing inflammatory disease with excessive occlusal force can amplify destruction and damage to the periodontium of affected teeth. If this conclusion is valid, the clinician has the responsibility to correlate the periodontal status of each tooth with its occlusal responsibilities and possible occlusal excesses.

Terminology

The following is a list of key descriptive terms, as used in this chapter, and their common synonyms:

Centric relation: Position of the mandible when both condyle–disk assemblies are in their most superior positions in their respective glenoid fossae and against the slope of the articular eminences of each respective temporal bone.

Disclusion: Separation of certain teeth caused by the guidance provided by other teeth during an excursion. When anterior guidance provides separation of posterior teeth during an excursion, posterior disclusion is achieved.

Excursive movement: Any movement of the mandible away from maximum intercuspation.

Guidance: The pattern of opposing tooth contact during excursive movements of the mandible.

Initial contact in centric relation: The first occlusal contact in the centric relation closure arc.

Interference: Any occlusal contact in the centric relation closure arc or in any excursion that prevents the remaining occlusal surfaces from achieving stable contact or functioning harmoniously or that encourages masticatory system disharmony; also called an *occlusal discrepancy.*

Lateral excursion: Movement of the mandible laterally to the right or to left from maximal intercuspation.

Maximal intercuspation: Position of the mandible when there is maximal interdigitation and occlusal contact between the maxillary and mandibular teeth; also called *centric occlusion* and *intercuspal position*.

Nonworking side: The side of either arch that corresponds with the side of the mandible moving toward the midline during a lateral excursion; also called the *balancing side.*

Protrusion: Movement of the mandible anteriorly from maximal intercuspation.

Retrusion: Movement of the mandible posteriorly relative to a more anterior position.

Working side: The side of either dental arch that corresponds with the side of the mandible moving away from the midline during a lateral excursion.

Occlusal Function and Dysfunction

Excellent sources for a comprehensive understanding of dental anatomy and function include textbooks by Ash and Nelson, McNeill, and Dawson. Trauma from occlusion is determined by whether the composite of all occlusal forces on a specific tooth exceeds the tolerance or adaptability of its periodontium. Identification of masticatory system disharmonies begins with an appreciation of physiologic norms; this allows the clinician to recognize dysfunctional relationships, which can influence the accuracy of the diagnosis.

Centric relation is a term used to describe the position of both condyles when they are fully seated in the fossae of their respective temporomandibular joints (TMJs). Rotation of the mandible around an axis through both condyles is called the *centric relation closure arc*. This is strictly a skeletal relationship until tooth contact occurs. Maximal intercuspation occurs when opposing teeth make contact, with optimal interdigitation, at the most stable endpoint of mandibular closure. Stability is enhanced by the simultaneous bilateral contact of multiple posterior teeth with occlusal forces in the long axis of most posterior teeth. If the initial tooth contact in the centric relation arc of closure occurs simultaneously with maximal intercuspation, the teeth do not displace the condyles. Conversely, if the teeth are firm and any contact occurs before maximal intercuspation, incline relationships of opposing occlusal surfaces guide the mandible into intercuspal position, thereby requiring one or both condyles to become dislocated from their fossa. If the teeth are mobile and contact first in the centric relation closure arc, then *they may move away from opposing teeth rather than cause condylar displacement.*

Cusp–fossa or cusp–marginal ridge relationships of the posterior teeth provide resistance to vertical loading and functional stability for the patient's dentition. When occlusal forces load teeth in their long axis, the periodontium is the most resistant and supportive. The anterior teeth can be stable with little occlusal loading in centric occlusion if they are favorably influenced by the oral musculature. If the anterior teeth are in contact in maximal intercuspation, they are coupled.

Movement of the mandible from centric occlusion is called an *excursion.* Movement forward is called a *protrusive excursion*, and movement to either side is called a *lateral excursion*. If the mandible can move posteriorly, it is called *retrusion*. There is evidence that the contact of posterior teeth in excursions can overload those teeth, which results in negative dental, periodontal, muscular, and TMJ consequences. The ideal relationship may be a light coupling of the anterior teeth in centric occlusion with immediate separation (i.e., disclusion) of all posterior teeth in all excursions.

During a lateral excursion, posterior teeth that make contact on the same side as the direction of mandibular movement are described as having a working contact. Posterior teeth that make contact on the side opposite the direction of the lateral excursion are described as having a nonworking contact. Although nonworking contacts are classically associated with negative consequences, the analysis of working contacts and the function of anterior teeth are critically important. Contacts that are disruptive to mandibular movement or stressful to individual teeth are called *occlusal interferences* or *discrepancies*. Dentists' ability to analyze the occlusion to identify contacts that can amplify a patient's periodontitis, thereby affecting certain teeth, is strategic to making the correct diagnosis.

Inflammation disrupts the integrity of the attachment apparatus, which results in less resistance to force from opposing teeth. When bone loss has occurred, less root surface area is supported, and there are fewer sensory fibers in the periodontal ligament, which limits the protective muscle modulation of the occlusal forces. The clinician must differentiate among inflammation-caused intolerance to occlusal forces, normal forces on teeth with reduced periodontal support, excessive occlusal forces, and well-tolerated forces on teeth affected by periodontitis.

Parafunction

Bruxism can cause occlusal forces on teeth that are susceptible to periodontitis to be increased in intensity or frequency, thereby magnifying the potential amplification of damage. Daytime or awake occlusal parafunction is commonly limited to clenching the teeth during incidents that require a person's focused effort or mental concentration. Patients can be engaged in identification of daytime teeth clenching, as was the case in a study of sleep bruxism and myofascial pain. Awake clenching was reported by 58 of the 60 participants. Selection criteria for a study must be very exacting because self-reports of sleep bruxism by patients is usually unreliable. Patients' identification of their parafunction can help them to understand its importance, and it supports the clinical experience that daytime clenching can be a frequent contributor to a patient's increased susceptibility to bone loss in sites of inflammatory periodontitis.

Nighttime or sleep bruxing of the teeth can take the form of grinding the teeth during various excursions or clenching the teeth. Sleep bruxism is probably an extension of the rhythmic masticatory muscle activity that is also observed in nonbruxers. Why nuclei in the brain stem allow bruxing to occur in some individuals while others are spared is unclear.

Bruxing is associated with the greater frequency and persistence of TMJ dysfunction, orofacial pain, and possibly periodontal attachment loss. The sensory input of teeth that are subject to bruxism is probably dampened, which may interfere with the diagnosis and treatment. There seems to be limited influence on bruxing tendencies from occlusal interferences. An exception was discovered in a clinical study of 30 bruxers and 30 nonbruxers; there was a significant difference in nonworking interferences in the bruxing population compared to their absence in the nonbruxing group. When these findings are viewed along with those reported by Youdelis and Mann decades ago, the correlation of bruxing and site-specific inflammatory bone damage appears meaningful.

Gerber and Lynd studied selective serotonin reuptake inhibitor-induced movement disorders. They found that selective serotonin reuptake inhibitors such as Prozac encouraged bruxism.

Evidence is emerging that sleep-disordered breathing can influence or be associated with inflammatory diseases such as periodontitis. Although a causal relationship between obstructive sleep apnea and sleep bruxism has not been firmly established, the reported data and observations support a definite association. A patient with periodontitis with clinical evidence of occlusal trauma may be experiencing the consequences of sleep-disordered breathing. If an occlusal appliance is being considered to address the periodontal implications of excessive occlusal force experienced by a periodontitis-susceptible patient, compliance may be problematic for a person with sleep-disordered breathing because the appliance can contribute to airway obstruction.

Clinical Examination

Before clinical evaluation, a conversation with the patient can help to provide a more complete diagnosis. With minimal symptoms, a patient may not associate loose teeth or significant dental wear with TMJ dysfunction or orofacial pain with occlusal function or parafunction. Comprehensive evaluation of occlusal anatomy and relationships is accomplished by the analysis of many factors in the clinical setting and by mounted diagnostic casts.

Clinical evaluation of the occlusion is sequenced to support the patient's learning. It should always include a clinical assessment of masticatory system function and identification of disharmonies.

Temporomandibular Disorders Screening and Evaluation

Complete assessment of the masticatory system and identification of temporomandibular disorders should be part of a patient's initial comprehensive examination. The temporomandibular disorder

BOX 39.1 Temporomandibular Disorder Screening Evaluation

1. Maximal interincisal opening (range, 40–50 mm)
2. Opening or closing pathway
3. Range of lateral and protrusive excursions (7–9 mm)
4. Auscultation for temporomandibular joint sounds
5. Palpation for temporomandibular joint tenderness or tissue displacement
6. Palpation for muscle tenderness
7. Load testing of the patient's temporomandibular joints

screening and clinical evaluation then become part of subsequent examinations.

The patient's range of motion is observed, maximal opening and the lateral and protrusive excursions are measured, and any deviation from the midline during opening and closing is defined. Light finger pressure applied over each TMJ can detect deflection of the tissue while the patient opens and closes the mouth; deflection suggests condyle–disk discoordination. Tenderness on palpation can indicate TMJ capsulitis. Listening to the joint with a stethoscope or a Doppler instrument during opening and closing can detect sounds that are consistent with uncoordinated condyle–disk relationships, arthritic changes, and other diagnostic sounds.

Palpation of the muscles of mastication and the related head and neck musculature can reveal muscle tension or spasm related to compensation for occlusal or TMJ disharmonies. Significant discoveries revealed during the screening examination summarized in Box 39.1 should lead the clinician to complete the comprehensive evaluation.

Testing for the Mobility of Teeth

Two basic methods are used to assess the firmness or looseness of a tooth. Classically, a dental instrument is used to exert pressure in the facial or lingual direction, and the dentist places his or her finger on the opposite side of the tooth to feel and see movement if it occurs. Recording a numeric value (range, 0–3) for the degree of mobility allows the clinician to track changes that may occur in response to therapy.

The other method is to test for the movement of teeth that are subject to pressure generated by the patient. Fremitus, vibration, or micromovement of a tooth can be felt when patients tap their teeth together. When the patient mimics clenching the teeth and then attempts to move the mandible in excursions, tooth movement can be observed. The patient placing a finger where the clinician felt tooth movement helps the patient to appreciate the looseness of his or her teeth (Fig. 39.2).

If the mobility of the teeth exceeds what is expected on the basis of the loss of support or the level of inflammation observed, trauma from occlusion is included in the diagnosis. The assimilation of all of the occlusal and periodontal diagnostic references can lead the clinician to conclude that even without mobility, there may be evidence of amplified periodontal damage as a result of unfavorable occlusal forces. Periodontitis susceptibility evidenced in previous or ongoing disease and damage and bruxism are both clearly identified as risk indicators for **peri-implantitis**. Partially dentate patients with dental implant tooth replacement restorations should have initial and ongoing tooth mobility carefully analyzed and documented to determine if implant fixtures might be excessively loaded, especially in the presence of any peri-implant inflammation.

Centric Relation Assessment

Bimanual manipulation of the mandible in the axis of rotation of the condyles in their respective glenoid fossae has become a standard method of assessing centric relation. This method is illustrated in Fig. 39.3, and it involves gentle guidance rather than the forced positioning of the mandible. This technique is essential for load testing of the TMJs, and it is effective for generating centric relation records for mounting diagnostic casts. Telling the patient that he or she will feel modest lifting pressure on the inferior borders of the mandible and a light depressing force in the mental region often allows for relatively free and comfortable hinging of the mandible. If hinging is uncomfortable or not repeatable, muscle deprogramming may be beneficial. Other methods for guiding the condyles toward a seated position (e.g., leaf gauges, anterior bite stops) can be effective.

Asking the patient to identify the first tooth to touch in the centric relation arc of closure may indicate that interferences to closure into maximal intercuspation exist. Asking the patient to close further may demonstrate a slide from centric relation to centric occlusion because teeth are firm enough to dislocate one or both condyles Drying the occlusal surfaces, positioning marking paper, and then guiding the patient to the initial contact in centric relation allows marking of occlusal contact points, thereby identifying any interference. Asking the patient to then close into maximal intercuspation marks the points or surfaces that contact during the slide. An early occlusal contact in centric relation before closure to centric occlusion is obtained that does not cause a slide may indicate the early contact that occurs on teeth that are mobile enough to move, allowing maximal intercuspation to be gained without condylar accommodation (Fig. 39.4). Confirmation of permissive intercuspation is a product of marking the teeth clinically and comparing the marks with the ones on mounted diagnostic casts, which demonstrates that mobile teeth can move out of the way to allow others to contact.

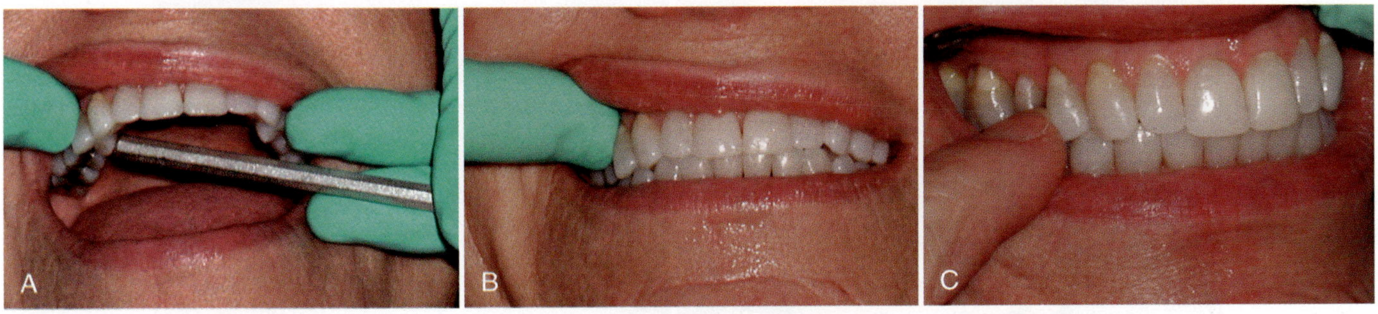

Fig. 39.2 A, Tactile and visual testing for mobility is done with a dental instrument by the dentist. B, Tactile and visual testing for mobility is done with the patient clenching and while beginning right lateral excursion by the dentist. C, The patient feels movement of her tooth when lateral excursion is attempted while the teeth are clenched.

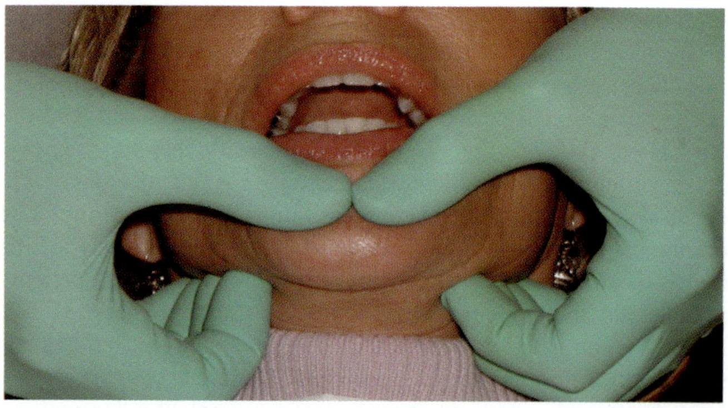

Fig. 39.3 Bimanual manipulation is used to hinge the mandible in centric relation and to load test the temporomandibular joints.

Evaluation of Excursions

Marking the teeth in all excursions reveals the pathways of contact of opposing occlusal or incisal surfaces during function, and it may identify interferences to harmonious function. Movement of any teeth during marking may lessen the intensity of the marks and the assessed severity of the forces experienced by the affected teeth.

Vectors of force and steepness of the opposing inclines are studied to determine whether the force is excessive. Interpreting contacts on a tooth-by-tooth basis can suggest or deny occlusal trauma as a contributing factor to the loss of attachment of each affected tooth. When patients are engaged in the evaluation of their occlusion, they can be given suggestions to observe certain habits, such as clenching their teeth during the day or sleeping with pressure on their mandible. As they contribute to their own diagnosis, patients become better prepared to make informed choices about treatment options.

Articulated Diagnostic Casts

When the maxillary diagnostic cast is mounted on an articulator with a facebow transfer technique, the occlusal surfaces become oriented to the axis of rotation of the patient's condyles. The centric relation transfer record orients the mandibular teeth to the maxillary teeth in centric relation. Study of the accurately mounted diagnostic casts can reveal occlusal discrepancies between initial contact in the centric relation closure arc and maximal intercuspation and occlusal disharmonies in excursions. Mobile teeth may produce a mark on a solid model but little or no mark in that patient's mouth during clinical assessment. Accuracy of the observations made on the models should be confirmed clinically to whatever degree possible.

Occlusal Therapy

Effective nonsurgical therapy usually reduces inflammation within the periodontium and results in some healing of attachment, which often results in mobile teeth becoming more stable. If the clinician concludes that inflammation has been optimally controlled and that occlusal forces on individual teeth still exceed the tolerance of the periodontium, the basis for intervention is established.

The harmonious function of both TMJs and their associated muscles is required for occlusal stability. When there is sufficient evidence of excessive occlusal forces on the patient's teeth or when masticatory system disharmony exists and the patient desires a more stable occlusion, an occlusal appliance is prescribed.

Occlusal Appliance Therapy

A well-designed and accurately fitted appliance can benefit masticatory system function while encouraging loose teeth in both arches to tighten as the supporting periodontium heals. The bilateral simultaneous contact of all opposing posterior teeth in centric relation, shallow anterior guidance, and the immediate disclusion of all posterior teeth in every excursion are essential elements of maxillary and mandibular occlusal appliances (Figs. 39.5 and 39.6).

Teeth that are opposing an appliance should be loaded as close as possible to their long axis. Maxillary appliances engage a portion of the hard palate, which provides substantial bracing of teeth and resistance to vertical and lateral forces. A horseshoe-shaped maxillary appliance relies on other, possibly compromised teeth to attempt to protect the most mobile teeth. Soft or partial coverage appliances are contraindicated for long-term protection and stabilization. The protective role of occlusal appliances was addressed in the 8-year study by McGuire. Occlusal appliances are not expected to cure bruxism, but they are often prescribed for patients with habitual parafunction as a compensating or protective intervention to limit masticatory system disharmony, damage to the teeth, and overstressing of implants.

Oral appliances fabricated and accurately fitted to address temporomandibular disharmonies and dysfunction and craniofacial pain, which may be associated with that diagnosis, have a favorable record of being helpful with a patient's symptoms. Physical therapy can usually be prescribed by a dentist addressing a painful temporomandibular situation, and that mode of treatment has proven to be an effective adjunct or a helpful stand-alone intervention. When persistence or magnitude of a patient's temporomandibular disorder, especially with pain, exceeds the knowledge and skill of a re-

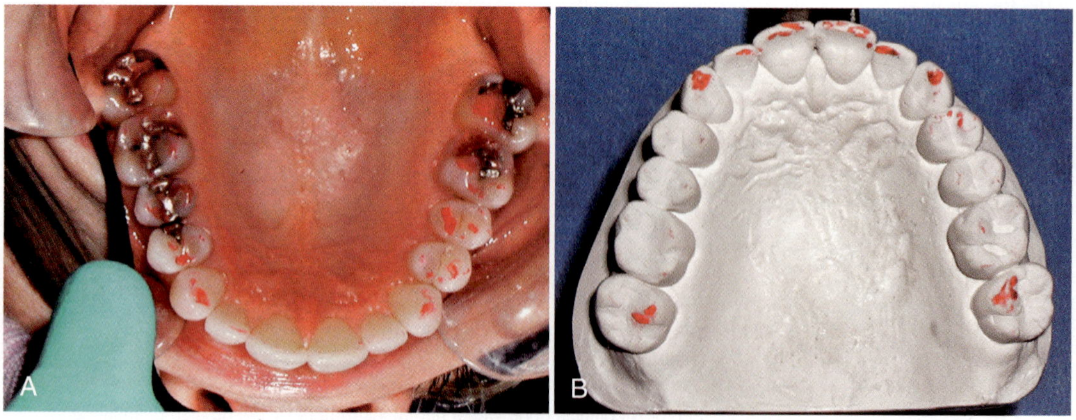

Fig. 39.4 A, Teeth are marked clinically in maximal intercuspation and in excursions while clenching. B, Teeth are marked in centric relation and maximal intercuspation on a diagnostic cast mounted in centric relation. Marks only on the second molars indicate that they were mobile and that they moved to permit the contact of other teeth.

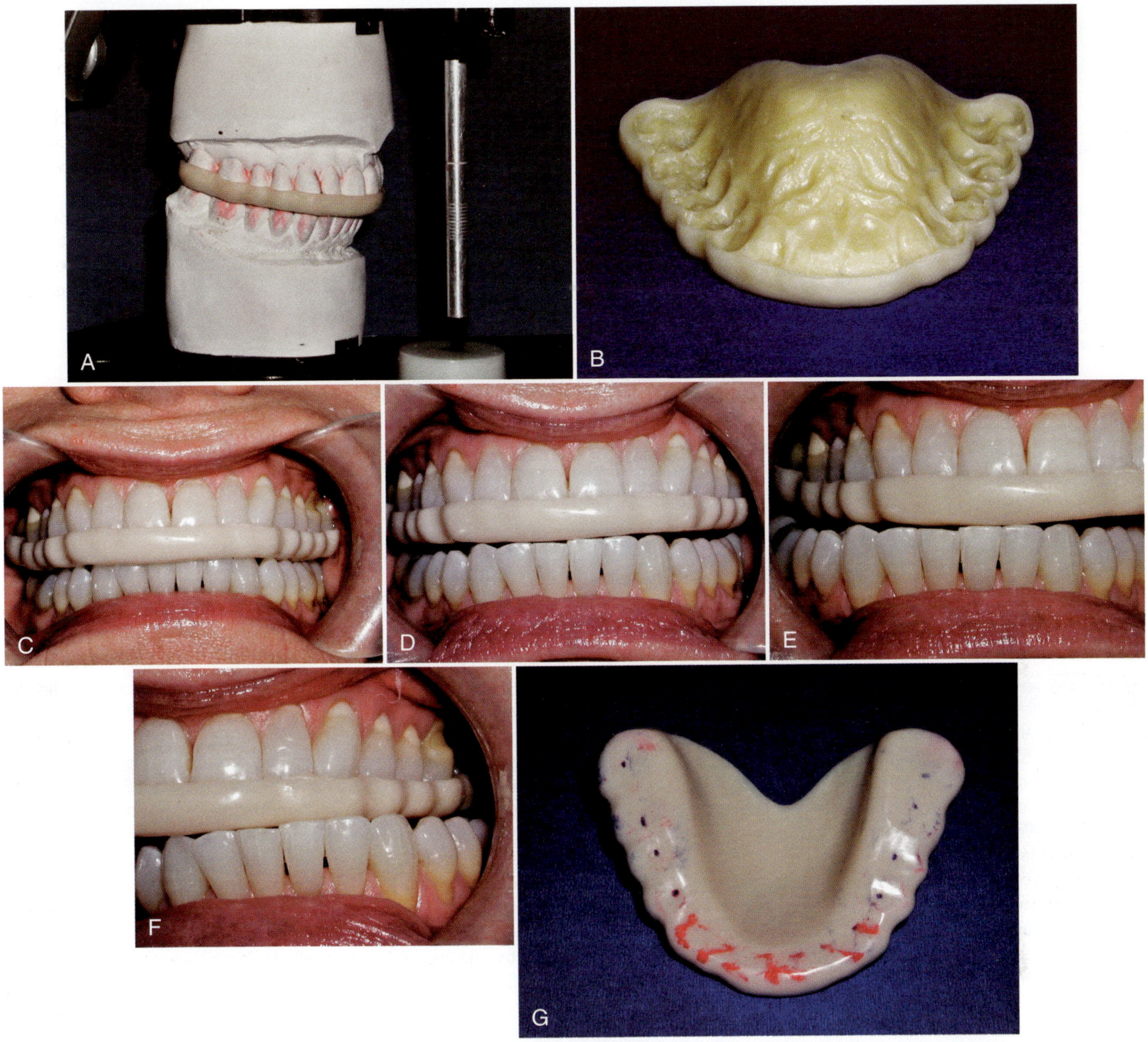

Fig. 39.5 A, An occlusal appliance is fabricated on accurately mounted diagnostic casts. B, The entire dental and palatal surface has been carefully relined to promote an optimal stabilizing influence on mobile teeth. C, There is bilateral, simultaneous contact of the cuspids and all posterior teeth in centric relation, fabricated to enhance axial loading of opposing mandibular teeth. D, There is smooth, relatively flat anterior guidance with immediate and sustained disclusion of all posterior teeth in protrusion. E, There is smooth, relatively flat anterior guidance with immediate and sustained disclusion of all posterior teeth in right lateral excursions. F, There is extreme left lateral excursion with smooth, harmonious transitions across the anterior teeth to maintain the disclusion of all posterior teeth. G, Marks created by the opposing dentition demonstrate bilateral, simultaneous contact in centric relation and the immediate disclusion of the opposing posterior teeth in all excursions.

storative dentist or a periodontist, referral to a temporomandibular disharmonies and dysfunction specialist or an oral surgeon may be indicated.

Occlusal Adjustment

As teeth tighten from consistent use of the appliance, occlusal interferences may become more evident, and greater discrepancy between the initial dental contact and maximal intercuspation may be observed. Interferences with harmonious excursive movement of the mandible may also become more obvious. When the clinician confirms that the interferences correlate with a greater than expected loss of attachment, direct intervention in the patient's occlusion is considered. With the patient's full understanding and consent, occlusal adjustment or selective reshaping of the occluding surfaces of the teeth can reduce the magnitude of occlusal interferences or direct the forces to be more compatible with the long axes of the affected teeth.

Clinical analysis of the occlusion should be combined with a detailed analysis of diagnostic casts mounted in centric relation on an adjustable articulator. Accurately mounted duplicate models can be used to accomplish a trial occlusal adjustment to determine safety and efficacy for a patient. Scheduling patients so that they

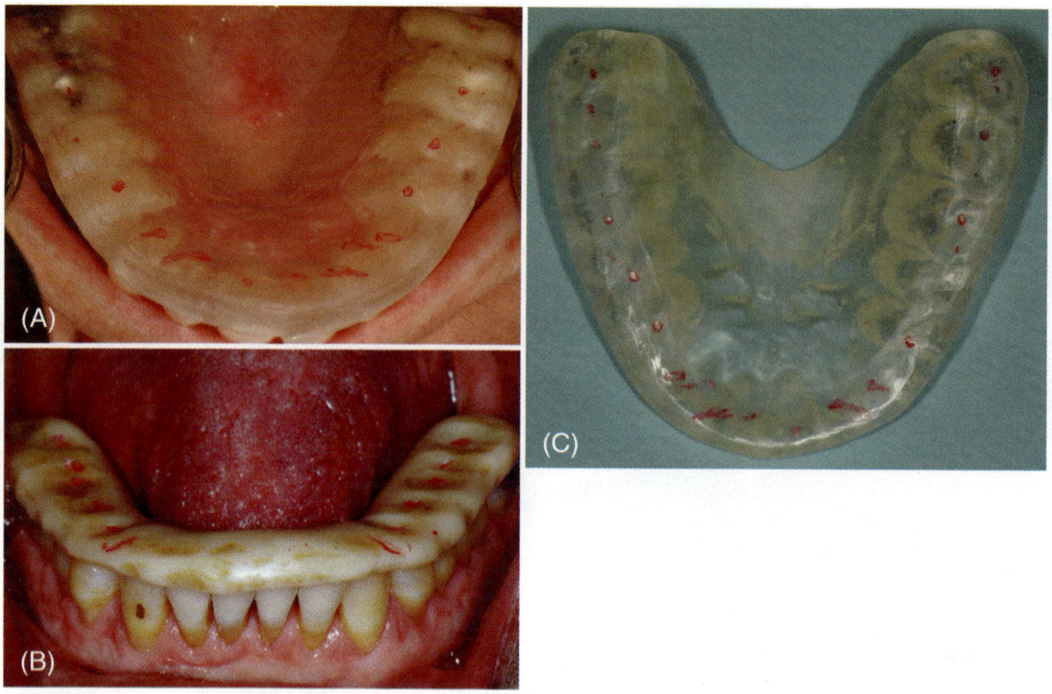

Fig. 39.6 A–C, A mandibular occlusal appliance is fabricated after surgery to provide a stabilizing influence for the incisors in particular and to demonstrate occlusal attributes similar to those of the maxillary appliance.

BOX 39.2 Requirements for Occlusal Stability

1. Forces on an individual tooth that do not exceed the support and resistance of the tooth's periodontium and that are vertically oriented to the long axis of each tooth as much as possible.
2. Even and simultaneous contact of all posterior teeth in the centric relation closure or in maximal intercuspation, with minimal difference between the two.
3. Little or no contact of the anterior teeth in centric occlusion, although such contact is readily available to provide guidance in excursion and to produce posterior disclusion.
4. Harmonious excursive movement of the mandible within the patient's envelope of function and with complete absence of occlusal interference.

leave their appliances on overnight and in place until they are seated in the dental chair allows assessment of their teeth at maximal firmness, when interferences are most readily identifiable. Teeth usually progressively tighten with continued compliance with the appliance and repeated careful occlusal adjustment.

Other methods that can be employed to alter occlusal relationships include orthodontics and restorative dentistry. Provisional restoration of teeth is another method of improving occlusal contacts and stability, and it often simplifies the process of occlusal adjustment and final restoration.

Occlusal Stability for Restorative Dentistry

A stable occlusion is considered a prerequisite for any restorative therapy (Box 39.2). Implants to replace the teeth of a partially dentate patient add to the occlusal considerations. Osseointegration of implants eliminates micromovement, which can allow teeth to accommodate occlusal forces. The extent and timing of occlusal loading and the guidance requirement for each tooth and for each implant must be carefully harmonized. This is especially critical if any of the teeth are mobile or the patient bruxes to a significant degree. If bruxism is suspected or the functional forces are considered to be excessive, the occlusal appliance as described may be a valuable application.

Splinting

Glossary of prosthodontic terms defines a splint as "a rigid or flexible device that maintains in position a displaced or movable part.; also used to keep in place and protect an injured part." It also defines splint as a "rigid or flexible material used to protect, immobilize, or restrict motion in a part." In regards to dentistry, it may be defined as "the joining of two or more teeth into a rigid unit by means of fixed or removable restorations or devices." A splint has also been defined as "any apparatus, appliance, or device employed to prevent motion or displacement of fractured or movable parts."

In the past, tooth mobility was thought to be directly associated to clinical attachment loss and splinting was hence performed to reduce the development and progression of periodontal disease. As a result, it was assumed that tooth stabilization had a direct impact on the periodontal healing and gain in attachment. However, it was later proven that excessive occlusal forces by themselves do not produce gingivitis, periodontitis, or pocket formation, and there is no direct correlation between tooth mobility and periodontal disease healing and hence the purpose behind doing splinting changed with time as periodontal clinical trials investigated these assumptions.

Now it is performed in cases of secondary trauma from occlusion where the weekend periodontium is unable to bear even the normal masticatory forces. In patients where tooth mobility becomes a functional limitation and interferes with eating and speaking, splinting improves patient's comfort during mastication by evenly distributing the masticatory and occlusal forces in the arch and assisting in phonetics. Splints stabilize the mobile teeth, aiding in better esthetics, improving masticatory comfort, and increasing the morale of the patient.

Management of tooth mobility is determined by the degree of damage to bone support. In cases where mobility is due to widening

BOX 39.3 Indications and Contraindications for Splint Therapy

Indications for splint therapy include:
- Facilitate periodontal instrumentation and occlusal adjustment of extremely mobile teeth.
- To control parafunctional or bruxing forces.
- Stabilization of mobile teeth during surgical, especially regenerative therapy since micromovement of the surgical site may inhibit repair to take place in the healing area.
- Stabilization of mobile teeth for masticatory comfort.
- Stabilization of a severely periodontally compromised tooth when more definitive treatment is not possible.
- Prevention of teeth tipping/drifting after orthodontic treatment or when a tooth is missing.
- Prevention of the eruption of an unopposed tooth.
- To restore the patients psychological and physical well-being.
- Prevention of mobility after acute trauma as in subluxation and avulsion.
- To protect the investing structures of the teeth.
- Restoration of the vertical dimension of occlusion in a case of posterior bite collapse.
- To protect the pulp.
- To control forces and stress.
- To establish physiologic occlusion.
- Cross-arch stabilization of an intact or virtually intact natural dentition or preservation of arch integrity.

Contraindications:
1. Insufficient number of nonmobile teeth to adequately stabilize mobile teeth.
2. Presence of occlusal interference and/or trauma.
3. Presence of untreated inflammatory periodontal disease.
4. Poor oral hygiene.
5. High caries activity.

of periodontal ligament as a result of adaptation of functional demands, treatment comprises periodontal therapy and occlusal adjustments. In cases of severe bone loss, successful treatment of inflammation only leads to a decrease in tooth mobility, not complete obliteration of it. The periodontally compromised teeth with poor prognosis may have to be removed. In such cases, splinting is the only way to completely stabilize the teeth and allow comfortable function for the patient. Few instances have been reported where the extracted periodontally compromised teeth were used as a natural tooth pontic after extraoral root canal and splinting with adjacent teeth. The treatment in such cases includes a combination of occlusal adjustments, periodontal therapy, and splinting. The indications and contraindications of splinting are listed in Box 39.3 and the requirements of an ideal splint in Box 39.4.

Types of Splints

Splints may be classified as:

On the basis of way of fabrication:
- Fixed
- Removable

On the basis of material:
- Metallic (stainless steel, chrome cobalt, and cast metals)
- Nonmetallic (acrylic and composites)
- Combination of metallic and nonmetallic

On the basis of location of the splinted teeth in the jaw:
- **Extracoronal**: Teeth are connected to each other by etching and bonding technique of composite resins. Wire, fiber-reinforced ribbons (commercially available as Ribbond-Ribbon, Interlig Fiber splint), or similar stabilization device is bonded to the outside of the teeth to reinforce the material (Figs. 39.7 and 39.8). These fiber-reinforced ribbons have been developed to chemically bind with the resin structure. The fibers used to reinforce the material are high strength color neutral fibers of either polyethylene or resin pre-impregnated glass fibers.,which are available in a variety of widths and sizes, can be braided ropes or woven/ unidirectional fibers.
- Splints can also be cast from metals, which are then cemented in place. Crowns placed on adjoining teeth (not involving any internal line angles) can be splinted together to function as a rigid splint. These splints have greater inherent strength than intracoronal splints.
- **Intracoronal:** Composite resin restorations placed in adjoining teeth and cured to eliminate interproximal separation are an example of intracoronal splints. Stabilizing devices such as wires, glass-reinforced fibers, or pins can be inserted into the slots in the affected teeth and bonded in place using

BOX 39.4 Requirements of an Ideal Splint

1. Should be esthetically acceptable and readily available.
2. Ease of fabrication and repair; relatively inexpensive.
3. Should not interfere with the occlusion.
4. Should be nonirritating to the oral soft tissues and permit good plaque control.
5. Should be simple in design without involving extensive tooth preparation.
6. It should incorporate as many firm teeth as is necessary (ideally for every mobile tooth, at least two firm teeth should be incorporated in the splint as per Ante's Law).
7. It should extend around the arch so that anteroposterior forces and faciolingual forces are counteracted.

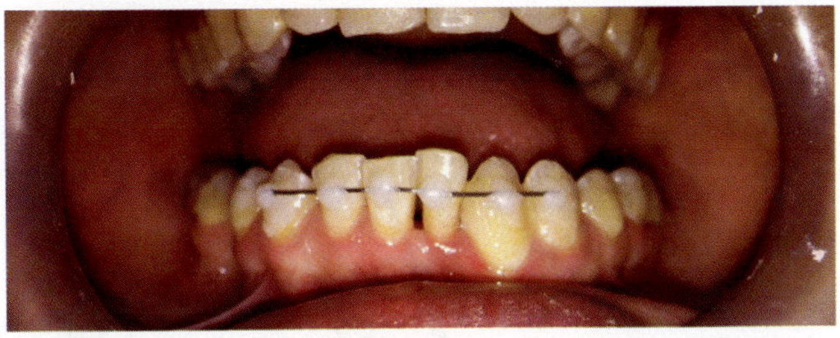

Fig. 39.7 Splinting with wire and composite without channel.

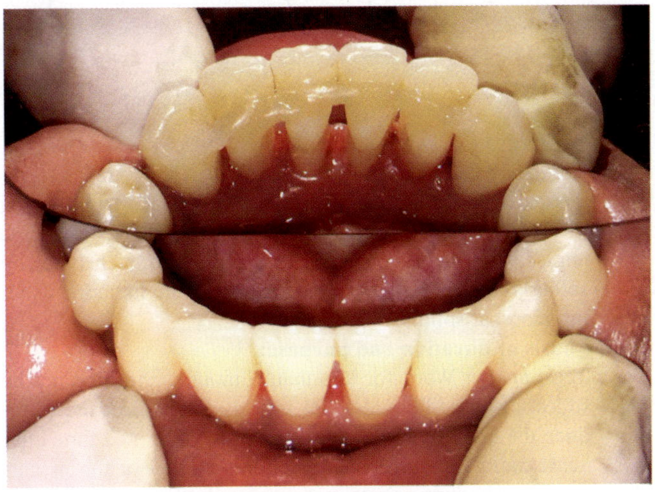

Fig. 39.8 Ribbond splint.

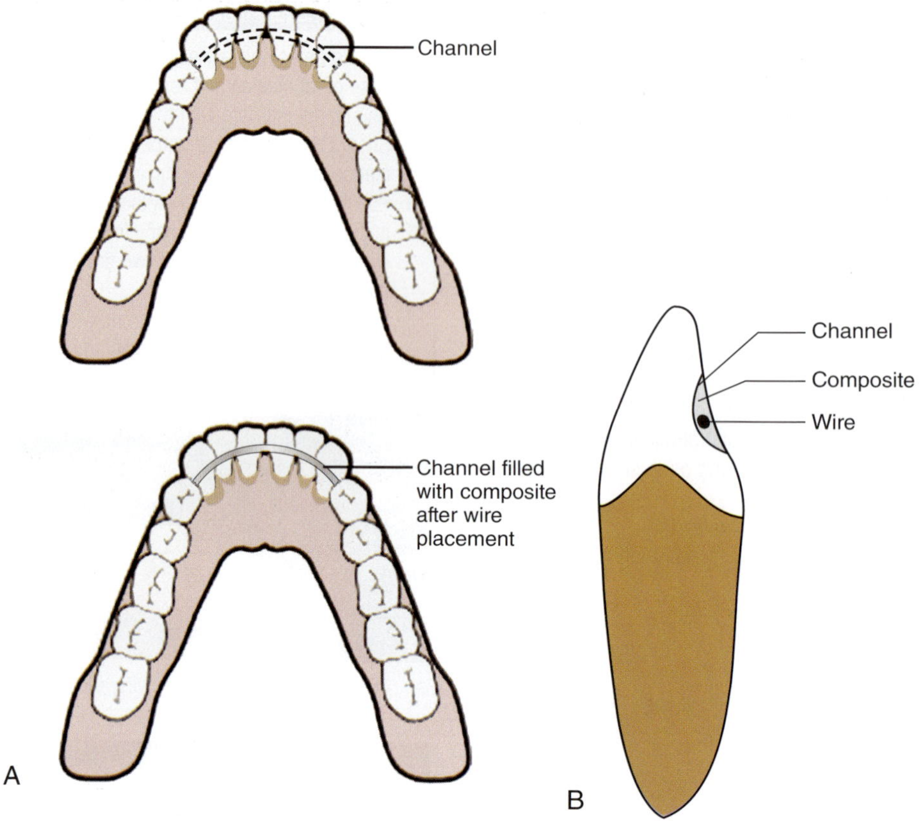

Fig. 39.9 A, Splinting with wire and composite with channel; B, cross-sectional view.

composite resin restorations (Fig. 39.9). They are more esthetically appealing than extracoronal splints. If restoration of mouth includes adjoining crowns involving internal line angles, crowns and/or inlays are splinted to each other by solder joints or precision attachments and are included under intracoronal splints.

On the basis of duration and purpose:

- **Temporary:** Worn for less than 6 months and may not be followed by additional splint therapy. They are used to reduce the unfavorable occlusal forces for a limited time after acute trauma, in advanced periodontitis cases or for anchorage in orthodontic therapy, for example, bite guards, Hawley's appliance, orthodontic bands welded together, and cast splints cemented to the teeth (Fig. 39.10).
- **Provisional**: Used for months to several years with a definitive end to the splint therapy. Can be internal/external. They may be used as an interim measure in cases where prognosis is bound to change after phase I therapy, for example, ligature wires, night guards (Fig. 39.11), composite resin splints, and interim fixed prosthesis.
- **Permanent**: Are worn indefinitely. Can be fixed/removable. They should be placed once the occlusion has been stabilized and periodontal treatment has been carried out, for example, clasp-supported partial denture.

Conclusion

Confirmation of the appropriateness of occlusal therapy is the product of a thorough evaluation of the patient's occlusion and his or her masticatory system. The sequence of occlusal treatment begins with antiinflammatory therapy and progresses through reversible appliance therapy before any irreversible options are considered. This

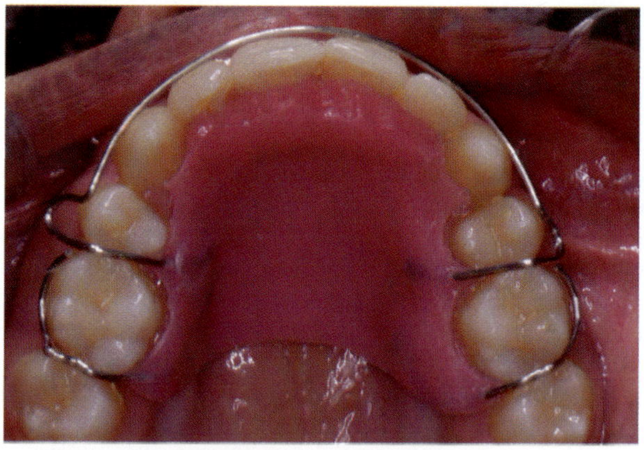

Fig. 39.10 Hawley's appliance.

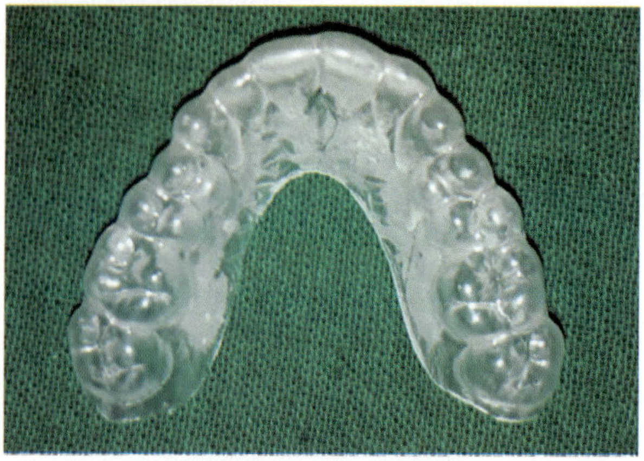

Fig. 39.11 Night guard.

provides the clinician with the most careful approach to assessing and treating the occlusion of a patient with periodontitis.

Splinting can be considered an adjunct in addition to cause-related therapy for periodontally compromised teeth with advanced mobility. Improvements in patient's self-esteem and masticatory functions are the major advantages of splinting. It also aids in healing in regenerative therapy cases by reducing the micromovements in the healing area. However, splinting by itself does not eliminate the cause behind tooth mobility and hence is only an aid in stabilizing the mobile tooth, and mobility may revert once the splints have been removed.

Key points

- The role of occlusal trauma and its possible influence on progression of periodontitis is tooth specific.
- Occlusal trauma can amplify (not cause) localized loss of attachment from inflammatory bone damage.
- Optimal resolution of inflammation is necessary to accurately interpret tooth mobility.
- Splint may be defined as "the joining of two or more teeth into a rigid unit by means of fixed or removable restorations or devices."
- Splints may be classified as fixed/removable; metallic/nonmetallic/combination of metallic and nonmetallic; extracoronal/intracoronal; temporary/provisional/permanent.

Suggested reading

Nelson SJ: *Wheeler's dental anatomy, physiology and occlusion: 1st SAE - e-book,* New Delhi, 2015, Elsevier Health Sciences.

Becker IM: *Comprehensive occlusal concepts in clinical practice*, New Jersey, 2011, John Wiley & Sons.

Gross MD, Gracis S, Gamborena I, et al: *The Science and Art of occlusion and oral Rehabilitation*, Quintessence: Berlin, 2015.

Wassell R, Naru A, Steele JG, Nohl F: *Applied occlusion*, London, 2015.

References

References and MCQs with answers for the chapter are available on the companion website www.medenact.com.

CHAPTER 40

Breath Malodor

M Quirynen | I Laleman | J Dadamio | SD Geest | B Vandekerckhove | W Teughels | A Jain | CD Hous | C Dekeyser

CHAPTER OUTLINE

Semantics and Classification

Breath odor can be defined as the subjective perception after smelling someone's breath. It can be pleasant, unpleasant, or even disturbing, if not repulsive. If unpleasant, the terms *breath malodor, halitosis, bad breath,* or *fetor ex ore* can be applied. These terms, however, are not synonymous with oral malodor. This term is restricted to halitosis with an origin in the oral cavity.

There are three main categories of halitosis: genuine halitosis, pseudo-halitosis, and halitophobia. *Genuine halitosis* is the term that is used when the breath malodor really exists and can be diagnosed organoleptically or by measurement of the responsible compounds. A distinction should be made between physiologic and a pathologic halitosis (Fig. 40.1). The transient disturbing odor caused by food intake (e.g., garlic, onions, and certain spices), smoking, or medication (e.g., metronidazole) do not reveal a health problem and are common examples of physiologic halitosis. The same is true for "morning" bad breath as habitually experienced on awakening. This malodor is caused by a decreased salivary flow and increased putrefaction during the night and spontaneously disappears after breakfast or after oral hygiene measures. A persistent breath malodor, by definition, does reflect some pathology (pathologic halitosis). The causes of this will be discussed later in the chapter. When an obvious breath malodor cannot be perceived, but the patient is convinced that he or she suffers from it, this is called *pseudo-halitosis*. If the patient still believes that there is bad breath after treatment of genuine halitosis or diagnosis of pseudo-halitosis, one considers halitophobia, which is a recognized psychiatric condition.

Important Terms for the Diagnosis of Bad Breath

Genuine halitosis	Malodor that can be verified objectively
Physiologic halitosis	Malodor that is transient and caused by physiologic factors, such as food intake or smoking
Oral malodor or intraoral halitosis	Obvious malodor originating from the oral cavity
Extraoral halitosis	Bad breath originating from pathologic conditions outside the oral cavity
Pseudo-halitosis	Malodor that cannot be perceived objectively even though the patient complains of its existence. This condition can be improved by oral hygiene instruction and counseling.
Halitophobia	No malodor that can be perceived objectively after treatment of halitosis or pseudo-halitosis even though the patient persists in believing that halitosis exists

Epidemiology

Only few studies have documented the prevalence of oral malodor. Moreover, these studies used different methodologies, ranging from self-reported breath malodor to more objective assessments such as measurement of volatile sulfur compounds (VSCs). Because self-reported halitosis correlates weakly with objective measurements and tends to overestimate the problem, data should be interpreted carefully. These studies have been performed in different parts of the world. Despite the different approaches of these studies, the results point out that about one in four to one in three subjects has persistent bad breath. If a VSC level of 75 ppb (limit for social acceptance) is used as a threshold for halitosis, the prevalence reported in the different populations can be calculated as 23% (late-morning group) and 20% for the Japanese and Chinese studies, respectively. In line with this, a prevalence of 27.5% and 29.8% for the Chinese and Israeli groups, respectively, can be calculated when an organoleptic score of at least 2 is considered as being representative for halitosis. With the same criterion, the calculated prevalence varied between 11.0% and 29.7% for different age groups in the Polish population.

From large-scale inventories in multidisciplinary outpatient clinics for breath odor, no sex predominance seems to exist for bad breath, although other studies indicate a higher prevalence in women. It has also been observed that women seek treatment more often than men. Age can range from 2 years to more than 80 years. No association was found between increased age and oral malodor. Most of the patients had been complaining about breath malodor for several years before seeking proper advice.

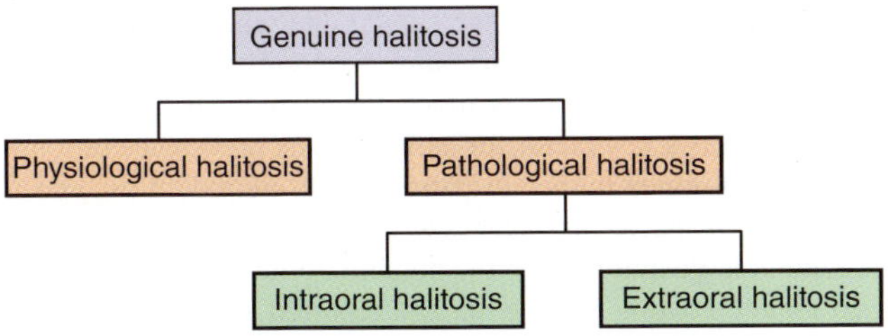

Fig. 40.1 Genuine halitosis: classification.

Etiology

In the vast majority, breath malodor originates from the oral cavity. Gingivitis, periodontitis, and especially tongue coating are the predominant causative factors.

In general, one can identify two pathways for bad breath. The first one involves an increase of certain metabolites in the blood circulation (e.g., due to a systemic disease), which will escape via the alveoli of the lungs during breathing (blood–breath exchange) and it is commonly referred as "extraoral halitosis." The second pathway (intraoral halitosis) involves an increase of either the bacterial load or the amount of substrate for these bacteria at one of the lining surfaces of the oropharyngeal cavity, the respiratory tract, or the esophagus. All types of infections, ulcerations, or tumors at one of the previously mentioned areas can thus lead to bad breath. Studies also suggest that oral malodor is associated with the total bacterial load of anaerobic bacteria in both saliva and tongue coating. The most commonly involved bacteria are *Porphyromonas gingivalis, Prevotella intermedia/nigrescens, Aggregatibacter actinomycetemcomitans* (previously *Actinobacillus actinomycetemcomitans), Campylobacter rectus, Fusobacterium nucleatum, Peptostreptococcus micros, Tannerella forsythia, Eubacterium* spp, and spirochetes. A study conducted by Niles and Gaffar made clear that these gram-negative species in particular cause an unpleasant smell by the production of sulfur compounds. However, because of the large species diversity found in patients with halitosis, it can be suggested that breath malodor is the result of complex interactions between several bacterial species. A recent study indicates that some gram-positive microorganisms, such as *Streptococcus salivarius*, also contribute to oral malodor production by deglycosylating salivary glycoproteins, thus exposing their protein core to further degradation by gram-negative microorganisms.

Recently, the presence of *Solobacterium moorei*, a gram-positive bacterium, has also been linked to oral malodor.

For oral malodor, the unpleasant smell of the breath mainly originates from VSCs, especially hydrogen sulfide (H_2S), methyl mercaptan (CH_3SH), and (less significantly) dimethyl sulfide [$(CH_3)_2S$], as first discovered by Tonzetich. However, in certain conditions (e.g., when the saliva dries out on the mucosal surfaces), other compounds in mouth air may also play a role such as diamines (e.g., putrescine, cadaverine), indole, skatole, and volatile organic acids like butyric or propionic acid. Most of these compounds result from the proteolytic degradation by oral microorganisms of peptides present in saliva (sulfur-containing or nonsulfur-containing amino acids), shed epithelium, food debris, gingival crevicular fluid, interdental plaque, postnasal drip, and blood. In particular, gram-negative, anaerobic bacteria possess such proteolytic activity.

For the extraoral causes of halitosis, other compounds besides the VSCs may be involved. Bad-smelling metabolites can be formed/absorbed at any place in the body (e.g., the liver, the gut) and transported by the bloodstream to the lungs. Exhalation of these volatiles in the alveolar air then causes halitosis, at least when the concentrations of the bad-smelling metabolites are sufficiently high. The crevicular fluid reflects the circulating molecules in the blood and can thus also play a relevant role but due to the small amount probably not a very dominant one. The extraoral causes are much more difficult to detect although they can sometimes be recognized by a typical odor. Uncontrolled diabetes mellitus can be associated with a sweet odor of ketones, liver disease can be revealed by a sulfur odor, and kidney failure can be characterized by a fishy odor because of the presence of dimethylamine and trimethylamine.

In a special patient category, subjects imagine they have breath malodor; this is called *imaginary breath odor* or *halitophobia.* The latter has been associated with obsessive–compulsive disorders and hypochondria. In a recent study of 2000 patients, 16% were diagnosed with pseudo-halitosis or halitophobia.

Intraoral Causes

Tongue and Tongue Coating

The dorsal tongue mucosa, with an area of 25 cm^2, shows a very irregular surface topography. The posterior part exhibits a number of oval cryptolymphatic units, which roughen the surface of this area. The anterior part is even rougher because of the high number of papillae: the filiform papillae with a core of 0.5 mm in length, a central crater, and uplifted borders; the fungiform papillae, 0.5–0.8 mm in length; the foliate papillae, located at the edge of the tongue, separated by deep folds; and the vallate papillae, 1 mm in height and 2–3 mm in diameter. These innumerable depressions in the tongue surface are ideal niches for bacterial adhesion and growth, sheltered from cleaning actions. Moreover, desquamated cells and food remnants also remain trapped in these retention sites and consequently can be putrefied by the bacteria. A fissurated tongue (deep fissures on dorsum, also called *scrotal tongue* or *lingua plicata*) and a hairy tongue (lingua villosa) have an even rougher surface (Fig. 40.2).

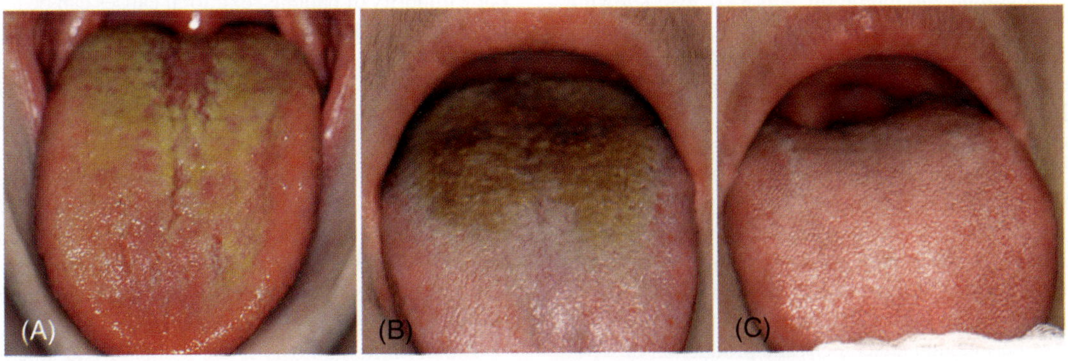

Fig. 40.2 A–C, Clinical pictures of heavily coated tongues.

The accumulation of food remnants intermingled with exfoliated cells and bacteria forms a coating on the tongue dorsum. The latter cannot be easily removed because of the retention offered by the irregular surface of the tongue dorsum (Fig. 40.2). As such, the two factors (bacteria and their nutrients) essential for putrefaction are united. Several investigators have identified the dorsal posterior surface of the tongue as the primary source of breath malodor. Indeed, high correlations have been reported between tongue coating and odor formation.

Both in healthy individuals and periodontitis patients with or without complaints of oral halitosis, a significant positive correlation was found between the presence or amount of tongue coating and levels of VSCs and/or organoleptic scores of the mouth odor. In a group of 2000 patients visiting a multidisciplinary halitosis clinic, significant correlations were found between the organoleptic scores and tongue coating ($R = 0.52$; $P < 0.001$). In another study, it was also observed that the amount of tongue coating was significantly greater in the halitosis-positive group compared to the halitosis-negative group.

Morita and Wang found that the volume of tongue coating and the percentile of sites with bleeding on probing were significantly associated with oral malodor. In 1992, Yaegaki and Sanada demonstrated that, even in patients with periodontal disease, 60% of the VSCs were produced from the tongue surface.

Recent research showed that the strongest determinant for the presence of tongue coating is suboptimal oral hygiene. Other influencing factors were periodontal status, presence of a denture, smoking, and dietary habits.

Periodontal Infections

A relationship between periodontitis and oral malodor has been shown. However, not all patients with gingivitis and/or periodontitis complain about bad breath, and there is some disagreement in the literature as to what extent oral malodor and periodontal disease are related. Bacteria associated with gingivitis and periodontitis are indeed able to produce VSCs.

Several studies have shown that the VSC levels in the mouth correlate positively with the depth of periodontal pockets (the deeper the pocket, the more the bacteria, particularly anaerobic species) and that the amount of VSCs in breath increases with the number, depth, and bleeding tendency of the periodontal pockets. It is important to realize that VSCs aggravate the periodontitis process by, for example, increasing the permeability of the pocket and mucosal epithelium and therefore exposing the underlying connective tissues of the periodontium to bacterial metabolites. Moreover, methyl mercaptan enhances interstitial collagenase production, interleukin-1 (IL-1) production by mononuclear cells, and cathepsin B production, thus further mediating connective tissue breakdown. It was also shown that human gingival fibroblasts developed an affected cytoskeleton when exposed to methyl mercaptan. The same gas alters cell proliferation and migration. VSCs are also known to impede wound healing. Thus, when periodontal surgery is planned, especially the insertion of implants, clinicians should recognize this pathologic role of VSCs. Furthermore, the reaction of hydrogen sulfide with collagen can alter the protein structure, thereby rendering the periodontal ligament and bone collagen more susceptible to destruction by proteases. Investigators have shown, in cases of gingivitis and periodontitis, a decrease in the content of acid-soluble and total collagen in the affected tissues. These findings suggest that increased production of VSCs may accelerate the progression of periodontal disease. Toxic VSCs are able to damage the periodontal tissues and create even more loss of attachment. A mutual reinforcement of the loss of periodontal attachment and production of VSCs occurs, resulting in a vicious cycle.

Some studies, however, have shown that when the presence of tongue coating is taken into account, the correlation between periodontitis and oral malodor is much lower, indicating that tongue coating remains a key factor for halitosis. The prevalence of tongue coating is six times higher in patients with periodontitis, and the same bacterial species associated with periodontal disease can also be found in large numbers on the dorsum of the tongue, particularly when tongue coating is present. The reported association between periodontitis and oral malodor may thus primarily be due to the effects of periodontal disease on tongue coating and may explain why other articles did not find a correlation.

A systematic review with a meta-regression analysis demonstrated the association between periodontitis and halitosis based on the evidence derived from five cross-sectional studies, with a collective sample size of 7184 subjects. Subjects with periodontitis have 3.2 times higher odds of oral malodor. Interestingly, the authors concluded that the magnitude of the association was greater in studies that used the organoleptic test for halitosis detection, but the association vanished in those that used the VSC test.

Other relevant malodorous pathologic manifestations of the periodontium are pericoronitis (the soft tissue "cap" being retentive for microorganisms and debris), major recurrent oral ulcerations, herpetic gingivitis, and necrotizing gingivitis/periodontitis. Microbiologic observations indicate that ulcers infected with gram-negative anaerobes (i.e., *Prevotella* and *Porphyromonas* species) are significantly more malodorous than noninfected ulcers.

Dental Disorders

Possible causes within the dentition are deep carious lesions with food impaction and putrefaction, extraction wounds filled with a blood clot, and purulent discharge leading to putrefaction process. The same applies to interdental food impaction in large interdental areas and crowding of teeth favor food entrapment and accumulation of debris. Acrylic dentures, especially when kept continuously in the mouth at night or not regularly cleaned, can also produce a typical smell. The denture surface facing the gingiva is porous and retentive for bacteria, yeasts, and debris, which are compounds needed for putrefaction.

Dry Mouth

Saliva has an important cleaning function in the oral cavity. Patients with xerostomia often present with large amounts of plaque on teeth and an extensive tongue coating. The increased microbial load and the escape of VSCs when saliva is drying up explain the strong breath malodor. Several studies link stress with VSC levels, but it is not clear whether this can simply be explained by a reduction of salivary flow. Other causes of xerostomia are medication, alcohol abuse, Sjögren syndrome (a common autoimmune rheumatic disease), and diabetes.

Extraoral Causes

For a minority of patients, extraoral causes can be identified, including ENT disorders, systemic disease (e.g., diabetes or kidney disease), metabolic or hormonal changes, hepatic or renal insufficiency, bronchial and pulmonary diseases, or gastroenterologic disorders. Moreover, multiple causes may be present at the same time, and over the course of time, the etiology may shift.

Extraoral halitosis can be subdivided into two types: non–blood-borne halitosis and blood-borne halitosis. Non–blood-borne halitosis is uncommon, and most information about it comes from case reports. Non–blood-borne halitosis encompasses, for example, throat infections, nasal infections, infections of the respiratory system, lung diseases, and stomach disorders.

Blood-borne halitosis is the result of bad-smelling metabolites that can be formed or absorbed at any place in the body (e.g., the liver, the gut) and transported by the bloodstream to the lungs. Exhalation of these volatiles in the alveolar air then causes halitosis, at least when the concentrations of the bad-smelling metabolites are sufficiently high. The crevicular fluid reflects the circulating molecules in the blood and can thus also play a relevant role, but due to the small amount, probably not a very dominant one.

The extraoral causes are much more difficult to detect, although they can sometimes be recognized by a typical odor. Uncontrolled diabetes mellitus can be associated with a sweet odor of ketones, liver disease can be revealed by a sulfur odor, and kidney failure can be characterized by a fishy odor because of the presence of dimethylamine and trimethylamine.

Ear, Nose, and Throat

During chronic or purulent tonsillitis, the deep crypts of the tonsils accumulate debris and bacteria, especially periopathogens, resulting in putrefaction. In the crypts, even calculus (e.g., subgingivally) can be formed (tonsilloliths or tonsil stones). Other examples include acute pharyngitis (viral or bacterial) and postnasal drip. The latter is a rather common condition, which is perceived by patients as a liquid flow in the throat originating from the nasal cavity. It is often associated with chronic sinusitis or regurgitation esophagitis, in which the acidic contents of the stomach reach the nasopharynx and cause mucositis. Ozena (caused by *Klebsiella ozaenae*) is a rare atrophic condition of the nasal mucosa, with the appearance of crusts that cause a very strong breath malodor. Finally, a foreign body in a nasal or sinus cavity can cause local irritation, ulceration, and subsequent putrefaction (e.g., children and mentally handicapped persons tend to put objects such as peas or wet paper in the nose).

Bronchi and Lungs

Pulmonary causes include chronic bronchitis, bronchiectasis (infection of standing mucus secretion in cystic dilations through walls of bronchioles), pneumonia, pulmonary abscess, bronchial carcinoma, and carcinoma of the lung. The relevance of an early diagnosis is evident.

Gastrointestinal Tract

Contrary to common public opinion, even among medical physicians, gastrointestinal disorders are rarely responsible for bad breath. The following may be responsible for less than 1% of malodor cases:

- A Zenker diverticulum (a hernia in the esophageal wall, allowing accumulation of food and debris and thus putrefaction) can cause significant breath odor because it is not separated from the oral cavity by a sphincter.
- A gastric diaphragmatic hernia (where the fundus of the stomach protrudes through the diaphragm, with relative sphincter insufficiency, allowing gases to escape or contents to flow back in the esophagus) can cause reflux of the gastric contents up to the oropharynx. This is sometimes combined with ructus, in which air from the stomach suddenly regurgitates.
- Regurgitation esophagitis (ulceration of the mucosal lining of the esophagus by acidic stomach contents flowing back because of improper functioning of the sphincter) may be a cause.
- Intestinal gas production: Some gases (e.g., dimethyl sulfide) are absorbed but not metabolized by the intestinal endothelium and thus transported by the blood. These gases can then be exhaled through the lungs.

Some disagreement exists in the literature over whether *Helicobacter pylori* infection is associated with halitosis. In one report, *H. pylori* was shown to produce hydrogen sulfide and methyl mercaptan, a finding suggesting that this microorganism can contribute to the development of halitosis. Tangerman and colleagues found no association between halitosis and *H. pylori* infection.

Liver

Patients with various degrees of hepatocellular failure and/or portosystemic shunting of blood may acquire a sweet, musty, or even slightly fecal aroma of the breath, termed *fetor hepaticus*, which has been mainly attributed to the accumulation of dimethyl sulfide. Moreover, if the metabolizing function of the liver fails, the concentrations of certain metabolites normally processed in the liver will increase, and they will enter the systemic circulation again and be exhaled.

Kidney

Kidney insufficiency, primarily caused by chronic glomerulonephritis, leads to an increase of the amines dimethylamine and trimethylamine, causing a typical fishy odor of the breath.

Systemic Metabolic Disorders

Uncontrolled diabetes mellitus results in the accumulation of ketones, which have a sweet smell, like the odor of rotten apples. Insulin resistance leads to an increase of triglycerides and free fatty acids, and ketones (e.g., acetone, acetoacetate, and hydroxybutyrate) are formed during lipolysis.

Trimethylaminuria

Trimethylaminuria is a hereditary metabolic disorder that leads to a typical fishy odor of the breath, urine, sweat, and other bodily secretions. Trimethylaminuria is an enzymatic defect that prevents the transformation of trimethylamine to trimethylaminoxide, resulting in abnormal amounts of this molecule.

Mutations in SELENBP1

Mutations in *SELENBP1* have been attributed to be the underlying cause of a novel autosomal recessive malodor syndrome. Blood-borne extraoral halitosis was diagnosed in five patients with breath smelling like cabbage. Increased levels of methyl mercaptan and dimethyl sulfide were the main odorous compounds in their breath and were responsible for the malodor.

Hormonal Causes

At certain moments during the menstrual cycle, a typical breath odor can develop. Evidence also indicates that VSC levels in the expired air are increased twofold to fourfold around the day of ovulation and in the perimenstrual period. Increases in VSCs are smaller in midfollicular phases.

Medications

At least nine medications have been identified as potential sources of blood-borne extraoral halitosis. Dimethyl sulfoxide, cysteamine, and suplatast tosilate are known to be metabolized to dimethyl sulfide. Nitrates used to treat or prevent heart disease are metabolized to nitrite by the anaerobic bacteria. Some of this nitrite will reduce to nitric oxide, which can react with VSCs. Carbon disulfide can arise as a product of the metabolism of disulfiram (Antabuse). For drugs such as chloral hydrate, paraldehyde, and phenothiazide, the mode of action responsible of their association with halitosis is unclear. More recently, a systematic review extended the list to include other drug types such as anticholinergics, antidepressants, antifungals, chemotherapeutic agents, and dietary supplements (fish oil, selenium, and rose hip powder) as potential sources of extraoral halitosis.

Pseudo-Halitosis or Halitophobia

If a patient presents with complaints but no objective halitosis can be detected, one speaks of pseudo-halitosis or *imaginary breath odor*, which can lead to *halitophobia*. The latter is the case when,

TABLE 40.1 Odor Threshold and Odor Power of Key Malodorous

	ODOR THRESHOLDS		ODOR POWER	VOLATILITY (HENRY'S CONSTANTS)
Compounds	Greenman (mol/dm^{-3})	Devos (mol/dm^{-3})	Greenman (× increase to "up" score 1 unit)	Volatility (K_{cc}) in H_2O at 20°C
Butyrate	2.3×10^{-10}	2.4×10^{-10}	10-fold	3.9×10^{4}
Isovalerate	1.8×10^{-11}	2.5×10^{-11}	42-fold	2.5×10^{4}
Skatole	7.2×10^{-13}	1.0×10^{-12}	8-fold	4.1×10^{5}
Trimethylamine	1.8×10^{-11}	1.5×10^{-11}	96-fold (low affinity)	2.0×10^{2}
Putrescine	9.1×10^{-10}	1.0×10^{-9}	27-fold	4.1×10^{1}
CH_3SCH_3	5.9×10^{-8}	5.0×10^{-8}	10-fold	1.7×10^{1}
H_2S	6.4×10^{-10}	5.0×10^{-10}	4.8-fold	1.7×10^{1}
CH_3SH	1.0×10^{-11}	1.0×10^{-11}	7.2-fold	1.7×10^{1}

CH_3SH, Methyl mercaptan; *CH_3SCH_3,* dimethylsulfide; *H_2S,* hydrogen sulfide; *K_{cc},* unit for Henry's Law constant.
(From Devos M, Patte F, Rouault J, et al: Standardized human olfactory thresholds, *Oxford, 1990, IRL Press at Oxford University Press.)*
(From Greenman J, Duffield J, Spencer P, et al: J Dent Res *83:81, 2004.)*

even after repeated diagnosis of an absence of bad breath, the patient cannot accept the absence of halitosis. This condition has been associated with obsessive-compulsive disorder and hypochondria. Well-established personality disorder questionnaires (e.g., Symptom Checklist 90) allow the clinician to assess the patient's tendency for illusional breath malodor. Having a psychologist or psychiatrist at the malodor consultation can be especially helpful for such patients. Because of the complexity of this disorder, a malodor consultation is thus preferably multidisciplinary, combining the knowledge of a periodontologist or dentist, an ENT specialist, an internist (if necessary), and a psychologist or psychiatrist.

Fundamentals of Malodor Detection

The breath of a person contains up to 150 different molecules. The characteristics of the expired molecules determine whether we can smell them or not. Some gases can cause a striking odor at very low concentrations, whereas others need to be present in much higher quantities. The perception of the molecules depends on the following factors:

1. The odor itself *(olfactory response)* can be pleasant, unpleasant, or even repulsive.
2. Each particular molecule has its specific concentration before it can be detected *(threshold concentration).*
3. The *odor power* is the extent of concentration that is necessary to increase the odor score with one unit.
4. The *volatility* of the compound: Malodorous molecules only express themselves when they become volatile.
5. The *substantivity:* The capacity of the molecule to stay present and thus to remain the cause of smell.

Table 40.1 provides an overview of these essential characteristics for the key malodorous compounds, clearly highlighting large interproduct variations. The odor power is the strongest for hydrogen sulfide and methyl mercaptan; if the concentration of these products increases 5- to 10-fold, the odor will receive a higher organoleptic rating. For some other compounds, increases of 25–100 times are needed to reach a similar effect. Skatole and methyl mercaptan are detected at the lowest concentrations (low threshold). The three sulfur molecules have the lowest volatility (i.e., will escape the liquid phase first).

In a study by Kleinberg and Codipilly, aqueous solutions of oral odoriferous volatiles were placed on the skin of the back of the hand. Afterward, odor scores were given (organoleptic score; see earlier). The results are shown in Table 40.2. All metabolites caused an explicit odor, which decreased in intensity over time. Some molecules disappeared very fast (e.g., hydrogen sulfide and methyl mercaptan), whereas others produced an unpleasant smell for a longer period of time (e.g., indole and skatole, for 10 min and longer).

TABLE 40.2 Odor Scores at the Back of the Hand

	Start	1 min	3 min	10 min
Hydrogen sulfide	3	1	0	0
Methyl mercaptan	3	1	0	0
Acetic acid	3	4	0	0
Propionic acid	3	4	0	0
Butyric acid	4	4	2	2
Valeric acid	4	4	3	2
Indole	4	4	4	2
Skatole	4	4	4	2
Putrescine	4	4	3	1
Cadaverine	4	4	2	1

The olfactory response, rated by an organoleptic scale, follows an exponential curve when correlated with the concentration of different gases. In other words, when the concentrations of the molecules were compared to their organoleptic outcomes, an optimal fit was obtained only when the concentrations of the gases were transformed to log values. The latter implies that all types of breath "measurements" [gas chromatography, portable breath analyzers (e.g., Halimeter, Interscan, Chatsworth, Calif)] require log transformation to be comparable with organoleptic scores.

Diagnosis of Malodor

Preconsultation Approach

A proper diagnostic approach starts with providing the right information to the patient before the appointment. It is recommended that the patient does not eat garlic, onions, or spices for 2 days before the consultation because they can cause bad breath and body odor that can last from several hours to 2 days. To remove confounding odors, the patient is also instructed to refrain from alcohol, coffee, and smoking during the 12-h period before the consultation. For the same reason, it is advisable not to use chewing gum, mints, drops, or mouthrinses during the 8 h preceding the appointment, both for the patient and for the oral malodor judge. The day of the consultation, the use of fragranced shampoo, body lotion, and perfume should also be avoided, so as not to disturb the organoleptic ratings. In most halitosis consultations, the patient is asked not to eat or drink on the morning of the examination. However, if breakfast is consumed, morning bad breath can be excluded.

Course of a Halitosis Consultation

Preconsultation patient information
Anamnesis
Organoleptic examination
Examination of the breath with portable sulfur monitor
Oropharyngeal examination
Explanation of halitosis and instructions for oral hygiene
If necessary, explanation of additional therapy

The patient should be encouraged to bring a confidant to the consultations who can identify whether the perceived odor is the one previously noticed. Some of these guidelines are crucial not only for the organoleptic evaluation but also for a correct interpretation of the results obtained with certain breath analyzers (see later).

Anamnesis

Each consultation should start with a thorough questioning about the breath malodor, eating habits, and medical and dental history. This can be done with a questionnaire that the patient fills out in the waiting room and/or orally at the beginning of the consultation, depending on the preferences of the examiner and the practical possibilities. To start with, the patient should be asked about the frequency of the halitosis (e.g., constantly, every day), the time of appearance during the day (e.g., after meals can indicate a stomach hernia), when the problem first appeared and whether others have identified the problem (to exclude imaginary breath odor). Also the medical history has to be recorded, with an emphasis on medication, and systemic diseases of the lungs, liver, kidneys, stomach, and pancreas. Concerning the ENT history, attention should be paid to the presence of nasal obstruction, mouth breathing, postnasal drip, allergy, tonsillitis, dysphagia, and previous ENT encounters. The dental history includes questions assessing the frequency of dental visits, the use of mouth rinses, the presence and maintenance of a dental prosthesis, and the frequency and the instruments used for tooth brushing, interdental cleaning, and tongue brushing and scraping. Finally, the patient is asked about his smoking, drinking, and dietary habits.

Examinations

After obtaining a thorough anamnesis, the clinician checks whether an unpleasant odor can be perceived and inspects the mouth to detect possible causes of bad breath. Different ways exist to examine the breath. The easiest and least expensive way is to smell the breath. However, several devices are on the market that mainly detect VSCs.

Organoleptic Rating

Even though devices are available, organoleptic assessment by a judge is still the gold standard in the examination of breath malodor. It is the easiest and most often used method because it gives a reflection of the everyday situation when halitosis is noticed. Moreover, the human nose can smell 10,000 different odors, many more than any device on the market. In an organoleptic evaluation, a trained and preferably calibrated "judge" sniffs the expired air and assesses whether it is unpleasant by using an intensity rating. Scoring is normally done according to the intensity scale of Rosenberg, where 0 represents the absence of odor, 1 is barely noticeable odor, 2 is slight malodor, 3 is moderate malodor, 4 is strong malodor, and 5 is severe malodor. In this six-point system, 0 indicates a concentration of odorant below a threshold, 1–4 are increasing occupancy of receptor binding sites, and 5 is assumed to be close to saturation. To avoid bias, it is advisable that the organoleptic assessment precedes all other measurements.

Before acting as a judge, clinicians must ensure they do not have *anosmia* (lost or impaired smelling capacity). A significant fraction of the adult population has partial loss of smelling acuity. After age 60, a decline of smelling acuity is common. Candidate odor judges should test their capacity to smell and recognize different odors (qualitative assessment), as well as to detect odors at low concentrations (quantitative assessment). The first aspect can be checked by using, for example, a commercially available test (Smell Identification Test, Sensonic) that establishes a response curve based on the capacity to recognize and discriminate among smells. After scratching an odorous surface in a booklet, several options of smells are proposed. If the candidate judge lacks the capacity to recognize certain odors, it will reveal partial anosmia. The second aspect is tested by sniffing a series of dilutions of substances such as isovaleric acid, phenethyl alcohol, thiophene, and pyridine, which are inexpensive organic components. These are presented to the candidate judge as dilutions, in one-log dilution steps from 1 to 10^{-1}. Concentrations of the odorous substances are presented in ascending order until the person detects the substance, then in descending order until he or she no longer detects it. This is the "psychophysical staircase method" for determining the threshold level. The threshold corresponds to the average between ascending and descending levels. Clinicians can thus find out whether their smelling threshold level is acceptable. Abnormalities in the capacity to judge or perceive odors can be caused by a viral infection of the nasal cavities, a concussion, or smoking. Whereas an infection can have a transient effect on olfactory performance, concussion and smoking have permanent effects.

In an organoleptic assessment, the judge smells a series of air samples (Fig. 40.3), as follows:

1. *Nasal breath odor:* The subject expires through the nose while keeping the mouth closed. When the nasal expiration is malodorous yet the air expired through the mouth is not, an ENT problem can be suspected.
2. *Oral cavity odor (passive):* The subject opens the mouth and refrains from breathing while the judge places his or her nose close to the mouth opening (approximately 10 cm from the patient's mouth).
3. *Oral cavity odor (active):* The patient counts from 1 to 10. This reveals the same as described earlier but favors oral malodor because of drying of the palatal and tongue mucosa.
4. *Tongue coating:* The judge smells a tongue scraping from the posterior part of the tongue, obtained with an odorless plastic spoon or tongue scraper, at a distance of approximately 5 cm from his or her nose. This odor resembles that emanating from the tongue dorsum.

Although the organoleptic assessment is still the gold standard for diagnosis of halitosis, the method also has some important drawbacks. The assessment can, for example, be influenced by several aspects, such as the position of the head, hunger, and the experience of the judge. Odor judges are also supposed to rest their nose for several minutes between tests to avoid habituation. The most important disadvantage of the method, however, is that it clearly has a degree of subjectivity. Researchers are trying to improve the reliability and reproducibility of the organoleptic method. When using a panel of odor judges instead of one judge, the reliability is already considered to increase. Furthermore, the agreement among judges may be

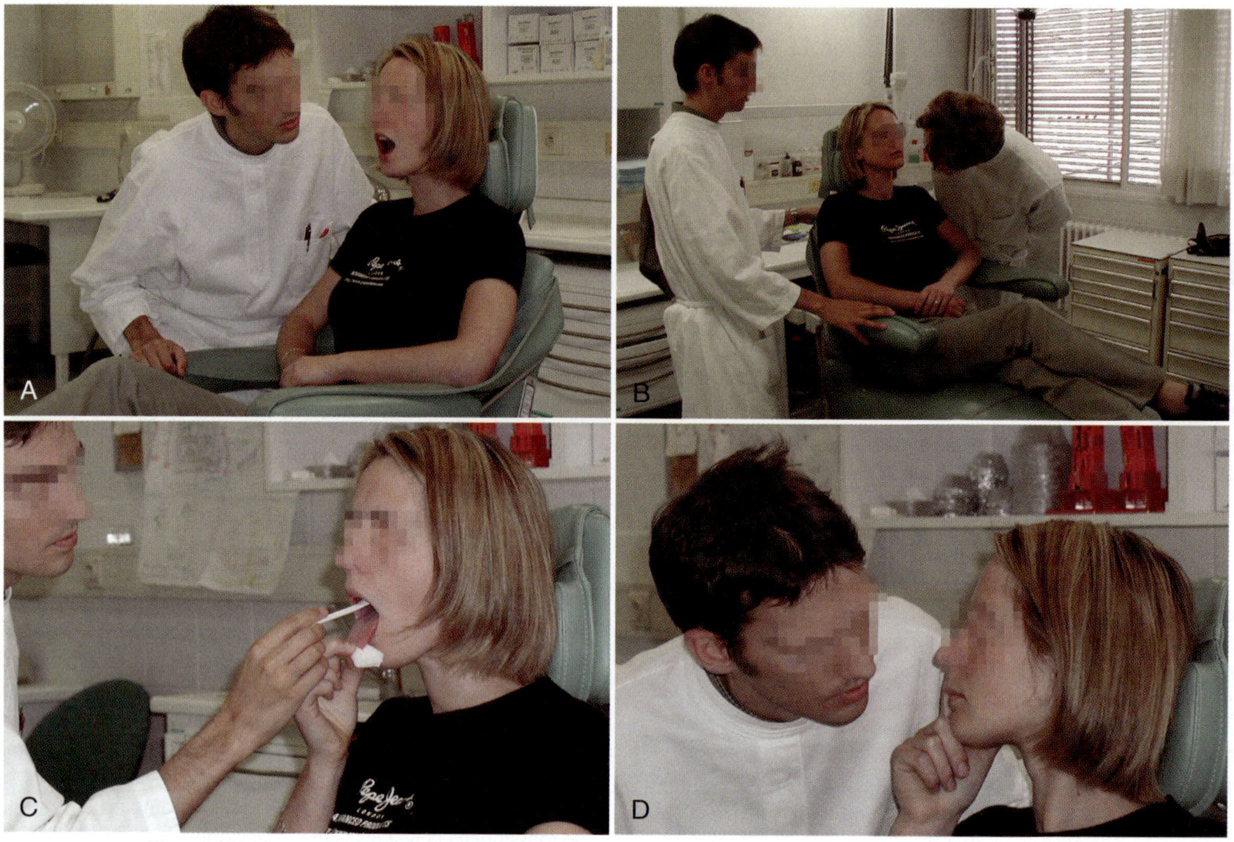

Fig. 40.3 A, Organoleptic assessment of the oral cavity odor while the patients refrains from breathing. B, Assessment of the oral cavity odor when the patient counts out loud from 1 to 10. C, A sample of the tongue coating is taken to smell afterward. D, The nasal odor is rated.

improved by standardization of the sense of smell using an odor solution kit for measuring the olfactory response. Training is also considered to reduce odor judges' errors.

Negative Pressure or Kim Method

The organoleptic method performed as described above can be a source of stress for the patients because of the proximity of the judge when sniffing the breath. In an attempt to improve this shortcoming, the use of a privacy screen or performing the test starting at a longer distance (1 m) have been used previously. Kim and colleagues have proposed a method for air sample collection that allows the organoleptic evaluation to be performed away from the patient. With this technique, a sample of mouth air is collected with a gas-tight syringe through negative pressure (hence, the given name of the procedure). The air sample is expelled into a plastic nonsmelling cup with the help of a needle. The judge holds the cup over the nose to rate the sample also according to the intensity scale of Rosenberg. The method also showed high sensitivity (80.1%) and specificity (94.2%). Even though the same considerations regarding minimizing odor interferences must be maintained, this method presents the advantage of being less affected by the presence of other odorants, as in case of body odor or the use of scented cosmetic products by the patient. Another relevant feature of the method is the possibility of assessing the exact same sample by more than one odor judge. A breath odor evaluation by an odor judge panel requires consecutive sampling and/or sequential measurements that might vary in concentration and even composition. The main disadvantage from this method is that it cannot be used for the evaluation of a sample of nasal air. Therefore, in the case of halitosis of extraoral origin, some relevant information could be overlooked.

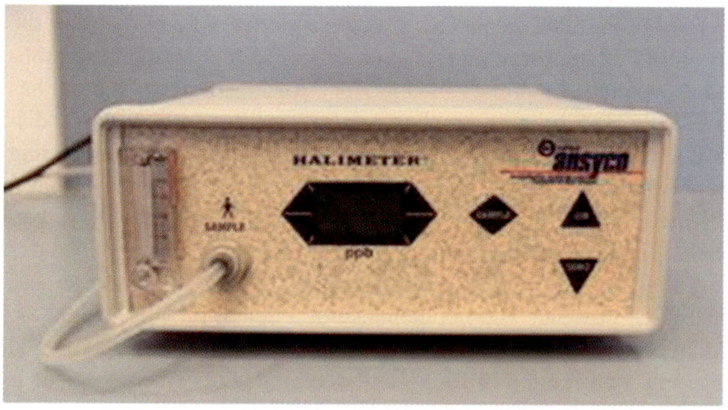

Fig. 40.4 Halimeter.

Portable Volatile Sulfur Monitor

The Halimeter (Interscan, Chatsworth, CA) is an electronic device that detects the presence of VSCs such as hydrogen sulfide and methyl mercaptan in breath. The instrument cannot discriminate among the different sulfur compounds. The sensitivity for methylmercaptan is five times lower than for hydrogen sulfide, and the device is almost insensitive to dimethyl sulfide. Moreover, ethanol and other compounds can disturb the measurements.

To allow an increase in concentration of VSCs, the patient has to keep his or her mouth closed for 2 to 3 min before sampling. The mouth air is aspirated by inserting a drinking straw fixed on the flexible tube of the instrument (Fig. 40.4). The straw is kept inside the mouth, preferably above the posterior part of the tongue dorsum, not touching the oral mucosa or the tongue, while the subject

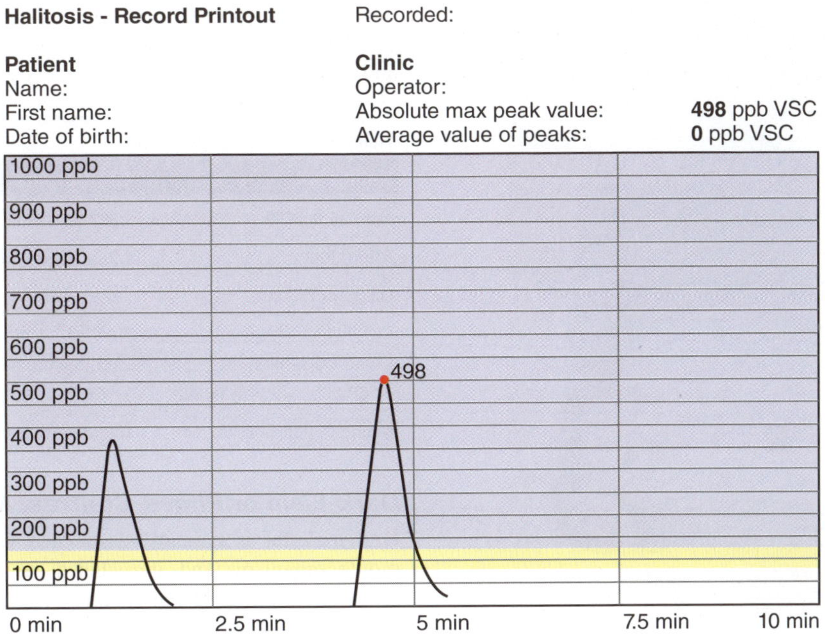

Fig. 40.5 Haligram.

keeps the mouth slightly open and breathes through the nose. The sulfur meter uses a voltametric sensor that generates a signal when exposed to sulfur-containing gases. Using a recorder or specific software, a graphic presentation can be obtained, called a *haligram* (Fig. 40.5), which gives the response as a function of time. For the most optimal results, the manufacturer recommends performing three measurements and using the average value. Between measurements, it is important to allow the meter to restabilize before repeating. The monitor needs regular calibration and replacement of the sensor biannually.

The Halimeter is easy to use as a chair-side test and is relatively inexpensive. Patients are usually less embarrassed by this examination than by organoleptic assessment. Moreover the absence of odor in cases of halitophobia can be more convincingly proven than by an organoleptic assessment. Several studies have shown good correlations between the organoleptic measurement and the Halimeter. An important drawback of the device is that it detects only sulfur compounds and thus is useful only for intraoral causes of halitosis. The absence of VSCs does not prove that no breath odor is present.

A wide range of threshold limits for halitosis has been proposed. Yaegaki and Sanade recommended a value of 75 ppb as the limit for social acceptance, whereas the Halimeter's manufacturer proposes 150 ppb. Following this recommendation, the sensitivity and specificity of the device for the organoleptic score have been calculated to be 63% and 98%, respectively. Previous studies from our group showed that a reduction in this threshold to 120 ppb improves the sensitivity of the device without detriment to specificity. In patients with oral malodor, VSC concentrations can easily reach 300–400 ppb.

Gas Chromatography

A gas chromatograph can analyze air, saliva, or crevicular fluid (Fig. 40.6). About 100 compounds have been isolated from the headspace of saliva and tongue coating, including ketones, alkanes, sulfur-containing compounds, and phenyl compounds. In the expired air of a person, at least 150 compounds can be found. The most important advantage of the technique is that when coupled with mass spectrometry, it can detect virtually any compound when using adequate materials and conditions. Moreover, it has very high sensitivity and specificity.

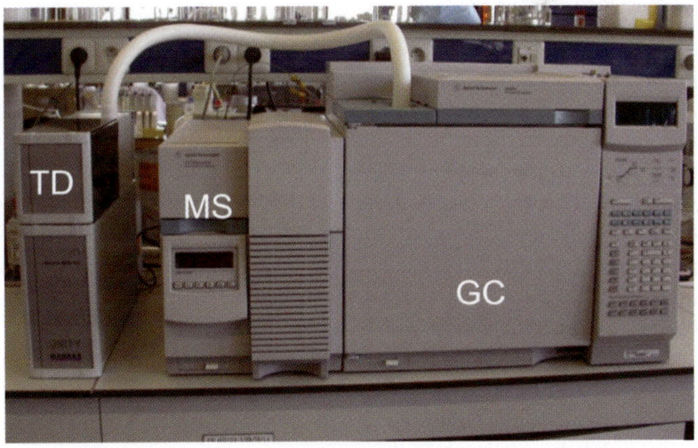

Fig. 40.6 Gas chromatography machinery, including thermal desorber *(TD)* to release molecules trapped in special collectors); gas chromatograph *(GC)* for separation of molecules; and mass spectrometer *(MS)* for identification of molecules.

Elaborate gas chromatography is available only in specialized centers but is especially useful for identifying nonoral causes. It is expensive and requires trained personnel.

A small, portable "gas chromatograph" (OralChroma, Nissha FIS, Inc., Japan) has been introduced, which makes this technique available for periodontal clinics (Fig. 40.7). More recently, the second generation of this portable gas chromatograph was introduced: the OralChroma CHM-2. The CHM-2 is a little bit smaller than the first-generation OralChroma, the measurements only take half the time, and it comes with optimized software. Sample collection is done by use of a disposable syringe, which is inserted two-thirds of the way into the oral cavity. The patient must close the mouth for 30 s before sample collection, and afterward the sample is injected into the gas chromatograph.

The analysis starts automatically. A software packet, OralChroma Data Manager, collects the data from the OralChroma and

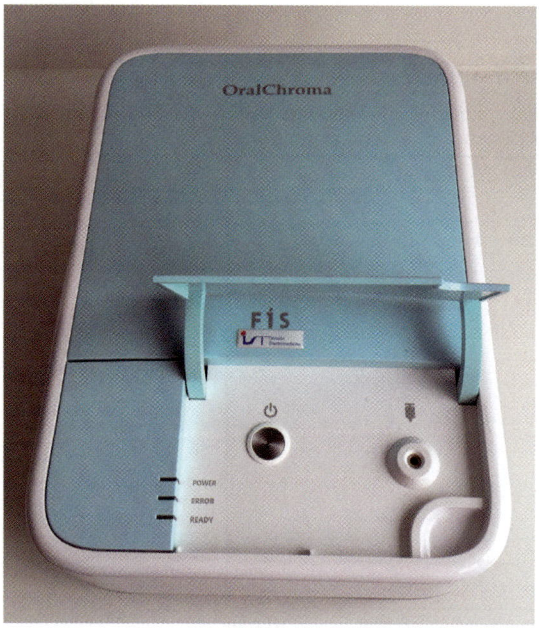

Fig. 40.7 Portable gas chromatograph (GC). A small amount of the breath sample, aspirated with a plastic syringe, is injected into the input port of the GC. The computer displays the detection and amount of the three important VSCs (in ppb) within 8 min.

graphically displays the sensor responses on a computer screen. After 4 min for the OralChroma CHM-2, the process is completed, and the concentrations of the three gases are displayed in either ng/10 mL or ppb (nmol/mol) (Fig. 40.8). The accompanying software packet gives a clear overview of the VSC measurement. However, with the OralChroma CHM-1, sometimes these graphics are not correct because the place of the VSCs is incorrectly assigned in the chromatogram. The latter can be corrected by analyzing the chromatograph.

The OralChroma has the capacity to measure the concentration of the three key sulfur compounds (hydrogen sulfide, methyl mercaptan, and dimethyl sulfide) separately. This can be helpful for a differential diagnosis. A high concentration of methyl mercaptan compared to hydrogen sulfide indicates, for example, periodontitis. If only hydrogen sulfide is increased, a problem with oral hygiene may exist. Dimethyl sulfide can indicate an extraoral cause. Just like the Halimeter, the OralChroma cannot detect compounds other than sulfur compounds, and some intraoral and extraoral causes can thus be overlooked. The apparatus needs calibration and the sensor and column need to be replaced every 2 years.

Halimeter Versus OralChroma

Halimeter	OralChroma
Easy to handle	Easy to handle
Affordable	More expensive
Displays results immediately	Takes 4 min (CHM-2) or 8 min (CHM-1) before measurements are shown
Cannot discriminate among different gases	Can discriminate among hydrogen sulfide, methyl mercaptan, and dimethyl sulfide
Maintenance needed	Maintenance needed

Dark-Field or Phase-Contrast Microscopy

Oral malodor is typically associated with a higher incidence of motile organisms and spirochetes, so shifts in their proportions allow monitoring of therapeutic progress. Another advantage of direct microscopy is that the patient becomes aware of bacteria present in plaque, tongue coating, and saliva. Too often, patients confuse plaque with food remnants.

Oropharyngeal Examination

The oropharyngeal examination includes inspection of deep carious lesions, interdental food impaction, wounds, bleeding of the gums, periodontal pockets, tongue coating, dry mouth, and the tonsils and pharynx (for tonsillitis and pharyngitis).

The tongue coating can be scored with regard to thickness and surface. Several methods have been proposed for thickness; Gross and coworkers, in 1975, proposed an index ranging from 0 (no coating) to 3 (severe coating). Miyazaki (Fig. 40.9A) assessed tongue-coating status according to area: 0 = none visible, 1 = less than one-third of the tongue dorsum covered, 2 = less than two-thirds, and 3 = more than two-thirds.

Winkel and coworkers considered both the extension and the thickness of the tongue coating. The dorsum of the tongue is divided into six areas, three in the posterior and three in the anterior of the tongue (see Fig. 40.9B). The tongue coating in each sextant is scored as follows: 0 = no coating, 1 = light coating, and 2 = severe coating. A score of 1 is given when the pink color underneath the coating is still visible; when this is not the case, 2 is given.

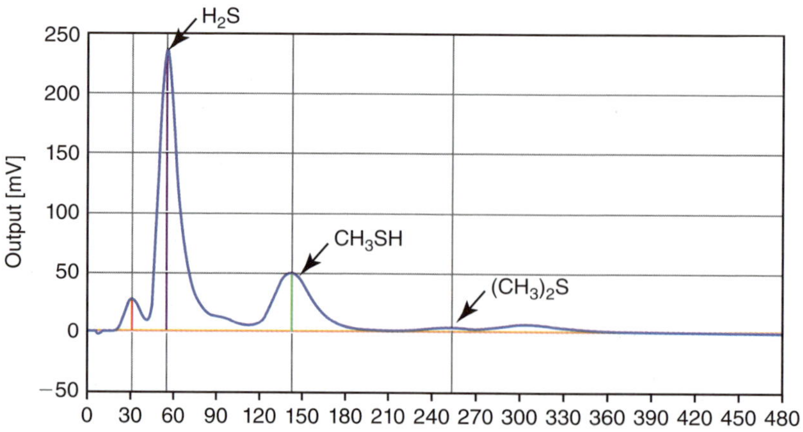

Fig. 40.8 Graphic from the OralChroma. The first peak indicates the level of hydrogen sulfide, the second of methyl mercaptan, and the third of dimethyl sulfide.

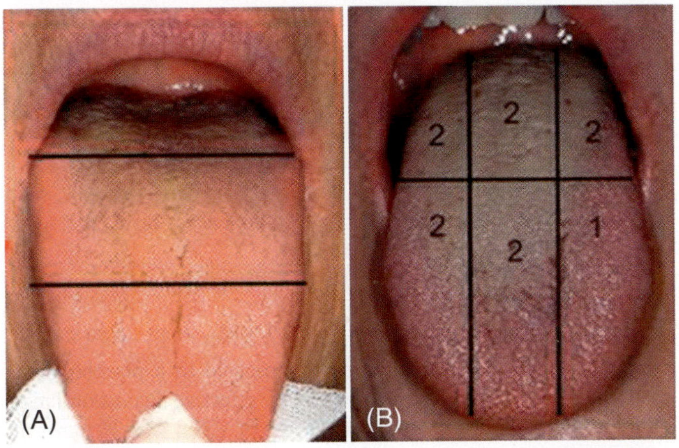

Fig. 40.9 A, Miyazaki tongue coating index. Score 0 = none visible, score 1 = less than one-third of the tongue dorsum covered, score 2 = less than two-thirds, and score 3 = more than two-thirds; here score 2 applies since less than two-thirds of the tongue dorsum is covered. B, Winkel tongue coating index. Divide the dorsum of the tongue is into six areas, that is, three in the posterior and three in the anterior part of the tongue. The tongue coating in each sextant is scored as 0 = no coating, 1 = light coating, and 2 = severe coating.

Attention should be paid to the morphology of the tongue. For example, the clinician should note whether the tongue looks normal or rough or has a deep sulcus or large papillae vallatae.

Self-Examination

Smelling one's own breath by expiring into the hands in front of the mouth is not relevant because the nose becomes used to the odor, and the smell of the skin and soap used for handwashing may interfere. Moreover, studies have shown that self-assessment of oral malodor is notoriously unreliable, and one should be careful with such information obtained from the patient.

Saliva Incubation Test

The analysis of the headspace above incubated saliva by gas chromatography reveals VSCs and other compounds such as indole, skatole, lactic acid, methylamine, diphenylamine, cadaverine, putrescine, urea, ammonia, dodecanol, and tetradecanol. By adding some proteins, such as lysine or cysteine, the production of cadaverine or hydrogen sulfide is dramatically increased. Organoleptic evaluation (or assessment of the VSCs) of the saliva headspace offers promising perspectives for monitoring treatment results. It is a less invasive test, especially for the patient, than smelling breath in front of the oral cavity. It is, however, impractical and time consuming and therefore only used for research purposes.

Electronic Nose

An electronic nose identifies the specific components of an odor and analyzes its chemical makeup. Also known as artificially intelligent olfaction, it consists of a mechanism for chemical detection, such as an array of electronic sensors, and a mechanism for pattern recognition. It is smaller, less expensive, and easier to use than, for example, gas chromatography, but can be developed only for specific applications if the important metabolites are already known. An artificial nose that has the same capacities as the human nose would be ideal. Currently, although significant improvements still need to be made, the first trials thus far have been promising.

Chair-Side Test

A salivary chair-side test may be an alternative for the general practitioner for diagnosing halitosis. Currently, several tests based on the detection of bacteria and metabolites involved in the process of oral malodor are commercially available. All these tests have reported acceptable correlation with the organoleptic ratings, some even with the VSC level. The BANA test is based on the ability of some bacterial species to hydrolyze a synthetic trypsin substrate (N-benzoyl-DL-arginine-2-naphthylamine). In this way, the test can detect three specific bacteria related to periodontal disease: *P. gingivalis*, *Bacteroides forsythus*, and *Treponema denticola*. As already mentioned, periodontitis is not the most common cause of oral malodor, given that not all patients with periodontitis have bad breath.

The β-galactosidase tests quantify, by means of chromogenic substrates, bacterial enzymes involved in the initial degradation of oral mucin. β-Galactosidase is one of the main enzymes responsible for the removal of carbohydrate side chains, a limiting step in the proteolysis of glycoproteins. It has been demonstrated that the presence of the enzyme accounts for the presence of oral malodor independent of the VSC level. The *ninhydrin* method is a colorimetric test to determine amino acids and low-molecular-weight amines. These compounds are, like VSCs, final products of bacterial proteolysis.

A newer colorimetric test offers the possibility of assessing amines in saliva by means of a simple color scale. In a first clinical study, the test appeared to be able to distinguish between volunteers with and without malodor. Besides the correlation of the test results with the organoleptic rating, the independent contribution to the odor of the amines in saliva has been demonstrated.

Treatment of Oral Malodor

The treatment of oral malodor (with an intraoral origin) should preferably because related therapy. Because oral malodor is caused by the metabolic degradation of available proteins to malodorous gases by certain oral microorganisms, the following general treatment strategies can be applied:

- Mechanical reduction of intraoral nutrients (substrates) and microorganisms.
- Chemical reduction of oral microbial load.
- Rendering malodorous gases nonvolatile.
- Masking the malodor.

Treatment should be centered on reducing the bacterial load and micronutrients by effective mechanical oral hygiene procedures, including tongue scraping. Periodontal disease should be treated and controlled, and as an auxiliary aid, oral rinses containing chlorhexidine and other ingredients may further reduce the oral malodor. If breath malodor persists after these approaches, other sources of the malodor, such as the tonsils, lung disease, gastrointestinal disease, or metabolic abnormalities (e.g., diabetes), should be investigated.

Mechanical Reduction of Intraoral Nutrients and Microorganisms

Because of the extensive accumulation of bacteria on the dorsum of the tongue, tongue cleaning should be emphasized. Previous investigations demonstrated that tongue cleaning reduces both the amount of coating (and thus bacterial nutrients) and the number of bacteria and thereby improves oral malodor effectively. Other reports indicated that the reduction of the microbial load on the tongue after cleaning is negligible and that the reduced malodor probably results from the reduction of bacterial nutrients.

Cleaning of the tongue can be done with a normal toothbrush but preferably with a tongue scraper if a coating is established. Tongue cleaning using a tongue scraper reduces halitosis levels by 75% after 1 week. This should be gentle cleaning to prevent soft tissue damage. It is best to clean as far backward as possible; the posterior portion of the tongue has the most coating. Tongue cleaning should be repeated until almost no coating material can be removed. The gagging reflex is often elicited, especially when using brushes; practice helps to prevent this. It can also be helpful to pull the tongue out with a gauze pad. Tongue cleaning has the additional benefit of improving taste sensation.

Interdental cleaning and toothbrushing are essential mechanical means of dental plaque control. Both remove residual food particles and organisms that cause putrefaction. Clinical studies have shown that the mechanical action of toothbrushing alone has no appreciable influence on the concentration of VSCs. In a short-term study, Tonzetich showed a short-term effect on bad breath after brushing with a sodium monofluorophosphate toothpaste. However, the effect was half of what was observed when combined with tongue brushing (73% and 30% reduction in VSCs, respectively).

When chronic oral malodor arises as a consequence of periodontitis, professional periodontal therapy is needed. A one-stage full-mouth disinfection, combining scaling and root planing with the application of chlorhexidine, reduced organoleptic malodor levels up to 90% in one study. In another study by the same investigators, initial periodontal therapy had only a weak impact on VSC levels, except when combined with a mouthrinse containing chlorhexidine.

Chewing gum may control bad breath temporarily because it can stimulate salivary flow. The salivary flow itself also has a mechanical cleaning capability. Not surprisingly, therefore, subjects with extremely low salivary flow rate have higher VSC ratings and tongue coating scores than those with normal saliva production. Waler showed that chewing gum without any active ingredient can reduce halitosis modestly.

Chemical Reduction of Oral Microbial Load

Together with toothbrushing, mouth rinsing has become a common oral hygiene practice. Formulations have been modified to carry antimicrobial and oxidizing agents, impacting the process of oral malodor formation. The active ingredients usually include antimicrobial agents such as chlorhexidine, cetylpyridinium chloride (CPC), essential oils, chlorine dioxide, triclosan, amine fluoride and stannous fluoride, hydrogen peroxide, and baking soda. Some of these agents have only a temporary effect on the total number of microorganisms in the oral cavity.

Chlorhexidine

Chlorhexidine is considered the most effective antiplaque and antigingivitis agent. Its antibacterial action can be explained by disruption of the bacterial cell membrane by the chlorhexidine molecules, thus increasing its permeability and resulting in cell lysis and death. Because of its strong antibacterial effects and superior substantivity in the oral cavity, chlorhexidine rinsing provides significant reductions in VSC levels and organoleptic ratings.

Rosenberg and associates showed that a 0.2% chlorhexidine regimen produced a 43% reduction in VSC values and >50% reduction in organoleptic mouth odor ratings. De Boever and Loesche reported that 1 week of rinsing with 0.12% chlorhexidine gluconate, in combination with tooth and tongue brushing, significantly reduced VSC levels, mouth odor, and tongue odor by 73%, 69%, and 78%, respectively. Morning halitosis was reduced up to 90%. Halita (Dentaid, Spain), a solution of 0.05% chlorhexidine, 0.05% CPC, and 0.14% zinc lactate, without alcohol, was even more efficient than chlorhexidine alone, suggesting that the other compounds are also important. This is explained by a synergistic effect between chlorhexidine and CPC, and between chlorhexidine and zinc (Zn^{++}). The latter was confirmed in a randomized controlled trial where amine fluoride/stannous fluoride solution showed improved outcomes when Zn^{++} was added.

Unfortunately, as mentioned in some trials, chlorhexidine at a concentration of 0.2% or greater also has some disadvantages, such as increased tooth and tongue staining, unpleasant taste, and some temporary reduction in taste sensation.

Essential Oils

Previous studies evaluated the short-term effect (3 h) of a Listerine rinse (which contains essential oils) compared to a placebo rinse. Listerine was found to be only moderately effective against oral malodor (±25% reduction vs 10% for placebo of VSCs after 30 min) and caused a sustained reduction in the levels of odorigenic bacteria. Similar VSC reductions were found after rinsing for 4 days.

Chlorine Dioxide

Chlorine dioxide (ClO_2) is a powerful oxidizing agent that can eliminate bad breath by oxidation of hydrogen sulfide, methyl mercaptan, and the amino acids methionine and cysteine. Studies demonstrated that a single use of a chlorine dioxide-containing oral rinse slightly reduced mouth odor.

Two-Phase Oil–Water Rinse

Rosenberg and colleagues designed a two-phase oil–water rinse containing CPC. The efficacy of oil–water-CPC formulations is thought to result from the adhesion of a high proportion of oral microorganisms to the oil droplets that is further enhanced by the CPC. A twice-daily rinse with this product (before bedtime and in the morning) showed reductions in both VSC levels and organoleptic ratings. These reductions were superior to those seen with Listerine and were significantly superior to placebo.

Triclosan

Triclosan, a broad-spectrum antibacterial agent, has been found to be effective against most oral bacteria and has good compatibility with other compounds used for oral home care. A pilot study demonstrated that an experimental mouthrinse containing 0.15% triclosan and 0.84% zinc (Zn^{++}) produced a stronger and more prolonged reduction in mouth odor than Listerine rinse. The anti-VSC effect of triclosan, however, seems strongly dependent on the solubilizing agents. Flavoring oils or anionic detergents and copolymers are added to increase the oral retention and decrease the rate of release in toothpaste formulations containing triclosan. The effects of these formulations in oral malodor have been illustrated in several studies. Significant reduction of breath scores were observed after a single use as well as after a week (28% and >50%, respectively), with a similar effect on VSC levels (57% reduction after 1 week of using the paste).

Amine Fluoride or Stannous Fluoride

The association of amine fluoride with stannous fluoride resulted in encouraging reductions of morning breath odor, even when oral hygiene was insufficient. More recent evidence supporting the use of this rinse has become available. The formulation showed not only short-term but also long-term effects on malodor indicators in patients with obvious malodor.

Stannous fluoride has also been shown to be effective in the management of oral malodor as a component of a dentifrice, reducing both organoleptic scores and VSC levels. A superior short-term and overnight benefit of a stannous-containing dentifrice versus a control dentifrice on morning bad breath was demonstrated in a meta-analysis.

Hydrogen Peroxide

Suarez and colleagues reported that rinsing with 3% hydrogen peroxide (H_2O_2) produced impressive reductions (±90%) in sulfur gases that persisted for 8 h.

Oxidizing Lozenges

Greenstein and associates reported that sucking a lozenge with oxidizing properties reduced tongue dorsum malodor for 3 h. This antimalodor effect may be caused by the activity of dehydroascorbic acid, which is generated by peroxide-mediated oxidation of ascorbate in the lozenges.

Baking Soda

Baking soda dentifrices have been shown to confer a significant odor-reducing benefit for up to 3 h. The mechanism by which baking soda produces its inhibition of oral malodor is related to its bactericidal effects.

Conversion of Volatile Sulfur Compounds

Metal Salt Solutions

Metal ions with an affinity for sulfur are efficient in capturing the sulfur-containing gases. Zinc is an ion with two positive charges (Zn^{++}), which will bind to the twice-negatively loaded sulfur radicals and thus reduce the expression of VSCs. The same applies for other metal ions such as stannous, mercury, and copper. Clinically, the VSC inhibitory effect was copper chloride > stannous fluoride > zinc chloride ($CuCl_2 > SnF_2 > ZnCl_2$). In vitro, the inhibitory effect was mercury chloride = copper chloride = cadmium chloride > zinc chloride > stannous fluoride > tin chloride > lead chloride ($HgCl_2 = CuCl_2 = CdCl_2 > ZnCl_2 > SnF_2 > SnCl_2 > PbCl_2$).

Compared to other metal ions, Zn^{++} is relatively nontoxic and noncumulative and gives no visible discoloration. Thus, Zn^{++} has been one of the most-studied ingredients for the control of oral malodor. Schmidt and Tarbet reported that a rinse containing zinc chloride was remarkably more effective than a saline rinse (or no treatment) in reducing the levels of both VSCs (±80% reduction) and organoleptic scores (±40% reduction) for 3 h.

As mentioned, Halita, a rinse containing 0.05% chlorhexidine, 0.05% CPC, and 0.14% zinc lactate, has been even more efficient than a 0.2% chlorhexidine formulation in reducing VSC levels and organoleptic ratings. The special effect of Halita may result from the VSC conversion ability of Zn^{++}, besides its antimicrobial action. The combination of Zn^{++} and chlorhexidine seems to act synergistically.

Similar observations have been reported for a chlorhexidine-free mouthrinse. The addition of zinc ions to a basic formulation containing amino fluoride and stannous fluoride caused short- and long-term reduction of oral malodor indicators in volunteers with morning bad breath as well as in volunteers with obvious halitosis.

In a study by Hoshi and van Steenberghe, a zinc citrate/triclosan toothpaste applied to the tongue dorsum appeared to control morning breath malodor for 4 h. If the flavor oil was removed, however, the antimalodor efficacy of the active ingredients decreased. Another clinical study reported up to a 41% reduction in VSC levels after 7 days' use of a dentifrice containing triclosan and a copolymer, but the benefit compared to a placebo was relatively small (17% reduction). Similar reductions were also found in two other more recent studies.

Chewing gum can be formulated with antibacterial agents, such as fluoride or chlorhexidine, helping to reduce oral malodor through both mechanical and chemical approaches. Tsunoda and associate investigated the beneficial effect of chewing gum containing tea extracts for its deodorizing mechanism. *Epigallocatechin* is the main deodorizing agent among the tea catechins. The chemical reaction between epigallocatechin and methyl mercaptan results in a nonvolatile product. Waler compared different concentrations of Zn^{++} in a chewing gum and found that a 2-mg Zn^{++} acetate-containing chewing gum that remained in the mouth for 5 min resulted in an immediate reduction in VSC levels of up to 45%, but the long-term effect was not mentioned.

Potential New Strategies to Alleviate Intraoral Halitosis

The number of products claiming to be able control, combat, or solve the problem of halitosis has increased significantly in the past decade, but with only limited research supporting their rationale of use, as pointed out in previous systematic reviews. Alternative therapies listed below, although promising, need to be evaluated in long-term follow-up studies before they can be taken into full consideration by professionals treating the condition.

Probiotics

Probiotics are "living organisms which, when administered in adequate amounts, confer a health benefit for the host." Their use has been approved by the World Health Organization (WHO) and the Food and Agriculture Organization of the United Nations (FAO). The rationale for probiotic use is to restore the microbial balance by adding beneficial species. Probiotics can modulate the host inflammatory response or have direct and indirect effects against pathogenic bacteria.

Herbal Substances

Green tea polyphenolic catechins have an impact on oral health via **antiseptic**, antioxidative, and antiinflammatory activity. *Epigallocatechin gallate* is the main deodorizing agent among the tea catechins. The chemical reaction between epigallocatechin and methylmercaptan results in a nonvolatile product. They are also able to suppress *mgl*, the **gene** encoding l-methionine-α-deamino-γ-mercaptomethane lyase, responsible for CH_3SH production by oral anaerobes.

Masking the Malodor

Treatment with rinses, mouth sprays, or lozenges containing volatiles with a pleasant odor has only a short-term effect. Typical examples are mint-containing lozenges and the aroma of rinses without antibacterial components.

Another pathway is to increase the solubility of malodorous compounds in the saliva by increasing the secretion of saliva; a larger volume allows the retention of larger volumes of soluble VSCs. The latter can also be achieved by ensuring proper liquid intake or using chewing gum; chewing triggers the periodontal-parotid reflex, at least when the lower (pre) molars are still present.

Conclusion

Breath malodor has important socioeconomic consequences and can reveal important diseases. A proper diagnosis and determination of the etiology allow initiation of the proper etiologic treatment. Although tongue coating and (less frequently) periodontitis and gingivitis are by far the most common causes of malodor, a clinician cannot take the risk of overlooking other, more challenging diseases. This can be done with a multidisciplinary consultation or, if this is not feasible, a trial therapy to deal quickly with intraoral causes (e.g., full-mouth one-stage disinfection, including the use of proper mouthrinses, tongue scrapers, and toothpastes).

Key points

- Three main categories of halitosis are genuine halitosis, pseudo-halitosis, and halitophobia.
- The bacteria most commonly involved with malodor are *Porphyromonas gingivalis, Prevotella intermedia/nigrescens, Aggregatibacter actinomycetemcomitans, Campylobacter rectus, Fusobacterium nucleatum, Peptostreptococcus micros, Tannerella forsythia, Eubacterium* spp, and spirochetes.
- Volatile sulfur compounds (VSCs), especially hydrogen sulfide (H_2S), methyl mercaptan (CH_3SH), and dimethyl sulfide [$(CH_3)_2S$] are the compounds most commonly associated with oral malodor.
- Hydrogen sulfide and methyl mercaptan have the strongest odor power.
- Organoleptic assessment by a judge is the gold standard in the examination of breath malodor. It is the easiest and most often used method.
- The portable volatile sulfur monitor (Halimeter) is an electronic device that detects the presence of volatile sulfur compounds in breath.
- Oral malodor can be treated by masking the malodor, mechanically reducing intraoral nutrients and microorganisms, by chemically reducing oral microbial load and by rendering malodorous gases nonvolatile.

Suggested Reading

Loesche WJ, Kazor C: Microbiology and treatment of halitosis, *Periodontol 2000* 28:256–279, 2002.

Quirynen M, Dadamio J, Van den Velde S, et al: Characteristics of 2000 patients who visited a halitosis clinic, *J Clin Periodontol* 36(11):970–975, 2009.

Rosenberg M, Sterer N: *Breath odors: origin, diagnosis, and management*, Berlin, 2011, Springer.

Sanz M, Roldán S, Herrera D: Fundamentals of breath malodour, *J Contemp Dent Pract* 2(4):1–17, 2001.

Scully C, Greenman J: Halitology (breath odour: aetiopathogenesis and management), *Oral Dis* 18(4):333–345, 2012.

Seemann R, Bizhang M, Djamchidi C, et al: The proportion of pseudo-halitosis patients in a multidisciplinary breath malodour consultation, *Int Dent J* 56(2):77–81, 2006.

van Steenberghe D, Rosenberg M: *Bad breath: a multidisciplinary approach*, Leuven, 1996, University Press.

Van Tornout M, Dadamio J, Coucke W, et al: Tongue coating: related factors, *J Clin Periodontol* 40(2):180–185, 2013.

References

References and MCQs with answers for the chapter are available on www.medenact.com.

CHAPTER 41

Phase II Periodontal Therapy

S Elangovan | HH Takei | CD Dwarakanath

CHAPTER OUTLINE

Therapy for **periodontal disease**, which encompasses many techniques and procedures, depends on the disease status and objective of the final outcome. Early problems can be corrected with successful nonsurgical (phase I) therapy, consisting of biofilm removal by the patient on a daily basis, **scaling**, and **root instrumentation** when necessary.

Many moderate to advanced cases cannot be resolved without surgically gaining access to the root surface for root instrumentation and reducing or eliminating **pocket** depth to help the patient remove biofilm. The surgical phase of periodontal therapy is also referred to as phase II therapy. This chapter provides an overview of the surgical techniques used for the following purposes:

- Controlling or eliminating periodontal disease.
- Correcting anatomic conditions that favor periodontal disease, impair esthetics, or impede placement of prosthetic appliances.
- Placing implants to replace lost teeth and improving the environment for their placement and function.

Many cases are successfully treated and maintained by phase I therapy. Following chapters will discuss the in-depth techniques and concepts used to treat periodontal diseases that require a surgical approach to reduce or eliminate pockets and obtain access to the root surface to remove accretions.

Objectives of the Surgical Phase

The surgical phase of periodontal therapy has the following objectives:

1. To improve the prognosis for teeth and their replacements.
2. To improve esthetics.

Surgical techniques are used for pocket therapy and for correction of related morphologic problems (i.e., **mucogingival defects**). In many cases, therapies are combined to provide one surgical intervention that fulfills both objectives but there will be scenarios in which attaining both objectives is not feasible.

Surgical techniques can do the following: (1) increase access to the root surface, allowing the clinician to remove all irritants; (2) reduce or eliminate pocket depth, making it possible for the patient to maintain the root surfaces free of biofilm; and (3) reshape soft and hard tissues to attain a harmonious topography. **Resective** or **regenerative surgery** or both is used to reduce pocket depth.

The second objective of phase II therapy is to correct anatomic defects that favor **plaque** or biofilm accumulation and pocket recurrence or impair esthetics. The aim of correcting anatomic problems is to alter defects of the **gingival** and mucosal tissues that predispose these areas to disease. Three types of techniques are performed on noninflamed tissues and in the absence of **periodontal pockets** (see Box 41.1):

- *Plastic surgery techniques* are used to create or widen the attached keratinized gingiva by placing soft tissue grafts of various types.
- *Esthetic surgery techniques* are used to cover denuded root surfaces resulting from recession and to re-create lost papillae.
- *Preprosthetic techniques* are used to modify the periodontal and neighboring tissues to receive prosthetic replacements. They include crown lengthening, ridge augmentation, and vestibular deepening.

Fig. 41.1 provides a three-tiered classification of the surgical procedures used in periodontics: pocket reduction surgery, periodontal plastic surgery, and preprosthetic surgery. Pocket reduction surgery consists of resective and/or regenerative procedures; periodontal plastic surgery includes esthetic and gingival augmentation (anatomic) procedures. Crown lengthening, ridge augmentation, and implant procedures are listed under preprosthetic surgery.

Periodontal surgical procedures also are available for the placement of dental implants. They include implant placement techniques and a variety of surgical procedures to modify neighboring tissues for the placement of implants. Bone augmentation of the sinus floor or for a narrow **edentulous** ridge is an example (see Box 41.1).

Surgical Pocket Therapy

Surgical pocket therapy can be used to gain access to the diseased root surface to ensure the removal of calculus located subgingivally before surgery and to eliminate or reduce the depth of the periodontal pocket.

Successful periodontal therapy completely eliminates calculus, plaque, or biofilm and diseased cementum from the tooth surface. Numerous investigations have shown that the difficulty of this task increases as the pocket becomes deeper. The irregularities and

BOX 41.1 Periodontal Surgery

Pocket Reduction Surgery
- Resective (e.g., gingivectomy, apically displaced flap, undisplaced flap with or without osseous resection)
- Regenerative (e.g., flaps with grafts, membranes)

Correction of Anatomic or Morphologic Defects
- Plastic surgery techniques used to widen attached gingiva (e.g., free gingival grafts)
- Esthetic surgery (e.g., root coverage, recreation of gingival papillae)
- Preprosthetic techniques (e.g., crown lengthening, ridge augmentation, vestibular deepening)
- Placement of dental implants, including techniques for site development for implants (e.g., guided bone regeneration, sinus grafts)

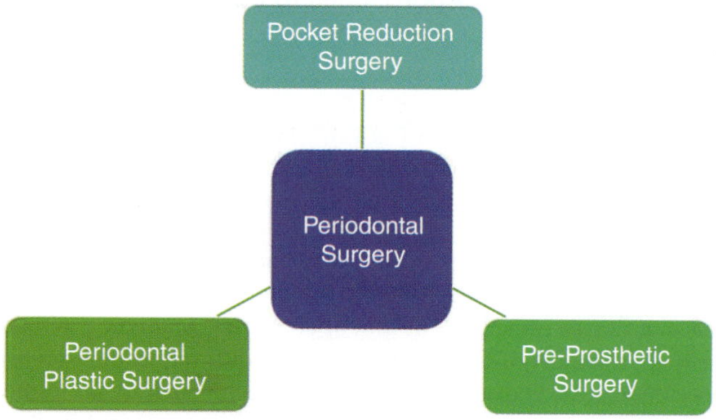

Fig. 41.1 Classification of periodontal surgery. The surgical procedures accomplished in periodontics are organized as pocket reduction surgery, periodontal plastic surgery, and preprosthetic surgery.

concavities on the root surface also increase, which adds to the difficulty of instrumenting the root surfaces.

Furcations also create problems for scaling and **subgingival root** instrumentation in these areas. Most of these problems can be rectified by resecting or displacing the soft tissue wall of the pocket, which increases the visibility and accessibility of the root surface. The surgical flap technique allows the clinician to overcome these problems of access to the root surface.

Pocket elimination is another important consideration. It consists of reducing the depth of the periodontal pocket to that of a physiologic sulcus to enable cleaning by the patient. By proper case selection, resective and/or regenerative techniques can be used to accomplish this goal. A pocket makes it impossible for the patient to remove biofilm, which is part of the vicious cycle depicted in Fig. 41.2.

Results of Pocket Therapy

A periodontal pocket can be in an active state or a period of inactivity or quiescence. In an active pocket, underlying bone is being lost (Fig. 41.3, top left). It often is diagnosed clinically by bleeding that occurs spontaneously or in response to probing. After phase I therapy, the inflammatory changes in the pocket wall subside, rendering the pocket inactive and reducing its depth (see Fig. 41.3, top *center*). The extent of this reduction depends on the depth before treatment and the degree to which the depth is the result of the edematous and inflammatory component of the pocket wall (i.e., pseudopocket).

Whether the pocket remains inactive depends on the depth, the individual characteristics of the plaque or biofilm components, and the host response. Recurrence of the initial activity is likely.

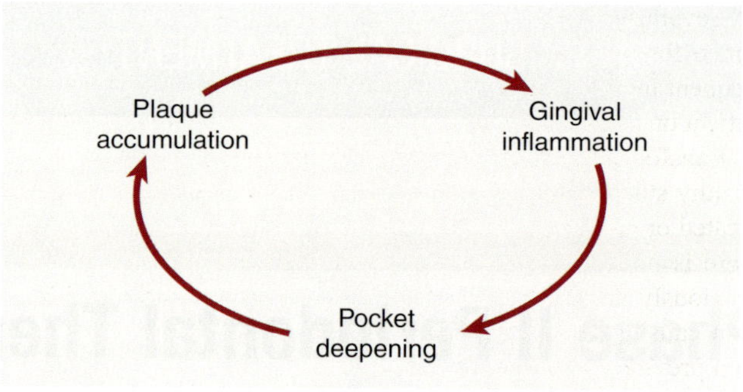

Fig. 41.2 Accumulation of plaque leads to gingival inflammation and pocket deepening, which increases the area of plaque accumulation.

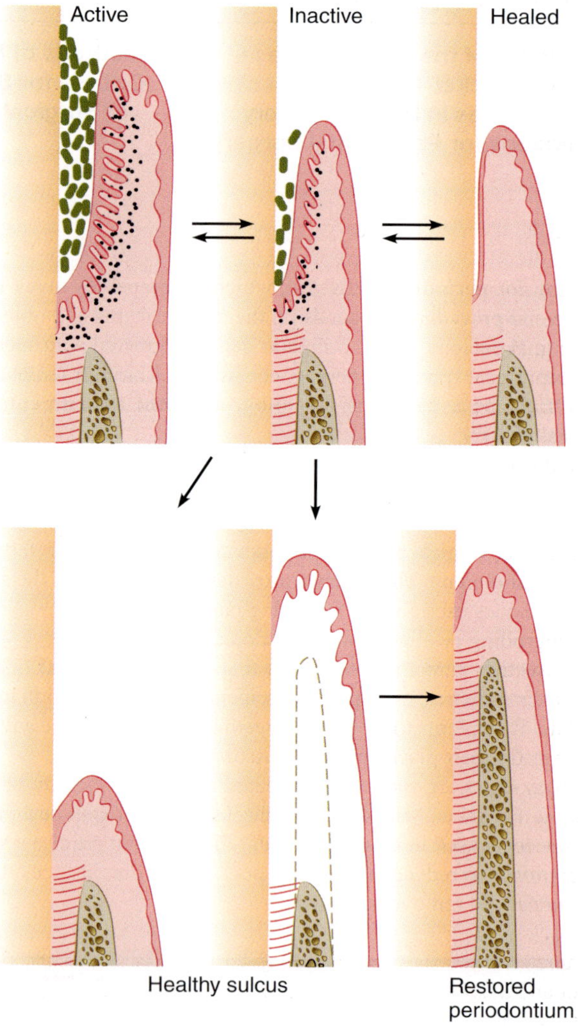

Fig. 41.3 Possible results of pocket therapy are shown. An active pocket can become inactive and heal by means of a long junctional epithelium. Surgical pocket therapy can result in a healthy sulcus, with or without gain of attachment. Improved gingival attachment promotes restoration of bone height, with re-formation of periodontal ligament fibers and layers of cementum.

Inactive pockets sometimes heal with a long **junctional epithelium** (see Fig. 41.3, *top right*). This condition can be unstable, and the chance of recurrence and re-formation of the original pocket remains because the epithelial union with the tooth is weak. However, one study in monkeys showed that the long junctional epithelial union could be as resistant to biofilm **infection** as a true connective tissue attachment.

Several studies reported that inactive pockets could be maintained for long periods with little loss of attachment by means of frequent therapy and by excellent plaque or biofilm removal by the patient on a daily basis. A more reliable and stable result is obtained by transforming the pocket into a healthy sulcus. The bottom of the healthy sulcus can be located where the bottom of the pocket was located or coronal to it. In the first case (see Fig. 41.3, *bottom left*), there is no gain of attachment, and the area of the root that was previously the tooth wall of the pocket becomes exposed. Rather than causing recession, periodontal treatment uncovers the recession previously caused by disease.

The healthy sulcus can be located coronal to the bottom of the preexisting pocket (see Fig. 41.3, *bottom center* and *right*). This is conducive to a restored marginal **periodontium**; the result is a sulcus of normal depth with a gain of attachment. The creation of a healthy sulcus and a restored periodontium entails total restoration of the status that existed before periodontal disease began, which is the ideal result of treatment. The bone regeneration diagram in Fig. 41.3 (*bottom center* and *right*) is for illustrative purpose only because bone regeneration without an osseous wall is seldom achieved.

Pocket Elimination Versus Pocket Maintenance

Pocket elimination (i.e., depth reduction to gingival sulcus levels) has traditionally been considered a type of periodontal therapy. It was considered vital because of the need to improve access to root surfaces for the therapist during treatment and for the patient after healing. Prevailing opinion considers that deep pockets after therapy represent a greater risk of disease progression than shallow sites. Individual **probing depths** are not good predictors of future clinical attachment loss. Conversely, the absence of deep pockets in treated patients is an excellent predictor of a stable periodontium.

Longitudinal studies of different therapeutic modalities over the past 30 years have produced conflicting results, probably because of problems created by the split-mouth design. After surgical therapy, pockets that rebound to a shallow or moderate depth can be maintained in a healthy state and without radiographic evidence of advancing bone loss by maintenance visits consisting of scaling and root instrumentation, with oral hygiene reinforcement performed at regular intervals of 3 months or less.

The findings emphasize the importance of the maintenance phase and close monitoring of the level of attachment and pocket depth, along with the other clinical variables (e.g., bleeding, **exudation**, tooth mobility). *Transformation of the initial deep, active pocket into a shallower, inactive, maintainable pocket requires some form of definitive pocket therapy and constant supervision thereafter.*

Pocket depth is an extremely useful and widely used clinical parameter, but it must be evaluated together with the level of attachment and degree of bleeding, exudation, and pain. The most important variable for evaluating whether a pocket is progressing is the *level of attachment*, which is measured in millimeters from the cementoenamel junction. Apical displacement of the level of attachment places the tooth in jeopardy, not the increase in pocket depth, which may be caused by coronal displacement of the gingival margin (as in gingival inflammation or gingival overgrowth).

Pocket depth remains an important clinical variable in making decisions about treatment. Lindhe and colleagues compared the effect of **root planing** alone or using a modified Widman flap with the resultant level of attachment and in relation to initial pocket depth. They reported that scaling and root planing procedures induced loss of attachment if performed in pockets shallower than 2.9 mm, whereas gain of attachment occurred in deeper pockets. The modified Widman flap induced loss of attachment if performed in pockets shallower than 4.2 mm but resulted in a greater gain of attachment than root planing in pockets deeper than 4.2 mm. The loss is a true loss of connective tissue attachment, whereas the gain can be considered a false gain because of the reduced penetrability of connective tissues apical to the bottom of the pocket after treatment.

Probing depths established about 6 months after active therapy and healing can be maintained, remain unchanged, or be reduced even further during a maintenance period involving careful reevaluation, plaque or biofilm removal, and root therapy as necessary every 3 months.

Ramfjord and Rosling and their colleagues reported that a certain pocket depth recurs regardless of the surgical technique used for pocket therapy. *Maintaining this depth without any further loss of attachment becomes the goal.*

Reevaluation After Phase I Therapy

Longitudinal studies found that all patients should be treated initially with subgingival root instrumentation (scaling and root planing) and plaque or biofilm control and that a final decision on the need for periodontal surgery should be made only after a thorough evaluation of the effects of phase I therapy. Assessment typically is made no less than 1–3 months and sometimes as much as 9 months after the completion of phase I therapy. Reevaluation of the periodontal condition includes repeat probing of the entire mouth. Calculus, root caries, defective restorations, and signs of persistent inflammation should also be evaluated.

Critical Zones in Pocket Surgery

Criteria for the selection of a surgical technique for pocket therapy are based on clinical findings in the soft tissue pocket wall, tooth surface, underlying bone, and attached gingiva.

Zone 1: Soft Tissue Pocket Wall

The clinician should determine the morphologic features, thickness, and topography of the soft tissue pocket wall and persistence of inflammatory changes in the wall.

Zone 2: Tooth Surface

The clinician should identify the deposits on and alterations of the cementum surface and determine the accessibility of the root surface to instrumentation. Phase I therapy should have solved many or all of the problems on the tooth surface. Evaluation of the results of phase I therapy can determine the need for further therapy and the method to be used.

Zone 3: Underlying Bone

The clinician should establish the shape and height of the alveolar bone next to the pocket wall through careful probing and clinical and radiographic examinations. The number of osseous walls—one, two, or three—helps determine whether resective or regenerative therapy can be used. Bony craters, **horizontal** or angular bone losses, and other bone deformities also are important criteria in selection of the treatment technique.

Zone 4: Attached Gingiva

The clinician should consider the presence or absence of an adequate band of keratinized attached gingiva when selecting the pocket treatment method. An inadequate attached gingiva can be caused by a high frenum attachment, marked gingival recession, or a deep pocket that reaches the level of the mucogingival junction. All these conditions should be explored and their influence on pocket therapy considered.

Indications for Periodontal Surgery

The following findings can indicate the need for a surgical phase of therapy:

1. Areas with irregular bony contours, deep craters, and other defects usually require a surgical approach.
2. Pockets around teeth where access to the root surface for complete removal of root irritants is not possible by nonsurgical means are an indication for surgery. These occur frequently around molars and premolars.
3. **Furcation involvement** of **grade** II or III may require a surgical approach to ensure the removal of irritants around root surfaces. If root resection or hemisection is necessary, surgical intervention will be needed.
4. Intrabony pockets distal to the last molars, which in many cases are complicated by mucogingival problems, often require surgery.
5. Areas with furcation involvements and intrabony defects that can be predictably treated by regenerative approaches require surgical intervention.
6. Persistent inflammation at sites with moderate to deep pockets that were treated nonsurgically in the past may require a surgical approach. These are usually areas where all the **subgingival calculus** could not be removed.
7. Cases with shallow pockets and good hygiene but bleeding on probing can be caused by mucogingival problems in areas where there is no keratinized tissue. Trauma to these areas can cause bleeding.

Methods of Pocket Therapy

The methods for pocket therapy can be classified as follows:

1. *New attachment techniques* offer the ideal result because they eliminate pocket depth by reuniting the attachment apparatus with the tooth at a position coronal to the bottom of the preexisting pocket. New attachment involves regeneration of bone, connective tissue, periodontal ligament, and cementum.
2. *Removal of the pocket wall* is the most common method. The wall of the pocket consists of soft tissue and can include bone in the case of intrabony pockets. It can be removed by the following methods:
   - Retraction or shrinkage, where plaque or biofilm removal by the patient and subgingival root instrumentation (scaling and root planing) resolve the inflammatory process, can occur. The gingival tissue shrinks, reducing the pocket depth.
   - Surgical removal of the pocket is done by gingivectomy or the undisplaced flap technique.
   - Apical displacement of the flap is performed with an apically positioned flap.
3. *Removal of the tooth side of the pocket*, which is accomplished by tooth extraction or by partial tooth extraction in the case of furcation involvement (i.e., hemisection or root resection).

Criteria for Selection of the Method of Surgical Therapy

Scientific criteria to establish indications for the use of each technique are difficult to determine. Criteria are based on longitudinal studies that follow a significant number of cases over a number of years, standardization of multiple factors, and long-term clinical experience. Selection of a technique for treating a particular periodontal lesion is based on the following considerations:

1. Characteristics of the pocket—depth, relation to bone, and configuration.
2. Accessibility to instrumentation, including furcation involvement.
3. Existence of mucogingival problems.
4. Response to phase I therapy.
5. Patient cooperation, including the ability to perform effective oral hygiene and quit smoking (smoking cessation).
6. Age and general health (e.g., diabetic status) of the patient.
7. Overall diagnosis of the case—various types of gingival enlargement and different **stages** and grades of **periodontitis**.
8. Esthetic considerations and patient expectations.
9. Previous periodontal treatments.

Each variable is analyzed in relation to the pocket therapy techniques available. A specific technique is then selected. The one most likely to solve the problem successfully, with the fewest undesirable effects, should be selected. Clinicians who adhere to one technique to solve all problems are not taking advantage of the wide repertoire of techniques that are at their disposal.

Approaches to Specific Pocket Problems

Therapy for Gingival Pockets

Gingival pockets do not have an osseous component (i.e., no attachment loss) and usually have edematous or fibrotic gingival tissue. Two factors are taken into consideration: the character of the pocket wall and accessibility of the pocket.

The pocket wall can be edematous or fibrotic. *Edematous tissue* shrinks after the elimination of local factors, reducing or totally eliminating pocket depth. Subgingival root instrumentation in the form of scaling and root planing is the technique of choice for these cases.

Pockets with a *fibrotic wall* are not appreciably reduced in depth after subgingival root instrumentation. These pockets are eliminated or reduced by surgical therapy. In the past, gingivectomy was frequently used to reduce these pockets. This solved the problem, but in cases of marked gingival enlargement (e.g., severe phenytoin-related enlargement), treatment could leave a large, open wound, and the patient had to endure a painful and prolonged healing process. Currently, a modified flap technique is used, and fewer postoperative problems are associated with primary closure of the wound. Some clinicians have advocated the use of laser therapy to manage gingival enlargement.

Therapy for Stage I Periodontitis (Incipient Disease)

In patients with slight or incipient periodontitis with minimal attachment and bone loss, the pocket depths are shallow or a moderate depth. In these patients, the conservative approach of good oral hygiene and subgingival root instrumentation (scaling and root planing), when necessary, usually suffices to control the disease. Incipient periodontitis that recurs in previously treated sites with good hygiene may require a thorough analysis of the recurrence, which may be caused by remnants of calculus that were missed during previous treatment or other factors such as open margins of a restoration located subgingivally. Occasionally, a surgical approach may be required to correct these problems.

Therapy for Stages II to IV Periodontitis (Moderate to Severe Disease) in the Anterior Sector

Because the maxillary anterior teeth are important esthetically, techniques that cause the least amount of visual root **exposure** should be considered. However, each patient has different expectations regarding the final result of therapy. The clinician must explain that the therapy may be a compromise between complete pocket elimination and achieving an esthetic result that is acceptable to the patient. The patient must be educated before therapy on the possibility of some degree of gingival recession and some loss of the interdental papilla.

The anterior dentition has two advantages for using a conservative (nonsurgical) approach: (1) the teeth are all single rooted and easily accessible for subgingival root instrumentation (scaling and root planing); and (2) patient compliance and thoroughness in plaque or biofilm control may be easier to attain. *Nonsurgical therapy is therefore the technique of choice for the maxillary anterior dentition.*

In some situations, surgical therapy may be necessary to improve accessibility for root instrumentation or regenerative therapy may be possible. The papilla preservation flap or modified papilla preservation flap can be used for both purposes and offers a better postoperative result, with less recession and reduced soft tissue crater formation interproximally.

When the interdental space is minimal, papilla preservation techniques may not be feasible. Instead, a technique that splits the papilla and retains as much of the papilla as possible is the appropriate surgical technique.

When the esthetic outcome is not the primary consideration and a flap procedure is necessary for root surface access, the *modified Widman flap* can be selected. This technique uses an internal bevel incision about 1–2 mm from the gingival margin without thinning the flap. This procedure may result in minor recession of the surrounding gingival tissue.

In cases with advanced osseous involvement, bone contouring may be needed, despite the resultant root exposure. The technique of choice is the *apically displaced flap with osseous bone contouring*. The clinician must educate the patient before therapy about the possibility of esthetic compromises due to the expected recession of gingival tissue.

Therapy for Stages II to IV Periodontitis (Moderate to Severe Disease) in Posterior Areas

Treatment for the maxillary and mandibular premolars and molars does not entail esthetic problems but frequently involves difficult access for root therapy. Bone defects occur more often in the posterior area than the anterior, with many areas having deep infrabony lesions and anatomic root problems with concavities, such as the mesial surface of the maxillary first premolar. A difficult problem encountered in the posterior area is the furcation lesion. Because this area can pose insurmountable problems for instrumentation unless a flap is reflected, surgery is frequently indicated.

Surgery is used in the posterior area for enhanced access to the root surface or for definitive pocket reduction requiring osseous surgery. Access can be obtained by an undisplaced or apically displaced flap.

Most patients with stage II to stage IV periodontitis have developed osseous defects that require some degree of bone remodeling or reconstruction. For osseous defects amenable to reconstruction, the *papilla preservation flap* or *modified papilla preservation flap* is the technique of choice because it better protects the interproximal areas where defects frequently occur. Second and third choices are the *sulcular flap* and *modified Widman flap*, maintaining as much of the papilla as possible.

For osseous defects with no possibility of reconstructive therapy, such as interdental craters, the technique of choice is an undisplaced or apically displaced flap with osseous contouring. It is important to note that in spite of the disease being present only in the posterior sextant, if severe and presenting with tooth loss or posterior bite collapse (stage IV), it can negatively affect the esthetics of the anterior dentition and warrants an **interdisciplinary** form of care.

Conclusion

Many steps are required to achieve and maintain a healthy periodontal status. After completion of phase I therapy, which consists of patient education, biofilm control, and thorough root therapy, the involved periodontal areas are reevaluated. The necessity of phase II therapy, which is the surgical phase of treatment, depends on the success of the initial phase and the severity of the periodontal condition. Periodontal surgery, which includes plastic, esthetic, resective, and regenerative procedures, becomes necessary when access for root therapy is required or correction of anatomic or morphologic defects is necessary. Placement of dental implants can be part of this therapy.

Key points

- Majority of periodontal cases are effectively treated by nonsurgical therapy.
- Persistence of disease even after phase I therapy, to regenerate lost periodontal tissues, to correct mucogingival problems and enhance esthetics, and to place dental implants to replace lost teeth calls for periodontal surgery.
- The main objective of surgical pocket therapy is to get access and visibility, thereby facilitating the elimination of pockets or reducing its depth.
- Inactive pockets may sometimes heal by long junctional epithelium but this may not be sustainable.
- The soft tissue pocket wall, tooth surface, underlying bone and attached gingiva are regarded as critical zones in pocket surgery.
- Decision to do surgery is taken 1–3 months after initial therapy.
- Choice of surgical technique depends upon many factors and is tailor-made for the particular patient.
- New attachment of regenerative techniques and respective techniques are the two main pocket elimination methods.

SUGGESTED READING

Lang NP. Indications and rationale for non-surgical periodontal therapy. *International dental journal*. 1983;33(2):127–36.

CHAPTER 42

Periodontal and Peri-Implant Surgical Anatomy

PR Klokkevold | JM Miller | FA Carranza | CD Dwarakanath

CHAPTER OUTLINE

A sound knowledge of the anatomy of the **periodontium** and the surrounding hard and soft tissue structures is essential to determine the scope and possibilities of periodontal and **implant** surgical procedures and to minimize their risks. The spatial relationship of bones, muscles, blood vessels, and nerves, as well as the anatomic spaces located in the vicinity of the periodontal or implant surgical field, are particularly important. Only those features with periodontal and implant surgery relevance are mentioned in this chapter; the reader is referred to oral and head and neck anatomy books for a more detailed and comprehensive description of these structures.

Mandible

The mandible is a horseshoe-shaped bone connected to the skull by the temporomandibular joints, stylomandibular and sphenomandibular ligaments, and the muscles of mastication (temporalis, masseter, medial, and lateral pterygoids). It presents several landmarks of great surgical importance for both periodontal and implant surgical procedures.

The *mandibular canal*, which is occupied by the inferior alveolar nerve and vessels, begins at the mandibular foramen on the medial surface of the mandibular ramus and curves inferiorly and anteriorly until it becomes **horizontal** below the apices of the molars (Fig. 42.1). The distance from the canal to the apices of the teeth is shortest in the third molar area. A significant percentage of mandibular canals (up to 27%) were found to bifurcate in a **systematic review** and **metaanalysis** of 15 studies of anatomic variation using samples of more than 300 individuals from different geographic regions. Trifid mandibular canals have also been documented. The mandibular canal status may have clinical significance in anesthesia failure, mandibular third molar extraction, implantation, and other surgical procedures. In the premolar area, the mandibular canal divides in two branches, with one exiting the mandible and the other continuing anteriorly—the *incisive canal*, which continues horizontally to the midline, and the *mental canal*, which turns superiorly and opens in the mental foramen.

The *mental foramen*, from which the mental nerve and vessels emerge, is located on the buccal surface of the mandible below the apices of the premolars, sometimes closer to the second premolar and usually halfway between the inferior border of the mandible and the alveolar margin (Fig. 42.2). It is often but not always visible on conventional radiographs. The opening of the mental foramen, which may be oval or round, typically faces superiorly and distally, with its posterior-superior border slanting gradually to the bone surface. An "anterior loop" of the mental foramen has been described, with the use of cadaver dissection, as a reverse turn and looping back of the mental nerve within the body of the mandible before its exit out of the mental foramen; the estimated length of the anterior loop ranges from 0.5 to 5.0 mm. A more recent evaluation of the anterior loop of the mental nerve involving the use of cone beam scans and cadaveric dissection reported this loop extension to range from 0.0 to 9.0 mm. The anterior loop of the mental nerve has a high **prevalence** (88%), symmetric occurrence, and mean length of 4.13 ± 1.08 mm. As it emerges, the *mental nerve* divides into three branches. One branch of the nerve turns anteriorly and inferiorly to supply the skin of the chin. The other two branches course anteriorly and superiorly to supply the skin and mucous **membranes** of the lower lip and the mucosa of the labial alveolar surface.

Surgical trauma (e.g., pressure, manipulation, postsurgical swelling) to the mental nerve can produce **paresthesia** of the lip, which recovers slowly. Partial or complete cutting of the nerve can result in permanent paresthesia, dysesthesia, or both. Familiarity with the location and appearance of the mental nerve reduces the likelihood of injury (Fig. 42.3).

In partially or totally edentulous jaws, the disappearance of the alveolar portion of the mandible brings the mandibular canal and mental foramen closer to the superior border (Figs. 42.4 and 42.5). When these patients are evaluated for the placement of implants, the distance between the canal and superior surface of the bone, as well as the location of the mental foramen, must be carefully determined to avoid surgical injury to the nerve.

The anterior extension of the inferior alveolar nerve or incisive nerve has been measured with the use of conventional radiography, computed tomography (CT) scans, cadaver dissections, and cone beam scans. This nerve, which is less evident on conventional radiographs and often unnoticed, extends beyond the anterior loop of the mental foramen in a horizontal direction toward the midline. The length of the incisive canal has been reported to be up to 21.45 mm from the mesial aspect of the mental foramen and to terminate just 4 mm from the midline.

The *lingual nerve*, along with the inferior alveolar nerve, is a branch of the posterior division of the mandibular nerve. It descends along the mandibular ramus medial and anterior to the inferior alveolar nerve. The lingual nerve lies close to the surface of the oral

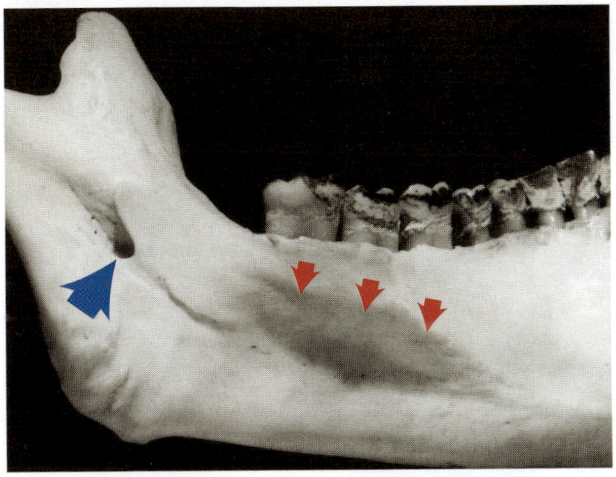

Fig. 42.1 Mandible, lingual surface view. Note the lingual or mandibular foramen *(blue arrow)*, where the inferior alveolar nerve enters the mandibular canal, and the mylohyoid ridge *(red arrows)*.

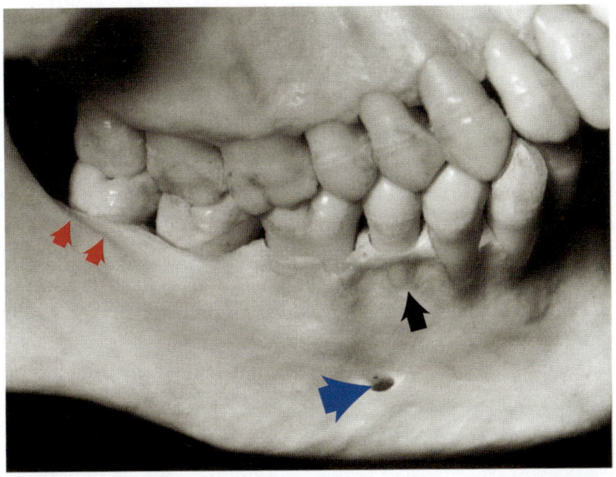

Fig. 42.2 Mandible, facial surface view. Note the location of the mental foramen *(blue arrow)*, which is slightly distal and apical to the apex of the second premolar, and the shelflike area in the region of the molars *(red arrows)*, which is created by the external oblique ridge. Note also the fenestration that is present in the second premolar *(black arrow)*.

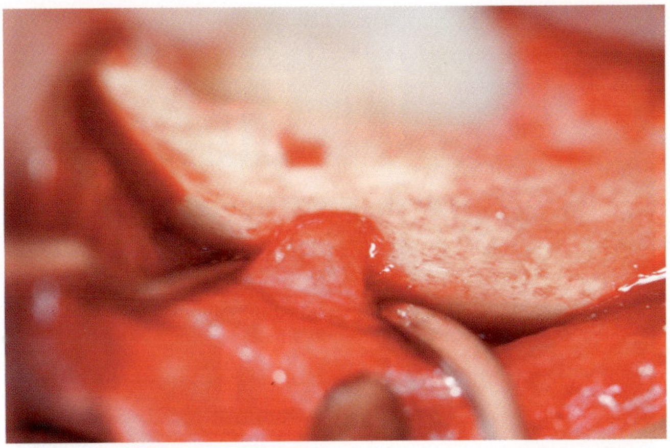

Fig. 42.3 Surgical view of the mental nerve emerging from the foramen in the premolar area.

mucosa in the third molar area and goes deeper as it travels anteriorly (Fig. 42.6). It can be damaged during anesthetic injections and during oral surgery procedures (e.g., third molar extractions). Less often, the lingual nerve may be injured when a periodontal partial-thickness flap is raised in the third molar region or when releasing incisions are made in the area.

The *alveolar process*, which provides the supporting bone to the teeth, has a narrower distal curvature than the body of the mandible (Fig. 42.7), thus creating a flat surface in the posterior area between the teeth and anterior border of the ramus. This results in the formation of the *external oblique ridge*, which runs inferiorly and anteriorly to the region of the second or first molar (Fig. 42.8) to create a shelflike bony area. **Resective** osseous therapy may be difficult or impossible in this area because of the amount of bone that must be removed distally toward the ramus to achieve resection of a periodontal osseous defect on the distal aspect of the mandibular second or third molar.

Distal to the third molar, the external oblique ridge circumscribes the *retromolar triangle* (see Fig. 42.8). This region is occupied by glandular and adipose tissue and covered by unattached, nonkeratinized mucosa. If sufficient space exists distal to the last molar, a band of attached **gingiva** may be present; only in such a case can a distal flap procedure be performed effectively.

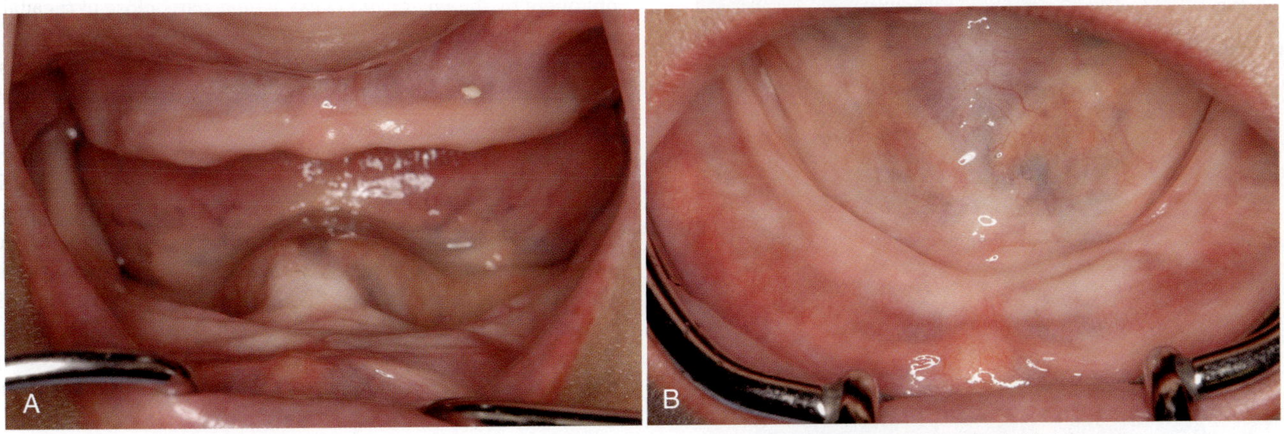

Fig. 42.4 Loss of the alveolar ridge in an edentulous patient brings the mental foramen and mandibular canal closer to the surface, which may lead to discomfort for the patient. A, Anterior view demonstrating a severe loss of vertical alveolar ridge height. B, Occlusal view of the same patient demonstrating a loss of vestibular depth with alveolar bone loss.

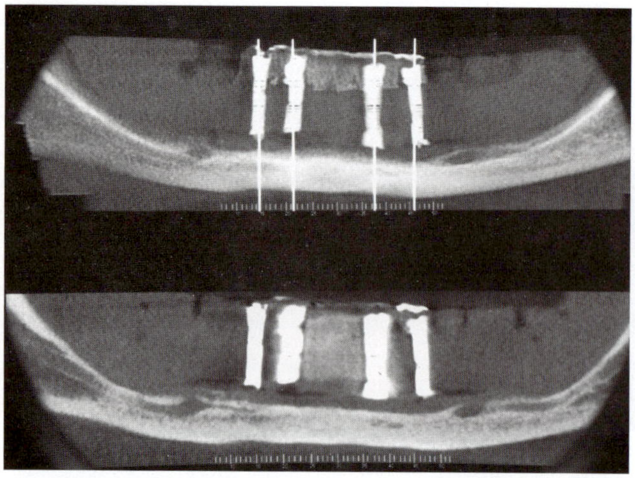

Fig. 42.5 Panoramic radiograph of an edentulous patient with a loss of alveolar bone height. This results in the mental foramen exiting the jaw at the superior aspect of the remaining bone (ridge crest), which is the denture-bearing surface. Pressure from the complete removable denture over this area causes pain.

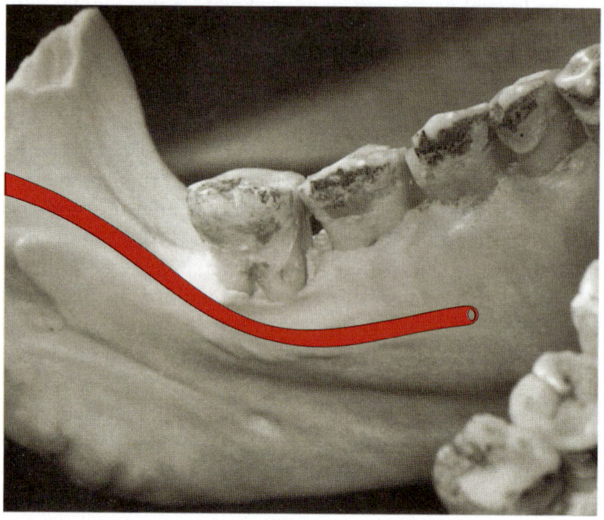

Fig. 42.6 Lingual view of the mandible showing the pathway of the lingual nerve *(red)*, which courses near the gingiva in the third molar area and then continues forward, running deeper and medially toward the tongue.

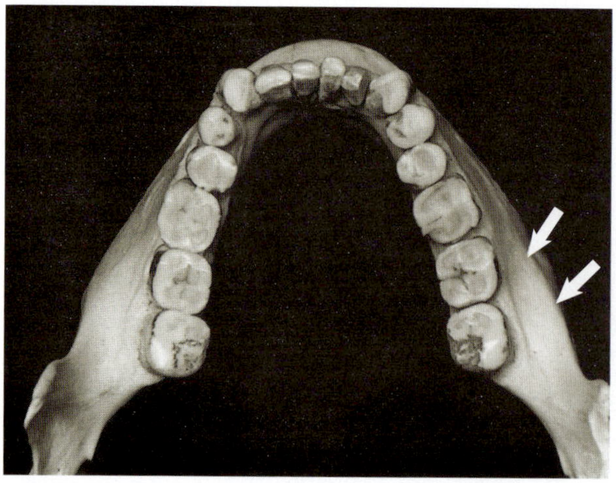

Fig. 42.7 Occlusal view of the mandible. Note the shelf that is created in the facial molar areas by the external oblique ridge. *Arrows* show the attachment of the buccinator muscle.

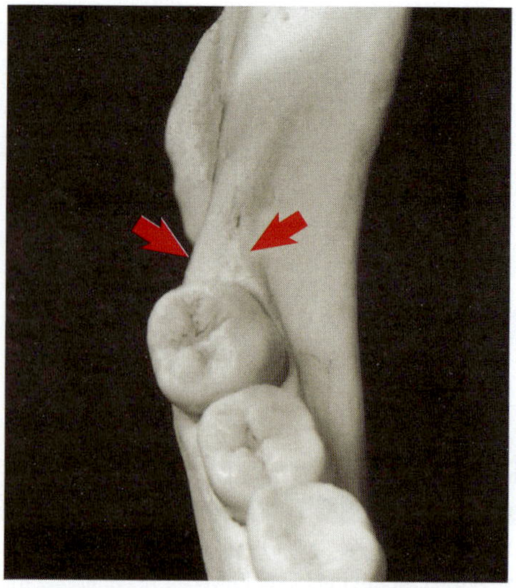

Fig. 42.8 Mandible; occlusal view of the ramus and molars. Note the retromolar triangle area distal to the third molar *(arrows)*.

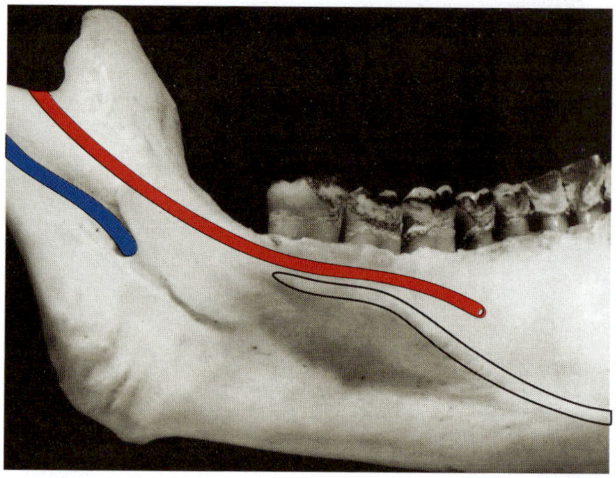

Fig. 42.9 Lingual view of the mandible showing the inferior alveolar nerve entering the mandibular canal *(blue)*, the lingual nerve traversing near the lingual surface of the third molar *(red)*, and the attachment of the mylohyoid muscle inferiorly *(outline)*.

The medial side of the body of the mandible is traversed obliquely by the *mylohyoid ridge*, which starts close to the alveolar margin in the third molar area and continues anteriorly in an apical direction, thereby increasing its distance from the osseous margin as it travels anteriorly (Fig. 42.9). The *mylohyoid muscle* inserts along this ridge and separates the *sublingual space*, which is located superiorly or more anteriorly and superiorly, from the submandibular space, which is located inferiorly or more posteriorly and inferiorly.

Maxilla

The maxilla is a paired bone that is hollowed out by the maxillary sinuses and the nasal cavity. The maxilla has the following four processes:

- The *alveolar process* contains the sockets for and supports the maxillary teeth.
- The *palatine process* extends horizontally from the alveolar process to meet its counterpart from the opposite maxilla at the midline intermaxillary suture, and it extends posteriorly with the horizontal plate of the palatine bone to form the hard palate.

- The *zygomatic process* extends laterally from the area above the first molar and determines the depth of the posterior vestibular fornix on the lateral aspect of the maxilla.
- The *frontal process* extends in an ascending direction and **articulates** with the frontal bone at the frontomaxillary suture.

The terminal branches of the nasopalatine nerve and vessels pass through the incisive canal, which opens in the midline anterior area of the palate (Fig. 42.10). The mucosa overlying the incisive canal presents a slight protuberance called the *incisive papilla.* Vessels that emerge through the incisive canal are of small caliber, and their surgical interference is of little consequence.

The *greater palatine foramen* opens 3–4 mm anterior to the posterior border of the hard palate (Fig. 42.11). The greater palatine nerve and vessels emerge through this foramen and run anteriorly in the submucosa of the palate, between the palatal and alveolar processes (Fig. 42.12). Palatal flaps and donor sites for **gingival** and connective tissue grafts should be carefully performed and selected to avoid invading these areas because profuse hemorrhage may ensue, particularly if vessels are damaged at the greater palatine foramen. Vertical incisions in the molar region should be avoided.

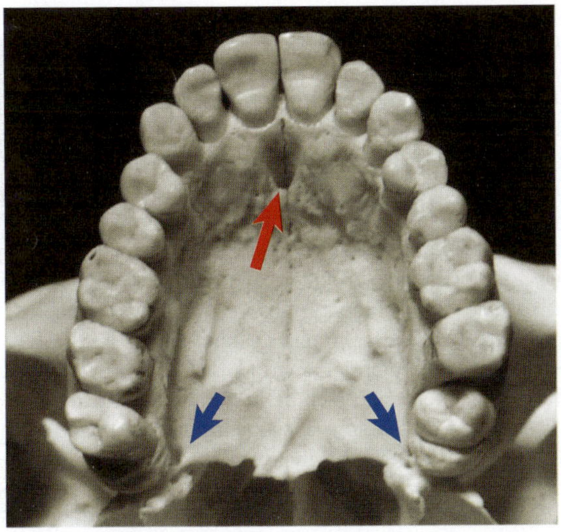

Fig. 42.10 Occlusal view of the maxilla and palatine bone. Note the opening of the incisive canal *(red arrow)* and the greater palatine foramina *(blue arrows).*

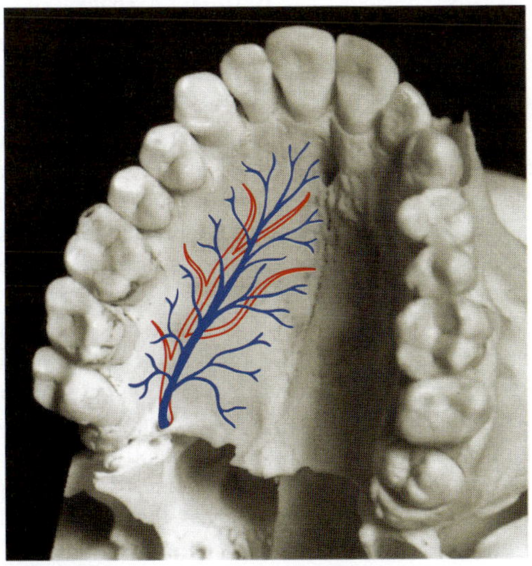

Fig. 42.11 Occlusal lateral view of the palate showing nerves *(red)* and vessels *(blue)* emerging from the greater palatine foramen and continuing anteriorly on the palate.

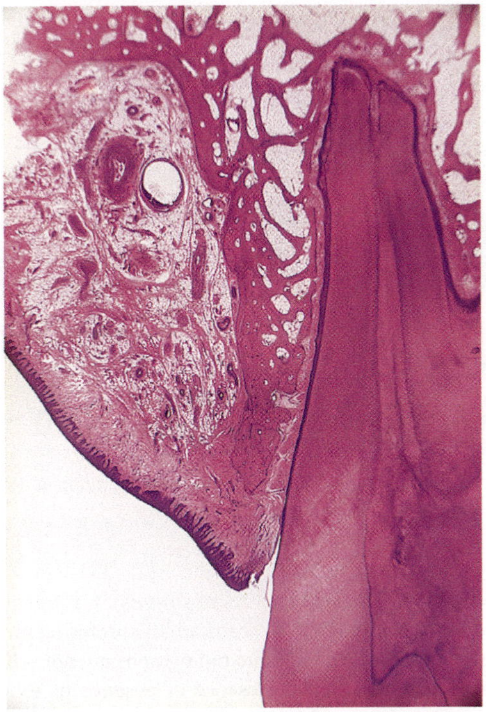

Fig. 42.12 Histologic frontal section of a human palate at the level of the first molar showing the location of the vessels and the nerve surrounded by adipose and glandular tissue. Hematoxylin and eosin stained tissues; 2× magnification.

The mucous membrane that covers the hard palate is firmly attached to the underlying bone. The submucosal layer of the palate posterior to the first molars contains the *palatal glands*, which are more compact in the soft palate and extend anteriorly, thereby filling the gap between the mucosal connective tissue and **periosteum** and protecting the underlying vessels and nerves (see Fig. 42.22, later).

The area distal to the last molar, called the *maxillary tuberosity*, consists of the posterior-inferior angle of the infratemporal surface of the maxilla. Medially it articulates with the pyramidal process of the palatine bone. It is covered by dense, fibrous connective tissue, and it contains the terminal branches of the lesser (middle and posterior) palatine nerves. Excision of the area for distal flap surgery may reach medially to the tensor veli palatini muscle. The tensor veli palatini muscle originates from the scaphoid fossa and spine of the sphenoid bone and ends by forming a tendon that winds around the pterygoid hamulus; it then expands medially to form the palatine aponeurosis, which then inserts onto the posterior border of the hard palate.

The body of the maxilla is occupied by the *maxillary sinus*, which is the largest of the paranasal sinuses. It is an air-filled cavity located in the posterior maxilla, superior to the teeth. The lateral wall of the nasal cavity borders the sinus medially; it is bordered superiorly by the floor of the orbit and laterally by the lateral wall of the maxilla, alveolar process, and zygomatic arch (Fig. 42.13). It is pyramidal, with its apex in the zygomatic arch and its base at the lateral wall of the nasal cavity. The size of the maxillary sinus varies from one individual to another (depending on the individual and his or her age) and from very small and narrow to quite large and expansive.

The maxillary sinus is frequently subdivided (incompletely) into recesses by one or more septa. Maxillary sinus septa vary in size and location. Clinical and radiographic examinations suggest that

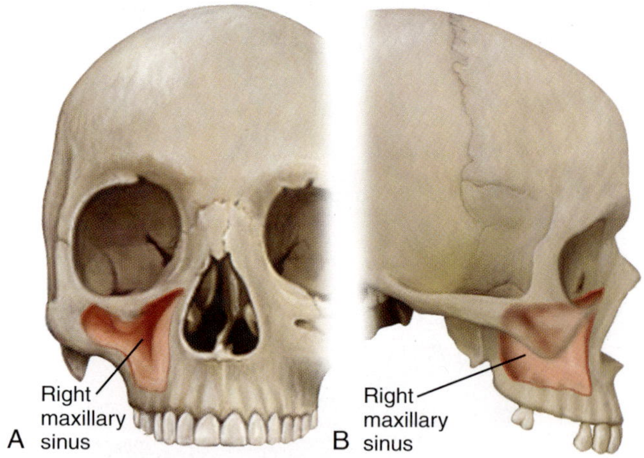

Fig. 42.13 Location and anatomy of the maxillary sinus. A, Frontal view. B, Lateral view.

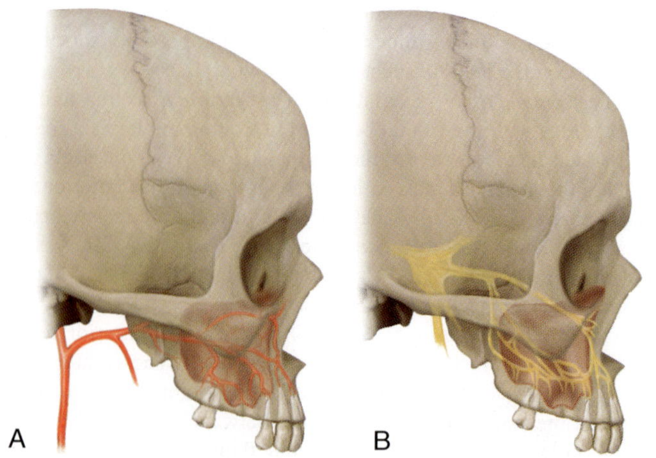

Fig. 42.14 Blood supply and innervation of the maxillary sinus. A, Arterial blood supply. B, Innervation of the maxillary sinus.

septa are frequently present (≤39% of sinuses). CT and cone-beam computed tomography (CBCT) scans are the preferred methods for detecting septa because panoramic radiographs are not reliable (i.e., 26.5% false diagnosis of the presence or absence of septa). Septa are found in the anterior (24%), middle (41%), and posterior (35%) aspects of the maxillary sinus, with the most common location being between the second premolar and first molar. The height of septa varies as well, ranging from 0 to 20.6 mm. Only 0.5% of septa form a complete separation of the sinus cavity into separate chambers.

The entire maxillary sinus is lined with a thin mucosal membrane called the **Schneiderian membrane**. This specialized structure of the respiratory mucous membrane, with its motile **cilia** and rich blood supply, is well adapted to purifying, moistening, and warming air to protect the lungs. The entrance to the maxillary sinus, through the orifice or maxillary duct, is located at the superior medial aspect of the sinus cavity. The orifice is relatively small, measuring only 3–6 mm in length and diameter. An accessory opening is occasionally found inferior and posterior to the main opening. The maxillary sinus drains into the middle meatus of the nasal cavity through the maxillary duct or **ostium**, which passes secretions medially to the semilunar hiatus. Normal amounts of secretion are moved from the sinus by the spiral pattern of the beating cilia that surround the orifice. If the maxillary sinus becomes infected or **chronically** inflamed, swelling of the mucosa around the orifice impairs drainage. The floor of the maxillary sinus extends inferiorly below the level of the nasal cavity into the alveolar process.

The roots of the maxillary first and second molars are often in close proximity to the floor of the sinus. Less frequently, the roots of the premolars and third molars may be observed in close proximity to the floor of the sinus. It has been suggested that the maxillary sinus expands or pneumatizes with age. It becomes more pneumatized down around the roots of the maxillary teeth, sometimes resulting in **exposure** of the roots through the bony floor into the sinus, with only the thin mucosal membrane covering the root surface. The ability to perform periodontal osseous surgery in the posterior maxilla may be limited when the sinuses are severely pneumatized. Extraction of teeth with roots exposed into the maxillary sinus (i.e., without bone to maintain integrity of the maxillary sinus floor) can result in an oroantral communication. A recent (2019) retrospective analysis using CBCT to assess maxillary sinus pneumatization has refuted the idea that it expands with age. Following CBCT evaluation of 50 dentate and 50 edentulous maxillae, the authors concluded that edentulism did not have an impact on maxillary sinus dimension, suggesting that there is no ongoing pneumatization in the sinus after tooth loss. Males had larger sinuses than females.

Blood supply to the maxillary sinus arises from the superior alveolar (anterior, middle, and posterior) branches of the maxillary artery (Fig. 42.14A). The maxillary artery, which is a large terminal branch of the external carotid artery, gives off many branches to supply the maxillary sinus, including the infraorbital artery, which travels superiorly and anteriorly and gives off the anterior superior alveolar artery. Branches of the greater palatine artery contribute to a lesser extent. Venous blood drains via the pterygoid plexus. Much of the vasculature travels through channels in the bony walls of the maxillary sinus, with many branches **anastomosing** with the highly vascularized Schneiderian membrane. Innervation of the maxillary sinus is supplied by the superior alveolar nerves (anterior, middle, and posterior) and branches of the maxillary nerve (see Fig. 42.14B).

Knowledge of the arterial blood supply is particularly important when considering a lateral window approach to sinus floor elevation and bone augmentation. Solar and colleagues found an intraosseous branch of the posterior superior alveolar artery anastomosing with the infraorbital artery in 100% of their human cadaver specimens (134 sinuses, all male cadavers). On average, the vessel was located 18.9 mm from the alveolar crest. By studying 50 CT scans from 625 patients (both male and female) who were undergoing sinus bone augmentation, Elian and colleagues found that the vessel was radiographically evident in 52.9% of sinuses. The vessel was located an average of 16.4 mm from the alveolar crest, a slightly shorter distance but consistent with the previous study. Human cadaver dissection and CT scan evaluations of the vessels running through the lateral wall of the maxillary sinus have revealed that intraosseous vessels are present in the lower two-thirds of the anterolateral wall in approximately 10.5% of cases (Fig. 42.15). In 57.1% of those cases (≈6% of all sinuses), the vessel diameter ranged in size from 1 to 2.5 mm. The location of the artery in relation to the position of the lateral window for sinus augmentation presents a risk for bleeding complications in 10%–20% of cases.

The floor of the maxillary sinus is frequently separated from the apices and roots of the maxillary posterior teeth by a thin bony plate (Fig. 42.16). In edentulous posterior areas, the maxillary sinus bony wall may only be a thin plate that is in intimate contact with the alveolar mucosa (Fig. 42.17). Adequate determination of the extension of the maxillary sinus into the surgical site is important to avoid creating an oroantral communication, particularly in relation

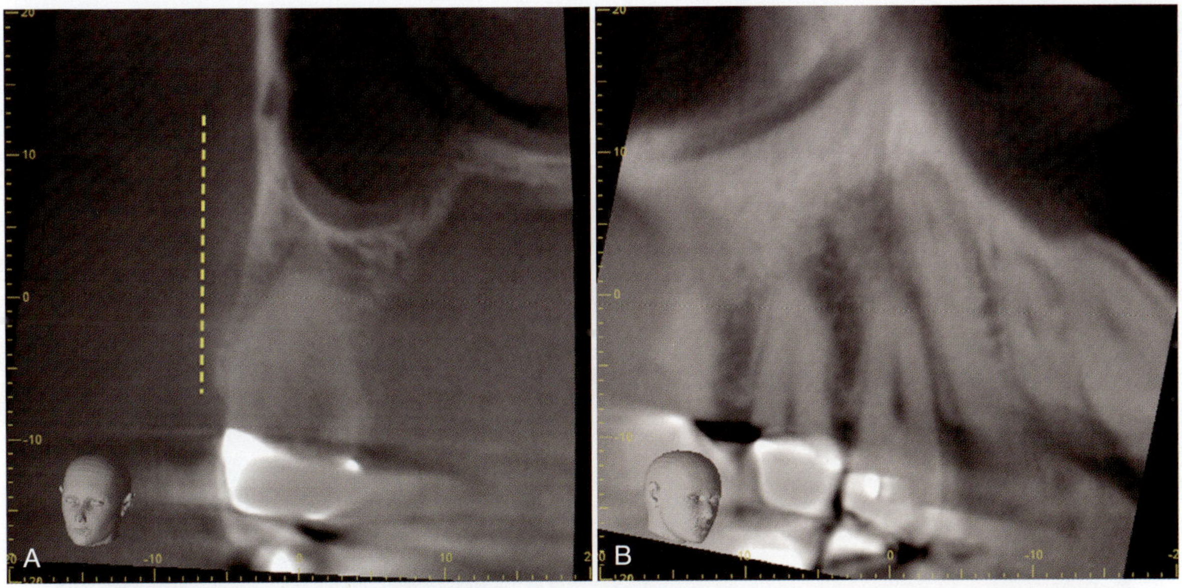

Fig. 42.15 A Cross-sectional image from a cone-beam computed tomography scan of the maxillary sinus demonstrating the presence of an intraosseous vessel in the lateral wall approximately 20 mm from the alveolar crest. B, Sagittal section through the maxillary sinus in the same patient demonstrating an intraosseous vessel extending along the maxillary sinus. The diameter of the intraosseous canal is 2 mm.

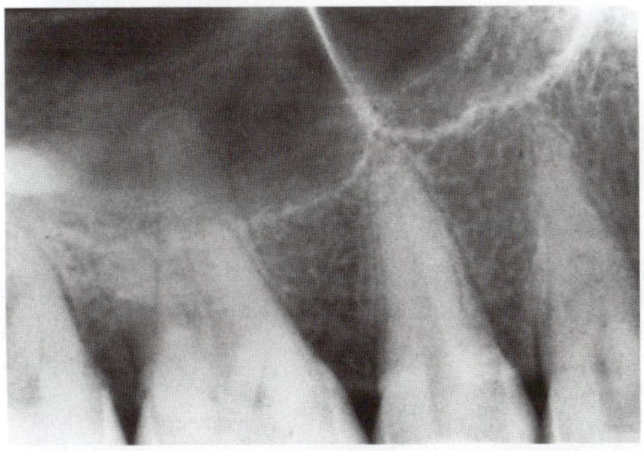

Fig. 42.16 Radiograph of the maxillary molars and premolars, with the maxillary sinus apparently near the apices. A radiopaque structure suggestive of a maxillary sinus septum is observed superior to the apex of the maxillary second premolar.

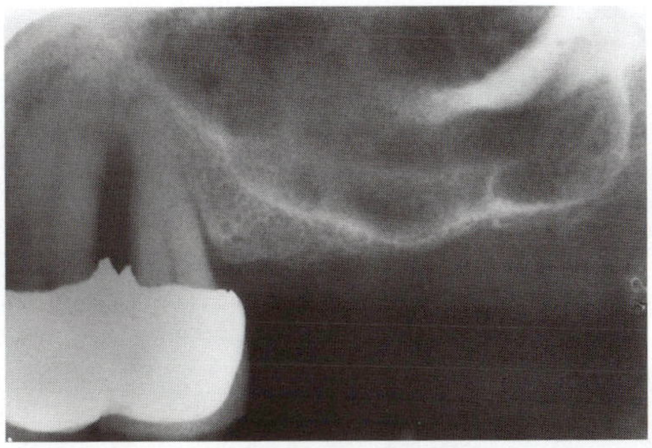

Fig. 42.17 Radiograph of an edentulous molar maxillary area demonstrating severe pneumatization of the maxillary sinus. Only a thin layer of cortical bone separates the sinus from the oral cavity.

to osseous reduction in periodontal surgery, surgical procedures for bone augmentation, or the placement of implants in edentulous areas. Determining the amount of available bone in the anterior area, inferior to the floor of the nasal cavity, is also critical for the placement of implants.

Exostoses

Both the maxilla and mandible may have exostoses or tori, which are considered to be within the normal range of anatomic variation. Sometimes these structures may hinder the daily **biofilm** removal by the patient and may have to be removed to improve the prognosis of adjacent teeth. Additional indications for the removal of exostoses include the inability to wear removable **prostheses** comfortably over these areas. The most common location of a mandibular torus is in the lingual area of the canines and premolars, superior to the mylohyoid muscle (Fig. 42.18). Mandibular tori can also be found on the buccal and labial surfaces of the mandibular teeth. Maxillary tori are usually located in the midline of the hard palate (Fig. 42.19). Smaller tori may be seen over the palatal roots of the maxillary molars, in the area inferior to the greater palatine foramen (see Fig. 42.19), or on the buccal and labial surfaces of the maxillary teeth (Fig. 42.20).

Muscles

Several muscles may be encountered when performing periodontal and implant placement flap surgery, particularly during **mucogingival** surgery and bone augmentation procedures. These are the mentalis, incisivus labii inferioris, depressor labii inferioris, depressor anguli oris (triangularis), incisivus labii superioris, and buccinator muscles. Their bony attachments are shown in Fig. 42.21. These muscles provide mobility to the lips and cheeks.

Anatomic Spaces

Several anatomic spaces or *compartments* are found close to the operative field of periodontal and implant surgery sites. These spaces contain loose connective tissue, but they can be easily distended by hemorrhage, inflammatory fluid, and infection.

Surgical invasion of these areas may result in dangerous hemorrhage (intraoperative) or infections (postoperative) and should be carefully avoided. Some of these spaces are briefly described in the following paragraphs. For more information, the reader is referred to other sources.

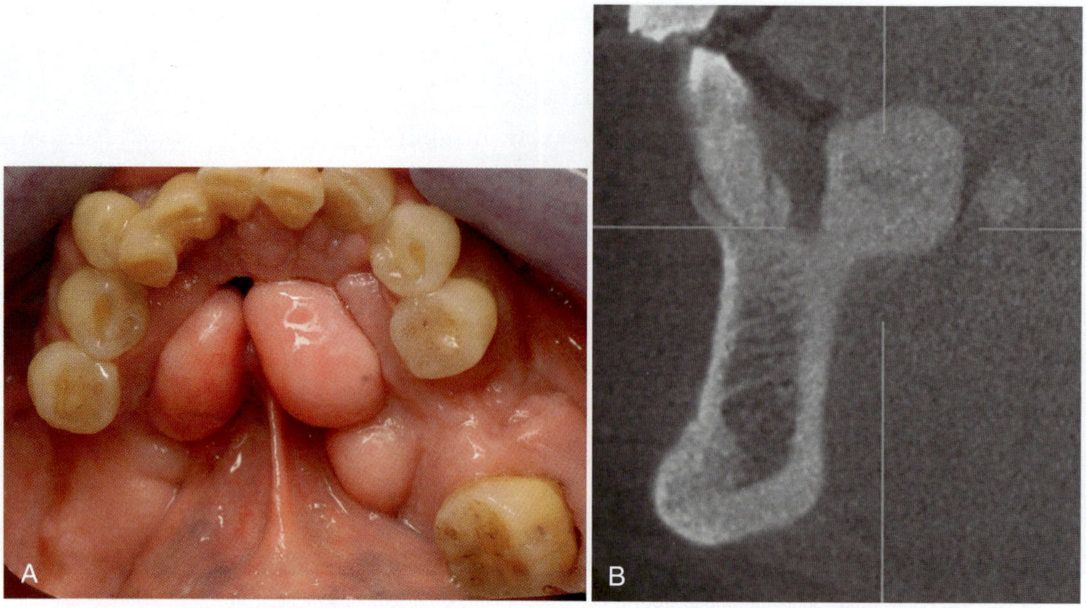

Fig. 42.18 A, Clinical photograph of large mandibular tori on the lingual aspect of both the right and left mandibles. B, Cross-sectional image of a mandibular torus in the premolar area in the same patient.

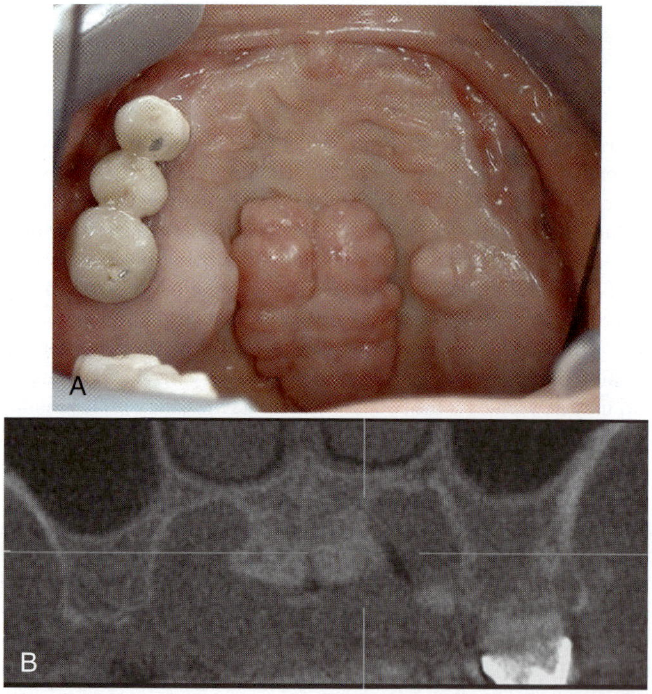

Fig. 42.19 A, Clinical photograph of a large palatal torus located in the midline of the palate. Note also the large tori on the palatal aspects of the maxillary alveolar ridge. B, Cross-sectional image of the maxillary midline torus in the same patient. Note also the torus located on the palatal aspect of the alveolar ridge.

The *canine fossa* contains varying amounts of connective tissue and fat. It is bounded superiorly by the levator (quadratus) labii superioris muscle, anteriorly by the orbicularis oris, and posteriorly by the buccinator. Infection of this area results in swelling of the upper lip, which obliterates the nasolabial fold, and possibly the upper and lower eyelids, resulting in closure of the eye.

The *buccal space* is located between the buccinator and masseter muscles. Infection of this area results in swelling of the cheek

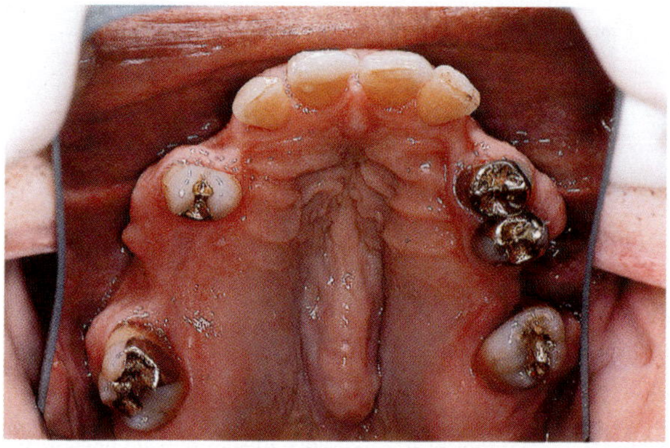

Fig. 42.20 Clinical photograph of large buccal exostosis in the maxillary arch. The patient also has a large midline palatal torus.

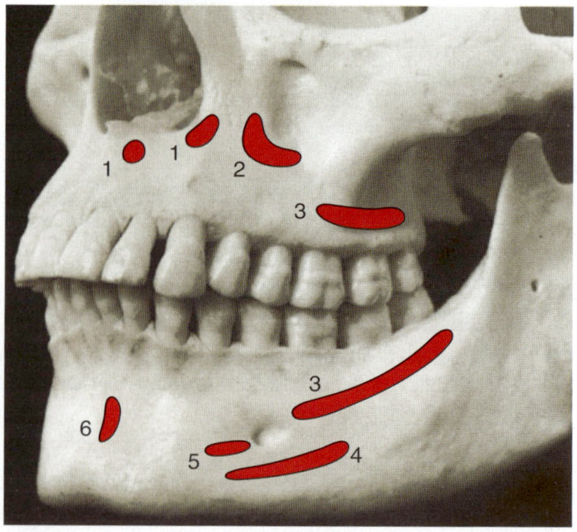

Fig. 42.21 Muscle attachments that may be encountered in mucogingival surgery. *1*, Nasalis; *2*, levator anguli oris; *3*, buccinator; *4*, depressor anguli oris; *5*, depressor labii inferioris; *6*, mentalis.

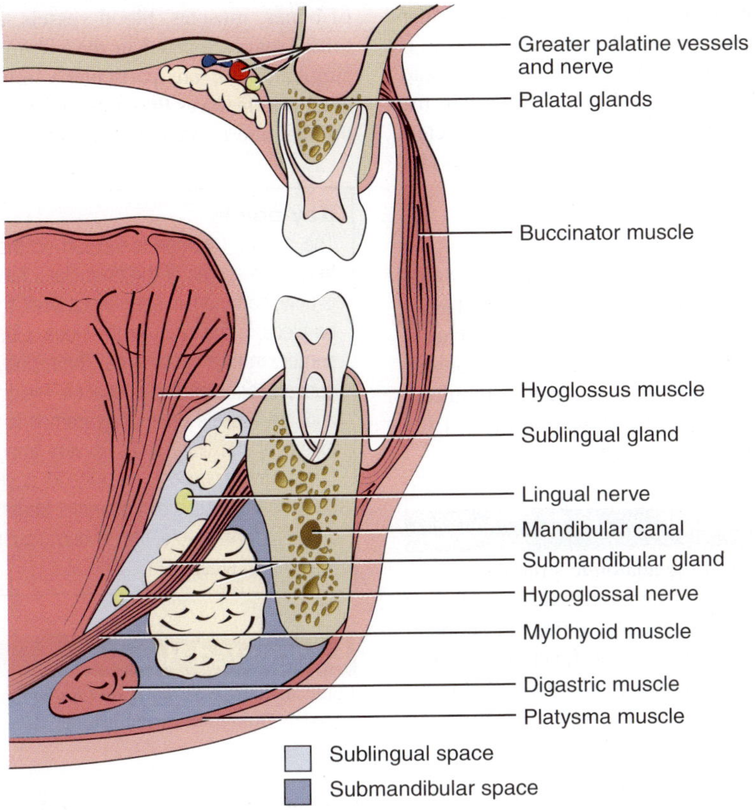

Fig. 42.22 Diagram of a frontal section of the human head at the level of the first molars depicting the most important structures in relation to periodontal surgery. Note the location of the sublingual space, submandibular space, and greater palatine nerve and vessels.

that may extend to the temporal or the submandibular spaces, with which the buccal space communicates.

The *mental* or *mentalis space* is located in the region of the mental symphysis, where the mentalis muscle, depressor labii inferioris, and depressor anguli oris are attached. Infection of this area results in large swelling of the chin, which extends inferiorly.

The *masticator space* contains the masseter muscle, pterygoid muscles, tendon of insertion of the temporalis muscle, mandibular ramus, and posterior part of the body of the mandible. Infection of this area results in swelling of the face, severe trismus, and pain. If the **abscess** occupies the deepest part of this compartment, facial swelling may not be obvious, but the patient may complain of pain and trismus. Patients may also complain of difficulty and discomfort when moving the tongue and swallowing.

The *sublingual space* is located below the oral mucosa in the anterior part of the floor of the mouth. It contains the sublingual gland and its excretory ducts and the submandibular (Wharton) duct. The sublingual space is traversed by the lingual nerve and vessels and by the hypoglossal nerve (Fig. 42.22). Its boundaries are the geniohyoid and genioglossus muscles medially, the lingual surface of the mandible inferiorly, and the mylohyoid muscle laterally and anteriorly (Fig. 42.23). Infection of this area raises the floor of the mouth and displaces the tongue, which results in pain and difficulty in swallowing but little facial swelling.

The *submental space* is found between the mylohyoid muscle superiorly and the platysma inferiorly. It is bounded laterally by the mandible and posteriorly by the hyoid bone. It is traversed by the anterior belly of the digastric muscle. Infections of this area arise from the region of the mandibular anterior teeth and result in swelling of the submental region; infections become more dangerous as they proceed posteriorly.

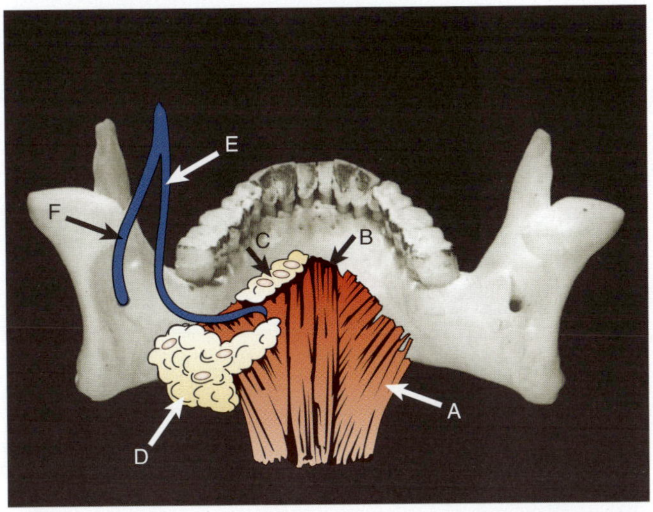

Fig. 42.23 Posterior view of the mandible showing the attachment of the mylohyoid muscles (A), geniohyoid muscles (B), sublingual gland (C), submandibular gland, which extends inferior to and also to some extent superior to the mylohyoid muscle (D), lingual nerve (E), and inferior alveolar nerve (F).

The *submandibular space* is found external to the sublingual space, inferior to the mylohyoid and hyoglossus muscles (see Figs. 42.22 and 42.23). This space contains the deep part of the submandibular gland, the superficial part of which extends partially superior to the mylohyoid muscle, thereby communicating with the sublingual space and numerous lymph nodes. Infections of this area originate in the molar or premolar area and result in swelling that obliterates the submandibular line and in pain with swallowing.

Ludwig angina is a severe form of infection of the submandibular space that may extend to the sublingual and submental spaces. It results in the hardening of the floor of the mouth and may lead to asphyxiation from edema of the neck and glottis. Although the bacteriology of these infections has not been completely determined, they are presumed to be mixed infections with an important **anaerobic** component.

Important Note

Ludwig angina is a life-threatening fascial space infection involving the submandibular, sublingual, and submental spaces. It is characterized by extraoral swelling and edema of the lower face and neck, with intraoral swelling that raises the floor of the mouth and tongue. If not treated urgently, it can lead to airway obstruction requiring tracheostomy. Infection can spread to other fascial spaces of the head and neck, including the retrosternal space.

Conclusion

Having a thorough understanding of the anatomic structures of the periodontium and the surrounding hard and soft tissues, including innervation and vasculature, is essential for periodontal and implant surgical procedures. Knowledge of anatomy and function is important for proper execution of surgical procedures, as well as to minimize the risk of injury and complications. The spatial relationship of bones, muscles, blood vessels, and nerves, as well as the anatomic spaces located in the vicinity of the periodontal or implant surgical field, are particularly important. This chapter describes anatomic features that are significant to clinicians performing periodontal and implant surgical therapy.

Key points

The mental foramen is located on the buccal surface of the mandible below the apices of the premolars. An anterior loop of the mental nerve is quite common. In edentulous jaws, the position of mental foramen may be close to the crest of the ridge. Lingual nerve may be injured during surgery in third molar area. The mylohyoid muscle separates the sublingual and submandibular spaces. The position of greater palatine foramen and the vessels emanating from it is very important. The location and extent of maxillary sinus is very important during implant placement. Canine fossa, buccal, masseteric, sublingual, submandibular, and post-pharyngeal spaces are potential targets of infection. Ludwig's angina is a severe form of infection involving submandibular, sublingual, and parapharyngeal spaces.

Suggested Reading

Louie Al-Faraje: *Surgical and Radiologic Anatomy for Oral Implantology*, ed 1, Quintessence Publishing, 2013.

CHAPTER 43

General Principles of Periodontal Surgery

PR Klokkevold | HH Takei | FA Carranza | CD Dwarakanath

CHAPTER OUTLINE

All periodontal surgical procedures must be carefully planned and executed. Clinicians must be knowledgeable and prepared for the surgical procedure as well as any untoward outcomes. Likewise, they need to prepare the patient medically, psychologically, and practically for all aspects of the surgical intervention. This chapter reviews general considerations that are common to all periodontal surgical procedures, including preparation of the patient, surgical instruments, intraoperative and postsurgical considerations, and management. Finally, although periodontal surgical procedures are usually performed in the dental office, an online section of this chapter briefly discusses situations that may require hospitalization and treatment using **general anesthesia** in the operating room.

Presurgical Patient Preparation

Reevaluation After Phase I Therapy

Most patients with **periodontitis** will have an initial or preparatory phase of therapy, which consists of patient education and thorough **root instrumentation** (**scaling** and **root planing**) to debride and remove all root surface accretions, **endotoxins**, or other irritants responsible for the periodontal **inflammation**. When these procedures are executed well and combined with good daily **biofilm** control, the results will: (1) eliminate some pockets entirely; (2) render the periodontal tissues firm and consistent, thereby facilitating the ability to perform more accurate and less invasive surgery; and (3) acquaint the patient with the office, the clinician, and the assistants, thereby reducing the patient's apprehension and fear.

The reevaluation phase consists of reprobing and reexamining all of the pertinent findings that previously indicated the need for surgery. The persistence of findings, such as deep pocket depth, confirms the indication for surgery. The number of surgical procedures, the anticipated outcome, and the postoperative care necessary should be determined and explained to the patient before scheduling treatment. Once the important information regarding the surgery is discussed, a final decision is made that incorporates any necessary adjustments to the original plan.

Premedication

For patients who are not medically compromised, the value of administering antibiotics for periodontal surgery has not been clearly demonstrated. Given the very low **incidence** of **infection** after periodontal surgery, there does not seem to be justification for the prophylactic use of antibiotics in healthy patients. Some older studies reported reduced postoperative complications, including reduced pain and swelling, when antibiotics are given before periodontal surgery and continued for 4–7 days after surgery.

The prophylactic use of antibiotics in patients who are otherwise healthy has been advocated for bone-grafting procedures and purported to enhance the results. Although the rationale for such use appears logical, published research to support it is scant. A **systematic review** of the literature assessing **randomized controlled clinical trials (RCTs)** and systematic reviews and **metaanalyses** that reported results of preventive antibiotic therapy for bone augmentation procedures in oral implantology found only one systematic review and four RCTs that met the inclusion criteria. The conclusion from this systematic review of bone augmentation for oral implantology recommended the prescription of 2 or 3 g of amoxicillin 1 h prior to surgery to reduce early failure of one-stage implants and to decrease bacterial loads in grafted bone. A survey of prescribing practices, among periodontists in California, for periodontal surgery confirmed there is a greater tendency for clinicians to prescribe antibiotics when bone grafts are used as opposed to when periodontal surgery is performed without the addition of bone grafts. In any case, the risks inherent in the administration of antibiotics should be evaluated together with the potential benefits.

Additional presurgical medications that may be administered include a nonsteroidal antiinflammatory drug such as ibuprofen (e.g., Motrin) 1 h before the procedure and rinsing with an **antimicrobial** mouthrinse such as 0.12% **chlorhexidine** gluconate (e.g., Peridex or PerioGard).

Smoking

The deleterious effect of smoking on the healing of periodontal wounds has been amply documented. Patients should be clearly informed about the adverse effect of smoking and advised to quit completely or to stop smoking for a minimum of 3–4 weeks after the procedure. For patients who are unwilling to follow this advice, an alternative **treatment plan** that does not include complex procedures (e.g., regenerative, **mucogingival**, esthetic) should be considered.

Informed Consent

Obtaining informed consent from the patient for surgical treatment is essential. The patient should be informed at the initial visit regarding the diagnosis, prognosis, and recommended treatment options that include explanations about expected outcomes. The pros and cons of each approach should be discussed prior to scheduling the surgery, and the patient should be encouraged to ask questions. On the day of surgery, the patient should again be reminded about the procedure to be performed, including the risks and expected outcomes. Patients should be given the opportunity to ask any additional questions, and, once their questions are answered, they should indicate their agreement to undergo the procedure by signing the informed consent.

Emergency Equipment

The clinician, all assistants, and office personnel should be trained to handle all possible medical emergencies that could arise. Each member of the team needs to know their role should an emergency situation present. Drugs and equipment for medical emergencies should be routinely checked for expiration and readily available at all times.

Syncope, which is a transient loss of consciousness caused by a reduction in cerebral blood flow, is the most common emergency. It is often precipitated by fear and anxiety. The syncope event is usually preceded by a feeling of weakness, and then the patient experiences pallor, sweating, coldness of the extremities, dizziness, and a slowing of the pulse. The patient should be placed in a supine position with the legs elevated, tight clothes should be loosened, and a wide-open airway should be ensured. Oxygen administration should be started. Unconsciousness may persist for a few minutes. A previous history of syncope during dental appointments should be explored before the treatment is started. If the patient has had other experiences with syncope, every effort should be made to minimize the patient's fear and anxiety. The use of oral sedatives should be considered as well.

Infection Control

Preventing the transmission of infections to the dental team or to other patients is a critical precaution that must be a part of every appointment in the dental office, especially with the threat of life-threatening infections, which are transmitted through body fluids. In the dental setting, blood-borne **viruses** including hepatitis B virus (HBV), hepatitis C virus (HCV), and **human immunodeficiency virus (HIV)**, along with respiratory **pathogens**, present the highest risks of cross-infection. Universal precautions, the use of personal protective equipment, and barrier techniques must be incorporated into the surgical protocol for every procedure. These include the use of disposable sterile gloves, gowns, caps, surgical masks, and protective eyewear. All surfaces that may be contaminated with blood or **saliva** but that cannot be sterilized (e.g., light handles, chairs) must be covered with sterile aluminum foil or plastic wrap. Aerosol-producing devices (e.g., ultrasonic scalers) should not be used on patients with suspected infections, and their use should be kept to a minimum in all other patients. This is especially true for preventing the spread of **contagious** infections, such as the SARS-CoV-2 coronavirus, which is an airborne pathogen and a concern for dental offices, but adhering to safe infection prevention practices, including screening patients for symptoms should mitigate the risk.

At the conclusion of each procedure, all instruments, handpieces, and burs must be properly cleansed of biologic debris in ultrasonic cleaners, dried, packaged, and sterilized. Excised tissues and contaminated gauze must be disposed as biohazard waste, and sharps (i.e., needles and blades) need to be carefully removed and disposed in special sharps containers.

Checklist before commencement of surgery:

Go through all the following criteria before starting surgery. The answers should be YES for all questions:

1. The patient
   a. Is the patient medically fit to undergo surgery?
   b. Have you ruled out the patients' allergy to local anesthetics, if any?
   c. Has the patient been duly explained about the need for surgery?
   d. Has informed consent been taken?
   e. Does the patient has any ailment today (like cold, cough, and diarrhea)?
   f. Has the patient taken meals?
   g. Have all necessary laboratory investigations been done and found to be within normal limits?
2. The periodontal status
   a. Is the surgery planned, indicated?
   b. Is the oral hygiene status satisfactory?
   c. Are the gingival tissues firm and well prepared?
   d. Is the oral cavity free of any acute inflammatory condition (such as aphthous ulcer and pulpitis)?
   e. Has root canal therapy been completed in case of endo-perio lesions?
3. The surgical plan
   a. Has the surgical plan been prepared?
   b. Are the presurgical photographs, models, and radiographs ready?
4. The surgical set-up
   a. Have all the required instruments been sterilized?
   b. Are all the components of the dental unit working?
   c. Are osseous management requirements present?
   d. Are the required suture materials available?
   e. Is the updated emergency medical kit available?

Intraoperative Surgical Considerations

Sedation and Anesthesia

Pain control during periodontal surgery is very important. Most procedures should be painless. The patient should be assured of this at the beginning and throughout the procedure. The most reliable means of providing painless surgery is the effective administration of local anesthesia. The area to be treated should be thoroughly anesthetized by means of regional block and local infiltration. Injections directly into the interdental papillae may also be helpful.

Apprehensive and neurotic patients may require special management with antianxiety or sedative-hypnotic agents. Modalities for the administration of these agents include inhalation, oral, intramuscular, and intravenous routes. The specific agents and the modality of administration are based on the desired level of sedation, the anticipated length of the procedure, and the overall condition of the patient. Specifically, the patient's medical history and physical and emotional status should be considered when determining the need for sedation, as well as the specific agents and techniques to be used.

Tissue Management

It is important to manage tissues well during surgery to optimize healing and minimize postoperative discomfort. There are some specific guidelines to follow including operating gently, ensuring that instruments are sharp and monitoring the patient at all times.

1. *Operate gently and carefully*. In addition to being most considerate to the patient, this is also the most effective way to operate. Tissue manipulation should be precise, deliberate, and gentle. It is essential to be thorough, but traumatic instrumentation and aggressive tissue manipulation must be avoided because it produces excessive tissue injury, causes postoperative discomfort, and delays healing.
2. *Be certain that the instruments are sharp*. Instruments must be sharp to be effective; a successful treatment outcome will be more likely when using sharp instruments. Dull instruments inflict unnecessary trauma as a result of inefficient cutting and

excessive forces applied to compensate for their ineffectiveness. A sterile sharpening stone should be available on the operating table at all times. Sharpening instruments during a procedure is essential and may be necessary.

3. *Observe the patient at all times*. It is important to pay careful attention to the patient's reactions. Facial expressions, pallor, and perspiration are distinct signs that may indicate when a patient is experiencing pain, anxiety, or fear. The clinician's responsiveness to these signs can be the difference between success and failure.

Root Instrumentation

Although root instrumentation (scaling and root planing) may have been performed previously as part of the initial phase I therapy, all exposed root surfaces should be carefully inspected, explored, and instrumented as needed during the surgical procedure. In particular, areas of difficult access (e.g., **furcations**, deep infrabony pockets) often have rough areas or residual calculus that was inaccessible or undetected during the preparatory sessions. The assistant who is retracting the tissues and using the aspirator should also check for the presence of calculus and the smoothness of each surface from a different angle.

Intrasurgical Complications

Despite extensive planning and precautions, sometimes complications occur during periodontal surgery. However, an alert and consummate clinician can manage to effectively overcome the situation.

1. Syncope and exhaustion

   Often patients complain of giddiness and a feeling of extreme tiredness during surgery. They may also go into syncope. The clinician should be well prepared to manage such adverse situations. This is more so in patients having medical problems like diabetes mellitus and hypertension. It is important to make sure that the patient had a restful night and proper meals before surgery. Prolonged surgery is also a common cause for patients to get exhausted. Ideally, surgery should be completed within an hour.

2. Pain during surgery

   It is not uncommon for patients to complain of pain during surgery, thereby making it difficult for proper instrumentation. Hence, it is important that adequate anesthesia is obtained prior to incision. If there is a possibility of the surgery prolonged, a long acting local anesthetic such as Bupivacaine is used. It is once again emphasized that surgical procedures should be completed within the stipulated time.

3. Hemorrhage

   Although bleeding occurs after the incisions, it usually is manageable as the surgery goes on. However, at times, excessive bleeding which is difficult to control occurs. This is mainly due to surgery done on unprepared tissues, perforation of flap, excess flap reflection, failure to remove granulation tissue or damage to vessels like greater palatine artery, mental artery, etc. A good suction system is vital for proper visibility of the surgical area. It is important to note that local hemostatics, such as Gelfoam and Botroclot, are ineffective when there is continuous bleeding. Of course, the clinician would have made sure that the patient does not suffer from any known bleeding disorder. A list of common absorbable hemostatic agents is given in Table 43.1.

TABLE 43.1 Absorbable Hemostatic Agents

Generic (Brand)	Directions	Adverse Effects	Precautions
Absorbable gelatin sponge (Gelfoam)	May be cut into various sizes and applied to bleeding surfaces	May form nidus for infection or abscess	Should not be overpacked into extraction site or wound—may interfere with healing
Oxidized cellulose (Oxycel)	Most effective when applied to wound dry as opposed to moistened	May cause foreign body reaction	Extremely friable and difficult to place; should not be used adjacent to bone—impairs bone regeneration; should not be used as a surface dressing—inhibits epithelialization
Oxidized regenerated cellulose (Surgicel Absorbable Hemostat)	May be cut to various shapes and positioned over bleeding sites; thick or excessive amounts should not be used	Encapsulation, cyst formation, and foreign body reaction possible	Should not be placed in deep wounds—may physically interfere with wound healing and bone formation
Microfibrillar collagen hemostat (Avitene)	May be cut to shape and applied to bleeding surface	May potentiate abscess formation, hematoma, and wound dehiscence; possible allergic reaction or foreign body reaction	May interfere with wound healing; placement in extraction sockets has been associated with increased pain
Collagen hemostat/ glycosaminoglycans (CollaCote, CollaTape, CollaPlug)	May be cut to shape and applied to bleeding surface	May become infected	Do not use on infected or contaminated wounds
Chitosan-based dressing (HemCon Dental Dressing Pro)	May be trimmed to fit; most effective in presence of blood to wet surface	Contains chitosan from shellfish.	Sutures may be used but not always required since dressing sticks to wound. Do not place into wound with primary closure.
Thrombin (Thrombostat)	May be applied topically to bleeding surface	Allergic reaction can occur in patients with known sensitivity to bovine materials	Must not be injected into tissues or vasculature—can cause severe (and possibly fatal) clotting

Postsurgical Management

Periodontal Dressings (Periodontal Packs)

At completion of the periodontal surgical procedure, clinicians may elect to cover the area with a periodontal dressing. In general, dressings have no curative properties but assist healing by protecting the tissue rather than providing "healing factors." The dressing minimizes the likelihood of postoperative infection, facilitates healing by preventing surface trauma during mastication, and protects the patient from pain induced by contact of the wound with food or with the tongue during mastication. For a complete literature review on this subject, see the article by Sachs and colleagues. In a study comparing the postoperative pain experienced by patients with and without periodontal dressings, Checchi and Trombelli reported no significant difference between treatment groups with respect to frequency of analgesic use. Most patients stated a psychological feeling of protection with the periodontal dressing.

Zinc Oxide–Eugenol Dressing

Dressings that are based on the reaction of zinc oxide and eugenol include the Wonder Pak, which was developed by Ward in 1923, and several other dressings that use modified forms of Ward's original formula. The addition of accelerators, such as zinc acetate, gives the material better working time.

Zinc oxide–eugenol dressings are supplied as a liquid and a powder that are mixed before use. Eugenol in this type of dressing may induce an allergic reaction that produces reddening of the area and burning pain in some patients.

Noneugenol Dressing

The reaction between a metallic oxide and fatty acids is the basis for Coe-Pak, which is the most widely used periodontal dressing in the United States. This is supplied in two tubes, the contents of which are mixed immediately before use until a uniform color is obtained. One tube contains zinc oxide, an oil (for plasticity), a gum (for cohesiveness), and lorothidol (a fungicide).

The other tube contains liquid coconut fatty acids that have been thickened with colophony resin (or rosin) and chlorothymol (a bacteriostatic agent). This dressing does not contain asbestos or eugenol, thereby avoiding the problems associated with these substances.

Other noneugenol dressings include cyanoacrylates and tissue conditioners (methacrylate gels). However, these products are not in common use.

Retention of Dressing

Periodontal dressings are usually kept in place mechanically by interlocking the dressing in interdental spaces and joining the lingual and facial portions of the dressing. In isolated teeth or when several teeth in an arch are missing, retention of the dressing may be difficult. Numerous reinforcements, splints, and stents for this purpose have been described. The placement of dental floss tied loosely around the teeth enhances retention of the dressing.

Antibacterial Properties of Dressing

Improved healing and patient comfort with less odor and foul taste have been obtained by incorporating antibiotics into the dressing. Bacitracin, oxytetracycline (Terramycin), neomycin, and nitrofurazone have been used. Care must be taken when any antibiotic products are used because they may produce hypersensitivity reactions. The emergence of resistant organisms and **opportunistic infections** has also been reported. The incorporation of tetracycline powder into the Coe-Pak is generally recommended, particularly when long and traumatic surgical procedures are performed.

Allergy

Contact allergies to eugenol and rosin have been reported.

Preparation and Application of Dressing

Zinc oxide dressings are mixed with eugenol or noneugenol liquids on a wax paper pad with a spatula or a wooden tongue depressor. The powder is gradually incorporated with the liquid until a thick paste is formed.

Coe-Pak is prepared by mixing equal lengths of paste from tubes that contain the accelerator and the base until the resulting paste is a uniform color (Fig. 43.1A–C). A capsule of tetracycline powder can be added at this time. The dressing is then placed in a cup of water at room temperature (see Fig. 43.1D). After 2–3 min, the paste loses its tackiness, and it can be handled and molded. The mixed dressing remains workable for 15–20 min. The working time can be shortened by adding a small amount of zinc oxide to the accelerator (pink paste) before spatulating.

The dressing is then rolled into two strips that are approximately the length of the treated area. The end of one strip is bent into a hook shape and fitted around the distal surface of the last tooth to approach that tooth from the distal surface (Fig. 43.2A). The remainder of the strip is brought forward along the facial surface to the midline and gently pressed into place along the **gingival** margin and interproximally. The second strip is applied from the lingual surface. It is joined to the dressing at the distal surface of the last tooth and then brought forward along the gingival margin to the midline and gently pressed (see Fig. 43.2B). The strips are joined interproximally by applying gentle pressure on the facial and lingual surfaces of the dressing (see Fig. 43.2C). For isolated teeth separated by **edentulous** spaces, the dressing should be made continuous from tooth to tooth to cover the edentulous areas (Fig. 43.3).

When split-thickness flaps have been performed, the area should be covered with a sterile tinfoil to protect the wound and sutures before the dressing is placed.

The dressing should cover the gingiva, but overextension onto uninvolved mucosa should be avoided. *Excess dressing irritates the*

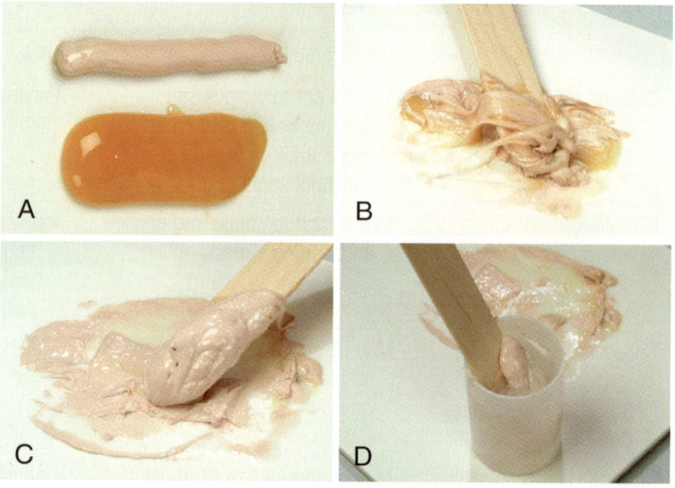

Fig. 43.1 Preparing the surgical pack (Coe-Pak). A, Equal lengths of the two pastes are placed on a paper pad. B, The pastes are mixed with a wooden tongue depressor for 2 or 3 min until (C) the paste loses its tackiness. D, The mixed paste is placed in a paper cup of water at room temperature. With lubricated fingers, it is then rolled into cylinders and placed on the surgical wound.

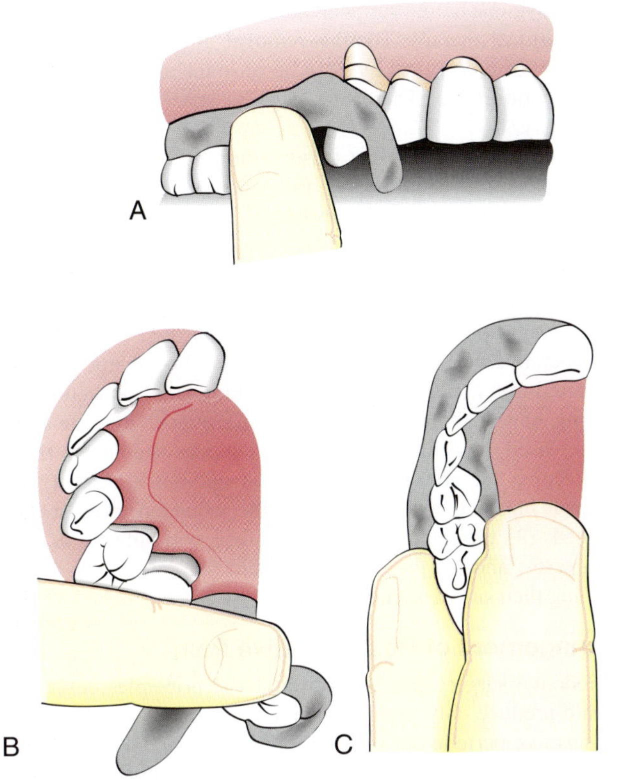

Fig. 43.2 Inserting the periodontal pack. A, A strip of pack is hooked around the last molar and pressed into place anteriorly. B, The lingual pack is joined to the facial strip at the distal surface of the last molar and fitted into place anteriorly. C, Gentle pressure on the facial and lingual surfaces joins the pack interproximally.

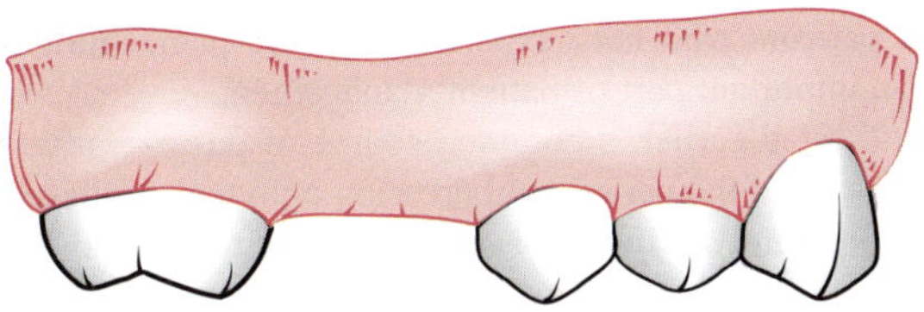

Fig. 43.3 Continuous pack covers the edentulous space.

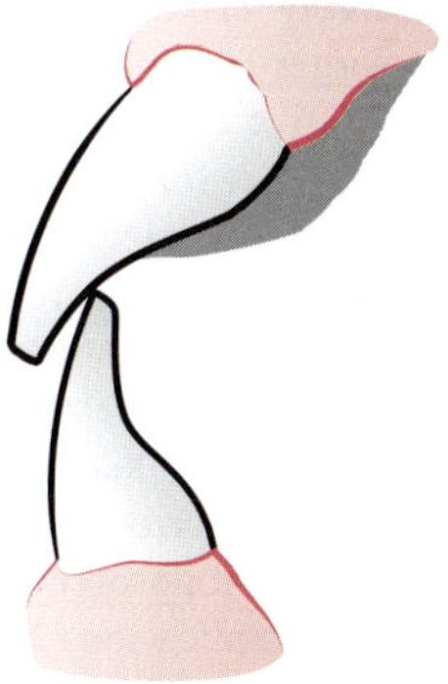

Fig. 43.4 Periodontal pack should not interfere with the occlusion.

mucobuccal fold and the floor of the mouth, and it interferes with the tongue. Overextension also jeopardizes retention of the dressing because the excess tends to break off and loosens the dressing from the operated area. *Dressing that covers occlusal surfaces or otherwise interferes with the occlusion should be removed before the patient is dismissed* (Fig. 43.4). Failure to do this causes discomfort and jeopardizes retention of the dressing.

The operator should ask the patient to move the tongue forcibly out and to each side, and the cheek and lips should be displaced in all directions to mold the dressing while it is still soft. After the dressing has set, it should be trimmed to eliminate all excess.

As a general rule, the dressing is kept on for 1 week after surgery. This guideline is based on the usual timetable of healing and clinical experience. It is not a rigid requirement; the period may be extended, or the area may be redressed for an additional week.

Portions of the dressing may not remain during the week, but this should not present a problem. If the dressing is lost from the operated area and the patient is uncomfortable, it is usually best to redress the area. The clinician should remove the remaining dressing, irrigate the area with warm water, and apply a topical anesthetic before replacing the dressing, which is then retained for another week. The excess dressing should be trimmed away with care taken to ensure that the new margin is not rough before the patient is dismissed.

Postoperative Instructions

After the dressing is placed, postoperative instructions are given verbally and in writing before the patient is dismissed from the chair.

First Postoperative Week

When the therapy is properly performed, periodontal surgery should present minimal postoperative problems. If biofilm control is compromised, patients can be instructed to rinse with 0.12% chlorhexidine gluconate (Peridex, PerioGard) immediately after the surgical procedure and twice daily thereafter until normal biofilm control can be resumed. The following complications may arise during the first postoperative week, although they are the exception rather than the rule:

1. *Persistent bleeding after surgery.* The dressing is removed, and local anesthesia may be needed before the bleeding areas are located. The bleeding is stopped with pressure, or if necessary, the area may have to be anesthetized and resutured. After the bleeding has been stopped, the area is again redressed.
2. *Sensitivity to percussion.* Extension of inflammation into the periodontal ligament may cause sensitivity to percussion. The patient should be questioned regarding the progress of the symptoms. Gradual diminishing discomfort is a favorable sign. The dressing should be removed and the surgical area checked for localized areas of infection or irritation. The area should be irrigated or incised to provide drainage if areas of localized **exudate** are present. Particles of calculus that may have been overlooked should be removed. Adjusting the occlusion can be helpful. Sensitivity to percussion may also be caused by excess dressing, which interferes with the occlusion. Removal of the excess usually corrects the condition.
3. *Swelling.* During the first 2 postoperative days, some patients may report a soft, painless swelling of the cheek in the surgical area. Lymph node enlargement may occur, and the temperature may be slightly elevated. The area of operation itself is usually symptom free. This type of involvement results from a localized inflammatory reaction to the surgical procedure. It generally subsides by the fourth postoperative day without necessitating the removal of the dressing. If swelling persists, enlarges, or is associated with increased pain, amoxicillin (500 mg) should be taken every 8 h for 1 week and moist heat can be applied intermittently to the area. The patient should be monitored closely until resolved.
4. *Feeling of weakness.* Occasionally, patients report having experienced a "washed-out," weakened feeling for about 24 h after surgery. This represents a systemic reaction to transient bacteremia

induced by the procedure. This reaction can be mitigated by premedication with amoxicillin (500 mg) every 8 h. This protocol should be started 24 h before the next procedure and continued for 5 days postoperatively.

Postoperative Visit and Removal of the Dressing

When the patient returns in 1 week, the periodontal dressing is removed by inserting a curette along the margin and exerting gentle lateral pressure. Pieces of the dressing retained interproximally and particles adhering to the tooth surfaces are also removed with curettes. Particles of dressing and debris may be enmeshed in the surgical surfaces and should be carefully removed with cotton pliers. The entire area is irrigated with peroxide or saline to remove the superficial debris.

Findings at the Time of Dressing Removal

Typical findings when the dressing is removed include the following:

- If *gingivectomy* has been performed, the incised surface is covered with a friable meshwork of new **epithelium**. This tissue should not be disturbed. If calculus has not been completely removed, red, beadlike protuberances of granulation tissue will persist. The granulation tissue must be removed with a curette to expose the calculus so the root can be planed. Granulation tissue will recur if the residual calculus is not completely removed.
- After a *flap operation*, the areas that correspond to the incisions are epithelialized, but they may bleed readily if irritated. These areas should not be disturbed nor probed.
- The facial and lingual mucosa may be covered with a grayish-yellow or white granular layer of debris that has entered under the dressing. This is easily removed with a moist cotton pellet or swab. The root surfaces may be sensitive to touch or to thermal change. The patient should be advised that these changes will diminish with time (4–6 weeks). The dentition that was beneath the dressing may be stained in a brownish-yellow color that can be removed by polishing at a later date.
- *Fragments of calculus delay healing.* Each root surface should be carefully rechecked visually to be certain that no calculus was missed during surgery. The grooves on proximal root surfaces and furcations are areas where calculus is likely to have been overlooked or missed.

Redressing

After the dressing is removed, it is usually not necessary to replace it. However, redressing for an additional week is advised for the following types of patients: (1) those with a low pain threshold who are particularly uncomfortable when the dressing is removed; (2) those with unusually sensitive root surfaces after surgery; or (3) those with an open wound where the flap edges have necrosed. Clinical judgment helps when deciding whether to redress the area or to leave the initial dressing for a longer period.

Tooth Mobility

Tooth mobility usually increases immediately after surgery. This is caused by edema in the periodontal ligament space from the inflammation that occurs following surgery. The mobility diminishes to the pretreatment level by the fourth week. The patient should be reassured before surgery that the increased tooth mobility after surgery is temporary.

Mouth Care Between Procedures

Care of the mouth by the patient between the treatments as well as after the surgery is extremely important. Biofilm control should begin after the dressing is removed. The patient has had instructions on oral hygiene before surgical therapy but must be instructed again after surgical therapy. Biofilm removal after surgery is different from that of presurgical hygiene because the areas are still healing and uncomfortable. There may also be spaces that did not exist previously.

Vigorous brushing is not feasible during the first week after the dressing is removed. However, the patient should be informed that biofilm and food accumulation impair healing and they should be advised to try to keep the area as clean as possible with the gentle use of an extra soft toothbrush and light water irrigation. Rinsing with a chlorhexidine mouthwash or applying such a rinse topically with cotton-tipped applicators may be indicated for the first few postoperative weeks, especially for those who are not effective or too timid to try. Return to normal brushing is introduced when the healing of the tissues permits, and the overall hygiene regimen is increased as healing progresses. Patients should be told that (1) keeping the area clean will aid in optimal healing; (2) some gingival bleeding will occur when the wounded areas are gently cleaned; (3) this bleeding is normal and will subside as healing progresses; and (4) the bleeding should not deter them from performing their oral hygiene regimen.

Management of Postoperative Pain

Periodontal surgery that follows the basic principles outlined here should produce only minimal pain and discomfort. A study of 304 consecutive periodontal surgical interventions revealed that 51.3% of the patients reported minimal or no postoperative pain, and only 4.6% reported severe pain. Of these, only 20.1% took five or more doses of analgesic. This is consistent with the finding of another study that reports a 4.1% incidence of severe pain following periodontal flap surgery. The previous study indicated that mucogingival surgery was 3.5 times more likely to cause pain than osseous surgery and 6 times more likely than plastic soft tissue surgery. For the few patients who may experience severe pain, **analgesia** becomes an important part of patient management.

As indicated earlier, a common source of postoperative pain is overextension of the periodontal dressing onto the soft tissue apical to the **mucogingival junction**, on a frenum, or beyond the vestibule. Overextended dressings cause localized areas of edema that are usually noticed 1–2 days after surgery. The removal of excess dressing is followed by resolution in about 24 h.

Extensive and excessively prolonged exposure of bone with poor irrigation during surgery induces greater pain. For most healthy patients, a preoperative dose of ibuprofen (600–800 mg) followed by one tablet every 8 h for 24–48 h is very effective for reducing discomfort after periodontal surgery. Alternatively, a preoperative dose of acetaminophen (500–1000 mg) may be taken followed by one tablet every 6 h for 24–48 h. Patients are advised to continue taking ibuprofen or acetaminophen thereafter, if needed. If pain persists, a narcotic such as acetaminophen plus codeine (Tylenol #3) can be prescribed. Caution should be used when prescribing or dispensing ibuprofen to patients with hypertension that is controlled by medications because it can interfere with the effectiveness of the medication. Ibuprofen should be avoided for patients with impaired kidney function. Patients experiencing severe postoperative pain should be seen on an emergency basis. The area should be anesthetized by infiltration, and the dressing should be removed to allow for the examination of the area in pain. Postoperative pain related to infection is accompanied by signs of infection (e.g., increased **erythema**, exudate, swelling), localized **lymphadenopathy**, and a slight elevation in temperature. This type of pain should be treated with systemic antibiotics and analgesics.

Dentin (Root) Hypersensitivity

Dentin or root hypersensitivity is a relatively common problem in dental and periodontal practices. It may occur spontaneously when the root becomes exposed as a result of gingival recession or pocket formation, or it may appear after root instrumentation (scaling and root planing) or periodontal surgical procedures. This type of sensitivity is manifested as pain that is induced by thermal changes (cold or hot temperature), by citrus fruits or sweets, or by contact with a toothbrush or a dental instrument.

Root sensitivity occurs more frequently in the cervical area of the root, where the **cementum** is extremely thin. Root instrumentation procedures remove this thin cementum, thereby inducing the hypersensitivity.

The transmission of stimuli from the surface of the dentin to the nerve endings located in the dental pulp or in the pulpal region of the dentin could result from the odontoblastic process or from a hydrodynamic mechanism (i.e., the displacement of dentinal fluid in the dentinal tubules). The latter process seems more likely and has been widely accepted as the mechanism, which would also explain the importance of burnishing desensitizing agents to obturate the dentinal tubule.

An important factor for reducing or eliminating hypersensitivity is adequate biofilm control. The problem is that hypersensitivity often prevents the patient from performing biofilm control, and therefore a vicious cycle of escalating hypersensitivity, avoidance, and biofilm accumulation ensues.

The patient should be informed about the possibility of root hypersensitivity *before* treatment. A patient who is educated about any potential adverse issues before surgery will be more understanding and less likely to complain because he or she is aware and expects the sensitivity may occur. The following information on how to cope with the problem should also be given to the patient:

1. Dentin hypersensitivity appears as a result of dentin exposure, which is inevitable if calculus, biofilm, and **endotoxins** are removed via root instrumentation.
2. Dentin hypersensitivity slowly disappears in a few weeks.
3. Biofilm control is an important factor in reducing dentin hypersensitivity.
4. Desensitizing agents do not produce immediate relief and must be used for at least 2 weeks to produce results.

Desensitizing Agents

Numerous desensitizing agents have been proposed to control dentin hypersensitivity. Clinical evaluation of these agents is difficult for the following reasons: (1) measuring and comparing pain among patients with different thresholds are difficult, (2) the time required for hypersensitivity resolution is different for each patient, and (3) each desensitizing agent acts differently both in terms of time and the level of relief it offers.

Desensitizing agents can be applied by the patient at home or by the dentist or hygienist in the dental office. The most likely mechanism of action is the reduction of the diameter of the dentinal tubules or blockage to limit the displacement of fluid. According to Trowbridge and Silver, this can be attained in the following ways: (1) by the formation of a smear layer produced by burnishing the exposed surface, (2) via the topical application of agents that form insoluble precipitates within the tubules, or (3) with the impregnation or sealing of tubules with plastic resins.

The most common agents used by the patient for oral hygiene are dentifrices. Although many dentifrice products contain stannous fluoride, which can help to decrease dentin hypersensitivity, additional active ingredients for desensitization are strontium chloride, potassium nitrate, sodium citrate, and arginine. The American Dental Association has approved several dentifrices for desensitizing purposes (Table 43.2). Fluoride rinsing solutions and gels can also be used after the usual biofilm control procedures.

TABLE 43.2 Common ADA Approved Dentifrices for Desensitization

Toothpaste	Active Ingredient(s)	Company
Sensodyne Original	Strontium chloride	GlaxoSmithKline Consumer Healthcare
Sensodyne Sensitivity and Gum	Stannous fluoride (0.454%) Sodium fluoride (0.072%)	GlaxoSmithKline Consumer Healthcare
Crest Pro-Health Gum and Sensitivity	Stannous fluoride (0.454%)	Proctor & Gamble Co.
Colgate Sensitive Prevent and Repair	Potassium nitrate (5.0%) Sodium fluoride (0.24%)	Colgate-Palmolive Co.
Colgate Sensitive Pro-Relief	Arginine (8.0%) Sodium fluoride (0.24%)	Colgate-Palmolive Co.

Note: This table is not intended to be an exhaustive or comprehensive list of dentrifrices for desensitization.
ADA, American Dental Association.

Patients should be aware that several factors must be considered during the treatment of dentin hypersensitivity, including the history and severity of the problem, as well as the physical findings of the tooth or teeth involved. A proper diagnosis is required before any treatment can be initiated so that pathologic causes of pain, such as dental **caries**, chipped or cracked tooth, fractured or leaking restoration, trauma from occlusion, and other pulpal problems can be ruled out before attempting to treat the dentin hypersensitivity. Desensitizing agents act through the precipitation of crystalline salts on the dentin surface that block dentinal tubules. Patients must be aware that their use will not prove to be effective unless they are used continuously for at least 2 weeks or longer. Consistent use over time may be necessary to control dentin hypersensitivity.

Table 43.3 lists various products used for the desensitization of dentin hypersensitivity. These products and treatments aim to decrease hypersensitivity by blocking dentinal tubules with either a crystalline salt precipitation or an applied coating (varnish or bonding agent) on the root surface.

Several agents have been used to precipitate crystalline salts on the dentin surface in an attempt to occlude the dentinal tubules. *Fluoride solutions* and *pastes* historically have been the agents of choice. In addition to their antisensitivity properties, fluoride agents have the advantage of anticaries activity, which is particularly important for patients with a tendency to develop root caries. Certain agents, such as chlorhexidine, decrease the ability of fluoride to bind with calcium on the root surfaces. Thus it is important to advise patients not to rinse or eat for 1 h after applying a fluoride-based desensitizing treatment.

Another method of treating hypersensitive dentin is the use of varnishes or bonding agents to occlude dentinal tubules. Newer restorative materials, such as glass-ionomer cements and the dentin bonding agents, are under investigation. These materials are considered for use when the tooth requires recontouring or when difficult cases do not respond to other treatments. Resin primers alone could

TABLE 43.3 Desensitizing Products

Name	Active Ingredient(s)	Usage/Instructions
Desensitizing Agents		
Sensitive Pro-Relief Desensitizing Paste with Pro-Argin	Arginine 8%, calcium carbonate, sodium monofluorophosphate	**Office**: Place paste in rotary cup; apply to area and polish at low to moderate speed for 3 s and repeat. **Home**: Patients advised to use paste as directed.
Bis-Block, Sensodyne Sealant, SuperSeal	Oxalate products	**Office**: Dry dentin surface; dispense 10–12 drops; apply with cotton pellet 1 min to area with light pressure; do not burnish; may require multiple 1 min applications. Expectorate after use.
Sultan Sodium Fluoride Paste	Sodium fluoride 33.50%	**Office**: Burnish onto sensitive area using orangewood stick for 1 min; followed by rinsing; sequential 1-min treatments may be required.
Many brands of over-the-counter toothpaste	Potassium nitrate, sodium fluoride	**Home**: Apply 1-inch toothpaste onto soft-bristled toothbrush; brush thoroughly at least 1 min twice a day or as recommended.
Gel-Kam Dentin Block	Sodium fluoride, stannous fluoride	**Office**: Dry dentin surface; dispense 10–12 drops; apply with cotton pellet for 1 min to area with light pressure; do not burnish; may require multiple 1-min applications. Expectorate after use.
Sealants/Adhesives/Resins/Bonding Agents		
Dentin Protect, Ivoclar Vivadent, Prime & Bond, Scotch Bond	Barrier dental sealant	**Office**: Apply chairside according to manufacturer's recommendations.
GC Tooth Mousse, MI Paste, Recaldent	Casein derivatives	**Office**: Apply chairside according to manufacturer's recommendations.
Seal & Protect, Vitrebond-Lite	Light-cured adhesives	**Office**: Apply chairside according to manufacturer's recommendations.
All-Bond DS, MicroPrime, Gluma Desensitizer, Glu/Sense, Hema Seal G	Methacrylate polymer	**Office**: Apply chairside according to manufacturer's recommendations.
Varnishes		
Cervitec Plus	Chlorhexidine dental varnish	**Office**: After isolating the area and drying, apply topically to all tooth surfaces and instruct patient to avoid eating for 3 h, and brushing teeth for 24 h, according to manufacturer's recommendations.
Cavity Shield, Durafluor, Duraphat, Fluoline, Fluor Protector, PreviDent Clear, Waterpik UltraThin	Sodium fluoride solutions	**Office**: Apply chairside according to manufacturer's recommendations.

Note: This table is not intended to be exhaustive or comprehensive. Clinicians are advised to read manufacturer's instructions and warnings.
(Excerpted from *ADA/PDR Guide to Dental Therapeutics*, 5th ed. Chicago, IL: American Dental Association; Physicians Desk Reference Inc.; 2009.)

be promising, but the effects are not permanent, and further investigations are ongoing. Despite some success with decreasing dentin hypersensitivity, these "dental office" treatments have not been predictable in resolving hypersensitivity, and the success that is achieved is often short lived. The crystalline salts, varnishes, and other sealants can be washed away over time, and the hypersensitivity may return. Repeated therapy will be necessary to help alleviate the hypersensitivity for these patients.

More recently, attempts have been made to improve the success and longevity of these treatments with the use of lasers. Low-level laser "melting" of the dentin surface appears to seal dentinal tubules without damage to the pulp. In a combined treatment modality, the neodymium:yttrium-aluminum-garnet (Nd:YAG) laser has been used to congeal fluoride varnish on root surfaces. This **in vitro** study demonstrated that the laser-treated fluoride varnish resisted removal by electric toothbrushing, with 90% of tubules remaining blocked. In the control subjects (i.e., those who did not undergo laser treatment), the fluoride varnish was almost completely brushed away. Despite these convincing preliminary results, further research is needed before laser treatment can be considered an effective and predictable means of desensitization.

Periodontal Surgery in the Hospital

For most patients, periodontal surgical procedures are managed well in the dental office with local anesthesia only or with some form of sedation. If multiple surgeries are indicated, they are typically performed by quadrant or sextant at biweekly or longer intervals. However, certain patients and procedures warrant treatment in the hospital operating room with general anesthesia. These include patients who are not well enough to undergo treatment in a dental office and procedures that are more extensive and difficult for patients to endure. Readers are referred to the online material for a discussion of indications and procedures in a hospital setting.

Conclusion

The majority of periodontal surgical procedures can be carried out with effective use of local anesthesia. Clinicians have the obligation to ensure a patient-centered approach that includes oral, intravenous, and inhalational sedation in their spectrum of available services for their patients.

The efficient, precise, and minimally traumatic management of tissues is necessary to achieve the most predictable and comfortable result and outcome for the patient. Most patients need oral analgesic support, and they should be given the necessary pain-relieving medications so that an effective level of analgesia is present during the immediate postsurgical period. The use of longer-acting local anesthetic agents (e.g., bupivacaine) and protective periodontal dressings also helps to reduce postsurgical pain.

During the immediate postsurgical weeks, biofilm control and healing can be facilitated with the use of antimicrobial mouthrinses such as chlorhexidine. Postsurgical root sensitivity is well controlled by ensuring that biofilm control is optimal, and occasionally desensitizing agents will be needed.

Key points

- A thorough and meticulous phase I therapy is vital for the success of any surgical procedure.
- Smokers should be encouraged to stop smoking for at least 3–4 weeks after surgery.
- Thorough scaling, root planing, and debridement enhance the outcome. Good initial therapy, correct incisions, and tissue handling reduce intrasurgical bleeding.
- Periodontal dressings merely protect the wound. They have no healing properties.
- Desensitizing agents are employed to tackle transient postoperative sensitivity.

Suggested Reading

Sachs HA, Farnoush A, Checchi L, et al: Current status of periodontal dressings. *J Periodontol* 55:689, 1984.

CHAPTER 44

Gingival Surgical Techniques

HH Takei | FA Carranza | K Shin | CD Dwarakanath

CHAPTER OUTLINE

Periodontal pocket reduction surgery limited to the gingival tissues only and not involving the underlying osseous structures, without the use of flap surgery, can be classified as *gingival curettage*, *gingivectomy*, and *gingivoplasty*. Both gingival curettage and gingivectomy have limited use currently because of the change in the understanding of etiology of periodontal disease.

Gingival Curettage

The word *curettage* is used in periodontics to mean the scraping of the gingival wall of a periodontal pocket to remove diseased soft tissue. *Scaling* refers to the removal of deposits from the root surface, whereas *planing* means smoothing the root to remove infected and necrotic tooth substance. Scaling and root planing may inadvertently include curettage to a certain degree. This is often called inadvertent curettage. However, they are different procedures with different rationales and indications. Both should be considered as separate parts of periodontal treatment.

This chapter refers to the intentional curettage performed during the same visit as scaling and root planing or as a separate procedure to reduce pocket depth by enhancing gingival shrinkage, new connective tissue attachment, or both.

Rationale

Curettage accomplishes the removal of the chronically inflamed granulation tissue that forms in the lateral wall of the periodontal pocket. This tissue, in addition to the usual components of granulation tissues (i.e., fibroblastic and angioblastic proliferation), contains areas of chronic inflammation, and it may also contain pieces of dislodged calculus and bacterial colonies. The latter may perpetuate the pathologic features of the tissue and hinder healing.

This inflamed granulation tissue is lined by epithelium, and deep strands of epithelium penetrate into the tissue. The presence of this epithelium is construed as a barrier to the attachment of new fibers in the area.

However, this rationale has been questioned because of the following reasons.

When the root is thoroughly planed, the major source of bacteria disappears, and the pathologic changes in the tissues adjacent to the pocket resolve with no need to eliminate the inflamed granulation tissue by curettage. The existing granulation tissue is slowly resorbed, and the bacteria present in the tissue without replenishment of their numbers from the plaque in the pocket are destroyed by the defense mechanisms of the host. It has been shown that scaling and root planing with additional curettage do not improve the condition of the periodontal tissues beyond the improvement that results from scaling and root planing alone.

The second reason is the fact that curettage may not remove pocket lining and junctional epithelium consistently.

Thirdly, it has also been shown that curettage done in an anterior esthetic zone may result in more shrinkage than compared to root planing alone.

Notwithstanding the above reservations curettage might be still indicated in following situations.

1. Curettage can be attempted as a nondefinitive procedure to reduce inflammation when aggressive surgical techniques (e.g., flaps) are contraindicated in patients as a result of their age, systemic problems, psychologic problems, or other factors. It should be understood that, in these patients, the goal of pocket elimination is compromised, and their prognosis is impaired. The clinician should attempt this approach only when the indicated surgical techniques cannot be performed and both the clinician and the patient have a clear understanding of its limitations.
2. Curettage is also frequently performed on recall visits as a method of maintenance treatment for areas of recurrent inflammation and pocket depth, especially where pocket reduction surgery has previously been performed. Careful probing should establish the extent of the required root planing and curettage.

Procedure

Basic Technique

Curettage does not eliminate the causes of inflammation (i.e., bacterial plaque and deposits). *Therefore, curettage should always be preceded by scaling and root planing*, which is the basic periodontal therapy procedure. The use of local infiltrative anesthesia for scaling and root planing is optional. However, gingival curettage will always require some type of local anesthesia.

The curette is selected so that the cutting edge is against the tissue. Curettage can be performed either by area specific Gracey curettes or Columbia Universal curettes. The instrument is inserted to engage the inner lining of the pocket wall, and it is then carried along the soft tissue, usually in a horizontal stroke (Fig. 44.1). The pocket wall may be supported by gentle finger pressure on the external surface. The curette is then placed under the most apical edge of the junctional epithelium to undermine it.

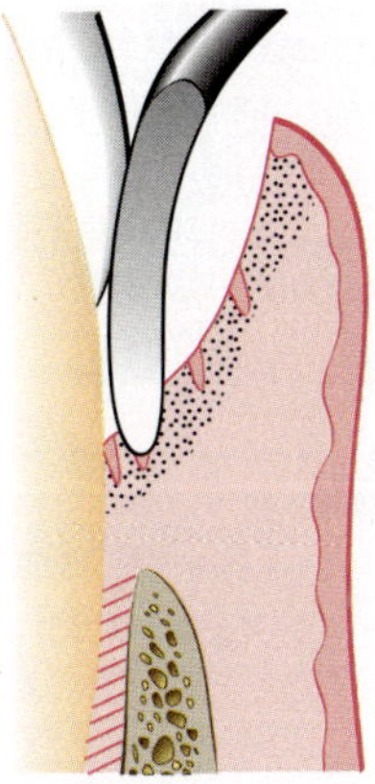

Fig. 44.1 Gingival curettage performed with a horizontal stroke of the curette.

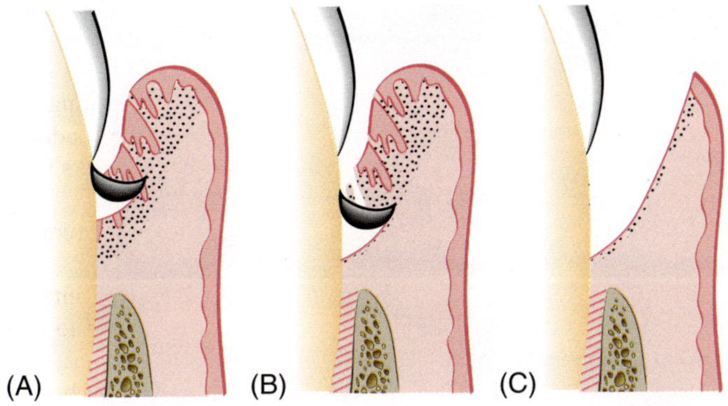

Fig. 44.2 Subgingival curettage. A, Elimination of pocket lining. B, Elimination of junctional epithelium and granulation tissue. C, Procedure completed.

During subgingival curettage, the tissues attached between the bottom of the pocket and the alveolar crest are removed with a scooping motion of the curette to the tooth surface (Fig. 44.2). The area is flushed to remove debris, and the tissue is partly adapted to the tooth by gentle finger pressure. In some cases, the suturing of separated papillae and the application of a periodontal pack may be indicated.

Other Techniques

Other techniques for gingival curettage include the excisional new attachment procedure, ultrasonic curettage, and the use of caustic drugs.

Excisional New Attachment Procedure

The excisional new attachment procedure which was developed and used by the US Naval Dental Corps is a definitive subgingival curettage procedure that is performed with a knife. Its usefulness is very limited today as it has been found that most of the time healing occurs by formation of long junctional epithelium rather than any true new attachment (Fig. 44.3).

Ultrasonic Curettage

The use of ultrasonic devices has been recommended for gingival curettage. When applied to the gingiva of experimental animals, ultrasonic vibrations disrupt tissue continuity, lift off the epithelium, dismember collagen bundles, and alter the morphologic features of fibroblast nuclei. Ultrasonics are effective for debriding the epithelial lining of periodontal pockets. This results in a narrow band of necrotic tissue (microcauterization), which strips off the inner lining of the pocket.

The Morse scaler-shaped and rod-shaped ultrasonic instruments are used for this purpose. Some investigators found ultrasonic instruments to be as effective as manual instruments for curettage and that such tools resulted in less inflammation and less removal of underlying connective tissue. The gingiva can be made more firm for ultrasonic curettage by injecting anesthetic solution directly into it.

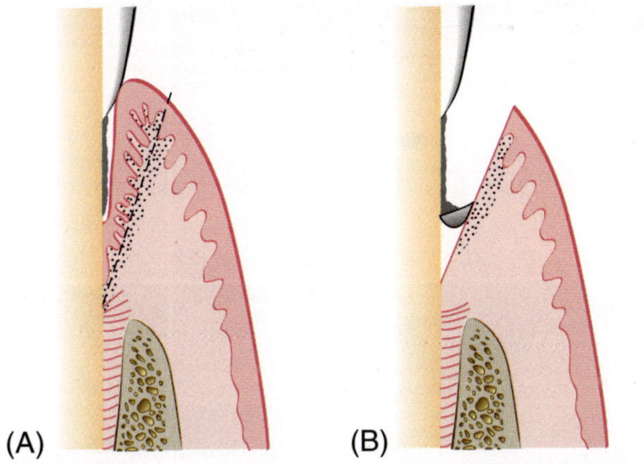

Fig. 44.3 Excisional new attachment procedure. A, Internal bevel incision to a point below the bottom of the pocket. B, After the excision of tissue, scaling and root planing are performed.

Caustic Drugs

These were used in the past and were by and large ineffective besides causing untoward damage to the tissues. They are outdated and have no place in current periodontal practice.

Healing After Scaling and Curettage

Immediately after curettage, a blood clot fills the pocket area, which is totally or partially devoid of epithelial lining. Hemorrhage is also present in the tissues with dilated capillaries and abundant polymorphonuclear leukocytes, which appear on the wound surface. This is followed by a rapid proliferation of granulation tissue with a decrease in the number of small blood vessels as the tissue matures.

The restoration and epithelialization of the sulcus generally require 2–7 days, and restoration of the junctional epithelium occurs in animals as early as 5 days after treatment. Immature collagen fibers appear within 21 days. Healthy gingival fibers that are inadvertently severed from the tooth and tears in the epithelium are repaired during the healing process. Several investigators have reported that, in monkeys and humans treated by scaling and curettage, healing results in the formation of a long, thin junctional epithelium with no new connective-tissue attachment. In some cases, this long epithelium is interrupted by "windows" of connective-tissue attachment.

Clinical Appearance After Scaling and Curettage

Immediately after scaling and curettage, the gingiva appears hemorrhagic and bright red. After 1 week, the gingiva appears reduced in height as a result of an apical shift in the position of the gingival margin. The gingiva is also darker red than normal, but it is much less red than it will have been on previous days. After 2 weeks and with proper oral hygiene, the normal color, consistency, surface texture, and contour of the gingiva are attained, and the gingival margin is well adapted to the tooth.

Gingivectomy

The word *gingivectomy* means "excision of the gingiva." By removing the pocket wall, gingivectomy provides visibility and accessibility for complete calculus removal and the thorough smoothing of the roots. This creates a favorable environment for gingival healing and restoration of a physiologic gingival contour.

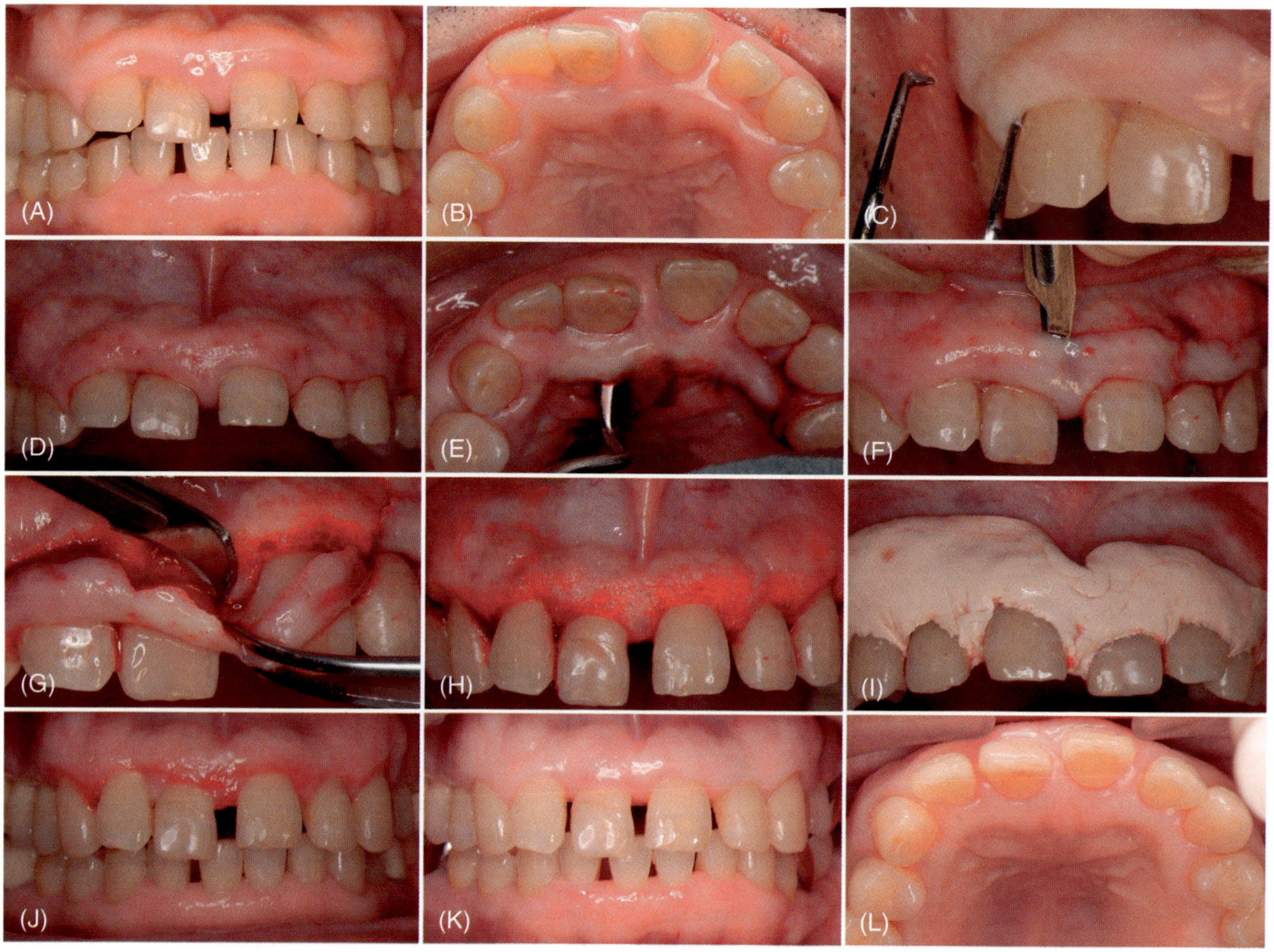

Fig. 44.4 Results obtained by treating a suprabony pocket with gingivectomy. A and B, Preoperative facial and palatal views. C, Marking of the depth of the suprabony pocket. D, The bottoms of the pockets are indicated by pinpoint markings. E, A beveled palatal incision with an Orban knife. F, A facial beveled incision with a Bard–Parker no. 15 blade extends apical to the perforations made by the pocket marker. Note that the beveled incision can also be made with a Kirkland knife. G, The interdental incision and excision of the pocket wall with a Bard–Parker no. 12 blade. H, A completed gingivectomy. I, The surgical site covered with periodontal dressing. J, One week after healing. K and L, Results 22 months after the operation.

The gingivectomy technique was widely performed in the past. Improved understanding of healing mechanisms and the development of more sophisticated flap methods have relegated the gingivectomy to a lesser role in the current repertoire of available techniques. However, it remains an effective form of treatment when indicated (Fig. 44.4).

Indications and Contraindications

The gingivectomy technique may be performed for the following indications:

1. Elimination of suprabony pockets, regardless of their depth, if the pocket wall is fibrous and firm.
2. Elimination of gingival enlargements.
3. Elimination of suprabony periodontal abscesses.

Contraindications to gingivectomy include the following:

1. The need for osseous surgery or examination of the shape and morphology of bone.
2. Situations in which the bottom of the pocket is apical to the mucogingival junction.
3. Esthetic considerations, particularly in the anterior maxilla.

The gingivectomy technique may be performed by means of scalpels, electrodes, lasers, or chemicals. All of these techniques are reviewed in this chapter, although the surgical method is the only technique that is recommended.

Surgical Gingivectomy

Step 1

The pockets on each surface are explored with a periodontal probe and marked with a pocket marker. Each pocket is marked in several areas to outline its course on each surface (Figs. 44.4C and D, 44.5, and 44.6).

Step 2

Periodontal knives (e.g., Kirkland knives) are used for incisions on the facial and lingual surfaces and on those distal to the terminal tooth in the arch. Orban periodontal knives are used for interdental incisions (Fig. 44.4E–G). Bard–Parker blades (nos. 12 and 15) as well as scissors are used as auxiliary instruments.

The incision is started apical to the points marking the course of the pockets, and it is directed coronally to a point between the base of the pocket and the crest of the bone. It should be as close as

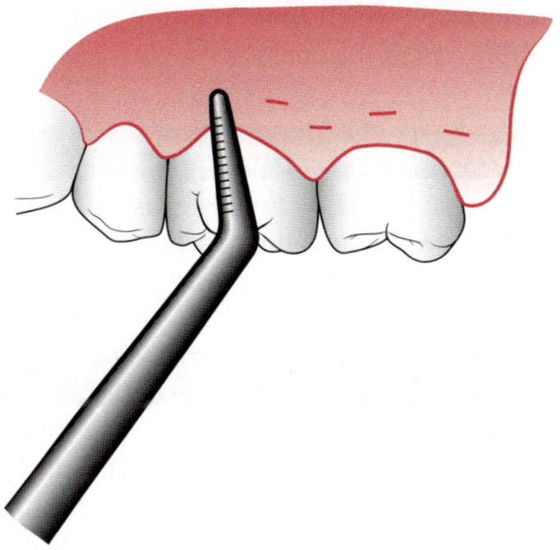

Fig. 44.5 The pocket marker makes pinpoint perforations that indicate pocket depth.

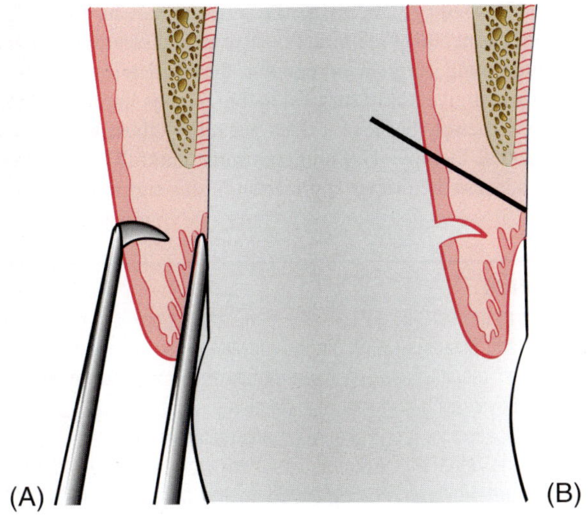

Fig. 44.6 Marking the depth of a suprabony pocket. A, A pocket marker in position. B, The beveled incision extends apical to the perforation made by the pocket marker.

possible to the bone without exposing it to remove the soft tissue coronal to the bone. Exposure of bone is undesirable. If this occurs, healing usually presents minimal complications if the area is adequately covered by the periodontal pack.

Either interrupted or continuous incisions may be used. The incision should be beveled at approximately 44 degrees to the tooth surface, and it should recreate the normal festooned pattern of the gingiva. Failure to bevel the incision will leave a broad, fibrous plateau that will take a longer time to develop a physiologic contour. During the interim, plaque and calculus may lead to the recurrence of pockets.

Step 3

Remove the excised pocket wall, clean the area, and closely examine the root surface. The most apical zone consists of a light, band-like zone where the tissues were attached. Coronally, calculus remnants, root caries, or resorption may be found. Granulation tissue may be seen on the excised soft tissue.

Step 4

Carefully curette the granulation tissue and remove any remaining calculus and necrotic cementum to leave a smooth and clean surface.

Step 5

Cover the area with a surgical pack (Fig. 44.4I).

Gingivoplasty

Gingivoplasty is similar to gingivectomy, but its objective is different. Gingivectomy is performed to eliminate periodontal pockets, and it includes reshaping as part of the technique. Gingivoplasty is a reshaping of the gingiva to create physiologic gingival contours with the sole purpose of recontouring the gingiva in the absence of pockets.

Gingival and periodontal disease often produces deformities in the gingiva that are conducive to the accumulation of plaque and food debris, which prolong and aggravate the disease process. Such deformities include the following: (1) gingival clefts and craters; (2) crater-like interdental papillae caused by acute necrotizing ulcerative gingivitis; and (3) gingival enlargements.

Gingivoplasty may be accomplished with a periodontal knife, a scalpel, rotary coarse diamond stones, or electrodes. The technique resembles that of the festooning of an artificial denture, which consists of tapering the gingival margin, creating a scalloped marginal outline, thinning the attached gingiva, creating vertical interdental grooves, and shaping the interdental papillae.

Healing After Surgical Gingivectomy

The *initial response* after gingivectomy is the formation of a protective surface blood clot. The underlying tissue becomes acutely inflamed with necrosis. The clot is then replaced by granulation tissue. In 24 h, there is an increase in new connective tissue cells, which are mainly angioblasts beneath the surface layer of inflammation and necrotic tissue. By the third day, numerous young fibroblasts are located in the area. The highly vascular granulation tissue grows coronally and creates a new free gingival margin and sulcus. Capillaries derived from the blood vessels of the periodontal ligament migrate into the granulation tissue, and, within 2 weeks, they connect with the gingival vessels.

After 12–24 h, epithelial cells at the margins of the wound begin to migrate over the granulation tissue, thereby separating it from the contaminated surface layer of the clot. Epithelial activity at the margins reaches a peak after 24–36 h.

The new epithelial cells arise from the basal and deeper spinous layers of the epithelial wound edge and migrate over the wound over a fibrin layer that is later resorbed and replaced by a connective tissue bed. The epithelial cells advance by a tumbling action, with the cells becoming fixed to the substrate by hemidesmosomes and a new basement lamina.

After 5–14 days, surface epithelialization is generally complete. During the first 4 weeks after gingivectomy, keratinization is less than it was before surgery. Complete epithelial repair takes about 1 month. Vasodilation and vascularity begin to decrease after the 4th day of healing, and they appear to be almost normal by the 16th day. Complete repair of the connective tissue takes about 7 weeks.

The flow of gingival fluid in humans is initially increased after gingivectomy, and it diminishes as healing progresses. Maximal flow is reached after 1 week, which coincides with the time of maximal inflammation.

Although the tissue changes that occur during postgingivectomy healing are the same in all individuals, the time required for complete healing varies considerably, depending on the area of the incised surface and interference from local irritation and infection. In patients with physiologic gingival melanosis, the pigmentation is diminished in the healed gingiva.

Gingivectomy by Electrosurgery

Advantage and Disadvantages

Electrosurgery permits an adequate contouring of the tissue and controls hemorrhage.

It cannot be used in patients who have incompatible or poorly shielded cardiac pacemakers. The treatment causes an unpleasant odor. If the electrosurgery point touches the bone, irreparable damage can be inflicted. Furthermore, the heat generated by injudicious use can cause tissue damage and a loss of periodontal support when the electrode is used close to bone. When the electrode touches the root, areas of cementum can be burned. *Therefore, the use of electrosurgery should be limited to superficial procedures such as the removal of gingival enlargements, gingivoplasty, the relocation of the frenum and muscle attachments, and the incision of periodontal abscesses and pericoronal flaps.* Extreme care should be used to avoid contacting the tooth surface. *Electrosurgery should not be used for procedures that involve proximity to the bone (e.g., flap operations) or for mucogingival surgery.*

Technique

The removal of gingival enlargements and gingivoplasty is performed with a needle electrode supplemented by a small ovoid loop or diamond-shaped electrodes for festooning. A blended cutting and coagulating (fully rectified) current is used. During all reshaping procedures, the electrode is activated and moved in a concise "shaving" motion.

For the treatment of acute periodontal abscesses, the incision to establish drainage can be made with the needle electrode without exerting pressure. The incision remains open because the edges are sealed by the current. After the acute symptoms subside, the regular procedure for the treatment of the periodontal abscess is followed.

For hemostasis, a ball electrode is used. Hemorrhage must first be controlled by direct pressure using air, a compress, or a hemostat; the surface is then lightly touched with a coagulating current. Electrosurgery is helpful for the control of isolated bleeding points. Bleeding areas located interproximally are reached with a thin, bar-shaped electrode.

Frenum and muscle attachments can be relocated to facilitate pocket elimination with the use of a loop electrode. For this purpose, the frenum or muscle is stretched and sectioned with the loop electrode and a coagulating current. For cases of acute pericoronitis, drainage may be obtained by incising the flap with a bent-needle electrode. A loop electrode is used to remove the flap after the acute symptoms subside.

Healing After Electrosurgery

Some investigators report no significant differences in gingival healing after resection by electrosurgery as compared to resection with periodontal knives. Other researchers find delayed healing, a greater reduction in gingival height, and more bone injury after electrosurgery. There appears to be negligible difference in the results obtained after gingival resection with electrosurgery and those obtained with periodontal knives. *However, when used for deep resections close to bone, electrosurgery can produce gingival recession, bone necrosis and sequestration, a loss of bone height, furcation exposure, and tooth mobility.* These problems do not occur with the use of periodontal knives.

Laser Gingivectomy

The lasers that are most often used in dentistry are the diode laser and the neodymium: yttrium-aluminum-garnet (Nd:YAG) laser, which have wavelengths of 910 and 1064 nm, respectively. They are both in the infrared range, so they must be combined with other types of visible lasers for the beam to be seen and aimed.

The diode laser has been used for the excision of gingival growths, although healing is delayed as compared to healing after conventional scalpel gingivectomy. The use of a laser for oral surgery requires precautionary measures to avoid reflecting the beam on instrument surfaces, which could result in injury to neighboring tissues and to the eyes of the operator.

Gingivectomy by Chemosurgery

Techniques to remove the gingiva with the use of chemicals such as 5% paraformaldehyde or potassium hydroxide have been described in the past, but they are not currently used.

Conclusion

The gingivectomy surgical technique has a long history of use in periodontal surgery. This technique has been attempted with the use of scalpels, electrosurgery, laser, and chemical cautery. Although this technique may have some use for the minimal reduction of redundant gingival tissue, many limiting factors must be considered. Current periodontal surgery must consider the following: (1) the conservation of keratinized gingiva; (2) minimal gingival tissue loss to maintain esthetics; (3) adequate access to the osseous defects for definitive defect correction; and (4) minimal postsurgical discomfort and bleeding by attempting surgical procedures that will allow for primary closure. The gingivectomy surgical technique has limited use in current surgical therapy because it does not satisfy these considerations for periodontal therapy. The clinician must carefully evaluate each patient to address the proper application of this surgical procedure.

Key points

- Scraping the soft tissue wall of a periodontal pocket to remove diseased soft tissue is called gingival curettage.
- However, results have not been shown to be superior to that performed by scaling and root planing alone.
- The indication for gingival curettage is quite limited.
- Curettage done with a knife is termed excisional new attachment procedure. However, healing occurs mainly by the formation of long junctional epithelium.
- Gingivectomy is the excision of the soft tissue wall of a periodontal pocket. Gingivoplasty is recontouring of gingiva and restoring its form so as to be conducive to maintenance of oral hygiene.
- Elimination of fibrous suprabony pockets and gingival enlargements are the main indications.
- The disadvantages of gingivectomy include creation of esthetic problems and loss of valuable keratinized tissue. After gingivectomy, healing occurs by secondary intention.

Suggested Readings

Engler WO, Ramfjord S, Hiniker JJ: Healing following simple gingivectomy: a tritiated thymidine radioautographic study. I. Epithelialization. *J Periodontol* 37:289, 1966.

Glickman I: The results obtained with the unembellished gingivectomy technique in a clinical study in humans. *J Periodontol* 27:247, 1956.

Lindhe J, Westfelt E, Nyman S, et al: Healing following surgical and non-surgical treatment of periodontal disease. *J Clin Periodontol* 9:115, 1982.

Moskow BS: The response of the gingival sulcus to instrumentation: a histologic investigation. II. Gingival curettage. *J Periodontol* 35:112, 1964.

Ramfjord SP, Costich ER: Healing after exposure of the periosteum on the alveolar process. *J Periodontol* 38:199, 1968.

Ramfjord SP, Engler WD, Hiniker JJ: A radiographic study of healing following simple gingivectomy. II. The connective tissue. *J Periodontol* 37:179, 1966.

Stahl S, Witkin G, Cantor M, et al: Gingival healing. II. Clinical and histologic repair sequences following gingivectomy. *J Periodontol* 39:109, 1968.

CHAPTER 45

The Periodontal Flap

HH Takei | FA Carranza | JH Do | K Shin | CD Dwarakanath

CHAPTER OUTLINE

Periodontal flap surgery is the most common type of surgery done in the oral cavity and is the basic requirement of several periodontal procedures. It has been in existence for over a century and many techniques and modifications have been evolved and practiced. This chapter covers the basic principles of flap surgery followed by different techniques for various situations such as pocket therapy, regeneration, and gingival enlargements.

Definition

A periodontal flap is a section of gingiva and/or mucosa that is surgically separated from the underlying tissues to provide visibility and access to the bone and root surface. The flap also allows the gingiva to be displaced to a different location in patients with mucogingival involvement.

Rationale

Removal of root surface noxious agents, inflamed tissue, and to have an ideal gingival and bone morphology without sacrificing investing and supporting tissues and compromising esthetics.

Indications

1. Presence of persistent moderate to deep pockets (more than 5 mm) even after a conscientious phase 1 therapy (Fig. 45.1).
2. Presence of osseous defects (Fig. 45.2).
3. Presence of inflammation and disease activity at the base of sulcus as seen by bleeding on probing (Fig. 45.3).
4. Furcation involvement (Fig. 45.4).
5. To regenerate periodontal tissues by the use of bone grafts, membranes, etc.
6. Gingival overgrowth and asymmetry (Fig. 45.5).
7. Periodontal pockets adjacent to distal molars (Fig. 45.6).
8. Other dental procedures such as crown lengthening and apicectomy (Fig. 45.7).

Contraindications

1. When optimal results can be obtained by nonsurgical periodontal therapy (Fig. 45.8).
2. Unprepared, soft, and edematous gingival tissues (Fig. 45.9).
3. Medically compromised patients where surgery is a risky proposition.
4. Patients presenting consistently with poor oral hygiene and who are noncompliant.
5. Teeth with hopeless prognosis (Fig. 45.10).
6. When surgery is likely to result in extreme esthetic disfigurement.

Classification of Flaps

Periodontal flaps are classified on the basis of the following criteria:

- Bone exposure after flap reflection.
- Placement of the flap after surgery.
- Management of the interdental papilla.

For bone exposure after reflection, the flaps are classified as either full-thickness (mucoperiosteal) or partial-thickness (mucosal) flaps (Fig. 45.11A and B).

In a **full-thickness flap,** all of the soft tissue, including the periosteum, is reflected to expose the underlying bone. This complete exposure of and access to the underlying bone is indicated when osseous surgery is contemplated.

The **partial-thickness flap** includes only the epithelium and a layer of the underlying connective tissue. The bone remains covered by a layer of connective tissue that includes the periosteum. This type of flap is also called the **split-thickness flap.** The partial-thickness flap is indicated when the flap is to be positioned apically or when the operator does not want to expose the bone as in the presence of fenestrations and dehiscences and in plastic surgical procedures.

For flap placement after surgery, flaps are classified as either (1) **nondisplaced flaps**, when the flap is returned and sutured in its original position, or (2) **displaced flaps**, which are placed apically, coronally, or laterally to their original position. These are commonly performed in mucogingival procedures. Both full-thickness and partial-thickness flaps can be displaced. However, to do so, the attached gingiva must be totally separated from the underlying bone, thereby enabling the unattached portion of the gingiva to be movable. Palatal flaps cannot be displaced because of the absence of unattached gingiva.

Apically displaced flaps have the important advantage of preserving the outer portion of the pocket wall and transforming it

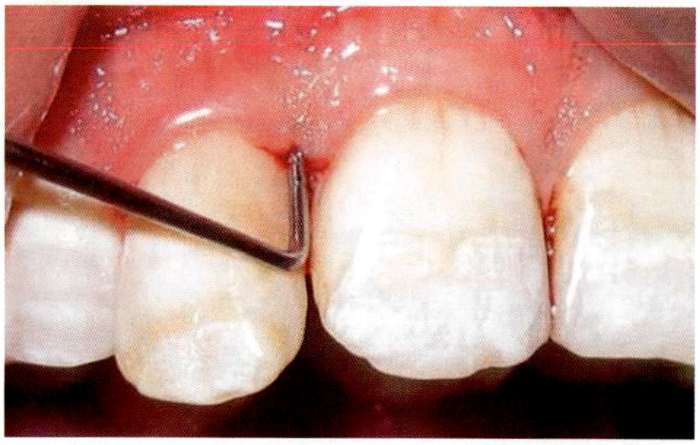

Fig. 45.1 Presence of persistent deep pocket.

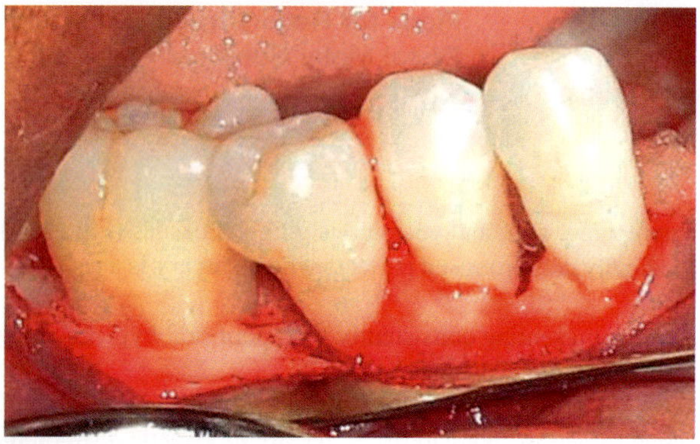

Fig. 45.2 Osseous defects showing inconsistent bone margin and reverse architecture.

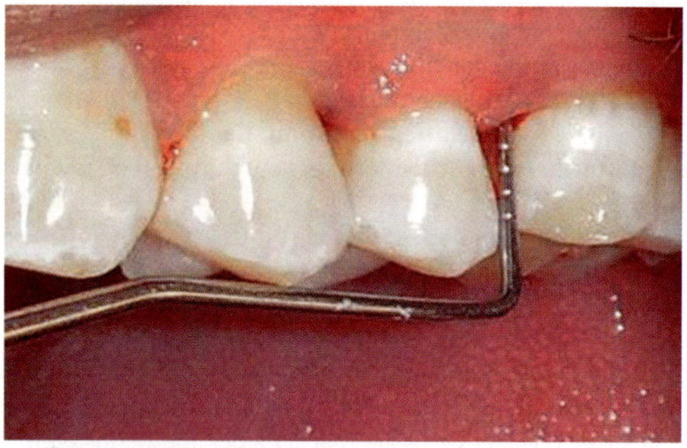

Fig. 45.3 Bleeding on probing the base of the pocket.

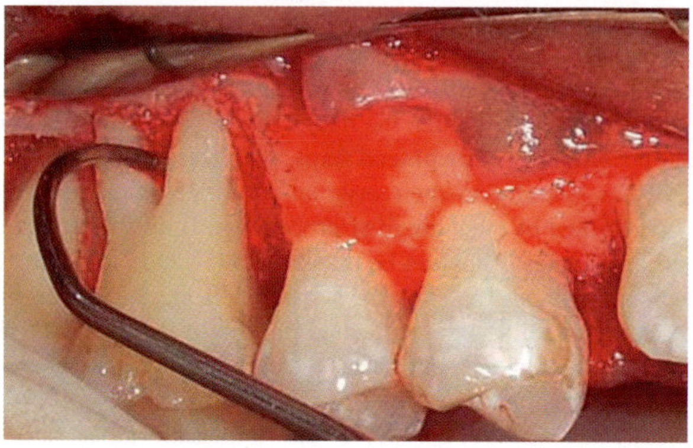

Fig. 45.4 Grade II furcation in maxillary molar.

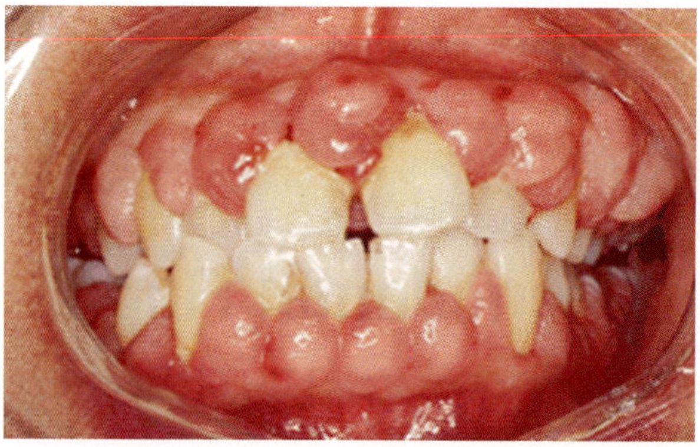

Fig. 45.5 Drug-induced gingival enlargement.

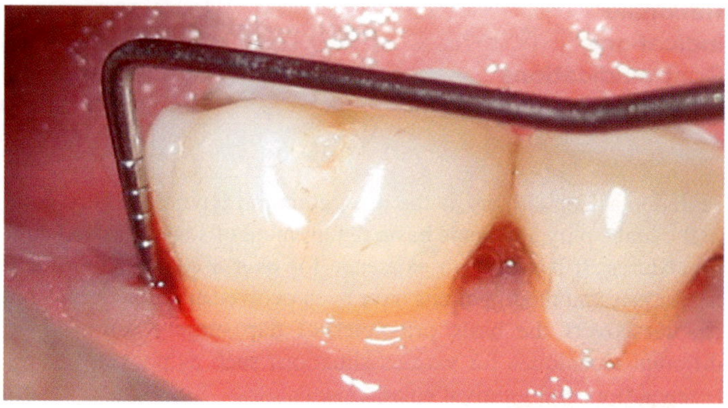

Fig. 45.6 Deep periodontal pocket on the distal surface of mandibular second molar.

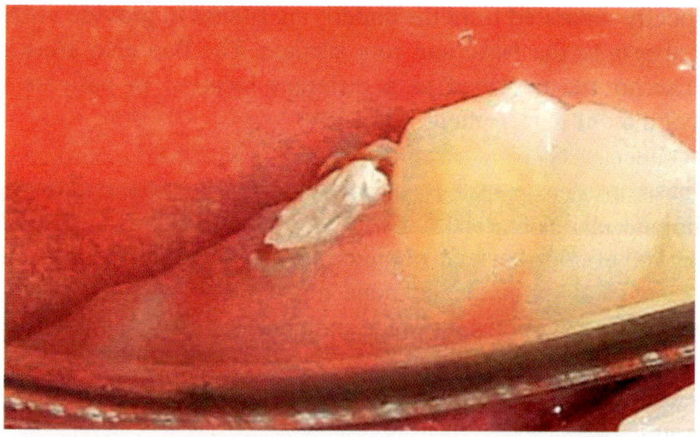

Fig. 45.7 Root canal treated molar requiring crown lengthening.

into attached gingiva. Therefore, these flaps accomplish the double objective of eliminating the pocket and increasing the width of the attached gingiva.

For the management of the papilla, flaps can be conventional and papilla preservation flaps. With the **conventional flap**, the interdental papilla is split beneath the contact point of the two approximating teeth to allow for the reflection of the buccal and lingual flaps. The incision is usually scalloped to maintain gingival morphology and to retain as much papilla as possible. The conventional flap is used (1) when the interdental spaces are too narrow, thereby precluding the possibility of preserving the papilla, (2) when the flap is to be displaced and (3) when there is break in continuity of the interdental papilla. This includes the modified Widman flap, the undisplaced flap, Kirkland flap (nowadays called

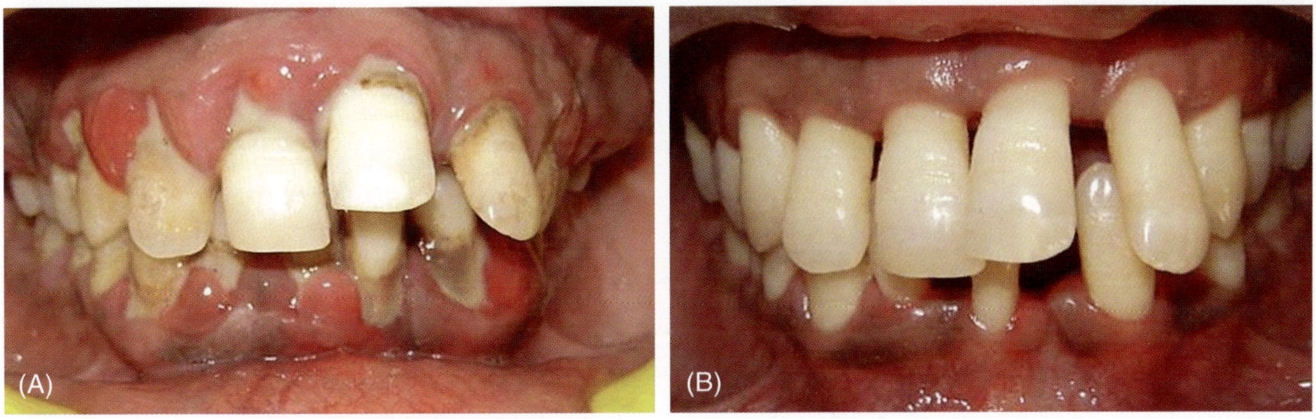

Fig. 45.8 A, Severe periodontitis with poor oral hygiene. B, Result after nonsurgical therapy.

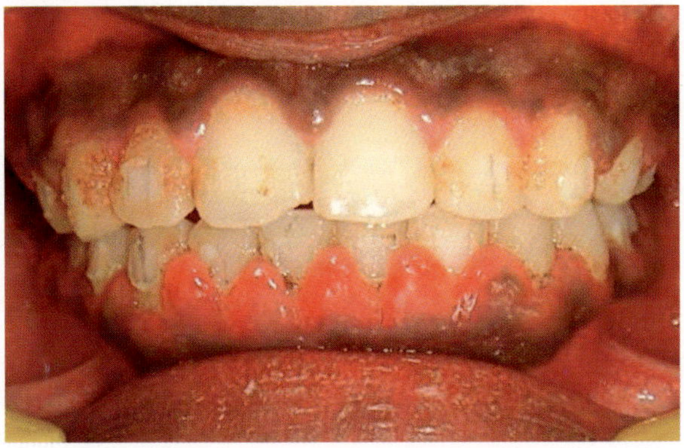

Fig. 45.9 Unprepared tissues showing soft and edematous gingiva.

the access flap), the apically displaced flap, and the flap for reconstructive procedures.

The **papilla preservation flap** incorporates the entire papilla in one of the flaps by means of crevicular interdental incisions to sever the connective tissue attachment as well as a horizontal incision at the base of the papilla to leave it connected to one of the flaps. This technique is indicated in esthetic zones and when bone grafts are going to be placed.

Flap Design

The design of the flap is dictated by the surgical judgment of the operator, and it may depend on the objectives of the procedure. The necessary degree of access to the underlying bone and root surfaces and the final position of the flap must be considered when designing the flap. The flap design may also be dictated by the esthetic concerns of the area of surgery. Preservation of good blood supply to the flap is another important consideration (Figs. 45.12 and 45.13).

The entire surgical procedure should be planned in every detail before the procedure is initiated. The surgical plan should include the type of flap, the exact location and type of incisions, the management of the underlying bone, and the final closure of the flap and sutures. Although some details may be modified during the actual performance of the procedure, detailed planning allows for a better clinical result.

Incisions

Periodontal flaps involve the use of horizontal (mesial–distal) and vertical (occlusal–apical) incisions.

Horizontal Incisions

Horizontal incisions are directed along the margin of the gingiva in a mesial or distal direction. Two types of horizontal incisions have been recommended: the **internal bevel incision**, which starts at a distance from the gingival margin and which is aimed at the bone crest, and the **crevicular incision**, which starts at the bottom of the pocket and which is directed to the bone margin. In addition, the interdental incision is performed after the flap is elevated to remove the interdental tissue.

The **internal bevel incision** is basic to most periodontal flap procedures. It is the incision from which the flap is reflected to expose the underlying bone and root. The internal bevel incision accomplishes three important objectives: (1) it removes the pocket lining; (2) it conserves the relatively uninvolved outer surface of the gingiva, which, if apically positioned, becomes attached gingiva;

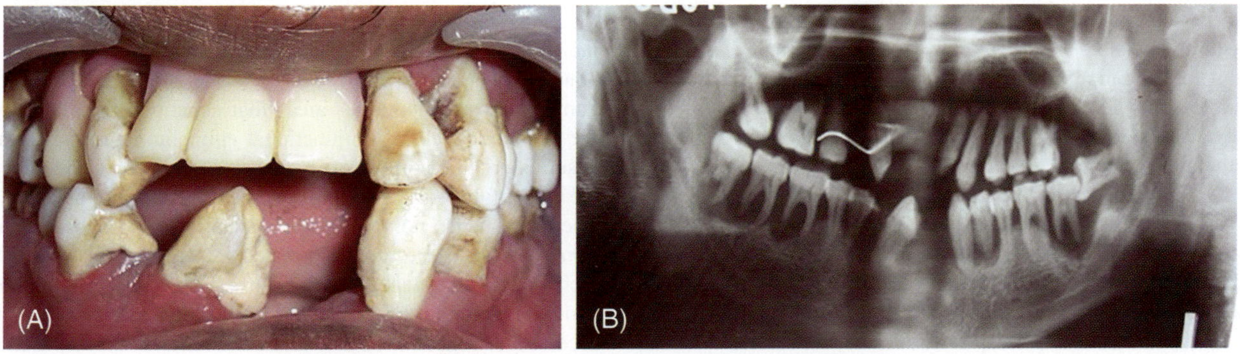

Fig. 45.10 A, Dentition with hopeless overall prognosis. B, OPG of the same case.

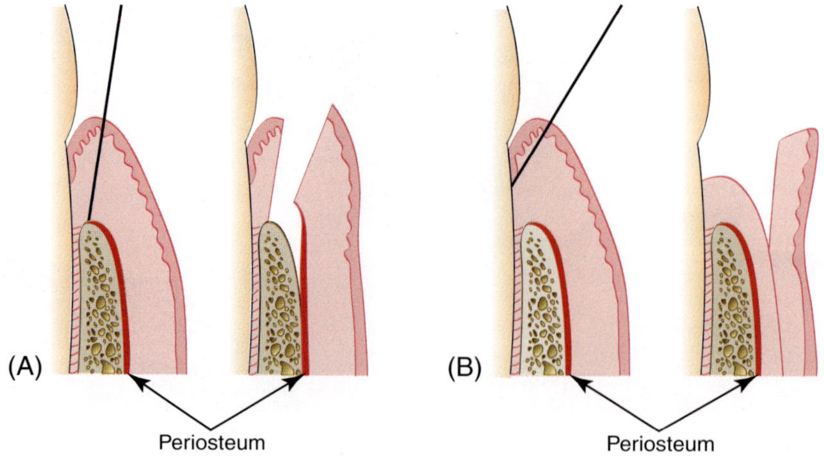

Fig. 45.11 A, Diagram of the internal bevel incision (first incision) to reflect a full-thickness (mucoperiosteal) flap. Note that the incision ends on the bone to allow for the reflection of the entire flap. B, Diagram of the internal bevel incision to reflect a partial-thickness flap. Note that the incision ends on the root surface to preserve the periosteum on the bone.

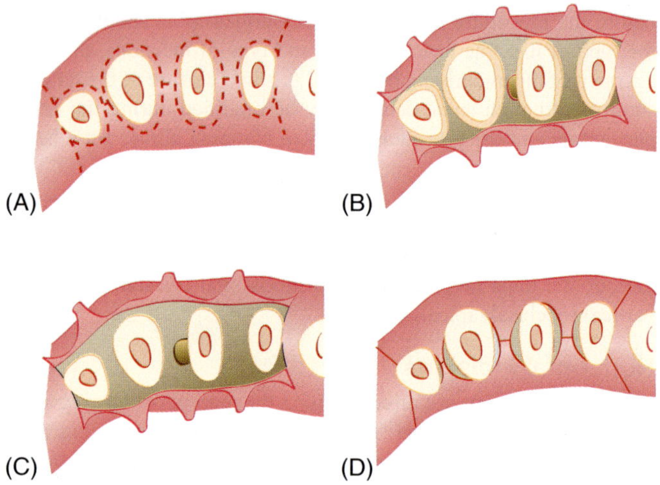

Fig. 45.12 Flap design for a conventional or traditional flap technique. A, Design of incisions: internal bevel incision, splitting the papilla, and vertical incisions are drawn in interrupted lines. B, The flap has been elevated, and the wedge of tissue next to the tooth is still in place. C, All marginal tissue has been removed to expose the underlying bone (see the defect in one space). D, The tissue has been returned to its original position. The proximal areas are not totally covered.

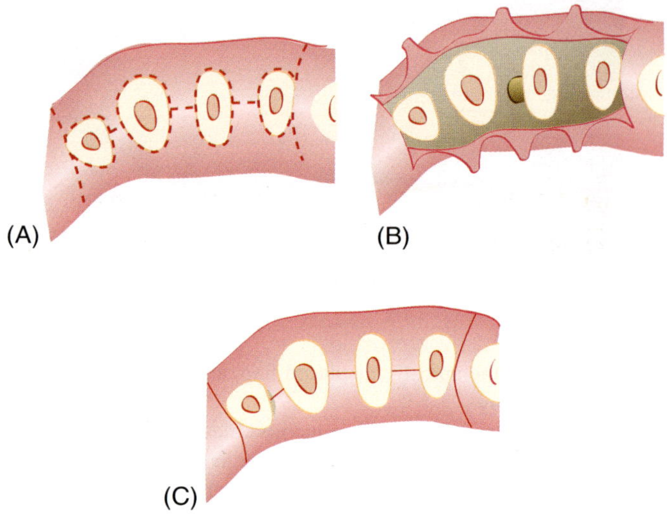

Fig. 45.13 Flap design for a sulcular incision flap. A, Design of incisions: sulcular incisions and vertical incisions are depicted by interrupted lines. B, The flap has been elevated to expose the underlying bone (see the defect in one space). C, The tissue has been returned to its original position to cover the interdental spaces.

and (3) it produces a sharp, thin flap margin for adaptation to the bone–tooth junction. This incision has also been termed the **first incision** because it is the initial incision for the reflection of a periodontal flap; it has also been called the **inverse** or **reverse bevel incision** because its bevel is in reverse direction from that of the gingivectomy incision. The no.11 or 15 BP surgical blade is used to make this incision in most areas of the mouth except in mandibular posterior region where a no. 12 blade might be preferred due to better access. That portion of the gingiva left around the tooth contains the epithelium of the pocket lining and the adjacent granulomatous tissue. It is discarded after the crevicular (second) and interdental (third) incisions are performed (Fig. 45.14).

The internal bevel incision starts from a designated area on the gingiva, and it is then directed to an area at or near the crest of the bone (Fig. 45.15). The starting point on the gingiva is determined by whether the flap is apically displaced or not displaced (Fig. 45.16). Ideally the incision should begin one tooth beyond the designated surgical area and from the most posterior tooth moving anteriorly.

The **crevicular incision**, which is also called the **second incision**, is made from the base of the pocket to the crest of the bone (Fig. 45.17). This incision, together with the initial reverse bevel incision, forms a V-shaped wedge that ends at or near the crest of bone (Fig. 45.18). This wedge of tissue contains most of the inflamed and granulomatous areas that constitute the lateral wall of the pocket as well as the junctional epithelium and the connective tissue fibers that still persist between the bottom of the pocket and the crest of the bone. The incision is carried around the entire tooth. The beak-shaped no. 12D blade is usually used for this incision.

A periosteal elevator is inserted into the initial internal bevel incision, and the flap is separated from the bone. The most apical end of the internal bevel incision is exposed and visible. With this access, the surgeon is able to make the *third incision*, which is also known as the *interdental incision*, to separate the collar of gingiva

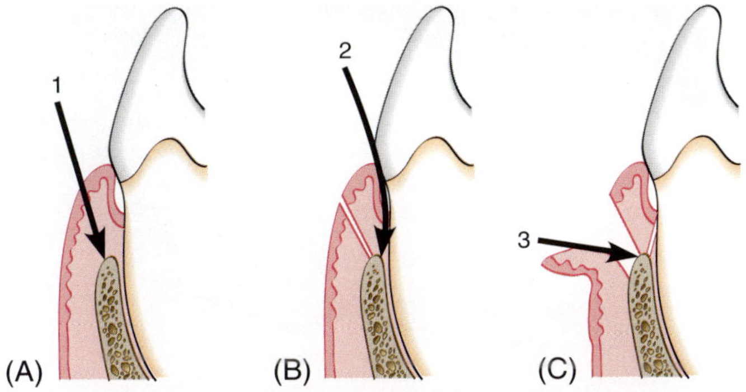

Fig. 45.14 The three incisions necessary for flap surgery. A, First (internal bevel) incision; B, second (crevicular) incision; and C, third (interdental) incision.

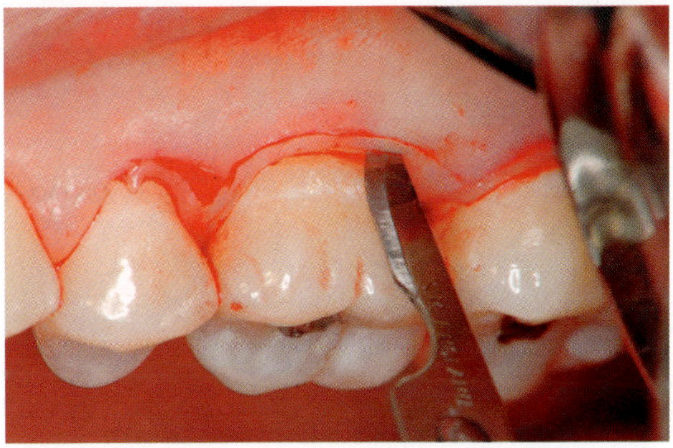

Fig. 45.17 Position of the knife to perform the crevicular (second) incision.

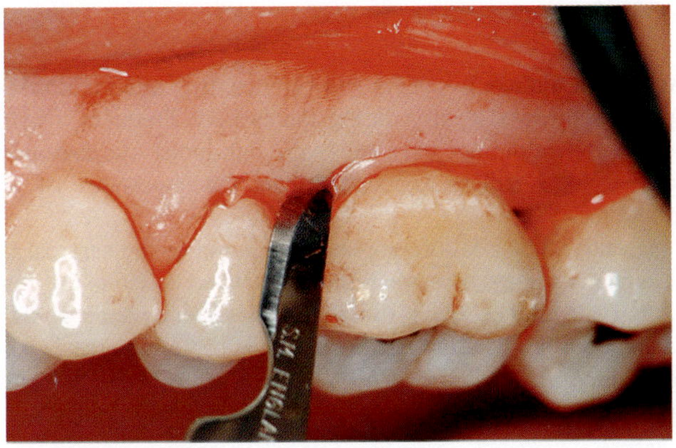

Fig. 45.15 Position of the knife to perform the internal bevel incision.

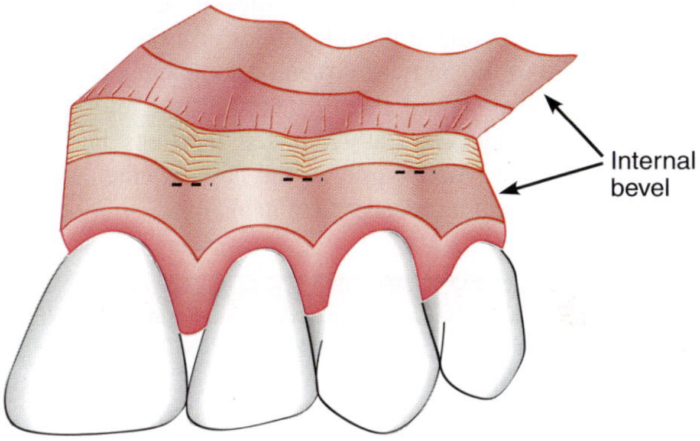

Fig. 45.18 After the flap has been elevated, a wedge of tissue remains on the teeth and is attached by the base of the papillae. An interdental (third) incision along the horizontal lines seen in the interdental spaces will sever these connections.

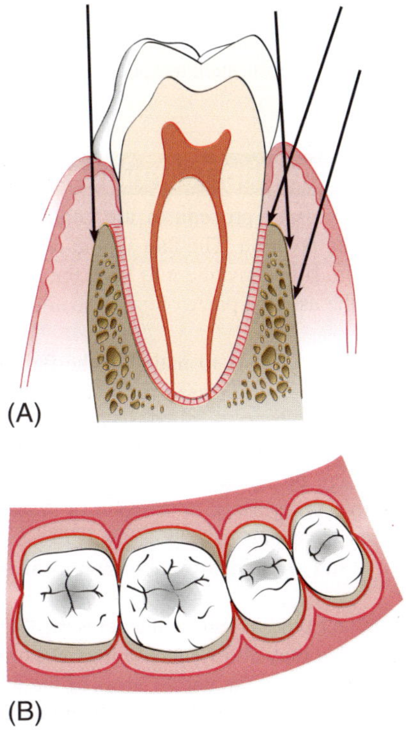

Fig. 45.16 A, The internal bevel (first) incision can be made at varying locations and angles according to the different anatomic and pocket situations. B, Occlusal view of the different locations in which the internal bevel incision can be made. Note the scalloped shape of the incisions.

that is left around the tooth. The Orban or the Buck knife is usually used for this incision. The incision is made not only around the facial and lingual radicular area but also interdentally, where it connects the facial and lingual segments to free the gingiva completely around the tooth (Figs. 45.14 and 45.18).

These three incisions allow for the removal of the gingiva around the tooth (i.e., the pocket epithelium and the adjacent granulomatous tissue). A surgical curette or a large scaler (Cumine) can be used for this purpose. After the removal of the large pieces of tissue, the remaining connective tissue in the osseous lesion should be carefully curetted and removed so that the entire root and the bone surface adjacent to the teeth can be observed.

Flaps can be reflected with the use of only the horizontal incision if sufficient access can be obtained in this way and if apical, lateral, or coronal displacement of the flap is not anticipated. If vertical incisions are not made, the flap is called an *envelope flap*.

Vertical Incisions

Vertical or oblique releasing incisions can be used on one or both ends of the horizontal incision, depending on the design and purpose of the flap. Vertical incisions at both ends are necessary if the flap is to be apically or coronally displaced. They are also preferred when the area of the surgery is limited to few teeth to prevent needless exposure of bone of uninvolved areas. These incisions must extend beyond the mucogingival line to reach the alveolar mucosa; this allows for the release of the flap to be displaced.

In general, vertical incisions in the lingual and palatal areas are avoided. Facial vertical incisions should not be made in the center

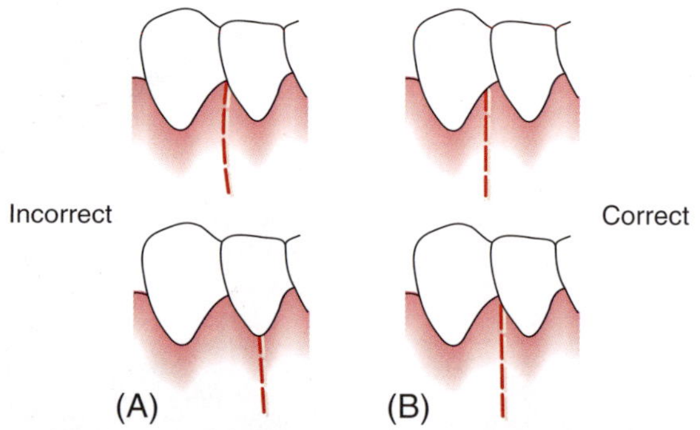

Fig. 45.19 A, Incorrect and, B, correct locations of a vertical incision. This incision should be made at the line angles to prevent the splitting of a papilla or incising directly over a radicular surface.

of an interdental papilla or over the radicular surface of a tooth. Incisions should be made at the line angles of a tooth either to include the papilla in the flap or to avoid it completely (Fig. 45.19). The vertical incision should also be designed to avoid short flaps (mesiodistal) with long, apically directed incisions because this could jeopardize the blood supply to the flap. In other words, the base of the flap should be broader than its margin.

Elevation of the Flap

When a full-thickness flap is desired, reflection of the flap is accomplished with a blunt dissection. A periosteal elevator is used to separate the mucoperiosteum from the bone by moving it mesially, distally, and apically until the desired reflection is accomplished. No more than 1–2 mm of bone needs to be exposed at most of the times (Fig. 45.20).

Sharp dissection is necessary to reflect a partial-thickness flap (Fig. 45.21). A combination of full-thickness and partial-thickness flaps may be indicated to obtain the advantages of both. The flap is started as a full-thickness procedure, and then a partial-thickness flap is made at the apical portion. In this way, the coronal portion of the bone—which may be subject to osseous remodeling—is exposed, whereas the remaining bone is protected by the periosteum.

Debridement

After the flap is reflected, the process of debridement begins. First the granulation tissue is removed by sharp Gracey curettes. Once this is done, the bleeding stops considerably allowing the operator to visualize the surgical field better. The root surface is carefully planed with ultrasonic scalers and curettes. It is important that the flap is not allowed to dry during the surgery. Frequent irrigation with normal saline not only keeps the flap moist but also aids in debridement. Needless to mention here the importance of good aspiration.

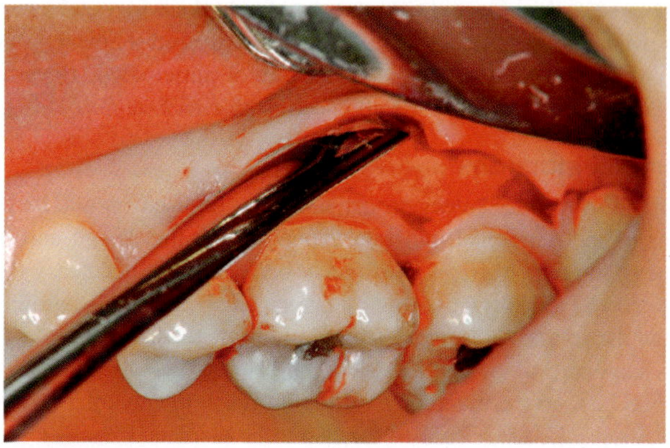

Fig. 45.20 Elevation of the flap with a periosteal elevator to obtain a full-thickness flap. Note the bone that is exposed with the full-thickness flap.

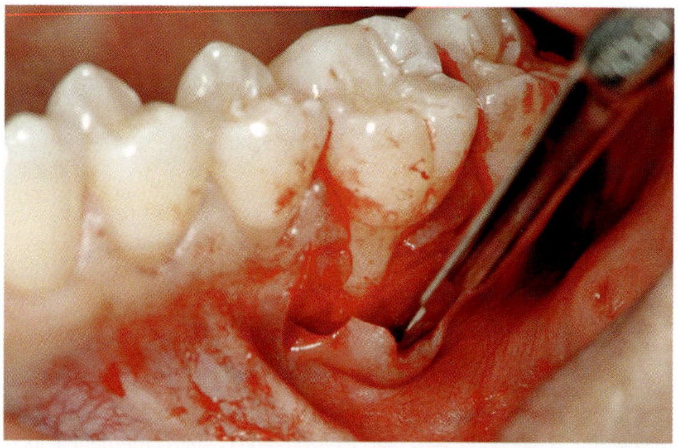

Fig. 45.21 Elevation of the flap with a Bard–Parker knife to obtain a split-thickness flap. Note that the bone is not exposed and that it is covered by periosteal tissue.

Recently, the need to completely degranulate the surgical field has been questioned by some researchers who claim that the granulation tissue may contain some growth factors which could be beneficial during healing. However, this is just a hypothesis which needs further investigation. Until now total removal of the granulation tissue has been the time tested concept and will remain so.

Osseous Management

The osseous shape and contour is examined, and the necessary osseous correction is accomplished. Often bony defects are discovered only after flap elevation. These are managed by either resective or additive osseous surgery.

The entire surgical area is thoroughly irrigated and re-examined for the presence of any debris such as specks of calculus prior to the flap replaced and sutured.

Sutures and Suturing Techniques

After all of the necessary procedures are completed, the flap is placed in the desired position. The flap should remain in this position without tension. It is convenient to keep the flap in place with light pressure via the use of a piece of gauze to allow the blood clot to form.

The purpose of suturing is to maintain the flap in the desired position until healing has progressed to the point at which sutures are no longer needed.

There are many types of sutures, suture needles, and materials. Suture materials may be either *nonresorbable* or *resorbable*, and they may be further categorized as *braided* or *monofilament*. The resorbable sutures have gained popularity because they enhance patient comfort and eliminate suture removal appointments (Box 45.1).

The monofilament type of suture alleviates the "wicking effect" of braided sutures that may allow bacteria from the oral cavity to be drawn through the suture to the deeper areas of the wound.

The braided silk suture was the most common nonresorbable suture used in the past because of its ease of use and low cost. It is still used in many countries around the world. However, the expanded polytetrafluoroethylene, synthetic, monofilament suture is an excellent nonresorbable suture that is preferred currently.

BOX 45.1 Suture Materials for Periodontal Flaps

Nonabsorbable (Nonresorbable)
- Silk: braided
- Nylon: monofilament
- ePTFE: monofilament
- Polyester: braided

Absorbable (Resorbable)
- Surgical: gut
- Plain gut: monofilament (30 days)
- Chromic gut: monofilament (45–60 days)

Synthetic
- Polyglycolic: braided (16–20 days)
- Vicryl
- Dexon
- Polyglycaprone: monofilament (90–120 days)
- Monocryl
- Polyglyconate: monofilament

The most common resorbable sutures used today are the plain and chromic gut sutures. Both are monofilaments, and both are processed from purified collagen of either sheep or cattle intestines. The chromic suture is a plain gut suture that has been processed with chromic salts to make it resistant to enzymatic resorption, thereby increasing the resorption time. The synthetic resorbable sutures are also often used (Box 45.1).

Technique

The needle is held with the needle holder, and it should enter the tissues at right angles and be no less than 2–3 mm from the incision. The needle is then carried through the tissue, where it follows the needle's curvature. The knot should not be placed over the incision.

The periodontal flap is closed either with independent sutures or with continuous, independent sling sutures. The latter method eliminates the pulling of the buccal and lingual or palatal flaps together and instead uses the teeth as an anchor for the flaps. The flaps are less likely to buckle, and the forces on the flaps are better distributed.

Sutures of any type that are placed in the interdental papillae should enter and exit the tissue at a point located below the imaginary line that forms the base of the triangle of the interdental papilla (Fig. 45.22). The location of sutures for the closure of a palatal flap depends on the extent of flap elevation that has been performed. The flap is divided into four quadrants as depicted in (Fig. 45.23).

If the elevation of the flap is slight or moderate, the sutures can be placed in the quadrant closest to the teeth. If the flap elevation is substantial, the sutures should be placed in the central quadrants of the palate.

The clinician may or may not use periodontal dressings. When the flaps are not apically displaced, it is not necessary to use dressings other than those needed for patient comfort.

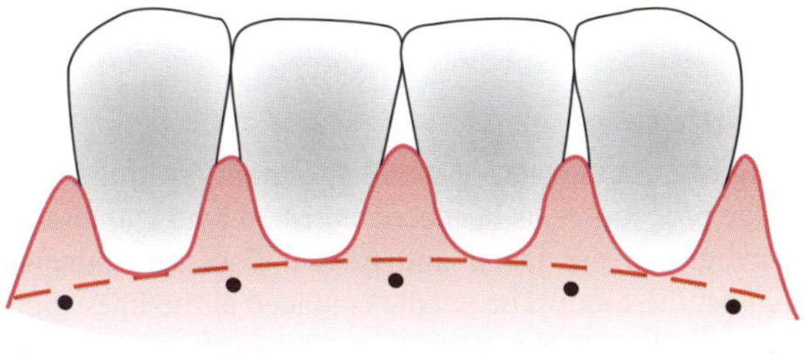

Fig. 45.22 Placement of sutures in the interdental space below the base of an imaginary triangle in the papilla.

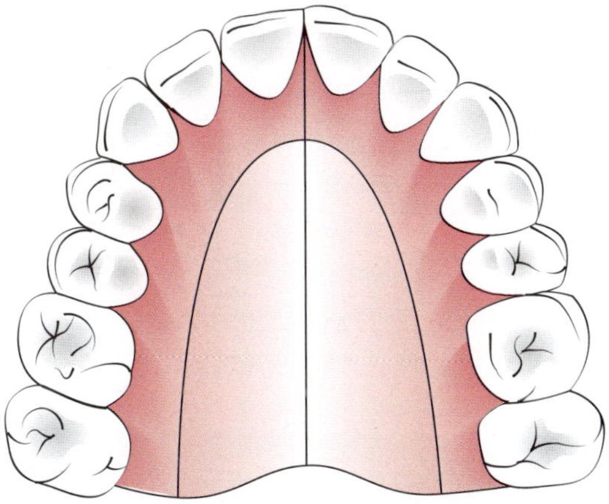

Fig. 45.23 Placement of sutures to close a palatal flap. For slightly or moderately elevated flaps, the sutures are placed in the shaded areas. For the more substantial elevation of the flap, the sutures are placed in the central (unshaded) areas of the palate.

Ligation

Interdental Ligation

Two types of interdental ligation can be used: the direct loop suture (Fig. 45.24) and the figure-eight suture (Fig. 45.25). With the figure-eight suture, thread is placed between the two flaps. This suture is used when the flaps are not in close apposition as a result of apical flap position or nonscalloped incisions. This is simpler to perform than the direct ligation. The direct suture allows for a better closure of the interdental papilla. It should be performed when bone grafts are used or when close apposition of the scalloped incision is required.

Sling Ligation

The sling ligation can be used for a flap on one surface of a tooth that involves two interdental spaces (Fig. 45.26).

Types of Sutures

Horizontal Mattress Suture

The horizontal mattress suture is often used for interproximal areas of diastemata or for wide interdental spaces to adapt the interdental papilla properly against the bone. Two sutures are often necessary. The horizontal mattress suture can be incorporated with the continuous, independent sling sutures (Fig. 45.27).

The penetration of the needle is performed in such a way that the mesial and distal edges of the papilla lie snugly against the bone. The needle enters the outer surface of the gingiva and crosses the undersurface of the gingiva horizontally. The mattress sutures should not be close together at the midpoint of the base of the papilla. The needle reappears on the outer surface at the other base of the papilla and continues around the tooth with the sling sutures.

Continuous, Independent Sling Suture

A sling suture is used when both a facial flap and a lingual flap are used and when they involve many teeth. The continuous, independent sling suture is initiated on the facial papilla closest to the midline because this is the easiest place to position the final knot. A continuous sling suture is laced for each papilla on the facial surface. When the last tooth is reached, the suture is anchored around it to prevent any pulling of the facial sutures when the lingual flap is sutured around the teeth in a similar manner. The suture is again anchored around the last tooth before the final knot is tied (Fig. 45.28).

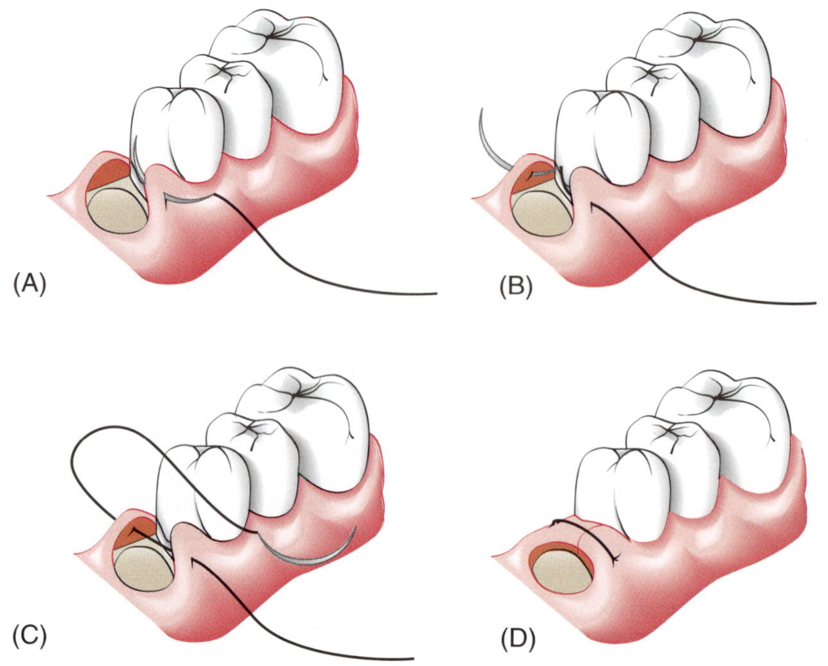

Fig. 45.24 Simple loop suture is used to approximate the buccal and lingual flaps. A, The needle penetrates the outer surface of the first flap. B, The undersurface of the opposite flap is engaged. C, The suture is brought back to the initial side, where, D, the knot is tied.

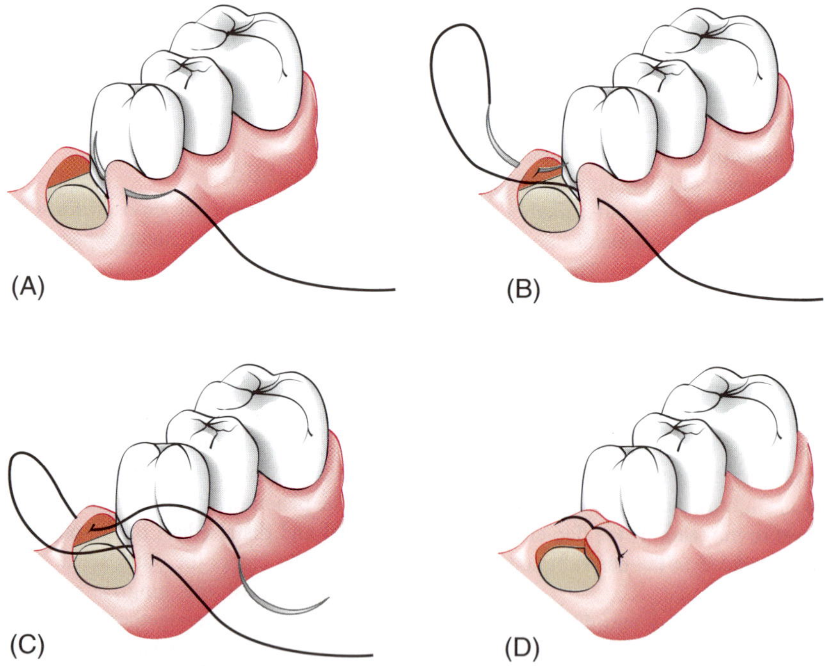

Fig. 45.25 Interrupted figure-eight suture is used to approximate the buccal and lingual flaps. A, The needle penetrates the outer surface of the first flap. B, The outer surface of the opposite flap. C, The suture is brought back to the first flap. D, The knot is tied.

This type of suture does not pull on the lingual flap when this flap is sutured. The facial and lingual flaps are completely independent of each other as a result of the anchoring around both the initial tooth and the final tooth. The flaps are tied to the teeth and not to each other because of the sling sutures.

Continuous, independent sling suturing is especially appropriate for the maxillary arch. This is true because the palatal gingiva is attached and fibrous, whereas the facial tissue is thinner and mobile.

Anchor Suture

The closing of a flap mesial or distal to a tooth, as in the mesial or distal wedge procedures, is best accomplished by the anchor suture. This suture closes the facial and lingual flaps and adapts them tightly against the tooth. The needle is placed at the line–angle area of the facial or lingual flap adjacent to the tooth, anchored around the tooth, passed beneath the opposite flap, and tied. The anchor suture can be repeated for each area that requires it (Fig. 45.29).

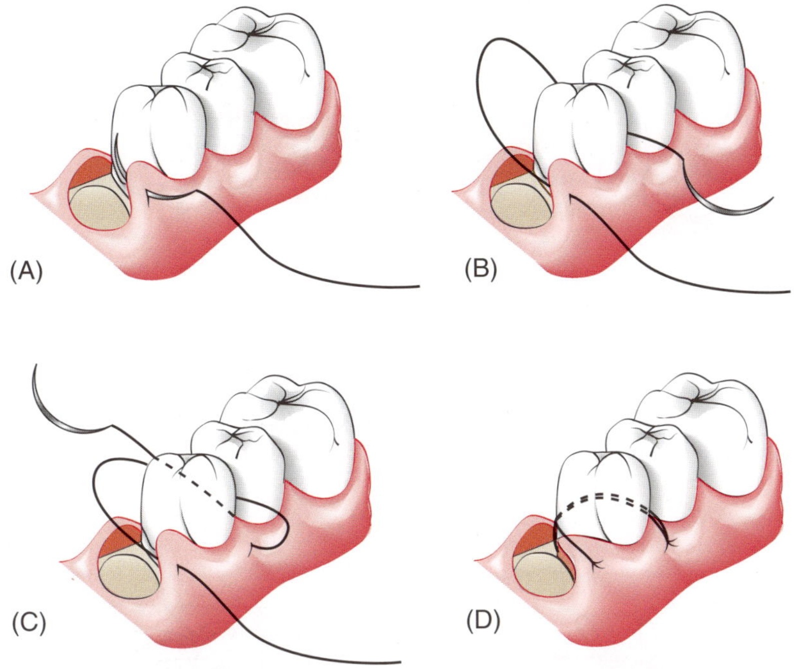

Fig. 45.26 Single, interrupted sling suture is used to adapt the flap around the tooth. A, The needle engages the outer surface of the flap and, B, encircles the tooth. C, The outer surface of the same flap of the adjacent interdental area is engaged. D, The suture is returned to the initial site, and the knot is tied.

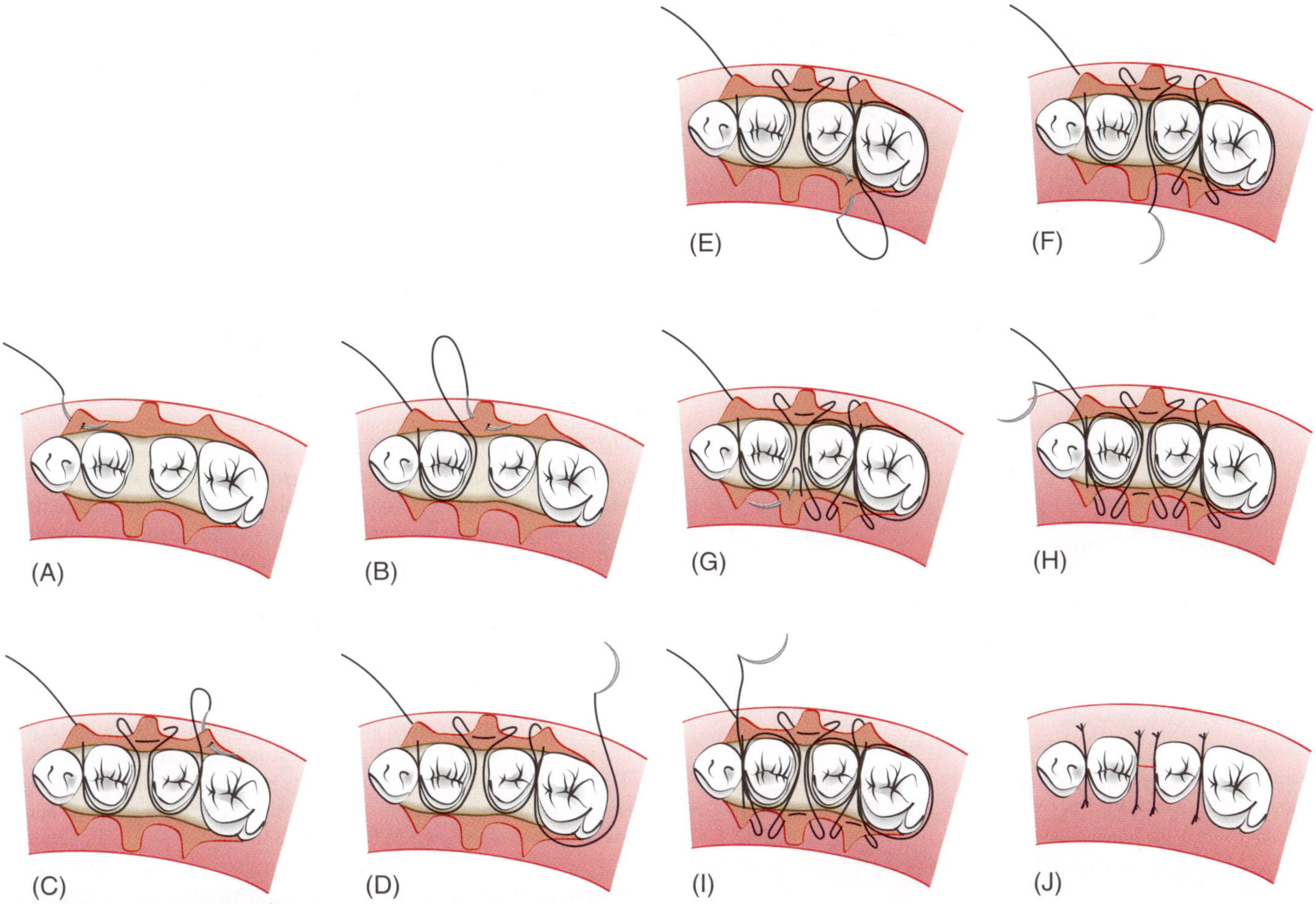

Fig. 45.27 A, Continuous, independent sling suture with the use of a horizontal mattress suture around, B, diastemata or, C, wide interdental areas. This mattress suture is used on both the, D, buccal and, E and F, lingual surfaces. G–I, Continuation of suture on the lingual surfaces. J, Completed suture.

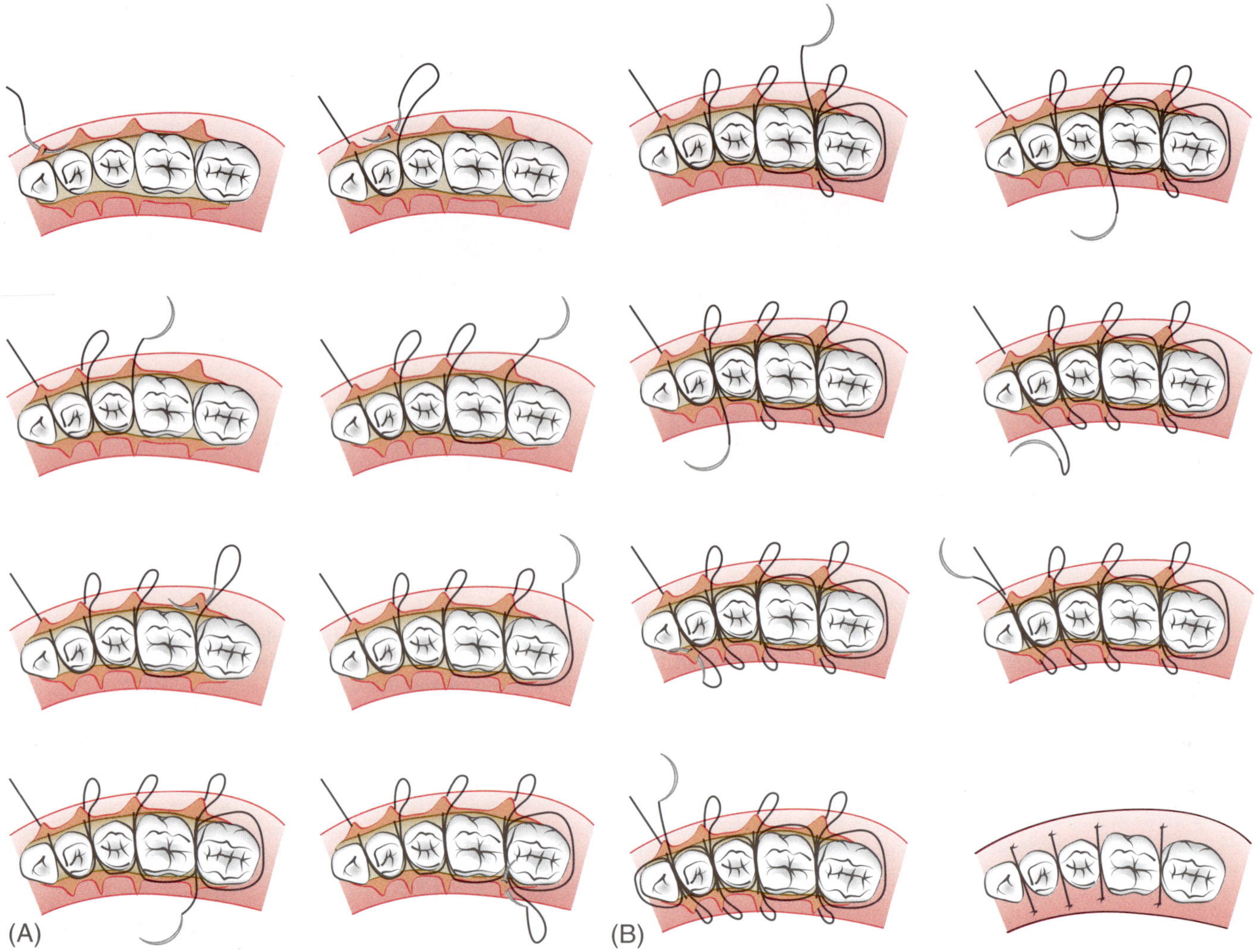

Fig. 45.28 (A & B) Continuous, independent sling suture is used to adapt the buccal and lingual flaps without tying the buccal flap to the lingual flap. The teeth are used to suspend each flap against the bone. It is important to anchor the suture on the two teeth at the beginning and end of the flap so that the suture will not pull the buccal flap to the lingual flap.

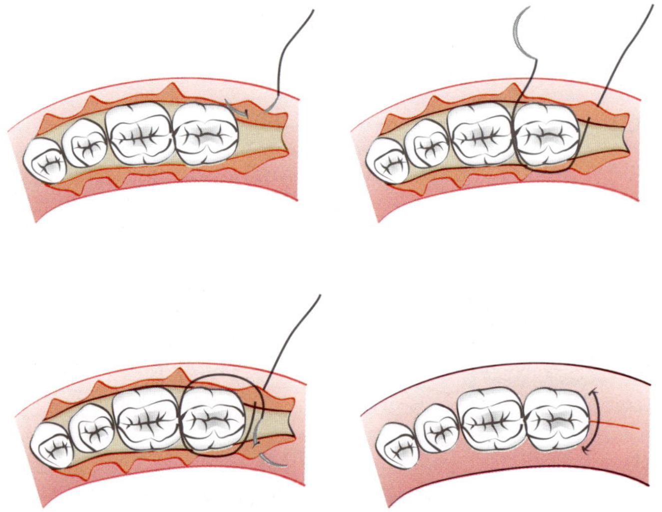

Fig. 45.29 Distal wedge suture. This anchor suture is also used to close flaps that are mesial or distal to a lone standing tooth.

Closed-Anchor Suture

Another technique to close a flap that is located in an edentulous area mesial or distal to a tooth consists of tying a direct suture that closes the proximal flap, carrying one of the threads around the tooth to anchor the tissue against the tooth, and then tying the two threads (Fig. 45.30).

Periosteal Suture

The periosteal suture is used to hold the apically displaced partial-thickness flaps on the periosteum. There are two types of periosteal sutures: the holding suture and the closing suture. The holding suture is a horizontal mattress suture that is placed at the base of the displaced flap to secure it into the new position. Closing sutures are used to secure the flap edges to the periosteum. Both types of periosteal sutures are shown in Figure 45.31.

Healing After Flap Surgery

Immediately after suturing (≤24 h), a connection between the flap and the tooth or bone surface is established by a blood clot, which

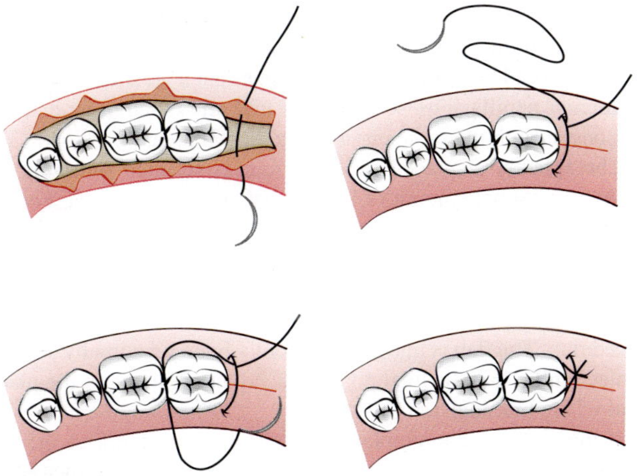

Fig. 45.30 The closed-anchor suture, which is another technique that can be used to suture distal wedges.

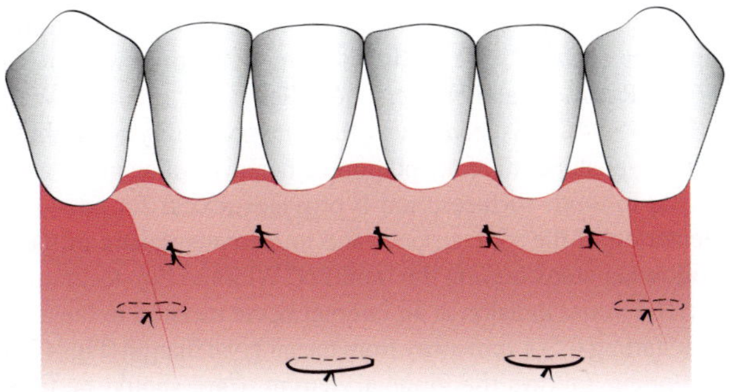

Fig. 45.31 Periosteal sutures for an apically displaced flap. Holding sutures, which are shown at the bottom, are placed first. This is followed by the closing sutures, which are shown at the coronal edge of the flap.

consists of a fibrin reticulum with many polymorphonuclear leukocytes, erythrocytes, debris of injured cells, and capillaries at the edge of the wound. Bacteria and an exudate or transudate also result from tissue injury.

One to three days after flap surgery, the space between the flap and the tooth or bone is thinner. Epithelial cells migrate over the border of the flap, and they usually contact the tooth at this time. When the flap is closely adapted to the alveolar process, there is a minimal inflammatory response.

One week after surgery, an epithelial attachment to the root has been established by means of hemidesmosomes and a basal lamina. The blood clot is replaced by granulation tissue derived from the gingival connective tissue, the bone marrow, and the periodontal ligament.

Two weeks after surgery, collagen fibers begin to appear parallel to the tooth surface. Union of the flap to the tooth is still weak because of the presence of immature collagen fibers, although the clinical aspect may be almost normal.

One month after surgery, a fully epithelialized gingival crevice with a well-defined epithelial attachment is present. There is a beginning functional arrangement of the supracrestal fibers.

Full-thickness flaps, which denude the bone, result in a superficial bone necrosis after 1–3 days. Osteoclastic resorption follows and reaches a peak at 4–6 days and then declines thereafter. This results in a loss of bone of about 1 mm^3; the bone loss is greater if the bone is thin.

A loss of bone occurs during the initial healing stages both in the radicular bone and in the interdental bone areas. However, in the interdental areas, which have cancellous bone, the subsequent repair stage results in total restitution without any loss of bone; in radicular bone (particularly if it is thin and unsupported by cancellous bone), bone repair results in the loss of marginal bone.

Different Flap Techniques

Whereas the basic principles of flap surgery remain the same slight variations and modifications are required to deal with different situations. The design of the flap and the extent to which tissues are resected/conserved, and the amount of flap reflection depends the purpose for which it is being performed and the final outcome the clinician desires. Accordingly, various clinicians have devised techniques over the period of time and several names have been given such as Newman flap, Kirkland flap, flap curettage, open flap curettage, and so on. But the most commonly practiced techniques today are the modified Widman flap, the Conventional or the Access flap, undisplaced flap (also called inverse bevel gingivectomy), and the apically displaced flap.

The **modified Widman flap** has been described for exposing the root surfaces for meticulous instrumentation and for the removal of the pocket lining. Again, it is not intended to eliminate or reduce pocket depth, except for the reduction that occurs during healing as a result of tissue shrinkage.

The **conventional or access flap** attempts to conserve the tissues as much as possible so as to ensure optimal coverage of graft materials and barrier membranes that might have to be placed for regenerating the periodontal tissues.

The **undisplaced (unrepositioned)** ***flap*** improves accessibility for instrumentation, but it also removes the pocket wall, thereby reducing or eliminating the pocket. This is essentially an excisional procedure of the gingiva.

The **apically displaced flap** provides accessibility and eliminates the pocket, but it does the latter by apically positioning the soft-tissue wall of the pocket. Therefore, it preserves or increases the width of the attached gingiva by transforming the previously unattached keratinized pocket wall into attached tissue. This increase in the width of the attached gingiva is based on the apical shift of the mucogingival junction, which may include the apical displacement of the muscle attachments.

Incisions

All three flap techniques that were just discussed involve the use of the basic incisions described earlier in this chapter. The internal bevel incision, the crevicular incision, and the interdental incision. However, there are important variations in the way these incisions are performed for the different types of flaps (Figs. 45.32 and 45.33). The internal beveled incision for the modified Widman flap closely follows the scalloped outline of the dentition to minimize the loss of the attached keratinized gingiva. This incision is made 1–2 mm from the teeth. The gingival margin is removed, and the flap is reflected to gain access for root therapy.

The technique that is used to achieve reconstructive and regenerative objectives is the *conventional flap with or without papilla preservation* which involves only the crevicular or second incision. This will allow the clinician to retain the maximum amount of gingival tissue, including the papilla, which is essential for graft or membrane coverage.

For the undisplaced flap, the internal bevel incision is initiated at or near a point just coronal to where the bottom of the pocket is projected on the outer surface of the gingival (Fig. 45.32). This

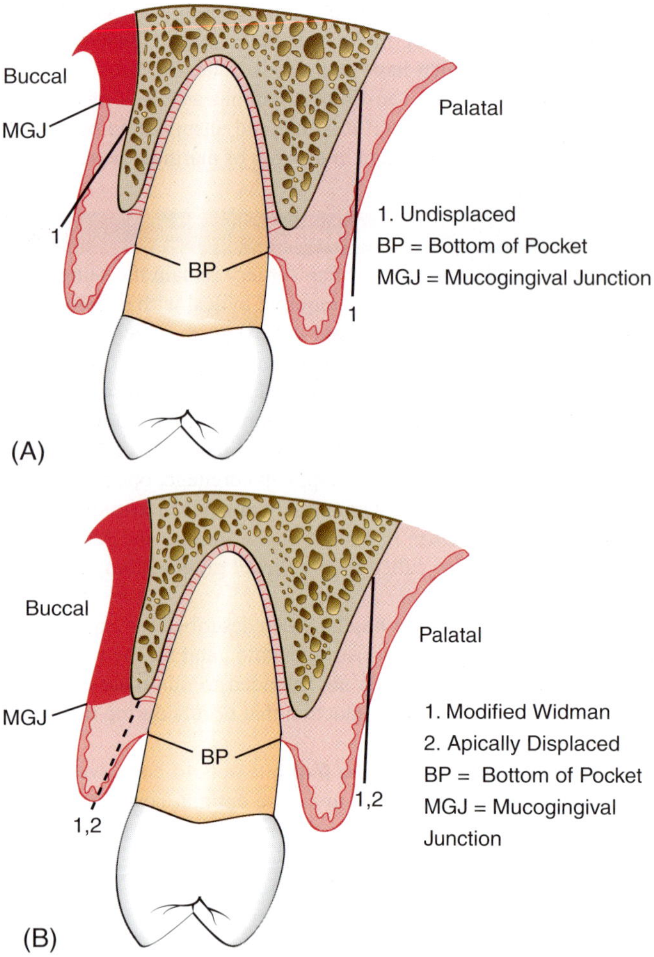

Fig. 45.32 (A & B) Locations of the internal bevel incisions for the different types of flaps.

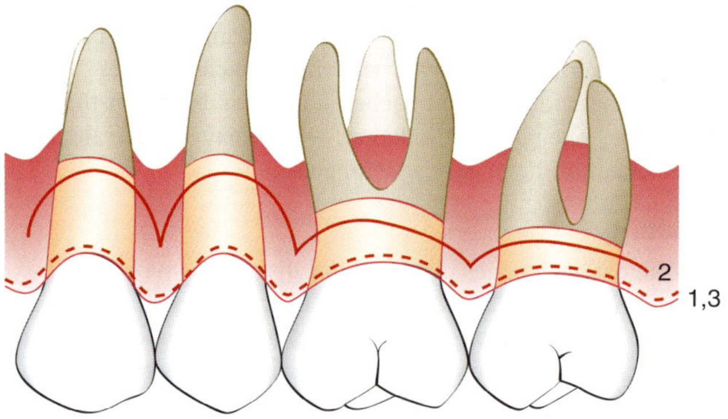

Fig. 45.33 Scalloping required for the different types of flaps.

incision can be accomplished only if sufficient attached gingiva remains apical to the incision. Therefore, the two anatomic landmarks—the pocket depth and the location of the mucogingival junction—must be considered to evaluate the amount of attached gingiva that will remain after the surgery has been completed. Because the pocket wall is not displaced apically, the initial incision should eliminate the pocket wall. Thus, an incision should not be made too close to the tooth because it will not eliminate the pocket wall, and it may result in the re-creation of the soft-tissue pocket. If the tissue is too thick, the flap margin should be thinned with the initial incision. The proper placement of the flap margin at the tooth–bone junction during closure is important to prevent either recurrence of the pocket or the exposure of bone. The internal bevel incision should be scalloped into the interdental area to preserve the interdental papilla (Fig. 45.33). This will allow better coverage of the bone at both the radicular and interdental areas.

The apically displaced flap technique is selected for cases that present a minimal amount of keratinized, attached gingiva. For this reason, the internal bevel incision should be made as close to the tooth as possible (i.e., 0.5–1.0 mm) (Fig. 45.32). There is no need to determine where the bottom of the pocket is in relation to the incision for the apically displaced flap as one would for the undisplaced flap. The flap is placed at the tooth–bone junction by apically displacing the flap. Its final position is not determined by the placement of the first incision.

If the surgeon contemplates osseous surgery, the first incision should be placed in such a way to compensate for the removal of the bone tissue so that the flap can be placed at the tooth–bone junction.

The Flap Technique for Pocket Therapy

Modified Widman Flap

In 1965, Morris revived a technique described early during the 20th century in the periodontal literature; he called it the "unrepositioned mucoperiosteal flap." Essentially, the same procedure was presented in 1974 by Ramfjord and Nissle, who called it the "modified Widman flap" (Fig. 45.34). This technique offers the possibility of establishing an intimate postoperative adaptation of healthy collagenous connective tissue to tooth surfaces, and it provides access for adequate instrumentation of the root surfaces and immediate closure of the area. The following steps outline the modified Widman flap technique:

Step 1: The initial incision is an internal bevel incision to the alveolar crest starting 0.5–1 mm away from the gingival margin (Fig. 45.34C). Scalloping follows the gingival margin. Care should be taken to insert the blade in such a way that the papilla is left with a thickness similar to that of the remaining facial flap. Vertical relaxing incisions are usually not needed.

Step 2: The gingiva is reflected with a periosteal elevator (Fig. 45.34D).

Step 3: A crevicular incision is made from the bottom of the pocket to the bone in such a way that it circumscribes the triangular wedge of tissue that contains the pocket lining.

Step 4: After the flap is reflected, a third incision is made in the interdental spaces coronal to the bone with a curette or an Orban knife, and the gingival collar is removed (Fig. 45.34E and F).

Step 5: Tissue tags and granulation tissue are removed with a curette. The root surfaces are checked and then scaled and planed, if needed (Fig. 45.34G and H). Residual periodontal fibers attached to the tooth surface should not be disturbed.

Step 6: Bone architecture is not corrected unless it prevents good tissue adaptation to the necks of the teeth. Every effort is made to adapt the facial and lingual interproximal tissue adjacent to each other in such a way that no interproximal bone remains exposed at the time of suturing. The flaps may be thinned to allow for close adaptation of the gingiva around the entire circumference of the tooth and to each other interproximally.

Step 7: Continuous, independent sling sutures are placed in both the facial and palatal areas (Fig. 45.34I and J) and covered with a periodontal surgical pack.

Ramfjord and Nissle performed an extensive longitudinal study that compared the Widman procedure (as modified by them) to the curettage technique and the pocket elimination methods, which include bone contouring when needed. The patients were assigned randomly to one of the techniques, and results were analyzed yearly for up to 7 years after therapy. The researchers reported similar results for each of the three methods tested. Pocket depth was

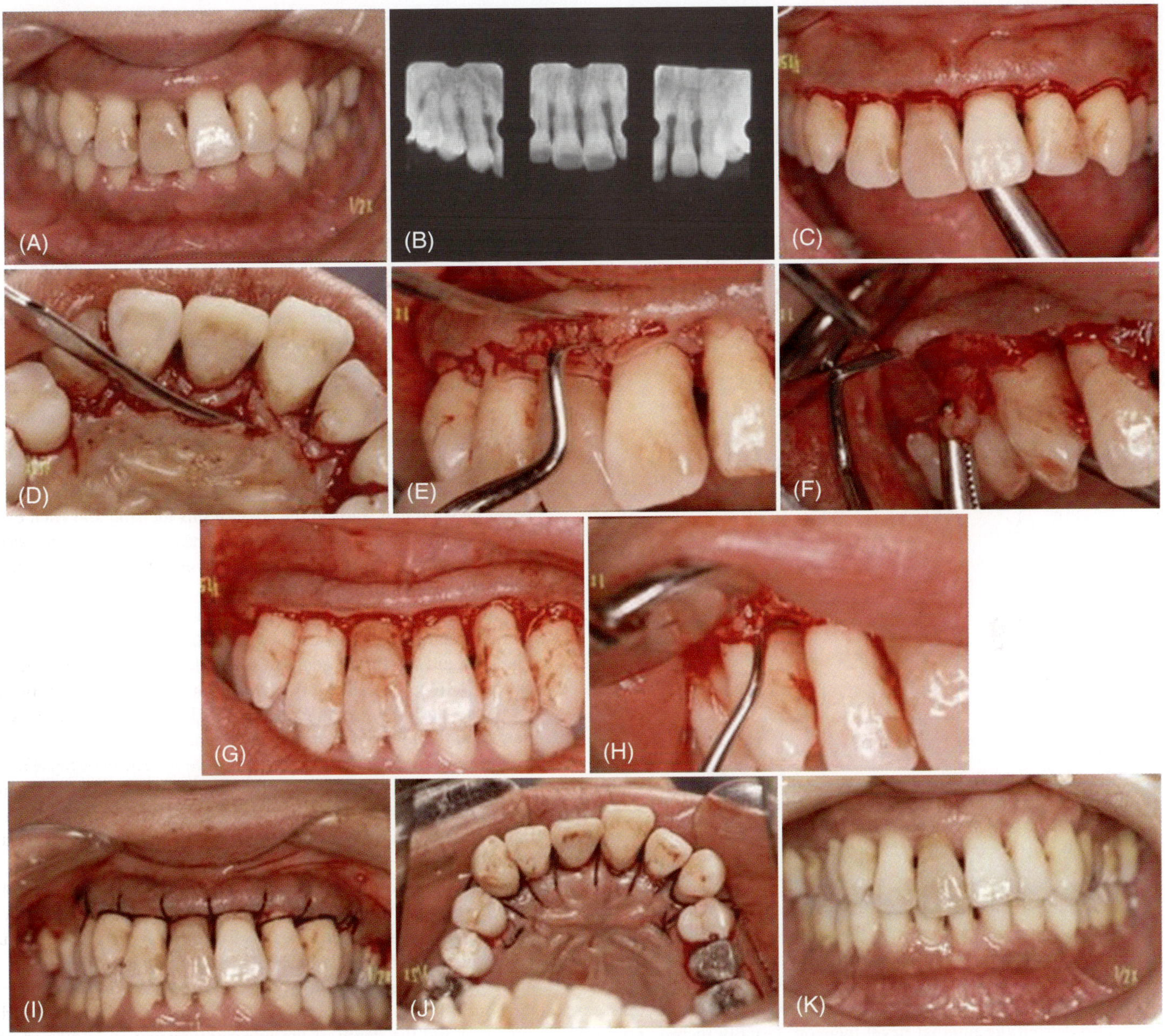

Fig. 45.34 Modified Widman flap technique. A, Facial view before surgery. The probing of pockets revealed interproximal depths that ranged from 4 to 8 mm and facial and palatal depths of 2–5 mm. B, Radiographic survey of the area. Note the generalized horizontal bone loss. C, Facial internal bevel incision. D, Palatal incision. E, Elevation of the flap, which left a wedge of tissue still attached to its base. F, Removal of tissue. G, Tissue removed and ready for scaling and root planing. H, Scaling and root planing of exposed root surfaces. I, Continuous, independent sling suture of facial portion of surgery. J, Continuous, independent sling suture of palatal portion of surgery. K, Postsurgical result. *(Courtesy: Dr. Kitetsu Shin, Saitama, Japan.)*

initially similar for all methods, but it was maintained at shallower levels with the Widman flap; the attachment level remained higher with the Widman flap.

Undisplaced Flap

Currently, the undisplaced flap may be the most frequently performed type of periodontal surgery. It differs from the modified Widman flap in that the soft-tissue pocket wall is removed with the initial incision; thus, it may be considered an "internal bevel gingivectomy." The undisplaced flap and the gingivectomy are the two techniques that surgically remove the pocket wall. To perform this technique without creating a mucogingival problem, the clinician should determine that enough attached gingiva will remain after removal of the pocket wall. The following steps outline the undisplaced flap technique.

Step 1: The pockets are measured with the periodontal probe, and a bleeding point is produced on the outer surface of the gingiva to mark the pocket bottom.

Step 2: The initial or internal bevel incision is made (Fig. 45.35) after scalloping the bleeding marks on the gingiva (Fig. 45.36). The incision is usually carried to a point apical to the alveolar crest, depending on the thickness of the tissue. The thicker the tissue is, the more apical the ending point of the incision (Fig. 45.35). In addition, thinning of the flap should be performed with the initial incision because it is easier to accomplish at this time than it is later with a loose, reflected flap that is

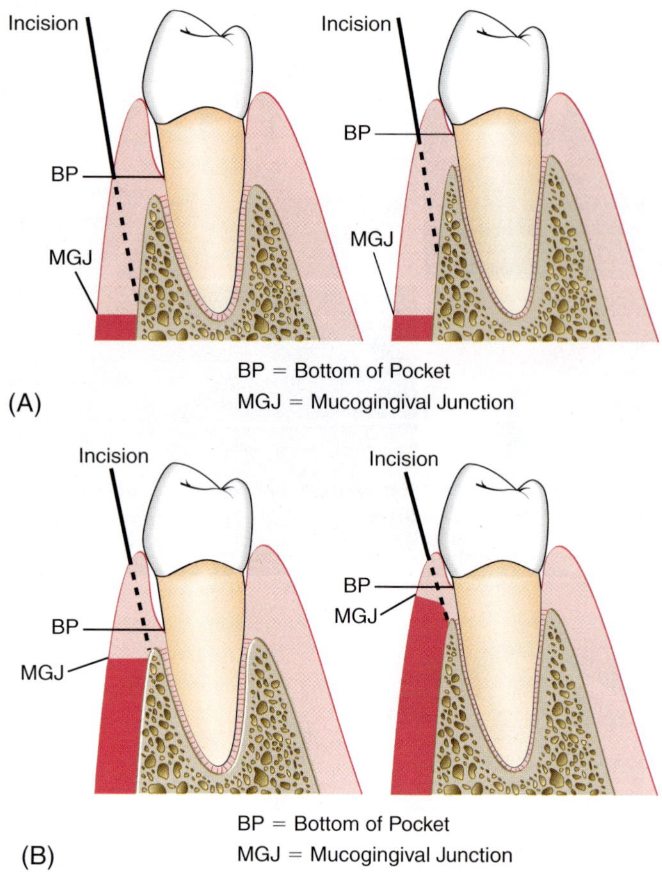

Fig. 45.35 (A & B) Diagram showing the location of two different areas where the internal bevel incision is made in an undisplaced flap. The incision is made at the level of the pocket to discard the tissue coronal to the pocket if there is sufficient remaining attached gingiva.

difficult to manage. (The use of this technique in palatal areas is considered in the discussion that follows this list.)

Step 3: The second or crevicular incision is made from the bottom of the pocket to the bone to detach the connective tissue from the bone.

Step 4: The flap is reflected with a periosteal elevator (blunt dissection) from the internal bevel incision. Usually there is no need for vertical incisions because the flap is not displaced apically.

Step 5: The third or interdental incision is made with an interdental knife to separate the connective tissue from the bone.

Step 6: The triangular wedge of tissue created by the three incisions is removed with a curette.

Step 7: The area is debrided to remove all tissue tags and granulation tissue with the use of sharp curettes.

Step 8: After the necessary scaling and root planing, the flap edge should rest on the root–bone junction. If this is not the case as a result of the improper location of the initial incision or the unexpected need for osseous surgery, the edge of the flap is scalloped again and trimmed to allow the flap edge to end at the root–bone junction.

Step 9: A continuous sling suture is used to secure the facial and lingual or palatal flaps. This type of suture, which makes use of the tooth as an anchor, is advantageous to position and hold the flap edges at the root–bone junction. The area is covered with a periodontal pack.

Palatal Flap

The surgical approach to the palatal area differs from that used for other areas as a result of the character of the palatal tissue and the anatomy of the area. The palatal tissue is all attached, keratinized tissue and has none of the elastic properties associated with other gingival tissues. Therefore, the palatal tissue cannot be apically displaced, and a partial-thickness (split-thickness) flap cannot be accomplished.

The initial incision for the palatal flap should allow the flap, when sutured, to be precisely adapted at the root–bone junction. The flap cannot be moved apically or coronally to adapt to the root–bone junction, as can be done with the flaps in other areas. Therefore, the location of the initial incision is important for the final placement of the flap.

The palatal tissue may be thin or thick, and it may or may not have osseous defects. The palatal vault may be high or low. These anatomic variations may require changes in the location, angle, and design of the incision.

The initial incision for a flap varies with the anatomic situation. As shown in Fig. 45.37, the initial incision may be the usual internal bevel incision, which will then be followed by crevicular and interdental incisions. If the tissue is thick, a horizontal gingivectomy incision may be made, and this may be followed by an internal bevel incision that starts at the edge of this incision and ends on the lateral surface of the underlying bone. The placement of the internal bevel incision must be done in such a way that the flap fits around the tooth without exposing the bone.

Before the flap is reflected to the final position for scaling and management of the osseous lesions, its thickness must be checked. Flaps should be thin to adapt to the underlying osseous tissue and provide a thin, knife-like gingival margin. Flaps—particularly palatal flaps—are often too thick; they may have a propensity to separate from the tooth, which may delay and complicate healing. It is best to thin the flaps before their complete reflection because a free, mobile flap is difficult to hold for thinning (Fig. 45.38). A sharp, thin papilla positioned properly around the interdental areas at the tooth–bone junction is essential to prevent the recurrence of soft-tissue pockets.

The purpose of the palatal flap should be considered before the incision is made. If the intent of the surgery is debridement, the internal bevel incision is planned so that the flap adapts at the root–bone junction when sutured. If osseous resection is necessary, the incision should be planned to compensate for the lowered level of the bone when the flap is closed. Probing and sounding of the osseous level and the depth of the intrabony pocket should be used to determine the position of the incision.

The apical portion of the scalloping should be narrower than the line–angle area because the palatal root tapers apically. A rounded scallop results in a palatal flap that does not fit snugly around the root. This procedure should be done before the complete reflection of the palatal flap because a loose flap is difficult to grasp and stabilize for dissection.

It is sometimes necessary to thin the palatal flap after it has been reflected. This can be accomplished by holding the inner portion of the flap with a mosquito hemostat or Adson forceps as the inner connective tissue is carefully dissected away with a sharp no. 15 scalpel blade. Care must be taken to not perforate or overthin the flap. The edge of the flap should be thinner than the base; therefore, the blade should be angled toward the lateral surface of the palatal bone. The dissected inner connective tissue is removed with a hemostat. As with any flap, the triangular papilla portion should be thin enough to fit snugly against the bone and into the interdental area (Fig. 45.39).

The principles for the use of vertical releasing incisions are similar to those for using other incisions. Care must be exercised so that the length of the incision is minimal to avoid the numerous vessels located in the palate.

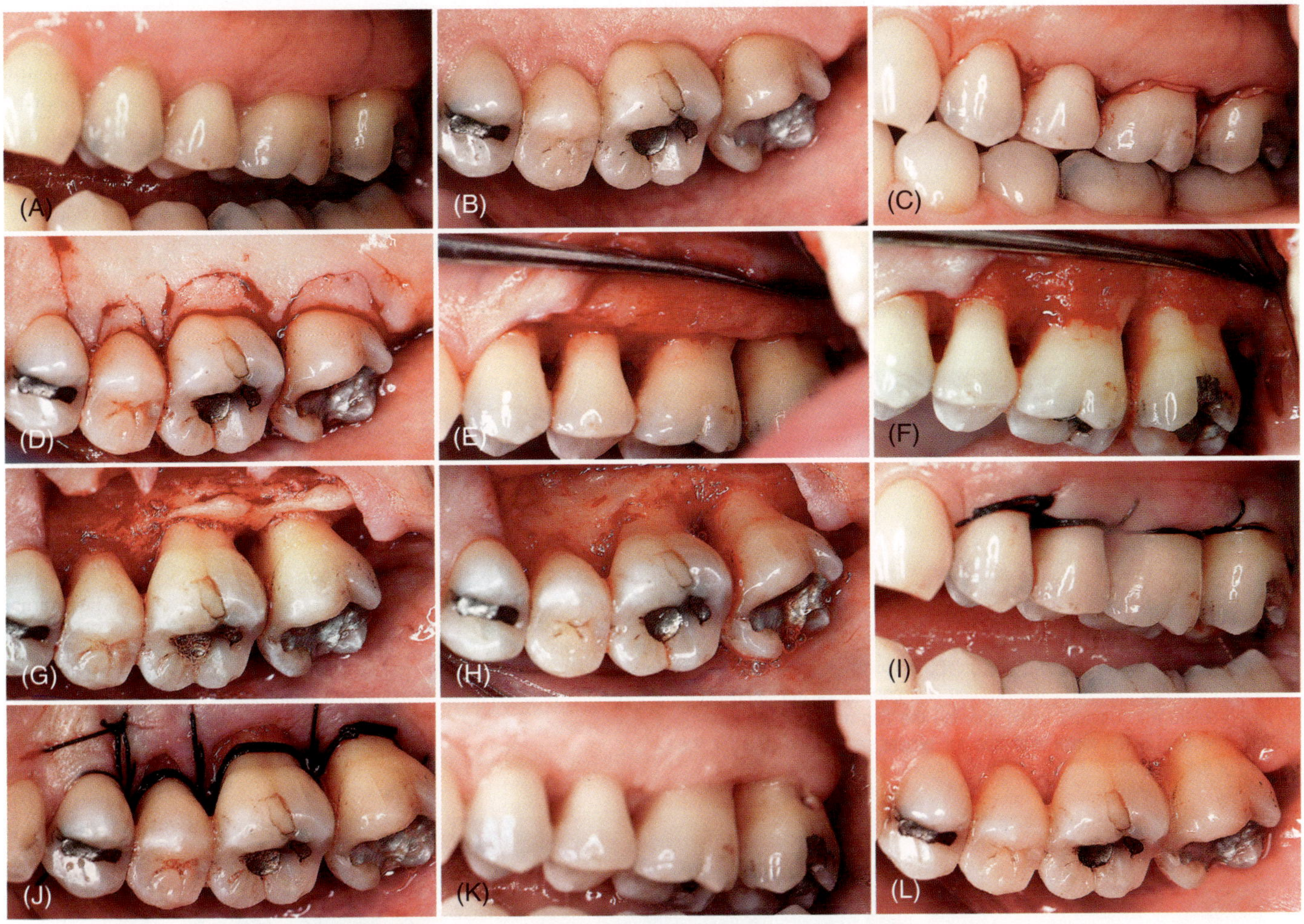

Fig. 45.36 Undisplaced flap. A and B, Preoperative facial and palatal views. C and D, Internal bevel incisions in the facial and palatal aspects. Note the deeper scalloping palatally for the replaced flap. E and F, Flap elevated to show osseous defects. G and H, Osseous surgery has been performed. I and J, Flaps have been placed in their original sites and sutured. K and L, Postoperative results. *(Courtesy: Dr. Paulo Camargo, University of California, Los Angeles.)*

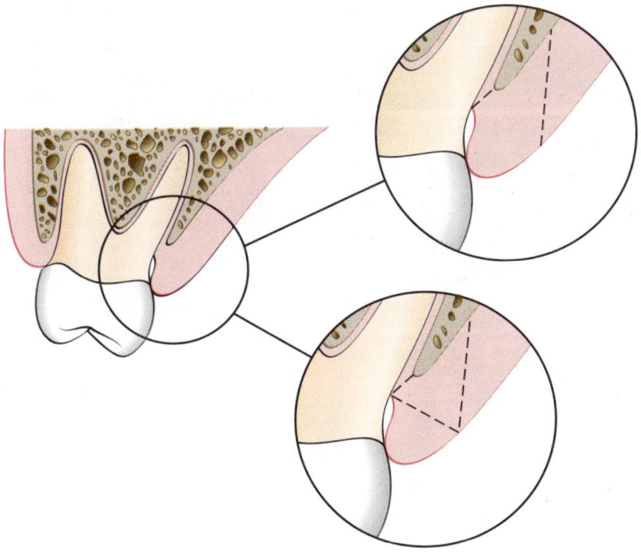

Fig. 45.37 Examples of two methods for eliminating a palatal pocket. One incision is an internal bevel incision made at the area of the apical extent of the pocket. The other procedure involves a gingivectomy incision, which is followed by an internal bevel incision.

Apically Displaced Flap

With some variants, the apically displaced flap technique can be used for pocket eradication, widening the zone of attached gingiva, or both. Depending on the purpose, the apically displaced flap can be a full-thickness (mucoperiosteal) flap or a split-thickness (mucosal) flap. The split-thickness flap requires more precision and time as well as a gingival tissue that is thick enough to split, but it can be more accurately positioned and sutured in an apical position with the use of a periosteal suturing technique, as follows.

Step 1: An internal bevel incision is made (Fig. 45.40). To preserve as much of the keratinized and attached gingiva as possible (Fig. 45.32), it should be no more than about 1 mm from the crest of the gingiva and directed to the crest of the bone. The incision is made after the existing scalloping, and there is no need to mark the bottom of the pocket in the external gingival surface because the incision is unrelated to pocket depth. It is also not necessary to accentuate the scallop interdentally because the flap is displaced apically and not placed interdentally.

Step 2: Crevicular incisions are made, and this is followed by the initial elevation of the flap. Interdental incisions are then performed, and the wedge of tissue that contains the pocket wall is removed.

Step 3: Vertical incisions are made extending beyond the mucogingival junction. If the objective is a full-thickness flap, it is

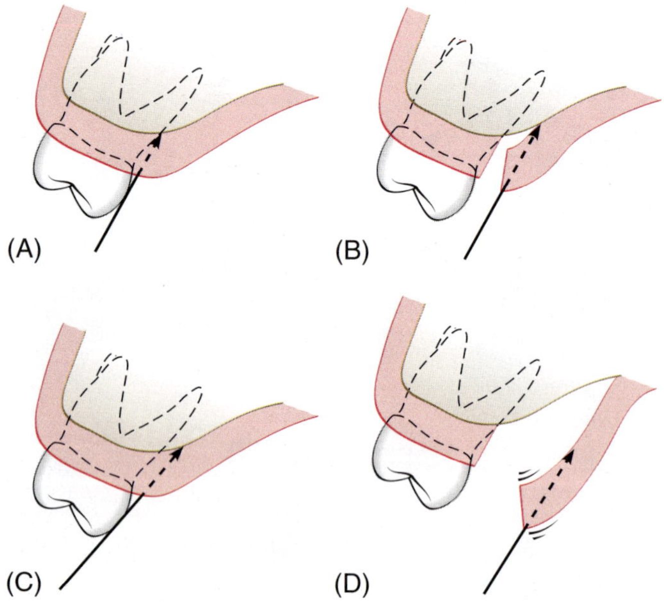

Fig. 45.38 Diagrams that illustrate the angle of the internal bevel incision in the palate and the different ways to thin the flap. A, The usual angle and direction of the incision. B, Thinning of the flap after it has been slightly reflected with a second internal incision. C, Beveling and thinning of the flap with the initial incision if the position and contour of the tooth allow. D, The problem encountered when thinning the flap after it has been reflected. The flap is too loose and free for proper positioning and for the making of the incision.

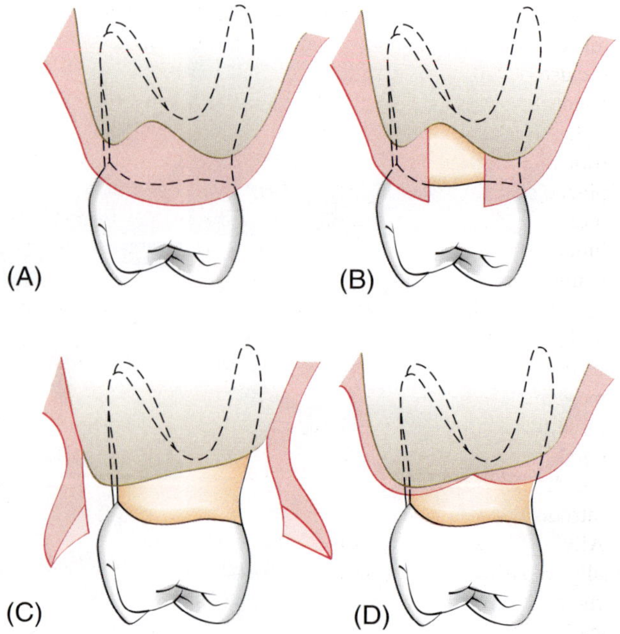

Fig. 45.39 A, Distal view of incisions made to eliminate a pocket distal to the maxillary second molar. B, Two parallel incisions and the removal of the intervening tissue. C, Thinning of the flap and contouring of the bone. D, Approximation of the buccal and palatal flaps.

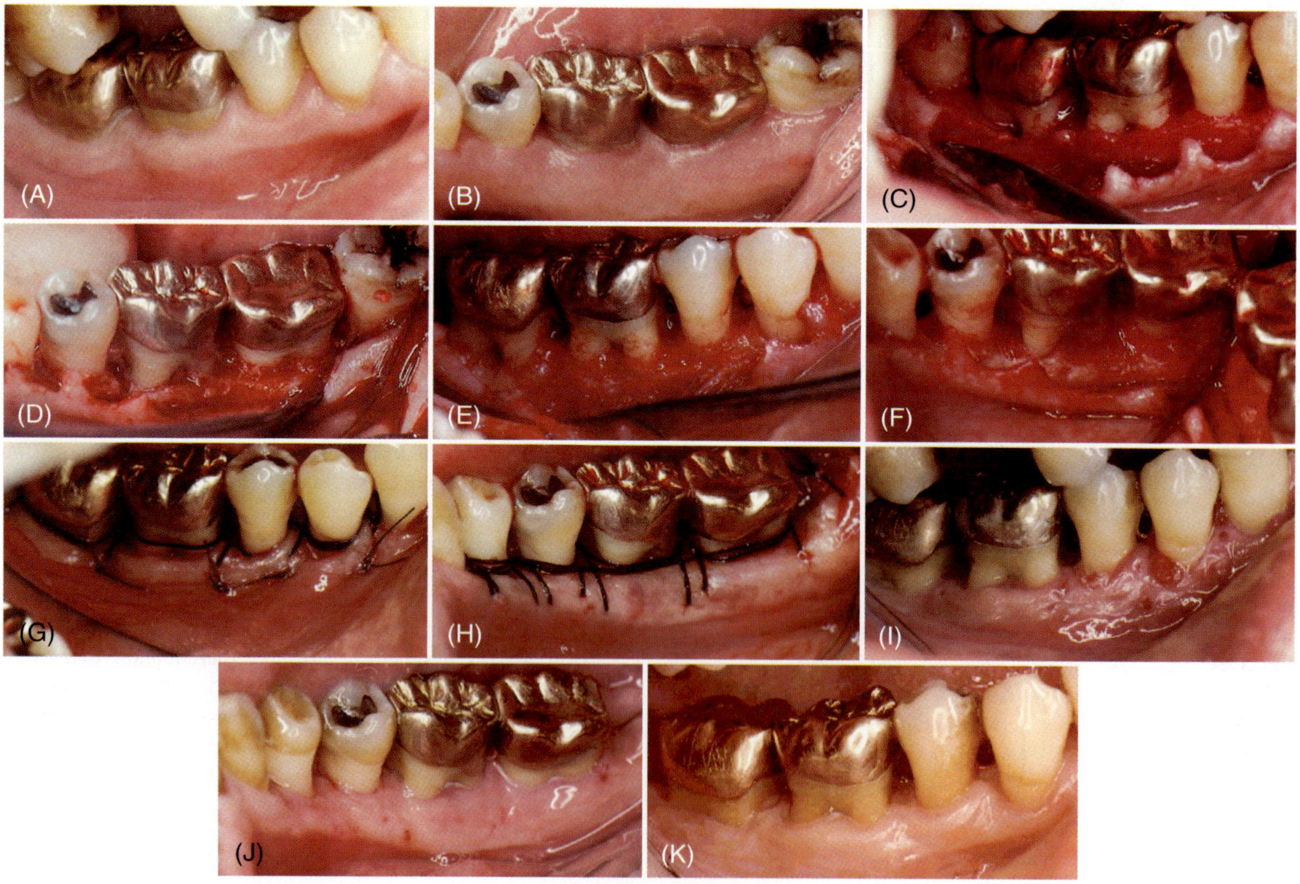

Fig. 45.40 An apically displaced flap. A and B, Facial and lingual preoperative views. C and D, The facial and lingual flaps have been elevated. E and F, After debridement of the areas. G and H, The sutures are in place. I and J, Healing after 1 week. K, Healing after 2 months. Note the preservation of attached gingiva displaced to a more apical position. *(Courtesy: of Dr. Thomas Han, Los Angeles, CA.)*

elevated by blunt dissection with a periosteal elevator. If a split-thickness flap is required, it is elevated via sharp dissection with the use of a Bard–Parker knife to split it. This leaves a layer of connective tissue, including the periosteum, on the bone.

Step 4: After the removal of all granulation tissue, scaling and root planing, and osseous surgery if needed, the flap is displaced apically. It is important that the vertical incisions—and therefore the flap elevation—reach past the mucogingival junction to provide adequate mobility to the flap for its apical displacement.

Step 5: If a full-thickness flap was created, a sling suture around the tooth prevents the flap from sliding to a position more apical than what is desired, and the periodontal dressing can avoid its movement in a coronal direction. A partial-thickness flap is sutured to the periosteum with the use of a direct loop suture or a combination of loop and anchor suture. A dry foil is placed over the flap before it is covered with the dressing to prevent the introduction of pack under the flap.

After 1 week, dressings and sutures are removed. The area is usually repacked for another week, after which the patient is instructed to use chlorhexidine mouth rinse or to apply chlorhexidine topically with cotton-tipped applicators for another 2 or 3 weeks.

Flaps for Reconstructive Surgery

In current reconstructive therapy, bone grafts, membranes, or a combination of these—with or without other agents—are used for a successful outcome. The flap design should therefore be set up so that the maximum amount of gingival tissue and papilla are retained to cover the material placed in the pocket.

Two flap designs are available for reconstructive surgery: the papilla preservation flap and the conventional flap with only crevicular incisions. *The flap design of choice is the papilla preservation flap*, which retains the entire papilla covering the lesion. However, to use this flap, there must be adequate interdental space to allow the intact papilla to be reflected with the facial or lingual/palatal flap. When the interdental space is very narrow, thereby making it impossible to perform a papilla preservation flap, a conventional flap with only crevicular incisions is made.

Papilla Preservation Flap

The technique for employing a papilla preservation flap is as follows (Figs. 45.41 and 45.42):

Step 1: A crevicular incision is made around each tooth, with no incisions across the interdental papilla.

Step 2: The preserved papilla can be incorporated into the facial or lingual/palatal flap, although it is most often integrated into the facial flap. In these cases, the lingual or palatal incision consists of a semilunar incision across the interdental papilla in its palatal or lingual aspect; this incision dips apically from the line angles of the tooth so that the papillary incision is at least 5 mm from the crest of the papilla.

Step 3: An Orban knife is then introduced into this incision to sever half to two-thirds of the base of the interdental papilla. The papilla is then dissected from the lingual or palatal aspect and elevated intact with the facial flap.

Step 4: The flap is reflected without thinning the tissue.

Conventional Flap/Access flap

The technique for employing a conventional flap for reconstructive surgery is as follows:

Step 1: With the use of a no. 12 blade, incise the tissue at the bottom of the pocket and to the crest of the bone to split the papilla below the contact point. Every effort should be made to retain as much tissue as possible to protect the area subsequently.

Step 2: Reflect the flap; keep it as thick as possible, and do not attempt to thin it as is done for resective surgery. The maintenance of a thick flap is necessary to prevent exposure of the graft or the membrane, which results from necrosis of the flap margins.

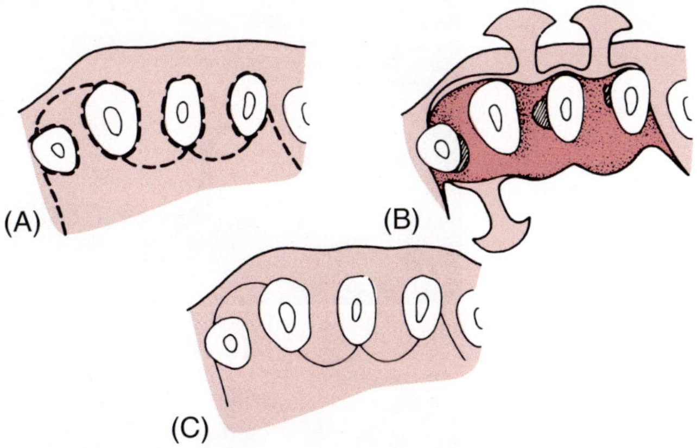

Fig. 45.41 Flap design for a papilla preservation flap. A, Incisions for this type of flap are depicted by interrupted lines. The preserved papilla can be incorporated into the facial or the lingual–palatal flap. B, The reflected flap exposes the underlying bone. Several osseous defects are seen. C, The flap has been returned to its original position, where it covers all of the interdental spaces.

Distal Molar Surgery

The treatment of periodontal pockets on the distal surface of terminal molars is often complicated by the presence of bulbous fibrous tissue over the maxillary tuberosity or prominent retromolar pads in the mandible. Deep vertical defects are also often present in conjunction with the redundant fibrous tissue. Some of these osseous lesions may result from incomplete repair after the extraction of impacted third molars (Fig. 45.43).

The gingivectomy incision is the most direct approach to the treatment of distal pockets that have adequate attached gingiva and no osseous lesions. However, the flap approach is less traumatic postsurgically because it produces a primary closure wound rather than the open secondary wound left by a gingivectomy incision. In addition, it results in attached gingiva. It also provides access for examination and, if needed, correction of the osseous defect. Procedures for this purpose were described by Robinson and Braden and modified by several other investigators. Some representative procedures are discussed in the following sections.

Maxillary Molars

The treatment of distal pockets on the maxillary arch is usually simpler than the treatment of a similar lesion on the mandibular arch because the tuberosity presents a greater amount of fibrous attached gingiva than does the area of the retromolar pad. In addition, the anatomy of the tuberosity that extends distally is more adaptable to pocket elimination than is that of the mandibular molar arch, where the tissue extends coronally. However, the lack of a broad area of attached gingiva and the abruptly ascending tuberosity sometimes complicate therapy (Fig. 45.44).

The following considerations determine the location of the incision for distal molar surgery: accessibility, amount of attached gingiva, pocket depth, and available distance from the distal aspect of the tooth to the end of the tuberosity or retromolar pad.

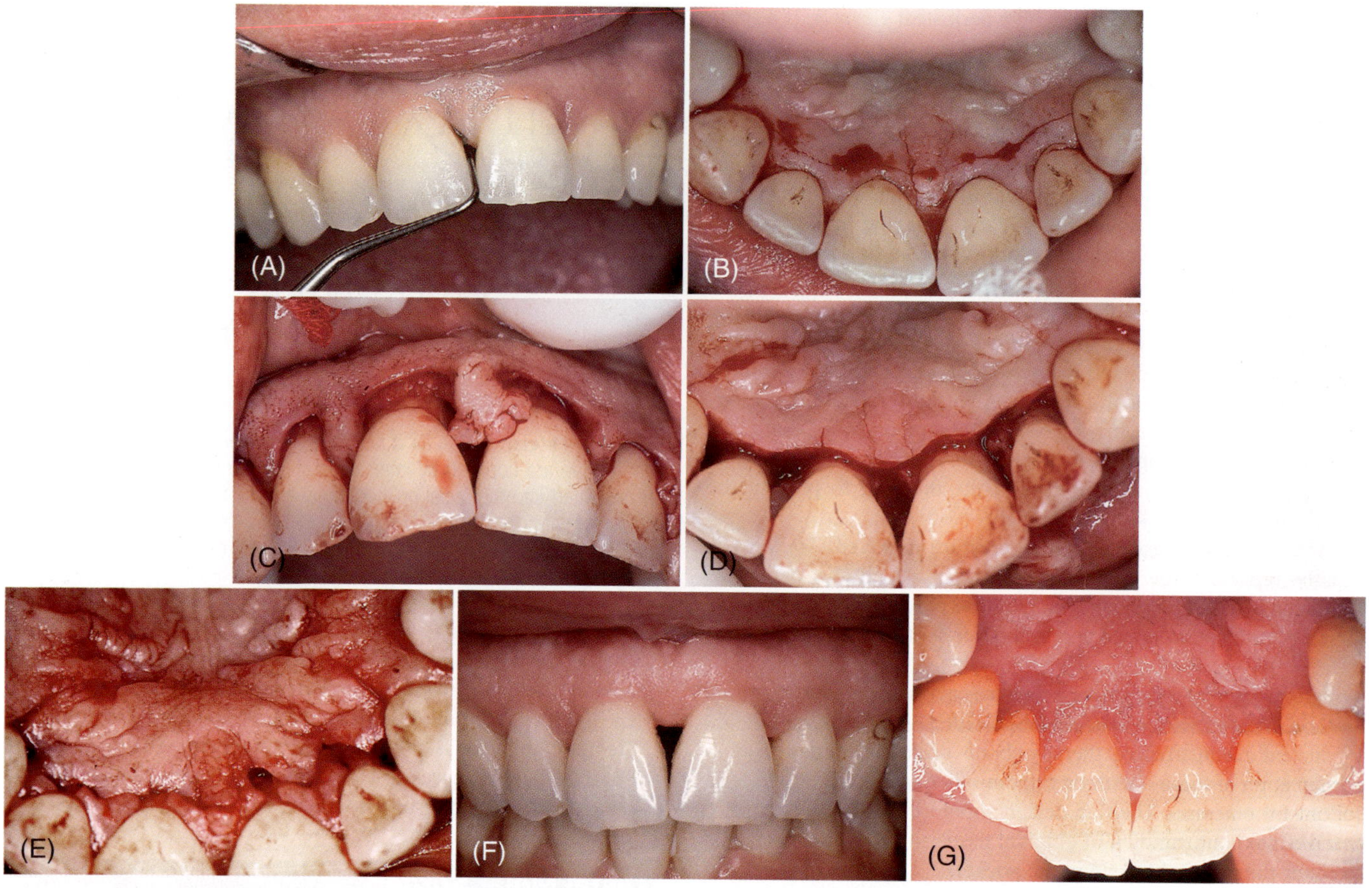

Fig. 45.42 Papilla preservation flap. A, Facial view after sulcular incisions have been made. B, Straight-line incision in the palatal area about 3 mm from the gingival margins. This incision is then connected to the margins with vertical incisions at the mid part of each tooth. C, Papillae are reflected with the facial flap. D, Lingual view after the reflection of the flap. E, Lingual view after the flap is brought back to its original position. It is then sutured with independent sutures. F, Facial view after healing. G, Palatal view after healing. *(Courtesy: of Dr. Thomas Han, Los Angeles, CA.)*

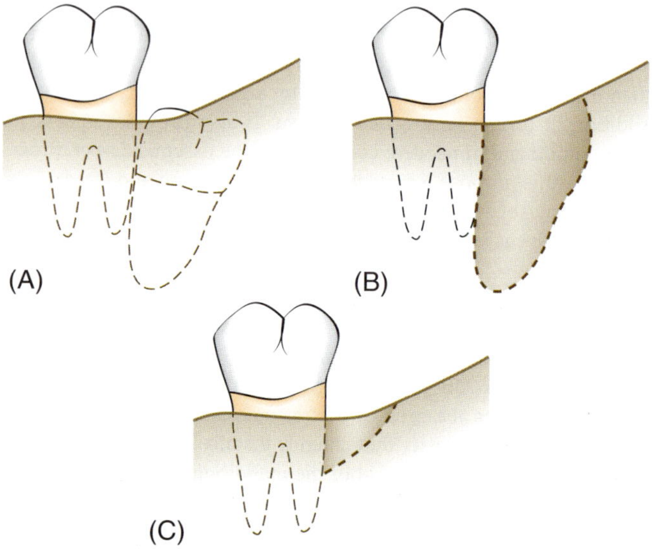

Fig. 45.43 A, Impaction of a third molar distal to a second molar with little or no interdental bone between the two teeth. B, Removal of the third molar creates a pocket with little or no bone distal to the second molar. C, This often leads to a vertical osseous defect distal to the second molar.

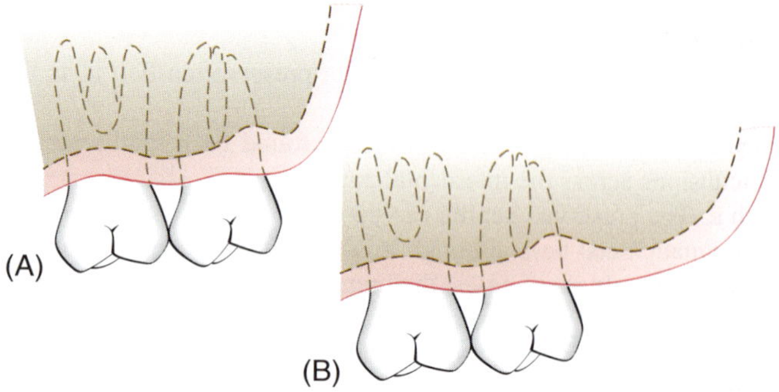

Fig. 45.44 A, Removal of a pocket distal to the maxillary second molar may be difficult if there is minimal attached gingiva. If the bone ascends acutely apically, the removal of this bone may make the procedure easier. B, A long distal tuberosity with abundant attached gingiva is an ideal anatomic situation for distal pocket eradication.

Technique

Two parallel incisions that begin at the distal portion of the tooth and extend to the mucogingival junction distal to the tuberosity or retromolar pad are made (Fig. 45.45). The faciolingual distance between these two incisions depends on the depth of the pocket and the amount of fibrous tissue involved. The deeper the pocket, the

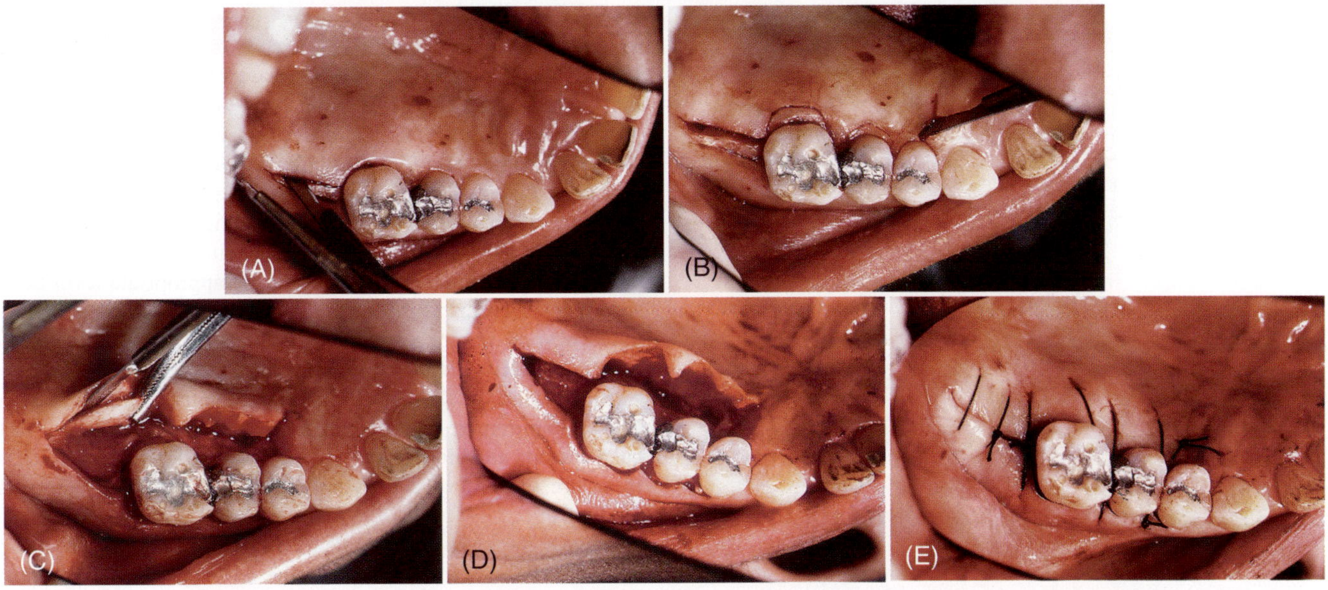

Fig. 45.45 A, A distal pocket eradication procedure with the incision distal to the molar. B, A scalloped incision around the remaining teeth. C, The flap has been reflected and thinned around the distal incision. D, The flap in position before suturing. It should be closely approximated. E, The flap sutured both distally and over the remaining surgical area.

greater is the distance between the two parallel incisions. It is important to note that, when the tissue between the two incisions is removed and the flaps are thinned, the two flap edges must approximate each other at a new apical position without overlapping.

When the depth of the pocket cannot be easily estimated, it is better to err on the conservative side to leave overlapping flaps rather than flaps that are too short and that result in the exposure of bone. When the two flaps overlap after the surgery is completed, they should be placed one over the other. The overlapping portion of one of them is grabbed with a hemostat, and a sharp knife or scissors is then used to cut the excess.

A transversal incision is made at the distal end of the two parallel incisions so that a long, rectangular piece of tissue can be removed. These incisions are usually interconnected with the incisions for the remainder of the surgery in the quadrant involved. The parallel distal incisions should be confined to the attached gingiva because bleeding and flap management become problems when the incision is extended into the alveolar mucosa. If access is difficult—especially if the distance from the distal aspect of the tooth to the mucogingival junction is short—then a vertical incision can be made at the end of the parallel incisions.

When treating the tuberosity area, the two distal incisions are usually made at the midline of the tuberosity (Fig. 45.46). In most cases, no attempt is made to undermine the underlying tissue at this time. These incisions are made straight down into the underlying bone, where access is difficult. A no. 12B blade is generally used. It is easier to dissect out the underlying redundant tissue when the flap is partially reflected. When the distal flaps are placed back on the bone, the two flap margins should closely approximate each other.

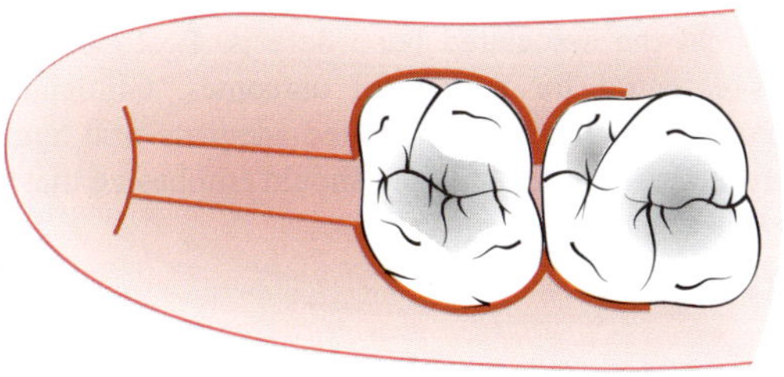

Fig. 45.46 Typical incision design for a surgical procedure distal to the maxillary second molar.

Mandibular Molars

Incisions for the mandibular arch differ from those used for the tuberosity as a result of differences in the anatomy and histologic features of the areas. The retromolar pad area does not usually present as much fibrous attached gingiva. The keratinized gingiva, if present, may not be found directly distal to the molar. The greatest amount may be distolingual or distofacial, and it may not be over the bony crest. The ascending ramus of the mandible may also create a short, horizontal area distal to the terminal molar. The shorter this area, the more difficult it is to treat any deep distal lesion around the terminal molar.

The two incisions distal to the molar should follow the area with the greatest amount of attached gingiva (Figs. 45.47 and 45.48). Therefore, the incisions could be directed distolingually or distofacially, depending on which area has more attached gingiva. Before the flap is completely reflected, it is thinned with a no. 15 blade. It is easier to thin the flap before it is completely free and mobile. After the reflection of the flap and the removal of the redundant fibrous tissue, any necessary osseous surgery is performed. The flaps are approximated similarly to those in the maxillary tuberosity area.

Newer Concepts

To minimize unpleasant postsurgical sequelae following flap operations, some modifications have been reported in the literature. These include modified papilla preservation flap and simplified papilla preservation flap in areas where interdental embrasures are too narrow. In conditions where angular defects are present which require the use of bone grafts, single flap approach wherein flap is reflected only on one side (usually facial or buccal surface) is recommended. Further, if the surgery is done under magnification, a minimally invasive approach has also been employed. But, the basic flap techniques and indications remain the same.

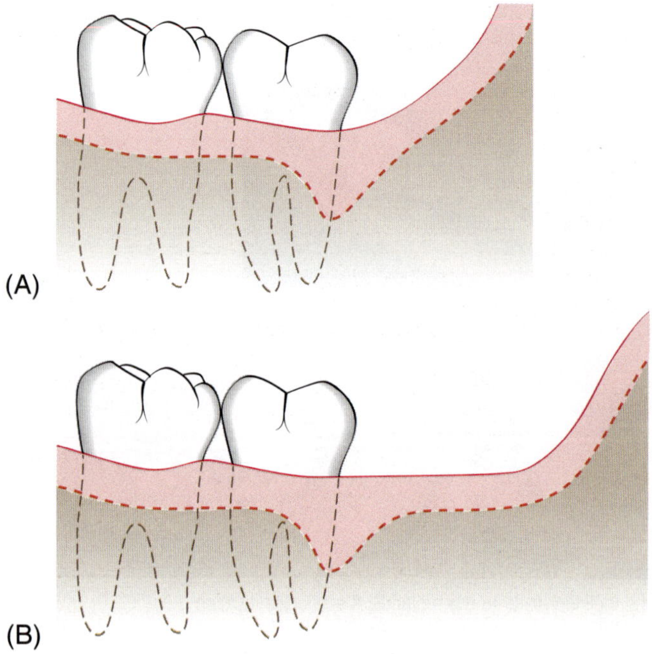

Fig. 45.47 A, Pocket eradication distal to a mandibular second molar with minimal attached gingiva and a close ascending ramus is anatomically difficult. B, For surgical procedures distal to a mandibular second molar, abundant attached gingiva and distal space are ideal.

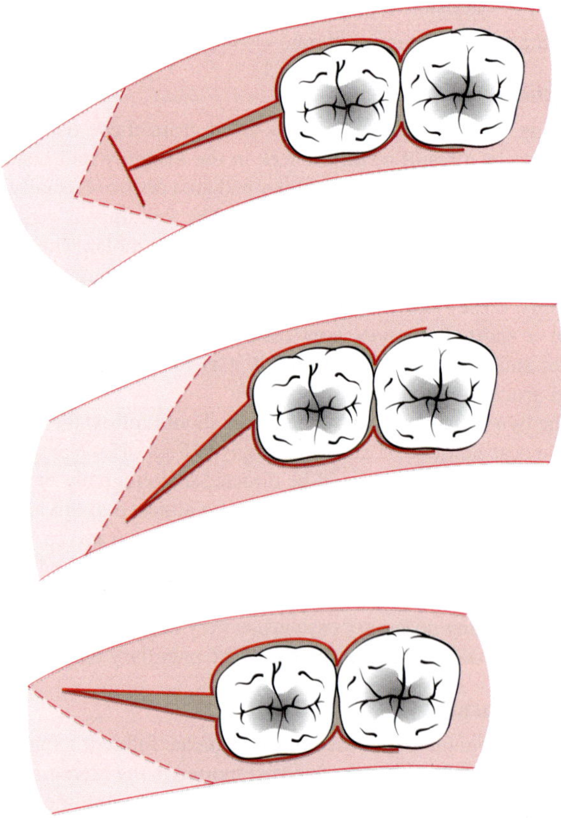

Fig. 45.48 Incision designs for surgical procedures distal to the mandibular second molar. The incision should follow the areas of greatest attached gingiva and underlying bone.

Conclusion

Periodontal flap surgery is the most widely used surgical procedure to treat pockets. Periodontal flaps are designed to preserve gingival integrity and to gain access to root surfaces for residual calculus removal and to thoroughly remove granulation tissue so that bone defects can be visualized and treated. Gentle and efficient procedures result in optimum healing and minimal postoperative pain. When flaps need to be repositioned apically or coronally, then they must sit passively at the appropriate level before suturing. To ensure this, buccal and lingual flaps need to be elevated beyond the mucogingival junction so that the elasticity of the mucosa allows for flap mobility. Sometimes it may be necessary to extend the flap elevation apically with a split incision approach to minimize the effect of the less elastic periosteum. Vertical incisions can aid in flap positioning by allowing the clinician to suture the flap at a different level to the adjacent untreated gingiva.

Palatal flaps are less mobile as a result of the absence of oral mucosa, so the apical position of the flap depends on how much marginal gingival tissue is discarded with the use of a reverse bevel incision. The more apical positioning desired, the more extensive is the reverse bevel cut. Palatal flaps are more difficult to position coronally than buccal or lingual flaps. Thus, if it is required to position flaps coronally or even at their original levels, then a sulcular incision is used. During osseous periodontal surgery, flaps are apically positioned to minimize postoperative pocket depth. During regenerative periodontal surgery, soft-tissue coverage of bony defects, graft materials, membranes, and biologic agents is important, so sulcular incisions and tight suturing techniques are crucial.

Periodontal flap procedures for pocket therapy include flaps that are created solely for access to root surfaces and bone margins, flaps for the precise processes of osseous surgery, and flaps for periodontal regeneration. All of these approaches have specific flap designs and step-by-step elements, and all of them include calculus removal and root planing as part of the essential treatment protocol. Flaps should allow for adequate access, and they should be reflected so that at least 3 mm of crestal bone is exposed. If the flaps are to be positioned apically, flap mobility is obtained by extending the facial and lingual flap elevation beyond the mucogingival junction, which enables the elasticity of the mucosa to be applied. Palatal flaps are much less mobile; thus, inverse bevel incisions are used to remove marginal gingival tissues so that, at the time of suturing, the flap margin is positioned apically, if so indicated.

Papilla preservation techniques with various modifications are applied to those areas in which gingival recession needs to be minimized. For some esthetic locations, nonsurgical therapy may be more appropriate than flap surgery.

Adjacent edentulous areas are incorporated into the flap design with the use of wedge incisions that enable access to adjacent root surfaces for complete root planing and that allow clinicians to visualize and treat the associated bone defects. Postoperative plaque control is essential for successful outcomes. Clinicians should ensure that patients have demonstrated adequate oral hygiene during the presurgical phase, and they should emphasize that this must continue this after surgery.

Key points

- Periodontal flap surgery is one of the most common surgical procedures in the oral cavity.
- It is indicated in persistent pockets, osseous defects, furcation defects, and whenever regeneration is attempted.
- The three basic horizontal incisions of periodontal flap are the internal bevel incision, crevicular incision, and the interdental incision. Occasionally vertical releasing incisions are needed.
- Papilla preservation is indicated in esthetic zone and when bone grafts are placed.
- Routine full thickness flaps are employed.
- Following flap reflection, a thorough debridement is performed.
- Osseous management is done either by additive or resective methods.
- Usually a nonabsorbable sutures made of either silk or ePTFE-Expanded Polytetrafluro Ethylene are used.
- Many types of suturing techniques are employed for different situations.
- Periodontal dressings may or may not be placed.
- The most common techniques for pocket reduction are modified Widman flap and undisplaced access flap.
- Apically displaced flap in addition to pocket eradication also aids in increasing the width of attached gingiva.

Suggested Readings

Ainamo A, Bergenholtz A, Hugoson A, et al: Location of the mucogingival junction 18 years after apically repositioned flap surgery. *J Clin Periodontol* 19:49, 1992.

Braden BE: Deep distal pockets adjacent to terminal teeth. *Dent Clin North Am* 13:161, 1969.

Caton J, Nyman S: Histometric evaluation of periodontal surgery. I. The modified Widman flap procedure. *J Clin Periodontol* 7:212, 1980.

Matelski DE, Hurt WC: The corrective phase: the modified Widman flap. In Hurt WC, editor: *Periodontics in general practice*, Springfield, IL, 1976, Charles C Thomas.

Morris ML: The unrepositioned mucoperiosteal flap. *Periodontics* 3:147, 1965.

Olsen C, Ammons WF, van Belle G: A longitudinal study comparing apically repositioned flaps, with and without osseous surgery. *Int J Periodontics Restorative Dent* 5:10, 1985.

Ramfjord SP: Present status of the modified Widman flap procedure. *J Periodontol* 48:558, 1977.

Ramfjord SP, Nissle RR: The modified Widman flap. *J Periodontol* 45:601, 1974.

Robinson RE: The distal wedge operation. *Periodontics* 4:256, 1966.

Takei HH, Han TJ, Carranza FA, et al: Flap technique for periodontal bone implants: papilla preservation technique. *J Periodontol* 56:204, 1985.

Tavtigian R: The height of the facial radicular alveolar crest following apically positioned flap operation. *J Periodontol* 41:412, 1970.

CHAPTER 46

Treatment of Gingival Enlargement

PM Camargo | FQ Pirih | HH Takei | FA Carranza | CD Dwarakanath

CHAPTER OUTLINE

The treatment of gingival enlargement is based on an understanding of the cause and underlying pathologic changes of this condition. Gingival enlargements are of special concern to the patient and the dentist because they pose problems that include biofilm control, impaired function (mastication, tooth eruption, and speech), and esthetics. Because gingival enlargements differ with regard to etiology, the treatment of each type is best considered individually.

Chronic Inflammatory Enlargement

Chronic inflammatory enlargements, which are characterized by gingival tissues that are soft and have an altered gingival color, are usually caused by edema and cellular infiltration. Typical therapy consists of scaling and root planing, provided the size of the enlargement does not interfere with the complete removal of deposits from the involved tooth surfaces.

When chronic inflammatory gingival enlargements include a significant fibrotic component that does not undergo shrinkage after scaling and root planning, or if the extent of the gingival enlargement is so severe that access to the deposits on the tooth surface is impossible, surgical removal is the treatment of choice. Two techniques exist for this purpose: gingivectomy and the flap operation. Before instituting surgical therapy, biofilm control, scaling, and root planing should always be completed, and sufficient time should be allowed to heal before reevaluating the periodontal status. It is important that the decision to implement surgical therapy should be made after this reevaluation.

Once the decision is made that surgical therapy is necessary, the selection of the appropriate surgical technique will depend on the extent of the enlargement and the status of the gingival tissues. When the enlarged gingiva remains soft and friable even after scaling and root planing, the gingivectomy technique may be preferable because management of the periodontal flap may be technically difficult on the friable tissues. If the gingival tissue is firm and fibrotic, preference is given to the flap operation, which is always the favorable choice because the healing is by primary intention and the keratinized tissue is better preserved. Therefore, conservation of the keratinized, attached gingiva must be considered along with removal of the excessive gingival tissue.

Tumor-like, localized, and severe inflammatory enlargements (Fig. 46.1) can be treated by gingivectomy as follows. With the patient under local anesthesia, the tooth surfaces beneath the mass are scaled to remove calculus and other debris. The lesion is separated from the mucosa at its base by using a surgical blade. If the lesion extends interproximally, the interdental gingiva is included in the incision to ensure the exposure of deposits. After the enlarged tissues are removed and access is sufficient, the root surfaces are scaled and planed, and the area is irrigated with saline solution. A periodontal dressing is applied and removed after a week, but in some cases, depending on the extent of the surgery, the postoperative appointment may have to be scheduled in 2 weeks to allow for further healing. It is important at this time that proper biofilm control is instituted.

Periodontal and Gingival Abscesses

Periodontal and gingival abscesses result in areas of gingival enlargement. However, the enlargement due to abscesses is usually localized around the area of the lesion, and the content of the enlarged area is purulent material, which must be drained and the area curetted.

Drug-Induced Gingival Enlargement

Gingival enlargement has primarily been associated with the administration of three different types of drugs: anticonvulsants, calcium channel blockers, and the immunosuppressant cyclosporine. Although the clinical presentation of the gingival enlargement induced by the three drug categories listed here may be similar, evidence suggests that their cellular and molecular mechanisms may differ. Limited evidence indicates that other drugs may also induce gingival enlargement, albeit at a lower prevalence and with a lesser severity.

The examination of cases of drug-induced gingival enlargement reveals the overgrown tissues to have two components: fibrotic, which is the result of the action of the drug on the physiologic gingival collagen turnover; and inflammatory, which is induced by the bacterial biofilm. Although the fibrotic and inflammatory components present in the enlarged gingiva are the result of distinct pathologic processes, they almost always are observed as gingival enlargement induced by the combination of drugs and biofilm. The role of bacterial biofilm in the overall pathogenesis of drug-induced

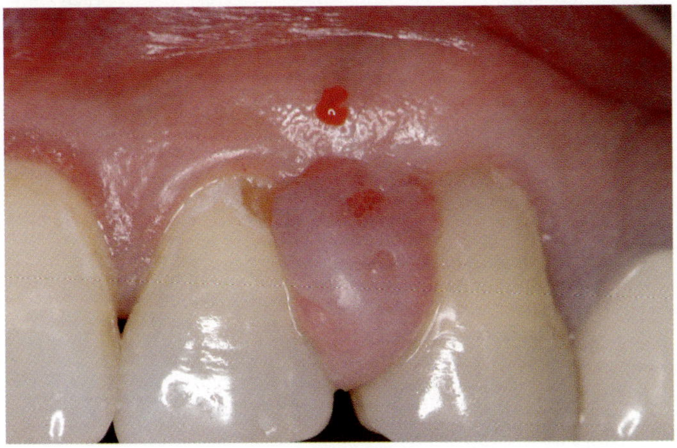

Fig. 46.1 Localized, fibrotic, tumor-like gingival enlargement on a female young adult. This lesion may be treated via gingivectomy.

gingival enlargement is not clear. Some studies indicate that biofilm is a prerequisite for gingival enlargement, whereas others suggest that the presence of biofilm is a consequence of biofilm accumulation caused by the enlarged gingiva. In patients taking calcium channel blockers, termination and/or substitution of the drug with another class of medication resulted in significant decreases in gingival enlargement, with no differences observed between patients with poor or good oral hygiene. These studies suggest that the gingival enlargement process is independent of biofilm-related inflammation.

Treatment Options

The treatment of drug-induced gingival enlargement should be based on the medication used and the clinical features of the case.

First, consideration should be given to the possibility of discontinuing the drug or changing the medication. These possibilities should be examined in consultation with the patient's physician. Simple discontinuation of the offending drug is often not practical, but substitution of the drug with another medication may be an option. If any drug substitution is attempted, it is important to allow a 6- to 12-month period to elapse between discontinuation of the offending drug and substitution with an alternative drug. The changes instituted with the drug should always be in combination with oral hygiene instructions, scaling, and root planing. Re-evaluation of the gingival enlargement after the alteration of drug therapy is necessary before any surgical treatment is planned.

Alternative medications to the anticonvulsant phenytoin include carbamazepine and valproic acid, both of which have been reported to induce gingival enlargement to a lesser degree. A murine study suggested that lovastatin may attenuate the onset of gingival enlargement induced by phenytoin. Further research is necessary to confirm the therapeutic value of lovastatin.

For patients who are taking nifedipine, which has a reported prevalence of gingival enlargement of up to 86%, other calcium channel blockers such as diltiazem or verapamil may be viable alternatives. The reported prevalence of inducing gingival enlargement is 20% for diltiazem and 4% for verapamil. In addition, consideration should be given to the use of another class of antihypertensive medications rather than calcium channel blockers. None of these drugs are known to induce gingival enlargement.

Drug substitutions for cyclosporine are more limited. Tacrolimus is another immunosuppressant that is used in organ transplant recipients. The incidence of gingival enlargement in patients receiving tacrolimus therapy is approximately 65% lower than that in individuals who are receiving cyclosporine. Clinical trials have also shown that the substitution of cyclosporine with tacrolimus results in a significant decrease in the severity of gingival enlargement as compared to patients who continue cyclosporine therapy. In another study, the same drug substitution resulted in a strong decrease or complete resolution of gingival enlargement in more than 70% of the patients who initially presented with cyclosporine-induced gingival enlargement. Therefore, the dental practitioner should consult with the treating physician to investigate the possibility of a change in immunosuppressant therapy as one of the steps in the treatment of cyclosporine-induced gingival enlargement. Patients who take cyclosporine in combination with a calcium channel blocker tend to have an overall lower prevalence of and less severe gingival enlargement if the antihypertensive drug is amlodipine as compared to nifedipine.

The administration of the antibiotic azithromycin has been shown to decrease the severity of gingival enlargement induced by cyclosporine. A 3-day course of systemic azithromycin significantly decreased gingival enlargement, and the effect was observed as early as 7–30 days after the initiation of antibiotic therapy. The use of azithromycin to decrease cyclosporine-induced gingival enlargement resulted in significantly greater changes than those observed with an improvement in oral hygiene. The topical administration of azithromycin in the form of a toothpaste also decreased the severity of cyclosporine-induced gingival enlargement

Second, the clinician should emphasize biofilm control as the first step in the treatment of drug-induced gingival enlargement. Although the exact role played by bacterial biofilm is not fully understood, evidence suggests that good oral hygiene, chemotherapeutic agents, and the frequent professional removal of biofilm decrease the degree of gingival enlargement and improve overall gingival health. The presence of drug-induced enlargement is associated with pseudo-pocket formation, frequently with abundant biofilm accumulation, which may lead to the development of periodontitis. Therefore, meticulous biofilm control helps to maintain attachment levels. In addition, adequate biofilm control may help to prevent the recurrence of gingival enlargement in surgically treated cases.

Third, in many patients, gingival enlargement persists after careful consideration of the previous two approaches. With these patients, surgical removal of the enlarged gingiva must be considered.

Fig. 46.2 is a decision tree that outlines the sequence of events and options for the treatment of drug-induced gingival enlargement.

Gingivectomy

The advantages of gingivectomy are the ease and simplicity of the procedure, but it has the disadvantages of more postoperative discomfort and an increased chance of postoperative bleeding. It also sacrifices keratinized tissue and does not allow for osseous recontouring. The flap operation, in contrast, is more technically demanding, but it tends to create less postoperative discomfort and bleeding, besides preserving keratinized tissue. The clinician's decision between the two surgical techniques available should include the extent of the area to be operated on, the severity of the enlargement, the presence of periodontitis and osseous defects, and the location of the base of the pockets in relation to the mucogingival junction.

In general, small areas (i.e., up to six teeth) of drug-induced gingival enlargement with no evidence of clinical attachment loss (and therefore no anticipated need for osseous surgery) can be effectively treated with the gingivectomy technique. An important consideration is the amount of keratinized tissue present. The removal of excessive amount of keratinized gingiva will create a mucogingival problem.

Fig. 46.3 depicts the gingivectomy procedure diagrammatically, and Fig. 46.4 illustrates a case of cyclosporine-induced gingival enlargement treated with the gingivectomy technique.

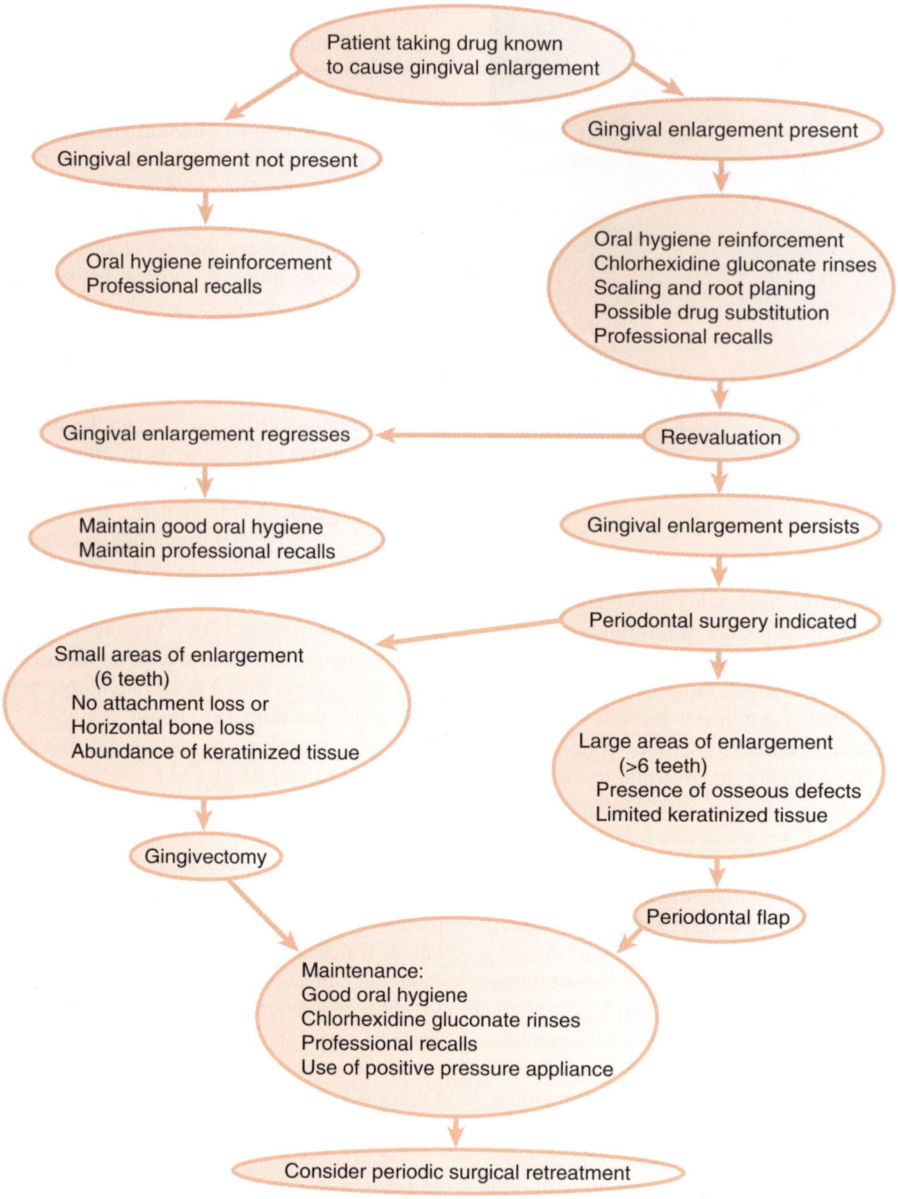

Fig. 46.2 Decision tree for treatment of drug-induced gingival enlargements.

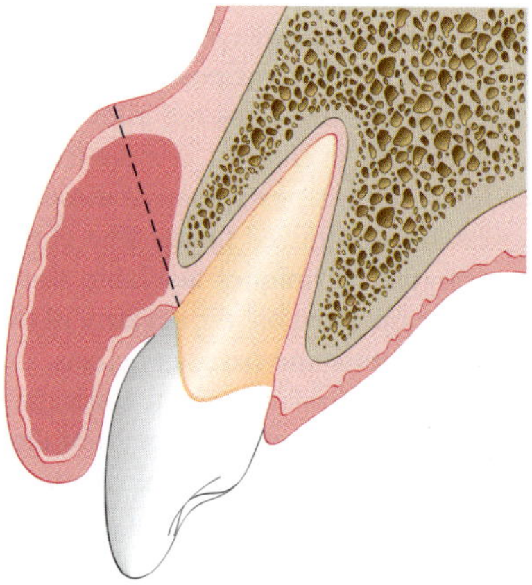

Fig. 46.3 Gingivectomy technique as used to treat patients with drug-induced gingival enlargement. The *dashed line* represents the external bevel incision, and the *shaded area* corresponds to the tissue to be excised. The gingivectomy incision may not remove the entire hyperplastic tissue *(shaded area)*. This may leave a wide wound of exposed connective tissue.

Gingivectomy or gingivoplasty can also be performed with electrosurgery or via a laser device. Some evidence indicates that recurrence of drug-induced gingival enlargement is reduced in patients treated via laser as compared to conventional gingivectomy or flap surgery.

Flap Operation

For larger areas of gingival enlargement (i.e., more than six teeth), and where attachment loss and osseous defects are present, flap surgery is recommended.

The periodontal flap technique used for the treatment of gingival enlargements is a simple variation of the one used to treat periodontitis. Fig. 46.5 shows the basic surgical steps in the use of the flap technique.

The flap surgical technique is as follows:

1. After anesthetizing the area, sounding of the underlying alveolar bone is performed with a periodontal probe to determine the presence and extent of the osseous defects.
2. On the buccal and lingual aspects, with a #15 surgical blade, the initial scalloped internal bevel incision is made at least 3 mm

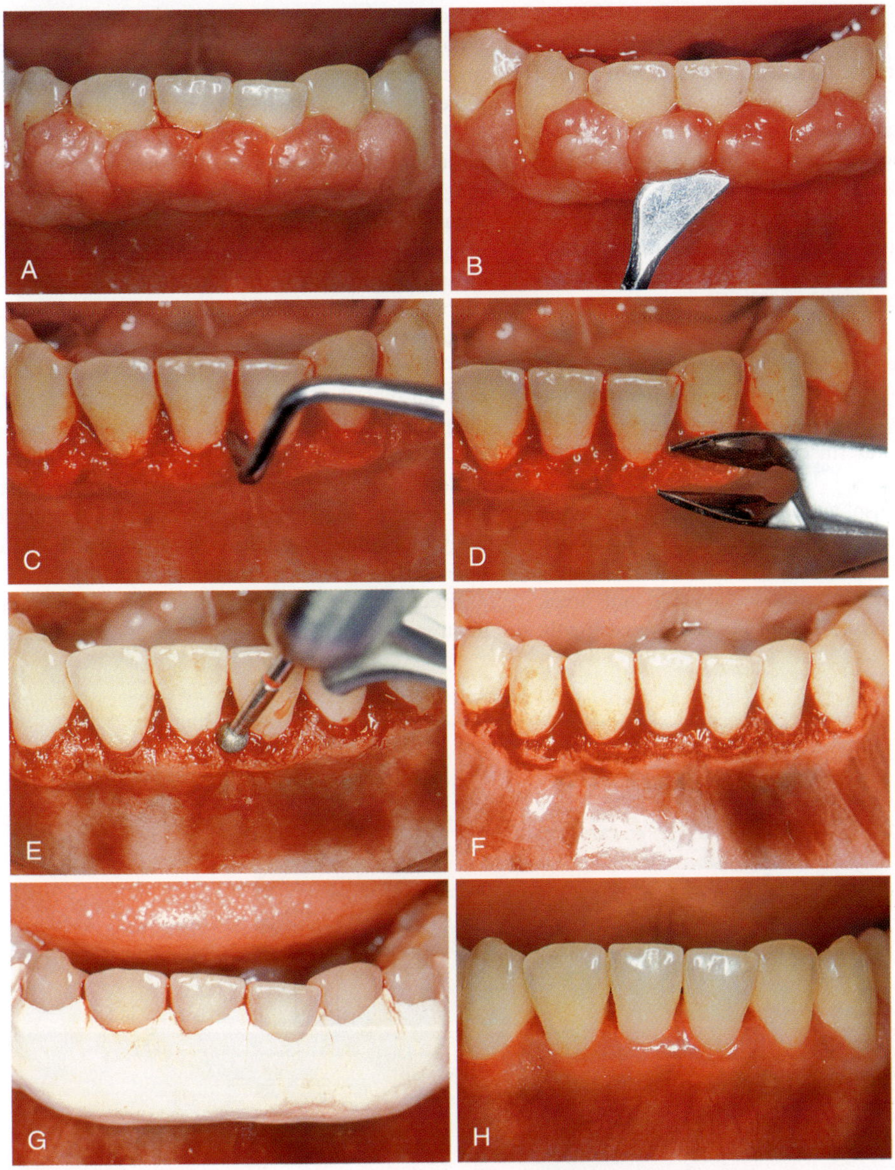

Fig. 46.4 Surgical treatment of cyclosporine-induced gingival enlargement with the use of the gingivectomy technique on a 16-year-old girl who had received a kidney allograft 2 years earlier. A, Enlarged gingival tissues and pseudo-pocket formation. No attachment loss or radiographic evidence of bone loss existed. B, Initial external bevel incision performed with a Kirkland knife. C, Interproximal tissue release achieved with an Orban knife. D and E, Gingivoplasty performed with tissue nippers and a round diamond at high speed with abundant cooling. F, Aspect of the surgical wound at conclusion of the surgical procedure. G, Placement of noneugenol periodontal dressing. H, The surgical area 3 months postoperatively. Note the successful elimination of the enlarged gingival tissue, the restoration of a physiologic gingival contour, and the maintenance of an adequate band of keratinized tissue.

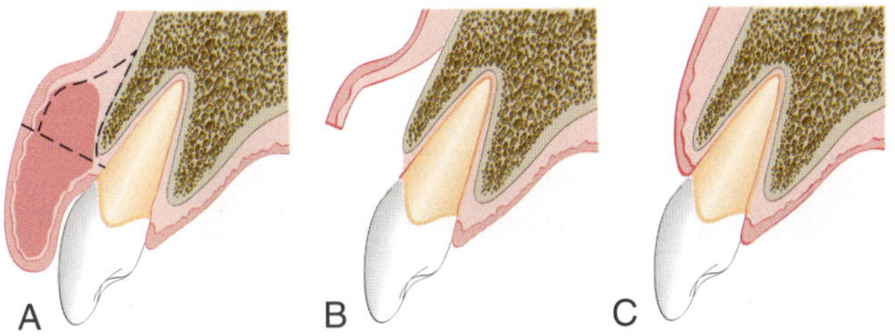

Fig. 46.5 Periodontal flap treatment for drug-induced gingival enlargement. A, Initial reverse bevel incision followed by thinning of the enlarged gingival tissue; *dotted lines* represent incisions, and the *shaded area* represents the tissue portion to be excised. B, After flap elevation, the enlarged portion of the gingival tissue is removed. C, The flap is placed on top of the alveolar bone and sutured.

coronal to the mucogingival junction, which includes the creation of new surgical interdental papillae in each interproximal space.

3. The same blade is used to thin the gingival tissues in the buccolingual direction to the mucogingival junction. At this point, the blade establishes contact with the alveolar bone, and a full-thickness or split-thickness flap is elevated.
4. On the palatal aspect, a scalloped internal bevel incision is made at the level of the intended postoperative gingival margin level, which is usually the cementoenamel or more apical in cases where periodontitis is combined with gingival enlargement. The whole extent of the palatal flap is thinned as needed in the apical direction. The base of the flap is then scored to bone and elevated.

5. With the use of an Orban knife, the base of each papilla that connects the facial and the lingual incisions is released.
6. Intrasulcular incisions are made on buccal, lingual, and palatal areas that are being treated to release the tissue collar.
7. The marginal and interdental tissues are removed with curettes.
8. After all tissue tags are removed, the roots are thoroughly scaled and planed, and the bone is recontoured as needed.
9. The flap is replaced or apically displaced and, if necessary, retrimmed to reach the bone–tooth junction exactly (palatal flaps). The flaps are then sutured with an interrupted or a continuous mattress technique, and the area is protected with periodontal dressing.

Sutures and periodontal dressing are removed after 1–2 weeks, depending on the extent of the surgery. The patient is instructed to begin biofilm control practices. Usually it is convenient for the patient to use chlorhexidine oral rinses once or twice daily for 2–4 weeks.

Fig. 46.6 shows a kidney transplant recipient who was receiving cyclosporine and nifedipine therapy and was treated with the flap technique. Fig. 46.7 depicts the treatment of a 9-year-old kidney transplant recipient whose upper anterior teeth could not break through the enlarged gingival tissues because of their overgrowth, which was induced by cyclosporine therapy; treatment via flap operation allowed for exposure of the anatomic crowns and for the maintenance of keratinized tissue, which could have been completely eliminated if the case had been treated with gingivectomy.

The recurrence of drug-induced gingival enlargement is a reality in surgically treated cases. The major cause of the recurrence of gingival enlargement is the difficulty with postsurgical oral hygiene. Meticulous home care, with a soft, postsurgical brush and chlorhexidine gluconate rinses, is indicated. Frequent professional cleanings can also help reduce the degree of recurrence. A hard, rubber, custom-fitted occlusal guard worn at night may also be helpful to control recurrence.

Although the periodontal flap approach may be technically more difficult than the gingivectomy procedure, as indicated previously, the postsurgical healing of the flap technique causes less discomfort and decreases the chances of postoperative bleeding. The primary closure of the surgical site with the flap procedure is a great advantage over the secondary open wound that results from the gingivectomy technique. In addition, postsurgical home care can be instituted earlier with the periodontal flap.

Recurrence may occur as early as 3–6 months after surgical treatment. In general, surgical results with minimal recurrence are

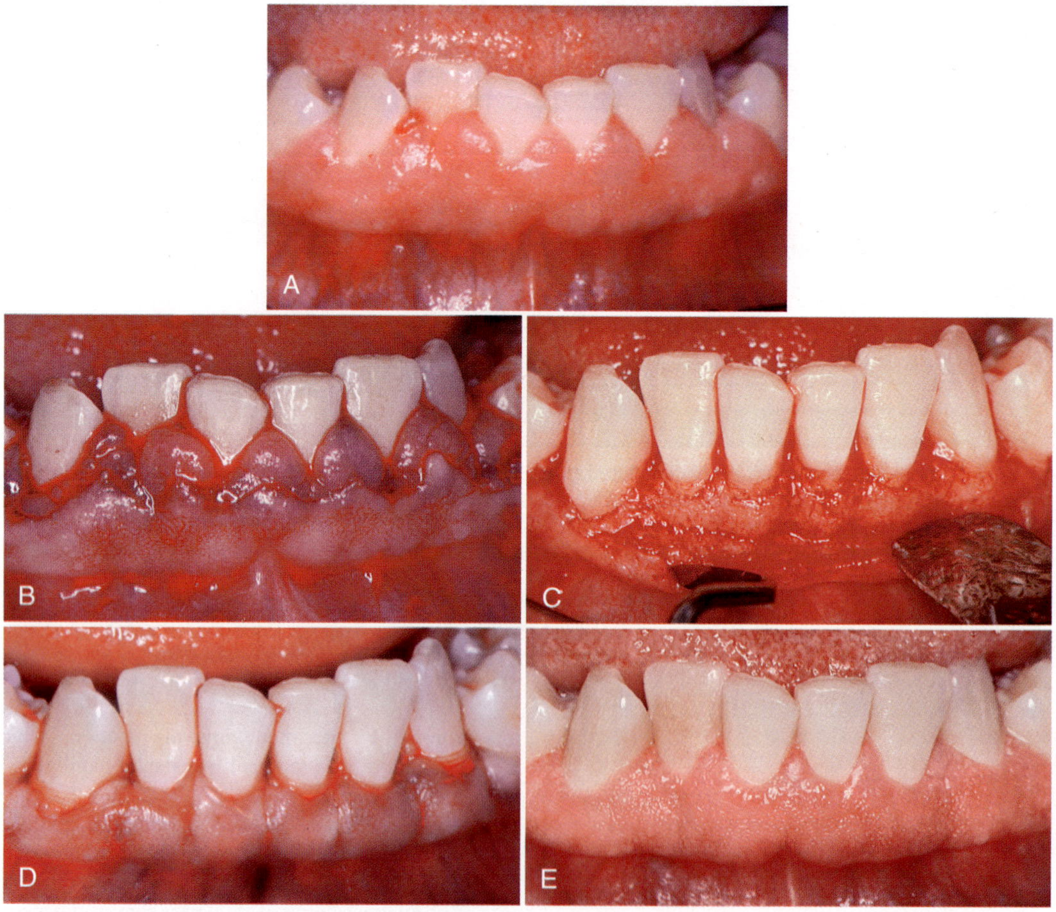

Fig. 46.6 Treatment of combined cyclosporine and nifedipine-induced gingival enlargement with a periodontal flap on a 35-year-old female patient who had received a kidney allograft 3 years earlier. A, Presurgical clinical aspect of the lower anterior teeth, showing severe gingival enlargement. B, Initial scalloped reverse bevel incision, including maintenance of keratinized tissue and creation of surgical papillae. C, Elevation of a full-thickness flap and removal of the inner portion of the previously thinned gingival tissue. After scaling and root planing, osseous recontouring can be performed if necessary. D, The flap is positioned on top of the alveolar crest. E, Postsurgical aspect of the treated area at 12 months. Note the reduction of enlarged tissue volume and acceptable gingival health.

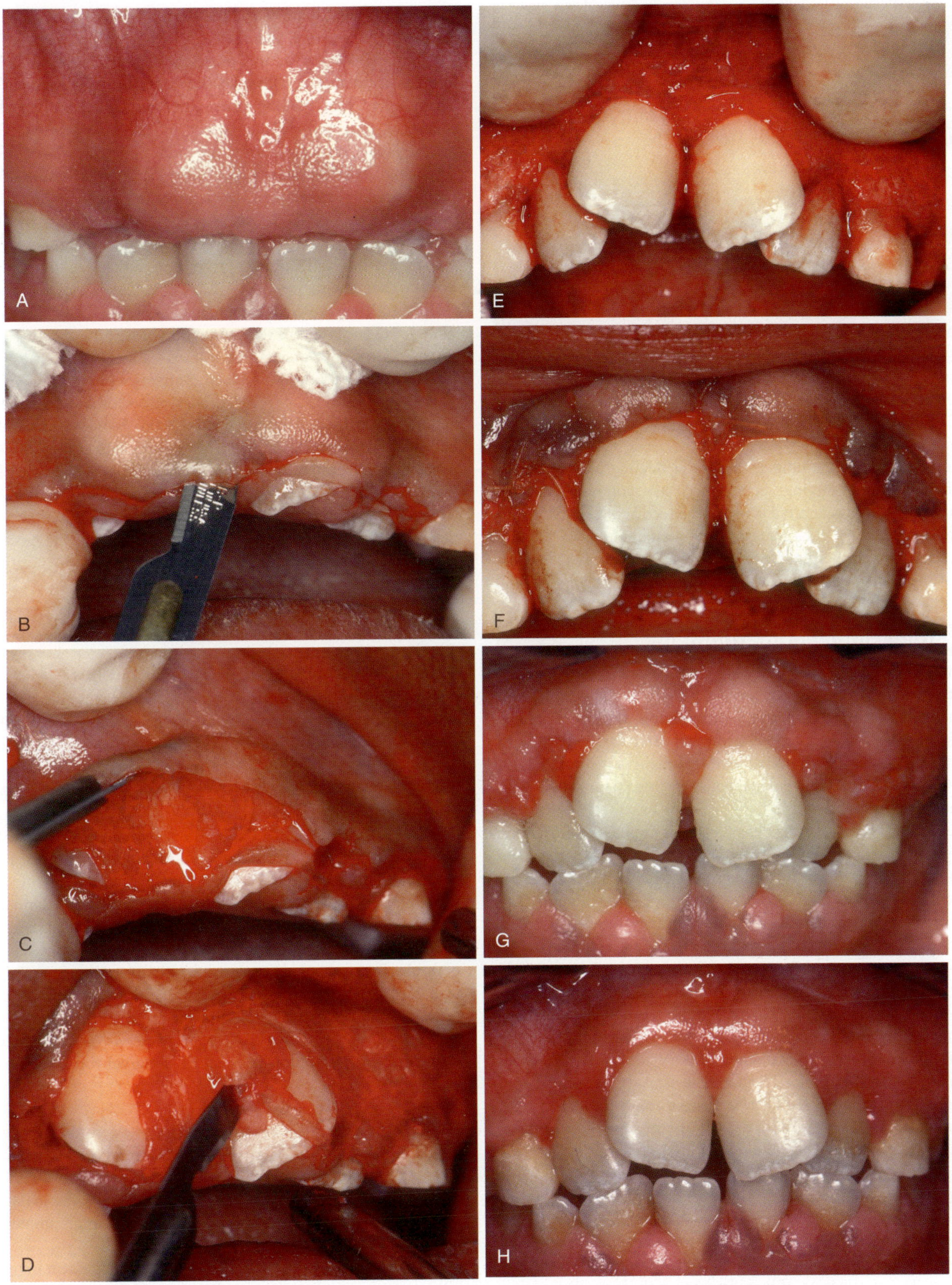

Fig. 46.7 Treatment of a 9-year old recipient of an allogeneic kidney transplant who had been receiving Cyclosporin A and nifedipine therapy for 2 1/2 years. Surgical treatment was with an apically positioned flap. A, Upper incisors were in an occluding position, but they did not erupt through the drug-enlarged gingival tissues. B, Crestal reversed bevel incision maintaining most of the buccal keratinized tissue. C, Flap thinning via split-thickness dissection. D, Removal of excess gingival connective tissue on the buccal surfaces of the anterior teeth and interproximal spaces. E, Clinical crowns fully exposed; periosteum preserved over alveolar bone. F, Flap was apically positioned and sutured to periosteum with 5-0 plain gut. G, Healing at 14 days after surgery. H, Healing at 3 months postoperatively with acceptable gingival health and presence of adequate buccal keratinized tissue.

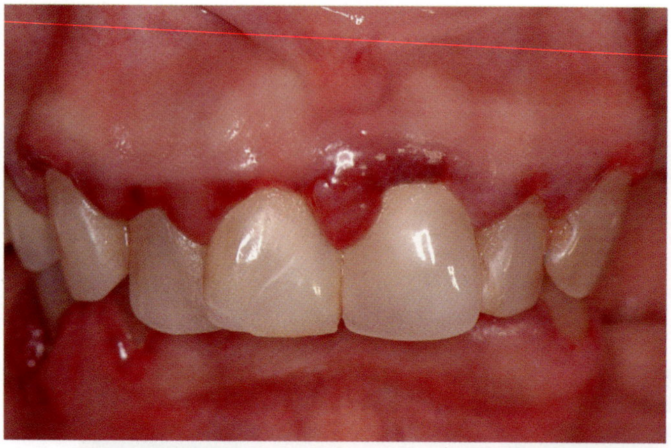

Fig. 46.8 A 74-year-old patient with acute leukemia. Gingival enlargement is observed in combination with a hemorrhagic appearance, which sometimes causes spontaneous bleeding.

possible for at least 12 months. In one study, healing of flap surgery was compared to that of gingivectomy after a 6-month postsurgical examination. This comparative study of the recurrence of cyclosporine-induced gingival enlargement after periodontal flap surgery compared to that of the gingivectomy technique indicated that the return of the pocket depth took longer with flap surgery.

Leukemic Gingival Enlargement

Leukemic enlargement occurs with acute or subacute leukemia (Fig. 46.8), and it is uncommon among patients in the chronic leukemic state. The patient's bleeding and clotting times and platelet count should be checked before treatment, and the hematologist should be consulted before periodontal treatment is instituted. Gingival bleeding, sometimes spontaneous, is often associated with leukemic gingival enlargement.

After acute symptoms subside, attention is directed to correction of the gingival enlargement. The rationale is to remove the local irritating factors to control the inflammatory component of the enlargement, and this is achieved by scaling and root planing. The initial treatment steps consist of gently removing all loose debris with cotton pellets, performing superficial scaling, and instructing the patient in oral hygiene for biofilm control. This hygiene should include, at least initially, the daily use of chlorhexidine mouthrinses. Oral hygiene procedures are extremely important for these patients and, if necessary, may require the assistance of a nurse.

Definitive scaling and root planing are carried out at subsequent visits using local anesthesia. Treatment sessions are confined to a small area of the mouth if hemostasis poses a challenge. Antibiotics are administered systemically the evening before and for a week after each treatment to reduce the risk of infection.

Gingival Enlargement During Pregnancy

Treatment requires the elimination of all local irritants that may be responsible for precipitating the gingival changes that occur during pregnancy. The elimination of local irritants early in pregnancy is a preventive measure against gingival disease, and prevention is preferable to treatment of gingival enlargement after it occurs. Marginal and interdental gingival inflammation and enlargement are treated by scaling and root planing. Treatment of tumor-like gingival enlargements consists of surgical excision, as well as the scaling and planing of the tooth surfaces adjacent to the lesion. The enlargement may recur unless all irritants are removed. Food impaction is frequently an inciting factor.

Gingival lesions during pregnancy should be treated as soon as they are detected, although not necessarily by surgical means. Scaling and root planing procedures and adequate oral hygiene measures may reduce the extent of the enlargement. Gingival enlargements do shrink after pregnancy, but they usually do not disappear. After pregnancy, the entire periodontal status of the patient should be reevaluated, and comprehensive treatment should be undertaken.

Lesions should be removed surgically during pregnancy if they interfere with mastication or produce an esthetic disfigurement that bothers the patient.

During pregnancy, the emphasis should be on (1) preventing gingival disease before it occurs and (2) treating existing gingival disease before it worsens. All patients should be seen as early as possible after becoming pregnant. Patients without gingival disease should be examined for potential sources of local irritation and should be instructed on meticulous oral hygiene procedures. In addition, patients who already have signs and symptoms of periodontal disease should be treated promptly, before the effect of pregnancy on the gingiva becomes manifest.

Every pregnant patient should be scheduled for periodic maintenance visits. The importance of such visits in the prevention of serious periodontal disturbances should be stressed.

Gingival Enlargement During Puberty

Gingival enlargement during puberty is treated by performing scaling and root planing, removing all sources of irritation, and controlling biofilm. Surgical removal may be required in severe cases. The most important problem in these young patients is recurrence, for which close maintenance therapy is recommended.

Neoplastic Gingival Enlargements (Gingival Tumors) and Other Solitary Overgrowths

Lesions such as peripheral giant cell granuloma, fibroma, and pyogenic granuloma are frequently encountered in practice. Such lesions have to be excised and subjected to histopathological examination to confirm the clinical diagnosis. While excising such lesions, care should be taken to maintain the periodontal architecture as much as possible. Rarely hemangiomas of the gingiva are seen and the clinician has to take appropriate measures during surgery in order to prevent potential bleeding complications.

Fig. 46.9A–D shows a case of pyogenic granuloma excised completely and resulting in excellent gingival form observed for a period of 2 years.

Recurrence of Gingival Enlargement

Recurrence after treatment is the most common problem in the management of gingival enlargement. Residual local irritation and systemic or hereditary conditions that cause noninflammatory gingival hyperplasia are the responsible factors.

The recurrence of chronic inflammatory enlargement immediately after treatment indicates that all irritants have not been removed. Contributory local conditions (e.g., food impaction, overhanging margins of restorations) are often overlooked. If the enlargement recurs after healing is complete and normal contour is attained, inadequate plaque control by the patient is the most common cause.

Recurrence during the healing period is manifested as red, beadlike, granulomatous masses that bleed with slight provocation. This

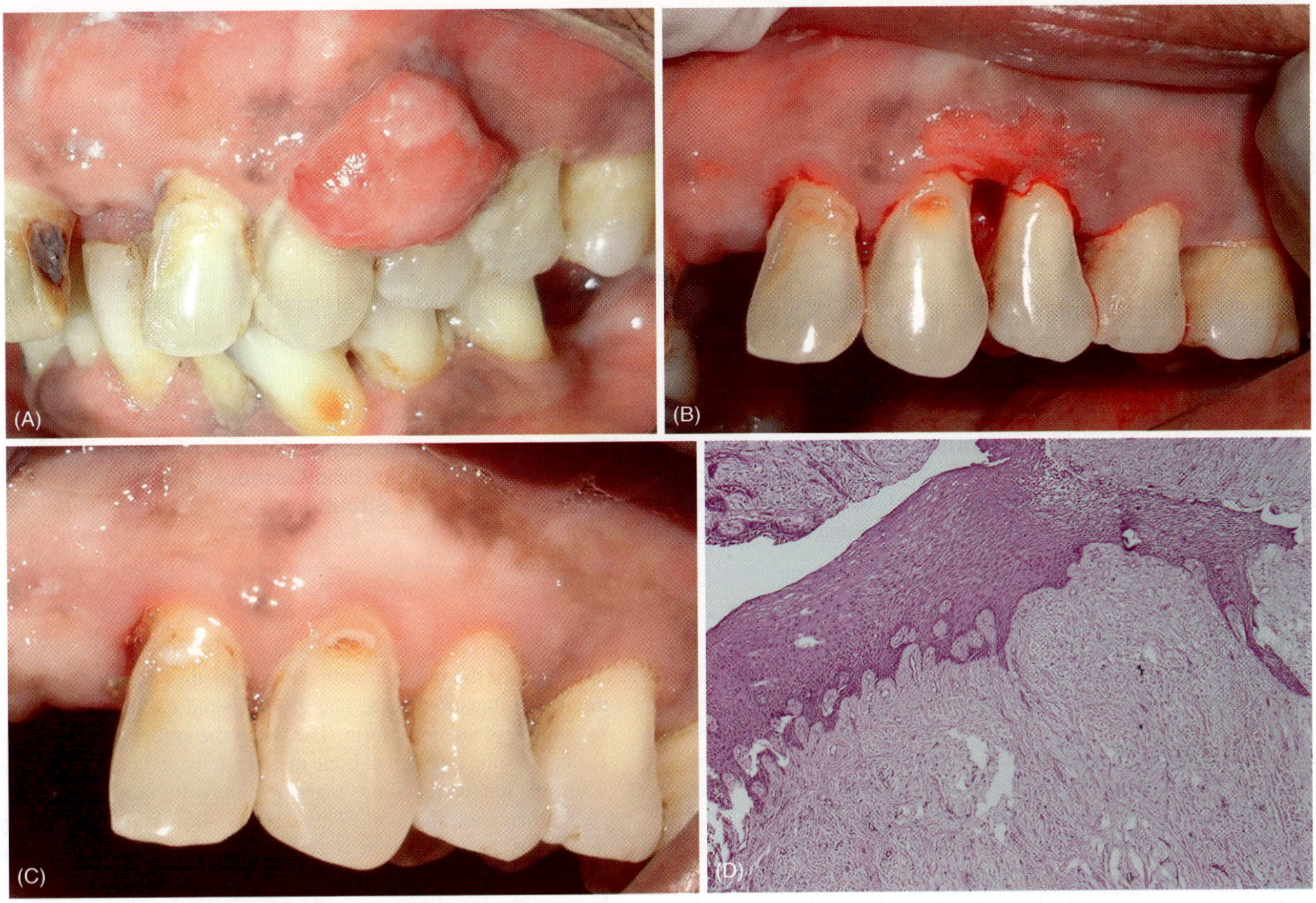

Fig. 46.9 Pyogenic granuloma treated by surgical excision. A, Preoperative photograph; B, lesion excised; C, Two year follow-up photograph showing excellent gingival contour; D, Photomicrograph confirming clinical diagnosis. *(From 2nd SA Edition, Chapter 46, Figs. 46.6A, B, C, D.)*

is a proliferative vascular inflammatory response to local irritation, which is usually a fragment of calculus on the root. The condition is corrected by removing the granulation tissue and scaling and planing the root surface. Also it should be noted that healing tissues are highly sensitive to plaque buildup and very quickly the gingiva increases in size. Hence optimal plaque control should be stressed to the patients. Further if the enlargement is predisposed by malalignment of teeth, orthodontic treatment should be instituted.

Familial, hereditary, or idiopathic gingival enlargement recurs after surgical removal even if all local irritants have been removed. The enlargement can be maintained at minimal size by preventing secondary inflammatory involvement.

Key points

- The most common type of gingival enlargement occurs due to chronic inflammation.
- Soft and edematous gingiva readily shrinks after scaling and root planing. But fibrotic enlargements may require surgical recontouring.
- Drug-induced gingival overgrowths may be managed either by discontinuation of the drug or change of medication if the consulting physician approves. Otherwise surgical recontouring is the choice.
- Gingivectomy/Gingivoplasty or an inverse bevel flap are the usual surgical procedures.

Suggested Reading

Camargo P, Melnick P, Pirih F, et al: Treatment of drug-induced gingival enlargement: aesthetic and functional considerations. *Periodontol 2000* 27:131, 2001.

CHAPTER 47

Resective Osseous Surgery

TN Sims | CD Dwarakanath

CHAPTER OUTLINE

The damage resulting from periodontal disease manifests in variable destruction of the tooth-supporting bone. Generally, bony deformities are not uniform; they are not indicative of the alveolar housing of the tooth before the disease process and do not reflect the overlying gingival architecture. Bone loss has been classified as either "horizontal" or "vertical," but in fact, bone loss is most often a combination of horizontal and vertical loss. Horizontal bone loss generally results in a relative thickening of the marginal alveolar bone because bone tapers as it approaches its most coronal margin.

The effects of this thickening and the development of vertical defects leave the alveolar bone with countless combinations of bony shapes. If these various topographic changes are to be altered to provide a more physiologic bone pattern, a method for osseous recontouring must be followed.

Osseous surgery may be defined as the procedure by which changes in the alveolar bone can be accomplished to rid it of deformities induced by the periodontal disease process or other related factors such as exostosis and tooth supraeruption.

Osseous surgery can be either additive or subtractive in nature. *Additive or regenerative osseous surgery* includes procedures directed at restoring the alveolar bone to its original level, whereas resective or *subtractive osseous surgery* is designed to restore the form of preexisting alveolar bone to the level present at the time of surgery or slightly more apical to this level (Fig. 47.1).

Additive osseous surgery brings about the ideal results of periodontal therapy. It implies regeneration of lost bone and reestablishment of the periodontal ligament, gingival fibers, and junctional epithelium at a more coronal level.

Resective osseous surgery procedures provide an alternative to additive methods and should be used when additive procedures are not feasible. These subtractive procedures are discussed in this chapter.

Normal Alveolar Bone Morphology

Knowledge of the morphology of the bony periodontium in a state of health is required to perform resective osseous surgery correctly. The characteristics of a normal bony form are as follows:

1. The interproximal bone is more coronal in position than the labial or lingual/palatal bone and pyramidal in form.
2. The form of the interdental bone is a function of the tooth form and the embrasure width. The more tapered the tooth, the more pyramidal is the bony form. The wider the embrasure, the more flattened is the interdental bone mesiodistally and buccolingually.
3. The position of the bony margin mimics the contours of the cementoenamel junction. The distance from the facial bony margin of the tooth to the interproximal bony crest is more flat in the posterior than the anterior areas. This "scalloping" of the bone on the facial surfaces and lingual/palatal surfaces is related to tooth and root form, as well as tooth position within the alveolus. Teeth with prominent roots or those displaced to the facial or lingual side may also have fenestrations or dehiscences. The molar teeth have less scalloping and a more flat profile than bicuspids and incisors.

Although these general observations apply to all patients, the bony architecture may vary from patient to patient in the extent of contour, configuration, and thickness. These variations may be both normal and healthy.

Terminology

Numerous terms have been developed to describe the topography of the alveolar housing, the procedure for its removal, and the resulting correction.

Procedures used to correct osseous defects have been classified into two: Osteoplasty and Ostectomy. *Osteoplasty* refers to reshaping the bone without removing tooth-supporting bone. *Ostectomy*, or *osteoectomy*, includes the removal of tooth-supporting bone. One or both of these procedures may be necessary to produce the desired result.

Terms that describe the bone form after reshaping can refer to morphologic features or to the thoroughness of the reshaping performed. Examples of morphologically descriptive terms include *negative, positive, flat*, and *ideal*. These terms relate to a preconceived standard of ideal osseous form.

Positive architecture and *negative architecture* refer to the relative position of interdental bone to radicular bone (Fig. 47.2). The architecture is "positive" if the radicular bone is apical to the interdental bone. The bone has "negative" architecture if the interdental bone is more apical than the radicular bone. *Flat architecture* is the reduction of the interdental bone to the same height as the radicular bone.

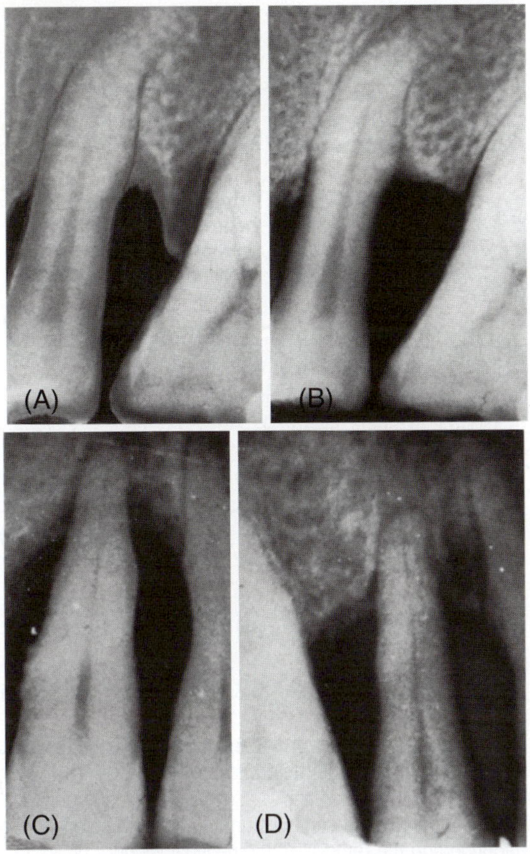

Fig. 47.1 Additive and subtractive osseous surgery. A, Before, and, B, immediately after subtractive osseous surgery; the osseous wall of the two adjoining infrabony pockets has been removed. C, Before, and, D, 1 year after additive osseous surgery; the area has been flapped and thoroughly instrumented, resulting in reconstruction of the interdental and periapical bone. *(Courtesy: Drs. E.A. Albano and B.O. Barletta, Buenos Aires, Argentina.) (From 2nd SA Edition.)*

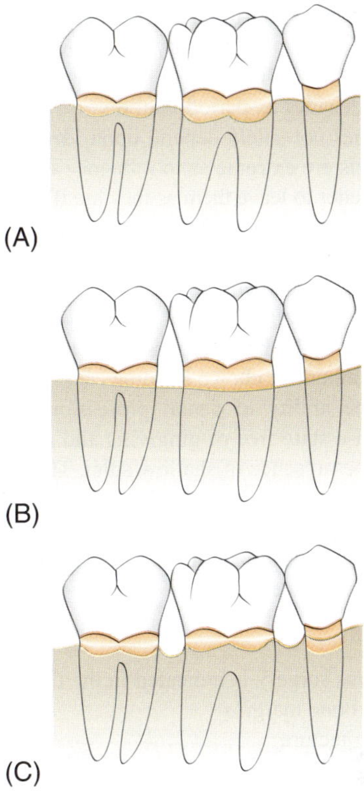

Fig. 47.2 Diagram of types of bony architecture. A, Positive bony architecture. B, Flat bony architecture. C, Reversed, or negative, bony form. *(From 2nd SA Edition.)*

Osseous form is considered to be "ideal" when the bone is consistently more coronal on the interproximal surfaces than on the facial and lingual surfaces. The ideal form of the marginal bone has similar interdental height, with gradual, curved slopes between interdental peaks (Fig. 47.3).

Terms that relate to the thoroughness of the osseous reshaping techniques include "definitive" and "compromise." *Definitive osseous reshaping* implies that further osseous reshaping would not improve the overall result. *Compromise osseous reshaping* indicates a bone pattern that cannot be improved without significant osseous removal that would be detrimental to the overall result.

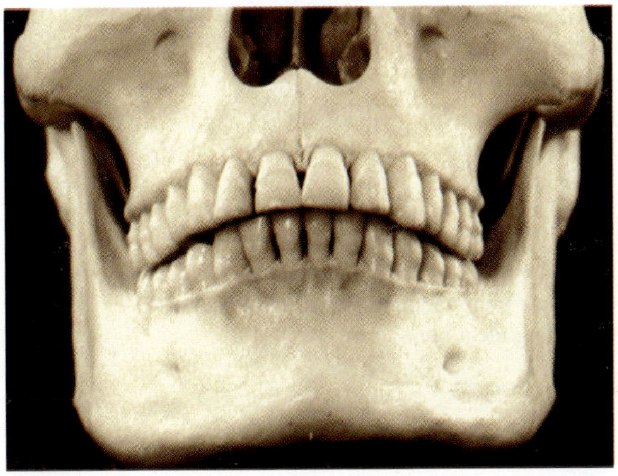

Fig. 47.3 Skull photograph of healthy periodontium. Note the shape of the alveolar bone housing. This bone is considered to have ideal form. It is more coronal in the interproximal areas, with a gradual slope around and away from the tooth. *(From 2nd SA Edition.)*

Selection of Treatment Technique

The morphology of the osseous defect largely determines the treatment technique to be used. *One-wall angular defects* usually need to be recontoured surgically. *Three-wall defects*, particularly if they are narrow and deep, can be successfully treated with techniques that strive for new attachment and bone reconstruction. *Two-wall angular defects* can be treated with either method, depending on their depth, width, and general configuration. Therefore, except for one-wall defects and wide, shallow two-wall defects, and interdental craters, osseous defects are treated with the objective of obtaining optimal repair by natural healing processes.

Rationale

Resective osseous surgery provides the surest method of reducing pockets and is based on the tenet that discrepancies in level and shapes of the bone and gingiva predispose patients to recurrence of pocket depth postsurgically. Its goal is to reshape the marginal bone to resemble that of the alveolar process undamaged by periodontal disease. The technique is performed in combination with apically positioned flaps and the procedure eliminates periodontal pocket depth and improves tissue contour to provide a more easily maintainable environment.

The conversion of the periodontal pocket to shallow gingival sulcus enhances the patient's ability to remove plaque and oral debris from the dentition. However, this concept has been questioned in the last two decades as periodontal disease pathogenesis is very complex and does not solely depend upon ideal bone form. Hence unless the defects are extreme as to influence the periodontal status markedly, it is better to leave them as they are if additive/regenerative techniques cannot be employed. Its value as a surgical approach is limited by the presence, quantity, and shape of the bony tissues and by the amount of attachment loss that is acceptable. Although this concept is not universally accepted and the procedure induces loss of radicular bone in the healing phase, recontouring of bone is the only logical treatment of choice in some cases.

Likewise, the ability of dental professionals to maintain the periodontium in a state free of gingivitis and periodontitis is more predictable in the presence of shallow sulci. The more effective the periodontal maintenance therapy, the greater is the longitudinal stability of the surgical result. The efficacy of osseous surgery therefore depends on its ability to affect pocket depth and to promote periodontal maintenance.

Indications

Resective osseous surgery is indicated in the following situations:

1. Inconsistent bone margins
2. Reverse architecture
3. One wall defects
4. Buttressing bone formation
5. Ledges and plateau
6. Shallow craters
7. Furcation defects
8. Crown lengthening for restorative dentistry

Contraindications

1. Extensive bone loss
2. High caries activity
3. Existing mobility
4. Esthetic zones

Advantages

1. Predictability
2. Complete elimination of periodontal pockets
3. Obtaining ideal bone form

Disadvantages

1. Loss of valuable supporting bone
2. Gingival recession and its sequelae
3. Often lengthy unpleasant postsurgical recovery
4. Postsurgical mobility

Factors in Selection of Resective Osseous Surgery

1. Depth and configuration of bony lesion to root morphology and the adjacent teeth (Fig. 47.4).
2. Amount of bone that requires removal.
3. The extent of attachment loss.
4. The number of remaining walls of bony defect.
5. The amount of soft tissue present interproximally.

Examination and Treatment Planning

In addition to the routine clinical and radiographic examination described earlier (Chapters 24 and 25). The following factors should be assessed.

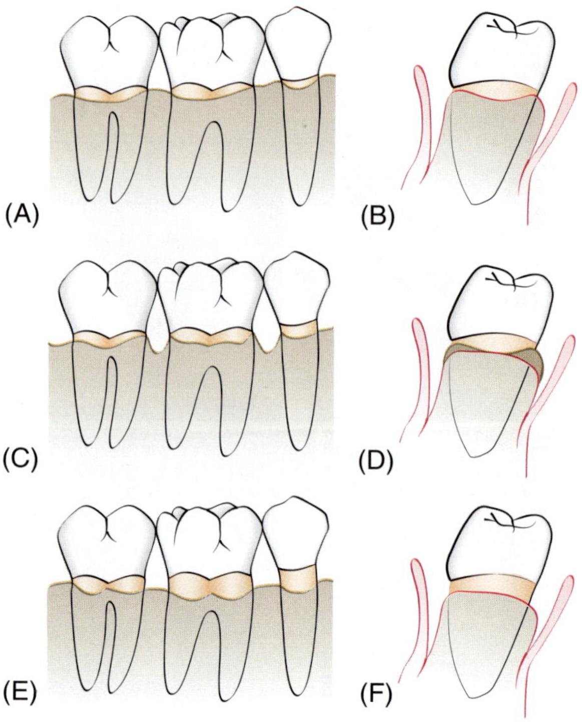

Fig. 47.4 Effect of correction of craters. A and B, Diagram of facial and interproximal bony contours after flap reflection. Note the loss of some interproximal bone and cratering. C and D, Line angles; this is only osteoplasty and has resulted in a reversed architecture. E and F, Ostectomy on the facial and lingual bone and the removal of the residual widow's peaks to produce a positive bony architecture. *(From 2nd SA Edition.)*

1. The type of bone loss and its configuration by sounding or transgingival probing under local anesthesia.
2. Evaluation of the esthetics.
3. Restorative/prosthodontic considerations.
4. Prognosis of the overall dentition.
5. The type of periodontitis.
6. Response to phase 1 therapy.

Treatment planning should provide solutions for active periodontal diseases and correction of deformities that result from periodontitis. Planning should also facilitate the performance of other dental procedures included in a comprehensive dental treatment plan. The extent of periodontal involvement can vary significantly from tooth to tooth in the same patient. The response to therapy from patient to patient may also vary, as may the treatment objectives for the patients. Therefore, a treatment plan may encompass a number of steps and combinations of procedures in the same surgical area.

After oral hygiene instruction, scaling and root planing, and other disease control procedures, the response of the patient to these treatment procedures is evaluated by re-examination and recording the changes in the periodontium. Because the extent of periodontal involvement can vary significantly from tooth to tooth in the same patient, the local response to therapy is also variable. The resolution of inflammation and decrease in edema and swelling may have resulted in a return to normal depth and configuration of some pockets, and additional therapy beyond periodic maintenance may not be required. However, notwithstanding conscientious efforts during phase 1 therapy, some probing depths may still remain. Further nonsurgical therapy has little effect on the bony deformities. In such cases, bone has to be exposed and its topography altered.

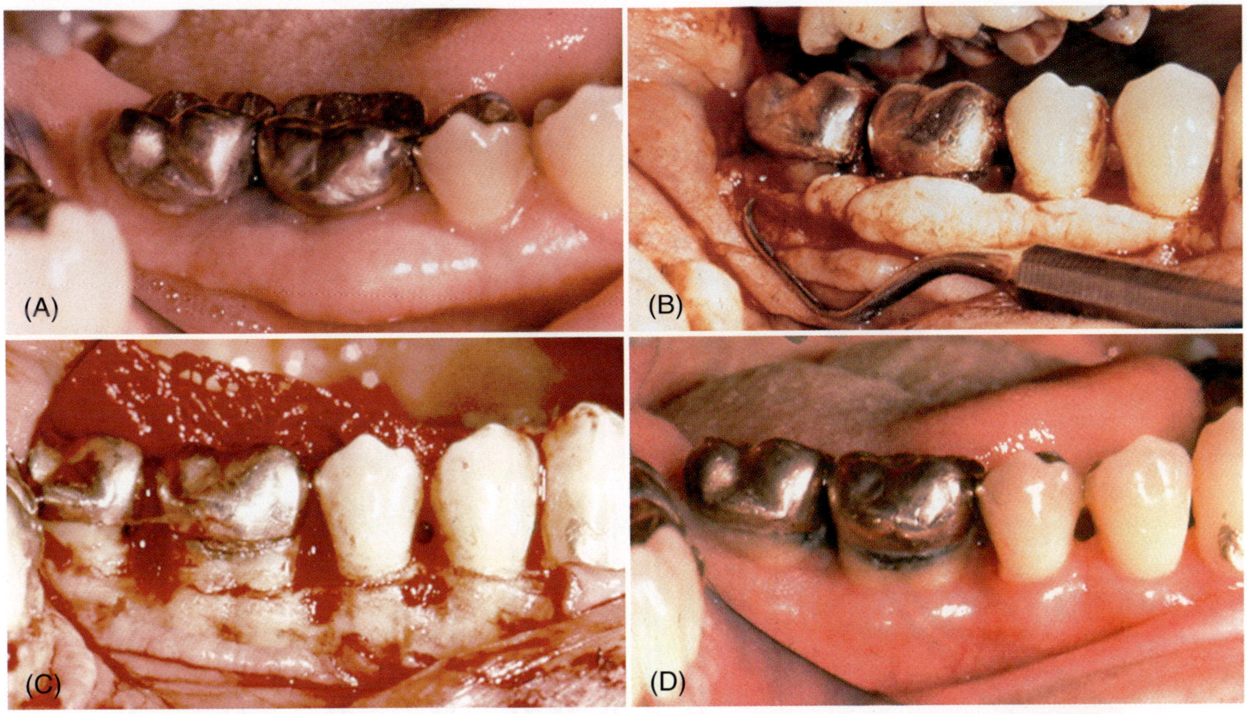

Fig. 47.5 Reduction of bony ledges and exposure of caries by osteoplasty. A, Buccal preoperative photograph showing two crowns, exostoses, and caries. B, Flap reflected to reveal caries on both molars at the restoration margins, interdental cratering, and a facial exostosis. C, After osseous surgery, the bulk of the bony removal was by osteoplasty, with minor ostectomy between the two molars. The caries is now exposed, and the crowns are lengthened for restoration. D, Postoperative photograph at 6 weeks. The plaque control is deficient, but the teeth should be readily restorable at this time. *(Courtesy: Dr. Joseph Schwartz, Portland, OR.) (From 2nd SA Edition.)*

Resective osseous surgery is also used to facilitate certain restorative and prosthetic dental procedures (Fig. 47.5). Dental caries can be exposed for restoration; fractured roots of abutment teeth can be exposed for removal; and bony exostoses and ridge deformities can be altered in contour to improve the performance of removable or fixed prostheses. Severely decayed teeth or teeth with short anatomic crowns can be lengthened by resection or by a combination of orthodontic tooth extrusion and osseous resection. Such procedures allow the therapist to expose more tooth for restoration, prevent an invasion of the biologic width of attachment, and create a periodontal attachment of normal dimension. Resection can also provide a means of producing optimal crown length for cosmetic purposes.

Osseous Resection Technique

Instrumentation

A number of hand and rotary instruments have been used for osseous resective surgery. Some excellent clinicians use only hand instruments and rongeurs, whereas others prefer a combination of hand and rotary instruments. Rotary instruments are useful for the osteoplasty, whereas hand instruments provide the most precise and safe results for ostectomy.

Recently piezoelectric surgical techniques have also been used with success for osseous surgical resection. Regardless of the type of instruments used, care and precision are required for each step of the procedure to prevent excessive bone removal or root damage, both of which are irreversible. Fig. 47.6 illustrates some of the instruments commonly used for osseous resection techniques.

To address the many clinical situations, the following sequential steps are suggested for resective osseous surgery (Fig. 47.7):

1. Vertical grooving
2. Radicular blending
3. Flattening interproximal bone
4. Gradualizing marginal bone

Not all steps are necessary in every case, but the sequencing of the steps in the order given is necessary to expedite the reshaping procedure, as well as to minimize the unnecessary removal of bone. Figure 47.8 illustrates bone reshaping in flap surgery for specific anatomic defects.

Vertical Grooving

Vertical grooving is designed to reduce the thickness of the alveolar housing and to provide relative prominence to the radicular aspects of the teeth. It also provides continuity from the interproximal surface onto the radicular surface. It is the first step of the resective process because it can define the general thickness and subsequent form of the alveolar housing. This step is usually performed with rotary instruments, such as round carbide burs or diamonds. The advantages of vertical grooving are most apparent with thick bony margins, shallow crater formations, or other areas that require maximal osteoplasty and minimal ostectomy. Vertical grooving is contraindicated in areas with close roots or thin alveolar housing.

Radicular Blending

Radicular blending, the second step of the osseous reshaping technique, is an extension of vertical grooving. Conceptually, it is an attempt to gradualize the bone over the entire radicular surface

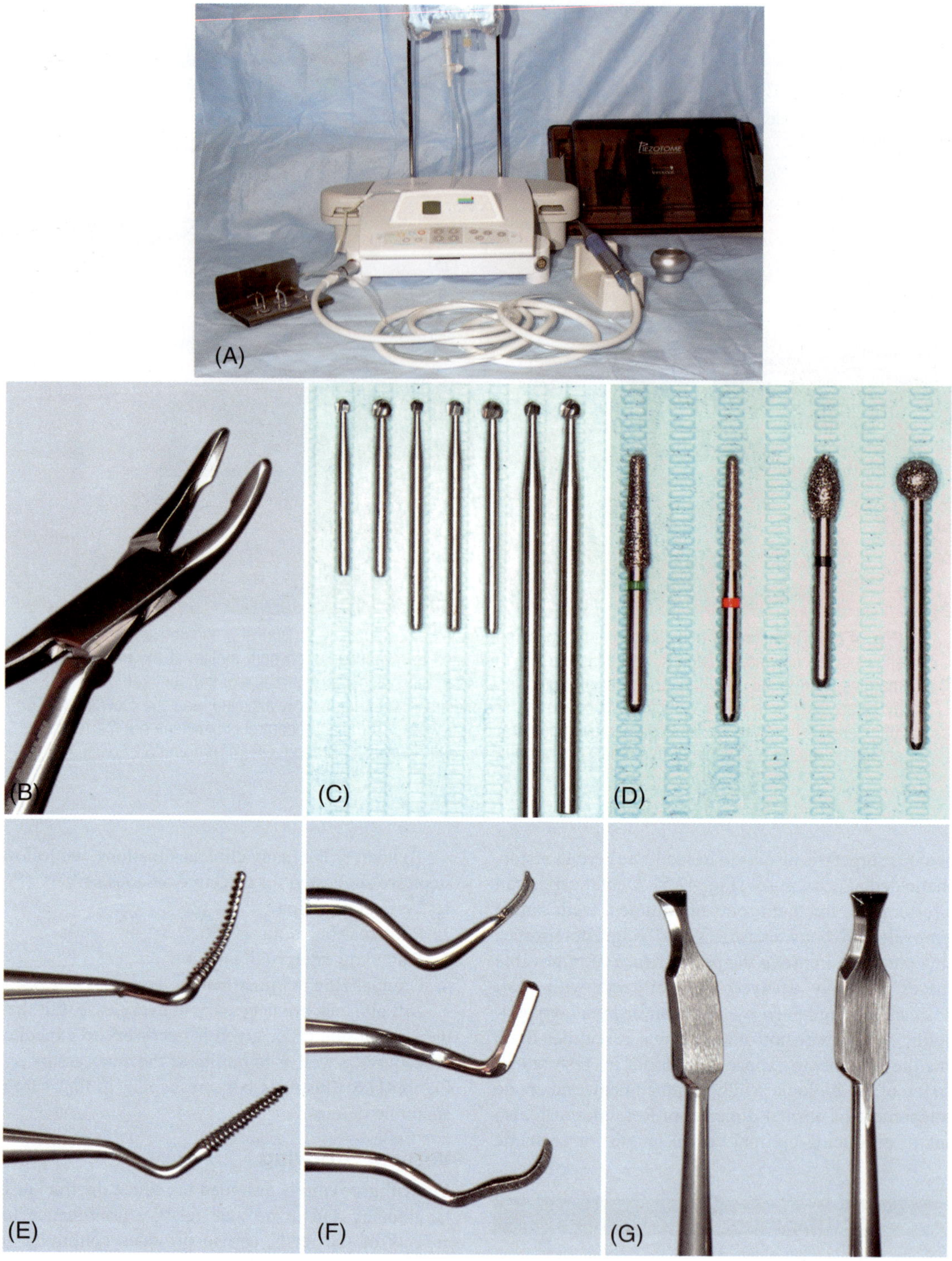

Fig. 47.6 Instruments often used in osseous surgery. A, Currently, the piezoelectric surgical instrument has been used successfully in osseous resective surgery. B, Rongeurs: Friedman *(top)* and 90-degree Blumenthal *(bottom)*. C, Carbide round burs. *Left to right*, Friction grip, surgical-length friction grip, and slow-speed handpiece. D, Diamond burs. E, Interproximal files: Schluger and Sugarman. F, Back-action chisels. G, Ochsenbein chisels. (*From 2nd SA Edition.*)

to provide the best results from vertical grooving. This provides a smooth, blended surface for good flap adaptation. The indications are the same as for vertical grooving (i.e., thick ledges of bone on the radicular surface, where selective surgical resection is desired). Naturally, this step is not necessary if vertical grooving is very minor or if the radicular bone is thin or fenestrated. Both vertical grooving and radicular blending are purely osteoplastic techniques that do not remove supporting bone. In most situations, these two procedures compose the bulk of resective osseous surgery. Classically, shallow crater formations, thick osseous ledges of bone on the radicular surfaces, and Class I and early Class II furcation involvements are treated almost entirely with these two steps.

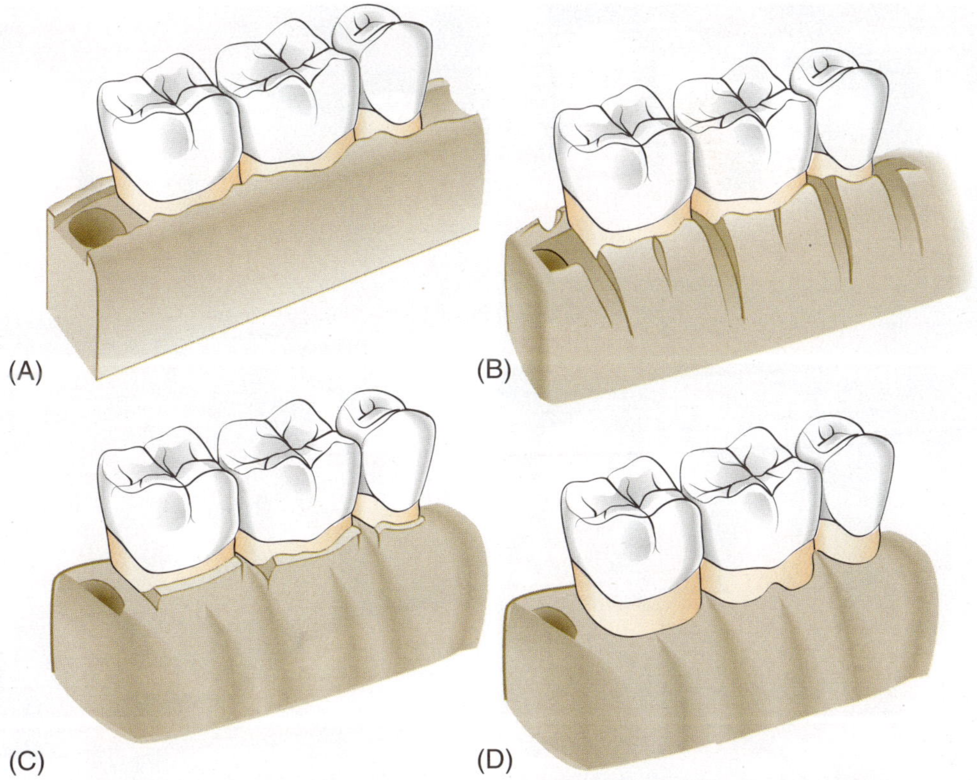

Fig. 47.7 A, Drawing of bony topography in moderate periodontitis with interdental craters. B, Vertical grooving, the first step in correction by osseous reshaping. C, Radicular blending and flattening of interproximal bone. D, Gradualizing the marginal bone. Note the area of the furcation on the first molar where the bone is preserved. *(From 2nd SA Edition.)*

Flattening Interproximal Bone

Flattening of the interdental bone requires the removal of very small amounts of supporting bone (Fig. 47.9). It is indicated when interproximal bone levels vary horizontally. By definition, most of the indications for this step are one-walled interproximal defects or hemiseptal defects. The omission of flattening in such cases results in increased pocket depth on the most apical side of the bone loss. This step is typically not necessary with interproximal crater formations or flat interproximal defects. It is best used in defects that have a coronally placed, one-walled edge of a predominantly three-walled angular defect, and it can be helpful in obtaining good flap closure and improved healing in the three-walled defect. The limitation of this step, as with resective osseous surgical therapy in general, is in the treatment of advanced lesions. Large hemiseptal defects would require removal of inordinate amounts of bone to provide a flattened architecture, and the procedure would be too costly in terms of bony support. Compromised osseous architecture is the only logical solution (Fig. 47.10).

Gradualizing Marginal Bone

The final step in the osseous resection technique is also an ostectomy process. Bone removal is minimal but necessary to provide a sound, regular base for the gingival tissue to follow. Failure to remove small bony discrepancies on the gingival line angles (widow's peaks) allows the tissue to rise to a higher level than the base of the bone loss in the interdental area. This may make the process of selective recession and subsequent pocket reduction incomplete. This step of the procedure also requires gradualization and blending on the radicular surface. The two ostectomy steps should be performed with great care so as not to produce nicks or grooves on the roots. When the radicular bone is thin, it is extremely easy to overdo this step, to the detriment of the entire surgical effort. For this reason, various hand instruments, such as chisels and curettes, are preferable to rotary instruments for gradualizing marginal bone.

Flap Placement and Closure

After performing resection, the clinician positions and sutures the flaps. Flaps may be replaced to their original position, to cover the new bony margin, or they may be apically positioned. Replacing the flap in areas that previously had deep pockets may result initially in greater postoperative pocket depth, although a selective recession may diminish the depth over time. Positioning the flap apically to expose marginal bone is one method of altering the width of the gingiva (denudation). However, such flap placement results in more postsurgical resorption of bone and patient discomfort than if the newly created bony margin were covered by the flap. Positioning the flap to cover the new margin minimizes postoperative complications and results in optimal postsurgical pocket depths (Fig. 47.11).

Suturing may be accomplished using a variety of different suture materials and suture knots. The sutures should be placed with minimal tension to coapt the flaps, prevent their separation, and maintain the position of the flaps. Sutures placed with excessive tension rapidly pull through the tissues.

Postoperative Maintenance

Sutures may be removed at various times after placement. Nonresorbable sutures such as silk are usually removed after 1 week of

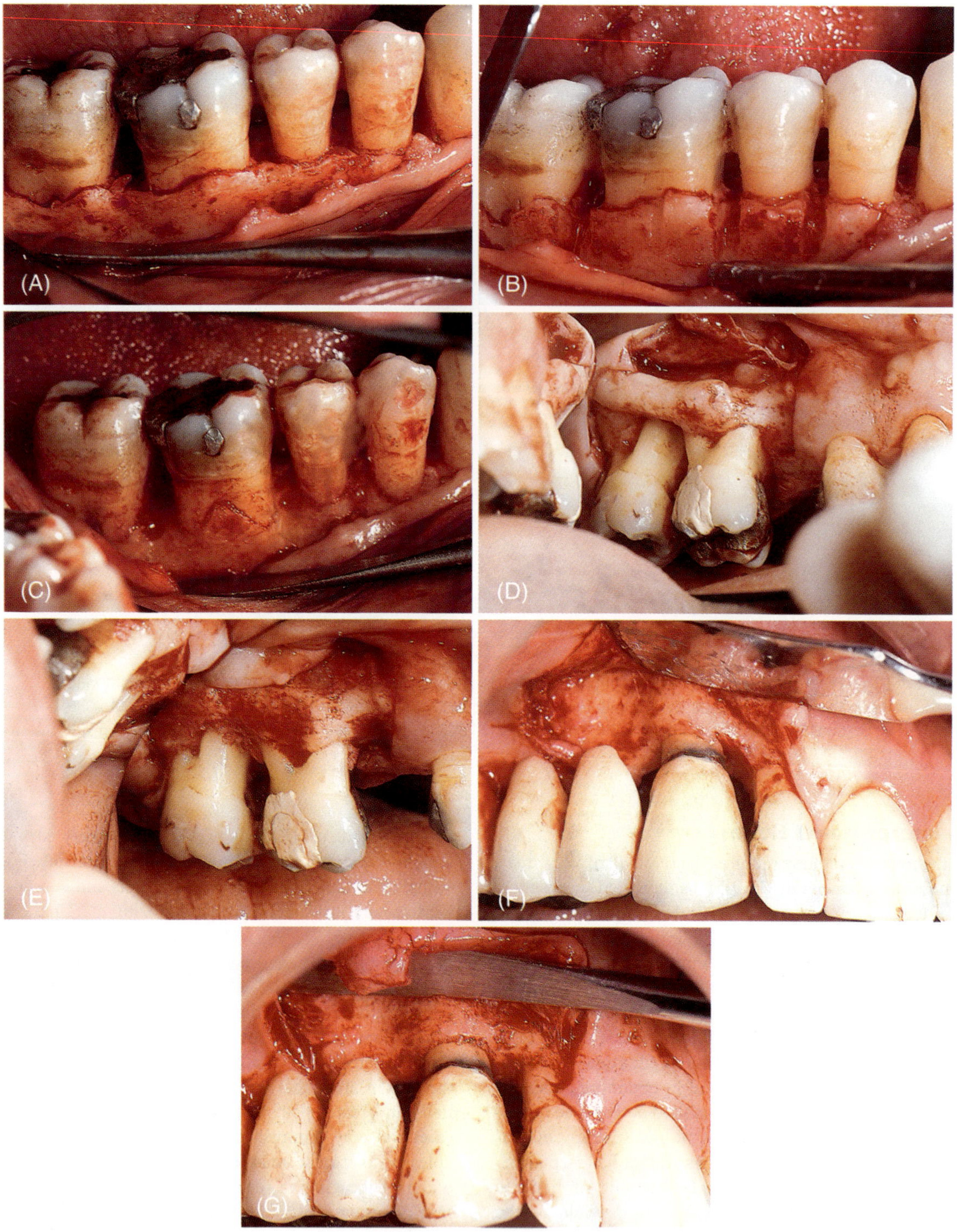

Fig. 47.8 Bone contouring in flap surgery. A–C, Bone contouring in interdental craters. D and E, Bone contouring in exostoses. F and G, Bone contouring in one-wall vertical defect.

healing, although some of the newer synthetic materials may be left for up to 3 weeks or longer without adverse consequences. Resorbable sutures maintain wound approximation for varying periods of 1–3 weeks or more, depending on the type of suture material. After suture removal, the surgical site is examined carefully, and any excessive granulation tissue is removed with a sharp curette. The patient is given instructions on optimal oral hygiene. Supersoft tooth brushes with chlorhexidine mouthrinse are generally prescribed.

Healing should proceed uneventfully, with the attachment of the flap to the underlying bone completed in 14–21 days. Maturation and remodeling can continue for up to 6 months. It is usually advisable to wait at least 6 weeks after completion of healing of the last surgical area before beginning dental restorations. For those patients with a major cosmetic concern, it is wise to wait as long as possible to achieve a postoperative soft tissue position and a stable sulcus.

Specific Osseous Reshaping Situations

The osseous corrective procedure previously described is classically applied to shallow craters with heavy faciolingual ledges (Fig. 47.12).

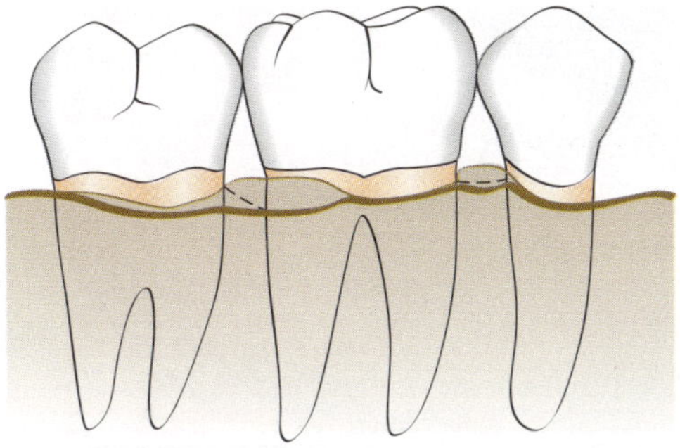

Fig. 47.9 Diagrammatic representation of bone irregularities in periodontal disease. The thick line is the proposed correction of the defect. Note the flattening of the interproximal bone between the molars and the protection of the furcal bone on the first molar. Facial crest height is reduced in both interproximal areas to the depth of the defect. *(From 2nd SA Edition.)*

The correction of other osseous defects is also possible; however, careful case selection for definitive osseous surgery is extremely important.

Correction of one-walled hemiseptal defects requires that the bone be reduced to the level of the most apical portion of the defect. Therefore, great care should be taken to select the appropriate case. If one-walled defects occur next to an edentulous space, the edentulous ridge is reduced to the level of the osseous defect (Fig. 47.13).

In the absence of ledges or exostoses, the elimination of the bony lesion begins with reduction of the interdental walls of craters, the one-walled component of angular defects, moats and grooving into sites of early involvement. The walls of the crater may be reduced at the expense of the buccal, lingual, or both (Fig. 47.14). The reduction should be made to remove the least amount of alveolar bone required to (1) produce a satisfactory form, (2) prevent the therapeutic invasion of furcations, and (3) blend the contours with

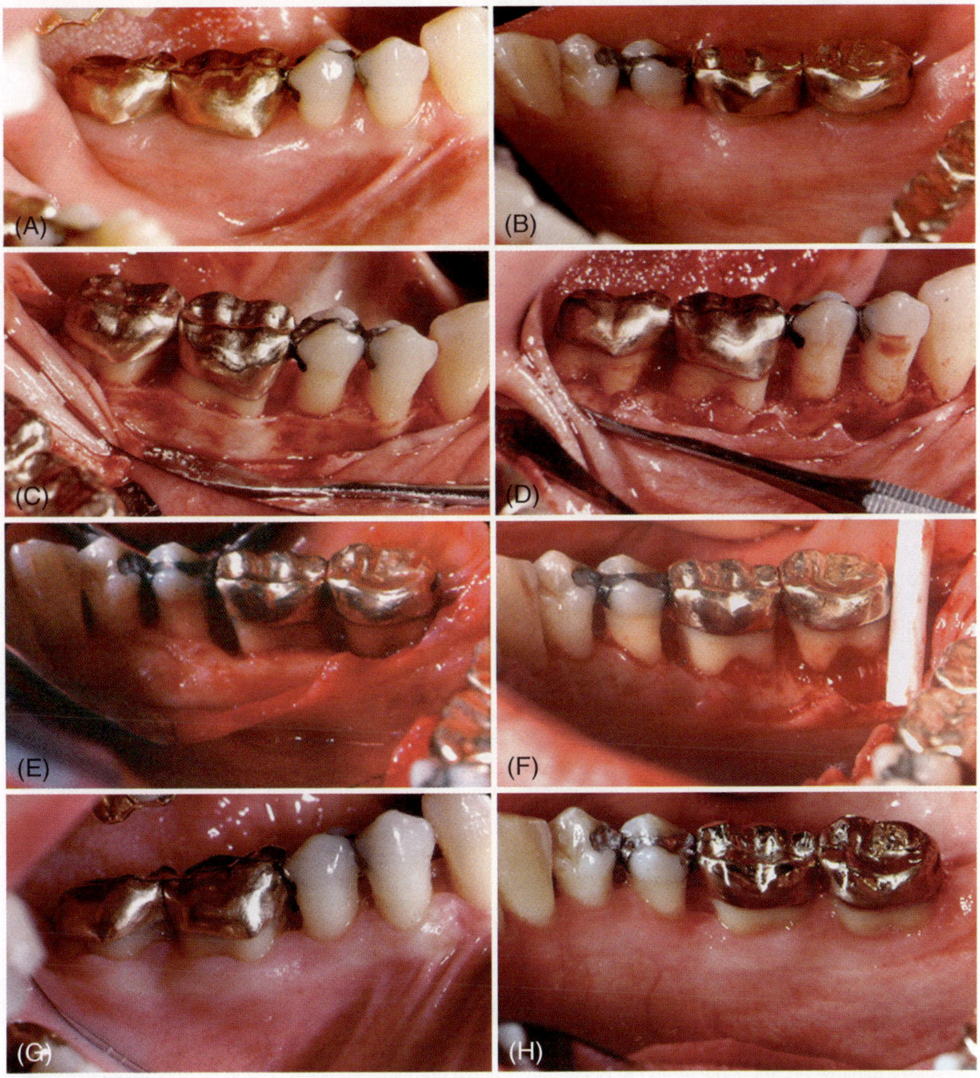

Fig. 47.10 Compromise osseous surgery. A and B, Preoperative views of the buccal and lingual surfaces. C and D, Preoperative and postoperative views of the buccal osseous recontouring of Class I buccal furcation defects, a moderate crater between the two molars, and a deep 1-2-3–walled defect at the mesial of the first involvements. D, Buccal aspects of these lesions were corrected with osteoplasty and a small amount of ostectomy. E and F, Preoperative and postoperative views of the lingual osseous management. In E, note the combination 1-2-3–walled defect between the second bicuspid and first molar, as well as the irregular pattern of bone loss with ledging. F, These defects were corrected by osteoplasty and ostectomy, except for the deep defect at the mesial surface of the molar. This area was resected until the residual defect was of two and three walls only and left to repair. G and H, Buccal and lingual 5-year postoperative views of tissue configuration. Note the residual soft-tissue defect between the bicuspid and first molar. *(From 2nd SA Edition.)*

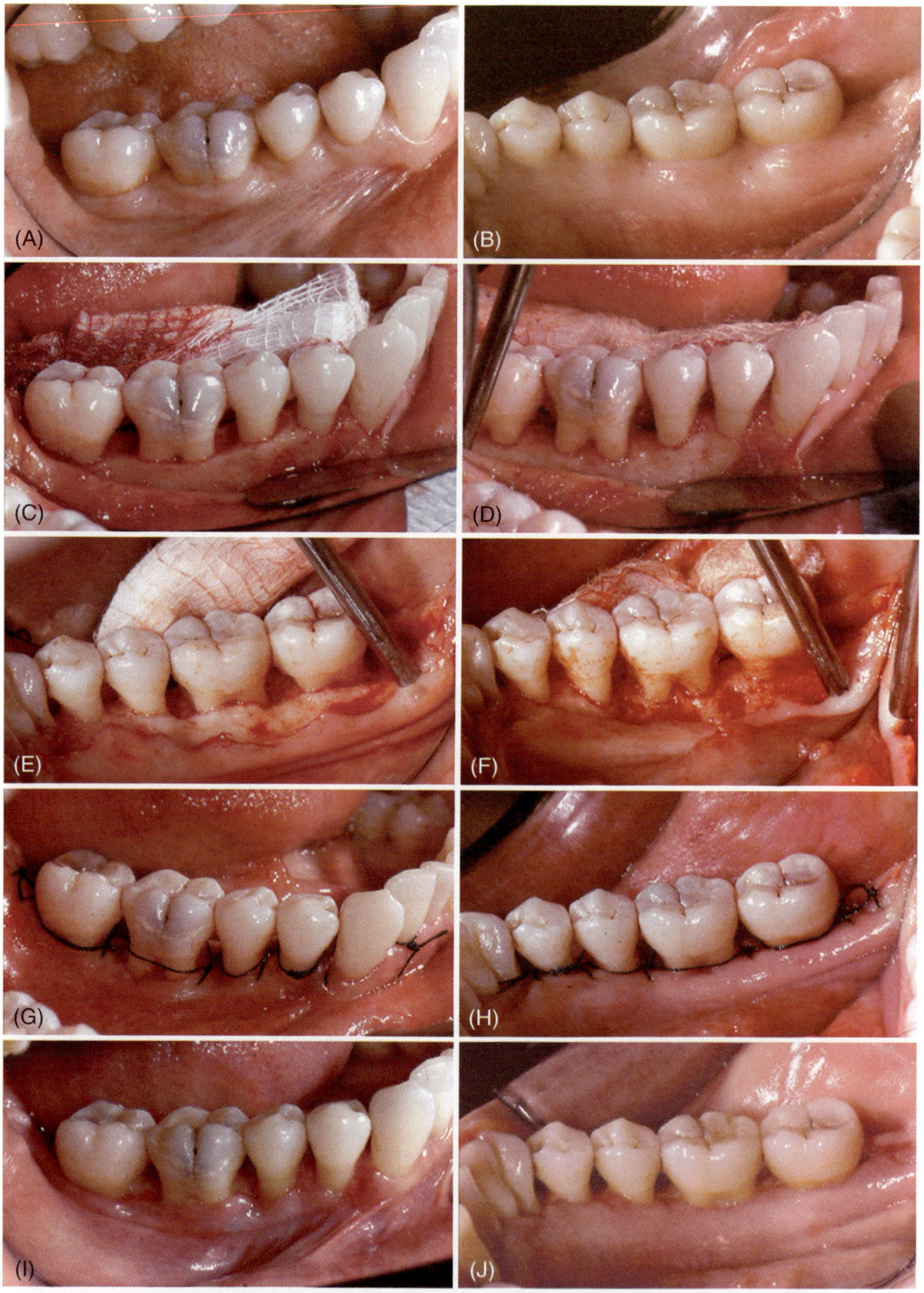

Fig. 47.11 Ostectomy and osteoplasty to a positive contour with flap placement at the newly created bony crest for minimal pocket depth. A and B, Buccal and lingual preoperative views. C and D, Buccal preoperative view and postoperative correction. Osteoplasty and ostectomy were used to produce a positive contour. Note the osteoplasty into the buccal furcation of the first molar. This is about the extent of craters that can be corrected to a positive contour in teeth with moderate root trunk length. E and F, Lingual preoperative view and postoperative correction. Osteoplasty and ostectomy were done to produce a positive contour. Note the lingual ledge, which was reduced. Such ledges are common in this area. G and H, Buccal and lingual flaps sutured with continuous sling sutures to allow placement of the flaps to cover the bony margins. Ostectomy and osteoplasty performed to a positive contour, with flap placement at the newly created bony crest for minimal pocket depth. Ostectomy and osteoplasty to a positive contour with flap placement at the newly created bony crest for minimal pocket depth. I and J, Buccal and lingual postoperative views at 1 week. Soft-tissue thickness is minimal, and the interdental areas are granulating in over the positive bony form. Minimal pocket depth results from such management. *(From 2nd SA Edition.)*

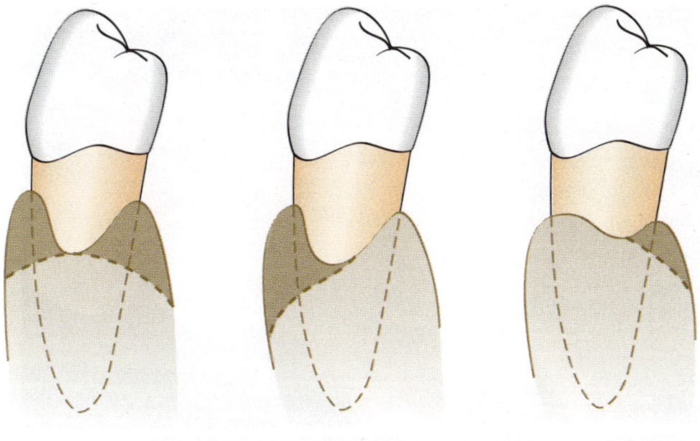

Fig. 47.12 Interproximal craters. The shaded areas illustrate different techniques for the management of such defects. The technique that reduces the least amount of supporting bone is preferable. (*From 2nd SA Edition.*)

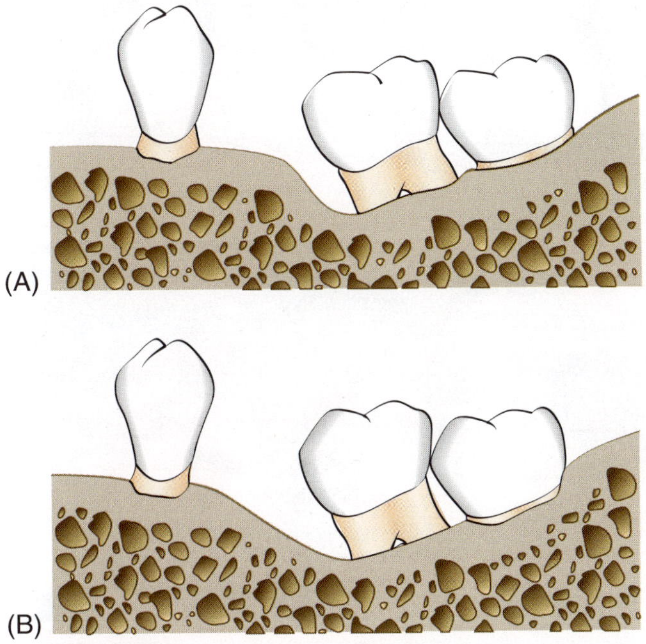

Fig. 47.13 Reduction of a one-wall angular defect. A, Angular bone defect mesial to the tilted molar. B, Defect reduced by "ramping" angular bone. (*From 2nd SA Edition.*)

the adjacent teeth. The selective reduction of bony defects by "ramping" the bone to the palatal or lingual to avoid involvement of the furcation can be done (Fig. 47.15).

In the presence of heavy ledges of bone, it is usually wise to do osteoplasty first to eliminate any exostoses or reduce the buccal/lingual bulk of the bone (Fig. 47.16). It is a common practice to

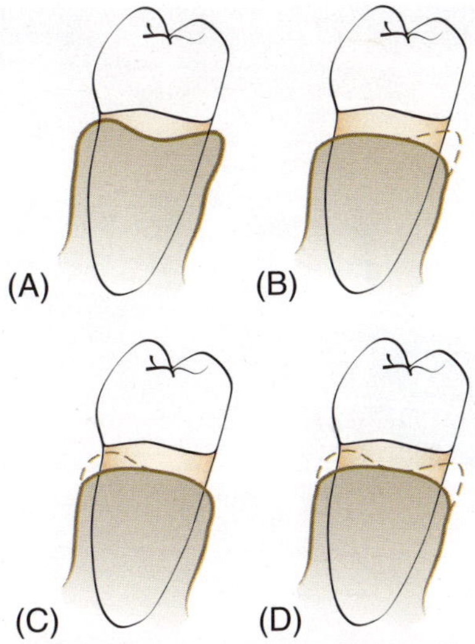

Fig. 47.14 Diagram of crater-reduction patterns. A, Preoperative bony form after flap reflection. B, Reduction of craters to the lingual wall. C, Reduction of craters to the facial wall. D, Reduction of craters to both the buccal and the lingual wall. (*From 2nd SA Edition.*)

incorporate a degree of vertical grooving during the reduction of bony ledges because this facilitates the process of blending the radicular bone into the interproximal areas at the next step.

One-walled or hemiseptal defects usually require the removal of some bone from the tooth with the greatest coronal bony height. This removal of bone may result in a significant reduction in attachment on relatively unaffected adjacent teeth to eliminate the defect. Hence, the clinician should take appropriate decision based on the correct judgment.

Conclusion

Osseous surgical techniques cannot be applied to every bony abnormality or topographic modification. However, judiciously advocated, they can eliminate and modify defects such as bony ledges, irregular alveolar bone, early furcation involvement, bony exostosis and circumferential defects. When properly performed, resective osseous surgery achieves a physiologic architecture of marginal alveolar bone conducive to gingival flap adaptation with minimal probing depth. The advantages of this surgical modality include a predictable amount of pocket reduction that can enhance oral hygiene and periodic maintenance. It also preserves the width of the attached tissue while removing granulomatous tissue and providing access for debridement of the radicular surfaces. In addition, the osseous resection technique permits recontouring of bony abnormalities, including hemiseptal defects, tori, and ledges. Its benefits also include facilitating restorative dentistry.

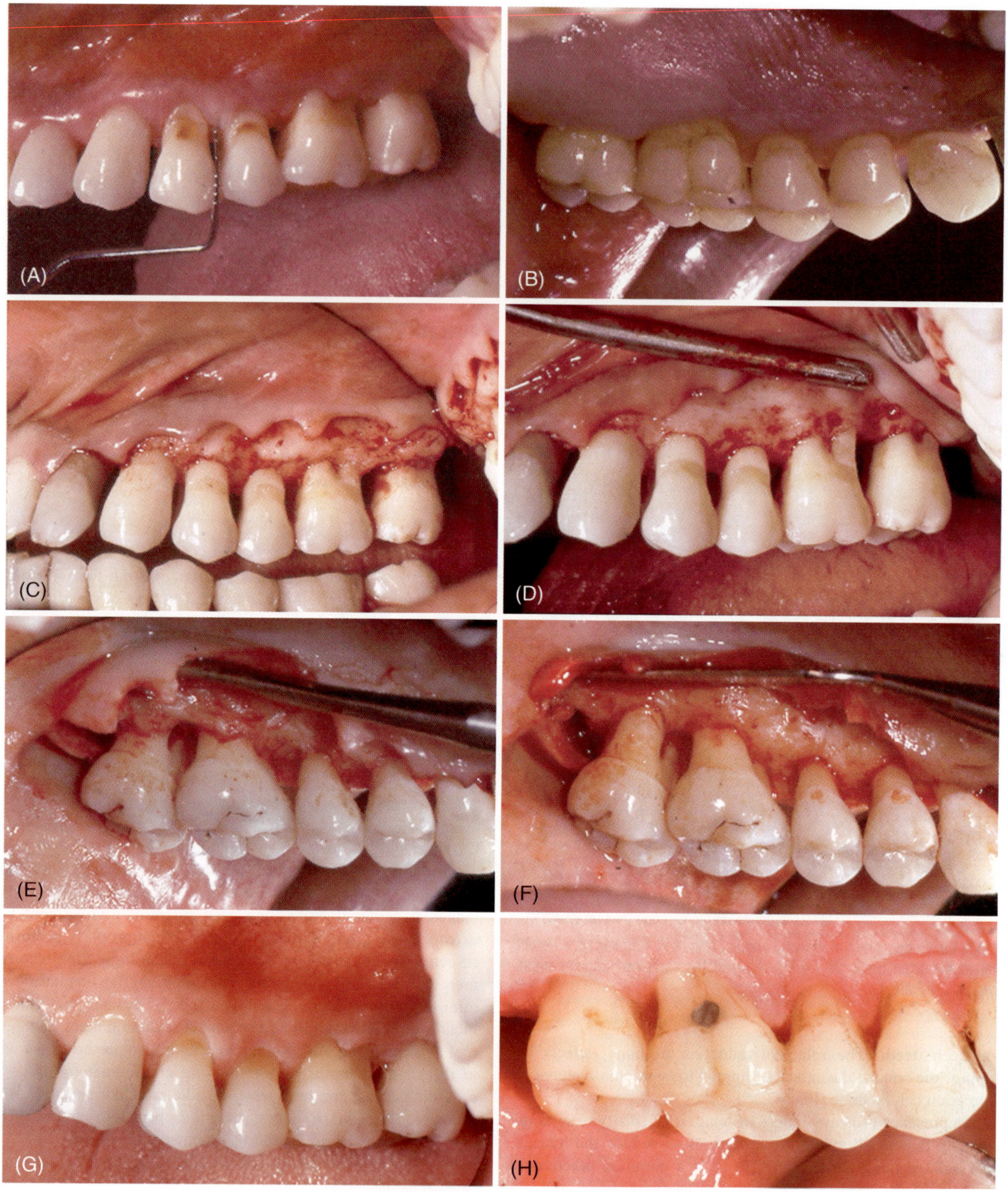

Fig. 47.15 Correction of osseous defects largely to the palatal wall. A and B, Buccal and palatal preoperative views, 6 weeks after completion of scaling and root planing. C and D, Buccal preoperative and postoperative views. In C, note the ledging on the facial wall of molars and the one-wall defects on both molars. D, Postoperative view shows the elimination of these defects by osteoplasty on the ledges and ostectomy of the one-wall defects to produce a positive buccal architecture. E and F, Palatal preoperative and postoperative views. In E, note the pattern of bony loss, which is more severe on the palatal wall. In addition to the facial one-wall defects, there is an incipient furcation defect at the mesial wall of the first molar and a Class II furcation at the mesial wall of the second molar. F, Configuration of the defects was such that ostectomy was performed on the palatal roots of both molars to produce a compromise architecture. G and H, Ten-year postoperative views of the buccal and palatal areas showing the pattern of soft-tissue adaptation to the surgically produced bony form. *(From 2nd SA Edition.)*

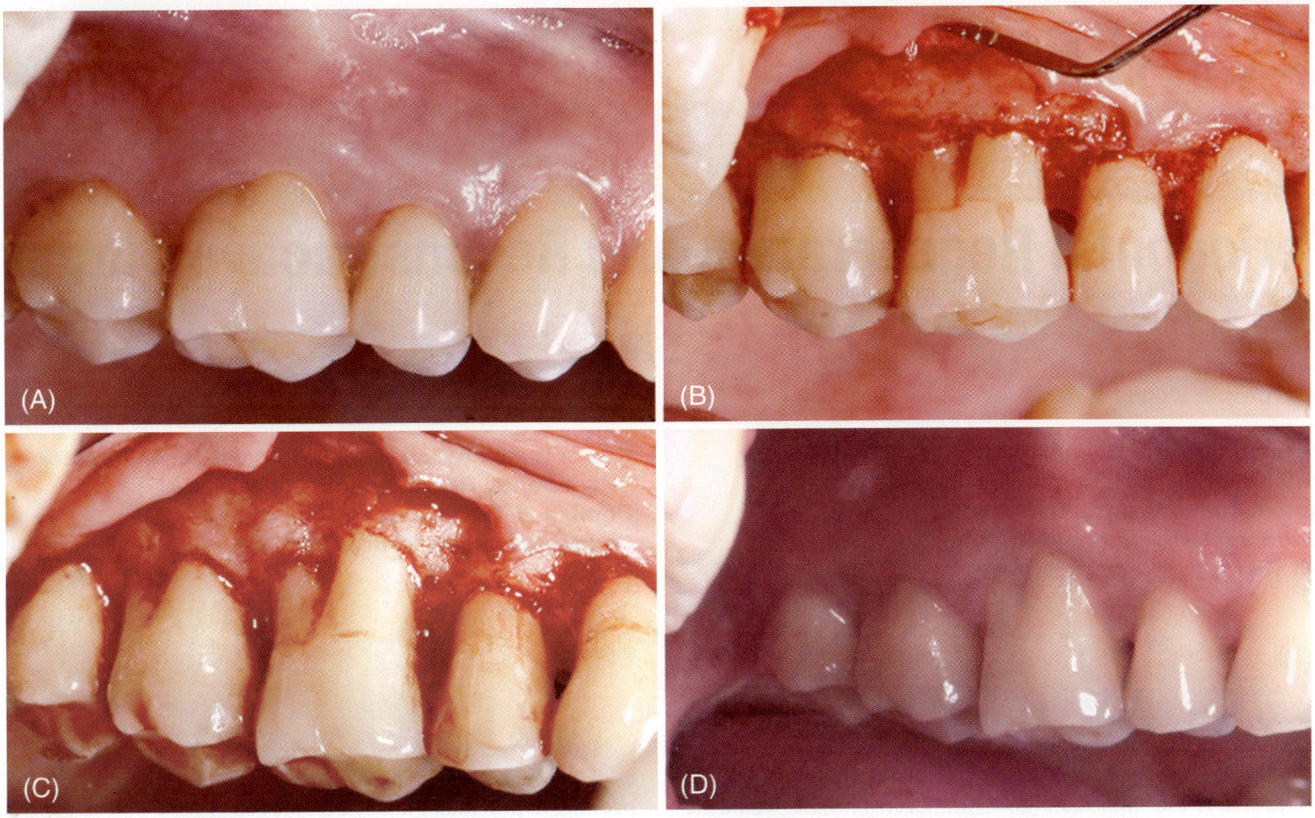

Fig. 47.16 Reduction of bony ledges by osteoplasty before correction of interdental defects. A, Buccal preoperative view. B, Buccal flap reflection. Note the buccal ledge and the Class II buccal furcation. C, Buccal correction largely by osteoplasty with minor ostectomy over the root prominence to produce a positive architecture. D, Ten-year postoperative view of soft-tissue form. Minimal pocket depth is present. *(From 2nd SA Edition.)*

Key points

- Periodontitis results in various types of osseous defects. The most common is the horizontal bone defect. However, defects such as buttressing bone formation, ledges, plateau, inconsistent bone margin, reverse architecture, etc. are frequently encountered, whereas two- or three-walled angular defects are amenable for regenerative procedures, other defects may require resective osseous surgery.
- Osteoplasty is the reshaping of bone without removing part of the supporting tissue, whereas ostectomy refers to recontouring by removing part of the bone that provides support.
- Properly and judiciously performed resective osseous surgery results in not only complete elimination of periodontal pockets but also tissue form conducive for maintenance of periodontal health.

Suggested Readings

Carnevale G, Kaldahl WB: Osseous resective surgery. *J Periodontol* 22:59–87, 2000.

Dibart S, Dibart J-P: *Practical osseous surgery in periodontics and implant dentistry*, 2011, Wiley-Blackwell.

CHAPTER 48

Periodontal Regeneration and Reconstructive Surgery

RT Kao | HH Takei | DL Cochran | ML Nevins | CD Dwarakanath

CHAPTER OUTLINE

Periodontal diseases result in the destruction of the attachment apparatus to a varying degree. Although arrest of further disease progression is the immediate goal, the ideal outcome would be regeneration and reconstruction of the lost tissues (Fig. 48.1A–C). In the last 3 decades, considerable research, both basic and clinical, has been done in an endeavor to obtain complete regeneration and reconstitution of periodontal structures.

Definition of terms such as repair, regeneration, and new attachment have been discussed in Chapter 28 (Fig. 48.2A–D).

Notwithstanding considerable progress in the direction of periodontal regeneration only three- and two-walled intrabony defects and grade 2 furcation involvements are amenable for predictable regeneration. The search for regeneration of supracrestal defects is still illusive.

Intrabony and **furcation** defects are sequelae of **periodontal disease**. Ideally, these defects are managed in a timely fashion through **periodontal** regeneration. In the past, the results of regenerative therapy were inconsistent and unpredictable. The current status of regenerative therapy has dramatically changed and improved due to research and a better understanding of the biology of the tissues that comprise the periodontal attachment. Various surgical approaches, including bone replacement grafts, guided tissue regeneration (GTR), and a better understanding of biologic mediators and tissue engineering have improved the predictability of regeneration. This chapter reviews the current strategies and clinical decision-making for optimizing regenerative success.

When the **periodontium** is damaged by **inflammation** or as a result of surgical treatment, the defect heals either through periodontal regeneration or repair. In periodontal regeneration, healing occurs through the reconstitution of a new periodontium, which involves the formation of **alveolar** bone, functionally aligned periodontal ligament, and new **cementum**. Alternatively, repair due to healing by replacement with epithelial and/or connective tissue that matures into various nonfunctional types of scar tissue is termed *new attachment*. Histologically, patterns of repair include long **junctional epithelium**, ankylosis, and/or new attachment. Although the stability of periodontal repair is not clear, the ideal goal of periodontal surgical therapy is periodontal regeneration.

Today, several highly reproducible regenerative approaches are used, as evidenced by clinical attachment gain, decreased pocket **probing depth**, radiographic evidence consistent with bone fill, and overall improvements in periodontal health. These clinical improvements can be maintained over long periods (often greater than 10 years).

Regeneration and Reconstructive Techniques

These techniques may be subdivided as follows.

1. Graft-assisted procedures using various types of bone grafts, enamel matrix derivatives, and so on.
2. Nongraft-associated techniques such as GTR, laser assisted new attachment procedures (LANAP), and root surface bio-modification.
3. Advanced techniques such as use of growth factors, stem cells, and tissue engineering.

Graft Materials and Procedures

Numerous bone grafts have been developed over the last three 3 decades and wealth of data has been generated. Many of them have become obsolete and are of only historical interest.

Classification of Bone Grafts

Based on the origin:

1. Autografts: wherein the bone is obtained from the same individual.
2. Allografts: which are obtained from different individuals of same species.
3. Xenografts: meaning bone obtained from different species usually bovine or porcine origin.
4. Alloplasts: which are synthetic graft materials/bone substitutes.

Bone grafts may also be classified by the mode of their action as under:

1. Osteogenic grafts where in the grafted tissue contains the cells necessary to form new bone. Only auto grafts have this capacity and hence are considered as gold standard.

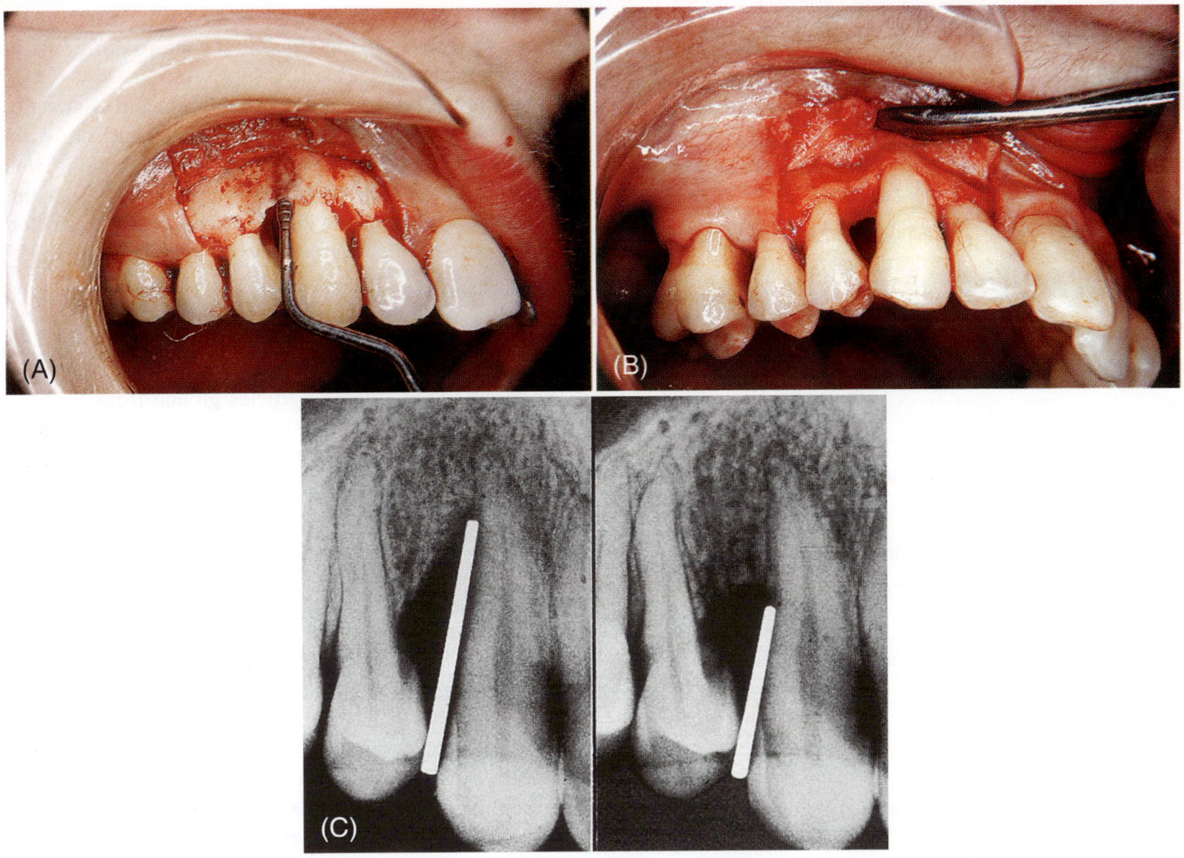

Fig. 48.1 A, Deep three-wall vertical osseous defect with measuring probe inserted. B, Reentry surgery 9 months after treatment shows repaired bone defect. C, Radiographs before and after treatment showing fill of angular osseous defect; gutta-percha points extend to base of pocket. *(From Glickman I: Clinical periodontology, ed 3, Philadelphia, 1964, Saunders.)*

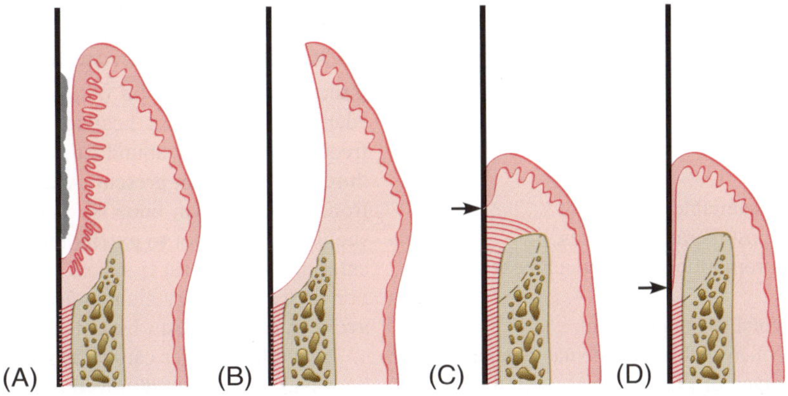

Fig. 48.2 A, Periodontal pocket preoperatively. B, Periodontal pocket immediately after scaling, root planing, and curettage. C, New attachment. The arrow indicates the most apical part of the junctional epithelium. Note regeneration of bone and periodontal ligament. D, Healing by long junctional epithelium. Again, the arrow indicates the most apical part of the junctional epithelium. Note that the bone is new, but the periodontal ligament is not.

2. Osteoinductive grafts which have the capacity to convert the surrounding tissue to form osteoblasts through the release of bone morphogenic proteins.
3. Osteoconductive which is a physical effect by which the matrix of the graft forms a scaffold that favors outside cells and blood vessels to penetrate graft and form new bone.
4. Osteoneutral graft is that which merely fills the bone defect without producing any effect and often gets encapsulated.

Depending on the rate of their bioresorption, grafts are classified as follows:

1. Fast resorbing wherein the graft gets resorbed within 8–10 weeks after placement.
2. Slow resorbing in which case the grafted material stays for many months.
3. Nonresorbing are those which do not resorb for years.

It is important for the clinician to understand the properties and origin of the materials and the purpose for which the graft material

TABLE 48.1 Commercially Available Biomaterials for Periodontal Regeneration

Biomaterial	Commercial Name
Allografts	
Demineralized freeze-dried bone allograft (DFDBA)	Distributed under various name by tissue banks
Freeze-dried bone allograft (FDBA)	Distributed under various name by tissue banks
Xenografts	
Anorganic bovine bone	Bio-Oss, OsteoGraf, Pep-Gen P-15
Hydroxyapatite (HA)	
Alloplasts	
Tricalcium phosphate	Synthograft
Hydroxyapatite	Periograf, Osteogen, ProOsteone
Bioactive glass polymers	PerioGlas, BioGran
Hard-tissue replacement polymer	Bioplant
Coralline calcium carbonate	Biocoral
Polymers and Collagens	
Collagen	CollaPlug, CollaCote, Gelfoam, Helistat
Poly(lactide-co-polyglycolide)	
Methylcellulose	
Hyaluronic acid ester	HY
Chitosan	

is intended to be used. Also it is the duty of the clinician to explain to his/her patients the source of the graft since the latter may have religious restrictions as to the type of the graft material that is been used in their mouth.

The properties of an ideal bone graft material:

1. Nontoxic.
2. Nonantigenic.
3. Resistant to infection.
4. Predictability.
5. Clinical feasibility.
6. Easy adaptability.
7. Readily and sufficiently available.
8. Minimal operative and postoperative hazards.
9. Adequate bone fill and promotion of new attachment including cementogenesis.
10. Cost-effective and acceptable to the patient.

Table 48.1 provides a list of available periodontal regeneration biomaterials. Regardless of the type of graft material used, the basic principles of approach are same. These include careful case selection and a meticulous phase 1 therapy and establishment of optimum plaque control. Trauma from occlusion may impair posttreatment healing of the supporting periodontal tissues, reducing the likelihood of new attachment. Occlusal adjustment, if needed, is therefore indicated. It is also preferable to splint mobile teeth before bone graft placement.

Systemic antibiotics are generally used after reconstructive periodontal therapy, although definitive information on the advisability of this measure is still lacking.

Graft Materials and Procedures

Autogenous Bone Grafts

Bone From Intraoral Sites

In 1923, Hegedüs attempted to use bone grafts for the reconstruction of bone defects produced by periodontal disease. The method was revived by Nabers and O'Leary in 1965 and numerous efforts have been made since that time to define its indications and technique.

Sources of bone include bone from healing extraction wounds, bone from edentulous ridges, bone trephined from within the jaw without damaging the roots, newly formed bone in wounds especially created for the purpose, bone removed from tuberosity or the ramus, bone removed during osteoplasty and ostectomy and the lingual surface of the mandible or maxilla at least 5 mm from the roots.

Osseous Coagulum. Robinson described a technique using a mixture of bone dust and blood that he termed "osseous coagulum." The technique uses small particles ground from cortical bone. The advantage of the particle size is that it provides additional surface area for the interaction of cellular and vascular elements (Fig. 48.3A–D).

Bone is removed with a carbide bur #6 or #8 at speeds between 5000 and 30,000 rpm, placed in a sterile dappen dish and used to fill the defect. The obvious advantage of this technique is the ease of obtaining bone from an area already exposed during surgery. The disadvantages are its relatively low predictability and the inability to procure adequate material for large defects. Although notable success has been reported by many individuals, studies documenting the efficacy of the technique are still inconclusive.

Bone Blend. Some disadvantages of osseous coagulum derive from the inability to use aspiration during accumulation of the coagulum. Another problem is the unknown quantity and quality of the bone fragments in the collected material. To overcome these problems, the "bone blend technique" has been proposed.

The bone-blend technique uses an autoclaved plastic capsule and pestle. Bone is removed from a predetermined site, triturated in the capsule to a workable, plastic-like mass, and packed into bony defects. Froum et al. found osseous coagulum–bone blend procedures to be at least as effective as iliac autografts and open curettage.

Cancellous Bone Marrow Transplants

Cancellous bone can be obtained from the maxillary tuberosity, edentulous areas, and healing sockets. The maxillary tuberosity frequently contains abundant cancellous bone, particularly if the third molars are not present. After a ridge incision is made distally from the last molar, bone is removed with a curved rongeur. Care should be taken not to extend the incision too far distally to avoid entering the mucosal tissue of the pharyngeal area. Also, the location of the maxillary sinus must be analyzed on the radiograph to avoid entering or disturbing it.

Edentulous ridges can be approached with a flap and cancellous bone and marrow are removed with curettes, back-action chisels, or trephine. Extraction sockets are allowed to heal for 8–12 weeks before re-entering and removing the newly formed bone from the apical portion, which is used as the donor material.

Bone Swaging

The bone swaging technique requires an edentulous area adjacent to the defect, from which the bone is pushed into contact with the root surface without fracturing the bone at its base. Bone swaging is technically difficult and its usefulness is limited.

Bone From Extraoral Sites

In 1923, Hegedüs also pioneered the use of extra oral sites as a source of bone for grafting into periodontal osseous defects, using bone from the tibia. Schallhorn and Hiatt revived this approach in the 1960s using the iliac crest (Fig. 48.4A–F).

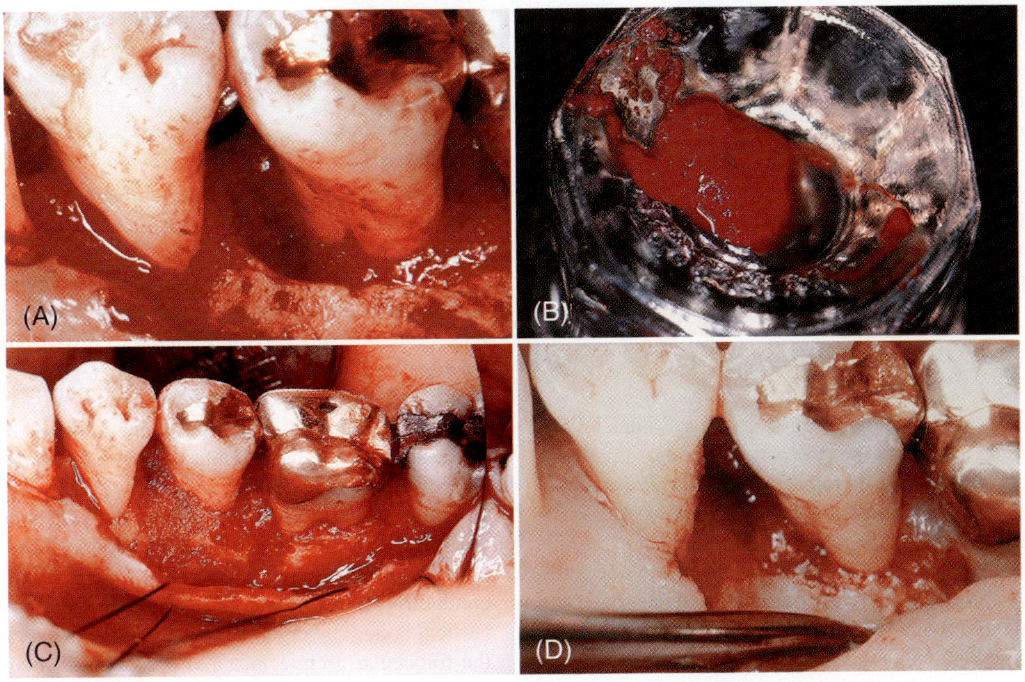

Fig. 48.3 A, Osseous defect mesial to a second premolar. B, Graft material placed in dappen dish before transfer to the graft site. C, Material in place. D, Reentry 6 months later. *(Courtesy: Dr. E. Earl Robinson.)*

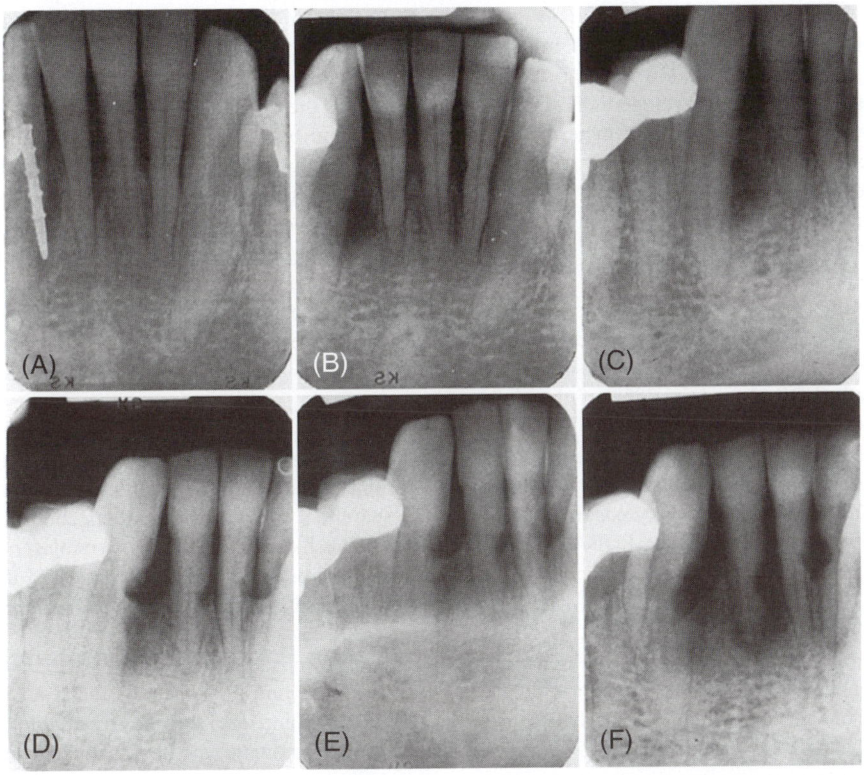

Fig. 48.4 A, November 1973: Radiograph of a patient immediately before placement of a fresh iliac autograft. B, Two months later, bone repair is evident. Note the early radiolucent areas on the mesial aspect of the canine. C, After 7 months, "bone fill" is occurring, but obvious root resorption is present. D, April 1975: Root resorption is apparent on all grafted teeth. Note the obvious degree of fill of the original bone defects. E, February 1976: Further involvement. F, October 1977: Four years later, root resorption has progressed into the pulp of the lateral incisor, causing a periosteal-endosteal complication.

The use of fresh or preserved iliac cancellous marrow bone has been extensively investigated. This material has been used by orthopedic surgeons for years. Data from human and animal studies support its use, and the technique has proved successful in osseous defects with various numbers of walls. It has also been successful in furcations and even supracrestally to some extent. However, because of numerous problems associated with its use, the technique is no longer in use. Some of the problems were postoperative infection, bone exfoliation, sequestration, varying rates of healing, root resorption, and rapid recurrence of the defect. Other problems were increased patient's expense and difficulty in procuring the donor material.

Bone Allografts

Obtaining donor material for autograft purposes necessitates inflicting surgical trauma on another part of the patient's body. Obviously, it would be to the patient's and therapist's advantage if a suitable substitute could be used for grafting purposes that would offer similar potential for repair and not require the additional surgical removal of donor material from the patient. However, both allografts and xenografts are foreign to the patient and, therefore, have the potential to provoke an immune response. Attempts have been made to suppress the antigenic potential of allografts and xenografts by radiation, freezing, and chemical treatment. Bone allografts are commercially available from tissue banks. They are obtained from cortical bone within 12 h of the death of the donor, defatted, cut in pieces, washed in absolute alcohol, and deep-frozen. The material may then be demineralized and subsequently ground and sieved to a particle size of 250–750 μm and freeze-dried. Finally, it is vacuum-sealed in glass vials.

Numerous steps are also taken to eliminate viral infectivity. These include exclusion of donors from known high-risk groups and various tests on the cadaver tissues to exclude individuals with any type of infection or malignant disease. The material is then treated with chemical agents or strong acids to inactivate the virus, if still present. The risk of human immunodeficiency virus (HIV) infection has been calculated as 1 in 1–8 million and is therefore characterized as highly remote.

Freeze-Dried Bone Allograft

Several clinical studies by Mellonig, Bowers, and coworkers reported bone fill exceeding 50% in 67% of the defects grafted with freeze-dried bone allograft (FDBA) and in 78% of the defects grafted with FDBA plus autogenous bone. FDBA, however, is considered an osteoconductive material, whereas demineralized FDBA (DFDBA) is considered an osteoinductive graft. Laboratory studies have found that DFDBA has a higher osteogenic potential than FDBA and is therefore preferred. However, FDBA being slow resorbing is often used in guided bone regeneration.

Demineralized Freeze-Dried Bone Allograft

Experiments by Urist have established the osteogenic potential of DFDBA. Demineralization in cold, diluted hydrochloric acid exposes the components of bone matrix, which are closely associated with collagen fibrils and have been termed *bone morphogenetic proteins* (BMPs).

Studies have provided strong evidence that DFDBA in periodontal defects results in significant probing depth reduction, attachment level gain, and osseous regeneration. The combination of DFDBA and GTR has also proved to be very successful. However, limitations of the use of DFDBA include the possible, although remote, potential of disease transfer from the cadaver.

A bone-inductive protein isolated from the extracellular matrix of human bones, termed *osteogenin* or *BMP-3*, has been tested in human periodontal defects and seems to enhance osseous regeneration.

Xenografts

Bone products from other species have a long history of use in periodontal therapy. Many of them, however, are no longer in use today.

Calf bone (Boplant), treated by detergent extraction, sterilized and freeze-dried, has been used for the treatment of osseous defects. Kiel bone is calf or ox bone denatured with 20% hydrogen peroxide, dried with acetone, and sterilized with ethylene oxide. Anorganic bone is ox bone from which the organic material has been extracted by means of ethylenediamine. It is then sterilized by autoclaving. These materials have been tried and discarded for various reasons.

Currently, an anorganic, bovine-derived bone marketed under the brand name Bio-Oss (Osteohealth) has been successfully used both for periodontal defects and in implant surgery. It is an osteoconductive, porous bone mineral matrix from bovine cancellous or cortical bone. The organic components of the bone are removed, but the trabecular architecture and porosity are retained. The physical features permit clot stabilization and revascularization to allow for migration of osteoblasts, leading to osteogenesis. Bio-Oss is biocompatible with the adjacent tissues, eliciting no systemic immune response.

Several studies have reported successful bone regeneration and new attachment with Bio-Oss in periodontal defects, as well as regeneration around implants and sinus grafting.

Periodontally, Bio-Oss has been used as a graft material covered with a resorbable membrane (Geistlich Bio-Gide). The membrane prevents the migration of fibroblasts and connective tissues into the pores and between the granules of the graft. Histologic studies of this technique have shown significant osseous regeneration and cementum formation.

Yukna et al. have used Bio-Oss in combination with a cell-binding polypeptide (P-15) that is a synthetic analog of a 15–amino acid sequence of type I collagen marketed as PepGen P-15 (Dentsply/CeraMed). This combination seems to enhance the bone-regenerative results of the matrix alone in periodontal defects.

Alloplasts (Synthetic Bone Graft Materials)

Risk of disease transmission albeit unlikely and religious constraints of the patients regarding the source of the grafts made the researchers to look for synthetic bone replacement grafts. Many materials like plaster of Paris, ceramics, polymers, bioactive glasses, and coral-derived materials came into the market. Many of them disappeared as quickly as they were introduced.

Calcium Phosphate Biomaterials

Several calcium phosphate biomaterials have been tested since the mid-1970s and are currently available for clinical use. Calcium phosphate biomaterials have excellent tissue compatibility and do not elicit any inflammation or foreign body response. These materials are osteoconductive and, therefore, act as a scaffold for blood clots to be retained to allow bone formation.

Two types of calcium phosphate ceramics have been used:

1. Hydroxyapatite (HA) has a calcium-to-phosphate ratio of 1.67, similar to that found in bone material. HA is generally nonbioresorbable.

2. Tricalcium phosphate (TCP), with a calcium-to-phosphate ratio of 1.5, is otherwise called whitlockite. TCP is at least partially bioresorbable.

Case reports and uncontrolled human studies have shown that calcium phosphate bioceramic materials are well tolerated and can result in clinical repair of periodontal lesions. Several controlled studies were conducted on the use of hydroxyl apatite (Periograf) and Calcitite. Clinical results were good, but histologically these materials appeared to be encapsulated by collagen.

Bioactive Glass

Bioactive glass consists of sodium and calcium salts, phosphates, and silicon dioxide. For its dental applications, it is used in the form of irregular particles measuring 90–170 μm (PerioGlas, Block Drug, Jersey City, NJ) or 300–355 μm (BioGran, Ortho Vita, Malvern, PA). When this material comes into contact with tissue fluids, the surface of the particles becomes coated with hydroxy-carbonate apatite, incorporates organic ground proteins such as chondroitin sulfate and glycosaminoglycans, and attracts osteoblasts that rapidly form bone.

Coral-Derived Materials

Two different coralline materials have been used in clinical periodontics: natural coral and coral-derived porous hydroxyapatite. Both are biocompatible, but whereas natural coral is resorbed slowly (several months), porous hydroxyapatite is not resorbed or takes years for resorption.

Clinical studies on these materials showed pocket reduction, attachment gain, and bone level gain. Coral-derived materials have also been studied in conjunction with membranes, with good results. Both materials have demonstrated microscopic cementum and bone formation, but their slow resorbability or lack of resorption has hindered clinical success in practice.

Nongraft Associated Reconstructive Procedures

The following sections discuss the rationale and techniques that must be considered for a successful outcome in achieving new attachment or periodontal bone regeneration in response to nongraft associated reconstructive surgical therapy. Of these procedures, GTR is the main procedure used in clinical practice. Recent evidences suggest that LANAP may also result in new attachment and regeneration but further clinical trial are needed to test its efficacy and parameter for success.

Guided Tissue Regeneration

GTR is used for the prevention of epithelial migration along the cemental wall of the pocket and maintaining space for clot stabilization. Derived from the classic studies of Nyman, Lindhe, Karring, and Gottlow, this method is based on the assumption that periodontal ligament and perivascular cells have the potential for regeneration of the attachment apparatus of the tooth. GTR consists of placing barriers of different types (membranes) to cover the bone and periodontal ligament, thus temporarily separating them from the gingival epithelium and connective tissue. Excluding the epithelium and the gingival connective tissue from the root surface during the postsurgical healing phase not only prevents epithelial migration into the wound but also favors repopulation of the area by cells from the periodontal ligament and the bone. It should be noted that in the United States, GTR is often performed with some type of bone graft as a scaffolding agent, so it is a combined therapy. In Europe and other parts of the world, where regulatory and religious constraints makes human graft materials unavailable, so it is performed as a traditional GTR procedure and may be occasionally used in conjunction with a other graft materials as a combined therapy.

Initial animal experiments using Millipore filters and Teflon membranes resulted in regeneration of cementum and alveolar bone and a functional periodontal ligament. Clinical case reports indicate that GTR results in a gain in attachment level. Histologic studies in humans provided evidence of periodontal reconstruction in most cases, even with horizontal bone loss. The use of polytetrafluoroethylene (PTFE) membranes has been tested in controlled clinical studies in mandibular molar furcations and has shown statistically significant decreases in pocket depths and improvement in attachment levels after 6 months, but bone level measurements have been inconclusive. A study on maxillary molar furcations did not result in significant gain in attachment or bone levels. With the regenerative success associated with the use of nonresorbable membrane, the advantage and disadvantage of this approach became apparent. Notably, problems such as membrane exposure, which resulted in no or limited regeneration and the need for a secondary procedure for surgical removal resulted in the development of biodegradable membranes. Today in clinical practice, most GTR procedures use biodegradable membranes while the nonresorbable membranes are used for implant site development. Nevertheless, the historical research using nonresorbable membranes and the development of various types of biodegradable membranes is valuable.

Nonresorbable Membranes

In classic animal and human studies demonstrating the efficacy of GTR, cellulose acetate filters were used. As this technique became more prevalent, the first commercial membrane was produced from expanded polytetrafluoroethylene (ePTFE). This membrane has all the properties necessary for GTR barriers in that it (1) is a cellular barrier; (2) is biocompatible; (3) provides space for the healing tissue; (4) permits tissue integration; and (5) is clinically manageable. Much of our current understanding of GTR is based on studies using ePTFE membranes. Although they are used less frequently now, they are still popular for guided bone regeneration and ridge preservation, so it is important to understand the clinical procedures for managing these membranes.

The clinical effectiveness of ePTFE membranes is dependent on technique. Preservation of the keratinized gingiva and a relatively thick overlying surgical flap are critical to avoid perforation of the flap by the membrane during healing. After the surgical area has been flapped, the defect is degranulated and the root surface scaled and root planed. The ePTFE membrane is trimmed to adapt to tooth configuration, secured by ePTFE sutures and the flap repositioned. It is interesting to note that, although much of the emphasis in the literature is on adapting the membrane to the defect, no membrane can ever be perfectly adapted. Despite gaps, these membranes seem to work. After membrane placement, healing is allowed to proceed for 4–6 weeks. Barring any membrane exposure, a second surgery is performed to remove the membrane. During this removal, the healing tissue appears reddish and granulomatous. After membrane removal, the area should not be probed for 3 months. Radiographic evidence of bone fill is usually present after 6 months and should continue over the course of 1 year.

Clinical studies have shown that ePTFE membranes used in GTR procedures are more effective than surgical debridement in correcting intrabony defects. In intrabony and furcation defects, there are gains in clinical attachment level (3–6 mm), improved bone levels (2.4–4.8 mm), and probing depth reductions (3.5–6 mm). Studies have demonstrated that these regenerative results can be maintained over the course of several years.

The advent of titanium-reinforced ePTFE allowed for the formation of larger spaces, thus permitting correction of larger defects. This resulted in significant clinical improvements using titanium-reinforced ePTFE compared to ePTFE.

To determine how regeneration can be enhanced with GTR technique, the prolonged retention of ePTFE membranes was evaluated. After allowing the membrane to be retained for 4 months, surgical re-entry after 1 year determined that the mean bone fill of intrabony defects was 95%. This suggests that prolonged retention of a barrier membrane is desirable if no tissue perforation is present. This is consistent with many clinical reports of the improved bone quality associated with guided bone regeneration in implant site development.

The major problem with using nonresorbable membranes is that the membrane is exposed to the oral environment during healing. Upon exposure, the membrane is contaminated and colonized by oral microflora. Several studies have shown that contamination of the surgical field can result in decreased formation of new attachment. If the membrane is exposed, the infection can be temporarily managed with topical application of chlorhexidine. This may minimize the infection and extend the time the membrane can be retained in place.

Biodegradable Membranes

Bioresorbable membranes have replaced the routine use of ePTFE membranes in GTR. There are basically three types of bioresorbable membranes: (1) polyglycoside synthetic polymers (i.e., polylactic acid, polylactate/polygalactate copolymers), (2) collagen, and (3) calcium sulfate. Polyglycoside membranes degrade as the result of random nonenzymatic cleavage of the polymer, producing polylactide and polyglycolide, which are converted to lactic acid and pyruvate, respectively, and metabolized by the enzymes of the Krebs cycle. Porcine collagen membranes are degraded by collagenases and subsequently by gelatinases and peptidases. There has been resurgence in the use of calcium sulfate as a regeneration material because it can be used as a pavable resorbable barrier when used in combination with bone or bone substitutes. The calcium sulfate is bioresorbed through a giant cell reaction. Several features make these bioresorbable membranes easier to manage clinically: (1) they are more tissue compatible than nonresorbable membranes, (2) the timing for resorption can be regulated by the amount of cross-linkage in the synthetic polymer and collagen membrane or the amount of heat-processed calcium sulfate chips in calcium sulfate barrier, and (3) a second surgical procedure is not required to retrieve the nonresorbable membrane.

A recent GTR study compared the use of bioresorbable membranes (polylactate/polygalactate copolymer) versus ePTFE membranes, with surgical debridement as a control. After 1 year, significant gains in clinical attachment level (CAL) were observed in all three groups (Fig. 48.5A–E). There was no difference in CAL gain between the two membrane groups, with both of them gaining 2 mm or more. In both membrane groups, 83% of the sites improved 4 mm or more, which was significantly better than the surgical debridement control group. These findings indicate GTR procedures are equally effective using resorbable and nonresorbable membranes. This finding has been confirmed by other investigators.

The search for resorbable membranes has included trials and tests with numerous materials and collagens from different species, such as bovine and porcine. Cargile membrane is derived from the cecum of an ox, polylactic acid, Vicryl (polyglactin 910), synthetic skin (Biobrane), and freeze-dried dura mater. Clinical studies with a mixture of copolymers derived from polylactic acid and acetyl tributyl citrate resorbable membranes (Guidor membrane, no longer on the market) and a poly-D, L-lactide-co-glycolide (Resolut membrane, also no longer on the market) have shown significant gains in clinical attachment and bone fill.

The potential of using autogenous periosteum as a membrane and also to stimulate periodontal regeneration has been explored in two controlled clinical studies, one of grade II furcation involvements in mandibular molars and another of interdental defects. The periosteum was obtained from the patient's palate by means of a window flap. Both studies reported that autogenous periosteal grafts can be used in GTR and result in significant gains in clinical attachment and osseous defect fill.

Laser-Assisted New Attachment Procedure

The role of laser in periodontal therapy has gained popularity. Nevertheless, the use of neodymium-yttrium-aluminum-garnet (Nd:YAG) to perform surgical LANAP has been reported for the management of chronic periodontitis and can potentially result in new attachment and periodontal regeneration.

Many questions remain about LANAP that need to be clarified. The first is the exact mechanism and parameter by which healing by new attachment versus regeneration occur with LANAP therapy. Additionally, a blinded split mouth study to compare LANAP protocol to other existing periodontal therapies is in progress and needs to be completed. This along with other randomized controlled trials will be needed for metaanalysis to determine if LANAP is equivalent or superior to other conventional therapy. As with all periodontal therapy, the long-term stability of the regeneration needs to be explored.

Biomodification of Root Surface

Changes in the tooth surface wall of periodontal pockets (e.g., degenerated remnants of Sharpey's fibers, accumulation of bacteria and their products, disintegration of cementum and dentin) interfere with new attachment. Although these obstacles to new attachment can be eliminated by thorough root planing, the root surface of the pocket can be treated to improve its chances of accepting the new attachment of gingival tissues.

Several substances have been proposed for this purpose including citric acid, fibronectin, and tetracycline.

Citric Acid. There has been a series of studies one of which applied citric acid to the roots to demineralize the surface, attempting to induce cementogenesis and attachment of collagen fibers.

The following actions of citric acid have been reported:

1. Accelerated healing and new cementum formation occur after surgical detachment of the gingival tissues and demineralization of the root surface by means of citric acid. Topically applied citric acid on periodontally diseased root surfaces has no effect on nonplaned roots, but after root planing, the acid produces a 4-μm-deep demineralized zone with exposed collagen fiber. Root planed, noncitric acid treated roots are left with a surface smear layer of microcrystalline debris. Citric acid application not only removes the smear layer, exposing the dentinal tubules, but also makes the tubules appear wider and with funnel-shaped orifices.
2. Citric acid has also been shown in vitro to eliminate endotoxins and bacteria from the diseased tooth surface.
3. An early fibrin linkage to collagen fibers exposed by the citric acid treatment prevents the epithelium from migrating over-treated roots.

This technique using citric acid has been extensively investigated in animals and humans. Studies in dogs have shown encouraging results, especially for the treatment of furcation lesions, but the results in humans have been contradictory.

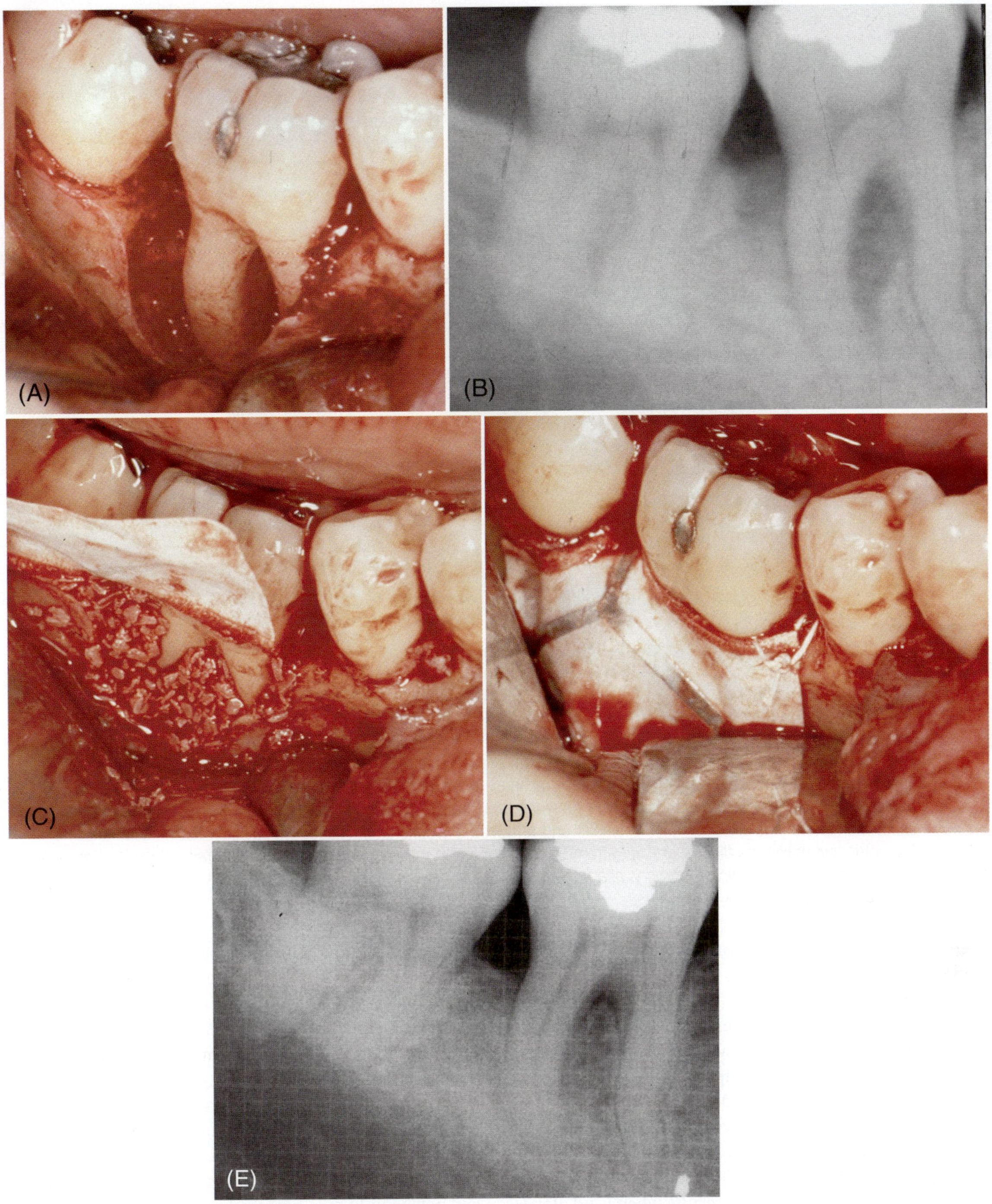

Fig. 48.5 Clinical photographs and radiographs of a guided tissue regeneration case using expanded polytetrafluoroethylene (ePTFE) with titanium-reinforced membrane. The osseous defect was along the distal interproximal area wrapping buccally over the furcation (A and B). To prevent the membrane from collapsing over the root surfaces, demineralized freeze-dried bone allograft (DFDBA) and adjusting the titanium membrane provide a larger space for regeneration (C and D). One year afterward, the radiographic and clinical signs are consistent with achieving regeneration in this defect (E). *(Courtesy: Rose L, et al, editor: Periodontics: medicine, surgery, and implants, Elsevier Mosby, 2004.)*

The recommended citric acid technique is as follows:

1. Raise a mucoperiosteal flap and thoroughly instrument the root surface, removing calculus and underlying cementum.
2. Apply cotton pledgets soaked in a saturated solution of citric acid (pH of 1.0) for 2–5 min.
3. Remove pledgets and irrigate root surface profusely with water.
4. Replace the flap and suture.

The use of citric acid has also been recommended in conjunction with coverage of denuded roots using free gingival grafts.

Fibronectin. Fibronectin is the glycoprotein that fibroblasts require to attach to root surfaces. The addition of fibronectin to the root surface may promote new attachment. However, increasing fibronectin above plasma levels produces no obvious advantages.

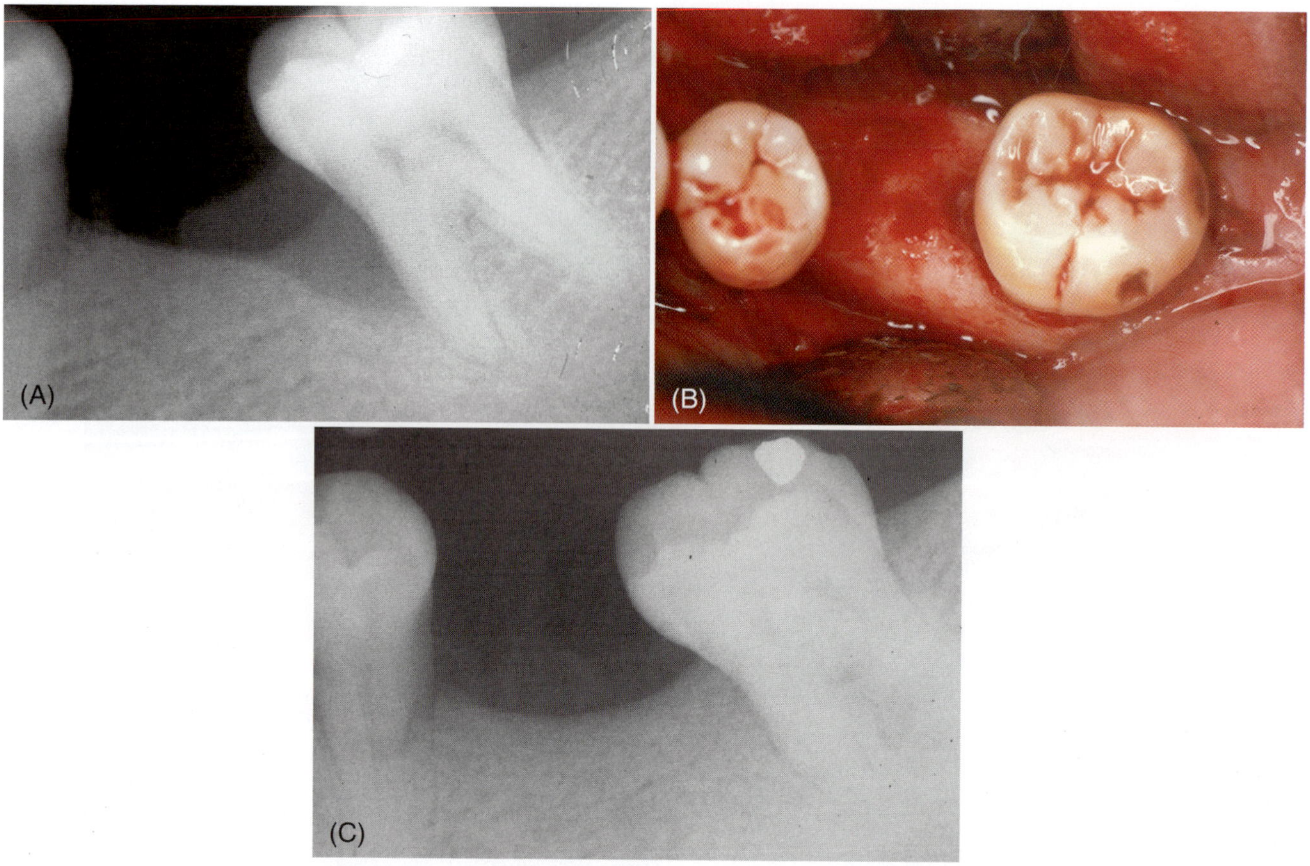

Fig. 48.6 Radiographs of a guided tissue regeneration (GTR) case using a nonresorbable expanded polytetrafluoroethylene (ePTFE) membrane. The mesially inclined molar is associated with a three-walled intraosseous defect (A and B). The defect was filled with demineralized freeze-dried bone allograft (DFDBA) and ePTFE was used. Membrane was exposed after 8 weeks and removed 2 weeks later. Radiographic "fill" was halfway after 6 months and maximum fill was present after 12 months (C) with minimal probing depth. *(Courtesy: Rose L, et al, editor: Periodontics: medicine, surgery, and implants, St Louis, Elsevier Mosby, 2004.)*

Adding fibronectin and citric acid to lesions treated with GTR in dogs did not improve the results.

Tetracycline. In vitro treatment of the dentin surfaces with tetracycline increases binding of fibronectin, which in turn stimulates fibroblast attachment and growth while suppressing epithelial cell attachment and migration. Tetracycline also removes an amorphous surface layer and exposes the dentin tubules. In vivo studies, however, have not shown favorable results. A human study showed a trend for greater connective tissue attachment after tetracycline treatment of roots. Tetracycline gave better results when used alone than when combined with fibronectin. It has been used as an adjunctive procedure in preparation of the root in regenerative procedures and is a recommended step for use with biologic mediators.

Other Techniques

Removal of junctional and sulcular epithelium, intentional interdental denudation, free gingival graft in the interproximal area, excisional new attachment procedure (ENAP), coronally advanced flap, etc. have been tried in the past to obtain periodontal regeneration but with little success and hence are not in vogue today.

Combined Techniques

Periodontal new attachment and bone reconstruction have been a challenge for the clinicians throughout the history of periodontal therapy. To take advantage of the different bone graft materials and biologic mediators, clinicians have combined these graft materials along with the use of membranes in an attempt to find a predictable technique to regenerate bone (Fig. 48.6A–C).

Several clinicians have proposed a combination of the techniques previously described in an attempt to enhance their results. A classic paper published by Schallhorn and McClain in 1988 described a combination technique using graft material, root conditioning with citric acid, and coverage with a nonresorbable membrane (the only available one at the time). More recently, with the advent of osteopromotive agents, such as the enamel matrix derivative (Emdogain) and osteoconductive bovine-derived anorganic bone (Bio-Oss) graft materials, other combination techniques have been advocated. The combined use of these products, along with autogenous bone with resorbable membrane coverage, has resulted in an increased percentage of cases with successful new attachment and periodontal reconstruction. Many of these combination techniques were reviewed in the previous sections of this chapter. Whereas the use of combination technique may be appealing, it is important for clinicians to remember that these added materials often escalate the cost of the procedure and should be balanced with the quality and the long-term stability of the clinical results.

Factors That Influence Therapeutic Success

Factors that adversely affect periodontal regeneration were reviewed at the 1996 World Workshop in Periodontics and 1997

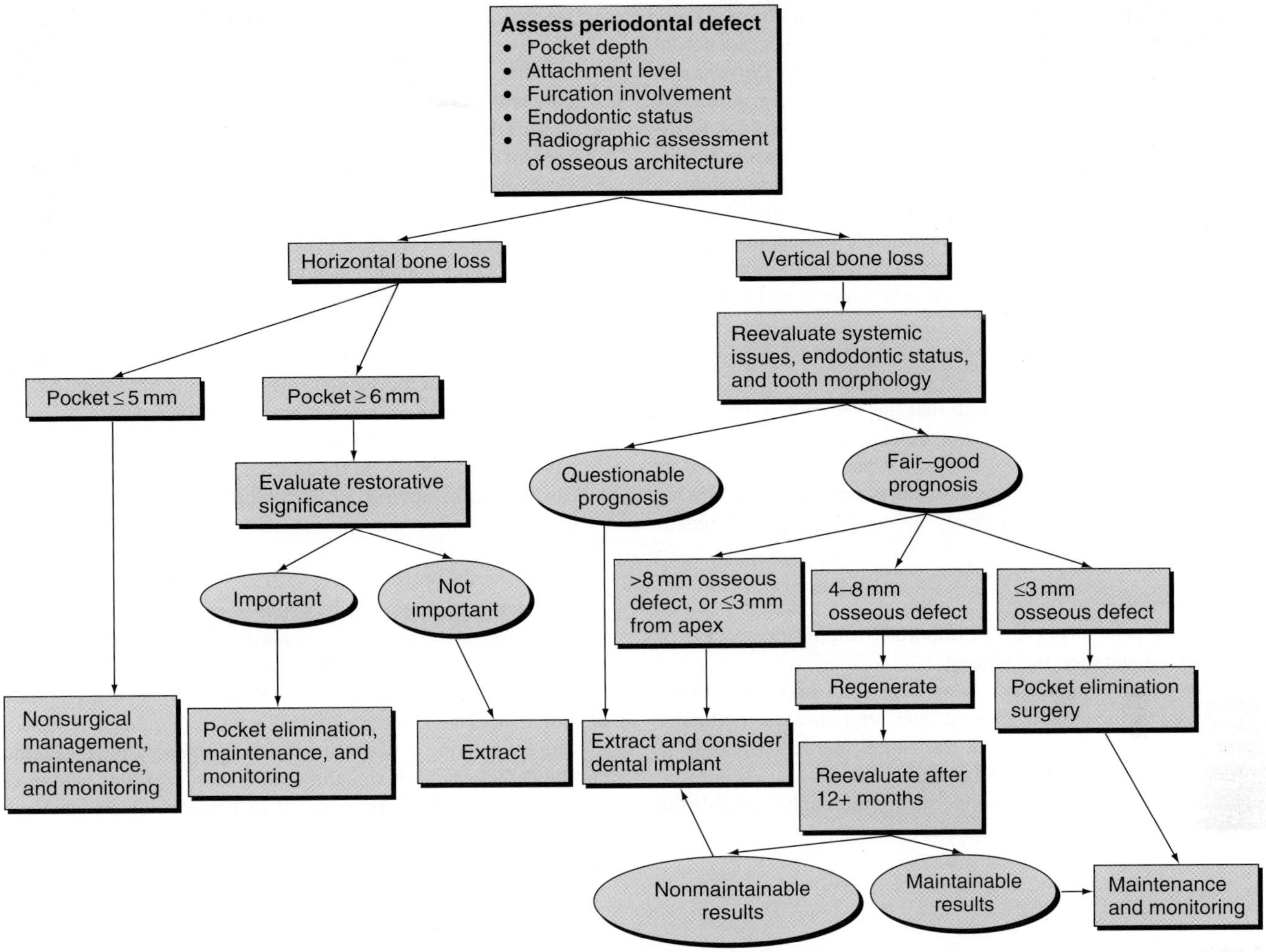

Fig. 48.7 Clinical decision tree for the management of advanced periodontitis.

Proceedings of the Second European Workshop on Periodontology. A number of factors have been implicated or shown to adversely influence periodontal regenerative therapy. These include site selection for reconstructive therapy, patient selection with consideration for compliance, and behavior habits such as smoking and surgical management.

Site Selection for Reconstructive Therapy

Therapeutic Selection

The selection of appropriate therapeutic approach is one that is based on accurate assessment of the periodontal defect, one's past clinical experience, and familiarity with the various regenerative and resective techniques. A clinical decision tree is provided to guide the clinician in deciding the appropriate situations (Fig. 48.7). As the new therapeutic approaches are developed, the clinical decision tree may need to be modified to accommodate for these advances.

Tooth and Defect Selection

Therapeutic success is influenced by the tooth's importance in the prosthetic rehabilitation, its endodontic status, and defect characteristics.

The critical question to be addressed is if the involved tooth is strategically important. If not, the strategic extraction may avoid potential technical difficulty, postsurgical complications, and expenses. Strategic extraction may also improve access of better patient oral hygiene and compliance.

Once a tooth is deemed essential, it is important to assess its endodontic status. If the tooth is endodontically healthy, regeneration may proceed. If not, then treatment of the endodontic component must be performed and resolution of the endodontic problem must be ascertained prior to the regenerative procedure. Given the expense for endodontic treatment, periodontal regenerative procedures, crown buildup and the crown, strategic extraction, and possible replacement with prosthesis or a dental implant should be seriously considered.

Characteristics of the defect, such as the overall defect depth, width, and walls, can influence clinical outcome in response to regenerative surgery. Studies have consistently shown that the deeper defect is correlated with increased clinical attachment level and probing depth. One is more likely to achieve improved regenerative results in narrow and circumferential, three- or two-walled configuration. Conversely, horizontal, one-walled, and wide defects are less amenable to regenerative procedures. Barring early reports on the use of iliac and autologous grafts, current regenerative approaches have not been consistently successful in regenerating horizontal and one-walled defects.

Patient Selection

Poor Plaque Control and Compliance

Classical studies on of poor plaque control and poor postoperative recall compliance have indicated that much of the therapeutic gain from periodontal surgery will deteriorate. Similarly, the positive results from GTR regenerative procedure have been shown to deteriorate with poor compliance. Progressive deterioration in these patients has been demonstrated to possess a higher incidence of infection with putative periodontal pathogens (*Porphyromonas gingivalis, Prevotella intermedia,* and *Aggregatibacter actinomycetemcomitans*). Areas that are difficult to maintain, such as furcation and root proximity situations, have also been shown to be difficult to be maintained. As a result, risk for deterioration is higher. It is important to remember that the patient came in with behavioral and anatomical issues, which resulted in the periodontal defect. After therapy, the hardest challenge is to continue to motivate patients to be highly enthusiastic about oral hygiene and compliant with periodontal maintenance.

Smoking

Smoking is a behavioral challenge that the therapist must always assess. Smoking not only promotes disease progression but also results in adverse therapeutic outcomes. It has been implicated as having a detrimental effect on periodontal wound healing following surgical procedures and to adversely influence periodontal regeneration.

Surgical Factors

The following principles play an important role in the success of periodontal regeneration techniques:

1. Correct incisions: Usually access flaps with maximum tissue conservation for optimal closure later are indicated. Particular care should be taken to retain the entire interdental papilla in order to obtain close approximation.
2. Thorough debridement: It is important to thoroughly debride the area free of diseased tissue and local irritants.
3. Decortication: Often following removal of granulation tissue, the osseous defects become dry. In such situations, healthy bleeding should be promoted by decortication using small round burs with copious irrigation.
4. Presuturing: It is always preferable to place presutures so as to prevent displacement of the graft material during suturing.
5. Graft placement: The bony defects should never be overfilled. The clinician has to be realistic as over enthusiastic placement of graft material results in poor outcome.
6. Optimal closure: Graft materials and membranes should be completely covered as exposure of the same leads to infections and consequently failure.
7. Periodontal dressing: It is recommended that periodontal dressings are avoided following GTR membrane placement as it may result in collapse of the membrane into the defect.
8. Postoperative care and maintenance: Ideally, the patients are advised not to brush on the grafted region for 3–4 weeks. They can instead be advised to use chlorhexidine mouth rinses. The importance of optimal plaque control need not be overemphasized.

Periodontal Regeneration Utilizing Biologics

A new approach for regeneration that departs from the use of grafting materials and/or bioexclusion with GTR membranes is the use of biologics. This category of regenerative approach is based on a tissue engineering concept of enhancing regeneration by augmenting the defect site with signaling molecules, scaffolds, and/or cells (Fig. 48.8). This appears to result in periodontal regeneration in a relatively more rapid pace of regeneration as well as faster

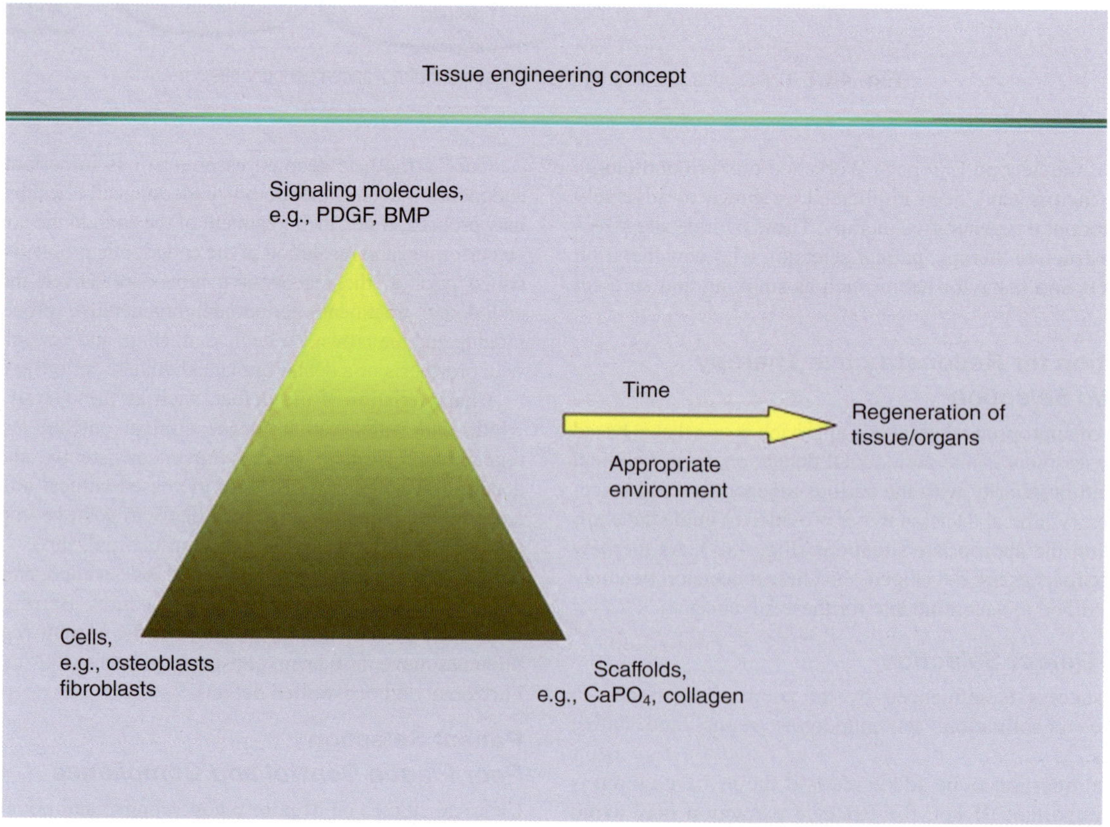

Fig. 48.8 Tissue engineering is the manipulation of one or more of the three elements: signaling molecules, scaffolds, or cells. *BMP*, Bone morphogenetic protein; *$CaPO_4$*, calcium phosphate; *PDGF*, platelet-derived growth factor. *(Courtesy Dr. Samuel Lynch.)*

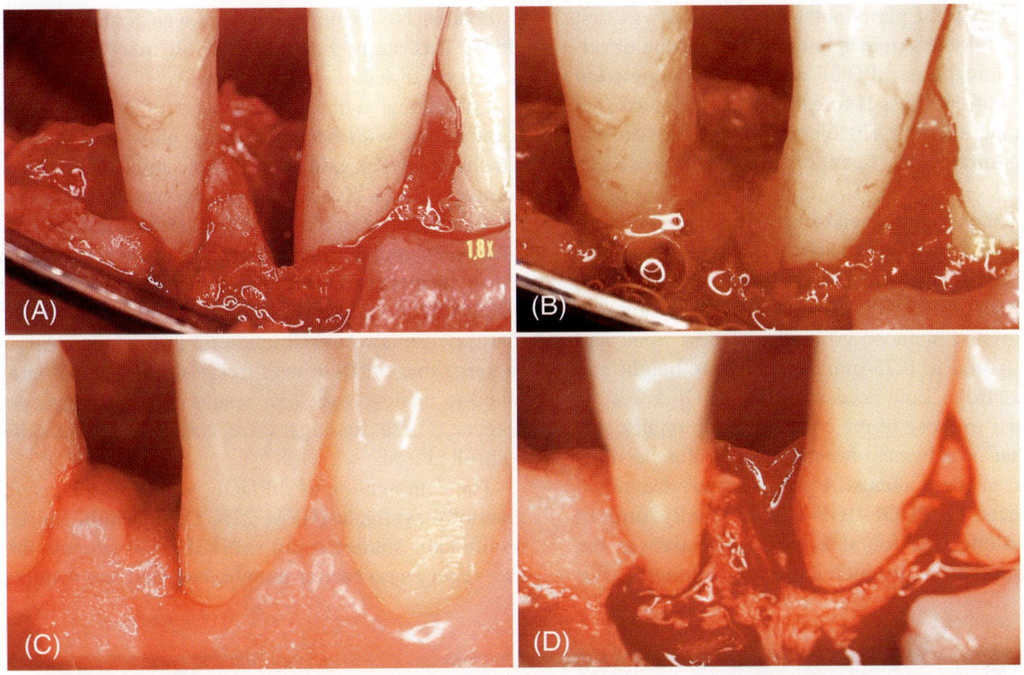

Fig. 48.9 A, Deep vertical bone loss distal to the lower left central incisor. B, Area flapped, root prepared, and defect filled with enamel matrix protein (Emdogain, Straumann, Andover, MA). C, Postoperative photograph 6 months later. D, Reentry surgery showing extensive bone fill. *(Courtesy Dr. Marco Orsini, Aquila, Italy.)*

response. This category consists of the use of enamel matrix derivative (EMD), recombinant human platelet-derived growth factor-BB (rhPDGF), osteogenic allograft, platelet rich plasma (PRP), and platelet rich fibrin (PRF). Other biologics, such as recombinant human bone morphogenetic protein (rhBMP) and recombinant fibroblast growth factor -2 (rhFGF), have undergone clinical trials but have not been FDA approved for clinical use and are discussed in the online material, *GTR membranes.*

Enamel Matrix Derivative

EMD has been available as a biologic periodontal regenerative material for 20 years. Several studies have provided human histologic evidence of intrabony regeneration associated with EMD therapy. EMD is present on root surfaces for ≥4 weeks after application, and early signs of periodontal wound regeneration can be observed after 2–6 weeks. Signs of clinical improvement are present as early as 6 months after treatment (Fig. 48.9).

Studies have evaluated the efficacy of EMD versus open flap debridement, with the majority confirming that debridement followed by EMD application resulted in substantial improvements in clinical measurements and bone fill in the management of intrabony defects. They also found that neither postoperative antibiotics nor EDTA root conditioning improved the clinical outcome of EMD therapy. In comparing EMD versus GTR, intrabony defect correction was comparable except in situations with deep, noncontained intrabony defects. In these defects, GTR with titanium reinforcement was superior. The latter results suggest that, in situations in which defect configuration is broad or lacking in wall containment, a supported barrier membrane may be critical to the success of EMD-associated regeneration. Additionally, no added clinical advantage was observed when EMD was combined with GTR.

There are several studies in which EMD has been used in combined therapy. Histologic evidence of periodontal regeneration has been demonstrated when EMD is used in combination with autogenous bone, allografts, a bovine-derived natural bone mineral (NBM), bioactive glass, NBM + PRP, or biphasic calcium phosphate. The majority of the studies indicated no added benefits in either clinical or radiographic gains when EMD is used with the addition of graft materials.

EMD remains a very intriguing biologic mediator. As we better understand the mechanism of action of the potpourri of proteins and **growth factors**, this may strengthen the biologic rationale for clinical use of this material. The concern remains whether commercial batches of EMD will be consistent and provide comparable clinical results in all cases. Perhaps the message is that the achievement of maximum regenerative response will require a mixture of biologic mediators. With further characterization of EMD, we may better develop a synergistic blend that will provide an optimal result.

In summary, EMD is a semipurified protein preparation from developing porcine teeth that contains a mixture of low-molecular-weight proteins. Although there were initial concerns about the poorly characterized nature of this preparation, recent reports suggest that the mixture may work synergistically on multiple levels to enhance periodontal regeneration. When applied to root surfaces, the proteins are absorbed into the hydroxyapatite and collagen fibers of the root surface, in which they induce cementum formation followed by periodontal regeneration. Clinical use of EMD can generally be characterized as safe, with excellent clinical healing and limited complications. EMD alone, or in combination with graft materials, provides clinical outcome and long-term clinical stability comparable with GTR. Although characterization of the EMD preparation remains incomplete, the challenge, as with allografts, is to provide a consistent batch of EMD, so the regenerative response is predictable.

Recombinant Human Platelet-Derived Growth Factor-BB for Periodontal Regeneration

Platelet-derived growth factor (PDGF) is one of the earliest growth factors studied for its effect on wound healing because it is a potent mitogenic and chemotactic factor for mesenchymal cells in cell

culture. Histologic evidence of periodontal regeneration was first reported in experimental defects in beagle dogs. During the development of PDGF for clinical use, rhPDGF was used in conjunction with allogenic bone to correct Class II furcations and interproximal intrabony defects on hopeless teeth. Histologic evidence of successful periodontal regeneration in the furcation lesion with excellent fill has been noted.

A human clinical trial was conducted using rhPDGF and recombinant human insulin-like growth factor 1 (rhIGF-1). Using a split-mouth design, defects were treated with either a low dose (50 μg/mL) or high dose (150 μg/mL) of rhPDGF–rhIGF-1. After 9 months, the high-dose rhPDGF–rhIGF-1 induced 2.08 mm of new bone and 43.2% defect fill, compared to 0.75-mm vertical bone height and 18.5% bone fill in controls. Low-dose rhPDGF–rhIGF-1 results were statistically similar to those of the controls. Additionally, this study demonstrated that no adverse immunologic or clinical reaction resulted from use of these agents. A primate study examined the regenerative effects of PDGF–IGF-1 individually and in combination. PDGF alone was found to be as effective as the PDGF–IGF-1 combination in producing new attachment after 3 months. No significant effect was found when IGF was used alone. This study suggests that IGF may not be important at the dose level tested.

Subsequently, the effectiveness of 0.3 mg/mL of rhPDGF in combination with beta tricalcium phosphate (β-TCP) to improve attachment level gain, bone level, and bone volume significantly compared to β-TCP alone was demonstrated after 6 months in a multicenter clinical trial. A subset of these patients was followed for 24 months, and a representative case series was reported to be stable, with increases in radiographic bone fill compared to the end results after 6 months (Fig. 48.10). A review of these cases indicates that the results were stable after 3 and 5 years. Another case series suggests that rhPDGF with freeze-dried bone allograft can be combined to achieve excellent results in severe periodontal intrabony defects. These findings were confirmed by another randomized controlled trial.

The combination of rhPDGF with a β-TCP carrier is now commercially available (GEM 21S, Osteohealth, Shirley, NY). These preliminary studies using rhPDGF-TCP suggest that it is easy to use, requires no barrier membranes, and has results comparable or

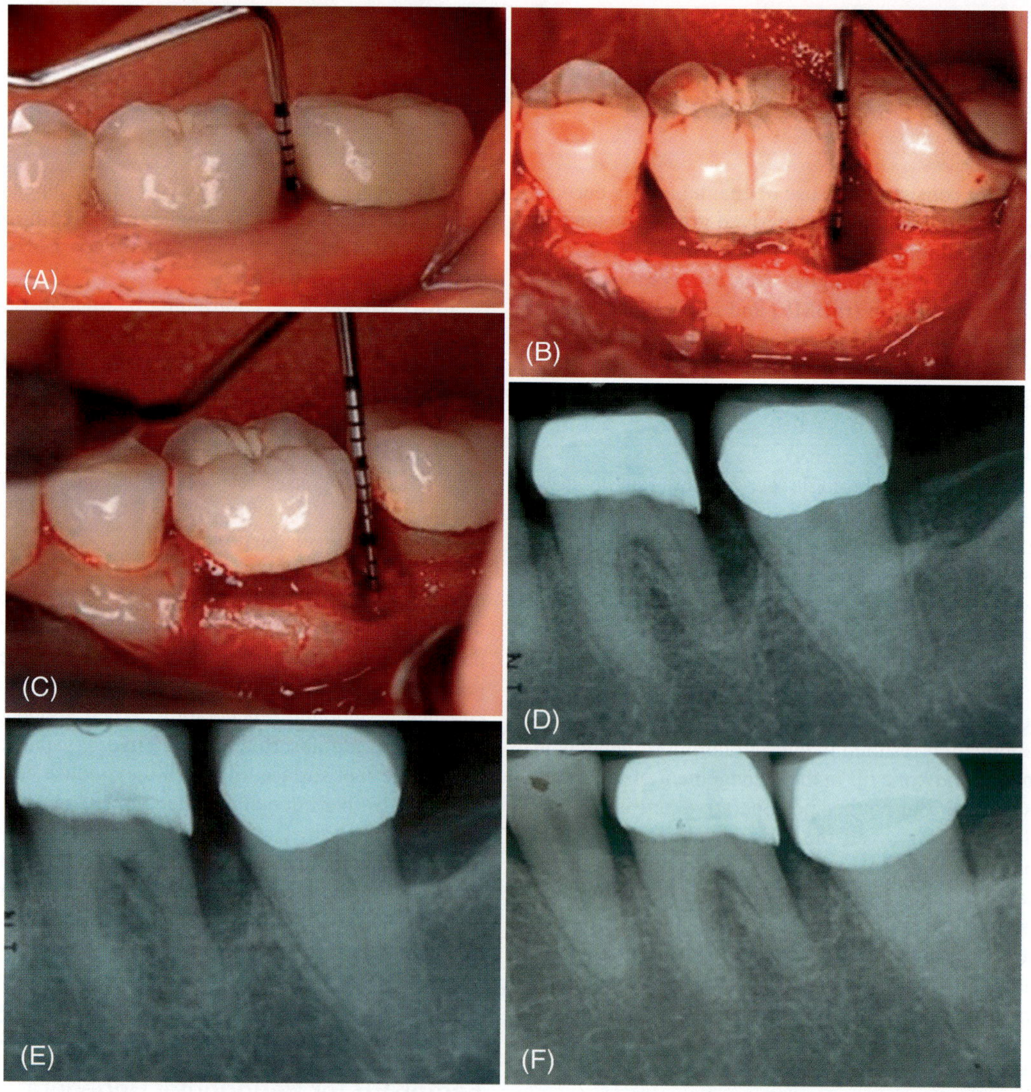

Fig. 48.10 A sample case of a patient treated in the pivotal trial. A–C, The pretreatment situation preoperatively, at surgical debridement, and at postsurgical reentry. D–F, The radiographic appearance after 12, 24, and 60 months. Surgical reentry after 12 months indicates good bone fill of the circumferential intrabony defect (C). The clinical pocket depth was 3 mm after 5 years.

superior to those of other regenerative graft materials. The potential for using rhPDGF for regeneration of furcation defects and implant site preparation still needs to be evaluated. Additionally, considerable clinical interest has been expressed in combining rhPDGF-BB with other bone replacement grafts, particularly bone allografts and xenografts.

Cell Therapy

Cell therapy has been used in periodontal surgery. Stem cells have the potential to improve current bone regeneration. These cells can expedite cell recruitment, act as target cells for growth factor delivery, and promote early extracellular matrix formation. All of these cellular activities increase the bioactivity of the graft. The concentration of multipotential stromal cells (MSCs) in a commercially available cellular bone allograft was compared to fresh age-matched iliac crest bone and bone marrow aspirate. Without cultivation or expansion, this allograft contains cells with cell surface markers called *cluster differentiation (CD) markers* that are found with immunotyping of osteoprogenitor cells and osteoblasts. These cells displayed an "osteoinductive" molecular signature and the presence of $CD45^+$, $CD271^+$, $CD73^+$, $CD90^+$, and $CD105^+$ MSC surface markers that were more than 100-fold of what are found in iliac crest bone. In comparison with bone marrow, MSC numbers enzymatically released from 1 g of cellular allograft were equivalent to approximately 45 mL of bone marrow aspirate. This MSC cellular allograft bone represents unique, nonimmunogenic material rich in MSCs, osteoblasts, and osteocytes. This osteoinductive cellular graft represents an attractive alternative to autograft bone by eliminating a secondary surgical harvest site and morbidity risk.

This stem cell preparation with bone scaffold has been used for implant site preparation by increasing alveolar ridge volume and sinus grafting. Additionally, this cellular allograft has been used successfully in regenerative treatment of periodontal defects in both a single-rooted tooth and a multirooted tooth. In the single-rooted case, a significant reduction in probing depth was obtained with radiologic evidence of approximately 4 mm of vertical bone fill at 6 months following grafting. In the multirooted case, clinical evidence showed decreased probing depths and radiographic bone improvement at 6 months. A cone-beam computed tomography scan taken at 14 months demonstrated three-dimensional bone fill. A similar result was presented in a case report, where this allograft cellular bone matrix was used in the successful treatment of a severe periodontal defect. These case reports indicate a potential resolution of periodontal defects using cellular allograft material.

Use of Platelet-Rich Plasma/Platelet-Rich Fibrin for Periodontal Regeneration

PRP and PRF are autologous blood concentrate products that have been utilized in a variety of regenerative surgical applications. While both products have unique preparation methods, both rely on concentrating the platelets of whole blood to produce a product that delivers the polypeptide growth factors associated with normal wound healing in a highly concentrated form to the surgical site.

The platelet-associated growth factors released from PRF and PRP include PDGF, VEGF, TGF-β, PDGEF, IGF-1, and bFGF. These growth factors have been shown to contribute to periodontal regeneration and were released in significantly higher concentrations from the PRF and PRP products compared to whole blood. In vitro studies have demonstrated that PRF and PRP can promote periodontal regeneration through the enhancement of cellular proliferation and differentiation of key progenitor cell populations. In addition, the clinical benefits of PRF and PRP in periodontal regeneration in humans have been well studied. Across multiple randomized controlled trials, the addition of PRF was effective for the treatment of intrabony defects and Class II furcation defects compared to open flap debridement alone, resulting in decreased PPD and increased CAL. The data have been inconclusive in terms of the benefit of adding PRF to bone graft material for the treatment of intrabony defects and Class II furcation defects. The addition of PRP to intrabony and furcation defects has demonstrated more heterogenous results with minimal to no clinical benefit demonstrated when comparing its effectiveness to open flap debridement. Proof of true periodontal regeneration using PRF or PRP via histological studies in humans is still lacking.

Miscellaneous Biologics Used for Periodontal Regeneration

Bone Morphogenetic Proteins for Periodontal and Implant Site Regeneration

Bone morphogenic proteins (BMPs) comprise a group of regulatory glycoproteins that are members of the transforming growth factor-beta (TGF-β) superfamily that function as differentiation factors. These proteins induce cellular differentiation of stem cells into chondroblastic and osteogenic cells. Several pathways that influence osteoblastogenesis and bone formation, including the Smad pathway, Hedgehog pathway, TGF-β pathway, and **cytokine**–cytokine **receptor** interaction, are involved. Much of the research interest has focused on BMP-2 (OP-2), BMP-3 (osteogenin), and BMP-7 (OP-1). BMP-2 target genes include a wide cohort of transcription factors located in the cell nucleus. The osteogenic effects of BMP-2 are mediated by the formation of Runx2-Smad complexes. BMP-2 promotes osteoblast maturation by increasing the expression of a series of transcription factors in the cell nucleus (RUNX2, OSX, DLX5), which lead to the expression of OSE2, the osteoblast marker **gene** that is responsible for osteoblast differentiation.

BMPs are present in FDBA and DFDBA, but the levels are so low that bovine bone yields only 2 μg of BMP. It is only through recombinant **DNA** technology (rhBMP) that BMP has been made available for clinical use.

Although early studies using crude preparations of BMP-2 and BMP-3 applied in surgically induced furcation defects appeared to stimulate periodontal regeneration, more recent studies with rhBMP-2 indicate that periodontal regeneration was associated with areas of ankylosis. Healing through ankylosis has been a concern, so most of the research using rhBMPs has involved correction of intrabony, supraalveolar, furcation, and fenestration defects, as well as implant site preparation.

More recently, BMP-7 has been utilized in an animal model to improve bone formation by incorporating BMP-7 into a patterned scaffold for the formation of PDL-like tissue and the overall integrity of the bone-PDL interface. Future translational and human studies are still needed to determine its clinical use in periodontal regeneration.

Use of Recombinant Human Fibroblast Growth Factor 2 for Periodontal Regeneration

The potential use of recombinant human FGF-2 (rhFGF-2) for periodontal regeneration has been reviewed. Preliminary beagle and nonhuman primate studies demonstrated that topical application of FGF-2 into intraosseous defects in alveolar bones induces significant periodontal tissue regeneration. Histologic observation revealed new cementum with Sharpey's fibers, new functionally oriented periodontal ligament fibers, and new alveolar bone. These findings suggest that topical application of FGF-2 may be efficacious in regeneration of human periodontal tissue that has been destroyed by **periodontitis**.

A randomized, controlled, double-masked Phase II clinical trial at 13 Japanese dental facilities compared the therapeutic response to varying doses of FGF-2 as compared to control. Eighty patients with a two- or three-walled vertical bone defect 3 mm or more from the alveolar crest were randomly divided into four groups: (group A) placebo control, (group B) 0.03% FGF-2, (group C) 0.1% FGF-2, and (group D) 0.3% FGF-2. The subjects underwent periodontal surgery during which 200 μL of the investigational drug or placebo carrier was applied to each test site. After 9 months, a significant increase ($P = 0.021$) in alveolar bone height was demonstrated by standardized radiographs between group A (23.92%) and group D (58.62%). No adverse effects were observed throughout this multicenter trial. This finding suggests that topical application of FGF-2 can be efficacious in regenerating periodontal tissue of patients with two- or three-walled intrabony defects.

Recently, a multicenter, double-blinded, dose-verification, clinical trial was conducted. This trial included 88 patients who needed surgical treatment for an infrabony periodontal defect. The participants were randomized into one of the four groups: β-TCP alone (control) and 0.1% rhFGF-2, 0.3% rhFGF-2, and 0.4% rhFGF-2 with β-TCP. At 6-month follow-up, the two higher-concentration groups showed a percentage of bone fill of 75% and 71%, compared to 48% and 61% in the control and lowest treatment group. In addition, no increases in specific antibody to rhFGF-2 were detected, and no significant adverse events related to the use of rhFGF-2 were identified. The findings from this clinical trial demonstrated that rhFGF-2/β-TCP can be used to enhance the regenerative outcomes of infrabony periodontal defects.

Combined Techniques

Periodontal new attachment and bone reconstruction have been challenges for clinicians throughout the history of periodontal therapy. To take advantage of the different bone graft materials and biologic mediators, clinicians have combined these graft materials with the use of membranes in an attempt to find a predictable technique to regenerate bone.

Several clinicians have proposed a combination of the techniques previously described in an attempt to enhance their results. A classic paper published by Schallhorn and McClain in 1988 described a combination technique using graft material, root conditioning with citric acid, and coverage with a nonresorbable membrane (the only available one at the time). More recently, with the advent of osteopromotive agents, such as the EMD (Emdogain, Straumann, Andover, MA) and osteoconductive bovine-derived anorganic bone (Bio-Oss) graft materials, other combination techniques have been advocated. The combined use of these products, along with autogenous bone with resorbable membrane coverage, has resulted in an increased percentage of cases with successful new attachment and periodontal reconstruction. Many of these combination techniques were reviewed in previous sections of this chapter. Whereas the use of combination techniques may be appealing, it is important for clinicians to remember that these added materials often escalate the cost of the procedure and should be balanced with the quality and the long-term stability of the clinical results.

Regenerative Supportive Graft Materials

Many of the commercial regenerative materials are provided along with osteoconducive materials, such as tricalcium phosphate, collagen, and calcium that function as carriers, supportive matrix, or support bioexclusive properties. Many of these are FDA-approved carriers but clinicians have been known to discard these carriers in favor of DFDBA/FDBA. Though these materials do not provide osteogenic properties, it is important for clinicians to be aware of how and when these materials are clinically applied.

Scaffold or Supporting Matrices

The use of scaffolding matrices to deliver growth factors to promote periodontal tissue regeneration has been an active area of research. Supporting matrices for engineering bone and soft tissue have included processed bone allografts, synthetic and natural polymers, synthetic ceramics, bovine type I collagen, and calcium sulfate (commercially available scaffolds are found in Table 48.1). The major roles for the supporting matrices are to:

1. Provide physical support for the healing area so that no collapse of the surrounding tissue into the wound site occurs. Examples of this would be bone allografts and synthetic ceramics, such as β-tricalcium phosphate (β-TCP).
2. Serve as a barrier to restrict cellular migration selectively. This is best exemplified by principles of GTR and guided bone regeneration where PTFE and resorbable polylactate, polyglycolic acid, and calcium sulfate are used. The exclusive properties of cell barrier membranes have been reviewed and are not addressed here.
3. Serve as a scaffold for cellular migration and proliferation. An example is the collagen matrix. Potentially, this scaffold can be further enhanced by selectively defining the types of cells permitted to attach to and proliferate on this matrix with the additions of **adhesins** and/or integrins.
4. Potentially serve as a time-release mechanism for signaling molecules.

Allogenic and Alloplastic Bone-Grafting Materials

The classic approach to orofacial regeneration since the 1980s has been the use of bone grafts or substitutes to repair periodontal and **maxillofacial** defects. The literature contains several excellent reviews on the use of autografts, allografts, and alloplastic graft materials.

Since 2000, mineralized and demineralized freeze-dried bone allografts (FDBA and DFDBA) have often been the regeneration material of choice. In addition to their availability and putative osteogenic potential, various clinical studies indicate that 2–3 mm of bone fill is possible with FDBA and DFDBA. However, other studies have questioned the osteogenic potential of bone allografts by suggesting that this may vary depending on the bone bank or batch, processing procedures used, and donor characteristics. These varying levels of osteoinductive properties have resulted in the US Food and Drug Administration not regulating nor formally approving commercially available FDBA and DFDBA. However, off-label use of this combination is common both in orthopedic and oral-periodontal surgical procedures.

Alternatively, a variety of xenograft and alloplastic grafting materials are available as scaffolding agents for tissue engineering. Alloplastic bone grafts consist of ceramics, such as hydroxyapatite (HA), porous HA, β-TCP, and biocompatible composite polymers (e.g., hard tissue replacement). Of these allografts, β-TCP is used in combination with rhPDGF-BB. In the development of rhPDGF-BB for clinical use, the biosynthetic β-TCP was used because it possessed defined and reproducible properties as required by the Food and Drug Administration. Allografts were not desirable because of varying osteogenic potential and properties. Extensive animal and human studies demonstrated biocompatibility of β-TCP with no reports of adverse reactions. This material physically fills bone defects, provides a scaffold for new bone formation, and prevents soft tissue collapse into the wound site. Clinically, β-TCP is osteoconductive and supports early healing. β-TCP resorbs at varying rates depending on the chemical structure, porosity, and particle size. Absorption, release, and bioactivity studies indicate that either β-TCP or calcium sulfate can be an effective carrier for PDGF-BB. Approximately 45% of the adsorbed PDGF-BB was released after 10 days. In clinical studies with rhPDGF-BB, this material resorbs and is replaced with regenerated periodontium. Superficial granules at the soft tissue interface appear to resorb at a slower rate. More recently, the use of β-TCP coated with recombinant human growth and differentiation factor-5 was evaluated for its osteoinductive and osteoconductive properties in an experimental rat calvarial critical size defect. Histomorphometric results suggest that this proprietary coating of growth factor on β-TCP achieved superior bone regeneration compared to conventional materials. These latter two studies indicate that the absorption and release kinetics of signaling agents are areas that require further elucidation if we are to achieve optimal regenerative response.

Collagen Carriers

Collagen is the main structural protein for tissue support. It also plays an essential role in wound healing by providing a biologic scaffold for cellular activities, such as cell attachment, migration, and proliferation. Collagen has been widely used in tissue engineering for seeding of mesenchymal stem cells, as well as incorporation of growth factors. Because most collagens are derived from bovine dermal or skeletal tissue, concerns related to the purity, quality, immunogenicity, and potential for prion transmission have been raised. Studies addressed these issues by further purifying bovine collagen and modifying the molecules to remove antigenic N- and C-terminal telopeptides. Two variations of this collagen were produced to create an atelocollagen scaffold where both constructs were effective in supporting rhBMP-induced bone formation.

Calcium Sulfate

Calcium sulfate is one of the oldest bone graft materials. Early clinical and animal studies indicate that calcium sulfate is biocompatible, degrades over time, is subsequently replaced with regenerated bone, and may be used in an infected area with no complications. More recent studies indicate that it also has barrier properties, enhances angiogenesis, and may be effective as a delivery vehicle for antibiotics and growth factors. Rosenblum and associates demonstrated that FGF was released at a rate directly proportional to the rate of calcium sulfate dissolution. A secondary benefit of calcium sulfate dissolution is a local decrease in pH. An interesting study in the orthopedic literature reported that when an experimental sheep distal femoral cancellous defect was filled with calcium sulfate, increased immunostaining for BMP-2, BMP-7, TGF-β, and PDGF-BB was observed. All of these growth factors have been demonstrated to stimulate bone formation and development. Calcium sulfate was found to be a suitable carrier for rhPDGF-BB with a longer release kinetic profile (;16 days) as compared to β-TCP. Because both materials are resorbable, the current debate centers on whether a longer sustained release of rhPDGF-BB would be more advantageous to periodontal and bone regeneration.

Other Carriers

Bioresorbable polymers of poly lactic-co-glycolic acid and polyglycolic acid have been considered as scaffolding agents for tissue engineering due to their biodegradable and tissue compatibility properties. Although these agents were promising as carriers for osteogenic factors in animals, variable tissue responses have made clinical application of these materials problematic. These tissue responses include inflammation, foreign body reaction, and local acid accumulation during polymer degradation.

Assessment of Periodontal Healing

It is difficult in clinical and experimental situations to determine accurately whether regeneration or new attachment has occurred and the extent to which it has occurred. The following methods are employed to determine the type of healing that has taken place:

Clinical Methods

Comparisons between pretreatment and posttreatment pocket probings and determinations of clinical **gingival** findings are used to confirm periodontal regeneration. The probe can be used to determine pocket depth, attachment level, and bone level. Clinical determinations of attachment level are more useful than probing pocket depths because the latter may change with the regenerative surgical procedure, which will result in changes in the level of the marginal **gingiva**.

Several studies have determined that the depth of penetration of a probe in a **periodontal pocket** varies according to the degree of inflammatory involvement of the tissues immediately beneath the pocket. Therefore, even though the forces used may be standardized with pressure-sensitive probes, an inherent margin of error in this method is difficult to overcome. Fowler and colleagues calculated this error to be 1.2 mm, but it is even greater when furcations are probed. Bone probing performed with the patient under anesthesia is not subject to this error and has been found to be as accurate as bone height measurements made on surgical reentry.

Measurements of the defect should be made before and after treatment from the same point within the defect and with the same angulation of the probe. This reproducibility of probe placement is difficult and may be facilitated in part by using a grooved stent to guide the introduction of the probe. Preoperative and postoperative comparability of probing measurements that do not use this standardized method may lead to questioning of the regenerative results.

Radiographic Methods

Radiographic evaluation of periodontal regeneration allows assessment of the bone tissue adjacent to the tooth. This technique also requires carefully standardized techniques for reproducible positioning of the film and the tube. Even with standardized techniques, the radiograph does not show the entire topography of the area before or after treatment. Furthermore, thin bone trabeculae may exist before treatment and may go undetected radiographically because a certain minimal amount of mineralized tissue must be present to register on the radiograph. Several studies have demonstrated that radiographs, even those taken with standardized methods, are less reliable than clinical probing techniques. A comparative study of pretreatment bone levels and posttherapy bone fill with 12-month reentry bone measurements showed that linear radiographic analysis significantly underestimates pretreatment bone loss and posttreatment bone fill.

Studies with subtraction radiography have enhanced the usefulness of radiographic evaluation. A comparative study of linear measurements, computer-assisted densitometric image analysis (CADIA), and a method combining the two, reported that the combination method offers the highest level of accuracy.

Surgical Re-entry

The surgical re-entry of a treated defect after a period of healing can provide a good view of the state of the bone crest that can be compared to the view taken during the initial surgical intervention and can also be subject to measurements. Models from impressions of the bone taken at the initial surgery, and later at reentry, can be used to assess the results of therapy.

This method is very useful but has two shortcomings: it requires a frequently unnecessary second procedure, and it does not show the type of attachment that exists (i.e., new attachment or long junctional epithelium):

1. Histological method: Through histologic analysis, one can accurately define the nature of reparative tissue. However, in humans, this is not applicable due to ethical considerations. A few human histologic studies are available after the tooth was extracted in conjunction with orthodontic or restorative therapy.

Conclusion

Over the past three decades, the periodontal literature has been filled with numerous reports related to periodontal regeneration. This therapeutic goal, although ideal, is difficult to achieve. A variety of graft materials and regenerative strategies are now available; however, they all have limitations. The surgical procedure can be technically demanding and when success is achieved, the maintenance of positive results is highly dependent on patients' oral hygiene habits and compliance with periodontal maintenance. Despite all these difficulties, periodontal regeneration is a clinical possibility that can be offered to patients. The clinician must carefully evaluate the various regenerative and reparative approaches and decide which technique may result in the best clinical outcome. With the advent of new regenerative approaches, such as biological modifiers like EMD and growth factors, one must critically evaluate how they may improve our ability to regenerate periodontal defects.

Treatment planning in periodontics also has changed dramatically in the past decade because of the acceptance of dental implants as a viable long-term option for replacing missing teeth. With the increased predictability of implants, the question arises as to when to treat severe periodontal defects with regenerative procedures and when to perform strategic extraction in preparation for implant placement. Sometimes the best management of a periodontal defect may be extraction in lieu of periodontal regeneration or when regenerative efforts have been unsuccessful. Extraction would minimize further bone loss and provide the maximum volume of bone at the future implant healing site. This paradigm shift has complicated our views about regeneration. With dental implants as a viable alternative, we need to redefine periodontal prognosis and consider strategic extraction more often. Conversely, heroic regenerative procedures would be contraindicated.

Periodontal regeneration continues to be one of the primary therapeutic approaches toward the management of periodontal defects. Although evidence suggests that present regenerative techniques can lead to periodontal regeneration, the use of GTR and biological modifiers can enhance these results. The crucial challenge for the clinician is to critically assess whether a periodontal defect can be corrected with a regenerative approach or whether it would be better managed with osseous resection for the slight periodontal defect and with strategic extraction for the advanced diseased state. In this assessment, the clinician should attempt to differentiate between techniques that have been studied in depth and with acceptable results and those that are still experimental and promising. Research papers must be critically evaluated for adequacy of controls, selection of cases, methods of evaluation, and long-term postoperative results. In addition, the clinician should remember that we treat patients on the basis of "clinical" success and not "statistical" success. A resulting clinical attachment gain of half a millimeter may be a "statistical" success, but it is meaningless for the patients whom we treat and manage over the long term.

Key points

- Periodontal regeneration attempts to reconstitute lost periodontal structures that include bone, periodontal ligament and cementum.
- At present, predictable periodontal regeneration is feasible in infrabony defects and grade 2 furcation involvement.
- Regeneration involves the use of various bone grafts, barrier membranes and biologic mediators.
- Various types of bone grafts are widely used in the management of periodontal osseous defects.
- Depending upon the source they are classified as autografts, allografts, xenografts and alloplasts. They may aid in bone formation by osteogenesis, osteoinduction or osteoconduction.
- While autografts are the gold standard in terms of the surgical outcome, their procurement is difficult as they require a second site often extra orally.
- Bone grafts best work in three walled infrabony and grade II furcation defects. Apart from providing about 50–70% bone fill, bone grafts also result in increased reduction of probing depth, gain in clinical attachment level and reduced gingival recession.

Suggested Readings

Alger FA, Solt CW, Vuddahanok S, et al: The histologic evaluation of new attachment in periodontally diseased human roots treated with tetracycline hydrochloride and fibronectin. *J Periodontol* 61:447, 1990.

Bowers GM, Chadroff B, Carnevale R, et al: Histologic evaluation of new attachment apparatus formation in humans. Part III. *J Periodontol* 60:683, 1989.

Camelo M, Nevins ML, Schenk RK, et al: Periodontal regeneration in human class II furcations using purified recombinant human platelet derived growth factor-BB (rhPDGF-BB) with bone allograft. *Int J Periodontics Restorative Dent* 23:213–225, 2003.

Caton JC: Overview of clinical trials on periodontal regeneration. *Ann Periodontol* 2:215, 1987.

Giannobile WV, Hollister SJ, Ma PX: Future prospects for periodontal bioengineering using growth factors. *Clin Ad Periodontics* 1:88, 2011.

Kao RT, Murakami S, Beirne OR: The use of biologic mediators and tissue engineering in dentistry. *Periodontol 2000* 20:127, 2009.

Murphy KG, Gunsolley JC: Guided tissue regeneration for the treatment of periodontal intrabony and furcation defects. A systematic review. *Ann Periodontol* 8:266–302, 2003.

Needleman I, Tucker R, Giedrys-Leeper E, et al: Guided tissue regeneration for periodontal intrabony defects—a Cochrane systematic review. *Periodontol 2000* 37:106–123, 2005.

Nevins M, Camelo M, Nevins ML, et al: Periodontal regeneration in humans using recombinant human platelet-derived growth factor BB (rhPDGF-BB) and allogenic bone. *J Periodontol* 74:1282, 2003.

Nevins M, Giannobile WV, McGuire MK, et al: Platelet-derived growth factor stimulates bone fill and rate of attachment level gain: results of a large multicenter randomized controlled trial. *J Periodontol* 76:2205, 2005.

Nevins M, Kao RT, McGuire MK, et al: PDGF promotes periodontal regeneration in localized osseous defects: 36 month extension results from a randomized, controlled, double-masked clinical trial. *J Periodontol* 84:456, 2013.

Reynolds MA, Aichelmann-Reidy EM, Branch-Mays GL, et al: The efficacy of bone replacement grafts in the treatment of periodontal osseous defects. A systematic review. *Ann Periodontol* 8:227–265, 2003.

Schallhorn RG, McClain PK: Combined osseous composite grafting, root conditioning, and guided tissue regeneration. *Int J Periodont Restor Dent* 8:8, 1988.

Sculean A, Alessandri R, Miron R, et al: Enamel matrix proteins and periodontal wound healing and regeneration. *Clin Adv Periodontics* 1: 101–117, 2011.

Susin C, Wikesjo UME: Regenerative periodontal therapy: 30 years of lessons learned and unlearned. *Periodontol* 2000 62:232–242, 2013.

Furcation Involvement and Treatment

TN Sims | HH Takei | CD Dwarakanath

CHAPTER OUTLINE

Inflammatory periodontal disease, if unabated, ultimately progresses to attachment loss sufficient to affect the bifurcation or trifurcation of multirooted teeth. The furcation is an area of complex anatomic morphology that may be difficult or impossible to debride by routine periodontal instrumentation. Routine home care methods may not keep the furcation area free of plaque.

The presence of furcation involvement is a clinical finding that can lead to a diagnosis of advanced periodontitis and potentially to a less favorable prognosis for the affected tooth or teeth. Thus, furcation involvement presents both diagnostic and therapeutic dilemmas.

Etiologic Factors

The primary etiologic factor in the development of furcation defects is *bacterial plaque* and the inflammatory consequences that result from its long-term presence. The extent of attachment loss required to produce a furcation defect is variable and related to local anatomic factors (e.g., root trunk length, root morphology) and local developmental anomalies (e.g., cervical enamel projections [CEPs]). Local factors may affect the rate of plaque deposition or complicate the performance of oral hygiene procedures, thereby contributing to the development of periodontitis and attachment loss. Studies indicate that prevalence and severity of furcation involvement increase with age. Dental caries and pulpal death may also affect a tooth with furcation involvement or even the area of the furcation. All of these factors should be considered during the diagnosis, treatment planning, and therapy of the patient with furcation defects.

Diagnosis and Classification of Furcation Defects

A thorough clinical examination is the key to diagnosis and treatment planning. Careful probing is required to determine the presence and extent of furcation involvement, the position of the attachment relative to the furca, and the extent and configuration of the furcation defect. The Nabors probe may be helpful to enter and measure difficult to access furcal areas (Fig. 49.1A and B). Transgingival sounding may further define the anatomy of the furcation defect. The goals of this examination are to identify and classify the extent of furcation involvement and to identify factors that may have contributed to the development of the furcation defect or that could affect treatment outcome. These factors include (1) the morphology of the affected tooth, (2) the position of the tooth relative to adjacent teeth, (3) the local anatomy of the alveolar bone, (4) the configuration of any bony defects, and (5) the presence and extent of other dental diseases (e.g., caries, pulpal necrosis).

The dimension of the furcation entrance is variable but usually quite small; 81% of furcations have an orifice of 1 mm or less, and 58% are 0.75 mm or less. The clinician should consider these dimensions, and the local anatomy of the furcation area, when selecting instruments for probing. A probe of small cross-sectional dimension is required if the clinician is to detect early furcation involvement.

Local Anatomic Factors

Clinical examination of the patient should allow the therapist to identify not only furcation defects but also many of the local anatomic factors that may affect the result of therapy (prognosis). Well-made dental radiographs, although not allowing a definitive classification of furcation involvement, provide additional information vital for treatment planning (Fig. 49.2). Important local factors include anatomic features of the affected teeth, as described next.

Root Trunk Length

A key factor in both the development and the treatment of furcation involvement is the root trunk length. The distance from the cementoenamel junction to the entrance of the furcation can vary extensively. Teeth may have very short root trunks, moderate root trunk length, or roots that may be fused to a point near the apex (Fig. 49.3). The combination of root trunk length with the number and configuration of the roots affects the ease and success of therapy. The shorter the root trunk, the less attachment needs to be lost before the furcation is involved. Once the furcation is exposed, teeth with short root trunks may be more accessible to maintenance procedures, and the short root trunks may facilitate some surgical procedures. Alternatively, teeth with unusually long root trunks or fused roots may not be appropriate candidates for treatment once the furcation has been affected.

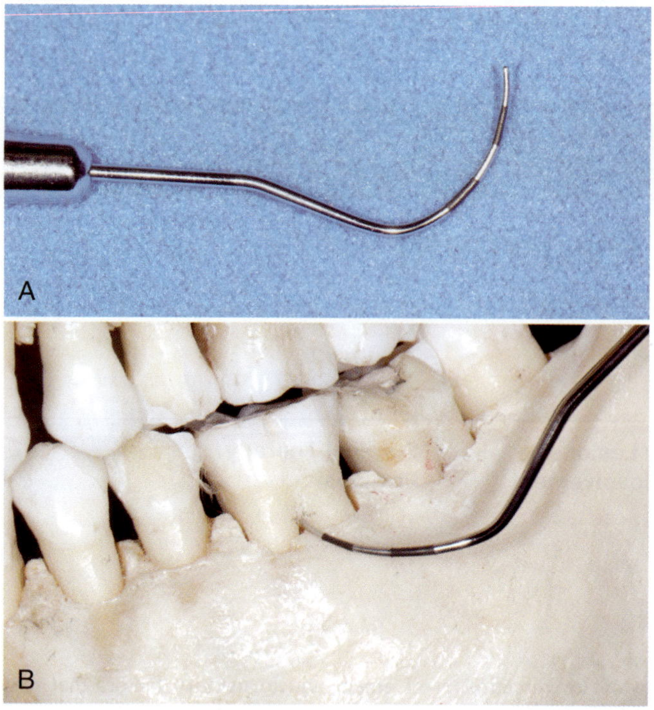

Fig. 49.1 A, The Nabers probe is designed to probe into the furcation. B, The probe placed into a Class II furcation of a dried skull.

Root Length

Root length is directly related to the quantity of attachment supporting the tooth. Teeth with long root trunks and short roots may have lost a majority of their support by the time that the furcation becomes affected. Teeth with long roots and short to moderate root trunk length are more readily treated because sufficient attachment remains to meet functional demands.

Root Form

The mesial root of most mandibular first and second molars and the mesiofacial root of the maxillary first molar are typically curved to the distal side in the apical third. In addition, the distal aspect of this root is usually heavily fluted. The curvature and fluting may increase the potential for root perforation during endodontic therapy or complicate postplacement during restoration. These anatomic features may also result in an increased incidence of vertical root fracture. The size of the mesial radicular pulp may result in removal of most of this portion of the tooth during preparation.

Interradicular Dimension

The degree of separation of the roots is also an important factor in treatment planning. Closely approximated or fused roots can preclude adequate instrumentation during scaling, root planing, and surgery. Teeth with widely separated roots present more treatment options and are more readily treated.

Anatomy of Furcation

The anatomy of the furcation is complex. The presence of bifurcational ridges, a concavity in the dome, and possible accessory canals complicates not only scaling, root planing, and surgical therapy but also periodontal maintenance. Odontoplasty to reduce or eliminate these ridges may be required during surgical therapy for an optimal result.

Cervical Enamel Projections

Cervical enamel projections (CEPs) are reported to occur on 8.6%–28.6% of molars. The prevalence is highest for mandibular and maxillary second molars. The extent of CEPs was classified by Masters and Hoskins in 1964 (Box 49.1). Fig. 49.4 provides an example of a grade III CEP. These projections can affect plaque removal, can complicate scaling and root planing, and may be a local factor in the development of gingivitis and periodontitis. CEPs should be removed to facilitate maintenance.

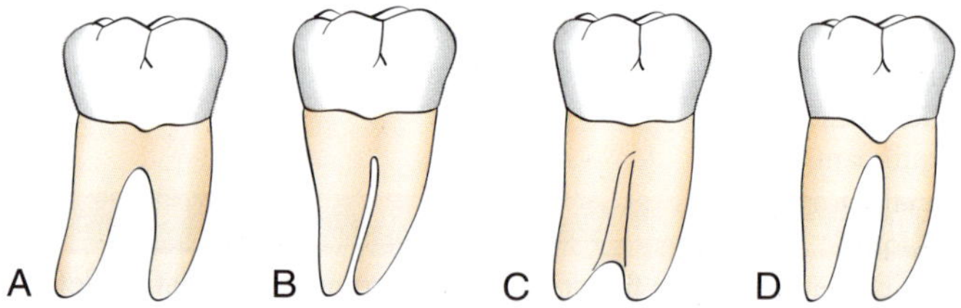

Fig. 49.3 Different anatomic features that may be important in prognosis and treatment of furcation involvement. A, Widely separated roots. B, Roots are separated but close. C, Fused roots separated only in their apical portion. D, Presence of enamel projection that may be conducive to early furcation involvement.

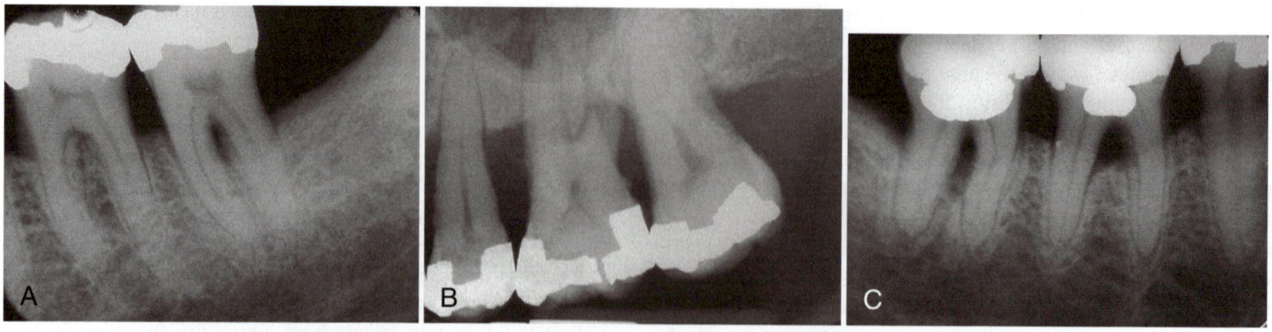

Fig. 49.2 Different degrees of furcation involvement in radiographs. A, Grade I furcation on the mandibular first molar and a grade III furcation on the mandibular second molar. The root approximation on the second molar may be sufficient to impede accurate probing of this defect. B, Multiple furcation defects on a maxillary first molar. Grade I buccal furcation involvement and grade II mesiopalatal and distopalatal furcations are present. Deep developmental grooves on the maxillary second molar simulate furcation involvement in this molar with fused roots. C, Grades III and IV furcations on mandibular molars.

BOX 49.1 Classification of Cervical Enamel Projections

Grade I: The enamel projection extends from the cementoenamel junction of the tooth toward the furcation entrance.

Grade II: The enamel projection approaches the entrance to the furcation. It does not enter the furcation, and therefore no horizontal component is present.

Grade III: The enamel projection extends horizontally into the furcation.

(From Masters DH, Hoskins SW: Projection of cervical enamel into molar furcations. *J Periodontol* 35:49, 1964.)

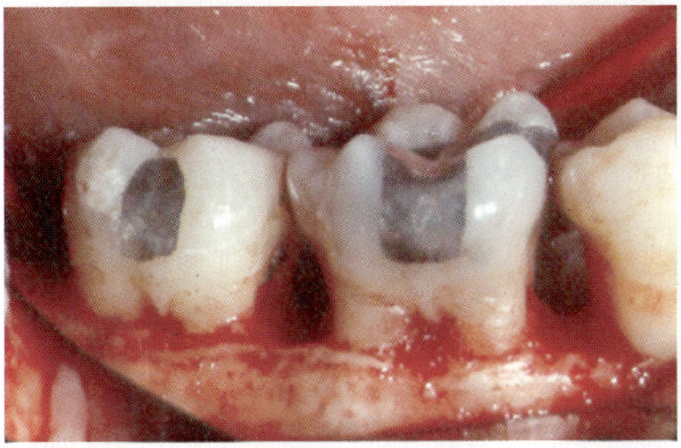

Fig. 49.4 Furcation involvement by grade III cervical enamel projections.

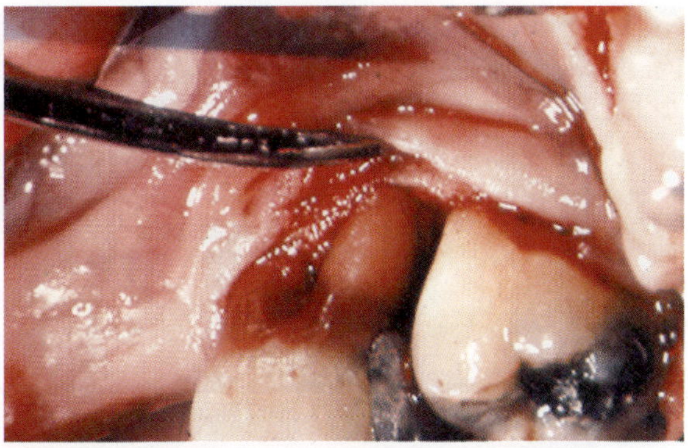

Fig. 49.5 Advanced bone loss, furcation involvement, and root approximation. Note the buccal furcation, which communicates with the distal furcation of a maxillary first molar that also displays advanced attachment loss on the distal root and approximation with the mesial root of the maxillary second molar. The patient with such teeth may benefit from root resection of the distobuccal root of the first molar or extraction of the molar.

Anatomy of the Bony Lesions

Pattern of Attachment Loss

The form of the bony lesions associated with the furcation can vary significantly. Horizontal bone loss can expose the furcation as thin facial or lingual plates of bone that may be totally lost during resorption. Alternatively, areas with thickened bony ledges may persist and predispose to the development of furcations with deep vertical components. The pattern of bone loss on other surfaces of the affected tooth and adjacent teeth must also be considered during treatment planning. The treatment response in deep, multiwalled bony defects is different from that in areas of horizontal bone loss. Complex multiwalled defects with deep, interradicular vertical components may be candidates for regenerative therapies. Alternatively, molars with advanced attachment loss on only one root may be treated by resective procedures.

Other Dental Findings

The dental and periodontal condition of the adjacent teeth must be considered during treatment planning for furcation involvement. The combination of furcation involvement and root approximation with an adjacent tooth represents the same problem that exists in furcations without adequate root separation. Such a finding may dictate the removal of the most severely affected tooth or the removal of a root or roots (Fig. 49.5).

The presence of an adequate band of gingiva and a moderate to deep vestibule will facilitate the performance of a surgical procedure, if indicated.

Indices of Furcation Involvement

The extent and configuration of the furcation defect are factors in both diagnosis and treatment planning. This has led to the development of a number of indices to record furcation involvement. These indices are based on the horizontal measurement of attachment loss in the furcation, on a combination of horizontal and vertical measurements, or a combination of these findings with the localized configuration of the bony deformity. Glickman classified furcation involvement into four grades (Fig. 49.6).

Grade I

A grade I furcation involvement is the incipient or early stage of furcation involvement (see Fig. 49.6A). The pocket is suprabony and primarily affects the soft tissues. Early bone loss may have occurred with an increase in probing depth, but radiographic changes are not usually found.

Grade II

A grade II furcation can affect one or more of the furcations of the same tooth. The furcation lesion is essentially a cul-de-sac (see Fig. 49.6B) with a definite horizontal component. If multiple defects are present, they do not communicate with each other because a portion of the alveolar bone remains attached to the tooth. The extent of the horizontal probing of the furcation determines whether the defect is early or advanced. Vertical bone loss may be present and represents a therapeutic complication. Radiographs may or may not depict the furcation involvement, particularly with maxillary molars because of the radiographic overlap of the roots. In some views, however, the presence of furcation "arrows" indicates possible furcation involvement.

Grade III

In grade III furcations, the bone is not attached to the dome of the furcation. In early grade III involvement, the opening may be filled with soft tissue and may not be visible. The clinician may not even be able to pass a periodontal probe completely through the furcation because of interference with the bifurcational ridges or facial-lingual bony margins. However, if the clinician adds the buccal and lingual probing dimensions and obtains a cumulative probing measurement that is equal to or greater than the buccal-lingual dimension of the tooth at the furcation orifice, the clinician must conclude that a grade III furcation exists (see Fig. 49.6C). Properly exposed and angled radiographs of early class III furcations display the defect as a radiolucent area in the crotch of the tooth.

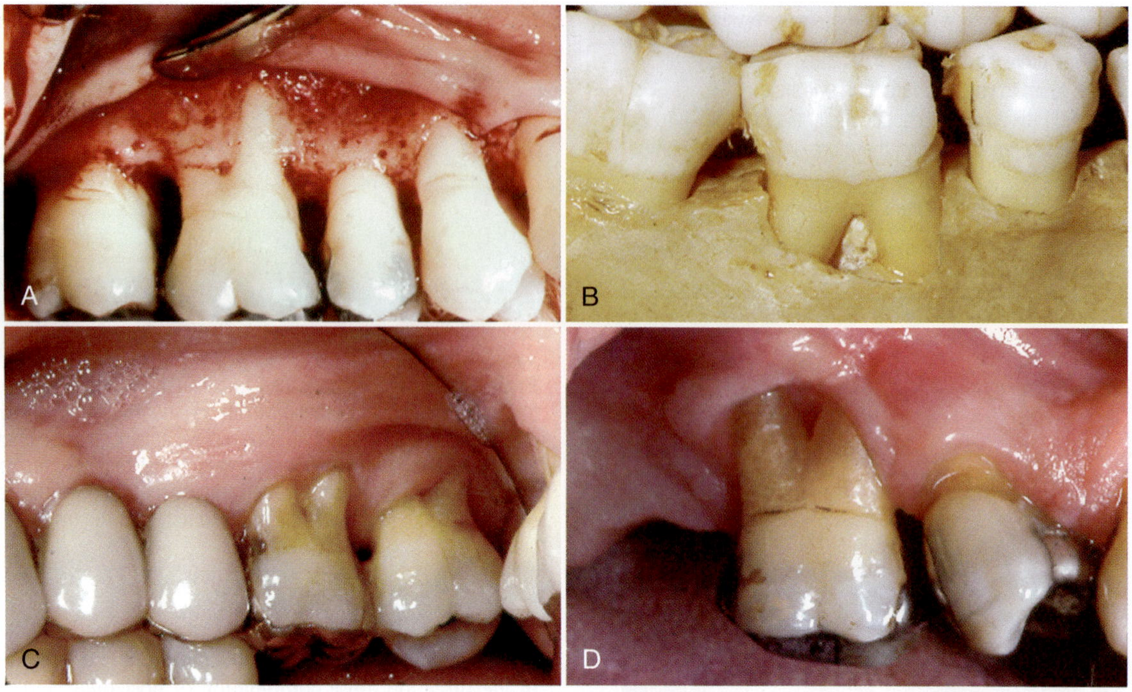

Fig. 49.6 Glickman's classification of furcation involvement. A, Grade I furcation involvement. Although a space is visible at the entrance to the furcation, no horizontal component of the furcation is evident on probing. B, Grade II furcation in a dried skull. Note both the horizontal and the vertical components of this cul-de-sac. C, Grade III furcations on maxillary molars. Probing confirms that the buccal furcation connects with the distal furcation of both these molars, yet the furcation is filled with soft tissue. D, Grade IV furcation. The soft tissues have receded sufficiently to allow direct vision into the furcation of this maxillary molar.

Grade IV

In grade IV furcations, the interdental bone is destroyed, and the soft tissues have receded apically so that the furcation opening is clinically visible. A tunnel therefore exists between the roots of such an affected tooth. Thus, the periodontal probe passes readily from one aspect of the tooth to another (see Fig. 49.6D).

Other Classification Indices

Hamp and associates modified a three-stage classification system by attaching a millimeter measurement to separate the extent of horizontal involvement. Easley and Drennan and Tarnow and Fletcher have described classification systems that consider both horizontal and vertical attachment loss in classifying the extent of furcation involvement. The Tarnow and Fletcher article uses a subclassification that measures the probeable vertical depth from the roof of the furca apically. The subclasses being proposed are: A, B, and C. "A" indicates a probeable vertical depth of 1–3 mm, "B" indicates 4–6 mm, and "C" indicates 7 or more mm of probeable depth from the roof of the furca apically. Furcations would thus be classified as IA, IB, and IC; IIA, IIB, and IIC; and IIIA, IIIB, and IIIC.

Consideration of defect configuration and the vertical component of the defect provides additional information that is useful in planning therapy.

Treatment

The objectives of furcation therapy are to (1) facilitate maintenance, (2) prevent further attachment loss, and (3) obliterate the furcation defects as a periodontal maintenance problem. The selection of therapeutic mode varies with the class of furcation involvement, the extent and configuration of bone loss, and other anatomic factors.

Therapeutic Classes of Furcation Defects

Class I: Early Defects

Incipient or early furcation defects (class I) are amenable to conservative periodontal therapy. Because the pocket is suprabony and has not entered the furcation, oral hygiene, scaling, and root planing are effective. Any thick overhanging margins of restorations, facial grooves, or CEPs should be eliminated by odontoplasty, recontouring, or replacement. The resolution of inflammation and subsequent repair of the periodontal ligament and bone are usually sufficient to restore periodontal health.

Class II

Once a horizontal component to the furcation has developed (class II), therapy becomes more complicated. Shallow horizontal involvement without significant vertical bone loss usually responds favorably to localized flap procedures with odontoplasty, osteoplasty, and ostectomy. Isolated deep class II furcations may respond to flap procedures with osteoplasty and odontoplasty (Fig. 49.7A and B). This treatment reduces the dome of the furcation and alters gingival contours to facilitate the patient's plaque removal.

Classes II to IV: Advanced Defects

The development of a significant horizontal component to one or more furcations of a multirooted tooth (late class II, class III, or class IV) or the development of a deep vertical component to the furca poses additional problems. Nonsurgical treatment is usually ineffective because the ability to instrument the tooth surfaces adequately is compromised. Periodontal surgery, endodontic therapy, and restoration of the tooth may be required to retain the tooth.

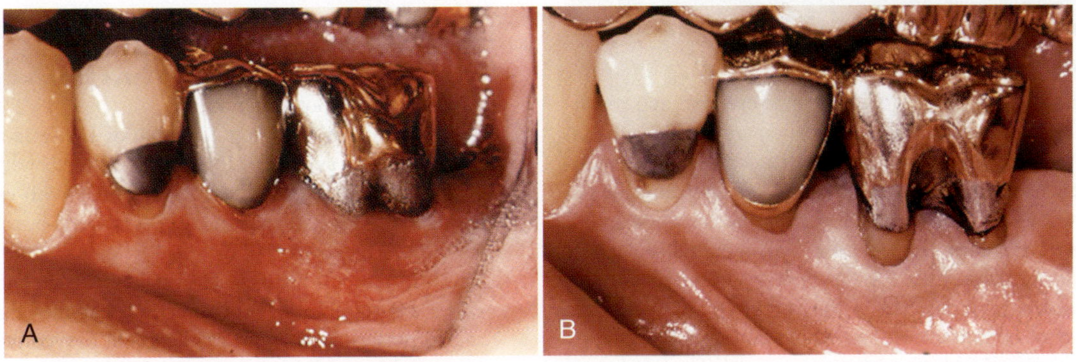

Fig. 49.7 Treatment of a grade II furcation by osteoplasty and odontoplasty. A, This mandibular first molar has been treated endodontically and an area of caries in the furcation has been repaired. A class II furcation is present. B, Results of flap debridement, osteoplasty, and severe odontoplasty 5 years postoperatively. Note the adaptation of the gingiva into the furcation area. *(Courtesy: Dr. Ronald Rott, Sacramento, CA.)*

Nonsurgical Therapy

Oral Hygiene Procedures

Furcal management is difficult at best. Therapeutic modalities for the treatment and maintenance of furcations have long been a dilemma for periodontists and restorative dentists. Nonsurgical therapy is a very effective way of producing a satisfactory stable result. Ideal results with furcations are impossible to obtain. Once furcation breakdown has begun, the clinical result is always somewhat compromised. Both surgical and nonsurgical therapies have been shown to work effectively over time. Nonsurgical therapy, a combination of oral hygiene instruction and scaling and root planing, has provided excellent results in some patients. The earlier the furcation is detected and treated, the more likely it will be that a good long-term result can be obtained. Nonetheless, even advanced furcation lesions can have successful long-term treatment. Several oral hygiene procedures have been used over time. All include access to the furcation. Obtaining access to the furcation requires a combination of the awareness of the furcation by the patient and an oral hygiene tool that facilitates that access. Many tools, including rubber tips, periodontal aids, both specific and general toothbrushes, and other aids have been used over time for access to the patient (Fig. 49.8A and B).

Scaling and Root Planing

Nonsurgical maintenance by the clinician has also improved over time as instrumentation has improved. In recent decades, instruments beyond simple curettes have been used to instrument the furcation. The frustration of instrumenting the furcation was illustrated beautifully by Bower in 1979 in his articles showing that only 58% of furcations could be entered by typically using curettes. Subsequently, other instrumentation has evolved, including DeMarco curettes, diamond files, Quétin furcation curettes, and Mini Five Gracey Curettes.

Svärdström and Wennström illustrated that in the long term, furcations could be maintained using nonaggressive techniques over a 10-year period in patients who were participants in consistent maintenance. Other studies also illustrate that maintenance therapy is useful for patients to facilitate furcation cleanliness. Chemotherapy has proven disappointing. Ribeiro and colleagues found that nonsurgical therapy can effectively treat class II furcation involvements but using povidone-iodine did not provide additional benefits to subgingival instrumentation.

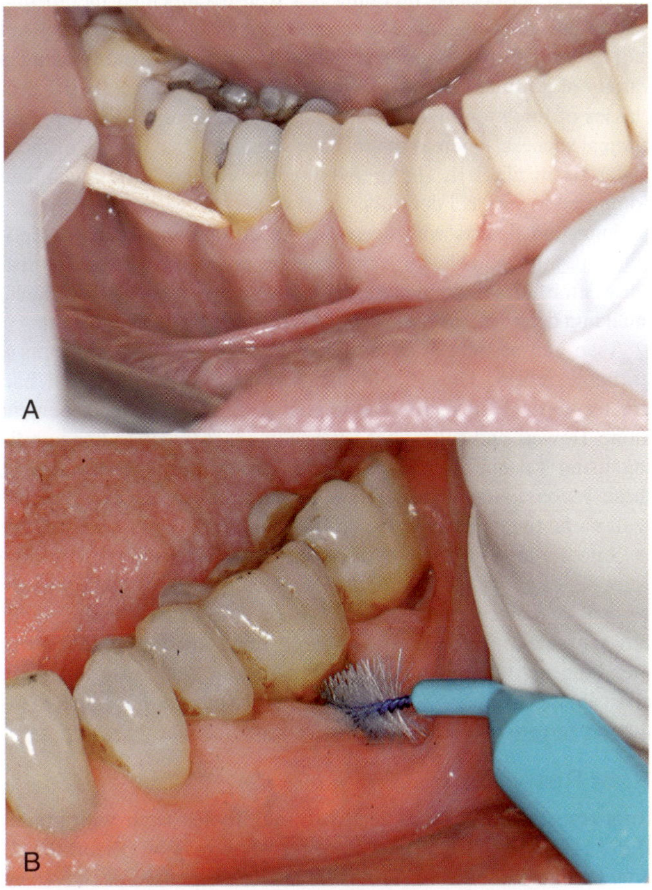

Fig. 49.8 A, The utilization of a Perio-Aid into the furcation for plaque removal. B, Proxy brush is used for plaque removal into the furcation lesion. *(Courtesy: Karen DeYoung, RDH, and Janet Shigekawa, RDH.)*

The area most critical in furcation management is maintaining a relatively plaque-free status to the furcation. Attaining access is a problem in this regard, but with the previously mentioned instruments and an effective nonsurgical approach, much can be accomplished. The most critical component of multirooted tooth maintenance is always the successful reduction or elimination of plaque retention areas from the furcation area; meticulous oral hygiene by the patient and effective nonsurgical therapy can play a major role in attaining this goal.

Surgical Therapy

Osseous Resection

Osseous surgical therapy can be divided into resective and regenerative therapy. This also applies to the furcation areas when surgical therapy is contemplated. For many years, osteoplasty and ostectomy have been used to make the furcation areas cleansable. In advanced cases, techniques were used to open the furcation into a class IV from a severe class II or III case. This would allow easier hygiene into the furcation area for the patient. These techniques have limited usefulness today, but in the compromised individual whose teeth cannot be extracted or in whom conservative therapy has failed, these surgical techniques have been used. The immediate goal with these surgical approaches is to create access for the patient to maintain good hygiene.

Regeneration

In furcal lesions, bone regeneration is often thought to be relatively futile. The periodontal literature has well-documented therapeutic efforts designed to induce new attachment and reconstruction on molars with furcation defects. Many surgical procedures using a variety of grafting materials have been tested on teeth with different classes of furcation involvement. Some investigators have reported clinical success, whereas others have suggested that the use of these materials in class II, III, or IV furcations offers little advantage compared to surgical controls.

Furcation defects with deep two-walled or three-walled components may be suitable for reconstruction procedures. These vertical bony deformities respond favorably to a variety of surgical procedures, including debridement with or without membranes and bone grafts.

Tsao and associates have shown that the furcation defect is a graftable lesion. They found that lesions that were grafted had greater vertical fill than areas treated with open flap debridement alone. Bowers and colleagues have shown that furcation bone grafting using various membranes can improve the clinical status of these lesions. Nonetheless, bone grafting remains an elusive goal with variable results in furcation lesions.

Another area of interest has been barrier membrane technology. Analysis of published studies demonstrated a great variability in the clinical outcomes in mandibular grade II furcations treated with different types of nonbioabsorbable and bioabsorbable barrier membranes. Although many barrier membrane studies show a slight clinical improvement after treatment in both maxillary and mandibular furcations, the results are generally inconsistent.

Root Resection

Root resection may be indicated in multirooted teeth with grades II–IV furcation involvement. Root resection may be performed on vital teeth or endodontically treated teeth. It is preferable, however, to have endodontic therapy completed before resection of a root or roots. If this is not possible, the pulp should be removed, the patency of the canals determined, and the pulp chamber medicated before resection. It is distressing for both patient and clinician to perform a vital root resection and subsequently have an unfavorable event occur, such as perforation, fracture of the root, or an inability to instrument the canal.

The indications and contraindications for root resection were well summarized by Bassaraba. In general, teeth planned for root resection include the following:

1. Teeth that are critically important to the overall dental treatment plan. Examples are teeth serving as abutments for fixed or removable restorations for which loss of the tooth would result in loss of the prosthesis and entail major prosthetic retreatment.
2. Teeth that have sufficient attachment remaining for function. Molars with advanced bone loss in the interproximal and interradicular zones, unless the lesions have three bony walls, are not candidates for root amputation.
3. Teeth for which a more predictable or cost-effective method of therapy is not available. Examples are teeth with furcation defects that have been treated successfully with endodontics but now have a vertical root fracture, advanced bone loss, or caries on the root.
4. Teeth in patients with good oral hygiene and low activity for caries are suitable for root resection. Patients unable or unwilling to perform good oral hygiene and preventive measures are not suitable candidates for root resection or hemisection. Root-resected teeth require endodontic treatment and usually cast restorations.

These therapies can represent a sizable financial investment by the patient in an effort to save the tooth. Alternative therapies and their impact on the overall treatment plan should always be considered and presented to the patient.

Which Root to Remove

A tooth with an isolated furcation defect in an otherwise intact dental segment may present few diagnostic problems. However, the existence of multiple furcation defects of varying severity combined with generalized advanced periodontitis can be a challenge to treatment planning. Careful diagnosis usually allows the therapist to determine the feasibility of root resection and the identification of which root to remove before surgery. Every attempt should be made to determine this before surgical exposure.

The following is a guide to determining which root should be removed in these cases:

1. Remove the root or roots that will eliminate the furcation and allow the production of a maintainable architecture on the remaining roots.
2. Remove the root with the greatest amount of bone and attachment loss. Sufficient periodontal attachment must remain after surgery for the tooth to withstand the functional demands placed on it such as bridge abutments and in bruxers. Teeth with uniform advanced horizontal bone loss are not suitable for root resection.
3. Remove the root that best contributes to the elimination of periodontal problems on adjacent teeth. For example, a maxillary first molar with a class III buccal-to-distal furcation is adjacent to a maxillary second molar with a two-walled intrabony defect between the molars and an early class II furcation on the mesial furcation of the second molar. Local anatomic factors affecting the teeth may or may not be present. The removal of the distobuccal root of the first molar allows the elimination of the furcation and management of the two-wall intrabony lesion and also facilitates access for instrumentation and maintenance of the second molar.
4. Remove the root with the greatest number of anatomic problems such as severe curvature, developmental grooves, root flutings, or accessory and multiple root canals.
5. Remove the root that least complicates future periodontal maintenance.

Hemisection

Hemisection is the splitting of a two-rooted tooth into two separate portions. This process has been called bicuspidization or separation because it changes the molar into two separate roots. Hemisection is most likely to be performed on mandibular molars with buccal and lingual class II or III furcation involvements. As with root resection, molars with advanced bone loss in the interproximal and interradicular zones are not good candidates for hemisection. After sectioning of the teeth, one or both roots can be retained. This decision is based on the extent and pattern of bony loss, root trunk and root length, ability to eliminate the osseous defect, and endodontic and restorative considerations. The anatomy of the mesial roots of mandibular molars often leads to their extraction and the retention of the distal root to facilitate both endodontic and restorative therapy.

The interradicular dimension between the two roots of a tooth to be hemisected is also important. Narrow interradicular zones can complicate the surgical procedure. The retention of both molar roots can complicate the restoration of the tooth because it may be virtually impossible to finish margins or to provide an adequate embrasure between the two roots for effective oral hygiene and maintenance. Therefore, orthodontic separation of the roots is often required to allow restoration with adequate embrasure form. The result can be the need for multiple procedures and extensive interdisciplinary therapy. In these patients, the availability of other treatment alternatives should be considered, such as guided tissue or guided bone regeneration or replacement by osseointegrated dental implants.

Root Resection or Hemisection Procedure

Procedures such as root resection, hemisection, and bicuspidization were popular in the past. They required a successful endodontic therapy and later crown and bridge dentistry for long-term maintenance. The results were not consistent and predictable. With the advent of dental implants, these procedures have become almost obsolete. They are discussed here mainly as a matter of historical interest.

The most common root resection involves the distobuccal root of the maxillary first molar. After appropriate local anesthesia, a full-thickness mucoperiosteal flap is elevated. Root resection or hemisection of teeth with advanced attachment loss usually requires opening both facial and lingual-palatal flaps. Typically, a root cannot be resected without elevating a flap. The flap should provide adequate access for visualization and instrumentation and minimize surgical trauma.

After debridement, resection of the root begins with the exposure of the furcation on the root to be removed. The removal of a small amount of facial or palatal bone may be required to provide access for elevation and facilitate root removal. A cut is then directed from just apical to the contact point of the tooth, through the tooth, and to the facial and distal orifices of the furcation. This cut is made with a high-speed, surgical-length fissure or crosscut fissure carbide bur. The placement of a curved periodontal probe into or through the furcation aids in orienting the angle of the resection. For hemisection, a vertically oriented cut is made faciolingually through the buccal and lingual developmental grooves of the tooth, through the pulp chamber, and through the furcation. If the sectioning cut passes through a metallic restoration, the metallic portion of the cut should be made before flap elevation. This prevents contamination of the surgical field with metallic particles.

If a vital root resection is to be performed, a more horizontal cut through the root is advisable. An oblique cut exposes a large surface area of the radicular pulp and/or dental pulp chamber. This can lead to postoperative pain and can complicate endodontic therapy. A horizontal cut, although it may complicate root removal, has fewer postoperative complications. This root stump can be removed by odontoplasty after the completion of endodontic therapy or at the time of tooth preparation.

After sectioning, the root is elevated from its socket. Care should be taken not to traumatize bone on the remaining roots or to damage an adjacent tooth. Removal of the root provides visibility to the furcation aspects of the remaining roots and simplifies the debridement of the furcation with hand, rotary, or ultrasonic instruments. If necessary, odontoplasty is performed to remove portions of the developmental ridges and prepare a furcation that is free of any deformity that would enhance plaque retention or adversely affect plaque removal.

Patients with advanced periodontitis often have root resection performed in conjunction with other surgical procedures. The bony lesions that may be present on adjacent teeth are then treated using resective or regenerative therapies. After resection, the flaps are then approximated to cover any grafted tissues or slightly cover the bony margins around the tooth. Sutures are then placed to maintain the position of the flaps. The area may or may not be covered with a surgical dressing.

The removal of a root alters the distribution of occlusal forces on the remaining roots. Therefore, it is wise to evaluate the occlusion of teeth from which roots have been resected and, if necessary, adjust the occlusion. Centric holds should be maintained, but eccentric forces should be eliminated from the area over the root that was removed. Patients with advanced attachment loss may benefit from temporary stabilization of the resected tooth to prevent movement.

Extraction

The extraction of teeth with through-and-through furcation defects (classes III and IV) and advanced attachment loss may be the most appropriate therapy for some patients. This is particularly true for individuals who cannot or will not perform adequate plaque control, who have a high level of caries activity, who will not commit to a suitable maintenance program, or who have socioeconomic factors that may preclude more complex therapies. Some patients are reluctant to accept periodontal surgery or even allow the removal of a tooth with advanced furcation involvement, even though the long-term prognosis is poor. The patient may elect to forego therapy, opt to treat the area with scaling and root planing or site-specific antibacterial therapies, and delay extraction until the tooth becomes symptomatic. Although additional attachment loss may occur, such teeth may survive a significant number of years.

Dental Implants

The advent of osseointegrated dental implants as an alternative abutment source has had a major impact on the retention of teeth with advanced furcation problems. The high level of predictability of osseointegration may motivate the therapist and patient to consider removal of teeth with a guarded or poor prognosis and to seek an implant-supported prosthetic treatment plan. Therefore, careful evaluation of the long-term periodontal, endodontic, and restorative prognosis must be considered before invasive surgical therapy is undertaken to save a tooth with an advanced furcated lesion (Fig. 49.9A–D).

Prognosis

For many years, the presence of significant furcation involvement meant a hopeless long-term prognosis for the tooth. Clinical research, however, has indicated that furcation problems are not as severe a complication as originally suspected if one can prevent the development of caries in the furcation. Relatively simple periodontal therapy is sufficient to maintain these teeth in function for long periods. Other investigators have defined the reasons for clinical failure of root-resected or hemisected teeth. Their data indicate that recurrent periodontal disease is not a major cause of the failure of these teeth. Investigations of root-resected or hemisected teeth have shown that such teeth can function successfully for long periods.

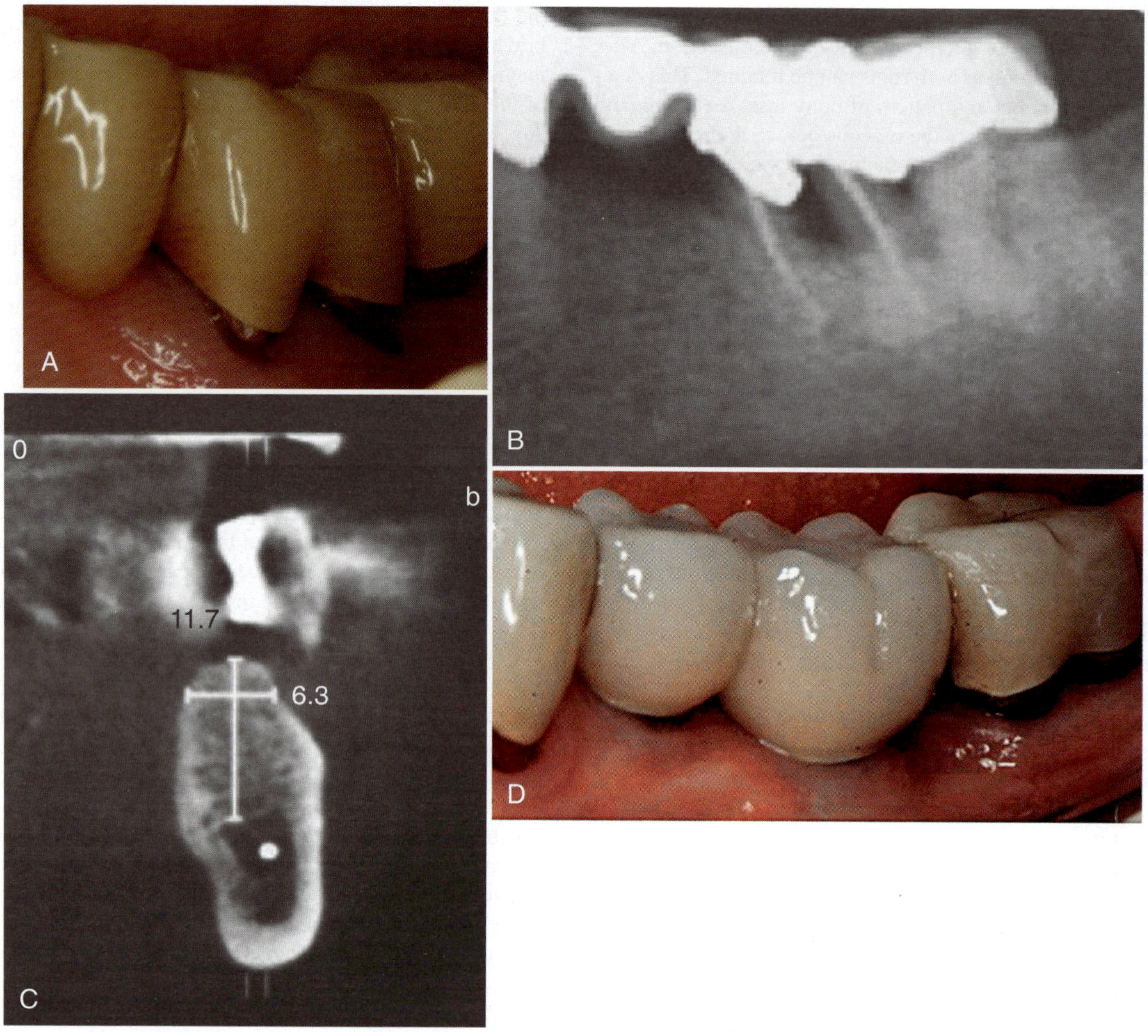

Fig. 49.9 A, Clinical picture of a class III furcation involvement. B, Radiographic appearance is far more grave than the clinical appearance. C, After the tooth is removed, a computed tomography image is taken to plan treatment for implant replacement. D, The implant restored. *(Courtesy: Dr. Sarvenaz Angha, Los Angeles, CA.)*

The keys to long-term success appear to be (1) thorough diagnosis, (2) selection of patients with good oral hygiene, (3) excellence in nonsurgical therapy, and (4) careful surgical and restorative management.

Key points

- Furcation involvement indicates advanced periodontitis and presents diagnostic and therapeutic problems.
- The primary etiologic factor of furcation involvement is bacterial plaque and related to other anatomical factors.
- Presence of cervical enamel projections and enamel pearls together with inadequate root separation complicates the treatment.
- Grade II furcations are good candidates for regeneration.
- Root resection and hemisection have limited indication. In cases of advanced furcation involvement, extraction of the tooth followed by replacement with a dental implant is a good alternative.

Suggested Readings

DeSanctis M, Murphy KG: The role of resective periodontal surgery in the treatment of furcation defects. *J Periodontol* 22:154–168, 2000.

Newell DH: The diagnosis and treatment of molar furcation invasions. *Dent Clin North Am* 42(2):301–337, 1998.

Periodontal Plastic and Esthetic Surgery

HH Takei | ET Scheyer | RR Azzi | EP Allen | TJ Han | CD Dwarakanath | JP George

CHAPTER OUTLINE

In the last three decades, the scope and ambit of periodontal therapy has gone far beyond arresting the disease and eliminating the pockets. Increasing patient awareness has resulted in a big demand for restoration and augmentation of esthetics. Further the periodontist is now an important member of the interdisciplinary team which aims at overall maintenance of the dentition in a state of health, function, and esthetic harmony.

Terminology

The term **mucogingival surgery** was initially introduced in the literature by Friedman to describe surgical procedures for the correction of relationships between the gingiva and the oral mucous membrane with reference to three specific problem areas: attached gingiva, shallow vestibule, and frenum interfering with the marginal gingiva. With the advancement of periodontal surgical techniques, the scope of nonpocket surgical procedures has increased, now encompassing a multitude of areas that were not addressed in the past. Recognizing this, the 1996 World Workshop in Clinical Periodontics renamed mucogingival surgery as "**periodontal plastic surgery**," a term originally proposed by Miller in 1993 and broadened to include the following areas:

- Periodontal-prosthetic corrections
- Crown lengthening
- Socket preservation
- Ridge augmentation
- Esthetic surgical corrections
- Coverage of the denuded root surface
- Reconstruction of papillae
- Esthetic surgical correction around implants
- Surgical exposure of unerupted teeth for orthodontics

Periodontal plastic surgery (PPS) is defined as "surgical procedures performed to prevent or correct anatomic, developmental, traumatic or disease-induced defects of the gingiva, alveolar mucosa or bone." Mucogingival therapy is a broader term that includes periodontal procedures for the correction of defects in the morphology, position, and/or amount of soft tissue and underlying bone support around teeth and implants such as papilla reconstruction by means of orthodontic or restorative therapy. PPS includes only the surgical procedures of mucogingival therapy. However, in common usage, clinicians use the terms PPS and mucogingival surgery interchangeably.

Objectives of Perioplastic Surgery
1. Widening the zone of attached gingiva.
2. Coverage of gingival recession.
3. Deepening of shallow vestibule.
4. Removal of aberrant frenum.
5. Various esthetic deformities of the gingiva.
6. Correction of esthetic deformities.

Source - Dr Joann Pauline George

This chapter discusses the periodontal plastic surgical techniques included in the traditional definition of mucogingival surgery: (1) widening of attached gingiva, (2) deepening of shallow vestibules, and (3) resection of the aberrant frenum. In addition, esthetic surgical therapy around the natural dentition and tissue engineering (biologic mediator) are included in this chapter. Other aspects of PPS, such as periodontal-prosthetic surgery, esthetic surgery around implants, and surgical exposure of teeth for orthodontic therapy are covered in other chapters of this book.

Problems Associated With Attached Gingiva

One of the goals of PPS is the creation or widening of attached gingiva around teeth and implants. The width of the attached gingiva varies in different individuals and on different teeth of the same individual. Attached gingiva is not synonymous with "keratinized gingiva" because the latter also includes the free gingival margin. The width of the attached gingiva is determined by subtracting the depth of the sulcus or pocket from the distance between the crest of the gingival margin and the mucogingival junction.

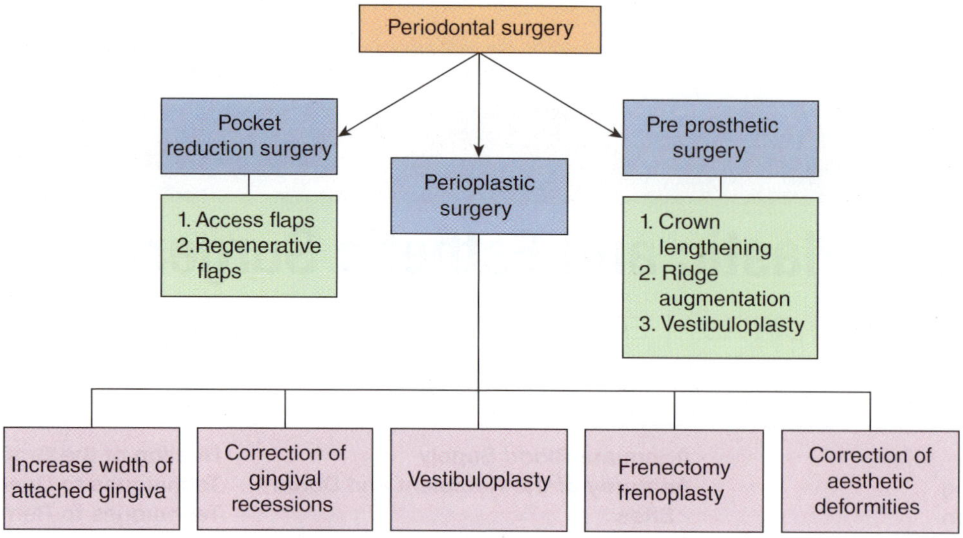

Classification of periodontal surgery
Source - Dr Joann Pauline George/Self

The original rationale for mucogingival surgery was predicated on the assumption that a minimal width of attached gingiva was required to maintain optimal gingival health. However, several studies have challenged the view that a wide, attached gingiva is more protective against the accumulation of plaque than a narrow or a nonexistent zone. No minimum width of attached gingiva has been established as a standard necessary for gingival health. People who practice good, atraumatic oral hygiene may maintain excellent gingival health with almost no attached gingiva. However, those individuals whose oral hygiene practices are less than optimal can be helped by the presence of keratinized gingiva and vestibular depth. Vestibular depth provides space for easier placement of the toothbrush and prevents brushing on mucosal tissue. To improve esthetics, the objective is the coverage of the denuded root surface. The maxillary anterior area, especially the facial aspect of the canine, often presents extensive gingival recession. In such cases, the covering of the denuded root surface not only widens the zone of attached gingiva but also creates an improved esthetic result. This recession and the resultant denuded root surface have special esthetic concerns for individuals with a high smile line. A wider zone of attached gingiva is also needed around teeth that serve as abutments for fixed or removable partial dentures, as well as in the ridge areas bearing a denture. Teeth with subgingival restorations and narrow zones of keratinized gingiva have higher gingival inflammation scores than teeth with similar restorations and wide zones of attached gingiva. In these cases, techniques for widening the attached gingiva are considered preprosthetic periodontal surgical procedures.

To summarize, widening the attached gingiva accomplishes the following objectives:

1. Enhances plaque removal around the gingival margin.
2. Improves esthetics.
3. Reduces inflammation around restorations, dental prostheses, implants, orthodontics, and future recession.
4. Gingival margin binds better around teeth and implants with attached gingiva.
5. Improves patient comfort.

Problems Associated With Shallow Vestibule

Another objective of PPS is the creation of vestibular depth when it is lacking. Gingival recession displaces the gingival margin apically, thus reducing vestibular depth, which is measured from the gingival margin to the bottom of the vestibule. As indicated previously, with minimal vestibular depth, proper hygiene procedures are jeopardized. The sulcular brushing technique requires the placement of the toothbrush at the gingival margin, which may not be possible with reduced vestibular depth. However, it is important to note that no minimal depth of vestibule has been defined. Minimal attached gingiva with adequate vestibular depth may not require surgical correction if proper atraumatic hygiene is practiced with a soft brush. Minimal amounts of keratinized attached gingiva with no vestibular depth benefit from mucogingival correction. Adequate vestibular depth is also necessary for the proper placement of removable prostheses.

Problems Associated With Aberrant Frenum

The frenum is a mucous membrane fold that attaches the lip and the cheek to the alveolar mucosa, the gingiva, and the underlying periosteum. A frenum is considered as aberrant when it is associated with a decreased vestibular depth and an inadequate width of the attached gingiva leading to esthetic problem, persistence of a midline diastema, gingival recession, and mechanical trauma during brushing.

Another important objective of PPS is to correct frenal or muscle attachments that may extend coronal to the mucogingival junction. If adequate keratinized, attached gingiva is present coronal to the frenum, it may not be necessary to remove the frenum. A frenum that encroaches on the margin of the gingiva may interfere with biofilm removal, and the tension on the frenum may tend to open the sulcus (Fig. 50.1). In such cases, surgical removal of the frenum is indicated.

Esthetic Deformities

The recession of the facial gingival margin will alter the acceptable gingival symmetry and result in an esthetic problem. Inconsistent gingival margin needs to be corrected to improve the smile profile of the patient. A missing interdental papilla creates a space that many address as a "black triangle." Reconstruction of the lost or reduced papilla is one of the most difficult goals in esthetic PPS.

Another area of concern is the patient who presents an excessive gingival display in the visible area. This condition is often addressed as a "gummy smile" and may be corrected surgically by

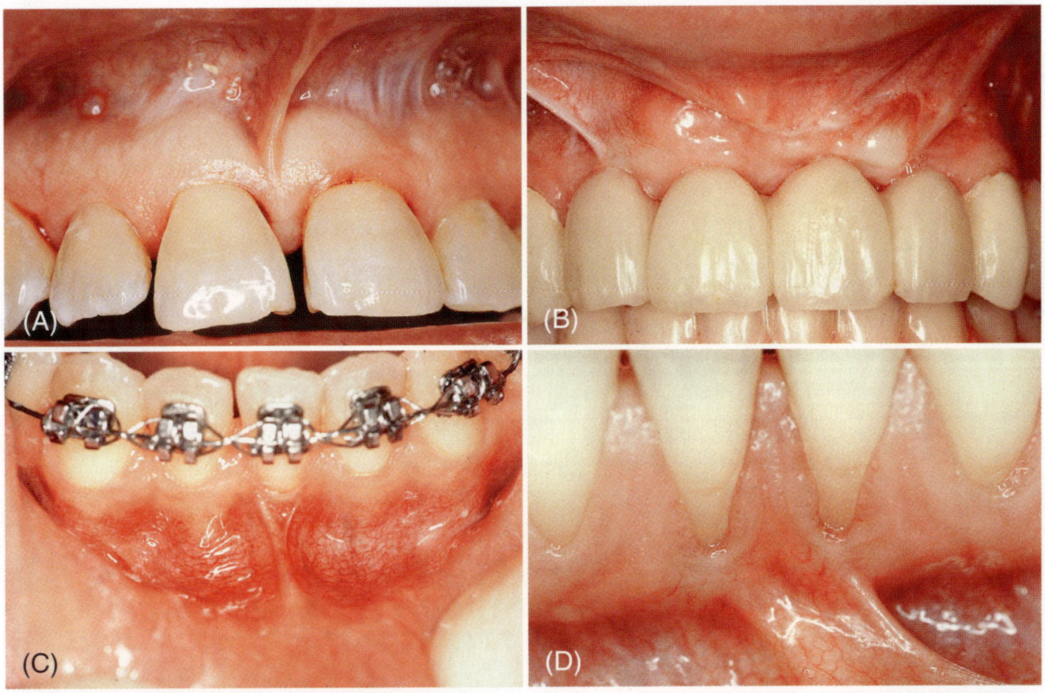

Fig. 50.1 (A) Abnormal frenal attachment (B) Lack of attached gingiva (C) Denuded roots (D) Shallow vestibule

crown lengthening. Gingival enlargement that result in pseudo pockets leads to esthetic and functional problems that require surgical correction. The correction of these anatomic defects has become an important part of PPS. The esthetic demands of the patients today have increased to such an extent that black or brownish discoloration of the gums—"physiologic hyper melanin pigmentation" is unacceptable. Gingival depigmentation, although provides only a temporary relief, is widely performed nowadays.

Tissue Engineering

The future of PPS will encompass the use of tissue-engineered products at the recipient site to reduce donor site morbidity. Results of numerous experimental and clinical studies support the clinician's use of a minimally invasive approach to PPS.

Gingival Recession

Exposed roots besides being unesthetic also cause additional problems, like dentinal hypersensitivity and pulpal hyperemia and are prone for caries.

Etiology of Marginal Tissue Recession

The most common cause of gingival recession and the loss of attached gingiva is abrasive and traumatic toothbrushing habits (Fig. 50.2). The bone and soft tissue anatomy of the buccal, radicular surface of the dentition is usually thin, especially around the anterior area. Teeth positioned buccally may have an even thinner bone and gingiva. The periodontal biotype that includes gingival thickness, width of keratinized tissue, and thickness of marginal bone plays an important role in predisposition to gingival recession. A thin periodontal biotype, absence of attached gingiva, and reduced thickness of the alveolar bone due to abnormal tooth position in the arch are considered risk factors for the development of gingival recession. In many instances, such areas may have a complete absence of bone beneath the thin overlying gingival tissue. Such defect in the bone is called a *dehiscence.* This anatomic status combined with external trauma from overzealous brushing can lead to the loss of gingival tissue. Recession of the gingival tissue and bone exposes the cemental surface of the root, which results in abrasion and "ditching" of the cemental surface apical to the cementoenamel junction (CEJ). The cementum is softer than enamel and will be destroyed before the enamel surface of the crown. Gingival recession may be associated with noncarious cervical lesion (NCCL) and cervical caries that leads to hypersensitivity.

Another cause for gingival recession is periodontal disease and chronic marginal inflammation. The loss of attachment caused by the inflammation is followed by the loss of bone and gingiva. Advanced periodontal involvement in areas of minimal attached gingiva results in the base of the pocket extending close to or apical to the mucogingival junction. Periodontal therapy of these areas also results in gingival recession caused by the loss of gingiva and bone (Fig. 50.2D and E).

Frenal and muscle attachments that encroach on the marginal gingiva can distend the gingival sulcus, which creates an environment for plaque biofilm accumulation. This condition increases the rate periodontal recession and will contribute to the recurrence of the recession even after treatment. These problems are more common on facial surfaces but may also occur on the lingual surface.

Orthodontic tooth movement through a thin buccal osseous plate may lead to a dehiscence beneath a thin gingiva, which can lead to recession.

Gingival recession can occur in three anatomically distinct areas, namely facial/buccal surfaces, papillary areas, and lingual surfaces.

Factors That Affect Surgical Outcome

Irregularity of Teeth

Abnormal tooth alignment is an important cause of gingival deformities that require corrective surgery and also an important factor in determining the outcome of treatment. The location of the gingival margin, width of the attached gingiva, and alveolar bone height and thickness are all affected by tooth alignment. On teeth that are tilted or rotated labially, the labial bony plate is thinner and located

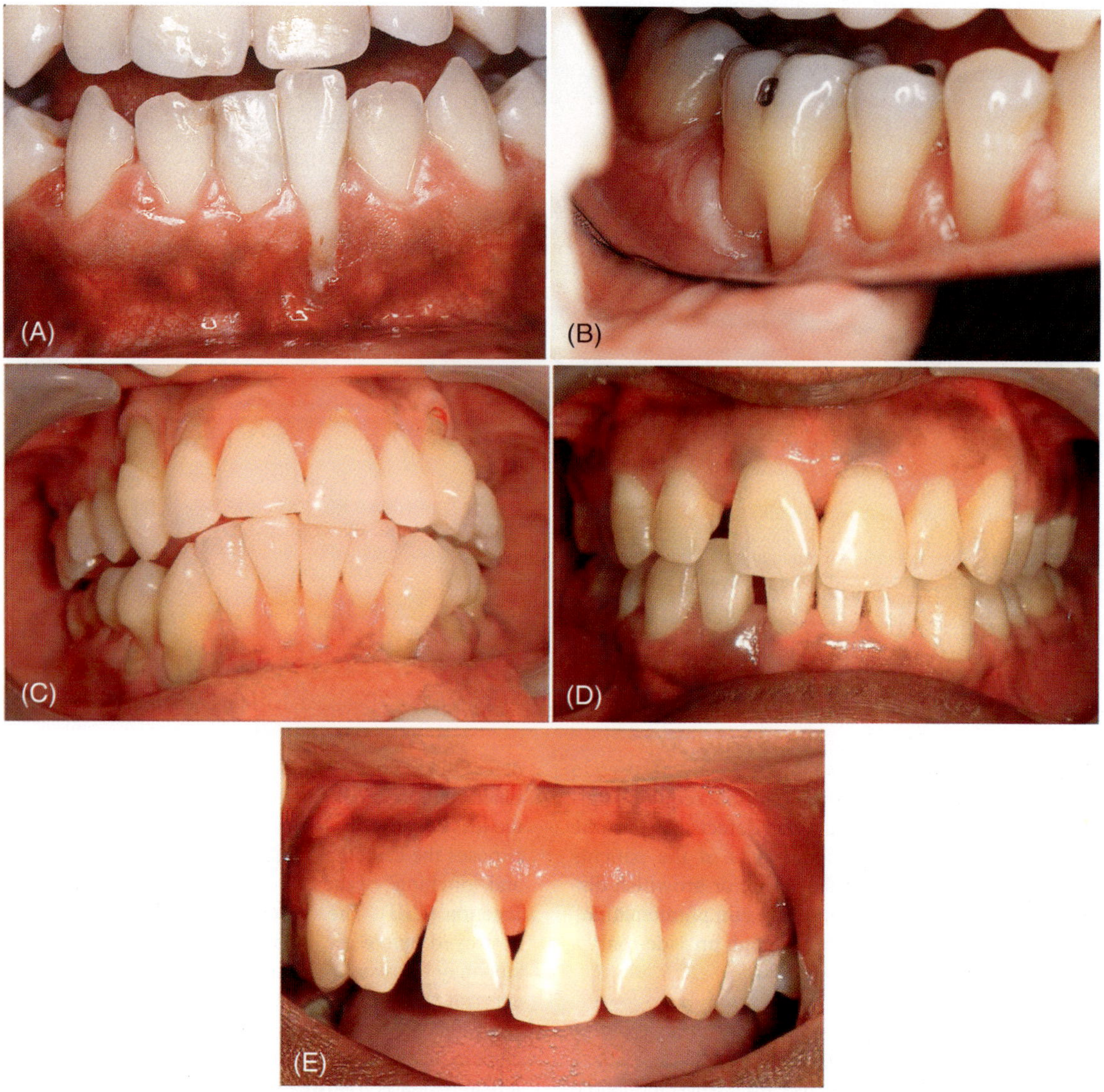

Fig. 50.2 A, Gingival recession and extreme inflammation around a lower central incisor. B, Advanced recession of mesial root of a first lower molar, C, Gingival recession caused by faulty tooth brushing. D, Preoperative view showing deep periodontal pocket between the maxillary central incisors. E, Recession following periodontal flap surgery.

farther apically than on the adjacent teeth; therefore, the gingiva is recessed so that the root is exposed. On the lingual surface of such teeth, the gingiva is bulbous and the bone margins are closer to the CEJ. The level of gingival attachment on root surfaces and the width of the attached gingiva after mucogingival surgery are affected as much by tooth alignment as by variations in treatment procedures.

Orthodontic correction is indicated when mucogingival surgery is performed on malposed teeth in an attempt to widen the attached gingiva or to restore the gingiva over denuded roots. If orthodontic treatment is not feasible, the prominent tooth should be reduced to within the borders of the alveolar bone, with special care taken to avoid pulp injury.

Roots covered with thin bony plates present a hazard in mucogingival surgery. Even the most protective type of flap, a partial-thickness flap, creates the risk of bone resorption on the periosteal surface. Resorption in amounts that ordinarily are not significant may cause loss of bone height when the bone plate is thin or tapered at the crest.

Mucogingival Line (Junction)

Normally, the mucogingival line in the incisor and canine areas is located approximately 3 mm apical to the crest of the alveolar bone on the radicular surfaces and 5 mm interdentally. In periodontal disease and on malposed disease free teeth, the bone margin is located farther apically and may extend beyond the mucogingival line. The distance between the mucogingival line and the CEJ before and after periodontal surgery is not necessarily constant. After inflammation is eliminated, the tissue tends to contract and draw the mucogingival line in the direction of the crown.

Periodontal Biotype

A thin periodontal biotype, absence of attached gingiva, and reduced thickness of the alveolar bone due to abnormal tooth position in the arch will play a decisive role in the management of mucogingival problems.

Factors That Affect Surgical Outcome
Irregularity of teeth
Mucogingival line (junction)
Periodontal biotype

Source - Dr Joann Pauline George

Criteria for Selection of Techniques

Numerous techniques are used for solving the mucogingival problems outlined in this chapter. Proper selection of a technique must be based on the predictability of success, which is based on specific criteria.

The following criteria are used for the selection of mucogingival techniques:

1. Surgical site free of biofilm, calculus, and inflammation.
2. Anatomy of the recipient and donor sites.
3. Minimal trauma to the surgical site.
4. Adequate flap mobility.
5. Adequate blood supply to the donor tissue.
6. Stability and passive adaptation of the flap/grafted tissue to the recipient site.

Surgical Site Free of Biofilm, Calculus, and Inflammation

Periodontal plastic surgical procedures should be undertaken in a biofilm-free and inflammation-free environment to enable the clinician to manage firm gingival tissue. Meticulous precise incisions and flap reflection cannot be achieved when tissue is inflamed and edematous. Thorough scaling and root planing and meticulous biofilm removal by the patient must be accomplished before any surgical procedure. The outcomes of perioplastic surgery depend on optimal oral hygiene standards than in conventional periodontal.

Adequate Blood Supply

To obtain the maximal amount of blood supply to the donor tissue, gingival augmentation apical to the area of recession provides a better blood supply than coronal augmentation because the recipient site is entirely periosteal tissue. Root coverage procedures involve a portion of the recipient site (i.e., denuded root surface) without blood supply. If esthetics is not a factor, gingival augmentation apical to the recession may be more predictable. A pedicle-displaced flap has a better blood supply than a free graft, with the base of the flap intact. If the anatomy is favorable, the pedicle flap or any of its variants may be the best procedure for root coverage. The Langer SECTG procedure and the pouch and tunnel techniques use a split flap with the connective tissue sandwiched between the flaps. This flap design maximizes the blood supply to the donor tissue. If large areas require root coverage, these sandwich-type recipient sites provide the best flap design for blood supply. This facilitates firm flap adaptation and provides a better vascular network within the pedicle flap. Keeping in mind the vascular supply of the flap, preparation should be done with an intent to avoid marginal and paramarginal incisions and place sulcular incisions instead, midcrestal incisions in edentulous areas, avoid releasing incisions, when releasing incision is placed it should be as short and as medially as possible and avoid releasing incisions on the buccal root prominences.

Anatomy of the Recipient and Donor Sites

The presence or absence of vestibular depth is an important anatomic criterion at the recipient site for gingival augmentation. If gingival augmentation is indicated apical to the area of recession, there must be adequate vestibular depth apical to the recessed gingival margin to provide space for a free or pedicle graft. If a vestibule is necessary, only a free graft can accomplish this objective apical to the recession.

Mucogingival techniques, such as free gingival grafts and free connective tissue grafts, can be used to create vestibular depth and widen the zone of attached gingiva. Other techniques require vestibular depth to be present before the surgery, including pedicle grafts (lateral and coronal), the Langer SECTG, and pouch and tunnel procedures.

Availability of donor tissue is another anatomic factor that must be considered. Pedicle displacement of tissue necessitates an adjacent donor site that has gingival thickness and width. Palatal tissue thickness is also necessary for the connective tissue donor autograft. Gingival thickness is required at the recipient site for techniques using a split-thickness, sandwich-type flap, or the pouch and tunnel techniques.

Stability of the Grafted Tissue to the Recipient Site

Good communication of the blood vessels from the grafted donor tissue to the recipient site requires a stable environment. This necessitates sutures that stabilize the donor tissue firmly against the recipient site. The stability of the grafted tissue to the recipient site with appropriate suturing appears to be a key prerequisite for optimal surgical outcomes. Minimal residual flap tension (approximately 0.4 g) improves recession reduction significantly. The suturing technique has a limited influence on the blood circulation in the healing wound. The least number of sutures and maximal stability should be achieved.

Minimal Trauma to the Surgical Site

As with all surgical procedures, PPS is based on the meticulous, delicate, and precise management of oral tissues. Unnecessary tissue trauma caused by poor incisions, flap perforations, tears or traumatic and excessive placement of sutures can lead to tissue necrosis. The proper selection of instruments, needles, and sutures is mandatory to minimize tissue trauma. Contoured blades, smaller diameter needles, and resorbable monofilament sutures are important factors in achieving atraumatic surgery. Finer suture diameters may be helpful owing to the fact that thinner sutures (6-0, 7-0) lead to thread breakage rather than tissue tear and breakage. A less traumatic approach in PPS by using magnification aids and fine suture materials ensures minimal trauma and passive wound closure in most surgical interventions.

Techniques to Increase Attached Gingiva

To simplify and better understand the techniques and the result of the surgery, the following classification is presented:

- **Gingival augmentation apical to the area of recession.** A donor graft tissue, either pedicle or free, is placed on a recipient bed apical to the recessed gingival margin. No attempt is made to cover the denuded root surface.
- **Gingival augmentation coronal to the recession (root coverage).** A donor graft tissue (either pedicle or free) is placed covering the denuded root surface. Both the apical and the coronal widening of attached gingiva enhance oral hygiene procedures, but only the latter can correct an esthetic problem. For preprosthetic purposes, the combination of widening keratinized gingiva apical and coronal to the recession would satisfy this objective. Consideration of the objectives as apical, coronal, or both provides a better understanding of the techniques required to achieve the goals.

Widening of the keratinized attached gingiva (apical or coronal to the area of recession) can be accomplished by numerous techniques, such as the free gingival autograft, free connective tissue autograft, and lateral pedicle flap, which can be used for either objective.

Gingival augmentation apical to the area of recession	1. Free gingival autografts	
	2. Alternative donor tissue	Acellular dermal matrix Extracellular matrix membrane Bilayer collagen matrix Living cellular construct
	3. Free connective tissue grafts	
	4. Apically displaced flap	Modified apically repositioned flap
Gingival augmentation coronal to the area of recession	1. Free gingival autograft	
	2. Free connective tissue autograft	
	3. Pedicle graft	Laterally or horizontally displaced flap Double papilla flap Semilunar pedicle graft (Tarnow)
	4. Coronally advanced flap	
	5. Subepithelial connective tissue graft (Langer)	
	6. Guided tissue regeneration (GTR)	
	7. Pouch and tunnel technique	Coronally advanced tunnel technique Modified coronally advanced tunnel Vestibular incision Subperiosteal tunnel access (VISTA) Pinhole technique (Fig. 50.3)
	8. Other techniques	Vestibular extension Fenestration operation

Techniques of Gingival Augmentation

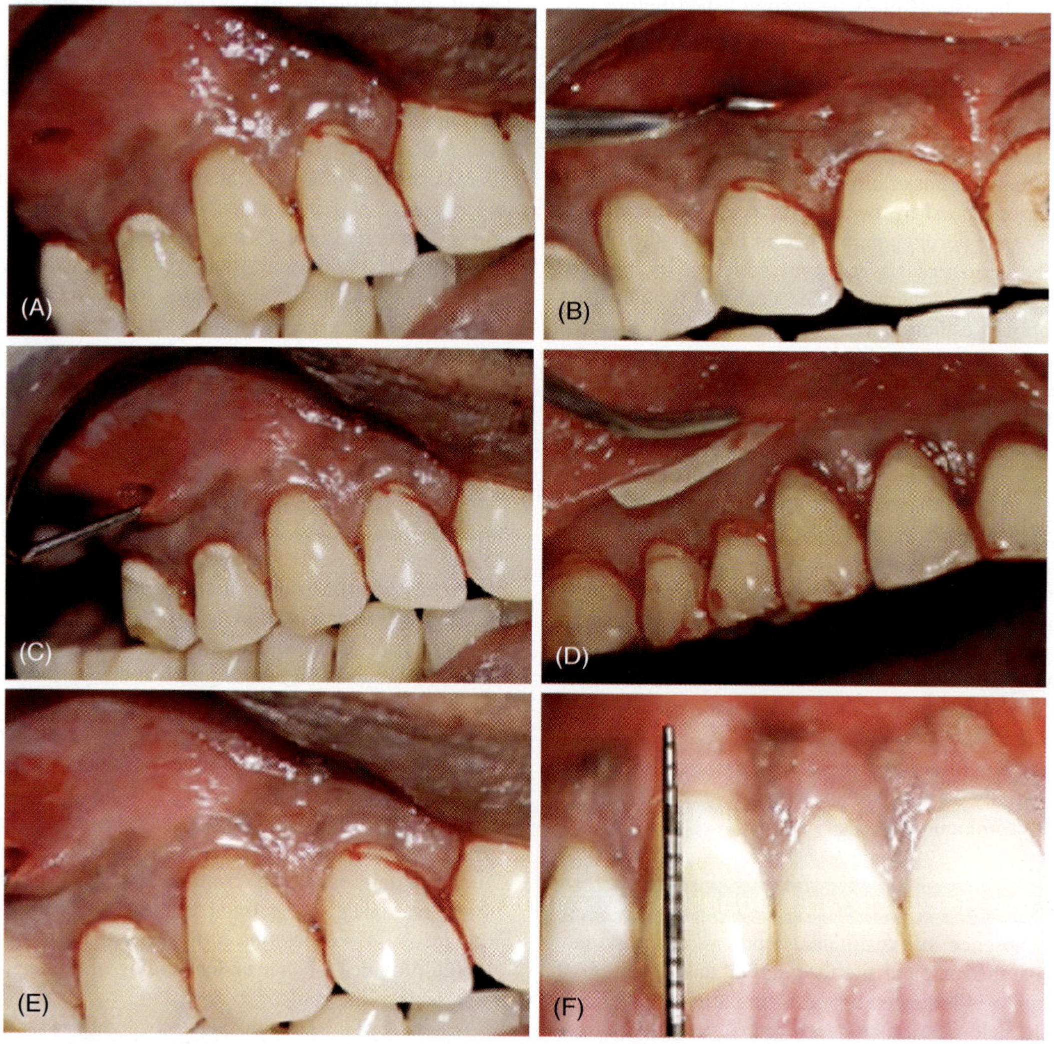

Fig. 50.3 A, 2-3 mm incision at mucogingival junction. B, Insertion of papilla elevator TKN2 for tunnel preparation. C, Passive tunnel advancement. D, Tucking of bioresorbable collagen membrane. E, Final position of gingival margin with passive advancement. F, 6-month post-operative appearance. *(Courtesy: Dr Joann Pauline George, India)*

Gingival Augmentation Apical to Recession

Free Gingival Autografts

Free gingival grafts are used to create a widened zone of attached gingiva. They were initially described by Bjorn in 1963 and have been extensively investigated since that time.

The Classic Technique (Fig. 50.4)

Step 1: Prepare the recipient site. The purpose of this step is to prepare a firm connective tissue bed to receive the graft.

i. The recipient site can be prepared by incising at the existing mucogingival junction with a #15 blade to the desired depth, blending the incision on both ends with the existing mucogingival line. Periosteum should be left covering the bone (Fig. 50.4A–C).

ii. Another technique consists of outlining the recipient site with two vertical incisions from the incised gingival margin into the alveolar mucosa. Extend the incisions to approximately twice the desired width of the attached gingiva, allowing for 50% contraction of the graft when healing is complete. The amount of contraction depends on the extent to which the recipient site penetrates the muscle attachments. The deeper the recipient site, the greater is the tendency for the muscles to elevate the graft and reduce the final width of the attached gingiva. The periosteum along the apical border of the graft is sometimes penetrated in an effort to prevent postoperative narrowing of the attached gingiva.

- The #15 blade is used to incise along the gingival margin to separate a flap consisting of epithelium and underlying connective tissue without disturbing the periosteum. Extend the flap to the depth of the vertical incisions. Suture the flap where the apical portion of the free graft will be located. Three to four independent gut sutures are placed. The needle is first passed as a superficial mattress suture perpendicular to the incision and then on the periosteum parallel to the incision.
- A sterile aluminum foil template of the recipient site can be made to be used as a pattern for the procuring the graft.
- Grafts can also be placed directly on bone tissue. For this technique, the flap should be separated by blunt dissection with a periosteal elevator. The advantages of this variant are less postoperative mobility of the graft, less swelling, better hemostasis and 1.5–2 times less shrinkage. However, there is a healing lag period that is observed for the first 2 weeks.

Step 2: Obtain the graft from the donor site. The classic or conventional free gingival graft technique consists of transferring a piece of keratinized gingiva approximately the size of the recipient site. To avoid the large wound that this procedure sometimes leaves in the donor site, some alternative methods have been proposed. The original technique is described first, followed by several of the most common variants.

i. For the classic technique, a partial-thickness graft is used. The palate is the usual site from which the donor tissue is removed. The graft should consist of epithelium and a thin layer of underlying connective tissue. Place the template over the donor site, and make a shallow incision around it with a #15 blade. Insert the blade to the desired thickness at one edge of the graft. Elevate the edge and hold it with tissue forceps. Continue to separate the graft with the blade, lifting it gently as separation progresses to provide visibility. Placing sutures at the margins of the graft helps control it during separation and transfer and simplifies placement and suturing to the recipient site.

ii. Proper thickness is important for survival of the graft. It should be thin enough to permit diffusion of fluid from the recipient site, which is essential in the immediate posttransplant period. A graft that is too thin may necrose and expose the recipient site. However, the thin graft carries the advantage of acceptable color matching with the surrounding tissues. If the graft is too thick, its peripheral layer is jeopardized because of the excessive tissue that separates it from new circulation and

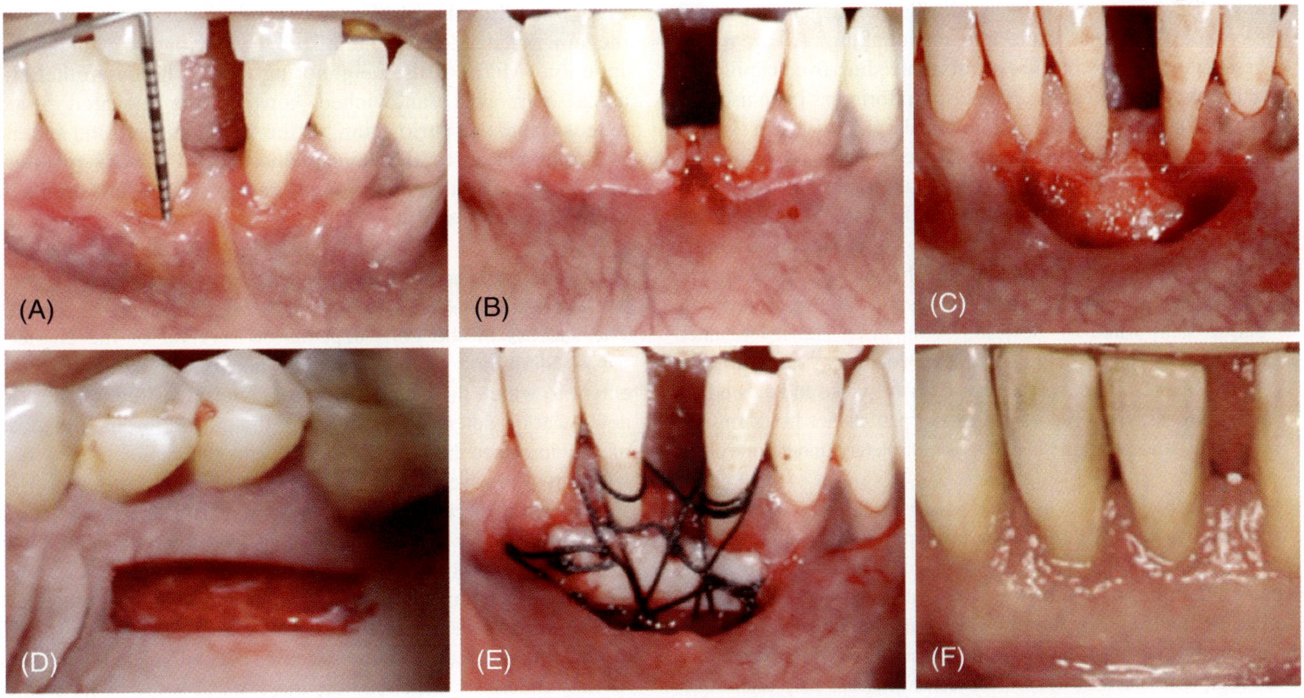

Fig. 50.4 Free gingival graft. A, and B, Preoperative view minimal keratinised gingiva. C, Recipient site prepared for free gingival graft. D, Donor tissue harvested from palate, E, Free gingival graft transferred to recipient site and sutured, F, At 6 months showing widened zone of attached gingiva. *(Courtesy: Dr. Joann Pauline George, India.)*

nutrients. Thick grafts may also create a deeper wound at the donor site, with the possibility of injuring major palatal arteries and an unesthetic tissue profile. The advantages of a thick graft is better functional resistance. After the graft is separated, remove the loose tissue tags from the undersurface. Thin the edge to avoid bulbous marginal and interdental contours. Special precautions must be taken with grafts from the palate.

iii. The submucosa in the posterior region is thick and fatty and should be trimmed so that it will not interfere with vascularization. Grafts tend to reestablish their original epithelial structure, so mucous glands may occur in grafts obtained from the palate.

iv. A thick graft can be thinned by holding it between two wet wooden tongue depressors and slicing it longitudinally with a sharp #15 blade.

Step 3: Transfer and immobilize the graft. Remove the sponge from the recipient site, reapply it with pressure if necessary until bleeding is stopped. Remove the excess clot. A thick clot interferes with vascularization of the graft. Position the graft and adapt it firmly to the recipient site. A space between the graft and the underlying tissue (dead space) impairs vascularization and jeopardizes the graft. Suture the graft at the lateral borders and to the periosteum to secure it in position. The graft must be immobilized. Any movement interferes with healing. Avoid excessive tension, which can distort the graft from the underlying surface. Every precaution should be taken to avoid trauma to the graft. Tissue forceps should be used delicately and a minimum number of sutures used to avoid unnecessary tissue perforation.

Step 4: Protect the donor site. The free gingival donor site is an open wound that cannot be sutured, preventing primary closure of the wound. If there is moderate or slight bleeding after pressure has been applied over the site at the completion of the surgery, several products can be placed over the wound, which can be covered with a periodontal dressing.

i. Hemostasis can be achieved with hemostatic agents such as absorbable gelatin sponge (Gelfoam), oxidized cellulose (Oxycel), oxidized regenerated cellulose (Surgicel Absorbable Hemostat), and microfibrillar collagen hemostat (Avitene, CollaCote, CollaTape, or CollaPlug). All are useful hemostatic agents for the control of bleeding from capillaries and small blood vessels. Platelet-rich fibrin has been used on the donor site to enhance wound healing.

ii. A sterile aluminum foil is placed over the wound before the periodontal dressing is used to cover the wound for 1 week and is repeated if necessary. Retention of the dressing on the donor site can be a problem. The dressing can be retained by locking it through the interproximal spaces onto the palatal surface. If there are no open interdental spaces, the dressing can be covered by a plastic stent wired to the teeth. A modified Hawley retainer should be prepared if the donor site wound is expected to be large. It is useful to cover the wound on the palate and over edentulous ridges. It is important that the patient not be dismissed from the office until the bleeding is completely under control.

Variant Techniques

The free gingival graft technique is a predictable procedure, but the donor site (palate) is left with an open wound that must heal by secondary intention. The following variant techniques attempt to minimize the donor site wound by removing the donor tissue in a different configuration and altering the shape to maximize coverage over the recipient site. The accordion technique, the strip technique (Fig. 50.5A–L), and the combination epithelial-connective tissue strip technique are modifications/variants of the free gingival graft.

Accordion technique, described by Rateitschak et al., attains expansion of the graft by alternate incisions in opposite sides of the graft. This technique increases the donor graft tissue by changing the configuration of the tissue.

The strip technique, developed by Han et al., consists of obtaining two or three strips of gingival donor tissue about 3–5 mm wide and long enough to cover the entire length of the recipient site. These strips are placed side by side to form one donor tissue and sutured on the recipient site. The area is then covered with aluminum foil and surgical dressing. The aluminum foil prevents the surgical dressing from sticking to the suture. The advantage of this technique is rapid healing of the donor site. The epithelial migration of the close wound edges (3–5 mm) allows rapid epithelialization of the open wound. The donor site usually does not require suturing and heals uneventfully in 1–2 weeks.

Combination of strip and connective tissue technique is a combination of deep strip graft that is taken from the palate and is split into an epithelial donor graft and undersurface portion of a connective tissue donor graft. The tissue is obtained by removing a strip of tissue from the palate that is about 3–4 mm thick. Place it between two wet tongue depressors, and split it longitudinally with a sharp #15 blade. Both are used as free grafts. The superficial portion consists of epithelium and connective tissue, and the deeper portion consists only of connective tissue. These donor tissues are placed on the recipient site as in the strip technique. The minimal donor site wound obtained by two donor tissues from one site is the advantage of this technique.

The connective tissue technique originally described by Edel has the advantage of healing by primary intention of the donor site and better color matching.

As FGGs are associated poor color match, tissue texture and alteration of the mucogingival junction alignment. To overcome this, a modified technique, the partly epithelialized free gingival graft (PE-FGG), with a de-epithelialized portion apically has been evaluated. The intent of this graft was to cover the recession area and 2–3 mm of bone apical to the dehiscence. The apical portion was de-epithelialized. The coronal edge of the graft was aligned with the CEJ and care was exercised to align the apical edge of epithelialized part with the Mucogingival Junction (MGJ) of the neighboring teeth. The de-epithelialized apical part was sandwiched between the elevated alveolar mucosa and the periosteum of the recipient bed and extended 2–3 mm apical to the bone dehiscence. PE-FGG resulted in favorable percentage of complete root coverage and satisfactory esthetic outcomes (Fig. 50.6).

Healing of the Graft

The success of the graft depends on survival of the connective tissue. Sloughing of the epithelium occurs in most cases, but the extent to which the connective tissue withstands the transfer to the new location determines the fate of the graft. Fibrous organization of the interface between the graft and the recipient bed occurs within two to several days.

1. Plasmatic circulation stage (2–3 days): The graft is initially maintained by a diffusion of fluid from the host bed, adjacent gingiva, and alveolar mucosa. The fluid is a transudate from the host vessels and provides nutrition and hydration essential for the initial survival of the transplanted tissues. During the first day, the connective tissue becomes edematous and disorganized and undergoes degeneration and lysis of some of its elements. As healing progresses, the edema is resolved, and degenerated connective tissue is replaced by new granulation tissue.

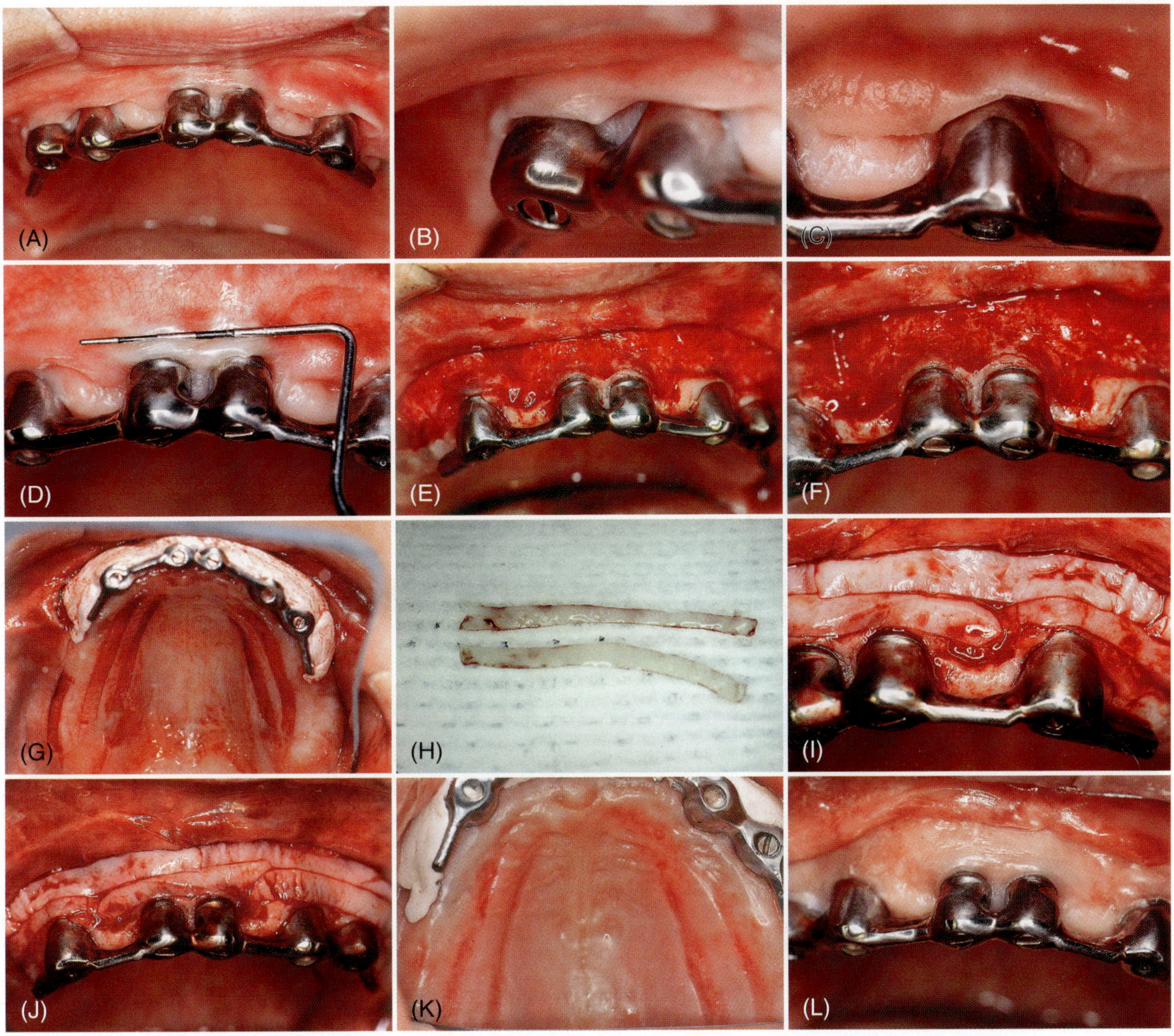

Fig. 50.5 Free gingival graft: strip technique. A–D, Mucosal tissue around implants. E and F, Recipient site prepared. G, Donor site with strips of free graft removed. H, Donor strips of free graft. I and J, Strips placed side by side on recipient site. K, Donor area 1 week after graft removal. L, Healing of recipient site after 3 months. Note good keratinized, attached gingiva. *(Courtesy: Dr. T. Han and Dr. P. Klokkevold, Los Angeles.)*

2. Capillary circulation stage (4–5 days): Revascularization of the graft starts by the second or third day. Capillaries from the recipient bed proliferate into the graft to form a network of new capillaries and anastomose with preexisting vessels. Many of the graft vessels degenerate and are replaced by new ones, and some of these participate in the new circulation. The central section of the surface is the last to vascularize, but this is complete by the 10th day.
3. Organization stage (10–14 days): The epithelium undergoes degeneration and sloughing, with complete necrosis occurring in some areas. It is replaced by new epithelium from the borders of the recipient site. A thin layer of new epithelium is present by the fourth day, with rete pegs developing by the seventh day. Heterotopically placed grafts maintain their structure (keratinized epithelium), even after the grafted epithelium has become necrotic and has been replaced by neighboring areas of nonkeratinized epithelium, which suggests that a genetic predetermination of the specific character of the oral mucosa exists that depends on stimuli originating in the connective tissue. This is the basis for the technique that uses grafts composed only of connective tissue obtained from areas in which it is covered by keratinized epithelium.

As seen microscopically, healing of a graft of intermediate thickness (0.75 mm) is complete by 10 weeks; thicker grafts (1.75 mm) may require 16 weeks or longer. The gross appearance of the graft reflects the tissue changes within it. At transplantation, the graft vessels are empty and the graft is pale. The pallor changes to an ischemic grayish white during the first 2 days until vascularization begins and a pink color appears. The plasmatic circulation accumulates and causes softening and swelling of the graft, which are reduced when the edema is removed from the recipient site by the new blood vessels. Loss of epithelium leaves the graft smooth and shiny. New epithelium creates a thin, gray, veil-like surface that develops normal features as the epithelium matures.

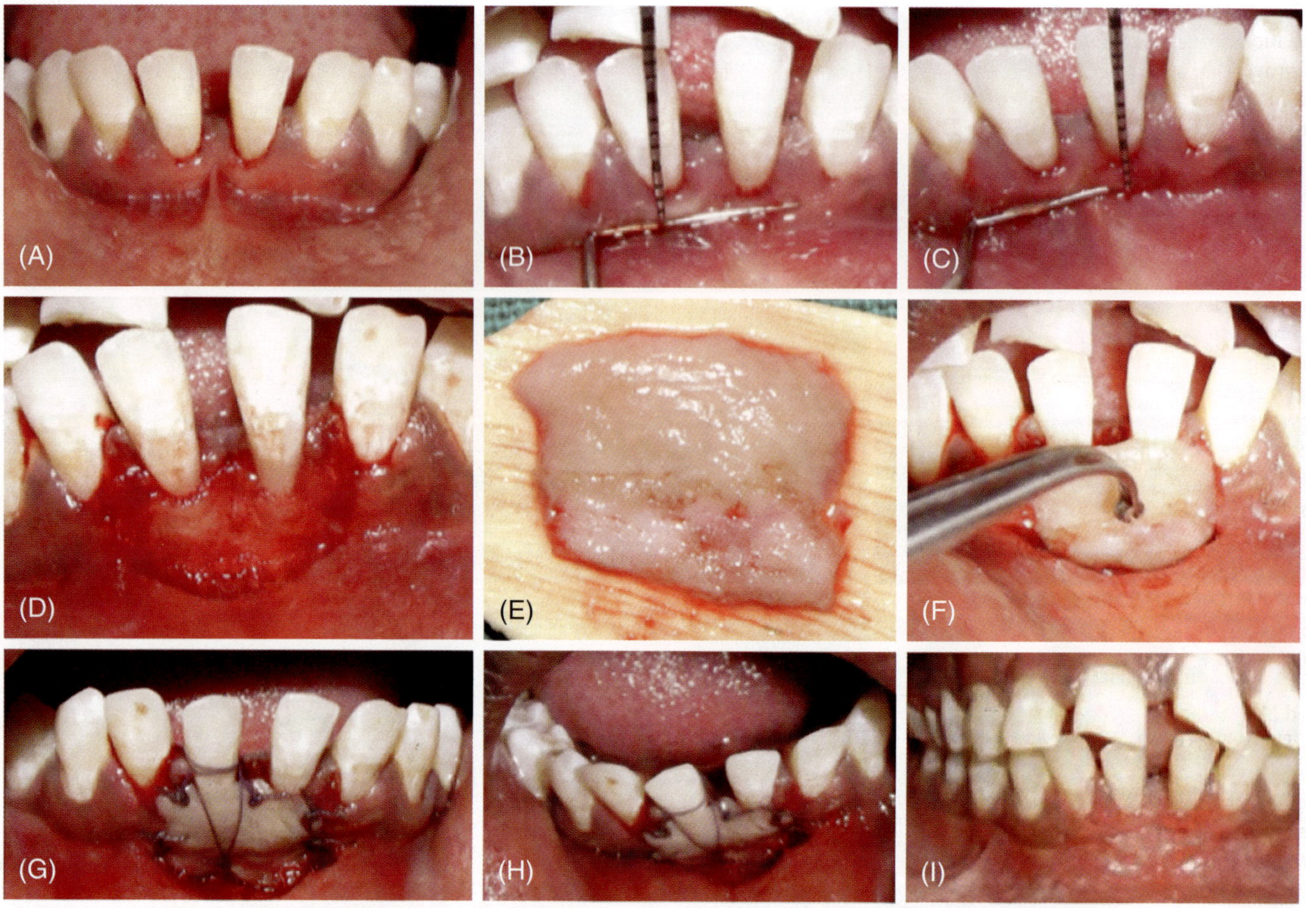

Fig. 50.6 Partially epthelialized free gingival graft. A, B, and C, Preoperative view of lack of attached gingiva and recession in mandibular central incisors. D, Recipient site prepared. E, The apical portion of the graft was de-epithelialized. F, The partially epithelialized FGG placed at recipient sir. G and H, The partially epithelialized FGG sandwiched between the elevated alveolar mucosa and the periosteum of the recipient bed and extended 2–3 mm apical to the bone dehiscence. I, Favorable root coverage and satisfactory aesthetic outcomes after 6 months. *(Courtesy: Dr Joann Pauline George, India.)*

Functional integration of the graft occurs by the 17th day, but the graft is morphologically distinguishable from the surrounding tissue for months. The graft eventually blends with adjacent tissues, but sometimes although pink, firm, and healthy, it is somewhat bulbous. This usually presents no problem, but if the graft traps plaque or is esthetically unacceptable, thinning of the graft may be necessary. Thinning the surface of the grafted tissue does reduce the bulbous condition because the surface epithelium tends to proliferate again. The graft should be thinned by making the necessary incisions to elevate it from the periosteum, removing tissue from its undersurface, and suturing it back in place.

Alternative Donor Tissue

The use of the palate as a donor site for gingival augmentation has numerous disadvantages, for not only are the patients fearful of palatal surgery from where the donor tissue is procured but there is also a limitation on the quantity of tissue that can be removed. Alternative donor tissue such as acellular dermal matrix, extracellular matrix membrane, bilayer collagen matrix, growth factors, living cellular construct, and other tissue engineered products are gaining importance.

Dermal substitute is commercially available under the name *AlloDerm* and is derived from donated human skin. ADM consists of a nondenatured three-dimensional arrangement of intact collagen fibers, ground substance, and vascular channels. Randomized, controlled clinical trials have demonstrated outcomes with ADM equivalent to palatal donor tissue in treatment of gingival recession. It acts as a three dimensional scaffold that allows cell colonization and repopulation of fibroblasts, blood vessels, and epithelium. No significant differences were observed with respect to percentage of root coverage and keratinized tissue width when compared to connective tissue graft (CTG). In addition to avoiding palatal donor surgery, ADM offers the advantage of availability of unlimited donor tissue for the treatment of multiple teeth in a single surgical appointment.

Accomplishments

Free gingival grafts effectively widen the attached gingiva. Several biometric studies have analyzed the width of the attached gingiva after the placement of a free gingival graft. After 24 weeks, grafts placed on denuded bone shrink 25%, whereas grafts placed on periosteum shrink 50%. The greatest amount of shrinkage occurs within the first 6 weeks. Considering that the average contraction of FGGs range from 25% to 50% in the vertical dimension, the surgeon should determine the graft size in lieu of the same. The reported keratinised tissue (KT) augmentation ranges from 3.1 to 5.6 mm. Due to the compromising outcomes of FGGs in periodontal plastic surgical procedures, they have been less frequently used and limited mainly for procedures aimed at increasing the width of keratinized tissue around teeth and implants in regions of less esthetic importance.

The limited donor tissue availability and mismatch in color are limitations of FGGs. The placement of a gingival graft does not "improve" the status of the gingiva. Therefore, the indication for a free gingival graft should be based on the presence of progressive gingival recession and inflammation. When recession continues to progress after a few months with good plaque control, a graft can be placed to prevent further recession and loss of attached gingiva.

Other materials have been used to replace gingival tissue in gingival extension procedures. The use of a porcine collagen matrix has also shown equivalent results when compared to a free gingival graft when augmenting keratinized gingiva.

Free autogenous gingival grafts have been found to be useful for covering nonpathologic dehiscences and fenestrations. Nonpathologic refers to openings of the bone through the tooth surface not previously exposed to the oral environment and found in the course of flap surgery.

The use of free gingival autografts to cover denuded roots is described later in this chapter.

Free Connective Tissue Autografts

The connective tissue autograft technique was originally described by Edel and is based on the fact that connective tissue carries the genetic message for the overlying epithelium to become keratinized. Only connective tissue from beneath a keratinized zone can be used as a graft.

The advantage of this technique is that the donor tissue is obtained from the undersurface of the palatal flap, which is sutured back in primary closure. Healing is by first intention. The patient has less discomfort postoperatively at the donor site. Another advantage of the free connective tissue autograft is that improved esthetics can be achieved because of a better color match of the grafted tissue to the adjacent areas.

Apically Displaced Flap

This technique uses the apically positioned flap, either partial thickness or full thickness, to increase the zone of keratinized gingiva (Fig. 50.7).

Accomplishments

The apically displaced flap technique increases the width of the keratinized gingiva but cannot predictably deepen the vestibule with attached gingiva. Adequate vestibular depth must be present before the surgery to allow apical positioning of the flap. The edge of the flap may be located in three positions in relation to the bone as follows:

1. **Slightly coronal to the crest of the bone.** This location attempts to preserve the attachment of supracrestal fibers. It may also result in thick gingival margins and interdental papillae with deep sulci and may create the risk of recurrent pockets.
2. **At the level of the crest.** This results in a satisfactory gingival contour, provided that the flap is adequately thinned.
3. **Two millimeters short of the crest.** This position produces the most desirable gingival contour and the same posttreatment level of gingival attachment as obtained by placing the flap at the crest of the bone. New tissue covers the crest of the bone to produce a firm, tapered gingival margin.

Placing the flap short of the crest increases the risk of a slight reduction in bone height, but the advantage of a well-formed gingival margin compensates for this.

Other Techniques

The vestibular extension technique, originally described by Edlan and Mejchar, produced statistically significant widening of attached nonkeratinized tissue. Currently, this technique is of historic interest only.

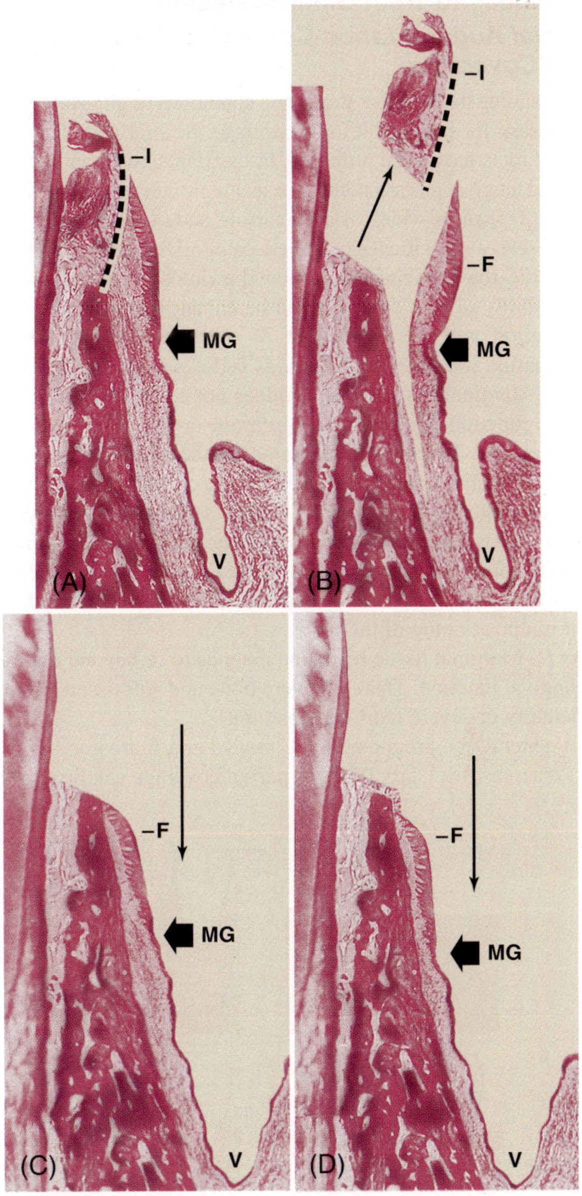

Fig. 50.7 Apically displaced partial-thickness flap. A, Internal bevel incision *(I)* separates inner wall of periodontal pocket. *MG*, Mucogingival junction; *V*, vestibular fornix. B, Partial-thickness flap *(F)* separated, leaving periosteum and a layer of connective tissue on the bone. The inner wall of the periodontal pocket *(I)* is removed, and the tooth is scaled and planed. C, Partial-thickness flap *(F)* displaced apically, with edge of the flap at crest of the bone. Note that the vestibular fornix is also moved apically. D, Partial-thickness flap *(F)* displaced apically, with edge of the flap several millimeters below crest of the bone.

The fenestration operation/periosteal separation technique was designed to widen the zone of attached gingiva with a minimal loss of bone height by using a partial thickness flap, except in a rectangular area at the base of the surgical field, where the periosteum is removed, exposing the bone. Its purpose is to create a scar that is firmly bound to the bone. It prevents soft tissue separation from the bone and postsurgical narrowing of the attached zone. Results obtained with this technique are not as predictable as with the free gingival graft, and it is therefore not widely performed, except for small isolated areas.

Techniques to Treat Gingival Recession

Gingival Augmentation Coronal to Recession (Root Coverage)

Understanding the different stages and conditions of gingival recession is necessary for predictable root coverage. Several classifications of denuded roots have been proposed. In the 1960s, Sullivan and Atkins classified gingival recession into four anatomic categories: (1) shallow-narrow, (2) shallow-wide, (3) deep-narrow, and (4) deep-wide.

This early classification helped categorize the lesion but did not enable the clinician to predict the outcome of therapy. The predictability of root coverage can be enhanced by the presurgical examination and the correlation of the recession by using the classification proposed by Miller, as follows (Fig. 50.8):

Class I. Marginal tissue recession does not extend to the mucogingival junction. There is no loss of bone or soft tissue in the interdental area. This type of recession can be narrow or wide.

Class II. Marginal tissue recession extends to or beyond the mucogingival junction. There is no loss of bone or soft tissue in the interdental area. This type of recession can be subclassified into wide and narrow.

Class III. Marginal tissue recession extends to or beyond the mucogingival junction. There is bone and soft tissue loss interdentally or malpositioning of the tooth.

Class IV. Marginal tissue recession extends to or beyond the mucogingival junction. There is severe bone and soft tissue loss interdentally or severe tooth malposition.

In general, the prognoses for Classes I and II are good to excellent. Whereas, for Class III, only partial coverage can be expected.

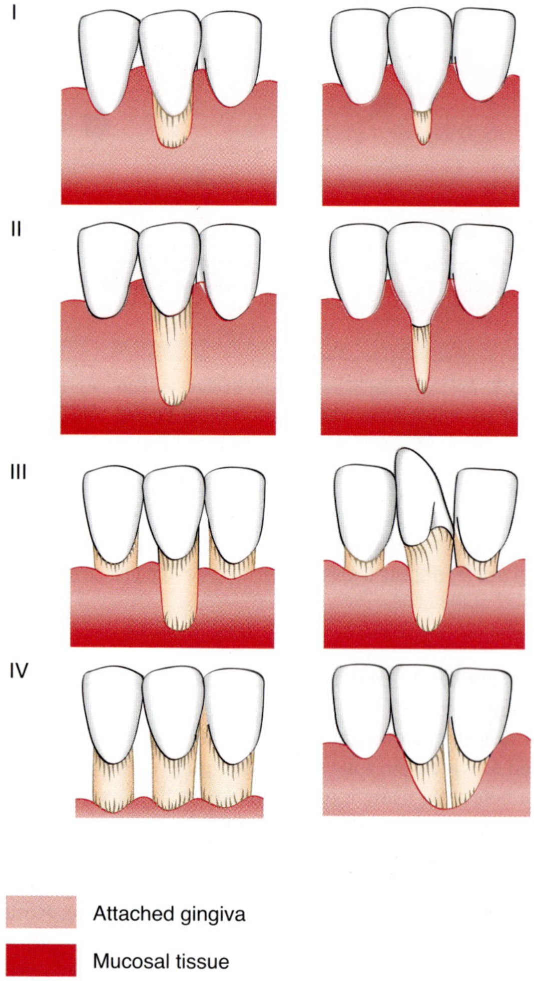

Fig. 50.8 P.D. Miller's classification of denuded roots.

Class IV has a very poor prognosis with current techniques. Miller's classification has certain limitations; to overcome this, Cairo et al. proposed a classification based on the interdental CAL measurement:

- Recession Type 1 (RT1): Gingival recession with no loss of interproximal attachment. Interproximal CEJ is clinically not detectable at both mesial and distal aspects of the tooth.
- Recession Type 2 (RT2): Gingival recession associated with loss of interproximal attachment. The amount of interproximal attachment loss (measured from the interproximal CEJ to the depth of the interproximal sulcus/pocket) is less than or equal to the buccal attachment loss (measured from the buccal CEJ to the apical end of the buccal sulcus/pocket).
- Recession Type 3 (RT3): Gingival recession associated with loss of interproximal attachment. The amount of interproximal attachment loss (measured from the interproximal CEJ to the apical end of the sulcus/pocket) is greater than the buccal attachment loss (measured from the buccal CEJ to the apical end of the buccal sulcus/pocket). This classification is a treatment-oriented classification and predicts the potential for root coverage through the assessment of interdental CAL. In the Cairo RT1 (Miller Class I and II), 100% root coverage can be predicted; in the Cairo RT2 (overlapping the Miller class III), some randomized clinical trials indicate the limit of interdental CAL loss within which 100% root coverage is predictable applying different root coverage procedures; in the Cairo RT3 (overlapping the Miller class IV), full root coverage is not achievable.

Some of the techniques used for widening the attached gingiva apical to the area of recession can also be used for root coverage. Both the free gingival and the connective tissue autograft used for apical widening can be used for coronal augmentation by incorporating some modifications. In using the free grafts for root coverage, the recipient bed surrounding the denuded root surface must be extended wider to allow for better blood supply to the donor free graft. This is necessary because a portion of the donor tissue overlies the root surface, which does not have blood supply.

Free Gingival Autograft

Successful and predictable root coverage has been reported using free gingival autografts.

The Classic Technique

Miller applied the classic free gingival autograft described previously with a few modifications.

Step 1: Root planing. Root planing is performed with the application of saturated citric acid for 5 min on the root surface. The application of this acid has not been validated by some studies, but numerous clinicians practice this technique. Root planing can also be carried out meticulously with manual instrumentation.

Step 2: Prepare the recipient site. Make a horizontal incision in the interdental papillae at right angles to create a margin against which the graft may have a butt joint with the incision. Vertical incisions are made at the proximal line angles of adjacent teeth and the retracted tissue is excised. Maintain an intact periosteum in the apical area.

Steps 3 and 4. Refer to the step-by-step technique described for the classic gingival graft earlier in this chapter. This technique results in predictable coverage of the denuded root surface but may present esthetic color discrepancies with the adjacent gingiva because of a lighter color.

Step 5: Transfer the graft. Transfer the graft to the recipient site and suture it to the periosteum with a gut suture. Good stability of the graft must be attained with adequate sutures.

Step 6: Cover the graft. Cover the grafted site with dry aluminum foil and periodontal dressing.

Free Connective Tissue Autograft

The free connective tissue technique was described by Levine in 1991. The difference between this technique and the free gingival autograft is that the donor tissue is connective tissue.

The following is a step-by-step surgical description of the free connective tissue autograft technique:

Step 1: Divergent vertical incisions. Divergent vertical incisions are made at the line angles of the tooth to be covered, creating a partial-thickness flap to at least 5 mm apical to the receded area.

Step 2: Suturing. The apical mucosal border is sutured to the periosteum using a gut suture.

Step 3: Scaling and root planing. Thoroughly scale and root plane the exposed root surface. The facial prominence on the root surface is also reduced, which is a favorable anatomy onto which the donor tissue is placed.

Step 4: Obtaining the graft. Obtain a connective tissue graft from the palate. The donor site is sutured after the graft is removed.

Step 5: Transferring the graft. Transfer the graft to the recipient site, and suture it to the periosteum with a gut suture. Good stability of the graft must be attained with the minimal number of sutures.

The grafted site should be covered with sterile foil before placing the dressing.

Pedicle Autograft

Laterally (Horizontally) Displaced Pedicle Flap

The displaced pedicle flap technique, originally described by Grupe and Warren in 1956, was the standard technique for many years and is still indicated in some cases. The laterally positioned flap can be used to cover isolated, denuded root surfaces that have adequate donor tissue laterally. Adequate vestibular depth must also be present.

Advantages	Disadvantages	Indications	Contraindications
• Single surgical site	• Dictated by keratinized tissue width of donor site	• Isolated recessions	• Presence of deep inter proximal tissues
• Adequate vascularity maintained by pedicle	• Possible recession at donor site	• Adequate keratinized tissue width of donor site	• Pronounced root concavity
	• Limited to isolated recessions	• Satisfactory vestibular depth	• Interdental papillary loss

The following is a step-by-step surgical description (Fig. 50.9):

Step 1: Prepare the recipient site. Epithelium is removed around the denuded root surface. The exposed connective tissue will be the recipient site for the laterally displaced flap. The root surface will be thoroughly scaled and root planed.

Step 2: Prepare the flap. The periodontium of the donor site should have a satisfactory width of attached gingiva and minimal loss

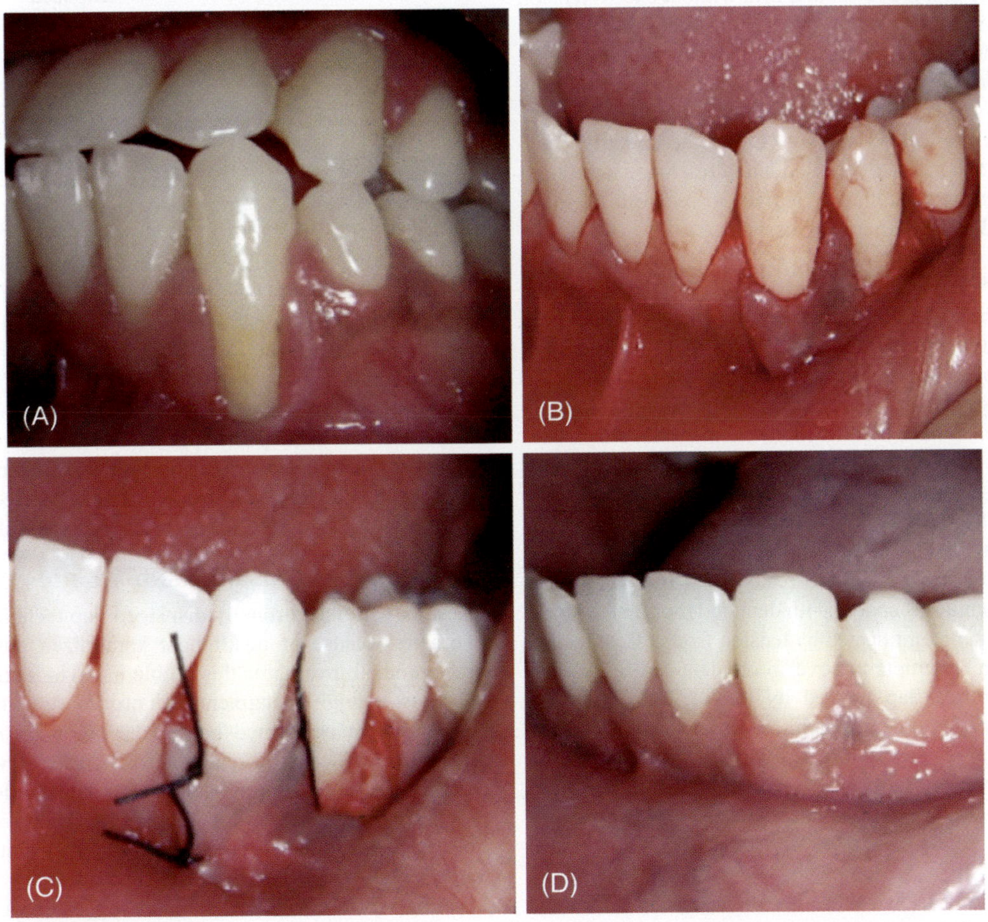

Fig. 50.9 Laterally displaced flap A, Preoperative of gingival recession on mandibular canine. B, Recipient site prepared and donor tissue laterally displaced. C, Donor flap sutured. D, Postoperative outcome after 2 years. *(Courtesy: Dr. Joann Pauline George, India.)*

of bone, without dehiscence or fenestration. A full-thickness or partial-thickness flap may be used, but the latter is preferable because it offers the advantage of rapid healing at the donor site and reduces the risk of loss of facial bone height. This is especially important if the bone is thin or a dehiscence or fenestration is suspected. However, if the gingiva is thin, even a partial-thickness flap may not be sufficient for flap survival.

- With a #15 blade, make a vertical incision from the gingival margin to outline a flap adjacent to the recipient site. Incise to the periosteum, and extend the incision into the oral mucosa to the level of the base of the recipient site. The flap should be sufficiently wider than the recipient site to cover the root and provide a broad margin for attachment to the connective tissue border around the root. The interdental papilla at the distal end of the flap, or a major portion of it, should be included to secure the flap in the interproximal space between the donor and the recipient teeth.
- Make a vertical incision along the gingival margin and interdental papilla, and separate a flap consisting of epithelium and a thin layer of connective tissue, leaving the periosteum on the bone.
- A releasing incision is sometimes needed to avoid tension on the base of the flap, which can impair the blood supply when the flap is moved. To do this, make a short oblique incision into the alveolar mucosa at the distal corner of the flap, in the direction of the recipient site.

Step 3: Transfer the flap. Slide the flap laterally onto the adjacent root, making sure that it lies flat and firm without excess tension on the base. Fix the flap to the adjacent gingiva and alveolar mucosa with interrupted sutures. A suspensory suture may be made around the involved tooth to prevent the flap from slipping apically.

Step 4: Protect the flap and donor site. Cover the operative field with aluminum foil and a soft periodontal dressing, extending it interdentally and onto the lingual surface to secure it. Remove the dressing and sutures after 1 week.

Variant Techniques

There are many variations in the incisions for the laterally displaced flap. A common alternative is the use of converging oblique incisions over the recipient site and a vertical or oblique incision at the distal end of the donor site so that the transposed flap is slightly wider at its base. In another modification, the marginal attachment at the donor site is preserved to reduce the likelihood of recession and marginal bone resorption, but this requires a donor site with a wider zone of attached gingiva.

Sliding partial-thickness grafts from neighboring edentulous areas (pedicle grafts) can be used to restore attached gingiva on teeth adjacent to edentulous spaces with denuded roots and a small, vestibular fornix, often complicated by tension from a frenum. The "double-papilla flap" attempts to cover roots denuded by isolated gingival defects with a flap formed by joining the contiguous halves of the adjacent interdental papillae. Results with this technique are unpredictable because blood supply is impaired by suturing the two flaps over the root surface which is devoid of a blood supply. Another variant is the laterally displaced coronally advanced flap.

Accomplishments of Pedicle Autograft

Coverage of the exposed root surface with the sliding-flap technique has been reported to be 60%, 61%, and 72%. Histologic studies in animals have reported 50% coverage.

The extent to which the flap establishes a new attachment to the root with the formation of new cementum and the embedding of new connective tissue fibers has not been established. New attachment on artificially denuded roots in experimental animals and in some clinical studies of humans has been reported, but it does not occur consistently enough to be predictable. In the donor site, there is uneventful repair and restoration of gingival health and contours, with some loss of radicular bone (0.5 mm) and recession (1.5 mm) reported with full-thickness flaps.

Coronally Advanced Flap

The purpose of the coronally displaced flap procedure is to create a split-thickness flap in the area apical to the denuded root and position it coronally to cover the root. Two techniques are available for this purpose.

Advantages	Disadvantages	Indications	Contraindications
• Multiple recession management	• Need for two surgical procedures	• Root coverage	• Lack of keratinized gingival apical to gingival margin
• Predictable outcome	• Lack of donor tissues	• Dentinal hyper-sensitivity due to exposed roots	• Muscle and frenal interferences
• Acceptable color match and contour			• Interdental papillary loss

Source - Dr Joann Pauline George

Classic Technique (Fig. 50.10)

Step 1. With two vertical incisions, delineate the flap. These incisions should go beyond the mucogingival junction. Make a crevicular incision from the gingival margin to the bottom of the sulcus. Elevate a mucoperiosteal flap using careful sharp dissection.

Step 2. Scale and plane the root surface.

Step 3. Return the flap and suture it at a level coronal to the pretreatment position. Cover the area with a periodontal dressing, which is removed along with the sutures after 1 week. The periodontal dressing is replaced for an additional week if it is necessary.

Variations to Classic Technique

Results with the coronally displaced flap technique are often unfavorable because of insufficient keratinized gingiva apical to the recession. To overcome this problem and to increase the chances of success, a gingival augmentation procedure with a free autogenous graft can be performed before the coronally positioned flap, as described earlier in this chapter. This creates several millimeters of attached keratinized gingiva apical to the denuded root.

Two months after this surgery, a second-stage procedure is performed, coronally positioning the flap that includes the free autogenous graft. The use of citric acid or tetracycline for conditioning the root surface has been suggested. A significant degree of reduction in recession treated by this double-step procedure was reported after 2 years by Bernimoulin et al. and confirmed by others.

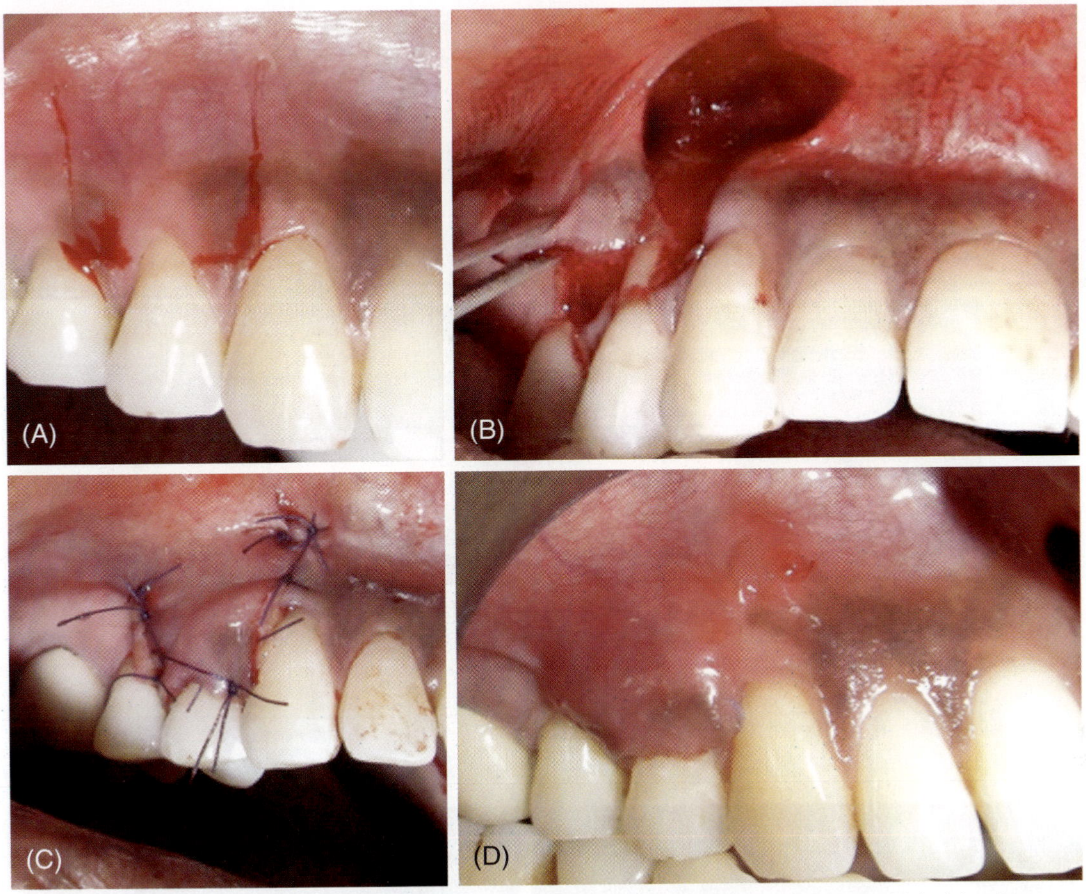

Fig. 50.10 Coronally displaced flap. A, Two vertical incisions extending beyond mucoginigival junction. B, Mucoperiosteal flap raised beyond mucoginigival junction. C, Flap passively advanced 1 mm coronal to CEJ and sutured. D, Postoperative view showing root coverage at 1 month. *(Courtesy: Dr Joann Pauline George, India.)*

Semilunar Flap Technique

Tarnow has described the semilunar coronally repositioned flap to cover isolated denuded root surfaces (Fig. 50.11).

Step 1. A semilunar incision is made following the curvature of the receded gingival margin and ending about 2–3 mm short of the tip of the papillae. This location is very important because the flap derives its blood supply from the papillary areas. The incision may need to reach the alveolar mucosa if the attached gingiva is narrow.

Step 2. Perform a split-thickness dissection coronally from the incision and connect it to an intrasulcular incision.

Step 3. The tissue will collapse coronally, covering the denuded root. It is then held in its new position for a few minutes with moist gauze. Many cases do not require either sutures or periodontal dressing. This technique is simple and predictably provides 2–3 mm of root coverage. It can be performed on several adjoining teeth. This technique is indicated where the recession is not extensive (3 mm) and the facial gingival biotype is thick. It is successful for the maxilla, particularly in covering roots left exposed by the gingival margin receding from a recently placed crown margin. It is not recommended for the mandibular dentition.

Subepithelial Connective Tissue Graft (Langer and Langer)

The subepithelial connective tissue procedure is indicated for larger and multiple defects with good vestibular depth and gingival thickness to allow a split-thickness flap to be elevated. Adjacent to the denuded root surface, the donor connective tissue is sandwiched between the split flap. This technique was described by Langer and Langer in 1985. Similar approaches had been previously reported by Perez-Fernandez and Raetzke.

Advantages	Disadvantages	Indications	Contraindications
• Multiple recession management	• Need for two surgical procedures	• Root coverage in esthetically demanding area	• Lack of keratinized gingival apical to gingival margin
• Predictable outcome	• Lack of donor tissues	• Dentinal hyper-sensitivity due to exposed roots	• Muscle and frenal interferences
• Acceptable color match and contour	• Technique sensitive	• Multiple recession management	• Interdental papillary loss

Source – Dr Joann Pauline George

The following is the step-by-step surgical description (Fig. 50.12).

Step 1. Raise a partial-thickness flap with a horizontal incision 2 mm away from the tip of the papilla and two vertical incisions

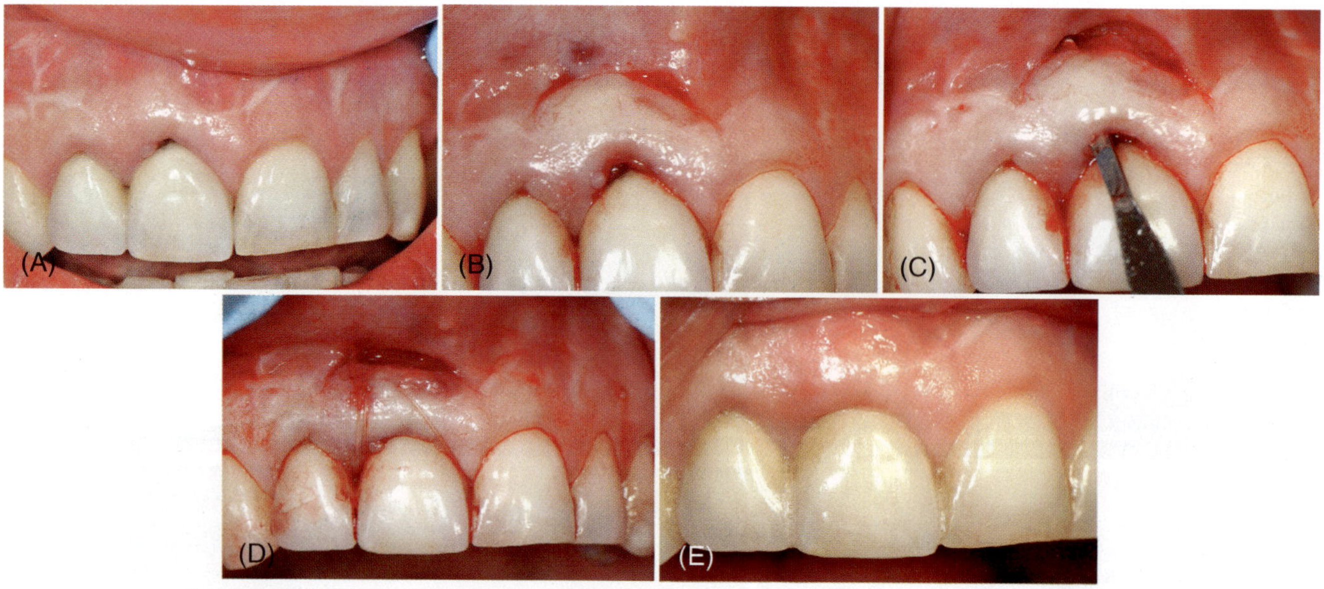

Fig. 50.11 Semilunar coronally positioned flap. A, Recession in facial aspect of the upper right central incisor. B, A semilunar incision and sulcular incision is made. C, The tissue separated from the underlying bone. D, The flap collapses, covering the recession. E, Postoperative at 6 months.

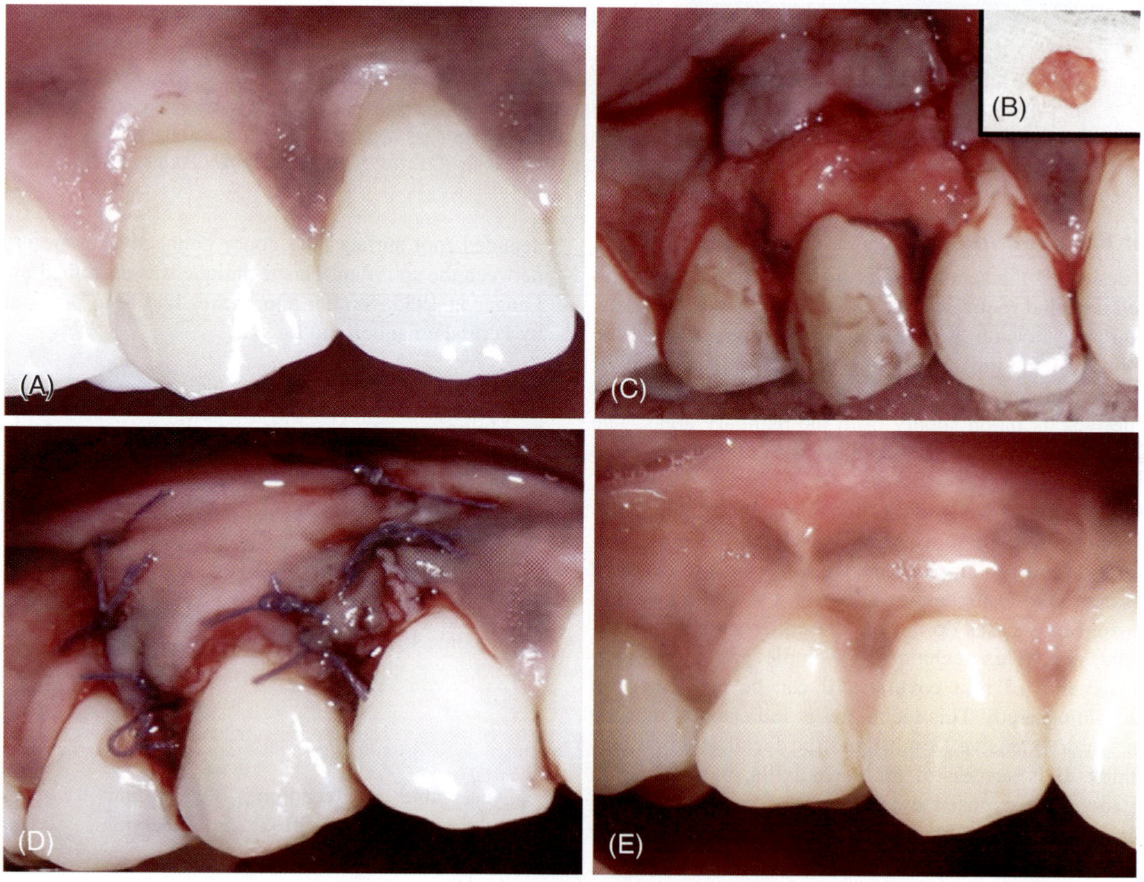

Fig. 50.12 Subepithelial connective tissue graft for root coverage, A, Preoperative view of recession. B, Harvested sub epithelial connective tissue graft. C, Graft placed and sutured in the recipient site. D, Flap coronally advanced and covered over the graft. E, 6 months post operative view showing complete root coverage *(Courtesy: Dr. Joann Pauline George, India.)*

1–2 mm away from the gingival margin of the adjoining teeth. These incisions should extend at least one tooth wider mesiodistally than the area of gingival recession. Extend the flap to the mucobuccal fold.

Step 2. Thoroughly plane the root, reducing its convexity.

Step 3. Obtain a connective tissue graft from the palate by means of a horizontal incision 5–6 mm from the gingival margin of molars and premolars. The palatal wound is sutured in a primary closure.

Step 4. Place the connective tissue on the denuded root(s). Suture it with resorbable sutures to the periosteum.

Step 5. Cover the graft with the outer portion of the partial-thickness flap and suture it interdentally.

Step 6. Cover the area with dry foil and surgical dressing. After 7 days, the dressing and sutures are removed.

The esthetic results are favorable with this technique since the donor tissue is connective tissue. The donor site heals by primary intention, with considerably less discomfort than after a free gingival graft.

A variant of the subepithelial connective tissue graft, called a *subpedicle (bilaminar) connective tissue graft*, was described by Nelson in 1987. This technique uses a pedicle over the connective tissue that covers the denuded root surface. Therefore, the blood supply is increased over the donor tissue and the gingival margin is

Techniques to Harvest Subepithelial Connective Tissue From the Palate	Techniques	Modifications
1. Trap door technique	1. Envelope technique	Vestibular incision subperiosteal tunnel access (VISTA)
2. Double incision technique	2. Langer's technique	The Pinhole approach
3. Single incision	3. Pouch and tunnel technique	Use of acellular dermal matrix
4. De-epithelialize FGG		Dento gingival transfer
		Periosteal transfer

Source - Dr Joann Pauline George

thickened for better marginal stability. Soft tissue substitutes such as porcine collagen matrices have also shown predictable outcomes (Fig. 50.13).

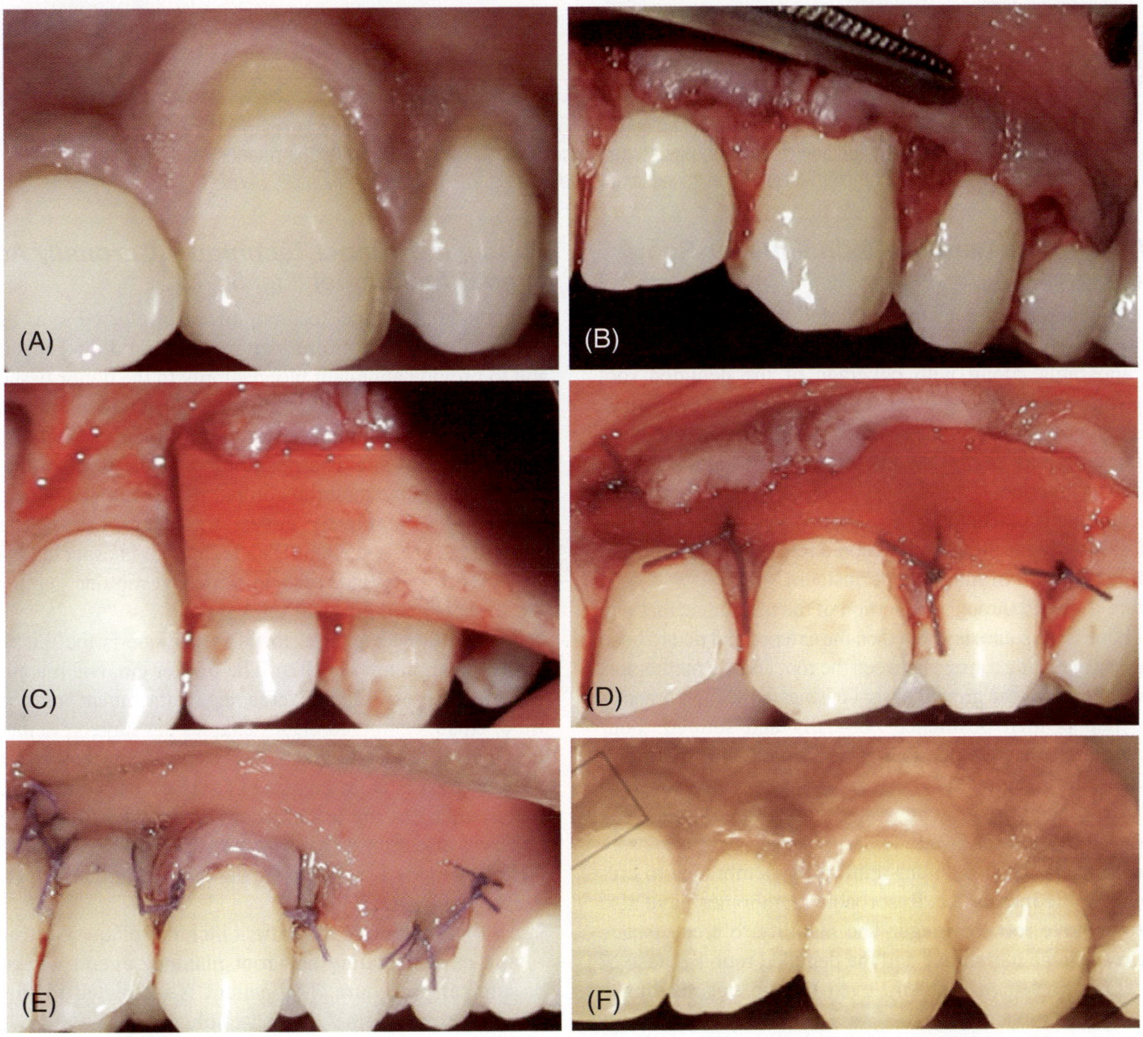

Fig. 50.13 Soft tissue substitute porcine collagen matrix for root coverage. A, Preoperative view of recession. B, Recipient site prepared and passive advancement of flap achieved. C, Collagen matrix trimmed and placed in recipient site. D, Collagen matrix stabilised with sutures. E, Flap coronally advanced and sutured. F, Post operative view at 15 months. *(Courtesy: Dr. Joann Pauline George, India.)*

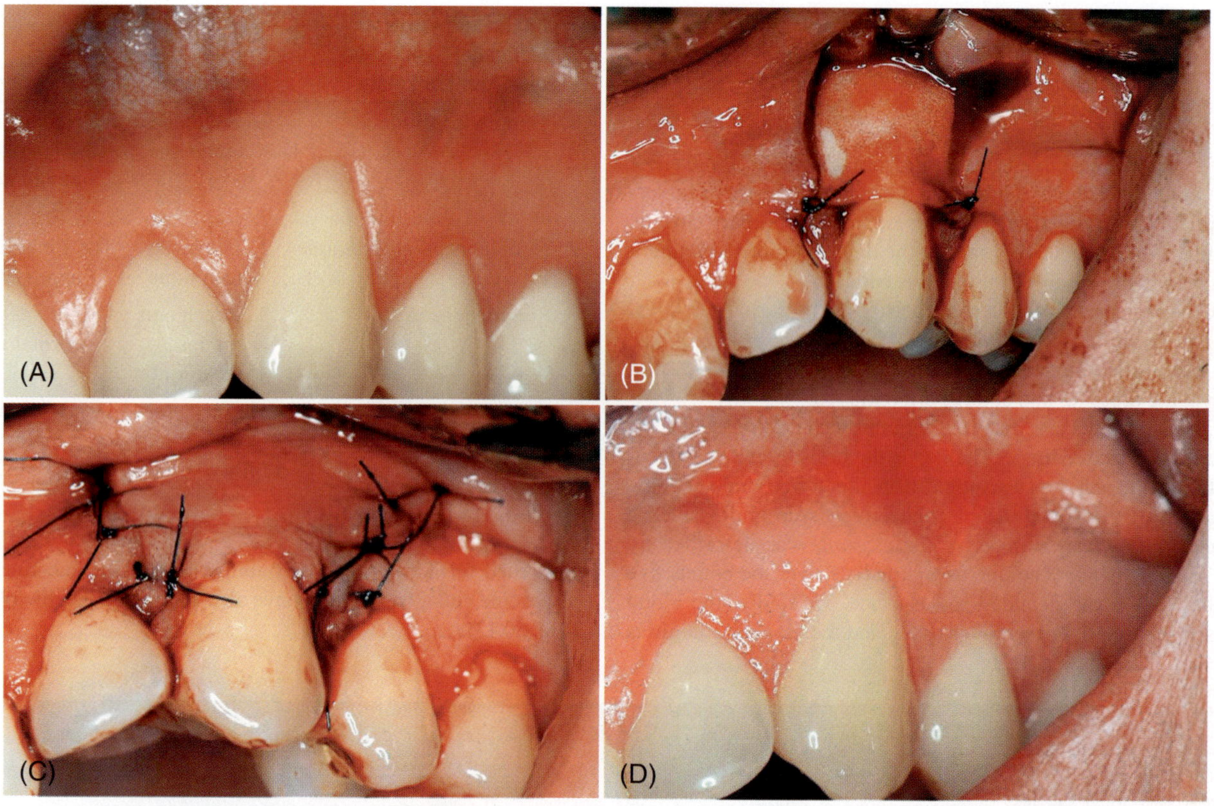

Fig. 50.14 Guided tissue regeneration technique for root coverage. A, Marked recession of maxillary left cuspid. B, Vertical incisions made and membrane placed over recession. C, Flap sutured over the membrane. D, Postoperative result. Note complete coverage of recession. *(Courtesy: Dr. Zoran Aleksic, Belgrade, Serbia.)*

Guided Tissue Regeneration Technique for Root Coverage (Fig. 50.14)

Pini Prato et al. described a technique based on the principle of GTR. Theoretically, GTR should result in reconstruction of the attachment apparatus, along with coverage of the denuded root surface. The following is a step-by-step description of the surgery:

Step 1. A full-thickness flap is reflected to the mucogingival junction, continuing as a partial-thickness flap 8 mm apical to the mucogingival junction.

Step 2. A membrane is placed over the denuded root surface and the adjacent tissue. It is trimmed and adapted to the root surface and covers at least 2 mm of marginal periosteum.

Step 3. A suture is passed through the portion of the membrane that will cover the bone. This suture is knotted on the exterior and tied to bend the membrane, creating a space between the root and the membrane. This space allows for the growth of tissue beneath the membrane.

Step 4. The flap is then positioned coronally and sutured. Four weeks later, a small envelope flap is performed, and the membrane is carefully removed. The flap is then again positioned coronally, to protect the growing tissue, and sutured. One week later these sutures are removed.

Tinti and Vincenzi used titanium-reinforced membranes to create space beneath the membrane. Resorbable membranes have also been used to achieve root coverage. The inability to create space between the resorbable membrane and the denuded root, because of its softness, may present a problem, even though not needing a second surgery is an advantage.

Clinical studies comparing this technique with the coronally displaced flap have shown that the GTR technique is better when the recession is greater than 4.98 mm apicocoronally. Histologically, one case reported 3.66 mm of new connective tissue attachment associated with 2.48 mm of new cementum and 1.84 mm of bone growth.

Pouch and Tunnel Technique (Coronally Advanced Tunnel Technique) (Fig. 50.15)

The pouch and tunnel technique is also referred to as the coronally advanced tunnel. To minimize incisions and the reflection of flaps and to provide abundant blood supply to the donor tissue, the placement of the subepithelial donor connective tissue into pouches beneath papillary tunnels allows for intimate contact of donor tissue to the recipient site The positioning of the graft in the pouch and through the tunnel and the coronal placement of the recessed gingival margins completely covers the donor tissue. Therefore, the esthetic result is excellent. The technique is especially effective for the anterior maxillary area in which vestibular depth is adequate and there is good gingival thickness.

One of the advantages to this technique is the thickening of the gingival margin after healing. The thicker gingival margin is stable to allow for the possibility of "creeping reattachment" of the margin. The use of small, contoured blades enables the surgeon to incise and split the gingival tissues to create the recipient pouches and tunnels. The work by Azzi et al. in this area of surgery has contributed to a better understanding of the technique and outcome of this procedure. This surgery is also referred to as the *coronally advanced tunnel technique*.

Following is a step-by-step description of the surgical procedure as outlined by Azzi:

Step 1. Preparation of the patient includes plaque control instruction and careful scaling and root planing several weeks before the surgical procedure. The patient is instructed to rinse for 3.0 s with chlorhexidine gluconate solution 0.12%.

Step 2. After adequate anesthesia of the region, the surgical procedure, as follows, is performed.

Step 3. Composite material stops are placed at the contact points (temporary) to prevent the collapse of the suspended sutures into the interproximal spaces before the surgery.

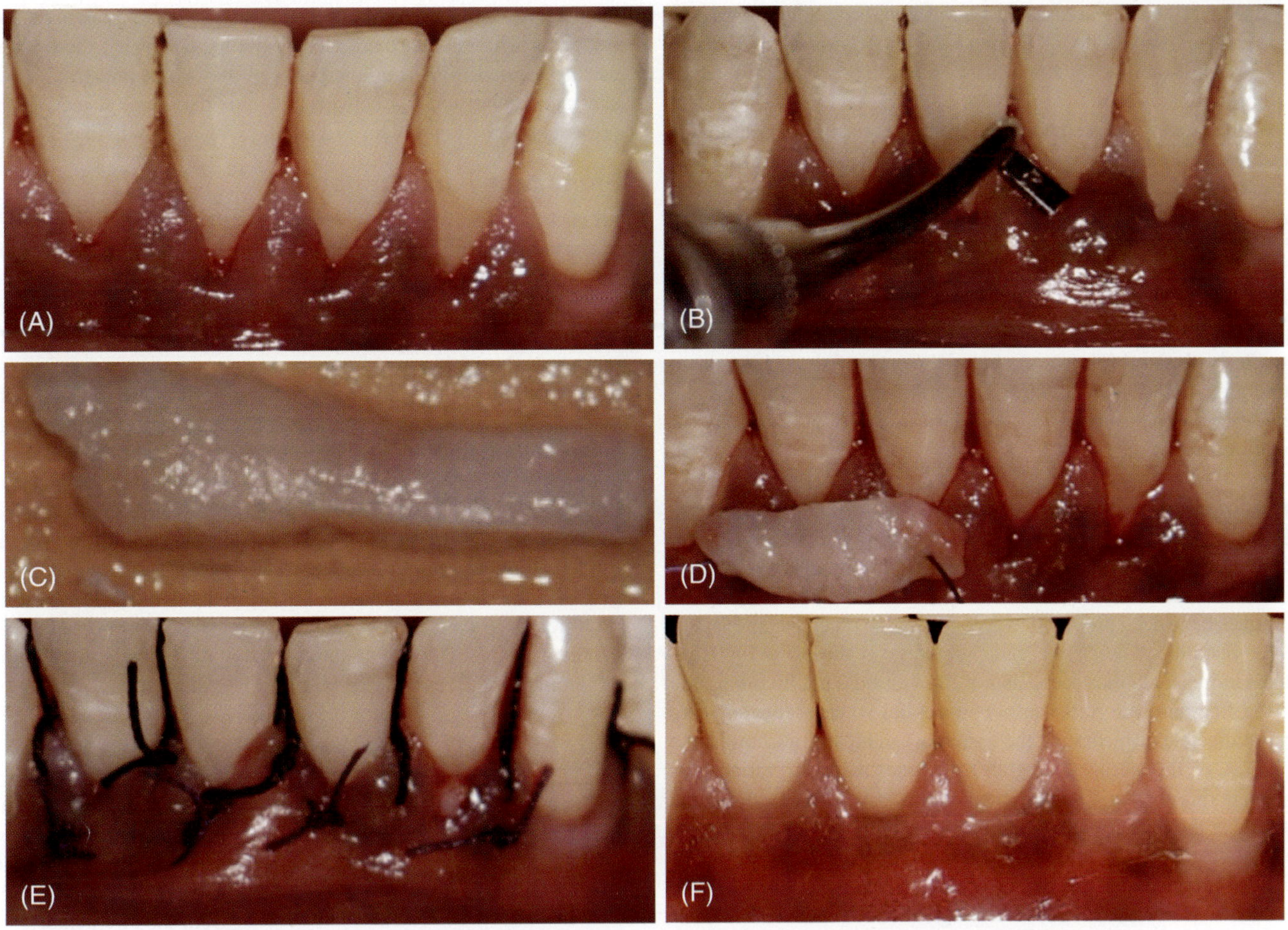

Fig. 50.15 Pouch and tunnel technique for root coverage. A, Preoperative view. Note gingival recession. B, Sulcular incision is made from the mesial to the facial line angles. A tunnel is made through the papilla using a blunt incision. C, A connective tissue graft is taken from the palate. D, The connective tissue is placed through the papillary tunnel and apically beneath the pouch. E, The facial gingival margin covers the connective tissue using horizontal mattress sutures interdentally. F, Postoperative view. Note complete root coverage and thickened gingival margin at 6 months. *(Courtesy: Dr. Joann Pauline George, India.)*

Step 4. Root planing of the exposed root surfaces is performed using Gracey curettes.

Step 5. Initial sulcular incisions are made using 15c and 12d blades. Small, contoured blades and mini curettes are used to create the recipient pouches and tunnels.

Step 6. On the buccal aspect, an intrasulcular incision is made around the necks of the teeth. The incision is extended to one adjacent tooth both mesially and distally using a 15c blade. This incision maintains the full height and thickness of the gingival component and enables access beneath the buccal gingiva with Gracey curettes. The cutting edge is directed toward the bone to dissect the connective tissue beyond the mucogingival line and free the buccal flap from its insertions to the bone around each tooth.

Step 7. Muscle fibers and any remaining collagen fibers on the inner aspect of the flap, which prevent the buccal gingiva from being moved coronally, are cut using Gracey curettes.

Step 8. The papillae are kept intact and undermined to maintain their integrity and carefully released from the underlying bone, which allows the coronal positioning of the papillae.

Step 9. An envelope, full-thickness pouch and tunnel are created and extended apically beyond the mucogingival line by blunt dissection for the insertion of the free connective tissue graft through the intrasulcular incision. Saline moistened gauze is placed over the recipient site.

Step 10. The size of the pouch, which includes the area of the denuded root surface, is measured so that an equivalent size donor connective tissue can be procured from the tuberosity.

Step 11. A second surgical site is created to obtain a connective tissue graft of adequate size and shape to be placed at the recipient site. The connective tissue harvested from the tuberosity area is contoured to fit into the recipient tunnel and pouch.

Step 12. A mattress suture placed at one end of the graft is helpful in guiding the graft through the sulcus and beneath each interdental papilla. The border of the tissue is gently pushed into the pouch and tunnel using tissue forceps and a packing instrument. The graft is pushed from the adjacent tooth on one side of the surgical area to the adjacent tooth on the other side.

Step 13. A mattress suture placed on one end of the graft will help maintain the graft in position while the buccal tissue covers the connective tissue graft. This connective tissue graft is anchored to the inner aspect of the buccal flap in the interdental papilla area. A vertical mattress suture is used to hold the connective tissue in position beneath the gingiva. The connective tissue graft is completely submerged beneath the buccal flap and the papillae.

Step 14. The entire gingivopapillary complex (buccal gingiva with the underlying connective tissue graft and papillae) is coronally positioned using a horizontal mattress suture anchored at the incisal edge of the contact area. The contact areas are splinted presurgically using a composite material.

Step 15. Other holding sutures may be placed through the overlying gingival tissue and donor tissue to the underlying periosteum to secure and stabilize the donor tissue and the overlying gingiva in a coronal position.

The area is not covered with periodontal dressing. The patient is instructed to rinse daily with chlorhexidine gluconate and to avoid touching the sutures during oral hygiene procedures. Antibiotics can be administered (Amoxicillin 500 mg three times a day) if deemed necessary.

Other Techniques

In the last few years, a number of new techniques have developed particularly for multiple root coverage. Some of them have been enumerated below. The reader is encouraged to go through the relevant literature from various standard international journals for detailed information.

Techniques to Deepen the Vestibule

The presence of adequate vestibular depth is important for both oral hygiene and retention of prosthetic appliances. Numerous surgical techniques have been proposed to accomplish the objective of deepening the vestibule. The classic clinical studies in the early 1960s by Bohannan indicated that deepening of the vestibule not involving the use of a free gingival graft was not successful when evaluated years later. Predictable deepening of the vestibule can only be accomplished by the use of free autogenous graft techniques and their variants, as covered in this chapter. The important clinical aspect in deepening the vestibule is the proper preparation of the recipient site. The recipient site must be covered by immobile periosteal tissue. If there is a lack of periosteal connective tissue, the donor tissue may be placed over bone. The donor tissue may be either free gingival or connective tissue, but it must be placed over a nonmobile recipient site.

Techniques	Subclassification	
Mucosal advancement vestibuloplasty	Closed submucosal vestibuloplasty	
	Open submucosal vestibuloplasty	Obwegeser technique
Secondary epithelialization	Kazanjian technique	
	Godwin's method	
	Lip-switch method	
	Clark's method	
Grafting vestibuloplasty	Mucosal graft	
	Skin graft	

Source - Dr Joann Pauline George

Techniques to Remove the Frenum

A frenum is a fold of mucous membrane, usually with enclosed muscle fibers, that attaches the lips and cheeks to the alveolar mucosa and/or gingiva and underlying periosteum. A frenum becomes a problem if the attachment is too close to the marginal gingiva. This anatomic situation may be a genetic condition of the individual or the result of recession of the gingival margin reaching the area of the frenum. Tension on the frenum may pull the gingival margin away from the tooth. This condition may be conducive to plaque accumulation and inhibit proper placement of the toothbrush at the gingival margin. These hygiene problems are most often encountered in the mandibular anterior areas. The maxillary anterior vestibule is deep and the frenum is usually located in the midline between the two central incisors. The aberrant frenum located between the maxillary central incisors may present an esthetic problem in a patient with a high lip line.

Frenectomy and Frenotomy

Frenectomy and frenotomy refer to surgical procedures that differ in degree. Frenectomy is complete removal of the frenum, including its attachment to underlying bone and may be required in the correction of an abnormal diastema between the maxillary central incisors. Frenotomy is the relocation of the frenum, usually in a more apical position.

Frenectomy and frenotomy can be performed in conjunction with other periodontal treatment procedures, such as during a free gingival graft procedure to deepen the vestibule in the mandibular anterior area but most often, they are accomplished as a separate surgical procedure. Frenal problems occur most often on the facial surface between the maxillary and mandibular central incisors and in the canine and premolar areas. They occur less often on the lingual surface of the mandible. Frenal problems in mandibular anterior facial regions mostly occur due to lack of attached gingiva. Whereas in the maxillary anterior region, it is usually developmental anomaly often associated with midline diastema.

Technique		
Miller's technique	Miller, 1985	Individuals with orthodontic relapse. The oral surgeon makes an incision on the frenum and separates it from the interdental gingiva. The frenum is removed from the gingiva
V-Y plasty	It is used to reattach the papillary type of frenum.	V- and Y-shaped incisions are made under the surface of the frenum, then it is detached from the interdental gingiva and repositioned.
Z-plasty (Fig. 50.17)	It is employed for the frenum attached very low in the gingiva and causes midline diastema (spacing between the front upper teeth).	The surgeon places two cuts in Z-shape to remove the frenum and close the suture site. Minimal scar formation and improved esthetics are the advantages of Z-plasty.
Classical frenectomy	Archer and Kruger, 1961 and 1964	The frenum and the interdental tissue are entirely detached from the periosteum and surgically removed.
Electro-surgery		The pros include minor bleeding from the surgical site, quick healing, and suturing not required
Laser		Treatment: produces heat on a localized area, minimizes the bleeding, and the surgical site heals fast.

Source - Dr Joann Pauline George

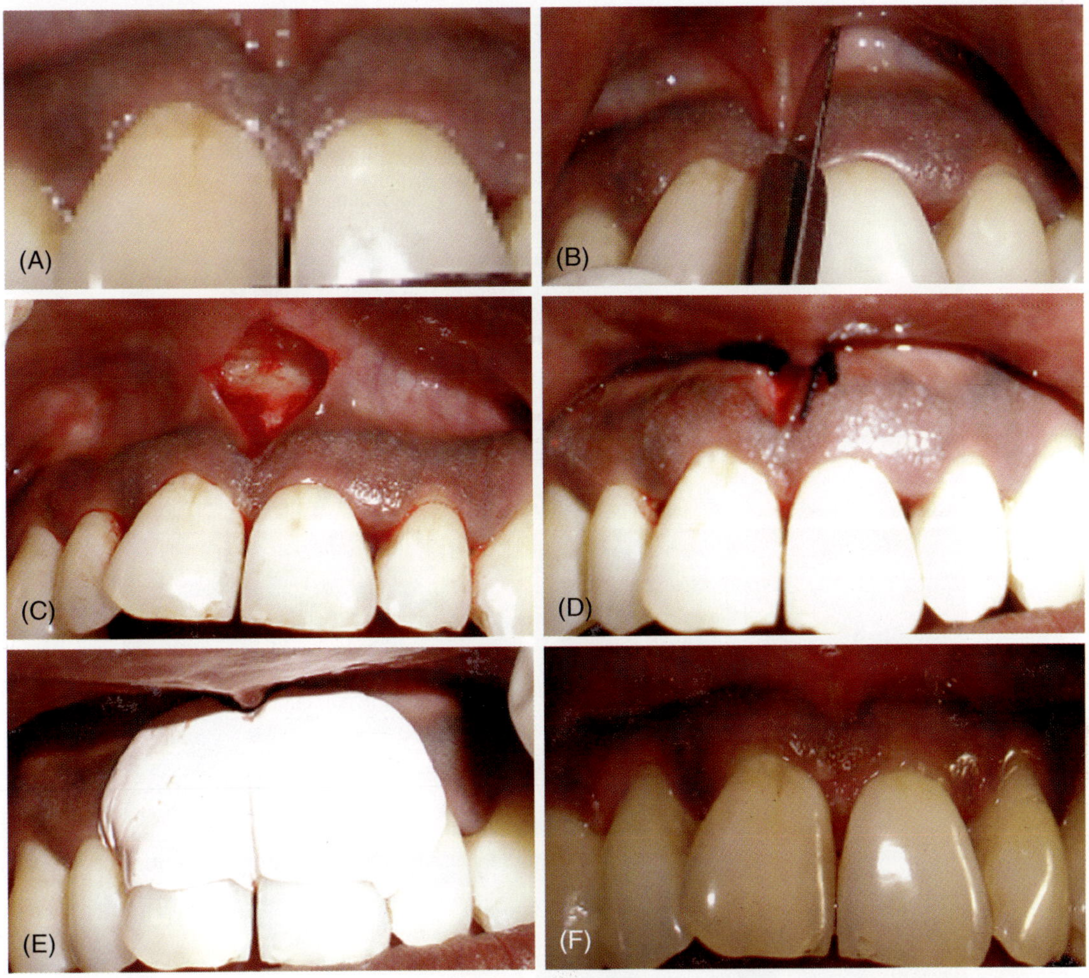

Fig. 50.16 Removal of the frenum. A, Preoperative view of frenum between the two maxillary central incisors. B, Placement of Incision. C, Removal of frenum D, Site is sutured. E, Periodontal dressing. F, Postoperative view at 4 weeks. *(Courtesy: Dr. Joann Pauline George, India.)*

Procedure (Fig. 50.16)

If the vestibule is deep, the procedure is confined to the frenum. It is often necessary to deepen the vestibule to provide space for the repositioned frenum.

This is accomplished as follows:

Conventional (Classical) Frenectomy Archer (1961) and Kruger (1964)

Step 1. After anesthetizing the area, engage the frenum with a hemostat inserted to the depth of the vestibule.

Step 2. Incise along the upper surface of the hemostat, extending beyond the tip.

Step 3. Make a similar incision along the undersurface of the hemostat.

Step 4. Remove the triangular resected portion of the frenum with the hemostat. This exposes the underlying fibrous attachment to the bone.

Step 5. Make a horizontal incision, separating the fibers and bluntly dissect to the bone.

Step 6. If necessary, extend the incisions laterally and suture the labial mucosa to the apical periosteum. A gingival graft or connective tissue graft is placed over the wound.

Step 7. Clean the surgical field with gauze sponges until bleeding stops.

Step 8. Cover the area with dry aluminum foil and apply the periodontal dressing.

Step 9. Remove the dressing after 2 weeks and redress if necessary. One month is usually required for the formation of an intact mucosa with the frenum attached in its new position.

Techniques to Correct Esthetic Deformities/ Improve Esthetics

The maxillary anterior area in a patient with a high lip line presents a visible area in which patients are concerned with the esthetic appearance of the gingival tissues. This area is addressed as the "esthetic zone," which requires special consideration in restorative, periodontal, and implant therapy. The symmetry of the facial gingival margin from canine to canine is altered with the recession of the gingival margin, the loss of the interdental papilla, or if there is excessive amount of gingival tissue creating a "gummy smile." The therapy to correct these gingival conditions is discussed under the following topics:

1. Root coverage.
2. Papilla reconstruction.
3. Therapy to correct excessive gingival display.
4. Procedure to correct gingival asymmetry.
5. Gingival depigmentation.

Root Coverage (Gingival Augmentation Coronal to the Recession)

The surgical correction of root coverage is discussed in detail in the section on gingival augmentation coronal to the recession.

Papilla Reconstruction

The loss of the interdental papilla is a major esthetic problem for many patients. It is often referred to as the "black triangle or hole"

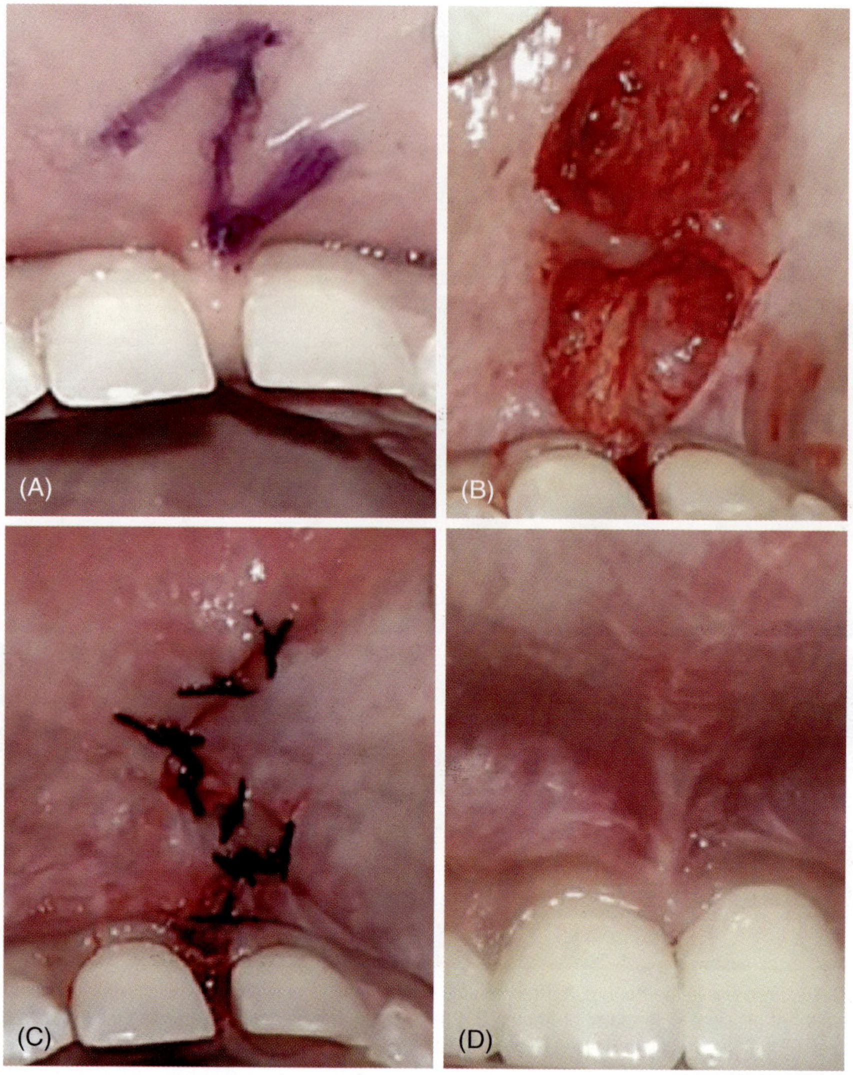

Fig. 50.17 Z-plasty. A,The planned incisions are marked out. B,The length of the frenum was incised and at each end, incisions at 60° angulation were made and submucosal tissues were dissected beyond the base of each flap. C, The resultant flaps were mobilized and transposed through 90° to close the vertical incisions horizontally and sutures were placed. D, At 1 month of follow-up satisfactory healing was found and composite restorations were done in the central incisors to close the diastema *(Courtesy: Dr. Joann Pauline George, India.)*

(Fig. 50.18). The reconstruction of the lost or reduced interdental papilla is the most difficult and unpredictable problem in esthetic periodontal therapy. The interdental papilla is gingival tissue supported and created by two adjacent teeth in contact and the underlying bone beneath this tissue. The loss of this bone as the result of periodontal disease or the loss of the contact alters the support of the interdental tissue, which can lead to the loss or the reduced height of the papilla.

Tarnow, in his study of this area, stated the distance from the crest of the interdental bone to the apical portion of the contact above this bone determines whether the interdental papilla is absent or present (Fig. 50.19). Therefore, the predictable reconstruction of the papilla is determined not only by the augmentation of the gingival tissue but also by the presence or absence of the underlying bone and the contact of the two adjacent teeth.

Orthodontics and restorative therapy also play an important role in the loss and reconstruction of the papilla since they can determine the location of the contact position in the dentition. We have also learned from experience that grafting bone or gingiva of minimal size to a small recipient site is unpredictable because of the lack of blood supply from the recipient site to the donor tissue. Therefore, bone grafting or free gingival grafting of interdental areas to reconstruct the papilla is not a predictable procedure.

There have been numerous case reports of different techniques to augment gingival tissue into the interdental area. All of these techniques must be based on the principle of adequate blood supply to the donor tissue. Of the many gingival grafting procedures used in periodontal therapy, the technique that offers the best blood supply to the donor tissue is the pedicle graft because it maintains a connection between the donor tissue and the origin of the graft. The pouch and tunnel surgical procedure also creates the ideal blood supply for the recipient site to accept the donor tissue.

Han et al. reported a technique using a semilunar pedicle graft and pouch to gain papillary height, but without bone support, this technique was able to only reduce the interdental space. Azzi et al. have also reported successful results with numerous cases using different surgical techniques to regain the lost papilla. All of these cases employ different grafting techniques, using not only connective tissue and bone but also a surgical flap design applying the principle of the pouch and tunnel to maximize the blood supply to the grafted tissue.

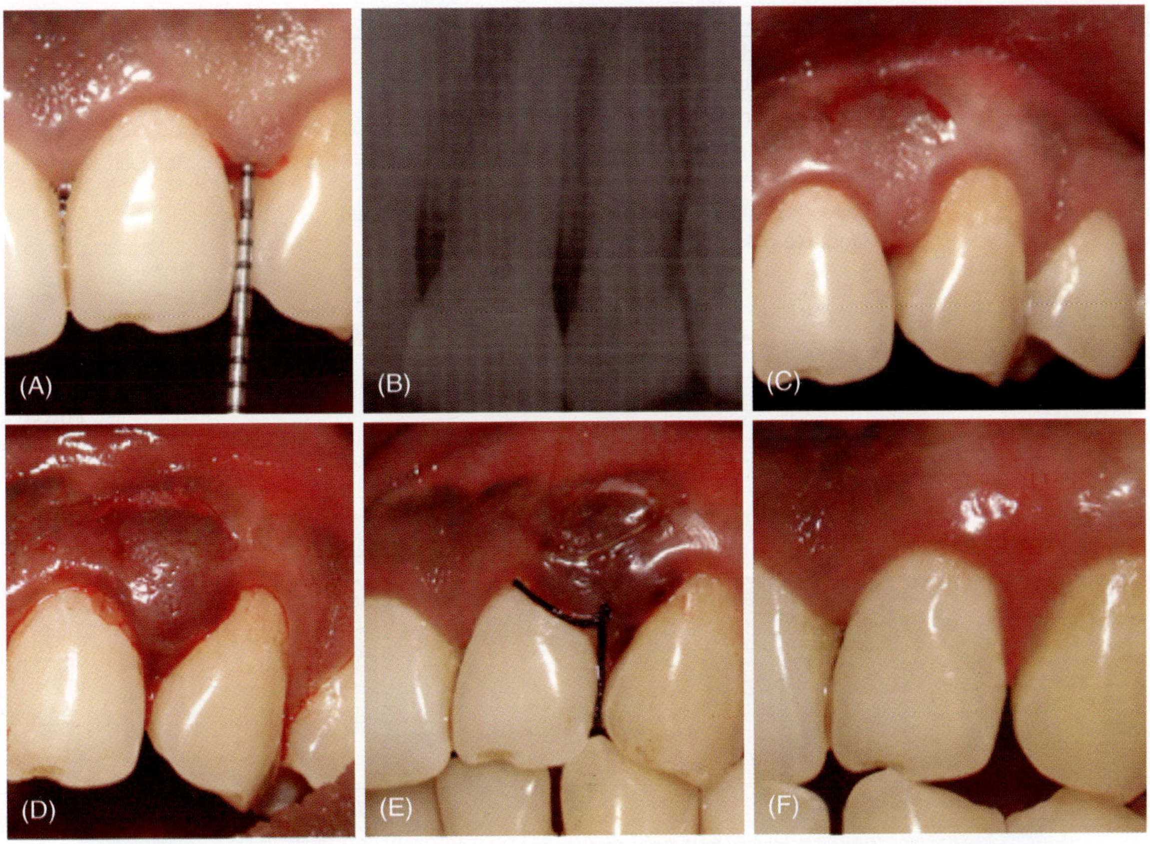

Fig. 50.18 A, Preoperative view. B, Radiograph. C, Split thickness semilunar buccal incision and intrasulcular releasing incisions made, papilla was undermined carefully, soft tissue was completely released from the root and the bone so that the whole flap was mobile. D, Donor tissue of 2 mm connective tissue was harvested and shaped to fit the interproximal area. E, Semilunar incision was sutured and entire gingivopapillary unit was advanced in the coronal position. F, Postoperative view at 6 months showing complete papillary fill. *(Courtesy: Dr. Joann Pauline George, India.)*

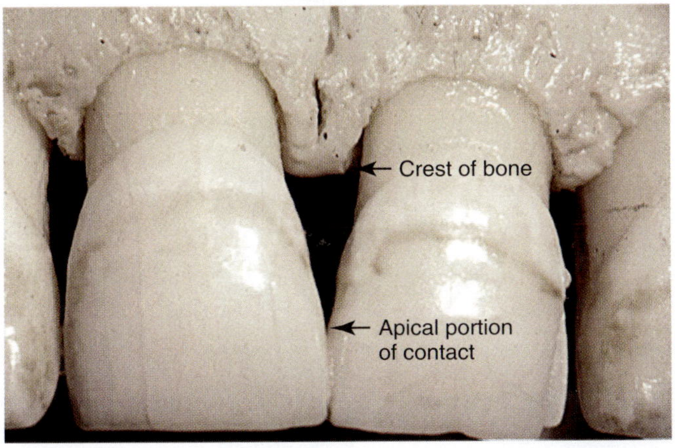

Fig. 50.19 The distance from the crest of the interdental bone to the apical portion of the contact, which determines the absence or presence of the papilla as indicated by Tarnow et al.

The case incorporates several of the concepts indicated earlier for papilla reconstruction. These concepts are (1) semilunar pedicle design, (2) both connective tissue (Fig. 50.20A and B) and bone grafting into the interdental area, and (3) the use of restorative dentistry to place the apical portion of the contact closer to the crestal bone.

The future of papilla reconstruction will involve techniques developed by tissue engineering using biologic mediators. In a study reported by McGuire and Scheyer, autologous fibroblasts were injected into the interdental papilla to atraumatically augment the deficient interdental papilla. The exciting field of tissue engineering will allow the clinician to use minimally invasive procedures to reconstruct the lost papilla. In the recent years dermal filler like hyaluronic acid have shown promising outcomes in minimally invasive approach.

Therapy to Correct Excessive Gingival Display

Excessive gingival display, commonly called a "gummy smile," represents an esthetic concern for many patients. This appearance may be caused by a skeletal problem called *vertical maxillary excess*, by dentoalveolar extrusion, or by incomplete exposure of the anatomic crown, often referred to as *altered passive eruption*. It may be associated with a short upper lip or excessive lip translation. There may be a combination of causative factors requiring more than one treatment option.

Even in patients with excessive gingival display, the primary esthetic feature is the appearance of the teeth. If the cause of the "gummy" appearance is incomplete exposure of the anatomic crown, the teeth will appear short and unattractive. This appearance is often noticed in adolescent patients during orthodontic treatment. It has been found that if there is a need for esthetic crown lengthening before orthodontic therapy, there will still be a need after orthodontic therapy and likely still a need 5 years later. Although patients may complain of the gummy exposure, the real esthetic issue is the altered tooth form. Surgical crown lengthening addresses both concerns, but its focus should be the exposure of a properly proportioned tooth.

Indications	Contraindications	Techniques		
• Delayed passive eruption	• Surgery would create an unesthetic outcome.	• Gingivectomy		
• Root perforation	• Deep caries or fracture would require excessive bone removal on contiguous teeth.	• Periodontal flap surgery		
• Root resorption	• The tooth is a poor restorative risk.	• Apically displaced flap		
• Inadequate clinical crown length for retention		• Apically displaced flap + osteotomy		
		• Orthodontic therapy	• Extrusive techniques	• Forced eruption + minor osseous resection
				• Forced eruption + fiberotomy
• Unequal or unesthetic gingival heights			• Intrusive techniques	

Source - Dr Joann Pauline George

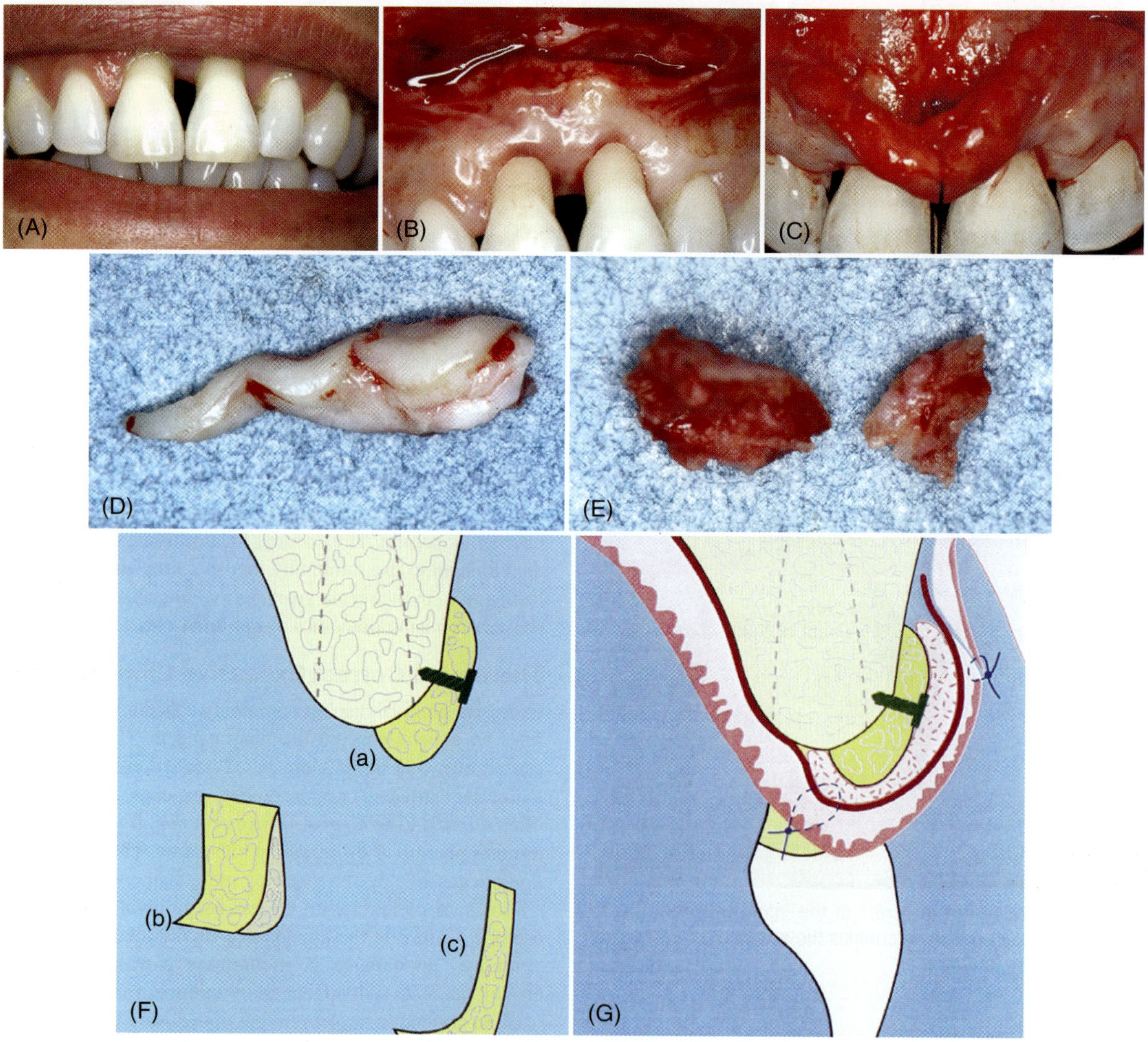

Fig. 50.20 A, Preoperative view. Note the loss of the interdental papilla and the extensive recession of the facial marginal gingiva. B, Intrasulcular incision is made around the neck of the right lateral incisor and central incisors. A horizontal incision starting at the mucogingival junction, extending into the alveolar mucosa and apically up to the labial fold, is performed to elevate a split-thickness flap. C, Mucogingival flap is elevated coronally and secured with a horizontal mattress suture anchored to the interdental contact point of the central incisors, exposing the interdental bone. D, Connective tissue removed from the tuberosity to be placed over the bone graft in the interdental area. E, Bone graft removed from the tuberosity, which will be grafted in the interdental area. F, Diagram of the bone fixed to the alveolar crest using a titanium screw. *(a)*, Saddle-shaped graft fits over the interdental bone crest. *(b)*, Internal view of the osseous graft. *(c)*, Profile view of the osseous graft. G, Diagram of the flap returned and sutured over the grafted materials to obtain complete closure.

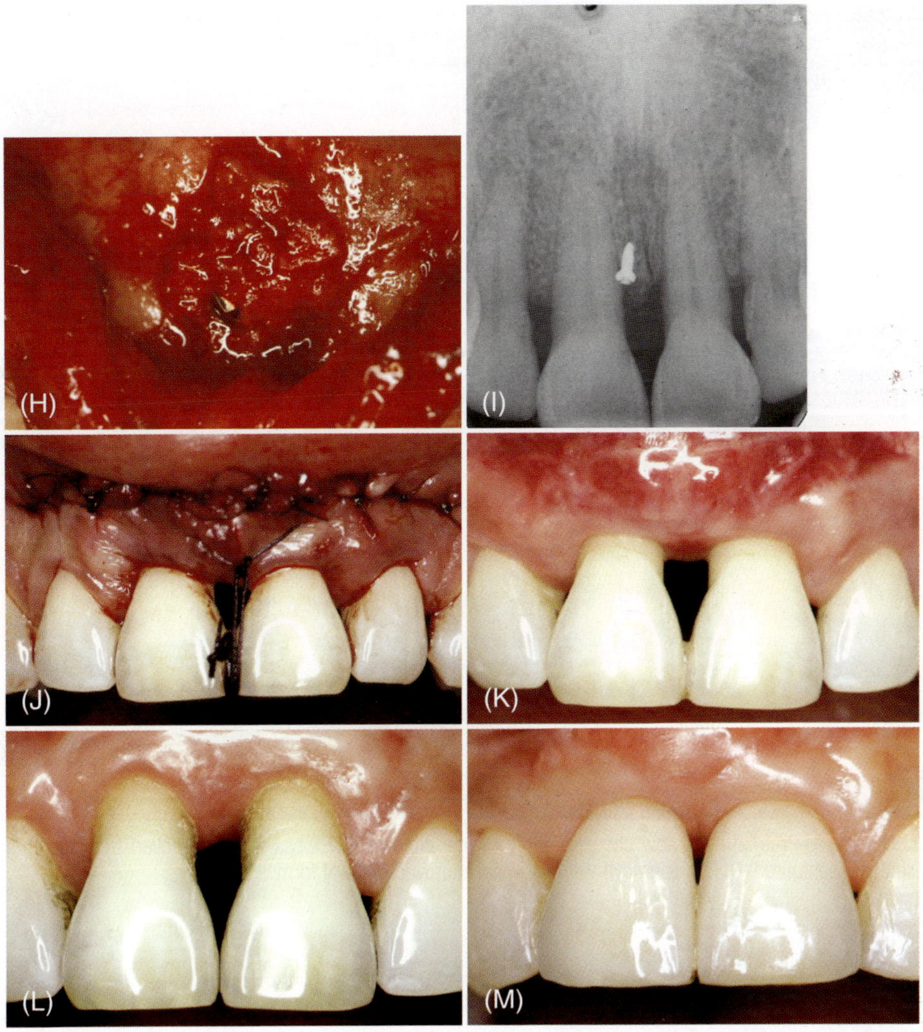

Fig. 50.20, cont'd H, Crushed cancellous bone is packed around the grafted bone in the shape of the reconstructed interdental bone. I, A radiograph indicating the titanium screw that is used to hold the grafted bone in place. J, Coronal positioning of the entire gingivopapillary unit by the use of a horizontal mattress suture anchored over the splinted incisal portion of the contact. The mucosal portion of the flap is approximated to the gingivopapillary edge of the flap and sutured using 4.0 sutures. K, Three-month postoperative healing. Normal anatomy and shape with complete root coverage on the right lateral incisor, partial root coverage on the central incisors, and reconstruction of the interdental papilla. L, Preoperative view. Compare with the reconstructed papilla. M, One-year postoperative view with two porcelain veneers bonded on the central incisors. The contact is placed apically to help reduce the interdental space. *(Courtesy: Dr R. Azzi, Paris.)*

Ideally, the width/length ratio of a maxillary central incisor clinical crown should fall between 0.78 and 0.85. Thus, a central incisor with a width of 8.5 mm should have a length between 10 and 11 mm. The length of the maxillary canine is equal to or slightly less than the central incisor and its gingival margin should be aligned with the central incisor gingival margin. The gingival margin of the lateral incisor is usually about 1.0 mm coronal to the margins of the adjacent teeth, although in patients with a high lip line, it is generally more pleasing to have the lateral incisor gingival margin equal to the central incisors and canines.

Surgical Techniques

Exposure of the full anatomic crown is necessary to achieve a smile with minimal gingival exposure. Measurements before surgery should include clinical crown width and length, anatomic crown length, and height of keratinized tissue.

Surgical crown lengthening may be accomplished by soft tissue excision alone or by flap surgery with or without osseous surgery. The determinants for choice of surgical procedure are (1) the need to leave a minimum of 3.0 mm of keratinized marginal tissue and (2) the possible need for osseous surgery. If excision of soft tissue for full anatomic crown exposure would leave at least 3.0 mm of keratinized marginal tissue and there is no need for osseous surgery, soft tissue excision alone is the treatment of choice. If less than 3.0 mm of keratinized marginal tissue would remain after the necessary excision, an apically positioned flap would be required.

The soft tissue level is determined by the thickness and level of the underlying alveolar bone. It is important to reduce the osseous crest so that the new position parallels the CEJ at each tooth facially and proximally. However, the height of the interdental crest is not reduced in esthetic crown lengthening.

Fig. 50.21 demonstrates a clinical case of esthetic crown lengthening to correct the "gummy appearance" in the maxillary esthetic zone.

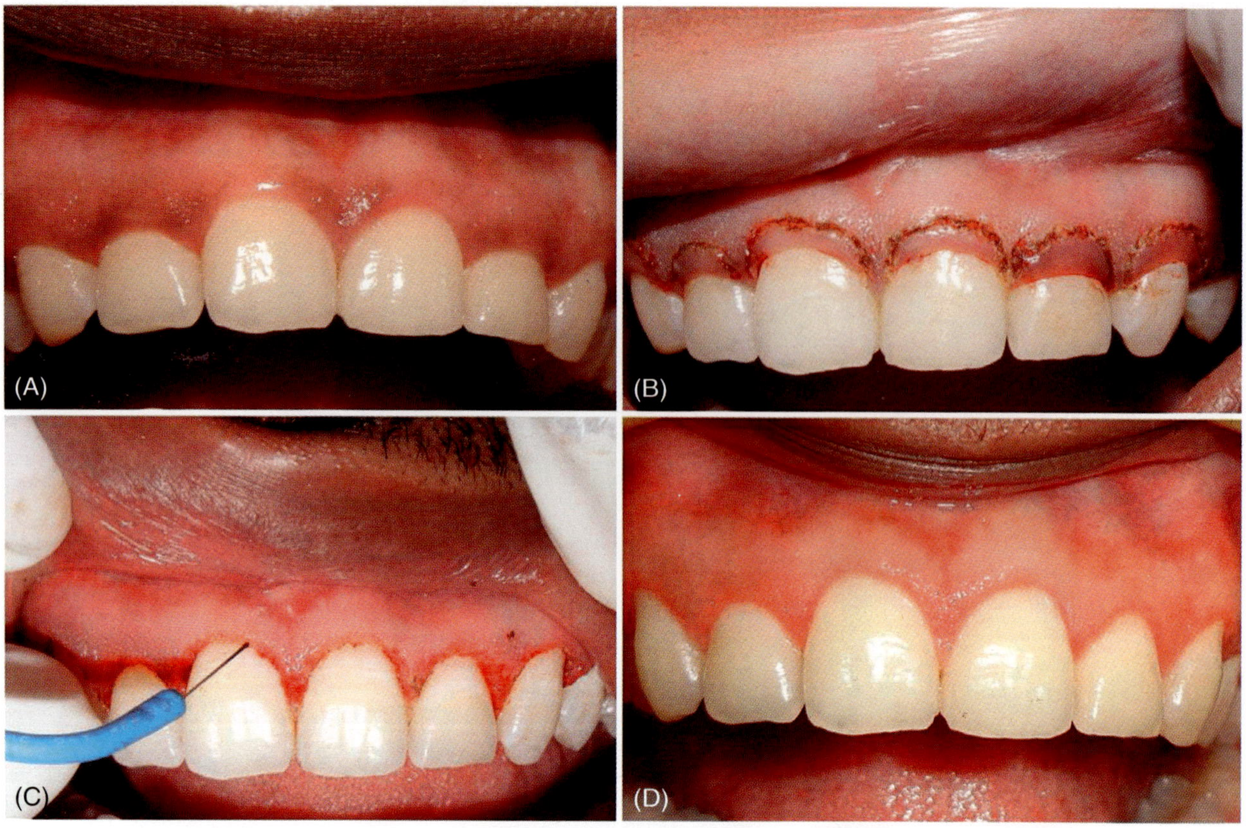

Fig. 50.21 A, Pretreatment view showing short clinical crowns. B, Excess tissue removed by a diode laser. C, Gingiva recontoured. D, Postoperative view showing improved gingival form.

Procedure to Correct Gingival Asymmetry

The clinician should have the precise idea of the normal contour, zenith, and curvature of the gingiva of the teeth in the esthetic zone. The gingiva can be reshaped either by gingivoplasty or minimally invasive flap surgery (Fig. 50.22).

Gingival Depigmentation

Gingival pigmentation is dependent on many factors including racial background. The activity of the melanocytes which are nonkeratinocytes present in the gingival epithelium varies among individuals. Physiological gingival hyperpigmentation can be treated albeit the fact that the results last for anywhere from 6 to 36 months (Fig. 50.23).

Gingival depigmentation involves the removal of the superficial epithelium by one of the following methods.

1. Mucosal excision/stripping by a BP blade
2. Rotary instruments
3. Electrosurgery
4. Cryosurgery
5. Lasers

Maximum care should be taken not to completely remove the gingiva and exposing the root and/or bone. This can happen particularly when the gingival biotype is thin.

The results obtained by cryosurgery and lasers appear to sustain for a longer time than surgery by scalpel blade. Rotary instruments produce the least satisfactory outcome, whereas electrosurgery is not indicated because of its inability to control the extent of tissue destruction.

It should be clearly understood that mentioned procedures are for only physiological hyperpigmented gingiva and not for pathologically discolored gums.

Tissue Engineering

Tissue engineering and the use of biologic mediators in PPS have become a reality as the result of research and the demand for noninvasive surgical procedures by patients and clinicians.

Passive engineering involves the following treatments and materials:

1. Therapies based on GTR-based therapies; barrier membranes.
2. Biologically based Acellular dermal matrix (ADM).

Active engineering involves the following treatments and materials:

1. Enamel matrix derivative (EMD).
2. Growth factors: recombinant human platelet-derived growth factor-BB (rhPDGF-BB) plus beta-tricalcium phosphate (β-TCP) plus collagen wound dressing.
3. Cell therapy:
   - Autologous fibroblast: Isolagen
   - Bilayered cell therapy (BLCT)—CelTx
   - Human fibroblast-derived dermal substitute (HFDDS): Dermagraft

At some point, recombinant growth factors could eliminate the need for donor sites and the use of exogenous materials inserted into the human body. Future research should focus on obtaining additional evidence for using growth factors and live cell technology during periodontal therapy to eliminate donor site morbidity.

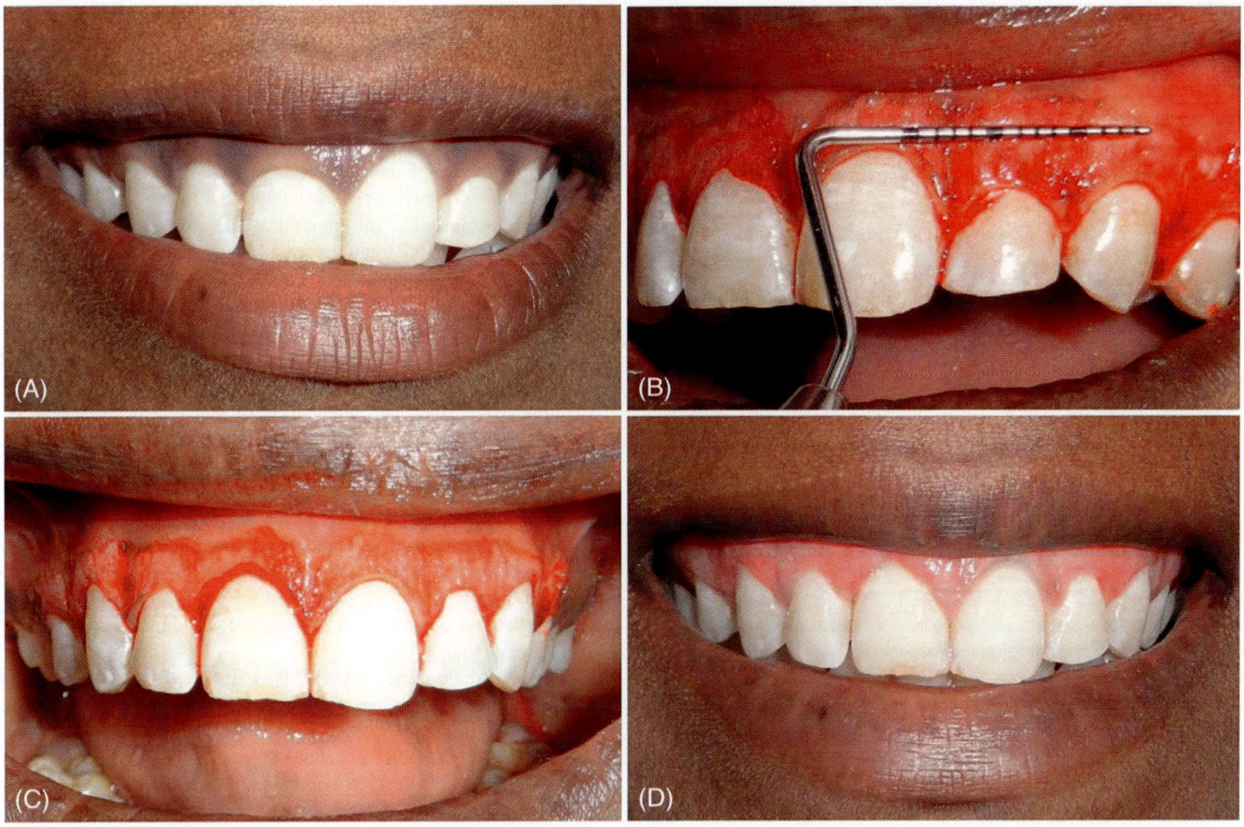

Fig. 50.22 A, Pretreatment view showing gingival asymmetry and hyper pigmentation. B, Superficial epithelium excised for de-pigmentation. C, Gingiva recontoured. D, Postoperative view showing pleasing gingival appearance.

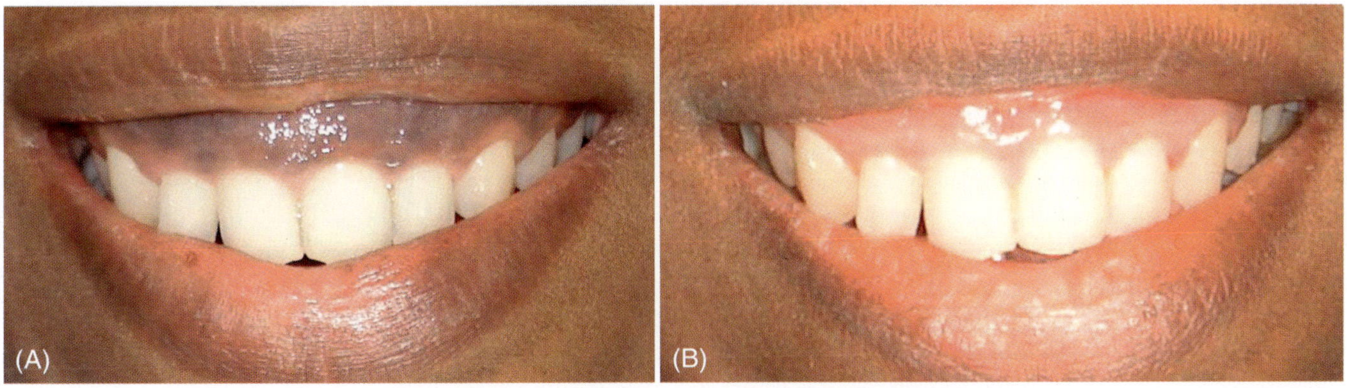

Fig. 50.23 A, Hyperpigmented gingiva. B, Following gingival depigmentation with cryosurgery.

Conclusion

As defined in this chapter, PPS refers to soft tissue relationships and manipulations. In all of these procedures, blood supply is the most significant concern and must be the underlying issue for all decisions regarding the individual surgical procedure. A major complicating factor is the avascular root surface, and many modifications to existing techniques are used to overcome this. Diffusion of fluids is short term and of limited benefit as tissue size increases. Thus, the formation of a circulation through anastomosis and angiogenesis is crucial to the survival of these therapeutic procedures. The formation of vascularity is based on growth molecules, such as vascular endothelial growth factor and cellular migration, proliferation, and differentiation. As tissue-engineering techniques improve, the success and predictability of mucogingival surgery should dramatically increase. Undoubtedly, all advancements will have adequate circulation and blood supply as their basis.

New techniques are constantly being developed and are slowly being incorporated into periodontal practice. The practitioner should be aware that, at times, new methods are published without adequate clinical research to ensure the predictability of the results and the extent to which the techniques may benefit the patient. Critical analysis of newly presented techniques should guide our constant evolution toward better clinical methods.

Key points

- Lack of keratinized gingiva, gingival recession, aberrant frenum, and esthetic deformities of gingiva constitute mucogingival problems.
- There is no prescribed minimum width of attached gingiva.
- A wider zone of attached gingiva is desirable before orthodontic treatment, and in teeth that serve as abutments as well as in ridge areas bearing an implant or a denture.
- Free gingival autograft is a more common procedure to augment the width of attached gingiva.
- Apically displaced flaps not only eliminate the pockets but also aid in increasing the width of attached gingiva.
- The subepithelial connective tissue graft and coronally advanced flap procedures are the most predictable techniques for root coverage.
- Pouch and tunnel technique, VISTA, pinhole approach, and use of allogenic grafts are the techniques used for multiple root coverage.
- Papilla reconstruction is the most challenging task in periodontal plastic surgery.
- Periodontal plastic surgery in smokers produce inferior results.

Suggested Readings

American Academy of Periodontology: *Glossary of periodontal terms*, ed 3, Chicago, 1992, American Academy of Periodontology.

Azzi R, Takei H, Etienne D, et al: Root coverage and papilla reconstruction using autogenous osseous and connective tissue grafts. *Int J Perio Rest Dent* 2:141–147, 2001.

Becker BE, Becker W: Use of connective tissue autografts for treatment of mucogingival problems. *Int J Periodont Restor Dent* 6:89, 1986.

Bertl K, Melchard M, Pandis N, Müller-Kern M, Stavropoulos A: Soft tissue substitutes in non-root coverage procedures: a systematic review and meta-analysis, *Clin Oral Investig* 21:505–518, 2017.

Burkhardt R, Lang NP: Fundamental principles in periodontal plastic surgery and mucosal augmentation–a narrative review, *J Clin Periodontol* 41:S98–S107, 2014.

Carranza FA, Jr, Carraro JJ: Mucogingival techniques in periodontal surgery. *J Periodontol* 41:294, 1970.

Chambrone L, Ortega MA, Sukekava F, et al: Root coverage procedures for treating single and multiple recession-type defects: an updated Cochrane systematic review, *J Periodontol* 90(12):1399–1422, 2019.

Cortellini P, Clauser C, Pini-Prato GP: Histologic assessment of new attachment following the treatment of a human buccal recession by means of a guided tissue regeneration procedure. *J Periodontol* 64:387, 1993.

Hawley CE, Staffileno H: Clinical evaluation of free gingival grafts in periodontal surgery. *J Periodontol* 41:105, 1970.

Langer B, Langer L: Subepithelial connective tissue graft technique for root coverage. *J Periodontol* 56:715, 1985.

McGuire MK, Nunn ME: Evaluation of human recession defects treated with coronally advanced flaps and either enamel matrix derivative or connective tissue. I. Comparison of clinical parameters. *J Periodontol* 74:1110–1125, 2003.

McGuire MK, Scheyer ET, Schupbach P: Growth factor-mediated treatment of recession defects: a randomized controlled trial and histologic and microcomputed tomography examination. *J Periodontol* 80:550–564, 2009.

Miller PD, Jr: A classification of marginal tissue recession. *Int J Periodont Restor Dent* 5:9, 1985.

Tatakis DN, Chambrone L, Allen EP, et al: Periodontal soft tissue root coverage procedures: a consensus report from the AAP Regeneration Workshop, *J Periodontol* 86:S52–S55, 2015.

Tavelli L, McGuire MK, Zucchelli G, et al: Biologics-based regenerative technologies for periodontal soft tissue engineering, *J Periodontol* 91(2):147–154, 2020.

Zucchelli G, Tavelli L, McGuire MK, et al: Autogenous soft tissue grafting for periodontal and peri-implant plastic surgical reconstruction, *J Periodontol* 91(1):9–16, 2020.

CHAPTER 51

Periodontal Microsurgery

DA Shanelec | LS Tibbetts | A McGregor | JD Cross | RT Kao | B Butler | CD Dwarakanath

CHAPTER OUTLINE

Many new technologies are being evolved to assist the clinician and to enhance the outcome of periodontal therapy. Microsurgeries, lasers, and piezosurgeries have been increasingly employed in periodontics. This chapter deals with the various applications of microsurgeries and lasers in periodontal therapy. By strict definition, microsurgery is defined as a surgery performed under magnification of 10× or more using a surgical microscope. However, periodontal microsurgery includes all the procedures done under magnification starting from 2.5× onwards either using surgical loupes or microscope. The hallmarks of microsurgery are increased visual acuity and improved manual dexterity when visibility is increased 10-fold, motor movement precision is increased from 1 to 10 mm. This is the approximate size of an epithelial cell. Large incisions for visibility are therefore not necessary. Small surgical instruments are used to advantage in the reduced surgical field (Fig. 51.1). This minimally invasive philosophy results in less injury, diminished morbidity, and rapid healing. Central to this approach are sharp microsurgical blades to create incisions at a virtual cellular level. These incisions are closed with meticulous apposition to eliminate wound edge gaps and dislocations, allowing healing by primary intention to begin within hours of microsurgical closure. This circumvents the need for an extensive secondary mitotic stage of wound healing to bridge wound gaps and fill surgical voids.

Philosophy of Periodontal Microsurgery

Microsurgery is a philosophy that embraces three core values. The first is enhanced motor skill for better surgical performance. This is accomplished through improved visual acuity and the use of a precise hand grip to increase accuracy and reduce tremor. The second is minimal tissue trauma, which is accomplished through smaller incisions and reduced surgical field (Fig. 51.2). The third value is primary passive wound closure. This is accomplished by microsuturing to eliminate gaps and dead spaces at the wound edge.

Advanced periodontics has an increasing need for clinical procedures that require intricate surgical skills. Regenerative procedures, periodontal plastic surgery, and dental implants are but a few of the surgical procedures that demand clinical performance that frequently challenges the skills of periodontal surgeons beyond the range of possibility with ordinary vision. Microsurgery establishes a minimally invasive surgical approach to periodontics exemplified by fewer vertical incisions and smaller surgical sites. Every field of microsurgery has noted the extent to which reduced incision size and less retraction directly relate to reduced postoperative morbidity and rapid healing (Fig. 51.3).

In addition to the use of magnification and reliance on atraumatic technique, microsurgery requires specially constructed instruments designed specifically to minimize trauma. An important characteristic of microsurgical instruments is their ability to create clean incisions that prepare wounds for healing by primary intention. Microsurgical incisions are established at a 90-degree angle to the surface using ophthalmic microsurgical scalpels. Microscopy permits easy identification of ragged wound edges for trimming and freshening. For primary wound closure, microsutures in the range of 6-0 to 9-0 are needed to approximate the wound edges accurately. Microsurgical wound apposition minimizes gaps or voids at the wound edges and encourages rapid healing with less postoperative inflammation and less pain (Figs. 51.4 and 51.5).

Advantages of Microsurgery

Periodontal microsurgery raises the treatment bar in many ways. Surgical decision making is enhanced because the quality and quantity of visual data reaching the cerebral cortex is increased by a square of the magnification level. Ergonomic and body posture advantages also occur when using the surgical microscope (Fig. 51.6). Issues, such as neuromuscular fatigue and occupational skeletal pathology, are reduced. Sitting comfort, good body posture, arm support, and controlled breathing are inherent to proper microscope use. Motor skills are enhanced through instruments designed for a precision grip of the hand. Titanium instruments are used for strength and lightness and are made with round handles to permit precise rotation. This reduces hand fatigue and tremor for precise surgical movement. Ergonomic benefit may be one of the most significant aspects of microscope use in periodontics.

An important aspect of periodontal microsurgery is technical improvement in surgical performance. Higher skill levels have been shown in many surgical disciplines and can be fully appreciated when a surgeon tries his or her hand under the microscope. Viewing surgery under the microscope impresses a surgeon with the coarseness of conventional surgical manipulation. What appears to the unaided eye as gentle surgery is revealed, under the microscope, as

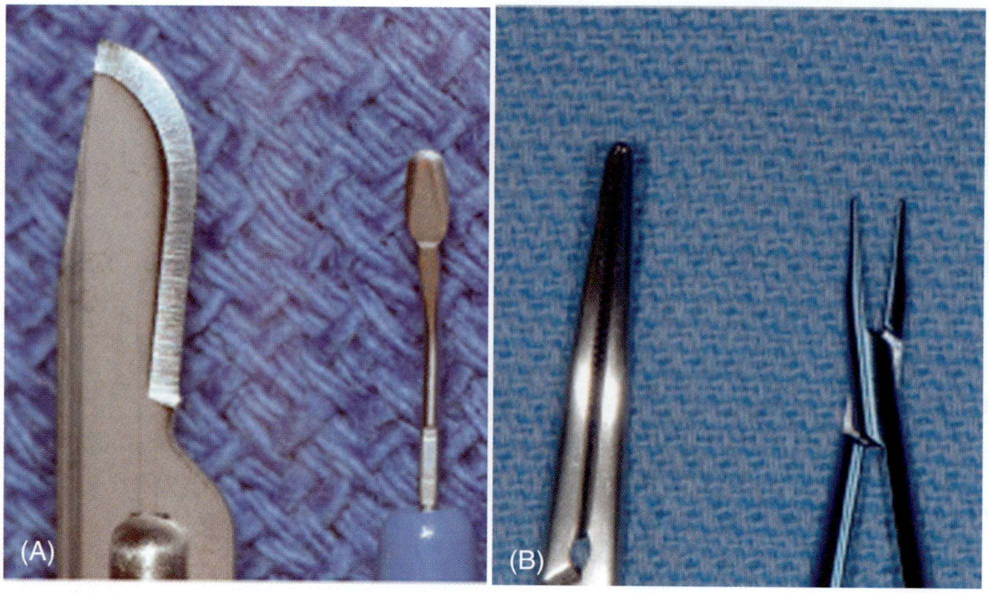

Fig. 51.1 Side-by-side dimensional comparison of commonly used conventional versus microsurgical instruments. A, No. 15 blade versus ophthalmic blade. B, Working tip of conventional needle holder versus McGregor microsuturing forceps.

gross crushing and tearing of delicate tissues. Periodontics has long advocated atraumatic surgery, but the limits of normal vision have made this goal unattainable.

Proprioceptive guidance is of little value at the microsurgical level. Visual guidance is used for midcourse correction of scalpels and instruments to achieve the finest level of skill and dexterity. Incisions can be accurately mapped, flaps elevated with minimal damage, and wounds closed accurately without tension. Periodontal microsurgery is a natural progression from conventional surgical principles to a surgical ethic in which the surgical microscope is employed for the most accurate and atraumatic handling of tissue.

The end-point appearance of microsurgery is superior to that of conventional surgery. The difference is self-evident and often startling (Fig. 51.7). As much as judgment and knowledge play a role in surgery, in the end surgery is a craft. Surgeons appreciate this, especially when microsurgery raises their work to the levels of artistic expression. Personal gratification in performing better surgery leads to acceptance of periodontal microsurgery by surgeons motivated to improve the quality of their work.

Another very important advantage of microsurgery is in the area of root preparation. The importance of root debridement is recognized universally as an essential component of periodontal therapy. Research in clinical dentistry has shown that microscope-enhanced vision more readily accomplishes the long-established clinical goals of endodontic and restorative dentistry. In periodontics, studies demonstrated that root debridement performed without magnification was incomplete. When debrided roots were examined with the aid of a microscope, substantial deposits remained. Even in the absence of clinical studies, it may be inferred that microscope-enhanced vision in periodontics permits more definitive root debridement.

The primary goals of periodontal surgery include visual access to the root surface for plaque and calculus removal and for removing pathologically altered tooth structure. Magnification greatly improves the surgeon's ability to create a clean, smooth root surface. The root surface represents one opposing edge of the periodontal wound. Root planing is therefore analogous to establishing a clean soft tissue incision. Magnification permits preparation of both hard and soft tissue wound surfaces so that they may be joined together according to the accepted microsurgical principle of butt joint wound approximation. This encourages primary wound healing and enhanced periodontal reconstruction. Wound healing studies show epithelial anastomosis of microsurgically joined surgical wounds in animals within 48 h.

With training, the average periodontal microsurgeon can consistently produce better crafted work than the most talented conventional surgeon.

Magnification Systems

A variety of simple and complex magnification systems are available to dentists, ranging from simple loupes to prism telescopic loupes and surgical microscopes. Each magnification system has its specific advantages and limitations. Although magnification improves the accuracy of clinical and diagnostic skills, it requires an understanding of optical principles that govern all magnification systems. The assumption that "more magnification is better" must always be weighed against the decrease in field of view and depth of focus that can occur as magnification increases, which is a problem more common with dental loupes than operating microscopes.

Magnifying Loupes

Dental loupes are the most common system of optical magnification used in periodontics. *Loupes* are fundamentally dual monocular telescopes with side-by-side lenses convergent to focus on the operative field. The magnified image formed has stereoscopic properties by virtue of their convergence. A convergent lens optical system is called a *Keplerian optical system.*

Although dental loupes are widely used, they have disadvantages compared to the microscope. The clinician's eyes must converge to view the operative field. This can result in eyestrain, fatigue, and even pathologic vision changes, especially after prolonged use.

Three types of Keplerian loupes are typically used in periodontics: simple or single-element loupes, compound loupes, and prism telescopic loupes. Each type may differ widely in optical sophistication and individual design.

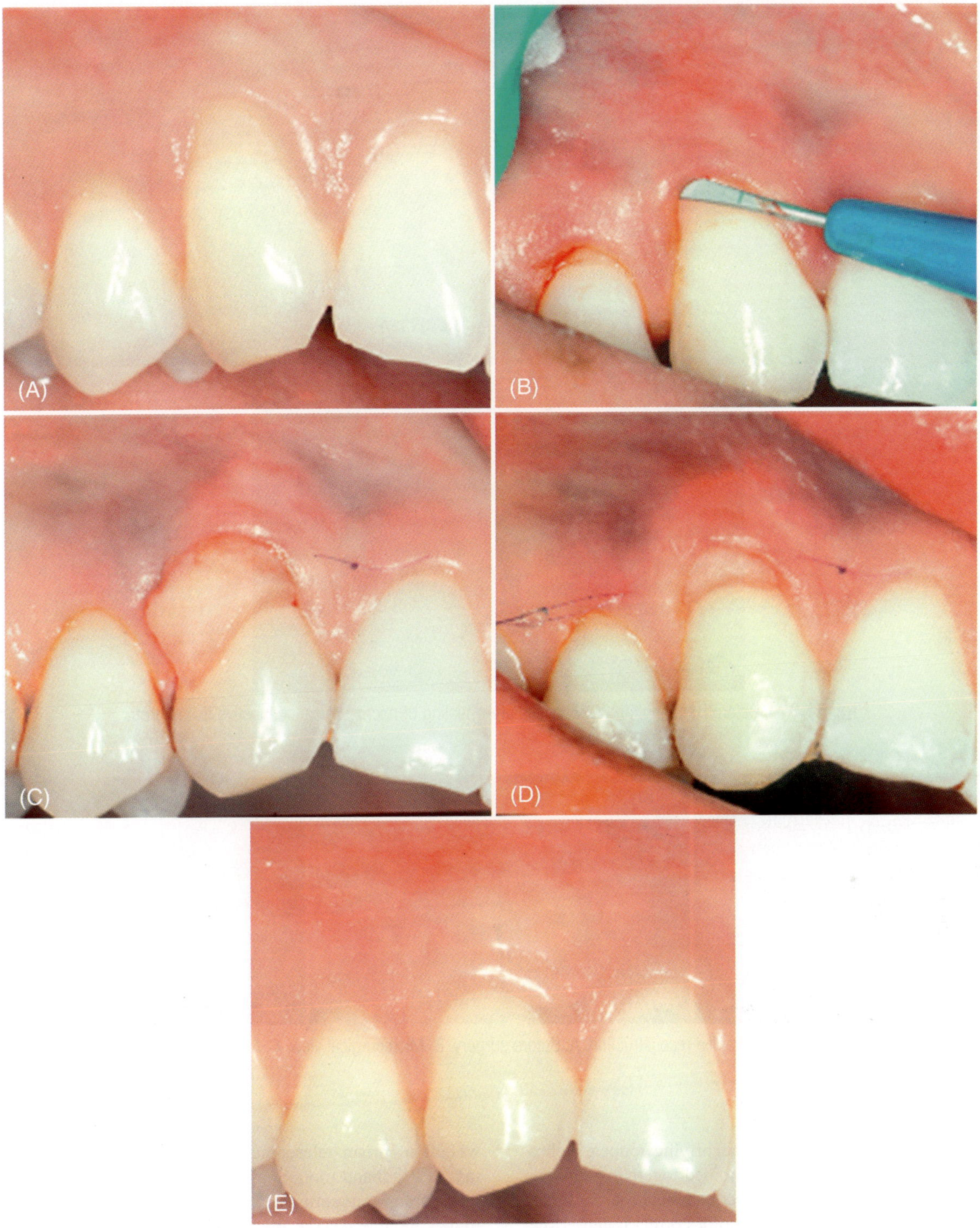

Fig. 51.2 A–E, Microsurgical connective tissue graft. Minimal tissue trauma during incisions, surgical manipulation, and suturing is accomplished after microsurgical principles.

Simple Loupes

Simple loupes consist of a pair of single meniscus lenses (Fig. 51.8). Simple loupes are primitive magnifiers with limited capabilities. Each lens is limited to only two refracting surfaces. Their magnification can only increase by increasing the lens diameter and thickness. Size and weight constraints make simple loupes impractical for magnification beyond 1.5×. Another disadvantage of simple loupes is that they are greatly affected by spherical and chromatic aberration. This distorts the image shape and color of objects being viewed.

Compound Loupes

Compound loupes use multielement lenses with intervening air spaces to gain additional refracting surfaces (Fig. 51.9). This allows increased magnification with more favorable working distance and depth of field. Magnification of compound loupes can be increased by lengthening the distance between lenses, thereby avoiding excessive size and weight.

In addition to offering improved optical performance, compound lenses can be *achromatic*, which is an optical feature that clinicians

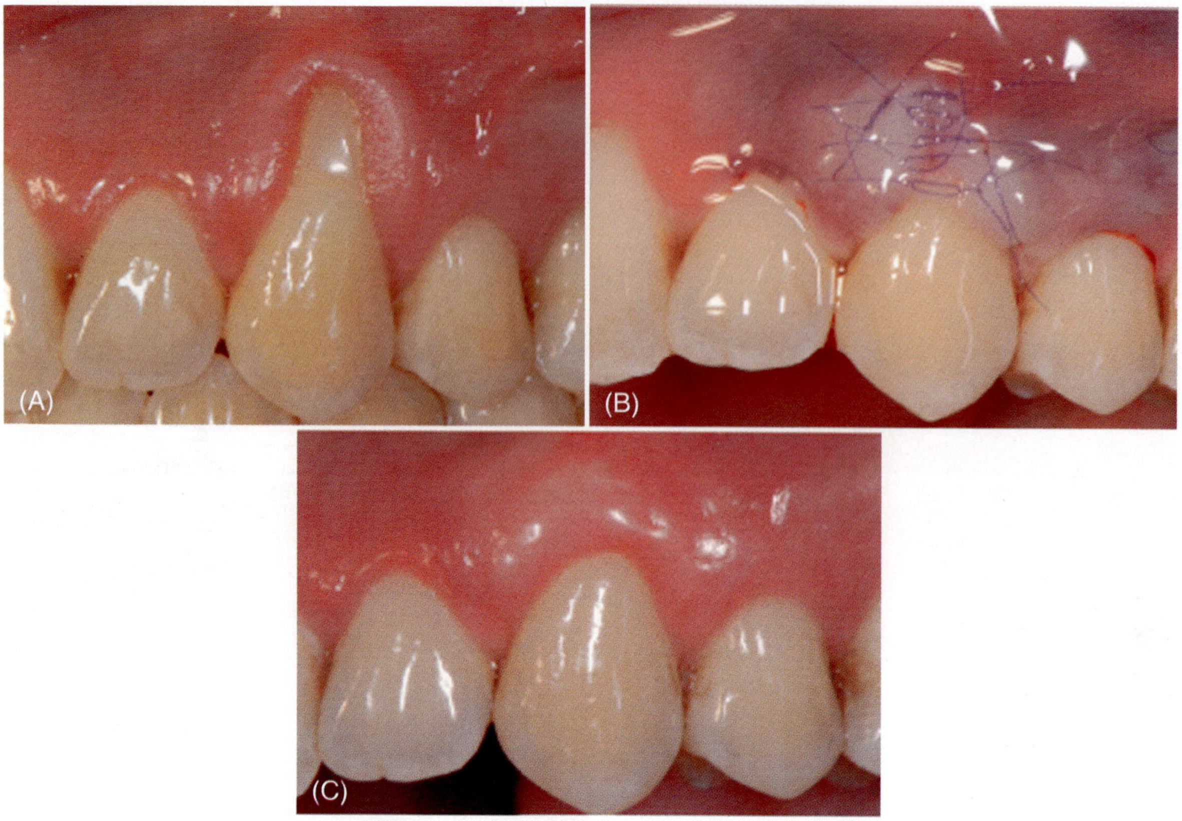

Fig. 51.3 A, Before B, during, and C, 8 weeks after healing of microsurgical connective tissue graft.

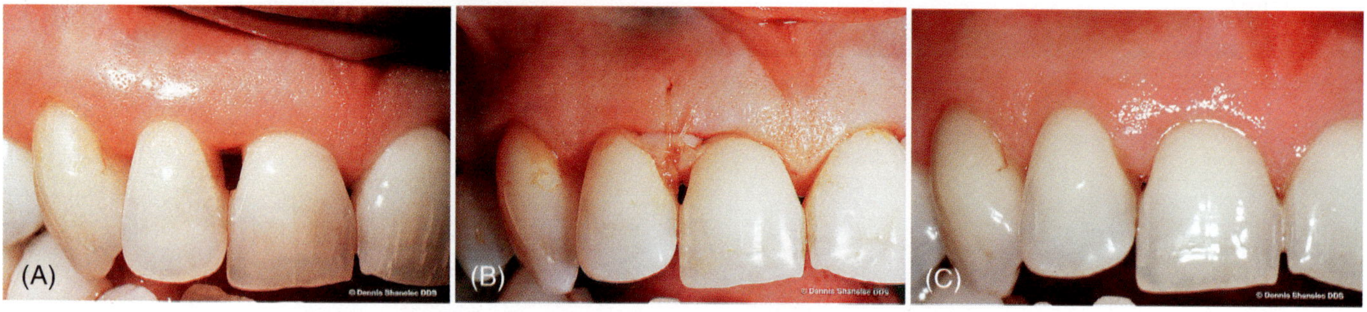

Fig. 51.4 Papilla reconstruction. A, Before surgery. B, Microsurgical view. C, After surgery.

should always choose when selecting magnifying loupes. Achromatic lenses consist of two glass lenses joined together with clear resin. The specific density of each lens counteracts the chromatic aberration of its paired lens to produce a color-correct image. However, multielement compound loupes become optically inefficient at magnifications above 3×.

Prism Telescopic Loupes

The most advanced loupe optical magnification currently available is the prism telescopic loupe (Fig. 51.10). Such loupes employ Schmidt or "rooftop" prisms to lengthen the light path through a series of switchback mirrors between the lenses. This arrangement folds the light so that the barrel of the loupes can be shortened. Prism loupes produce better magnification, wider depths of field, longer working distances, and larger fields of view than other types of loupes. The barrels of prism loupes are short enough to be mounted on either eyeglass frames or headbands. However, increased weight of prism telescopic loupes with magnification above 4× makes headband mounting more comfortable and stable than eyeglass frame mounting. Recent innovations in prism telescopic loupes include coaxial fiber optic lighting incorporated in the lens elements to improve illumination (Fig. 51.11).

Magnification Range of Surgical Loupes

Dental loupes provide a limited range of magnification, 1.5× to 6×. Loupes delivering magnification of less than 3× are usually inadequate for the visual acuity necessary for clinical periodontics. Surgical loupes providing magnification of more than 4× are impractical because of their small field of view, shallow depth of focus, and excessive weight. Excessively heavy loupes can make it difficult to maintain a stable visual field.

For some periodontal procedures, prism telescopic loupes with magnification of 4× provide an adequate combination of magnification, field of view, and depth of focus. However, the surgical

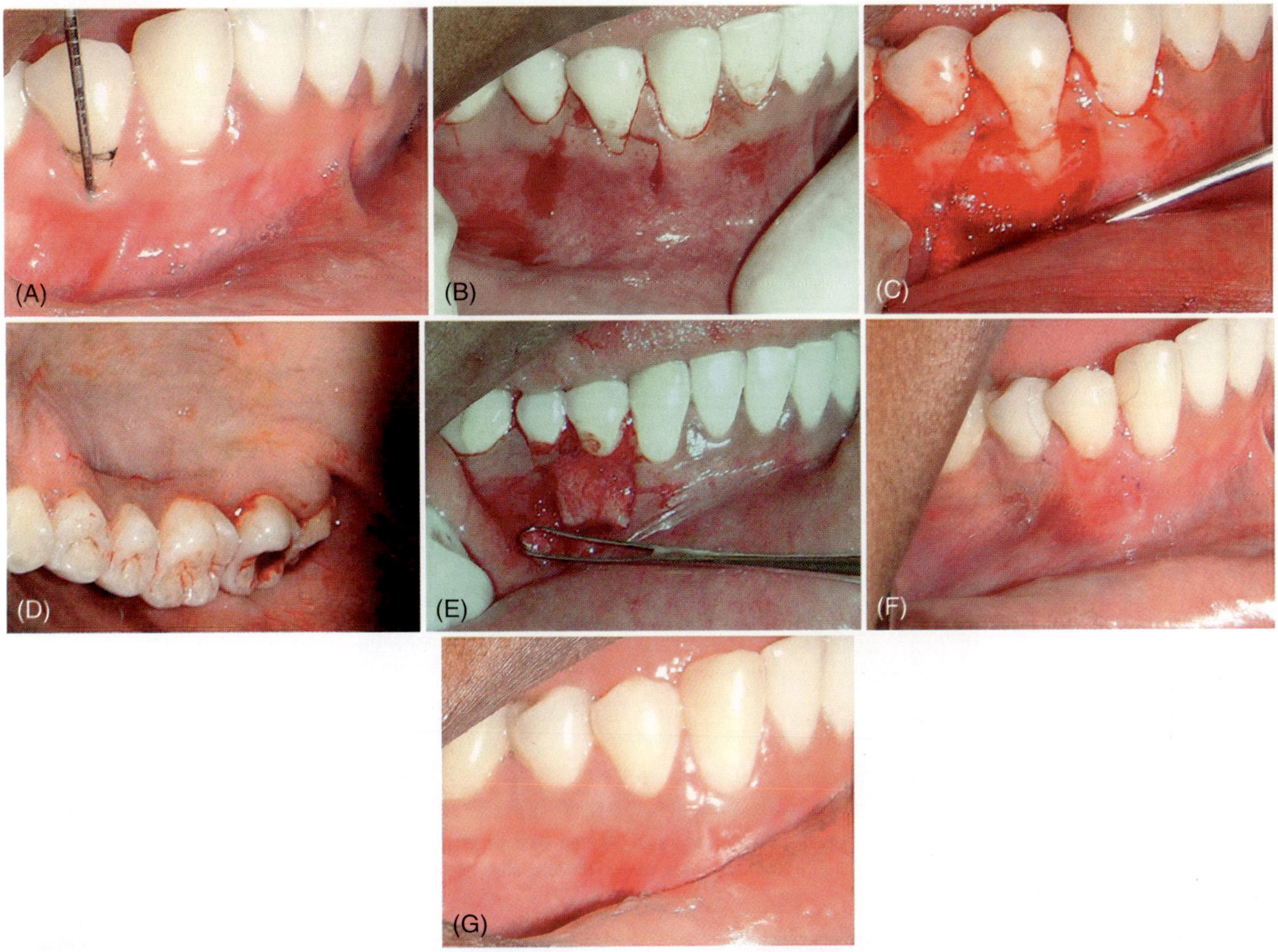

Fig. 51.5 A, Mandibular first bicuspid showing class II gingival recession. B, Incisions placed. C, Partial thickness flap reflected. D, Palatal incision. E, Harvested graft in place. F, 1-week postoperative showing microsutures. G, Result after 6 months showing complete root coverage. *(Photographs presented by Dr Geetha Priyadarshini and Dr CD Dwarakanath.)*

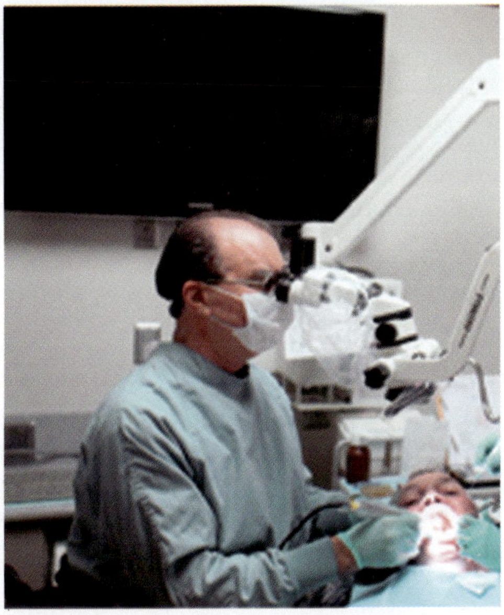

Fig. 51.6 Muscle strain and potential career-ending injuries can be prevented through a more ergonomic position facilitated by the proper use of a microscope.

microscope offers much higher magnification and superior optics compared to any of the loupe optical systems mentioned.

The Surgical Microscope

The surgical microscope offers greater versatility than dental loupes by providing a range of magnification with superior optical performance. A surgical microscope can last an entire career, making its long-term expense practical. Proficient use of the microscope requires training and practice. Surgical microscopes designed for dentistry employ Galilean optics, which have binocular eyepieces joined by offset prisms, to establish a parallel optical axis and permit stereoscopic vision without eye convergence or eyestrain. An additional binocular eyepiece can aid the microsurgical assistant.

Surgical microscopes have coated achromatic lenses and high optical resolution, as well as a rotating magnification element that allows the microsurgeon to easily change magnification to a value appropriate for the surgical task at hand. Since the optical elements of surgical microscopes are more advanced than those in loupes, depth-of-focus and field-of-view characteristics are greatly enhanced. Surgical microscopes have objective lenses with various working distances. A useful range in dentistry is 250–350 mm. For practical use, a surgical microscope must have both maneuverability and stability. Mountings are available for the ceiling, wall, or

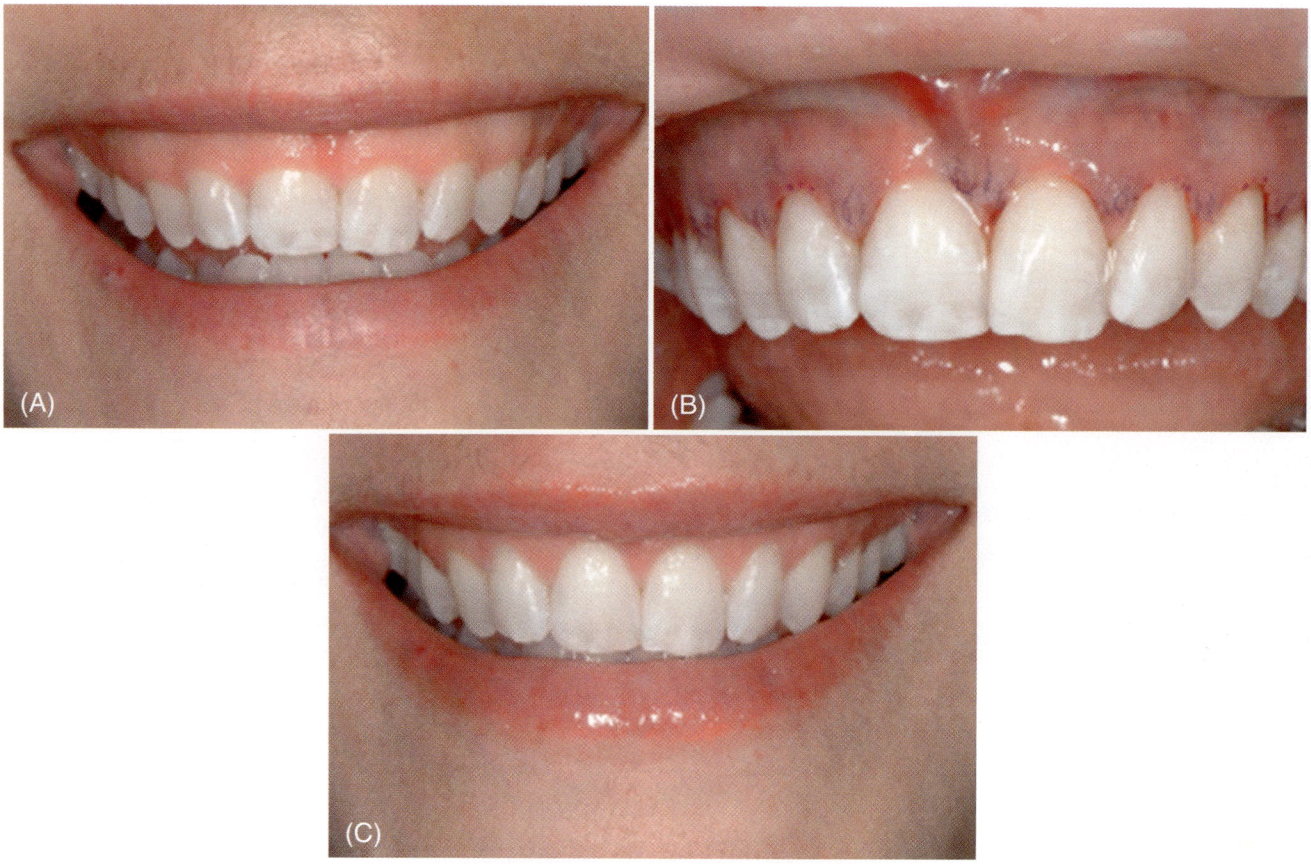

Fig. 51.7 Microsurgical crown-lengthening procedure. A, Altered passive eruption covering teeth crowns. B, Immediate microsurgical postoperative result. C, Three weeks' postoperative healing.

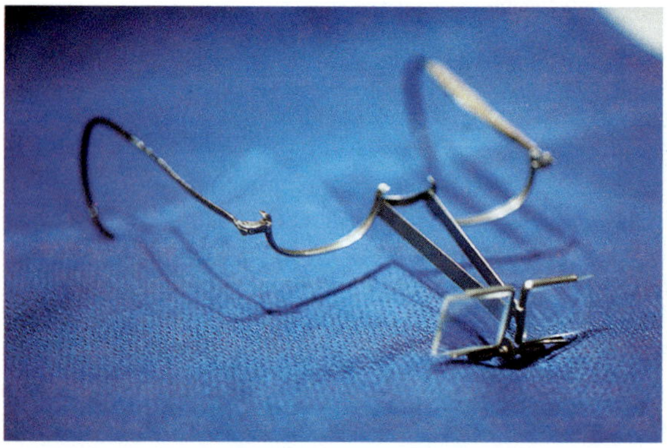

Fig. 51.8 Simple loupes.

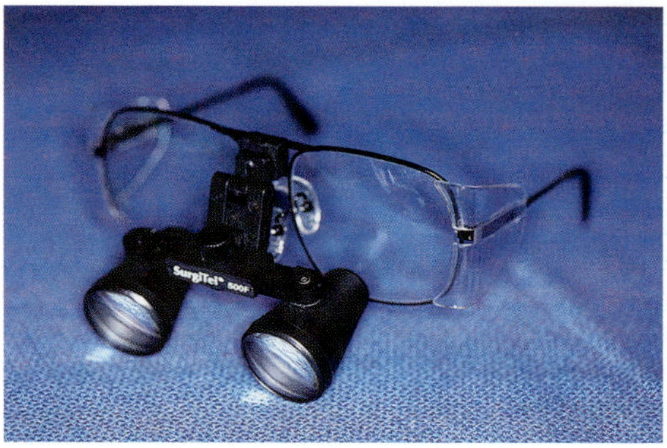

Fig. 51.9 Compound loupes.

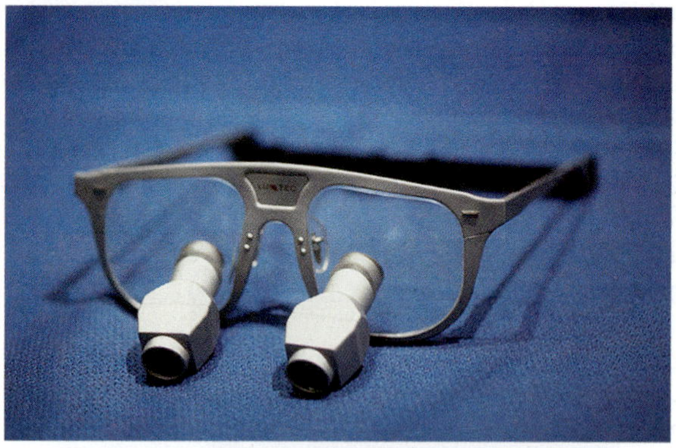

Fig. 51.10 Eyeglass-mounted prism loupes.

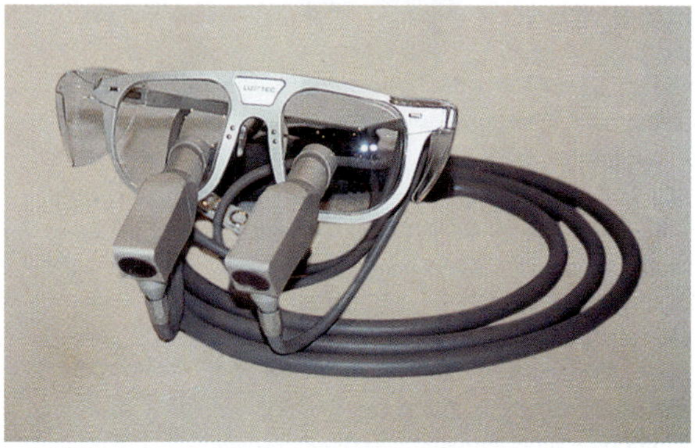

Fig. 51.11 Coaxial lighted prism loupes.

floor. Adjustable inclining eyepieces enhance postural flexibility for various procedures. This maneuverability provides visual access to every area of the mouth and is an important factor in choosing to use a surgical microscope.

Illumination of the microsurgical field is also an important consideration. Dentists are accustomed to working with lateral illumination from side-mounted dental lights or headlamps. Fiberoptic coaxial illumination is a major advantage because it focuses light parallel to the microscope's optical axis, which eliminates shadows. Surgeons can visualize the deepest reaches of the oral cavity, including subgingival pockets and angular bony defects. Definitive visualization of the root surface to detect deposits and irregularities is possible. Surgeons can view anatomy to make clinical decisions based on the accurate assessment of pathology rather than blind, educated guesses.

Documentation is important for patient and professional education and for dental legal reasons. The surgical operating microscope is an ideal platform for documenting periodontal pathology and clinical procedures. Digital images can be captured using a beam splitter and camera attachment. A foot control switch permits a surgeon to record, as the procedure unfolds, without interrupting surgery. These images represent the surgical field exactly as the surgeon sees it, as opposed to a camera view over the surgeon's shoulder. High-definition video cameras capture both still and video images simultaneously to permit documentation of periodontal procedures for educational purposes.

Microsurgical Sutures

To achieve ideal microsurgical wound closure, a surgeon depends on how the incisions were planned and executed, how the surgery was performed, and the suturing technique. Selection of proper suture needles and materials is essential for successful microsurgical wound closure. The choice of suture and needle size is critical for atraumatic tissue passage. Suture material must maintain wound closure until healing is sufficiently advanced to withstand functional stress.

Sutures are classified according to structure as monofilament or braided, according to surface as coated or uncoated, and according to biologic properties as absorbable or nonabsorbable. The suture of choice in microsurgery is a monofilament suture material such as polypropylene or polydioxanone. These materials are bacteriostatic and noninflammatory, hold a knot extremely well, and are easily removed. The purpose of sutures is to provide initial wound support. They are chosen to appropriate wounds based on the fragility of the tissue. The smallest suture capable of supporting the wound produces the least tissue trauma and the least interruption of the blood supply.

In periodontal microsurgery, the suture size ranges from 6-0 (diameter of a human hair) to 9-0. The size and shape of the needle used is essential for the atraumatic passage of the suture. The needle diameter is ideally slightly larger than the suture size. Sutures used in microsurgery are swaged, making the needle and the suture continuous. Penetration and passage of the needle depends on the angle of entry of needle point. Cutting needles pass through gingival tissue easily but can tear tissue. Tapered needles are less traumatic and less likely to tear tissue.

An important component to needle design is the chord distance. The chord of a needle is the length of a line drawn between the cutting point and the swaged end. The radius of a needle is the arc of its circumference. A one-half round needle has an arc of 180 degrees. The chord determines the ease in passing a suture between adjacent teeth. The arc determines the bite size and angle of entry taken by the needle. These needle dimensions are important when selecting sutures for periodontal microsurgery.

Esthetic Periodontal Microsurgery

Esthetic periodontal microsurgery to reconstruct gingival tissue over denuded roots is routine and predictable using subepithelial connective tissue grafting. The color match, esthetic appearance, and lack of scarring of these grafts are ideal. Microsurgical closure of the palatal donor site allows healing by primary intention without a painful period of open granulation. This greatly reduces postoperative pain.

To achieve optimal wound healing, three basic microsurgical principles are needed: (1) precision tailoring, (2) delicate tissue manipulation, and (3) passive primary wound closure.

Precise Tailoring

An important feature of microsurgery is the ability to create clean incisions. Design of incisions has a significant impact on how the wound edges fit together. A fundamental principle of microsurgery is making incisions perpendicular to the tissue surface, creating "butt joint" edges that easily approximate for wound-edge stability and maintain blood supply patency.

Delicate Tissue Manipulation

The microsurgical philosophy is based on minimal invasiveness and minimal trauma. This premise extends to the manipulation of gingival tissues during surgery. Gentle handling is necessary to reduce cellular injury and subsequent necrosis and inflammation. It is also necessary to maintain tissue hydration and color to maximize healing.

Passive Primary Wound Closure

After precision tailoring and gentle tissue manipulation, the final and critical element of microsurgery is achieving passive primary wound closure. There is a specific geometry of the suturing required, with the following six well-defined components:

1. *Angle of entry and angle of exit.* The needle should penetrate the tissue at a 90-degree angle, perpendicular to the tissue surface. Passing the needle at an oblique angle causes tearing when the knot is tied.
2. *Bite size.* Proper bite size is between 1 and 1.5 times the tissue thickness. Too small a bite size can tear the wound edges. Too large a bite size can cause underriding or overriding of wound edges. Both outcomes result in impaired healing and unsightly scarring.
3. *Direction of passage.* Once the needle has penetrated one edge of the wound, it must exit the opposing side of the wound with a direction of passage perpendicular to the incision line. This directs the suture force vectors at 90 degrees and prevents lateral dislocation at the wound edge.
4. *Tension.* Suturing should be accomplished with minimal tension. Gentle passage of the suture, in a perpendicular direction of passage, sets the stage for a microsurgical knot that does not cause tissue strangulation through ligation. Good suturing, however, will never save poor tailoring.
5. *Symmetry.* The distance between the bite sizes on either side of the wound edge should be the symmetrical as should the distance between sutures.
6. *Frequency.* Smaller suture material and smaller bite size makes it necessary to place more microsutures at frequent intervals along the wound edge. This supports wound closure and avoids stress breakage of sutures or tissue tearing.

Microsurgical Knots

Two basic knots are employed in microsurgery. The square knot, or reef knot, is composed of two single loops thrown in opposite directions. The reef knot has more internal stability than any other knot. For this reason, it has been employed for centuries in nautical applications. It lies flat when tied well and is ideal for passive wound closure. As postsurgical edema occurs, the reef knot opens slightly then becomes self-locking. It maintains wound-edge support without ligation caused by excessive tension. If, in tying a knot, both loops are thrown in opposite directions, it becomes the granny knot and unties easily. The English surgeon's knot is composed of two double loops thrown in opposite directions. The first double throw is less likely to loosen when performing the second throw, making it is easier to control tissue apposition. The English surgeon's knot requires, however, a larger bite size. Both knots are tied with instruments.

Conclusion

As medicine and dentistry continue the pursuit of minimally invasive treatment, periodontal microsurgery and its principles will emerge as the methodology to meet both professional and public demand. The microscope provides a tremendous platform from which the microsurgical clinician can gather and observe detailed and precise amounts of information for the diagnosis and treatment of patients with skill and accuracy. Microsurgery leads to improved esthetics, rapid healing, reduced morbidity, and enhanced patient acceptance.

Key points

- Periodontal microsurgery has several advantages such as improved surgical decision making, ergonomics and body posture, excellent handling of tissues leading to enhanced surgical outcome
- Various magnification systems are available such as magnifying loupes (simple, compound, Prism, Telescopic etc.) and surgical microscope.
- The surgical instruments and sutures employed in microsurgery are very specific and specially designed for precise handling of tissues.

Suggested Readings

Barraquer JI: The history of microsurgery in ocular surgery, *J Microsurg* 1:288, 1980.

Hoerenz P: Optical principles, illumination systems and support systems, *J Microsurg* 1:367, 1980.

Shanelec D: Current trends in soft tissue grafting, *J Calif Dent Assoc* 19:57, 1991.

Shanelec D: Optical principles of dental loupes, *J Calif Dent Assoc* 20:25, 1992.

Shanelec D, Tibbetts L: An overview of periodontal microsurgery, *Curr Sci* 2:187, 1994.

References

References and MCQs with answers for the chapter are available on www.medenact.com.

CHAPTER 52

Lasers in Periodontal and Peri-Implant Therapy

PR Klokkevold | B Butler | RT Kao | CD Dwarakanath

CHAPTER OUTLINE

The first working laser was made in 1960 by Theodore H. Maiman at Hughes Research Laboratories, a subdivision of Hughes Aircraft in Malibu, California. Maiman created the laser by pumping very high energy from a flashtube into a solid state ruby medium, which emitted a monochromatic beam of deep red visible light with a wavelength of 694.3 nm. Almost immediately thereafter, researchers began investigating the use of lasers for dental applications. Early uses focused on removal of hard tissues and caries, but these lasers offered little benefit over standard rotary instruments. Consequently, interest in the use of lasers for dentistry faded. Laser activity for dental applications remained nominal until the 1990s when advances in new wavelengths, delivery units, and power maximums refocused the use of lasers for soft tissue as well as hard tissue procedures (Table 52.1). More recently, there has been an increased interest in the use of lasers for periodontal therapy including both surgical and nonsurgical applications. In addition to their application as a cutting device, lasers have been advocated in antimicrobial photodynamic therapy mode for biofilm disruption to reduce or eliminate pathogens from the periodontal pocket. Yet another potential laser application in periodontics is the use of low-level laser therapy (LLLT) to stimulate cellular activity for enhanced wound healing and tissue regeneration.

As with the introduction of most new technologies, advocates of laser therapy for periodontics hope it will be able to replace or enhance traditional therapies. It is important to recognize that making the determination of whether a new technology should be incorporated into practice requires evidence from clinical studies to demonstrate equivalence or superiority to accepted therapies. The sample size required to statistically test superiority versus equivalence is generally much larger than what has been tested in clinical trials evaluating lasers to date. Hence, the only reasonable conclusions will state that lasers are equivalent, at best, as compared to conventional therapies. The limited number of longitudinal clinical trials and cohort studies for each laser type along with the fact that different exposure settings and various protocols are used in these studies make justification to implement this new technology for periodontal applications difficult. Published studies to date are too small and heterogeneous to make definitive conclusions. Nonetheless, if a new therapy is found to be equivalent, albeit not superior to a conventional therapy, there may be other reasons such as safety, cost, or ease of use that warrant utilization of the new technology. Systematic reviews and metaanalyses of available reports have attempted to define whether lasers provide additional benefits for periodontal applications. Unfortunately, there is a lack of well-designed randomized controlled clinical trials (RCTs), which is the optimal type of study needed for metaanalyses, and those studies that exist are often heterogeneous with regard to laser type, settings, and exposure. As such, the conclusions should be interpreted with caution. This chapter describes some of the clinical applications of lasers for periodontal therapy and discusses the currently available literature.

Laser Physics and Biologic Interactions

Laser is an acronym for "*L*ight *A*mplification by *S*timulated *E*mission of *R*adiation." Lasers function by stimulating the emission of light energy from a given medium in a collimated, focused monochromatic ray of light. The energy beam reacts with a target tissue by being absorbed, reflected, or scattered depending on wavelength and absorption characteristics (Fig. 52.1). Some lasers (e.g., Nd:YAG lasers) may be transmitted through surface tissues to interact with deeper tissues. When the laser is well absorbed, the energy explodes the target tissue cells and extracellular matrix in a process called *ablation.* The efficiency of ablation is related to the wavelength and the affinity of the laser beam for the target tissue. Laser beams may also be reflected or bounced off the target (e.g., reflected off a metal surface) without interaction. This is typically an undesirable effect because there is no effect on the target tissue and the reflected beam can interact with unintended targets. If the wavelength is not well absorbed, there can be scattering and a thermal reaction in the adjacent tissues with carbonization, charring, and melting. Clinicians must understand and appreciate not only how this energy is affecting the target tissues but also how it affects the adjacent tissues as well.

Production of a laser requires a medium, an optical chamber or laser tube, and an externally applied energy source to create an emitted monochromatic energy beam (Fig. 52.2). When energy is applied to the medium, electrons are "excited" to a higher energy orbit. When they return to the normal orbit, a photon (particle of light) is emitted. Because the photons are all the same wavelength, the laser beam is "coherent." The medium, which can be a gas, a solid, or a semiconductor, determines the laser wavelength. Lasers

TABLE 52.1 Types of Lasers Currently Used in Dentistry

Laser Medium	Wavelength (nm)	Dental Uses
Argon	488–514	Tooth bleaching and advanced curing lights
Diode	655–980	Gingivectomy/gingivoplasty, oral medicine uses (aphthous ulcer therapy, biopsies, dentinal desensitizing), second-stage implant exposure, periodontal curettage (advocated but not evidence based)
Neodymium:yttrium-aluminum-garnet (Nd:YAG)	1064	Gingivectomy/gingivoplasty, oral medicine uses (aphthous ulcer therapy, biopsies, dentinal desensitizing), second-stage implant exposure, periodontal curettage (advocated but not evidence based)
Erbium, chromium:yttrium-scandium-gallium-garnet (Er,Cr:YSGG)	2780	Gingivectomy/gingivoplasty, oral medicine uses (aphthous ulcer therapy, biopsies, dentinal desensitizing), second-stage implant exposure, periodontal curettage (advocated but not evidence based), hard tissue cutting (dentin and osseous)
Erbium:yttrium-aluminum-garnet (Er:YAG)	2940	Gingivectomy/gingivoplasty, oral medicine uses (aphthous ulcer therapy, biopsies, dentinal desensitizing), second-stage implant exposure, periodontal curettage (advocated but not evidence based), hard tissue cutting (dentin and osseous)
Carbon dioxide (CO_2)	10,600	Gingivectomy/gingivoplasty, second-stage implant exposure, periodontal curettage (advocated but not evidence based)

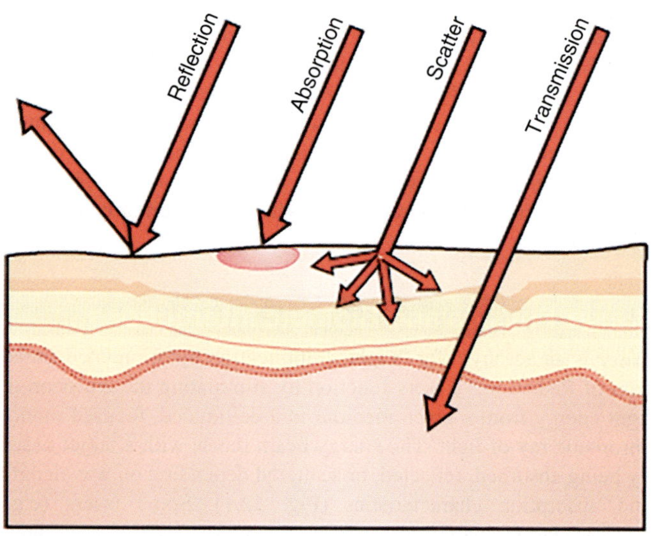

Fig. 52.1 Four potential laser-tissue interactions. The laser beam may be reflected, absorbed, scattered, or transmitted. *(From Convissar RA: Principles and practice of laser dentistry, ed 2, St. Louis, 2016, Mosby.)*

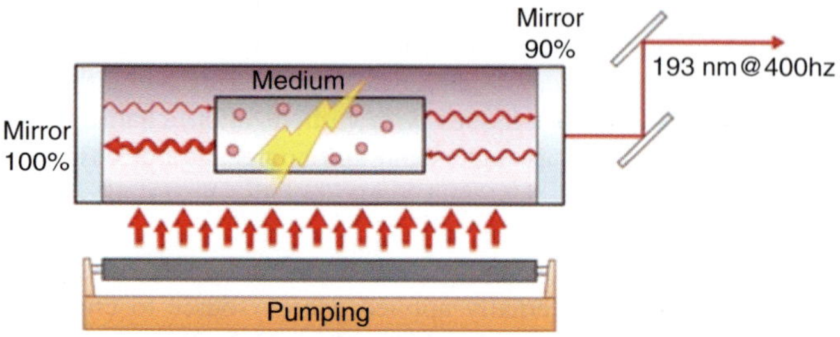

Fig. 52.2 Diagrammatic presentation of the main components of a laser device. Lasers require a medium, an optical chamber or laser tube, and an externally applied energy source to create an emitted monochromatic energy beam. *(From Spaeth GL, Danesh-Meyer H, Goldberg I, et al: Ophthalmic surgery: principles and practice, ed 4, Edinburgh, 2012, Saunders.)*

are named in relationship to the active element(s) that, when stimulated, generates the energy beam. Typical lasers used in dentistry include argon, GaAs (diode), Nd:YAG, Er:YAG, Er,Cr:YSGG, and CO_2 lasers. Wavelengths are delivered either in a continuous, pulsed (gated), or in a running pulse waveform. Argon lasers have wavelengths in the ultraviolet and visible light range with primary dental applications in composite resin placement, enamel and dentin bonding, preventive therapies, and endodontic procedures. Reported periodontal applications for the other lasers include soft tissue incision, ablation, depigmentation, subgingival curettage, scaling of root surfaces, calculus removal, bacterial killing, osteoplasty, and ostectomy.

Each laser has a unique wavelength spectrum resulting in specific absorption characteristics that must be understood and appreciated for the desired purpose (Figs. 52.3 and 52.4). When applied to the various periodontal tissues such as the gingiva, periodontal ligament, cementum, dentin, and bone, the biologic interactions will be unique for that wavelength. Tissues are composite structures of inorganic and organic elements with various constituents. Gingiva is composed of fibrous connective tissue, extracellular matrix components (including melanin pigmentation), and 70% water. Bone is composed of 67% inorganic minerals (calcium hydroxyapatite) and 33% organic elements (collagen, noncollagenous proteins, and water). Other factors to consider are the textures, compositions, and densities of these structures. For example, the varying percentages of mineralized structures, blood vessels, and fluid found in cortical bone versus cancellous bone will result in the laser energy beam encountering differing fluctuations in absorption and scattering, regardless of the wavelength, due to these differences. Blood contains 55% plasma (water) and 45% cells including red blood cells with hemoglobin, white blood cells, and platelets. Thus, when considering the use of lasers for a given clinical application, it is important to appreciate not only the type of laser being used and the target tissue but also the composition of that tissue.

The affinity of a laser wavelength for the target tissue (absorption coefficient) is critical to its effectiveness for the procedure (Fig. 52.5). The relatively short wavelengths of the diode (655–980 nm) and Nd:YAG (1064 nm) are well absorbed by pigment and are better suited for soft tissue procedures than for hard tissue procedures. The CO_2 laser, which has a very long wavelength (10,600 nm), has an

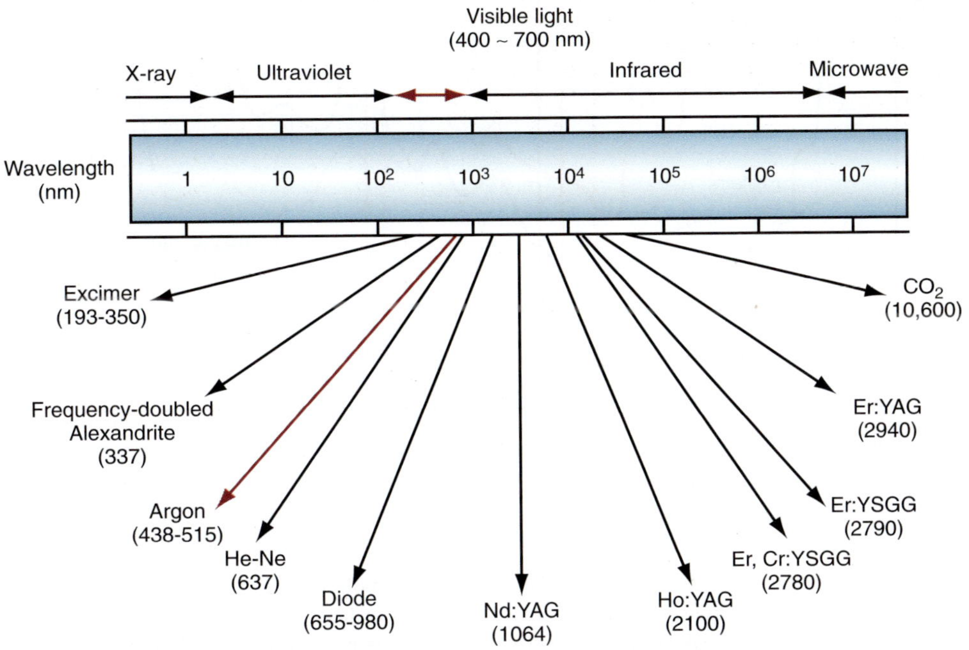

Fig. 52.3 Laser wavelengths. Each laser has a unique wavelength spectrum resulting in specific absorption characteristics. The wavelength of most of the lasers used in dentistry/periodontics is in the red and near-infrared spectrum.

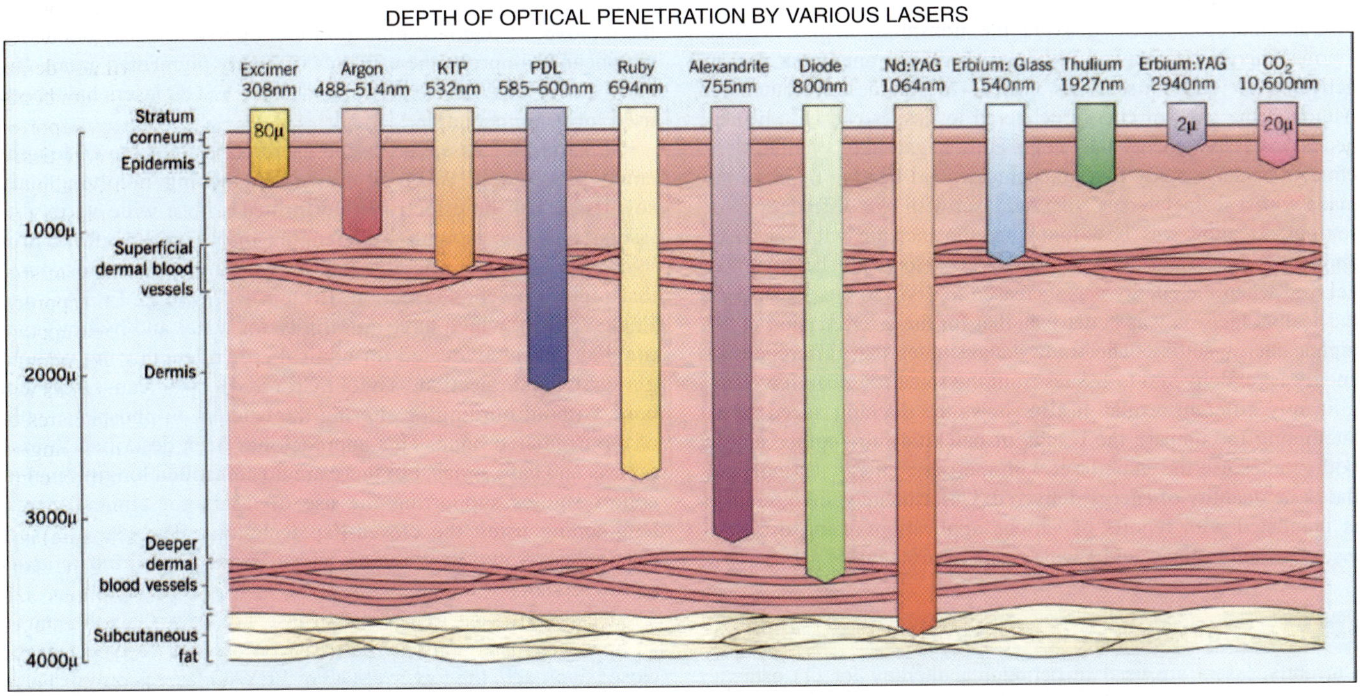

Fig. 52.4 Depth of optical penetration by various lasers. Tissue penetration is a function of laser wavelength and absorption characteristics. It should be noted that the treatment depth can greatly exceed the optical penetration depth for ablative lasers. On the face, the fat can be present at depth of 2–3 mm. For example, the depth of optical penetration for CO_2 lasers is only 20 microns, but fractional CO_2 lasers can vaporize nearly full-thickness microchannels through the dermis. *KTP*, Potassium titanyl phosphate; *Nd*, neodymium; *PDL*, pulsed dye laser; *YAG*, yttrium aluminum garnet. *(From Bolognia JL, Jorizzo JL, Schaffer JV: Dermatology, two-volume set, ed 3, Philadelphia, 2012, Saunders.)*

affinity for water and is best suited for soft tissue procedures. Diode and Nd:YAG wavelengths are not absorbed by hydroxyapatite and thus are not effective for hard tissues such as cementum, dentin, and bone. The wavelengths of Er:YAG (2940 nm) and Er,Cr:YSGG (2780 nm) lasers have a positive affinity for both water and hydroxyapatite. The specificity for hydroxyapatite allows erbium lasers to cut hard tissues including bone, dentin, and enamel. The selective absorption by water also makes erbium lasers effective for soft tissue procedures.

Selection of the laser type is ultimately based on the amount of energy transmitted to the tissue during a procedure. Photothermal energy is measured in watts (W = joules/second) and hertz

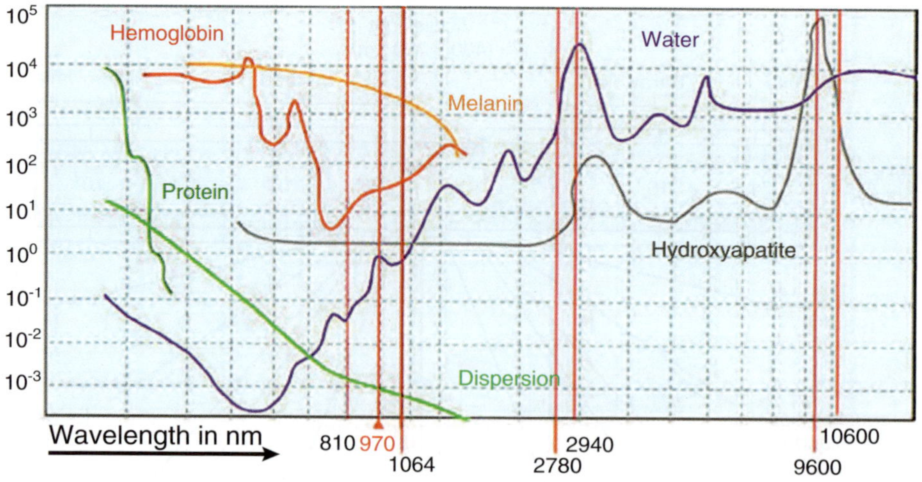

Fig. 52.5 Laser absorption coefficient of various tissue constituents as a function of wavelength.

(Hz = cycles/second). The energy beam can be delivered in a continuous or pulsed manner. A continuous laser transmits more energy than a pulsed laser, as there are momentary breaks or cooling periods in the latter. When comparing outcomes of different laser therapies, it is imperative to consider the type of laser, the wavelength, *and* the amount of energy delivered to tissues including watts, hertz, and total time of exposure.

Care must be taken to avoid the transmission of excessive thermal energy to target and adjacent tissues. The amount of energy delivered to target tissues is critical to the desired outcome. Although the optimal energy delivered to tissues can be advantageous, excessive energy may completely negate the potential benefits. Consider a study that compared wound healing of incisions made with a scalpel versus Nd:YAG laser with two different power settings. Healing was best following the incision with the laser applied with settings of 1.75 W, 20 Hz. However, healing was delayed when the energy was increased to 3 W, 20 Hz. Healing of the scalpel incision was better than that for the laser incision at the higher energy setting. The study demonstrates that differences in energy level delivered to tissues from the same laser can have significantly different results. It also shows the dilemma faced when attempting to compare the results of one study to another unless both studies use the same laser with the same energy settings and the same quantity of energy delivered. Unfortunately, the literature is inundated with reports of various applications using different lasers, varied settings, and a wide range of protocols.

Laser Applications in Periodontics

Currently, lasers are used in periodontal therapy for (1) esthetic surgical procedures such as gingivoplasty and gingivectomy, crown lengthening without osseous involvement, and depigmentation; (2) nonsurgical therapy; (3) decontamination and antimicrobial therapy; (4) excision of solitary lesions such as pyogenic granuloma; (5) operculectomy and frenectomy; and (6) biomodulation.

Esthetic and Preprosthetic Surgical Applications

Several types of laser wavelengths have been used for soft tissue surgical procedures. Appropriate use of lasers for procedures such as frenectomy, gingivectomy/gingivoplasty, reshaping of drug-induced gingival overgrowth, exposure of short crowns associated with altered passive/delayed eruption, and management of excess mucosal tissue such as pericoronitis situations distal of mandibular second molars have been well documented. Some of the positive aspects of laser therapy are good visibility during the surgical procedure as a result of coagulation, hemostasis, and minimal tissue damage adjacent to the laser wound. Additionally, laser therapy can offer extreme precision and may be easier than using a scalpel.

Esthetic applications for gingivectomy and gingivoplasty procedures allow delicate tissue reshaping. The laser is effective for the removal of pigmentation from the gingival tissues, which can significantly improve the esthetics of highly pigmented areas. The CO_2, diode, Nd:YAG, Er:YAG, and Er,Cr:YSGG lasers have been used for depigmentation.

Some clinicians advocate the use of lasers for crown-lengthening procedures. Whereas crown lengthening involving only soft tissue can be effectively performed with a wide variety of lasers, only lasers with wavelengths that have an affinity for hydroxyapatite are effective for crown-lengthening procedures that require osseous resection. Erbium lasers (e.g., Er:YAG and Er,Cr:YSGG), which have an affinity for water and hydroxyapatite, have been advocated for clinical crown lengthening without gingival flap reflection. The Er,Cr:YSGG laser can safely cut bone without burning or altering the calcium-to-phosphate ratio of the irradiated bone. This approach has been described in case reports and case series, but there are no controlled longitudinal or cohort studies supporting the use of lasers for clinical crown lengthening using the closed-flap technique. The use of lasers for flapless crown lengthening with osseous contouring remains controversial.

Decision making for the use of lasers in crown lengthening in an open or closed approach is based on osseous biotypes. In the closed approach, the Er,Cr:YSGG or Er:YAG laser is only feasible in medium biotype cases with an osseous crest that is approximately 1 mm in thickness and may be limited to situations where only 1–2 mm of osseous removal is required. In this technique, bone sounding with a probe is used after the external gingivectomy to determine the thickness of the osseous biotype and to determine the amount of bone removal required. The laser tip is aligned parallel to the root surface in contact with the bone and fired for 1–2 s. The tip is moved slowly around the tooth, firing intermittently while in contact with the bone until the desired osseous reduction is achieved. The osseous removal is verified by sounding, and detailing is performed with a small chisel (Fig. 52.6). This technique can be surgically conservative and result in symmetric gingival levels in the esthetic zone.

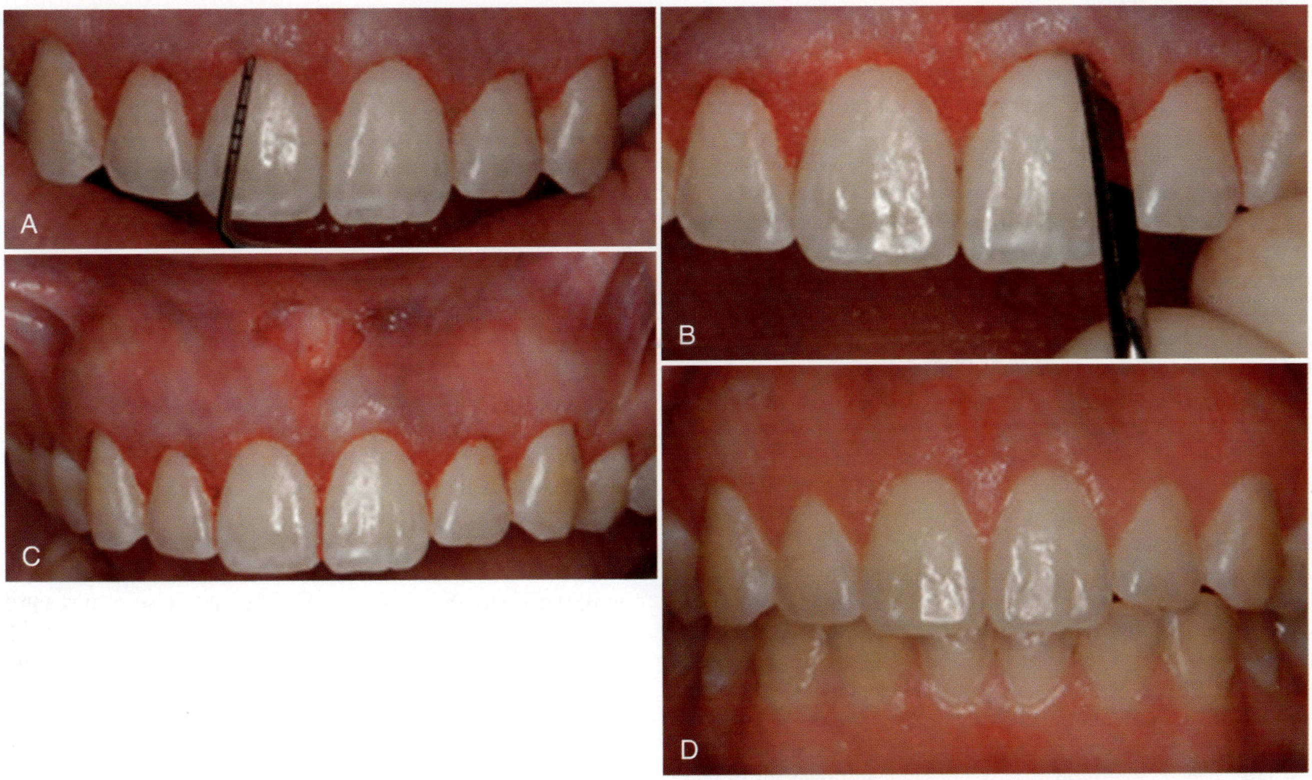

Fig. 52.6 Crown-lengthening procedure performed using a closed approach with a laser. A, Periodontal sounding after the initial gingivectomy, which indicated the need for osseous contouring to achieve biologic width. B, The osseous contouring was done via intrasulcular access. Sounding confirms 3 mm from the gingival to osseous crest. Final small fragments of bone are checked and removed with a small chisel. C, Final surgical photograph shows minimal bleeding with no need for sutures. A frenectomy was also completed at the time of surgery. D, Smile at 3 months postsurgery. *(Case courtesy: Dr. Bobby Butler, Seattle, Washington.)*

Case selection based on osseous biotypes is critical for the success of this closed approach for crown lengthening. In a thick biotype, the laser will likely create a "trough" or an intrabony defect. Because inadequate bone removal is performed, the soft tissue will often rebound soon after the procedure. An open-flap approach with direct vision of bone is indicated for cases with a thick osseous biotype so definitive osseous contouring can be performed. Closed or flapless laser crown lengthening should absolutely be avoided in all cases of thin biotype. Using laser therapy in an ablative mode for osseous removal in thin biotype cases poses a high risk for overheating tissues and adversely affecting the healing response, leading to unfavorable or possibly disastrous clinical outcomes.

Further issues of concern include the limited ability to assess the appropriateness of osseous recontouring and the inability to avoid or detect damage to root surfaces. These concerns and the possible need for retreatment because of tissue rebound or poor healing suggest that this is not a superior or equivalent technique as compared to traditional functional crown lengthening that requires osseous contouring.

Nonsurgical Periodontal Therapy

One of the more prevalent applications of lasers in periodontics is the nonsurgical treatment of moderate to advanced chronic periodontitis. Lasers have been used as a monotherapy or as an adjunct to scaling and root planing. The purported benefits of lasers for nonsurgical periodontal therapy include subgingival curettage, minimally invasive access for scaling and root planning, and calculus removal, as well as detoxification and killing of subgingival periodontal pathogens.

BOX 52.1 Questions to Consider When Evaluating the Effectiveness of Laser Therapy

1. Do the in vivo studies demonstrate a reduction in pathogenic bacteria as compared to conventional therapy [e.g., scaling and root planing (SRP)]?
2. Are positive microbial changes sustained, or do the periodontal pathogens return and recolonize the sites?
3. Are there any differences in clinical parameters following laser-assisted versus conventional therapy SRP? When evaluating nonsurgical periodontal therapy, gain in clinical attachment level (CAL) represents the gold standard. Pocket depth (PD) and levels of subgingival microbes are important because they correlate with changes in CAL.
4. Are there changes in root surface condition based on in vitro or in vivo studies?

In the clinical situation, periodontal pathogenic bacteria exist within a protective biofilm in a periodontal pocket. Consequently, it is difficult for conventional periodontal therapies to completely eliminate them. Laser therapy is proposed to improve access to areas that are difficult for instruments to reach and to facilitate killing bacteria. Indeed, lasers with various wavelengths have been shown to effectively kill periodontal pathogens. See the *Photodynamic Therapy* section.

When assessing the effectiveness of any particular laser type used for nonsurgical periodontal therapy, several questions need to be considered, as listed in Box 52.1.

Photodynamic Therapy

Photodynamic therapy (PDT) involves the use of a photosensitizer (photoactive dye) that is activated by exposure to a specific wavelength of light in the presence of oxygen. The activated photosensitizer transitions to an excited state and subsequently reacts with oxygen to create singlet oxygen and free radicals, which are damaging to proteins, lipids, nucleic acids, and other vital elements causing destruction of the target tissues. In the case of biofilm and periodontal pathogens, antimicrobial photodynamic therapy (aPDT) may *appear* to offer a magic bullet effect of target killing bacteria. PDT may be an effective means of disrupting the biofilm. Most studies evaluating PDT have been conducted in Europe. The US Food and Drug Administration does not yet approve PDT.

The use of lasers for PDT has been reviewed. aPDT for periodontitis uses a photosensitizer dye that specifically targets microorganisms and is activated by low-level laser light. Photosensitizer activation can be achieved with low-level energy exposure from various laser light sources including but not limited to argon, Nd:YAG, and diode. The introduction of a photosensitizer can greatly increase the bactericidal ability of a laser. This is supported by an in vitro study using methylene blue with a diode laser to destroy black-pigmented bacteria (*Porphyromonas gingivalis* and *Prevotella intermedia*; 99%–100% of bacteria were eliminated). However, it is important to recognize that pathogenic bacteria within the protective biofilm that exists in vivo may not be killed to the same degree observed during in vitro studies. Laboratory analysis of laser bactericidal properties is not clinically relevant in that these bacteria do not exist as a suspension or monolayer in vivo.

To date, the results of clinical studies evaluating the effectiveness of aPDT are mixed and not convincing. A systematic review including 17 clinical studies found that 4 studies demonstrated significantly reduced bacteria with laser PDT, whereas 13 studies showed equivalent effectiveness as compared to conventional scaling root planing (SRP) alone. The authors concluded that the bactericidal efficacy of aPDT as an adjunct to SRP against periodontal pathogens remains debatable. The incomplete elimination of periodontal pathogens and the protective nature of the biofilm environment may be responsible for the observed persistence and recolonization of microbial pathogens in this microniche. Several individual clinical studies have been published on the use of aPDT as adjunct to SRP. A majority of these studies reported significant clinical and microbiologic improvements in the PDT + SRP combination as compared to SRP alone. One study found the results to be comparable. A clinical and microbiologic evaluation of the effectiveness of PDT in the nonsurgical treatment of aggressive periodontitis, using a split-mouth design (PDT + SRP vs SRP only), found no additional benefits from PDT as compared to SRP alone. A metaanalysis evaluating the effectiveness of aPDT as an adjunct to nonsurgical periodontal therapy in patients with diabetes included four RCTs reporting clinical and metabolic parameters. Although aPDT with SRP was shown to be effective in treating chronic periodontitis, no difference was observed between the test (aPDT + SRP) and control (SRP only) groups. The authors concluded that aPDT has no additional benefit. More clinical trials are required prior to clinical implementation.

Low-Level Laser Therapy

The use of LLLT for photobiomodulation is prevalent in medicine. Soon after the discovery of lasers in the 1960s, it was recognized that laser "light" therapy had the potential to reduce pain, inflammation, and swelling and to improve wound healing. The term *low-level laser therapy* refers to the therapeutic application of light to tissues with the goal of reducing pain or stimulating healing. The wavelengths of light used for LLLT are in the red to near-infrared range (600–1070 nm). It is referred to as "low level" because the density of light energy is low compared to other lasers, which are used for ablation, cutting, and thermally heating tissue. The power of low-level light (energy) is typically in the range of 1–1000 mW. LLLT is thought to promote wound healing by reducing inflammation, increasing the formation of granulation tissue, enhancing epithelialization, fibroblast proliferation, and matrix synthesis, as well as neovascularization.

Although LLLT is widely used in medicine, it continues to be controversial because the biologic mechanism(s) are not understood and the parameters of use (i.e., wavelength, power, pulse, and timing or exposure duration) are not defined. As with other laser investigations, there is heterogeneity of experimental protocols, parameters used, and results reported. Some published reports are positive, whereas others are negative. In the case of LLLT, perhaps more than other forms of laser therapy, the therapeutic effectiveness greatly depends on the optimal parameters being applied, and those details have yet to be defined.

LLLT has been shown to reduce inflammation and enhance nonsurgical periodontal treatment in healthy subjects as well as subjects with diabetes. In a metaanalysis of eight publications (seven RCTs) evaluating the effectiveness of LLLT as an adjunct to nonsurgical periodontal therapy, short-term (1–2 months) improvements in probing pocket depth and crevicular fluid levels of IL-1ß were shown. However, LLLT failed to show significant intermediate-term (3–6 months) effects in terms of clinical parameters.

Case reports and case controlled series have suggested that LLLT *may* improve the effects of periodontal regenerative procedures. One clinical study evaluated the effectiveness of enamel matrix derivative (EMD, Emdogain) with or without the application of a low-level laser (diode) to treat intrabony defects in 22 periodontitis patients. The EMD + LLLT sites healed with less gingival recession, less swelling, and less visual analog scale pain scores as compared to the EMD-only sites. More research, preferably well-designed RCTs, is needed to assess the effectiveness of LLLT on periodontal therapy.

Lasers in the Management of Periodontitis

The role of laser therapy in the surgical management of periodontitis remains controversial. At the center of this controversy is the apparent potential for the Nd:YAG laser to result in new attachment and regeneration when used with the laser-assisted new attachment procedure (LANAP) protocol. The patented LANAP procedure consists of a first pass with the Nd:YAG laser at a setting of 4.0 W and energy density of 1965 mJ/mm^2, 100-µs pulse duration, and 20 Hz applied. The first pass is purported to de-epithelialize the sulcular/pocket epithelium while sparing the underlying connective tissue and killing pigmented bacteria. The teeth are then scaled and root planed with piezo ultrasonic instrumentation. A second pass is performed with similar output but with a 650-µs pulse duration and 20 Hz with the objective of creating a blood clot that presumably, if kept stable, acts as the foundation for periodontal wound healing.

Since the initial description of LANAP, most evidence was based on case reports. Some publications suggest that this protocol may have merits. This is based on two histologic studies that report new attachment and periodontal regeneration following treatment with the LANAP protocol. More recently, the effectiveness of LANAP was examined in the treatment of 107 consecutive patients presenting with moderate-to-advanced chronic periodontitis. The main criterion for determining treatment success over time was tooth loss. A significant criticism is that there were no controls in this study. Data were compared with published studies of tooth loss over time. Tooth loss per patient treated by LANAP was 0.43 of a tooth over an average of 6.2 years posttreatment. Although a direct comparison with classic studies is not possible due the shorter time frame for posttreatment evaluation, the trend suggests that LANAP compares favorably with conventional surgical treatment modalities and may be a less invasive treatment alternative.

There are limited studies on the surgical management of chronic periodontitis with other laser types. Given the positive histologic evidence of new attachment and regeneration associated with LANAP performed with the Nd:YAG, the question remains: Can the Er:YAG or the Er,Cr:YSGG laser produce similar results? If proved to be effective, erbium lasers may be advantageous due to the lower risk and greater versatility associated with this wavelength. In a case report, periodontal regeneration (radiographic bone fill) of a maxillary intrabony defect following Er,Cr:YSGG treatment has been described. In a case series that included 46 patients with 79 angular intrabony defects, Er,Cr:YSGG laser treatment resulted in significant pocket depth reduction and significant radiographic bone fill. Although these results are promising, the difficulty is that there are no controls, and periodontal regeneration requires histologic evidence of new pulsed dye laser, cementum, and bone formation. Because this has not been demonstrated with this wavelength, one can only state that the finding is suggestive of radiographic bone fill of the intrabony defects that is consistent with *possible* periodontal regeneration. In a split-mouth design, the use of the ER,Cr:YSGG laser versus open-flap debridement was compared. The laser-assisted pocket therapy was found to provide similar clinical attachment level gains with similar reduction in pocket depth, gingival index, and the sulcular bleeding index. These findings were similar to the findings that compared a split-mouth design with three closed approaches, which included SRP, diode laser curettage with SRP, and laser-assisted curettage with SRP and laser sealing, versus an open approach of papilla reflection with SRP and flap closure. On comparing these open and closed protocols, all treatments resulted in a reduction of pocket depth and bleeding on probing. Consistent with the previous study, closed protocols all resulted in less gingival recession. These authors concluded that if esthetics is a concern, laser curettage is a viable option. Because this is an issue of concern in the maxillary anterior region, the caveat is that the clinician must be appropriately trained and familiar with the laser being used. There are clinical instances where mismanagement with laser resulted in irreversible hard and soft tissue damage (Fig. 52.7).

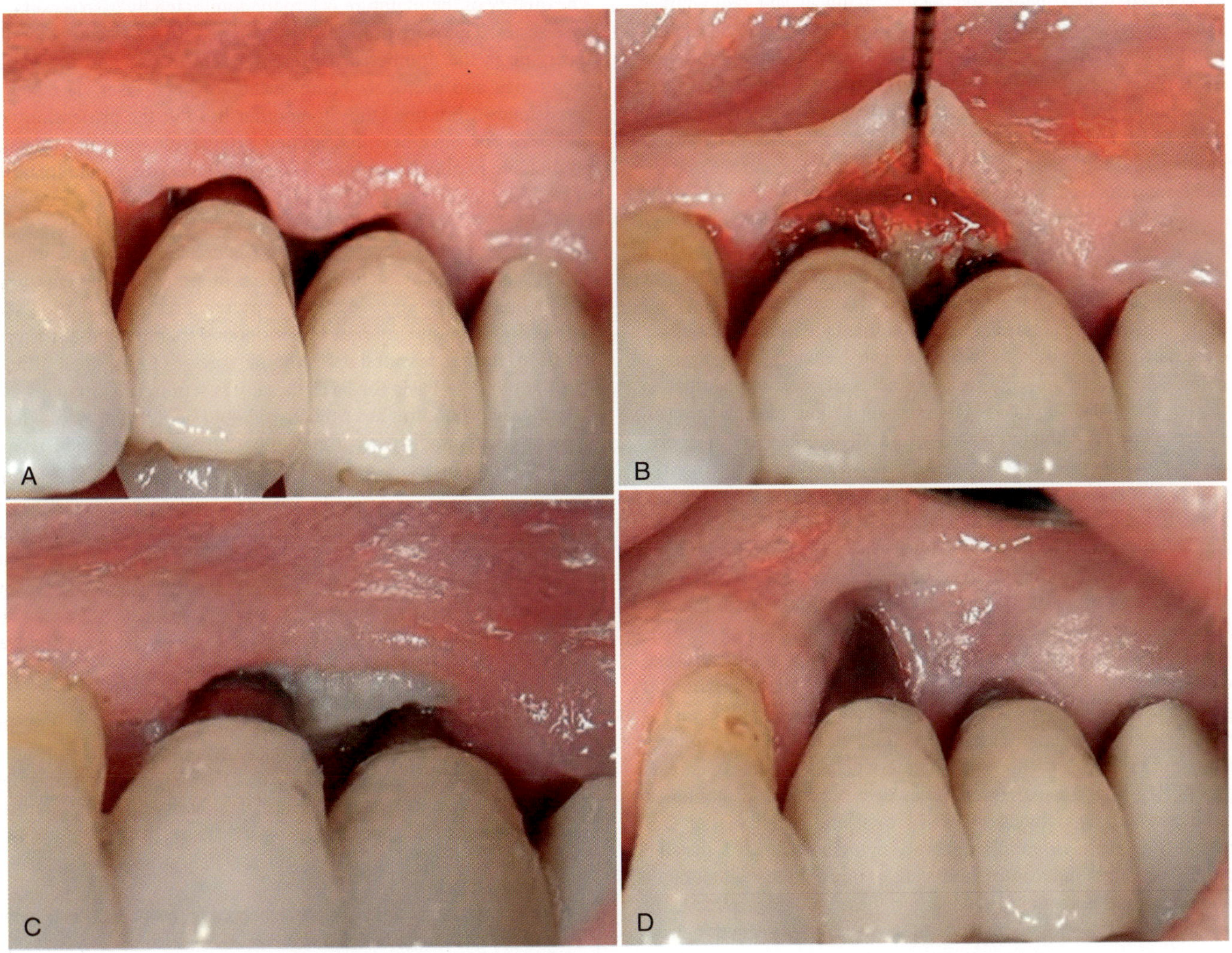

Fig. 52.7 Interproximal soft tissue cratering with underlying bone necrosis around two dental implants following laser treatment of peri-implantitis using inappropriate energy density and duration of exposure. Photos in sequence: A and B, One-month post laser treatment. C, Sequestration of necrotic interproximal and facial bone at 2 months posttreatment. D, Healing at 3 months posttreatment. *(Courtesy: Dr. Charles Cobb, University of Missouri, Kansas City.)*

Lasers in the Management of Peri-Implantitis

There is increased interest in the use of laser to manage peri-implantitis. This is due to anecdotal reports of cession and reversal of radiographic changes associated with bone damages surrounding peri-implantitis cases. This clinical phenomenology, although interesting, is not a consistent finding, and there is no clear biologic basis for when and why this phenomenology happens. In the Sixth European Workshop on Periodontology, the surgical treatment of peri-implantitis recognized the use of Er:YAG for implant surface decontamination. In a dog study, surface decontamination of experimental peri-implantitis was compared with closed- and open-approach debridement using Er:YAG laser and an ultrasonic scaler or plastic curettes and local metronidazole gel application. The authors found both open-flap submerged approaches (Er:YAG and ultrasonic scaling) resulted in higher clinical attachment gain (bone implant contact), with the laser therapy having a higher degree of reosseointegration (44.8%) as compared to ultrasonic (8.7%) and plastic curette/metronidazole gel debridement (14.8%). Similar but more modest results were found with the use of the CO_2 laser to decontaminate implant surfaces. Subsequently, in a case series of 15 patients with failing implants, the CO_2 laser was used to decontaminate implant surfaces in conjunction with bone augmentation (autogenous bone or xenogenic bone covered with collagen membrane). Clinical and radiographic evaluation after 27 months revealed almost complete bone fill of peri-implant bony defects. Further in vitro investigation defined the optimal Er:YAG laser parameters for debridement of implant surfaces without damaging the implant surface. Although the experimental findings of Er:YAG are encouraging, the use of this laser in two clinical trials found the healing response to be similar to controls, and the clinical improvements were limited. This suggests that the long-term stability of clinical outcomes may be influenced by factors other than the method used for surface debridement and decontamination. In a case report, a soft laser was successfully used to decontaminate the implant surface before regenerating the defect with autogenous bone and the use of an expanded polytetrafluoroethylene membrane, but this approach has not been further investigated. Finally, a laser-photodynamic approach for the management of peri-implantitis in 15 patients with IMZ implants (cylindrical titanium plasma sprayed) has been reported. Although there was significant decrease in *Aggregatibacter actinomycetemcomitans*, *P. gingivalis*, and *P. intermedia*, complete elimination was not achieved.

The biologic basis of peri-implant bone regeneration, reosseointegration, and reversal of peri-implantitis using laser therapy is being elucidated. Crevicular fluid analysis of patients and osteoblasts in cell culture treated with laser therapy demonstrate an increase in the levels of cytokines associated with tissue regeneration including platelet-derived growth factor, basic fibroblast growth factor, insulin-like growth factor 1, and bone morphogenic protein 2. These growth and differentiation factors are associated with tissue healing and regeneration. Conversely, proinflammatory cytokines associated with inflammation and tissue destruction such as interleukin-1-β, tumor necrosis factor (TNF)-α, and metalloproteinases decreased. The combination of an increase in reparative associated growth and differentiation factors and a decrease in proinflammatory cytokines suggests that the biologic mediators induced by lasers are of a profile that encourages tissue repair and regeneration. Although these studies provide early clues for a possible biologic basis, further research is needed.

Complications and Risks of Laser Therapy

The primary disadvantage of laser therapy is the potential for unintended tissue damage, as lasers can easily generate excessive temperatures. The exposure of bone to temperatures ≥47°C (116.6°F) can induce cellular damage and osseous resorption. Extreme temperature levels of ≥60°C (140°F) result in tissue necrosis.

Overexposure of laser energy has been the basis for complications, reports of tissue damage, and destruction of the periodontium. New, inexperienced operators as well as more seasoned, "cutting-edge" clinicians may encounter disastrous results from their initial treatments (Fig. 52.7). To avoid these negative outcomes, knowledge of the laser mechanics and technique is essential to minimize tissue damage. Once mastery of the information has been achieved, it is critical to identify the desired laser application and the fashion in which it will be used.

Conclusion

There are many potential advantages to using laser therapy, including better visualization of cutting, patient acceptance, wound detoxification, less invasive surgical access, and minimal wound contraction with less scarring. Although these laser applications hold promise, many require more well-designed, controlled research to validate their effectiveness

The literature has numerous positive findings for the use of lasers in the management of periodontal and peri-implant disease. The quality of the literature is largely dominated by case reports and case series. There are limited well-designed RCTs. Further clouding the issue is the number of different lasers in use and the variety of settings and protocols being tested for each laser. The lack of consistency from one study to another has left the profession with no lasers that have been researched extensively enough to provide predictable parameters of use. Therefore, laser use for the treatment of periodontal or peri-implant disease continues to have numerous unknowns.

As in all professions, technology is constantly advancing with new research to provide the clinician with better equipment, drugs, and techniques to improve the therapy rendered to patients. Lasers may become an integral part of periodontal therapy, but at the present time, further research as to the parameters for clinical efficacy and the biologic basis for laser therapy is required. Clinicians considering incorporating laser therapy should be familiar with what is known, understand the appropriate parameter for use, and receive adequate training to master the laser of interest.

Key points

- Laser is an acronym for light amplification by stimulated emission of radiation and functions by transmitting light energy to tissues. It is a collimated monochromatic ray of light. There are different types of lasers depending on the active element used, such as CO_2, Nd:YAG, diode, Er:YAG, and Er:Cr:YSGG.
- Lasers are applied in periodontics for procedures such as soft tissue excision and ablation, viz. gingivectomy/gingivoplasty, crown lengthening, frenectomy, gingival depigmentation, subgingival curettage, root scaling, photodynamic therapy, laser-assisted new attachment procedure, and in implantology.
- Each laser has its own wavelength, spectrum, absorption, and other characteristics.
- As of now, lasers are excellent adjuncts of conventional periodontal therapy but cannot replace the same.

Suggested Readings

Cobb CM: Lasers in periodontics: a review of the literature. *J Periodontol* 77(4):545–564, 2006.

de Paula Eduardo C, De Freitas PM, Esteves-Oliveira M, et al: Laser phototherapy in the treatment of periodontal disease. A review. *Lasers Med Sci* 25:781–792, 2010.

Harris DM, Gregg RH, McCarthy DK, et al: Laser-assisted new attachment procedure in private practice. *Gen Dent* 52:396–403, 2004.

Nevins ML, Camelo M, Schubach P, et al: Human clinical and histologic evaluation of laser-assisted new attachment procedure. *Int J Periodontics Restorative Dent* 32:497, 2012.

Schwarz F, Jepsen S, Herten M, et al: Influence of different treatment approaches on non-submerged and submerged healing of ligature induced periimplantitis lesions: an experimental study in dogs. *J Clin Periodontol* 33:584–595, 2006.

Sgolastra F, Petrucci A, Gatto R, et al: Efficacy of Er:YAG laser in the treatment of chronic periodontitis: systematic review and meta-analysis. *Lasers Med Sci* 27:661–673, 2012.

Sgolastra F, Severino M, Petrucci A, et al: Effectiveness of diode laser as adjunctive treatment to scaling root planning in the treatment of chronic periodontitis: a meta-analysis. *Lasers Med Sci* 28(5): 1393–1402, 2013. doi: 10.10007/s10103-102-1181-5. [Epub August 16, 2012].

Sgolastra F, Severino M, Petrucci A, et al: Nd:YAG laser as an adjunctive treatment to nonsurgical periodontal therapy: a meta-analysis. *Lasers Med Sci* 2013. doi: 10.1007/s10103-013-1293-6. [Epub March 10, 2013].

Tilt LV: Effectiveness of LANAP over time as measure by tooth loss. *Gen Dent* 60:143–146, 2012.

Yukna RA, Carr RL, Evans GH: Histologic evaluation of an Nd:YAG laser-assisted new attachment procedure in humans. *Int J Periodontics Restorative Dent* 27(6):577–587, 2007.

References

References and MCQs with answers for this chapter are found on www.medenact.com.

CHAPTER 53

Diagnosis and Management of Endodontic-Periodontic Lesions

MK Kang | S Mehrazarin | KC Trabert | N Ambalavanan

CHAPTER OUTLINE

Anatomic Considerations of the Pulpal and Periodontal Continuum

Periodontium and pulpal spaces represent the two primary sites of dental infection from oral bacteria. These two spaces are separated by hard shell of dentin, but they may communicate through various portals, such as root canal foramina, dentinal tubules, and even crack lines, through which bacteria and microbial irritants may trigger inflammatory responses in surrounding tissues. At the clinical level, compound dentoalveolar infections involving both periodontium and pulpal spaces are common and present challenges for diagnosis and treatment. Persistent infection in the pulp tissue leads to secondary infection and breakdown of tissues in the periodontium. Conversely, severe periodontal disease may initiate or exacerbate inflammatory changes in the pulp tissue. This mutuality of infection between pulp and periodontium is mediated through anatomic routes, allowing for communication between the two spaces. The main and obvious routes of communication are the apical foramina. Advanced pulpitis leads to pulp necrosis, which often is accompanied by inflammatory bone resorption at the root apex, as found in cases of apical periodontitis or an apical abscess (Fig. 53.1). This is also known as *retrograde periodontitis* because it represents periodontal tissue breakdown from an apical to a cervical direction and is the opposite of *orthograde periodontitis*, which results from a sulcular infection. This condition is typically identified as a periapical radiolucency (PARL) (Fig. 53.2). Retrograde periodontitis is the most common example of pulpal diseases leading to secondary periodontal breakdown. The presence of patent apical foramina may also lead to inflammatory changes in the pulp secondary to severe periodontitis in cases where the periodontal defect reaches the apical foramina.

Alternatively, lateral or accessory canals may comprise the route of periodontal and pulpal communication. The prevalence of accessory root canals in various human teeth and their contribution to the complexity of the root canal system have been well established. Accessory canals are found along the length of the root canals, albeit at varying frequencies depending on their location. By using the "clearing technique" for transparent root canal visualization, prior studies showed that 59.5% of maxillary second premolars possess lateral canals; 78.2% of those canals are located in the apical regions of the root canals. Notably, accessory canals were also found in both midroot and cervical regions, albeit at reduced frequencies, at 16.2% and 4.0%, respectively. A subsequent study showed that 28.4% of permanent molars exhibit patent accessory canals in furcation regions, a finding suggesting that these accessory canals allow a pulpal and periodontal communication to exist. Root canal therapies frequently fail in maxillary molars because of unidentified second mesiobuccal canals. These canals are found in a surprisingly high percentage (80.8%) of teeth. Clearly, accessory canals can lead to asymptomatic apical periodontitis resulting from chronic pulpal diseases. This condition can be readily detected in periapical radiographs (Fig. 53.3), and the periodontal lesions usually heal after successful completion of endodontic therapy. However the likelihood of primary periodontal infections reaching the dental pulp through accessory canals is highly remote.

The third route of communication between the periodontium and the pulp is through the dentinal tubules. **Dentinal tubules** maintain a tapered structure along the length from the pulpodentinal complex to the dentinoenamel junction with a diameter of 2.5 μm at the pulpodentinal complex and 0.9 μm at the dentinoenamel junction. It is therefore conceivable that dentinal permeability changes at different locations along the root surface according to the size and density of the dentinal tubules. Bacterial colonization in the tubules from infected root canals has been well documented. In addition, bacterial invasion into dentinal tubules from the periodontal pocket has been demonstrated, suggesting that dentinal tubules may allow pulpal irritation from chronic periodontal infections. Periodontal pathogens penetrating into the dentinal tubules also may be the source of persistent periodontal infection. Subgingival root instrumentation

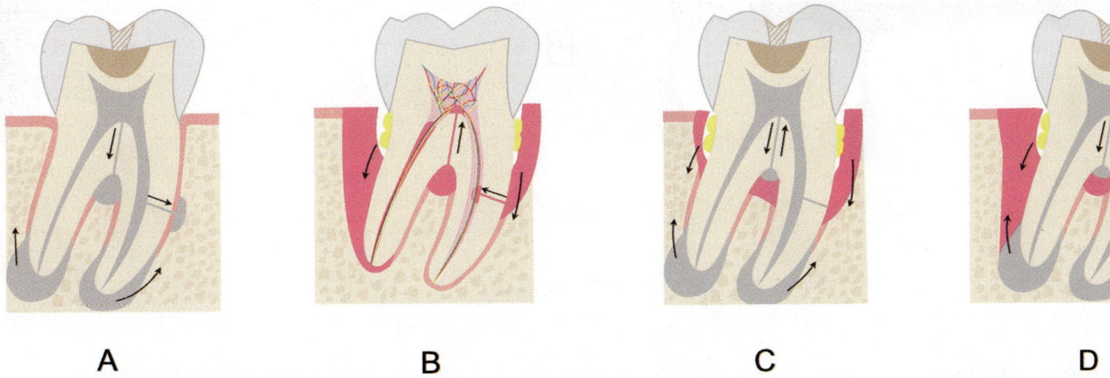

Fig. 53.1 Classification of endodontic-periodontic lesions. A, Primary pulpal infection can lead to chronic periradicular periodontitis by which a periapical radiolucency can develop and migrate cervically. Mandibular molars can also have accessory canals in lateral orientation or in the furcation area. These accessory canals can allow migration of the primary pulpal infection and cause secondary breakdown of the periodontium at their respective loci. B, Primary periodontal infection can lead to extensive breakdown of alveolar crest bone that migrates from the cervical area to the apex. In these lesions, one would find generalized bone loss around a single tooth or that often could involve multiple adjacent teeth. Because of the pulpal-periodontal continuum through main root canal foramina or through accessory canals, extensive periodontal infection can cause irritation in the pulp tissues. C, Both primary pulpal infection and primary periodontal infection can occur simultaneously in an "independent" endo-perio lesion, exhibiting the characteristics of both. D, Primary pulpal and primary periodontal infections can occur extensively in this "combined" endo-perio lesion.

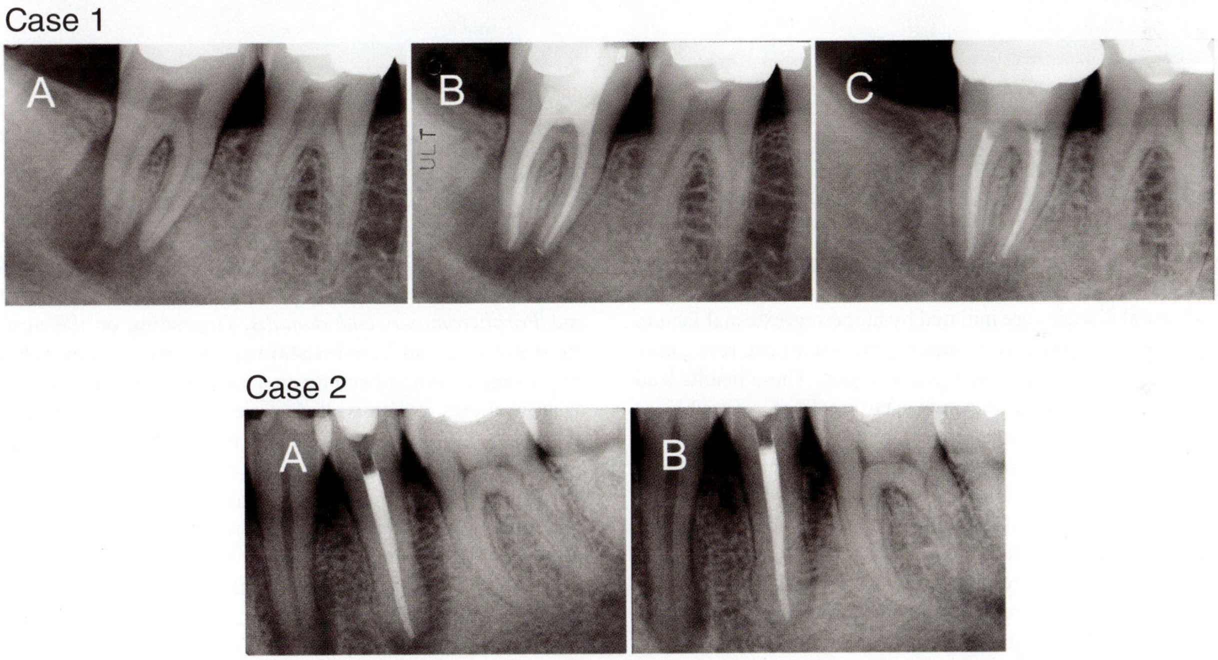

Fig. 53.2 Retrograde periodontitis. Case 1. A, Large periapical lesion extending around the periapex of tooth #47. No visible fractures were detected on the mesial or distal marginal ridges. The tooth tested nonvital. A sinus tract was visible on the buccal gingiva. B, Endodontic therapy was completed in two visits, and the canals were obturated. C, Healing of the periradicular bone is evident at 6 months, and a crown providing complete coverage has been placed. Case 2. A, Tooth #35 had a broad periradicular lesion extending from the apex to the distal root surface that resembled a J-shaped lesion. Conventional root canal therapy was completed. B, Healing of periradicular bone lesion after 6-month recall. *(Case 1, Courtesy: Dr. Thomas Rauth.)*

in the form of root planing is shown to decrease dentin permeability and result in the formation of a smear layer that is acid-labile. However, dentin permeability may increase on the removal of the smear layer, resulting in tubular penetration of oral pathogens and subsequent pulpal irritation. Further study is needed to delineate the role of dentinal tubules in causing secondary infection in pulpal or periodontal tissues.

In addition to the foregoing routes of anatomic communication between pulpal and periodontal tissues, in some instances, communication is established between the pulp and periodontium by iatrogenic defects such as vertical root fractures and tooth perforations. Both of these situations represent nonanatomic communication between the pulp and periodontium and result in the spread of infection from one compartment to the other.

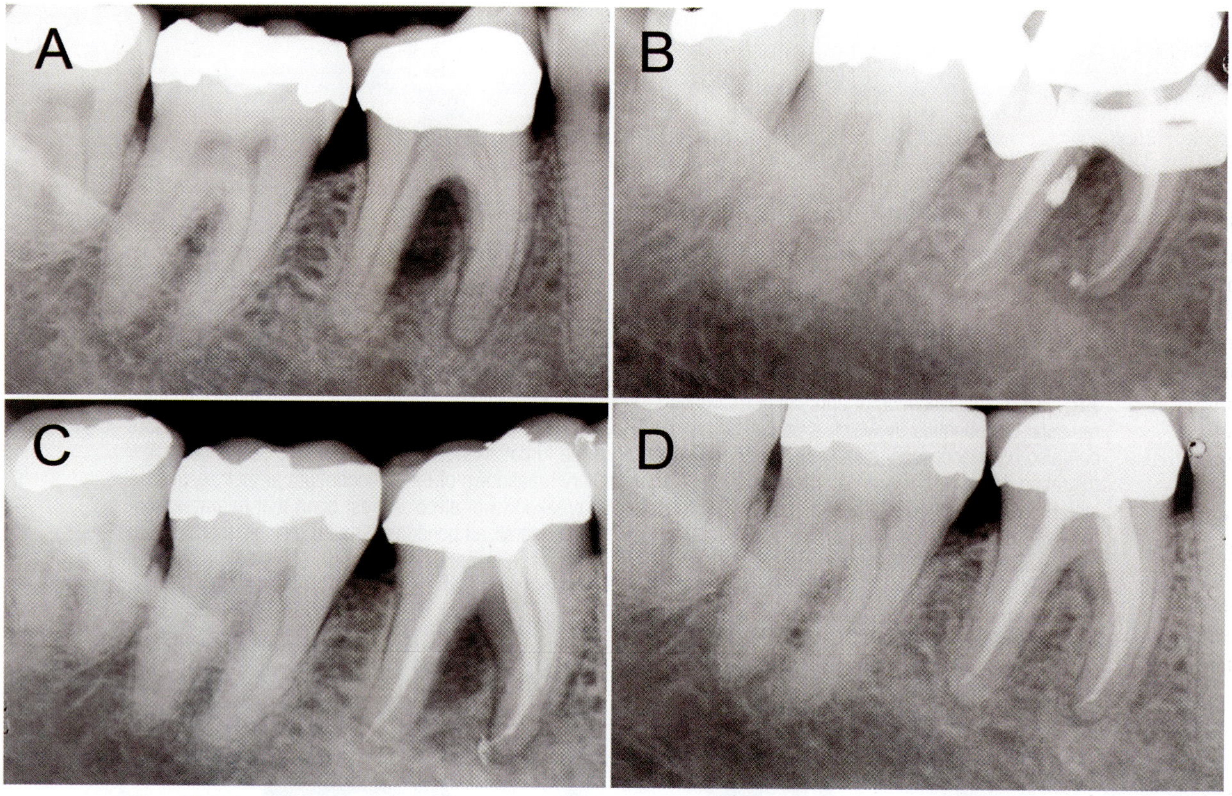

Fig. 53.3 Lateral canal-led periodontal defect from a primary endodontic infection. A, Bone loss is present in the furcation with sinus tract present on the buccal mucosa. Tooth # 46 tested nonvital. B, During condensation, a large amount of sealer was expressed through a large lateral canal in the distal root. C, Sealer was removed after obturation by curettage of the furcation and irrigation with anesthetic solution through the sinus tract. D, Healing at 12 months demonstrates complete repair of periradicular bone. *(Courtesy: Dr. Thomas Rauth.)*

Factors Initiating Pulpal and Apical Diseases

Pulpal and apical diseases are initiated by numerous external factors that may include microorganisms, trauma, excessive heat, restorative procedures, restorative agents, and malocclusion. These insults lead to inflammatory changes in the pulp, starting from reversible or irreversible pulpitis and ultimately progressing to pulpal necrosis and subsequent breakdown of the periodontium. Dental caries is a prominent cause of pulpal disease, and bacterial infection is the primary form of microbial insult to the pulp. Local invasion of the **cariogenic** bacteria or a shift in the bacterial content of biofilm can lead to inflammatory changes in the dental pulp. This frequently happens in the absence of caries extension into the pulp chamber. Bacterial by-products relevant to pulpitis include lactic acid, ammonia, urea, **lipopolysaccharide** (LPS), and lipoteichoic acid. It is notable that the dental pulp is capable of managing numerous microbial insults because of its extensive intrapulpal lymphatic system. However, an overwhelming pulpal inflammatory response may be induced through various mechanisms and numerous microbial challenges. In particular, tumor necrosis factor-alpha (TNF-α), **interleukin**-1 (IL-1), IL-8, IL-12, and chemokines CCL2 and CXCL2 are well described for their role in pulpitis. IL-1 is known to be released from **macrophages** after stimulation with LPS and is responsible for bone resorption leading to apical periodontitis. During **acute** pulpitis, the inflammatory mediators trigger vasodilation, transient increase of pulpal blood flow, inflammatory cell infiltration, increased intrapulpal pressure, and finally, ischemic necrosis of the pulp.

In an acute apical abscess, **anaerobic** bacteria are predominant over aerobic strains and **anaerobes**, and **microaerophiles** were predominant in 82% of the cases studied. The most prevalent isolated bacteria are *Fusobacterium nucleatum, Parvimonas micra,* and *Porphyromonas endodontalis*. Depending on the virulence of the organisms and host **resistance**, a lesion that has been chronic may exacerbate and become an acute apical abscess. The presence of **spirochetes** is also well documented in apical and **periodontal abscesses**. Spirochetes most often isolated in root canal infections are *Treponema denticola* and *Treponema maltophilium*. When comaparing chronic and acute apical abscesses, Baumgartner found that there was a significantly higher **incidence** of spirochetes in acute abscesses or cellulitis than in asymptomatic infected root canals. *Treponema socranskii* was the most frequently encountered species.

Thermomechanical irritants can induce altered pulpal circulation and pulp tissue damage. Earlier studies demonstrated that thermal changes caused by dental procedures such as tooth preparation led to a marked diminution of pulpal blood flow and plasma extravasation, resulting in an inflammatory response. Extreme heat caused by dry tooth preparation triggers vascular stasis and hemorrhage in the subodontoblastic vascular plexus. Investigators noted that even a small increase in pulpal temperature (5°C–6°C) is capable of inducing necrotic changes in the pulp. Pulpal necrosis eventually leads to apical periodontitis. Similarly, chemical irritants impose measurable changes in the pulp status. Etching the dentin surface with high phosphoric acid content causes deleterious effects on dental pulp. In addition, bonding resins used as pulp capping materials led to acute pulpitis and varying degrees of necrosis in human teeth. Root canal overfills with gutta-percha and sealers invariably cause severe inflammatory reactions in the apical tissues, even though patients may be completely asymptomatic. Thus, dental materials often contain chemical irritants that affect both the pulpal and periodontal tissues, and one must be aware of the potential iatrogenic endodontic pathosis associated with their misuse.

Classification of Pulpal and Periapical Diseases

The diagnosis of endodontic lesions that may often have a periodontal component can be confusing. The diagnostic terminology used in various dental schools and textbooks further compounds the confusion for students and practitioners alike. In an attempt to simplify and unify a standardized diagnostic terminology, the American Association of Endodontists established new endodontic diagnosis terminology in 2009. Throughout this chapter, we refer to this new terminology, which is also summarized in Table 53.1.

To make a proper endodontic diagnosis, the clinician must evaluate the symptoms of the patient, the radiographic and clinical findings, and the presence or absence and location of any swelling or drainage. Given all these variables, it is easy to understand why a lack of clarity exists and mistakes are made about whether the lesion is primarily endodontic or periodontal, or a true combined lesion.

The classification of diseases of the dental pulp depends on the extent of pulpal injury and its ability to repair. Many factors influence whether a tooth will be classified as normal, or whether it will develop reversible pulpitis or irreversible pulpitis, or will become necrotic.

Previous studies have found little correlation between the histologic features of pulpal disease and the symptoms that the patient experienced before treatment. A review of the diagnosis of pulpal pain found that 80% of patients who gave a previous history of odontogenic pain manifested histopathologic evidence of pulpitis and partial necrosis in the dental pulp. Controversy still remains, however, regarding the degree of correlation between pulpal symptoms and the histopathologic features of the pulpal tissues. Apical pathoses of endodontic origin are inflammatory processes occurring in periradicular tissues surrounding root apices. They result from various microbial agents that originate from root canal infection and create a series of inflammatory and immunologic responses. These agents exit through the apical foramen, lateral canals, or dentinal tubules. It is an infectious process caused by a large number of microbial species, unlike classic infectious diseases occurring elsewhere in the body that may be caused by only one or two specific organisms. These species reside in ecologically balanced communities discussed previously and constitute the *biofilm.* The different characteristics of pulpal and periodontal lesions are summarized in Table 53.2.

TABLE 53.1 Classification of Pulpal Diseases

Pulpal State	Symptom	Vitality	Response to Cold[a]
Normal pulp	Asymptomatic	Vital	Within normal limits
Reversible pulpitis	Sensitive to pressure or temperature[b]	Vital	Hypersensitive to cold
Symptomatic irreversible pulpitis[c]	Spontaneous throbbing pain	Vital	Hypersensitive to cold and lingering response
Asymptomatic irreversible pulpitis[d]	None	Vital	Within normal limits
Pulp necrosis[e]	Asymptomatic[e]	Nonvital	No response
Previously treated	Variable	Nonvital	No response
Previously initiated therapy	Variable	Variable	Variable

[a]Different pulpal conditions cannot be discerned by periapical radiographs. Symptoms and responses to cold explained herein are the general findings, but there can be exceptions.
[b]Patients' response to pressure may be due to hyperocclusion in reversible pulpitis cases. In the absence of such factors, patients' complaints mainly revolve around thermal sensitivity.
[c]Symptomatic irreversible pulpitis may be symptomatic and painful as described or may be asymptomatic and nonpainful.
[d]Asymptomatic irreversible pulpitis is based on the presence of pulpal inflammation (e.g., extensive caries, hyperemia, or traumatic injury) in the absence of patients' subjective symptoms.
[e]Necrotic pulp may cause acute exacerbation of symptoms, including spontaneous throbbing pain. However, such sensitivity results from periradicular inflammation.
(Diagnostic terminology based on the recommendations of the American Association of Endodontists consensus conference, as shown in Glickman GN: AAE consensus conference on diagnostic terminology: background and perspectives. *J Endod* 35:1634, 2009.)

TABLE 53.2 Different Characteristics of Pulpal and Periodontal Lesions[a]

	Primary Pulpal	Primary Periodontal	Independent Endodontic-Periodontic	Combined Endodontic-Periodontic
Patient symptom	Varies[b]	Mild discomfort	Varies[b]	Varies[b]
Coronal integrity	Compromised	Intact	Compromised	Compromised
Radiographic lesions	Periapical radiolucency	Crestal bone loss	Separate periapical radiolucency and crestal lesions	Continuous bony lesions from alveolar crest to apex
Vitality	Nonvital	Vital	Nonvital	Nonvital
Periodontal probing	Narrow probing to apex[c]	Generalized bone loss	Generalized bone loss	Generalized bone loss with narrow probing to apex

[a]These are generalized summaries, and there can be deviations.
[b]Patients' symptoms of pulpal lesions may vary, depending on the type of pathosis. Chronic lesions can be completely asymptomatic, whereas acute pain symptoms can be triggered without any radiographic lesions.
[c]Primary pulpal lesions may not manifest with any periodontal defect. Narrow probing in pulpal lesions may indicate a sinus tract through the sulcus.

Biologic Effects of Endodontic Infection on Periodontal Tissues

The effects of pulpal disease on the surrounding periodontal tissues are widely accepted by clinicians and researchers, and these effects have been studied since the 1960s. Early inflammatory changes in the pulp exert very little effect on the periodontium. Even a pulp that is significantly inflamed may have little or no effect on the surrounding periodontal tissues. Investigators believe that this initial pulpal inflammatory response is an attempt to prevent the spread of infection to the apical tissues.

When the pulp becomes necrotic, however, it produces a significant inflammatory response involving extremely complex inflammatory and immune reactions. This response can traverse the apical foramen, the furcation, lateral canals, dentinal tubules, and areas of trapped necrotic tissue along the surface of the root that extend past the periodontal ligament and into the surrounding apical tissues. This initial inflammatory response of the pulp and subsequent necrosis that permeates the numerous spaces of the canal system include various bacterial strains, spirochetes, fungi, yeasts, and viruses. The nature and extent of the periodontal destruction that follows depend on the virulence of the pathogens in the root canal system, the chronicity of the disease, and the defense mechanism of the host.

Bacterial infection plays a pivotal role in endodontic-periodontic lesions in the form of bacterial biofilm. Proteolytic bacteria predominate in early root canal infections and then change over time to a flora that contains a greater number of anaerobes.

Several nonliving irritants have also been implicated in the inflammatory process. These include foreign bodies, epithelial rests, cholesterol crystals, Russell bodies, Rushton hyaline bodies, and Charcot-Leyden crystals. In addition, these irritants may also be responsible for the lack of healing of apical lesions in teeth that have received appropriate endodontic treatment. If the growth of epithelial cells is stimulated by any of these living or nonliving pathogens, the integrity of the periodontal tissues also may be affected.

As the degree of pulpal inflammation becomes more extensive, a greater amount of destruction of the periodontal tissues ensues. Extension of the infection through the periodontal ligament space, tooth socket, and surrounding bone occurs, and the patient begins to experience a localized or diffuse swelling that may result in cellulitis that invades the various facial spaces. Most often, however, the infection erupts through the labial, buccal, or lingual mucosa and results in a draining sinus tract. In cases where the path of least resistance for the infectious process is along the attached gingiva, the infection may dissect the periodontal ligament space, resulting in the formation of a deep but narrow periodontal pocket. This pocket usually extends to the main site of the infection (e.g., root apex) when probed or traced with a gutta-percha point. Confusion often results among both general dentists and specialists about whether the probing defect is the result of an endodontic or periodontal problem or the result of vertical root crack. Generally, a narrow probing defect combined with a nonvital pulpal response indicates that the problem is usually of endodontic rather than periodontal origin. In addition, a probing defect associated with vertical root crack generally extends to the level of the crack, as opposed to the root apex. Vertical root crack is generally detected during access into the pulp chamber under high-power magnification or by using transillumination. If vertical root crack is not detected, it should be ruled out as a potential cause of the narrow probing defect.

In a few situations, adjacent teeth, their root surfaces, or furcation areas may also probe deeply. Care must be taken to test all maxillary and mandibular teeth thoroughly to assess correctly whether the problem is endodontic or periodontal. Once the correct diagnosis is made, only then should the treatment plan be formulated and discussed with the patient. When endodontic therapy is the main cause of the swelling or breakdown of the periodontium, successful endodontic treatment usually results in healing of both the periapical and periodontal tissues. At times, however, trauma to the tooth, severe loss of adjacent periodontal tissues, continued tooth mobility, and occlusal trauma do not provide an environment that allows for apical healing to occur. In these cases, splinting is sometimes necessary to help stabilize the tooth and allow for potential repair of the apical tissues

If an endodontic infection is left untreated, the progression of periodontal disease continues. Untreated and unresolved infections of endodontic origin can sustain the growth of various endodontic pathogens that may lead to increased pocket formation, bone loss, calculus deposition, osteoclastic activity, and subsequent bone and tooth resorption. They may additionally impair wound healing and aggravate the development and progression of the periodontal disease state.

The ability of the periodontium to regenerate and heal the lost attachment apparatus has been controversial. This is especially true when the teeth have been endodontically treated and the cement layer is no longer present. Studies need to be done to understand more clearly the relationship between the presence of endodontic infection and the increased loss of marginal bone and attached tissue in patients prone to periodontal disease.

It is evident that endodontium and periodontium are closely related from the structural, functional, and pathogenic perspective and that microorganisms and nonliving irritants play important roles in the disease progression of both structures. Proper diagnosis of endodontic-periodontic lesions therefore is critically important and will dictate the appropriate course of treatment.

Biologic Effects of Periodontal Infection on the Dental Pulp

Effects of periodontal disease on the dental pulp appear to be more controversial compared to the effects of pulpal disease on the periodontium. Not all studies agree about the effects of periodontal disease on the pulp. Even though inflammation and localized pulpal necrosis have been observed next to lateral canals exposed by periodontal diseases, other studies have not confirmed a correlation between periodontal disease and changes within the pulp. Langeland and colleagues indicated that when pathologic changes do occur in the pulp as a result of advanced periodontal disease, the pulp does not usually undergo degenerative changes as long as the main canal has not been involved. If the vasculature of the pulp remains vital, no inflammatory reaction occurs and no symptoms of pulpal pathosis develop.

However, the spread of advanced periodontal lesions that extend to the apical foramen and result in pulpal necrosis has been observed. This retrograde infection may proliferate through large accessory canals on the lateral surfaces of the tooth, canals positioned closer to the apical foramen, and the area where the main canal exits the tooth apex. Protection and preservation of the cementum and dentin surrounding the tooth are also important in preserving the health of the pulp and preventing the ingress of periodontal pathogens. The presence of an intact layer of cementum is important in protecting the pulp from dental plaque and other periodontal pathogens that migrate along the root surface during the development of advanced periodontal disease. Excessive root planing and curettage that remove the cementum and dentin from the root surface encourage narrowing of the pulp canals. This process is

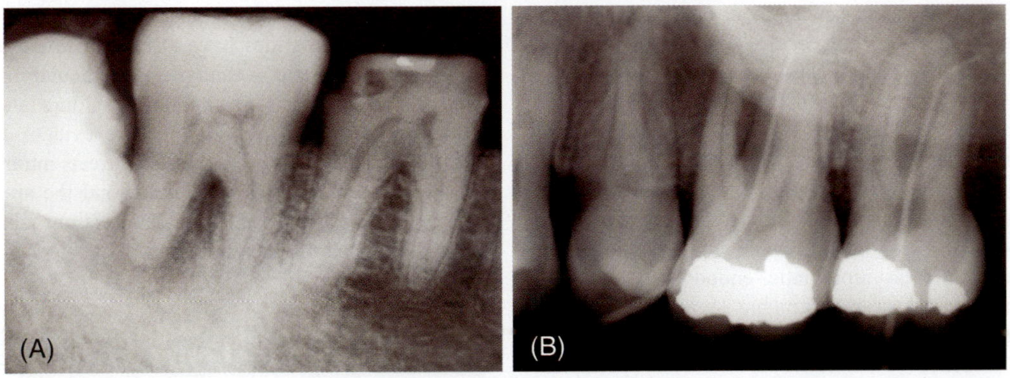

Fig. 53.4 Primary periodontal defects causing periradicular bony lesions and pulpal irritation. A, Primary periodontal lesion is evident on the distal surface of tooth #47. The defect was probed to a depth of 7 mm, and the tooth tested vital to both thermal and electrical pulp testing. The defect was most likely the result of the impacted third molar and formation of a chronic periodontal abscess. B, Primary periodontal lesions both probing 12 mm into the furcation. Teeth #26 and #27 tested vital to thermal and electrical testing. The patient's chief complaint was discomfort to cold, thus exemplifying pulpitis secondary to the primary periodontal infection. *(B, Courtesy: Dr. Gregory Kolber.)*

thought to be reparative rather than inflammatory. Several studies have also suggested that periodontal disease is degenerative to pulpal tissues and results in continued calcification, fibrosis, collagen resorption, and inflammation.

Dentin thickness also contributes to the protection of the pulp. Stanley stated that if a 2-mm thickness of dentin remains between the pulp and an irritating stimulus, little chance of pulpal damage exists. Some precautions that can be taken during the course of periodontal therapy are as follows: (1) Avoid using irritating chemicals on the root surface, (2) minimize the use of ultrasonic scalers when less than 2 mm of dentin remains, and (3) allow minor pulpal irritations to subside before completing additional procedures. When these precautions are not followed and the microvasculature of the pulp is damaged during periodontal procedures that involve deep curettage or periodontal surgical efforts to save the tooth, necrosis may result.

The healing success and failure rates after endodontic microsurgery were studied in teeth that had lesions of only endodontic origin compared to those teeth that had lesions of a combined endodontic-periodontal origin. Lesions only of endodontic origin had a successful outcome of 95.2%, whereas those teeth with combined lesions had a successful outcome of only 77.5%. This suggests that bone and tissue healing are negatively affected after endodontic surgery with lesions of combined origin.

It appears, therefore, that the pulp and periodontal compartments influence each other. Periodontal disease, however, seems to have less of an influence on the pulpal tissues compared to the influence of pulpal disease on the periodontium. Clearly, advanced periodontal disease has some biologic effects on the pulpal state (Fig. 53.4). Unless the microvasculature of the pulp is compromised during aggressive periodontal procedures or excessively deep curettage severs the apical vessels, most periodontal interventions result in only a localized pulpal response and dentin hypersensitivity.

Endo-Perio Lesions With Vertical Tooth Defects

Vertical tooth defects are very common. Vertical tooth defects can be either coronal tooth crack or Vertical Root Fracture (VRF). There are several clear differences between coronal tooth crack and VRF. First, the location is different. A coronal tooth crack initiates within the coronal dentin and migrates apically, while VRF affects primarily radicular dentin. Secondly, the orientation of the defect is different. The tooth crack extends mesiodistally. It is most frequently found at the distal marginal ridge of mandibular second molars, followed by the mesial marginal ridge of maxillar first molars. These coronal cracks would then migrate mesiodistally and apically. On the contrary, VRF is almost always found at the buccolingual root surfaces, often initiated from the radicular dentin. Finally, the prognosis is different. An earlier study reported 2-year survival of endodontically treated teeth with a coronal crack at 85%. One of the most important factors that influence the prognosis of a cracked tooth after endodontic therapy is the probing defect at the location of the crack. The 2-year survival of teeth with more than 6 mm probing defect was 74.1%, while those with less than 6 mm probing defect were 94.8%. On the other hand, teeth with VRF exhibit a very poor prognosis and account for a significant portion of endodontically treated teeth that are extracted. Therefore, it is critically important for clinicians to recognize Endo Perio Lesion (EPLs) with vertical tooth defects and identify whether it is coronal tooth crack or VRF.

Effects of Endodontic Pathosis on Development of Retrograde Peri-Implantitis

The management and resolution of adjacent endodontic and periapical infection are important considerations when planning the placement of a dental implant. Persistence of endodontic bacteria and inflammatory cells commonly facilitates the development of retrograde peri-implantitis or a radiographically evident periapical lesion at the apex of an osseointegrated implant, accompanied by swelling, pain, tenderness, and sinus tract formation. Although retrograde peri-implantitis can occur as a result of overloading or premature loading on the implant or contamination of the external surface of the implant upon placement, the presence of preexisting periapical inflammation, endodontic bacteria, or inflammatory cells at, near, or adjacent to the site of implant placement has also been shown to play an important role in the development of this condition.

Two scenarios exist in which the interaction between the implant and the adjacent tooth may lead to retrograde peri-implantitis. Under circumstances where complications arise during implant placement, such as overheating of bone during preparation of the implant osteotomy, placement of the implant too close to the adjacent tooth, or altering of the blood supply of the adjacent tooth during implant surgery, the implant placement itself may result in devitalization of the adjacent tooth and subsequent development of peri-implantitis. More common, however, is the presence of existing or recurrent periapical disease from an endodontically treated tooth resulting in contamination of the adjacently placed implant, which may also lead to peri-implantitis.

Root canal therapy is critical for resolution of intraradicular or periapical infection. Although radiographic evidence of periapical lesion healing may be noted on endodontic treatment, periapical inflammation may persist and be detectable only histologically, implants placed adjacent to asymptomatic, endodontically treated teeth exhibiting no clinical or radiographic signs of periapical disease resulted in peri-implantitis, which resolved with surgical intervention. The presence of persistent or refractory periapical inflammation adjacent to the implant may increase the risk of developing retrograde peri-implantitis.

Certain treatment considerations should be taken into account when planning implant placement adjacent to an endodontically involved tooth. First and foremost, conventional root canal therapy should be performed to resolve underlying symptomatic or radiographic endodontic and periapical disease, and endodontic retreatment should be performed to address failure of endodontic therapy. Delaying the placement of an implant after completion of endodontic treatment on an adjacent tooth or increasing the distance between the implant and the adjacent endodontically treated tooth may reduce the likelihood of peri-implantitis. The use of nonmachined surfaced implants may also decrease the chances of implant failure because machined-surfaced implants placed adjacent to or at the site of previous endodontic infection are more likely to result in the development of retrograde peri-implantitis.

Under circumstances where endodontic infection results in peri-implantitis, surgical debridement and disinfection of the implant surface and resolution of the endodontic pathosis are critical to continued success of the implant. Implant stability is also an important consideration when planning for treatment of retrograde peri-implantitis. Affected implants exhibiting poor stability require removal of the implant, debridement of granulation tissue within the implant osteotomy site, and either placement of bone graft and subsequent implant or immediate placement of a longer or wide implant.

Interactions Between Extraradicular Infection and the Periodontium

Although failure of endodontic therapy and persistence of periapical pathology are typically the result of persistent or secondary infection arising from incomplete obturation or abnormal root canal anatomy, in some instances, extraradicular infection is to blame. This bacterial infection occurs periapically along the external surface of the root apex and can lead to or exacerbate acute periapical abscess development. Extraradicular infection can occur either as a result of or independent of intraradicular infection.

Although intraradicular infection is the predominant source of extraradicular infection, far less common external factors also propagate extraradicular pathosis. One such source is the accumulation of calculus on the external surface of the root apex, which is associated with failed periapical lesion healing, persistent sinus tract formation, and refractory apical periodontitis. Several case reports have identified the presence of calculus along the root apex upon removal by apicoectomy and found that persistent sinus tract and periapical disease resolved on calculus removal. The formation of calculus around the root apex is thought to be the result of accumulation and calcification of plaque from the external oral environment and periodontium by means of the open persistent sinus tract present in these cases.

In addition to calculus, bacterial biofilms held together by extracellular polysaccharides have also been found along the external surface of the root tip. Although extraradicular infection is not common, its implications in endodontic failure and management of refractory periapical periodontitis are evident. Although conventional root canal therapy successfully treats intraradicular infection, the presence of microorganisms beyond the apical foramen often makes extraradicular periapical infections difficult to resolve without surgical intervention.

Differential Diagnosis of Endodontic and Periodontal Infection

Acute infections of the periodontium and the pulp must be differentiated from each other for clinicians to be able to establish a correct diagnosis with reasonable certainty and initiate appropriate therapy. A thorough understanding of both disease processes and the correct interpretation of clinical and radiographic findings will aid the dentist in establishing a diagnosis that results in the rapid relief of acute and painful condition.

When pulpal and periodontal abscesses are separate from one another, most clinicians believe that the diagnosis is usually easier. In some instances, however, the primary diseases may have similar clinical characteristics that make the diagnosis more difficult. In other situations, no demarcation may exist between the two areas of pathosis that clinically and radiographically appear as one large and continuous lesion, with extreme pain and swelling. When this occurs, the clinician must avoid classifying these continuous lesions as true combined lesions. One must rely on all available clinical testing methods to help clarify the correct clinical diagnosis before beginning treatment.

Accurately differentiating between pulpal and periodontal lesions can be challenging. If the lesion originates from a pulpal infection yet was treated by extensive periodontal therapy, it will not resolve. Conversely, performing endodontic therapy on a tooth that has an extensive periodontal defect and a vital pulp will result in persistence of the periodontal infection. Thus, identifying the primary cause of infection is a critical determinant of treatment outcome. Perhaps the most important consideration when making such a distinction is to base the diagnosis on multiple findings. These findings include the patient's symptoms, coronal integrity, shape and size of the radiographic lesions, periodontal probing, and tooth vitality. It is possible that one or more of these findings will suggest a pulpal or periodontal infection, whereas others may point to the contrary. For instance, a tooth may exhibit extensive failing restorations, recurring decay, and radiographic lesions, suggesting probable pulpal involvement. However, the tooth may test completely vital and lack any evidence of an irreversible pulpitis on thermal testing. Under these circumstances, one would rule out primary pulpal infection and examine the patient for periodontal involvement. Thus, making the distinction between pulpal and periodontal infection requires collectively dissecting the multiple findings and synthesizing the most probable diagnosis (see Table 53.2).

Patients' Subjective Symptoms

Patients in the acute phase of pulpal infection present with symptoms that are generally absent in chronic periodontal infection. During the initial stage of pulpitis, patients may complain about sensitivity and pain exacerbated by certain stimuli, including temperature changes, pressure, and/or biting. If the symptoms result from reversible pulpitis, they will usually resolve spontaneously with time as the result of various mechanisms, such as closure of dentinal tubules, clearance of microbial irritants and toxins, and reparative dentin formation. Persistent inflammation leads to symptomatic irreversible pulpitis, which is often associated with sharp and spontaneous pain, although asymptomatic irreversible pulpitis may also occur, as described previously. Acute pain in response to thermal stimulus may subside after several days as the pulp becomes necrotic and the bacteria and their byproducts migrate down the complex canal system. As the infection extends to and then past the apical foramen or a lateral root canal, the tooth becomes particularly sensitive to bite pressure and percussion. After several days, the necrotic tooth may develop an acute apical abscess, which results in elevation of the tooth from the dentoalveolar complex. Patients frequently report that the tooth feels "high" on occlusion. However, patients with irreversible pulpitis or necrotic pulp may be asymptomatic. Thus, making the diagnosis of primary pulpal infection must be based on multiple objective findings, such as the patient's responses to percussion, palpation, biting, periodontal probing, and vitality testing, as well as a thorough evaluation of his or her subjective symptoms.

In apical and periodontal abscesses, the extent of pain may vary. Generally, an acute apical abscess causes extreme pain on pressure, bite, percussion, and, at times, palpation if the infection has penetrated the cortical bone. Periodontal abscesses are thought to cause less pain because little or no elevation of the periosteum occurs. Edema and swelling are characteristics that may be shared by both conditions. The swelling and edema with a periodontal abscess are generally confined to the cervical portion of the tooth. An apical abscess is usually more sensitive to palpation around the tooth apex if the infection has penetrated the bony cortical plate. Redness and a smooth appearance of the marginal gingival tissues are more common with abscesses of periodontal origin, whereas redness can be detected more apically if a pulpal abscess has started to swell and elevate surrounding tissues. Objective findings in periodontal abscesses include bleeding on probing, suppuration, increased pocket depth, increased tooth mobility, and occasionally lymphadenopathy. Abscesses of endodontic origin usually probe normally but may also display increased mobility, depending on the amount of bone loss. Patients may describe the tooth as feeling longer or higher than the adjacent teeth.

Suppuration and drainage from periradicular and periodontal abscesses may also differ. Periodontal abscesses are associated with severe periodontal destruction. Some patients also suffer from lymphadenopathy. Aspects of periodontal therapy that correlate highly with the development of acute periodontal abscesses are (1) patients undergoing current periodontal treatment, (2) incomplete removal of calculus, (3) a history of a previous abscess at the same site, and (4) previous use of antibiotics for dental or nondental reasons.

Drainage from apical abscesses usually comes from one of two sites. The most prevalent area of drainage is a sinus tract that develops when the area of swelling breaks through the mucoperiosteum and exits the mucosal tissue either near or at some distance from the site of infection. Additionally, the path of least resistance may be along the periodontal ligament, and the infection may dissect the ligament along the surface of the root and exit the tooth at the height of the epithelial attachment. This results in a periodontal defect that probes along a narrow path to the apex of the root, as previously discussed. Both the sinus tract and narrow sulcular lesions can usually be traced to the infected tooth or offending root by using a gutta-percha point.

Coronal Integrity

Periodontal infection without pulpal involvement may manifest with an intact crown structure and the absence of coronal defects. Conversely, endodontic infection is almost always associated with loss of coronal integrity such as caries, failing restorations, extensive restorations, and cracks or fractures that extend to the pulpal tissues. However, this does not mean that all periodontal infections are devoid of coronal defects or that all endodontic lesions exhibit loss of coronal integrity. When pulp tissue is severed by trauma, for example, one could expect to find necrotic pulp in the absence of coronal defects. If left untreated, such lesions originating from primary pulpal infection lead to the breakdown of the periodontium, as in asymptomatic apical periodontitis or apical abscess. Of course, primary periodontal lesions can develop in teeth with coronal defects. Furthermore, combined lesions (so-called endo-perio lesions) would manifest with a periodontal infection and extensive coronal destruction. However, careful inspection of the coronal status during either the intraoral or radiographic examination can provide supportive information in deciding whether the lesion originates from an endodontic or a periodontal infection.

Radiographic Appearance

Periapical radiographs can provide distinguishing information on whether the lesion is of pulpal or periodontal origin. Although radiographic findings are objective data, *interpretation* of radiographs can be highly subjective, depending on who reads the radiograph. Thus, it is important to focus on specific entities on a radiograph. These should include the coronal status, crestal bone height and shape, presence of an apical or lateral radiolucency, bony trabeculation, integrity of the lamina dura, and careful evaluation of the obturation of the root canal if present. Coronal status as revealed on a radiograph can also help in the differential diagnosis, as described previously. In addition, apical lesions originating from a primary pulpal infection lead to retrograde periodontitis that migrates from the root apex in a cervical direction. On the contrary, periodontal infections lead to the loss of crestal bone from the cervical area of the tooth in an apical direction. Thus, radiographic lesions appear different in endodontically treated teeth than periodontal lesions, and the shape of the bony lesions can help distinguish between the two. For example, radiographic lesions representing severe periodontitis appear wider at the cervical end than the apical portion of the lesion. Apical or lateral radiolucencies may also result from differences in trabeculation patterns not associated with pulpal infection. For this reason, it is critical to consider the integrity of the lamina dura. A break in the lamina dura accompanied by an apical or lateral radiolucency is usually indicative of a chronic or acute pulpal infection. If the tooth had been endodontically treated, assessment of the previous obturation qualities (e.g., voids, short fills or overfills, missed canals) is also important. These radiographic features provide very useful and often distinguishing information to make the differential diagnosis between pulpal and periodontal lesions more accurate.

Vitality

Testing of tooth vitality is often one of the most important methods to differentiate between periodontal and endodontic infection. Teeth with periodontal infection usually test vital to thermal testing, unless the acute condition is a combined lesion in which both endodontic and periodontal compartments have become diseased. Teeth with both endodontic infection and periodontal abscess usually test nonvital. Exceptions to this are teeth with extremely calcified canals, extensively restored teeth, or multirooted teeth where canals may be partly necrotic as a result of either pulpal or periodontal disease. Other canals may still retain vital tissue that responds to thermal or electric pulp testing. Thermal testing is usually the most reliable way to determine pulpal health or disease. Patients with symptomatic irreversible pulpitis often report a lingering painful response to thermal stimulus. In later stages of pulpitis, heat exacerbates the symptom more than cold, and the application of cold may even cause short-term pain relief. Although thermal testing can be informative about the status of the pulp, a patient's response to thermal stimulus may be confused with hypersensitivity resulting from exposed dentin and patent dentinal tubules in the absence of pulpitis. Therefore, thermal testing must be combined with other diagnostic criteria, as discussed previously, to distinguish between lesions originating from pulpal or periodontal infection.

Classification of Endodontic-Periodontic Lesions

A simple classification of perio-endo lesions was given by Simon, Glick, and Frank in 1972 as follows:

1. Primary endodontic lesions.
2. Primary periodontal lesions.
3. Primary endodontic lesion with secondary periodontal involvement.
4. Primary periodontal lesion with secondary endodontic involvement.
5. True combined lesion.

Treatment Considerations

In managing lesions of pulpal or periodontal origin, making an accurate diagnosis of the source of infection is a critical determinant of treatment outcome. *Primary* pulpal pathoses combined with *secondary* periodontal defects completely resolve by conventional root canal therapy alone. Fig. 53.3 shows a chronic pulpal infection associated with a necrotic pulp that led to a periodontal defect through the apical foramen. This is a classic example of primary pulpal infection causing a secondary periodontal defect. In this case, root canal therapy alone led to complete resolution of the chronic apical periodontitis involving the furcal defect. In fact, this type of lesion and healing pattern are observed in almost all secondary periodontal defects resulting from root canal infection.

Lesions originating from pulpal infections require endodontic therapy and do not resolve from periodontal treatment alone. This is exemplified in Fig. 53.5, a preoperative radiograph of an "independent" endo-perio lesion that shows an apical radiolucency spanning the entire length of the distal root of tooth #19 and moderate bone loss at the mesial aspect. On completion of root canal therapy, the periodontal breakdown around the distal root completely resolved, whereas the mesial bony defect remained unchanged. Case 2 shows a "combined" endo-perio lesion involving extensive apical defects around the apices of tooth #19 and a periodontal defect in the bifurcation. After successful endodontic therapy alone, the apical lesions and furcation defect resolved, but incomplete healing is noted in the coronal aspect of the furcation. This finding presumes that the unhealed defect originated from a primary periodontal infection.

Therefore, endo-perio lesions require both endodontic and periodontal therapy for complete healing to occur. This is true whether the lesions are independent or combined. One important consideration is the sequence of therapies: Which of the two should be performed first? As discussed earlier, endodontic lesions are often associated with more pronounced symptoms than periodontal lesions. More importantly, in combined endo-perio lesions, some periodontal defects will resolve on completion of the endodontic treatment, whereas the opposite would not be the case. After resolution of the secondary periodontal defect stemming from a primary pulpal infection, the residual periodontal disease may be more accurately and predictably managed. These considerations indicate that combined endo-perio lesions are best treated by performing the necessary endodontic treatment first, followed by periodontal therapy.

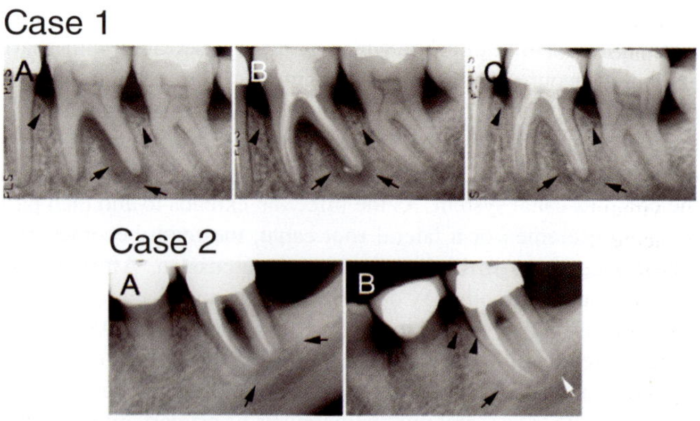

Fig. 53.5 Case 1. "Independent" endo-perio lesion. A, "Truly independent" endo-perio lesions. Vertical periodontal bone loss can be seen at the mesial surface of teeth #37 and #36. A large endodontic lesion extends around the apex and into the bifurcation. An apical and furcal defect is evident radiographically (black arrows). Interproximal periodontal bone loss is also evident (black arrowheads). B, Final condensation film 2 weeks after initiating treatment. C, Nearly complete healing of the endodontic lesion at 6 months and restoration of the tooth with a porcelain-fused-to-metal crown. The areas of vertical bone loss from the periodontal lesions are still present. Case 2. "Combined" endo-perio lesion. A, Nonvital tooth with a narrow 9-mm probing defect in the bifurcation of tooth #36 and a large periapical lesion (black arrows). B, At 9 months, healing demonstrates significant bone repair in the furcation and periapical areas (white arrow). A small amount of bone loss in the furcation still remains (black arrowheads) because of a persistent periodontal defect. *(Case 1, Courtesy: Dr. Thomas Rauth.)*

When patients present with an abscess, periodontal and apical abscesses are managed differently. Previous studies suggested that treating patients with acute periodontal abscesses should be done in two stages. The first stage consists of management of the acute lesion. In the second stage, more comprehensive treatment of the original and any residual lesions is accomplished. Management of acute periodontal abscesses involves establishing drainage through the periodontal pocket and subgingival scaling and root planing.

Curettage of the epithelium lining, the pocket, and the surrounding connective tissue is then accomplished, followed by compression of the pocket wall. If the swelling is large and fluctuant, flap surgery or incision and drainage may be necessary to relieve the pressure. In cases in which the bone loss is extensive and the prognosis for the tooth is hopeless, extraction may be required.

Rational use of antibiotics should be considered in acute periodontal abscesses. The use of systemic antibiotics may be indicated when a patient has elevated temperature, cellulitis, or systemic disease and is immunocompromised. The abscess should be drained by incision and drainage and/or root canal debridement. Depending on the maturity of the abscess, incision and drainage may not establish draining exudate from the periapical tissues. However, it is highly recommended to initiate root canal therapy to debride the root canal and eliminate the source of infection. An incision and drainage procedure is efficient and relieves the pressure that has accumulated under the subperiosteal tissues, resulting in a fluctuant, swollen, and painful lesion. Pulpectomy removes the infected pulp tissues and microorganisms within the canal system, and calcium hydroxide is placed into each of the canals. Its use has proved to be a suitable intracanal medicament because of its stability and bactericidal effect in a limited space. Substantial evidence indicates that systemic antibiotic therapy may not be beneficial for patients with acute apical abscess unless they present with systemic complications such as fever, lymphadenopathy, or cellulitis, or are immunocompromised.

Penicillin V and amoxicillin are still the antibiotics of choice for the majority of bacteria isolated from acute endodontic infections. If penicillin V therapy is ineffective, the combination of penicillin V with metronidazole or amoxicillin–clavulanate potassium is recommended. Pain associated with acute apical periodontitis is well controlled by systemic nonsteroidal antiinflammatory drugs with or without paracetamol. Narcotics are usually unnecessary unless an acute flare-up occurs. The correct diagnosis of periodontal and apical abscesses is the most critical step in resolving the disease process. Failing to properly diagnose and treat these often encountered conditions results in progression of the disease, continued loss of bone and periodontal attachment apparatus, a poor prognosis, and possible loss of the tooth.

Conclusion

Bacteria-induced inflammations of the pulpal and periodontal tissues often occur together. Endodontic lesions are more likely to spread to surrounding periodontal tissues, with subsequent bone and tissue destruction, compared to the less frequent involvement of periodontal infections in the pulpal tissues that result in retrograde pulpitis.

Understanding the etiology and making the diagnosis of dental abscess are based on the patient's history and clinical and radiographic findings. Pulpal pathosis often results in significant pain to thermal stimulus or tissue swelling, or it may be totally asymptomatic. Radiographic evaluation may demonstrate a circumscribed periapical lesion when the tooth tests necrotic and the origin of the lesion is pulpal. Vitality testing can detect changes of sensation caused by pulpal inflammation and necrosis. If evidence indicates pulpal disease and the possibility of associated periodontal bone loss, the endodontic treatment should be completed first, and then the patient should be reevaluated. In many cases, apparent periodontal disease, including bone loss, suppuration, and pocket depth, resolves if a pulpal lesion has been successfully treated endodontically.

Residual periodontal problems can be treated after completion of successful endodontic treatment, and in many cases, successful regeneration of periodontal defects is possible in endodontically treated teeth. Knowledge of these two disciplines is necessary for successful treatment outcomes.

Key points

- The main route of communication between the pulp and periodontium is through apical foramina, lateral or accessory canals, and through the dentinal tubules.
- A narrow probing defect combined with a nonvital pulpal response indicates that the problem is usually of endodontic origin rather than periodontal.
- When endodontic therapy is the main cause of the swelling or breakdown of the periodontium, successful endodontic treatment usually results in healing of both the periapical and periodontal tissues.
- Untreated and unresolved infections of endodontic origin can sustain the growth of various endodontic pathogens that may lead to increased pocket formation, bone loss, calculus deposition, osteoclastic activity, and subsequent bone and tooth resorption.
- Some precautions that can be taken during the course of periodontal therapy are: (1) avoidance of the use of irritating chemicals on the root surface, (2) minimization of the use of ultrasonic scalers when there is less than 2 mm of remaining dentin, and (3) subsidence of minor pulpal irritations before completion of additional procedures.
- Teeth with periodontal infection usually test vital to thermal testing unless the acute condition is a combined lesion in which both endodontic and periodontal compartments have become diseased.
- Teeth with both endodontic infection and periodontal abscess usually test nonvital.
- Combined endodontic-periodontic lesions are best treated by first performing the necessary endodontic treatment followed by periodontal therapy.
- Teeth with vertical root fractures exhibit a very poor prognosis and account for a significant portion of endodontically treated teeth that are extracted.

Suggested Readings

Bender IB, Seltzer S: The effect of periodontal disease on the pulp, Oral Surg *Oral Med Oral Pathol* 33: 458–474, 1972.

Chen SY, Wang HL, Glickman GN: The infl uence of endodontic treatment upon periodontal wound healing, *J Clin Periodontol* 24: 449–456, 1997.

Czarnecki RT, Schilder H: A histological evaluation of the human pulp in teeth with varying degrees of periodontal disease, *J Endod* 5: 242–253, 1979.

González-Moles MA, González NM: Bacterial infections of pulp and periodontal origin, *Med Oral Patol Oral Cir Bucal* 9 (Suppl 34-6): 32–36, 2004.

Herrera D, Roldán S, González I, et al: The periodontal abscess (I). Clinical and microbiological fi ndings, *J Clin Periodontol* 27: 387–394, 2000.

Jansson LE, Ehnevid H, Lindskog S, et al: The infl uence of endodontic infection on progression of marginal bone loss in periodontitis, *J Clin Periodontol* 22: 729–734, 1995.

Jaramillo A, Arce RM, Herrera D, et al: Clinical and microbiological characterization of periodontal abscesses, *J Clin Periodontol* 32: 1213–1218, 2005.

Kerns DG, Glickman GN: Endodontic and periodontal interrelationships. In Cohen S, Hargreaves K, editors: *Pathways of the pulp*, ed 9, St. Louis, 2006, Elsevier Mosby.

Kobayashi T, Hayashi A, Yoshikawa R, et al: The microbial fl ora from root canals and periodontal pockets of non-vital teeth associated with advanced periodontitis, *Int Endod* J 23: 100–106, 1990.

Nair PN: Pathogenesis of apical periodontitis and the causes of endodontic failures, *Crit Rev Oral Biol Med* 15: 348–381, 2004.

Rothstein I, Simon JH: The endo–perio lesion: a critical appraisal of the disease condition, *Endod Topics* 13: 34–56, 2006.

Simon JH, Glick DH, Frank AL: The relationship of endodontic–peridontic lesions, *J Periodontal* 43(4), 1972.

Whyman RA: Endodontic–periodontic lesions. Part II: management, *New Zeal Dent* J 84: 109–111, 1988. C0260.

References

References and MCQs with answers for the chapter are available on www.medenact.com.

CHAPTER 54

Periodontal–Restorative Interrelationships

FM Spear | JP Cooney | TR Schoenbaum | J Mitchell | HH Takei | N Ambalavanan

CHAPTER OUTLINE

Preparation of the Periodontium for Restorative Dentistry

Periodontal health is a prerequisite for successful comprehensive dentistry. To achieve the long-term therapeutic targets of comfort, good function, treatment predictability, longevity, and ease of restorative and maintenance care, active periodontal infection must be treated and controlled before the initiation of restorative, esthetic, and implant dentistry. In addition, the residual effects of periodontal disease or anatomic aberrations inconsistent with realizing and maintaining long-term stability must be addressed. More recently, this phase of treatment includes techniques performed in anticipation of esthetic or implant dentistry, such as clinical crown lengthening, covering denuded roots, alveolar ridge retention or augmentation, and implant site development.

The relationship between periodontal health and the restoration of teeth is intimate and inseparable. For restorations to survive long term, the periodontium must remain healthy so that the teeth are maintained. For the periodontium to remain healthy, restorations must be critically managed in several areas so that they are in harmony with their surrounding periodontal tissues. To maintain or enhance the patient's esthetic appearance, the tooth–tissue interface must present a healthy natural appearance, with gingival tissues framing the restored teeth in a harmonious manner.

Rationale for Therapy

The many reasons for establishing periodontal health before performing restorative dentistry include the following:

1. Periodontal treatment is undertaken to ensure the establishment of stable gingival margins before tooth preparation. Noninflamed, healthy tissues are less likely to change (e.g., shrink) as a result of subgingival restorative treatment or postrestoration periodontal care. In addition, tissues that do not bleed during restorative manipulation allow for a more predictable restorative and esthetic result.
2. Certain periodontal procedures are designed to provide for adequate tooth length for retention, access for tooth preparation, impression making, tooth preparation, and finishing of restorative margins in anticipation of restorative dentistry. Failure to complete these procedures before restorative care can add to the complexity of treatment and introduce unnecessary risk of failure.
3. Periodontal therapy should antecede restorative care because the resolution of inflammation may result in the repositioning of teeth or in soft-tissue and mucosal changes. Failure to anticipate these changes may interfere with prosthetic designs planned or constructed before periodontal treatment.
4. Traumatic forces placed on teeth with ongoing periodontitis may increase tooth mobility, discomfort, and possibly the rate of attachment loss. Restorations constructed on teeth free of periodontal inflammation, synchronous with a functionally appropriate occlusion, are more compatible with long-term periodontal stability and comfort.
5. Quality, quantity, and topography of the periodontium may play important roles as structural defense factors in maintaining periodontal health. Orthodontic tooth movement and restorations completed without the benefit of periodontal treatment designed for this purpose may be subject to negative changes that complicate construction and future maintenance.
6. Successful esthetic and implant procedures may be difficult or impossible without the specialized periodontal procedures developed for this purpose.

Sequence of Treatment

Treatment sequencing should be based on logical and evidenced-based methodologies, taking into account not only the disease state encountered but also the psychologic and esthetic concerns of the patient. Because periodontal and restorative therapy is situational and specific to each patient, a plan must be adaptable to change depending on the variables encountered during the course of treatment. For example, teeth initially determined to be salvageable may be judged "hopeless," thus altering the established treatment scheme.

Generally, the preparation of the periodontium for restorative dentistry can be divided into two phases: (1) control of periodontal inflammation with nonsurgical and surgical approaches and (2) preprosthetic periodontal surgery (Box 54.1).

BOX 54.1 Sequence of Treatment in Preparing Periodontium for Restorative Dentistry

Control of Active Disease
1. Emergency treatment
2. Extraction of hopeless teeth
3. Oral hygiene instructions
4. Scaling and root planing
5. Reevaluation
6. Periodontal surgery
7. Adjunctive orthodontic therapy

Preprosthetic Surgery
1. Management of mucogingival problems
2. Preservation of ridge morphology after tooth extraction
3. Crown-lengthening procedures
4. Alveolar ridge reconstruction

Control of Active Disease

Periodontal therapy is intended to control active disease. In addition to the removal of root surface accretions that are primary etiologic agents, secondary local factors, such as plaque-retentive overhanging margins and untreated caries, must be addressed.

Emergency Treatment

Emergency treatment is undertaken to alleviate symptoms and stabilize acute infection. This includes endodontic as well as periodontal conditions.

Extraction of Hopeless Teeth

Extraction of hopeless teeth is followed by provisionalization with fixed or removable prosthetics. Retention of hopeless teeth without periodontal treatment may result in bone loss on adjacent teeth. Restorative margins are refined and provisional restorations refitted after the completion of active periodontal therapy.

Oral Hygiene Measures

Oral hygiene measures, when properly applied, have been shown to reduce plaque scores and gingival inflammation (see Chapter 34). However, in patients with deep periodontal pockets (>5 mm), plaque control measures alone are insufficient in resolving subgingival infection and inflammation.

Scaling and Root Planing

Scaling and root planing combined with oral hygiene measures have been demonstrated to significantly reduce gingival inflammation and the rate of progression of periodontitis. This applies even to patients with deep periodontal pockets.

Re-evaluation

After 4 weeks, the gingival tissues are evaluated to determine oral hygiene adequacy, soft-tissue response, and pocket depth (see Chapter 33). This permits sufficient time for healing, reduction in inflammation and pocket depths, and gain in clinical attachment levels. In deeper pockets (>5 mm), however, plaque and calculus removal is often incomplete, with risk of future breakdown. As a result, periodontal surgery to access the root surfaces for instrumentation and to reduce periodontal pocket depths must be considered before restorative care may proceed.

Periodontal Surgery

Periodontal surgery may be required for some patients. This should be undertaken with future restorative and implant dentistry in mind. Some procedures are intended to treat active disease successfully, and some are aimed at the preparation of the mouth for restorative or prosthetic care.

Adjunctive Orthodontic Therapy

Orthodontic treatment has been shown to be a useful adjunctive to periodontal therapy. It should be undertaken only after active periodontal disease has been controlled. If nonsurgical treatment is sufficient, definitive periodontal pocket therapy may be postponed until after the completion of orthodontic tooth movement. This allows for the advantage of the positive bone changes that orthodontic therapy can provide. However, deep pockets and furcation invasions may require surgical access for root instrumentation in advance of orthodontic tooth movement. Failure to control active periodontitis can result in acute exacerbations and bone loss during tooth movement. As long as they are periodontally healthy, teeth with preexisting bone loss may be moved orthodontically without incurring additional attachment loss.

Soft tissue-grafting procedures are often indicated in anticipation of orthodontic therapy to increase the dimension of attached tissue.

The Role of the Periodontal Phenotype

A patient's periodontal phenotype may play an essential role in the success of restorative dentistry and, by extension, complementary therapies, such as orthodontics and implant dentistry. An organism's phenotype is its observable characteristics influenced both by its genotype and its environment. The periodontal phenotype has been defined as the combination of gingival phenotype (three-dimensional gingival volume—e.g., gingival thickness, keratinized tissue width) and thickness of the buccal bone plate (bone morphotype).

The gingival thickness may be estimated by detecting a periodontal probe showing through the gingival tissue after insertion into the gingival sulcus: (1) probe visible, thin (≤1 mm), (2) probe not visible, thick (>1 mm). The keratinized tissue width is measured from the gingival margin to the mucogingival junction. Cone-beam computed tomography can estimate bone thickness; however, the risk of radiation exposure versus the benefit of acquiring these data should be considered.

Periodontal Phenotype and Restorative Dentistry

Patients with a thin periodontal phenotype, including those with minimal or no attached gingiva, can be maintained in periodontal health. However, the risk of inflammation and recession increases when oral hygiene is suboptimal and thin periodontal tissues are subjected to restorative dentistry. This would include routine occurrences such as trauma from gingival retraction, placement of intracrevicular restorative margins, and restorations with large restorative overhangs. In patients with a thin periodontal phenotype and no gingival recession, treating clinicians should correct potential harmful environmental influences and concentrate on prevention and monitoring. However, in situations of an extremely thin phenotype, current gingival recession, minimal (≤2 mm), or no attached gingiva, an appropriate surgical gingival augmentation procedure should be considered in anticipation of potentially traumatic procedures and intracrevicular restorative dentistry.

Periodontal Phenotype and Orthodontics

With appropriate oral hygiene, healthy gingiva of any dimension is considered sufficient to maintain periodontal health. However, during orthodontic tooth movement, the three-dimensional adequacy of periodontal hard and soft tissues is critical to preventing gingival recession. Tooth movement within the alveolar envelope, irrespective of gingival thickness or quality, is considered a lower risk of a future recession. If, however, the tooth is moved outside the alveolar process, resulting in a bony dehiscence, there is an increased potential for gingival recession. In that event, the gingival thickness is more likely to be a critical factor in preventing future gingival recession. Therefore, sites showing thin periodontal tissues (<2 mm) are potential candidates for periodontal surgical soft tissue augmentation (grafting) and fastidious preventive measures in advance of orthodontic treatment and in preparation for future restorative dentistry.

Preprosthetic Surgery

Management of Mucogingival Problems

Periodontal plastic surgical procedures may be undertaken for a variety of reasons. The most common techniques include those that increase gingival dimensions and achieve root coverage. These procedures are often indicated before restoration for prosthetic reasons and in conjunction with orthodontic tooth movement. Root coverage procedures may also be undertaken for purposes of comfort and esthetics (Fig. 54.1).

At least 2 months of healing is recommended after soft tissue-grafting procedures before initiating restorative dentistry.

Surgical Modification of Periodontal Phenotype

A thick periodontal phenotype is more resistant to gingival inflammation and recession. Conversely, sites with a thin periodontal phenotype are more suspectable to gingival recession when subjected to plaque-associated inflammation, restorative procedures, and orthodontic tooth movement. Thus, the clinician needs to identify the deficiencies in patient-performed oral hygiene and periodontal phenotype and plan the most appropriate therapies, including surgical techniques, best suited to enhance the quality of soft tissue to support periodontal health and stability. Autogenous free gingival grafts to increase the dimension of attached gingiva and bilaminar tissue grafts to enhance gingival thickness are considered the gold standard for gingival augmentation. The gingival tissues will normally regenerate to their full dimension after correctly performed osseous surgery, including crown lengthening. This takes on special significance when planning for restorative dentistry. The healing period after surgical crown lengthening can vary and may be affected by several factors, including the patient's periodontal phenotype. Whereas a thin phenotype may regrow and mature sufficiently within 6–12 weeks to allow for the restorative process, a thick phenotype may take as long as 6–12 months to regenerate completely. Consequently, tooth preparation and restoration in advance of healed and stable gingival tissues can invite placement of the restorative margin within the supracrestal attachment zone.

Preservation of Ridge Morphology After Tooth Extraction

Alveolar ridge resorption is a common consequence of tooth loss. Ridge preservation procedures have been shown to be useful in anticipation of the future placement of a dental implant or pontic, as well as in cases where unaided healing would result in an unesthetic deformity.

Crown-Lengthening Procedures

Surgical crown-lengthening procedures are performed to provide retention form to allow for proper tooth preparation, impression procedures, and placement of restorative margins (Fig. 54.2) and to adjust gingival levels for esthetics. It is important that crown-lengthening surgery is done in such a manner that the biologic width is preserved. The *biologic width* is defined as the physiologic dimension of the junctional epithelium and connective tissue attachment. This measurement has been found to be relatively constant at approximately 2 mm (±30%). The healthy gingival sulcus has shown an average depth of 0.69 mm (Fig. 54.3). It has been theorized that infringement on the biologic width by the placement of a restoration within its zone may result in gingival inflammation, pocket formation, and alveolar bone loss (Fig. 54.4). Consequently, it is recommended that there be at least 3.0 mm between the gingival margin and bone crest. This allows for adequate biologic width when the restoration is placed 0.5 mm within the gingival sulcus (Fig. 54.5).

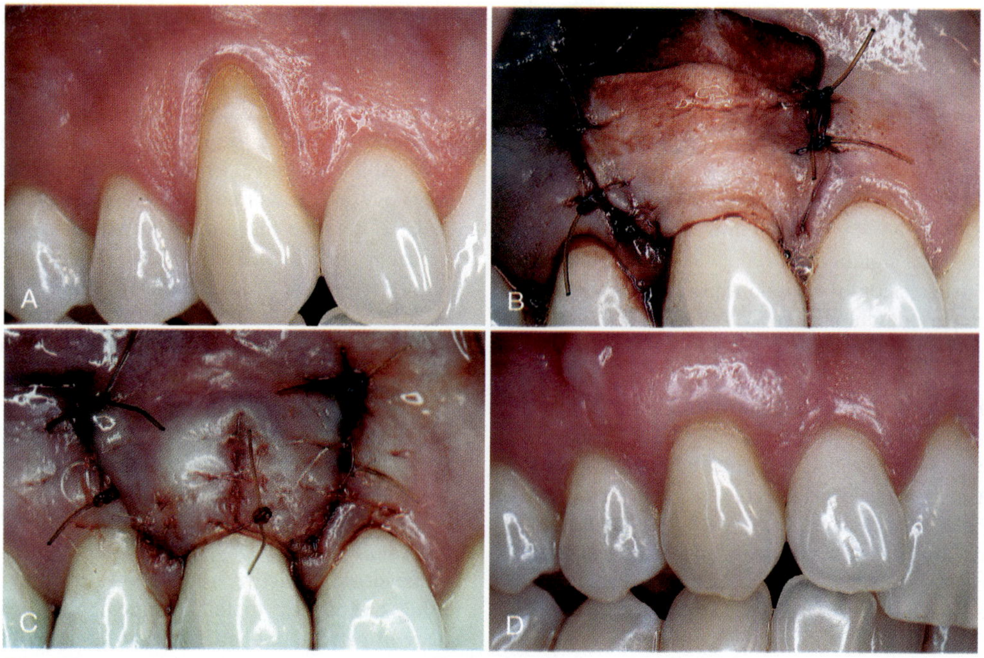

Fig. 54.1 Connective tissue graft placed under a double-papilla flap has been used to provide root coverage for a maxillary right canine. A, Maxillary canine before therapy. B, Connective tissue graft placed over denuded root surface. C, Papilla placed over connective tissue. D, Final result.

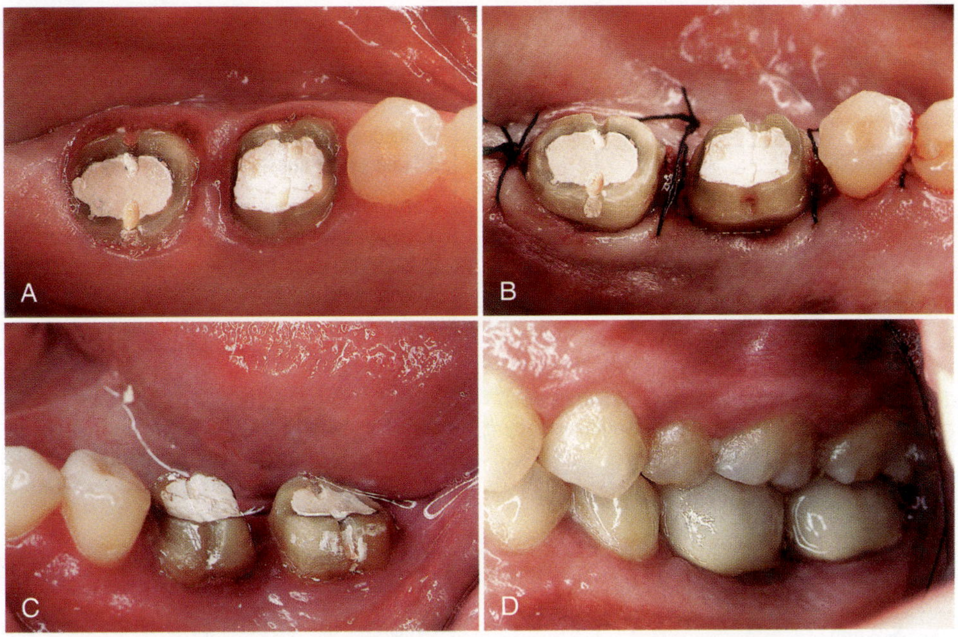

Fig. 54.2 Surgical crown lengthening has provided these otherwise unrestorable mandibular molars with improved retention and restorative access for successful restorations. A, Before crown lengthening. B, Crown-lengthening surgery completed. Note increased clinical crown. C, Buccal view after surgery. D, Final restorations.

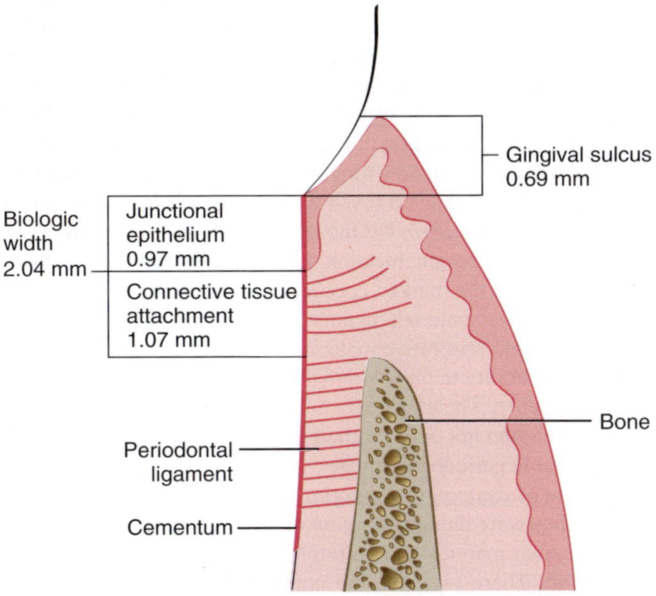

Fig. 54.3 Estimation of supracrestal tissue attachment (biologic width) that comes out to be about 2 mm. Efforts should be made to preserve its integrity.

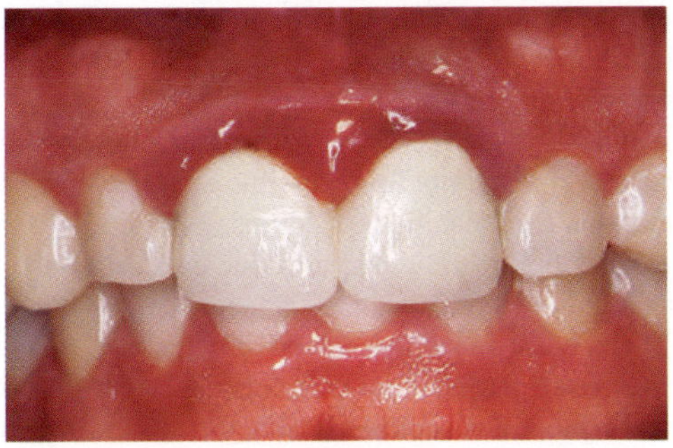

Fig. 54.4 Importance of considering infringement of supracrestal tissue attachment (biologic width) is must, even though gingival inflammation around crowns may have a variety of causes.

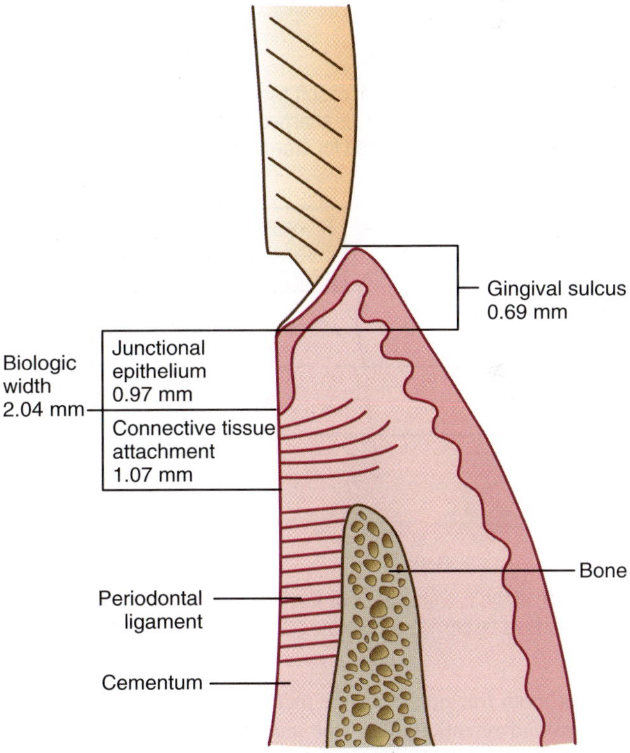

Fig. 54.5 Placement of the restorative margin 0.5 mm into the sulcus, which allows for the maintenance of the supracrestal tissue attachment (biologic width).

Surgical crown lengthening may include the removal of soft tissue or both soft tissue and alveolar bone. Reduction of soft tissue alone is indicated if there is adequate attached gingiva and more than 3 mm of tissue coronal to the bone crest (Fig. 54.6). This may be accomplished by either gingivectomy or flap technique. Inadequate attached gingiva and less than 3 mm of soft tissue require a flap procedure and bone recontouring (Fig. 54.7). In the case of

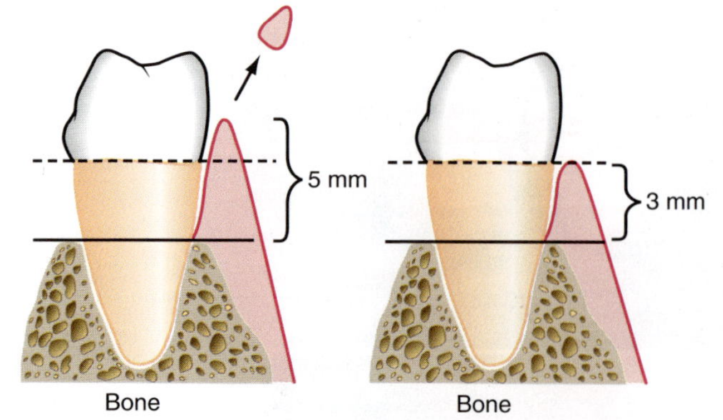

Fig. 54.6 Greater than 3 mm of soft tissue between the bone and gingival margin, with adequate attached gingiva, allowing crown lengthening by gingivectomy.

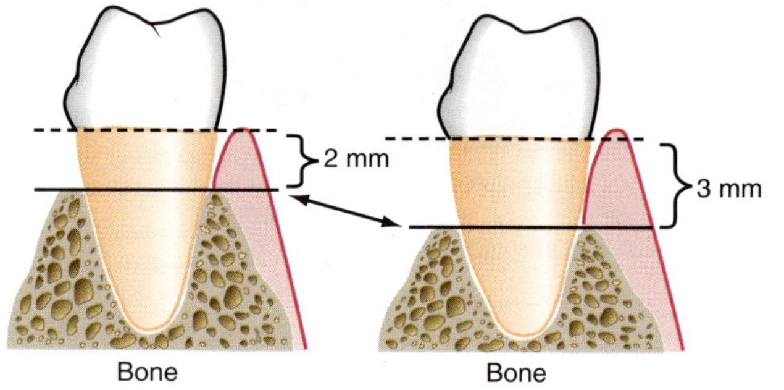

Fig. 54.7 With less than 3 mm of soft tissue between the bone and gingival margin, or less-than-adequate attached gingiva, a flap procedure and osseous recontouring are required for crown lengthening.

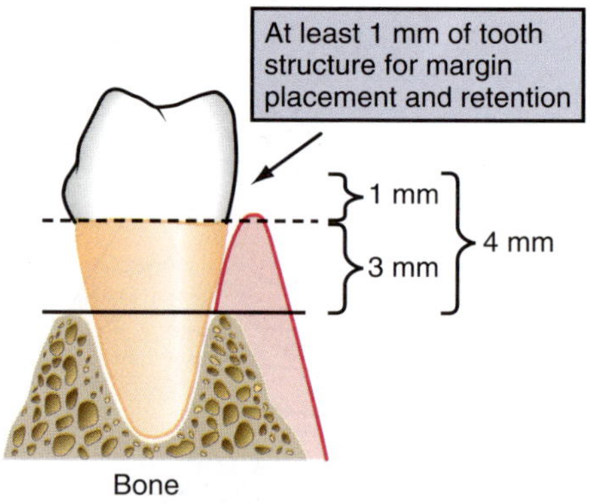

Fig. 54.8 In the case of caries or fracture, at least 1 mm of sound tooth structure should be provided above the gingival margin for proper restoration.

caries or tooth fracture, to ensure margin placement on sound tooth structure and retention form, the surgery should provide at least 4 mm from the apical extent of the caries or fracture to the bone crest (Fig. 54.8).

With the advent of predictable implant dentistry, it is important to weigh carefully the value of crown lengthening for restorative ease as opposed to tooth removal and replacement with a dental implant (Box 54.2).

Alveolar Ridge Reconstruction

Patients are frequently seen after tooth loss and alveolar ridge resorption have occurred. To provide for adequate anatomic dimensions for the construction of an esthetic pontic or the placement of dental implants, alveolar ridge reconstruction is undertaken. In the case of esthetic pontic construction, small defects may be treated with soft-tissue ridge augmentation (Fig. 54.9). For larger defects and in those sites receiving dental implants, hard tissue modalities are used.

BOX 54.2 Surgical Crown Lengthening

Indications

1. Subgingival caries or fracture.
2. Inadequate clinical crown length for retention.
3. Unequal or unesthetic gingival heights.

Contraindications

1. Surgery would create an unesthetic outcome.
2. Deep caries or fracture would require excessive bone removal on contiguous teeth.
3. The tooth is a poor restorative risk.

Biologic Considerations

Margin Placement and Supracrestal tissue attachment (Formerly Biologic Width)

One of the most important aspects of understanding the periodontal–restorative relationship is the location of the restorative margin to the adjacent gingival tissue. Restorative clinicians must understand the role of biologic width in preserving healthy gingival tissues and controlling the gingival form around restorations. They must also apply this information in the positioning of restoration margins, especially in the esthetic zone where a primary treatment goal is to mask the junction of the margin with the tooth.

A clinician is presented with three options for margin placement: supragingival, equigingival (even with the tissue), and subgingival. The *supragingival margin* has the least impact on the periodontium. Classically, this margin location has been applied in unesthetic areas because of the marked contrast in color and opacity of traditional restorative materials against the tooth. With the advent of more translucent restorative materials, adhesive dentistry, and resin cements, the ability to place supragingival margins in esthetic areas is now a reality. Therefore, whenever possible, these restorations should be chosen not only for their esthetic advantages but also for their favorable periodontal impact.

The use of *equigingival margins* traditionally was not desirable because they were thought to retain more plaque than supragingival or subgingival margins and therefore result in greater gingival inflammation. There was also the concern that any minor gingival recession would create an unsightly margin display. These concerns are not valid today not only because the restoration margins can be esthetically blended with the tooth but also because restorations can be finished easily to provide a smooth, polished interface at the gingival margin. From a periodontal viewpoint, both supragingival and equigingival margins are well tolerated.

The greatest biologic risk occurs when placing *subgingival margins*. These margins are not as accessible as supragingival or equigingival margins for finishing procedures. In addition, if the margin is placed too far below the gingival tissue crest, it violates the gingival attachment apparatus.

The dimension of space that the healthy gingival tissues occupy between the base of the sulcus and the underlying alveolar bone comprises the junctional epithelial attachment and the connective tissue attachment. The combined attachment width is now identified as the *biologic width*. It was found that, in the average human, the connective tissue attachment occupies 1.07 mm of space above the

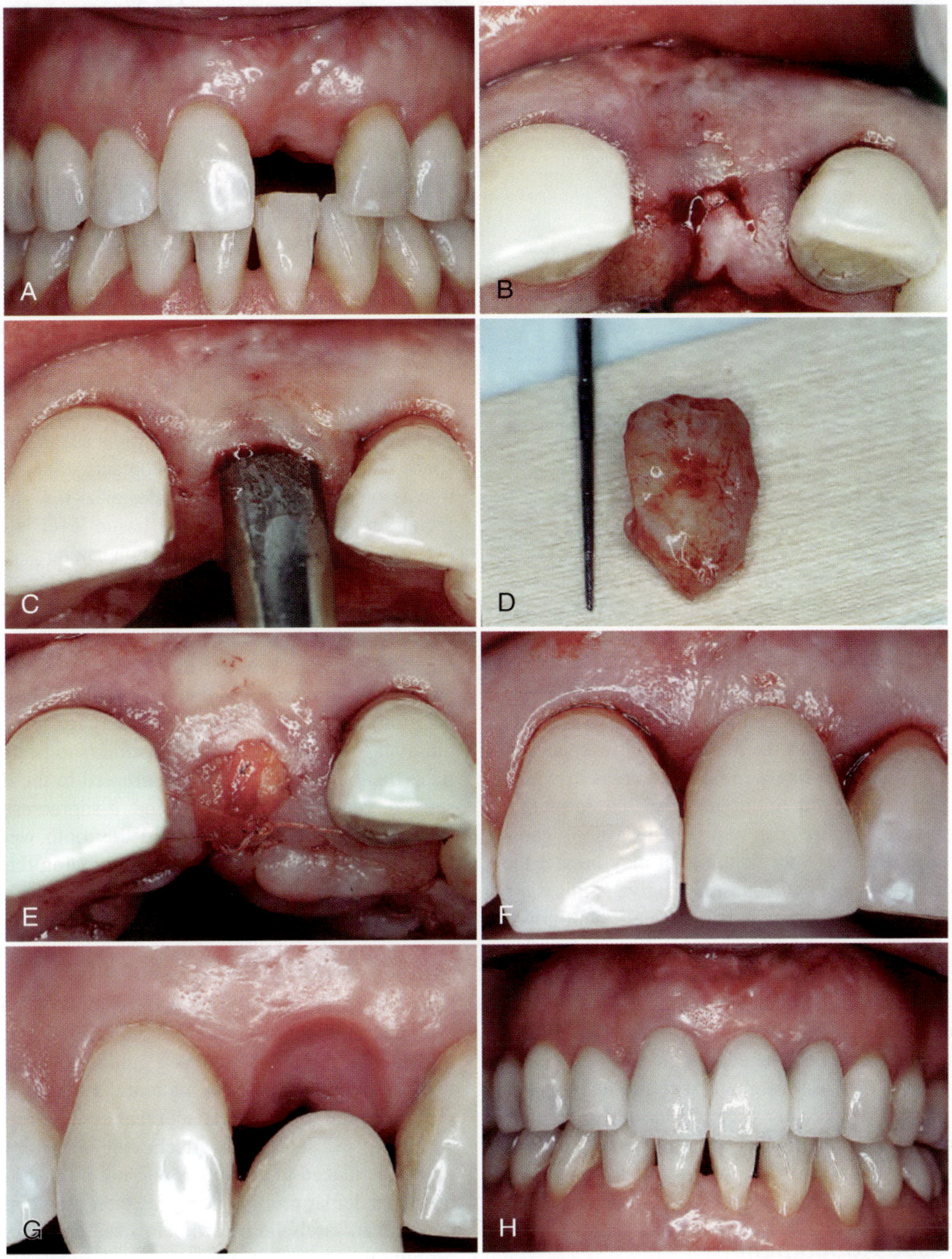

Fig. 54.9 A, Loss of the maxillary left central incisor has resulted in an unesthetic alveolar ridge defect. B–E, An incision is made at ridge crest, a pouch is created, and a soft tissue graft harvested from the palate is placed into the pouch. F–H, A removable appliance with an ovate pontic is placed in light contact with the grafted site. Swelling around the pontic apex results in a tissue concavity from which the more natural-appearing final restoration emerges.

crest of the alveolar bone and that the junctional epithelial attachment below the base of the gingival sulcus occupies another 0.97 mm of space above the connective tissue attachment. The combination of these two measurements, averaging approximately 1 mm each, constitutes the supracrestal tissue attachment (biologic width).

The supracrestal tissue attachment (biologic width) can be identified for the individual patient by probing to the bone level (referred to as "sounding to bone") and subtracting the sulcus depth from the resulting measurement. This measurement must be done on teeth with healthy gingival tissues and should be repeated on more than one tooth to ensure an accurate assessment. The technique allows the variations in sulcus depths found in individual patients to be assessed and factored into the diagnostic evaluation. The information obtained is then used for definitive diagnosis of biologic width violations, the extent of correction needed, and the parameters for placement of future restorations.

Restorative considerations frequently dictate the placement of restoration margins beneath the gingival tissue crest. Restorations may need to be extended gingivally (1) to create adequate resistance and retentive form in the preparation, (2) to make significant contour alterations because of caries or other tooth deficiencies, or (3) to mask the tooth-restoration interface by locating it subgingivally.

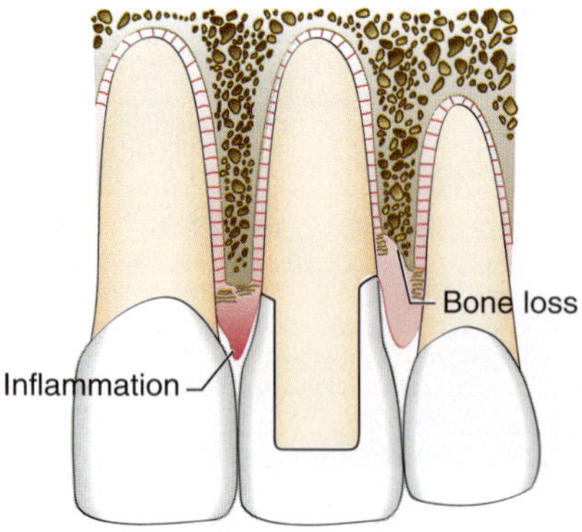

Fig. 54.10 Ramifications of a supracrestal tissue attachment (biologic width) violation if a restorative margin is placed within the zone of the attachment. On the mesial surface of the left central incisor, bone has not been lost, but gingival inflammation occurs. On the distal surface of the left central incisor, bone loss has occurred, and a normal biologic width has been reestablished.

When the restoration margin is placed too far below the gingival tissue crest, it impinges on the gingival attachment apparatus and creates a violation of biologic width. Two different responses can be observed from the involved gingival tissues (Fig. 54.10).

One possibility is that bone loss of an unpredictable nature and gingival tissue recession occurs as the body attempts to recreate room between the alveolar bone and the margin to allow space for tissue reattachment. This is more likely to occur in areas in which the alveolar bone surrounding the tooth is very thin in width. Trauma from restorative procedures can play a major role in causing this fragile tissue to recede. Other factors that may impact the likelihood of recession include (1) whether the gingiva is thick and fibrotic or thin and fragile and (2) whether the periodontium is highly scalloped or flat in its gingival form. It has been found that highly scalloped, thin gingiva is more prone to recession than a flat periodontium with thick fibrous tissue.

The more common finding with deep margin placement is that the bone level appears to remain unchanged, but gingival inflammation develops and persists. To restore gingival tissue health, it is necessary to establish space clinically between the alveolar bone and the margin. This can be accomplished either by surgery to alter the bone level or by orthodontic extrusion to move the restoration margin farther away from the bone level.

Supracrestal Tissue Attachment (Biologic Width) Evaluation

Radiographic interpretation can identify interproximal violations of supracrestal tissue attachment (biologic width). However, with the more common locations on the mesiofacial and distofacial line angles of teeth, radiographs are not diagnostic because of tooth superimposition. If a patient experiences tissue discomfort when the restoration margin levels are being assessed with a periodontal probe, it is a good indication that the margin extends into the attachment and that a supracrestal tissue attachment (biologic width) violation has occurred.

A more positive assessment can be made clinically by measuring the distance between the bone and the restoration margin using a sterile periodontal probe. The probe is pushed through the anesthetized attachment tissues from the sulcus to the underlying bone. If this distance is less than 2 mm at one or more locations, a diagnosis of supracrestal tissue attachment (biologic width) violation can be confirmed. This assessment is completed circumferentially around the tooth to evaluate the extent of the problem.

Correcting Supracrestal Tissue Attachment (Biologic Width) Violations

Biologic width (now termed as supracrestal tissue attachment or supracrestal attached tissue) violations can be corrected either by surgically removing bone away from proximity to the restoration margin (by apically displaced flap) or by orthodontically extruding the tooth and thus moving the margin away from the bone. Surgery is the more rapid of the two treatment options. It is also preferred if the resulting crown lengthening creates a more pleasing tooth length. In these situations, the bone should be moved away from the margin by the measured distance of the ideal biologic width for that patient, with an additional 0.5 mm of bone removed as a safety zone.

There is a potential risk of gingival recession after removal of bone. If interproximal bone is removed, there is a high likelihood of papillary recession and the creation of an unesthetic triangle of space below the interproximal contacts. If the biologic width violation is on the interproximal side, or if the violation is across the facial surface and the gingival tissue level is correct, orthodontic extrusion is indicated. The extrusion can be performed in two ways. (1) By applying low orthodontic extrusion force, the tooth will erupt slowly, bringing the alveolar bone and gingival tissue with it. The tooth is extruded until the bone level has been carried coronal to the ideal level by the amount that needs to be removed surgically to correct the attachment violation. The tooth is stabilized in this new position and then is treated with surgery to correct the bone and gingival tissue levels. Another option is to perform rapid orthodontic extrusion where the tooth is erupted to the desired amount over several weeks. During this period, a supracrestal fibrotomy is performed circumferentially around the tooth weekly in an effort to prevent the tissue and bone from following the tooth. The tooth is then stabilized for at least 12 weeks to confirm the position of the tissue and bone, and any coronal creep can be corrected surgically.

Margin Placement Guidelines

When determining where to place restorative margins relative to the periodontal attachment, it is recommended that the patient's existing sulcular depth be used as a guideline in assessing the biologic width requirement for that patient. The base of the sulcus can be viewed as the top of the attachment, and therefore the clinician accounts for variations in attachment height by ensuring that the margin is placed in the sulcus and not in the attachment. The variations in sulcular probing depth are then used to predict how deep the margin can safely be placed below the gingival crest. With shallow probing depths (1.0–1.5 mm), extending the preparation more than 0.5 mm subgingivally risks violating the attachment. This assumes that the periodontal probe will penetrate into the junctional epithelial attachment in healthy gingiva an average of 0.5 mm. With shallow probing depths, future recession is unlikely because the free gingival margin is located close to the top of the attachment. Deeper sulcular probing depths provide more freedom in locating restoration margins farther below the gingival crest. In most circumstances, however, the deeper the gingival sulcus, the greater is the risk of gingival recession.

Clinical Procedures in Margin Placement

The first step in using sulcus depth as a guide in margin placement is to manage gingival health. Once the tissue is healthy, the following three rules can be used to place intracrevicular margins:

Rule 1: If the sulcus probes 1.5 mm or less, place the restoration margin 0.5 mm below the gingival tissue crest. This is especially important on the facial aspect and will prevent a biologic width violation in a patient who is at high risk in that regard.

Rule 2: If the sulcus probes more than 1.5 mm, place the margin half the depth of the sulcus below the tissue crest. This places the margin far enough below tissue, so that it will still be covered if the patient is at higher risk of recession.

Rule 3: If a sulcus greater than 2 mm is found, especially on the facial aspect of the tooth, evaluate to see if a gingivectomy could be performed to lengthen the teeth and create a 1.5-mm sulcus. Then the patient can be treated using Rule 1.

The rationale for Rule 3 is that deep margin placement is more difficult and the stability of the free gingival margin is less predictable when a deep sulcus exists. Reducing the sulcus depth creates a more predictable situation in which to place an intracrevicular margin. The clinician cannot be sure that the tissue will remain at the corrected level, however, because some gingival rebound can occur after gingivectomy. However, sulcular depth reduction ensures that the restorative margins will not be exposed and visible in the patient's mouth (Figs. 54.11–54.15).

The placement of supragingival or equigingival margins is simple because it requires no tissue manipulation. With regard to overall tooth preparation, the amount reduced incisally or occlusally, facially, lingually, and interproximally is dictated by the choice of restorative materials. Before extending subgingivally, the preparation should be completed to the free gingival margin facially and interproximally. This allows the margin of the tooth preparation to be used as a reference for subgingival extension once the tissue is retracted.

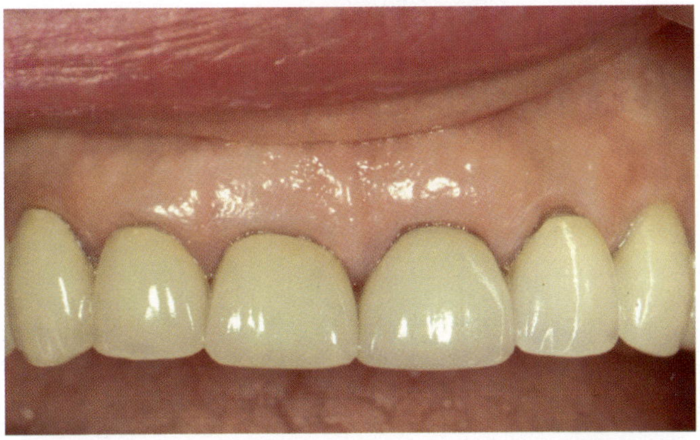

Fig. 54.11 A 78-year-old woman presents with the maxillary anterior restorations placed 6 months earlier. She is unhappy with the exposed margins and notes that the margins were covered the day the restorations were placed (see Figs. 54.11–54.15).

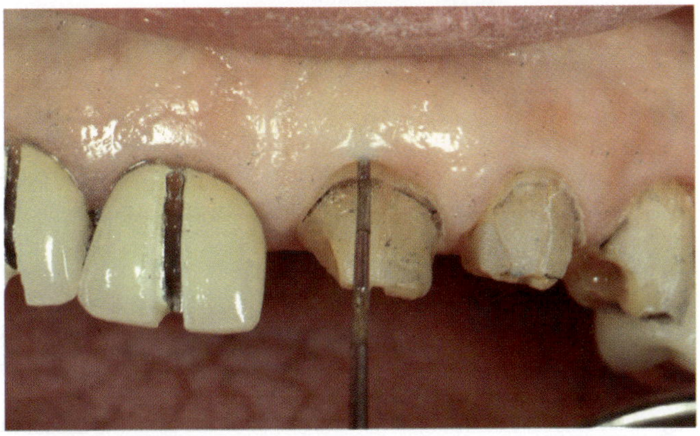

Fig. 54.12 Depth from the attachment to the level of the preparation margin is greater than 3 mm. This patient in Fig. 54.11 had an altered eruption pattern and a sulcus depth of more than 3 mm when these restorations were placed.

Tissue Retraction

Once the supragingival portion of the preparation is completed, it is necessary to extend below the tissue. The preparation margin must now be extended to the appropriate depth in the sulcus, applying the guidelines presented previously. In this process, the tissue must be protected from abrasion, which will cause hemorrhage and can

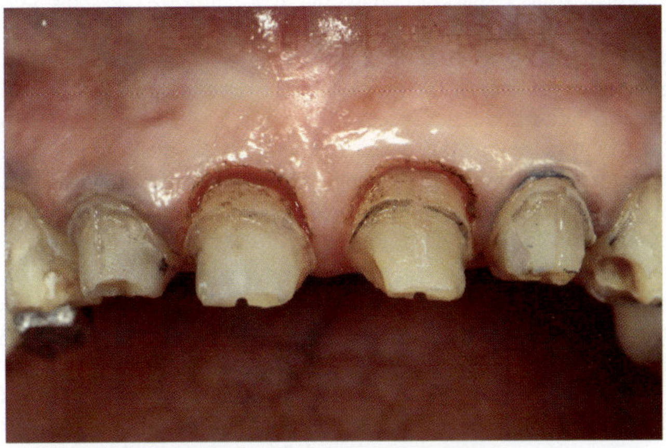

Fig. 54.13 Two available options to manage treatment appropriately. (1) Place the original margins to half the depth of the sulcus, in which case the recession that occurred would not have exposed them. (2) Perform a gingivectomy, creating a 1- to 1.5-mm sulcus. The second option was chosen when the restorations were redone. The margins were then placed 0.5 mm below the tissue after the gingivectomy (see Figs. 54.12 and 54.14).

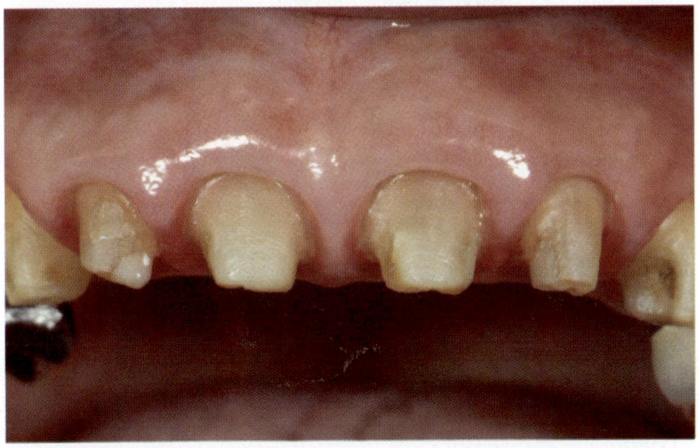

Fig. 54.14 At 6 weeks after the gingivectomy and preparation of the teeth. Note the tissue level and that the tissue is rebounding coronally over the margins. This is a common finding when a pure gingivectomy is done.

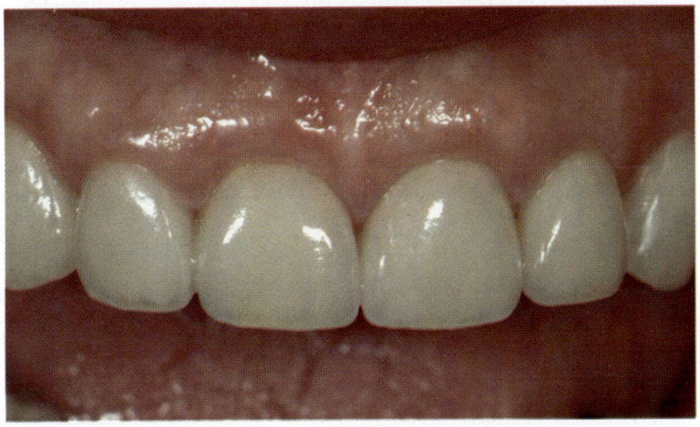

Fig. 54.15 A 4-year recall photograph after placement of the final restorations for patient in Fig. 54.11. Note the tissue level has been maintained, with a sulcus depth of 2 mm on the facial surface.

adversely affect the stability of the tissue level around the tooth. Access to the margin is also required for the final impression, with a clean, fluid-controlled environment. Tissue management is achieved with gingival retraction cords using the appropriate size to achieve the displacement required. Thin, fragile gingival tissues and shallow sulcus situations usually dictate that smaller diameter cords be chosen to achieve the desired tissue displacement.

For a Rule 1 margin (sulcus depth 1.5 mm or less), the cord should be placed so that the top of the cord is located in the sulcus at the level in which the final margin is to be established, which will be 0.5 mm below the previously prepared margin (Fig. 54.16). On the interproximal aspects of the tooth, the cord is usually 1.0–1.5 mm below the tissue height because the interproximal sulcus is often 2.5–3.0 mm in depth. With this initial cord in place, the preparation is extended to the top of the cord, with the bur angled to the tooth so that it does not abrade the tissue (Fig. 54.17). This process protects the tissue, creates the correct axial reduction, and establishes the margin at the desired subgingival level. To create space and allow access for a final impression, it is now necessary to pack a second retraction cord. The second cord is pushed so that it displaces the first cord apically and sits between the margin and the tissue (Fig. 54.18). For the final impression, only the top cord is removed, leaving the margins visible and accessible to be recorded with the impression material (Fig. 54.19). The initial cord remains in place in the sulcus until the provisional restoration is completed.

As an alternative to additional retraction cords, electrosurgery can be used to remove any overlying tissue in the retraction process. A fine-wire electrode tip is held parallel to the tooth and against the margin in the sulcus and moved through the overhanging tissue, opening up the margin and the retraction cord to visual access (Figs. 54.20–54.23). The electrosurgery tip sits on top of the retraction cord in place in the sulcus. This controls the vertical position of the tip and results in the removal of the least tissue needed for access.

For Rule 2 situations in which the sulcus is deeper, two larger diameter cords are used to deflect the tissue before extending the margin apically (Figs. 54.24–54.26). The top of the second cord is placed to identify the final margin location at the correct distance below the previously prepared margin, which was at the gingival tissue crest level. The margin is lowered to the top of the second cord (Fig. 54.27), then a third cord is placed in preparation for the impression (Figs. 54.28 and 54.29). In the patient with a deep sulcus in which the margin may be 1.5–2.0 mm below the tissue crest, electrosurgery is often required to remove overhanging tissue. To avoid altering the gingival tissue height, it is important to hold the electrosurgery tip parallel to the preparation (Fig. 54.30).

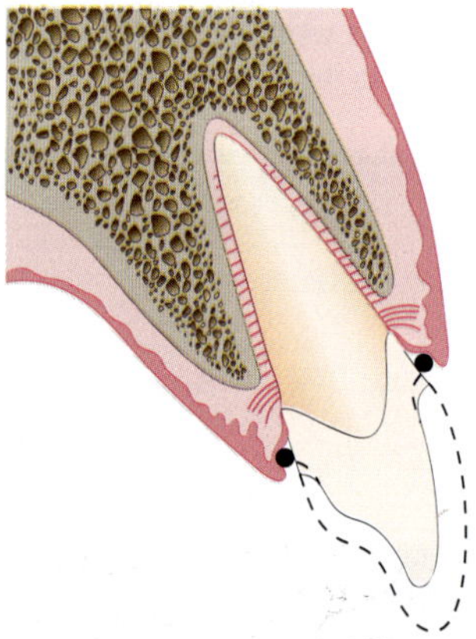

Fig. 54.16 Second step in margin placement. This step includes placing a single layer of deflection cord below the previously prepared margin to the desired final margin level. Here, a single cord has been placed 0.5 mm below the previously prepared margin.

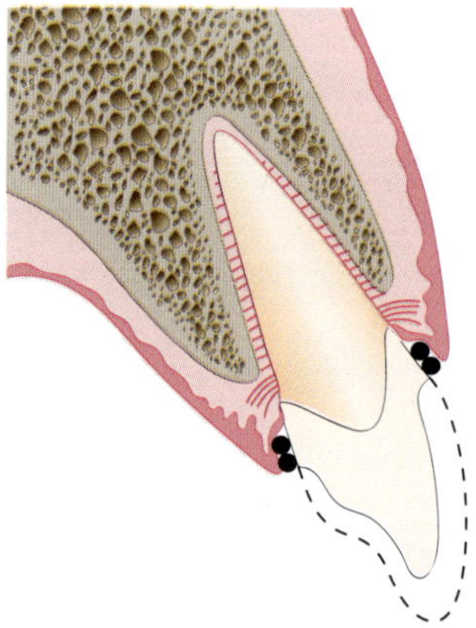

Fig. 54.18 Placing a second impression cord on top of the first deflection cord to provide space for impression material. This impression cord is placed so that it is between the margin of the preparation and the gingiva to create adequate space for impression material after removal of the cord.

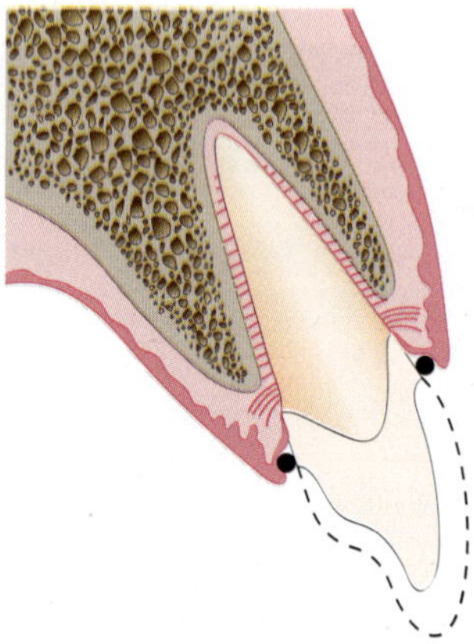

Fig. 54.17 Margin of the preparation extended apically to the top of the retraction cord. This represents the correct placement of the margin below the previously nonreflected, free gingival margin.

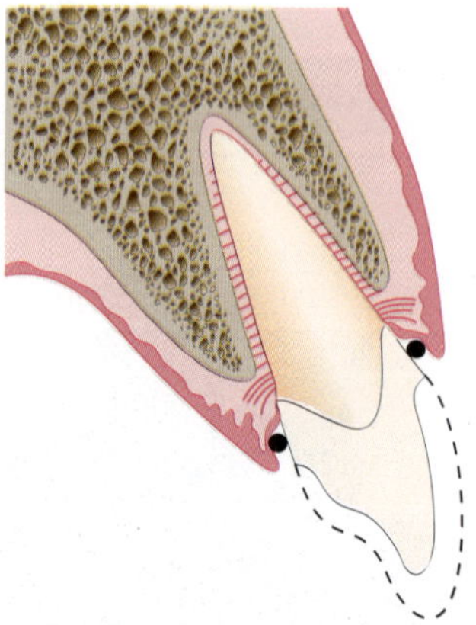

Fig. 54.19 Ideal situation after removal of impression cord. The deflection cord is still in place maintaining the open sulcus but has been displaced apically another 0.5 mm by the placement of the impression cord, exposing tooth structure apical to the margin so that it can be captured in the impression.

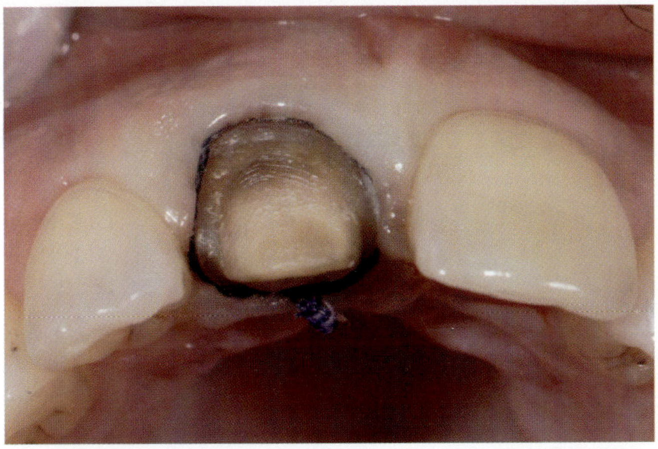

Fig. 54.20 Deflection cord and impression cord are in place. The soft tissue is falling over the margins of the preparation. In this situation, if the impression cord were removed, the impression would not capture the margins in the areas in which the tissue is overhanging.

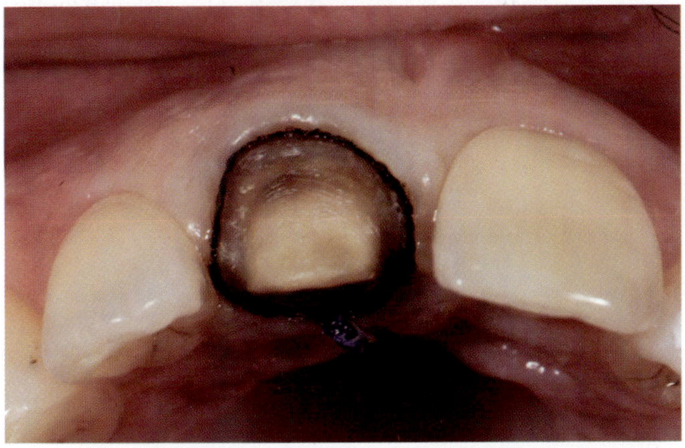

Fig. 54.21 Overhanging tissue has been removed and space created for the impression material with electrosurgery. Note that the deflection cord and the impression cord are still in place. The impression cord is now visible completely around the tooth, allowing easy access for the impression material to the margin after removal of the impression cord.

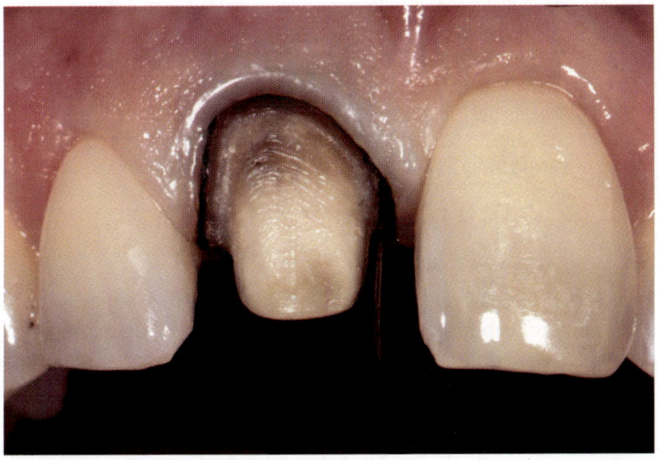

Fig. 54.22 Using electrosurgery, the fine-wire electrode tip held parallel to the tooth preparation and rests on the cord as the tip is moved around the tooth.

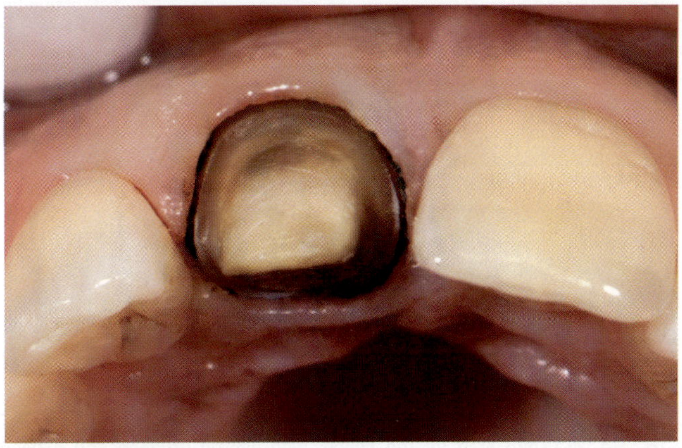

Fig. 54.23 After removal of the impression cord, an adequate space is created for the impression material, with no soft tissue overhanging the margins to trap or tear the impression material. Note the first cord, or deflection cord, is still in place.

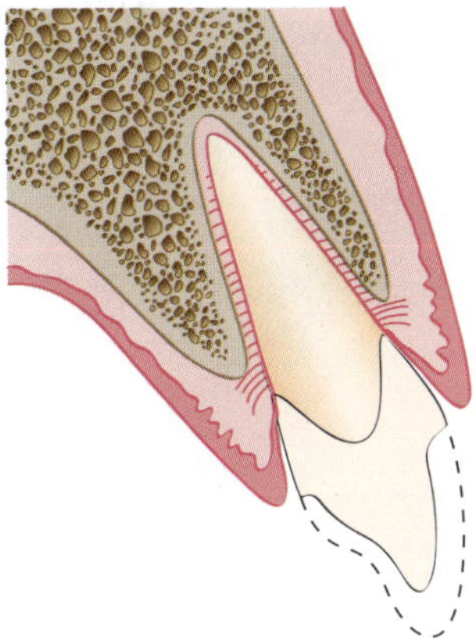

Fig. 54.24 First step in margin placement for the patient with altered eruption or a deep sulcus is to prepare to the existing free gingival margin, as in the "Rule 1" patient (see text).

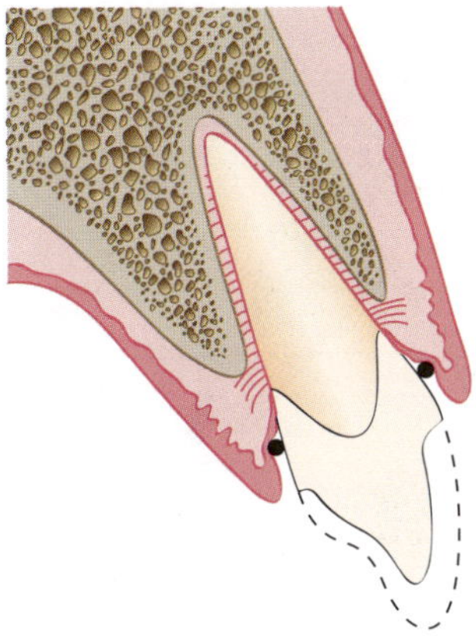

Fig. 54.25 Second step for the patient with altered eruption is to place the deflection cord. Note that the placement of a single deflection cord does not provide adequate deflection of the tissue to allow the margin to be carried below tissue without abrading the gingiva with the bur.

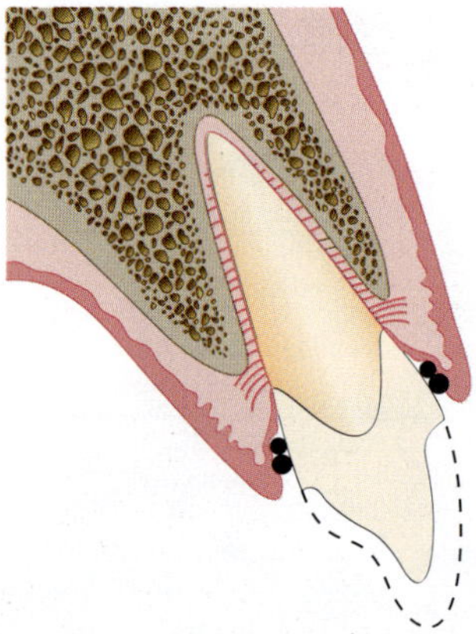

Fig. 54.26 Third step for the patient with altered eruption and a deep sulcus is to place a second, larger diameter deflection cord on top of the first deflection cord. Combined, these two cords allow adequate deflection to open up the sulcus so that the margin can be carried below tissue without abrading the gingiva.

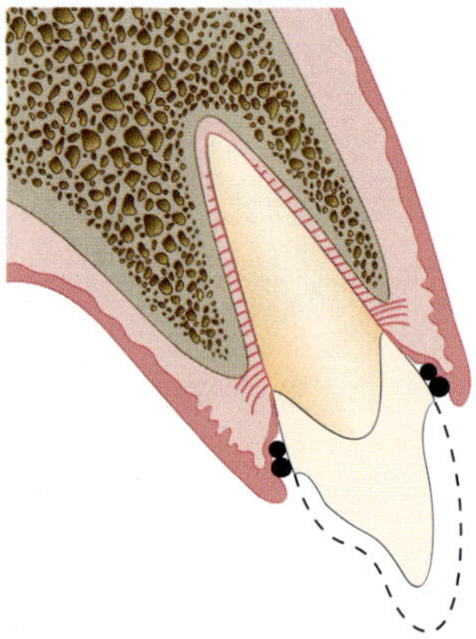

Fig. 54.27 Preparation is now extended to the top of the second deflection cord, finalizing margin location.

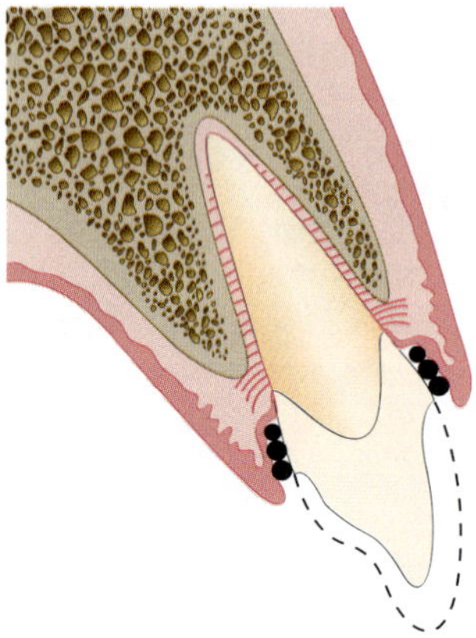

Fig. 54.28 After extension of the margin to the top of the deflection cord, a third layer of cord is applied that will act as the impression cord. This impression cord should be placed so that it fits between the free gingival margin and the margin of the preparation. Its placement will also apically displace the two previously positioned deflection cords.

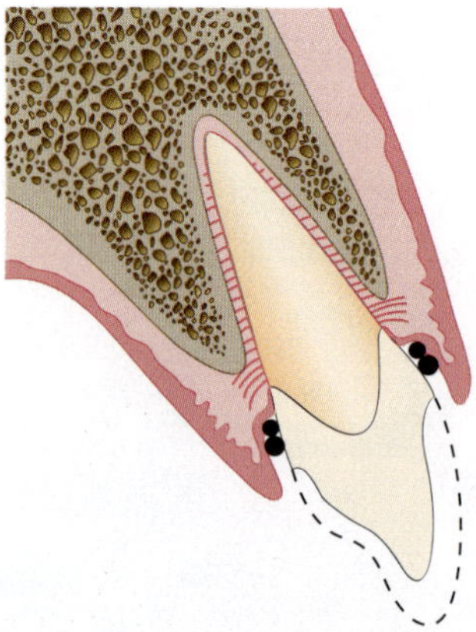

Fig. 54.29 Removal of the impression cord creates an adequate space for the impression material to capture the margin and 0.5 mm of tooth structure below the margin in which the impression cord had displaced the first two cords.

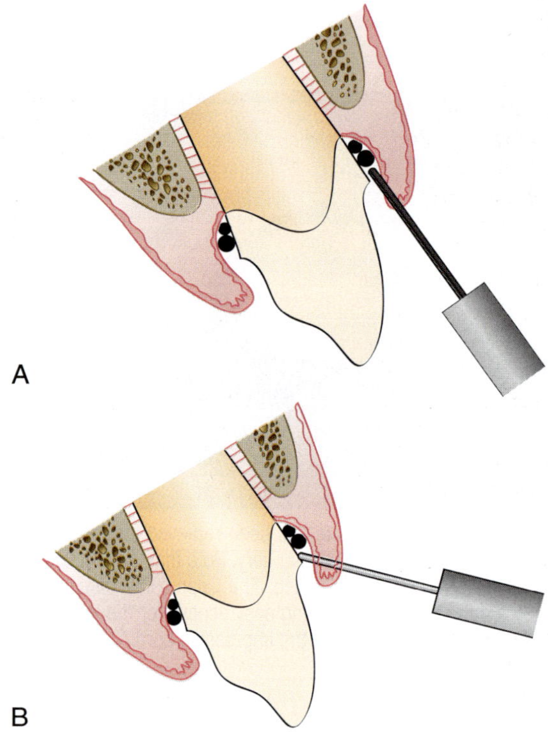

Fig. 54.30 If it is necessary to use electrosurgery, either in the normal or altered-eruption patient, the correct inclination of the electrosurgery tip is important. A, Electrosurgery tip being held parallel to the preparation and resting on the previously placed retraction cord. This removes a minimal amount of tissue, and the presence of the retraction cord protects the attachment from the electrosurgery. B, Incorrect inclination of electrosurgery tip. The tip is leaning away from the preparation. This inclination results in excess tissue removal.

Provisional Restorations

Three critical areas must be effectively managed to produce a favorable biologic response to provisional restorations. The marginal fit, crown contour, and surface finish of the interim restorations must be appropriate to maintain the health and position of the gingival tissues during the interval until the final restorations are delivered. Provisional restorations that are poorly adapted at the margins, that are overcontoured or undercontoured, and that have rough or porous surfaces can cause inflammation, overgrowth, or recession of gingival tissues. The outcome can be unpredictable, and unfavorable changes in the tissue architecture can compromise the success of the final restoration.

Marginal Fit

Marginal fit has clearly been implicated in producing an inflammatory response in the periodontium. It has been shown that the level of gingival inflammation can increase corresponding with the level of marginal opening. Margins that are significantly open (several tenths of a millimeter) are capable of harboring large numbers of bacteria and may be responsible for the inflammatory response seen. However, the quality of marginal finish and the margin location relative to the attachment are much more critical to the periodontium than the difference between a 20- and a 100-μm fit.

Restoration Contour

Restoration contour has been described as extremely important to the maintenance of periodontal health. Ideal contour provides access for hygiene, has the fullness to create the desired gingival form, and has a pleasing visual tooth contour in esthetic areas. Evidence from human and animal studies clearly demonstrates a relationship between overcontouring and gingival inflammation, whereas undercontouring produces no adverse periodontal effect. The most frequent cause of overcontoured restorations is inadequate tooth preparation by the dentist, which forces the technician to produce a bulky restoration to provide room for the restorative material. In areas of the mouth in which esthetic considerations are not critical, a flatter contour is always acceptable.

Subgingival Debris

Leaving debris below the tissue during restorative procedures can create an adverse periodontal response. The cause can be retraction cord, impression material, provisional material, or either temporary or permanent cement. The diagnosis of debris as the cause of gingival inflammation can be confirmed by examining the sulcus surrounding the restoration with an explorer, removing any foreign bodies, and then monitoring the tissue response. It may be necessary to provide tissue anesthesia for patient comfort during the procedure.

Hypersensitivity to Dental Materials

Inflammatory gingival responses have been reported related to the use of nonprecious alloys in dental restorations. Typically, the responses have occurred to alloys containing nickel although the frequency of these occurrences is controversial. Hypersensitivity responses to precious alloys are extremely rare, and these alloys provide an easy solution to the problems encountered with the nonprecious alloys. More importantly, tissues respond more to the differences in surface roughness of the material rather than to the composition of the material. The rougher the surface of the restoration subgingivally, the greater are the plaque accumulation and gingival inflammation. In clinical research, porcelain, highly polished gold, and highly polished resin all show similar plaque accumulation. Regardless of the restorative material selected, a smooth surface is essential on all materials subgingivally.

Esthetic Tissue Management

Managing Interproximal Embrasures

Current restorative and periodontal therapy must consider a good esthetic result, especially in the maxillary anterior "esthetic zone." The interproximal papilla is a very important part in creating this esthetic result. The interproximal embrasure created by restorations and the form of the interdental papilla have a unique and intimate relationship. The ideal interproximal embrasure should house the gingival papilla without impinging on it and should also extend the interproximal tooth contact to the top of the papilla so that no excess space exists to trap food and to be esthetically displeasing.

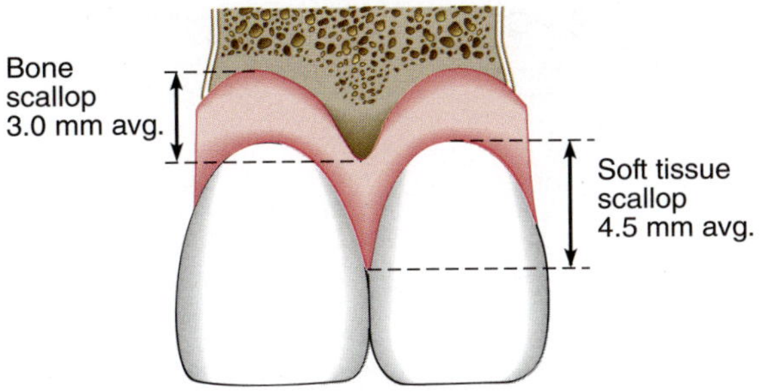

Fig. 54.31 Comparison of the behavior of the interproximal papilla relative to bone and the free gingival margin relative to bone in the average human. There is a 3-mm scallop from the facial bone to the interproximal bone. However, on average, a 4.5- to 5.0-mm gingival scallop exists between the facial tissue height and the interproximal papilla height. This extra scallop of 1.5–2.0 mm of gingiva compared to bone is the result of the extra soft-tissue height above the attachment interproximally.

Papillary height is established by the level of the bone, the biologic width, and the form of the gingival embrasure. Changes in the shape of the embrasure can impact the height and form of the papilla. The tip of the papilla behaves differently than the free gingival margin on the facial aspect of the tooth. The free gingival margin averages 3 mm above the underlying facial bone, whereas the tip of the papilla averages 4.5–5.0 mm above the interproximal bone (Fig. 54.31). This means that if the papilla is farther above the bone than the facial tissue but has the same biologic width, the interproximal area will have a sulcus 1.0–1.5 mm deeper than that found on the facial surface.

When the gingival level of the interproximal tooth contacts measured 5 mm or less to the alveolar bone, the papilla always filled the space. When the contact was 6 mm from bone, only 56% of the papillae could fill the space. Finally, when the contact was 7 mm from bone, only 37% of the papillae could fill the spaces.

Knowing that there is individual variability to the required biologic width, this information relative to the papilla is applied by locating the lowest point of the interproximal contact in relation to the top of the epithelial attachment. The ideal contact should be 2–3 mm coronal to the attachment, which coincides with the depth of the average interproximal sulcus. As in assessing the facial tissues for margin location, this technique requires that the tissue is healthy to allow accurate probing. If the sulcus measures greater than 3 mm, there is some risk of papillary recession with restorative procedures.

The clinician most frequently confronts a normal or shallow sulcus with a papilla that appears too short rather than a tall papilla with a deep sulcus. Management of this situation is best approached by viewing the papilla as a balloon of a certain volume that sits on the attachment. This balloon of tissue has a form and height dictated by the gingival embrasure of the teeth. With an embrasure that is too wide, the balloon flattens out, assumes a blunted shape, and has a shallow sulcus (Fig. 54.32).

If the embrasure is the ideal width, the papilla assumes a pointed form, has a sulcus of 2.5–3.0 mm, and is healthy. If the embrasure is too narrow, the papilla may grow out to the facial and lingual, form a col, and become inflamed. This information is applied when evaluating an individual papilla with an open embrasure. The papilla in question is compared to the adjacent papillae. If the papillae are all on the same level, and if the other areas do not have open embrasures, the problem is one of gingival embrasure form. If the

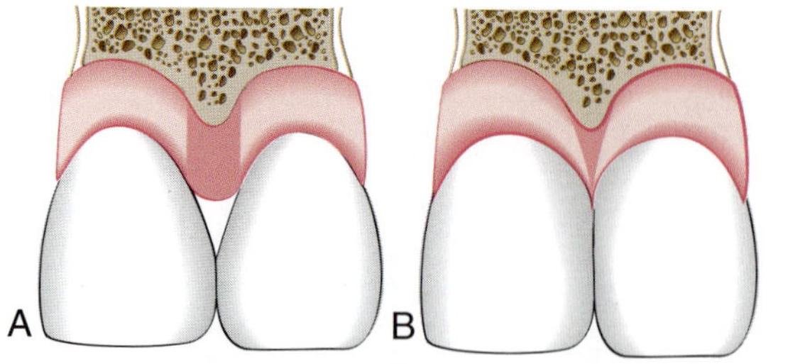

Fig. 54.32 Relationship between gingival embrasure volume and papillary form. A, Gingival embrasure of the teeth is excessively large as the result of a tapered tooth form. Because of the large embrasure form, the volume of tissue sitting on top of the attachment is not molded to the shape of a normal papilla but rather has a blunted form and a shallower sulcus. B, Ideal tooth form in which the same volume of tissue sits on top of the attachment as in A. Because of the more closed embrasure form from the teeth in B, however, the papilla completely fills the embrasure and has a deeper sulcus, averaging 2.5–3.0 mm. Note that the ideal contact position is 3 mm coronal to the attachment.

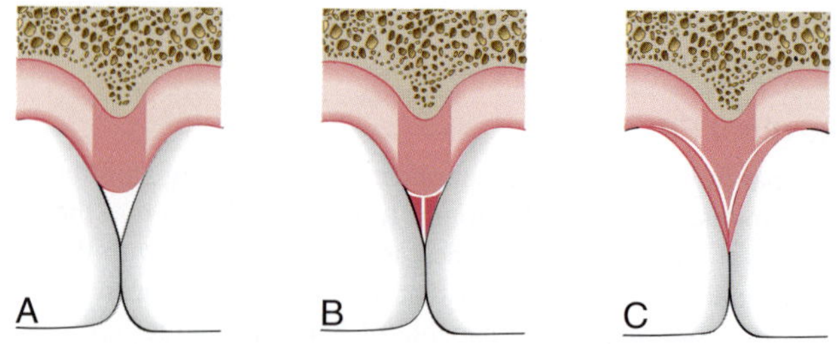

Fig. 54.33 Methods of altering gingival embrasure form. A, Typical open gingival embrasure caused by excessively tapered tooth form. B, Common method employed by restorative dentists to correct the embrasure, in which material is added supragingivally. This closes the embrasure by moving the contact to the tip of the papilla but results in overhangs that cannot be cleaned using dental floss. Removing these overhangs restoratively reopens the embrasure. C, Correct method of closing the gingival embrasure, in which the margins of the restoration are carried 1.0–1.5 mm below the tip of the papilla. Note that this does not encroach on the attachment because the average interproximal sulcus probes 2.5–3.0 mm. This allows easy cleaning because of the convex profile. It also reshapes the papilla to a more pleasing profile esthetically.

papilla in the area of concern is apical to the adjacent papillae, however, the clinician should evaluate the interproximal bone levels. If the bone under that papilla is apical to the adjacent bone levels, the problem is caused by bone loss. If the bone is at the same level, the open embrasure is caused by the embrasure form of the teeth and not a periodontal problem with the papilla.

Correcting Open Gingival Embrasures Restoratively

There are two causes of open gingival embrasures: (1) the papilla is inadequate in height because of bone loss or (2) the interproximal contact is located too high coronally. If a high contact has been diagnosed as the cause of the problem, there are two potential reasons. If the root angulation of the teeth diverges, the interproximal contact is moved coronally, resulting in the open embrasure. However, if the roots are parallel, the papilla form is normal, and an open embrasure exists, then the problem is probably related to tooth shape, specifically an excessively tapered form. Restorative dentistry can correct this problem by moving the contact point to the tip of the papilla. To accomplish this, the margins of the restoration must be carried subgingivally 1.0–1.5 mm, and the emergence profile of the restoration is designed to move the contact point toward the papilla while blending the contour into the tooth below the tissue (Fig. 54.33). This can be accomplished easily with direct bonded restorations because the soft tissue can clearly be seen. For indirect restorations, the desired restoration contours and embrasure form should be established in the provisional restorations, and the gingival tissues are allowed to adapt for 4–6 weeks before the tissue contour information is relayed to the laboratory for use in the final restorations.

Managing Gingival Embrasure Form for Patients With Gingival Recession

Management of the gingival embrasure form for patients who have experienced gingival recession varies, depending on whether the treatment is in the anterior or posterior regions of the mouth. In esthetic areas, it is necessary to carry the interproximal contacts apically toward the papilla to eliminate the presence of large, open embrasures. With multiple-unit restorations, it is also possible with tissue-colored ceramics to bake porcelain papillae directly on the restoration. In the posterior areas where the interroot widths are significantly greater, it is often impossible to carry the proximal contacts to contact the tissue without creating large overhangs on the restorations. In these situations, the contact should be moved far enough apically to minimize any large food traps while still leaving an embrasure of a convenient size to be accessed with an interdental brush for hygiene. It should be noted that developing excessively long interproximal contacts, whether on anterior or posterior teeth, always creates rectangular, somewhat unesthetic, tooth forms.

Pontic Design

Classically, there are four options to consider in evaluating pontic design: sanitary, ridge-lap, modified ridge-lap, and ovate designs (Fig. 54.34). Regardless of design, the pontic should provide an occlusal surface that stabilizes the opposing teeth, allows for normal mastication, and does not overload the abutment teeth. The restorative material for all four designs can be glazed porcelain, polished gold, or polished resin. The biologic response of the tissue in contact with the restoration is no different in regard to the material chosen, as long as it has a smooth surface finish.

The key differences between the four pontic designs relate to the esthetics and access for hygiene procedures. The primary method for cleaning the undersurface of pontics is to draw dental floss mesiodistally along the undersurface. The shape of this undersurface determines the ease with which plaque and food debris can be removed in the process. The sanitary and ovate pontics have convex undersurfaces, which makes them easiest to clean. The ridge-lap and modified ridge-lap designs have concave surfaces, which are more difficult to access with the dental floss. Although the sanitary pontic design provides the easiest access for hygiene procedures, it is rarely used because of its unesthetic form and a variable acceptance of the open contour by patients.

The ovate pontic is the ideal pontic form. It is created by forming a receptor site in the edentulous ridge with a diamond bur or by electrosurgery. The site is shaped to create either a flat or a concave contour so that when the pontic is created to adapt to the site, it will have a flat or convex outline. The depth of the receptor site depends on the esthetic requirements of the pontic. In highly esthetic areas such as the maxillary anterior region, it is necessary to create a receptor area that is 1.0–1.5 mm below the tissue on the facial aspect. This creates the appearance of a free gingival margin and produces optimal esthetics (Fig. 55.35). This site can then be tapered to the height of the palatal tissue to facilitate hygiene access from the

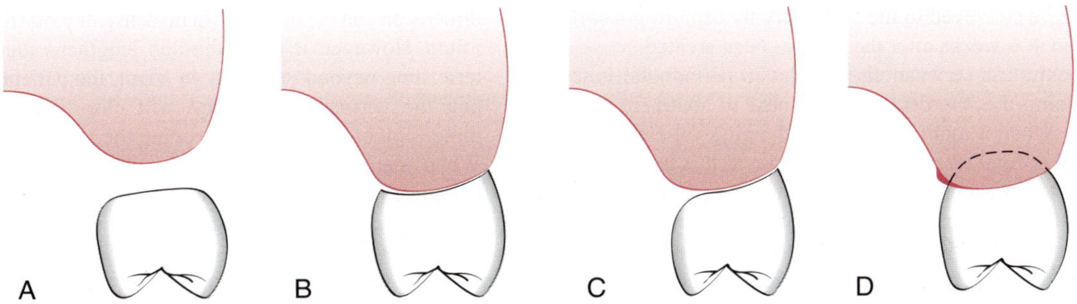

Fig. 54.34 Four options to designing the shape of a pontic. A, Sanitary pontic tissue surface of the pontic is 3 mm from the underlying ridge. B, Ridge-lap pontic. Tissue surface of the pontic straddles the ridge in saddlelike fashion. The entire tissue surface of the ridge-lap pontic is convex and very difficult to clean. C, Modified ridge-lap pontic. Tissue surface on the facial is concave, following the ridge. However, the lingual saddle has been removed to allow access for oral hygiene. D, Ovate pontic. The pontic form fits into a receptor site within the ridge. This allows the tissue surface of the pontic to be convex and also optimizes esthetics.

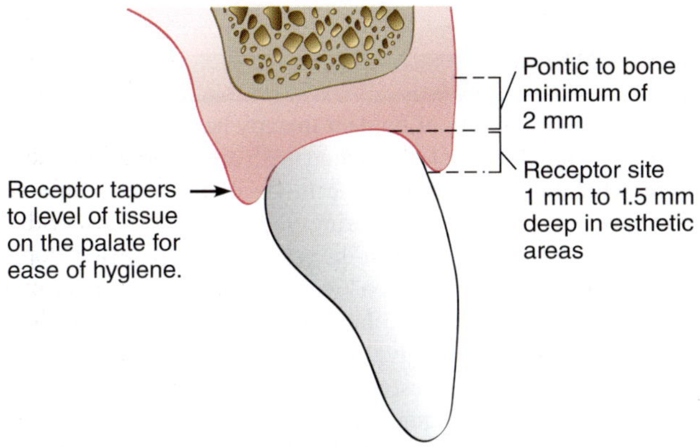

Fig. 54.35 Ideal shape and form of an ovate pontic in the esthetic area. The receptor site has been created 1.0–1.5 mm apical to the free gingival margin on the facial aspect. This creates the illusion of the pontic erupting from the tissue. On the palatal side, the pontic is tapered so that the receptor site is not extended below tissue; this allows easier access for oral hygiene. Note that when the receptor site is created, the bone must be a minimum of 2 mm from the most apical portion of the pontic.

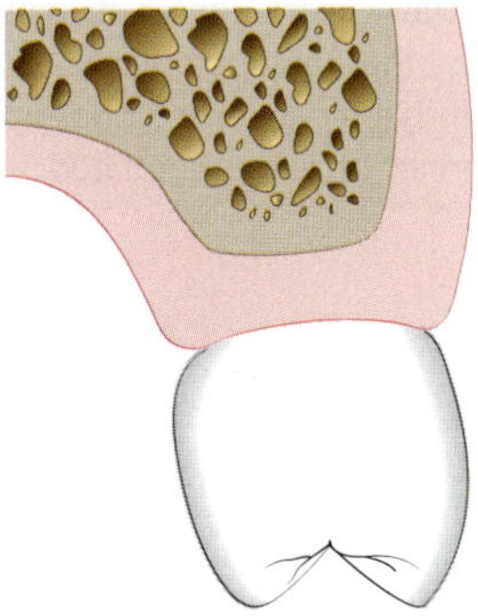

Fig. 54.36 Option for creating an ovate pontic receptor site in less esthetic areas of the mouth. Rather than creating the receptor site so that the pontic extends into the ridge, it is possible to create a flattened receptor site in which the pontic sits flush with the ridge. This facilitates oral hygiene.

palatal side. In the posterior areas, a deep receptor site can complicate hygiene access. In these situations, the ideal site has the facial portion of the pontic at the same level as the ridge, and then the site is created as a straight line to the lingual side of the pontic. This removes the convexity of the ridge and produces a flat, easily cleanable tissue surface on the pontic (Fig. 54.36).

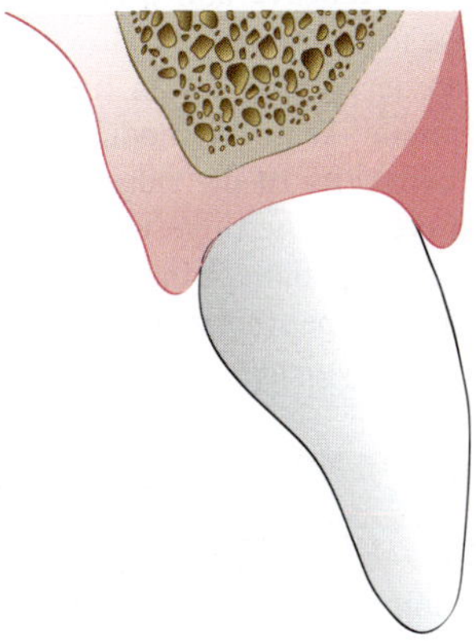

Fig. 54.37 Ridge considerations when an ovate pontic is desired. For an ovate pontic to be properly created, the soft-tissue ridge must be labial to the desired cervical portion of the pontic. When the pontic is facial to the ridge, it is not possible to create what appears to be a "free gingival margin" correctly. The shaded area represents the necessary amount of tissue that would be augmented to produce an ideal ovate pontic in this particular site.

Ridge Modification Procedures for Ideal Pontic Contours

When the ridge is being surgically modified, it is important to know the thickness of soft tissue above the bone. This measurement is obtained by probing to the bone through the anesthetized tissue. If the tissue is removed to less than 2 mm in thickness, significant rebound in ridge height may occur. If it is necessary to reduce the tissue height to less than 2 mm above the bone to create the desired pontic form, some bone will need to be removed to achieve the desired result.

It is important when considering an ovate pontic to realize that certain soft-tissue ridge parameters must exist to optimize the ovate pontic form. First, the ridge height needs to match the ideal height of the interproximal papillae where interproximal embrasures are planned, either between pontics or next to abutment teeth. Second, the gingival margin height must also be at the ideal level, or the pontic will appear too long. Third, the ridge tissue must be facial to the ideal cervical facial form of the pontic so that the pontic can emerge from the tissue. If any of these three areas is inadequate, some form of ridge augmentation is needed to produce a ridge that can have an adequate receptor site created (Fig. 54.37). Any ridge augmentation procedures should be completed before, or in conjunction with, fabricating an ovate pontic. When constructing the final restorations, the contours of the developed ovate pontic receptor site can be conveyed to the laboratory by capturing a soft-tissue impression 4–6 weeks after the site has been created.

The ovate pontic can serve another important periodontal function by maintaining the interdental papilla next to abutment teeth after extraction. When a tooth is removed, the gingival embrasure form is lost. The normal response of the papilla to this loss of embrasure form is to recede 1.5–2.0 mm, which corresponds to the additional soft tissue that exists above bone on the interproximal versus the facial aspect. However, this recession can be prevented. By inserting the correct pontic form 2.5 mm into the extraction site the day the tooth is removed, the gingival embrasure form and papilla can be maintained. At 4 weeks, the 2.5-mm extension can be reduced to a 1.0–1.5 mm extension to facilitate hygiene. This procedure can maintain the papilla next to the abutment teeth as long as the bone on the abutment tooth is at a normal level.

The "full ridge-lap pontic" is an outdated design that straddles the convexity of the ridge buccolingually and creates an undersurface that is entirely concave and cannot be cleaned. It is not recommended for use in any situations. However, a *modified ridge-lap pontic* can be an acceptable design if inadequate ridge exists to create an ovate pontic. With the modified ridge-lap design, the pontic follows the convexity of the ridge on the facial aspect but stops on the lingual crest of the ridge without extending down the lingual side of the ridge. Although the facial aspect of the undersurface has a concave shape, the more open lingual form allows adequate access for oral hygiene.

Occlusal Considerations in Restorative Therapy

Occlusion plays an important role in restorative dentistry. The increased use of dental implants and nonmetallic cosmetic restorations has resulted in greater concern over force management. These restorations are more sensitive to occlusal trauma, with subsequent structural failure, than are traditional restorations on teeth. Consequently, for the restorative dentist wanting a high degree of predictability in the final result, understanding occlusion is critical. The clinician must know how to create an occlusion, with the following guidelines as a goal:

1. There should be even, simultaneous contacts on all teeth during centric closure. This distributes the force of closure over all the teeth instead of the few teeth that may touch first.
2. When the mandible moves from centric closure, some form of canine or anterior guidance is desirable, with no posterior tooth contacts. This combination of anterior guidance and posterior disclusion reduces the ability of the elevator muscles to contract and distributes the force of the movement onto the anterior teeth, which receive less force because of the Class-III lever system being applied in this situation. It has been shown that, as a result of the Class-III lever action, the anterior teeth receive approximately one-ninth the force of a second molar.
3. The anterior guidance needs to be in harmony with the patient's neuromuscular envelope of function. Harmony of this relationship is demonstrated by a lack of fremitus and mobility on the anterior teeth, by the ability of the patient to speak clearly and comfortably, and by the patient's general sense of comfort with the overbite, overjet, and guidance created during chewing and when holding the head upright.
4. The occlusion should be created at a vertical dimension that is stable for the patient. It is generally accepted that the patient's existing vertical dimension is at equilibrium between the eruptive forces of the teeth and the repetitive contracted length of the elevator muscles. It has been demonstrated that vertical dimension can be altered with no sense of pain from muscles and joints. However, if this alteration lengthens the pterygomasseteric sling beyond its ability to adapt, the patient will not maintain the vertical change and will close the occlusal vertical dimension back down by intruding the teeth.
5. When managing a pathologic occlusion or when restoring a complete occlusion, the clinician needs to work with a repeatable condylar reference position. Centric relation, defined as the most superior condylar position, provides such a starting point. Centric relation has been shown to be reproducible over multiple appointments, allowing the clinician to create the occlusion indirectly on an articulator and return it to the same reference position in the mouth. It is the only position that has been shown to shut off lateral pterygoid muscle contraction. Because it is a border position, any mandibular movement will result in the condyle moving inferiorly. Therefore, centric relation is the only position from which an interference-free occlusion can be created.

Root-Resected Teeth

Although the availability of implant therapy has greatly reduced the frequency with which root-amputated teeth are saved, restoration of root-resected teeth is still a viable mode of treatment. Structural challenges are created in restoring these teeth because of the amount of tooth structure lost in the resection process (Fig. 54.38). Conservative tooth preparation will maintain as much of the remaining tooth as possible, but the resulting supragingival or minimally prepared subgingival finish lines will require additional metal display in the final restoration. A cast post and core may be indicated to create an adequate foundation for the final restoration. Because the remaining roots are often very thin mesiodistally, it is difficult to cement premade posts and have adequate bulk to place a foundation core on the mesial and distal surfaces of the post. This problem is avoided with the one-piece cast post and core restoration. Another area of concern when restoring root-resected teeth is the development of appropriate contours for hygiene access. The primary concern is to avoid any excessively heavy convexities of contour that would prevent access. Facially and lingually, the contours should be essentially a straight line from the margin coronally, while interproximally, the contour emerges from the margin as a straight line or is slightly convex as it slopes up to the contact point. The interproximal areas of root-amputated and hemisected teeth

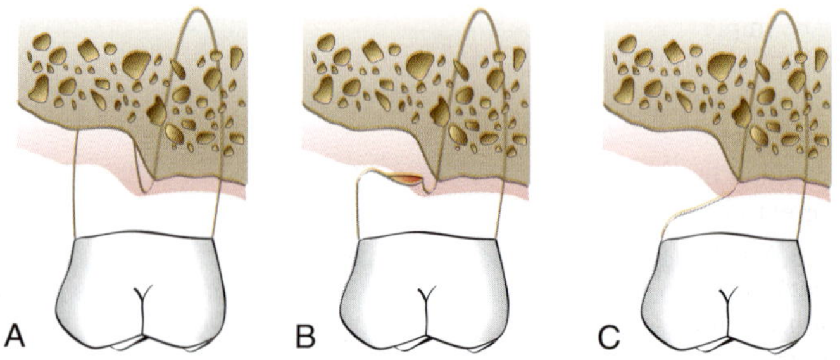

Fig. 54.38 A, Maxillary molar with a class III furcation and bone loss surrounding the distal buccal root. B, Contour created when the distal buccal root is removed, but the coronal contour has not yet been reshaped. Note the overhang, which can trap food and plaque and create gingival inflammation. C, Correct contour after the restoration or reshaping of the tooth. Note this illustration is only of the facial portion of the tooth. The palatal portion of the crown and the palatal root do not appear. Note how the contour has been altered to allow easy access for an interdental brush to the gingival tissue and the tooth in the area in which the root was removed.

often present with surface concavities on the root trunk, and these areas cannot be adequately cleaned with floss because it will bridge across the concavity. The gingival embrasure form created in the restoration must be fluted into these areas so that the surfaces can be accessed with an interdental brush.

Esthetics is usually not a major concern unless the tooth in question is a maxillary molar with a mesiobuccal root amputation and the patient has a broad smile. The solution is to create an artificial mesiobuccal root with normal crown contour coronal to it and a furcation made of restorative material that is easily cleanable with an interdental brush.

Special Restorative Considerations

Splinting

Splinting therapy may be applied with bonded external appliances, intracoronal appliances, or indirect cast restorations to connect multiple teeth, with the goal of improving tooth stability. Unstable teeth may be caused by a lack of periodontal support from bone loss, a lack of support from tooth loss, or the need to splint abutment teeth to support pontics. Indications for splinting are (1) mobility of teeth that is increasing or that impairs patient comfort, (2) migration of teeth, and (3) **prosthetics** in which multiple abutments are necessary.

Before considering splinting, the clinician must identify the etiology of the instability. Excessive occlusal forces from parafunction or deflective tooth contacts are frequent causes of excessive mobility. Whenever the occlusion is the cause, occlusal therapy is always performed first. The mobility is then evaluated over time to determine if it resolves before splinting is considered. In addition, any inflammation of the periodontal supporting apparatus must be controlled before making a decision on splinting because inflammation can produce mobility in the presence of normal occlusal forces and normal periodontal support. When the teeth are splinted, all the teeth in the splint share the occlusal load to some extent. The rigidity of the splint and the number of teeth used determine how the forces are distributed.

The most common indication to splint mobile teeth is to improve patient comfort and to provide better control of the occlusion. If the anterior teeth are mobile, adequate crown length on the teeth being splinted is critical so that the interproximal connectors do not impinge on the interdental papilla. Also, adequate space must exist between the connector and the papilla for access with dental floss anteriorly and with an interproximal brush on posterior teeth.

Anterior Esthetic Surgery

The importance of gingiva in relation to anterior esthetics has been well documented. Various methods for altering gingival levels have been described, including gingivectomy, apically positioned flaps with osseous recontouring, and the use of orthodontic therapy to position the gingival tissue level apically or coronally by intruding or extruding the teeth

Whenever an alteration in gingival levels is contemplated, the expected outcome must be communicated to the patient to determine if the planned surgery is acceptable. A wide variety of computer design and virtual imaging programs can be used to provide the patient with a visual plan for the final esthetic result. Digital design can be converted into three-dimensional (3D)-printed wax-up, or a conventional stone model wax-up may be used to confirm the desired final outcome. However, this design process may not allow the dentist or patient to include the dynamics of lip movement in the evaluation of the proposed changes.

When the surgery will involve many or all of the anterior teeth and will result in moving gingiva several millimeters, to the extent that a flap will be raised and bony levels altered, an esthetic template guide is desirable. Before constructing the guide, treatment planning is completed as described above to determine the desired incisal edge position and the desired gingival level of the tissues. This will establish the amount of tooth display at rest and at full smile. For a patient who is undergoing both periodontal and restorative esthetic procedures to change the architecture of the smile, this step is critical.

Once the conventional or digital wax-up is completed and accepted by the patient, a mock-up procedure using composite or acrylic resin may be performed using direct putty technique to evaluate intraorally the desired incisal edge position. From there, the gingival positions are confirmed and an esthetic template guide can be made on the patient's initial cast to be used at the time of surgery. This guide can be made of either clear thermoplastic material or the same composite or acrylic used for the mock-up.

When the patient approves the gingival levels established with the guide, the desired gingival correction can be completed using the esthetic guide as a surgical template. In addition to locating the initial incisions at the correct level, the guide can also be employed after flap reflection to aid in the bony recontouring to ensure adequate supracrestal attached tissue and sulcus depth at the new gingival position. The surgeon replaces the flap at closure to the gingival level established with the guide. Employing an esthetic template in this manner optimizes the predictability of the surgical therapy and establishes the ideal tissue framework to complete the esthetic restorations. It is also common practice to place provisionals at the time of suturing/surgery to guide healing and maintain tissue levels. Absolute care and attention to detail must be paid to ensure highly polished, closed margins on provisionals.

Conclusion

The therapeutic goals of patient comfort, function, esthetics, predictability, longevity, and ease of restorative and maintenance care are attainable only by a carefully constructed interdisciplinary approach, with accurate diagnosis and comprehensive treatment planning serving as cornerstones. The complex interaction between periodontal therapy and successful restorative dentistry only serves to underscore this premise.

Key points

- To maintain or enhance the patient's esthetic appearance, the tooth–tissue interface must present a healthy natural appearance, with gingival tissues framing the restored teeth in a harmonious manner.
- Periodontal treatment is undertaken before restorative dentistry to ensure the establishment of stable gingival margins before tooth preparation.
- The preparation of the periodontium for restorative dentistry can be divided into two phases: (1) control of periodontal inflammation with nonsurgical and surgical approaches and (2) preprosthetic periodontal surgery.
- The dimension of space that the healthy gingival tissues occupy between the base of the sulcus and the underlying alveolar bone comprises the junctional epithelial attachment and the connective tissue attachment. The combined attachment width is now identified as suprcrestal tissue attachment (biologic width).
- The connective tissue attachment occupies 1.07 mm of space above the crest of the alveolar bone and that the junctional epithelial attachment below the base of the gingival sulcus occupies another 0.97 mm of space giving a biological width of 2.04 mm.

- The biologic or attachment width can be identified for the individual patient by probing to the bone level (referred to as "sounding to bone") and subtracting the sulcus depth from the resulting measurement.
- In highly esthetic areas, such as the maxillary anterior region, it is necessary to create a receptor area that is 1.0–1.5 mm below the tissue on the facial aspect. This creates the appearance of a free gingival margin and produces optimal esthetics.
- Occlusion plays an important role in restorative dentistry. There should be even, simultaneous contacts on all teeth during centric closure.
- When managing a pathologic occlusion or when restoring a complete occlusion, the clinician needs to work with a repeatable condylar reference position.
- *Splinting* therapy may be applied with bonded external appliances, intracoronal appliances, or indirect cast restorations to connect multiple teeth, with the goal of improving tooth stability.

MCQs

MCQs with answers for the chapter are available on www.medenact.com.

Suggested Readings

Camargo PM, Melnick PR, Camargo LM: Clinical crown lengthening in the esthetic zone, *J Calif Dent Assoc* 35(7):487–498, 2007.

Felton DA, Kanoy Be, Bayne SC, et al: Effect of in vivo crown margin discrepancies on periodontal health, *J Prosthet Dent* 65:357, 1991.

Fradeani M: *Esthetic rehabilitation in fixed prosthodontics, volume 2: prosthetic treatment: a systematic approach to esthetic, biologic, and functional integration*, Chicago, 2004, Quintessence.

Gracis S, Fradeani M, Celletti R, et al: Biological integration of esthetic restorations: factors influencing appearance and long-term success, *Periodontol 2000* 27:29–44, 2001.

Günay H, Seeger A, Tschernitschek H, et al: Placement of the preparation line and periodontal health: a prospective 2-year clinical study, *Int J Periodont Restor Dent* 20:173, 2000.

Kois JC: The restorative-periodontal interface: biological parameters, *Periodontol 2000* 11:29, 1996.

Kois JC: Clinical techniques in prosthodontics: relationship of the periodontium to impression procedures, *CompendContinEduc Dent* 21:684, 2000.

Kois JC, Spear FM: Periodontal prosthesis: creating successful restorations, *J Am Dent Assoc* 123:108, 1992.

Kokich VG: Esthetics: the orthodontic-periodontic restorative connection, *Semin Orthodont* 2:21, 1996.

Melnick PR, Camargo PM: Alveolar bone reservation following tooth extraction in the esthetic zone. In Fugazzotto P, editor: *Implant and regenerative therapy in dentistry: a guide to decision making*, Hoboken, 2009, Wiley-Blackwell.

Spear FM: Maintenance of the interdental papilla following anterior tooth removal, *Pract Periodontics Aesthet Dent* 11:21, 1999.

Studer S, Zellweger U, Scharer P: The esthetic guidelines of the mucogingival complex for fixed prosthodontics, *Pract Periodontics Aesthet Dent* 8:333, 1996.

Tarnow DP, Magner AW, Fletcher P: The effects of the distance from the contact point to the crest of bone on the presence or absence of the interproximal dental papilla, *J Periodontol* 63:995, 1992.

Vacek JS, Gher ME, Assad DA, et al: The dimensions of the human dentogingival junction, *Int J Periodont Restor Dent* 14:155, 1994.

Van der Veldon U: Regeneration of the interdental soft tissue following denudation procedures, *J Clin Periodontol* 9:455, 1982.

CHAPTER 55

Adjunctive Role of Orthodontic Therapy

F Celenza | VG Kokich† | C Martin | N Ambalavanan

CHAPTER OUTLINE

Orthodontic tooth movement may be of substantial benefit to the adult periorestorative patient. Many adults who seek routine restorative dentistry have problems with tooth malposition, which compromises their ability to clean and maintain their dentition. If these individuals also are susceptible to periodontal disease, tooth malposition may be an exacerbating factor that could cause premature loss of specific teeth.

Orthodontic appliances have become smaller, less noticeable, and easier to maintain during orthodontic therapy. Many adults are taking advantage of the opportunity to have their teeth aligned to improve the esthetics of their smile. Underlying gingival or osseous periodontal defects often can be improved during orthodontic therapy if the orthodontist is aware of the situation and designs the appropriate tooth movement. In addition, implants have become a major part of the treatment plan for many adults with missing teeth. If adjacent teeth have drifted into edentulous spaces, orthodontic therapy is often helpful to provide the ideal amount of space for implants and subsequent restorations.

Benefits of Orthodontic Therapy

Orthodontic therapy can provide several benefits to adult periodontal patients. The following seven factors should be considered:

1. Aligning crowded or malpositioned maxillary or mandibular anterior teeth permits adult patients better access to clean all surfaces of their teeth. This could be a tremendous advantage for patients who are susceptible to periodontal disease or do not have the dexterity to maintain oral hygiene.
2. Vertical orthodontic tooth repositioning can improve certain types of osseous defects in periodontal patients. Often, moving the tooth eliminates the need for resective osseous surgery.
3. Horizontal orthodontic tooth movement undertaken immediately after tooth extraction can counteract the resultant physiologic alveolar ridge contraction, and thus develop an appropriately sized alveolar ridge.
4. Orthodontic treatment can improve the esthetic relationship of the maxillary gingival margins before restorative dentistry. Aligning the gingival margins orthodontically avoids gingival recontouring, which could also entail bone removal and exposure of the roots of the teeth.
5. Orthodontic therapy also benefits the patient with a severe fracture of a maxillary anterior tooth that requires forced eruption to permit adequate restoration of the root. Erupting the root allows the crown preparation to have sufficient resistance form and retention for the final restoration.
6. Orthodontic treatment allows open gingival embrasures to be corrected to regain lost papillae. If open gingival embrasures are located in the maxillary anterior region, this can present an esthetic problem. In most patients, these areas can be corrected with a combination of orthodontic root movement, tooth reshaping, and restoration.
7. Orthodontic treatment could improve adjacent tooth positioning before implant placement or tooth replacement. This is especially true for the patient who has been missing teeth for several years and has drifting and tipping of the adjacent dentition.
8. A common tooth malalignment problem that results in periodontal pockets is the mesially tipped molar. Orthodontic uprighting of tipped molars corrects the deep gingival contours and eliminates or reduces the mesial periodontal pocket (Fig. 55.3).

Effects of Orthodontic Therapy on the Periodontium

A systematic review about the effect of orthodontic treatment on periodontal outcomes concluded that orthodontic treatment with fixed appliances has little to no clinically relevant effect on periodontal clinical attachment levels.

In some patients with poor oral hygiene, the fixed orthodontic appliances may promote gingival enlargement, which further enhances plaque accumulation. In these situations, subgingival instrumentation is indicated to resolve the inflammation, and reinstatement of efficient oral hygiene practices are mandatory. Sometimes the marginal tissues do not revert to their appropriate position with only subgingival instrumentation, and surgical removal of the excessive gingival tissue is needed.

Orthodontic Therapy in Severe Periodontitis Patients

A recent systematic review concluded that in stable, treated stage IV periodontitis patients, orthodontic therapy had no significant impact on periodontal outcomes. In those studies in which periodontal

†Deceased

outcomes were reported before periodontal therapy, combined periodontal and orthodontic therapy had a significant benefit on clinical attachment level, probing pocket depth, and radiographic bone level.

In fact, many clinical studies have clearly shown that with adequate plaque control, orthodontic treatment in patients with a reduced but healthy periodontium achieves the orthodontic objectives without aggravating their periodontal condition, and the risk of periodontal recurrence in these patients had not increased during orthodontic therapy. When periodontal inflammation is not fully controlled during orthodontic treatment, however, these inflammatory processes may accelerate the progression of periodontal destruction, leading to further loss of attachment. The timing of initiating orthodontic treatment after periodontal therapy in periodontitis patients is still controversial. Three main time points were found in the literature: less than 2 weeks, 1–2 months, or more than 3 months after periodontal surgeries. The best results were observed when the active force was applied 2 months after the patients were periodontally controlled.

Preorthodontic Osseous Surgery

The extent of periodontal osseous surgery depends on the type of defect (e.g., crater, hemiseptal defect, three-wall defect, or furcation lesion).

Osseous Craters

An osseous crater is an interproximal, two-wall defect that does not improve with orthodontic treatment. Some shallow craters (4–5 mm pocket) may be maintained nonsurgically during orthodontic treatment. However, if surgical correction is necessary, this type of osseous lesion can easily be eliminated by reshaping the defect and reducing the pocket depth. This in turn enhances the ability to maintain these interproximal areas during orthodontic treatment. The need for surgery is based on the patient's response to initial root planing, the patient's periodontal resistance, the location of the defect, and the predictability of maintaining defects nonsurgically while the patient is wearing orthodontic appliances.

Three-Wall Intrabony Defects

Three-wall osseous defects are amenable to pocket reduction with regenerative periodontal therapy. Bone grafts using either autogenous bone from the surgical site or allografts, along with resorbable membranes, have been successful in regenerating three-wall defects. If the result of periodontal therapy is stable 3–6 months after periodontal surgery (Fig. 55.1), orthodontic treatment may be initiated.

Orthodontic Treatment of Osseous Defects

Hemiseptal Defects

Hemiseptal defects are one- or two-wall osseous defects that often are found around mesially tipped teeth or teeth that have supererupted (Fig. 55.2). Usually, these defects can be eliminated with the appropriate orthodontic treatment. In the case of the tipped tooth, uprighting and eruption of the tooth levels the bony defect. If the tooth is supererupted, intrusion and leveling of

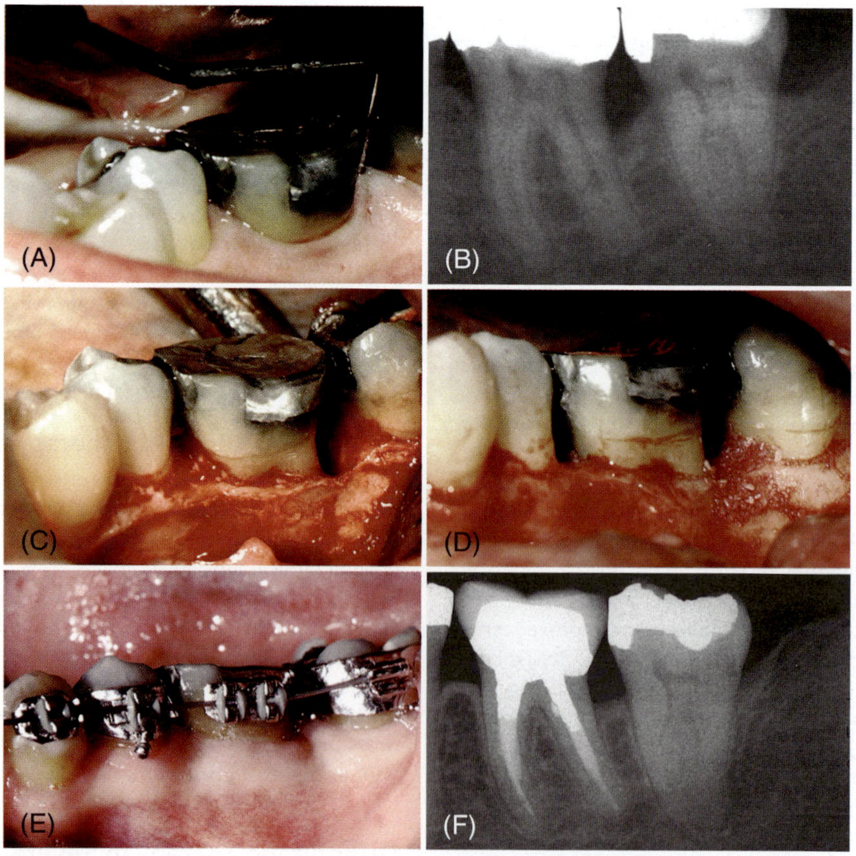

Fig. 55.1 This patient had a significant periodontal pocket (A) distal to the mandibular right first molar. Periapical radiograph (B) confirmed the osseous defect. A flap was elevated (C), revealing a deep, three-wall osseous defect. Freeze-dried bone (D) was placed in the defect. Six months after the bone graft, orthodontic treatment was initiated (E). The final periapical radiograph shows that the preorthodontic bone graft helped regenerate bone and eliminate the defect distal to the molar (F).

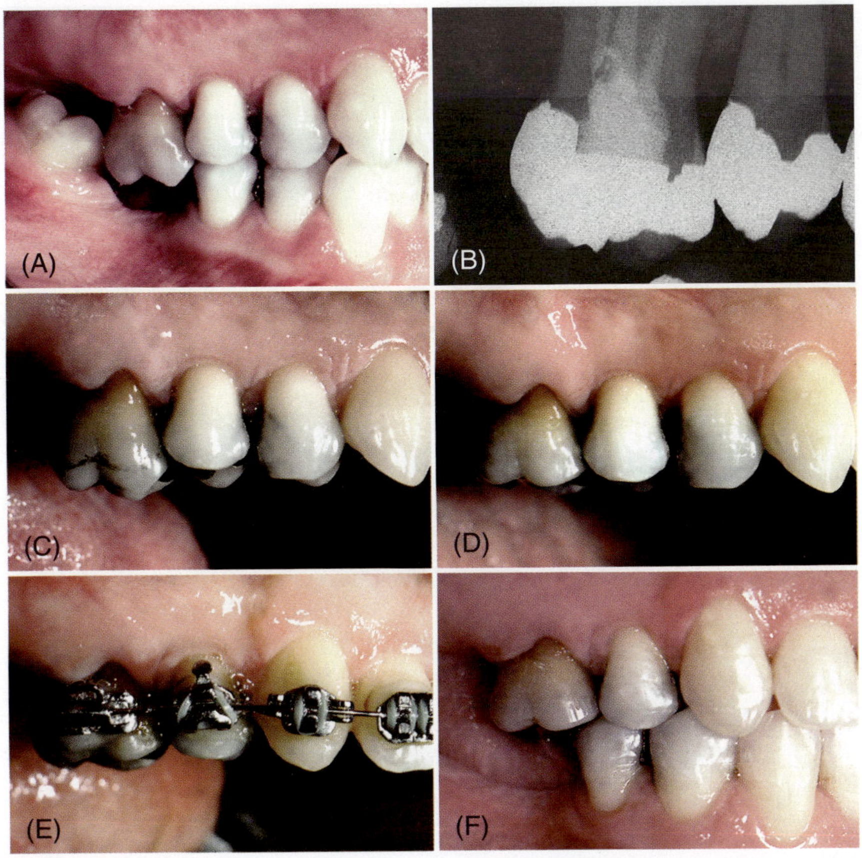

Fig. 55.2 This patient showed overeruption of the maxillary right first molar and a marginal ridge defect between the second premolar and first molar (A). The pretreatment periapical radiograph (B) showed that the interproximal bone was flat. To avoid creating a hemiseptal defect, the occlusal surface of the first molar was equilibrated (C and D), and the malocclusion was corrected orthodontically (E and F).

the adjacent cementoenamel junctions (CEJs) can help level the osseous defect.

It is imperative that periodontal inflammation be controlled before orthodontic treatment. This usually can be achieved with patient education regarding biofilm control, initial debridement, and scaling and root planing. After the completion of orthodontic treatment, these teeth should be stabilized for at least 6 months and reassessed periodontally. Often, the pocket has been reduced or eliminated and no further periodontal treatment is needed. It would be injudicious to perform preorthodontic osseous corrective surgery on such lesions if orthodontics is part of the overall treatment plan.

In the periodontally healthy patient, orthodontic brackets are positioned on the posterior teeth relative to the marginal ridges and cusps. However, some adult patients may have marginal ridge discrepancies caused by uneven tooth eruption. When marginal ridge discrepancies are encountered, the decision as to where to place the bracket or band is not determined by the anatomy of the tooth. In these patients, it is important to assess these teeth radiographically to determine the interproximal bone level.

If the bone level is oriented in the same direction as the marginal ridge discrepancy, leveling of the marginal ridges will level the bone. However, if the bone level is flat between adjacent teeth and the marginal ridges are at significantly different levels, orthodontic correction of the marginal ridge discrepancy produces a hemiseptal defect in the bone. This could cause a periodontal pocket between the two teeth.

If the bone is flat and a marginal ridge discrepancy is present, the orthodontist should not level the marginal ridges orthodontically. In these situations, it may be necessary to equilibrate the crown of the tooth (see Fig. 55.2). For some patients, the latter technique may require endodontic therapy and restoration of the tooth because of the required amount of reduction of the length of the crown. This approach is acceptable if the treatment results in a more favorable bone contour between the teeth.

Some patients have discrepancies between both the marginal ridges and the bony levels between two teeth. However, these discrepancies may not be of equal magnitude; orthodontic leveling of the bone may still leave a discrepancy in the marginal ridges (Fig. 55.3). In these patients, the crowns of the teeth should not be used as a guide for completing orthodontic therapy. The bone should be leveled orthodontically, and any remaining discrepancy between the marginal ridges should be equilibrated. This method produces the best occlusal result and improves the patient's periodontal health.

During orthodontic treatment, when teeth are being extruded to level hemiseptal defects, the patient should be monitored regularly. Initially, the hemiseptal defect has a greater sulcular depth and is more difficult for the patient to clean. As the defect is ameliorated through tooth extrusion, interproximal cleaning becomes easier. The patient should be recalled every 2–3 months during the leveling process to control inflammation in the interproximal region.

Advanced Horizontal Bone Loss

After orthodontic treatment has been planned, one of the most important factors that determine the outcome of therapy is the location of the bands and brackets on the teeth. In a periodontally healthy

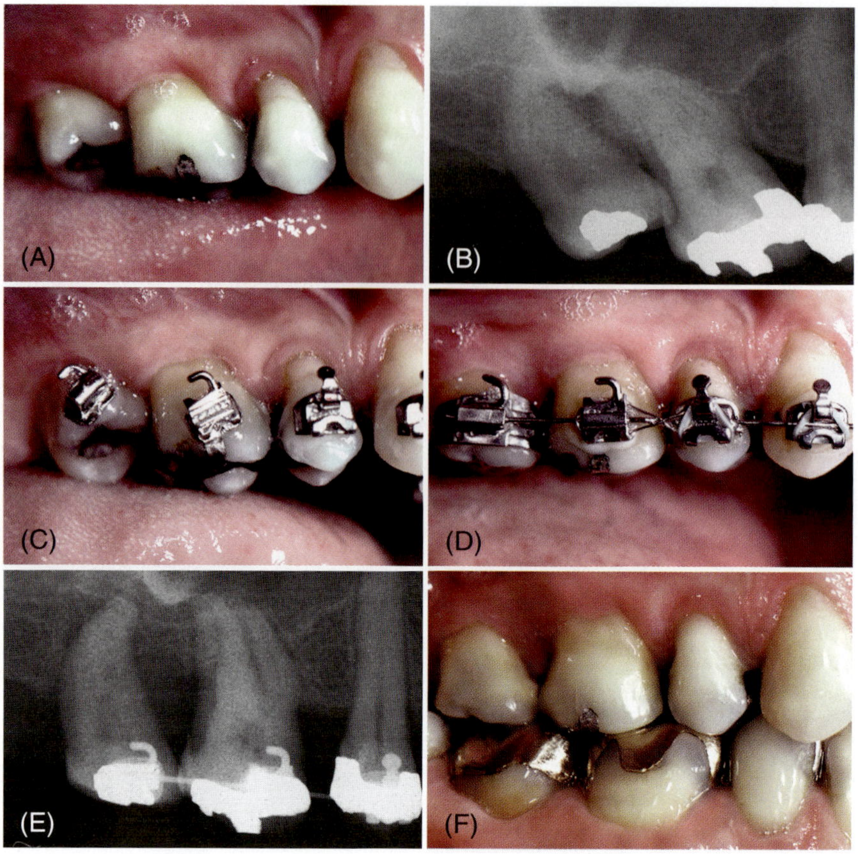

Fig. 55.3 Before orthodontic treatment, this patient had significant mesial tipping of the maxillary right first and second molars, causing marginal ridge discrepancies and deep periodontal pockets (A). The tipping produced root proximity between the molars as well as a disruption of the normal gingival anatomy (B). To eliminate the root proximity, the brackets were placed perpendicular to the long axes of the teeth (C). This method of bracket placement facilitated root alignment and elimination of the root proximity, as well as leveling of the marginal ridge discrepancies (D through F).

individual, the position of the brackets is usually determined by the anatomy of the crowns of the teeth. Anterior brackets should be positioned relative to the incisal edges. Posterior bands or brackets are positioned relative to the marginal ridges. If the incisal edges and marginal ridges are at the correct level, the CEJ will be at the same level. This relationship creates a flat, bony contour between the teeth. However, if a patient has underlying periodontal problems and significant alveolar bone loss around certain teeth, it is not appropriate to use the anatomy of the crown to determine bracket placement.

In a patient with advanced horizontal bone loss, the bone level may have receded several millimeters from the CEJ. As this occurs, the crown-to-root ratio becomes less favorable. By aligning the crowns of the teeth, the clinician may perpetuate tooth mobility by maintaining an unfavorable crown-to-root ratio. In addition, aligning the crowns of the teeth and disregarding the bone level lead to significant bone discrepancies between healthy and periodontally diseased roots. This could require periodontal surgery to ameliorate the discrepancies.

Many of these problems can be corrected by using the bone level as a guide to position the brackets on the teeth. In these situations, the crowns of the teeth may require considerable equilibration. If the tooth is vital, the equilibration should be performed gradually to allow the pulp to form secondary dentin and insulate the tooth during the equilibration process. The goal of equilibration and creative bracket placement is to provide a more favorable bony architecture and a more favorable crown-to-root ratio. In some of these patients, the periodontal defects that were apparent initially may not require periodontal surgery after orthodontic treatment.

Furcation Defects

Furcation defects can be classified as *incipient* (class I), *moderate* (class II), or *advanced* (class III). discusses furcation problems in detail.). These lesions require special attention in patients undergoing orthodontic treatment. Often, the molars require bands with tubes and other attachments that impede access to the buccal furcation for home care and instrumentation at the time of recall.

Furcation lesions require special consideration because they are the most difficult lesions to maintain and can worsen during orthodontic therapy. These patients should be maintained on a 2- to 3-month recall schedule. Detailed periodontal instrumentation and biofilm control of these furcation lesions will help to minimize further periodontal breakdown.

If a patient with a class III furcation defect will be undergoing orthodontic treatment, a possible method for treating the furcation is to eliminate it by hemisecting the crown and root of the tooth (Fig. 55.4). However, this procedure requires endodontic, periodontal, and restorative treatment. If the patient will be undergoing orthodontic treatment, it is advisable to perform the orthodontic treatment first. This is especially true if the roots of the teeth will not be moved apart. In these patients, the molar to be hemisected remains intact during orthodontic therapy. These patients require recall visits every 2 or 3 months to ensure that the furcation defect does not lose bone during orthodontic treatment. Keeping the tooth

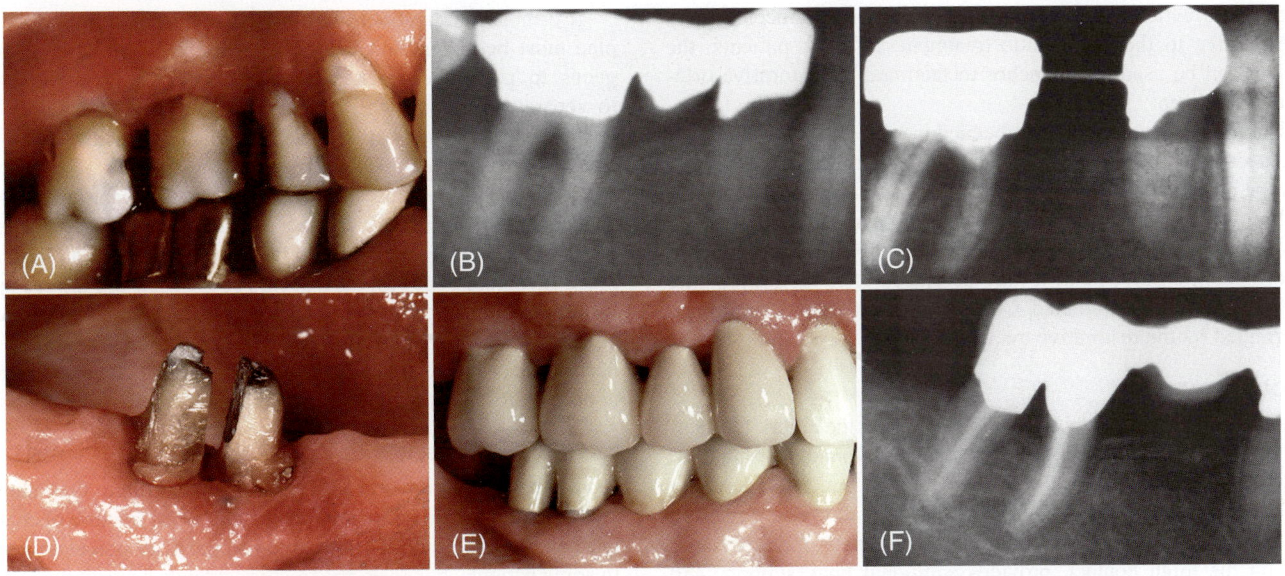

Fig. 55.4 This patient had a class III furcation defect before orthodontic treatment (A and B). Orthodontic treatment was performed (C), and the furcation defect was maintained by the periodontist with 2-month recalls until after orthodontic treatment. After appliance removal, the tooth was hemisected (D), and the roots were restored and splinted together (E). The final periapical radiograph (F) shows that the furcation defect was eliminated by hemisection and restoration of the two root fragments.

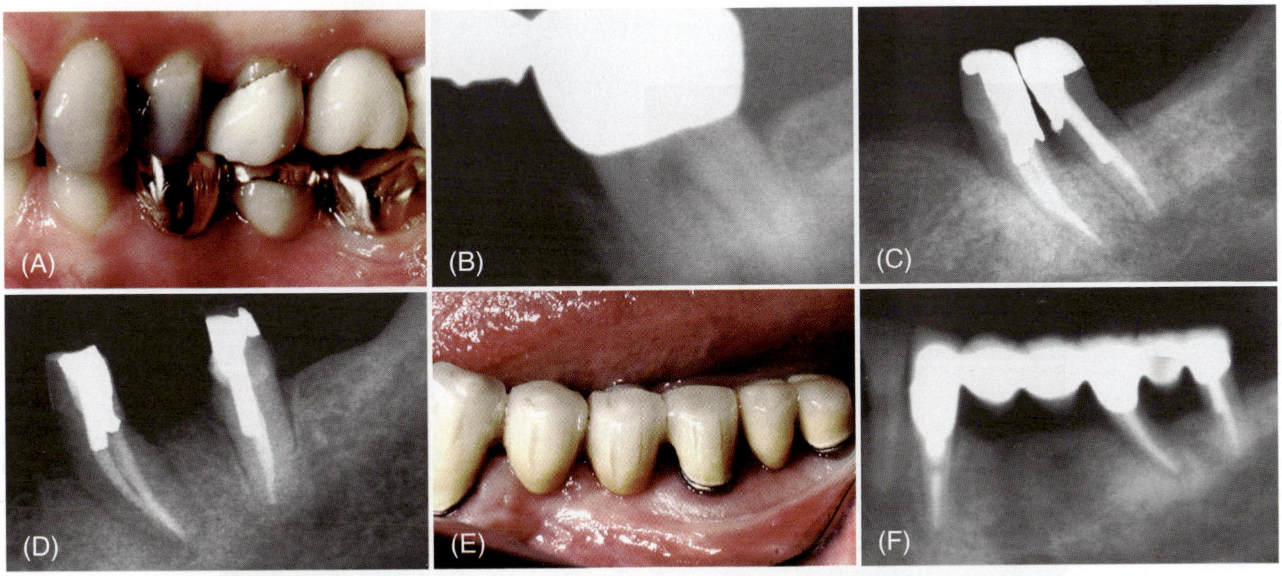

Fig. 55.5 Before orthodontic treatment, this patient had a class III furcation defect in the mandibular left second molar (A and B). Because the patient had an edentulous space mesial to the molar, the tooth was hemisected (C), and the root fragments were separated orthodontically (D). After orthodontic treatment, the root fragments were used as abutments to stabilize a multiunit posterior bridge (E and F).

intact during orthodontic therapy simplifies the concentration of tooth movement for the orthodontist. After orthodontic treatment, endodontic therapy is required, followed by periodontal surgery to divide the tooth.

In some patients requiring hemisection of a mandibular molar with a class III furcation, moving the roots apart during orthodontic treatment may be advantageous (Fig. 55.5). If the hemisected molar will be used as an abutment for a bridge after orthodontics, moving the roots apart orthodontically permits a favorable restoration and splinting across the adjacent edentulous spaces. In these patients, hemisection, endodontic therapy, and periodontal surgery must be completed before the start of orthodontic treatment. After completion of these procedures, bands or brackets can be placed on the root fragments, and coil springs can be used to separate the roots. The amount of separation is determined by the size of the adjacent edentulous space and the occlusion in the opposing arch. About 7 or 8 mm may be created between the roots of the hemisected molar. This process eliminates the original furcation problem and allows the patient to clean the area with greater efficiency.

In some molars with class III furcation defects, the tooth may have short roots, advanced bone loss, fused roots, or other problems that prevent hemisection and crowning of the remaining roots. In these patients, extracting the root with a furcation defect and placing an implant may be more advisable. If this type of plan has been adopted, extraction and placement of the implant can occur at any time relative to the orthodontic treatment. In some patients, the implant can be used as an anchor to facilitate prerestorative orthodontic treatment.

The implant must remain embedded in bone for 4–6 months after placement before it can be loaded as an orthodontic anchor. It must be placed precisely so that it not only provides an anchor for tooth movement but also may be used as an eventual abutment for a crown or fixed bridge. If the implant will not be used as an anchor for orthodontic movement, it may be placed after the orthodontic treatment has been completed. Considerations regarding timing are determined by the restorative treatment plan.

Root Proximity

When roots of posterior teeth are close together, the ability to maintain periodontal health and accessibility for restoration of adjacent teeth may be compromised. However, for the patient undergoing orthodontic therapy, the roots can be separated and bone will form between adjacent roots (see Fig. 55.3). This opens the embrasure beneath the tooth contact, provides additional bone support, and enhances the patient's access to the interproximal region for hygiene. This approach generally improves the periodontal health of this area.

If orthodontic treatment will be used to separate the roots, this plan must be understood before bracket placement. It is advantageous to place the brackets so that the orthodontic movement to separate the roots will begin with the initial archwires (see Fig. 55.3). Brackets must be placed obliquely to facilitate this process. Radiographs are needed to monitor the progress of orthodontic root separation. In general, 2–3 mm of root separation provides adequate bone and embrasure space to improve periodontal health. During this time, patients should be maintained on recall to ensure that a favorable bone response occurs as the roots are moved apart. In addition, these patients need occasional occlusal adjustment to recontour the crown because the roots are moving apart. As this occurs, the crown may develop an unusual occlusal contact with the opposing arch. This should be equilibrated to improve the occlusion.

Extrusive Movements

Occasionally, children and adolescents fall and injure their anterior teeth. If the injury is minor and results in a small fracture of enamel, this can be restored with light-cured composite or porcelain veneer. In some patients, however, the fracture extends beneath the level of the gingival margin and terminates at the level of the alveolar ridge (Fig. 55.6). Restoration of the fractured crown is impossible

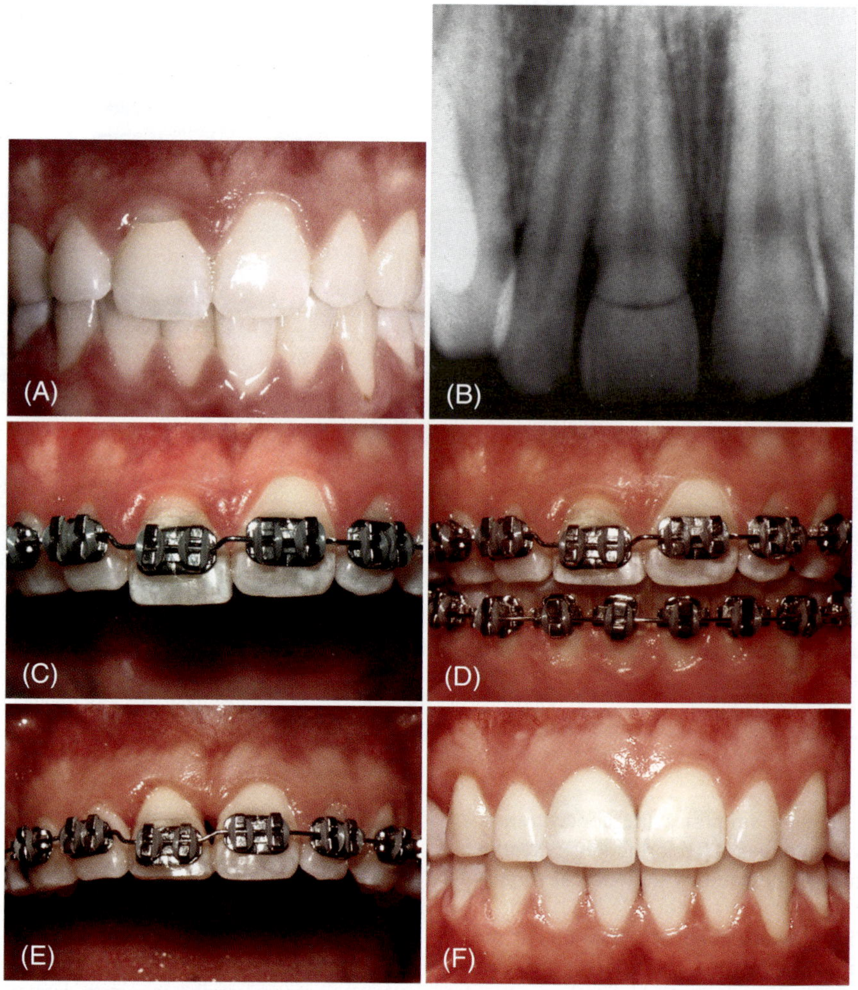

Fig. 55.6 This patient had a severe fracture of the maxillary right central incisor (A) that extended apical to the level of the alveolar crest on the lingual side (B). To restore the tooth adequately and avoid impinging on the periodontium, the fractured root was extruded 4 mm (C). As the tooth erupted, the gingival margin followed the tooth (D). Gingival surgery was required to lengthen the crown of the central incisor (E), so that the final restoration had sufficient ferrule for resistance and retention as well as the appropriate gingival margin relationship with the adjacent central incisor (F).

because the tooth preparation would extend to the level of the bone. This overextension of the crown margin could result in an invasion of the biologic width of the tooth and cause persistent inflammation of the marginal gingiva. It may be beneficial in such cases to erupt the fractured root out of the bone and move the fracture margin coronally by extrusive movements so that it can be properly restored. However, if the fracture extends too far apically, it may be better to extract the tooth and replace it with an implant or bridge. The following six criteria are used to determine whether the tooth should be forcibly erupted or extracted:

1. *Root length*. Is the root long enough so that a one-to-one crown-to-root ratio can be preserved after the root has been erupted? To answer this question, the clinician must know how far to erupt the root. If a tooth fracture extends to the level of the bone, it must be erupted 4 mm. The first 2.5 mm moves the fracture margin far enough away from the bone to prevent a biologic width problem. The other 1.5 mm provides the proper amount of ferrule for adequate resistance form of the crown preparation. Therefore, if the root is fractured to the bone level and must be erupted 4 mm, the periapical radiograph must be evaluated and 4 mm subtracted from the end of the fractured tooth root. The length of the residual root should be compared to the length of the eventual crown on this tooth. The root-to-crown ratio should be about 1:1. If the root-to-crown ratio is less than that, there may be too little root remaining in the bone for stability. In this situation, it may be prudent to extract the root and place a bridge or implant.
2. *Root form*. The shape of the root should be broad and nontapering rather than thin and tapered. A thin, tapered root provides a narrower cervical region after the tooth has been erupted 4 mm. This could compromise the esthetic appearance of the final restoration. The internal root form is also important. If the root canal is wide, the distance between the external root surface and the root canal filling will be narrow. In these patients, the walls of the crown preparation are thin, which could result in early fracture of the restored root. The root canal should not be more than one-third of the overall width of the root, so that the root can still provide adequate strength for the final restoration.
3. *Level of the fracture*. If the entire crown is fractured 2–3 mm apical to the level of the alveolar bone, it is difficult, if not impossible, to attach to the root to erupt it.
4. *Esthetics*. If the patient has a high lip line and displays 2–3 mm of gingiva when smiling, any type of restoration in this area will be more obvious. Keeping the patient's own tooth would be much more esthetic than any type of implant or prosthetic replacement.
5. *Endodontic/periodontal prognosis*. If the tooth has a significant periodontal defect, it may not be possible to retain the root. In addition, if the tooth root has a vertical fracture, the prognosis would be poor, and extraction of the tooth would be the proper course of therapy.

If all these factors are favorable, forced eruption of the fractured root is indicated. The orthodontic mechanics necessary to erupt the tooth can vary from elastic traction to orthodontic banding and bracketing. If a large portion of the tooth is still present, orthodontic bracketing is necessary. If the entire crown has fractured, leaving only the root, elastic traction from a bonded bar may be possible. The root may be erupted rapidly or slowly. If the movement is performed rapidly, the alveolar bone will be left behind temporarily, and a circumferential fiberotomy may be performed to prevent bone from following the erupted root. However, if the root is erupted slowly, the bone follows the tooth. In this situation, the erupted root requires crown lengthening to expose the correct amount of tooth to create the proper ferrule, resistance form, and retention for the final restoration.

After the tooth root has been erupted, it must be stabilized to prevent it from intruding back into the alveolus. The reason for *reintrusion* is to orient the principal fibers of the periodontium. During forced eruption, the periodontal fibers become oriented obliquely and stretched as the root moves coronally. These fibers eventually reorient themselves after about 6 months. Before this occurs, the root can reintrude significantly. Therefore, if this type of treatment is performed, an adequate period of stabilization is necessary to avoid significant relapse and reintrusion of the root.

As the root erupts, the gingiva moves coronally with the tooth. As a result, the clinical crown length becomes shorter after extrusion. In addition, the gingival margin may be positioned more incisally than the adjacent teeth. In these patients, gingival surgery is necessary to create ideal gingival margin height. The type of surgery varies, depending on whether bone removal is necessary. If the bone has followed the root during eruption, a flap is elevated and the appropriate amount of bone is removed to match the bone height of the adjacent teeth. If the bone level is flat between adjacent teeth, a simple excisional gingivectomy corrects the gingival margin discrepancy.

After gingival surgery, an open gingival embrasure may exist between the erupted root and adjacent teeth. The space occurs because the narrower root portion of the erupted tooth has been moved into the oral cavity. This space may be closed in two ways: (1) overcontouring of the replacement restoration or (2) reshaping of the crown of the tooth and movement of the root to close the space. The second method often helps improve the overall shape of the final crown on the restored tooth.

Intrusive Movements

Intrusive tooth movements can be attempted even in situations of reduced periodontal support provided the periodontal tissues are free of inflammation and plaque control is excellent. It is important to use light forces during these intrusive movements to prevent root resorption, mainly in teeth with an increased crown–root ratio due to reduced periodontal support. There is controversy whether this orthodontic tooth movement should be recommended in the presence of angular or intrabony defects. These movements, however, are not always predictable and some authors have recommended that intrabony defects are first treated with surgical periodontal regenerative procedures, followed by intrusive tooth movement. In the presence of shallow circumferential bony lesions, orthodontic intrusive movements may resolve the defect, but if these defects are deep, they should be treated first with periodontal regenerative procedures.

Hopeless Teeth Maintained for Orthodontic Anchorage

Patients with advanced periodontal disease may have specific teeth that are diagnosed as hopeless and would be extracted before orthodontic therapy (Fig. 55.7). However, these teeth may be useful for orthodontic anchorage if the periodontal inflammation can be controlled. In moderate to advanced cases, some periodontal surgery may be indicated around a hopeless tooth. Flaps are reflected for debridement of the roots to control inflammation around the hopeless tooth during the orthodontic process. The important factor is to maintain the health of the bone around the adjacent teeth. Periodontal recall is imperative during this process.

After orthodontic treatment, there is a 6-month period of stabilization before reevaluation of the periodontal status. Occasionally, the hopeless tooth may be so improved after orthodontic treatment

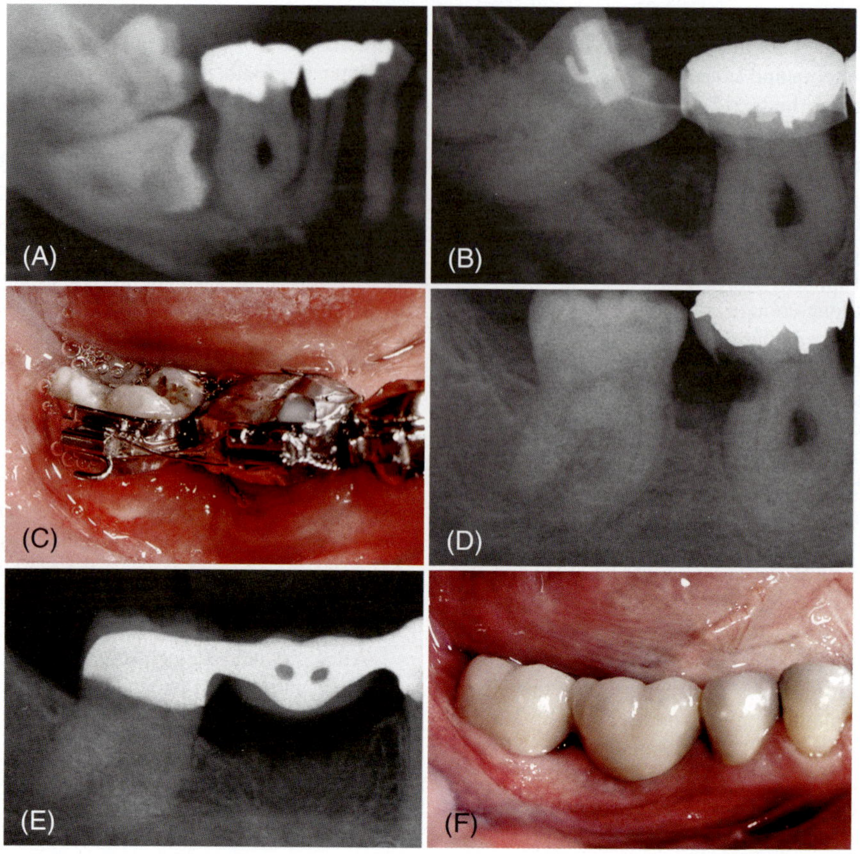

Fig. 55.7 This patient had an impacted mandibular right second molar (A). The mandibular right first molar was periodontally hopeless because of an advanced class III furcation defect. The impacted second molar was extracted, but the first molar was maintained as an anchor to help upright the third molar orthodontically (B through D). After orthodontic uprighting of the third molar, the first molar was extracted and a bridge was placed to restore the edentulous space (E and F).

that it is retained. In most cases, however, the hopeless tooth requires extraction, especially if other restorations are planned in the segment. Again, these decisions require reevaluation by the clinician.

Orthodontic Treatment of Gingival Discrepancies

Uneven Gingival Margins

The relationship between the gingival margins of the six maxillary anterior teeth plays an important role in the esthetic appearance of the crowns. The following four factors contribute to ideal gingival form:

1. The gingival margins of the two central incisors should be at the same level.
2. The gingival margins of the central incisors should be positioned more apically than the lateral incisors and at the same level as the canines.
3. The contour of the labial gingival margins should mimic the CEJs of the teeth.
4. A papilla should exist between each tooth, and the height of the tip of the papilla is usually halfway between the incisal edge and the labial gingival height of contour over the center of each anterior tooth. Therefore, the gingival papilla occupies half of the interproximal contact and the adjacent teeth form the other half.

However, some patients have gingival margin discrepancies between adjacent teeth. These discrepancies may be caused by abrasion of the incisal edges or by delayed migration of the gingival margins. When gingival margin discrepancies are present, the proper solution for the problem must be determined: orthodontic movement to reposition the gingival margins or surgical correction of the discrepancies.

To make the correct decision, it is necessary to evaluate four criteria. First, the relationship between the gingival margin of the maxillary central incisors and the lip line should be assessed when the patient smiles. If a gingival margin discrepancy is present but is not exposed, it does not require correction.

If a gingival margin discrepancy is apparent, the second step is to evaluate the labial sulcular depth over the two central incisors. If the shorter tooth has a deeper sulcus, excisional gingivectomy may be appropriate to move the gingival margin of the shorter tooth apically. However, if the sulcular depths of the short and long incisors are equivalent, gingival surgery does not correct the problem.

The third step is to evaluate the relationship between the shortest central incisor and the adjacent lateral incisors. If the shortest central incisor is still *longer* than the lateral incisors, the other possibility is to extrude the longer central incisor and equilibrate the incisal edge. This moves the gingival margin coronally and eliminates the gingival margin discrepancy. However, if the shortest central incisor is *shorter* than the lateral incisors, this technique would produce an unesthetic relationship between the gingival margins of the central and lateral incisors.

The fourth step is to determine whether the incisal edges have been abraded. This is best accomplished by evaluating the teeth from an incisal perspective. If one incisal edge is thicker labiolingually than on the adjacent tooth, this may indicate that it has been abraded and the tooth has overerupted. In such cases, the best method of correcting the gingival margin discrepancy is to intrude the short central incisor. This method moves the gingival margin apically and permits restoration of the incisal edges. The intrusion should be accomplished at least 6 months before appliance removal. This allows reorientation of the principal fibers of the periodontium and avoids reextrusion of the central incisor or incisors after appliance removal.

Significant Abrasion and Overeruption

Occasionally, patients have destructive dental habits, such as protrusive bruxing, that can result in significant wear of the maxillary and mandibular incisors and compensatory overeruption of these teeth. The restoration of these abraded teeth is often impossible because of the lack of crown length to achieve adequate retention and resistance form for the crown preparations. Two options are available. One option is extensive crown lengthening by elevating a flap, removing sufficient bone, and apically positioning the flap to expose adequate tooth length for crown preparation. However, this procedure is contraindicated in the patient with short, tapered roots because it could adversely affect the final root-to-crown ratio and potentially open gingival embrasures between the anterior teeth.

The other option for improving the restorability of these short abraded teeth is to intrude the teeth orthodontically and move the gingival margins apically. It is possible to intrude up to four maxillary incisors by using the posterior teeth as anchors during the intrusion process. This is accomplished by placing the orthodontic brackets as close to the incisal edges of the maxillary incisors as possible. The brackets are placed in their normal position on the canines and remaining posterior teeth. The patient's posterior occlusion resists the eruption of the posterior teeth, and the incisors gradually intrude and move the gingival margins and the crowns apically. This creates the space necessary to restore the incisal edges of these teeth temporarily and eventually to place the final crowns.

When abraded teeth are significantly intruded, it is necessary to hold these teeth for at least 6 months in the intruded position with orthodontic brackets or archwires (or both) or some type of bonded retainer. The principal fibers of the periodontium must accommodate to the new intruded position, a process that takes a minimum of 6 months in most adult patients. Orthodontic intrusion of severely abraded and overerupted teeth usually carries a distinct advantage compared to periodontal crown lengthening, unless the patient has extremely long and broad roots or has had extensive horizontal periodontal bone loss.

Open Gingival Embrasures

The presence of a papilla between the maxillary central incisors is a key esthetic factor in any individual. Occasionally, adults have open gingival embrasures or lack gingival papillae between their central incisors. These unesthetic areas are often difficult to resolve with periodontal therapy. However, orthodontic treatment can correct many of these open gingival embrasures. This open space is usually caused by (1) tooth shape, (2) root angulation, or (3) periodontal bone loss.

The interproximal contact between the maxillary central incisors consists of two parts: the tooth contact and the papilla. The papilla/contact ratio is 1:1. Half the space is occupied by papilla, and half is formed by the tooth contact. If the patient has an open embrasure, the first factor that must be evaluated is whether the problem is caused by the papilla or the tooth contact. If the papilla is the problem, the cause is usually a lack of bone support for the papilla due to an underlying periodontal problem.

In some situations, a deficient papilla can be improved with orthodontic treatment. By closing open contacts, the interproximal gingiva can be squeezed and moved incisally. This type of movement may help create a more esthetic papilla between two teeth despite alveolar bone loss. Another possibility is to erupt adjacent teeth when the interproximal bone level is positioned apically.

Most open embrasures between the central incisors are caused by problems with tooth contact. The first step in the diagnosis of this problem is to evaluate a periapical radiograph of the central incisors. If the root angulation is divergent, the brackets should be repositioned so that the root position can be corrected. In these patients, the incisal edges may be uneven and require either composite or porcelain restoration. If the periapical radiograph shows that the roots are in their correct relationship, the open gingival embrasure is caused by a triangular tooth shape (Fig. 55.8).

If the shape of the tooth is the problem, two solutions are possible: (1) restore the open gingival embrasure or (2) reshape

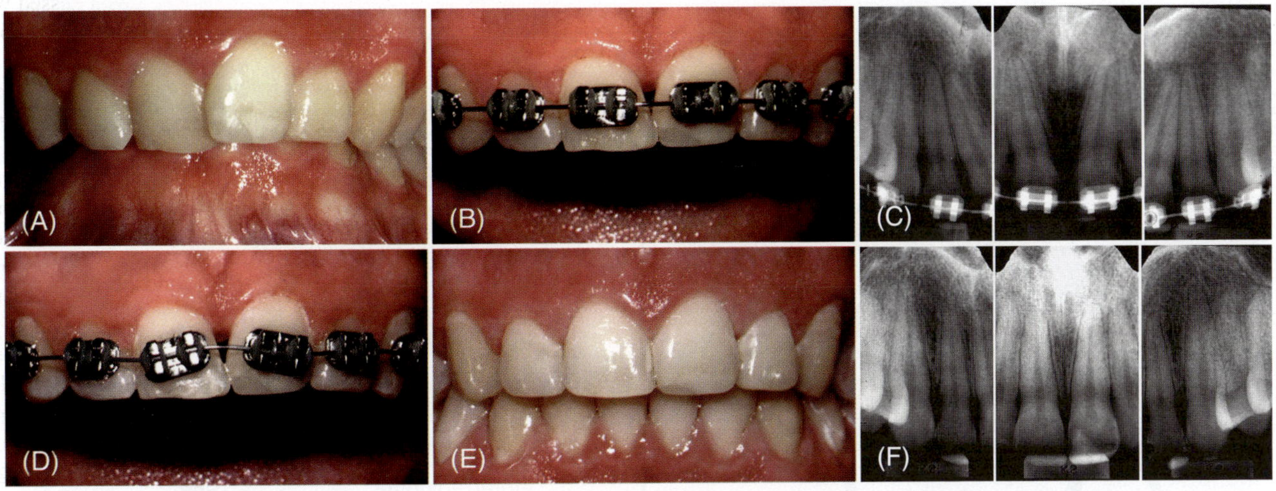

Fig. 55.8 This patient initially had triangular-shaped central incisors (A and B), which produced an open gingival embrasure after orthodontic alignment (C). Because the roots of the central incisors were parallel to one another, the appropriate solution for the open gingival embrasure was to recontour the mesial surfaces of the central incisors (D). As the diastema was closed (E), the tooth contact moved gingivally and the papilla moved incisally, resulting in the elimination of the open gingival embrasure (F).

the tooth by flattening the incisal contact and closing the space (Fig. 55.8). This second option results in lengthening of the contact until it meets the papilla. In addition, if the embrasure space is large, closing the space squeezes the papilla between the central incisors. This helps create a 1:1 ratio between the contact and the papilla and restores uniformity to the height between the midline and adjacent papillae.

Implant Anchorage in Orthodontics

The inclusion of implants in orthodontic mechanotherapy has resulted in the advent of a new class of anchorage, termed absolute anchorage. Among other features, the implications of absolute anchorage are that the predictability of the outcome rises dramatically, mechanotherapy can be simplified and streamlined, and, perhaps most importantly, compliance dependency is eliminated.

With conventional orthodontic anchorage strategies, movement is generally controlled by embracing anchor segments of teeth that outnumber the active segments of the teeth. In this way, the combined root surface area of the anchor units is collectively greater than that of the active segments and consequently is less likely to lead to movement under orthodontic load. The desired movement is theoretically achieved with minimal or no reciprocal movement. When the anchor segment includes an implant or miniscrew, the active units can actually outnumber the anchor units because anchorage preservation is no longer an issue. For this reason, en masse movement is quite easily achieved. The implication is that sequencing of orthodontic movement for the purpose of anchor preservation is no longer required, both saving time and significantly simplifying the orthodontic mechanotherapy (Box 55.1).

BOX 55.1 eLearning

The nature of attachment of an implant or miniscrew is very different than that of a tooth to alveolar bone. Whereas a dentoalveolar attachment features a ligamentous insertion, implants or miniscrews either osseointegrate or rely upon skeletal fixation. Consequently, Wolff's law of pressure and tension stimuli to remodel bone and allow tooth movement does not apply to fixtures. When properly fixated, implants and miniscrews can withstand orthodontic force application without incurring movement and thus can be used to overpower teeth, which respond very efficiently when proper mechanotherapy is designed.

Treatment Phase (See Fig. 55.9)

Direct Anchorage

In one form of direct anchorage, distalization is achieved through temporary anchorage device (TAD) placement and activation. In other cases, implants are placed in dental locations to provide orthodontic anchorage and eventual tooth replacement (see Fig. 55.10).

Indirect Anchorage

Indirect anchorage can utilize the buccal cortex (see Fig. 55.11) or a palatal location.

Space Management

An orthodontic fixed appliance may be utilized to restore space for implant replacement. Space is created not just at the coronal level but also at the interradicular level through proper root parallelism (see Fig. 55.12A and B).

Orthodontic Acceleration

Periodontally accelerated osteogenic orthodontics (PAOO) was the first such surgical endeavor; it has also been termed "Wilckodontics," after its pioneers. The technique involves elevation of full-thickness mucoperiosteal flaps and cortical cuts or perforations. This, in turn, recruits cellular responses that promote bone healing and remodeling, thereby accelerating bone turnover and tooth movement. PAOO is often combined with particulate bone grafting techniques that seemingly incorporate very effectively.

An apparently less intrusive surgical technique of piezocision was later developed that obviates the need for mucoperiosteal flaps by providing a similar decortication through gingival incisions. Healing and discomfort with this method are reportedly improved while it provides a similar effect. The ability to deliver bone grafting material is lost, however.

The next development was micro-osteoperforation. In this technique, a surgical-grade screw device is used transmucosally to provide the cortical injury. This device, manufactured by Propel Orthodontics, is the least invasive of the surgical modalities. Propel's Alveocentesis procedure features the option of localized delivery, as might be indicated in the case of a recalcitrant tooth that needs to be stimulated. The depth of the micro-osteoperforation can be controlled to accommodate various locations through clever design of the device.

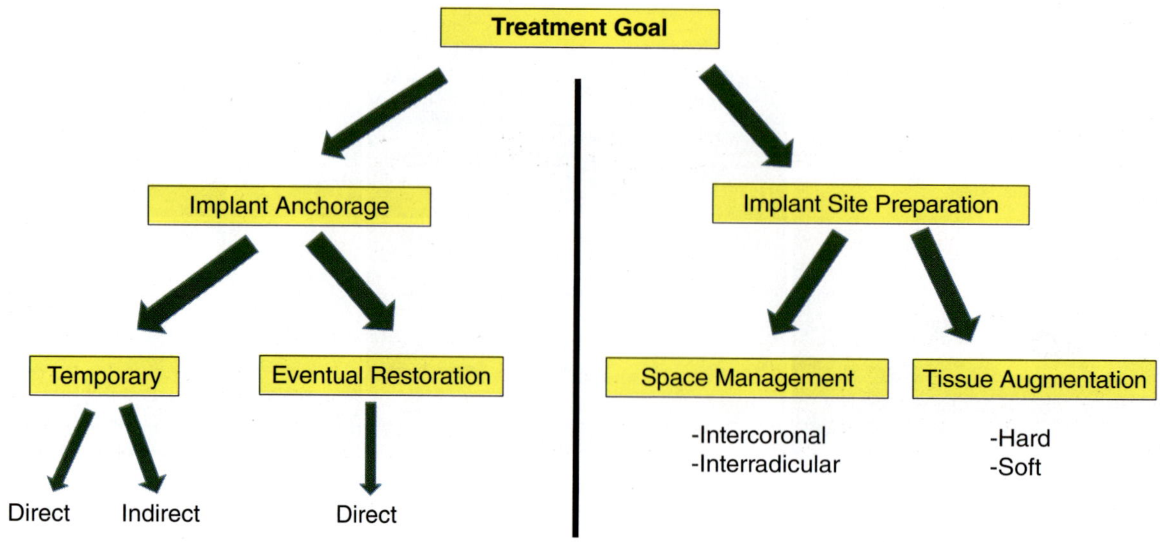

Fig 55.9 Flowchart for treatment plan.

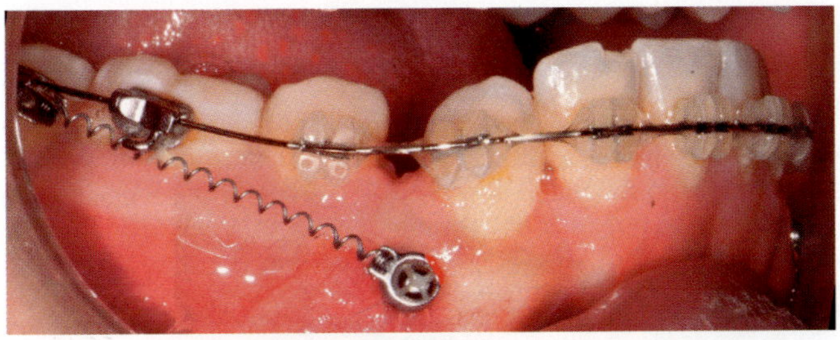

Fig 55.10 In this example of direct anchorage, a miniscrew (or temporary anchorage devices [TAD]) is placed between the roots of the mandibular bicuspid and cuspid teeth and is activated through by a nickel titanium coil spring from the TAD to the molar bracket. In this way, the posterior teeth are protracted by direct force application to the TAD.

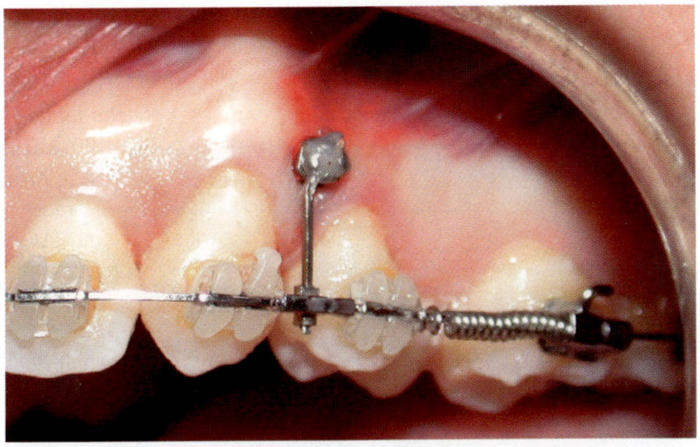

Fig 55.11 Indirect anchorage. Here an orthodontic miniscrew is placed in the buccal cortex between the maxillary left cuspid and first premolar. The temporary anchorage device is used to stabilize the orthodontic archwire and prevent unwanted mesial movement by employing a T-bar. This allows an open coil spring to be placed on the orthodontic archwire for distal driving of the upper left posterior teeth into a class I relation, thereby creating space to eliminate the crowding that the patient presented with. The upper left bicuspid tooth is considered as an indirect anchor because it is attached to the temporary anchorage devices, which serves to stabilize it.

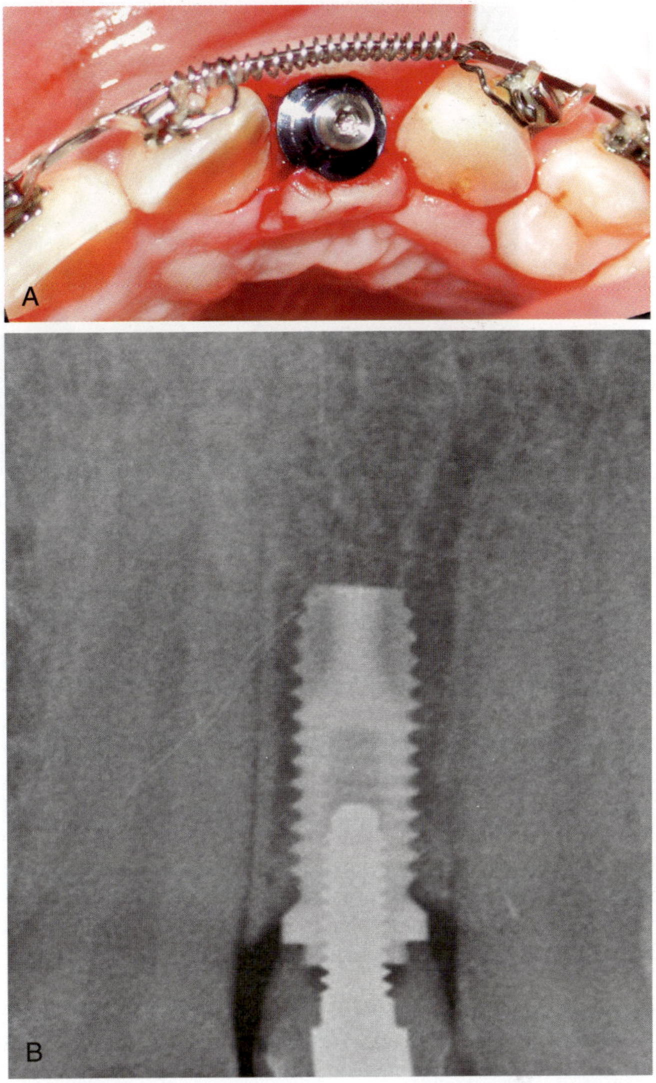

Fig 55.12 In this case, an orthodontic fixed appliance was utilized to restore space for the implant replacement of a maxillary left lateral incisor. A, Implant placement after correcting tooth position and root parallelism is achieved with the archwire in place to facilitate proper orientation. B, Radiograph of restored implant shows proper interradicular management to permit ideal implant placement.

Stimulatory Devices

Electronic stimulatory devices have also been developed. These methods attempt to harness the same healing cascade that surgical endeavors attempt to initiate, but, rather than accomplishing this through actual injury, they rely on micropulsation, or vibratory stimulus. This technology has been explored and successfully employed in orthopedic science. The first of these devices is the AcceleDent by OrthoAccel. It features a microprocessor that delivers a micropulsation stimulus to the dentition through a bite block. It is worn for 20 min every 24 h and delivers its pulse at a frequency and amplitude that are reportedly most conducive to cytokine recruitment, which is necessary for accelerated bone turnover.

A similar device is the VPro5 by Propel, which functions in similar fashion but delivers its pulse at a higher frequency. It is reportedly equally effective as the AcceleDent device but requires just 5 min/day.

Aligner Therapy

Unlike the removable orthodontic appliances, aligners (Fig. 55.13) do not work by single point contact, instead they function by very intimately and accurately grasping the entire clinical crown of a tooth and can even be programmed (using sophisticated software and digital manufacturing technology) to apply forces in exact locations upon the crown of the tooth, to effect very intricate and exact movements. When combined with accurate impressioning of the dentition, achieved through digital impression technology, virtual treatment mapping, three-dimensional printing manufacture and advanced thermoforming, these movements and desired outcomes can be planned and achieved with great predictability and reliability. The absence of potentially plaque-retentive brackets and auxiliaries (attachments notwithstanding) is clearly advantageous, as is the ease of cleaning the unobstructed dentition when aligners are removed. Improved patient comfort is almost uniformly reported and expected when compared to fixed appliances, not to mention the near elimination of emergency appointments due to appliance breakage or discomfort. Treatment duration is often reduced, owing

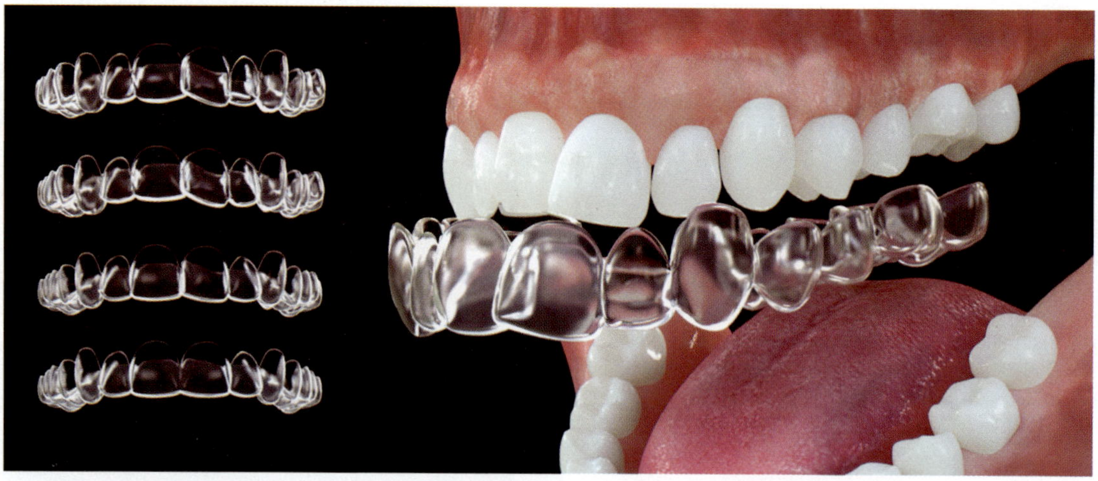

Fig 55.13 Graphical illustration showing maxillary aligners and their use in maxillary dentition to treat malocclusion (PerioPixel).

to immediate appliance activation (obviating the need to ramp up appliance mechanotherapy) as well as the ability to effect multiple movements simultaneously. Fewer appointments with longer intervals between appointments can be attractive to many patients (and practitioners), and even the feasibility of "teledentistry" clearly contributes to enhanced convenience.

Most notable in terms of disadvantages of aligner therapy would be patient compliance. As these appliances are removable by design, consistent and nearly compulsive application of the appliance and its protocols is required of the patient, and so a less than motivated patient, or a patient lacking in dexterity or ability, might not be considered a good candidate for this modality.

A Note Regarding Retention

Retention is an essential part of orthodontic therapy, for long-term stability, and is frequently more important than the active treatment. The design of retainers should be custom tailored to each case, and a common philosophy is that any tooth that is moved orthodontically needs to be retained, by some means. Of course, the first decision regards the choice of fixed or removable retainer designs. Selecting fixed retainers has certain advantages and is most frequently employed for lower anterior teeth.

Advantages of fixed retention:

- Full time
- No concern for patient compliance
- Elimination of mobility
- Disadvantage of fixed retention
- Hygienic concerns
- Occasional breakage
- Possible discomfort

The purpose of this discussion is to point out some untoward side effects of certain fixed retention designs, specifically, twisted wire retainers. Clinicians are cautioned that the twisted (or "spun down") fixed bonded retainers have recently shown detrimental effects in that they can unwind gradually over time, exerting unwanted torquing force on a tooth resulting in a root malposition and often an associated dehiscence, if not recession. Preferable designs would be flat braided wires, rigid wires, or, most recently, laser-etched nickel titanium examples (Figs. 55.14 and 55.15).

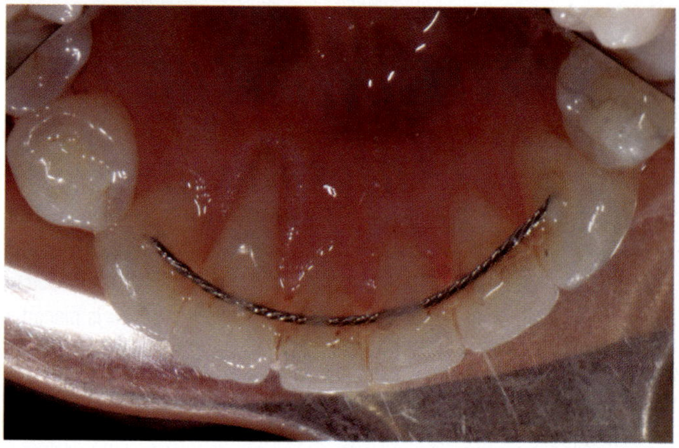

Fig 55.14 Example of a bonded (fixed) lower lingual retainer and the undesirable effect of the twisted wire design. Over time (in this case 6 years), the twisted wire apparently unravels applying torque forces to the teeth resulting in a lingual dehiscence of the right central incisor.

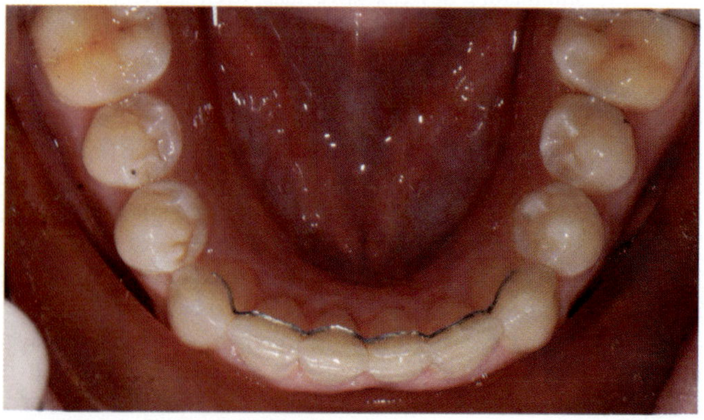

Fig 55.15 Laser-etched nickel titanium fixed lingual retainer (Memotain). Observe how the wire contours accurately to the crown contours, yet is inactive because it is not bent from wire but rather is laser etched from a sheet of material and, consequently, has no "memory."

Conclusion

There are many benefits to integrating orthodontics and periodontics in the management of adult patients with underlying periodontal defects. The key to treating these patients is communication and proper diagnosis before orthodontic therapy, as well as continued dialog during treatment. Not all periodontal problems are treated in the same way. This chapter provides a framework for the integration of orthodontics to solve periodontal problems.

Key points

- Hemiseptal defects can be eliminated with appropriate orthodontic treatment. In the case of the tipped tooth, uprighting and eruption of the tooth levels the bony defect. If the tooth is supererupted, intrusion and leveling of the adjacent cementoenamel junctions (CEJs) can help level the osseous defect.
- Furcation defects can be classified as *incipient* (class I), *moderate* (class II), or *advanced* (class III). These lesions require special attention in the patient undergoing orthodontic treatment.
- If a patient with a class III furcation defect will be undergoing orthodontic treatment, a possible method for treating the furcation is to eliminate it by hemisecting the crown and root of the tooth.
- In some patients requiring hemisection of a mandibular molar with a class III furcation, pushing the roots apart during orthodontic treatment may be advantageous.
- For a patient undergoing orthodontic therapy, the roots can be moved apart and bone formation will occur between the adjacent roots, which opens the embrasure beneath the tooth contact, provides additional bone support, and enhances the patient's access to the interproximal region for hygiene.
- Patients with advanced periodontal disease may have specific teeth diagnosed as hopeless, which would be extracted before orthodontic therapy. However, these teeth can be useful for orthodontic anchorage if the periodontal inflammation can be controlled.
- Treatment options for restoration of abraded anterior teeth due to destructive dental habits are extensive crown lengthening or to intrude the teeth orthodontically and move the gingival margins apically.

Suggested Readings

Adjunctive Role of Orthodontic Therapy

Aimetti M, Garbo D, Ercoli E, Grigorie MM, Citterio F, Romano F: Long-term prognosis of severely compromised teeth following combined periodontal and orthodontic treatment: a retrospective study, *Int J Periodontics Restor Dent* 40(1):95–102, 2020.

Alpan D: A review of accelerated orthodontics, Orthod Pract US 7:44, 2016.

Amato F, Mirabella AD, Macca U, et al: Implant site development by orthodontic forced extraction: a preliminary study, *Int J Oral Maxillofac Implants* 27:411, 2012.

Attia MS, Hazzaa HH, Al-Aziz FA, Elewa GM: Evaluation of adjunctive use of low-level diode laser biostimulation with combined orthodontic regenerative therapy, *J Int Acad Periodontol* 21(2):63–73, 2019.

Baloul SS: Osteoclastogenesis and osteogenesis during tooth movement, *Front Oral Biol* 18:75, 2016.

Bowman SJ: The effect of vibration on the rate of levelling and alignment, *J Clin Orthod* 48:678, 2014.

Brown IA: The effect of orthodontic therapy on certain types of periodontal defects. 1. Clinical findings, *J Periodontol* 44:742, 1973.

Carnio J, Carnio AT: Papilla reconstruction: interdisciplinary consideration for clinical success, *J Esthet Restor Dent* 30(6):484–491, 2018.

Ingber J: Forced eruption. Part I. A method of treating isolated one and two wall infrabony osseous defects. Rationale and case report, *J Periodontol* 45:199, 1974.

Kokich V: Enhancing restorative, esthetic and periodontal results with orthodontic therapy. In Schluger S, Youdelis R, Page R, et al, editors: *Periodontal therapy*, Philadelphia, 1990, Lea and Febiger.

Kokich V: Esthetics and vertical tooth position: the orthodontic possibilities, *Compend Contin Edu dent* 18:1225, 1997.

Kokich V, Nappen D, Shapiro P: Gingival contour and clinical crown length: their effects on the esthetic appearance of maxillary anterior teeth, *Am J Orthod* 86–89, 1984.

References

References and MCQs with answers for the chapter are available on www.medenact.com.

CHAPTER 56

Supportive Periodontal Treatment

RL Merin | A Uppoor

CHAPTER OUTLINE

Preservation of the periodontal health of the treated patient requires a supportive program that is just as important as the therapy used to treat the periodontal disease. After phase I therapy has been completed, patients are placed on a schedule of periodic recall visits for maintenance care to prevent the recurrence of the disease (Figs. 56.1 and 56.2).

KEY FACT

The long-term preservation of the dentition is closely associated with the frequency and quality of recall maintenance.

Transfer of the patient from active treatment status to a maintenance program is a definitive step in total patient care that requires time and effort on the part of the dentist and staff. Patients must understand the purpose of the maintenance program, and the dentist must emphasize that preservation of the teeth depends on maintenance therapy. Patients who are not maintained in a supervised recall program subsequent to active treatment show obvious signs of recurrent periodontitis (e.g., increased pocket depth, bone loss, or tooth loss). The more often patients present for recommended supportive periodontal treatment (SPT), the less likely they are to lose teeth. One study indicated that treated patients who do not return for regular recall have a 5.6 times greater risk for tooth loss than compliant patients. Another study showed that patients with inadequate SPT after successful regenerative therapy have a 50-fold increase in risk of probing attachment loss compared to those who have regular recall visits.

KEY FACT

Patients who do not return for SPT lose five to six times more teeth than compliant patients.

Motivational techniques and reinforcement of the importance of the maintenance phase of treatment should be considered before performing definitive periodontal surgery. Studies show that few patients display complete compliance with recommended maintenance schedules (Fig. 56.3). *It is meaningless simply to inform patients that they are to return for periodic recall visits without clearly explaining the significance of these visits and describing what is expected of patients between visits.*

The maintenance phase of periodontal treatment starts immediately after the completion of phase I therapy (see Figs. 56.1 and 56.2). While the patient is in the maintenance phase, the necessary surgical and restorative procedures are performed. This ensures that all areas of the mouth retain the degree of health attained after phase I therapy.

Rationale for Supportive Periodontal Treatment

Studies indicate that even with appropriate periodontal therapy, some progression of disease is possible. One likely explanation for the recurrence of periodontal disease is incomplete subgingival plaque/biofilm and calculus removal. If subgingival biofilm is left behind during scaling, it regrows within the pocket. The regrowth of subgingival biofilm is a slow process compared to that of supragingival biofilm. During this period (perhaps months), the subgingival biofilm may not induce inflammatory reactions that can be discerned at the gingival margin. The clinical diagnosis may be further confused by the introduction of adequate supragingival biofilm control because the inflammatory reactions caused by the biofilm in the soft-tissue wall of the pocket are not likely to manifest clinically as gingival erythema and edema. Thus, inadequate subgingival biofilm control can lead to continued loss of attachment, even without the presence of clinical gingival inflammation. Scaling and root planing are generally not effective at sites with probing depths of 6 mm or greater.

Bacteria are present in the gingival tissues in chronic and aggressive periodontitis cases. Eradication of intragingival microorganisms may be necessary for a stable periodontal result. Scaling, root planing, and even flap surgery may not eliminate intragingival bacteria in some areas. These bacteria may recolonize the pocket and cause recurrent disease.

Bacteria associated with periodontitis can be transmitted between spouses and other family members. Patients who appear to be successfully treated can become infected or reinfected with potential pathogens. This is especially likely in patients with remaining pockets.

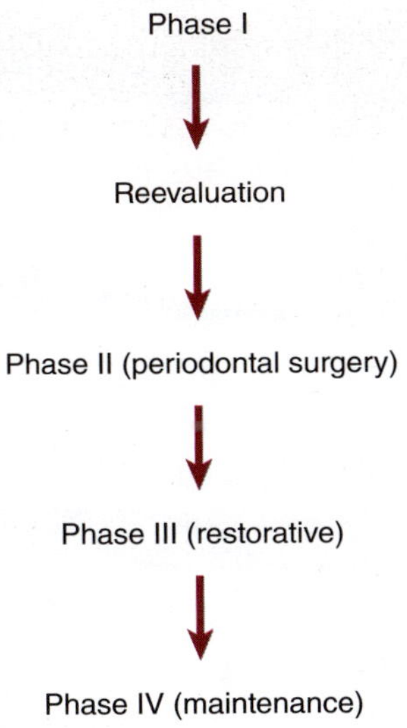

Fig. 56.1 Incorrect sequence of periodontal treatment phases. Maintenance phase should be started immediately after the reevaluation of phase I therapy.

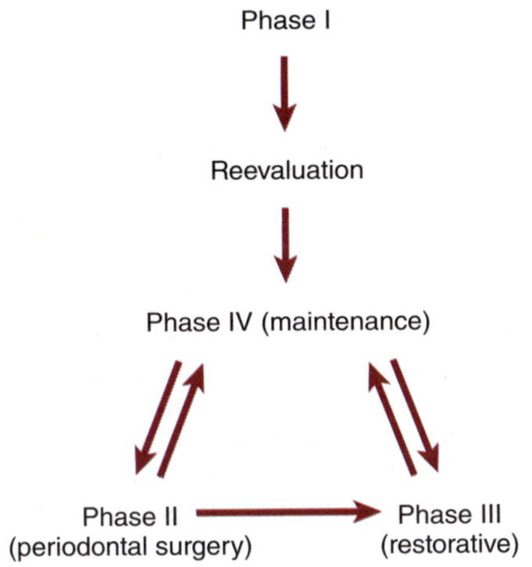

Fig. 56.2 Correct sequence of periodontal treatment phases.

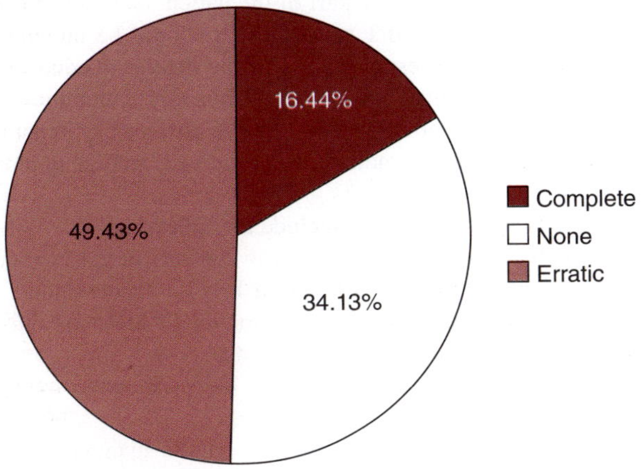

Fig. 56.3 Compliance with maintenance therapy in 961 patients studied for 1–8 years. *(Modified from Wilson TG Jr, Glover ME, Schoen J, et al.: Compliance with maintenance therapy in a private periodontal practice.* J Periodontol *55:468, 1984.)*

Another possible explanation for the recurrence of periodontal disease is the microscopic nature of the dentogingival unit healing after periodontal treatment. Histologic studies have indicated that after periodontal procedures, tissues usually heal by the formation of a long junctional epithelium instead of new connective tissue attachment to root surfaces. It has been speculated that this type of dentogingival unit may be weaker and that inflammation may rapidly separate the long junctional epithelium from the tooth. Thus, treated periodontal patients may be predisposed to recurrent pocket formation if maintenance care is not optimal.

Subgingival scaling alters the microflora of periodontal pockets. In one study, a single session of scaling and root planing in patients with chronic periodontitis resulted in significant changes in subgingival microflora. Reported alterations included a decrease in the proportion of motile rods for 1 week, a marked elevation in the proportion of coccoid cells for 21 days, and a marked reduction in the proportion of spirochetes for 7 weeks.

Although pocket debridement suppresses components of the subgingival microflora associated with periodontitis, periodontal pathogens may return to baseline levels within days or months. The return of pathogens to pretreatment levels generally occurs in approximately 9–11 weeks but can vary dramatically among patients

KEY FACT

Scaling and root planing are generally not effective at sites with probing depths of 6 mm or greater.

Both the mechanical debridement performed by the therapist and the motivational environment provided by the appointment seem to be necessary for good maintenance results. Patients tend to reduce their oral hygiene efforts between appointments. Knowing that their hygiene will be evaluated motivates them to perform better oral hygiene in anticipation of the appointment.

In one study, the proportion of spirochetes obtained in baseline samples of subgingival flora was highly correlated with clinical periodontal deterioration over 1 year. However, subsequent reports in the same longitudinal study concluded that the arbitrary assignment of treated periodontitis patients to 3-month maintenance intervals appears to be as effective in preventing recurrences of periodontitis as assignment of recall intervals based on microscopic monitoring of the subgingival flora. Microscopic monitoring was found not to be a reliable predictor of future periodontal destruction in patients on 3-month recall programs, presumably because of the alteration of subgingival flora produced by subgingival instrumentation.

In conclusion, there is a sound scientific basis for recall maintenance because subgingival scaling alters the pocket microflora for variable but relatively long periods.

Maintenance Program

Periodic recall visits form the foundation of a meaningful long-term prevention program. The interval between visits is initially set at 3 months but may vary according to the patient's needs.

Periodontal care at each recall visit comprises three parts (Box 56.1). The first part involves examination and evaluation of the patient's current oral health. The second part includes the necessary maintenance treatment and oral hygiene reinforcement. The third part involves scheduling the patient for the next recall appointment, additional periodontal treatment, or restorative dental

BOX 56.1 Maintenance Recall Procedures

Part I: Examination
(Approximate time: 14 min)
Patient greeting
Medical history changes
Oral pathologic examination
Oral hygiene status
Gingival changes
Pocket depth changes
Mobility changes
Occlusal changes
Dental caries
Restorative, prosthetic, and implant status

Part II: Treatment
(Approximate time: 36 min)
Oral hygiene reinforcement
Scaling
Polishing
Chemical irrigation or site-specific antimicrobial placement

Part III: Report, Cleanup, and Scheduling
(Approximate time: 10 min)
Write report in chart.
Discuss report with patient.
Clean and disinfect operatory.
Schedule next recall visit.
Schedule further periodontal treatment.
Schedule or refer for restorative or prosthetic treatment.

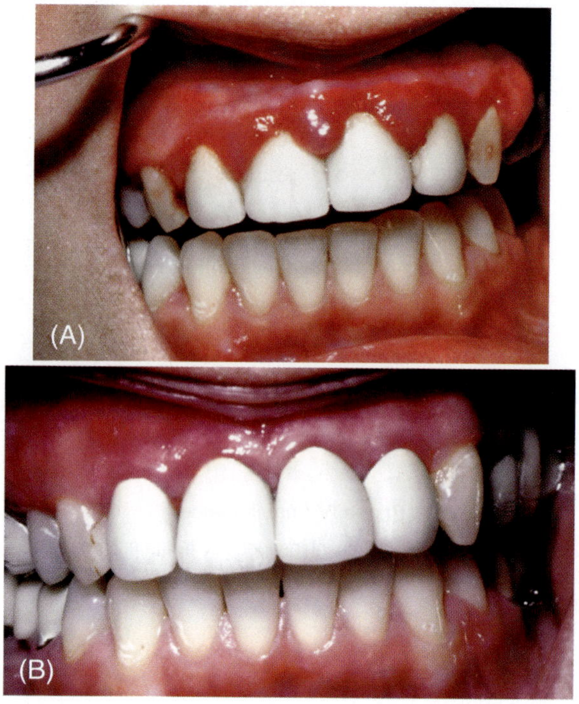

Fig. 56.4 A, Hyperplastic gingivitis related to crown margins and plaque accumulation in a 27-year-old woman. B, Four months after treatment, there is significant improvement. However, some inflammation around crown margins still exists, which cannot be resolved without replacing the crowns.

procedures. The time required for a recall visit for patients with multiple teeth in both arches is approximately 1 h.

Examination and Evaluation

The recall examination is similar to the initial evaluation of the patient (see Chapter 31). However, because the patient is not new to the office, the dentist or hygienist primarily looks for changes that have occurred since the last evaluation. Analysis of the current oral hygiene status of the patient is essential. Updating of changes in the medical history and evaluation of restorations, caries, prostheses, occlusion, tooth mobility, gingival status, and periodontal and periimplant probing depths are important parts of the recall appointment. The oral mucosa should be carefully inspected for pathologic conditions (Figs. 56.4–56.9).

Radiographic examination must be individualized depending on the initial severity of the case and the findings during the recall visit (Table 56.1). These are compared with findings on previous radiographs to check the bone height and look for repair of osseous defects, signs of trauma from occlusion, periapical pathologic changes, and caries.

Checking of Plaque/Biofilm Control

To assess the effectiveness of their plaque control, patients should perform their hygiene regimen immediately before the recall appointment. Plaque/biofilm control must be reviewed and corrected until the patient demonstrates the necessary proficiency, even if additional instruction sessions are required. A motivational interviewing technique of teaching may help to produce positive results. Patients instructed in plaque/biofilm control have less biofilm and gingivitis than uninstructed patients, and because the amount of supragingival plaque/biofilm is less, there is a decrease in the number of subgingival anaerobic organisms.

Treatment

Following consultation, examination, consultation, and oral hygiene instruction, the required scaling and root planing are performed (see Chapter 49). Care must be taken not to instrument healthy sites with shallow sulci (1–3 mm deep) and an absence of gingival inflammation because studies have indicated that repeated subgingival scaling and root planing of sites not periodontally involved result in significant loss of attachment and gingival recession, which will affect esthetics. Irrigation with antimicrobial agents or placement of site-specific antimicrobial devices may be performed in maintenance patients with remaining pockets.

Recurrence of Periodontal Disease

Occasionally, lesions may recur, which is often due to inadequate plaque/biofilm control on the part of the patient or failure to comply with recommended SPT schedules. It should be understood, however, that it is the responsibility of the dentist to educate and motivate patients to improve their oral hygiene techniques. Surgery should not be undertaken unless the patient participates in disease prevention and demonstrates proficiency in plaque/biofilm control.

Other causes for recurrence include the following:

1. Inadequate or insufficient treatment that has failed to remove all of the potential factors favoring biofilm accumulation (see Fig. 56.4). Incomplete calculus removal in areas of difficult access is a common source of problems.
2. Inadequate restorations placed after the periodontal treatment was completed.
3. Failure of the patient to return for periodic maintenance care (see Fig. 56.6). This may be a result of the patient's conscious or unconscious decision not to continue treatment or the failure of the dentist and staff to emphasize the need for periodic supportive therapy.

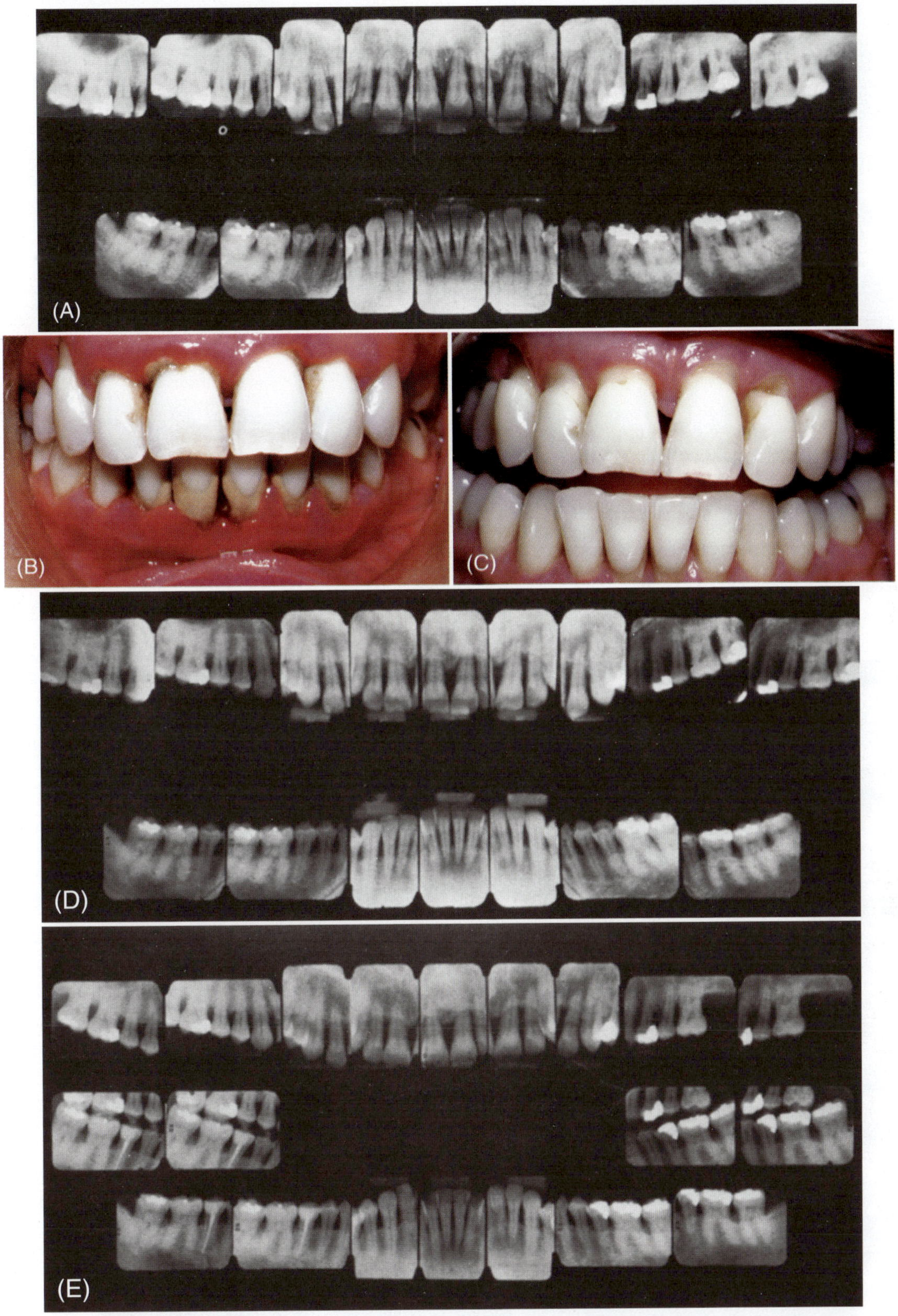

Fig. 56.5 A, Patient was 38 years old when these original radiographs were taken and was treated with a combination of surgical and nonsurgical therapy. This individual is a classic class C maintenance patient. B, Pretreatment photograph. Note the inflammation and heavy calculus deposits. C, Photograph taken 10 years after treatment. D, Radiographs taken 5 years after treatment. E, Radiographs taken 10 years after treatment. The radiographic appearance is as good as can be expected in such a severe case. Teeth #15 and #17 were extracted 8 years after treatment.

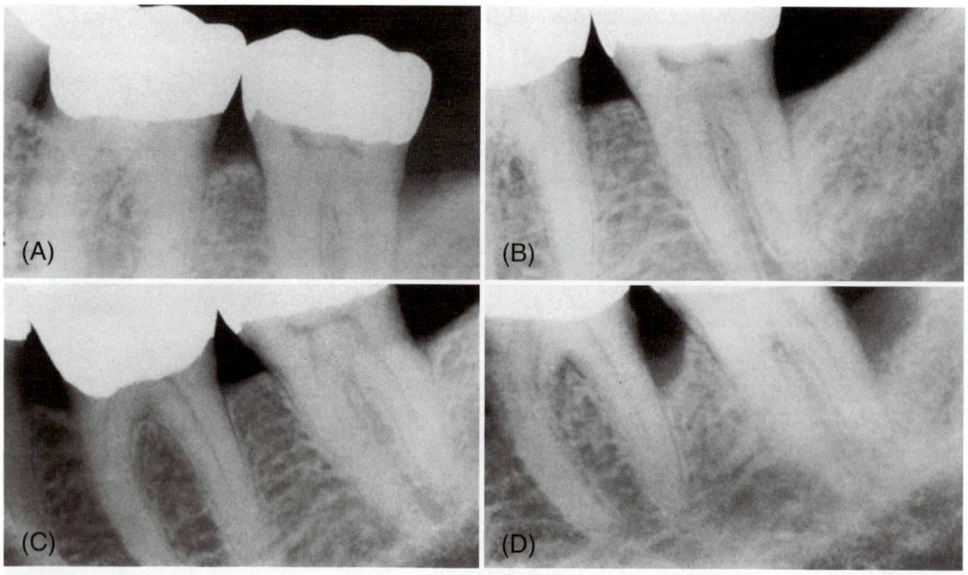

Fig. 56.6 This series of radiographs clearly shows the importance of maintenance therapy. A, Original radiograph of a 58-year-old male. Note the deep distal bone loss on tooth #18 and the moderate distal lesion of tooth #19. Surgical treatment included osseous grafting. B, Radiograph 14 months after surgical therapy. The patient had recall maintenance performed every 3–4 months. C, Appearance 3 years after surgery, with regular recalls every 3— 4 months. D, Appearance after 2 years without recalls (7 years after surgery). Note the progression of the disease on the distal surfaces of teeth #18 and #19.

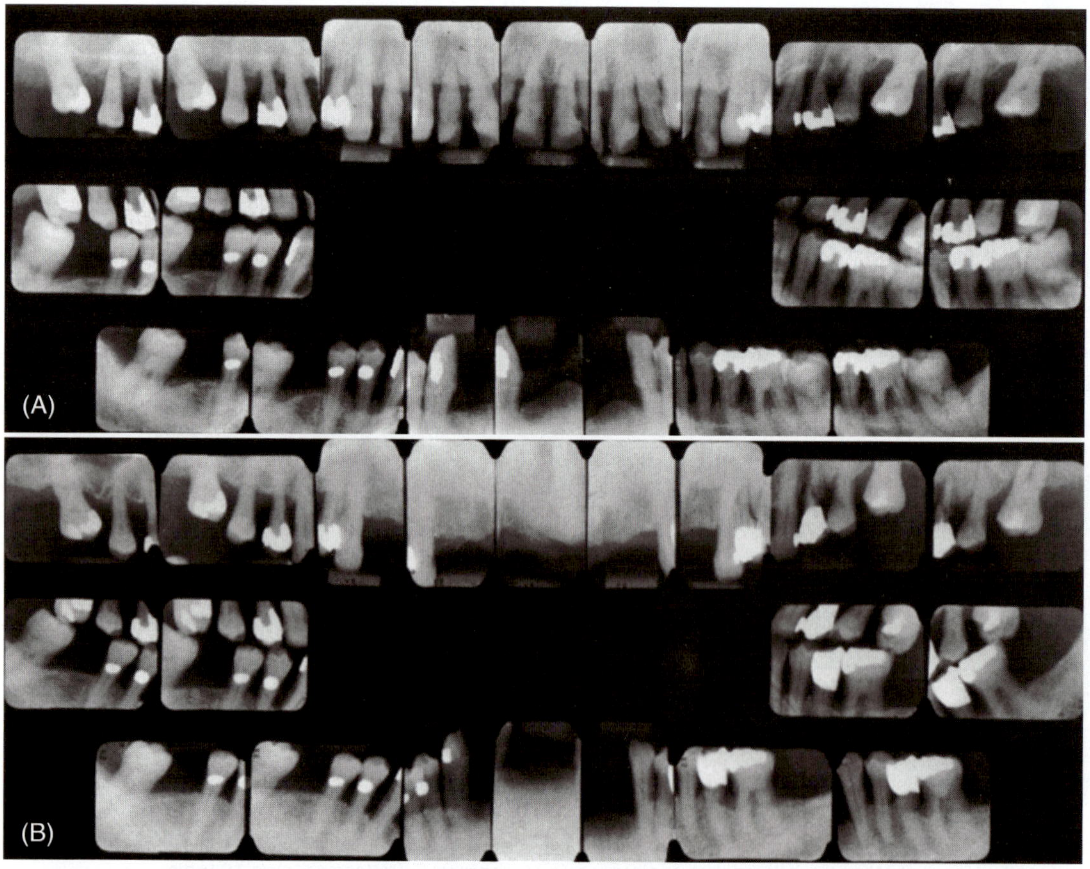

Fig. 56.7 Advanced cases sometimes do better than expected when the patient complies with maintenance therapy. A, Initial radiographs showing an advanced case. The maxillary arch had extractions and nonsurgical treatment. A plastic partial denture was placed and was expected to grow into a full denture within a few years. The mandibular arch was treated with periodontal surgery, and a permanent, metal and plastic, removable partial denture was placed. B, Radiographs taken 8 years later. The patient performed good oral hygiene and had 3-month recalls. Teeth #12 and #15 required extraction.

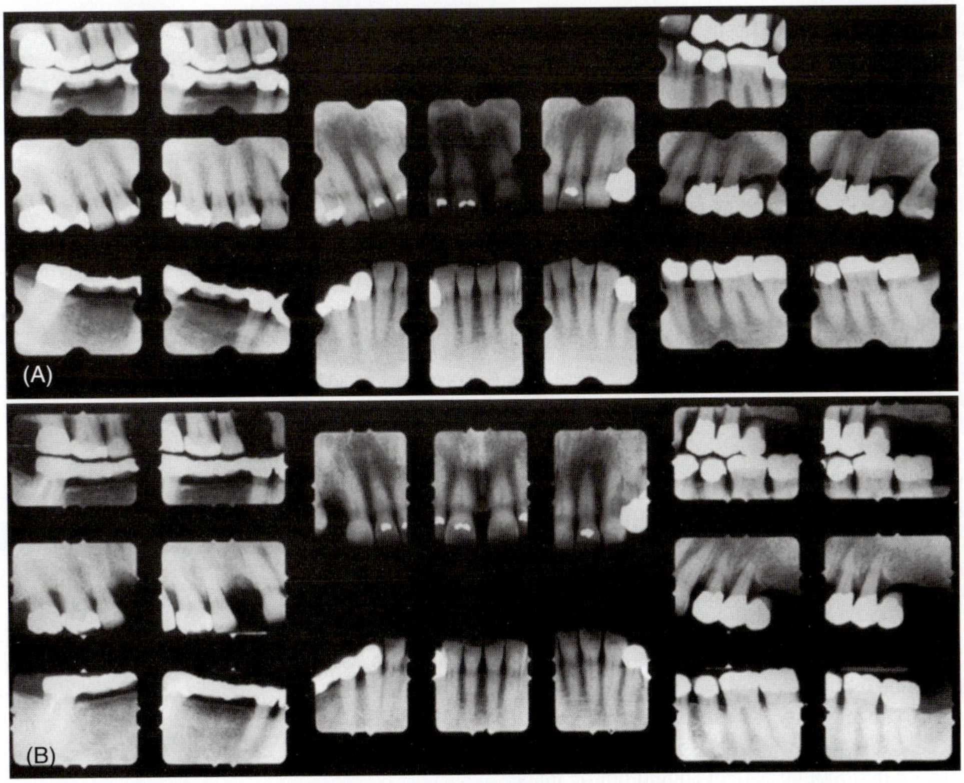

Fig. 56.8 A, Initial radiographs. The patient was advised to have localized areas of periodontal surgery and periodontal recall every 3 months. However, the patient did not comply and only had dental cleanings once or twice yearly. B, Radiographs 4 years later. Note the loss of teeth #5 and #15 and the increased bone loss of several premolars and molars.

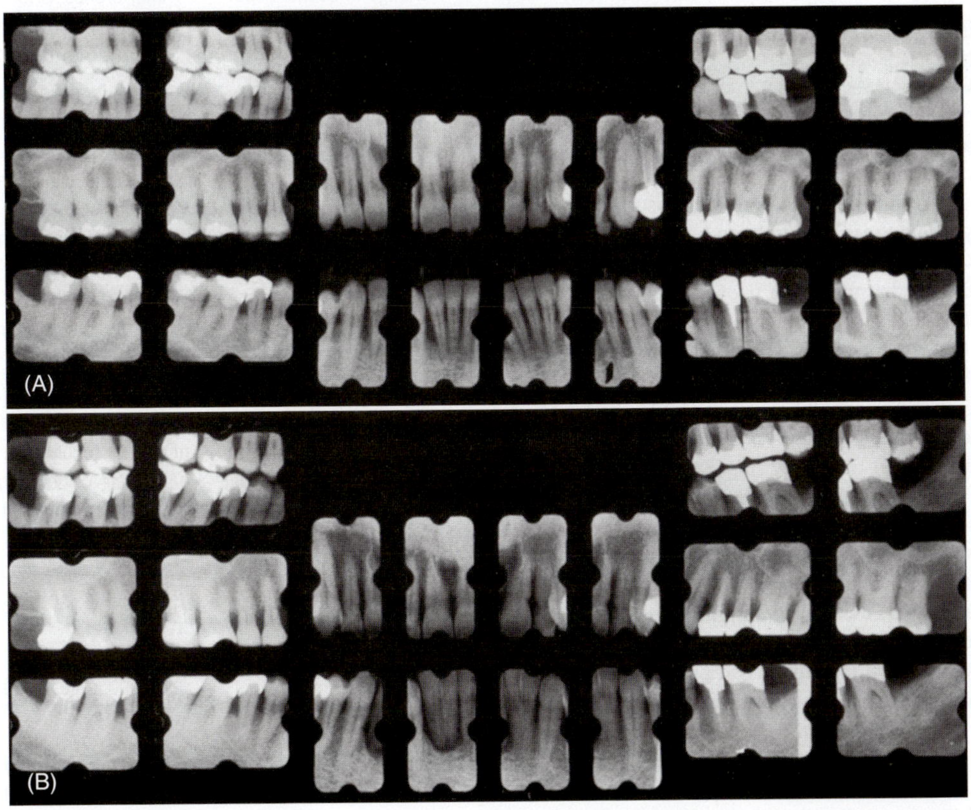

Fig. 56.9 A, Initial radiographs. The patient was advised to have localized areas of periodontal surgery and periodontal recall every 3 months. However, the patient did not comply and had no treatment other than emergency care and occasional dental cleanings. B, Radiographs 7 years later. Note the advanced bone loss and caries on many teeth.

TABLE 56.1 Radiographic Examination of Recall Patients for Supportive Periodontal Treatment

Patient Condition/Situation	Type of Examination
Clinical caries or high-risk factors for caries	Posterior bitewing examination at 6- to 18-month intervals
No clinical caries and no high-risk factors for caries	Posterior bitewing examination at 24- to 36-month intervals
Periodontal disease not under good control	Periapical or vertical bitewing radiographs of problem areas every 12–24 months
History of periodontal treatment with disease under good control	Bitewing examination every 24–36 months
Root form dental implants	Periapical or vertical bitewing radiographs after prosthetic placement and at 12 and 24 months, then every 24–36 months unless clinical problems arise
Transfer of periodontal or implant maintenance patients	Full-mouth series if a current set not available; if full-mouth series has been taken within 24 months, radiographs of implants and periodontal problem areas should be taken

Radiographs should be taken when they are likely to affect diagnosis and patient treatment. The recommendations in this table are subject to clinical judgment and may not apply to every patient. (Adapted from Guide to Patient Selection and Limiting Radiation Exposure. American Dental Association website, http://ada.org/2760/aspx, 2013.)

4. Presence of some systemic diseases that may affect host resistance to previously acceptable levels of biofilm.

A failing case can be recognized by the following:

1. Recurring inflammation revealed by gingival changes and bleeding of the sulcus on probing.
2. Increasing depth of sulci, leading to the recurrence of pocket formation.
3. Gradual increases in bone loss, as determined by radiographs.
4. Gradual increases in tooth mobility, as ascertained by clinical examination.

The decision to retreat a periodontal patient should not be made at the preventive maintenance appointment but should be postponed for 1–2 weeks. Often, the mouth appears improved at that time because of the resolution of edema and the resulting improved tone of the gingiva. Table 56.2 summarizes the symptoms of the recurrence of periodontal disease and their probable causes.

TABLE 56.2 Symptoms and Causes of Recurrence of Disease

Symptom	Possible Causes
Increased mobility	Increased inflammation Poor oral hygiene Subgingival calculus Inadequate restorations Deteriorating or poorly designed prostheses Systemic disease modifying host response to plaque
Recession	Toothbrush abrasion Inadequate keratinized gingiva Frenum pull Orthodontic therapy
Increased mobility with no change in pocket depth and no radiographic change	Occlusal trauma caused by lateral occlusal interference, bruxism, high restoration Poorly designed or worn-out prosthesis Poor crown-to-root ratio
Increased pocket depth with no radiographic change	Poor oral hygiene Infrequent recall visits Subgingival calculus Poorly fitting partial denture Mesial inclination into edentulous space Failure of new attachment surgery Cracked teeth Grooves in teeth New periodontal disease Gingival overgrowth caused by medication
Increased pocket depth with increased radiographic bone loss	Poor oral hygiene Subgingival calculus Infrequent recall visits Inadequate or deteriorating restorations Poorly designed prostheses Inadequate surgery Systemic disease modifying host response to plaque Cracked teeth Grooves in teeth New periodontal disease

Classification of Posttreatment Patients and Risk Assessment

The first year after periodontal therapy is important in terms of indoctrinating the patient in a recall pattern and reinforcing oral hygiene techniques. In addition, it may take several months to evaluate accurately the results of some periodontal surgical procedures. Consequently, some areas may have to be retreated because the results may not be optimal. Furthermore, the first-year patient often has etiologic factors that may have been overlooked and may be amenable to treatment at this early stage. For these reasons, the recall interval for first-year patients should not be longer than 3 months.

Patients who are on a periodontal recall schedule are a varied group. Table 56.3 lists several categories of maintenance patients and a suggested recall interval for each group. Patients can improve or may relapse to a different classification, with a reduction in or exacerbation of periodontal disease. When one dental arch is more involved than the other, the patient's periodontal disease is classified by the arch with the worse condition.

Table 56.3 is a traditional method of assigning the risk of a recurrence of periodontal destruction. A practitioner uses the listed risk factors and his or her own diagnostic and prognostic gestalt to assign a risk category and maintenance schedule. New risk factor assessment tools for the prevention of periodontal destruction have been developed. The Periodontal Risk Assessment (PRA) (Fig. 56.10) and the Periodontal Risk Calculator (PRC) have the most studies documenting their ability to predict the progression of periodontitis and tooth loss. The PRC is marketed by the PreViser Corporation and offers a web-based system for periodontal risk analysis and prognosis. The PRA is offered free of charge by the Clinical Research Foundation and the University of Bern at http://www.perio-tools.com/PRA/en/index.asp. Patient data are entered into the online form, and the program automatically calculates whether the patient is at low risk, moderate risk, or high risk; an appropriate

TABLE 56.3 Recall Intervals for Various Classes of Recall Patients

Merin Classification	Characteristics	Recall Interval
First year	First-year patient: routine therapy and uneventful healing. First-year patient: difficult case with complicated prosthesis, furcation involvement, poor crown-to-root ratios, or questionable patient cooperation	3 months 1–2 months
Class A	Excellent results well maintained for 1 year or longer Patient displays good oral hygiene, minimal calculus, no occlusal problems, no complicated prostheses, no remaining pockets, and no teeth with less than 50% of alveolar bone remaining	6 months to 1 year
Class B	Generally good results maintained reasonably well for 1 year or more, but patient displays some of the following factors: 1. Inconsistent or poor oral hygiene 2. Heavy calculus formation 3. Systemic disease that predisposes to periodontal breakdown 4. Some remaining pockets 5. Occlusal problems 6. Complicated prostheses 7. Ongoing orthodontic therapy 8. Recurrent dental caries 9. Some teeth with less than 50% of alveolar bone support 10. Smoking 11. Positive family history or genetic test 12. More than 20% of pockets bleed on probing	3–4 months (decide on a recall interval based on the number and severity of negative factors)
Class C	Generally poor results after periodontal therapy or several negative factors from the following list: 1. Inconsistent or poor oral hygiene 2. Heavy calculus formation 3. Systemic disease that predisposes to periodontal breakdown 4. Many remaining pockets 5. Occlusal problems 6. Complicated prostheses 7. Recurrent dental caries 8. Periodontal surgery indicated but not performed for medical, psychological, or financial reasons 9. Many teeth with less than 50% of alveolar bone support 10. Condition too far advanced to be improved by periodontal surgery 11. Smoking 12. Positive family history or genetic test 13. More than 20% of pockets bleed on probing	1–3 months (decide on a recall interval based on the number and severity of negative factors; consider retreating some areas or extracting severely involved teeth)

recall interval is then suggested. Because the different assessment tools use different risk factors and algorithms, they will not be in complete agreement. In one study, 57 patients were assessed with the PRC and PRA. The PRC classified 14 as low risk, 17 as medium risk, and 26 as high risk, whereas the PRA classified 8 as low risk, 28 as medium risk, and 21 as high risk.

Currently, there is no universally accepted objective method of predicting periodontitis progression, and there has been little research to determine if the risk calculators are more accurate than good clinical judgment. In summary, maintenance care is a critical phase of therapy. The long-term preservation of the dentition is closely associated with the frequency and quality of recall maintenance.

KEY FACT

The therapist should use risk assessment to determine SPT frequency.

Referral of Patients to the Periodontist

A general dentist can properly manage many periodontal patients, as a greater number of people retain their teeth throughout their lifetime. Another important fact to consider is that as the proportion of older people in the population increases, more teeth will be at risk for periodontal disease. Numerous studies indicate possible links between periodontal disease and systemic diseases, such as heart disease, stroke, diabetes, and adverse pregnancy outcomes. Therefore, the prevalence of patients requiring SPT is likely to increase in the future.

This expected increase in the number of periodontal patients will necessitate a greater understanding of periodontal problems and an increased level of expertise for the solution of such problems on the part of the general practitioner. General dentists must know when comanagement with a periodontist is indicated. Specialists are needed to treat difficult periodontal cases, patients with systemic health problems, dental implant patients, and those with a complex prosthetic construction that requires predictable results.

The criteria for cases to be treated in the general dental office and cases to be referred to a specialist vary for different practitioners and patients. The American Academy of Periodontology has issued guidelines to help the general practitioner decide when comanagement with a periodontist is indicated. The diagnosis will indicate the type of periodontal treatment required. If periodontal destruction necessitates surgery on the distal surfaces of second molars, extensive osseous surgery, or complex regenerative procedures,

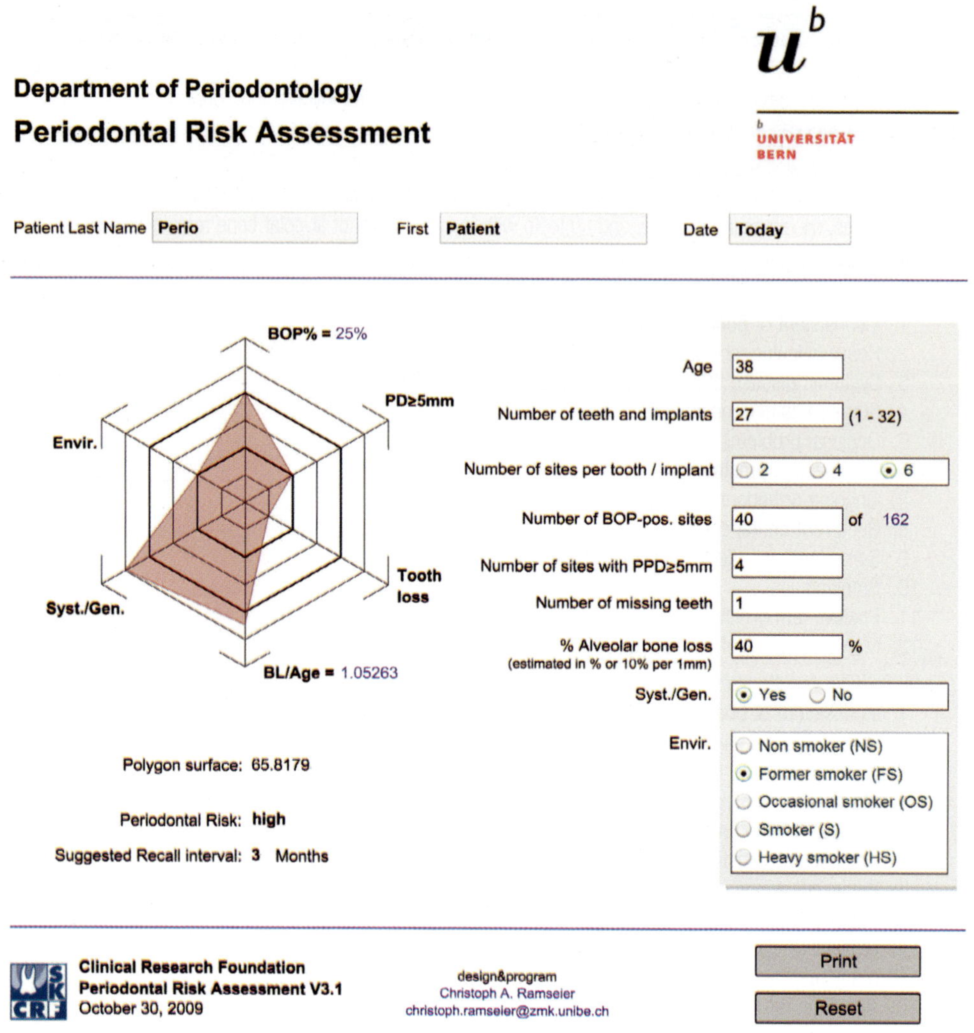

Fig. 56.10 Sample Periodontal Risk Assessment (PRA) report completed and downloaded from http://www.perio-tools.com/PRA/en/index.asp.

the patient is usually best treated by a specialist. Patients who require localized nonsurgical therapy or minor flap surgery can usually be managed by the general practitioner. General dentists have a primary responsibility to do what is best in the interest of the patient. According to Christensen, quality dentistry for a complex case requires a team effort partnering with a periodontal specialist to provide optimal care for the patient.

The decision to have the general practitioner treat a patient's periodontal disease should be guided by consideration of the risk that the patient will lose a tooth or teeth due to periodontal involvement or the periodontal disease negatively affecting the patient's systemic health.

The most important factors in the decision to refer a patient to a periodontist are the severity and location of the periodontal disease. Teeth with pockets of 5 mm or more, as measured from the cementoenamel junction, may have a questionable prognosis, as do teeth with furcation invasions even when more than 50% of bone support remains. Therefore, patients with strategically important teeth that have moderate to severe attachment loss or furcation invasions are usually best treated by specialists.

An important question remains: Should the maintenance phase of therapy be performed by the general practitioner or the specialist? This should be determined by the extent and severity of periodontal

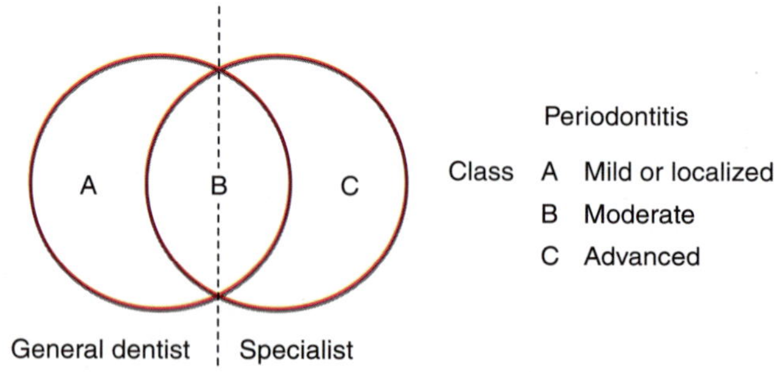

Fig. 56.11 Scheme for determining which practitioner should perform periodontal maintenance in patients with different degrees of periodontitis.

disease present. Class A recall patients should be maintained by the general dentist, whereas class C patients should be maintained by the specialist (see Table 56.3). Class B patients can alternate recall visits between the general practitioner and the specialist (Fig. 56.11). The suggested rule to decide who should maintain the recall therapy is determined by the initial category of the patient's disease and the result of the therapy. Patients with moderate to severe initial bone loss, advanced grades 2 or 3 furcation invasions, or pockets that could not be completely eradicated are those who should be seen by the periodontist. The specialist and the general dentist must work together, respect the other's knowledge and skills, and decide on a maintenance schedule that is in the best interest of the patient.

KEY FACT

Quality dentistry for a complex case requires a team effort partnering with a periodontal specialist to provide optimal care for the patient.

Tests for Disease Activity

Periodontal patients, even though they have received effective periodontal therapy, are at risk of disease recurrence for the remainder of their lives. In addition, pockets in and around the furcation areas are difficult to eliminate even with surgical therapy. These areas with pockets may continue to lose attachment. Comparison of sequential probing measurements, which may be facilitated by a dental practice management software, gives the most accurate indication of the rate of loss of attachment. A number of other clinical and laboratory variables have been correlated with disease activity.

No accurate method exists to predict disease activity, and clinicians rely on the information obtained from evaluating multiple risk factors. Patients whose disease is clearly refractory are candidates for bacterial culturing and antibiotic therapy in conjunction with additional mechanical therapy.

New methods will undoubtedly be developed in the future to help predict disease activity. The clinician must be able to interpret whether a test may be useful in determining disease activity and future loss of attachment. Tests should be adopted only when they are based on research that includes a critical analysis of the sensitivity, specificity, disease incidence, and predictive value of the proposed test

Conclusion

The long-term preservation of the dentition is closely associated with the frequency and quality of recall maintenance. The therapist should use risk assessment and educate the patient on the need for periodontal maintenance. Supportive periodontal therapy is a lifetime effort to prevent the disease from recurring. Patients who do not return for supportive periodontal therapy lose more teeth than compliant patients.

Suggested Readings

American Academy of Periodontology: Position paper: periodontal maintenance, *J Periodontol* 74:1395, 2003.

American Academy of Periodontology: Peri-implant mucositis and peri-implantitis: a current understanding of their diagnoses and clinical implications, *J Periodontol* 84:436, 2013.

Becker W, Becker BE, Berg LE: Periodontal treatment without maintenance: a retrospective study in 44 patients, *J Periodontol* 155:505, 1984.

Costa FO, Lages EJ, Cota LO, et al: Tooth loss in individuals under periodontal maintenance therapy: 5-year prospective study, *J Periodontal Res* 49:121, 2014.

Hirschfeld L, Wasserman B: A long-term survey of tooth loss in 600 treated periodontal patients, *J Periodontol* 49:225, 1978.

Lang NP, Joss A, Orsanic T, et al: Bleeding on probing, *J Clin Periodontol* 13:590, 1986.

Lindhe J, Nyman S, Karring T: Scaling and root planing in shallow pockets, *J Clin Periodontol* 9:415, 1982.

Wilson TG Jr, Glover ME, Malik AK, et al: Tooth loss in maintenance patients in a private periodontal practice, *J Periodontol* 58:231, 1987.

Wilson V: An insight into peri-implantitis: a systematic literature review, *Prim Dent J* 2:69, 2013.

MCQs

MCQs with answers for the chapter are available on www.medenact.com.

CHAPTER 57

Biological Aspects of Dental Implants

JP Fiorellini | K Wada | PG Stathopoulou | PR Klokkevold | A Jain | HL Sarmiento

CHAPTER OUTLINE

Attempts to replace lost dentition by means of implanted materials can be traced back to the ancient Egyptians, who hammered shaped seashells directly into the jaws for the purpose of replacing teeth. Over the past few centuries, a variety of materials have been implanted into jaws in an attempt to replace missing teeth. The success of these early implants was extremely poor primarily because they never achieved a stable state of integration with the supporting tissues. The typical outcome, regardless of material or design, was healing with a soft tissue layer interposed between the implant and bone (i.e., fibrous encapsulation). Consequently, implants became mobile, infected, and painful, which led to failure.

The history of modern implant dentistry began with the introduction of titanium implants. In the 1950s, Per-Ingvar Brånemark, a Swedish professor of anatomy, had a serendipitous finding while studying blood circulation in bone that became a historical breakthrough in medicine. He discovered an intimate bone-to-implant apposition with titanium that offered sufficient strength to cope with load transfer. He called the phenomenon "*osseointegration*" and developed an implant system with a specific protocol to predictably achieve it. The implants were used to anchor prosthetic replacement teeth in the edentulous jaw, and the first patient was successfully treated in 1965. Subsequent clinical studies proved that commercially pure (CP) titanium implants, placed with a strict protocol, including an unloaded healing period, could predictably achieve osseointegration and retain a full-arch prosthesis in function with a long-term success (15 years). Since that time, millions of patients worldwide have had missing teeth replaced with implants based on this original concept. Over the years, implant systems with variations in design (geometric and surface characteristics) and modified protocols have been developed and used with equal or better long-term success.

Today, implant designs, surgical placement techniques, healing times, and restorative protocols continue to evolve with the goal of improving outcomes. It is important for clinicians to know peri-implant anatomy, to understand the biology, and to appreciate the functional capacity of osseointegrated implants. This chapter reviews implant geometry and surface characteristics, as well as the anatomical and biological relationship of peri-implant tissues.

Implant Geometry (Macrodesign)

Numerous implant systems with various geometric (macrodesign) designs have been developed and used before the current implant systems in use today. Previous implant designs included blade vents (narrow, flat shape; tapped into boney trough prepared with rotary burs), press-fit cylindrical (bullet shape; pressed or tapped into prepared hole), subperiosteal (custom-made framework; adapted to the surface of jawbone), and transmandibular (long rods or posts; placed through the anterior mandible). Some of these implant systems were initially stable and appeared to be successful over short-term periods (e.g., 5 years) but failed to remain stable, became symptomatic and/or loose, and failed over longer periods. Lacking predictability, these implant systems are no longer used.

Since the time of the Brånemark studies, millions of patients have been treated worldwide using variations of these techniques with implants of different geometries and surface characteristics. Similar research including that of André Schroeder in Switzerland in the mid-1970s contributed to the success of endosseous dental implants. The serendipitous finding of Brånemark was that when a hole is prepared into the bone without overheating or otherwise traumatizing the tissues, an inserted biocompatible implantable device would predictably achieve an intimate bone apposition, as long as micromovements at the interface were prevented during the early healing period. The history of the research endeavors in Sweden provides a better understanding of the relevant biologic parameters involved.

The macroscopic configuration of implants has varied widely; the most common types are listed in Box 57.1. Currently, most endosseous implants have a cylindrical or tapered, screw-shaped/threaded design. The disastrous results with other implant configurations were largely responsible for the evolution toward the current popular designs.

Endosseous Implants

Blade Implants

Blade implants were designed and developed by Linkow and used clinically in 1960s and 1970s. Blade implants were inserted into the jawbone after mucoperiosteal flap elevation and preparation of

BOX 57.1 Implant Geometry (Macrodesign)

1. Endosseous implants
   - Blade-like
   - Pins
   - Cylindrical (hollow and full)
   - Disk-like
   - Screw shaped
   - Tapered and screw shaped
2. Subperiosteal frame-like implants
3. Transmandibular implants

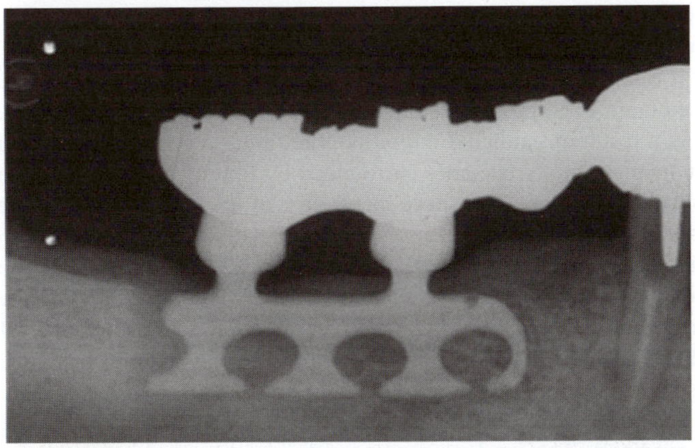

Fig. 57.1 Blade implant shows a large radiolucency, indicating that the fibrous encapsulation has led to deep pocketing and subsequent bone loss. Neighboring teeth bear the load of the implant restoration.

a channel with a high-speed rotary bur. They were tapped into the narrow trench. One or several posts pierced through the mucoperiosteum after suturing of the flaps. After a few weeks of healing, a fixed prosthesis was fabricated by a classic method and cemented on top of it.

Since the high-speed drilling leads to extensive bone necrosis at the histologic level, fibrous scar tissue formation occurs. This allows downgrowth of the epithelium, which leads to marsupialization of the blade implants (Fig. 57.1). If a bacterial infection occurs, it can lead to an intractable peri-implantitis with ample bone loss. More importantly, removal of such implants after complications implies sacrificing the surrounding jawbone. Due to its retentive geometry, the blade implant cannot simply be extracted or removed by a trephine, as with a cylindrical or screw-shaped implant.

The interface between blade vent implant and bone was called *fibroosseous integration*, which was defined as a tissue-to-implant contact: interposition of healthy dense collagen fibers at the interface between the implant and bone. At that time, the fibrous tissue was thought to be the replacement of the periodontal ligament; however, it was fibrous scar tissue produced following the bone necrosis initiated by high-speed drilling. This allows epithelial downgrowth around the post caused by the bacterial infection, which leads to encapsulation of blade implant with the fibrous scar tissue.

Most of the studies reported less than 50% success rate for 5-year duration with the complication of pocket formation exceeding 6 mm, followed by the significant alveolar bone loss around the implant. It was also a more complicated and invasive surgery to remove the failed implant, which was sacrificing significant surrounding jawbone. As a result of the poor long-term success, as well as the high complication rate, the use of blade vent implants has been significantly reduced. Removal of failed blade implants often requires significant cutting and bone removal despite being mobile.

Pins

Although seldom used at present, in the classic technique, three diverging pins were inserted either transgingivally or after reflection of mucoperiosteal flaps in holes drilled by spiral drills. At the point of convergence, the pins were interconnected with cement to ensure the proper stability because of their divergence. On top of this arrangement, a single tooth could be installed. In edentulous jaws, several of these pin triads could be used to interconnect with a fixed prosthesis.

As with blade implants, the bone necrosis during drilling leads to fibrous encapsulation, marsupialization, and loss of the implants because of infections. A positive aspect, however, is that when such implants must be removed, removing the connection at the place of convergence is sufficient to allow easy extraction of each individual pin. Thus, bone loss from removal is minimal.

Disk Implants

Disk implants are rarely used at present. The concept developed by Scortecci is based on the lateral introduction into the jawbone of a pin with a disk on top. Once introduced into the bone, the implant has strong retention against vertical extraction forces. Implants have been used with one, two, and even three disks. Unfortunately, as mentioned previously for blade implants, the cutting of the bone by means of high-speed drills leads to a fibrous scar tissue surrounding the implant, as revealed frequently by peri-implant radiolucencies. Data on the clinical success of disk implants are mostly anecdotal.

Root Form (Cylindrical) Implants

The first implant in this category, designed and developed by Schroeder and coworkers between 1974 and 1985, was called *ITI* (International Team for Implantology) *hollow-cylinder, plasma-sprayed, one-stage implant* (Fig. 57.2). It was thought that the hollow geometry should provide large bone-to-implant contact and holes would be favorable for the additional fixation of the implant. However, the survival rates were less favorable compared to the other system. Thus, this system was withdrawn from clinical use.

When discussing cylindrical implants, it is important to distinguish between hollow and full cylindrical implants. Straumann and coworkers introduced hollow cylinders in the mid-1970s with the ITI system. The idea was that implant stability would benefit from

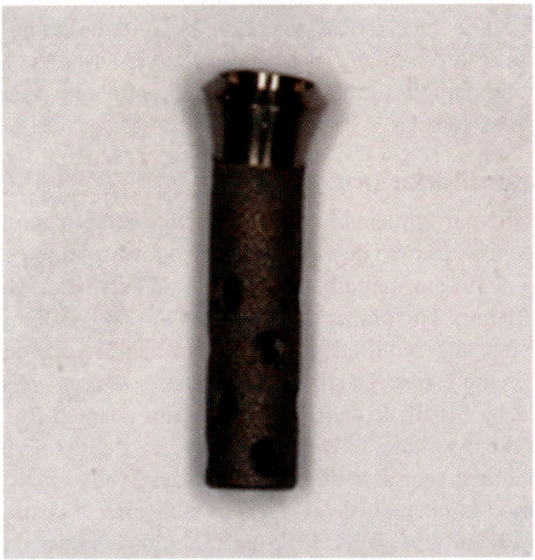

Fig. 57.2 International Team for Implantology (ITI) hollow cylinder implant. Note the hollow geometry, which should provide large bone-to-implant contact, and holes that theoretically should be favorable for the additional fixation of the implant.

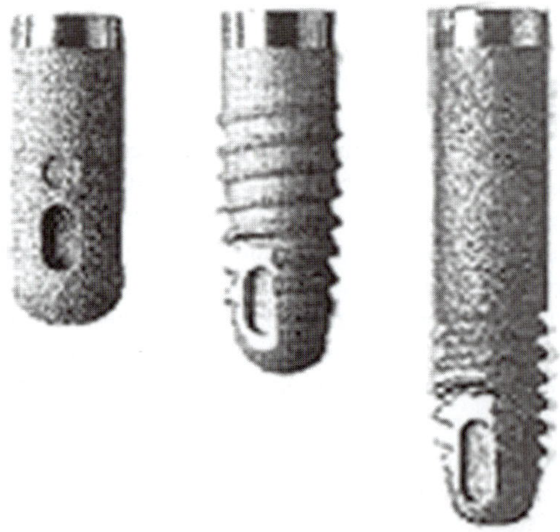

Fig. 57.3 The IMZ implants. The roughened surface of the fixture had an advantage of higher integration of bone. Conversely, the surface characteristic added to the high frequency of peri-implantitis in long-term use.

the large bone-to-implant surface provided by means of the hollow geometry. It was also thought that the holes (vents) would favor the ingrowth of bone to offer additional fixation. The same concept was used in the Core-Vent system developed by Niznick. Although it was not clarified whether the cause was geometry or the associated surface characteristics (titanium plasma–sprayed surface, titanium alloy), survival statistics were disappointing for hollow cylinder implants.

Solid cylindrical implants were used by Kirsch and became available under the name IMZ, referring to the *internal mobile shock absorber*. The IMZ system, developed by Kirsch, prevailed in the market (Fig. 57.3). The characteristic function of this system was the *internal mobile element* (IME) shock absorber, which was able to connect with the adjacent natural tooth. The system presented successful results in the short term, but long-term success rates were unacceptable (38% in 10 years), leading to the limited use of this implant design. For this reason, this implant is rarely seen in the market.

Even when an intimate bone apposition is achieved, extraction forces on such cylindrical implants lead to strong shear forces at the bone-to-implant interface. Only the microscopic surface irregularities offer some mechanical retention by interdigitation of bone growing onto the implant surface. With a screw-based geometry, forces acting parallel to the long axis of the implants are dispersed in many directions.

Transmandibular Implants

Transmandibular implants were developed to retain dentures in the edentulous lower jaw. They were indicated for use in the extremely resorbed edentulous mandible with a minimal alveolar ridge height less than 10 mm. The implant was inserted through a submandibular skin incision and required general anesthesia. Two models were available in the 1960s. The first, called the *staple-bone implant*, was developed by Small. It consisted of a splint adapted to the lower border of the mandible, to which it is fixed by stabilizing pins. Two transmandibular screws were driven transgingivally into the mouth. The reported implant survival rate was 93% after 5 years and continued to exceed 90% after 15 years. The other model, introduced by Bosker, has two metal splints, one below the lower border of the mandible and one intraorally to connect the four posts piercing through the soft tissues. The Bosker implant seemed less reliable than the staple-bone implant, achieving only 70% survival after 5 years in the mandibular symphyseal area. Both transmandibular implants presented with the gingival hyperplasia or infection with the incidence of 10%–15% of all cases. Despite the good long-term survival data reported (especially for the staple implant), the high incidence of complications and the necessity of using general anesthesia for implant placement, the transmandibular implant design is rarely used today.

Subperiosteal Implants

Subperiosteal implants are customized according to a plaster model derived from an impression of the exposed jawbone, before the surgery planned for implant insertion. The implant was designed with several posts, typically four or more for an edentulous jaw, which passed through the gingival tissues.

Subperiosteal implants are designed to retain an overdenture although fixed prostheses have also been cemented onto the posts. As a result of epithelial migration, the framework of subperiosteal implants usually becomes surrounded by fibrous connective tissue (scar), including the space between the implant and the bone surface. The marsupialization, as described earlier, often leads to infectious complications, which often necessitates removal of the implant. Furthermore, while being loaded by jaw function, jawbone resorption occurs rapidly, resulting in a lack of adaptation of the frame to the bone surface. As a result of this type of outcome, subperiosteal implants are now rarely used.

The subperiosteal implant was used in the treatment of atrophic mandibles. The implant is custom designed to fit the mandibular jaw bone using a plaster model obtained from an impression of the exposed mandible. It consisted of a cast metal framework with a subperiosteal component in contact with the bone and a transgingival component (posts), which were used to retain the dental prosthesis. The number of transgingival posts on the implants depends on the number of missing teeth, averaging four to six for the totally edentulous jaw. Several clinical studies reported poor survival rates of less than 50% for 5–10 years, with the frequent complication of gingival inflammation, involving tissue reaction around the post caused by the lack of soft tissue attachment to the metal post. These complications led to the development of sinus tract resorption of the cortical bone and exposure of framework. As a result of this higher rate of failure, as well as the significant complications and surgical invasion, subperiosteal implants are rarely used.

The most common implant design being used today is the screw-shaped or threaded cylindrical implant (Fig. 57.4A). A threaded implant design is preferred because it engages bone well and is able to achieve good primary stabilization. Even systems that started with cylindrical press-fit (nonthreaded) designs progressively evolved to a threaded geometry. The (longitudinal) shape of implants may be parallel or tapered (Fig. 57.4B). Although a vast majority of all implants have been parallel walled, the use of a tapered implant design has recently been advocated because it requires less space in the apical region (i.e., better for placement between roots or in narrow anatomic areas with labial concavities). Tapered implants have also been advocated for use in extraction sockets (Fig. 57.5).

Implant Surface Characteristics (Microdesign)

Implant surface characteristics (microtopography) have been shown to positively influence the healing process. Accordingly, modification of implant surface characteristics has been a major area of research interest and development over the past 15–20 years. Modifications in surface energy, chemical composition, and surface topography are known to influence cellular activity and tissue

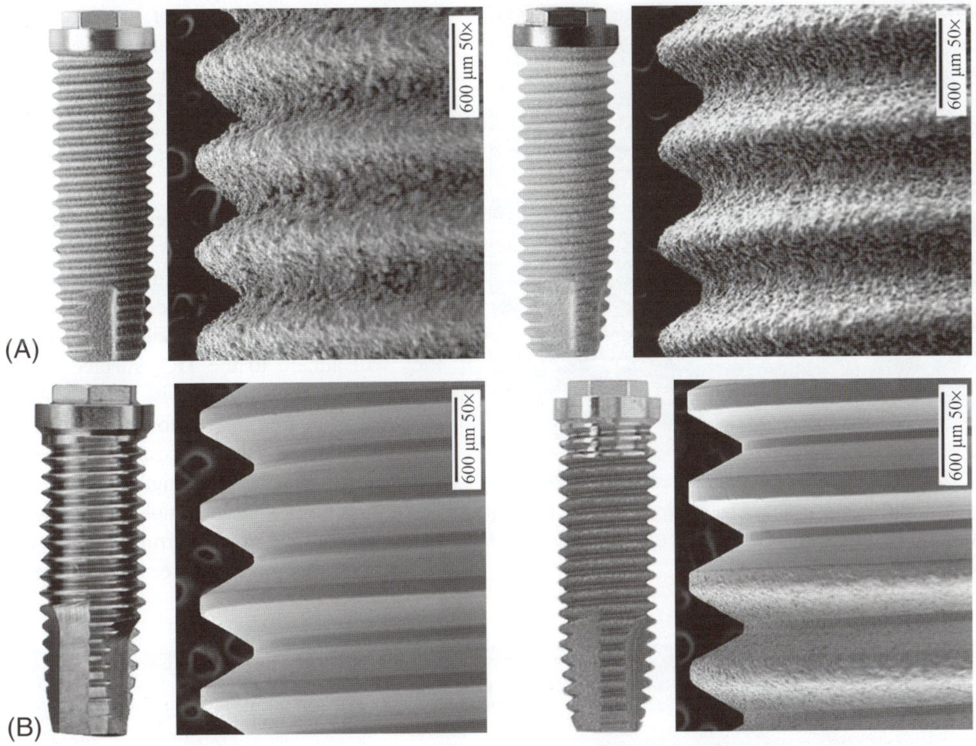

Fig. 57.4 A, Illustration of a parallel, threaded implant. B, Illustration of a tapered, threaded implant. *(Copyright 2012 BIOMET 3i, LLC. Used by permission, all rights reserved.)*

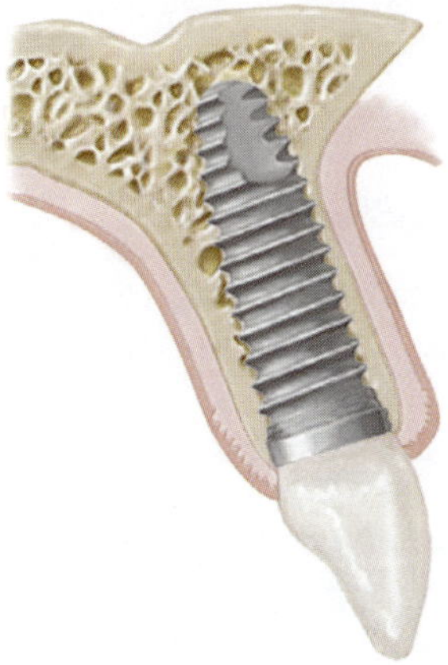

Fig. 57.5 A tapered, threaded implant design is helpful to minimize apical bone fenestration in areas such as the anterior maxilla, as the result of the presence of labial concavities. Tapered implant designs are also advantageous for immediate implant placement into extraction sockets.

responses leading to enhanced osteogenesis. At the molecular level, modified implant surfaces increase adsorption of serum proteins, mineral ions, and cytokines, which subsequently promote cellular migration and attachment. Implant surface characteristics can also aid in the retention of a fibrin clot, thus providing a migratory pathway for the differentiating osteogenic cells to reach the implant surface. Today, implants are treated with a variety of technologies to modify surface characteristics (microscale or nanoscale) to enhance bone formation.

Additive Processes

The additive process modifies the microstructure/macrostructure and chemical nature of the implant surface by adding materials or chemicals to the existing surface. There are several methods used to add materials and/or chemicals to the implant surface, such as inorganic mineral coatings, plasma spraying, biocoating with growth factors, fluoride, and particulates or cements containing calcium phosphates, sulfates, or carbonates (Fig. 57.6). The addition of materials, such as hydroxyapatite, to the implant surface has been shown to enhance or accelerate the initial bone cells adaptation or proliferation. In general, additive surface modifications tend to increase the surface texture greater than subtractive surface modifications, which results in topographically "rougher" implant surfaces. Surface roughness can also be increased by oxidizing or adding an oxide layer (see Fig. 57.14A–D).

Subtractive Processes

The subtractive process modifies the microstructure and chemical nature of the implant surface by removing or altering the existing surface. The roughness of implant surface can be modified by machining, acid etching, blasting, or a combination of these processes to enhance the amount or speed of osseointegration. The changes are most notable at the microscopic level (Fig. 57.7). Implant surfaces that are modified at the microscopic level with techniques such as acid-etching are thought to promote favorable cellular responses and increased bone formation in close proximity to the surface.

Implant Surface Chemical Composition

There have been unsuccessful trials with oral implants made of carbon or hydroxyapatite. The lack of resistance, because of material properties, to occlusal forces led to frequent fractures. The so-called noble metals or alloys, however, do not resist corrosion and have thus been abandoned. Today, the vast majority of oral implants are made of CP titanium or titanium alloys. The following discussion relates to titanium implants.

Titanium is a very reactive metal that oxidizes within nanoseconds when exposed to air. Due to this passive oxide layer, the titanium

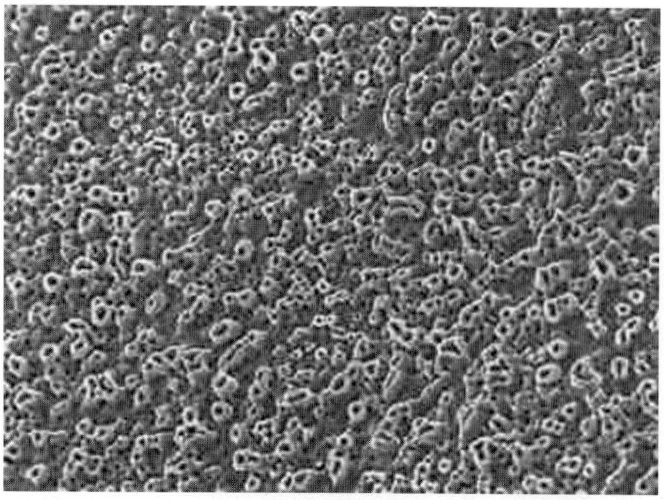

Fig. 57.6 Roughened surfaces are achieved by plasma spraying, by acid etching, or as shown here by oxidizing (TiUnite surface). *(Courtesy: Nobel Biocare Services AG, Zurich, Switzerland.)*

then becomes very resistant to corrosion in its CP form. Some alloys, such as titanium-aluminum 6% and vanadium 4% (Ti6Al4V), are known to provoke bone resorption as the result of leakage of some toxic components. The oxide layer of CP titanium reaches 10 nm of thickness. It grows over the years when facing a bioliquid. It consists mainly of titanium dioxide (TiO_2).

All titanium oxides have dielectric constants, which are higher than most other metal oxides. This factor may explain titanium's tendency to adsorb biomolecules, as seen during surgery when the blood creeps up the surface during implant insertion. The biomolecules normally appear as folded-up structures to hide their insoluble parts, while putting water-soluble radicals on their surface. Thus, they will adhere to the TiO_2 surface after displacing the original water molecules sitting on its surface. Although initially attracted by weak van der Waals forces, the high dielectric constant of titanium oxides and the polarizability of the molecules after adsorption will lead to high bond strengths, which are considered irreversible when they surpass 30 kcal/mol. In fact, because of its propensity for being covered by an uninterrupted oxide layer, which has ceramic-like properties similar to other metal oxides (e.g., aluminum oxides),

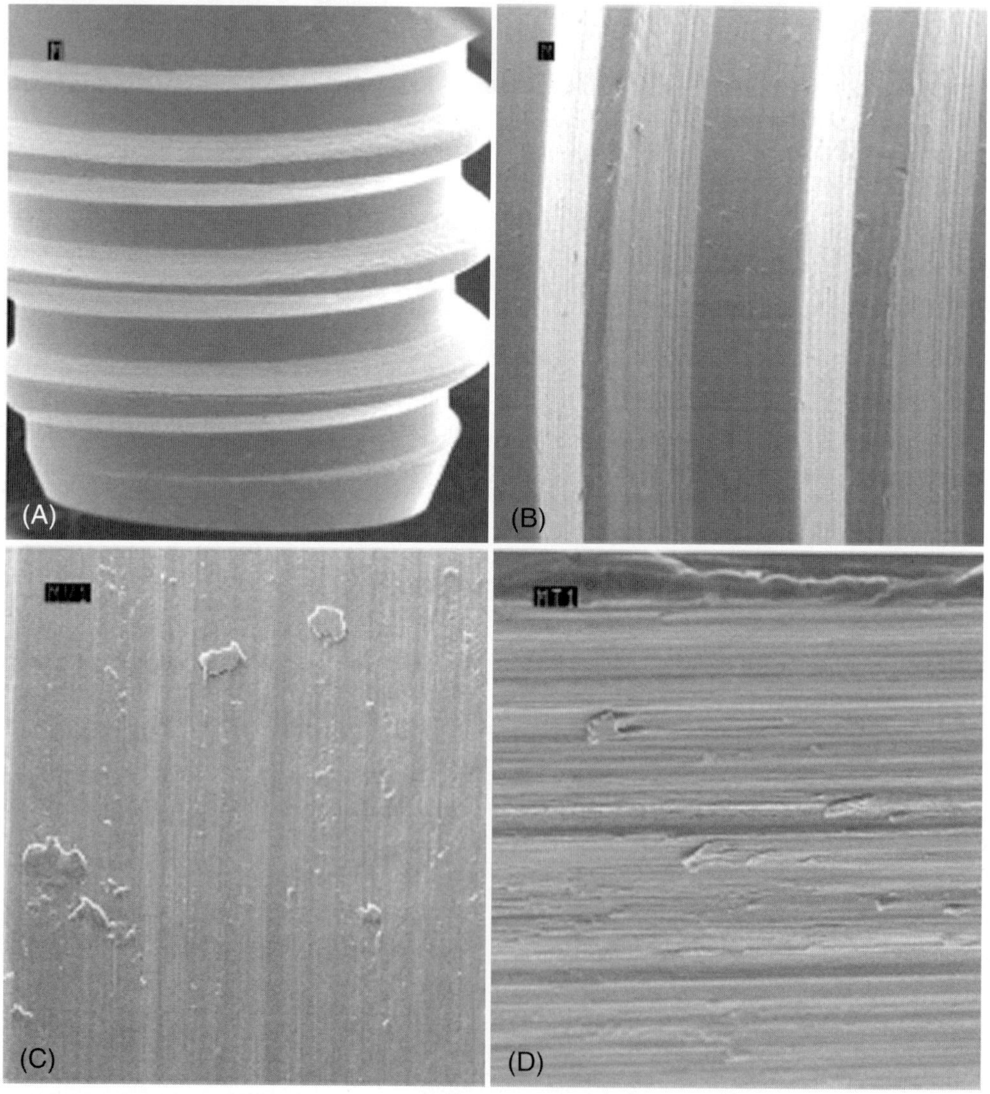

Fig. 57.7 SEM image of machined surface implant with characteristic grooved pattern. A, Implant with machined surface (×40). B, Grooved pattern apparent on machined surface (×100). C, Machined surface with distinct ridges and grooves (×500). D, Machined surface with distinct ridges and grooves (×1000). *(Courtesy: Nobel Biocare Services AG, Zurich, Switzerland.)*

titanium makes the coating of implants superfluous. This should be stressed because many authors hope for even better osseointegration potential with calcium phosphate (CaP)-coated surfaces and strongly advocate their use. To date, clinical results with CaP-coated implants have not been encouraging in a long-term perspective.

Thus, the overall view of potential advantages for different implant surface characteristics is complex, and only clinical observations can determine their validity. For good-quality bone, after 15 years of follow-up, clinical success rates of 99% have been reported for implants with a turned surface. Enhanced implant surface characteristics are likely to be most beneficial for the more challenging situations, such as poor quality bone and early and immediate loading.

Implant Surface Free Energy and Micro-Roughness

When an implant is brought into contact with bodily tissues and fluids, in this case mostly bone, it faces a "bioliquid," an aqueous environment. Within milliseconds, water, ions, and small biomolecules are absorbed. One could imagine that this absorbed layer renders all surfaces equal. However, the large molecules and the cells that will subsequently adhere to this surface are influenced by the surface characteristics of this pellicle layer. The composition and structure of the initial layer are largely determined by the underlying surface. Thus, the three-dimensional shape of the molecules will be modified during their adherence to this pellicle layer and will unveil different radicals, depending on this metamorphosis.

The surface free energy, often called *wettability*, is an important parameter for these interactions. It can be assessed through the shape of a standardized drop of liquid put on the clean implant surface. The angle of this drop toward the underlying surface reveals that the cohesive forces between liquid molecules are stronger than the adhesive forces between the liquid and the surface. Thus, a ball-shaped drop would reveal a low surface free energy.

Surface topography at the cellular and molecular level means microscopic roughness. Surface roughness can be measured with a profilometer, a stylus that follows the surface and measures the peak-to-valley dimensions (expressed as R_a values) or the spacing between irregularities (expressed as *S*cx values). Wennerberg and Albrektsson provide guidelines for topographic evaluation of implant surfaces. No implant surface is smooth although several reports have incorrectly referred to the "turned" (machined) implant surface as "smooth" (see Fig. 57.9). Roughened implant surfaces speed up the bone apposition; as demonstrated in vitro, more prostaglandin E_2 (PGE_2) and transforming growth factor beta 1 (TGF-β_1) are produced on rough than on smooth surfaces. Rough surfaces may show some disadvantages, such as increased ion leakage and increased adherence of macrophages and subsequent bone resorption.

It was also reported that in vitro adsorption of fibronectin was higher on smooth than on rough, CP titanium surfaces. Fibronectin is a glycoprotein quickly adhering on hard surfaces and known to determine subsequent cell adhesion. Microtopography also influences the number and morphology of cell adhesion pseudopods and cell orientation. Grooves in an implant surface will guide the cell migration along their direction. Bone growth can enter altered microtopographic features such as pits and porosities with internal dimensions that are only a few microns.

Lack of load can also be detrimental and can lead to cortical bone resorption. This is well documented in orthopedics and is termed *stress shielding*. This phenomenon has not been properly evaluated for oral implants in which marginal bone resorption is thought to be associated with chronic inflammation of the overlying soft tissues.

The use of finite element analysis (FEA) has become popular but lacks value by itself; invalid assumptions, such as the isotropic nature of the bone, must be used in the modeling. The deviation of FEA data from in vivo data has been well documented. FEA data should be considered as "descriptive" models that require confirmation by biologic data. However, as with photoelastic studies, FEA analyses do provide some insight on stress concentrations and their relation to implant geometry and the prosthetic superstructures.

Osseointegration

The primary goal of implant installation is to achieve and maintain a stable bone-to-implant connection (i.e., osseointegration). Histologically, osseointegration is defined as the direct structural and functional connection between ordered, living bone and the surface of a load-bearing implant without intervening soft tissues (Fig. 57.8). Clinically, osseointegration is the asymptomatic rigid fixation of an alloplastic material (implant) in bone with the ability to withstand occlusal forces. The hard tissue interface is a fundamental requirement for and an essential component of implant success.

Initial Bone Healing

The osseointegration process observed after implant insertion can be compared to bone fracture healing. Implant site osteotomy preparation (bone wounding) initiates a sequence of events, including an inflammatory reaction, bone resorption, release of growth factors, and attraction by chemotaxis of osteoprogenitor cells to the site. Differentiation of osteoprogenitor cells into osteoblasts leads to bone formation at the implant surface. Extracellular matrix proteins, such as osteocalcin, modulate apatite crystal growth. Specific conditions, optimal for bone formation, must be maintained at the healing site to achieve osseointegration.

Immobility of the implant relative to the bone must be maintained for bone formation at the surface. A mild inflammatory response enhances the bone healing, but moderate inflammation or movement above a certain threshold is detrimental. When micromovements at the interface exceed 150 μm, the movement will impair differentiation of osteoblasts, and fibrous scar tissue will form between the bone and implant surface. Therefore, it is important to avoid excessive forces, such as occlusal loading, during the early healing period.

Bone tissue damage and debris created by the osteotomy site preparation must be cleared up by osteoclasts for normal bone healing. These multinuclear cells, originating from the blood, can resorb bone at a pace of 50–100 μm per day. There is a coupling between bone apposition and bone resorption (Fig. 57.9). Preosteoblasts, derived from primary mesenchymal cells, depend on a favorable oxidation-reduction (redox) potential of the environment. Thus, a proper vascular supply and oxygen tension are needed. If oxygen tension is poor, the primary stem cells may differentiate into fibroblasts, form scar tissue, and lead to implant failure (nonintegration).

If bone is overheated or crushed during preparation, it will become necrotic and may lead to nonmineralized (soft tissue) scar formation or be sequestered. The critical temperature for bone cells that should not be exceeded is 47°C (116.6°F) at an exposure time of 1 min. Thus, preparation of implant osteotomy sites require profuse irrigation (cooling) along with gentle, intermittent, moderate-speed drilling using sharp drills. Another complicating factor, well recognized from open wound fractures, is that microbial contamination jeopardizes the normal bone healing. Accordingly, strict aseptic techniques should be maintained.

New bone formation follows a specific sequence of events. Woven bone is quickly formed in the gap between the implant and

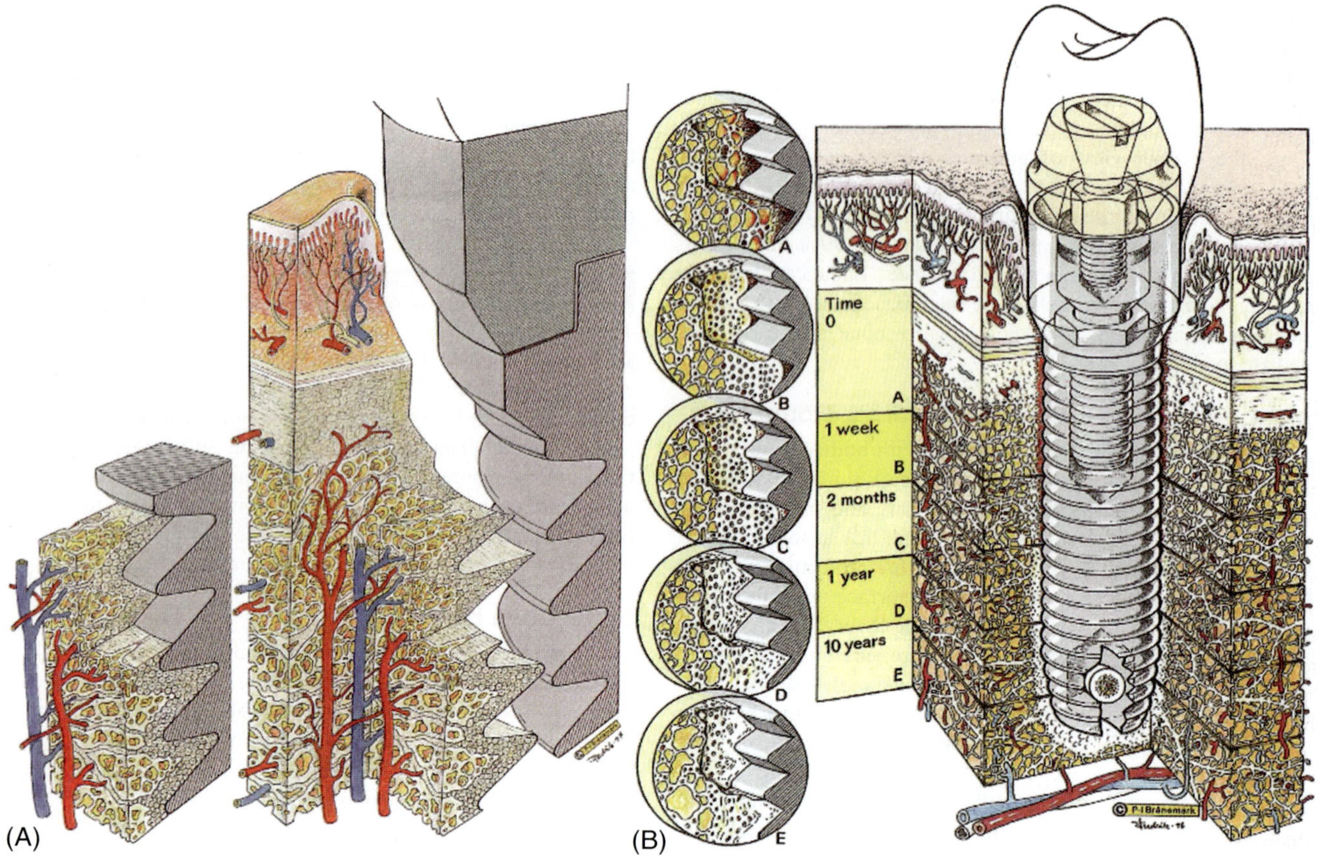

Fig. 57.8 A, Three-dimensional diagram of the tissue and titanium interrelationship showing an overall view of the intact interfacial zone around the osseointegrated implant. B, Physiologic evolution of the biology of the interface over time.

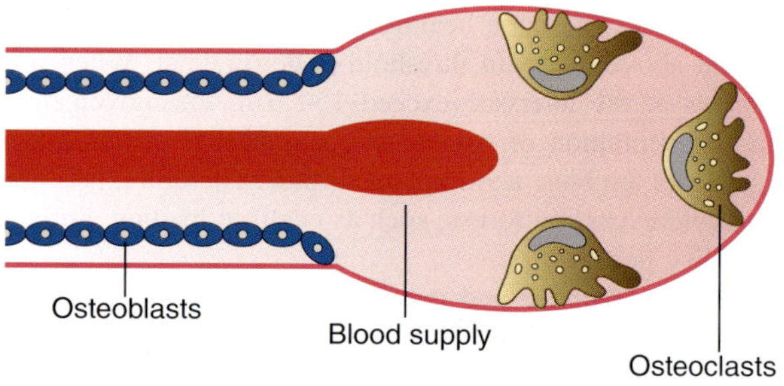

Fig. 57.9 The basic multicellular unit is the basic remodeling process for bone renewal. Osteoclasts are imported by the vascular supply, and the resorption lacunae are soon filled by the lining osteoblasts.

the bone; it grows fast, up to 100 μm per day, and in all directions. Characterized by a random orientation of its collagen fibrils, high cellularity, and limited degree of mineralization, the biomechanical capacity of woven bone is poor (Fig. 57.10A). Thus, any occlusal load should be well controlled or avoided in the early phase of healing. After several months, woven bone is progressively replaced by lamellar bone with organized, parallel layers of collagen fibrils and dense mineralization. Contrary to the fast-growing woven bone, lamellar bone formation occurs at a slow pace (only a few microns per day). Ultimately, after 18 months of healing, a steady state is reached where lamellar bone is continuously resorbed and replaced (Fig. 57.10B). At the light microscopic level, an intimate bone-to-implant contact has been extensively reported. Once the bone-to-implant interface has reached a steady state, it can maintain itself over decades, as ascertained by human histology from implants retrieved because of hardware fractures.

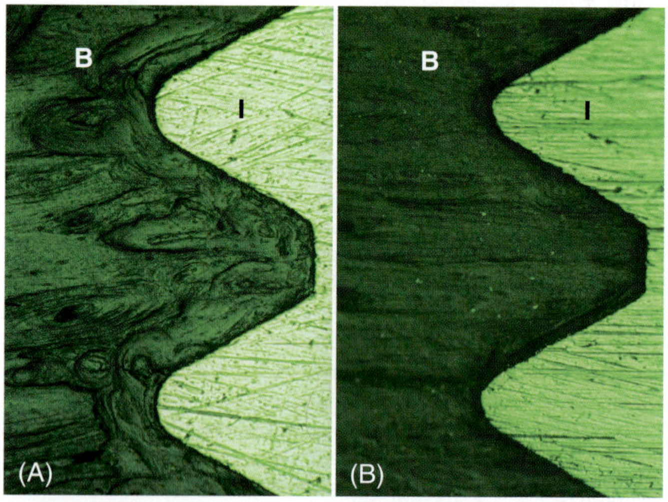

Fig. 57.10 A, After initial healing, woven bone, as characterized by its irregular pattern, is laid down. B, After weeks or months, progressively a lamellar bone is laid down, with regular concentric lamellae. *B*, Bone; *I*, implant. *(Courtesy: Professor T. Albrektsson, Gothenburg, Sweden.)*

Bone Remodeling and Function

Clinically, both primary and secondary stability of an implant are critical to success. Primary stability, achieved at the time of surgical placement, depends on the implant geometry (macrodesign), as well as the quality and quantity of bone available for implant anchorage at a specific site. Secondary stability, achieved over time with healing, depends on the implant surface (microdesign), as well as the quality and quantity of adjacent bone, which will determine the percentage of contacts between the implant and bone. For example, areas such as the anterior mandible have dense cortical bone and provide rigid primary stabilization and good support throughout the healing process. Conversely, areas such as the posterior maxilla have thin cortical bone and large marrow spaces provide less primary stability. For this reason, the posterior maxilla has been associated with lower success rates compared to other sites with greater bone density and support.

Once osseointegration is achieved, implants can resist and function under the forces of occlusion for many years. Longitudinal biomechanical assessments seem to indicate that during the first weeks after placement of one-stage implants, decreased rigidity is observed. This may be indicative of bone resorption during the initial phase of healing. Subsequently, rigidity increases and continues to increase for years. Thus, when a prosthesis is installed immediately (in 1 day) or early (in 1–2 weeks), care must be taken to control against overload. It is important to recognize that sites with limited primary stability or less bone-to-implant contact (e.g., posterior maxilla) will likely go through a period of even less bone support in the early stages of bone healing due to the initial phase of bone resorption.

Assessment of implant biomechanics can easily be done at the clinical level by noninvasive devices such as the Periotest (Fig. 57.11A and B) and the Ostell (Fig. 57.12). The Periotest (Gulden, Bensheim, Germany) projects a rod against the implant or abutment using a magnetic pulse at a certain speed. The apparatus measures the deceleration time needed before the rod comes to a standstill. This is transformed in an arbitrary unit, which reflects that the rigidity of the bone-to-implant continuum values should be below +7, the minimum with the most rigid being −8. Osseointegrated implants are thought to demonstrate an increased rigidity over time. The *resonance frequency analysis* (RFA) offers an alternative measurement. With the Ostell device, a small transducer attached to the implant imposes a series of frequencies and measures the overall resonance frequency and because the transducer and the structure are constant, any change in the resonance frequency reveals a change in the implant-bone interface, either in quality or in quantity. Primary stability measurements reveal a frequency range of 6–9 kHz, with higher values in the mandible. The measures are transformed into arbitrary values where measurements should exceed 56, which indicate a level of bone support that is consistent with osseointegration (Fig. 57.13). These noninvasive tests reflect the *rigidity* of the bone to implant interface.

The *strength* of the bone to implant interface cannot be clinically assessed. Some investigators have measured the force needed to undo the tight adhesion of bone tissues. This has often been done by counter torque force measurements to determine the threshold at which loosening, or often fracturing, is observed. This methodology is questionable because it does not reveal the strength of the biologic interface as such, but rather the *congruency* of the implant surface irregularities with the surrounding bone. Indeed, a very roughened surface, such as that achieved with a titanium plasma-sprayed implant, will demonstrate a higher torque resistance than a turned one, where the grooves are much smaller in scale and run parallel to the applied removal force. When the surface roughness is microscopic, such as that achieved with an acid-etched or blasted implant, the bone adaptation to the microtopography will increase the shear strength needed to fracture the bone from the surface to a level that is greater than a turned surface but lesser than a plasma-sprayed surface.

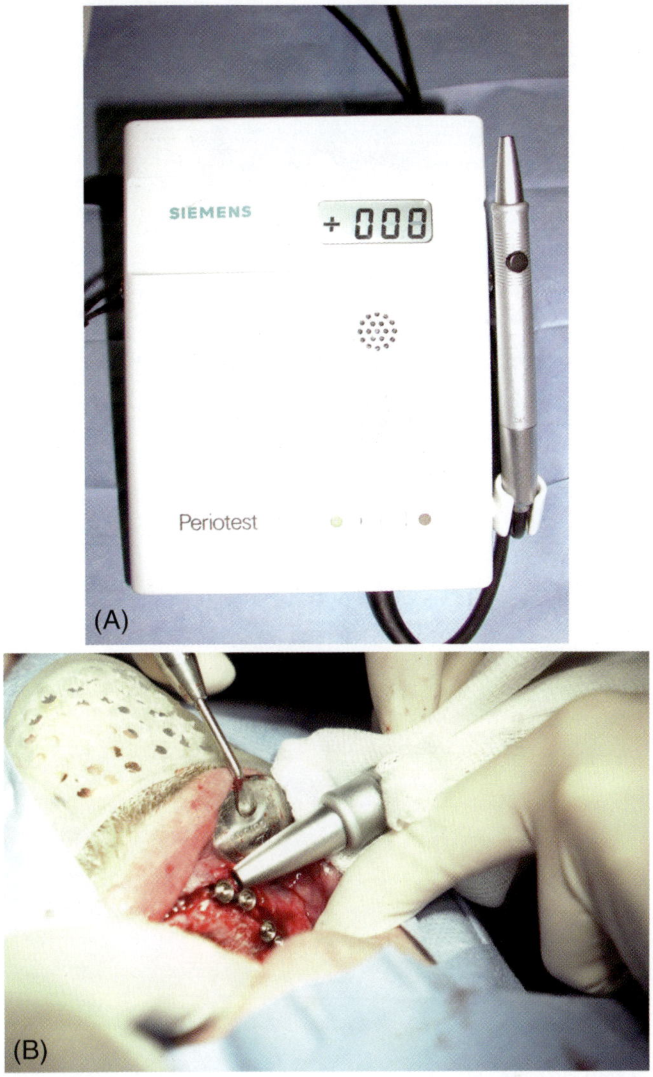

Fig. 57.11 A, Periotest electronic apparatus (presently made by Gulden, Bensheim, Germany) provides objective means to measure endosseous implant rigidity. B, Periotest measurement performed at surgery to evaluate the increasing rigidity at future control visits.

Others have used pullout tests of the implants as a whole in a coronal direction. For screw-shaped implants, which are very retentive in this axis because of the threads, this approach apparently cannot assess the biologic adhesion force. The real test should be "pull-off" test in which a nonretentive surface is detached from the adhering bone. This is a difficult experimental model that is seldom used.

Soft Tissue Considerations

Not surprisingly, for two decades, research and clinical interest focused on the bone-to-implant interface of osseointegrated implants and the overlying soft tissues were largely ignored. Except for a few descriptive sentences, the classic handbook by Brånemark et al. presented no data or information about the soft tissue interface. This may be due in part to the fact that most patients were fully edentulous and the Brånemark system implants had turned (machined) surfaces, which are less likely to be associated with soft tissue inflammatory problems. Today, there is greater interest in and appreciation for peri-implant soft tissues and the soft tissue-to-implant interface as a function of esthetics and maintenance of a seal or barrier against microbial invasion.

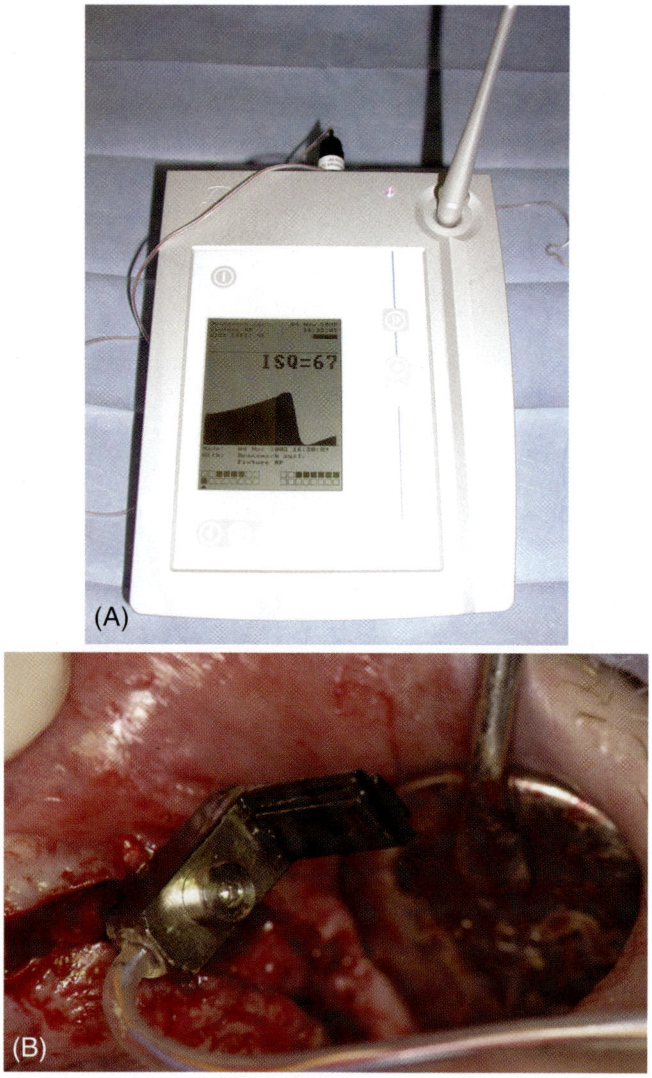

Fig. 57.12 A, Ostell device measures changes in resonance frequency over time. B, Stimulator is fixed on the implant or abutment to transmit energy in a series of frequencies. Use of the Ostell allows measurement of the primary stability at surgery.

Time	At Abutment Connection	1 year	2 years	3 years	4 years	5 years	6 years
Mean	−2.16	−2.80	−2.92	−3.30	−3.90	−4.75	−5.50
	*---------	---------*					
		*--------	--------*				
		*--------	----------	--------*			
			*--------	--------*			
				*--------	--------*		
					*--------	--------*	
					*--------	----------	--------*
						*--------	--------*

Fig. 57.13 Over time, Periotest values (PTVs, arbitrary units) indicate increasing rigidity, which parallels the increased bone density over time.

Peri-implant soft tissues are similar in appearance and structure to periodontal soft tissues (see Chapter 1). Clearly, both implants and teeth emerge through the soft tissues on the alveolar ridge. The soft tissues consist of connective tissue covered by epithelium. There is a gingival/mucosal sulcus, a long junctional epithelial attachment, and a zone of connective tissue above the supporting bone (Fig. 57.14A and B). Despite the apparent similarities in soft tissues around teeth and implants, the presence of a periodontal ligament around teeth and not around implants is an important, distinct difference. Whereas natural teeth have a periodontal ligament with connective tissue fibers suspending them in the alveolar bone, osseointegrated implants do not. There are no inserting collagen fibers anywhere along the interface of osseointegrated implants. Bone is in direct contact with the implant surface without intervening soft tissues.

Clinically, the thickness of the peri-implant soft tissues varies from 2 to several millimeters (Fig. 57.15). An animal study determined the total height of the peri-implant "biologic width" to be approximately 3–4 mm, where about 2 mm is the epithelial attachment, and about 1–2 mm is the supracrestal connective tissue zone. Consistent with this finding, a human histologic study determined the height of the peri-implant "biologic width," consisting of an epithelial attachment and supracrestal connective tissue, to be about 4–4.5 mm (Fig. 57.16).

Epithelium

As in the natural dentition, the oral epithelium around implants is continuous with a sulcular epithelium that lines the inner surface of the gingival sulcus; the apical part of the gingival sulcus is lined with long junctional epithelium(JE). Ultrastructural examination of the long junctional epithelial attachment adjacent to dental implants has demonstrated that epithelial cells attach with a basal lamina and hemidesmosomes. Histologic studies indicate that these epithelial structures and the surrounding lamina propria cannot be distinguished from those structures around teeth. In health, the dimension of the sulcular epithelium is about 0.5 mm, and the dimension of the epithelial attachment is about 2 mm, which is higher than that of the periodontal epithelial attachment.

The apical edge of the epithelial attachment is about 1.5–2.0-mm above the bone margin. In healthy peri-implant tissues, progressive epithelial downgrowth does not occur, indicating that factors other than inserted collagen fiber bundles (i.e., Sharpey's fibers in natural dentition) prevent it.

Connective Tissue

Peri-implant connective tissue morphology closely resembles that of the natural dentition except that it lacks a periodontal ligament, cementum, and inserting fibers. No significant differences were found at the biochemical level between the peri-implant and the periodontal soft tissues, while the dimension of the peri-implant connective tissue is 1–2 mm, which is higher than that of the periodontal connective tissue.

The zone of supracrestal connective tissue has an important function in the maintenance of a stable soft tissue–implant interface and as a seal or barrier to the "outside" oral environment. The orientation of connective tissue fibers adjacent to an implant differs from that of periodontal connective tissue fibers. In the absence of cementum and inserting connective tissue fibers (i.e., as in a natural tooth), most peri-implant connective tissue fibers run in a direction more or less parallel to the implant surface. Even when the fiber bundles are oriented perpendicularly, which occurs more often in the gingiva than in the mucosa surrounding implants, the bundles are never embedded in the implant surface.

The fiber bundles can also have a "cuff-like" circular orientation. The role of these fibers remains unknown, but it appears that their presence helps to create a soft tissue "seal" around the implant. The adaptation of the connective tissue to an implant surface may also be affected by the mobility of the soft tissue around the implant. The connective tissue in direct contact with the implant

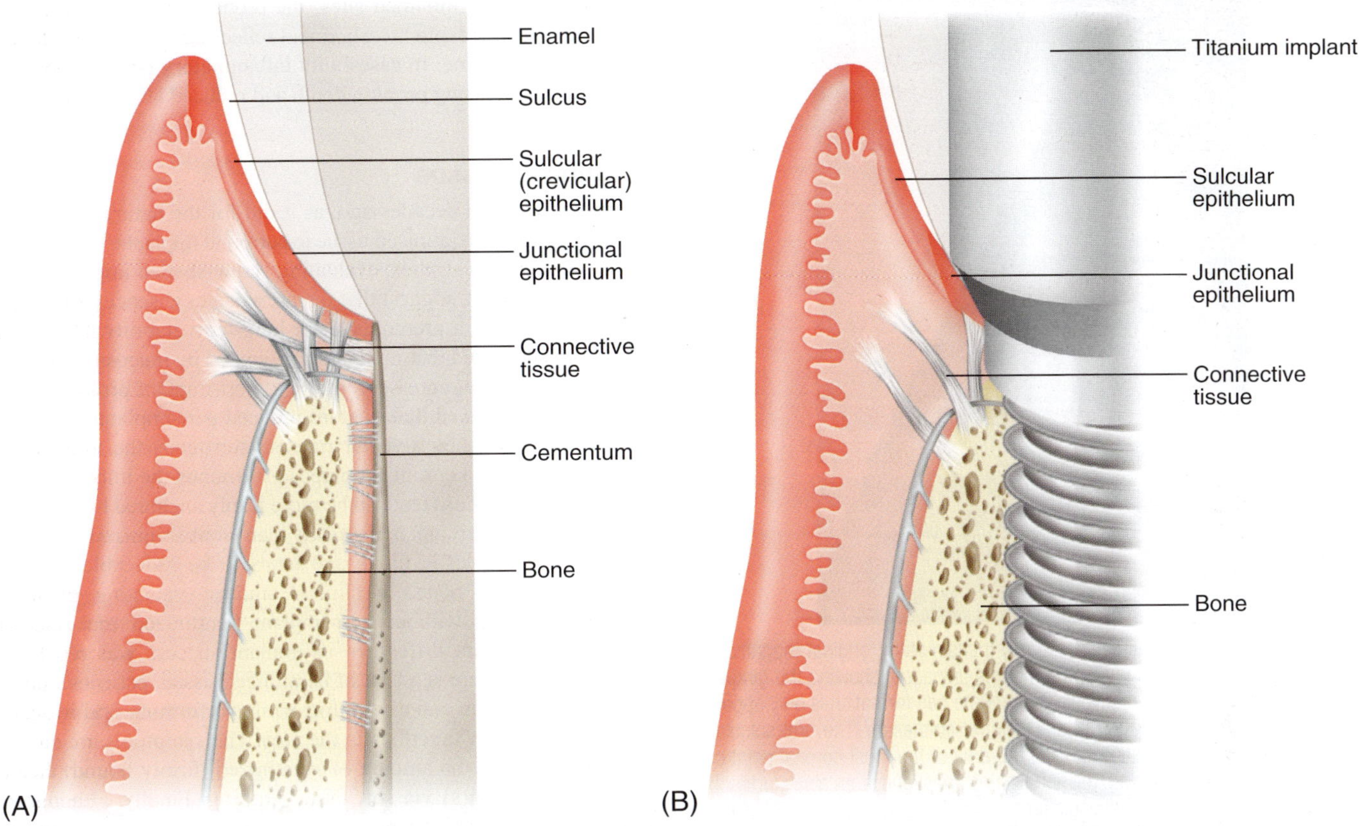

Fig. 57.14 Schematic illustration of hard and soft tissue around a tooth and an implant. A, Hard and soft tissue anatomy around a natural tooth demonstrates bone support with a periodontal ligament, a connective tissue zone above the crest of bone with connective tissue fibers (Sharpey) inserting into dentin, a long junctional epithelial attachment, a gingival sulcus lined with sulcular epithelium, and oral gingival epithelium (outer surface of gingiva). B, Hard and soft tissue anatomy around an implant demonstrates some similarities and some distinct differences. There is supporting bone in direct approximation to the implant surface without any intervening soft tissues (i.e., no periodontal ligament). A connective tissue zone is present above the level of bone with fibers running parallel to the implant surface and no inserting fibers. There is a long junctional epithelial attachment, a gingival/mucosal sulcus lined with sulcular epithelium and oral gingival/mucosal epithelium (outer surface of soft tissue). *(From Rose LF, Mealey BL:* Periodontics: medicine, surgery, and implants, *St. Louis, 2004, Mosby.)*

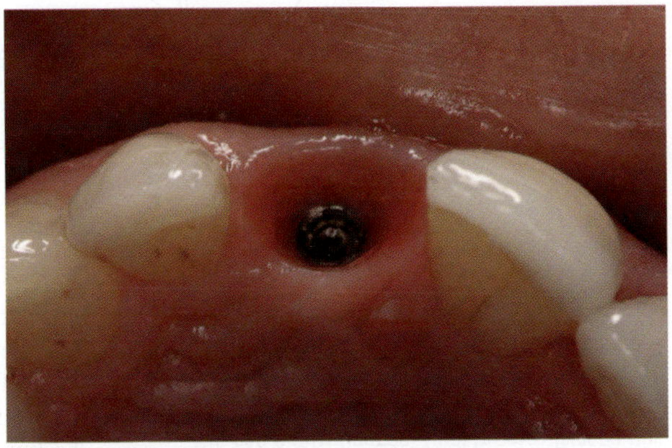

Fig. 57.15 Clinical appearance of normal, healthy peri-implant tissue with implant restoration removed. Soft tissue thickness varies from site-to-site, depending on quantity and quality of tissue, as well as the anatomy of the surrounding area (e.g., adjacent to natural teeth with healthy periodontal attachment vs adjacent to a space). Note that the intrasulcular tissue appears more erythematous as the result of the thin, nonkeratinized layer of epithelium overlying the connective tissue. *(Courtesy: Dr Stuart Froum, New York, NY.)*

surface is characterized by an absence of blood vessels and an abundance of fibroblasts interposed between collagen fibers. Several animal and human studies have shown that the alignments of connective fibers were circular and horizontal around the implants (Fig. 57.17).

More recent studies have shown histologic evidence of connective tissue attachment perpendicular to the microgrooved implant surface on both animal and human studies. This laser-microtextured grooves (Fig. 57.18) have been shown to be able to stop the epithelial downgrowth and establish connective tissue insertion right at the most coronal part of the laser microgrooved area (Fig. 57.19). A prospective controlled clinical study showed that laser-grooved surface resulted in shallower probing depth and lesser peri-implant crestal bone loss than that seen around implants with machined collars.

This connective tissue interface has been examined by probing attachment level measurements in patients. Probing attachment levels were consistently found coronal to the alveolar crest in patients with peri-implant tissue health, indicating the presence of a zone of direct connective tissue contact to the implant surface. This means that the probing depth measurement performed with a periodontal probe may be about 1.5-mm higher above the bone level in

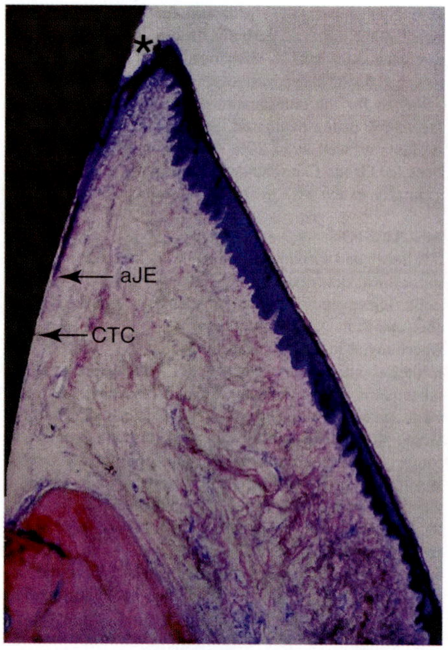

Fig. 57.16 Buccolingual section (basic fuchsin stain; original magnification ×12.5; one-part SLA implant, 3 months unloaded) showing the gingiva and the most coronal part of alveolar bone. Rete peg formation is only apparent in the area of the keratinized oral gingival epithelium. The oral sulcular epithelium exhibits no keratinization. In the area of the most coronal point of the junctional epithelium (cJE), the soft tissues are slightly torn away (artifact) because of nondecalcified histologic processing. The most apical point of the junctional epithelium (JE) is indicated (aJE). No rete peg formation is evident adjacent to the basal cell layer of the JE, all showing healthy and physiologic soft tissue structures. In addition, the area of connective tissue contact (CTC) adjacent to the machined titanium surface is marked. A slight round cell infiltrate in the connective tissue indicates a mild inflammation. Note bone remodeling/new bone formation in the crestal bone region indicated by saturated, *dark-red* stained areas.

healthy tissues. At inflamed sites, the probe may penetrate to the bone with probing depth measurement reflecting the total soft tissue thickness above bone. In cases with inflammatory peri-implant tissue disease, increasing probing depth and reduced attachment levels have been reported.

Keratinized Tissue

Questions emerged decades ago, as it did for the natural dentition, about the need for keratinized tissue to surround implants. Prospective and cross-sectional studies, evaluating screw-shaped implants with a machined surface, suggest that the presence or absence of keratinized gingiva is not a prerequisite for long-term stability. However, it has been suggested that implants surrounded by mucosa only (i.e., nonkeratinized) are more susceptible to peri-implant problems. An animal study observed that ligature-induced peri-implantitis occurs more frequently when alveolar mucosa surrounds the implant as compared to when keratinized mucosa surrounds the implant.

Keratinized mucosa tends to be more firmly anchored by collagen fibers to the underlying periosteum than nonkeratinized mucosa, which has more elastic fibers and tends to be moveable relative to the underlying bone. In clinical studies evaluating intraoral implants, with or without peri-implant keratinized mucosa, no clinically significant difference in implant success was reported. However, when there is a lack of keratinized tissue, patients tend to complain about pain and discomfort while performing oral hygiene procedures or other functions in the area. The symptoms are alleviated by increasing the amount of keratinized (firmly bound) tissue around the implant(s) via soft tissue grafting. Finally, although it may not be comparable to intraoral implants, mobility of soft tissues surrounding extraoral implants is associated with a higher incidence of implant failure.

Vascular Supply and Inflammation

The vascular supply of the peri-implant gingival or alveolar mucosa may be limited, as compared to periodontal gingiva, due to the lack

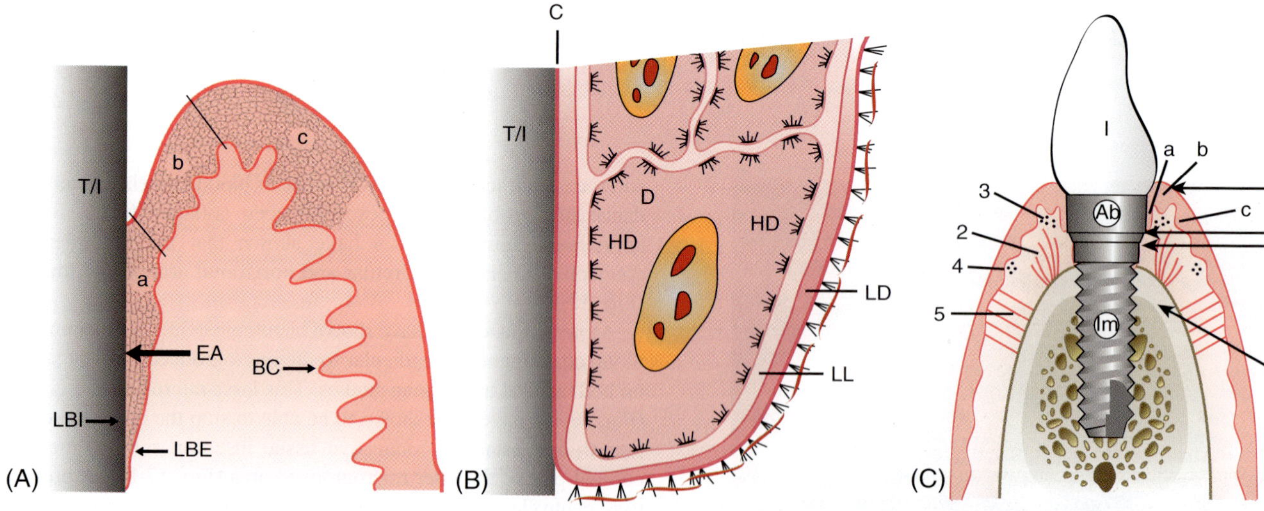

Fig. 57.17 A, Histologic scheme of epithelial attachment (EA) (identical for tooth and implant). *T/I*, Titanium implant; *BC*, basal complex; *LBI*, lamina basalis interna; *LBE*, lamina basalis externa (only location where cell divisions occur); *a*, long junctional epithelial attachment zone; *b*, sulcular epithelial zone; *c*, oral epithelial zone. B, At electron microscopic level, basal complex at epithelial attachment (three most apical cells) and connection with stroma. *HD*, Hemidesmosomes; *D*, desmosome; *LL*, lamina lucida; *LD*, lamina densa; *C*, cuticle. C, Implant, abutment (Ab), and crown within alveolar bone and soft tissues. *Im*, Endosseous part of implant; *MR*, margin of gingiva/alveolar mucosa; *Bo*, marginal bone level; *1*, implant crown; *2*, vertical alveolar-gingival connective tissue fibers; *3*, circular gingival connective tissue fibers; *4*, circular gingival connective tissue fibers; *5*, periosteal-gingival connective tissue fibers; *a*, junctional epithelium; *b*, sulcular epithelium; *c*, oral epithelium; *A/I*, abutment/implant junction; *aAE*, apical (point) of attached epithelium.

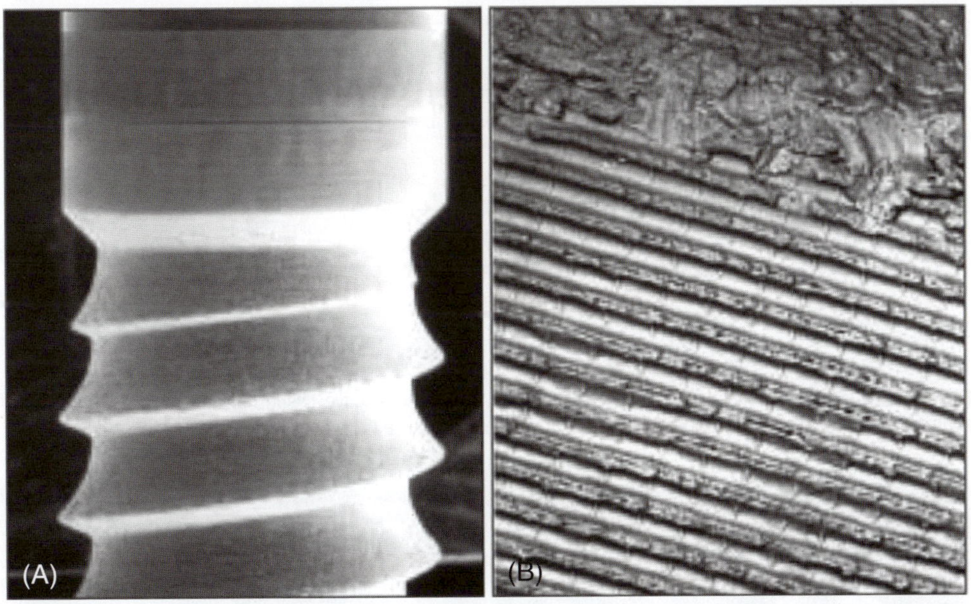

Fig. 57.18 A, Laser-microtextured surface; B, machined collar, 500×. *(Botos et al:* Int J Oral Maxillofac Implants *26:492–498, 2011. With the permission of Dr Spyros Botos.)*

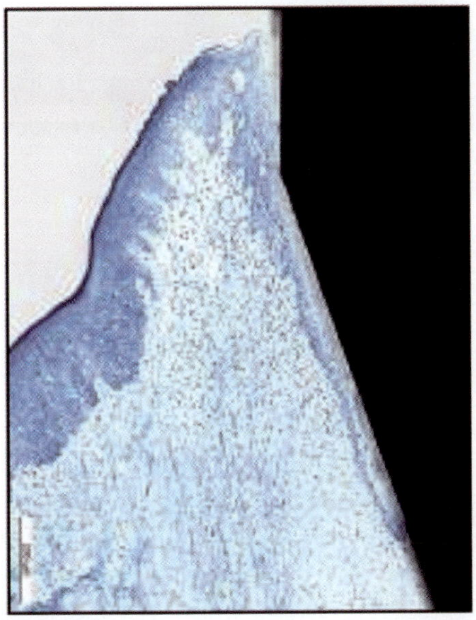

Fig. 57.19 Laser-ablated surface: epithelial downgrowth was stopped right at the coronal-most microgrooved area *(arrow).* Apical to the JE, healthy connective tissue fibers attached perpendicularly to the laser-ablated channels. *(Courtesy: Dr Myron Nevins.)*

of a periodontal ligament (Fig. 57.20). This is especially true in the tissue immediately adjacent to the implant surface. However, capillary loops in the connective tissue under the junctional and sulcular epithelium around implants appear to be anatomically similar to those found in the normal periodontium (Fig. 57.21A and B).

Emerging knowledge indicates that the peri-implant gingival or alveolar mucosa has the same morphology as the corresponding tissues around teeth. These soft tissues also react the same way to plaque accumulation. Studies investigating the histology (light microscopic and ultrastructural) of healthy and inflamed tissues surrounding implants in humans have indicated that the inflammatory response to plaque is similar to that observed in periodontal tissues. Polymorphonuclear cells and mononuclear cells transmigrate normally through the peri-implant sulcular epithelium (Fig. 57.22A and B).

Clinical Comparison of Teeth and Implants

Although the soft tissue-to-implant (abutment) interface offers striking similarities with tissue surrounding the natural dentition, some differences should be considered. At the bone level, the lack of a periodontal ligament is the most striking difference. The following discussion elaborates on the clinical perspectives of these similarities and differences.

At the bone level, the absence of the periodontal ligament surrounding an implant has important clinical consequences. This means that no resilient connection exists between implants and supporting bone. Implants cannot intrude or migrate to compensate for the presence of a premature occlusal contact (as teeth can). Implants and the rigidly attached implant restorations do not move. Thus, any occlusal disharmony will have repercussions at either the restoration-to-implant connection, the bone-to-implant interface, or both.

Proprioception in the natural dentition comes from the periodontal ligament. The absence of a periodontal ligament around implants reduces tactile sensitivity and reflex function. This can become even more challenging when osseointegrated, implant-supported, fixed prostheses are present in both jaws.

The lack of a periodontal ligament and inability of implants to move contraindicates their use in growing individuals. Natural teeth continue to erupt and migrate during growth while implants do not. Implants placed in individuals prior to the completion of growth can lead to occlusal disharmonies with implants. Likewise, it may be problematic to place one or more implants in a location adjacent to teeth that are very mobile from the loss of periodontal support because as the teeth move in response to or away from the occlusal forces, the implant(s) will bear the entire load.

Overload, because of improper superstructure design, parafunctional habits, or excessive occlusal load may cause microstrains and microfractures in the bone, which will lead to bone loss and a fibrous inflammatory tissue at the implant interface.

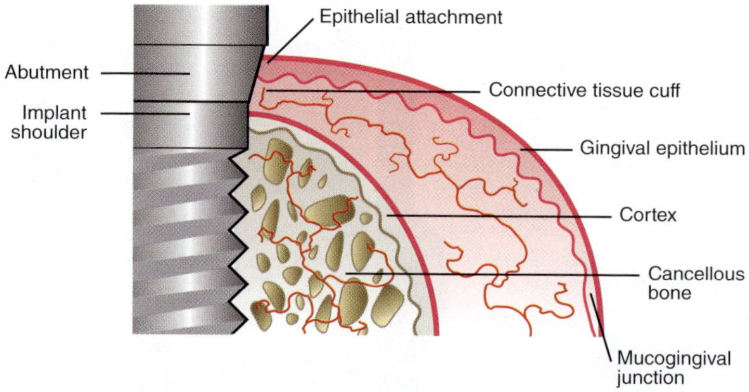

Fig. 57.20 Schematic illustration of the blood supply in the connective tissue cuff surrounding the implant/abutment is scarcer than in the gingival complex around teeth because none originates from a periodontal ligament.

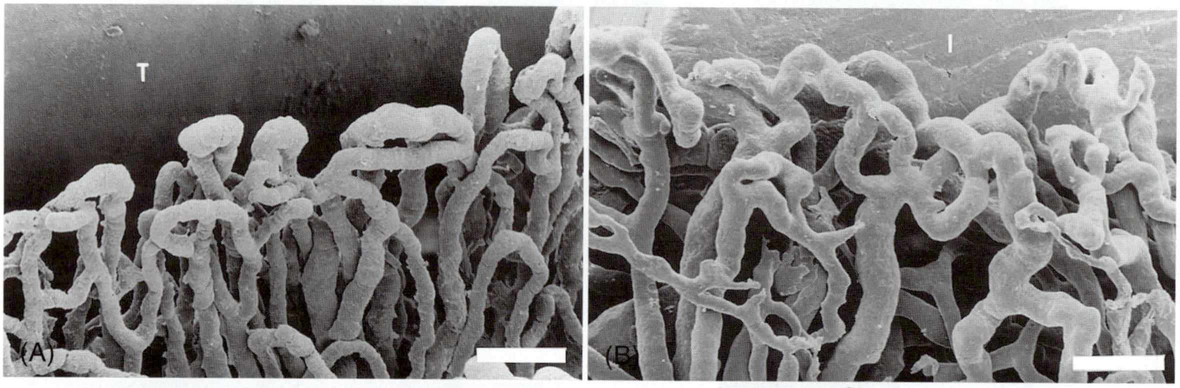

Fig. 57.21 A, Microvascular topography surrounding a tooth. B, Microvascular topography surrounding an implant. Bar = 5 μm. *(Courtesy: Dr N. Selliseth and Dr K. Selvig, Bergen, Norway.)*

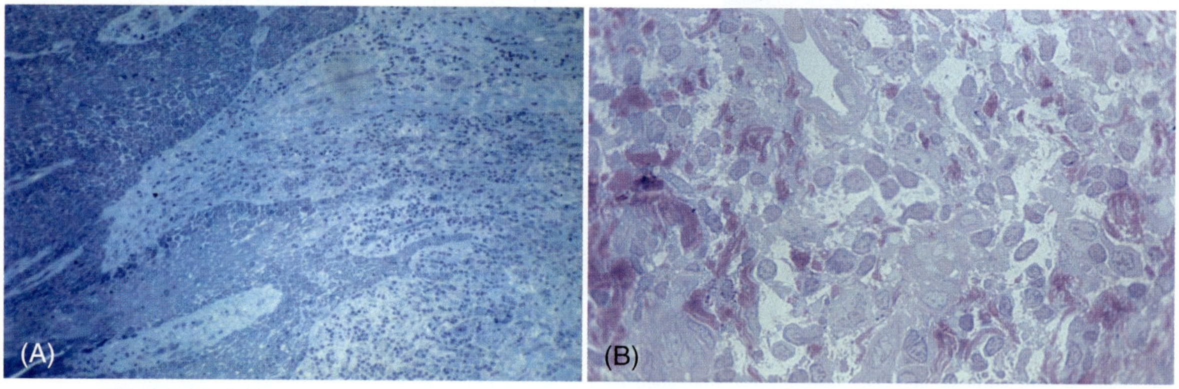

Fig. 57.22 A, Histologic slide from healthy gingiva surrounding a well-functioning implant in human patient. No morphologic characteristics differentiate tissue around implant from that around teeth. B, When gingivitis occurs, a profuse migration of inflammatory cells through the pocket epithelium can be observed. *(Courtesy: Professor Mariano Sanz, Madrid.)*

Conclusion

Appreciating the osseointegration process is facilitated by a good knowledge and understanding of bone healing. Many factors can interfere with the predictable establishment of a permanent rigid connection between an implant surface and the surrounding bone that is able to sustain occlusal loads. The bone-to-implant interface and its rigidity are a predominant biomechanical aspect of coping with the time and intensity of loading. The soft tissue-to-implant interface also plays an important role in the long-term maintenance of stable marginal bone levels around implants. Clinicians must familiarize themselves with the underlying molecular and cellular events to evaluate the future evolution of implant design and implant protocols, including surgical placement, restoration, and maintenance.

Key points

- The phenomenon of osseointegration was a serendipitous finding of Per-Ingvar Brånemark.
- Implants according to their macrodesign can be endosseous implants (blade-like, pins, cylindrical, disk-like, screw shaped), subperiosteal frame-like implants, and transmandibular implants.

- Implants microdesign can be modified by additive processes like addition of materials, such as hydroxyapatite, inorganic mineral coatings, plasma spraying, biocoating with growth factors, fluoride, cements containing calcium phosphates, sulfates, carbonates or by adding an oxide layer, or by subtractive processes like machining, acid etching, blasting, or a combination of these processes.
- Osteoclasts resorb bone at a pace of 50–100 μm per day.
- The critical temperature for bone cells that should not be exceeded during implant osteotomy is 47°C (116.6°F) at an exposure time of 1 min.
- Resonance frequency analysis measurements exceeding 56 kHz indicate a level of bone support that is consistent with osseointegration.
- According to a human histologic study, the height of the peri-implant "biologic width," consisting of an epithelial attachment and supra-crestal connective tissue, is about 4–4.5 mm.
- The lack of a periodontal ligament and inability of implants to move contraindicates their use in growing individuals.

Suggested Readings

Abrahamsson I, Soldini C: Probe penetration in periodontal and peri-implant tissues. An experimental study in the beagle dog, *Clin Oral Implants Res* 17:601–605, 2006.

Botos S, Yousef H, Zweig B, et al: The effects of laser microtexturing of the dental implant collar on crestal bone levels and peri-implant health, *Int J Oral Maxillofac Implants* 26 (3):492–498, 2011.

Buser D, Schenk RK, Steinemann S, et al: Influence of surface characteristics on bone integration of titanium implants. A histomorphometric study in miniature pigs, *J Biomed Mater Res* 25:889–902, 1991.

Davies JE: Mechanisms of endosseous integration, *Int J Prosthodont* 11:391–401, 1998.

Hermann JS, Buser D, Schenk RK, et al: Biologic width around titanium implants. A physiologically formed and stable dimension over time, *Clin Oral Implants Res* 11:1–11, 2000.

Nevins M, Nevins ML, Camelo M, et al: Human histologic evidence of a connective tissue attachment to a dental implant, *Int J Periodontics Restorative Dent* 28:111–121, 2008.

Nevins M, Kim DM, Jun SH, et al: Histologic evidence of a connective tissue attachment to laser microgrooved abutments: a canine study, *Int J Periodontics Restorative Dent* 30:245–255, 2010.

Nevins M, Camelo M, Nevins ML, et al: Connective tissue attachment to laser-microgrooved abutments: a human histologic case report, *Int J Periodontics Restorative Dent* 32:385–392, 2012.

Pecora GE, Ceccarelli R, Bonelli M, et al: Clinical evaluation of laser microtexturing for soft tissue and bone attachment to dental implants, *Implant Dent* 18:57–66, 2009.

Quirynen M, van Steenberghe D, Jacobs R, et al: The reliability of pocket probing around screw-type implants, *Clin Oral Implants Res* 2:186–192, 1991.

References

References and MCQs with answers for the chapter are available on www.medenact.com.

CHAPTER 58

Diagnosis and Treatment Planning in Implantology

PR Klokkevold | DL Cochran | S Tetradis | SM Mallya | E Chung | T-L Chang | TR Schoenbaum | A Jain

CHAPTER OUTLINE

Clinical Evaluation of the Implant Patient

Endosseous dental implants and their retained prostheses have had a great success over the past few decades following the landmark research and development of osseointegrated implants by Brånemark et al. Initially, most prosthetic reconstructions with osseointegrated implants were limited to use in the edentulous patients, with many reports documenting their excellent long-term success of implant-retained prostheses.

Following much success with implants in edentulous patients, the original implant treatment protocols were adapted for use in partially edentulous patients. Although some transitional problems were associated with the early use of dental implants in them, successes were eventually achieved. Subsequently, modifications in implant design, procedural techniques, and treatment planning greatly improved implant therapy for the partially edentulous patient. Currently, the long-term success of dental implants used to replace single and multiple missing teeth in the partially edentulous patient is very good. Additionally, with the implementation of bone augmentation procedures, even patients with inadequate bone volume have a good opportunity to be successfully restored with implant-retained prostheses. Virtually any patient with an edentulous space is a candidate for endosseous implants, and studies suggest that greater than 90%–95% success rates can be expected in healthy patients with good bone health and normal healing capacity.

The ultimate goal of dental implant therapy is to satisfy the patient's desire to replace one or more missing teeth in an esthetic, secure, functional, and long-lasting manner. To achieve this goal, clinicians must accurately diagnose the current dentoalveolar condition, as well as the overall mental and physical well-being of the patient, to determine whether implant therapy is possible or practical and, perhaps most importantly, whether it is indicated for a particular patient. Local evaluation of potential jaw sites for implant placement (e.g., measuring available alveolar bone height, width, and spatial relationship) and prosthetic restorability is an essential part of determining whether an implant(s) is possible. However, determining whether the patient is a good candidate for implants is an equally important aspect of the evaluation process. This aspect of the patient evaluation includes identifying factors that might increase the risk of failure or complications, as well as determining whether the patient's expectations are reasonable.

This chapter presents an overview of the clinical aspects of dental implant therapy, including an assessment of possible risk factors and contraindications. It also provides guidelines for the pretreatment evaluation of potential implant patients and the posttreatment evaluation of patients with implants.

Case Types and Indications

Edentulous Patients

The patients who seem to benefit most from dental implants are those with fully edentulous arches. These patients can be effectively restored, both esthetically and functionally, with an implant-assisted removable prosthesis or an implant-supported fixed prosthesis.

The original design for the edentulous arch was a fixed-bone-anchored bridge that used five to six implants in the anterior area of the mandible or the maxilla to support a fixed, hybrid prosthesis. The design is a denture-like complete arch of teeth attached to a substructure (metal framework), which in turn is attached to the implants with cylindrical titanium abutments (Fig. 58.1). The prosthesis is fabricated without flange extensions and does not rely on any soft-tissue support. It is entirely implant supported. Usually, the prosthesis includes bilateral distal cantilevers, which extend to replace posterior teeth (back to premolars or first molars).

Another implant-supported design used to restore an edentulous arch is the ceramic–metal fixed bridge (Fig. 58.2A–C). Some

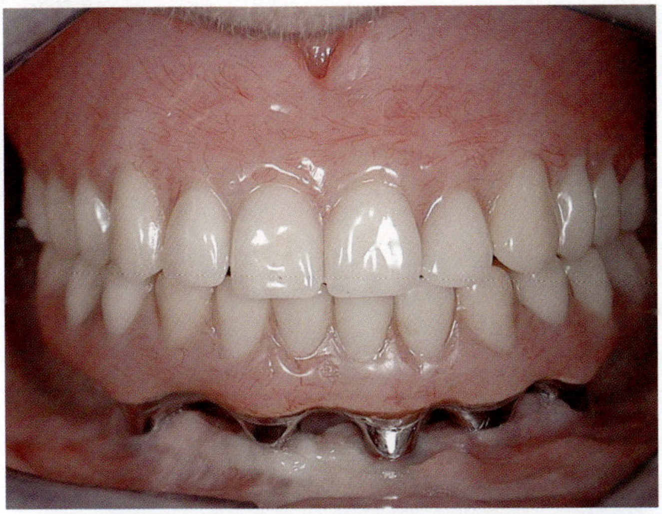

Fig. 58.1 Clinical photograph of patient with a complete maxillary denture opposing a full-arch implant-supported fixed prosthesis in the mandibular arch.

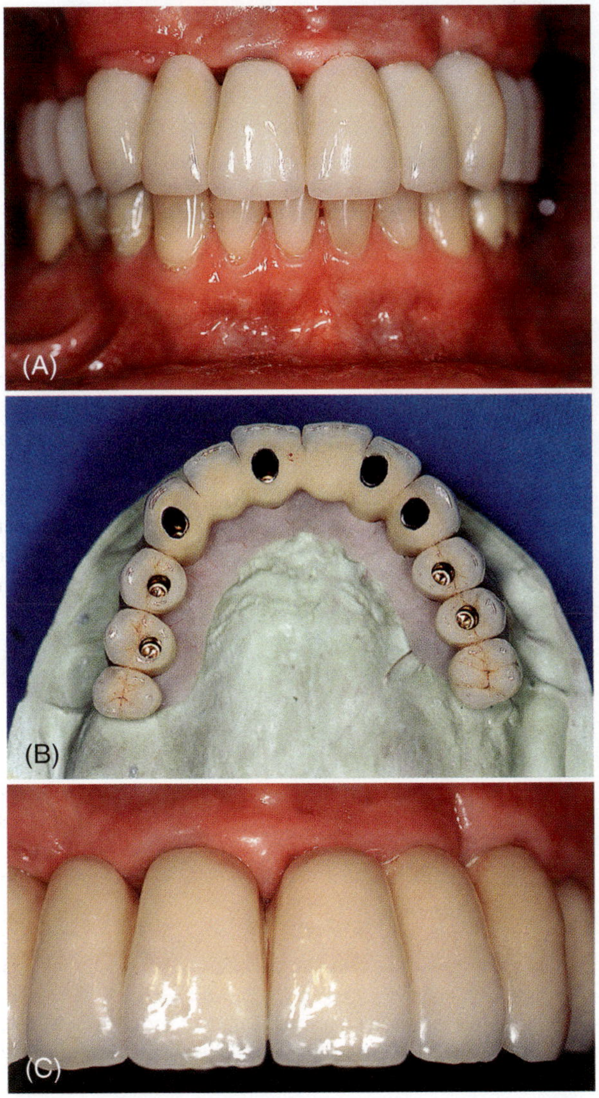

Fig. 58.2 A, Clinical photograph of acrylic provisional fixed full-arch prosthesis in the maxilla. B, Clinical photograph of the final ceramometal restoration, anterior view. C, Occlusal view of final restoration on master cast. *(Courtesy: Dr Russell Nishimura, Westlake Village, CA.)*

patients prefer this design because the ceramic restoration emerges directly from the gingival tissues in a manner similar to the appearance of natural teeth.

One limitation of both hybrid and ceramometal implant-supported fixed prostheses is that they provide very little lip support and thus may not be indicated for patients who have lost significant alveolar dimension. This is often more problematic for maxillary reconstructions because lip support is more critical in the upper arch. Furthermore, for some patients, the lack of a complete seal (i.e., spaces under the framework) allows air to escape during speech, thus creating phonetic problems.

Depending on the volume of existing bone, the jaw relationship, the amount of lip support, and phonetics, some patients may not be able to be rehabilitated with an implant-supported fixed prosthesis. For these patients, a removable, complete-denture type of prosthesis is a better choice because it provides a flange extension that can be adjusted and contoured to support the lip and there are no spaces for unwanted air escape during speech. This type of prosthesis can be retained and stabilized by two or more implants placed in the anterior region of the maxilla or mandible. Methods used to secure the denture to the implants vary from separate attachments on each individual implant to clips or other attachments that connect to a bar, which splints the implants together (Fig. 58.3A–D). Although the stability of the implant-retained overdenture does not compare to the rigidly attached, implant-supported fixed prosthesis, the increased retention and stability over conventional complete dentures is an important advantage for denture wearers. Additionally, implant-assisted and implant-supported prostheses are thought to protect alveolar bone from additional bone loss caused by the long-term use of removable prostheses that are bearing directly on the alveolar ridges.

Partially Edentulous Patients

Multiple Teeth

Partially edentulous patients with multiple missing teeth represent another viable treatment population for osseointegrated implants but the remaining natural dentition (occlusal schemes, periodontal health status, spatial relationships, and esthetics) introduces additional challenges for successful rehabilitation. The juxtaposition of implants with natural teeth in the partially edentulous patient presents the clinician with challenges not encountered with implants in the edentulous patient. As a result of distinct differences in the biology and function of implants compared to natural teeth, clinicians must educate themselves and use a prescribed approach to the evaluation and treatment planning of implants for partially edentulous patients. In general, endosseous dental implants can support a freestanding fixed-partial denture. Adjacent natural teeth are not necessary for support, but their close proximity requires special attention and planning. The major advantage of implant-supported restorations in partially edentulous patients is that they replace missing teeth without invasion or alteration of adjacent teeth. Preparation of natural teeth becomes unnecessary and larger edentulous spans can be restored with implant-supported fixed bridges. Moreover, patients who previously did not have a fixed option, such as those with Kennedy Class I and II partially edentulous situations, can be restored with an implant-supported fixed restoration (Fig. 58.4A–C).

Early attempts to use endosseous implants to replace missing teeth in the partially edentulous patient were a challenge partly because the implants and armamentarium were designed for the edentulous patient and did not have much flexibility for adaptation and use in the partially edentulous patient. Today, clinicians have many choices in terms of implant length, diameter, and abutment

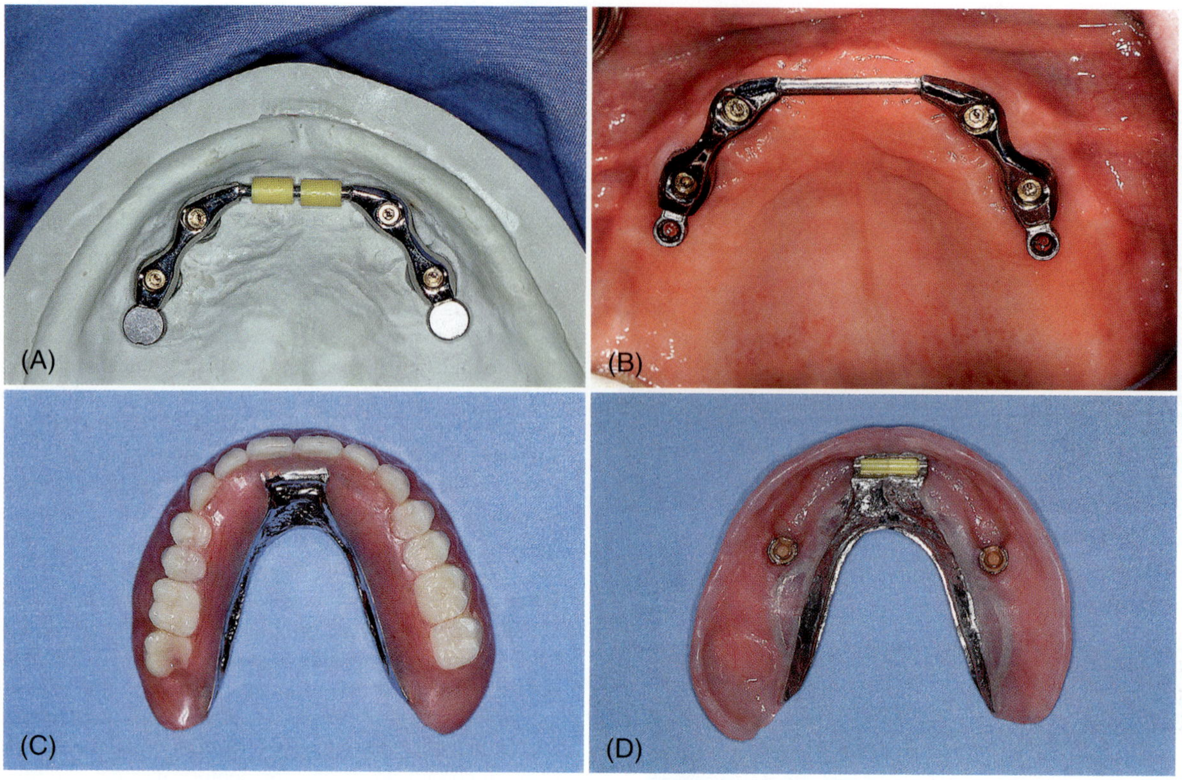

Fig. 58.3 A, Laboratory view of maxillary overdenture bar attached to four implants with anterior clips and posterior extracoronal resilient attachments (ERAs). B, Clinical view of maxillary overdenture bar. C, Palateless maxillary complete overdenture. D, Tissue surface of same maxillary implant-assisted overdenture showing clips and ERAs. *(Courtesy: Dr John Beumer, UCLA Maxillofacial Prosthodontics, Los Angeles.)*

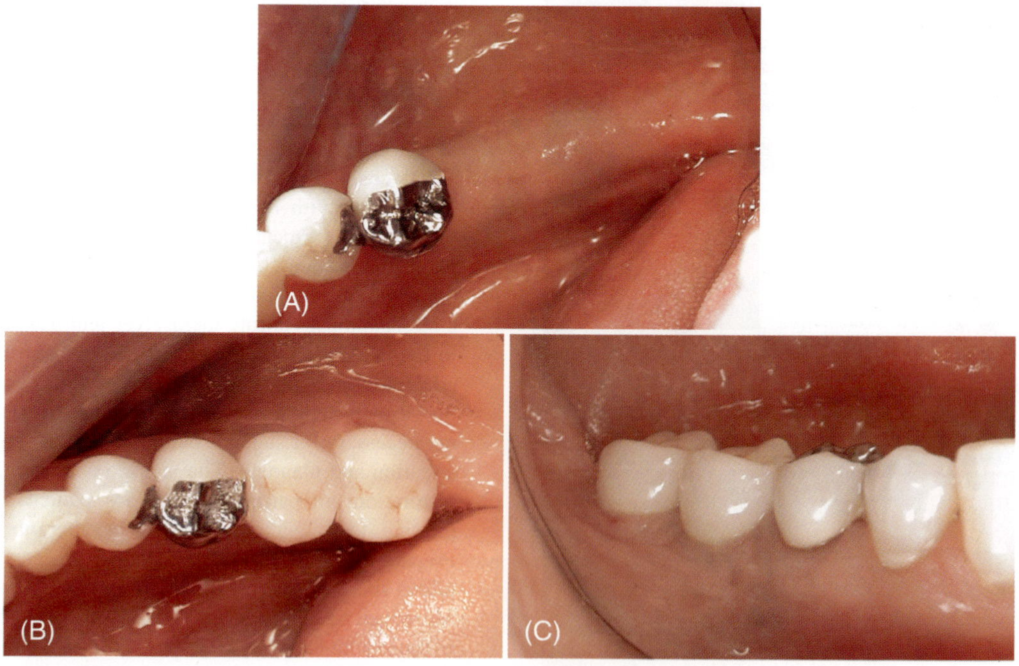

Fig. 58.4 A, Clinical view of partially edentulous posterior mandible (Kennedy Class II distal extension). B, Occlusal view of same patient in A restored with implant-supported fixed restoration replacing teeth #18 and #19. Note that the dimensions of the crowns are smaller than typical mandibular molars (i.e., closer to bicuspid size). C, Buccal view of same restorations.

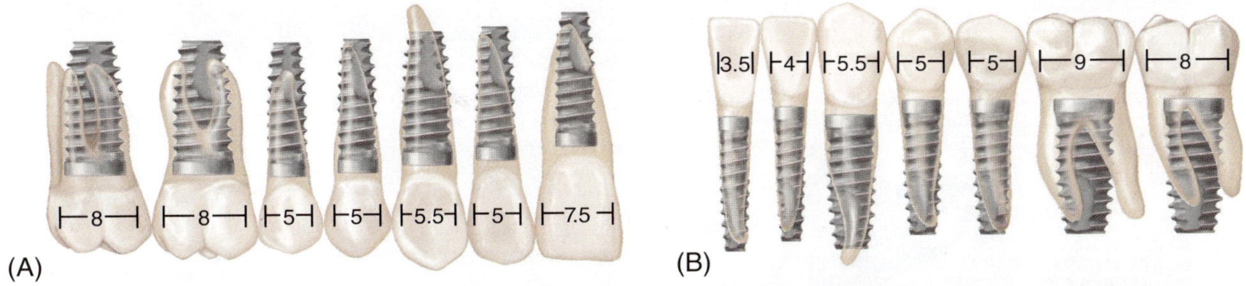

Fig. 58.5 Diagram representing the use of wide-, narrow-, and standard-diameter implants for molars, mandibular incisors, and other teeth (different-sized implants superimposed over various teeth). A, Maxillary teeth. B, Mandibular teeth.

connection to choose for the optimal replacement of any missing tooth, large or small (Fig. 58.5A and B).

The primary challenge with partially edentulous cases is an underestimation of the importance of treatment planning for implant-retained restorations with an adequate number of implants to withstand occlusal loads. For example, one problem that required correction was the misconception that two implants could be used to support a long-span, multiunit fixed bridge in the posterior area. Multiunit fixed restorations in the posterior jaw are more likely to experience complications or failures (mechanical or biologic) when they are inadequately supported either in terms of the number of implants, quality of bone, or strength of the implant material. The use of implants of adequate width and length and better treatment planning (more implants used to support more restorative units), particularly in areas of poor-quality bone, has solved many of these problems.

Single Tooth

Patients with a missing single tooth (anterior or posterior) represent another type of patient who benefits greatly from the success and predictability of endosseous dental implants. Replacement of a single missing tooth with an implant-supported crown is a much more conservative approach than preparing two adjacent teeth for the fabrication of a tooth-supported fixed-partial denture. It is no longer necessary to "cut" healthy or minimally restored adjacent teeth to replace a missing tooth with a nonremovable prosthetic replacement (Fig. 58.6A and B). Reported success rates for single-tooth implants are excellent.

Replacement of an individual missing posterior tooth with an implant-supported restoration has been successful as well. The greatest challenges to overcome with the single-tooth implant restorations were screw loosening and implant or component fracture. Due to the increased potential to generate forces in the posterior area, the implants, components, and screws often failed. Both these problems have been addressed with the use of wider-diameter implants and internal fixation of components (Fig. 58.7A and B). Wide-diameter implants often have a wider platform (restorative interface) that resists tipping forces and thus reduces screw loosening. The wide-diameter implant also provides greater strength and resistance to fracture as a result of increased wall thickness (the thickness of the implant between the inner screw thread and the outer screw thread). Implants with an internal connection are inherently more resistant to screw loosening and thus have an added advantage for single-tooth applications.

Esthetic Considerations

Anterior single-tooth implants present some of the same challenges as the single posterior tooth supported by an implant but they also

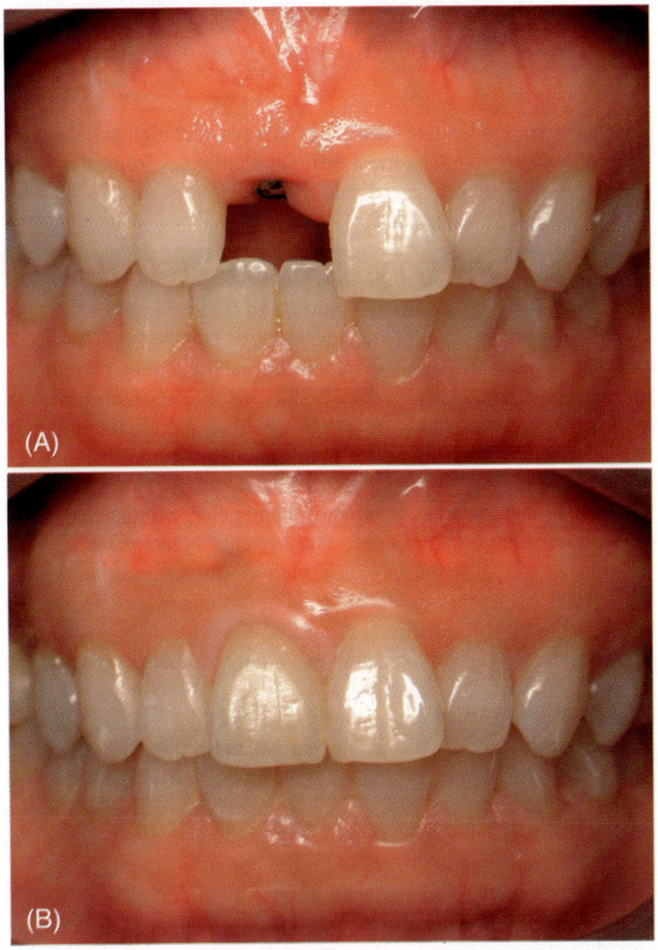

Fig. 58.6 Single-tooth replacement. A, Implant in place. B, Metalloceramic crown.

are an esthetic concern for patients. Some cases are more esthetically challenging than others because of the nature of each individual's smile and display of teeth. The prominence and occlusal relationship of existing teeth, the thickness and health of periodontal tissues, and the patient's own psychologic perception of esthetics, all play a role in the esthetic challenge of the case. Cases with good bone volume, bone height, and tissue thickness can be predictable in terms of achieving satisfactory esthetic results (see Fig. 59.6). However, achieving esthetic results for patients with less-than-ideal tissue qualities poses difficult challenges for the restorative and surgical team. Replacing a single tooth with an implant-supported crown in a patient with a high-smile line, compromised or thin

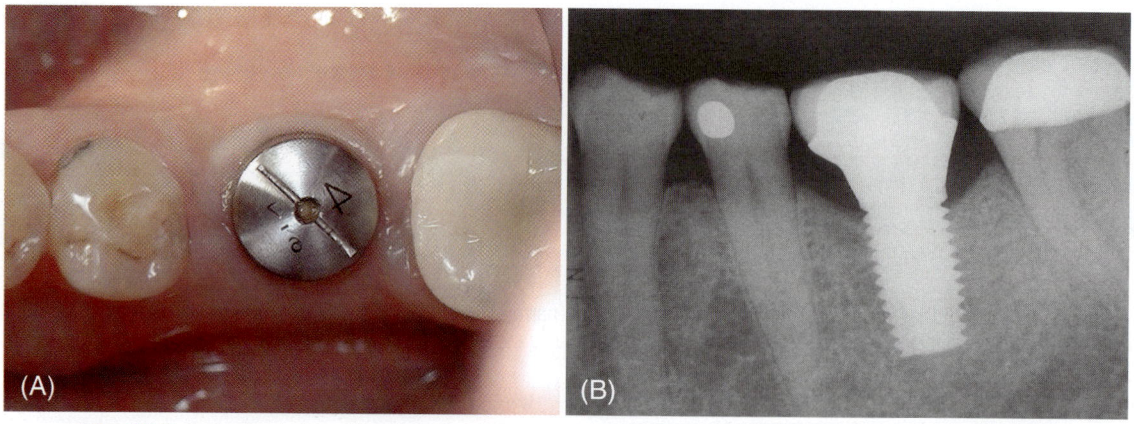

Fig. 58.7 A, Occlusal view of healing abutment, which is attached to a wide-diameter implant used to replace a single missing molar. B, Radiograph of same patient depicted in A, showing the wide-diameter implant supporting the final restoration (molar replaced with a single-tooth implant-supported crown).

periodontium, inadequate hard or soft tissues, and high expectations are probably some of the most difficult challenges in implant dentistry and should not be attempted by novice clinicians.

Pretreatment Evaluation

A comprehensive evaluation is indicated for any patient who is being considered for dental implant therapy. The evaluation should assess all aspects of the patient's current health status, including a review the patient's past medical history, medications, and medical treatments. Patients should be questioned about parafunctional habits, such as clenching or grinding teeth, as well as any substance use or abuse, including tobacco, alcohol, and drugs. The assessment should also include an evaluation of the patient's motivations, level of understanding, compliance, and overall behavior. For most patients, this involves simply observing their demeanor and listening to their comments for an impression of their overall sensibility and coherence with other patient norms.

An intraoral and radiographic examination must be done to determine whether it is possible to place implant(s) in the desired location(s). Properly mounted diagnostic study models and intraoral clinical photographs are a useful part of the clinical examination and treatment-planning process to aid in assessment of spatial and occlusal relationships. Once the data collection is completed, the clinician will be able to determine whether an implant therapy is possible, practical, and indicated for the patient.

Conducting an organized, systematic history and examination is essential in obtaining an accurate diagnosis and creating a treatment plan that is appropriate for the patient. Each treatment plan should be comprehensive and provide several treatment options for the patient, including periodontal and restorative therapies. Then, in consultation, the clinician can agree on the final treatment plan with the patient. Information gathered throughout the process will help the clinician's decision-making process and determine whether a patient is a good candidate for dental implants. A thoughtful and well-executed evaluation can also reveal deficiencies and indicate what additional surgical procedures may be necessary to accomplish the desired goals of therapy (e.g., localized ridge augmentation, sinus bone augmentation, etc.). Each part of the pretreatment evaluation is briefly discussed here.

Chief Complaint

What is the problem or concern in the patient's own words? What is the patient's goal of treatment, and how realistic are the patient's expectations? The patient's chief concern, desires for treatment, and vision of the successful outcome must be taken into consideration. The patient will measure implant success according to personal criteria. The overall comfort and function of the implant restoration are often the most important factors, but satisfaction with the appearance of the final restoration will also influence the patient's perception of success. Furthermore, patient satisfaction may be influenced simply by the impact that the treatment has on the patient's perceived quality of life. Patients will evaluate for themselves whether the treatment helped them to eat better, look better, or feel better about themselves.

The clinician could consider an implant and the retained prosthesis a success using standard criteria of symptom-free implant function, implant stability, and lack of peri-implant infection or bone loss. At the same time, however, the patient who does not like the esthetic result or does not think the condition has improved could consider the treatment as a failure. Therefore, it is critical to inquire, as specifically as possible, about the patient's expectations before initiating implant therapy and to appreciate the patient's desires and values. With this goal in mind, it is often helpful and advisable to invite patients to bring their spouses or family members to the consultation and treatment-planning visits to add an independent "trusted" observer to the discussion of treatment options. Ultimately, it is the clinician's responsibility to determine if the patient has realistic expectations for the outcome of therapy and to educate the patient about realistic outcomes for each treatment option.

Medical History

A thorough medical history is required for any patient in need of dental treatment, regardless of whether implants are part of the plan. This history should be documented in writing by the patient's completion of a standard health history form and verbally through an interview with the treating clinician. The patient's health history should be reviewed for any condition that might put the patient at risk for adverse reactions or complications.

Patients must be in reasonably good health to undergo surgical therapy for the placement of dental implants. Any disorder that may impair the normal wound-healing process, especially as it relates to bone metabolism, should be carefully considered as a possible risk factor or contraindication to implant therapy (see section: Risk Factors and Contraindications).

A thorough physical examination is warranted if any questions arise about the health status of the patient. Appropriate laboratory tests (e.g., coagulation tests for a patient receiving anticoagulant therapy) should be requested to further evaluate any conditions that may affect the patient's ability to undergo the planned surgical and restorative procedures safely and effectively. If any questions remain about the patient's health status, a medical clearance for surgery should be obtained from the patient's treating physician.

Dental History

A review of a patient's past dental experiences can be a valuable part of the overall evaluation. Does the patient report a history of recurrent or frequent abscesses, which may indicate a susceptibility to infections or diabetes? Does the patient have many restorations? How compliant has the patient been with previous dental recommendations? What are the patient's current oral hygiene practices?

The individual's previous experiences with surgery and prosthetics should be discussed. If a patient reports numerous problems and difficulties with past dental care, including a history of dissatisfaction with past treatment, the patient may have similar difficulties with implant therapy. It is essential to identify past problems and to elucidate any contributing factors. The clinician must also assess the patient's dental knowledge and understanding of the proposed treatment, as well as the patient's attitude and motivation toward implants.

Intraoral Examination

The oral examination is performed to assess the current health and condition of existing teeth, as well as to evaluate the condition of the oral hard and soft tissues. It is imperative that no pathologic conditions are present in any of the hard or soft tissues in the maxillofacial region. All oral lesions, especially infections, should be diagnosed and appropriately treated before implant therapy. Additional criteria to consider include the patient's habits, level of oral hygiene, overall dental and periodontal health, occlusion, jaw relationship, temporomandibular joint condition, and ability to open wide.

After a thorough intraoral examination, the clinician can evaluate potential implant sites. All sites should be clinically evaluated to measure the available space in the bone for the placement of implants and in the dental space for prosthetic tooth replacement (Box 58.1). The mesial–distal and buccal–lingual dimensions of edentulous spaces can be approximated with a periodontal probe or other measuring instrument. The orientation or tilt of adjacent teeth and their roots should be noted as well. There may be enough space in the coronal area for the restoration but not enough space in the apical region for the implant if roots are directed into the area of interest (Fig. 58.8A and B). Conversely, there may be adequate space between roots but the coronal aspects of the teeth may be too close for emergence and restoration of the implant. If either of these conditions is discovered, orthodontic tooth movement may be indicated. Ultimately, edentulous areas need to be precisely measured using diagnostic study models and imaging techniques to determine whether space is available and whether adequate bone volume exists to replace missing teeth with implants and implant restorations. Fig. 58.9 diagrams the minimal space requirements for standard-, wide-, and narrow-diameter implants placed between natural teeth, and the minimal interocclusal space needed to restore implants.

Diagnostic Study Models

Mounted study models are an excellent means of assessing potential sites for dental implants. Properly articulated models with diagnostic wax-up of the proposed restorations allow the clinician to evaluate the available space and to determine potential limitations of the planned treatment (Fig. 58.10A–E). This is particularly useful when multiple teeth are to be replaced with implants or when a malocclusion is present.

BOX 58.1 How Much Space Is Required for the Placement of One or More Implants?[a]

Alveolar Bone

Assuming an implant is 4 mm in diameter and 10 mm long, the minimal width of the jawbone needs to be 6–7 mm, and the minimal height should be 10 mm (minimum of 12 mm in the posterior mandible where an additional margin of safety is required over the mandibular nerve). This dimension is desired to maintain at least 1.0–1.5 mm of bone around all surfaces of the implant after preparation and placement.

Interdental Space

Edentulous spaces need to be measured to determine whether enough space exists for the placement and restoration with one or more implant crowns. The minimal space requirements for the placement of one, two, or more implants are illustrated diagrammatically in Fig. 59.9. The minimal mesial–distal space for an implant placed between two teeth is 7 mm. The minimal mesial–distal space required for the placement of two standard-diameter implants (4-mm diameter) between teeth is 14 mm. The required minimal dimensions for wide-diameter or narrow-diameter implants will increase or decrease incrementally according to the size of the implant. For example, the minimal space needed for the placement of an implant 6 mm in diameter is 9 mm (7 mm + 2 mm). Whenever the available space between teeth is greater than 7 mm and less than 14 mm, only one implant, such as placement of a wide-diameter implant, should be considered. Two narrow-diameter implants could be positioned in a space that is 12 mm. However, the smaller implant may be more vulnerable to implant fracture.

Interocclusal Space

The restoration consists of the abutment, the abutment screw, and the crown (it may also include a screw to secure the crown to the abutment if it is not cemented). This restorative "stack" is the total of all the components used to attach the crown to the implant. The dimensions of the restorative stack vary slightly depending on the type of abutment and the implant–restorative interface (i.e., internal or external connection). The minimum amount of interocclusal space required for the restorative "stack" on an external hex-type implant is 7 mm.

[a]All the minimal space requirements discussed here are generic averages. The actual space limitations for any particular implant system must be determined according to the manufacturer's specifications.

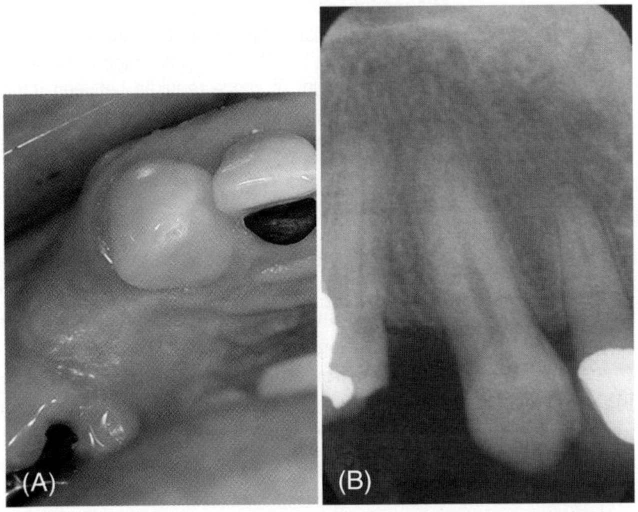

Fig. 58.8 A, Clinical photograph of maxillary premolar space with apparently adequate space between the remaining teeth for an implant-supported crown. B, Radiograph clearly shows a lack of space between the roots of the adjacent teeth as a result of convergence into the space (same patient as in A).

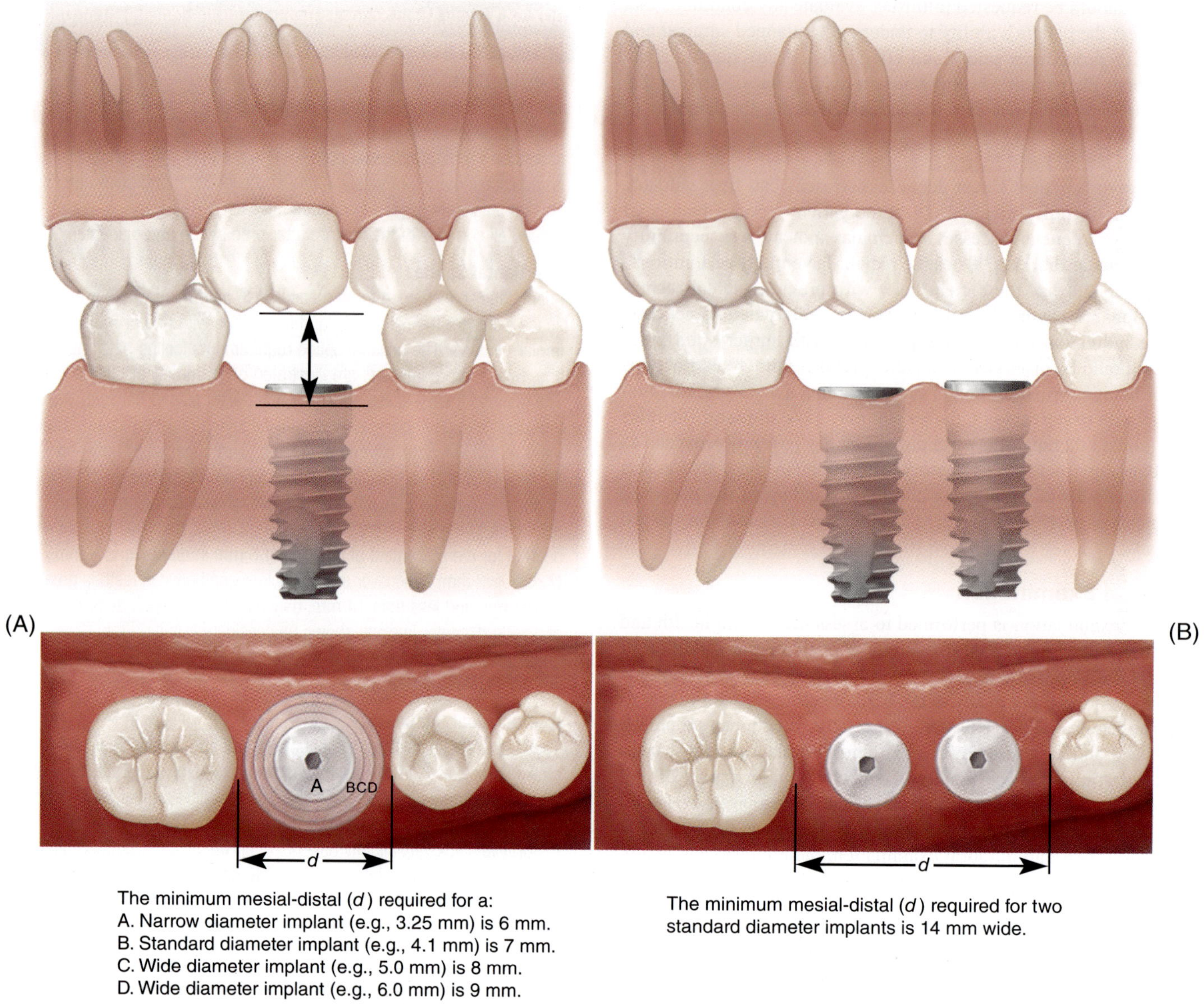

Fig. 58.9 A, Minimum amount of mesial–distal space (d) required for placement of single-tooth implant between natural teeth: (A) 6 mm for narrow-diameter implant (3.25 mm); (B) 7 mm for standard-diameter implant (4.1 mm); (C and D) 8 mm and 9 mm, respectively, for wide-diameter implants (5.0 mm and 6.0 mm). B, Minimum amount of mesial–distal space (d) required for placement of two standard-diameter (4.1 mm) implants between natural teeth is 14 mm. This allows approximately 2 mm between teeth/implants and between implant/implant. Minimum amount of space required between implant/restoration interface and opposing occlusal surfaces for restoration of an implant. This dimension will vary, depending on implant design and manufacturer component dimensions. The minimal dimension of 7 mm is based on an externally hexed implant and UCLA abutment.

Hard-Tissue Evaluation

The amount of available bone is the next criterion to evaluate. Wide variations in jaw anatomy are encountered, and it is therefore important to analyze the anatomy of the dentoalveolar region of interest both clinically and radiographically.

A visual examination can immediately identify deficient areas (Fig. 58.11A–D), whereas other areas that appear to have good ridge width will require further evaluation (Fig. 58.12A–D). Clinical examination of the jawbone consists of palpation to feel for anatomic defects and variations in the jaw anatomy, such as concavities and undercuts. If desired, it is possible with local anesthesia to probe through the soft tissue (intraoral bone mapping) to assess the thickness of the soft tissues and measure the bone dimensions at the proposed surgical site.

The spatial relationship of the bone must be evaluated in a three-dimensional (3D) view because the implant must be placed in the appropriate position relative to the prosthesis. It is possible that an adequate dimension of bone is available in the anticipated implant site (Box 58.1), but that the bone and thus the implant placement might be located too lingual or too buccal for the desired prosthetic tooth replacement. Bone augmentation procedures may be necessary to facilitate the placement of an implant in an acceptable prosthetic position despite the availability of an adequate quantity of bone (i.e., the bone is in the wrong location).

Radiographic Examination

Radiographic assessment of the quantity, quality, and location of available alveolar bone in potential implant sites ultimately

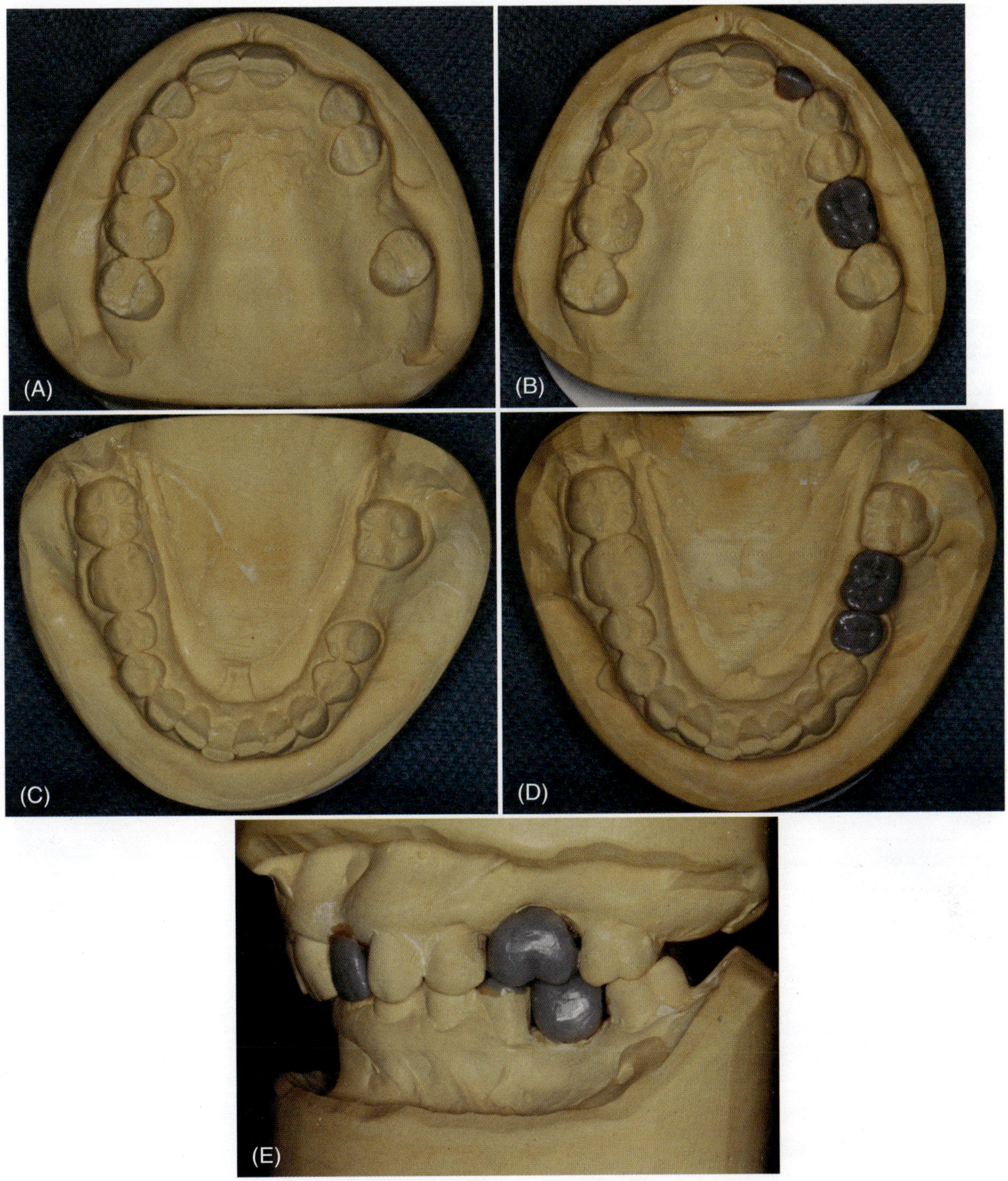

Fig. 58.10 Photographs of a diagnostic model with proposed lateral incisor and first molar tooth replacement waxed-up to evaluate the amount of space and contours. A, Diagnostic cast of maxillary arch with missing left lateral incisor and left first molar. B, Diagnostic wax-up of lateral incisor and first molar in the maxillary arch. C, Diagnostic cast of mandibular arch with missing left first molar. D, Diagnostic wax-up of first molar. E, Articulated maxillary and mandibular diagnostic models with wax-up of lateral incisor and first molars to evaluate dimensions and contours. *(Courtesy: Dr Stacy Yu, University of California, Los Angeles.)*

determines whether a patient is a candidate for implants and if a particular implant site needs bone augmentation. Appropriate radiographic procedures, including periapical radiographs, panoramic projections, and cross-sectional imaging, can help identify vital structures, such as the floor of the nasal cavity, maxillary sinus, mandibular canal, and mental foramen. In addition to the absolute dimensional measurement of the alveolar bone, it is important to determine whether the volume of bone radiographically (as well as clinically) is located in a position to allow for the proper position of the implant to facilitate restoration of the tooth/teeth in proper esthetic and functional relationship with the adjacent and opposing dentition. The best way to evaluate the relationship of available bone to the dentition is to image the patient with a diagnostically accurate guide using radiopaque markers that are positioned at the proposed prosthetic locations, ideally with appropriate restorative contours (Fig. 58.13).

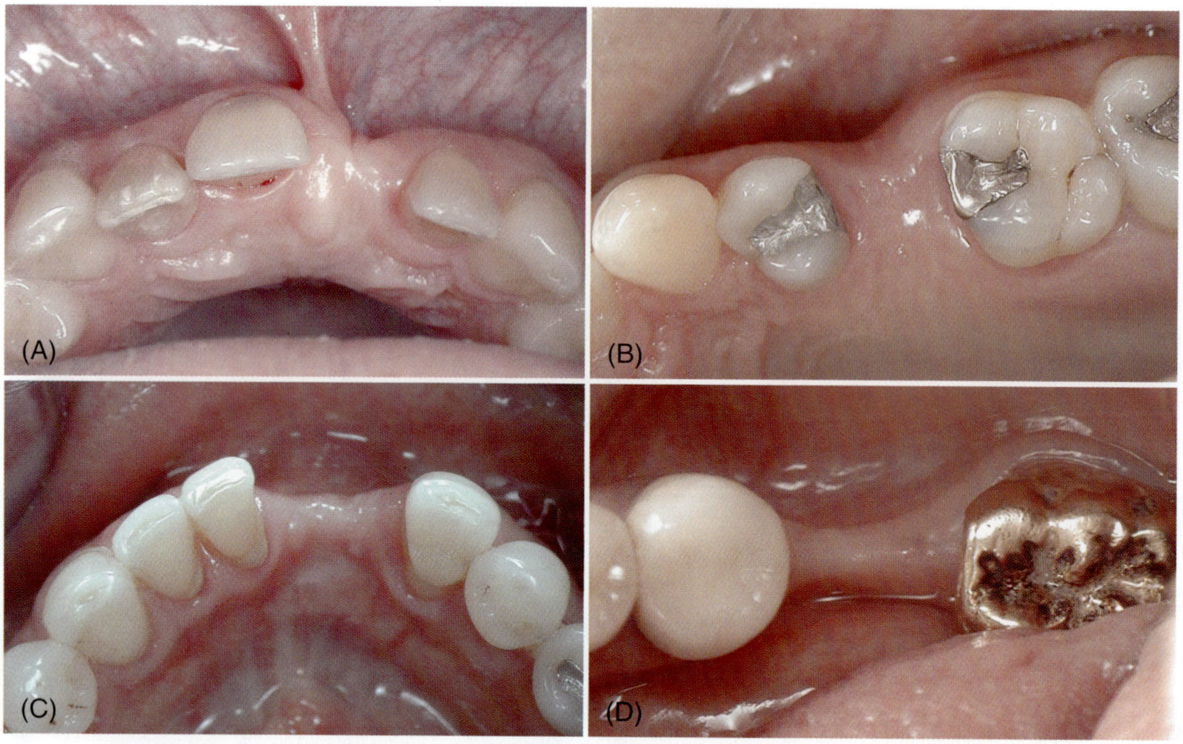

Fig. 58.11 Clinical photographs of edentulous areas with obvious deficient areas of alveolar dimension noted on visual examination. A, Anterior maxilla; B, Posterior maxilla; C, Anterior mandible; D, Posterior mandible. These clinical images all represent buccal–lingual deficiencies in the alveolar dimensions.

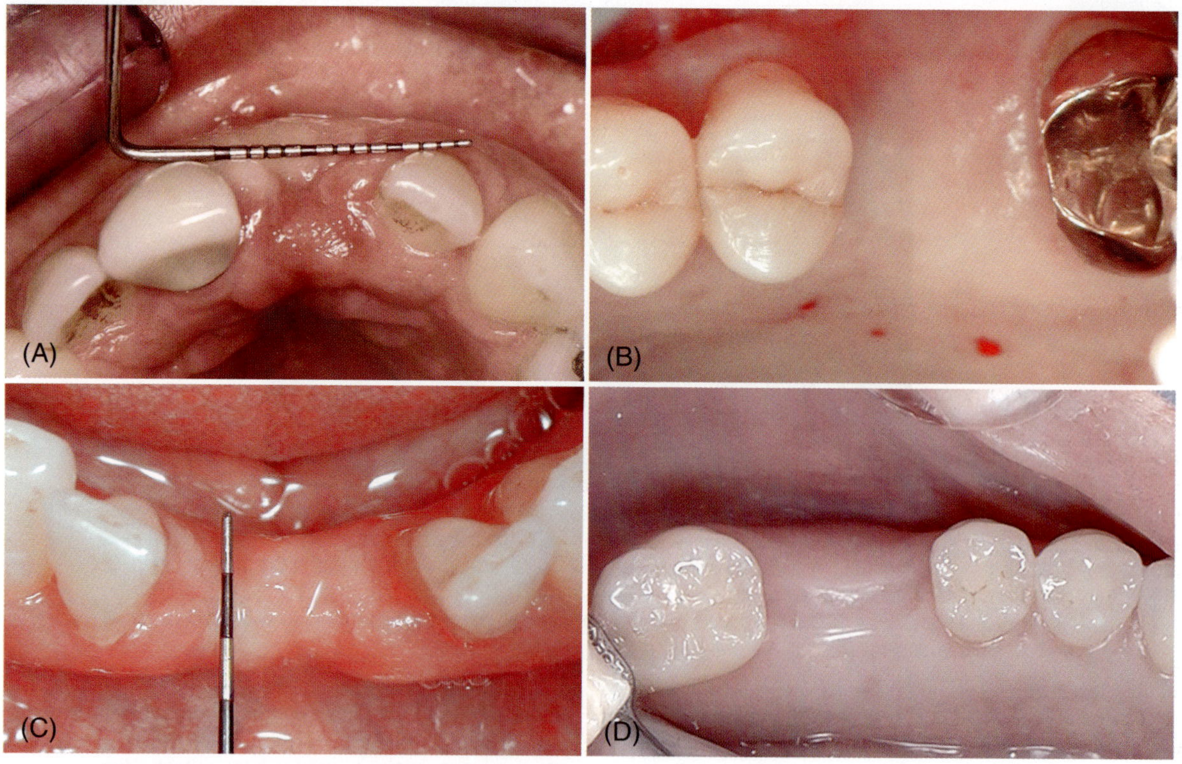

Fig. 58.12 Clinical photographs of edentulous areas with apparent good alveolar dimension noted on visual examination. A, Anterior maxilla; B, Posterior maxilla; C, Anterior mandible; D, Posterior mandible. It is likely that these sites have adequate bone volume for implant placement. However, it is also possible to find alveolar deficiencies despite the appearance of wide ridges.

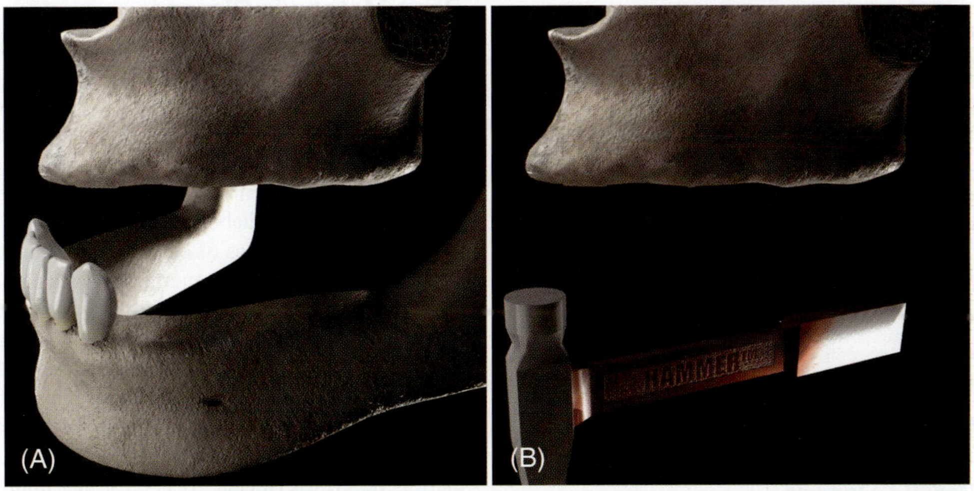

Fig. 58.13 The hammer-and-anvil effect is a useful analogy for the clinician to keep in mind, evoking the combination syndrome, when planning treatment for an edentulous maxilla opposing a partially dentate mandible. A, Illustration of an edentulous maxilla opposing a mandible that is missing posterior teeth. The lack of posterior occlusion leads to overclosure of the mandible and results in increased forces being applied to the anterior maxilla by the mandibular anterior natural dentition. B, Illustration of the hammer-and-anvil effect of combination syndrome.

BOX 58.2 How Much Keratinized Tissue Is Required for Health and Maintenance of Implants?

The debate about whether it is necessary to have a zone of keratinized tissue surrounding implants continues. Despite strong opinions and beliefs about the need for keratinized mucosa around implants versus this mucosa being unnecessary, neither argument has been proved.

Some studies have concluded that, in the presence of good oral hygiene, a lack of keratinized tissue does not impair the health or function of implants. Others strongly believe that keratinized mucosa has better functional and esthetic results for implant restorations. Keratinized mucosa is typically thicker and denser than alveolar mucosa (nonkeratinized). It forms a strong seal around the implant with a cuff of circular (parallel) fibers around the implant, abutment, or restoration that is resistant to retraction with mastication forces and oral hygiene procedures. Implants with coated surfaces [i.e., hydroxyapatite or titanium-plasma spray coating] demonstrate greater peri-implant bone loss and failures in the absence of keratinized mucosa.

Soft-Tissue Evaluation

Evaluation of the quality, quantity, and location of soft tissue present in the anticipated implant site helps to anticipate the type of tissue that will surround the implant(s) after treatment is completed (keratinized vs nonkeratinized mucosa). For some cases, depending on the clinician's view of keratinized tissue, evaluation may reveal a need for soft-tissue augmentation (Box 58.2). Areas with minimal or no existing keratinized mucosa may be augmented with gingival or connective tissue grafts. Other soft tissue concerns, such as frenum attachments or pulls, should be thoroughly evaluated as well.

Risk Factors and Contraindications

Clearly, there are numerous indications for the use of endosseous dental implants to replace missing teeth. Most patients who are missing one or more teeth can benefit from the application of an implant-retained prosthesis provided they meet the requirements for surgical and prosthetic rehabilitation. Edentulous patients who are unable to function with complete dentures and who have adequate bone for the placement of dental implants can be especially good dental implant candidates. Partially edentulous patients are increasingly being treated with dental implant restorations. Many patients, whether they are missing one, several, or all of their teeth, can be predictably restored with implant-retained prostheses.

In this era of high implant success and predictability and thus possible complacency, it is imperative for clinicians to recognize risk factors and contraindications to implant therapy so that problems can be minimized and patients can be accurately informed about risks. As such, the clinician must be knowledgeable in this area and inform patients about risk factors and contraindications before initiating treatment. Contraindications for the use of dental implants, although relatively few and often not well defined, do exist. Some conditions are probably best described as "risk factors" rather than "contraindications" for treatment because implants can be successful in almost all patients; implants may be less *predictable* in some situations, and this distinction should be recognized. Ultimately, it is the clinician's responsibility with the patient to make decisions as to when implant therapy is not indicated.

Table 58.1 lists some conditions and factors that are thought to increase the risk for implant failure or otherwise deem the patient a poor candidate for implant therapy. Some of these conditions are briefly discussed online under the following heads:

- Medical and systemic health-related issues like diabetes mellitus, bone metabolic disease, bisphosphonate therapy, immune compromise and immune suppression, radiation therapy (e-only).
- Psychological and mental conditions (e-only).
- Habits and behavioral considerations like smoking and tobacco use, parafunctional habits, and substance abuse (e-only).

Medical and Systemic Health-Related Issues

Although few absolute medical contraindications to implant therapy exist, some relative contraindications are important to consider. The clinician must consider medical and health-related conditions that affect bone metabolism or any aspect of the patient's capacity to heal normally. This category includes conditions, such as diabetes, osteoporosis, immune compromise, medications, and medical treatments such as chemotherapy and irradiation.

TABLE 58.1 Risk Factors and Contraindications for Implant Therapy

	Risk Factor	Contraindication
Medical and Systemic Health-Related Issues		
Diabetes (poorly controlled)	??—Possibly	Relative
Bone metabolic disease (e.g., osteoporosis)	??—Probably	Relative
Radiation therapy (head and neck)	Yes	Relative/Absolute
Bisphosphonate therapy [intravenous (IV)]	??—Probably	Relative/Absolute
Bisphosphonate therapy (oral)	??—Possibly	Relative
Immunosuppressive medication	??—Probably	Relative
Immunocompromising disease (e.g., HIV and AIDS)	??—Possibly	Relative
Psychologic and Mental Conditions		
Psychiatric syndromes (e.g., schizophrenia and paranoia)	No	Absolute
Mental instability (e.g., neurotic and hysteric)	No	Absolute
Mentally impaired and uncooperative	No	Absolute
Irrational fears and phobias	No	Absolute
Unrealistic expectations	No	Absolute
Habits and Behavioral Considerations		
Smoking and tobacco use	Yes	Relative
Parafunctional habits	Yes	Relative
Substance abuse (e.g., alcohol and drugs)	??—Possibly	Absolute
Intraoral Examination Findings		
Atrophic maxilla	Yes	Relative
Current infection (e.g., endodontic)	Yes	Relative
Periodontal disease	??—Possibly	Relative

Diabetes Mellitus

Diabetes is a metabolic disease that can have significant effects on the patient's ability to heal normally and resist infections. This is particularly true for patients whose diabetes is not well controlled. Poorly controlled diabetics often have impaired wound healing and a predisposition to infections, whereas diabetic patients whose disease is well controlled experience few, if any, problems.

There is concern about the success and predictability of implants in patients with diabetes. Several studies have reported moderate failure rates in patients with diabetes, with implant success ranging from 85.6% to 94.3%. A prospective study demonstrated 2.2% early failures and 7.3% late failures in diabetic patients. After 5 years, the overall success rate for this group of diabetic patients was 90%. None of these studies were able to correlate gender, age, smoking, diabetes type, or level of diabetic control with implant failure. In a metaanalytical review of implant failures in patients who were not diabetics, the early implant failure rate was 3.2% and the late implant failure rate 5.2%. The finding that patients with diabetes experience slightly more late failures may be related to less tissue integrity caused by reduced tissue turnover and impaired tissue perfusion. These results suggest that diabetes may be a risk factor for implants, particularly for late failures. However, the risk does not appear to be particularly high.

Bone Metabolic Disease

Osteoporosis is a skeletal condition characterized by decreased mineral density. The two main classifications are primary (three types) and secondary (multiple types) osteoporosis. *Primary osteoporosis* has been attributed to menopausal changes (type I), age-related changes (type II), or idiopathic causes (type III). *Secondary osteoporosis* has been attributed to many different diseases and conditions, including diabetes, alcoholism, malnutrition, and smoking.

All the various types of osteoporosis share the same fundamental problem of decreased bone-mineral density, and the concern that this condition may impair the patient's ability to achieve and maintain implant osseointegration. The premise that implants will not perform as well in a patient with osteoporosis is reasonable, given that osseointegration depends on bone formation adjacent to the implant surface and that success rates are highest in dense bone and lowest in poor-quality, loose trabecular bone. However, to date, there is no clear evidence to suggest that implants will not be successful in patients with osteoporosis, so the issue continues to be debated. On the positive side, although the evidence is weak, case reports have demonstrated successful implant treatment in patients with osteoporosis. Some investigators advocate the use of longer healing times for osseointegration to occur before loading the implants in patients with osteoporosis. Conversely, in a retrospective analysis of 49 patients who received sinus-bone augmentation, individuals (11 patients) with lower bone mass density had significantly lower implant success rates as compared to age- and sex-matched controls. Other parameters evaluated in this study did not demonstrate any significant differences.

Interestingly, there is a trend in aging adults (men over 50 years and postmenopausal women) for bone mass to decrease progressively through bone demineralization at a rate of 1%–2% per year and in some individuals as much as 5%–8% per year throughout their later life. If one considers this decline in bone mass with aging along with a continually increasing life expectancy in the population, the number of individuals with osteopenia or osteoporosis will continue to increase, and the concern about this condition's influence on implant success will become increasingly more important for clinicians.

Bisphosphonate Therapy

Some prescribed medications, including steroids and bisphosphonates, may be cause for concern relative to the potential implant patient. Corticosteroid therapy, whether used for hormone replacement, cancer treatment, immune suppression, or other chronic condition may suppress the immune response, impair wound healing, or compromise the normal adrenal response to stress. Although there is heightened awareness and great concern about risk of bisphosphonate-related osteonecrosis of the jaw (BRONJ), the causal relationship and pathogenesis of the problem has not been defined. A review of available literature offers information that will help to guide clinicians in their decision-making, but it is far from definitive. The prevalence and incidence remains uncertain. In general, the risk of BRONJ is between 1 in 10,000 and 1 in 100,000 but may increase to 1 in 300 after an oral surgical procedure. The great majority of BRONJ cases will likely remain in the IV population. Cofactors, such as smoking, steroid use, anemia, hypoxemia, diabetes, infection, and immune deficiency, have not been firmly established but may be important. Rarely does BRONJ in the oral bisphosphonate patient appear to progress beyond stage 2 and many cases reverses with discontinuation of oral medication. Procedures reported to have contributed to the development of BRONJ include extractions, periodontal surgery, root-canal treatment, and dental implant surgery. Dental implant therapy, as well as other surgical procedures, should be avoided in individuals who have been treated with IV bisphosphonate therapy and carefully considered with caution in patients treated with oral bisphosphonate therapy, particularly those with a history of more than 3 years of use.

Immune Compromise and Immune Suppression

Individuals undergoing chemotherapy or taking medications that impair healing potential (e.g., steroids) are probably not good candidates for implant therapy because of the effects these agents have on normal healing. This is especially true for cancer chemotherapy. A lowered resistance to infection may also be problematic for these patients. Past history of chemotherapy or immunosuppressive therapy may not be problematic if the patient has recovered from the side effects of treatment.

Patients with an immunocompromising disease, such as HIV infection or AIDS, are not good candidates for implants when their immune system is seriously impaired. Patients with very low or undetectable viral loads and normal immune function (T-cell counts) may be candidates for implant therapy

Radiation Therapy

Patients with a history of radiation treatment to the head and neck region may not heal well after surgery. Soft tissue dehiscence may follow surgical manipulation, which may lead to osteoradionecrosis (ORN), a serious condition of nonhealing exposure and infection of bone. This is especially problematic for patients who have received radiation dosages greater than 60 Gy. Surgical procedures, or any procedure that may initiate a wound, are generally avoided in patients with a history of radiation therapy. If deemed necessary, surgical procedures can be done in conjunction with hyperbaric oxygen (HBO) therapy to reduce the risk of ORN.

Several studies have documented poor success rates for implants in patients with a history of radiation therapy. In a literature review, Sennerby and Roos found irradiation to be associated with high failure rates, as did Esposito et al. in their review. Beumer et al. reported success rates as low as 60.4% in the irradiated maxilla. Granstrom et al. reported a significant improvement in survival rates for implants in patients treated with HBO. However, in a systematic review, Coulthard et al. concluded that the evidence is lacking to support the clinical effectiveness of HBO in irradiated patients receiving implants. The application of implants in patients with a history of irradiation, with or without the use of HBO, is not resolved and continues to be debated. Clearly, irradiation is a risk factor for implant success and may be a contraindication.

Psychologic and Mental Conditions

In general, any type of psychologic abnormality can be considered a contraindication to dental implant treatment because of the patient's uncooperativeness, lack of understanding, or behavioral problems. Physiologically, there is no reason to suspect that implants could not become osseointegrated in these patients. However, the patient's ability to tolerate the number and type of treatment appointments required for implant placement, restoration, and maintenance could be problematic. All psychologic conditions have the potential to be absolute contraindications to implant treatment depending on the severity of the condition. The exception might be individuals who demonstrate good cooperative behavior with only mild psychologic or mental impairment. The clinician should take great care before accepting a mentally or psychologically impaired individual for treatment with implants.

Habits and Behavioral Considerations

Patients have a variety of habits and behaviors that may increase the risk of failure for dental implants. Smoking, clenching or grinding of teeth, and drug or alcohol abuse are among the most well-known habits that should be identified because of the increased risk for implant failure or complications.

Smoking and Tobacco Use

Moderate to heavy smoking has been documented to result in higher rates of early implant failure and adversely affect the long-term prognosis of dental implant restorations. This is particularly true for implants placed in poor quality bone, such as the posterior maxilla. The mechanisms of action responsible for higher implant failures associated with smoking are not understood. Plausible explanations include the effect of smoking on white-blood cells, vasoconstriction, wound healing, and osteoporosis. Smoking is a known risk factor for osteoporosis and thus may adversely affect implant success through its effect on bone metabolism. Smoking cessation may improve the success rate of implants. In a metaanalytical review, Bain et al. found that implants with an altered surface microtopography (Biomet 3i, Osseotite; dual acid-etched surface) seemed to significantly lessen the adverse effects of smoking on implant success.

Parafunctional Habits

Parafunctional habits, such as clenching or grinding of teeth (consciously or unconsciously), has been associated with an increased rate of implant failure (e.g., failure to integrate, loss of integration, and implant fracture). Repeated lateral forces (i.e., parafunctional habits) applied to implants can be detrimental to the osseointegration process, especially during the early healing period. Patients with known parafunctional habits should be advised of an increased risk of complications or failures as a result of their clenching or grinding. Many consider bruxism to be a contraindication to implant treatment, especially in the case of a short-span, fixed-partial denture or a single-tooth implant. If implants are planned for a patient with parafunctional habits, protective measures should be employed, such as creating a narrow occlusal table with flat cusp angles, protected occlusion, and the regular use of occlusal guards.

Substance Abuse

Drug and alcohol abuse should be considered a contraindication for implant therapy for reasons similar to the psychologic problems discussed earlier. Patients with drug or alcohol addictions can be irresponsible and noncompliant with treatment recommendations. Depending on the severity and duration of an individual's addiction, some patients may be malnourished or may even have impaired organ function and therefore may not be good surgical candidates because of poor healing capacity. All elective treatments, including implant therapy, should be refused until addictions are treated and controlled.

Posttreatment Evaluation

Periodic posttreatment examination of implants, the retained prosthesis, and the condition of the surrounding peri-implant tissue is an important part of successful treatment. Aberrations and complications can often be treated if discovered early but many problems will go unnoticed by the patient. Thus, periodic examination is essential in discovering problems early and to intervene and prevent problems from getting worse. Several parameters are available to evaluate the condition of the prosthesis, the stability of the implant(s), and the health of surrounding peri-implant tissues after implant integration and prosthetic restoration. Intraoral radiographs should be taken at the time of placement (baseline), at the time of abutment connection (confirm seating and serve as another baseline), at the time of final restoration delivery (loading), and subsequently to monitor marginal or peri-implant bone changes. Periapical radiographs have excellent resolution and provide adequate details for evaluating bone support around implants if taken at a perpendicular direction.

The long-term success of dental implants is dependent on the health and stability of supporting peri-implant tissues. Good oral hygiene and regular professional care are essential in maintaining peri-implant health and the importance of good oral hygiene should be stressed as early as possible. Patients should be taught to maintain good oral hygiene. Their performance should be monitored and reinforced at each visit.

Hence concluding, dental clinicians can now predictably replace missing teeth with endosseous dental implants. Most patients, whether missing a single tooth, several teeth, or all their teeth, can be candidates for dental implant therapy. However, many factors influence the outcome; the clinician must consider the quantity, quality, and location of available bone; the patient's mental and physical health; as well as risk factors and contraindications. Patients should be advised about risk factors and be provided treatment options, both with and without dental implants. Periodic evaluation, good oral hygiene, and regular maintenance are important aspects of care for the long-term success and the prevention of complications with dental implants.

Diagnostic Imaging for the Implant Patient

Several radiographic imaging options are available for diagnosis and treatment planning of patients receiving dental implants. Options range from standard projections routinely available in the dental office to more complex radiographic techniques typically available only in radiology centers. Standard projections include intraoral (periapical and occlusal) and extraoral (panoramic and lateral cephalometric) radiographs. More complex imaging techniques include cone-beam computed tomography (CBCT) and multislice computed tomography (MSCT). The CBCT and MSCT image data files can be reformatted and viewed on a personal computer using simulation software, making the diagnosis and treatment-planning process interactive and visually more meaningful. Often, combinations of various modalities are used because no single modality can provide all information pertinent to the radiographic evaluation of the implant patient. Familiarity with the benefits, limitations of various techniques, and awareness of the specific clinical questions that need to be answered should guide the decision-making process and selection of radiographic examinations for individual patients.

Multiple factors influence the selection of radiographic technique(s) for a particular case, including cost, availability, radiation exposure, and case type. The decision is a balance between these factors and the desire to minimize risk of complications for the patient. Accurately identifying vital anatomic structures and being able to perform implant placement surgery without injury to these structures are critical to treatment success. Diagnostic imaging techniques must always be interpreted in conjunction with a good clinical examination.

Common imaging techniques used for the evaluation of the implant patient are briefly discussed below. Indications for each technique are outlined, along with the advantages and limitations of each technique.

Standard Projections

Standard diagnostic imaging modalities include periapical, panoramic, lateral cephalometric, and occlusal radiographs. Table 58.2 summarizes the advantages and disadvantages of each modality. Individual modalities are discussed below in detail under the following subheadings:

Periapical radiographs (e-only)
Occlusal radiographs (e-only)
Panoramic radiographs (e-only)
Lateral cephalometric radiographs (e-only)
Cross-sectional imaging

- Cone-beam computed tomography
- Multislice computed tomography

Interactive "Simulation" software programs (e-only)

Periapical Radiographs

Periapical radiographs offer great advantages for the evaluation of the implant patient. They provide an overall assessment of the quantity and quality of the edentulous alveolar ridge and the adjacent teeth. They are easy to obtain in the dental office, are inexpensive, and deliver low radiation to the patient (Table 58.3). Dentists are familiar with the depicted anatomy and possible pathology. Since these direct-exposure projections do not use intensifying screens, intraoral radiographs offer the highest detail and spatial resolution of all radiographic modalities (eFig. 58.14). Thus, intraoral radiographs are the projection of choice when subtle pathology, such as a retained root tip, needs to be detected and evaluated.

The most significant disadvantage of periapical radiographs is their susceptibility to unpredictably magnify anatomic structures, which does not allow reliable measurements. Foreshortening or elongation can be minimized by the use of paralleling technique.

TABLE 58.2 Advantages and Disadvantages of the Various Radiographic Projections

Modality	Advantages	Disadvantages
Periapical and occlusal radiography	High resolution and detail, easy acquisition, low exposure, and inexpensive	Unpredictable magnification, small imaged area, and 2D representation of anatomy
Panoramic radiography	Easy to acquire, images whole ridge, low exposure, and inexpensive	Unpredictable magnification, unequal magnification in vertical and horizontal dimensions, and 2D representation of anatomy, not detailed
Lateral cephalometric radiography	Easy to acquire, predictable magnification, low exposure, and inexpensive	Limited use in area of midline and 2D representation of anatomy
MSCT	3D representation, predictable magnification, sufficient detail, digital format, and images whole arch	Requires special equipment, is expensive, and has a high-exposure dose
CBCT	3D representation, predictable magnification, sufficient detail, digital format, images whole arch, and low dose	Requires special equipment and is expensive

TABLE 58.3 Radiation Dose (Effective Dose in μSv) Received From Common Projections During Evaluation of the Implant Patient Data

Modality	Effective Dose (μSv)
Full-mouth X-ray (FMX) series	177
Panoramic	20
Limited field-of-view CBCT	47
Medium field-of-view CBCT	98
Large field-of-view CBCT	117
MSCT, Maxillofacial	913

CBCT, Cone-beam computed tomography; *CT*, computed tomography; *MSCT*, multislice computed tomography.

(Adapted from Mallya SM: Principles of cone beam computed tomography. In Fayad M, Johnson BR, editors: *3D imaging in endodontics: a new era in diagnosis and treatment.* Median effective doses for standard exposure protocols were derived from collation of data from several reports in the literature.)

However, distortion is particularly accentuated in edentulous areas where missing teeth and resorption of the alveolus necessitate receptor placement at significant angulation in relation to the long axis of the teeth and the alveolar bone. Additionally, periapical radiographs are two-dimensional (2D) representations of 3D objects and do not provide any information of the buccal–lingual dimension of the alveolar ridge. Structures that are distinctly separated in the buccal–lingual dimension appear to be overlapping. Also, the periapical image is limited by the size of film or sensor being used. Often, it is not possible to image the entire height of the remaining alveolar ridge, and when extensive mesial–distal areas need to be evaluated, multiple periapical radiographs are required.

In summary, periapical radiographs are useful screening images that offer a detailed view of a small area of the alveolar arch. Limitations that must be considered include the possibility of distortion and the 2D representation of anatomic structures.

Occlusal Radiographs

Occlusal radiographs are intraoral projections that offer easy, economic, low-dose, and high-resolution images covering a larger area than periapical projections. Depending on receptor placement and the angulation of the X-ray tube, occlusal radiographs can provide an image of the mandibular width or can depict an extended area of the edentulous ridge. Occlusal radiographs have the same limitations of distortion and overlapping anatomy as periapical radiographs.

In summary, occlusal radiographic projections are good screening images as compared to periapical radiographic projections as they provide an overview of the mandibular width and can visualize larger areas of alveolar ridge.

Panoramic Radiographs

Panoramic radiographs are often used in the evaluation of the implant patient because they offer several advantages over other modalities. Panoramic radiographs deliver low radiation (Table 58.3) to provide a broad picture of both arches and thus allow assessment of extensive edentulous areas, angulation of existing teeth and occlusal plane, and important anatomy in implant treatment planning, such as the maxillary sinus, nasal cavity, mental foramen, and mandibular canal (eFig. 58.15). Panoramic units are widely available and easy to operate and dentists are familiar with the anatomy and pathology depicted by the images. Similar to intraoral projections, panoramic images are 2D and thus do not offer diagnostic information for the buccal–lingual width of the alveolar arch.

Panoramic images appear intuitively familiar. However, they combine characteristic physical and radiographic principles that make them distinct from other intraoral and extraoral radiographs. Although outside the scope of this chapter, familiarity with the principles underlying panoramic radiography is central in understanding, and thus compensating for, the limitations and constraints of the images. The reader is referred to other textbooks for detailed discussion of this topic. Briefly, the existence of ghost shadows, unpredictable horizontal and vertical magnification, distortion of structures outside the focal trough, projection geometry generated by the negative vertical angulation of the X-ray beam, and propensity to patient-positioning errors do not allow consistent detailed and accurate measurements to be generated. As a result, panoramic radiographs do not provide the highly detailed images that are generated by intraoral radiographs.

Measurement distortion is more prevalent and varies across the radiographic image. On average, panoramic radiographs are 25% magnifications of actual size. Implant manufacturers often provide transparency sheets with implant size outlines of 25% magnification. However, it is important to appreciate that the 25% magnification is an estimate. The actual magnification may range from 10% to 30% in different areas within the same image and depends greatly on patient positioning during panoramic radiography. For this reason, precise measurements on panoramic projections are not possible. Nonetheless, panoramic radiographs offer an overall view of the maxilla and mandible that can be used to estimate bone measurements and evaluate the approximate relationships between teeth and other anatomic structures. More precise diagnostic imaging should be used to measure the proximity of critical anatomic structures, such as the maxillary sinus, the mandibular canal, or proposed implant positions.

In summary, panoramic projections are useful screening images of the jaws for approximations and relative spatial relationships. However, because of magnification and distortion errors, panoramic radiographs should not be used for detailed measurements of proposed implant sites.

Lateral Cephalometric Radiographs

Lateral cephalometric radiographs are occasionally used to evaluate potential implant patients. These projections provide useful information for the cortical thickness, height, and width of the alveolar ridge at the midline, as well as the skeletal relationship between maxilla and mandible and facial profile. Lateral cephalometric radiographs are low in cost, readily available, easy to interpret, and have a predictable magnification of the depicted structures. However, their use for the implant patient is limited to structures at the midline, with minimal usefulness for other areas of the jaws.

In summary, lateral cephalometric radiographs have a limited use in implant treatment planning.

Cross-Sectional Imaging

Cross-sectional diagnostic imaging modalities include MSCT and CBCT. Conventional tomography also provides cross-sectional images with predictable magnification and has been used in the assessment of the implant patient. However, with the introduction and expansion of CBCT imaging, conventional tomography is becoming progressively infrequent and is not described in this chapter.

Cone-Beam Computed Tomography

CBCT is an imaging modality that offers significant advantages for the evaluation of implant patients. CBCT was introduced to dentistry in the late 1990s, and several CBCT units are commercially available for imaging of the craniofacial complex. The X-ray source and the detector are diametrically positioned and make a 180- to 360-degree rotation around the patient's head within the gantry. The X-ray beam is collimated and the resultant beam is cone or pyramid shaped. Typically, a single complete rotation, 180–500 basis projections of the region of interest, is generated. The computer uses these images to generate a digital, three-dimensional map of the face. Once this map is generated, multiplanar reconstructions—axial, coronal, sagittal, or oblique sections of various thicknesses—can be reconstructed from the data.

An important feature of the various CBCT units is the field of view (FOV) describing the extent of the imaged volume. CBCT units are typically categorized as large FOV (greater than 15 cm), medium FOV (8–15 cm), and limited FOV systems (less than 8 cm). Fig. 58.16 depicts schematically the anatomic area covered by large, medium, and limited FOV scans. In general, large FOV units image a more extensive anatomic area, deliver a higher radiation exposure to the patient, and produce lower-resolution images (Fig. 58.17). Conversely, limited FOV units image a small area of the face, deliver less radiation, and produce a higher-resolution image (Fig. 58.18).

CBCT scans offer several advantages for evaluation of the implant patient, compared to two-dimensional (2D) imaging. True cross-sections offer a precise and detailed evaluation of the height and width of the alveolar ridge. The images can be adjusted and printed without magnification, facilitating measurements directly on the prints or films with standard rulers (i.e., not magnified). Vertical and horizontal rulers adjacent to each section allow the clinician to check for magnification and make direct measurements. The digital format allows for image enhancement tools, rapid communication between the radiologist and the surgeon, and generation of multiple copies of the images. Various anatomic structures can be visualized and analyzed at all three coordinate axes, so that their superoinferior, anteroposterior, and

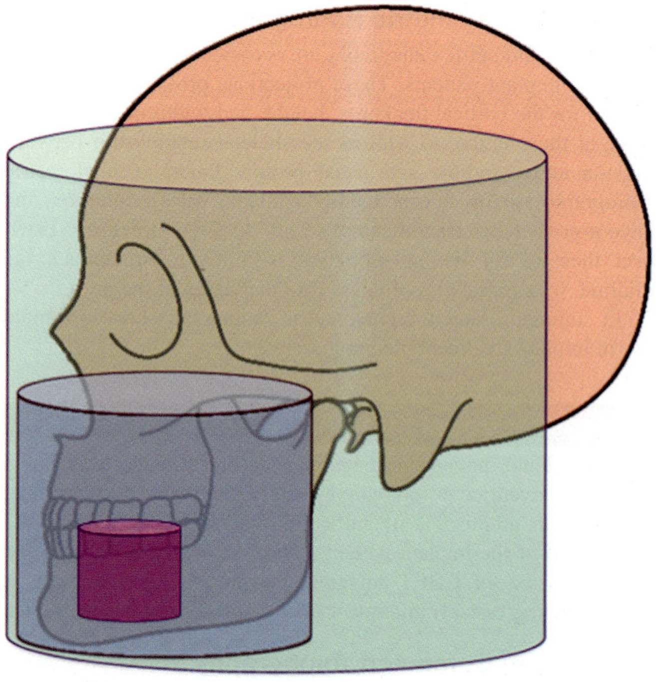

Fig. 58.16 Schematic diagram of the anatomic area imaged with large *(green)*, medium *(blue)*, and limited *(magenta)* field of view cone-beam computed tomography.

buccolingual location can be identified with precision. CBCT images the entire arch, or even both arches, so several edentulous areas can be visualized with a single examination. The bone and soft-tissue contrast and resolution are appropriate for the diagnostic task.

In summary, CBCT scanning is a valuable imaging modality for three-dimensional and cross-sectional evaluation of the implant patient. It has similar advantages and disadvantages as CT scanning. The most significant difference is that CBCT imaging delivers much less radiation exposure to the patient.

Multislice Computed Tomography

MSCT was widely used in the evaluation of the implant patient. However, with the advent of CBCT, utilization of MSCT has been reduced significantly. However, MSCT is an excellent choice for evaluation of the implant patient if CBCT scanning is not available.

Typical dental views reconstructed from a MSCT scan include a scout view (see Fig. 58.19A) as well as axial (Fig. 59.19B), panoramic (Fig. 59.19C), and cross-sectional (Fig. 59.19D) views of the jaws. Appropriate axial slices through the alveolar ridge of interest are selected as scout views. The curvature of the maxillary or mandibular ridge is then drawn on the axial slices, and panoramic images along the drawn line are created. Finally, cross-sectional slices, typically at every 1–2 mm and perpendicular to the drawn curvature, are created. In addition to these flat, two-dimensional views, complex, three-dimensional images with surface rendering can also be generated from the CT data (Fig. 58.19E). These images can provide useful information about the alveolar ridge defects that are easy to comprehend.

MSCT offers the same advantages and disadvantages as MSCT. However, the two modalities have basic differences that result from the different physical principles used during image acquisition. MSCT scans offers a greater *contrast resolution*, or the ability to distinguish two objects with small density differences. In contrast, CBCT scans have a limited capacity to separate muscle from fat or connective tissue compared to MSCT scans. Fortunately, the diagnostic tasks in implant treatment planning do not require high-contrast resolution. Because bone has a much higher radiodensity than surrounding soft tissues, both CBCT and MSCT clearly depict bone morphology and internal trabecular architecture. One of the most significant advantages of CBCT scanning versus MSCT scanning is the significantly lower radiation dose delivered to the patient (Table 58.3).

MSCT scanning requires specialized equipment and setting. Radiologists and technicians need to be knowledgeable of the anatomy, anatomic variants, and pathology of the jaws, as well as considerations pertinent to implant treatment planning, so that optimal views will be provided. An MSCT scan delivers a much higher radiation dose to the patient than the other modalities used during implant treatment planning (Table 58.3). Because a CT scan images the whole arch, radiation is delivered to the entire imaged area, regardless of how many or how few sites are actually needed. Metallic restorations can cause beam-hardening artifacts that impair the diagnostic quality of the images. This is particularly challenging in patients with heavily restored dentition. In general, the cost of MSCT is significantly higher than that of CBCT or the other standard intraoral and extraoral projections.

In summary, MSCT scanning offers many advantages during implant treatment planning, including accurate cross-sectional imaging and three-dimensional visualization of anatomic structures. High dose to the patient and artifacts caused by metallic restorations are concerns that should be considered.

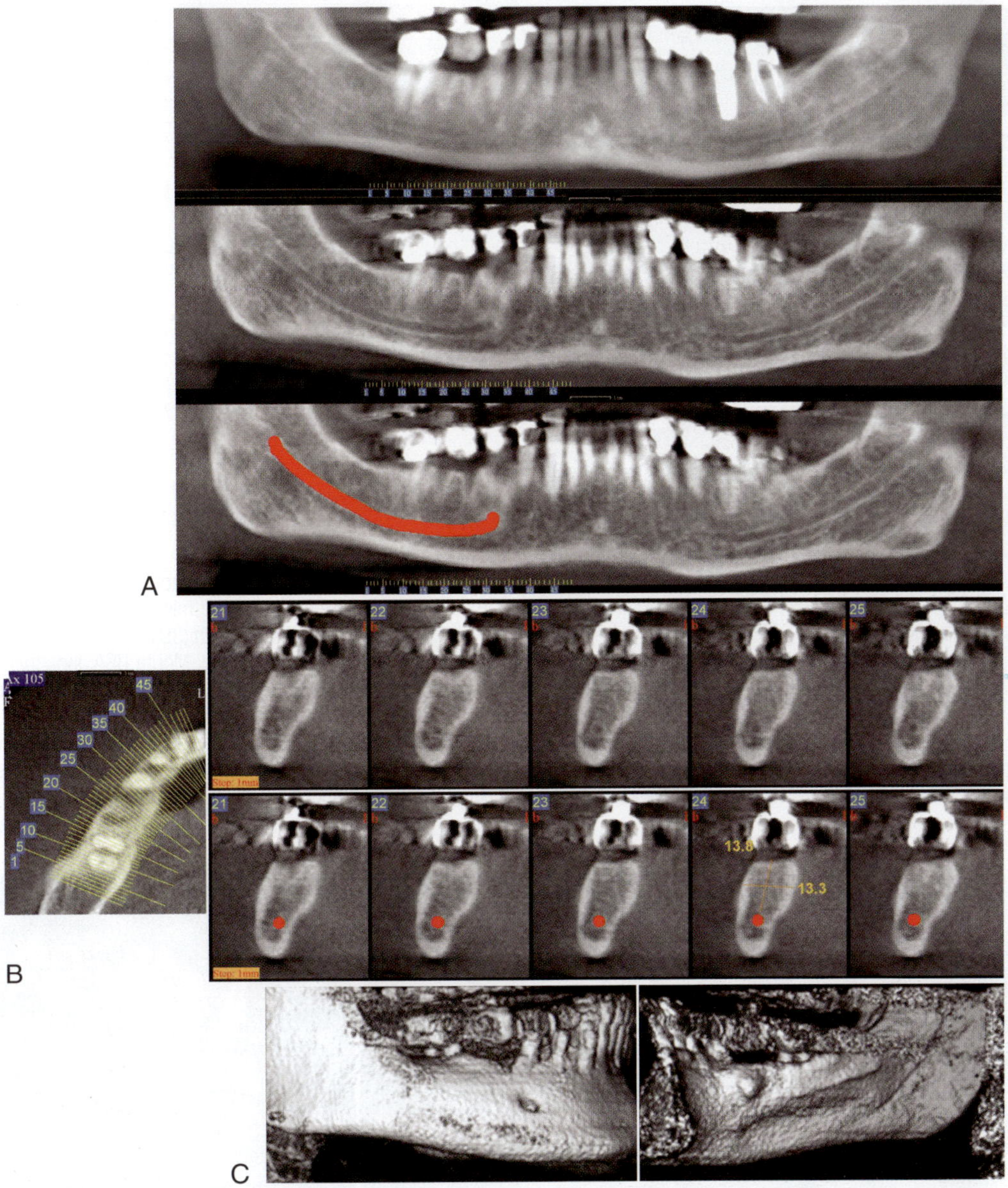

Fig. 58.17 Cone-beam computed tomography images for the evaluation of the edentulous space at the area of missing tooth #30 before implant placement using a large field-of-view unit (NewTom 3G, Verona, Italy, distributed by AFP Imaging, Elmsford, New York). Note the tooth-shaped marker used. A, A series of "panoramic" reconstructions through the alveolar ridge reveals the relationship of the marker to the adjacent teeth. The top "panoramic" view is 12 mm thick so as to depict most of the extent of the alveolar ridge and adjacent teeth. The middle "panoramic" image is 1 mm thick through the area of the mandibular canal. Note that adjacent teeth are out of the plane of the section and thus not depicted on the image. The bottom "panoramic" view is the same as the middle one, but the position of the mandibular canal has been depicted by the *red line*. B, Scout axial view and series of cross sections through the area of the marker. The bottom row shows the same axial slices as the top row. However, the position of the *red line* drawn on the panoramic view is also depicted to help localization of the mandibular canal. The height and width of the alveolar ridge have been measured in a selected section. C, Three-dimensional reconstructions provide an overall impression of the bone contours and shape of the alveolar ridge. Note the small exostosis on the lingual surface of the alveolar ridge.

Interactive "Simulation" Software Programs

Implant treatment planning can be greatly enhanced by the use of specialized software. In addition to measuring the quantity and quality of bone in potential implant sites, these programs use CT- or CBCT-scan data to simulate placement of implant and restorations. Using a database of commercially available implant images, the length, width, angulation, and position of implants can be "simulated" in the desired positions and evaluated relative to other structures in 3D. In cases of alveolar ridge deficiency or defects or when sinus-bone augmentation is indicated, the additional bone volume needed can be evaluated and quantified. The restoration of the implants can also be simulated and the distribution of mechanical forces onto the implant and adjacent bone predicted.

Software programs specialized in implant treatment planning, such as SIM/Plant (Materialise/Columbia Scientific, Glen Burnie, MD), can reformat CBCT- or CT-scan data. The clinician can use

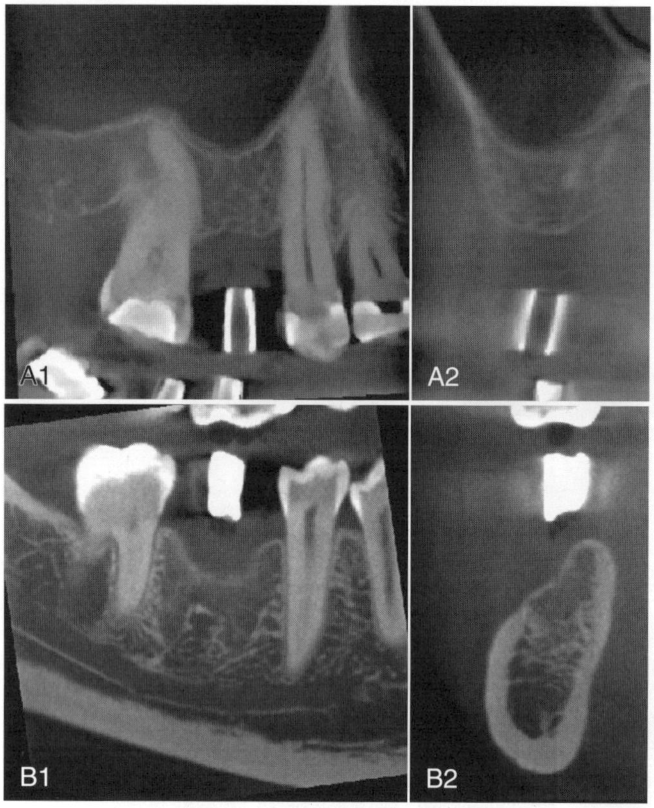

Fig. 58.18 Cone-beam computed tomography images for the evaluation of the edentulous space at the area of missing tooth #4 (A) and missing tooth #30 (B) using a limited field-of-view scan (3D Accuitomo, J. Morita Corporation, Suita City, Osaka, Japan, distributed by J. Morita USA, Inc., Irvine, California). Sagittal and cross-sectional slices are shown. Although the anatomic area imaged is limited, the resolutions of the images are high. (A) Implant site #4 (maxillary right second premolar) in anterior–posterior (A1) and buccolingual (A2) cross-sectional views. (B) Implant site #30 (mandibular right first molar) in anterior–posterior (B1) and buccolingual (B2) cross-sectional views.

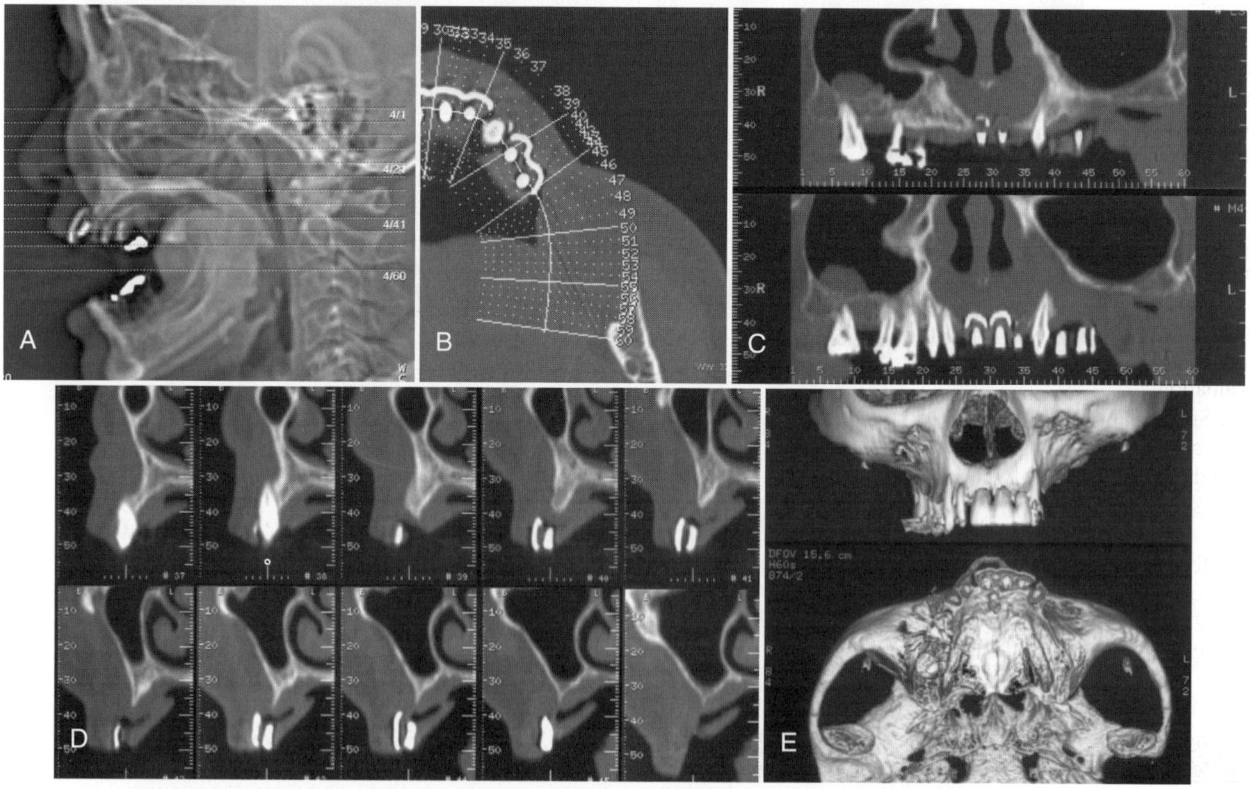

Fig. 58.19 Multislice computed tomography (MSCT) examination for evaluation of edentulous maxilla before implant placement. A, Scout view of the patient's head; axial sections through the area of interest are indicated. B, Axial slice through the markers is used to display the orientation of the panoramic and cross-sectional images through the alveolar ridge. C, Panoramic views through the alveolar ridge demonstrate the relation of the markers to adjacent teeth. D, Cross-sectional slices through the area of the markers reveal the height and buccolingual dimension of the alveolar ridge, as well as the relation of the markers to the ridge. E, Three-dimensional reconstructions provide an overall impression of the bone contours and shape of the alveolar ridge.

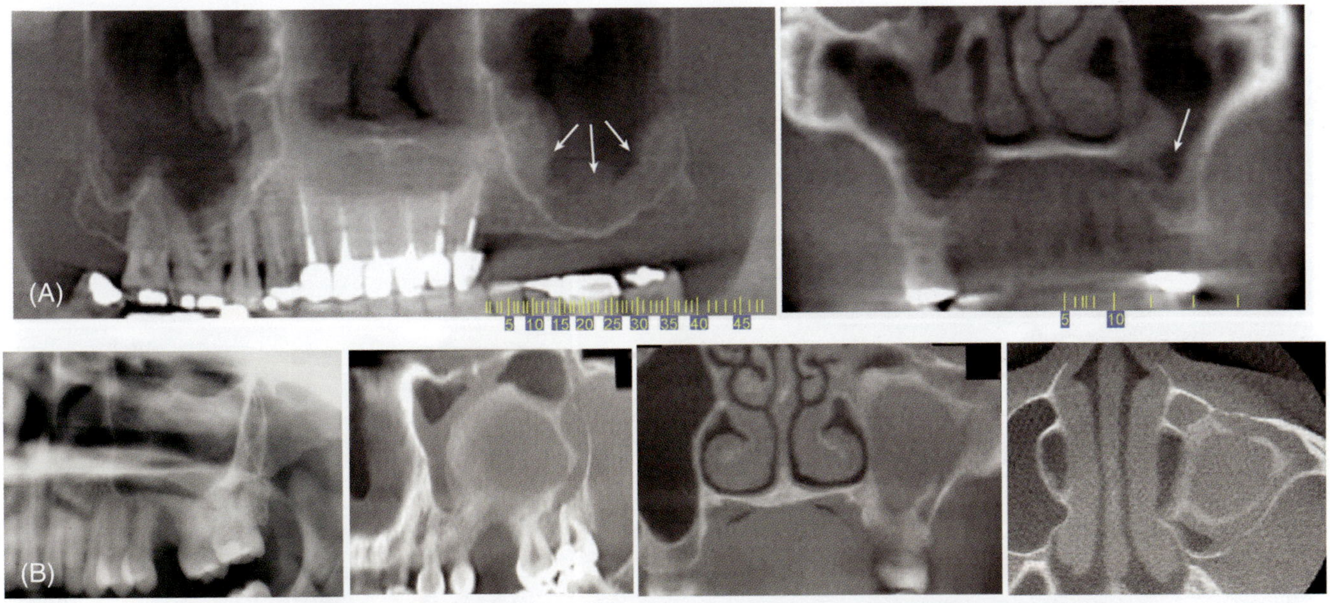

Fig. 58.22 CBCT examination of the posterior left maxilla. A, Top row shows reconstructed "panoramic" and coronal sections of the alveolar ridge. Note the thickened mucoperiosteal lining of the floor of the left maxillary sinus *(white arrow).* The patient has chronic maxillary sinusitis. B, Bottom row shows conventional panoramic, reconstructed "panoramic," coronal and axial sections of the alveolar ridge at the area of missing first maxillary molar. A large radiolucent lesion at the edentulous alveolar ridge elevates the floor of the maxillary sinus and occupies most of the sinus. Biopsy revealed a keratocystic odontogenic tumor that was an incidental finding in this asymptomatic patient.

the reformatted images on a personal computer in an interactive manner to identify anatomic structures, simulate implant placement positions, and better appreciate relationships between planned implant positions and teeth or anatomic structures (eFig. 58.20). InVivo5 planning software (Anatomage, San Jose, CA) acquires data directly from CBCT- or CT-scan DICOM (Digital Imaging and Communications in Medicine) files without the need for reformatting. Once implant positions are confirmed, a computer-generated surgical guide is produced to facilitate the surgical placement of implants in the planned positions (eFig. 58.21).

BOX 58.3 Anatomic Structures Pertinent to Treatment Planning of the Implant Patient

Maxilla

1. Maxillary sinus (floor and anterior wall)
2. Nasal cavity (floor and lateral wall)
3. Incisive foramen
4. Canine fossa
5. Canalis sinuosus

Mandible

1. Mandibular canal
2. Anterior loop of the mandibular canal
3. Anterior extension of the mandibular canal
4. Mental foramen
5. Submandibular fossa
6. Retromolar canal
7. Lingual inclination of the alveolar ridge

Patient Evaluation

Evaluation of the implant patient should be disciplined and objective. Specific questions that can affect implant placement and outcome should be considered and examined carefully and explicitly. The advantages and disadvantages of various radiographic projections should be considered and radiographic modalities chosen based on necessary information for the particular patient. The objectives for any radiographic evaluation, regardless of imaging technique used, should include an evaluation to (1) exclude pathology, (2) identify anatomic structures, and (3) measure the quantity, quality, and location of available bone.

Exclude Pathology

Healthy bone is a prerequisite for successful osseointegration and long-term implant success. The first step in the radiographic evaluation of the implant site is to establish the health of the alveolar bone and other tissues imaged within a particular projection. Local and systemic diseases that affect bone homeostasis can preclude, modify, or alter placement of implants. Retained root fragments, residual periodontal disease, cysts, and tumors should be identified and resolved before implant placement. Systemic diseases, such as osteoporosis and hyperparathyroidism, alter bone metabolism and might affect implant osseointegration. Areas of poor bone quality should be identified and if indicated, adjustments to the treatment plan incorporated. Maxillary sinusitis, polyps, or other sinus pathology should be diagnosed and treated when implants are considered in the posterior maxilla, especially if sinus-bone augmentation procedures are planned (Fig. 58.22).

Identify Anatomic Structures

Several important anatomic structures are found close to desired areas of implant placement in the maxilla and mandible (Box 58.3). Familiarity with the radiographic appearance of these structures is important during treatment planning and implant placement. Their exact localization is central to prevent unwanted complication and unnecessary morbidity. Important anatomic structures in the maxilla

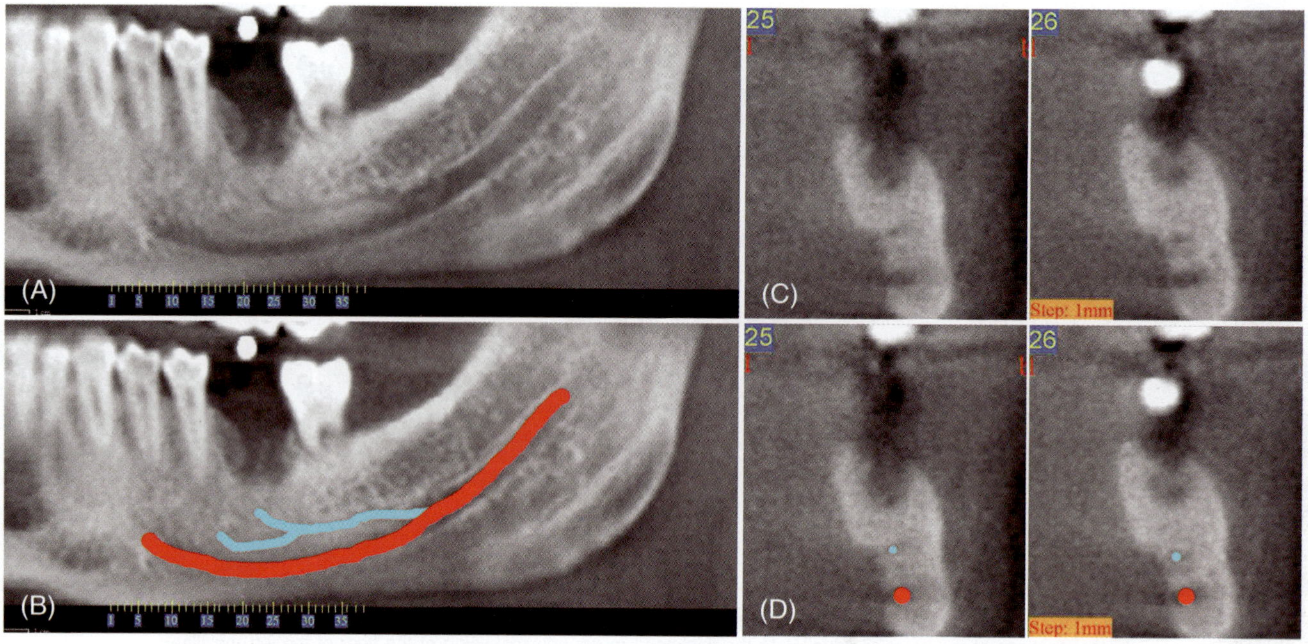

Fig. 58.23 CBCT examination of the area of missing tooth #19 before implant placement. A, Panoramic view of the area of interest depicts an accessory mandibular canal. B, Same panoramic view with the accessory mandibular canal colored *blue* and the main canal *red*. C, Cross-sectional views through the area of missing tooth #19. D, Same cross-sectional images depicting the *blue* and *red* markings. Note that the position of the markings coincides with the position of the accessory and main mandibular canals (compare C and D).

include the floor and anterior wall of the maxillary sinus, incisive foramen, floor and lateral wall of the nasal cavity, and canine fossa. Important anatomic structures in the mandible that should be recognized include the mandibular canal, anterior loop of the mandibular canal, mental foramen, anterior extension of the canal, and submandibular fossa. The existence of anatomic variants, such as incomplete healing of an extraction site, sinus loculation, division of mandibular canal (Fig. 58.23), or absence of a well-defined corticated canal, should also be recognized.

Assess Bone Quantity, Quality, and Volume

The primary goal of diagnostic imaging for potential implant patients is to evaluate the available bone volume for implant placement in desired anatomic locations. The clinician wants to estimate and verify exact adequate height, width, and density to the recipient bone while avoiding damage to critical anatomic structures. Failure to accurately assess the location of important anatomic structures can lead to unnecessary complications. For example, inadvertent penetration and damage to the inferior alveolar nerve can result in serious immediate-term (profuse bleeding), short-term, and long-term (nerve paresthesia/anesthesia) complications. The height and width of the alveolar bone should be accurately detailed. Depending on the technique, diagnostic imaging can estimate or measure the coronal–apical height, the buccal–lingual width, and the mesial–distal spacing available for implants that will be placed in proximity to teeth or relative to other planned implants.

This task can be simple in cases with good bone quality and sufficient bone volume in the desired implant location(s). However, in cases with moderate–severe bone resorption, alveolar defects, or recent extraction sites, obtaining a clear and accurate diagnostic image can be more challenging. The diagnostic imaging may reveal inadequate bone volume for the proposed implant(s) and indicate a need for bone augmentation or depending on the severity of the deficiency, preclude the patient from the possibility of implant therapy (Fig. 59.24). When ridge augmentation is deemed necessary,

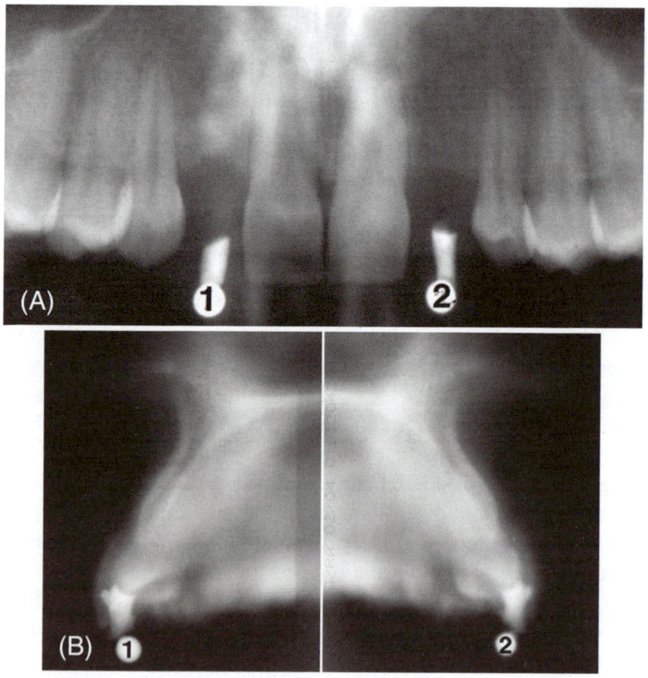

Fig. 58.24 Radiographic evaluation of a patient with congenitally missing maxillary lateral incisors before implant placement. A, Panoramic radiograph reveals sufficient height and mesial–lateral width of the alveolar ridge. B, Cross-sectional conventional tomography of the edentulous areas reveals a narrow (<4 mm) buccal–lingual width of the alveolar ridge that needs to be addressed by modifications in the treatment planning, such as bone augmentation.

radiographic evaluation prior and postsurgery informs treatment planning and ensures grafting integrity and quality (Fig. 58.25).

In addition to the amount, the quality of the available bone should also be evaluated. A uniform, continuous cortical outline and a lacy, well-defined trabecular core reflect the normal bone homeostasis necessary for appropriate bone response around the implant. Thin or discontinuous cortex, sparse trabeculation, large marrow spaces, and altered trabecular architecture should be noted because they might predict poor implant stabilization and a less desirable response of the bone. Poor bone quality may necessitate modifications of the treatment planning, such as waiting longer for healing (osseointegration) to maximize bone-to-implant contact before loading.

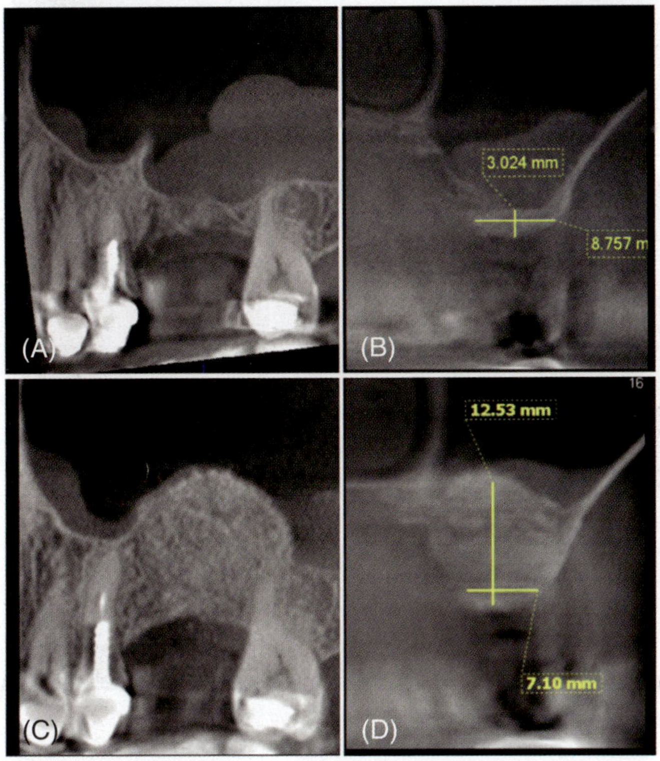

Fig. 58.25 Radiographic evaluation of a patient with missing left maxillary second premolar and first molar. Initial CBCT reveals A, an atrophic alveolar ridge with, B, an inadequate height for implant placement. Also note the thickened mucoperiosteum at the floor of the maxillary sinus. CBCT after sinus grafting for ridge augmentation shows, C, uniformly opaque grafting area blending with alveolar trabeculation and a smooth sinus floor elevation, which provides, D, adequate dimensions for implant placement.

Evaluate Relation of Alveolar Ridge with Existing Teeth and Desired Implant Position

Accurate placement (spatial position and angulation relative to adjacent teeth and occlusal plane) will greatly affect the restorative success and long-term prognosis of the implant. A significant variable during the preimplant evaluation is the relation of the desired implant position relative to the existing teeth, alveolar crest, and occlusal plane. Angled or custom abutments can accommodate slight variations in implant position and implant inclination. However, more significant deviations should be avoided.

Prolonged tooth loss is usually associated with atrophy of the alveolar ridge and in the case of the maxilla, with pneumatization of the sinus floor toward the alveolar crest. Traumatic extractions can compromise the buccal or lingual cortex and alter the shape and buccolingual ridge dimension. Anatomic variants, such as lingual inclination of the alveolus or narrow ridges, should be considered during treatment planning of the implant patient (Fig. 58.26).

An important part of diagnostic imaging must include an evaluation of the available bone relative to the "prosthetically driven" implant position. This aspect of the patient evaluation is best accomplished with diagnostic models, wax-up of planned tooth replacement, and radiographic markers in the desired tooth positions during imaging. Steel balls, brass tubes, and gutta–percha have all been used to establish the proposed tooth positions relative to the existing alveolar bone. The use of these nonanatomic markers is helpful for evaluating bone height and width in specific anatomic locations. However, they do not accurately represent the tooth contours and do not allow the clinician to estimate variations in implant position and angulation relative to the position and emergence of the planned tooth replacement. Therefore, it is more desirable and beneficial to use radiopaque "tooth-shaped" markers so that the existing alveolar bone can be evaluated relative to the entire tooth position/contours (Fig. 58.27). This is particularly important for anterior, esthetic implant cases. Patients should always be imaged with radiographic guides (markers).

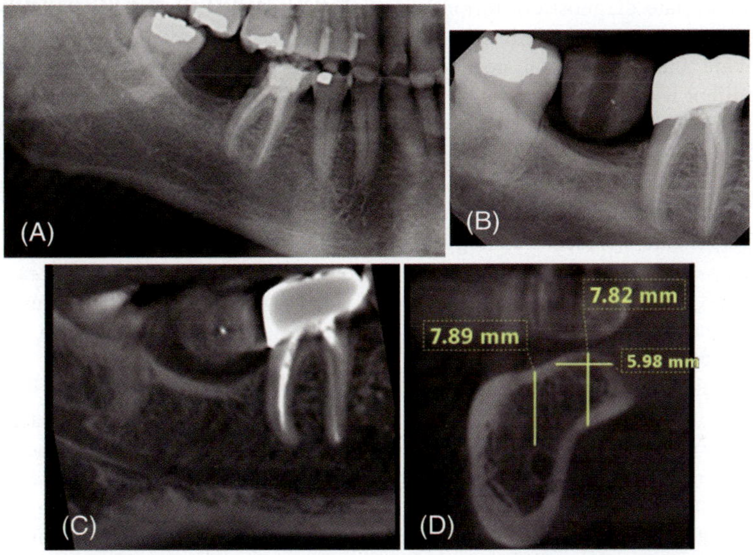

Fig. 58.26 Radiographic evaluation of a patient with edentulous posterior left mandible before implant placement. A and B, Panoramic and periapical radiographs demonstrate sufficient height of the alveolar ridge with little or no resorption. C and D, CBCT sections reveal significant lingual inclination of the alveolar ridge with lingual concavity that is not depicted on conventional radiographs.

(A)

(B)

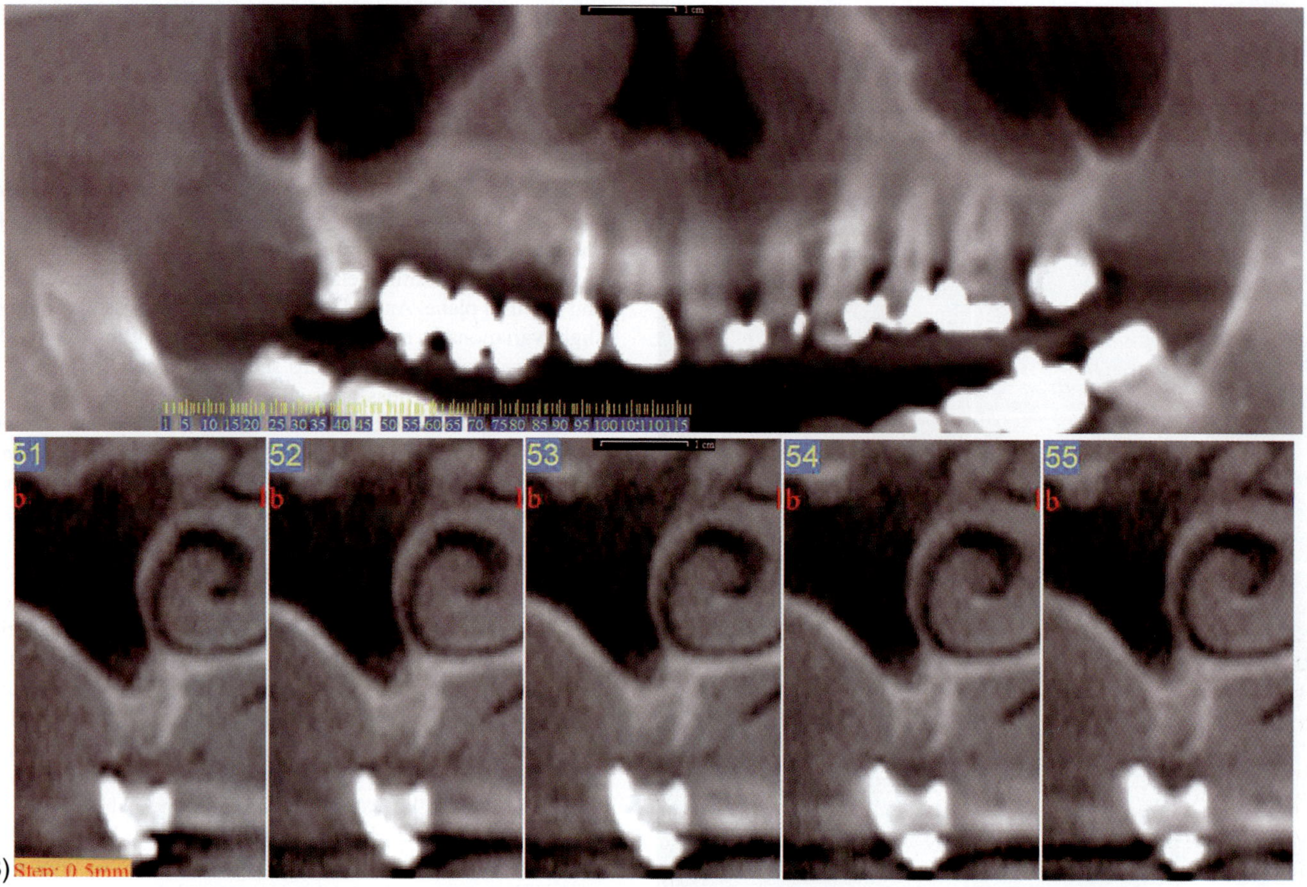

Fig. 58.27 A, Panoramic view of partially edentulous maxilla with tooth shaped markers in areas of missing teeth (potential implant sites). B, Cross-sectional views from a CBCT examination before implant placement in the right maxilla. Appropriately sized and shaped tooth markers placed in the prosthetically desired locations of the planned restorations for the missing teeth help evaluate the existing alveolar ridge relative to the prospective tooth positions and contours.

Clinical Selection of Diagnostic Imaging

Radiography is an important diagnostic tool for the evaluation of the implant patient. However, radiographic imaging alone is insufficient. It is important to correlate diagnostic information with a good clinical examination. Conversely, a clinical examination is insufficient to provide the information needed to plan implant treatment for a patient without some radiographic imaging.

Clinical Examination

Before taking any radiographs, a complete clinical examination of the implant patient is required. This should include the etiology and duration of tooth loss, any history of traumatic extraction, and a review of records and radiographs, if available. Clinical assessment of the edentulous area, covering mucosa, adjacent and opposing teeth, and occlusal plane should be performed. Temporomandibular function, mandibular maximal opening, and protrusive and lateral movements should be evaluated.

Screening Radiographs

At this point, an overall assessment of the health of the jaws should be performed. Periapical radiographs provide a high-resolution image of the alveolus and the surrounding structures, including adjacent teeth. For extended edentulous areas, panoramic, lateral cephalometric, and occlusal radiographs can be used to estimate bone height and width. Any pathology of the bone at the prospective implant site, as well as of the surrounding structures, should be identified and treated as indicated.

Fabrication of Radiographic and Surgical Guides

Once the health of the soft and hard tissues is established, casts should be taken and detailed analysis performed. The clinician should decide on the number of implants and their desired location. Next, a radiographic guide should be fabricated, usually with clear acrylic. The position of the desired implants is indicated by the use of radiopaque objects such as metallic balls, cylinders, or rods; gutta–percha; or composite resin. If CT imaging might be performed, the use of metallic markers should be avoided. The design of such a guide greatly enhances the diagnostic information provided by the radiographs because it correlates the radiographic anatomy with the exact position of the proposed implant location.

Cross-Sectional Tomography

Some type of cross-sectional imaging, such as conventional tomography, CT, or CBCT, should be performed before implant placement in any site of the jaws. The potential morbidity of a compromised anatomic structure and the poor performance and potential failure of a misplaced implant, combined with the wide availability of tomographic facilities, favor the use of cross-sectional imaging in most cases of implant-treatment planning. It is crucial that the cross-sections are perpendicular to the curvature of the mandible and parallel to the planned implant. Improper patient positioning

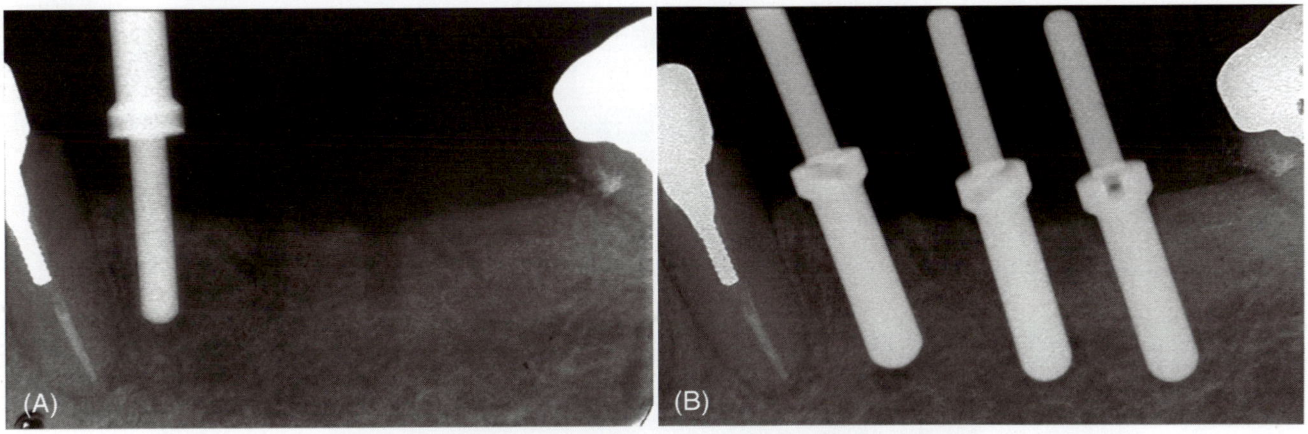

Fig. 58.28 Intraoperative periapical radiographs are valuable in assessing the proximity of adjacent teeth. A, The 2-mm guide pin is used to determine direction of the osteotomy site and its proximity to the adjacent root. B, After angle correction, the osteotomy sites are completed to length with the final drill. Here the 3-mm guide pins confirm the correct angulation and spacing of the final osteotomy site preparation before implant placement.

can lead to an overestimation of the height and width of the available bone. If the surgeon believes that sections were performed at the wrong angulation, new images should be requested. This might necessitate re-exposure of the patient.

Intraoperative and Postoperative Radiographic Assessment

Various radiographic modalities can provide valuable information during implant placement. Due to the ease of acquisition and high resolution, periapical radiographs are most commonly used. Intraoperative radiographs can be taken during surgery to evaluate proximity to important anatomic structures. Sequential periapical radiographs guide the clinician to visualize changes in direction and depth of the drilling procedure and parallelism to adjacent teeth and other implants (Fig. 58.28). Digital radiographs are particularly advantageous during intraoperative assessment of implant placement; images appear on the screen almost instantaneously and can be manipulated to extract the most pertinent diagnostic information.

Implant osseointegration and the level of peri-implant-alveolar bone are major determinants of implant prognosis. Panoramic and periapical radiographs offer a fast, easy, and low-radiation depiction of the implant and surrounding tissues and aid in assessment of implant success. To obtain an accurate assessment of peri-implant-bone height, the X-ray beam should be directed perpendicular to the implant. In the case of threaded implants, the implant threads should be distinguishable and not overlapping (Fig. 58.29A).

A 1.2-mm marginal bone loss during the first year after implant placement and 0.1 mm/year afterwards are expected; however, further bone loss is considered abnormal. Pathologic bone loss could be localized along the full extent of the implant (peri-implant-bone loss) or around the crestal part of the implant ("saucerization") and could reflect poor osseointegration, peri-implantitis, and/or unfavorable stress distribution (Fig. 58.29B and C).

In select cases, when poor implant placement (Fig. 58.30) or compromise of vital anatomic structures (Fig. 58.31) are suspected, advanced imaging (CBCT, CT, or conventional tomography) provides a 3D evaluation of the oral structures in relation to the implants. Such information can be very important for proper assessment and treatment planning. The treating dentist should recognize relevant signs and symptoms and order appropriate imaging as soon as possible after implant placement. Implant removal, if necessary, would be less complicated before advanced osseointegration.

Conclusion

Many radiographic projections are available for the evaluation of implant placement, each with advantages and disadvantages. The clinician must follow sequential steps in patient evaluation, and radiography is an essential diagnostic tool for implant design and successful treatment of the implant patient. Selection of appropriate radiographic modalities will provide the maximum diagnostic information, help avoid unwanted complications, and maximize treatment outcomes while delivering "as low as reasonably achievable" radiation dose to the patient.

Prosthetic Considerations for Implant Treatment

- **Implant considerations**
- **Abutment/Prosthesis considerations for single units**
- **Management of partially edentulous implant treatment in the esthetic zone**
- **Fully edentulous: prosthetic considerations (e-only)**

Ultimately, successful implant treatment requires a team of clinicians dedicated to excellence in surgical and the prosthetic aspects of the process. This chapter reviews the critical aspects of prosthetic implant treatment proven to maximize long-term functional, biologic, and esthetic success.

Implant Considerations

Understanding the Anticipated Load on the System and Its Relation to Implant Diameter

Selecting the appropriate implants for the partially edentulous patient depends in part on the anticipated loads of that particular tooth location. The larger the anticipated loads, the more robust the implant must be to properly support the prosthesis. Notably, for any given implant design, larger-diameter implants result in stronger prostheses. However, the prosthetic advantages of a larger-diameter implant must be balanced with the surgical needs for sufficient (~1.5 mm) surrounding bone.

The anticipated load on the implant is affected by its position in the arch. The more posterior the implant is in the arch, the higher the anticipated load. However, first molar implant with good second molars will receive significantly less force than that same molar with no other molar support.

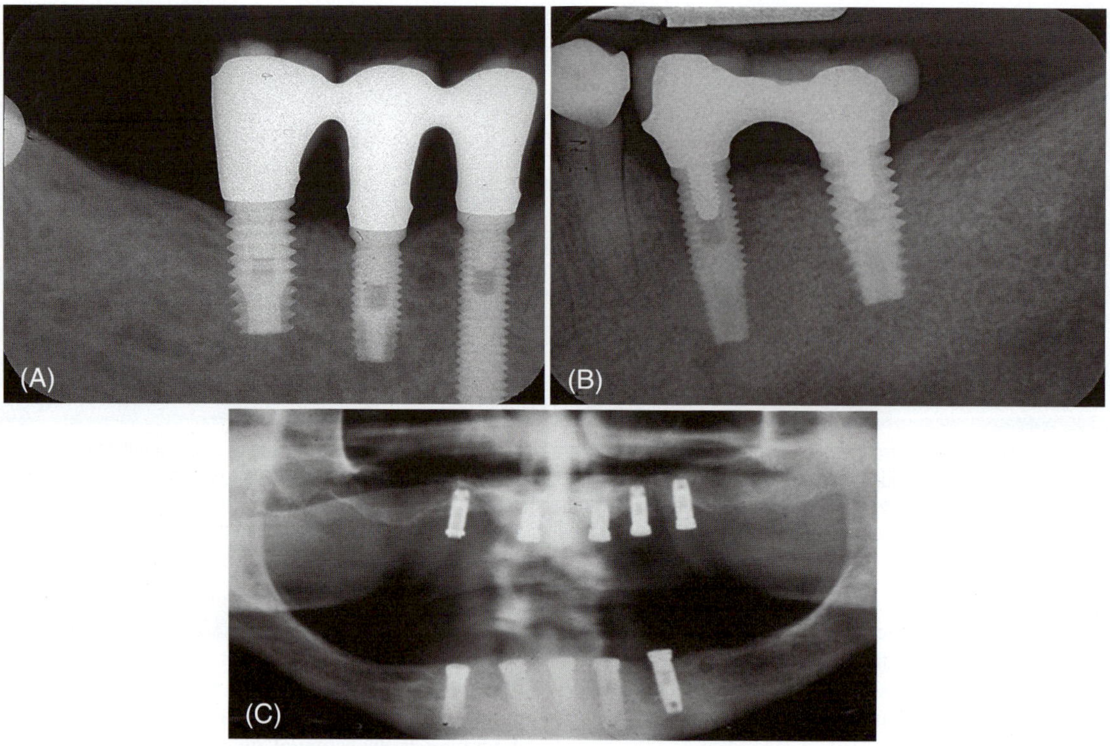

Fig. 58.29 Radiographic follow-up after implant placement in three different patients. A, Periapical radiograph of three implants in the posterior right mandible. "Normal" bone remodeling around anterior two implants and slight horizontal bone loss/remodeling around the molar/posterior implant is present. B, Periapical radiograph of two implants in the left posterior mandible. Severe bone loss (50% of implant length) is seen around anterior implant, while mild bone loss/bone remodeling is observed around posterior implant. A moderate buccal cantilever in the restoration likely contributed to an adverse occlusal load and the resultant bone loss observed in this case. C, Panoramic radiograph of maxillary and mandibular implants in an edentulous patient prior to implant loading. The mandibular implants do not show signs of bone loss and appear to be osseointegrated. All maxillary show signs of moderate-to-severe peri-implant bone loss and the success of osseointegration is questionable.

Often overlooked, the size of the muscles of mastication can provide cursory evidence regarding just how much force a patient is able to produce on his or her dentition. Patients with very large muscles will generate greater forces on their teeth and implants. Patients with a history of cracked or broken teeth and crowns should be expected to place heavier loads on the implants used to replace them.

In the evaluation of the implant patient, special attention should be given to the arch opposing the location of expected implant treatment. If the opposing dentition is a removable appliance, then the implant will receive significantly lower forces. Conversely, if the opposing dentition is implant-supported fixed restorations, the forces are likely to be quite high. This phenomenon is largely due to the lack of a periodontal ligament (PDL) around the implants.

Larger-diameter implants create stronger prosthetics and are less likely to fracture. The use of larger implants becomes more important under the following circumstances: enlarged masseter/temporalis muscles, a history of broken teeth and crowns, distal-most tooth in the arch, opposing other implants, and patients unwilling to wear an occlusal guard. However, the prosthetic advantages of larger platform implants must be balanced with the realities of the surgical site. In locations with space constraints, other prosthetic modalities may be employed to mitigate the anticipated risks.

Number of Implants

Partially edentulous patients with multiple adjacent missing teeth can present some unique challenges. If we use 4 mm as the diameter of a "regular" implant, and the guideline of 1.5 mm of circumferential peri-implant bone, we can quickly estimate the amount of space required for implants by multiplying 7 mm times the number of missing teeth. Or more simply, one tooth requires 7 mm of mesiodistal space; two teeth require 14 mm, three teeth require 21 mm, and so on (Fig. 58.32). This is an oversimplification of the planning process but makes initial estimations of treatment options easier.

When space constraints push the clinician to select smaller and riskier implants, alternative options should be seriously considered: orthodontics, tooth-borne full denture prosthesis (FDPs) (Fig. 58.33), bone augmentation, and additional extractions. Though the last option may sound overly aggressive, it can be the best choice in scenarios where adequate space cannot be created. This most commonly presents as a single missing mandibular incisor. The two missing incisors can then be replaced with a single implant. In this scenario, the implant can be placed centrally between the two missing teeth or off to one side with a larger cantilever (Fig. 58.34). The centrally located implant will reduce the stress due to the decreased length of the cantilever, but the offset implant may allow for the creation of a more natural gingival architecture around the pontic.

Implant-Abutment Connection

Of all the variations in implant designs, perhaps none is as important to prosthetic success as the connection design. The design of an implant abutment junction (IAJ) will influence everything from incidence of screw loosening, to maintenance of the hard and

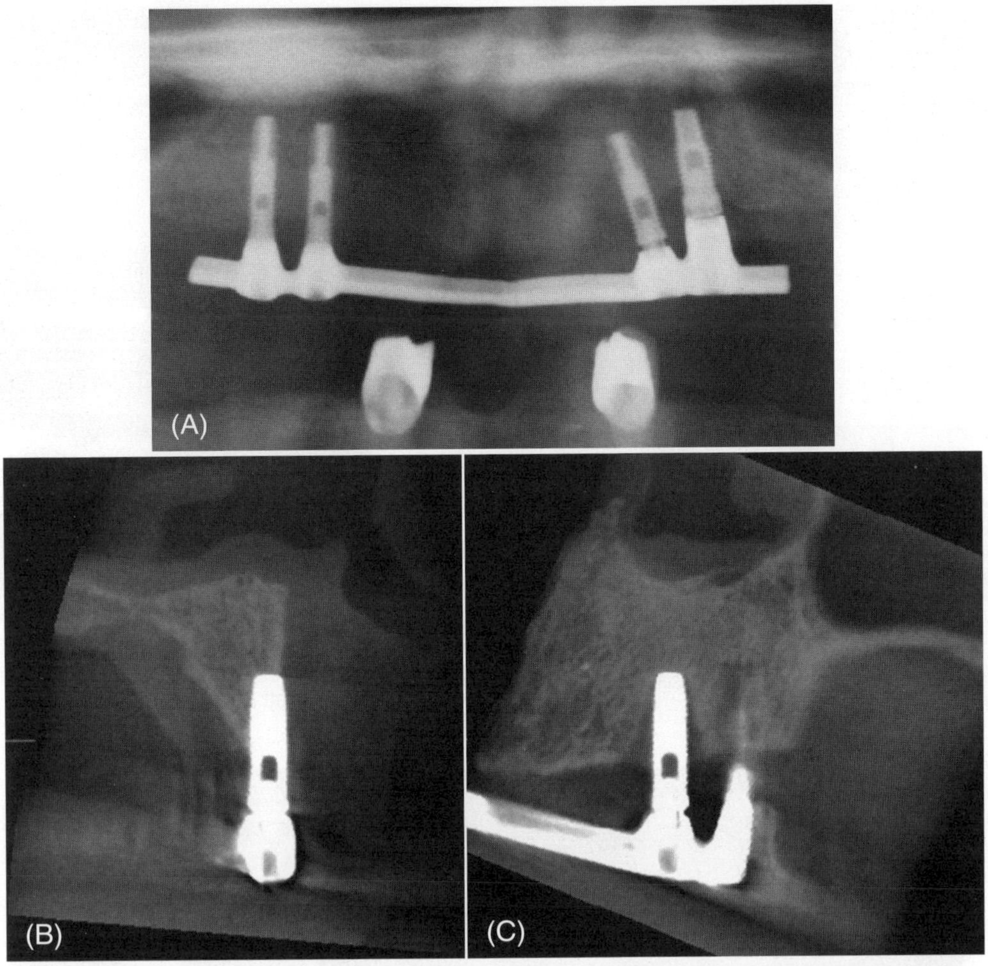

Fig. 58.30 Radiographic follow-up after implant placement. A, Panoramic radiograph suggests mild-to-moderate bone loss around the neck of all implants. This is especially true for the implants in the left maxilla. These implants appear to be angled and the distal implant is positioned more apical. The overdenture bar is not completely seated on the left implants. Note superimposed overlapping anatomic structures in this panoramic radiograph impair the ability to clearly visualize and assess bone loss around implants. B and C, Cross-sectional and sagittal CBCT images of the anterior implant in the left maxilla. Poor implant placement beyond the buccal cortex of the alveolar ridge (cross-section) and peri-implant bone loss (sagittal) are revealed.

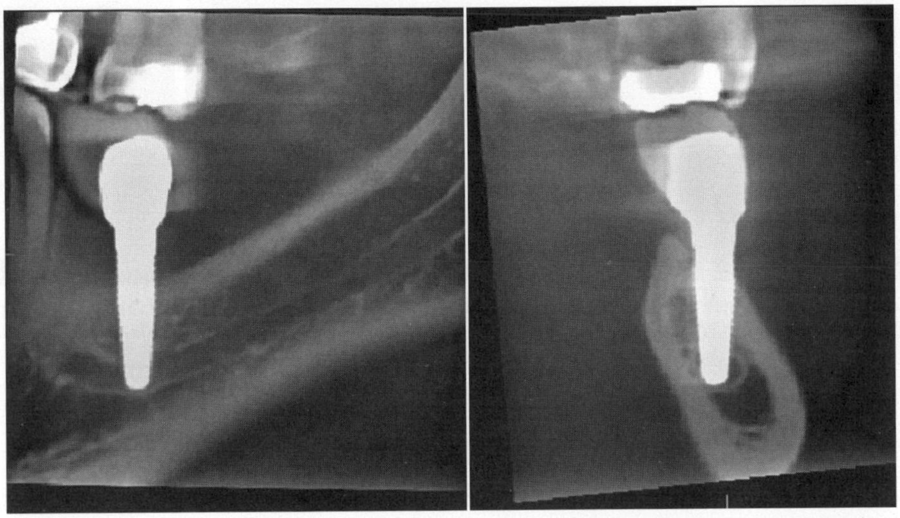

Fig. 58. 31 CBCT sagittal and cross-sectional images clearly demonstrate penetration of the implant into the mandibular canal.

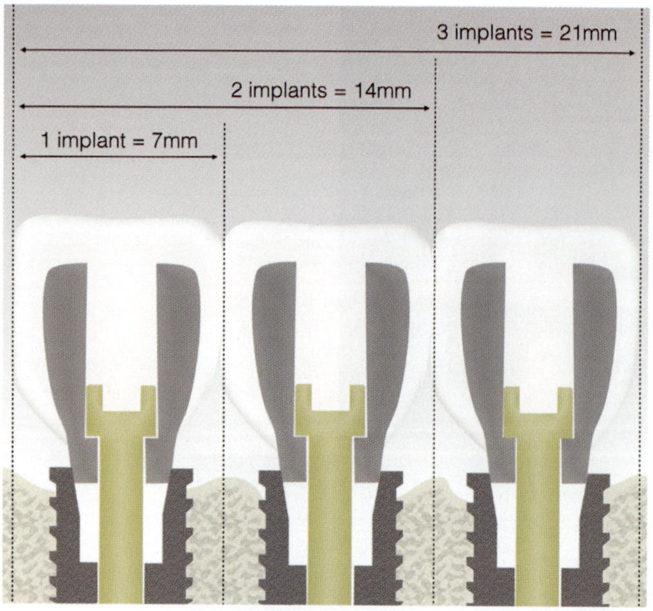

Fig. 58.32 Implants benefit from the presence of 1.5 mm of bone circumferentially. A "normal" diameter implant is ~4 mm. For treatment planning purposes, each implant should have 7 mm of space mesial–distally at the bone crest, two implants would need 14 mm, and so on.

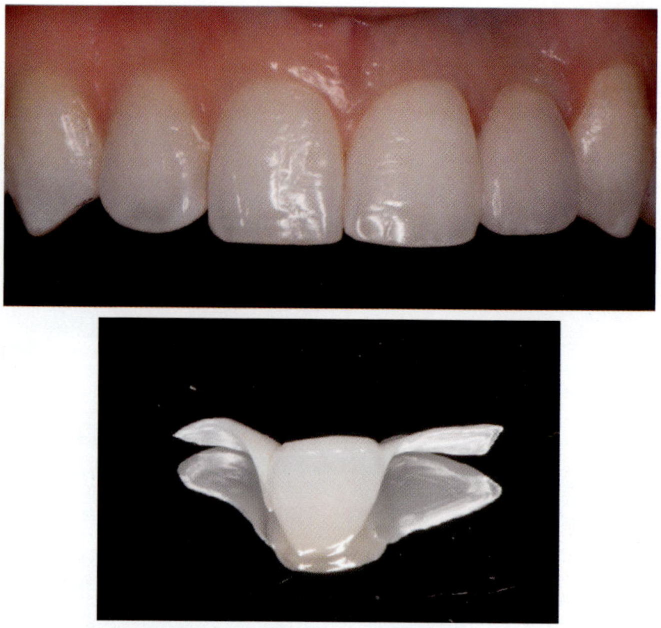

Fig. 58.33 It is important to understand that implants are not the only way to replace missing teeth. In this example, a ceramic Maryland bridge is used to replace the upper left lateral incisor.

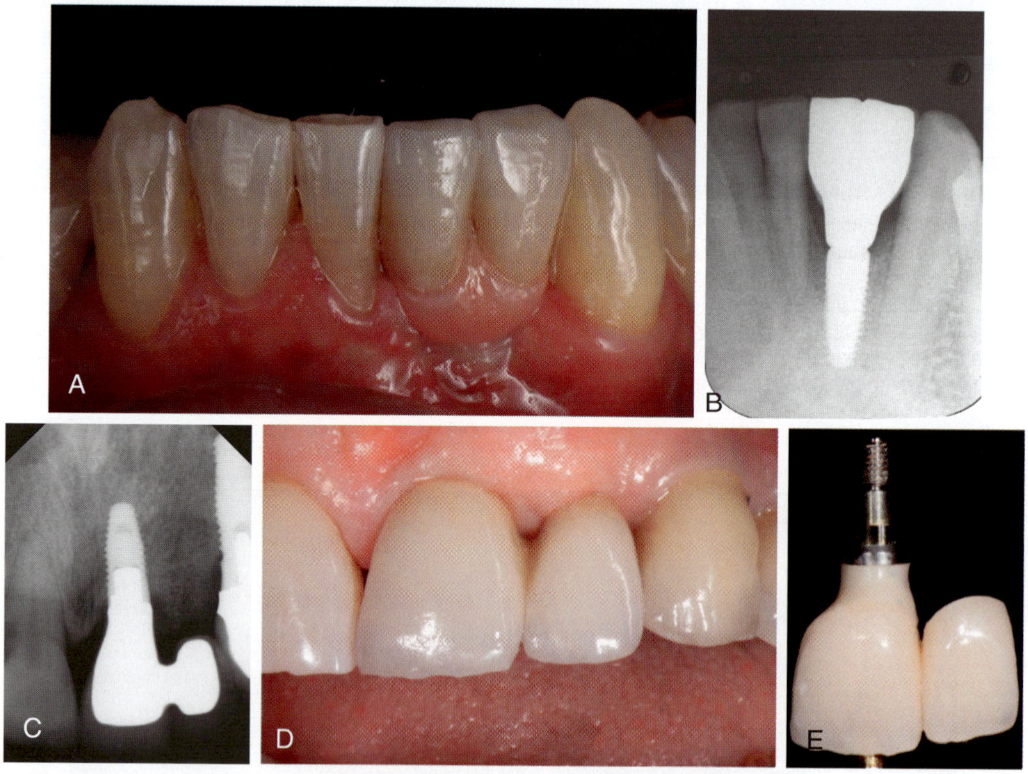

Fig. 58.34 Replacement of two consecutive missing teeth presents a unique challenge. Mesial–distal space requirements often preclude the use of two adjacent implants. The implant can be placed centrally (A–B) or in the position of one of the missing roots (C–E).

soft tissues, to leakage *inside* the implant. The implant(s) should be selected for a particular scenario based on a thorough consideration of the connection that best suits the case. There is no "one size fits all" solution.

Currently available dental implants are classified into three types (Fig. 58.35) based on their abutment connection design: external connection, internal connection, and solid body (the abutment is contiguous with the implant body).

The external connection implant is commonly referred to as an "external hex" implant due to the presence of a raised hexagon connection on most versions of this design. The external connection is one of the older connection designs still in common use today. It

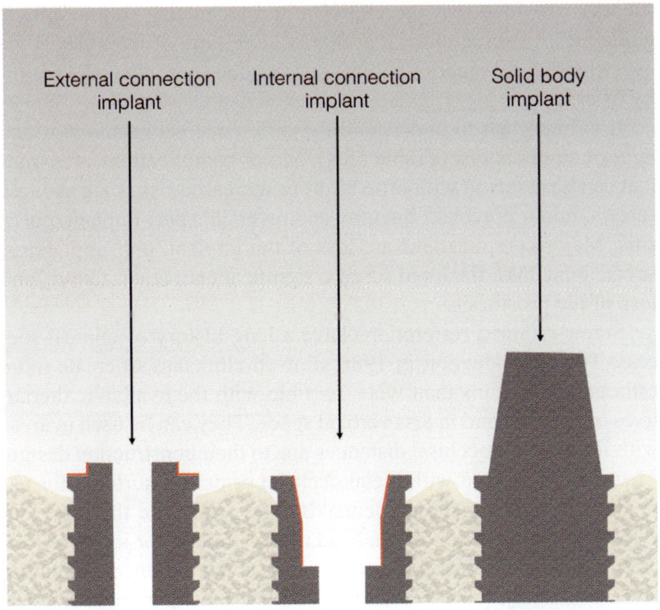

Fig. 58.35 Most currently available implants can be classified as one of three types: external connection, internal connection, or solid body. The external hex connection is primarily indicated for full-arch treatments. The solid body implant must be placed in the ideal position, as there is no way to correct the position with the abutment. The internal connection implant (of which there are many varieties) is indicated for most partially edentulous treatments. Note the abutment engagement areas, as highlighted in *red*.

offers the advantages of an extremely extensive array of prosthetic products to address even the most complicated of clinical presentations. It is a robust implant and rarely suffers from fracture of the implant body itself. This is a well-tested and widely accepted implant design. It is well suited to the restoration of fully edentulous patients desiring a fixed restoration. The wide platform of the implant creates a stable base, whereas the relatively short connection (0.7 mm tall) allows for easy correction of nonparallel implants.

The primary drawback of the external connection implant is screw loosening. The short connection height does little to share the forces between the abutment and the implant body. Even if the hex portion is engaged, there is still very little vertical wall height to transfer the oblique forces of the prosthesis. Inevitably, these forces are transferred largely to the abutment screw, which stretches and deforms under load. Over time, this will result in the need to tighten and replace the screws. This problem is significantly reduced with prostheses supported by multiple implants. It is primarily a problem with single tooth replacements on the external connection implant.

The internal connection (in all its variations) has become the implant of choice for most partially edentulous rehabilitations due to improved reliability compared to the external hex design. For most systems, it is a misnomer to call it an "internal hex." The geometry of the connection itself comes in many variations including hexagons, octagons, 12-pointed stars, trilobes, circles with four flat sides, seven-splines, and others. The number of sides to the connection allows the user various positions from which to orient a stock manufacturer abutment. Some manufacturers prescribe which lobe or point of the implant connection should be oriented buccally to address this. Although more sides on the connection allow for more flexibility in positioning a stock abutment, this does increase the difficulty of correctly aligning a custom abutment.

Many implant systems have begun to incorporate a tapered element into the implant abutment connection. The rationale for incorporating a taper into the connection is to further stabilize the IAJ, thus minimizing leakage, abutment movement, and loosening of screws. This concept comes from the world of machining tools, like lathes and drill presses. For some unknown reason, the dental profession has taken to referring to any tapered connection implant as a "Morse taper," though few implant designs meet the very specific specifications of any Morse taper variation (~1.5-degree taper). "Platform switched" connection term has come to encompass any implant that has an abutment that is narrower than the implant neck. The concept of platform switching has been discussed online.

"Platform Switched" Connection

Regardless, upon fully torquing the abutment screw, implants with a very narrow taper do create a better seal and will have better long-term stability of the abutment and the screw. Both are advantages in terms of maintenance and persevering the peri-implant tissues at a maximum level. Some tapered connection implant systems even require a special tool to remove the abutments, as after screw removal, the components can have such a strong friction fit.

When wide diameter external connection implants were introduced, they remained compatible with the abutments from the narrower implants. Some clinicians and scientists began experimenting with using these narrow abutments on wider implants; they referred to these connections as "platform switched." This term has come to encompass any implant that has an abutment that is narrower than the implant neck (eFig. 58.36). The preponderance of evidence suggests that the platform-shifted design maintains bone at a higher level than that of a nonplatform switched design. The reasons for this effect are less leakage at the IAJ (most are tapered connections), less screw loosening, less stress on the peri-implant bone, and movement of the nonosseointegrating surface of the abutment away from the bone. The latter concept creates a horizontal space on the implant for supracrestal connective tissue to establish a circumferential peri-implant seal, thereby allowing the bone to maintain its position at a higher level without having to remodel to a lower position.

The only potential downside to a platform-switched implant system is that the abutment is narrower and therefore more prone to breakage. Data on this concern are sparse, but it stands to reason that for any material (in particular zirconia), the thinner it is, the more easily it will suffer fracture. Many manufacturers have begun to address this problem by offering their zirconia abutments with a titanium insert that interfaces with the implant body (eFig. 58.37). This has the benefit of placing the more fragile zirconia outside the implant and prevents the possibility of the zirconia wearing the implant connection prematurely.

The last type of implant connection to address is the "solid body" implant, or an implant in which the abutment and the implant are one contiguous piece. Such implants have been available for some time but have never gained significant popularity. The challenge with solid body implants is not surgical, and they may in fact be better for the peri-implant tissues because there is no microgap and no leakage. The problem is prosthetic. For these implants, there is no screw-retained option for the prosthesis, and the cement margin is determined at the time of placement. The abutment can be prepped to move the margin apically if absolutely necessary, but there is no reasonable way to move the margin coronally. This presents a serious problem when the gingiva has any significant papilla adjacent to the implant, as the cement margin that is placed perhaps 1 mm subgingival on the facial aspect may now be 3–7 mm subgingival at the mesial and distal aspect (Fig. 58.38). With no option for a screw-retained restoration, the restoring clinician is now tasked with fully removing cement far too deep subgingival and will inevitably leave cement behind. This residual cement is likely to

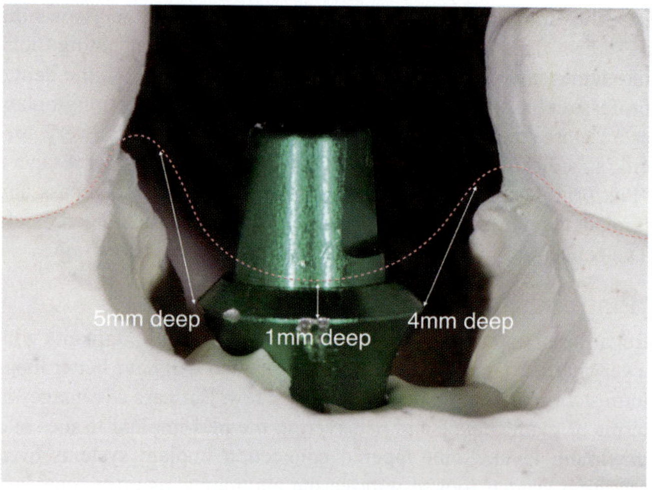

Fig. 58.38 Solid body (and tissue-level) implants present a unique prosthetic challenge due to the margin being on the implant body itself. This often results in mesial and distal margins that are far too deep to reliably remove cement. As such, restorations for tissue-level implants should generally be screw retained. Unfortunately, restorations on solid body implants can only be cemented. Extreme care must be used with solid body implants.

induce inflammatory reactions and loss of bone, soft tissue, and perhaps the implant itself.

Abutment/Prosthesis Considerations for Single Units

Retention method for partially edentulous treatment: cemented prostheses, screw-retained porcelain-fused-to-metal options, screw-retained full contour zirconia, and hybrid designs (e-only)
Abutment material selection (e-only)
Abutment design and emergence profile (e-only)
Covering the screw access (e-only)
Splinting adjacent implants (e-only)

Abutment/Prosthesis Considerations for Single Units

Retention Method for Partially Edentulous Treatment: Cemented Prostheses, Screw-Retained Porcelain-Fused-to-Metal Options, Screw-Retained Full Contour Zirconia, and Hybrid Designs

When treatment planning a partially edentulous case for restoration with an implant, one of the major prosthetic decisions to be made is whether to have a crown that is cemented to an abutment or a crown that is contiguous with the abutment and screwed directly to the implant. For the sake of discussion here, the screw-retained option will be defined as a cast gold alloy abutment with appropriate support of feldspathic porcelain that will be layered directly on it (sometimes referred to as UCLA abutments). Variations of the screw-retained crown will be discussed later. Many clinicians have developed personal preferences for screw or cement-retained crowns based on their experiences and failures. Much of an individual clinician's anecdotal experience likely has much to do with the skill of his or her technician when considering screw-retained Porcelain fused metal crowns (PFMs). Here we will consider the peer-reviewed evidence to determine the evidence-based advantages and disadvantages of each type of retention.

For *most* single tooth replacements, either screw or cement-retained crowns have proven to have very high levels of long-term success, provided that the clinician and technician follow critical guidelines. In some clinical scenarios, one type of retention is the overwhelmingly superior choice, but this does not reflect the majority of cases.

It is important to understand the difference between *major* and *minor* complications (eTable 58.4). Minor complications are issues that can be resolved with little effort or increased risk, such as loose screws, minor porcelain fracture, and reversible peri-implant mucositis. Major complications are loss of the implant, peri-implantitis, severe bone loss, fractured screws, significant porcelain failure, and loss of the prosthesis.

Screw-retained restorations have a long history of clinical success. Their introduction in 1988 allowed clinicians to create more esthetic restorations than were possible with the available alternatives of the time and in less vertical space. They can be used in areas with limited interocclusal distances due to their construction design. They can be created with metal occlusal or palatal surfaces for patients with high functional demands. They can have the porcelain carried to within 1 mm of the head of the implant for improved esthetics. The primary disadvantages of the screw-retained restoration are significantly more prosthetic complications: porcelain fracture (eFig. 58.39), screw loosening, increased bone loss, increased lab costs, and the need for ideal implant angulation. Minor areas of porcelain fracture can be predictably remedied with contouring and polishing. Larger fractures will require replacement of the entire prosthesis, as porcelain cannot be repaired after prolonged exposure to the oral environment. A dedicated technician could strip all the porcelain off the metal framework in an attempt to save the costs of a new abutment and alloy, but it may very well be that the reason for the fracture in the first place was a poorly designed framework. As such, it is advisable to fabricate an entirely new prosthesis should the porcelain fail. Screw loosening has been established repeatedly as significantly more common in screw-retained restorations, in spite of the fact that cemented restorations generally use the same screw and torque specifications. The reason for this phenomenon is not exactly known, though it is likely due to poorly casted abutment interfaces, increased preload due to nonpassive frameworks, the historic use of weaker gold alloy screws, or damage to the interface during divestment (eFig. 58.40) or finishing. Technicians must exercise care when creating a screw-retained restoration to ensure the integrity of the abutment interface. The UCLA abutment should have a machined interface made by the manufacturer to ensure the integrity of the fit between the abutment and the implant. Because the screw access channel must exit the crown, this option is best reserved for when the implant angulation exits directly through the occlusal surface in posterior regions and through the palatal/lingual surface in the anterior regions.

The common alternative to the screw-retained crown is the cement-retained crown. This system is made up of an abutment (titanium, gold alloy, or zirconia) that is screwed into the implant and a crown that will be cemented to the abutment. The cement-retained crown allows the restoration of implants that are not placed ideally without having to manage a screw access channel exiting through a crucial esthetic or functional area. This situation is most common in the esthetic zone. When implants are placed angled such that and their line of draw exits through the facial surface of the crown, it becomes esthetically prohibitive to use a "normal" screw-retained crown (eFig. 58.41). There are some workarounds that will be discussed briefly later.

Some clinicians prefer cement-retained restorations because the cementation process is familiar and comfortable. However, the cementation process is not to be taken lightly, as residual cement is one of the major causes (but not the only cause) of peri-implantitis.

Cementation details will be discussed later, but note that no attempt should be made to cement an implant crown when margins are more than 1 mm subgingival (eFig. 58.42). Cement-retained implant crowns have the main advantage of being far more durable than the screw-retained alternative, a fact confirmed in multiple reviews. Porcelain failure of screw-retained crowns has been reported to be as high as 38%, compared to just 4% for cement-retained crowns at an average of 5 years. For this reason cement-retained implant crowns are indicated in scenarios of higher loads (i.e., molars, patients with enlarged masseters). Should the patient break the cemented crown, retrieval of the remaining abutment is greatly simplified. Drilling through even an intact cemented crown to access the screw channel is a relatively simple matter, akin to endodontic access. Lastly, there is the issue of lab cost. The cemented restorations typically lead to far less expensive lab bills compared to the screw-retained PFM options, though the cost of the latter varies significantly with the market price for gold alloy.

One of the reasons cited for selecting a screw-retained restoration is the ease of retrievability. There is a valid concern that should something fail, the cemented crown is more difficult to remove. Although it may seem obvious, removal of the cemented crown is hardly more difficult than for a screw-retained crown (eFig. 58.43). The differences are drilling the access through porcelain or metal instead of composite and the location of access may be difficult to discern. Most clinicians are fairly adept at cutting through porcelain, but locating the access channel can be a slight challenge. Most often, the access is fairly easy to locate based off simple radiographs. More sophisticated approaches to recording the location of the access have been proposed, from stents, to guides, to occlusal markings (eFig. 58.44). During the era of weaker abutment screws and external connection implants, screw loosening was a common problem. As such, replacement of the screws was a common maintenance requirement and a screw-retained restoration was ideal. Modern implant connections rarely suffer from loose screws, even for single-unit implants.

There are a few other crown retention variations that should be mentioned. One is the full-contour zirconia, screw-retained crown. This crown is similar in design to the cast gold, screw-retained crown, but it has no feldspathic layering porcelain, and the substructure is zirconia. Though relatively new to market, these restorations may prove to maintain many of the advantages of the screw-retained system while eliminating its major complication—porcelain fracture. Not all manufacturers offer this restoration, and some variants do not offer a titanium insert to protect the implant from wear and zirconia failure. The titanium insert should be used whenever possible. Some manufacturers offer this restoration with a screw channel that can be angled up to 25 degrees to allow for screw-retained restorations even when the implant is not in the long access of the crown. The screw-retained zirconia option is relatively new and not fully tested in clinical trials. Implement with caution.

Another option is the hybrid crown (sometimes referred to as a screwmentable crown). This system consists of a crown that is cemented to a stock titanium abutment (eFig. 58.45), but the cementation is performed in the laboratory where excess cement can be easily removed. The screw access is predrilled into the crown. This system offers the advantages of minimal risk of retained cement, minimal risk of porcelain fracture when stronger ceramics are used, and a lower lab cost than cast gold alloys. This system is relatively new and not fully tested; in clinical trials, implement with caution.

Lastly, there is the option of lingual set screws. This system is most commonly employed in the anterior areas of the mouth when the implants are angled too far toward the facial for a traditional screw-retained restoration and the clinician is uncomfortable with a cemented option. The challenges with lingual set screws are increased lab costs, difficulty in locating technicians competent in the technique, leakage between the crown and the abutment, and challenging screw access.

Abutment Material Selection

In most bone-level implant designs, the junction between the abutment and the implant is near the crestal bone. In this area, the connective tissue and the junctional epithelium may be in intimate contact with the abutment. As such, the abutment material and accuracy of the fit play a critical role in preserving the peri-implant bone and soft tissue. Some abutments better preserve the peri-implant tissues than others. The most relevant options for currently available definitive abutment materials are titanium, titanium with a titanium nitride coating, full-contour zirconia, zirconia with a titanium base, and gold alloy (eFig. 58.46). Other less common options include lithium disilicate and chrome-cobalt alloys.

The most rigorous study examining bone and soft tissue reactions to abutment materials found histologic evidence that titanium preserved 1.5 mm more soft tissue and 1 mm more bone compared to the fully cast gold alloy abutment. However, it should be noted that this study was performed in the canine mandible and that when a titanium interface was used in conjunction with a cast gold abutment, there was less bone loss than with the gold alone. It stands to reason that some of the bone and soft tissue loss with gold abutments may have more to do with the less accurate fit of a cast restoration than to the influence of the material itself. More recent clinical studies and reviews have questioned these findings, with gold and titanium showing an equivalent biologic response. However, the latter were done with radiographic analysis rather than the histologic measurements of the former. As a whole, the data are not yet conclusive on the biocompatibility of the abutment material and its clinical effects on the tissues. Titanium has been repeatedly shown to perform better on a histologic level than gold alloys, but the difference may be of little clinical significance. What is clear is that the interface between the abutment and the implant must be as accurate as possible. This will ensure minimal leakage, minimal screw loosening, and better maintenance of the peri-implant tissues. Abutments that require casting of the implant interface portion cannot match the fit accuracy of the machined interface.

The strength of the abutment is critical in maintaining long-term success with minimal technical complications. Titanium and gold alloy abutments have a long track record of outstanding strength. Some studies have even shown failure of the implant before failure of the titanium abutment. The primary concern regarding strength is related to zirconia abutments.

Zirconia abutments can be used with little risk of fracture in many clinical scenarios, but there are a few caveats. The zirconia abutment should have an implant interface component made of titanium (eFig. 58.47). This minimizes the risk of wear to the implant body, and should the zirconia fracture, it is outside the implant where it is much easier to treat. The zirconia abutment should not be used in cases with extreme loads (i.e., molars, patients with enlarged muscles of mastication, long span FDPs). The zirconia abutments should be made by a reputable manufacturer. Evidence has shown that the manufacturer can have a huge impact on the strength of the material. The abutment walls should be sufficiently thick, no less than 0.7 mm. Every effort should be made to avoid cutting the zirconia after it has been sintered.

Lastly, we must consider the effect of the abutment material on the color of the soft tissue. Gray-colored metallic abutments will darken the tissue more than zirconia abutments, but the effect is not as great as might be expected. Zirconia abutments still cause a significant and perceptible darkening of the soft tissue, confirmed in multiple studies. Some manufacturers and clinicians have developed techniques to anodize or coat titanium abutments to create gold or pink shades. These may offer some improvement of soft tissue esthetics. The gold-colored abutments (eFig. 59.48) allow predictable use of semitranslucent ceramics with minimal shade change. The thickness of the overlying tissue has been shown to have a greater influence on the perceived color of the gingiva over an implant than the material used. Thick tissues have an almost nonperceptible color shift, whereas with thin tissues, the shift is always perceptible, even with zirconia abutments.

Abutment Design and Emergence Profile

The design and contours of the abutment play a key role in the shape and dimensions of the peri-implant tissues. If the abutment is overcontoured, it will ultimately lead to a loss of bone and soft tissue. This is a common problem when technicians design and shape the abutment without the soft tissue mask on the model. Such overcontoured abutments may require surgery to deliver because the tissue prevents complete seating of the restoration. Alternatively, the restoration can be reshaped to reduce or eliminate impingement on tissues.

The emergence profile of the abutment is the area of the abutment between the head of the implant and the soft tissue margins. More data are showing that undercontouring the emergence profile helps to protect and maintain the peri-implant bone and soft tissue. The "platform switch" style implant helps to create the narrowed abutment design due to the smaller diameter of the connection interface. In most scenarios, the abutment should be designed to emerge from the implant in a narrowed hourglass shape. The narrowed design may allow for increased blood flow around the implant and provide sufficient room for the soft tissues without bone remodeling.

Understanding the effects the emergence profile has on the shape and position of the soft tissue is critical for implant treatment in the esthetic zone. By selectively over- or undercontouring the emergence zone, the soft tissue can be positioned with a high degree of accuracy. More on this technique will be described in the next section with the use of esthetic zone provisional restoration.

For cement restorations, arguably the most critical aspect of the abutment design is the placement of the margins. The peri-implant soft tissue is never perfectly flat, and as such custom abutments are almost universally indicated to avoid deep subgingival margins with the risk of retained cement and the resulting peri-implantitis. The only way for a stock abutment to be used with minimal risk is to select one with completely supragingival margins, but this can be esthetically unacceptable. If a common stock abutment is selected to hide the titanium, with a facial margin 1 mm subgingival, in most scenarios, the margin at the mesial and distal papilla will be 4 mm or more subgingival. Both in vitro and in vivo studies have shown that for margins beyond 1 mm subgingival, significant amounts of cement will always be left behind. No attempt should ever be made to cement restorations on implants with margins more than 1 mm subgingival (eFig. 58.49). A custom abutment can be easily designed to address the natural scalloping of the gingiva. It is fabricated by milling or casting, though casting of custom abutments for cement-retained crowns is no longer the best option due to increased costs, increased screw loosening, and the less accurate fit at the implant.

Milled custom abutments can be made out of titanium or zirconia. When prescribing these abutments, it is critical to communicate to the technician where the margins should be placed. If left unstated, many technicians will opt to place them deep subgingivally. Several studies have clearly shown that cement cannot be predictably removed at depths greater than 1 mm subgingival. If the margins are any deeper than 1 mm, significant amounts of cement will be left behind and will likely start the process of peri-implantitis (eFig. 58.50). It is common for clinicians and technicians to place the margins deeper than 1 mm subginival in esthetic cases in an attempt to hide the titanium abutment if recession should occur. This strategy is unwise and will inevitably result in retained cement. The correct approach is to shape the tissue with a provisional, allow it to mature, and place the margin no deeper than 1 mm. The abutment could also be made of zirconia and stained to resemble the root surface. Clinicians should be aware of the significant strength variations in zirconia abutments based on the manufacturer.

Covering the Screw Access

After placement and proper torquing of the abutment screw, there is the need to cover the screw access channel. The ideal material for this is one that does not inhibit future access to the abutment screw and provides a seal to inhibit leakage into the abutment. Traditionally, this has been done with a cotton pellet, a technique adapted from the temporary procedure used in endodontics. However, unlike a root canal temporary, the screw cover in an implant abutment will be left in place for many years.

The challenge in implants is that the internal aspect of the implant and the abutment are hollow, body temperature, dark, and oxygen free. Upon functioning, the abutment will move slightly in the implant, and the fluids and bacteria from the oral environment will fill this hollow chamber. Ultimately, proliferation of certain bacterial strains inside the implant may play a role in the presence of peri-implantitis. Obviously, placing a cotton pellet into this environment for any extended period of time is a poor idea. It provides no seal and is an ideal environment for the proliferation of pathogenic bacteria (i.e., *Parvimonas micra*) (eFig. 58.51).

Reasonable and tested alternatives include gutta-percha, polytetrafluoroethylene (PTFE) tape (also known as Teflon or "plumber's" tape), and polyvinyl siloxane (PVS) impression material. Gutta-percha has been shown to provide a good seal but can be challenging to remove without the use of an endodontic heat instrument. PTFE tape and PVS look to be reasonable alternatives, but further testing is needed to determine their long-term success and clinical effects. To use PTFE tape, a long portion (~10 cm) is sterilized then rolled up and condensed into the screw access (eFig. 58.52). Alternatively, light body PVS impression material can be injected into the screw access (eFig. 58.53). With either technique, 3–4 mm of space must be left coronally in screw-retained restorations to allow space for a robust composite seal. For cement-retained restorations, either material can be placed to the top of the abutment screw. It is advisable to clean the screw access beforehand with a strong chlorhexidine solution (eFig. 58.54) and dry thoroughly.

Splinting Adjacent Implants

The rational for splinting adjacent implants (eFig. 58.55) stems from various finite element analysis (FEA) and photo-elastic gel (PEG) experiments. These in vitro studies repeatedly confirm that multiple implants produce less acute forces in the peri-implant bone when splinted compared to multiple individual restorations. However, we do not have a clear notion of how much stress is acceptable for the peri-implant bone and at what threshold we might expect pathologic bone loss. The clinician must consider the length and diameter of the implants as well as the quality and quantity of the bone when determining if multiple implants should be splinted together.

Splinted restorations are advisable when the foundation is compromised (i.e., short or narrow implants, compromised bone). This will allow the stronger or better supported implants to "assist" the others. The compromise here is that if the weaker implant fails, an entirely new prosthesis may need to be fabricated, usually at a significant expense.

The rationale for splinting adjacent implants involves the intention of "sharing the forces," a concept derived from the in vitro studies of the early 2000s cited earlier. The implication is that clinically we would see fewer implant failures and less bone loss over extended use with splinted restorations. Long-term in vivo randomized controlled trials (RCTs) have tested this hypothesis in order to quantify the differences in bone loss and implant failure with splinted versus nonsplinted restorations. In the partially edentulous RCT, at 10 years, the mean difference in bone loss between splinted and nonsplinted restorations for 132 implants was a mere 0.1 mm. This could hardly be considered clinically significant under most scenarios. In the fully edentulous study with two mandibular implants retaining a full denture, the differences at 3 years were statistically insignificant at most sites and only about 0.5 mm at the most significantly different sites. A prospective split mouth, in vivo trial examining bone levels around splinted and nonsplinted restorations showed no significant difference at 36 months. Until better evidence shows otherwise, "sharing forces" in an attempt to reduce bone loss is not a proper consideration for whether or not adjacent implants should be splinted. These data are not necessarily in conflict with the early in vitro experiments, they simply illustrate that higher forces do not necessarily result in more bone loss and that it is difficult to extrapolate data from FEAs and PEGs to clinical realities. Depending on the type of bone and implant, there is likely a threshold below which increased forces will not result in significant bone loss over extended use. Conversely, despite the lack of significance found in these studies, there may be scenarios in which clinical judgment warrants splinting adjacent implants such as multiple implants placed in the posterior maxilla in type IV bone opposing an intact natural dentition or implants.

The downside to splinted restorations is largely related to long-term repair and replacement costs. With patients having implants that must maintain a prosthesis for 30, 40, or 50 years, it is appropriate to consider that the prosthesis will require replacement throughout its life. Most commonly, this is related to porcelain failure on screw-retained PFM FDPs. After a PFM restoration has been in the mouth for any significant period of time, porcelain failure cannot simply be repaired. The restoration must be fully stripped or replaced. Practically speaking, it can be a challenge to find a laboratory willing and able to strip and restack porcelain, and most will opt for complete replacement of the prosthesis. Essentially this has doubled, tripled, or quadrupled the cost of replacement. If an individual unit suffers the same complication, only the unit affected needs to be replaced. Issues related to patient autonomy and desires need to be considered in the replacement of multiple adjacent missing teeth. Some patients may tolerate splinted restorations, whereas others may desire individual units. Oral hygiene techniques and ease of cleansibility will vary between restoration types as well.

Indications for splinting adjacent implants include significant off-axis forces (i.e., canine replacement), multiple adjacent external hex implants, poor bone, and diminutive implants.

Management of Partially Edentulous Implant Treatment in the Esthetic Zone

Diagnosis and treatment planning
Implant-retained provisional restorations (e-only)
Tissue shaping and management
Customized impression copings (e-only)

Diagnosis and Treatment Planning

Treatment of the partially edentulous patient in the esthetic zone is one of the more challenging prosthetic scenarios. The "esthetic zone" is not simply canine to canine in the maxilla. Each patient must be individually evaluated for lip position and movement (Fig. 58.56) to determine the appropriate level of esthetic consideration necessary.

The primary challenge in this treatment is the peri-implant soft tissues. If patients show soft tissue during lip movement, then particular attention should be paid to the creation and preservation of natural appearing gingiva. First, there must be sufficient thickness of the gingiva. Thin tissue biotypes are more prone to recession, peri-implant mucositis, papilla loss, and graying. The surgical team may need to employ various techniques prior to, or at the time of, implant placement to increase the tissue thickness.

During the treatment planning phase, the clinical team should consider the shape and position of the soft tissue on all teeth or implants in the area. If any of these positions are planning to be modified, the corresponding implant position may change as well.

Management of potential changes to the tissue color can be challenging, as there is a shift in the gingiva around implants to a gray tone. This can be somewhat managed with the use of UCLA or zirconia abutments, though research has clearly shown that there can still be a perceptible color shift with these more esthetic materials (delta E >3.9). Though zirconia abutments are weaker than titanium, they have shown comparable survival rates for single units in vivo. Some technicians have begun experimenting with the use of fluorescing glazes over the emergence zone of zirconia abutments to decrease the color shift. Some manufacturers and clinicians have coated the titanium abutments with a gold or pink color, again in an attempt to mitigate color changes.

The greatest challenge of implants in the esthetic zone is papilla management. Implants, even with contemporary designs (i.e., platform switch, conical connections), cannot maintain crestal bone height as much as a healthy tooth. The implant is very different than the natural tooth because it does not have periodontal ligament (and its blood supply) or supracrestal inserting connective tissue fibers. The clinical appearance (i.e., height and fullness) of the papilla between an implant and a tooth ultimately depends on the periodontal attachment level of the adjacent tooth and not the level of bone adjacent to the implant. Should the papilla fail to meet desires and expectations, the open gingival embrasure is generally best managed through additional surgery or closing the space with restorations. Although there have been good attempts to solve the problem of deficient papilla with pink prosthetics, it is all but impossible to resolve it in a manner that is both esthetically convincing and hygienic in the partially edentulous patient.

Although there will be variations in papilla height adjacent to or between implants, the average papilla height adjacent to a single implant is 4.2 mm. Between adjacent, unrestored natural teeth, the average papilla height is at least 5 mm. Between adjacent (external hex) implants, the average papilla is only 3.4 mm (Table 58.5).

The preceding figures are averages and do not represent the actual value for what is possible for any given patient. The key to predictable, successful treatment in the esthetic zone is the implant-retained provisional restoration. This will allow the clinical team and the patient to truly test the four key criteria of esthetics, phonetics, function, and hygiene. Revisions and alterations are much easier to accomplish with provisionals as compared to the definitive prosthesis.

Implant-Retained Provisional Restorations

The implant-retained provisional restoration is a critical tool in the treatment of partially edentulous patients. It can be fabricated in the

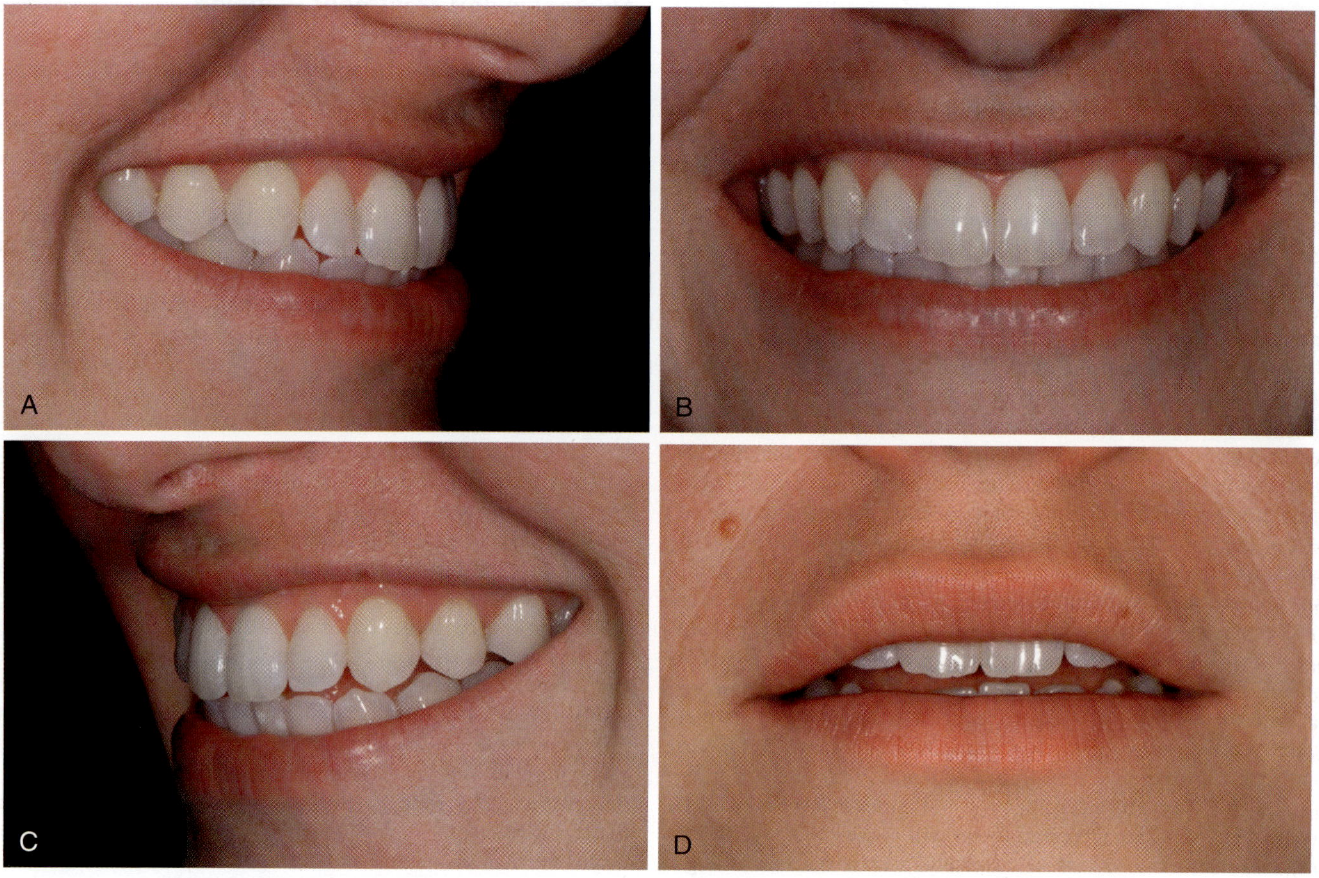

Fig. 58.56 Implant treatment in the esthetic zone is more challenging than in the functional zone. It is important to keep in mind that the esthetic zone differs for each patient. It should be evaluated though a series of basic photos: right, center, and left at maximum smile (A–C), and with lips at rest (D). In this patient, the esthetic zone clearly includes the anterior teeth and all premolars.

TABLE 58.5 Anticipated Papilla Height

	Between Natural Teeth	Between Tooth and Implant	Between Adjacent Implants
Average expected papilla height (from crest of bone)	≥5 mm (Tarnow, 1992)	4.2 mm (Kan, 2003)	3.4 mm (Tarnow, 2003)

laboratory or directly in the mouth (eTable 58.6). As stated previously, the provisional restoration allows the clinical team and the patient to determine if the proposed treatment will meet expectations. Regardless of the definitive restoration design, the implant provisional should be screw retained because the use of cement should be avoided in fresh surgical sites, and the ability to remove, modify, and replace the restoration is essential. The emergence zone of the provisional must be smooth and well-polished. The apical most 2 mm of the provisional should be clean titanium (not polyether ether ketone [PEEK], composite, or acrylic) (eFig. 58.57) due to its well-proven effects on the soft tissues and minimal risk of breakage.

The main advantage of the implant-retained provisional restoration is its use in *preserving* and supporting the peri-implant tissue contours. This scenario presents itself when an implant is placed and restored with the provisional immediately at the time of extraction—a technique commonly called "immediate provisionalization" or "immediate loading." Immediate loading requires sufficient stability of the implant, the ability to keep the restoration out of occlusion/excursion, stable maximum intercuspal position (MIP), and patient cooperation. There appears to be little change in implant failure when these criteria are carefully followed. The main advantage of immediate loading is the preservation of the papilla and decreased bone loss. It is much easier to preserve papilla than to regenerate.

At the time of implant placement, the provisional should be designed with the goals of protecting the surgical site and maximizing the potential volume of the peri-implant tissues. To accomplish these goals, it should have a smooth, titanium emergence that is no wider than the implant itself. This will help to promote blood supply to the area and any graft that may have been placed. It should not blanch the tissue or compress the papilla at this stage. It should emerge from the implant narrow and gradually transition to the contour of the crown near the gingival margin. Should the implants be angled to the facial, a screw-retained provisional can still be predictably used.

To fabricate the restoration, the following items are needed (eFig. 58.58):

- Titanium provisional abutment (not PEEK)
- Abutment screw
- Crown form (composite, natural tooth, or crown)

Prior to the appointment, the titanium abutment should be sandblasted with 50 micron aluminum oxide, covered with an appropriate opaquing resin (generally A1), and polymerized.

Some titanium temporary abutments are incorrectly designed with a flared portion directly exiting from the junction with the implant. This puts unnecessary pressure on the per-implant tissues and will force the peri-implant bone to remodel to a more apical position. This area of the abutment can and should be removed prior to the procedure (eFig. 58.59).

The crown form can be fabricated from composite resin in the laboratory on a model. Alternatively, the patient's existing natural tooth or current crown may be used. Material-specific bonding procedures should be implemented to ensure adhesion. Acrylic materials could be used as well, but delivery and manipulation can be difficult in the surgical environment.

Following the placement and stability check of the implant, the provisional abutment is attached, checked for full seating, and hand tightened. The crown form is then adjusted to fit over or around the provisional abutment (eFig. 58.60). If the angulation is through the facial, the abutment itself must be marked, removed, cut, and repositioned. It is critical that the crown form easily fits into the exact desired position over or around the abutment. Both the crown and the abutment are cleaned, bonding agent applied, and both are lined with flowable composite (eFig. 58.61). The crown is then positioned and the composite polymerized. Upon removal, there will be sharp, unfilled, and undercut areas (eFig. 58.62). The provisional is thoroughly cleaned and fresh bonding agent applied. Composite is then used to fill and shape the emergence area (eFig. 58.63). It should now be placed back onto the implant to ensure there is no blanching and that there is some degree of open gingival embrasures to allow for swelling and papilla migration (eFig. 58.64). The provisional should be removed, polished, and carefully examined. At this stage, the surgeon may opt to complete the grafting procedure, prior to delivery of the provisional. It should be checked to ensure that there is absolutely no contact in MIP or throughout the excursive movements (eFig. 58.65).

Tissue Shaping and Management

Following integration of the implant and maturation of the soft tissue, there may be the need to correct slight malpositions of the peri-implant tissues. This can be done through modification of the implant abutment, but it should not be done repeatedly to avoid increased tissue changes that lead to bone loss. Significant deficiencies of tissue may be difficult to correct, whereas others may be able to be addressed with additional surgery.

The emergence profile of the provisional restoration can be added to or contoured back to manipulate the soft tissue position. Applying additional contour will move the gingiva apically, whereas undercontouring will allow the tissue to drape more coronally. The abutment can also be modified to apply pressure to the base of the papilla, thus forcing the tip coronally, but this technique should be used with caution around implants due to a diminished blood supply and fragility of the soft tissue. The clinician should minimize the number of reattachments to the head of the implant, as this will weaken the integrity of the tissues and create additional bone loss.

Ideally all contours of the soft tissues should be designed in the patient's mouth, and the four keys (esthetics, phonetics, function, and hygiene) should be tested and approved. If done correctly, the transition from the patient to the technician is seamless with the provisional serving as a blueprint for the definitive prosthesis.

Fully edentulous: prosthetic considerations are discussed online under the following subheads:

- *Edentulous maxilla (e-only)*
- *Edentulous mandible (e-only)*

Customized Impression Copings

To ensure that the technician is fabricating the definitive abutment and crown on a model that *exactly* replicates the current patient condition, a customized impression coping should be used (eTables 58.7 and 58.8). The customized impression coping replicates or preserves the existing tissue contours in the final impression. Without the use of a custom impression coping, the soft tissue will collapse and deform during the impression, leaving the technician guessing about where to put margins or how to shape the emergence zone.

Fully Edentulous: Prosthetic Considerations

Edentulous Maxilla

Prosthetic options for the patient with an edentulous maxilla include a conventional complete denture, an implant-assisted denture, or an implant-supported fixed prosthesis. However, a conventional complete denture does not provide the comfort and quality of life that many patients desire. An implant-assisted or implant-supported prosthesis can provide stability, retention, and comfort and can restore the patient's confidence, especially in patients with one or more of the following conditions:

1. *Poor ridge form with a marginally stable conventional maxillary denture.* Two or four implants provide greater stability and security of a maxillary denture in function when the maxillary ridge is severely resorbed and lacks resistance to lateral forces.
2. *Lack of posterior support with an intact mandibular anterior dentition.* Implants in the maxilla can offset the potentially destructive effects on the premaxillary region when a mandible with natural anterior teeth and missing posterior teeth opposes an edentulous maxilla. In this situation, the lack of posterior support leads to a condition often referred to as *combination syndrome*, in which overclosure of the jaws with mandibular anterior teeth causes destruction of the edentulous anterior maxilla.
3. *Palatal coverage is not tolerated.* Some patients prefer a palateless denture, which may enhance their sensations of taste and texture or may simply provide a psychological advantage. Some patients prefer a palateless denture because the proximity of the denture with the soft palate induces a gag reflex. Patients with large palatal tori can also benefit from a palateless maxillary denture. A minimum of four implants with adequate anterior-posterior (A-P) spread allows the fabrication of an implant-assisted overdenture without palatal coverage.
4. *High functional expectations and strong preference on fixed prosthodontic tooth replacement treatment option.* Patients with a failing natural dentition, especially those who have never used a removable prosthesis, often strongly prefer the implant-supported fixed prosthesis treatment modality to meet their specific expectations and to allow a smoother transition. With modern rough surface implants and computer-aided design/computer-assisted manufacture (CAD/CAM) technology, immediate restoration of function and esthetics with implant-supported fixed prostheses offers great benefits and patient satisfaction in carefully selected cases.

The design of a maxillary implant-retained prosthesis is greatly influenced by the anatomy of the maxilla. Most notably, the maxillary sinus limits the height of bone available for implant placement in the posterior region. As a result, implant placement is confined to the anterior region, and the A-P spread that can be achieved is often limited (eFig. 58.66). If the A-P spread is inadequate to provide support, a full-palatal-coverage overlay denture is recommended.

Most edentulous patients are best served with an implant-assisted overlay denture. Lower cost, improved hygiene access, better lip support, and predictable speech articulation are additional benefits that favor the use of an overlay denture in the edentulous maxilla over an implant-supported fixed prosthesis. The four-implant–assisted, palateless overlay denture ideally addresses the needs of most patients (eFig. 58.67). Many patients who are edentulous in the maxilla have lost a significant amount of structure in the premaxillary region resulting in a lack of support for the upper lip. An implant-assisted maxillary overdenture is preferred over an implant-supported fixed prosthesis for this patient population because the labial flange can provide the needed lip support to optimize the esthetic outcomes. The usual resorption pattern of the alveolus places the gingival margin of a fixed restoration too far superiorly, too far palatally, or both. Even if the patient has a low enough smile line to hide the appearance of long crowns and deficient soft tissue height, a lack of lip support just beneath the nose can be unsightly with fixed prostheses.

For patients who prefer an implant-supported fixed prosthesis (and do not require additional lip support), six or more implants arranged in an appropriate arc of curvature with at least 2 cm of A-P spread are required (see eFig. 59.66). In this situation, the fixed prosthesis can be fabricated with distal extension cantilevers up to half the A-P spread, provided it does not exceed 10 mm.

Transition from terminal dentition to complete edentulism always presents the biggest challenge for patients with failing remaining teeth. In the past, many patients were reluctant and unable to benefit from the dental implants due to multiple surgeries, lengthy treatment time, and the psychological fears of losing all their natural teeth and getting used to an immediate removable prosthesis. However, advances in modern implant designs, implant surfaces, and CAD/CAM technology have broadened the implant applications due to high primary stability, precision planning, and optimal implant placement. Emerging evidence showed high patient-reported satisfaction and a comparable implant success rate of immediate implant placement and immediate loading compared to the delayed loading protocols. With careful patient selection and appropriate training, the experienced clinician can shorten the treatment time, provide immediate restoration of function and esthetics, and mitigate the psychological impact of complete edentulism with immediate loading of implant-supported fixed prostheses (eFig. 58.68A and B).

That being stated, caution should be exercised in choosing immediate treatment until methods have proven successful, especially in the maxillary arch. Parel and Phillips identified several common primary factors in maxillary implant failure scenarios based on a retrospective study of the all-on-four implant concept. They found the number of maxillary implant failures was about five to six times the number of failed mandibular implants. Through this process of patient profiling, they concluded that opposing natural dentition, male gender, lack of bone density, the distal implant site, and parafunctional habits were sufficiently frequent occurrences in failure situations to suggest that either the use of additional implants or delayed loading and the provision of a complete denture as an interim prosthesis may be more appropriate in the management of patients identified as being high risk. Secondary factors such as bone availability (volume) and smoking were less common in failure situations. These factors, when considered and evaluated presurgically, can be helpful in treatment planning with regard to the appropriate number of implants necessary and the possible loading sequence for optimal integration and prosthesis success.

The use of CAD/CAM technologies for digital workflow from the virtual implant treatment planning, image-guided implant surgery, to the manufacturing prosthetic frameworks on dental implants is noticeably increasing. While embracing the exciting technology advancement in implant dentistry, clinicians must be mindful of the limitations, and the overall possible accuracy of the CAD/CAM technology depends on the accuracy of the individual steps of the production process. Flügge and colleagues showed that the registration accuracy in commercial virtual implant planning software is significantly influenced by the preprocessing of imported data, by the user, and by the number of restorations resulting in clinically nonacceptable deviations encoded in image-guided implant surgery drilling guides. This study emphasized that the automatic segmentation in the implant planning software was significantly less accurate compared to the manual segmentation by the users, especially in patients with multiple preexisting dental restorations.

Edentulous Mandible

Similar to the edentulous maxilla, prosthetic options for patients with an edentulous mandible include a conventional complete denture, an implant-assisted denture, or an implant-supported prosthesis. A mandibular complete denture is more problematic for patients than a maxillary complete denture, especially for patients with a severely resorbed (atrophic) mandibular ridge. The lack of stability and retention makes it challenging for patients to control the denture. The addition of implants offers unprecedented control (i.e., stability and retention) for a complete, removable prosthesis.

Implant-assisted overlay dentures are designed so that most of the masticatory load is borne by the primary denture-support areas (i.e., retromolar pad, buccal shelf). A common practice is to place two implants in the anterior mandible with a connecting bar. One or two clips retain the denture to the bar (eFig. 58.69). When occlusal forces are applied, the denture rotates around the bar (anterior axis of rotation) and depresses slightly in the posterior aspect, directing the forces to the primary denture-bearing areas (eFig. 58.70). The implants provide stability and retention while bearing minimal stress from occlusal loads. Individual attachments secured to each implant can also offer a simple prosthetic alternative (eFig. 58.71) to the bar and clip design. However, it is more critical for implants with individual attachments to be parallel to one another to facilitate a proper path of insertion and to minimize stress during prosthetic seating and function.

For patients who prefer an implant-supported fixed prosthesis, four, five, or six implants arranged in an appropriate arc of curvature with at least 1 cm of A-P spread are required (see eFig. 59.66). In this situation, the fixed prosthesis can be fabricated with distal extension cantilevers up to twice the A-P spread (eFig. 58.72).

Many patients prefer a fixed option for psychological reasons, but the mastication efficiency provided by a fixed versus removable prosthesis does not appear to be significant. Evidence suggests that such fixed restorations tend to stop the resorption of the body of the posterior mandible and, in some cases, enable regeneration of the bone in this region.

Conclusion

Successful implant treatment requires a team of clinicians and technicians dedicated to excellence in surgical and prosthetic aspects. A thorough understanding of the prosthodontic restoration of implants from implant-abutment connections to hard and soft tissue interfaces and compatibility with the implant/abutment/restoration is essential. This chapter reviewed the critical aspects of prosthetic implant treatment proven to maximize long-term functional, biologic, and esthetic success.

Key points

- It is desired to maintain at least 1.0–1.5 mm of bone around all surfaces of the implant after preparation and placement.
- Assuming an implant is 4 mm in diameter and 10 mm long, the minimal width of the jawbone needs to be 6–7 mm, and the minimal height should be 10 mm (minimum of 12 mm in the posterior mandible where an additional margin of safety is required over the mandibular nerve).
- The minimal mesial–distal space for an implant placed between two teeth should be 7 mm.
- The minimal mesial–distal space required for the placement of two standard-diameter implants (4-mm diameter) between teeth is 14 mm.
- Whenever the available space between teeth is greater than 7 mm and less than 14 mm, only one implant, such as placement of a wide-diameter implant, should be considered. Two narrow-diameter implants could be positioned in a space that is 12 mm.
- The minimum amount of interocclusal space required for the restorative "stack" on an external hex-type implant is 7 mm.
- Anatomic structures pertinent to treatment planning of the implant patient in maxilla are maxillary sinus (floor and anterior wall), nasal cavity (floor and lateral wall), incisive foramen, canine fossa, and canalis sinuosus.
- Anatomic structures pertinent to treatment planning of the implant patient in mandible are mandibular canal, anterior loop of the mandibular canal, anterior extension of the mandibular canal, mental foramen, submandibular fossa, retromolar canal, and lingual inclination of the alveolar ridge.

Suggested Readings

Angelopoulos C, Aghaloo T: Imaging technology in implant diagnosis, *Dent Clin North Am* 55 (1): 141–158, 2011.

Baxter JC, Fattore L: Osteoporosis and osseointegration of implants, *J Prosthodont* 2: 120–125, 1993.

Beikler T, Flemmig TF: Implants in the medically compromised patient, *Crit Rev Oral Biol Med* 14: 305–316, 2003.

Benson BW, Shetty V: Dental Implants. In White SC, Pharoah MJ, editors: *Oral radiology: principles and interpretation*, ed 6, St. Louis, 2009, Mosby.

Brånemark PI, Hansson BO, Adell R, et al: Osseointegrated implants in the treatment of the edentulous jaw. Experience from a 10-year period, *Scand J Plast Reconstr Surg Suppl* 16: 1–132, 1977.

Brunski JB, Puleo DA, Nanci A: Biomaterials and biomechanics of oral and maxillofacial implants: current status and future developments, *Int J Oral Maxillofac Implants* 15: 15–46, 2000.

DeBruyn H, Collaert B: The effect of smoking on early implant failure, *Clin Oral Implants Res* 5: 260, 1994.

Eckert SE, Meraw SJ, Cal E, et al: Analysis of incidence and associated factors with fractured implants: a retrospective study, *Int J Oral Maxillofac Implants* 15: 662–667, 2000.

Esposito M, Hirsch JM, Lekholm U, et al: Biological factors contributing to failures of osseointegrated oral implants. (I). Success criteria and epidemiology, *Eur J Oral Sci* 106: 527–551, 1998a.

Esposito M, Hirsch JM, Lekholm U, et al: Biological factors contributing to failures of osseointegrated oral implants. (II). Etiopathogenesis, *Eur J Oral Sci* 106: 721–764, 1998b.

Fiorellini JP, Chen PK, Nevins M, et al: A retrospective study of dental implants in diabetic patients, *Int J Periodontics Restorative Dent* 20: 366–373, 2000.

Hagi D, Deporter DA, Pilliar RM, et al: A targeted review of study outcomes with short (< or = 7 mm) endosseous dental implants placed in partially edentulous patients, *J Periodontol* 75: 798–804, 2004.

Hatcher DC, Dial C, Mayorga C: Cone beam CT for pre-surgical assessment of implant sites, *J Calif Dent Assoc* 31: 824, 2003.

Iplikcioglu H, Akca K: Comparative evaluation of the effect of diameter, length and number of implants supporting three-unit fixed partial prostheses on stress distribution in the bone, *J Dent* 30: 41–46, 2002.

Klokkevold PR, Han TJ: How do smoking, diabetes, and periodontitis affect outcomes of implant treatment? *Int J Oral Maxillofac Implants* 22 (Suppl): 173–202, 2007.

Lang NP, Pjetursson BE, Tan K, et al: A systematic review of the survival and complication rates of fixed partial dentures (FPDs) after an observation period of at least 5 years. II. Combined tooth–implant-supported FPDs, *Clin Oral Implants Res* 15: 643–653, 2004.

Marx RE, Sawatari Y, Fortin M, et al: Bisphosphonate-induced exposed bone (osteonecrosis/osteopetrosis) of the jaws: risk factors, recognition, prevention, and treatment, *J Oral Maxillofac Surg* 63: 1567–1575, 2005.

Pjetursson BE, Tan K, Lang NP, et al: A systematic review of the survival and complication rates of fixed partial dentures (FPDs) after an observation period of at least 5 years, *Clin Oral Implants Res* 15: 667–676, 2004.

Sahin S, Cehreli MC, Yalin E: The influence of functional forces on the biomechanics of implant-supported prosthesis–a review, *J Dent* 30 (7–8): 271–282, 2002.

Tyndall DA, Price JB, Tetradis S, et al: Position statement of the American Academy of Oral and Maxillofacial Radiology on selection criteria for the use of radiology in dental implantology with emphasis on cone beam computed tomography, *Oral Surg Oral Med Oral Pathol Oral Radiol* 113 (6): 817, 2012.

Wennstrom JL, Bengazi F, Lekholm U: The influence of the masticatory mucosa on the peri-implant soft tissue condition, *Clin Oral Implants Res* 5: 1–8, 1994.

White SC, Mallya SM: Update on the biological effects of ionizing radiation, relative dose factors and radiation hygiene, *Aust Dent J* 57 (Suppl 1): 2, 2012.

References

References and MCQs with answers for the chapter are available on www.medenact.com.

CHAPTER 59

Surgical Concepts of Implant Therapy

PR Klokkevold | IA Urban | DL Cochran | TJ Han | K-B Park | DA Shanelec | LS Tibbetts | T Vercellotti | DH Etienne | RR Derycke | A Jain | G Vercellotti

CHAPTER OUTLINE

The surgical procedures for the placement of nearly all endosseous dental implants currently used are based on the original work of Professor Per-Ingvar Brånemark and coworkers in Sweden in the 1960s and 1970s. Their landmark research evaluated the biologic, physiologic, and mechanical aspects of the titanium screw-shaped implant, subsequently known commercially as the Nobelpharma "Brånemark" implant system and currently manufactured by Nobel Biocare. The original Brånemark implant was a parallel-walled, cylindrically shaped, threaded implant with an external hex connection and a machined surface. In the past few decades, many different designs of root form implants have been developed, modified, and studied. The same fundamental principles of atraumatic, precise implant site preparation applies to all implant systems. In brief, this includes a gentle surgical technique and progressive, incremental preparation of the bone for a precise fit of the implant at the time of placement.

This chapter outlines the basic surgical procedures for the placement of endosseous dental implants using either one-stage or two-stage protocols. The principles described here are intentionally generic and designed to serve as guidelines and to be applicable to most of the common implant systems. Each implant system is designed with specific armamentarium and recommendations for use (e.g., drilling speeds), and it is advisable to follow the detailed protocols provided by the manufacturer.

General Principles of Implant Surgery

Patient Preparation

Most implant surgical procedures can be done in the office using local anesthesia. Conscious sedation (oral or intravenous) may be indicated for some patients. The risks and benefits of implant surgery specific to the patient's situation and needs should be thoroughly explained prior to surgery. A written, informed consent should be obtained for the procedure.

Implant Site Preparation

Some basic principles must be followed to achieve osseointegration with a high degree of predictability (Box 59.1). The surgical site should be kept aseptic, and the patient should be appropriately prepared and draped for an intraoral surgical procedure. Prerinsing with chlorhexidine gluconate for 1–2 min immediately before the procedure will aid in reducing the bacterial load present around the surgical site. Every effort should be made to maintain a sterile surgical field and to avoid contamination of the implant surface. Implant sites should be prepared using gentle, atraumatic surgical techniques with an effort to avoid overheating the bone.

When these clinical guidelines are followed, successful osseointegration occurs predictably for submerged and nonsubmerged dental implants. Well-controlled studies of patients with good plaque control and appropriate occlusal forces have demonstrated that root form, endosseous dental implants show little change in bone height around the implant over years of function. After initial bone remodeling in the first year (1.0–1.5 mm of resorption described as "normal remodeling around an externally hexed implant"), the bone level around healthy functioning implants remains stable for many years. The average annual crestal bone loss after the first year in function is expected to be 0.1 mm or less. Hence, implants offer a predictable solution for tooth replacement.

Regardless of the surgical approach, the implant must be placed in healthy bone with good primary stability to achieve osseointegration, and an atraumatic technique must be followed to avoid damage to bone. Drilling of the bone without adequate cooling generates excessive heat, which injures bone and increases the risk of failure. The anatomic features of bone quality (dense compact vs loose

BOX 59.1 Basic Principles of Implant Therapy to Achieve Osseointegration

1. Implants must be sterile and made of a biocompatible material (e.g., titanium).
2. Implant site preparation should be performed under sterile conditions.
3. Implant site preparation should be completed with an atraumatic surgical technique that avoids overheating of the bone during preparation of the recipient site.
4. Implants should be placed with good initial stability.
5. Implants should be allowed to heal without loading or micromovement (i.e., undisturbed healing period to allow for osseointegration) for 2–4 or 4–6 months, depending on the bone density, bone maturation, and implant stability.

trabecular) at the recipient site influence the interface between bone and implant. Compact bone offers a much greater surface area for bone-to-implant contact than cancellous bone. Areas of the jaw exhibiting thin layers of cortical bone and large cancellous spaces, such as the posterior maxilla, have lower success rates than areas of dense bone. The best results are achieved when the bone-to-implant contact is intimate at the time of implant placement.

One-Stage Versus Two-Stage Implant Placement Surgery

Currently, most threaded endosseous implants can be placed using either a one-stage (nonsubmerged) or a two-stage (submerged) protocol. In the one-stage approach, the implant or the abutment emerges through the mucoperiosteum/gingival tissue at the time of implant placement, whereas in the two-stage approach, the top of the implant and cover screw are completely covered with the flap closure (Fig. 59.1). Implants are allowed to heal, without loading or micromovement, for a period of time to allow for osseointegration. In two-stage implant surgery, the implant must be surgically exposed following a healing period. Some implants are specifically designed with the coronal portion of the implant positioned above the crest of bone and extending through the gingival tissues at the time of placement in a one-stage protocol (Fig. 59.1A). Other implant systems are designed to be placed at the level of bone and require a healing abutment to be attached to the implant at the time of placement to be used in a one-stage approach (Fig. 59.1B).

A one-stage surgical approach simplifies the procedure because a second-stage exposure surgery is not necessary. The two-stage, submerged approach is advantageous for situations that require simultaneous bone augmentation procedures at the time of implant placement because membranes can be submerged, which will minimize postoperative exposure. Mucogingival tissues can be augmented if desired at the second-stage surgery in a two-stage protocol or as part of the one-stage protocol. Fundamental differences in flap management for these two surgical techniques are described separately.

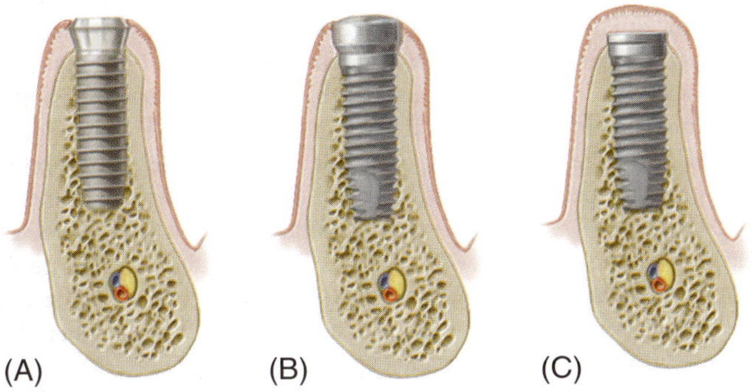

Fig. 59.1 One-stage implant versus two-stage implant surgeries. A, One-stage surgery with the implant designed so that the coronal portion of the implant extends through the gingiva. B, One-stage surgery with implant designed to be used for two-stage surgery. A healing abutment is connected to the implant during the first-stage surgery. C, In the two-stage surgery, top of the implant is completely submerged under gingiva.

Two-Stage "Submerged" Implant Placement

In the two-stage implant surgical approach, the first-stage or implant placement surgery ends by suturing the soft tissues together over the implant cover screw so that it remains submerged and isolated from the oral cavity. In areas with dense cortical bone and good initial implant support, the implants are left to heal undisturbed for a period of 2–4 months, whereas in areas of loose trabecular bone, grafted sites, and sites with lesser implant stability, implants may be allowed to heal for periods of 4–6 months or more. Longer healing periods are indicated for implants in sites with less bone support. During healing, osteoblasts migrate to the surface and form bone adjacent to the implant (osseointegration). Shorter healing periods are indicated for implants placed in good quality (dense) bone and for implants with an altered surface microtopography (e.g., acid etched, blasted, or etched and blasted). Readers are referred to online material and other resources for more information about implant surface microtopography.

In the second-stage (exposure) surgery, the implant is uncovered and a healing abutment is connected to allow emergence of the abutment through the soft tissues. Once healed, the restorative dentist then proceeds with the prosthodontic aspects of the implant therapy (impressions and fabrication of prosthesis).

The following paragraphs describe the steps for osteotomy preparation and the first-stage implant placement surgery of the two-stage protocol. Figs. 59.2 and 59.3 illustrate the procedures via diagrams, and Fig. 59.4 depicts the procedures with clinical photographs.

Flap Design, Incisions, and Elevation

Flap management for implant surgery varies slightly, depending on the location and objective of the planned surgery. There are different incision/flap designs but the most common is the crestal flap design. The incision is made along the crest of the ridge, bisecting the existing zone of keratinized mucosa (Figs. 59.2A and 59.4B).

A remote incision with a layered suturing technique may be used to minimize the incidence of bone graft exposure when extensive bone augmentation is planned. The crestal incision, however, is preferred in most cases because closure is easier to manage and typically results in less bleeding, less edema, and faster healing.

A full-thickness flap is raised (buccal and lingual) up to or slightly beyond the level of the mucogingival junction, exposing the alveolar ridge of the implant surgical sites (Figs. 59.2B and 59.4C). Elevated flaps may be sutured to the buccal mucosa or the opposing teeth to keep the surgical site open during the surgery. The bone at the implant site(s) must be thoroughly debrided of all granulation tissue.

For a "knife-edge" alveolar process with sufficient alveolar bone height and distance from vital structures (e.g., inferior alveolar nerve), a large round bur is used to recontour or flatten the bone to provide a wider, level surface for the implant site preparation (Fig. 59.2B). However, if the vertical height of the alveolar bone is limited (e.g., $<$10 mm), the knife-edge alveolar bone height should be preserved. Bone augmentation procedures can be used to increase the ridge width while preserving alveolar bone height.

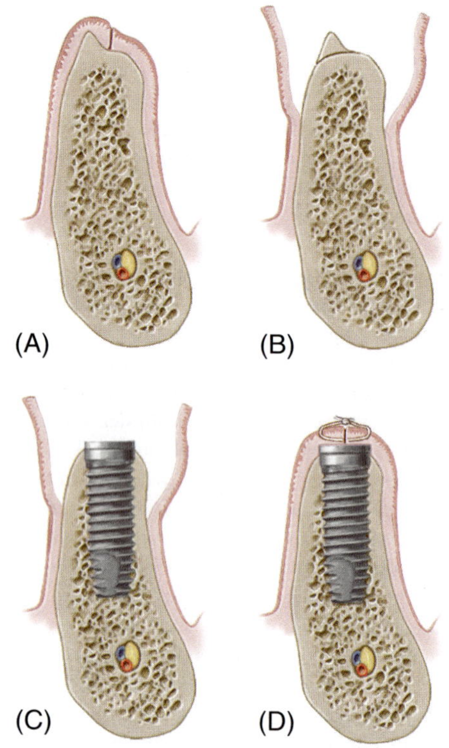

Fig. 59.2 Tissue management for a two-stage implant placement. A, Crestal incision made along the crest of the ridge, bisecting the existing zone of keratinized mucosa. B, Full-thickness flap is raised buccally and lingually to the level of the mucogingival junction. A narrow, sharp ridge can be surgically reduced/contoured to provide a reasonably flat bed for the implant. C, Implant is placed in the prepared osteotomy site. D, Tissue approximation to achieve primary flap closure without tension.

Implant Site Preparation

Once the flaps are reflected and the bone is prepared (i.e., all granulation tissue removed and knife-edge ridges flattened), the implant osteotomy site can be prepared. A series of drills are used to prepare the osteotomy site precisely and incrementally for an implant (Fig. 59.5). A surgical guide or stent is inserted, checked for proper positioning, and used throughout the procedure to direct the proper implant placement (Fig. 59.4E).

Round Bur

A small round bur (or spiral drill) is used to make the initial penetration into bone for the implant site(s). The surgical guide is removed, and the initial marks are checked for their appropriate buccal-lingual and mesial-distal location, as well as the positions relative to each other and adjacent teeth. Slight modifications may be necessary to adjust spatial relationships and to avoid minor ridge defects. Any changes should be compared to the prosthetically driven surgical guide positions. Each marked site is then prepared to a depth of 1–2 mm with a round drill, breaking through the cortical bone and creating a starting point for the 2-mm twist drill (Fig. 59.3A).

The 2-mm Twist Drill

A small twist drill, usually 2 mm in diameter and marked to indicate various lengths (i.e., corresponding to the implant sizes), is used next to establish the depth and align the long axis of the implant recipient site (Fig. 59.3B). This drill may be externally or internally irrigated. In either case, the twist drill is used at a speed of approximately 800–1500 rpm, with copious irrigation to prevent overheating of the bone. Additionally, drills should be intermittently and repeatedly "pumped" or pulled out of the osteotomy site while drilling to expose them to the water coolant and to facilitate clearing bone debris from the cutting surfaces. In other words, clinicians should pump the drill (up and down) intermittently and avoid using a constant "push" of the drill in the apical direction only.

When multiple implants are being placed next to one another, a guide pin should be placed in the prepared sites to check alignment, parallelism, and proper prosthetic spacing throughout the preparation process (Fig. 59.3C). The relationship to neighboring vital structures (e.g., nerve and tooth roots) can be determined by taking a periapical radiograph with a guide pin(s) or radiographic marker(s) in the osteotomy site(s). Implants should be positioned with approximately 3 mm between one another to ensure sufficient space for interimplant bone and soft-tissue health and to facilitate oral hygiene procedures. Therefore, the initial marks should be separated by at least 7 mm (center to center) for 4 mm standard-diameter implants. Incrementally more space is needed for wide-diameter implants.

The 2-mm twist drill is used to establish the final depth of the osteotomy site corresponding to the length of each planned implant. The clinician should also evaluate the bone quality (density) with this drill while preparing the osteotomy to assess the need for modification of subsequent drills used (Box 59.2). If the vertical height of the bone was reduced during the initial ridge preparation, this must be taken into account when preparing the site for a predetermined implant length. For example, if it appears that the implant will be too close to a vital structure, such as the inferior alveolar nerve canal, the depth of the implant osteotomy site, and length of the implant may need to be reduced.

The next step is to use a series of drills to incrementally increase the width of the osteotomy site to accommodate the planned implant diameter. The styles, shapes, and final diameter of the drills will differ slightly among different implant systems, but their general purpose is to prepare a recipient site with a precise diameter (and depth) for the selected implant without unduly traumatizing the surrounding bone. It is important to use copious irrigation and a "pumping" action for all drilling.

Pilot Drill

Following the 2-mm twist drill, a pilot drill with a noncutting 2-mm diameter "guide" at the apical end and a cutting 3-mm diameter (wider) midsection is used to enlarge the osteotomy site at the coronal end, thus facilitating the insertion of the subsequent drill in the sequence (Fig. 59.3D).

The 3-mm Twist Drill

The final drill in the osteotomy site preparation for a standard-diameter (4.0 mm) implant is the 3-mm twist drill. It is the last drill used to widen the site along the entire depth of the osteotomy from the previous diameter (2 mm) to final diameter (3 mm). This final drill in the sequence finishes preparing the osteotomy site and consequently is the step that dictates whether the implant will be stable or not (Fig. 59.3E). It is critically important that the final diameter drilling be accomplished with a steady hand, without wobbling or changing direction so that the site is not overprepared. Finally, depending on bone density, the diameter of this final drill may be slightly increased or decreased to enhance implant support (Box 59.2).

Countersink Drill (Optional)

When it is desirable to place the cover screw at or slightly below the crestal bone, countersink drilling is used to shape or flare the crestal aspect of the osteotomy site allowing the coronal flare of the implant head and cover screw to fit within the osteotomy site (Fig. 59.3F). As

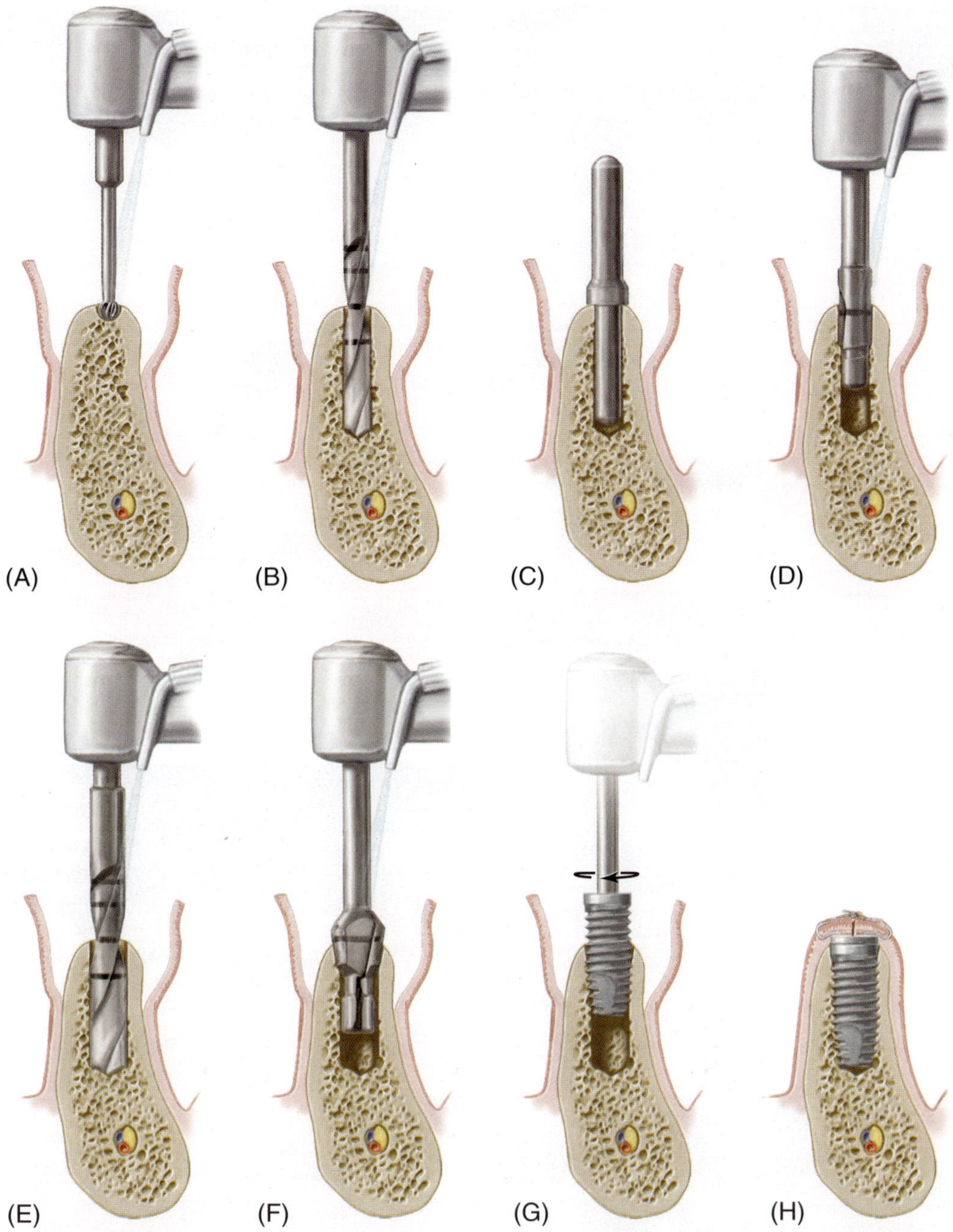

Fig. 59.3 Implant site preparation (osteotomy) for a 4.0-mm diameter, 10-mm length screw-type, threaded (external hex) implant in a subcrestal position. A, Initial marking or preparation of the implant site with a round bur. B, Use of a 2-mm twist drill to establish depth and align the implant. C, Guide pin is placed in the osteotomy site to confirm position and angulation. D, Pilot drill is used to increase the diameter of the coronal aspect of the osteotomy site. E, Final drill used is the 3-mm twist drill to finish preparation of the osteotomy site. F, Countersink drill is used to widen the entrance of the recipient site and allow for the subcrestal placement of the implant collar and cover screw. *Note:* An optional tap (not shown) can be used following this step to create screw threads in areas of dense bone. G, Implant is inserted into the prepared osteotomy site with a handpiece or handheld driver. *Note:* In systems that use an implant mount, it would be removed prior to placement of the cover screw. H, Cover screw is placed and soft tissues are closed and sutured.

with all drills in the sequence, copious irrigation and gentle surgical techniques are used.

Bone Tap (Optional)

As the final step in preparing the osteotomy site in dense cortical bone, a tapping procedure may be necessary (not shown). With self-tapping implants being almost universal, there is less need for a tapping procedure in most sites. However, in dense cortical bone or when placing longer implants into moderately dense bone, it is prudent to tap the bone (create threads in the osteotomy site) before implant placement to facilitate implant insertion and to reduce the risk of implant binding (Fig. 59.3G).

When faced with a very soft, poor-quality bone (e.g., loose trabecular bone in the posterior maxilla), tapping is not necessary or

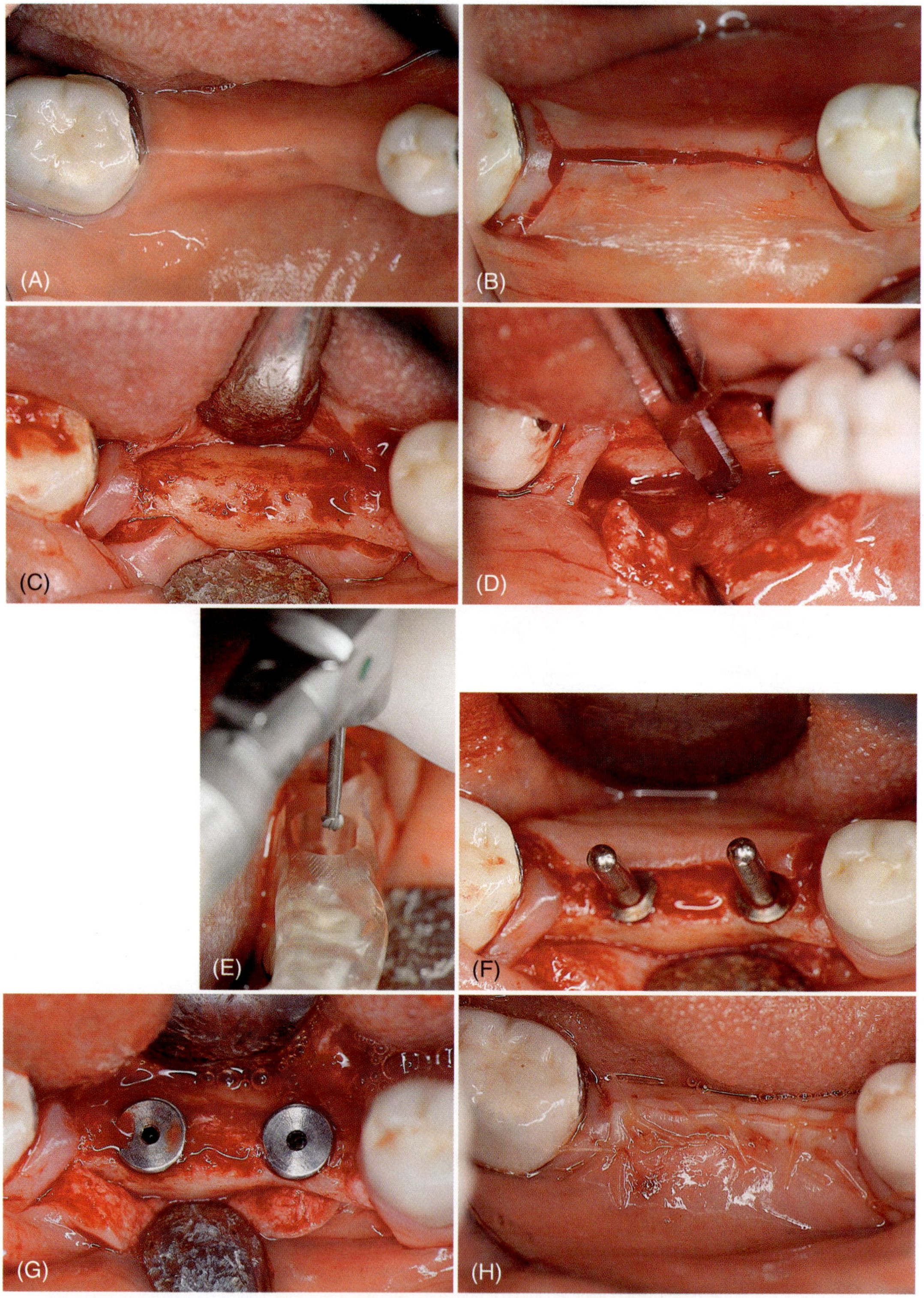

Fig. 59.4 Clinical view of stage one implant placement surgery. A, Partial edentulous ridge; presurgical and prosthodontic treatment has been completed. B, Mesial sulcular and distal vertical incisions are connected by a crestal incision. Notice that bands of gingival collars remain adjacent to the distal molar tooth. C, Minimal flap reflection is used to expose the alveolar bone. Sometimes a ridge modification is necessary to provide a flap recipient bed. D, Buccal flap is partially dissected at the apical portion to provide a flap extension. This is a critical step to ensure a tension-free closure of the flap after implant placement. E, It is important to use the surgical stent to determine the mesial-distal and buccal-lingual dimensions and proper angulation of the implant placement. F, Frequent use of the guide pins ensures parallelism of the implant placement. G, After placement of two Nobelpharma implants, the cover screws are placed. The cover screws should be flushed with the rest of the ridge to minimize the chance of exposure. This is especially important if the patient will wear a partial denture during the healing phase. H, Suturing completed. Both regular interrupted and inverted mattress sutures are used intermittently to ensure tension-free, tight closure of the flaps.

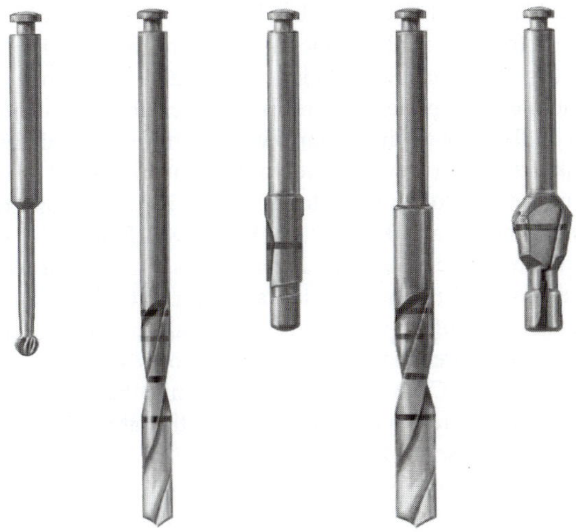

Fig. 59.5 Sequence of drills used for standard-diameter (4.0 mm) implant site osteotomy preparation: round, 2-mm twist, pilot, 3-mm twist, and countersink. Bone tap (not shown here) is an optional drill that is sometimes used in dense bone before implant placement.

BOX 59.2 Clinical Advice to Enhance Precision of Final Implant Site Preparation

Clinical Situation 1

If the final drill hits the bottom of the recipient site before reaching the desired depth, the added hand pressure necessary to achieve the proper depth often causes wobbling and funneling of the recipient site. This is especially true with "cannon" drills (used for cylindrical implants). To minimize this effect, a smaller-diameter drill should be used to prepare the site slightly deeper (e.g., 0.5 mm or less). This narrower drill allows the desired depth to be reached without affecting the side walls and facilitates a more precise osteotomy preparation with the final drill.

Clinical Situation 2

If the final drill is inserted at an inaccurate angle, the result is funneling of the coronal portion of the implant site. To minimize this potential problem, when drilling multiple implant sites, the operator should always keep a direction indicator in an adjacent site. For single-implant sites, the adjacent teeth and surgical guide should serve as direction indicators. When dealing with dense bone, a precise recipient site can be achieved more predictably if there is minimal diameter change from drill to drill. For example, switching from 3.0 to 5.0 mm is much less precise than proceeding from 3.0–3.3 to 4.2–5.0 mm.

Clinical Situation 3

If the bone is "soft" (e.g., loose trabecular bone), it may be advantageous to underprepare the osteotomy site. A slightly underprepared site can be accomplished by using the final drill to a shallower depth than the previous drill (e.g., half the depth of the osteotomy site). This avoids removing too much bone and increases the implant stability or tightness at the time of placement. Another method to achieve an underprepared site is to use a drill with a slightly smaller diameter as the final drill in the preparation (e.g., a 2.75-mm drill as the final drill rather than a 3.0 or a 3.25 mm as the final drill for a 4.0-mm implant).

recommended (Box 59.2). It is better to allow the threaded implant to "cut" its own path into the osteotomy site.

Bone tapping and implant insertion are both done at very slow speeds (e.g., 20–40 rpm). All other drills in the sequence are used at higher speeds (800–1500 rpm).

It is important to create a recipient site that is very accurate in size and angulation. In partially edentulous cases, limited jaw opening or proximity to adjacent teeth may prevent appropriate positioning of the drills in posterior edentulous areas. In fact, implant therapy may be contraindicated in some patients because of a lack of interocclusal clearance, lack of interdental space, or a lack of access for the instrumentation. Therefore, a combination of longer drills and shorter drills, with or without extensions, may be necessary. Anticipating these needs before surgery facilitates the procedure and improves the results.

Implant Placement

Implants are inserted with a handpiece rotating at slow speeds (e.g., 25 rpm) or by hand with a wrench. Insertion of the implant must follow the same path or line as the osteotomy site. When multiple implants are being placed, it is helpful to use guide pins in the other sites to have a visual guide for the path of insertion.

Flap Closure and Suturing

Once the implants are inserted and the cover screws secured (Fig. 59.4G), the surgical sites should be thoroughly irrigated with sterile saline to remove debris and clean the wound. Proper closure of the flap over the implant(s) is essential. One of the most important aspects of flap management is achieving good approximation and primary closure of the tissues in a tension free manner (Fig. 59.3H). This is achieved by incising the periosteum (innermost layer of full-thickness flap), which is nonelastic. Once the periosteum is released, the flap becomes very elastic and is able to be stretched over the implant(s) without tension. One suturing technique that consistently provides the desired result is a combination of alternating horizontal mattress and interrupted sutures (Fig. 59.4H). Horizontal mattress sutures evert the wound edges and approximate the inner, connective tissue surfaces of the flap to facilitate closure and wound healing. Interrupted sutures help to bring the wound edges together, counterbalancing the eversion caused by the horizontal mattress sutures.

The clinician should choose an appropriate suture for the given patient and procedure. For patient management, it is sometimes simpler to use a resorbable suture that does not require removal during the postoperative visit (e.g., 4–0 chromic gut suture). However, when moderate-to-severe postoperative swelling is anticipated, a nonresorbable suture is recommended to maintain a longer closure period (e.g., 4–0 monofilament suture). These sutures require removal at a postoperative visit.

Postoperative Care

Simple implant surgery in a healthy patient usually does not require antibiotic therapy. However, antibiotics [e.g., amoxicillin, 500 mg three times a day (tid)] can be prescribed if the surgery is extensive, or if the patient is medically compromised. Postoperative swelling is likely after flap surgery. This is particularly true when the periosteum has been incised (released). As a preventive measure, patients should apply cold packs over the first 24–48 h. Chlorhexidine gluconate oral rinses can be prescribed to facilitate plaque control, especially in the days after surgery when oral hygiene is typically poorer. Adequate pain medication should be prescribed (e.g., ibuprofen, 600–800 mg tid).

Patients should be instructed to maintain a relatively soft diet after surgery. Then, as healing progresses, they can gradually return to a normal diet. Patients should also refrain from tobacco and alcohol use after surgery. Provisional restorations, whether fixed or removable, should be checked and adjusted to minimize trauma to the surgical area.

Second-Stage Exposure Surgery

For implants placed using a two-stage "submerged" protocol, a second-stage exposure surgery is necessary. Box 59.3 lists the objectives for second-stage implant exposure surgery. The need for a zone of keratinized tissue surrounding implants is desirable, as one long-term study indicated that the presence of keratinized tissue is strongly correlated with soft- and hard-tissue health.

Simple Circular "Punch" or Crestal Incision

In areas with sufficient zones of keratinized tissue, the gingiva covering the head of the implant can be exposed with a circular or "punch" incision (Fig. 59.6). Alternatively, a crestal incision through the middle of the keratinized tissue and full-thickness flap reflection can be used to expose implants.

Partial-Thickness Repositioned Flap

If a minimal zone of keratinized tissue exists at the implant site, a partial-thickness flap technique can be used to fulfill the objective of the second-stage surgery (exposing the implant) while increasing the width of keratinized tissue. The initial incision is made within the zone of keratinized tissue so that it becomes the outer edge of the reflected split-thickness flap. Vertical releasing incisions are used on both the mesial and the distal end of the flap (Fig. 59.7A and B). A partial-thickness flap is then raised in such a manner that a nonmobile, firm periosteum remains attached to the underlying bone. The flap, containing a narrow band of keratinized tissue, is then repositioned to the facial side of the emerging head of the implant and sutured to the periosteum with a fine needle and resorbable suture such as a 5–0 gut suture (Fig. 59.8). If the initial amount of keratinized tissue is less than 2 mm, the flap may be started at the labial edge of the keratinized tissue, allowing that zone to remain on the lingual aspect of the implant. A partial-thickness flap is apically displaced and sutured to the periosteum without exposing the alveolar bone (Fig. 59.7C). A free gingival graft may be harvested from the palate and sutured to the periosteum on the labial surface of the implants to increase the zone of keratinized tissue (not shown).

After the flap is repositioned and secured with periosteal sutures, the excess tissue coronal to the cover screw is excised, usually with a surgical blade (Fig. 59.8B). However, if removal of this tissue would jeopardize the amount of remaining keratinized tissue around the lingual aspect of the implant(s), a similar partial-thickness flap can be elevated and repositioned on the lingual side as well. Extra care must be taken when creating a split-thickness flap on the lingual surface of mandibular sites because the tissue is often very thin. Alternatively, a full-thickness lingual flap will be safer and will serve a similar purpose of preserving keratinized tissue on the lingual surface of the implant(s).

When the excess tissue over the cover screw is removed or displaced, the outline of the cover screw is visible. A sharp blade is used to eliminate all tissues coronal to the cover screw (Fig. 59.7D). The cover screw is then removed, the head of the implant is thoroughly cleaned of any soft- or hard-tissue overgrowth, and the healing abutments or standard abutments are placed on the implant

BOX 59.3 Objectives of Second-Stage Implant Surgery

1. To expose the submerged implant without damaging the surrounding bone.
2. To control the thickness of the soft tissue surrounding the implant.
3. To preserve or create attached keratinized tissue around the implant.
4. To facilitate oral hygiene.
5. To ensure proper abutment seating.
6. To preserve soft-tissue esthetics.

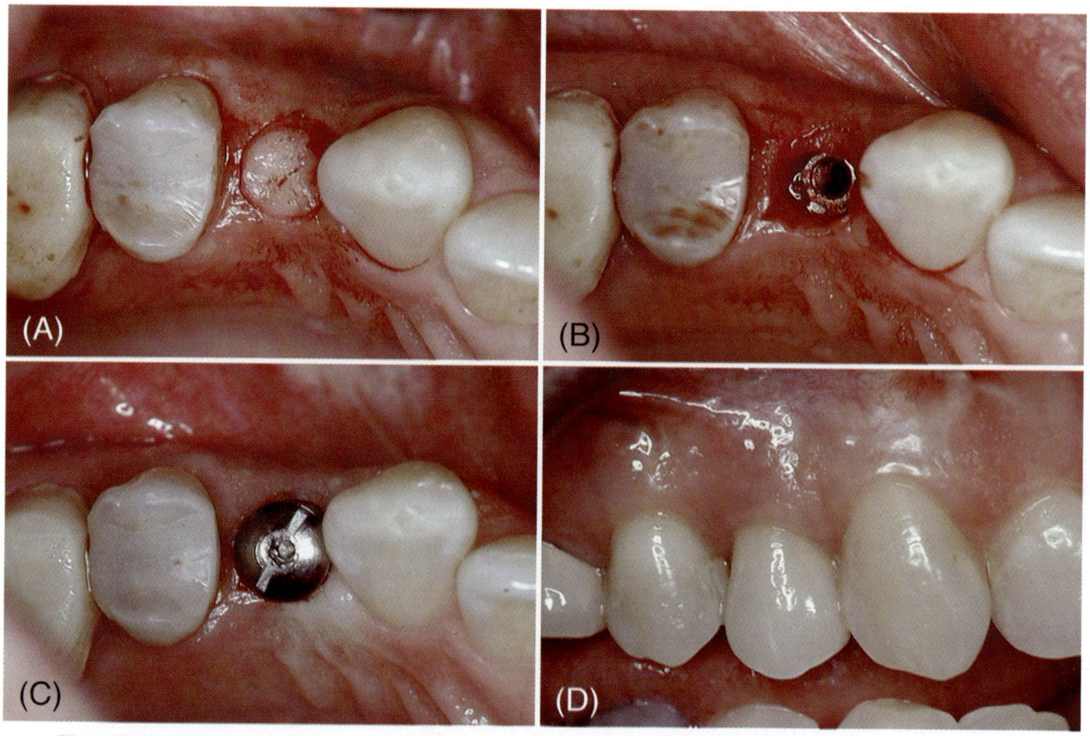

Fig. 59.6 Clinical view of second-stage implant exposure surgery in a case with adequate keratinized tissue. A, Simple circular "punch" incision used to expose implant when sufficient keratinized tissue is present around the implant(s). B, Implant exposed. C, Healing abutment attached. D, Final restoration in place, achieving an esthetic result with a good zone of keratinized tissue.

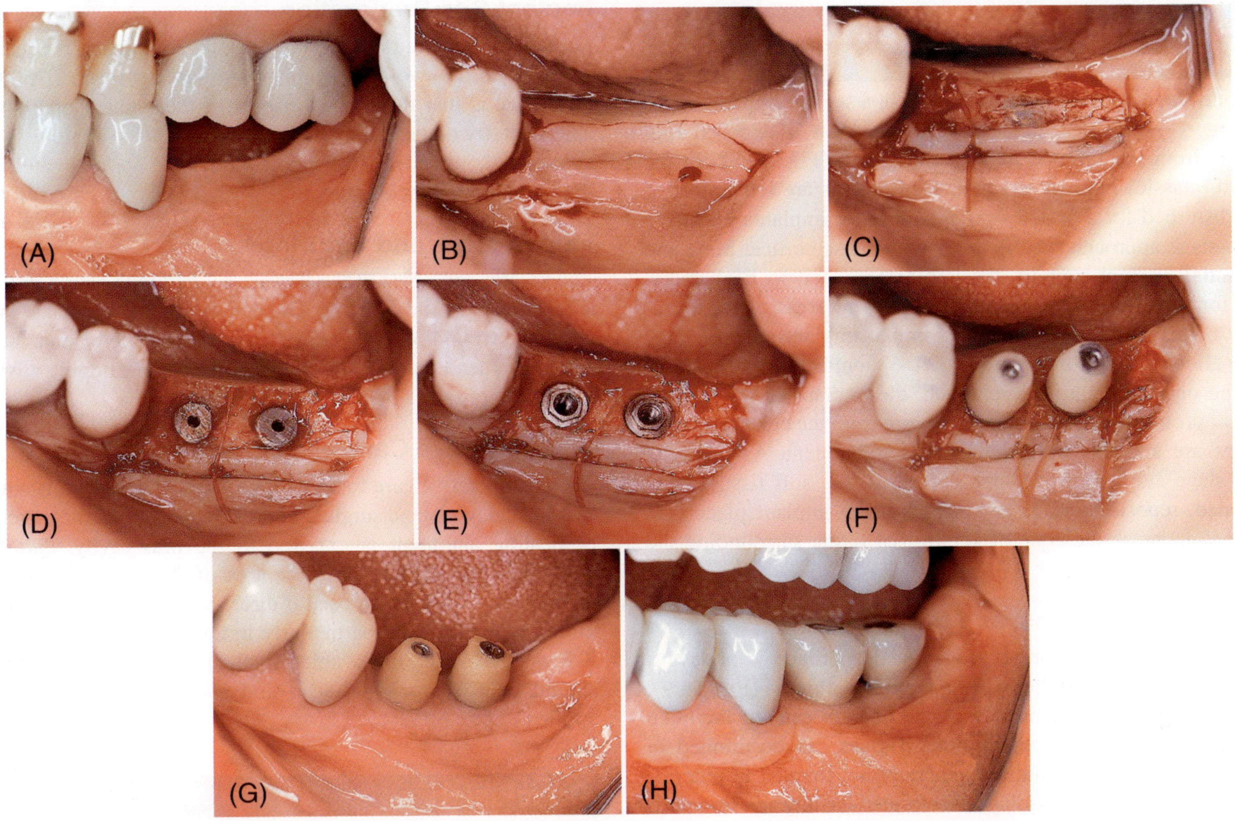

Fig. 59.7 Clinical view of second-stage implant exposure surgery in a case with inadequate keratinized tissue. A, Two endosseous implants were placed 4 months previously and are ready to be exposed. Note the narrow band of keratinized tissue. B, Two vertical incisions are connected by crestal incision. If facial keratinized tissue is insufficient, it is necessary to locate the crestal incision more lingually so that there is at least 2–3 mm of keratinized band. C, Buccal partial-thickness flap is sutured to the periosteum apical to the emerging implants. D, Gingival tissue coronal to the cover screws is excised using the gingivectomy technique. E, Cover screws are removed, and heads of the implants are cleared. F, Abutments are placed. Visual inspection ensures intimate contact between the abutments and the implants. G, Healing at 2–3 weeks after second-stage surgery. H, Four months after the final restoration. Note the healthy band of keratinized attached gingiva around the implants.

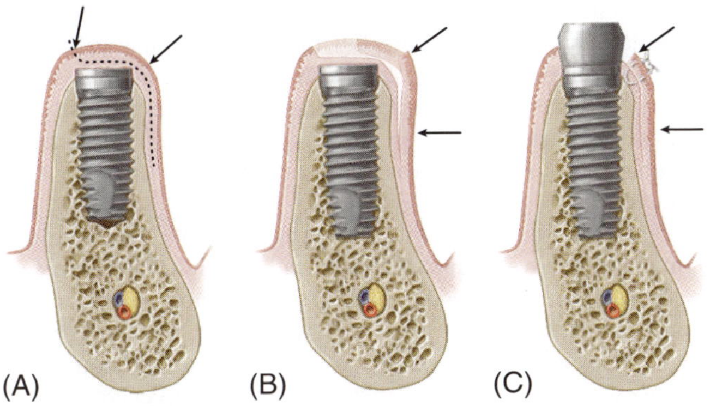

Fig. 59.8 Illustration depicting the use of a split-thickness flap that is repositioned to the labial surface in order to preserve and increase the amount of keratinized tissue. A, Partial-thickness flap is created from the lingual aspect of the crest toward the labial surface in order to preserve the keratinized tissue on the crest (over the implant). *Note:* This tissue might be excised in a simple implant exposure. B, The split-thickness flap is repositioned to the labial surface. C, The flap is sutured to the periosteum at a more apical position preserving the amount of keratinized tissue *(arrows)*. Finally, the remaining connective tissue over the cover screw (B) is excised with a sharp blade to expose the implant. Care should be taken to avoid removing keratinized tissue from the lingual aspect of the implant.

(Fig. 59.7E and F). The fit of the healing abutments to the implants can often be visually evaluated. However, if it is not possible to visualize clearly the intimate connection between the implant and the abutment, an intraoral periapical X-ray film should be taken to confirm complete seating. Bone may need to be removed around the top of the implant to get the abutment to seat properly. Readers are referred to online material for a discussion of bone profiling.

Postoperative Care

Once the implant is exposed and soft tissues are sutured, it is important to remind the patient of the need for good oral hygiene around the implant and adjacent teeth. Care should be taken during oral hygiene procedures to avoid dislodging any repositioned or grafted soft tissues. Direct pressure or movement directed toward the soft tissue from a provisional prosthesis can delay healing and should be avoided. Tissues should be monitored regularly and the provisional prosthesis should be adjusted as needed. Impressions for the final prosthesis fabrication can begin about 2–6 weeks after implant exposure surgery, depending on healing and maturation of soft tissues. Fig. 59.7G and H show the postoperative results in a clinical case after 2–3 weeks and 4 months, respectively.

One-Stage "Nonsubmerged" Implant Placement

In the one-stage implant surgical approach, a second implant exposure surgery is not needed because the implant is exposed (per gingival) from the time of implant placement (Fig. 59.9). In the standard (classic) implant protocol, the implants are left unloaded and undisturbed for a period similar to that for implants placed in the two-stage approach (i.e., in areas with dense cortical bone and good initial implant support, the implants are left to heal undisturbed for a period of 2–4 months, whereas in areas of loose trabecular bone, grafted sites, and/or minimal implant support, they may be allowed to heal for periods of 4–6 months or more).

In the one-stage surgical approach, the implant or the healing abutment protrudes approximately 2–3 mm from the bone crest, and the flaps are adapted around the implant/abutment. As with the second-stage surgical procedures described, the soft tissues may be thinned, repositioned, or augmented at the implant placement surgery to increase the zone of keratinized tissue surrounding the implant(s).

Flap Design, Incisions, and Elevation

The flap design for the one-stage surgical approach is always a crestal incision bisecting the existing keratinized tissue (Fig. 59.9). Vertical incisions may be needed at one or both ends to facilitate access to the bone or osteotomy site. Tissues can be thinned in posterior areas if desired but are generally not thinned in anterior esthetic areas. Full-thickness flaps are elevated facially and lingually.

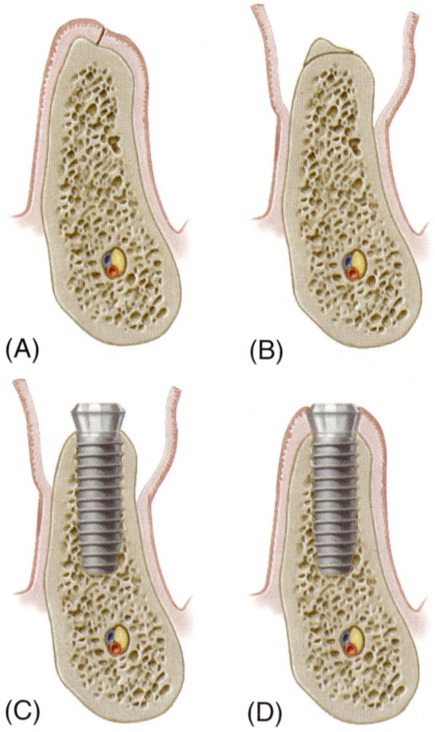

Fig. 59.9 Tissue management for a one-stage implant placement. A, Crestal incision made along the crest of the ridge, bisecting the existing zone of keratinized mucosa. B, Full-thickness flap is raised buccally and lingually to the level of the mucogingival junction. A narrow, sharp ridge can be surgically reduced or contoured to provide a reasonably flat bed for the implant. C, Implant is placed in the prepared osteotomy site. D, Tissues are adapted around the neck of the implant to achieve flap closure with the implant protruding through the soft tissues.

Implant Site Preparation

Implant site preparation for the one-stage approach is identical in principle to the two-stage implant surgical approach. The primary difference is that the coronal aspect of the implant or the healing abutment (two-stage implant) is placed approximately 2–3 mm above the bone crest and the soft tissues are approximated around the implant/implant abutment.

Flap Closure and Suturing

The keratinized edges of the flap are sutured with single interrupted sutures around the implant. Depending on the clinician's preference, the wound may be sutured with resorbable or nonresorbable sutures. When keratinized tissue is abundant, scalloping around the implant(s) provides better flap adaptation.

Postoperative Care

The postoperative care for one-stage surgical approach is similar to that for the two-stage surgical approach except that the cover screw or healing abutment is exposed to the oral cavity. Patients are advised to avoid chewing in the area of the implant(s). Prosthetic appliances should not be used if direct chewing forces can be transmitted to the implant, particularly in the early healing period (first 4–8 weeks). When removable prosthetic appliances are used, they should be adequately relieved and a soft-tissue liner should be applied.

Conclusion

It is essential to understand and follow basic guidelines to predictably achieve osseointegration. Fundamental protocols must be followed for implant placement (stage 1) and implant exposure surgery (stage 2). These fundamentals apply to all implant systems.

Localized Bone Augmentation and Implant Site Development

One of the most critical aspects of creating an esthetic implant restoration is surgical placement of the implant in a "prosthetically driven" position to restore the tooth in a natural position and to emulate the natural emergence of the tooth from the soft tissues. Implants placed without regard for prosthetic position often lead to dental restorations that are functionally and esthetically compromised, and patients are left with a less-than-optimal reconstruction. Placement of dental implant(s) in an esthetically and functionally optimal position requires reconstruction of deficient alveolar ridges (or preservation of ridges when teeth are to be extracted).

Periodontal bone loss, gingival recession, tooth loss, and long-term use of removable appliances typically result in alveolar defects that prevent the placement of implants in an optimal prosthetic position. It also leads to soft-tissue deficiencies that are unacceptable. Fortunately, continuous innovations in surgical techniques and advances in the biologic understanding of bone-regenerative techniques have led to advanced implant procedures and an increased predictability in the reconstruction of alveolar ridge defects.

Standard implant placement surgery, as described in this chapter, is based on adequate bone volume and quality in the desired implant location. The time-tested standard protocol allows for adequate remodeling and maturation of bone, with healing periods of 3–6 months. Recent implant procedures often challenge these original conventions by placing implants in areas with inadequate bone volume, simultaneous with bone augmentation, and restoring or loading implants after shorter healing periods. This chapter presents an overview of surgical bone augmentation procedures used to correct or to prevent alveolar ridge deficiencies for the optimal placement of dental implants and is discussed under the following heads:

Guided Bone Regeneration
Barrier membranes (e only)
Bone graft materials (e only)
Localized ridge augmentation
 Flap management (e only)
Horizontal bone augmentation
 Particulate bone graft (e only)
 Monoblock block graft (e only)
Simultaneous implant placement
Complications
Alveolar ridge preservation (e only)
Delayed implant placement (e only)
Staged implant placement (e only)
Immediate implant placement (e only)
Conclusion

Guided Bone Regeneration

Much of what can be achieved with implant surgery and specifically with bone augmentation procedures is directly related to the achievements and understanding of guided bone regeneration (GBR). Historically, augmentation or "regeneration" of alveolar bone that was lost following tooth removal, or from alveolar bone resorption or traumatic injury, presented a significant challenge for clinicians. Allowed to heal without the intervention of regenerative procedures, extraction site defects (especially those lacking a self-supporting bone structure) heal with fibrous connective tissue or scar formation and often did not fill completely with bone. The surrounding soft tissues collapsed into the bone defect, leaving an alveolar ridge deficiency with respect to the natural tooth position and jaw shape. Over time, the alveolar ridge continued to resorb, especially when removable prosthetic appliances are used.

Periodontal studies during the past several decades have led to new techniques and a new treatment approach referred to as guided tissue regeneration (GTR). In brief, this concept is based on the principle that specific cells contribute to the formation of specific tissues. Exclusion of the faster-growing epithelium and connective tissue from a periodontal wound for a minimum of 6–8 weeks allows the slower-growing tissues to occupy the space adjacent to the tooth. Osteoblasts, cementoblasts, and periodontal ligament cells then afforded the opportunity to regenerate a new periodontal attachment (defined by new bone and new connective tissue fibers inserted into newly formed cementum) on the previously diseased root surface. Chapter 48 includes a discussion on the concepts of GTR as related to periodontal regeneration.

The same basic principle of GTR has been applied to alveolar bone defects to regenerate new bone. Using a canine model, Schenk et al. demonstrated with histology that bone regeneration in membrane-protected defects healed in a sequence of steps that simulated bone formation after tooth extraction. They found that after blood clot formation, bone regeneration was initiated by the formation of woven bone initially along new blood vasculature at the periphery of the defect. The new vascular supply emanated from the existing bone bed (recipient site). Cortical perforations surgically created in the recipient site are thought to enhance the blood supply and cellular access to the bone grafted area. The woven bone, which is formed quickly with a disorganized, immature structure, was subsequently replaced by lamellar bone with an organized, mature structure. Over time, bone remodeling continued with new, secondary osteons being formed.

TABLE 59.1 Biologic Requirements for Bone Regeneration

Requirement	Surgical Procedure
Blood supply	Cortical perforations
Stabilization	Fixation screws, membrane tacks
Osteoblasts	Autogenous bone (graft or recipient site)
Confined space	Barrier membrane
Space maintenance	Tenting screws, bone graft materials
Wound coverage	Flap management, tension-free suturing

This concept employed the same principles of specific tissue exclusion but was not associated with teeth. Rather, it was bone that was being isolated from the surrounding soft tissues. Thus the term applied to this technique was GBR. Since the objective of GBR is to regenerate a single tissue, namely bone, it is theoretically easier to accomplish than GTR, which strives to regenerate multiple tissues simultaneously in a complex relationship.

Interestingly, long before the current concepts of GBR were introduced, Murray and coworkers demonstrated that when a cavity with a source of osteoblasts and a blood supply was isolated from adjacent soft tissues, it could fill with bone, whereas if the space were not protected, it would fill with fibrous connective tissue. In addition to this observation, they suggested that a bone graft placed in the space might interfere with bone formation because the graft would need to be resorbed before bone could occupy the space.

Bone is a unique tissue that has the capacity to regenerate itself completely. Due to its rigid calcified structure, however, bone has specific requirements that must be respected to achieve regeneration. Since the calcified structure of bone is not conducive to perfusion, new bone formation is critically dependent on establishing an adequate blood supply through the ingrowth of new vasculature while maintaining rigid fixation or stabilization for bone formation. Any movement of the segments of bone relative to one another (even micromotion) during healing results in disruption of the blood supply and a change in the type of tissue formed in the site from mineralized bone to fibrous connective tissue. Table 59.1 lists the biologic requirements for bone regeneration and the associated component of GBR surgical procedures needed to accomplish bone regeneration.

Localized Ridge Augmentation

Patients often present for implant planning after tooth loss and alveolar ridge resorption. In these cases, the clinician is obligated to perform augmentation procedures to reconstruct lost bone and place implants in a prosthetically driven position.

Surgical reconstructive procedures for the preparation and placement of dental implants have become more numerous and complex. Depending on the size and morphology of the defect, various augmentation procedures can be used. These procedures have been categorized according to the deficient dimension: horizontal or vertical. Methods used to augment horizontal, as well as vertical, bone deficiencies include particulate bone grafts and monocortical block grafts. Barrier membranes can be used with bone grafts to reconstruct all types of alveolar bone defects. See further in this chapter for a review of procedures used to achieve vertical augmentation. All the proven principles of GBR and flap management must be followed to achieve good results. These include an adequate blood supply; maintaining a stable, protected space for bone growth; and achieving tension-free flap wound closure.

Horizontal Bone Augmentation

A deficiency in the horizontal dimension of bone may be minimal, such as a dehiscence or fenestration of an implant surface, or it may be more significant, such that the implant would have more than one axial surface exposed while having some bone along the entire vertical length. Dehiscence defects can usually be managed during implant placement because most of the implant is covered and stabilized by native bone. If the horizontal deficiency is large and the implant placement would result in significant exposure (i.e., implant body is significantly outside the alveolar bone), it may be better to reconstruct the bone first, in a staged approach, with a subsequent surgery for implant placement.

Although reconstruction of deficient ridges with bone grafts alone (i.e., without barrier membrane) has proved to be effective, variable resorption of the grafted bone has been reported. Preliminary results in a 1- to 3-year study using autografts harvested from the maxillary tuberosity showed an increased ridge width, but resorption of 50% of the graft volume was also noted. Buser et al. investigated the lateral ridge augmentation procedure using an autograft from the retromolar or symphysis area covered by a membrane in 40 consecutively treated patients and noted no clinical signs of resorption of the block graft. The researchers emphasized a remote incision technique, perforation of the cortex, stable placement of corticocancellous autografts, precise adaptation and stabilization (with miniscrews) of the ePTFE membranes, and a tension-free primary soft tissue closure. After 7–13 months, the sites were reopened for membrane removal and implant placement. Of the 40 patients, 38 exhibited excellent ridge augmentation, whereas 2 sites showed some soft tissue encapsulation of the grafted bone.

Nevins and Mellonig and Doblin et al. reported an increased amount of new bone using freeze-dried bone allografts (FDBAs) with membranes, even in the presence of membrane exposure. The biopsies showed viable bone cells and visible osteocytes in lacunae, and a 9-month specimen showed no remaining allograft material.

On the other hand, there are some contradictory results using DFDBA and membrane combinations. In a human study, seven paired extraction sockets were grafted with either DFDBA or autologous bone. Sites were reentered and biopsied after 3–13 months to evaluate bone formation. Histologic specimens revealed dead particles of DFDBA with no evidence of bone formation on the surface and no evidence of osteoclastic resorption. Conversely, the autogenous sites revealed vascular channels with woven and lamellar bone. Some nonvital, cortical bone chips were observed with osteoclastic resorption.

Fig. 59.10 shows an example of the lack of bone formation around DFDBA particles used in a ridge augmentation procedure after more than 20 months of healing under a nonresorbable ePTFE barrier membrane.

Simultaneous Implant Placement

Large alveolar bone defects need to be augmented before implant placement and require a healing period of 6 months or longer. In selected cases, it is possible to perform a bone augmentation procedure simultaneously with the implant placement. It is essential to achieve good implant stability in the existing native bone so that endosseous integration can occur.

A very predictable osseous defect to manage with simultaneous implant placement is the implant dehiscence or fenestration defect. *Fenestration* defects are exposures of the implant's axial surface that do not include the coronal aspect of the implant (Fig. 59.14). *Dehiscence* defects expose a part of the axial surface, including the coronal aspect of the implant, while maintaining sufficient bone volume around all remaining implant surfaces (Fig. 59.15). In a dehiscence defect, the implant remains within the confines of the existing bone.

Fenestration and dehiscence defects have been managed with barrier membranes or simply with flap closure. Bone grafts have also been used. The only controlled comparison studies between membrane treatment and periosteal flap coverage of exposed implant surfaces in humans demonstrated that the membrane treatment was far superior with regard to bone fill. Another controlled study in humans showed better results in the membrane groups; four of six sites (67%) treated with a membrane resulted in 95%–100% elimination of the dehiscence and total coverage of the threads. In the control sites, only two of six sites (33%) showed moderate-to-complete bone fill. All other clinical studies are in the form of case reports. Fig. 59.16M demonstrates coverage of an implant dehiscence using a barrier membrane. Admittedly, without a biopsy, it cannot be determined whether the tissue covering the implant is bone or firm connective tissue.

A 1-year multicenter study evaluating 55 Brånemark implants (i.e., machined-surface, external hex) with bone dehiscence in 45 patients, treated by ePTFE membrane alone, demonstrated an average bone fill of 82%. The average initial defect height was 4.7 mm. The 1-year follow-up of these implants demonstrated a favorable response to loading. Of the 55 implants, a total of 6 failed, corresponding to a cumulative survival rate of 84.7% in the maxilla and 95.0% in the mandible, which is similar to previously published results for this implant design.

A clinical report on the use of TR membranes demonstrated the biologic potential to fill a large protected space in four patients. Bone dehiscence at implant sites ranged from 5 to 12 mm (mean: 8.2 mm). They were covered with a TR membrane alone (no graft). Reentry after 7–8 months of submerged healing found complete bone coverage over all implants. Radiographic evaluation demonstrated the implants functioning with normal crestal bone support after 1 year.

No clinical comparisons are available in the literature evaluating the placement of bone grafts with or without barrier membranes on implant dehiscence defects. Most evidence supports the use of graft materials in conjunction with membrane treatment, especially the use of FDBA in conjunction with GBR. In a study with 40 patients, 110 implants were placed in conjunction with barrier membranes and FDBA; a success rate of 96.8% was achieved with complete bone fill (defined as >90% fill of dehiscence). This study reported a membrane exposure rate of 29% but noted little adverse effect on the bone regeneration.

With respect to ridge preservation, Becker et al. reported the effect of barrier membranes and autogenous bone grafts on the preservation of ridge width around implants. They evaluated the ridge width around 76 implants in 61 patients from a case series database. Three groups were compared, including 34 implants treated with GBR (barrier membranes), 27 implants treated with autogenous bone grafts, and 15 implants placed without the need for ridge preservation/augmentation procedures (control group). The results revealed that implant sites treated with barrier membranes and autogenous bone grafts lost an average of 0.1 and 0.8 mm, respectively, more than the no augmentation group.

Another study evaluated the possibility of regenerating bone around implants placed in extraction sockets. Bone augmentation was achieved with human DFDBA particles mixed with tetracycline packed around the exposed implant surfaces. Implants and graft material were covered with ePTFE barrier membranes with

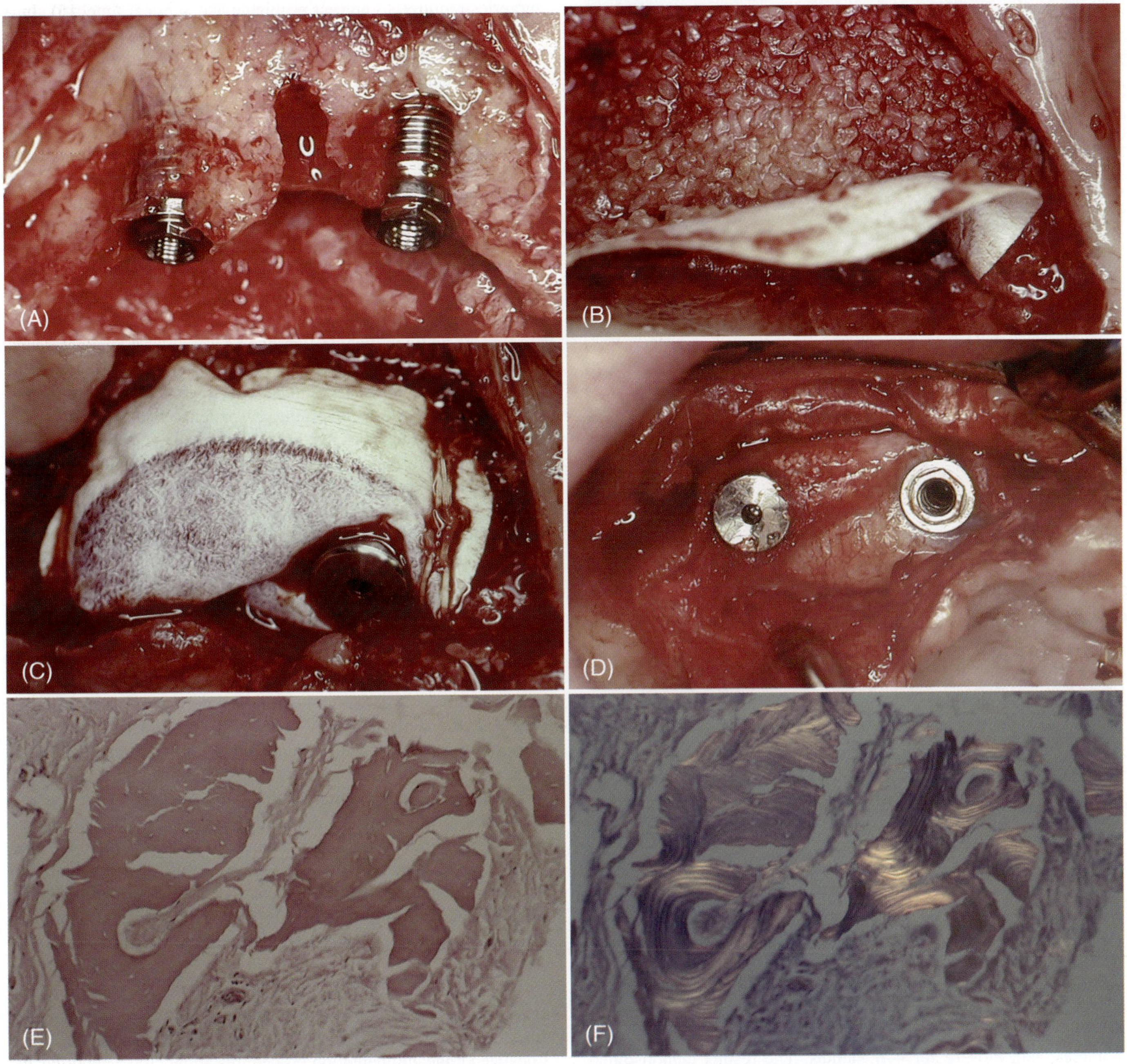

Fig. 59.10 A, Clinical view of maxillary alveolar ridge after removal of a failed implant (center defect) and placement of two implants in the bone adjacent to this site. B, The narrow ridge was grafted with decalcified freeze-dried bone allograft (DFDBA) particulate bone graft material. The graft material was completely covered by a nonresorbable, expanded polytetrafluoroethylene (ePTFE) barrier membrane. C, The ePTFE barrier membrane was secured with the cover screw of one implant and sutures that were secured to the periosteum. D, Clinical view of DFDBA-augmented ridge after more than 20 months healing under a nonresorbable ePTFE barrier membrane. The membrane remained submerged throughout the entire healing period. E, Hematoxylin–eosin (H&E) light microscopic view of specimen harvested from the DFDBA-augmented ridge. Note there are no bone cells (osteoblasts, osteoclasts, or osteocytes), no bone formation, and no osteoclastic resorption of DFDBA particles. There is no evidence of inflammation. Fibroblasts and connective tissue surround the "dead" DFDBA particles. F, Polarized light microscopic view of the same specimen (E) harvested from the DFDBA-augmented ridge. Note the appearance of lamellar layers demonstrating the presence of the DFDBA particles.

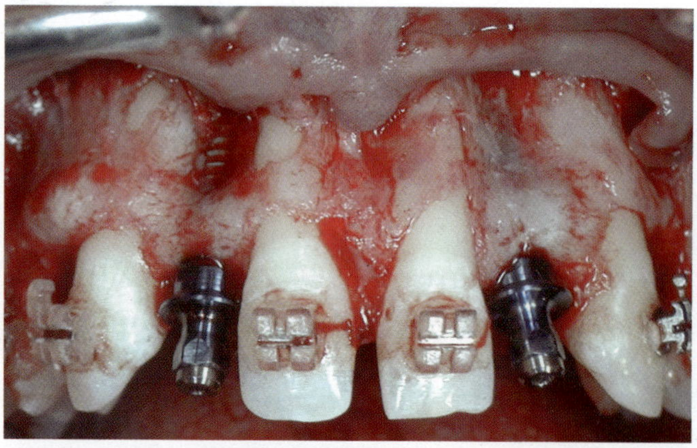

Fig. 59.14 Fenestration defect observed in very thin maxillary anterior sites. Implants placed in the maxillary lateral incisor positions demonstrating fenestration defects caused by the concavities in the apical area. Notice that the natural teeth (centrals and cuspids) also demonstrate fenestrations. Bone will grow across this type of defect in a very predictable manner because the implants are stable; the defect is small and surrounded by bone.

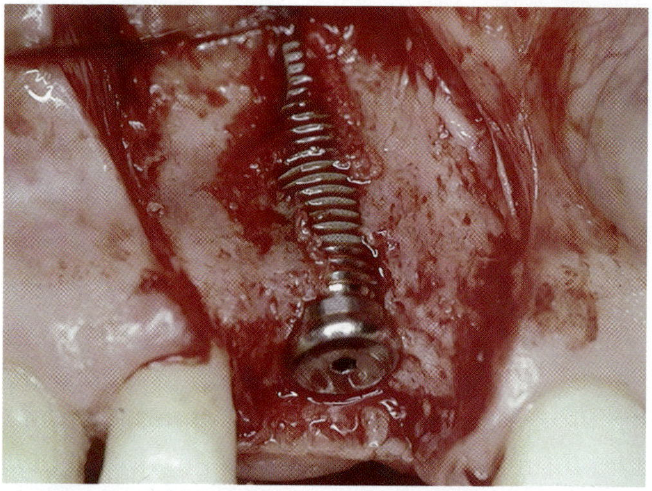

Fig. 59.15 Dehiscence defect observed during placement of an implant in the maxillary central incisor position. Note that the implant is completely surrounded by existing native bone except for the facial surface, which is exposed. Bone will grow across this type of defect in a very predictable manner because the implant is stable and the exposed surface is relatively flat with bone on all surfaces.

complete flap closure for 4–6 months. The results demonstrated complete bone regeneration in all cases except when barrier membranes were prematurely exposed and removed. One-year posttreatment histologic evaluation of regenerated bone revealed remnants of the DFDBA graft particles in direct contact with vital bone tissue (woven and lamellar bone). Osteoblasts were observed and appeared to be actively engaged in bone formation adjacent to graft particles. Fig. 59.16L and M demonstrate a simultaneous GBR and implant placement in a dehiscence defect.

Complications

Bone augmentation procedures used to increase the bone volume in deficient alveolar ridges have been successful and have enabled the placement of implants into prosthetically driven positions. Unfortunately, these augmentation procedures carry an increased risk of morbidity and can require secondary surgeries to correct problems resulting from the procedure. The subsequent corrective surgeries required to correct problems add surgical time and complexity to the implant therapy.

Surgical complications are reported for a variety of bone reconstructive techniques. A review assessed the number and types of complications associated with bone reconstructive procedures for endosseous implants. The review of literature (1976–1994) included 2315 implants in 733 autogenous blocks, particulate, and various other bone graft materials. Complications reported included bleeding, postoperative infection, bone fracture, nerve dysfunction, perforation of the mucosa, loss of a portion of the bone graft, pain, decubital ulcers, sinusitis, and wound dehiscence. Wound dehiscence seemed to have the most deleterious effect on implant survival. This finding emphasizes the importance of flap management.

Typical findings include less bone fill with early exposure and membrane removal versus retaining the membrane without exposure for 6–8 months. Buccolingual ridge deficiencies were treated in a prospective study involving 19 patients using ePTFE membranes and miniscrews as fixation and tenting devices. The group of defects, which healed uneventfully, yielded on reentry 90%–100% bone regeneration compared to the maximal volume of the space defined by the membrane placement. In the exposed-membrane group, the percentage of regenerated bone ranged from 0% to 62%. When a late membrane removal was performed (3–5 months postsurgically), the regeneration varied between 42% and 62%. The authors concluded that the length of membrane healing and size of the defect played a significant role in the amount of new bone formation.

Other authors have reported successful bone fill in situations in which the membranes had to be removed because of an early exposure. A significantly greater fill of the osseous defects at the grafted sites was noted. The authors concluded that the regeneration of bone around the implants appeared most dependent on the anatomy of the bony defect at the time of implant placement.

Although the effect or amount of regenerated bone with regard to membrane exposure is somewhat contradictory, the goal should be to keep the membranes covered during the healing period so that the risk of infection and soft tissue and esthetic problems can be minimized or eliminated. Again, the importance of flap management for ridge augmentation procedures should be stressed.

Conclusion

Localized bone augmentation procedures allow clinicians to reconstruct horizontal alveolar ridge deficiencies and replace missing teeth with dental implants in a prosthetically driven position with natural appearance and function. In many cases, implants can be placed simultaneously with the augmentation procedure. In cases of advanced bone resorption, ridge augmentation before implant placement may be a better choice. Bone augmentation procedures can also be used to preserve alveolar dimensions following tooth extraction. If adequate bone exists to stabilize an implant, these procedures may be combined. The predictable outcome of these procedures depends on several biologic principles that must be followed. Diagnosis, treatment planning, careful execution of the surgical treatment, postoperative follow-up, and appropriate implant loading are all important factors in achieving success.

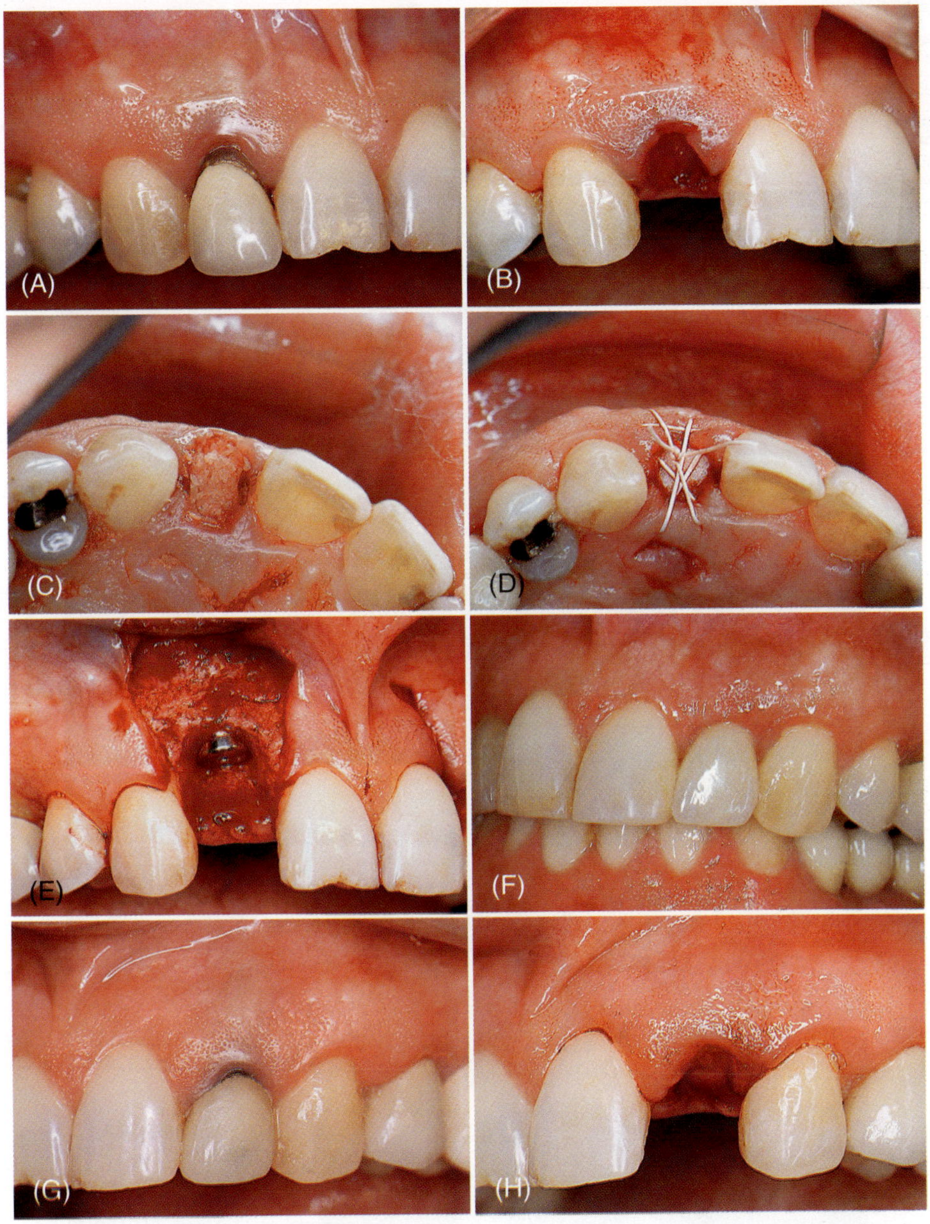

Fig. 59.16 Use of staged (A–H) and delayed (I–O) implant placement after extraction of two maxillary lateral incisors in one individual. A, Preoperative photograph of tooth #7 with gingival recession and marginal inflammation. B, Atraumatic extraction or tooth #7 without tissue incision or tissue elevation. Palpation reveals no facial bone present at the time of extraction. C, Decalcified freeze-dried bone allograft condensed into extraction site. D, Expanded polytetrafluoroethylene (ePTFE) barrier membrane positioned over graft and held in place with sutures. E, Six months after the extraction/graft, the implant is placed. Notice the implant is completely covered with bone. F, Final restoration. G, Preoperative photograph of tooth #10 with exposed gingival margin. H, Atraumatic extraction of tooth #10 without tissue incision or tissue elevation. Palpation reveals no facial bone present, and dehiscence is expected.

Continued

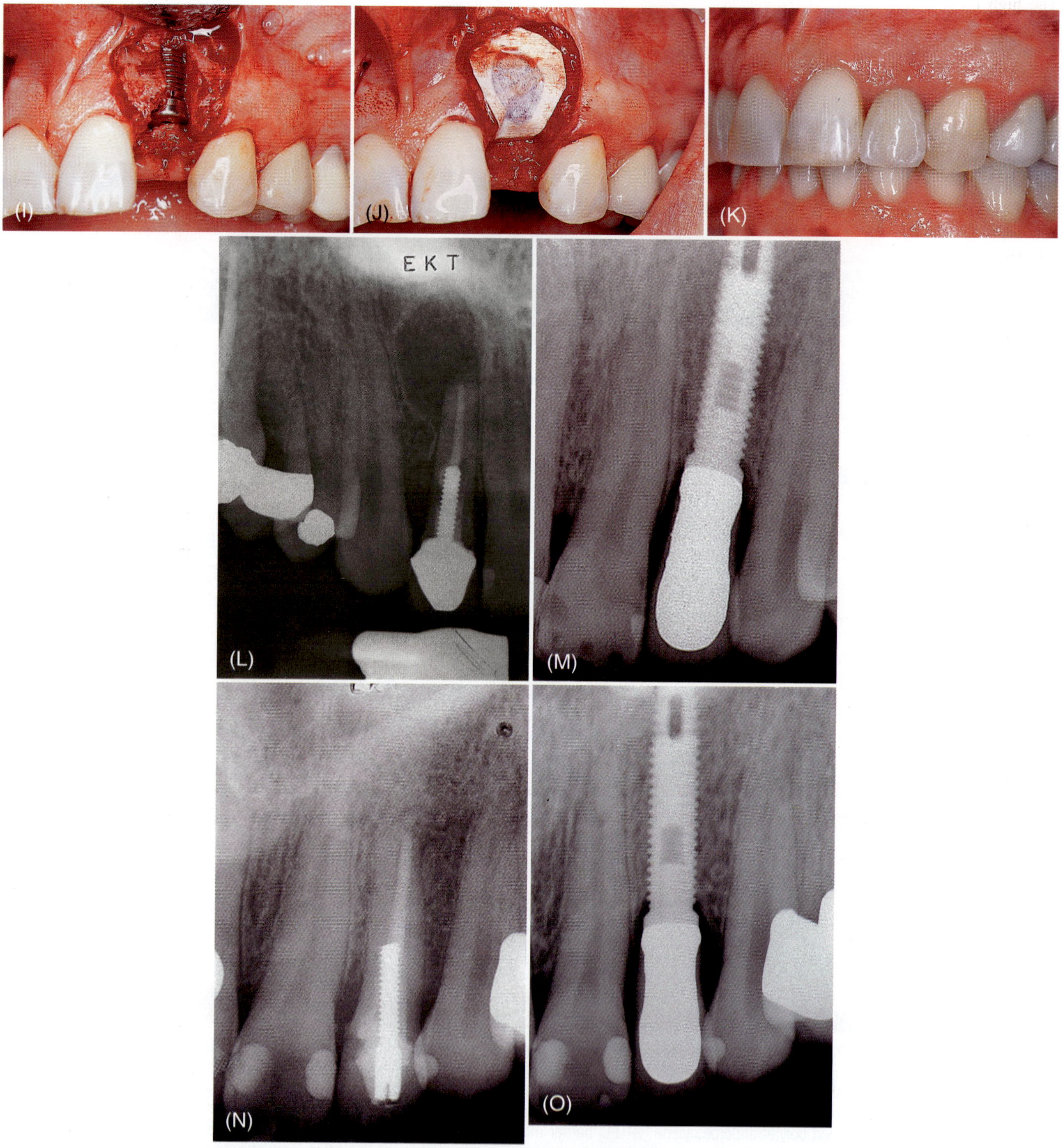

Fig. 59.16, cont'd I, Two months after extraction, the implant is placed with dehiscence defect. J, Guided bone regeneration accomplished with ePTFE barrier membrane positioned over the dehiscence. K, Final restoration. L, Periapical radiograph of tooth #7 with a large radiolucent lesion around the apex and periodontal bone loss along the distal interproximal area. M, Final radiograph of delayed implant placement. N, Periapical radiograph of tooth #10. O, Final radiograph. *(Figs. A, B, C, F, G, J, M, N, and O from Klokkevold PR, Han TJ, Camargo PM.: Esthetic management of extractions for implant site development: delayed versus staged implant placement.* Pract Periodontics Aesthet Dent *11:603, 1999.)*

Advanced Implant Surgical Procedures

The high predictability of endosseous dental implants has led to routine use and an expectation for success. However, the ultimate success for any patient or any particular implant relies on several factors, the most important of which is the *availability of bone*. The loss of teeth, whether caused by disease or trauma, can result in severe deficiency of the alveolar bone. Horizontal bone deficiencies are managed quite predictably with localized bone augmentation procedures. However, vertical bone deficiencies are much more challenging. The edentulous posterior maxilla is challenging as the result of a general lack of bone volume and the omnipresent poor bone quality of the area; that is, posterior maxillary bone often consists of a thin cortical shell filled with sparse trabecular bone. Edentulous sites, in any anatomic location, that have suffered significant vertical alveolar bone loss are especially challenging to reconstruct.

This part of the chapter reviews advanced surgical procedures used to treat the most challenging type of bone loss, which is *a deficiency in vertical bone height.* Topics reviewed are:

- Maxillary sinus elevation and bone augmentation
  - Indications and contraindications
  - Surgical procedures for sinus elevation (e only)
    - Crestal osteotomy technique (e only)
    - Lateral window technique (e only)
  - Risks and complications
- Vertical bone augmentation
- Guided bone regeneration (e only)
- Distraction osteogenesis (e only)
- Growth factors in bone augmentation
  - Bone morphogenetic proteins (e only)
  - Autologous platelet concentrates (e only)
- Conclusion

Maxillary Sinus Elevation and Bone Augmentation

Rehabilitation of the edentulous posterior maxilla with endosseous dental implants often represents a clinical challenge because of insufficient bone volume resulting from *pneumatization* of the maxillary sinus and resorption or loss of alveolar crestal bone. Before the utilization of bone augmentation procedures, patients with missing teeth and deficient bone in the posterior maxilla could only be rehabilitated with removable prostheses, short implants, or cantilevered restorations (i.e., supported by adjacent teeth or implants). Historically, the failure rate for implants in the posterior maxilla has been significantly higher than failure rates for implants in all other anatomic locations. Consequently, procedures such as the maxillary sinus elevation and bone augmentation are needed to increase the amount of vertical bone height in the posterior maxilla for the placement of implants.

In 1980, Boyne and James first described a procedure to graft the maxillary sinus floor with autogenous marrow and bone for placing an implant (blade type). Access to the maxillary sinus was gained through a "Caldwell-Luc" procedure (i.e., an opening into the maxillary sinus created at the anterior–superior aspect). Since then several other techniques have been described, including variations on the lateral window osteotomy and a variety of techniques to lift the sinus floor from a crestal approach.

Various bone graft materials have been used to augment the maxillary sinus. The 1996 Consensus Conference on Maxillary Sinus Bone Grafting reviewed available data and concluded that allografts, alloplasts, and xenografts, alone or in combination with autogenous bone, can be effective as bone substitute graft materials for sinus bone augmentation. More importantly, it was concluded that the sinus graft procedure with implant placement is a highly predictable and effective therapeutic modality for the rehabilitation of the posterior maxilla. Sinus floor elevation with bone augmentation of the maxillary sinus is now a well-accepted procedure used to increase bone volume in the posterior maxilla. Numerous reports have validated the safety and efficacy of this procedure. Implant success rates are equal to or better than that of implants placed in nongrafted maxillary bone (i.e., areas of the posterior maxilla with adequate height of existing native bone). Thus, bone augmentation of the maxillary sinus is a viable option for the vertically deficient posterior maxilla in which the interocclusal dimension is normal or only moderately increased.

Indications and Contraindications

As with any therapeutic procedure, treatment success depends on appropriate patient selection, careful evaluation of the anatomy, identification and management of any pathology, sound surgical procedures, and appropriate postsurgical management. The primary indication for maxillary sinus elevation and bone augmentation, specific for the placement of endosseous dental implants, is an alveolar bone height in the posterior maxilla that is deficient (e.g., less than 7 mm of existing vertical bone height). Other factors that must be considered include the health of the patient, the condition of the remaining dentition, and the likelihood of a beneficial outcome. A thorough evaluation of the patient and the judgment of the clinician ultimately determine whether the procedure is indicated for any particular individual.

Contraindications to maxillary sinus elevation and bone augmentation are similar to contraindications for other surgical procedures, with the added consideration of the maxillary sinus (Box 59.4). Patients must be in good general health and free of diseases that affect the maxilla or maxillary sinus. Local factors that are considered contraindications to maxillary sinus elevation and bone augmentation include the presence of tumors, maxillary sinus infection, severe chronic sinusitis, scar or deformity of the sinus cavity from previous surgery, dental infection, severe allergic rhinitis, and chronic use of topical steroids. Systemic contraindications to treatment include radiation therapy, uncontrolled metabolic disease (e.g., diabetes), excessive tobacco use, drug or alcohol abuse, and psychologic or mental impairment.

Risks and Complications

The maxillary sinus elevation and bone augmentation procedure is technique sensitive, requiring meticulous surgical skills. Risks and complications of the procedure include tearing or perforation of the Schneiderian membrane, intraoperative/postoperative bleeding, postoperative infection, and loss of bone graft or implants.

The reported incidence of perforation or tearing of the Schneiderian membrane varies greatly (up to 60%) and depends largely on the anatomy of the sinus and the skill and experience of the operator. The presence of septa in the maxillary sinus increases the likelihood of membrane perforation.

Positioning of the sinus window within 2–4 mm from the anterior and inferior borders of the sinus makes it easier to get direct access to the bony walls. This may lessen the amount of membrane perforation during the elevation of the sinus membrane.

If the perforation is small, it can often be managed with a resorbable barrier membrane placed over the opening, followed by careful packing of the bone augmentation material. If a perforation or tear

BOX 59.4 Contraindications for Maxillary Sinus Elevation and Bone Augmentation

Local Factors

1. Tumors or pathologic growth in the sinus
2. Maxillary sinus infection
3. Severe chronic sinusitis
4. Surgical scar/deformity of sinus cavity
5. Dental infection involving or in proximity to sinus
6. Severe allergic rhinitis/sinusitis
7. Chronic topical steroid use

Systemic Factors

1. Radiation therapy involving the maxillary sinus
2. Metabolic disease (e.g., uncontrolled diabetes mellitus)
3. Excessive tobacco use
4. Drug/alcohol abuse
5. Psychological/mental impairment

is extensive, it may be necessary to abort the procedure, close the wound, and attempt it again at a later date.

Infections have been reported in a small but significant number of cases (up to 10%) after maxillary sinus elevation and bone augmentation procedures. Prevention of infection is crucial for bone augmentation procedures. Surgery should always be performed using sterile technique. Patients should use a presurgical antimicrobial mouth rinse (e.g., chlorhexidine), and postoperative antibiotics should be prescribed. The signs and symptoms of sinus graft infection as well as a detailed protocol for its treatment was described in a recent clinical study.

Opening a window through the lateral wall is accomplished by completely cutting through the bone of the lateral wall up to the Schneiderian membrane. The membrane is highly vascularized and may bleed significantly. However, a more serious bleeding problem can arise if an intraosseous artery is severed in the process. Bone wax and topical hemostatic agents must be available to manage such an urgent surgical complication. If a medium-to-large vascular channel is identified (with CT or CBCT scan) presurgically, it can usually be avoided.

Supracrestal/Vertical Bone Augmentation

Supracrestal or vertical bone augmentation presents one of the greatest challenges of bone regeneration in implant dentistry. This is primarily a result of the difficulty of the surgical procedure and its potential complications. Since vertical augmentation can be a very challenging procedure with a relatively high rate of complications, it is necessary to justify this particular treatment for each patient. The rate of complications associated with vertical bone augmentation procedures, including membrane exposure and/or postoperative infection, is reported to range from 2.78% to 17%. Alternative treatment options, albeit with limited outcomes, need to be considered. For example, regenerating a vertically deficient defect may not be necessary if (1) implants can be placed in adjacent sites, (2) short implants can be used, or (3) pink ceramic can be used to create an illusion of "normal" soft-tissue anatomy.

Historical attempts to vertically increase alveolar bone height using modalities such as onlay bone grafting have failed. More recent treatment modalities developed for vertical bone growth include distraction osteogenesis and vertical GBR. The techniques and evidence of success are presented online.

Growth Factors in Bone Augmentation

Current research is exploring the use of various growth factors to induce bone formation. These bone-inductive mediators are powerful modifiers of the healing process. Incorporation of osteoinductive mediators into bone graft material or other carriers can be applied to sites in conjunction with conventional bone augmentation procedures to enhance the outcome.

Most of the clinical techniques available to try and stimulate new bone growth at such sites use some type of bone replacement graft, including autograft, allograft, xenograft, or alloplast. These bone graft materials have both advantages and limitations. Consequently, attempts have been made to improve bone grafting by either using growth factors alone or growth factors combined with a bone replacement graft. The rationale is that bone formation can be further enhanced when a growth factor is used to stimulate osteoblast precursor or osteoblast cells and hence to push the bone formation/bone resorption balance in favor of bone formation.

Conclusion

Bone augmentation and advanced implant surgery procedures allow clinicians to reconstruct vertical alveolar bone deficiencies and replace missing teeth with endosseous dental implants. As stated in this chapter, the predictable outcome of these procedures depends on several biologic principles that must be followed. Diagnosis, treatment planning, careful execution of the surgical treatment, postoperative follow-up, and appropriate implant loading are all important factors in achieving success. Sinus elevation and bone augmentation have become a widely used and predictable procedure to augment the deficient posterior maxilla (i.e., pneumatized maxillary sinus). Reconstruction of vertically deficient ridges remains a significant challenge despite the reported progress and success of new techniques.

Esthetic Management of Difficult Cases (Minimally Invasive Approach)

In recent years, implant dentistry has been increasingly influenced by esthetic considerations. In addition to successful osseointegration, harmonious soft and hard tissues must surround the implant restorations so that they look natural and healthy. A major challenge in implant dentistry is that, in many instances, dental implants need to be placed in an esthetic zone in which there is extensive alveolar bone deficiency from tooth loss, dentoalveolar infection, or other pathology (Fig. 59.27A–C). Gingival morphology follows the shape of the underlying bone, and it is difficult to build esthetically acceptable gingiva in areas with deficient supporting bone. Furthermore, using conventional surgical approaches to accomplish the goal in a patient-friendly manner with minimal trauma and clinical predictability is an extremely demanding task.

Treatment planning in a complex implant case today is often confusing because there are many different surgical and restorative approaches to solve the same problem. Many times these procedures seem to conflict. When considering the surgical placement of implants, clinicians must consider the approach (conventional two-stage approach vs a one-stage approach) and the timing of implant placement (immediate vs delayed or staged placement). For bone augmentation procedures, there is the more conventional approach of augmenting the ridge first and placing the implant(s)

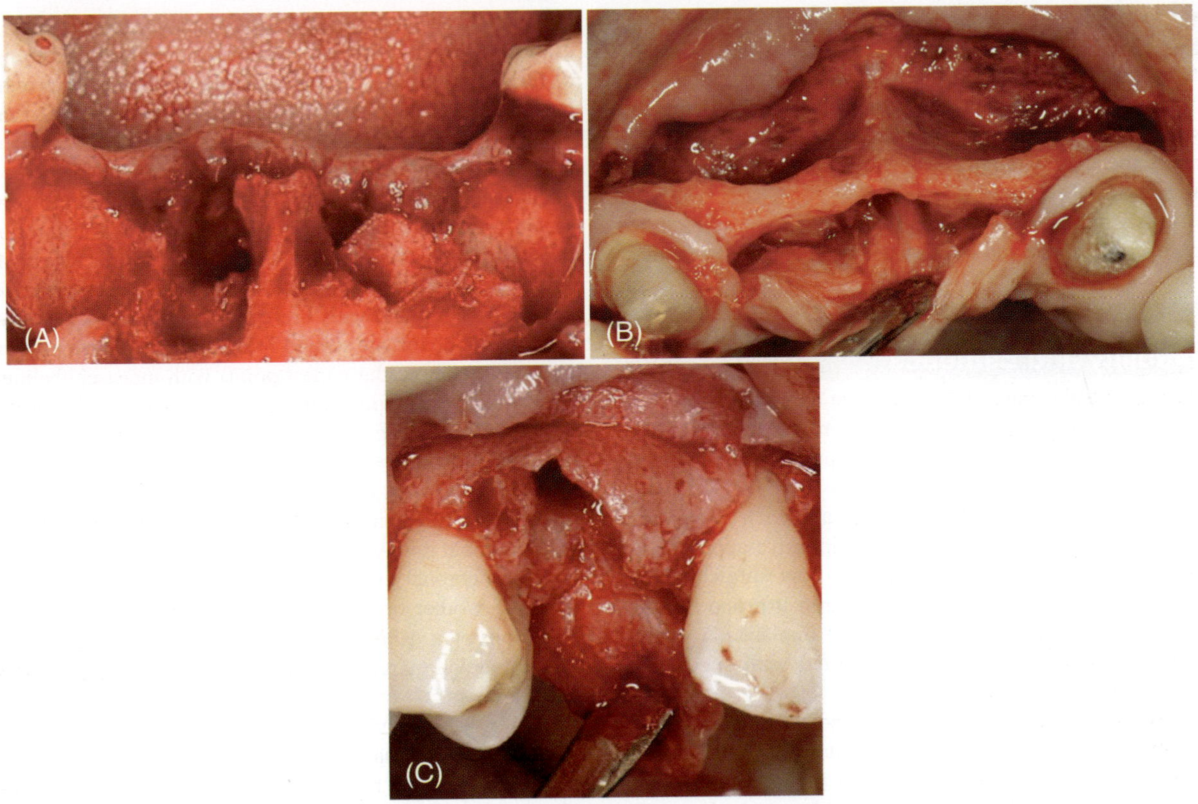

Fig. 59.27 Implant sites in the anterior, esthetic zone with extensive bone loss. A, Anterior mandibular site showing extensive bone loss following extraction of hopelessly infected mandibular incisors. B, Extremely narrow (labial–palatal) ridge width in the anterior maxilla that was missing centrals and laterals for many years. C, Moderate bone loss associated with the extraction socket of a maxillary cuspid.

after healing, or the simultaneous implant placement with bone augmentation approach in which bone grafting is done at same time as implant placement. All of these approaches can provide a successful outcome if patient selection is appropriate and techniques are performed properly. However, depending on the situation, some of these techniques are more advantageous than others in achieving esthetic results with better predictably and less patient discomfort.

It is easy for a clinician to "dogmatically" choose one approach, usually choosing the one that the clinician feels most comfortable with, and to treat all patients with the same approach. However, with heightened expectations of esthetics pushing the art and science of dentistry, it is necessary more than ever for clinicians to fully understand all the available options of treatment and decide appropriately which, where, when, and how to use these options for each patient.

An important recent clinical development in dental implant surgery is the concept of "minimally invasive" approaches to treatment. Specifically, there is a new drive toward minimally invasive implant placement. With advances in technologies, materials, and biologic sciences in dentistry, this approach to implant surgery is becoming more popular among clinicians and will most likely dominate the way dental implants will be placed in the near future.

Minimally invasive surgery in implant dentistry implies a surgical approach that minimizes the extent and number of surgeries while providing esthetics, predictability, and longevity with minimal surgical morbidity and discomfort to patients. The surgical approach most often required to achieve these goals for anterior implant therapy involves immediate implant placement, one-stage surgical approach, with or without flap, and simultaneous bone grafting. Furthermore, these surgical techniques need to be guided by a consistent surgical strategy that provides predictable esthetic results in implant dentistry. A minimally invasive approach to implant therapy in posterior sextants in which esthetics is not a major concern can be predictably achieved with the use of short wide implants.

This part of the chapter introduces surgical strategies that enhance the esthetic predictability in implant dentistry. The minimally invasive surgical approach to manage difficult esthetic and anatomically deficient cases is discussed with examples. The one-stage, immediate implant placement technique, which is the foundation of a patient-friendly approach to esthetic implant dentistry, is presented in detail. The thought processes involved in case selection, their scientific rationale, and proper techniques of soft and hard tissue management are described with cases. Topics are reviewed under the following heads:

- Surgical strategy for predictable esthetics
- Determine the level of surgical esthetic goal to be achieved (e only)
- Visualize the final outcome (e only)
- Preserve existing tissues important for esthetics (e only)
- Always overbuild bone and soft tissue in augmentation surgeries (e only)
- Immediate implant placement for predictability and esthetics
- Surgical management of difficult cases (minimally invasive approach (e only))
- Conclusion

Surgical Strategy for Predictable Esthetics

Observation of and adherence to the following surgical strategies enhance predictability and outcomes for esthetic dental implant surgeries with minimal discomfort to patients:

1. Determine the level of surgical esthetic goal to be achieved.
2. Visualize the final outcome.
3. Preserve existing tissues important for esthetics.
4. Always overbuild bone and soft tissue in augmentation surgeries.

Immediate Implant Placement for Predictability and Esthetics

Immediate implant placement in a one-stage approach, in which a healing abutment or provisional restoration is attached to the implant and remains exposed, provides more predictable preservation of the interproximal peri-implant gingival tissue with less patient discomfort and treatment time. This approach to implant placement is the foundation of a minimally invasive approach to esthetic implant dentistry. However, as with any surgical technique, it takes learning and practice to perform it properly. The criteria and techniques for proper immediate implant placement have previously been established and reported with successful long-term outcomes.

One of the more difficult aspects of immediate implant placement is positioning the implant with sufficient primary stability in an extraction socket, often without elevating a flap. The alveolar architecture in relation to the angle of the implant to be inserted; the presence or absence of a bone concavity apical to the extracted tooth; the amount of existing bone apical and palatal to the extraction socket, which can provide primary stability for the immediate implant; and the quality of the bone and soft tissues of the ridge should all be thoroughly evaluated clinically and radiographically before surgery. Many clinicians perform successful immediate implant placement without the aid of 3D scans [e.g., computed tomography (CT) or cone-beam CT (CBCT)]. However, if the tooth involved is long and large or if there is an alveolar concavity or other anatomic variations, the use of a CT/CBCT scan is advised.

A major disadvantage of placing implants immediately in the changing alveolar bone of an extraction socket is that it may result in progressive recession of the gingival labial margin over the implant restoration. Therefore, when placing an immediate implant with one-stage surgical approach in an esthetic zone, a prudent strategy would be to improve the quality and quantity of labial gingival tissue, which seems to be vital for the stability of the labial gingival margin involving immediate implants. One of the most effective ways to keep the implanted socket from collapsing and improve the labial gingival biotype is to simultaneously fill the labial socket void with particulate bone and augment the labial gingival tissue with soft tissue.

An effective bone and gingival tissue augmentation technique used with flapless immediate implant placement in a one-stage approach is the bone and crescent-shaped free gingival grafting technique. In this technique, the space between the inner surface of the labial bony wall and the labial surface of the implant is filled with slow-resorbing mineralized, freeze-dried particulate bone allograft or particulate xenograft to help preserve the horizontal dimension of the ridge (Fig. 59.31A). Then, a crescent-shaped soft-tissue graft is harvested from the ipsilateral palate (Fig. 59.31B) and transplanted into the labial recipient site coronal to the particulate bone graft (Fig. 59.31C). To provide/maintain the blood supply to the donor tissue, it is important that the outer surface of the crescent graft fits with an intimate contact with the bleeding lamina propria of the labial gingiva. Proper suturing ensures good proximity and prevents the graft from being displaced coronally out of the recipient site (Fig. 59.31D).

The advantage of this approach to gingival augmentation is simplicity and minimal surgical morbidity. In addition to providing a sealed protection for the bone graft, it prevents resorption of the sensitive labial crestal bone. Preparation of the recipient site involves no surgical manipulation other than deepithelialization as described. Gingival walls are completely intact with a full blood supply. The donor site wound is small (approximately 3 mm depth × 3 mm height at the widest point) with intact epithelium around the wound, which epithelializes within a week and causes minimal discomfort for the patient. Since each donor tissue graft is small, multiple grafts can be harvested from a single palate so that multiple immediate implants can be augmented at same time. Furthermore, this gingival augmentation technique frequently improves an unfavorable initial gingival margin because the grafted gingival margin is always coronal to the existing gingival margin. This minimizes a need for other time-consuming techniques, such as orthodontic extrusion, or a delayed approach to implant placement when the initial gingival margin is not esthetic or ideal, as recommended by many authors.

The risk-to-benefit ratio of the crescent grafting technique is favorable enough that if the graft does not survive, or if more than expected horizontal resorption of the ridge occurs, traditional techniques (e.g., subepithelial connective tissue graft) can be performed to augment the results. This is usually possible without refabrication of the implant restoration because the vertical height of the interdental papilla is sufficiently preserved with immediate implant placement in a one-stage approach.

Conclusion

The clinical science in dentistry has evolved to where placement of dental implants and restoring them requires sufficient knowledge in several disciplines of dentistry. In addition to mastering surgical objectives and techniques, periodontists must be able to evaluate and accurately diagnose (and treat or refer) a wide range of related "restorative" issues including but not limited to esthetics, occlusion, temporomandibular joint function, vertical dimension, and dental–skeletal relationships. These "other" aspects of diagnosis are essential for the development of an appropriate treatment plan, which is necessary for a successful outcome in esthetic implant dentistry.

In addition, with heightened expectations of esthetics pushing the art and science of dentistry, it is necessary more than ever for clinicians to fully understand all the available treatment options and to be able to appropriately determine which option to choose, when to use certain techniques, and how to apply them for each patient scenario.

The minimally invasive approach and techniques presented in this chapter are not the only ways to manage difficult esthetic cases, and some may consider them controversial. Certainly, these techniques require learning and practice to make them effective in each clinician's hands. However, they present a sound approach to what is possible in hard- and soft-tissue management for esthetic implant surgery and provide effective strategies and techniques for solving many difficult esthetic cases in a patient-friendly manner.

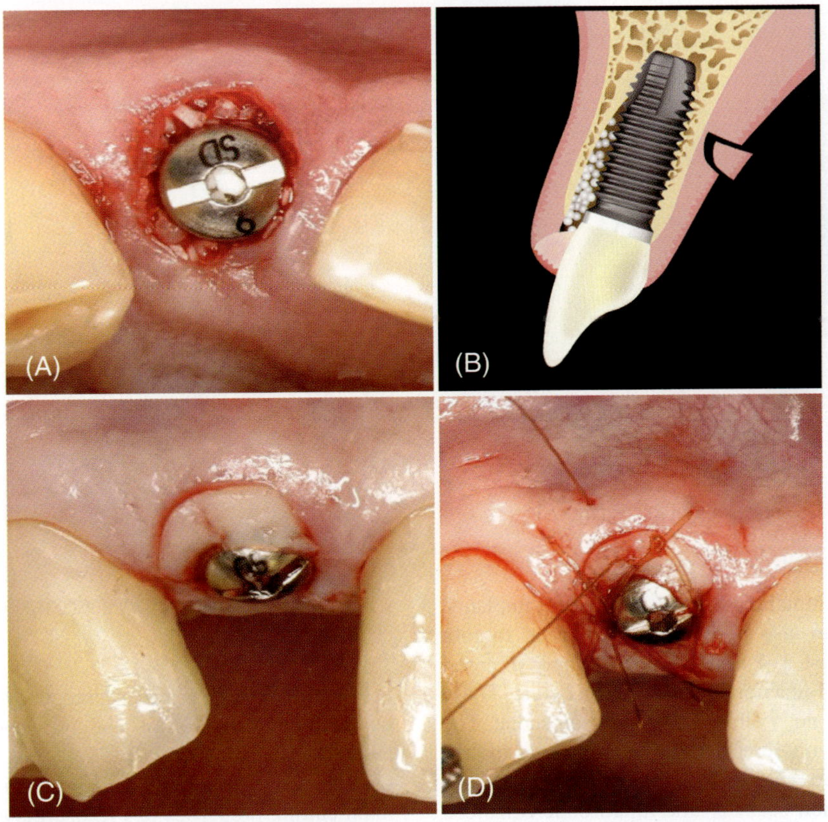

Fig. 59.31 A, Bone graft material is lightly packed into the extraction socket gap between the labial wall and the implant surface. B, Diagram of crescent-shaped, free gingival graft tissue being harvested from the palate. C, Clinical photograph of crescent-shaped, free gingival graft tissue positioned over the bone graft to fit snuggly in the gap between the gingival wall and the implant surface. D, Crescent-shaped, free gingival graft is sutured in place using 5–0 gut sutures. The sutures pass through the gingival graft toward the labial gingival margin and are tied. Then, without cutting the ends, the suture is passed over the graft and tied to the palatal gingival tissue. Three sutures are needed to keep the graft in position.

Dental Implant Microsurgery—Immediate Placement

The success of dental implants in extraction sites combined with immediate provisionals for newly placed dental implants has brought a convergence in restorative and surgical practice for treatment planning of dental implants. This convergence reaches its summit in the approach to failing teeth in the maxillary esthetic zone. For anatomic reasons, maxillary anterior teeth are at high risk for traumatic injury (Fig. 59.35). Traumatized teeth frequently receive endodontic treatment that may be followed by horizontal or vertical root fracture. Dentistry's historic answer to tooth loss has been the fixed bridge. Tooth preparation necessary for a fixed bridge often results in significant reduction of tooth structure. Inherent esthetic limitations of fixed bridges include loss of gingival papillae and resorption of the buccal alveolar plate. For these reasons, dental implants are a preferred choice for tooth replacement in the maxillary esthetic zone.

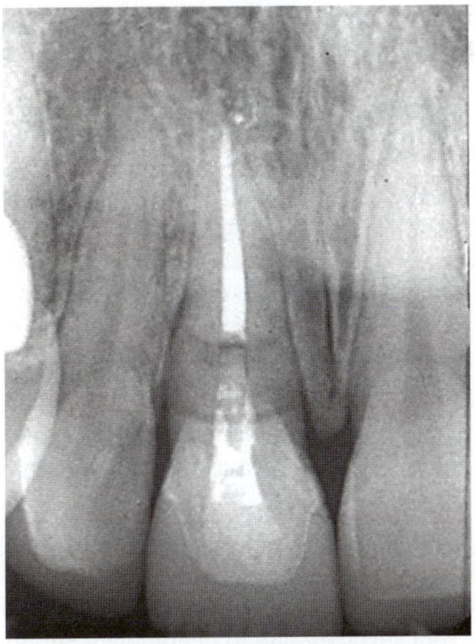

Fig. 59.35 X-ray of typical fractured central incisor.

Implant Microsurgery

Microsurgery is associated with enhanced soft-tissue procedures and fine suturing. This is part of the scope of implant microsurgery but additional benefits include dental implant drilling precision. The ability to discern minute dimensional differences permits implant osteotomy preparations centered exactly between reference points such as adjacent teeth, adjacent implants, or buccal and lingual ridge anatomy. More profoundly, the microscope allows immediate detection of subtle changes in drill position so appropriate feedback corrections can be applied to the handpiece. Enhanced angular perception is also important. The drill's angular position can be oriented relative to small landmarks such as the implant platform surface level or the angle of adjacent implant healing caps. This

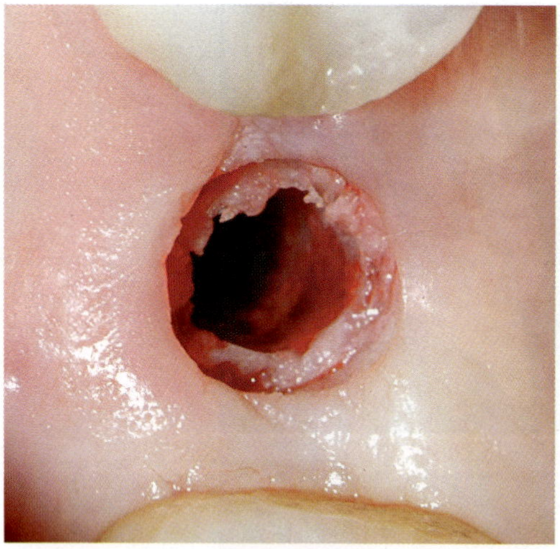

Fig. 59.36 Flapless dental implant microsurgery.

permits optimal parallel positioning and depth of adjacent implants. The implant drill angle can also be accurately oriented to root surface angulation using just 3–4 mm of root anatomy exposed between the cementoenamel junction and the osseous crest. These reference points are simply not visible without a microscope. The detection of subtle angulation reference points and changes in drill position permit feedback correction, which is important for osteotomy preparation in extraction sockets. The microscope-enhanced accuracy of osteotomy microsurgery permits socket implant placement in an ideal position followed by an esthetic implant-supported provisional (Fig. 59.36). As a flapless procedure, this is accomplished with minimal patient morbidity. The details of the procedure are given online under the following heads:

Microsurgical tooth extraction (e only)
Implant drilling in the extraction site (e only)
Bone grafting (e only)
Buccal gingival grafting (e only)
Immediate provisional fabrication (e only)
Immediate implant occlusion (e only)
Custom impression transfer coping (e only)
Final implant restoration (e only)

Conclusion

Some of the advantages of microsurgery for extraction and implant placement have been described with an emphasis on tissue management and the ability to enhance visualization of details, which translates into better results. This microsurgery protocol advances dentistry from an era of traumatic tooth extraction to one of seamless immediate tooth replacement using implant microsurgery.

Piezoelectric Bone Surgery

Ultrasound has been used for many years in periodontics to remove tartar, debride root surfaces, and to degranulate periodontal defects. In the past decade, a novel family of ultrasonic-powered devices has been developed that is revolutionizing maxillofacial bone surgery.

A new surgical technique, known as *Piezosurgery*, was invented by Vercellotti and developed by Mectron Medical Technology. The Piezosurgery device (Fig. 59.50) consists of a piezoelectric ultrasonic transducer powered by an ultrasonic generator, capable of driving a range of specially designed cutting inserts. The Piezosurgery device employs ultrasonic vibrations to cut mineralized

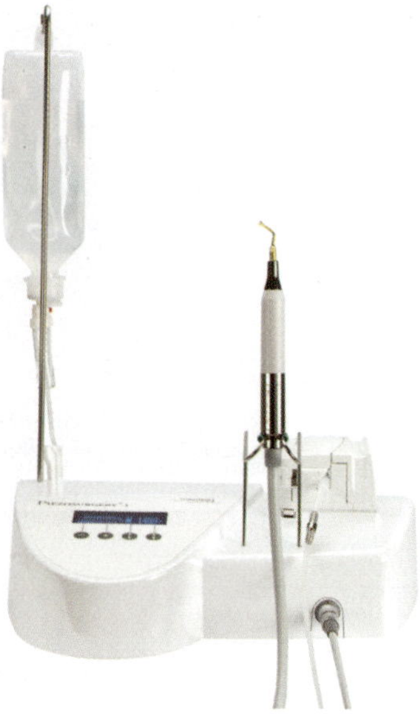

Fig. 59.50 Piezosurgery device by Mectron Medical Technology.

tissues. To this end, a primary frequency at 30 kHz is overmodulated by the superimposition of a sound wave (30–60 Hz) to generate a hammering action that effectively cuts bone without harming soft tissues and with minimal heat production. Box 59.6 describes the main cutting properties of Piezosurgery by Mectron, and Box 59.7 describes Piezosurgery inserts. Piezoelectric bone surgery techniques have been developed for clinical applications in dentistry and are becoming state of the art for a variety of procedures. Recently, Piezosurgery Medical expanded development of clinical applications to other fields of medicine. The extraordinary cutting properties of piezoelectric bone surgery have been introduced and applied in maxillofacial surgery, facial plastic surgery, otolaryngologic surgery, cranial and spinal neurosurgery, and minute orthopedic surgery.

The most compelling characteristics of piezoelectric bone surgery are low surgical trauma, exceptional control during surgery, and a fast healing response of tissues. Clinical studies demonstrate that the specificity of operation and the techniques employed with piezoelectric bone surgery make it possible to advantageously

BOX 59.6 Description and Cutting Properties of Piezosurgery by Mectron

Bone Operating Mode

Cortical Bone

The basic low ultrasonic frequency (30 kHz) is overmodulated by sound waves for cutting and removing small cortical bone fragments.

Spongy Bone

The basic low ultrasonic frequency is overmodulated by sound waves that are slower than those for cortical bone, which is better for cutting and removing cancellous bone fragments.

Root Operating Mode

Periodontal Surgery

The low ultrasonic frequency without overmodulation is set at an ideal power level for scaling, debridement, and root planing.

Endodontic Surgery

The ultrasonic frequency is set at an ideal power level for retrocanal and intracanal debridement after root canal treatment.

BOX 59.7 Description of Piezosurgery Inserts

The mechanical action of bone cutting takes place thanks to the linear microvibrations of inserts with a variable range from 20 to 80 μm, depending on efficiency. Piezosurgery inserts are classified based on their functional and clinical characteristics.

Functional Classification

1. Sharp: These inserts have sharp ends for osteotomy and osteoplasty. They are made of nitride titanium steel and they are gold in color.
2. Smoothing: These nitride titanium inserts are diamond coated and gold in color. Their different granulometry produces a smoothening action that is generally used to complete the cut near soft tissue.
3. Blunt: These steel color inserts are characterized by rounded ends and are generally used to refine the cut in contact with soft tissue.

The inserts described in the functional classification as sharp, smoothing, and blunt have clinical classification codes that relate to their specific use.

Clinical Classification

1. OT: The identification code for inserts used to perform osteotomy is *OT* followed by a number.
2. OP: The identification code for inserts used to perform osteoplasty is *OP* followed by a number.
3. EX: The identification code for inserts used to perform extraction is *EX* followed by a number.
4. IM: The identification code for inserts used to perform implant site preparation is *IM* followed by a number.

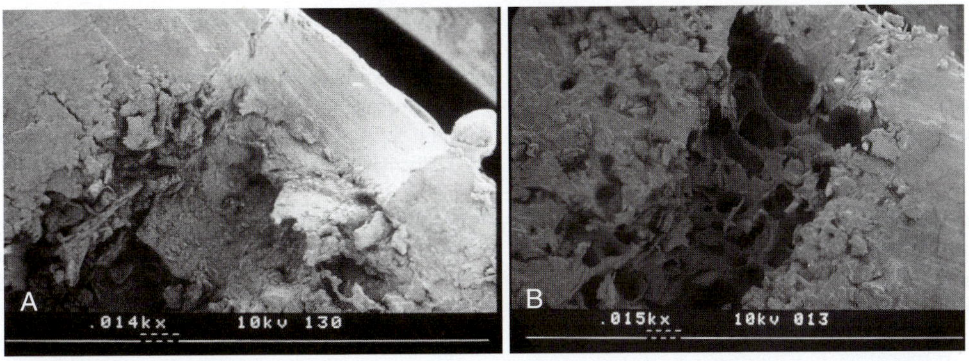

Fig. 59.51 Comparison of bone surfaces prepared with rotary instrumentation and Piezosurgery (Mectron Medical Technology, Carasco, Italy). A, Rotary technique: in vitro photograph of the implant site following preparation with twist drill of 3.15 mm. The site is ready to receive the implant. Note the compact surface of the cortical bone where no vascular canals are visible. The underlying spongiosa is irregular due to the presence of bone debris in the endosteal spaces. B, Piezoelectric technique: in vitro image of implant site preparation with 3-mm ultrasonic inserts. The site is ready to receive the implant. Note the cortical bone microporosity where open vascular canals are clearly visible. The underlying spongiosa is intact and free from bone debris. *(Courtesy: Dr. Alberto Rebaudi, Genoa, Italy.)*

exploit differences in hard- and soft-tissue anatomy. This not only increases treatment effectiveness but it also improves postoperative recovery and healing. Experimental studies on animals have shown faster tissue healing when compared to traditional cutting instruments.

Ideally, surgical trauma should be minimized to obtain the optimal healing, which depends on gentle management of soft and hard tissues. Surgery, by definition, alters normal physiology by interrupting the vascular supply of tissues. The degree of surgical invasiveness is extremely important for the quality of tissue healing and may effect whether wounds heal by repair or regeneration. Indeed, when surgical trauma is kept to a minimum, it generates enough stimulation to favor healing mechanisms that lead to regeneration. On the other hand, surgical techniques that are more traumatic often lead to greater inflammatory responses with slow healing that may lead to repair and scarring rather than regeneration. For this reason, it is desirable to choose the least-traumatic surgical instruments and techniques for any surgical procedure. Piezoelectric bone surgery was conceived and developed precisely to overcome the limits of traditional bone-cutting instruments and to achieve the most effective treatment with the least morbidity.

From a mechanical standpoint, the effect of burs or twist drills on bone is characterized by lamellar fracturing in areas adjacent to the cut surface and the deposition of large bone fragments and debris in the endosteal spaces. This finding is thought to be, at least in part, responsible for the inflammatory process that takes place in the immediate postsurgical wound healing and for the delay of osteogenesis observed in these wounds. In contrast, the micromechanical cutting action of piezoelectric bone surgery results in micronization of the cut bone and does not cause lamellar fracturing in adjacent bone, which may favor exposure and release of BMPs and be responsible for the early onset of osteogenesis at these sites. Furthermore, there may be a diminished inflammatory response since there is little or no need to remove damaged bone and surgical debris as compared to conventional rotary-drilled sites (Fig. 59.51).

Clinical Characteristics of Ultrasonic Cutting

The primary clinical characteristics of the Piezosurgery cutting action include microprecision, selective cutting, maximum visibility, and excellent healing.

Microprecision

Piezosurgery cuts mineralized tissues with microprecision and extraordinary surgical control. Piezoelectric osteotomies are easy to create, but it is important to recognize that the technique and instrument handling are different from the technique using a traditional handpiece with rotary instruments. The Piezosurgery insert is

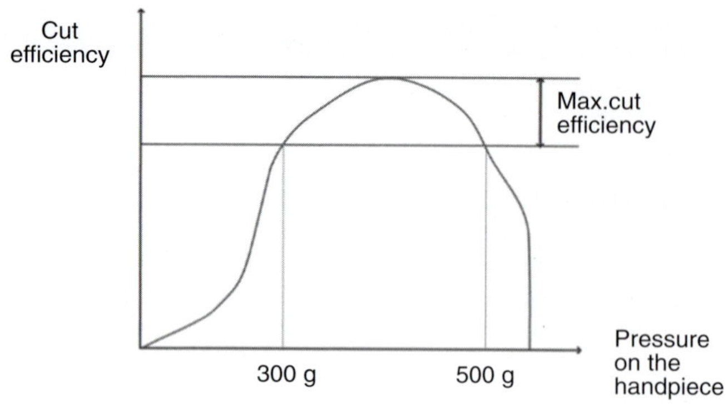

Fig. 59.52 Graph illustrating the relationship between Piezosurgery (Mectron Medical Technology, Carasco, Italy) cutting efficiency and pressure applied on the handpiece. Note that optimal cutting efficiency is found between 300 and 500 g; pressure in excess of 500 g leads to a sudden and complete loss of cutting efficiency. *Max.*, Maximum.

applied to the bone with a relatively light stroke similar to the smooth precision used to draw a picture. Heavy pressure or force is not required and can, in fact, antagonize the ultrasonic frequency, thus reducing efficiency and transforming mechanical energy into thermal energy (Fig. 59.52). The microprecision of this instrument is made possible by the ultrasonic frequency, which produces mechanical microshock waves at a linear range of approximately 80 µm. The extraordinary surgical control that characterizes Piezosurgery is due to the fact that its microvibrations require only light pressure (approximately 300 g) to be applied to the handpiece. Indeed, the pressure applied by the surgeon to the Piezosurgery handpiece is much lower than the pressure typically applied to a rotary or oscillating type handpiece (approximately 5000 g), which uses mechanical macrovibrations for cutting. This characteristic provides maximum control during surgery and makes this technique unique, especially in areas with delicate anatomy.

Selective Cutting

Piezosurgery ultrasonic microvibrations are low frequency and selective for cutting mineralized tissue only. These microvibrations are physically unable to cut soft tissue. Clearly, the most significant demonstrated benefit of Piezosurgery selective cutting is the ability to preserve the integrity of soft tissues, such as the alveolar nerve, the infraorbital nerve, the maxillary sinus membrane, and the dura mater, while effectively cutting the mineralized tissue (bone) in close proximity to these tissues.

Maximum Visibility

Piezosurgery allows maximum visibility by creating a surgical field that is blood free during cutting because of the cavitation of the cooling irrigation solution. Cavitation is a physical phenomenon that, from a clinical standpoint, happens with the nebulization of the saline solution when it contacts the insert vibrating at ultrasonic frequency. The slight hydropneumatic pressure applied by the nebulized irrigation fluid induces hemostasis in both hard and soft tissues. An important advantage of the cavitation effect is the thorough debridement of the surgical site at the time of the mechanical removal of inflammatory tissue by means of dedicated Piezosurgery inserts. This effect is only temporary, and bleeding resumes shortly after the cutting (and cavitation) action is stopped. Clinically, it is important to ensure proper irrigation and intermittent cutting action to maintain optimal surface microcirculation, especially for long surgical procedures. An added benefit of the temporary hemostasis induced by the cavitation effect is the notably reduced blood loss, especially during longer procedures, which leads to decreased postoperative edema.

Excellent Healing

Clinical studies comparing use of piezoelectric bone surgery with traditional rotary instruments for third molar extractions and periodontal surgery have reported better recovery and fewer postoperative symptoms in those treated with Piezosurgery. Postoperative healing after piezoelectric bone surgery is characterized by minimal swelling and little bleeding and postoperative morbidity is lower compared to traditional techniques.

Improved hard and soft tissue healing are discussed online.

Clinical Applications

The clinical use of Piezosurgery in osseous surgery advantageously promotes all the benefits of microsurgery, especially when working under optical magnification. Piezosurgery has become an essential instrument in dentistry and in periodontal daily practice to minimize patients' morbidity and increase overall clinical predictability. Piezoelectric bone surgery has many important clinical applications in dentistry. In fact, nearly all techniques previously performed with burs, twist drills, chisels, or oscillating saws have the potential to be performed with Piezosurgery. For 18 consecutive years, one of the authors (T.V.) has used Piezosurgery on a daily basis for oral, periodontal, and implant surgical procedures, thus enabling him to develop techniques and protocols for each. Readers are referred to online materials and other publications for detailed descriptions and step-by-step instructions on these Piezosurgery protocols. A brief overview of basic clinical applications using piezoelectric surgery is described online under the following heads:

- Use of Piezosurgery in periodontal surgery, crown lengthening, tooth extraction, implant site preparation.
- Advanced clinical applications of piezosurgery like in sinus lift, ridge expansion using both particulate and block bone grafts.

Conclusion

Piezosurgery is a new surgical technique for bone surgery with many clinical applications in dentistry. The extraordinary cutting properties and applications of piezoelectric bone surgery were described. The most compelling characteristics of piezoelectric bone surgery are low surgical trauma, exceptional precision, and fast healing response. As a result, Piezosurgery has the ability to increase treatment effectiveness while improving postoperative recovery and healing.

Although a great deal of scientific research focuses on new products for tissue engineering and bone regeneration, the importance of minimal surgical trauma for optimal bone healing and regeneration should not be overlooked. A new appreciation for the effectiveness of Piezosurgery has the potential to redefine the concept of minimally invasive surgery in osteotomy and osteoplasty procedures.

Key points

- Threaded endosseous implants can be placed using either a one-stage (nonsubmerged) or a two-stage (submerged) protocol.
- In one-stage approach, the implant or the abutment emerges through the mucoperiosteum/gingival tissue at the time of implant placement.
- In two-stage approach, the top of the implant and cover screw are completely covered with the flap.

- Tapping is not necessary or recommended in a very soft, poor quality bone (e.g., loose trabecular bone in the posterior maxilla).
- The biologic mechanisms that support the use of bone graft materials are osteoconduction, osteoinduction, and osteogenesis.
- Bone grafts can be autografts, allografts (derived from the same species), xenografts (derived from a different species), and alloplasts or synthetic graft materials.
- Bone graft particles in the range of 1001000 μm are conducive to neovascularization and ingrowth of bone.
- Depending on the quantity, quality, and support of existing bone, as well as the preferences of the clinician and patient, the placement of implants after tooth extraction can be immediate, delayed, or staged.
- Immediate implant placement occurs at the time of extraction.
- Delayed implant placement is performed approximately 2 months after extraction to allow for soft tissue healing.
- Staged implant placement allows for substantial bone healing within the extraction site, which typically requires 4–6 months or longer.

Suggested Readings

Attard N, Barzilay I: A modified impression technique for accurate registration of peri-implant soft tissues, *J Can Dent Assoc* 69:80–83, 2003.

Bahat O, Handelsman M: Periodontal reconstructive flaps—classification and surgical considerations, *Int J Periodontics Restorative Dent* 11: 480–487, 1991.

Becker W, Becker BE, Caffesse R: A comparison of demineralized freeze-dried bone and autologous bone to induce bone formation in human extraction sockets, *J Periodontol* 65:1128–1133, 1994a.

Becker W, Becker BE, Polizzi G: Autogenous bone grafting of bone defects adjacent to implants placed into immediate extraction sockets in patients: a prospective study, *Int J Oral Maxillofac Implants* 9:398, 1994b.

Becker W, Dahlin C, Becker BE, et al: The use of e-PTFE barrier membranes for bone promotion around titanium implants placed into extraction sockets: a prospective multicenter study, *Int J Oral Maxillofac Implants* 9:31–40, 1994c.

Becker W, Schenk R, Higuchi K, et al: Variations in bone regeneration adjacent to implants augmented with barrier membranes alone or with demineralized freeze-dried bone or autologous grafts: a study in dogs, *Int J Oral Maxillofac Implants* 10:143–154, 1995.

Becker W, Hujoel P, Becker BE: Effect of barrier membranes and autologous bone grafts on ridge width preservation around implants, *Clin Implant Dent Relat Res* 4:143–149, 2002.

Boyne PJ, Lilly LC, Marx RE, et al: De novo bone induction by recombinant human bone morphogenetic protein-2 (rhBMP-2) in maxillary sinus floor augmentation, *J Oral Maxillofac Surg* 63:1693–1707, 2005.

Breeding LC, Dixon DL: Transfer of gingival contours to a master cast, *J Prosthet Dent* 75:341–343, 1996.

Brief J, Edinger D, Hassfeld S, et al: Accuracy of image-guided implantology, *Clin Oral Implants Res* 16:495–501, 2005.

Buser D, Dula K, Hirt HP, et al: Lateral ridge augmentation using autografts and barrier membranes: a clinical study with 40 partially edentulous patients, *J Oral Maxillofac Surg* 54:420–432, 1996.

Chen ST, Darby IB, Reynolds EC, et al: Immediate implant placement postextraction without flap elevation, *J Periodontol* 80:163–172, 2009.

Cochran DL, Wozney JM: Biological mediators for periodontal regeneration, *Periodontol 2000* 19:40–58, 1999.

Covani U, Barone A, Cornelini R, et al: Soft tissue healing around implants placed immediately after tooth extraction without incision: a clinical report, *Int J Oral Maxillofac Implants* 19:549–553, 2004.

De Bruyn H, Koole S, Mattheos N, et al: A survey on undergraduate implant dentistry education in Europe, *Eur J Dent Educ* 13(Suppl 1):3–9, 2009.

Del Fabbro M, Testori T, Francetti L, et al: Systematic review of survival rates for implants placed in the grafted maxillary sinus, *Int J Periodontics Restorative Dent* 24:565, 2004.

Derycke R, Tracol JJ, Mongeot M, et al: La chirurgie Implantaire mini-invasive: un nouvel environnement clinique et de communication, *Clinic*, 2012, 6–19 November Special Issue.

Fitzpatrick JM, West JB, Maurer CR Jr: Predicting error in rigid-body point-based registration, *IEEE Trans Med Imaging* 17:694–702, 1998.

Fortin T, Coudert JL, Champleboux G, et al: Computer-assisted dental implant surgery using computed tomography, *J Image Guid Surg* 1:53–58, 1995.

Geurs NC, Wang IC, Shulman LB, et al: Retrospective radiographic analysis of sinus graft and implant placement procedures from the Academy of Osseointegration Consensus Conference on Sinus Grafts, *Int J Periodontics Restorative Dent* 21:517–523, 2001.

Grunder U: Stability of the mucosal topography around single-tooth implants and adjacent teeth: 1-year results, *Int J Periodontics Restorative Dent* 20:11–17, 2000.

Han TJ, Jeong CW: Bone and crescent shaped free gingival grafting for anterior immediate implant placement: technique and case report, *J Implant Adv Clin Dent* 1(5):23–33, 2009.

Hinds KF: Custom impression coping for an exact registration of the healed tissue in the esthetic implant restoration, *Int J Periodontics Restorative Dent* 17:584–591, 1997.

Ilizarov GA: Clinical application of the tension-stress effect for limb lengthening, *Clin Orthop Relat Res* 250:8–26, 1990.

Jensen OT, Shulman LB, Block MS, et al: Report of the Sinus Consensus Conference of 1996, *Int J Oral Maxillofac Implants* 13(Suppl):11–45, 1998.

Kai J, Shiomi H, Sasama T, et al: Optical high-precision three-dimensional position measurement system suitable for head motion tracking in frameless stereotactic radiosurgery, *Comput Aided Surg* 3:257–263, 1998.

Kan JY, Rungcharassaeng K, Lozada J: Immediate placement and provisionalization of maxillary anterior single implants: 1-year prospective study, *Int J Oral Maxillofac Implants* 18:31–39, 2003.

Kan JY, Rungcharassaeng K, Lozada JL: Bilaminar subepithelial connective tissue grafts for immediate implant placement and provisionalization in the esthetic zone, *J Calif Dent Assoc* 33:865–871, 2005.

Kawachi H, Kawachi Y, Ikeda C, et al: Oral and maxillofacial surgery with computer-assisted navigation system, *Bull Tokyo Dent Coll* 51:35–39, 2010.

Klein M, Abrams M: Computer-guided surgery utilizing a computer-milled surgical template, *Pract Proced Aesthet Dent* 13:165–169, 2001.

Klokkevold PR: Implant education in the dental curriculum, *J Calif Dent Assoc* 29(11):747–755, 2001.

Klokkevold PR, Han TJ, Camargo PM: Esthetic management of extractions for implant site development: delayed versus staged implant placement, *Pract Periodontics Aesthet Dent* 11:603–610, 1999.

Lazzara RJ, Porter SS: Platform switching: a new concept in implant dentistry for controlling postrestorative crestal bone levels, *Int J Periodontics Restorative Dent* 26:9–17, 2006.

Malamas E, Petrakis E, Zervakis M, et al: A survey of industrial vision systems: applications and tools, *Image Vis Comput* 21:171–188, 2003.

Mattheos N, Albrektsson T, Buser D, et al: Teaching and assessment of implant dentistry in undergraduate and postgraduate education: a European consensus, *Eur J Dent Educ* 13(Suppl 1):11–17, 2009.

Mellonig JT, Nevins M: Guided bone regeneration of bone defects associated with implants: an evidence-based outcome assessment, *Int J Periodontics Restorative Dent* 15:168–185, 1995.

O'Sullivan D, Sennerby L, Meredith N: Influence of implant taper on the primary and secondary stability of osseointegrated titanium implants, *Clin Oral Implants Res* 15:474–480, 2004.

Park KB, Ryu KH: *The short implant (5 mm and 6 mm in length)*, Seoul, Korea, 2007, Narae Publishing, Inc.

Park KB, Ryu KH: *Super wide diameter implants. The rescue system (from 6. 0 mm to 8. 0 mm in diameter)*, Seoul, Korea, 2008, Narae Publishing, Inc.

Pennec X, Thirion JP: A framework for uncertainty and validation of 3D registration methods based on points and frames, *Int J Comput Vis* 25:203, 1997.

Petropoulos VC, Arbree NS, Tarnow D, et al: Teaching implant dentistry in the predoctoral curriculum: a report from the ADEA Implant Workshop's survey of deans, *J Dent Educ* 70(5):580–588, 2006.

Preti G, Martinasso G, Peirone B, et al: Cytokines and growth factors involved in the osseointegration of oral titanium implants positioned using piezoelectric bone surgery versus a drill technique: a pilot study in minipigs, *J Periodontol* 78(4):716, 2007.

Rosano G, Taschieri S, Gaudy JF, et al: Maxillary sinus vascular anatomy and its relation to sinus lift surgery, *Clin Oral Implants Res* 22:711–715, 2011.

Saadoun AP: Immediate implant placement and temporization in extraction and healing sites, *Compend Contin Educ Dent* 23, 2002, 309–312, 314–306, 318 passim, quiz 326.

Schaeren S, Jaquiéry C, Heberer M, et al: Assessment of nerve damage using a novel ultrasonic device for bone cutting, *J Oral Maxillofac Surg* 66:593, 2008.

Shanelec DA: Anterior esthetic implants: microsurgical placement in extraction sockets with immediate provisionals, *J Calif Dent Assoc* 33:233–240, 2005.

Simion M, Dahlin C, Trisi P, et al: Qualitative and quantitative comparative study on different filling materials used in bone tissue regeneration: a controlled clinical study, *Int J Periodontics Restorative Dent* 14: 198–215, 1994.

Simion M, Fontana F, Rasperini G, et al: Vertical ridge augmentation by expanded-polytetrafluoroethylene membrane and a combination of intraoral autogenous bone graft and deproteinized anorganic bovine bone (Bio Oss), *Clin Oral Implants Res* 18:620–629, 2007.

Small BW: Achieving and maintaining periodontal health and esthetics following the extraction of a central incisor, *Gen Dent* 51:396–398, 2003.

Summers RB: A new concept in maxillary implant surgery: the osteotome technique, *Compendium* 15, 1994, 152, 154–156, 158 passim, quiz 162.

Touati B, Guez G, Saadoun A: Esthetic soft tissue integration and optimized emergence profile: provisionalization and customized impression coping, *Pract Periodontics Aesthet Dent* 11:305–314, 1999, quiz 316.

Urban IA, Lozada JL: Implants placed in augmented sinuses with minimal and moderate residual crestal bone: results after 1 to 5 years, *Int J Oral Maxillofac Implants* 25:1203–1212, 2010.

Vercellotti T: Piezoelectric surgery in implantology: a case report—a new piezoelectric ridge expansion technique, *Int J Periodontics Restorative Dent* 20(4):359, 2000.

Vercellotti T: Technological characteristics and clinical indications of piezoelectric bone surgery, *Minerva Stomatol* 53(5):207, 2004.

Vercellotti T: *Essentials in piezosurgery. Clinical advantages in dentistry*, Hanover Park, IL, 2009, Quintessence.

Vercellotti T, Crovace A, Palermo A, et al: The piezoelectric osteotomy in orthopedics: clinical and histological evaluations (pilot study in animals), *Medit J Surg Med* 9:89, 2001a.

Vercellotti T, De Paoli S, Nevins M: The piezoelectric bony window osteotomy and sinus membrane elevation: introduction of a new technique for simplification of the sinus augmentation procedure, *Int J Periodontics Restorative Dent* 21(6):561, 2001b.

Vercellotti T, Nevins ML, Kim DM, et al: Osseous response following resective therapy with a piezosurgery, *Int J Periodontics Restorative Dent* 25(6):543, 2005.

Wallace SS, Froum SJ: Effect of maxillary sinus augmentation on the survival of endosseous dental implants. A systematic review, *Ann Periodontol* 8:328, 2003.

References

References and MCQs with answers for the chapter are available on www.medenact.com.

CHAPTER 60

Results and Complications of Implant Therapy

SJ Froum | PR Klokkevold | SC Cho | SH Froum | A Jain

CHAPTER OUTLINE

The landmark Göteborg study and the replica study at the University of Toronto supported expectations for the success and predictability of root-form dental implants. The study, conducted over a 15-year period at the University of Göteborg, Sweden, by P.I. Bränemark and coworkers, began in 1965 and concluded in 1980. The results, which were reported in several articles, defined the concept of osseointegration, described protocols for success, and shared clinical experiences.

The most significant article from the study, published in 1981, was on osseointegrated implants in the treatment of the edentulous jaw. The Göteborg study included 2768 root-form implants placed into 410 edentulous jaws in 371 consecutive patients. The data were most often reported in subsets according to the three study phases (i.e., initial, developmental, and routine). Cases treated in the routine period with standardized procedures and an observation time of 5–9 years were thought to reflect the potential of the method and were the basis of data reported in that historic publication. The subset consisted of 895 implants placed in 130 jaws. The implant survival rate was 81% in the maxilla and 91% in mandible. The prosthesis survival (i.e., continuous stability) rate was 89% in the maxilla and 100% in the mandible.

The replica study, which was conducted at the University of Toronto, demonstrated that comparable results could be predictably achieved using the same implant design and treatment protocols. Together, these studies demonstrated that implant survival of 81% or more and prosthesis survival of 89% or more could be expected in the edentulous patient.

In the decades since the landmark discovery of osseointegration and the documentation of its clinical effectiveness, clinicians have had tremendous success in replacing missing teeth with endosseous root-form dental implants in both partially edentulous and edentulous patients. Despite the high level of success and long-term predictability, a 100% success rate cannot be achieved. Complications and implant failures do occur. Some implants fail to achieve osseointegration; some achieve osseointegration but lose bone progressively over time, leading to failure; and other implants rapidly lose bone and fail in a short time. Some implants achieve and maintain osseointegration but fail because they do not meet the esthetic expectations of the patient or clinician.

The reporting of implant success varies widely in the literature, which makes defining an absolute implant success rate impractical. This chapter considers implant treatment results in light of the factors that influence implant survival and success. The intent is to outline important aspects that need to be considered in evaluating implant outcomes and offer guidelines for understanding published results.

Defining Implant Outcomes

Implant outcomes are reported in a variety of ways in the literature. Various levels of implant success and failure are described in case reports, case series, retrospective studies, controlled studies, and prospective studies. The type of study and method of reporting are decided by the authors and often influenced by the data collected and the study objectives. Each type of study or report has recognized limitations, but because of tremendous variation that exists in the ways individual investigators measure, interpret, and report implant outcomes, differences in the results from one study to another may not be obvious.

Some implant outcomes are reported as the presence or absence of the implant at the time of the last examination, regardless of whether the implant was functional, suffered from bone loss, or had other problems. This type of assessment is a measure of implant *survival* and should not be confused with implant *success*. In contrast to such an overly simplified assessment, some investigators report implant outcomes using specific criteria to determine implant success.

Implant success is defined by specific criteria used to evaluate the condition and function of the implant. Criteria for implant success have been proposed in the literature but have not been used consistently. The problem is that a universally accepted definition of implant success has not been established. In the classic definition, Albrektsson and colleagues defined success as an implant with no pain, no mobility, no radiolucent peri-implant areas, and less than 0.2 mm of bone loss annually after the first year of loading. Bone loss in the first year was recognized, but it was not defined or quantified as part of the success criteria until later in a separate definition by Roos and associates.

The challenge in comparing reported data between studies is that investigators use different criteria for success in their work. As a result, it is difficult or impossible to make comparisons between studies, and drawing conclusions about implant success or failure from data reported in different studies is tenuous.

Success rates are dramatically affected by variations in the criteria used to define them. In strict terms, if implant success is considered to be an outcome without adverse effects or problems, the treatment would be performed as planned, implants would remain stable and functioning without problems, peri-implant tissues would be stable and healthy, and the patient and treating clinician would be pleased with the outcome (Fig. 60.1A–D). Use of strict criteria would produce implant success rates lower than those determined using less stringent criteria.

Table 60.1 illustrates the powerful effect that small changes in success criteria have on reported success rates. The data demonstrate that changing the criteria of success to include a probing pocket depth (PPD) of 5 mm or less to 6 mm or less changed the implant success rates from 52.4% to 62% and from 79.1% to 81.3% for patients with and without a history of periodontitis, respectively. This also shows that implant survival is quite different from implant success.

Implant survival is defined as an implant that remains in place at the time of evaluation, regardless of untoward signs and symptoms or a history of problems. Extant implants that are healthy and functioning under an implant-retained restoration are different from those that are suffering from peri-implant bone loss or those that are not connected to a restoration and not functioning (Fig. 60.2), but these operational differences do not affect calculations of implant survival. Implants that are osseointegrated but not functional are referred to as sleepers and should not be

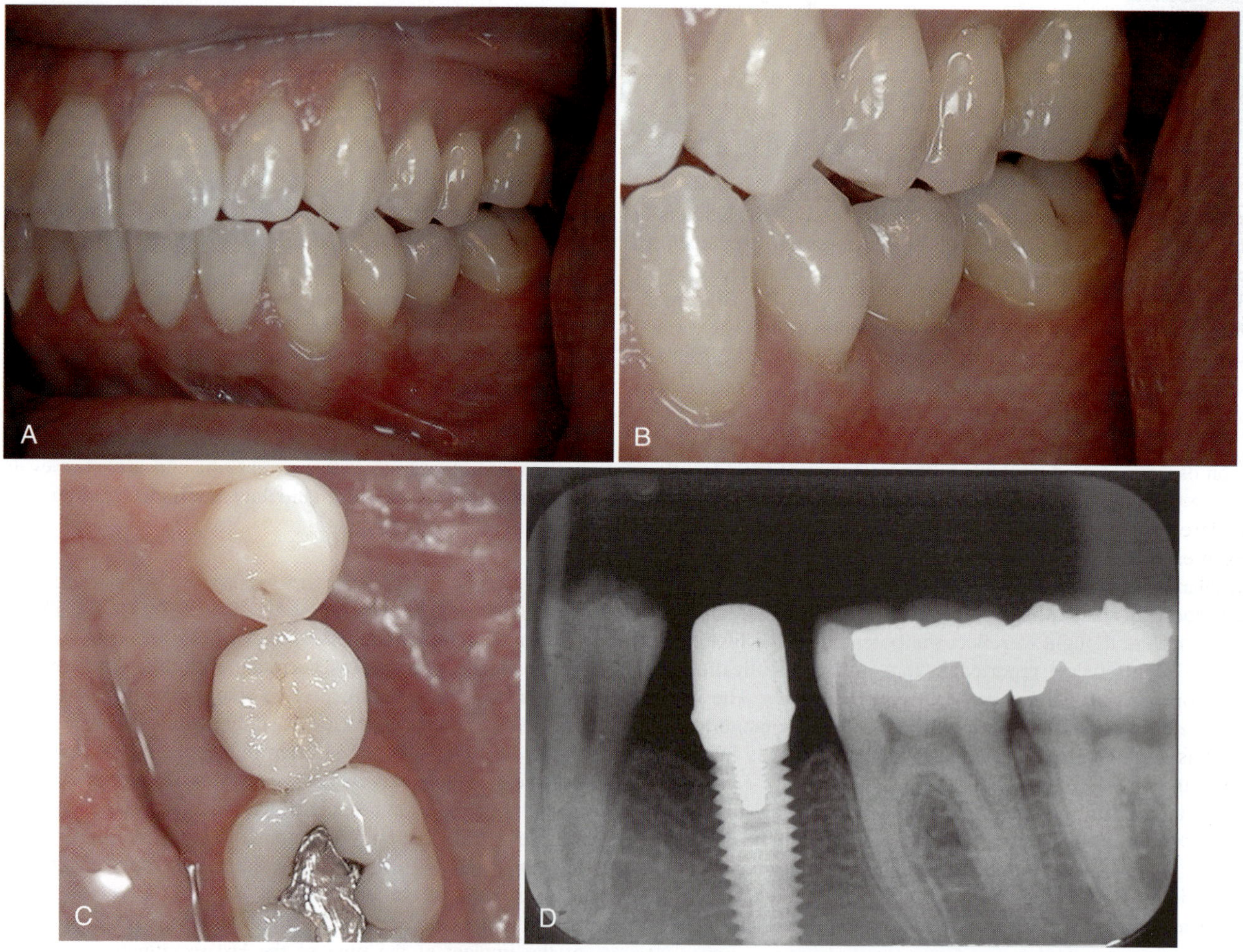

Fig. 60.1 Clinical implant success was demonstrated when a single implant was placed in the mandible to replace the lower second premolar (as planned). The implant osseointegrated and function was successfully restored. The patient and clinicians were pleased with the outcome. A, Photograph of the dentition in occlusion (from the left side). B, Close-up photograph of the dentition in occlusion. The mandibular second premolar is an implant-supported crown. C, Occlusal view of an implant-supported crown in the second premolar position. Replacement of the mandibular second premolar with an implant is a conservative treatment, obviating the need to prepare adjacent teeth. D, Periapical radiograph of the posterior mandibular teeth and implant in the second premolar position. Bone support is good, and bone loss is minimal and consistent with expectations for this implant design.

TABLE 60.1 Effect of Slight Modifications of Implant Success Criteria on Successful Outcomes[a]

Group	PPD ≤5 mm, No BOP, BL <0.2 mm/yr (%)	PPD ≤6 mm, No BOP, BL <0.2 mm/yr (%)	PPD ≤5 mm, No BOP (%)	PPD ≤6 mm, No BOP (%)	Implant Survival (%)
Group A	52.4	62	71.4	81	90.5
Group B	79.1	81.3	94.5	96.7	96.5

[a]The initial success criteria at 10 years were set as a PPD ≤5 mm, no BOP, and BL <0.2 mm annually. The implant success rates for group A (i.e., patients with a history of periodontitis) and group B (i.e., patients with periodontal health) using these initial criteria are listed in the first column. Notice how dramatically the success rates change when the criteria used to define success are modified to include PPD ≤6 mm (i.e., second column). The next two columns show the success rates for each group using PPD ≤5 mm and ≤6 mm when the criteria are modified to omit bone loss as a determinant. The last column shows the implant survival rate for each group, which demonstrates that the survival rate is different than the success rate.

PPD, Probing pocket depth; *BOP*, bleeding on probing; *BL*, bone loss.

(Data from Karoussis IK, Salvi GE, Heitz-Mayfield LJ, et al: Long-term implant prognosis in patients with and without a history of chronic periodontitis: a 10-year prospective cohort study of the ITI Dental Implant System. *Clin Oral Implant Res* 14:329–339, 2003.)

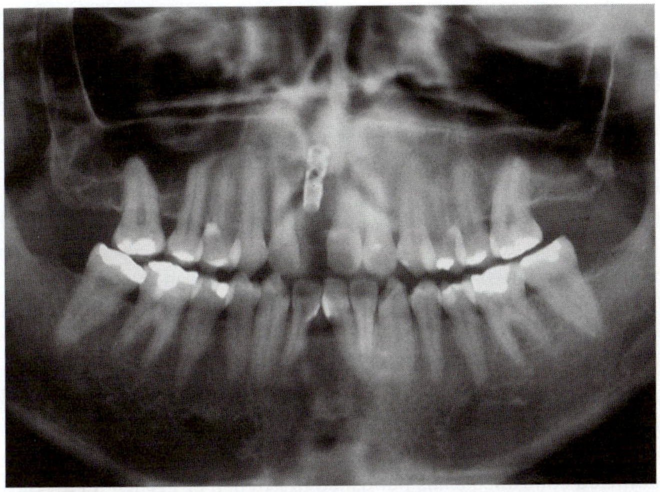

Fig. 60.2 Panoramic radiograph shows an implant placed in the position of a missing maxillary right central incisor. The implant appears to be placed in a nonrestorable position. It is osseointegrated and could technically be counted as a surviving implant, but it must be considered a failure because it does not meet the intended goal and function has not been restored.

considered successful merely because they are present and osseointegrated.

Implant survival and implant success are different outcome measures. Consider the dramatic difference between survival and success rates for implants reported in a systematic review (21 studies included) of implants supporting fixed partial dentures. The 5-year implant survival rate was 95.4%, whereas the overall 5-year success rate (individual implant success rates were not calculated), defined as free of complications, was only 61.3%.

In a 10-year retrospective study of 397 fixed implant reconstructions in 300 patients, the observed mechanical complication rate was 24.7%. The most frequent complication was ceramic chipping (20.31%), followed by occlusal screw loosening (2.57%) and loss of retention (2.06%). Although relatively uncommon, occlusal screw loosening can result in a subgingival gap at the implant–abutment junction that retains plaque and stimulates an inflammatory reaction in the soft and hard tissues, leading to bone loss around the implant. Although surviving, these implants would fail to meet optimal success criteria.

Defining implant results in absolute terms is difficult and confusing. Strictly defined, implant success is any implant-retained restoration in which (1) the original treatment plan is performed as intended without complications, (2) all implants that were placed remain stable and functioning without problems, (3) the peri-implant hard and soft tissues are healthy, and (4) the patient and treating clinicians are pleased with the results.

Implant survival, which typically is reported in studies, can overestimate good implant outcomes. Implant success, which is less often reported, could offer a better measure if specific success criteria were universally defined, accepted, and used. Implant success is difficult or impossible to compare across studies because of differences in evaluation criteria used by investigators. Implant success in a single study or series of studies using the same success criteria is meaningful only in the context of that study or series.

An additional criterion of implant success that is not typically reported but should be considered is the esthetic success or patient satisfaction with the outcome. Several methods have been proposed to evaluate esthetic results. A restorative index was proposed by Jensen and coworkers to appraise the esthetics of the final restoration. The index uses a scale of 1–10, with 1 being an extremely poor result and 10 being a superlative esthetic result. Based on subjective and objective criteria, the index evaluates the size and shape of the implant restoration compared to the equivalent contralateral tooth, how well it blends into the arch, and the papillae, gingival form, color, and other factors considered essential in determining an esthetic result. The pink esthetic score is an index proposed by Furhauser and colleagues that considers seven soft tissue parameters, including evaluation of the color, contour, and texture of the surrounding soft tissues (i.e., papilla and facial mucosa). Each parameter is given a score of 0, 1, or 2, which allows the best score of 14 to determine the highest level of esthetics.

Other indices were proposed for single-tooth implant restorations in the esthetic zone. Proposed by Belser and colleagues, one index combines a modified pink esthetic score with a white esthetic score that focuses on the visible part of the implant restoration. Scoring includes five parameters: general tooth form, hue, value, surface texture, and translucency. The maximum white esthetic score is 10. These indices are aimed at quantifying the esthetic result, which can provide an objective method of judging implant esthetic success.

Currently, the usefulness of implant success rates from different studies is limited. Implant survival is important but is only an indicator of surviving implants and does not reveal whether they are functioning or had problems associated with them over time. The incidence of peri-implant problems is more significant than once thought. A systematic review of the literature evaluating the prevalence of peri-implant disease reported that peri-implant mucositis and peri-implantitis occurred in 19%–65% and 1%–47% of cases, respectively.

Factors That Influence Implant Outcomes (e only)

Many issues influence implant outcomes, including available bone, implant design, placement and loading protocols, and host-related factors.

Anatomic Location

Implant Design

Placement and Loading Protocols

Immediate Implant Placement

Immediate Occlusal Loading

Bone Augmentation

Risk Factors

Smoking

Diabetes

Periodontitis

Esthetic Results and Patient Satisfaction

The ultimate goal of treatment is to achieve natural-appearing, optimally functioning, implant-supported tooth replacements. Proper tooth dimensions and contours, and ideal soft tissue support are key factors for successful esthetic outcomes. If crown form, dimension, and shape and gingival harmony around the implants are not ideal, the patient may consider the implant restoration unacceptable because the result does not represent a natural dental profile (Fig. 60.3). For some patients, such as those with severe alveolar deficiency, an ideal esthetic outcome may be impossible because reconstructive surgical procedures are complex, require extensive time, and remain unpredictable. For others, a less-than-ideal esthetic outcome may be acceptable.

Esthetic problems and patient dissatisfaction happen when results are inferior to what was expected. Satisfaction with the esthetic outcome of the implant prosthesis varies from patient to patient, depending on a number of factors. The risk for esthetic failure is increased for patients with high esthetic expectations. The risk is also higher when patients present with patient-related risk factors such as a high smile line, thin periodontal soft tissues, and compromised bone support. Two recent systematic reviews reported that the patient's perceptions and desires greatly influence and determine how well he or she accepts the implant outcome.

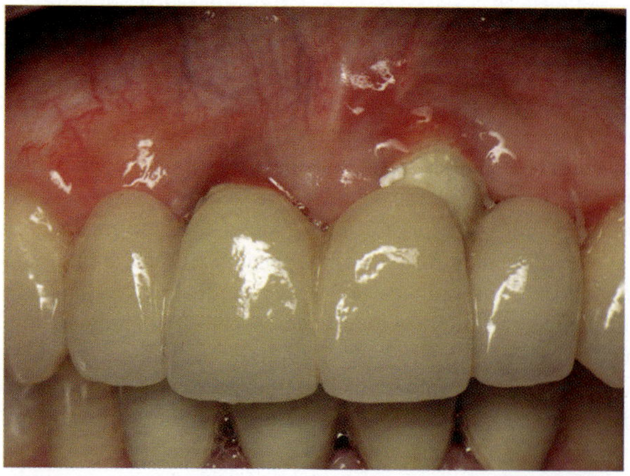

Fig. 60.3 Clinical photograph shows a maxillary anterior fixed restoration supported by two malpositioned implants in the central incisor positions. The patient was dissatisfied with the esthetic outcome. The left implant was positioned between the central and lateral incisor and angled toward the facial surface at a level above the gingival margin. A tooth-colored material was used to mask the exposed framework in the gingival area.

Although infrequently reported, esthetic success and patient satisfaction need to be included when considering the results of implant therapy. Despite several proposed methods for evaluating esthetic results, reports of esthetic parameters in the scientific literature are scarce. A restorative index appraises the white esthetics of the final restoration, a soft tissue or pink esthetic score considers soft-tissue parameters, and an esthetic index uses a combination of pink and white esthetic scores, focusing on the visible part of the implant restoration. These indices quantify the esthetic result, providing an objective method of judging esthetic success.

In a survey of patient satisfaction, more than 90% of patients were completely satisfied in terms of function and esthetics. A questionnaire was given to 104 patients 5–15 years (mean, 10.2 years) after implant placement to assess subjective perceptions of treatment. Of these patients, 48% were treated with single implant crowns and 52% were treated with fixed partial dentures. The survival rate for all implants was 93%. Most patients had favorable responses to the questions regarding function, esthetics, hygiene, and cost. Table 60.2 lists the percentage of patients responding as highly satisfied or satisfied for each category. Comparing chewing comfort for teeth or implants, 72.1% perceived no difference, 17.3% felt more secure chewing on teeth, and 7.7% felt more secure chewing on implants.

In another survey, patient satisfaction with implant-supported prostheses in totally edentulous jaws was evaluated. Experience with an implant-supported prosthesis was assessed over a period of 10 years, and 97% of the 135 patients reported overall satisfaction with treatment. Chewing satisfaction was reported as good or very good by all but one patient (99.3% positive response rate). Improved lifestyle and greater self-confidence in public were reported by 75% and 82% of patients, respectively.

A systematic review of the literature, which included all randomized controlled trials published in English or French up to April 2007 comparing conventional mandibular dentures and implant overdentures in adult edentulous patients, identified eight publications for metaanalysis. The study reported that patients were more satisfied with implant overdentures than with conventional mandibular dentures. However, there was a lack of evidence to show a patient's perception of the impact of mandibular implant overdentures on general health.

TABLE 60.2 Patient Satisfaction With Implant Treatment

Implant Experience	Highly Satisfied or Satisfied (%)[a]
Function or chewing	97
Phonetics	96
Esthetics	97
Oral hygiene ease	93
Complete fulfillment	92
Would do treatment again	94
Would recommend to friend or relative	89
Reasonable or justified cost	87

[a]Percentage of patients subjectively responding with *highly satisfied* or *satisfied* to survey questions about their implant experience. More than 90% responded favorably and thought implant treatment was a positive experience.

(Data from Pjetursson BE, Karoussis I, Burgin W, et al: Patients' satisfaction following implant therapy. A 10-year prospective cohort study. *Clin Oral Implants Res* 16:185–193, 2005.)

Conclusion

The use of dental implants to replace missing teeth is highly predictable, advantageous, and beneficial for patients. Because of variations in implant designs, study protocols, and populations studied, results are difficult to compare and an absolute definition of implant success remains elusive. The results of implant treatment are reported using a wide range of criteria from being present (i.e., survival) to being functional without complications (i.e., success).

It is challenging to compare the results of studies because the number of variables continues to change. Clinical research suggests that certain risk factors can decrease success rates for some patients. Understanding what is being reported in the literature helps patients and clinicians appreciate implant treatment results.

Implant-Related Complications and Failures

Patients have experienced much success with endosseous dental implants. Yet, despite the long-term predictability and success of implants, complications do occur in a percentage of cases. Some complications are relatively minor and easy to correct, but others are more significant, resulting in loss of implants, failure of prostheses, and occasionally in severe loss of tissues in the area of implant failure. Complications may be surgical, biologic, mechanical, or esthetic.

Biologic complications are those that involve the peri-implant supporting hard and soft tissues. Changes in the peri-implant soft tissues may be minor, such as inflammation and proliferation, or more significant, involving progressive bone loss. The ultimate biologic complication is implant loss or failure, which may also result in soft and hard-tissue defects. Biologic loss of implants may be caused by a lack of osseointegration in the early stages before restoration or by a loss of osseointegration as a result of bone loss after the restoration is installed and functioning.

Surgical complications are those problems or adverse outcomes that result from surgery, including procedures used for implant placement, implant exposure, and augmentation procedures. One of the more prevalent types of implant complications are those arising from implant malposition or those arising from an implant being placed in a nonideal position. Malpositioned implants, which usually are the result of poor presurgical treatment planning and/or surgical technique, can lead to an array of implant problems ranging in severity from minor to major. These complications include compromised esthetic and/or prosthetic results, soft-tissue and bone dehiscences, impingement on anatomic structures, and possibly implant failure. Unfortunately, the extent of the problems that arise from implant malposition are often not recognized until the time of implant restoration or years after insertion.

Prosthetic or mechanical complications and failures typically occur in the form of material failure such as abutment and prosthetic screw loosening or fractures. The patient can recover from many of these mechanical problems if they are minor and recognized early. However, some complications, such as implant fractures, are not salvageable.

Esthetic complications arise when patient expectations are not met. Patient satisfaction with the esthetic outcome of the implant prosthesis will vary from patient to patient, depending on several factors. The risk for esthetic complications is increased for patients with high esthetic expectations and less-than-optimal patient-related factors (e.g., high smile line, thin gingival tissues, or inadequate bone quantity and quality).

Types and Prevalence of Implant Complications

The prevalence of implant-related complications has been reported in several reviews. However, until recently, a systematic review of the incidence of biological and technical complications in studies of at least 5 years revealed that biological complications were considered in only 40%–60% and technical complications in only 60%–80% of the studies. One of the few conclusions of this review indicated that the incidence of technical complications related to implant components and suprastructures was higher in overdentures than in fixed restorations. In a systematic review of reports on the survival and complication rates of implant-supported fixed partial dentures (FPDs), Pjetursson et al. found that the most common technical complication was fracture of veneers (13.2% after 5 years), followed by loss of the screw access hole restoration (8.2% after 5 years), abutment/occlusal screw loosening (5.8% after 5 years), and abutment/occlusal screw fracture (1.5% after 5 years; 2.5% after 10 years). Fracture of implants occurred infrequently (0.4% after 5 years; 1.8% after 10 years). A retrospective evaluation of 4937 implants by Eckert et al. found that implant fractures occur more frequently in partially edentulous restorations (1.5%) than in restorations of completely edentulous arches (0.2%), and all observed implant fractures occurred with commercially pure 3.75-mm diameter threaded implants.

In a literature review that included all types of implant-retained prostheses, Goodacre et al. found that the most common technical complications were loosening of the overdenture retentive mechanism (33%), resin veneer fracture with FPDs (22%), overdentures needing to be relined (19%), and overdenture clip/attachment fracture (16%). Their review, with the inclusion of edentulous patients having overdentures, seemed to indicate a significantly higher percentage of complications than Pjetursson systematic review of patients with implant-supported FPDs. Goodacre et al. found it impossible to calculate an overall prosthesis complication rate because most studies included in their review did not report on several of the complication categories.

The most common complication reported for single crowns was abutment or prosthesis screw loosening. Abutment screw loosening varied dramatically from one study to another, ranging from 2% to 45%. The highest rate of abutment screw loosening was associated with single crowns, followed by overdentures. The rate of prosthesis screw loosening was similar, ranging from 1% to 38% in various studies. A higher frequency was reported for single crowns in the posterior areas (premolar and molar) than in the anterior region.

Implant fracture is an uncommon but significant complication. Goodacre et al. reported a 1.5% incidence in their literature review. The incidence of implant fracture was higher in FPDs supported by only two implants. Consistent with this finding, Rangert et al. reported that most fractured implants occurred in single- and double-implant–supported restorations. They also indicated that most of these fractures were in posterior partially edentulous segments, in which the generated occlusal forces can be greater, as opposed to anterior segments (Fig. 60.4).

In a systematic review of prospective longitudinal studies (minimum of 5 years) reporting both biologic and technical complications associated with implant therapy (all restoration types included), Berglundh et al. found that the incidence of technical complications was consistent with Pjetursson findings, with implant fracture occurring in less than 1% (0.08%–0.74%) of cases. Interestingly, consistent with the findings in Goodacre review, technical complications were higher for implants used in overdenture therapy than implants supporting fixed prostheses.

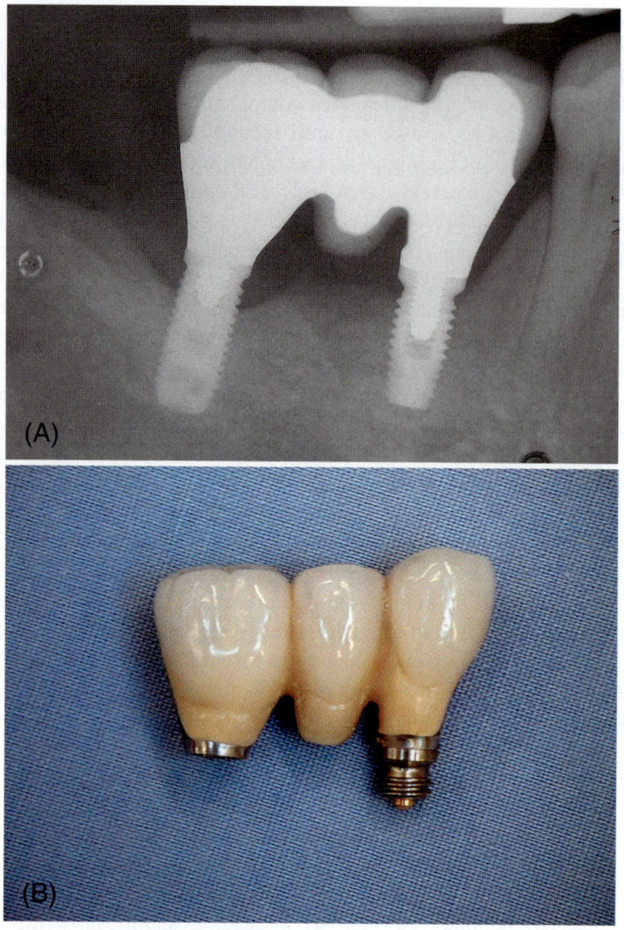

Fig. 60.4 A, Radiograph of a three-unit, posterior, FPD supported by two standard-diameter, screw-shaped threaded implants. Notice long crown height, relatively short implant length, and bone loss around posterior implant. B, Photograph of the ultimate implant-supported restoration failure. The anterior implant fractured between the second and third threads, which resulted in loss of the restoration.

In Pjetursson systematic review of survival and complication rates for implant-supported FPDs, biologic complications, such as peri-implantitis and soft-tissue lesions, occurred in 8.6% of implant-supported FPDs after 5 years. However, in a more recent literature review of the prevalence of peri-implant diseases, Zitzmann and Berglundh reported that although cross-sectional studies are rare, data from the only two studies available showed that peri-implant mucositis occurred in 80% of the subjects and 50% of implant sites. Peri-implantitis, conversely, was identified in 28% and 56% or more of subjects and in 12% and 43% of implant sites in the two studies that followed subjects with implants in function at least 5 years. A critical review of the literature by Esposito et al. included 73 publications reporting early and late failures of Brånemark implants; biologically related implant failures were relatively low at 7.7%. The treatments involved all anatomic areas and all types of prosthetic design. The authors concluded that the predictability of implant treatment was especially good for partially edentulous patients compared to totally edentulous patients, with failures in the latter population being twice as high. Also, the incidence of implant failure was three times higher for the edentulous maxilla than for the edentulous mandible, whereas failure rates for the partially edentulous maxilla were similar to those for the partially edentulous mandible.

Risk factors, such as smoking, diabetes, and periodontal disease, may contribute to implant failure and complications. Several studies with numerous implants and years of follow-up have concluded that smoking is a definite risk factor for implant survival. A systematic review of the effect of risk factors on implant outcomes concluded that smoking has an adverse effect on implant survival and success, with the effects being more pronounced in areas of loose trabecular bone (i.e., posterior maxilla). The review suggested that type 2 diabetes may have an adverse effect on implant survival rates but did not have enough studies to permit a definitive conclusion. Finally, the same review also concluded that while patients with a history of treated periodontitis did not show any decrease in implant survival, they did experience more biologic implant complications and lower success rates.

Types of Dental Implants (e only)

Analysis of the data on the prevalence of implant complications (i.e., failure, fracture, and peri-implantitis) in published systematic reviews should consider the fact that many of these studies reported on implants with earlier designs (i.e., machined surfaces and external connections). Most current implant systems feature surfaces with an altered microtopography (i.e., rough), and many have internal connections. The prevalence and type of complications associated with the newer implant designs may be different.

Many modifications have been developed to try to improve the long-term success rates of implants. More than 1300 types of dental implants are available with different materials, shapes, sizes, lengths, and surface characteristics or coatings. Although it has been suggested that machined surfaces are more resistant to plaque accumulation and peri-implantitis, there is limited evidence to show that implants with relatively smooth surfaces (i.e., machined) are less prone to bone loss from chronic infection than implants with rough surfaces. To date, there is no evidence showing that any particular type of dental implant has superior long-term success.

Different implant designs and surfaces must be studied in prospective human trials over long periods. Until those data become available, clinicians should be aware that historical data reporting success rates for earlier implant designs may not reflect the outcomes for current implants. Moreover, new implant surfaces and designs are commonly introduced with limited or no data available on potential complications.

Surgical Complications

As with any surgical procedure, there are risks involved with implant surgery. Proper precautions must be taken to prevent the risk of injury resulting from surgical procedures, including but not limited to (1) a thorough review of the patient's past medical history, (2) a comprehensive clinical and radiographic examination, and (3) good surgical techniques. Surgical complications include perilous bleeding, damage to adjacent teeth, injury to nerves, and iatrogenic jaw fracture. Postoperative complications include bleeding, hematoma, and infection. They may be minor, transient, and easily managed or more serious and require postoperative treatment.

Hemorrhage and Hematoma (e only)

Neurosensory Disturbances (e only)

Implant Malpostion (e only)

Biologic Complications

Biologic complications involve pathology of the surrounding peri-implant hard and soft tissues. Frequently, soft-tissue problems are an inflammatory response to bacterial accumulation. The cause of bacterial accumulation around implants is key to understanding the problem. For example, bacteria may accumulate at the junction of an ill-fitting implant-abutment or abutment-crown connection. Some of the highly textured, macroscopically rough implant surfaces [e.g., titanium plasma-sprayed (TPS) or hydroxyapatite (HA) coated] may also perpetuate the accumulation of bacteria on the implant surface.

Inflammation and Proliferation

Inflammation in the peri-implant soft tissues has been found to be similar to the inflammatory response in gingival and other periodontal tissues. Not surprisingly, the clinical appearance is similar as well. Inflamed peri-implant tissues demonstrate the same erythema, edema, and swelling seen around teeth. Occasionally, however, the reaction of peri-implant soft tissues to bacterial accumulation is profound, almost unusual, with a dramatic inflammatory proliferation (Fig. 60.11). This type of lesion is somewhat characteristic around implants and is indicative of either a loose-fitting implant to abutment connection or trapped excess cement that remains buried within the soft-tissue space or "pocket." The precipitating local factor ultimately becomes infected with bacterial pathogens, leading to mucosal hypertrophy or proliferation and possible abscess formation (Fig. 60.12). Correction of the precipitating factors (e.g., loose connection, retained cement) may effectively resolve the lesion. Another type of lesion resulting from a loose abutment connection is the fistula (Fig. 60.13). Again, correcting the etiologic factor can quickly resolve the fistula.

Dehiscence and Recession

Dehiscence or recession of the peri-implant soft tissues occurs when support for those tissues is lacking or has been lost. Recession is a common finding after implant restoration and should be anticipated especially when soft tissues are thin and not well supported (Fig. 60.14). Improper implant positioning also predisposes peri-implant tissues to recession. As noted earlier, placement or angulation

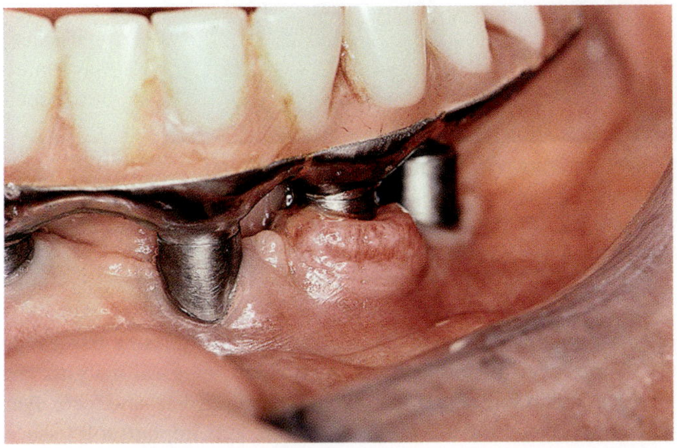

Fig. 60.11 Inflammatory proliferation caused by a loose-fitting connection between the abutment and the implant. *(Courtesy: Dr John Beumer, UCLA Maxillofacial Prosthetics, Los Angeles, CA.)*

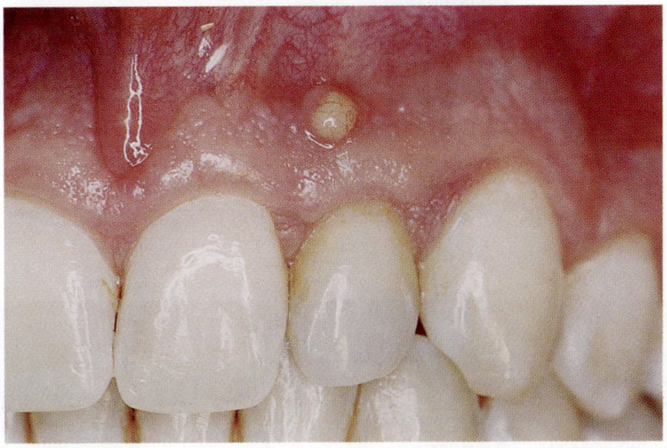

Fig. 60.13 Fistula caused by loose implant-abutment connection (maxillary left lateral incisor).

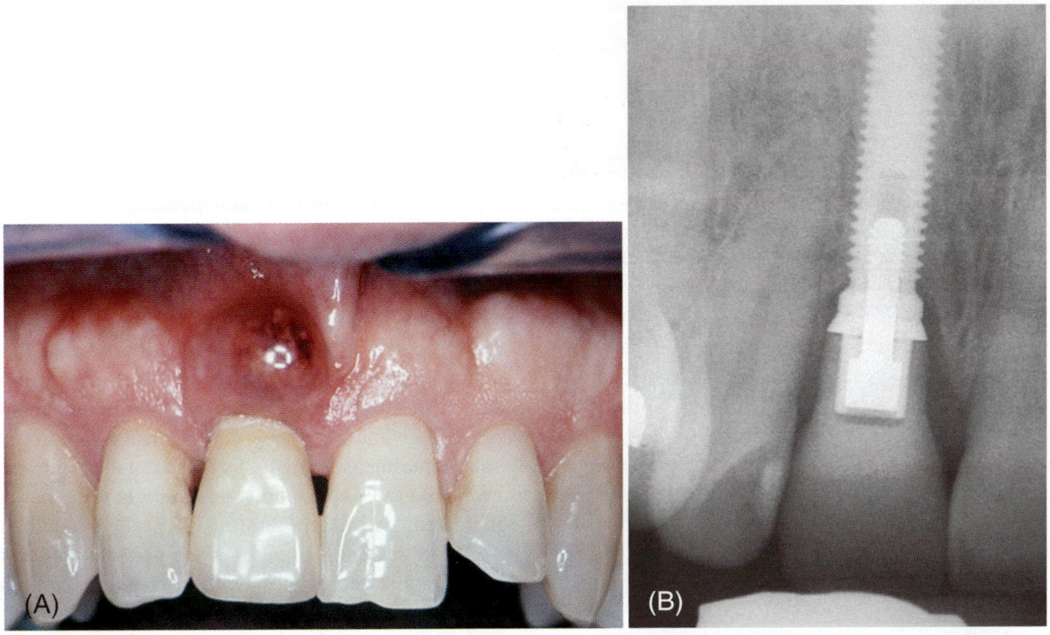

Fig. 60.12 A, Clinical photograph of abscess caused by excess cement trapped within the soft tissues. B, Radiograph of implant with cemented crown (same patient as in A). Notice the subgingival depth of the crown-abutment (cement line) junction, which is below the level of the adjacent interproximal bone and therefore impossible to adequately access with explorer to remove excess cement. *(Courtesy: Dr John Beumer, UCLA Maxillofacial Prosthetics, Los Angeles, CA.)*

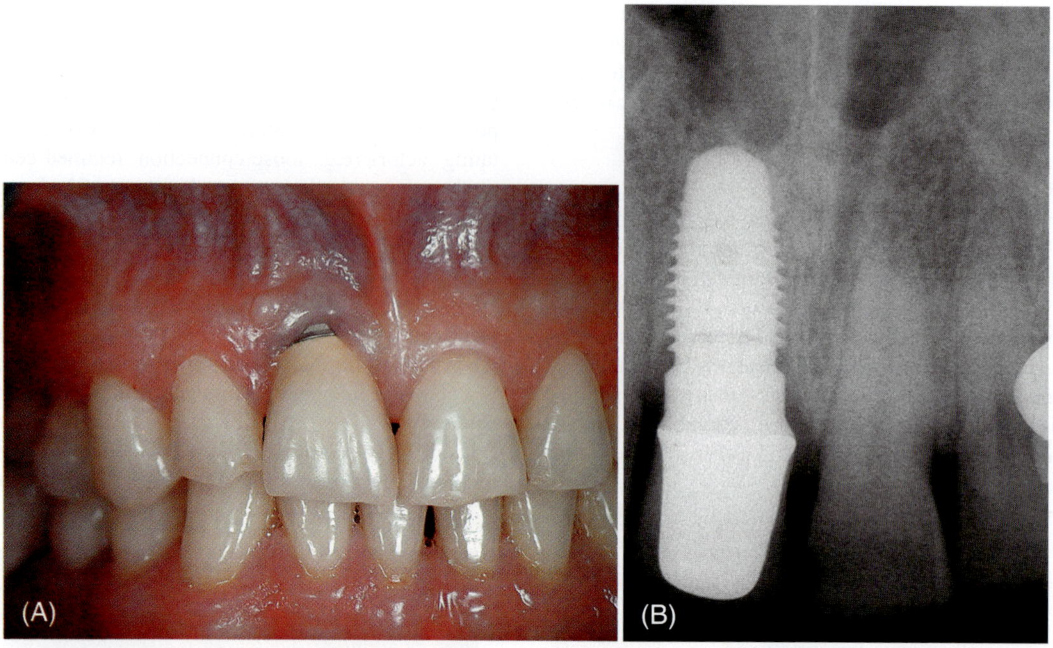

Fig. 60.14 A, Clinical photograph of single-tooth implant crown (maxillary right central) with moderate recession that occurred 1-year after delivery of final restoration. Recession, in this case, most likely occurred because the labial bone around this wide-diameter implant was very thin or nonexistent. B, Radiograph of wide-diameter (6 mm) implant supporting maxillary central incisor crown (same patient as in A).

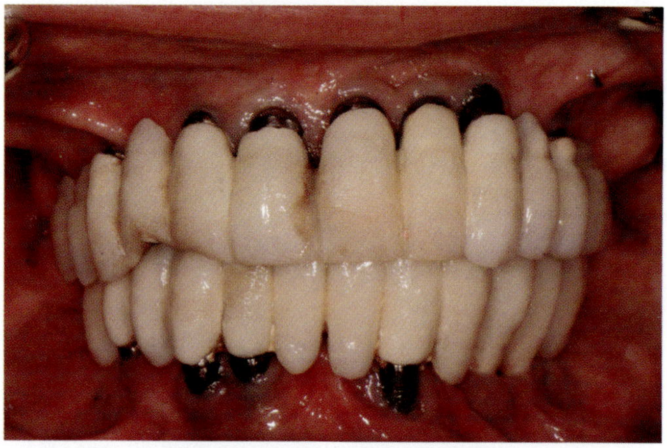

Fig. 60.15 Poor esthetics resulting from gingival recession and exposure of crown margins, implant collars, and threads of several maxillary and mandibular implants supporting full-arch FPDs. Notice the thin labial tissues and erythema (especially around mandibular implant sites).

of the implant too far to the buccal causes the buccal plate to resorb and has been shown to result in greater recession. Another factor to consider is the thickness of the buccal plate of bone. Spray et al. recommended this thickness to be 2 mm or greater to support the buccal soft tissue. If this thickness is not present, presurgical or simultaneous site development using guided bone regeneration (GBR) is indicated. Recession is a problem that is particularly disconcerting in anterior esthetic areas. Patients with a high smile line or high esthetic demands consider such recession a failure (Fig. 60.15).

The anatomy and soft-tissue support around implants is different than that around teeth. Specifically, periodontal tissues have the distinct advantage of soft-tissue support from circumferential and transseptal connective tissue fibers that insert into the cementum at a level that is more coronal than the supporting bone. In the absence of inflammation, these fibers support periodontal soft tissues far above the level of crestal bone. As a result, gingival margins and interdental papillae are supported and maintained around teeth even when the periodontal tissues are very thin. Peri-implant soft tissues, however, are entirely dependent on the surrounding bone for support. Soft-tissue thickness accounts for some soft-tissue height, but there are no supracrestal inserting connective tissue fibers to aid in the soft-tissue support around an implant. Therefore, soft-tissue height around implants typically does not exceed about 3–4 mm, and bone loss around implants often leads to recession.

Peri-implantitis and Bone Loss

Peri-implantitis is defined as an inflammatory process affecting the tissues around an osseointegrated implant in function, resulting in loss of supporting bone. The prevalence of peri-implantitis has been reported to be controversial depending on the criteria used to define the amount of marginal bone loss necessary to be present, together with the evidence of soft-tissue inflammation to determine the existence of the disease. Reports of prevalence of peri-implantitis have varied from approximately 7% to 37% of implants in various studies. Recently, a proposed classification for early, moderate, and advanced peri-implantitis based on the degree of bone loss was presented in an attempt to improve communication when describing prevalence and treatment. To diagnose a compromised implant site, soft-tissue measurements using manual or automated probes have been suggested. Although some reports state that probing is contraindicated, careful monitoring of probing depth over time seems useful in detecting changes of the peri-implant tissue. Standardized radiographic techniques, with or without computerized analysis, have been well documented and found to be useful in evaluating peri-implant bone levels. Together with periodic evaluation of tissue appearance, probing depth changes and radiographic assessment are the best means of detecting changes in bone support. Clinicians should monitor the surrounding tissues for signs of peri-implant disease by monitoring changes in probing depth and radiographic

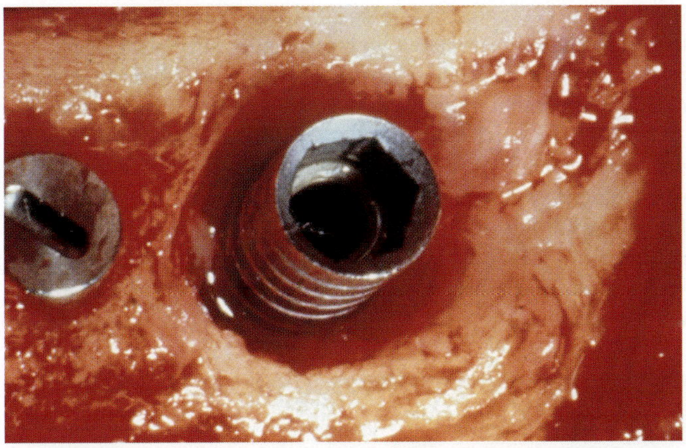

Fig. 60.16 Moderately advanced bone loss around an implant with the typical circumferential trough type of boney defect. *(From Garg AK:* Implant dentistry: a practical approach, *ed 2, Mosby, St. Louis, 2010.)*

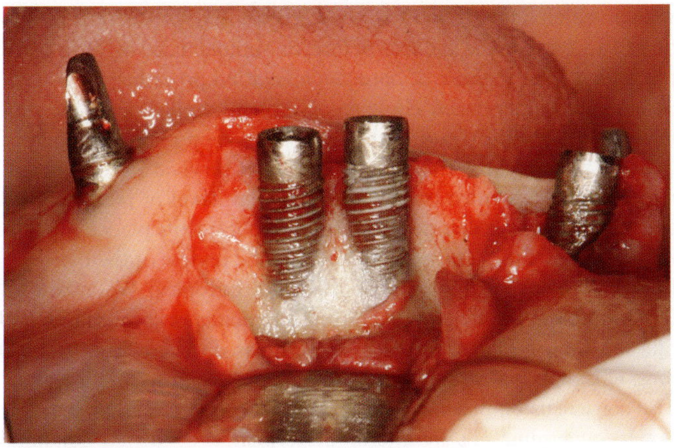

Fig. 60.17 Severe horizontal and vertical bone loss around several mandibular implants.

evidence of bone destruction, suppuration, calculus buildup, swelling, color changes, and bleeding. Peri-implantitis may be perpetuated by bacterial infection that has contaminated a rough (e.g., TPS, HA-coated) implant surface and by excessive biomechanical forces. A classic trough-type defect is typically associated with peri-implantitis (Fig. 60.16). In cases with severely reduced bone support extending into the apical half of the implant (Fig. 60.17) or in cases demonstrating mobility, implant removal should be considered. The number and distribution of implants and the occlusal relationships influence the biomechanical forces applied to implants. A recent review by Lindhe and Meyle from the Consensus Report of the Sixth European Workshop on Periodontology concluded that risk indicators for peri-implantitis included (1) poor oral hygiene, (2) a history of periodontitis, (3) diabetes, (4) cigarette smoking, (5) alcohol consumption, and (6) implant surface. Most of these risk factors (1–4) have been recognized and reported in the literature. The report suggests that although data for the latter two risk factors (5 and 6) are limited, they appear to be relevant to peri-implantitis. Another risk factor that has been proposed involves gene polymorphism related to an individual's genotype. More research is needed to study the relationship of this potential risk factor to the development of peri-implantitis.

Other risk factors, including excess and retained cement, have been implicated in peri-implantitis. One article said that excess dental cement was associated with signs of peri-implant disease in 81% of cases evaluated using a dental endoscope. The radiopacity of some commonly used cements affects their detectability. This emphasizes the importance of proper cementation, use of screw-retained rather than cemented restorations when possible, and careful clinical examination after final crown cementation on implants.

Other proposed peri-implantitis predisposing factors include the presence of aggressive bacteria, excessive mechanical stress, and corrosion. Each was documented as a factor that could act synergistically with biofilm or existing peri-implantitis to worsen the condition.

Nine systematic reviews concluded that no predicable method of treatment for peri-implantitis could be recommended. However, a clinical study of 170 consecutively treated implants with peri-implantitis using a regenerative protocol reported a more than 98% success rate.

Implant Loss or Failure

Implant loss or failure is generally considered relative to the time of placement or restoration. Early implant failures occur before implant restoration. Late implant failures occur after the implant has been restored. When an implant fails before restoration, it probably did not achieve osseointegration, or the integration was weak or jeopardized by infection, movement, or impaired wound healing (Fig. 60.18A and B). Late implant failures occur after prosthesis installation for a variety of reasons, including infection and implant overload (Fig. 60.19A–C). In a review of the literature to evaluate biologic causes for implant failure, Esposito et al. found that infections, impaired healing, and overload were the most important contributing factors. Two systematic reviews of the literature concluded that a single dose of preoperative antibiotic therapy may decrease the failure rate of dental implants.

The risk of implant failure varies among patients and patterns of loss tend to cluster within subjects. A second attempt at dental implant placement should be approached cautiously when attempting to place the implant in the same site as the one that previously failed. Oftentimes, it is challenging to achieve adequate diameter,

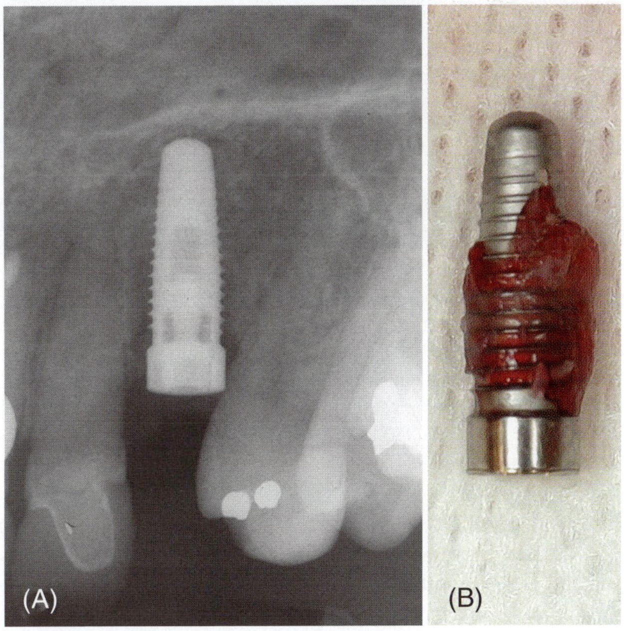

Fig. 60.18 A, Radiograph of early failed implant caused by lack of osseointegration. In addition to the crestal bone loss, notice the radiolucency along the sides of the implant. B, Photograph of the failed (nonintegrated) implant (shown in A) that was easily removed along with surrounding connective tissue.

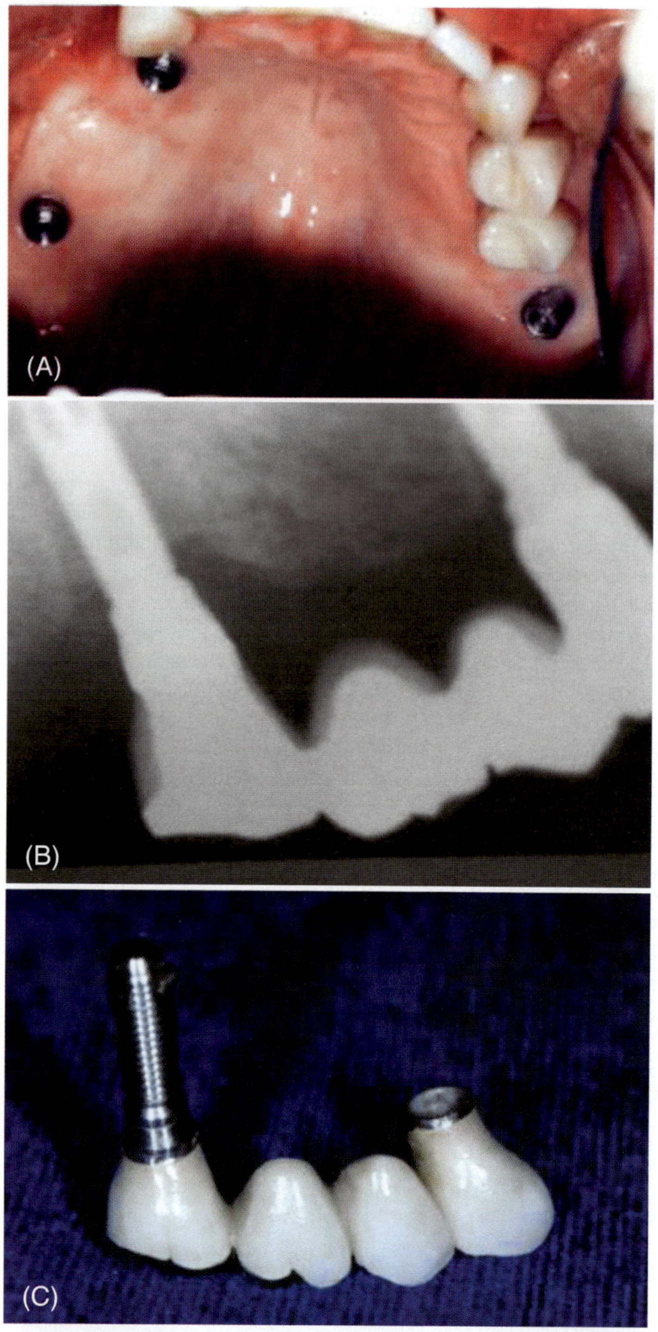

Fig. 60.19 Four-unit FPD in the posterior maxilla supported by only two implants. A, Clinical photograph of implant abutments in the posterior maxilla. B, Radiograph taken 30-months after restoration. Note the bone loss around the distal implant. C, Failed distal implant attached to failed prosthesis. The biologic failure of one (posterior) implant resulted in a long-span cantilever extension from the other (anterior) implant that ultimately led to its mechanical failure (i.e., abutment screw fracture). *(Courtesy: Dr John Beumer, UCLA Maxillofacial Prosthetics, Los Angeles, CA.)*

length, and stability of replacement implants due to the residual defect created by removal of the failed implant. In 2007, Grossmann and Levin reported an overall survival rate of 71% for dental implants that were placed in sites of previously failed single implants. In that study, all of the original implants failed during the early healing phase (mean 2.3–3.2 months postplacement). In a similar study in 2008, Machtei reported an overall survival rate of 83.5% for the second attempt of dental implants. They concluded that replacing failed implants resulted in implants with a lower survival rate compared to implants placed in pristine sites. A factor that could not be associated with conventional implant or patient-related implant failures. They suggested a possible site-specific negative effect that might be associated with this phenomenon.

In 2011, Machtei reported a lower survival rate of 60% for the third reimplanted sites. This outcome represents a further diminished prognosis compared to implants in original sites in or even following the first re-do. Their findings demonstrated that the replacement of a failed implant presents a challenge in achieving osseointegration in a healed bone site and may result in a decline in the survival rate.

Complications Related to Augmentation Procedures

A common problem encountered in implant dentistry is insufficient bone quantity to allow implant placement according to standard procedures. Deficiencies in alveolar bone result from developmental defects, periodontal disease, tooth loss, and trauma. For most cases with alveolar ridge resorption, bone regenerative procedures are required to correct the defects before or simultaneous with implant placement. The success of bone augmentation procedures has been assessed by experienced clinicians in several workshops. One systematic review of literature (the 2003 Workshop on Contemporary Science in Clinical Periodontics) found that survival rates of dental implants in augmented bone achieved a high level of predictability and showed that these rates were similar to implants placed in natural bone. However, a more-recent systematic review of the literature (the 2008 Consensus Report of the Sixth European Workshop on Periodontology) concluded that bone augmentation procedures can fail and that implants placed in these areas do not enjoy the high long-term survival rates of dental implants placed in pristine sites. The consensus emphasized that research is needed to answer questions concerning (1) long-term performance of dental implants placed in augmented bone, (2) the clinical performance of dental implants placed in augmented or pristine sites, and (3) the clinical benefits of bone augmentation with respect to alternative treatments.

The procedures most often used to regenerate bone include autogenous bone harvesting and grafting, GBR, and sinus bone augmentation. The most common complications related to these three augmentation procedures are:

- Autogenous Bone Harvesting and Grafting (e only)
- **Guided Bone Regeneration** (e only)
- **Sinus Bone Augmentation** (e only)
  - i. Lateral Window Sinus Lift
  - ii. Crestal (Osteotome) Sinus Lift

Complications Related to Placement and Loading Protocols

The traditional implant placement protocol required a healed edentulous ridge into which implants were placed and allowed to osseointegrate for a period of 3–6 months without occlusal loading. In contrast to these early standards, some current protocols advocate dramatically different approaches, including (1) implant placement immediately after tooth extraction, (2) implant loading immediately after placement, and (3) flapless implant placement surgery. Each of these approaches has distinct advantages but are also accompanied by specific risks of complications. The most common complications associated with these newer, developing protocols are discussed online.

- Immediate Implant Placement (e only)
- Immediate Loading After Implant Placement (e only)
- Implant Placement Using a Flapless Approach (e only)

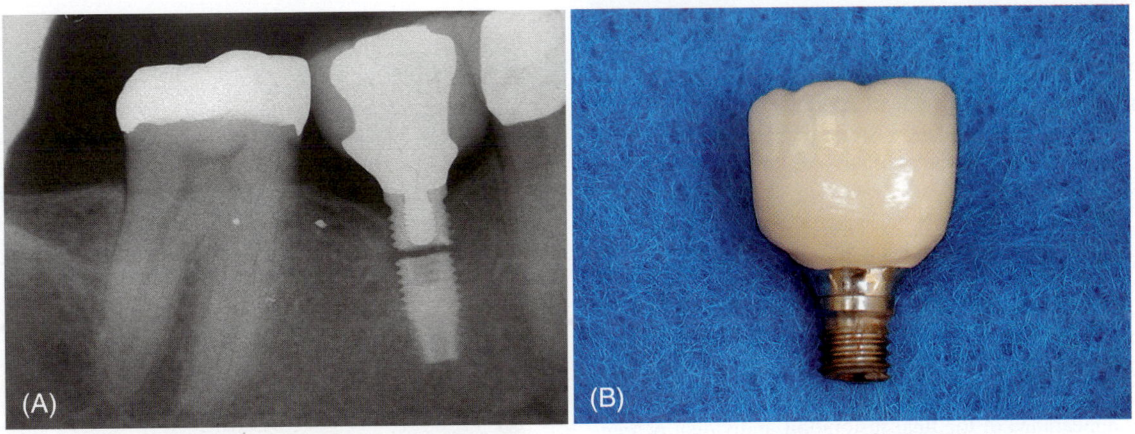

Fig. 60.26 A, Radiograph of fractured implant (standard diameter) used to support a molar-sized single crown in the posterior mandible. B, Crown and coronal portion of implant (same as that shown in A) that fractured between the third and fourth threads.

Prosthetic or Mechanical Complications

Prosthetic or mechanical complications occur when the strength of materials is no longer able to resist the forces that are being applied. As materials fatigue, they begin to stretch and bend; ultimately, depending on the applied forces, they will fracture. Material failures, in turn, lead to prosthetic complications such as loose, broken, and failed restorations.

Screw Loosening and Fracture

Screw loosening has been reported to occur quite frequently in screw-retained FPDs. Screw-retained single crowns attached to externally hexed implants (i.e., those with narrow- or standard-diameter restorative interface connection surfaces) are particularly prone to this type of mechanical complication. Studies have reported screw loosening in 6%–49% of cases at the first annual checkup. Screw loosening was a more prevalent problem with earlier designs. For example, abutment screws were previously made with titanium, which did not offer the clamping forces of current materials. Newer abutment designs and improved abutment screws allow for an increased clamping force to be achieved without excessive torque levels, which has helped to reduce the rate of screw loosening.

Abutment or prosthesis screw loosening is often corrected by retightening the screws. Over time, however, if screws continue to be stretched, they become fatigued and eventually fracture. This problem is evident in the patient with a loose single crown. However, in the patient with a prosthesis retained by multiple implants, the ability to detect a loose screw is greatly diminished and the problem may go unnoticed until additional screws stretch, fatigue, and fracture. In either case, the biomechanical support (and resistance) for the restoration must be evaluated and, if possible, changed to prevent recurrence of the problem.

Implant Fracture

The ultimate mechanical failure is implant fracture because it results in loss of the implant and possibly the prosthesis (Fig. 60.26A and B). Furthermore, removal of a fractured implant creates a large osseous defect. Factors such as fatigue of implant materials (Fig. 60.27) and weakness in prosthetic design or dimension are the usual causes of implant fractures. Balshi listed three categories of causes that may explain implant fractures: (1) design and material, (2) nonpassive fit of the prosthetic framework, and (3) physiologic or biomechanical overload. Patients with bruxism seem to be at higher risk for such events and therefore need to be screened, informed, and managed accordingly. These patients should be fitted with occlusal guards in conjunction with placement of the final prostheses.

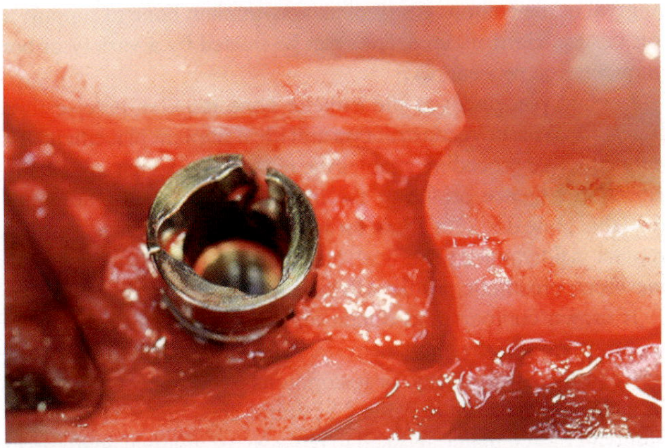

Fig. 60.27 Implant fractured at internal connection collar resulting from fatigue. This collar fracture was caused by rotational forces applied to the implant at the time of placement into dense bone. The fracture was likely the result of a combination of material weakness and density of the prepared site.

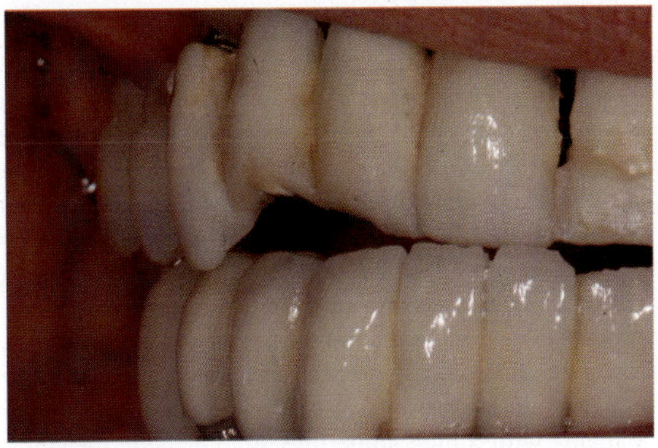

Fig. 60.28 Fractured porcelain from incisal edges of implant-supported FPD.

Fracture of Restorative Materials

Fracture or failure of materials used for implant-retained restorations can be a significant problem. This is particularly true for veneers (acrylic, composite, or ceramic) that are attached to superstructures (Fig. 60.28).

Esthetic and Phonetic Complications

Esthetic Complications

The challenge of modern implant dentistry is achieving an esthetic, as well as a functional, implant restoration. Harmonious tooth shape, size, and ideal soft-tissue contours are key factors for successful esthetic outcomes.

Esthetic complications arise when patient expectations are not met. Patient satisfaction with the esthetic outcome of the implant prosthesis vary from patient to patient, depending on a number of factors. As mentioned earlier, the risk for esthetic complications is increased for patients with high esthetic expectations and less-than-optimal patient-related factors (e.g., high smile line, thin periodontal soft tissues, or inadequate bone quantity and quality). In addition to the actual appearance of the final restoration, individual perceptions and desires determine the acceptance of the results. Esthetic complications result from poor implant position and deficiencies in the existing anatomy of the edentulous sites that were reconstructed with implants. An important prerequisite for achieving optimal gingival tissue contour is sufficient peri-implant bone to support the soft tissues. Hard-tissue defects can be treated by a variety of bone augmentation procedures.

Implant placement in the esthetic zone requires precise three-dimensional tissue reconstruction and ideal implant placement. This reconstructive procedure enables the restorative dentist to develop a natural emergence profile of the implant crown. If the amount of available bone does not allow for ideal implant placement and if the implant is positioned too apical, buccal, or in the proximal space, an unesthetic prosthetic profile will be developed (Fig. 60.29A–C).

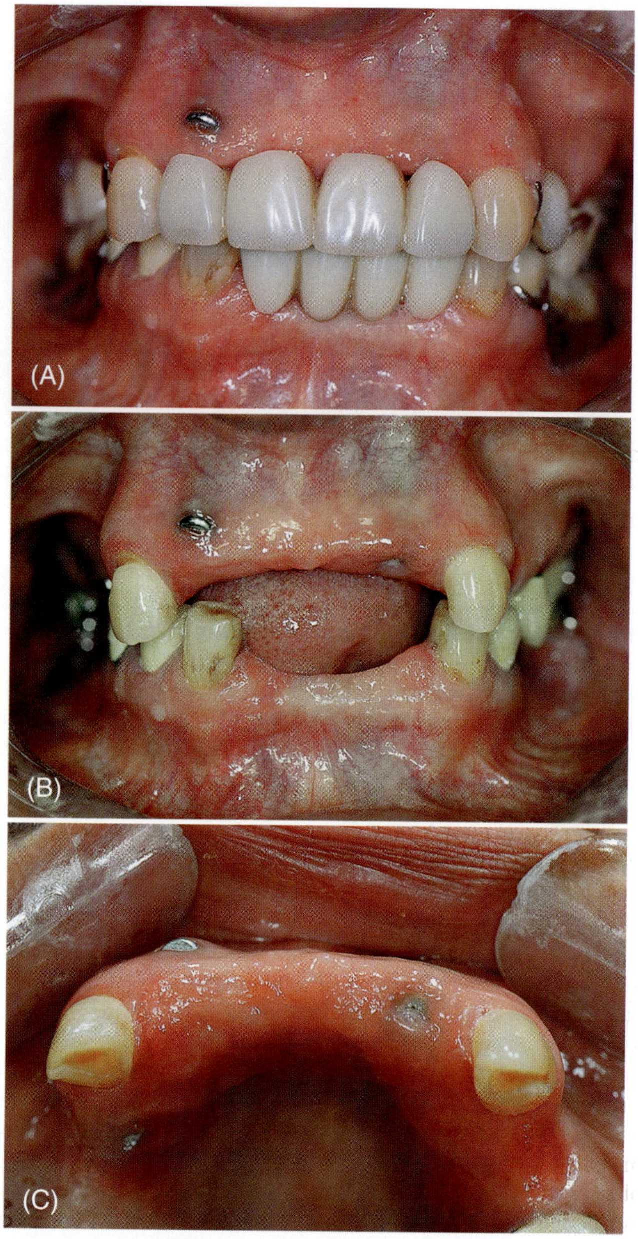

Fig. 60.29 Poor implant position makes it impossible to restore with an esthetic, "natural appearing" restoration. A, Anterior view with removable partial dentures inserted. B, Anterior view without removable partial dentures. Notice the high level of implant cover screw/head exposure (maxillary right lateral incisor) that is significantly apical to the level of the adjacent natural tooth (cuspid) gingival margin. C, Occlusal view of same patient. Again, notice the labial projection of same implant (maxillary right lateral incision), as well as the palatal position of the implant in premolar area. Any attempt to restore the anterior implants would not be esthetically acceptable.

If crown contours and dimensions are not ideal or if gingival harmony around the implant restoration is unesthetic, the patient may consider the implants or restorations as complications because the outcome does not represent a natural appearance (Fig. 60.30). Gingiva-colored materials used to replace lost gingival anatomy can offer an alternative to surgical augmentation in patients undergoing implant therapy (Fig. 60.31). These restorations provide numerous advantages over conventional restorations, including improved lip support, masking of interproximal spaces, and restoration of gingival symmetry in selected cases.

If the patient is truly dissatisfied with the esthetic result and there is a problem with the position of the implants that can be corrected (i.e., the patient's expectations are reasonable), the implants could be removed; the case could be reevaluated and possibly retreated. However, the clinician should consider prosthetic solutions before implant removal. Use of angulated abutments, superstructures, and gingiva-colored materials may result in an acceptable esthetic result, thus avoiding multiple surgeries necessary to rebuild hard and soft tissue if an integrated implant is removed.

Careful patient evaluation and treatment planning along with a solid understanding and appreciation for the predictability and limitations of implant procedures will minimize esthetic complications. Patients with a high smile line, high esthetic demands, thin periodontium, or lack of hard- and soft-tissue support in the anterior esthetic region are some of the most difficult cases to treat and should only be treated after extensive planning by experienced clinicians.

Phonetic Problems

Implant prostheses that are fabricated with unusual palatal contours (e.g., restricted or narrow palatal space) or that have spaces under and around the superstructure can create phonetic problems for the patient. This is particularly problematic when full-arch, implant-supported, fixed restorations are fabricated for patients who have a severely atrophied maxilla. These patients are probably best served with an implant-assisted maxillary overdenture because the design facilitates replacement of missing alveolar structure and avoids creating spaces that allow air to escape during speech.

Conclusion

Although implants offer a highly predictable treatment option for the replacement of single and multiple missing teeth, there are a variety of potential complications that may be surgical, biologic,

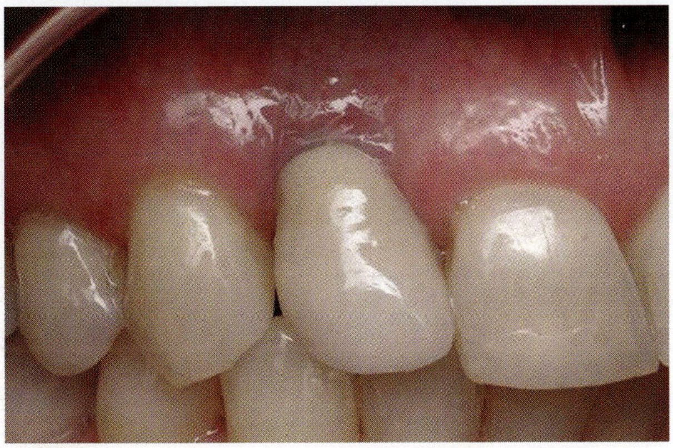

Fig. 60.30 High gingival margin on single-tooth implant crown in the maxillary lateral incisor position. Notice the discrepancy between gingival margin levels of the implant and the adjacent natural teeth.

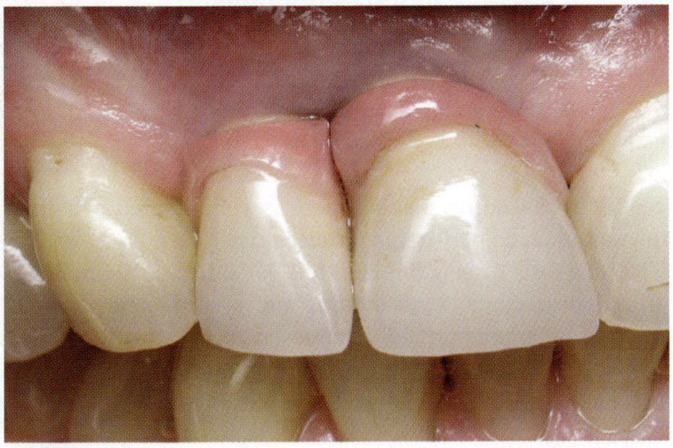

Fig. 60.31 Pink porcelain used on implant-supported fixed restoration to mask the high gingival margin and long implant crowns resulting from an uncorrected alveolar ridge defect.

mechanical, prosthetic, or esthetic. Careful diagnosis and treatment planning, along with the use of diagnostic imaging, surgical guides, meticulous techniques, and adherence to proven principles can prevent many of the problems discussed in this chapter. A thorough understanding of anatomy, biology, and wound healing can reduce the incidence of complications. However, there is no substitute for training, knowledge, and clinical experience for preventing, recognizing, and successfully managing complications. This chapter is a start. The clinician who places and/or restores implants must be aware of techniques and procedures for early intervention should a complication arise.

Key points

- Implant-related complications may be surgical, biologic—complications related to augmentation procedures, complications related to placement and loading protocols, prosthetic or mechanical complications, esthetic and phonetic complications.
- Implant survival is defined as any implant that remains in place at the time of evaluation, regardless of any untoward signs, symptoms, or history of problems. Implant success, conversely, is defined not only by the presence of the implant but also by the criteria evaluating the condition and function of the implant at the time of examination.
- Sleepers are implants that are present in the oral cavity but not connected to any restoration and not providing support or function.
- Smoking is a definite risk factor for implant survival.
- Early implant failures occur before implant restoration. Late implant failures occur after the implant has been restored.
- Guided bone regeneration (GBR) is a procedure that uses a barrier membrane to isolate an area for bone growth.

Suggested Readings

Berglundh T, Persson L, Klinge B: A systematic review of the incidence of biological and technical complications in implant dentistry reported in prospective longitudinal studies of at least 5 years, *J Clin Periodontol* 29 (Suppl 3):197–212, 2002, discussion 232–233.

Del Fabbro M, Testori T, Francetti L, et al: Systematic review of survival rates for immediately loaded dental implants, *Int J Periodontics Restorative Dent* 26:249–263, 2006.

den Hartog L, Slater JJ, Vissink A, et al: Treatment outcome of immediate, early and conventional single-tooth implants in the esthetic zone: a systematic review to survival, bone level, soft-tissue, esthetics and patient satisfaction, *J Clin Periodontol* 35:1073–1086, 2008.

Esposito M, Hirsch J, Lekholm U, et al: Differential diagnosis and treatment strategies for biologic complications and failing oral implants: a review of the literature, *Int J Oral Maxillofac Implants* 14:473–490, 1999.

Goodacre CJ, Bernal G, Rungcharassaeng K, et al: Clinical complications with implants and implant prostheses, *J Prosthet Dent* 90:121–132, 2003.

Lang NP, Pjetursson BE, Tan K, et al: A systematic review of the survival and complication rates of fixed partial dentures (FPDs) after an observation period of at least 5 years. II. Combined tooth–implant-supported FPDs, *Clin Oral Implants Res* 15:643–653, 2004.

Pjetursson BE, Tan K, Lang NP, et al: A systematic review of the survival and complication rates of fixed partial dentures (FPDs) after an observation period of at least 5 years, *Clin Oral Implants Res* 15:667–676, 2004.

Roos-Jansaker AM, Lindahl C, Renvert H, et al: Nine to fourteen-year follow-up of implant treatment. Part II: presence of peri-implant lesions, *J Clin Periodontol* 33:290–295, 2006.

References

References and MCQs with answers for the chapter are available on www.medenact.com.

CHAPTER 61

Peri-implant Disease, Management, and Supportive Implant Therapy

J Do | PR Klokkevold | A Jain

CHAPTER OUTLINE

Classification of Peri-implant Diseases and Conditions

A new classification for peri-implant health, peri-implant mucositis, and peri-implantitis was developed by the 2017 World Workshop on the Classification of Periodontal and Peri-implant Diseases and Conditions. An organizing committee from the American Academy of Periodontology (AAP) and the European Federation of Periodontology (EFP) commissioned 19 review papers and four consensus reports covering relevant areas in periodontology and implant dentistry. Their proceedings regarding dental implants classified peri-implant diseases and conditions into:

1. Peri-implant health
2. Peri-implant mucositis
3. Peri-implantitis
4. Peri-implant soft and hard tissue deficiencies

Peri-implant health: Peri-implant health is defined both clinically and histologically. Clinically, peri-implant health is characterized by an absence of visual signs of inflammation and bleeding on probing. Peri-implant health can exist around implants with normal or reduced bone support. It is, however, not possible to define a range of probing depths compatible with peri-implant health. The healthy peri-implant mucosa, at the microscopic level, comprises a core of connective tissue covered by either a keratinized (masticatory mucosa) or nonkeratinized epithelium (lining mucosa).

Diagnosis of peri-implant health hence requires:

- Absence of clinical signs of inflammation.
- Absence of bleeding and/or suppuration on gentle probing.
- No increase in probing depth compared to previous examinations.
- Absence of bone loss beyond crestal bone level changes resulting from initial bone remodeling.

Peri-implant mucositis: Peri-implant mucositis is an inflammatory lesion of the soft tissues surrounding an endosseous implant in the absence of loss of supporting bone or continuing marginal bone loss.

Peri-implant mucositis is characterized by bleeding on probing and visual signs of inflammation (erythema, swelling, and/or suppuration). An increase in probing depth is often observed in the presence of peri-implant mucositis due to swelling or decrease in probing resistance. While there is strong evidence that peri-implant mucositis is caused by plaque, there is very limited evidence for nonplaque-induced peri-implant mucositis.

The diagnosis of peri-implant mucositis, hence, requires:

1. Visual inspection demonstrating the presence of peri-implant signs of inflammation: red as opposed to pink, swollen tissues as opposed to no swelling, soft as opposed to firm tissue consistency;
2. Presence of profuse (line or drop) bleeding and/or suppuration on probing;
3. An increase in probing depths compared to baseline; and
4. Absence of bone loss beyond crestal bone level changes resulting from the initial remodeling.

Peri-implant mucositis can be reversed with measures aimed at eliminating the plaque. Biofilm-induced peri-implant mucositis is reversible at the host biomarker level once biofilm control is reinstituted. Reversal of the clinical signs of inflammation may take longer than 3 weeks. Factors identified as risk indicators for peri-implant mucositis include biofilm accumulation, smoking, and radiation. Further evidence is required for potential risk factors, including diabetes, lack of keratinized mucosa, and presence of excess luting cement.

Peri-implantitis: Peri-implantitis was defined as a plaque-associated pathologic condition occurring in the tissue around dental implants, characterized by inflammation in the peri-implant mucosa and subsequent progressive loss of supporting bone. Peri-implant mucositis is assumed to precede peri-implantitis. Peri-implantitis is associated with poor plaque control and with patients with a history of severe periodontitis. The onset of peri-implantitis may occur early following implant placement as indicated by radiographic data. Peri-implantitis, in the absence of treatment, seems to progress in a nonlinear and accelerating pattern.

Peri-implantitis sites exhibit clinical signs of inflammation and increased probing depths compared to baseline measurements. At the histologic level, compared to periodontitis sites, peri-implantitis sites often have larger inflammatory lesions. Surgical entry at peri-implantitis sites often reveals a circumferential pattern of bone loss. There is strong evidence that there is an increased risk of developing peri-implantitis in patients who have a history of chronic periodontitis, poor plaque control skills, and no regular maintenance care after implant therapy. Data identifying "smoking" and "diabetes" as potential risk factors/indicators for peri-implantitis are inconclusive. There is some limited evidence linking peri-implantitis to other factors such as postrestorative presence of submucosal cement, lack of peri-implant keratinized mucosa, and positioning of implants that make it difficult to perform oral hygiene and maintenance. Progressive crestal bone loss around implants in the absence of clinical signs of soft tissue inflammation is a rare.

Peri-implant soft and hard tissue deficiencies: Normal healing following tooth loss leads to diminished dimensions of the alveolar process/ridge that result in both hard and soft tissue deficiencies. Larger ridge deficiencies can occur at sites associated with severe loss of periodontal support, extraction trauma, endodontic infections, root fractures, thin buccal bone plates, poor tooth position, injury, and pneumatization of the maxillary sinuses. Other factors affecting the ridge can be associated with medications and systemic diseases reducing the amount of naturally formed bone, tooth agenesis, and pressure from prostheses. Factors affecting hard- and soft-tissue deficiencies at dental implants have further been grouped as:

Hard tissue deficiencies prior to implant placement:

- Tooth loss
- Trauma from tooth extraction
- Periodontitis
- Endodontic infections
- Longitudinal root fractures
- General trauma
- Bone height in the posterior maxilla (area of the sinus floor)
- Systemic diseases

Hard-tissue deficiencies after implant placement:

- Defects in healthy situations
- Malpositioning of implants
- Peri-implantitis
- Mechanical overload
- Soft-tissue thickness
- Systemic diseases

Soft-tissue deficiencies prior to implant placement:

- Tooth loss
- Periodontal disease
- Systemic diseases

Soft-tissue deficiencies after implant placement:

- Lack of buccal bone
- Papilla height
- Keratinized tissue
- Migration of teeth and lifelong skeletal changes

When more than one factor leading to hard and/or soft tissue deficiencies appear together, the severity of the resulting condition may increase. Efforts should be made to better identify the relative importance of these etiological factors and to develop strategies to counteract their negative effects.

Management of Peri-implant Diseases

Examination of Implants and Peri-implant Tissues

Examination of Implants

The supportive implant-treatment appointment should include an inquiry of any new concerns, problems, or pain; review of changes in the patient's medical and oral status; evaluation and reinforcement of oral hygiene; examination and evaluation of soft and hard tissue health; evaluation of implants and the associated implant restorations' stability and integrity; and professional supportive treatment. Finally, assessment should be made to determine the appropriate recall interval and plan for the next visit.

Examination begins with visual inspection for plaque and calculus accumulation; signs of inflammation and swelling; peri-implant soft-tissue quality, color, consistency, and contour; and aberrations in the implant prosthesis. Peri-implant soft tissue can be digitally palpated to detect edema, tenderness, exudation, or suppuration. Peri-implant probing can be used to assess the condition and level of soft and hard tissues surrounding implants. When indicated, radiographic images can be obtained to help verify the level of the peri-implant crestal bone. Determination of implant stability (mobility) and percussion testing can help verify implant osseointegration (Fig. 61.1).

Peri-implant Probing

Probing of implants can be done with light force (0.25 N) using a traditional steel probe without adverse effects to the peri-implant mucosa. Implant probing should be recorded at the time of final restoration delivery as the baseline measurement and at least annually thereafter.

Clinicians should use caution when evaluating peri-implant probing because these measures cannot be interpreted the same as probing depths around teeth. While periodontal probing around natural teeth is very useful to assess the health of periodontal tissues, the sulcus or pocket depth, and the level of attachment, probing around implants may not provide comparable results. Due to distinct differences in the tissues that surround and support teeth compared to those that surround and support implants, the probe inserts and penetrates differently. Around teeth, the periodontal probe is resisted by the health of the periodontal tissues and, perhaps most importantly, by the insertion of supracrestal connective tissue fibers into the cementum of the root surface. These fibers, unique to teeth, are the primary source of resistance to the probe. There is no equivalent fiber attachment around implants. Connective tissue fibers around implants generally run parallel to the implant or restorative surface and do not have perpendicular or inserting fibers. The primary source of resistance to the probe around an implant will differ depending on the conditions surrounding the implant. At noninflamed sites, the most coronal aspect of connective tissue adhesion to the implant will resist the probe. At inflamed sites, the probe tip consistently penetrates farther into the connective tissue until less inflamed connective tissue is encountered, which is often close to or at the level of bone.

The value of peri-implant probing is different than periodontal probing and offers very limited information by comparison. Probing around implants can measure the level of the mucosal margin relative to a fixed position on the implant or restoration and can also measure the depth of tissue around the implant. The peri-implant probing depth is often a measure of the thickness of the surrounding connective tissues and correlates most consistently with the level of surrounding bone. However, peri-implant probing is affected by several conditions, including the size of the probe, the force and direction of insertion, the health and resistance of peri-implant tissues, the level of bone support, the features of the implant, abutment, and prosthesis design (Fig. 61.2). A comparison of probing pocket depth of implants with peri-implantitis before and after the removal of the prosthetic restorations reported similar probing depths in only 37% of sites. In 39% of sites, the difference was ±1 mm, in 15% of sites, it was ±2 mm, and in 9% of sites, it was ±3 mm. In other words, probing measurements can be an accurate measure of soft-tissue thickness around an implant (i.e., peri-implant soft tissue above the bone level), but in many cases or sites, the inability to properly angle and direct the probe alongside the implant may lead to the inaccurate assessment of soft-tissue thickness. In these situations, the clinician must appreciate the

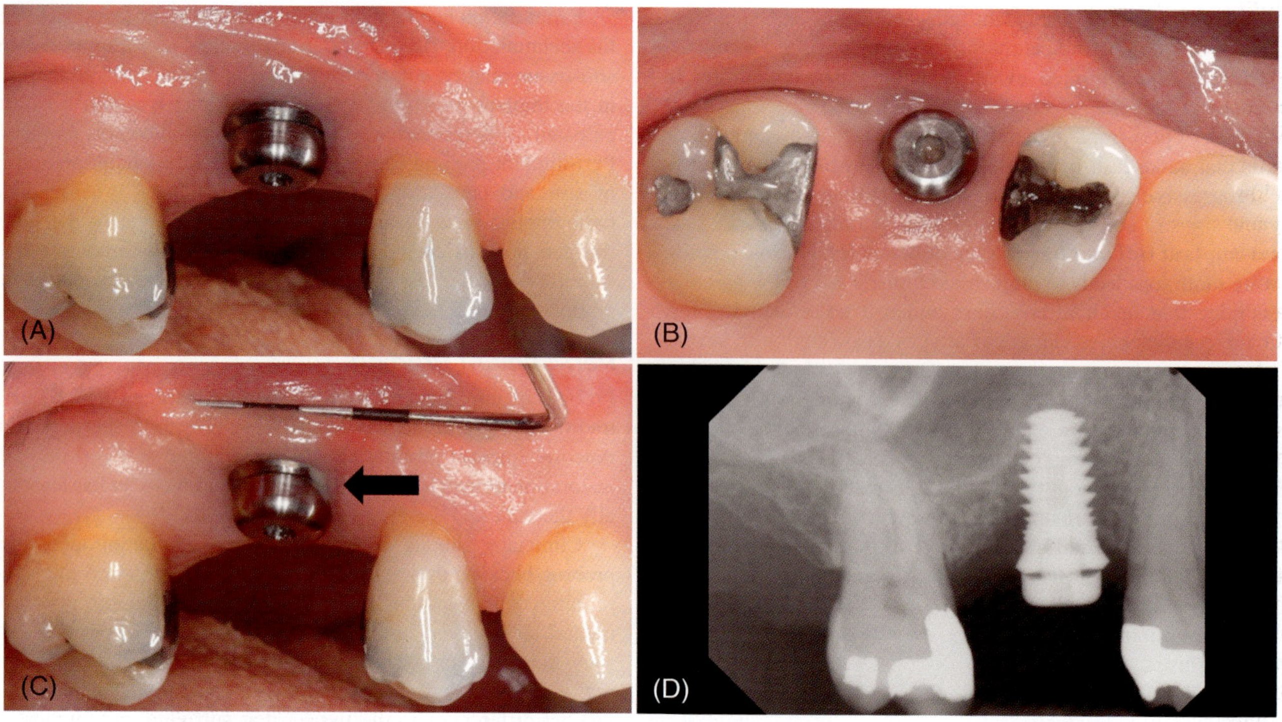

Fig. 61.1 Peri-implantitis. A and B, Minimal plaque accumulation. Peri-implant mucosa exhibits minimal erythema and edema. Note: buccal placement of implant in B. C, Manipulation of tissue indicates lack of buccal keratinized attached gingiva and exudation from peri-implant sulcus (arrow). D, Periapical radiograph shows peri-implant bone loss to the apex of the implant.

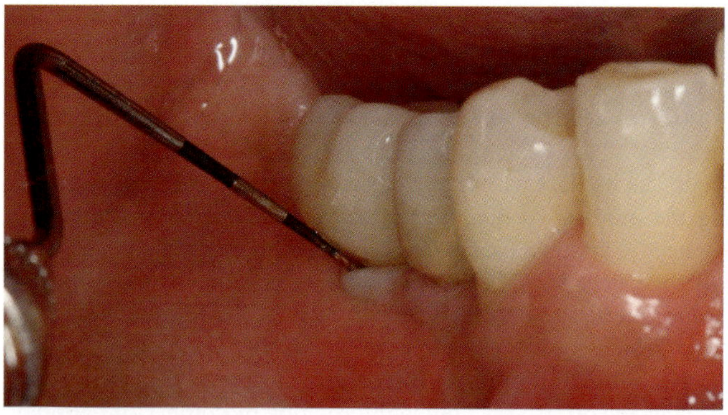

Fig. 61.2 Buccal probing of implant impeded by implant restoration.

limitations and know that other clinical parameters and radiographs are required to help evaluate peri-implant condition. Furthermore, probing around implants is likely to be more variable than around teeth; studies have shown that a change in probing force around implants results in more dramatic changes than a similar change in probing force around teeth. The probing depth around implants presumed to be "healthy" (and without bleeding) has been documented to be about 3 mm around all surfaces. The absence of bleeding on probing around teeth has been established as an indicator of health and a predictor of periodontal stability. Studies comparing bleeding on probing around teeth and implants in the same patient have reported that bleeding around implants occurs more frequently. The presence of bleeding on probing at implant sites may indicate inflammation in the peri-implant mucosa. However, the ability to use bleeding on probing as an indicator of assessing diseased versus healthy sites around implants has not been established. Due to the potential for false-positive bleeding (i.e., provoked-bleeding) with probing, the use of marginal bleeding, which is a more sensitive indicator of inflammation and is less likely to elicit false-positive bleeding, has been proposed to assess peri-implant inflammation. Marginal bleeding can be evaluated by running a probe circumferentially along the coronal portion in the implant sulcus. Overall, the value of peri-implant probing is in monitoring changes in the probing pocket depth over time rather than the initial value as some implants may be placed apically for esthetics.

Microbial Testing

Studies in animals and humans have demonstrated the development of peri-implant mucosal inflammation in response to the accumulation of bacterial plaque. Microbiologic studies suggest that greater probing depths or "pockets" around implants harbor higher levels of pathogenic microorganisms. Studies have also documented similarities in the microbial composition of plaque in healthy periodontal sites compared to healthy peri-implant sites. Likewise, evidence indicates that the microbiota of diseased periodontal pockets harbor the same periodontal pathogenic microorganisms as those observed in inflamed peri-implant sites (peri-implantitis). However, there is no evidence to prove that periodontal pathogens cause peri-implant disease and the pathogenesis of inflammatory disease around implants has not been defined. A recent report now generally accepts the belief that peri-implant disease, like periodontal disease, occurs primarily as a result of an overwhelming bacterial insult and subsequent host response. Furthermore, human biopsies indicate that peri-implantitis and periodontitis exhibit similar histologic features including an inflammatory cell infiltrate in the connective tissue dominated by B lymphocytes and plasma cells, as well as upregulation of inflammatory biomarkers. No convincing evidence indicates that laboratory tests for the identification of suspected periodontal pathogens are of any use in the evaluation of implants. The usefulness of microbial testing may be limited to the evaluation of peri-implant sites that show signs of infection and bone loss, so the clinician can prescribe appropriate antibiotics.

Stability Measures

The assessment of implant stability (or mobility) is an important measure for determining whether osseointegration is being maintained. Important as it is, however, this measure has extremely low sensitivity but high specificity; that is, an implant may exhibit significant bone loss and remain stable. Stability measure in this case has a low sensitivity for the detection of any bone loss. Conversely, if any implant mobility is detected, it is likely that the implant is not surrounded by bone; mobility is highly specific for the detection of implant failure or lack of osseointegration. Mobility must be differentiated between loss of implant osseointegration and loose implant restoration.

There is a great interest in evaluating the stability of the bone-to-implant contact in a noninvasive manner. Two noninvasive techniques that have been used for evaluating implant stability are impact resistance (e.g., Periotest) and resonance frequency analysis (RFA). Originally designed to evaluate tooth mobility quantitatively, the Periotest (Gulden, Bensheim, Germany) is a noninvasive, electronic device that provides an objective measurement of the reaction of the periodontium to a defined impact load applied to the tooth crown. The Periotest value depends to some extent on tooth mobility but mainly on the dampening characteristics of the periodontium. Despite the dependence on the periodontium, the Periotest has been used to evaluate implant stability as well. However, unlike teeth, the movement of implants and the surrounding bone are minuscule and therefore the Periotest values fall within a much smaller range compared to the range found with teeth. Detection of horizontal mobility may be a significant advantage for the use of the Periotest because it is much more sensitive to horizontal movement than similar detection by other means, such as manual assessment. Another noninvasive method used to measure the stability of implants is with RFA. This method uses a transducer that is attached to the implant or abutment. A steady-state signal is applied to the implant through the transducer and a response is measured. The RFA value is a function of the stiffness of the implant in the surrounding tissues. The stiffness is influenced by the implant, the interface between the implant and bone and soft tissues, as well as the surrounding bone itself. Additionally, the height of the implant or abutment above the bone will influence the RFA value. Unlike the Periotest, however, the RFA is not dependent on movement in only one direction. Thus, the absolute RFA values vary from one implant design to another and from one site to another but there is high consistency for any one implant or location. The value of RFA is most appreciated with repeated measures of the same implant over time because it is very sensitive to changes in the bone–implant interface. Small changes in tissue support can be detected using RFA. An increase in the RFA value indicates increased implant stability, whereas a decrease indicates loss of stability. However, this is a relative measure and it has not been determined whether RFA is capable of detecting impending failure before the implant actually fails. Currently, much interest and research have focused on the use of noninvasive methods to evaluate implant stability. Mobility remains the cardinal sign of implant failure and detecting mobility is, therefore, an important parameter.

Implant Percussion

Tapping of an implant-healing abutment or restoration with an instrument will produce a sound that can help determine implant osseointegration. A solid resonating sound and the absence of pain usually indicate implant osseointegration. A dull sound may indicate the implant is fibrous encapsulated; radiographic and other clinical findings are needed for diagnosis.

Radiographic Examination

Perpendicular intraoral–periapical radiographs should be taken at implant placement, at abutment connection, at final restoration delivery for baseline documentation of bone levels, and annually thereafter to monitor marginal or peri-implant bone changes. In the presence of peri-implant inflammation, a periapical radiograph is indicated for peri-implant bone evaluation and disease diagnosis. Periapical radiographs have excellent resolution and, when taken perpendicular to an implant, can provide valuable details of the implant–abutment junction, mesial and distal crestal bone level relative to the implant platform, and bone-to-implant interface along the length of the implant (Fig. 61.3). The limitation of periapical radiographs is that they are difficult to standardize and great variability is inherent in the acquisition process. However, periapical radiographs are relatively simple, inexpensive, and readily available in the dental office. It is diagnostically important to obtain images that clearly show implant threads (i.e., not blurred by nonperpendicular angulation) and the restorative-implant abutment connection.

The objective of the radiographic examination is to measure the height of bone adjacent to the implant(s) and to evaluate the presence and quality of bone along the length of the implant, as well as to detect any peri-implant radiolucencies. Although the predictive

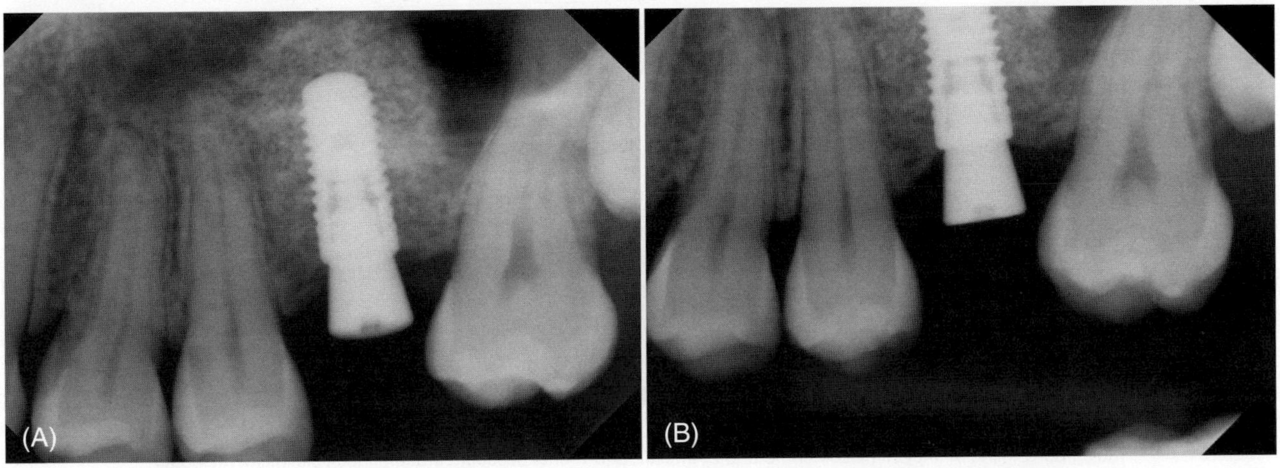

Fig. 61.3 A, Periapical radiograph capturing the whole implant. B, A second perpendicular periapical is necessary to assess crestal bone level. Note: platform-switching at implant–abutment junction.

value of assessing implant stability with radiographs is low, films do offer a reasonable method to measure changes in bone levels. The predictive value of detecting implant failure or loss of stability is good when radiolucent lesions are discovered with periapical radiographs. Radiographic identification of unstable implants is reliable when performed as part of annual examinations and when examining patients on a routine, long-term basis.

The radiographic examination remains one of the primary tools for detecting failed or failing implants in routine clinical evaluation, even though it is not as accurate as mobility tests. In one study designed to evaluate the accuracy and precision of radiographic diagnosis of mobility, the probability of predicting implant mobility in a population with a low prevalence of implant failures was found to be low. Other studies, however, have demonstrated much higher predictive value for radiographic diagnosis of implant mobility. The authors concluded that the most important factors for making an accurate radiographic diagnosis are the quality of the radiograph and the experience of the clinician.

Evaluation of Biofilm Control

Impeccable plaque control or removal of biofilm is crucial for peri-implant tissue health. Poor plaque control is associated with peri-implant diseases with an odds ratio of 14:3. It is advantageous to evaluate plaque control prior to any tissue manipulation. The amount and location of plaque and calculus accumulation should be assessed visually. Poor plaque control is typically associated with plaque and calculus retention and erythematous and edematous gingival tissue. When plaque control is inadequate, the patient should be asked to demonstrate his or her oral hygiene routine in front of a mirror so that the clinician can evaluate the patient's oral hygiene techniques. If the patient fails to remove plaque in any areas, the patient's attention should be directed to the location of the plaque. An instrument can be used to remove the plaque under the attention of the patient so that he or she can see its color and consistency. At this time, oral hygiene instruction should be demonstrated and reinforced.

Evaluation of Peri-implant Health and Disease

Peri-implant mucosal health is characterized by pink, firm, and well-adapted gingival tissue. Peri-implant disease is associated with clinical erythema, edema, and loss of tissue tightness around the implant. Peri-implant mucosa can be nonkeratinized unattached (Fig. 61.1C) or keratinized attached (Fig. 61.4C). In the presence of keratinized attached mucosa, a gingival seal or gingival cuff is established around the implant. The gingival cuff has the potential to protect the underlying bone and reduce subgingival plaque formation. Due to the mobile nature of oral mucosa, the protective function of nonkeratinized unattached peri-implant mucosa may not be as effective. However, the presence of keratinized attached gingiva, which can facilitate oral hygiene, is not a requisite for peri-implant health if plaque is well controlled. Nonetheless, sites deficient in keratinized attached tissue typically exhibit vertical and/or horizontal ridge deficiencies, shallow

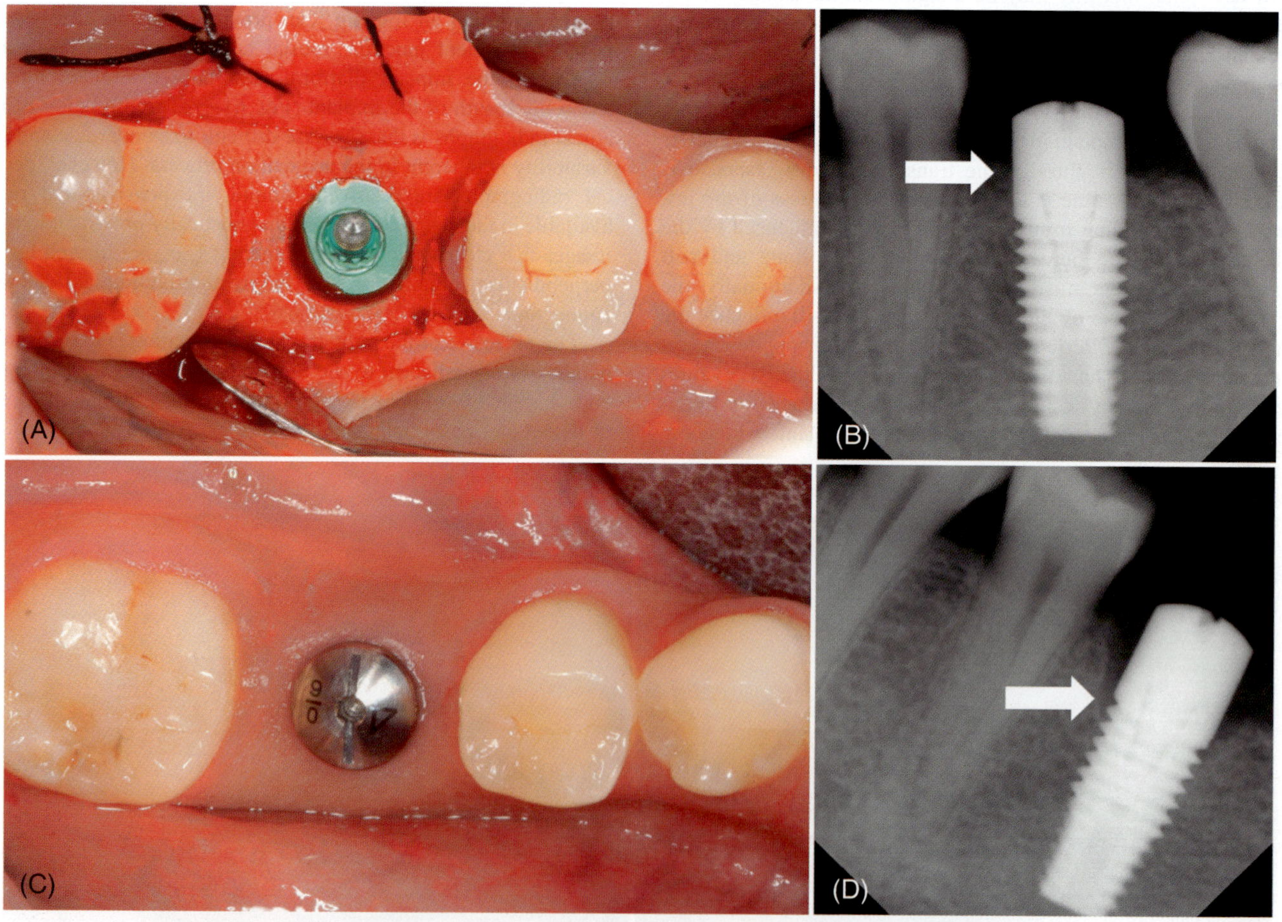

Fig. 61.4 A, Subcrestal placement of implant with adequate buccal and lingual bone thickness. B, Periapical radiograph at time of implant placement. C and D, Implant at 5-month osseointegration check exhibiting adequate peri-implant keratinized attached tissue and crestal bone remodeling to the first thread. Arrows indicate mesial–crestal bone level.

vestibular depths, and long or bulky restorations. All of these factors can impede oral hygiene access and contribute to plaque accumulation and peri-implant inflammation.

In the presence of peri-implant inflammation, the peri-implant tissue must be palpated for tenderness and suppuration, the implant must be probed, and periapical radiographs must be obtained and compared to baseline radiographs to determine peri-implant bone loss. The presence of suppuration often indicates peri-implantitis. Radiographic crestal bone loss beyond the implant baseline level at the time of final prosthesis delivery in conjunction with bleeding on probing is a characteristic of peri-implantitis; due to potential measurement errors, a threshold of detectable bone loss of 1.0–1.5 mm is recommended for diagnosis of peri-implantitis. In the absence of a baseline radiograph, a vertical distance of 2 mm from the expected marginal bone level following the initial crestal bone remodeling is recommended as the threshold for diagnosing peri-implantitis. The amount of initial marginal bone remodeling can vary depending on the design of the implant–abutment junction. Platform-switched implants (Figs. 61.5C and 61.3), in which the abutment is internally offset relative to the implant fixture at the implant–abutment junction, may exhibit less crestal bone remodeling than nonplatform-switched implants (Fig. 61.4), in which the abutment is flush or even with the implant fixture at the implant–abutment junction.

Evaluation of Implant Osseointegration

Implant osseointegration must be determined prior to the fabrication and delivery of the final implant prosthesis. Implant osseointegration can only be definitively determined histologically, which would require the implant and the surrounding bone to be removed. Thus, a combination of radiographic and clinical parameters is used to make an assessment of implant osseointegration or to rule out lack of osseointegration. These include absence of peri-implant inflammation and pain to palpation and percussion, presence of a solid resonating sound to percussion, complete radiographic bone-to-implant contact along the implant surface (i.e., absence of radiolucencies along the bone–implant interface), and implant stability.

Evaluation of Implant Restorations

Implant superstructures, frameworks, and restorations should be fabricated to accommodate and facilitate oral hygiene (e.g., embrasure spaces should be made to allow the passage of a proxy brush) (Fig. 61.4). Occlusal schemes of implant restorations should provide adequate posterior support, maximize axial loading, and minimize incline contacts, nonaxial loading, and interferences in excursive movements. During delivery, radiographs perpendicular to the implant should be obtained for baseline documentation and to verify complete seating of the restorations. Following delivery, cement-retained implant restorations should be thoroughly evaluated for residual excess cement, which must be removed. During follow-up visits, implant restorations should be carefully examined for heavy contacts, fractures, loose screws, and in removable prostheses, worn-out retentive components (i.e., Hader clips and locator–attachment inserts). Occlusion should be adjusted accordingly to prevent implant overload and fractures of implant parts. Loose abutment and setscrews must be evaluated, possibly replaced and properly torqued down. Worn-out retentive components must be replaced periodically to ensure proper retention, stability, and function of the removable prostheses. Occlusal wear of teeth and fit of tissue-borne surfaces of the implant–tissue-borne prostheses should be assessed and corrected as indicated. In patients with oral parafunctions and heavy occlusal forces, occlusal guards are recommended to protect implants and restorations.

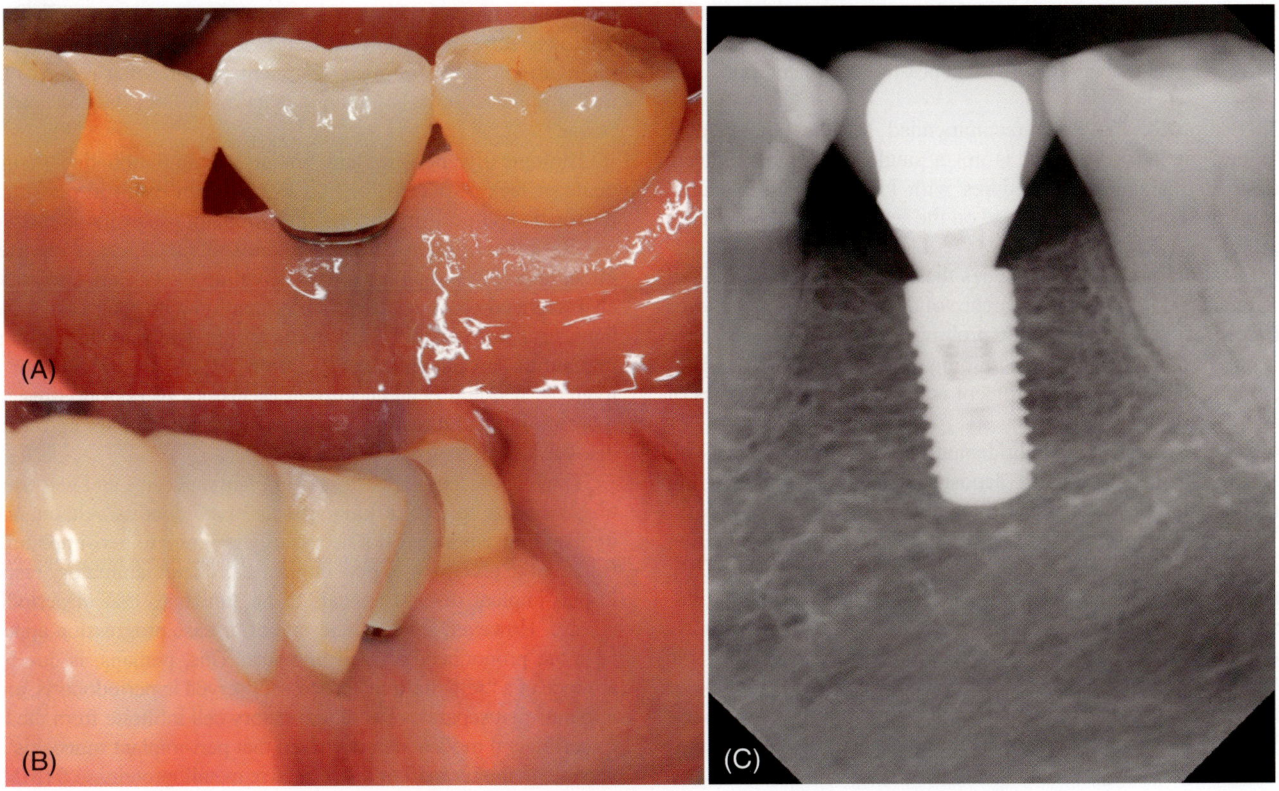

Fig. 61.5 Restoration designed with adequate hygiene access. A, Lingual view. B, Mesial view of buccal contour. C, Periapical radiograph showing gradual transition from implant fixture to restoration. Note: platform-switching at implant–abutment junction.

Treatment of Peri-implant Diseases

The goals of peri-implant disease treatment are the elimination of all peri-implant infectious and inflammatory processes, prevention of disease progression, and preservation and restoration of function and esthetics. Treatment begins with patient education in the etiology, disease process, prevention of peri-implant diseases, and oral hygiene instruction. Although bacteria are the main etiologic factor, systemic (e.g., smoking and poorly controlled diabetes) and local factors (e.g., residual excess cements and poorly designed restorations that inhibit hygiene access) should be identified and modified.

Peri-implant Mucositis

Peri-implant mucositis can be effectively treated with nonsurgical mechanical therapy. Treatment requires complete removal of supramucosal and submucosal plaque, calculus, and deposits using curettes, ultrasonic scalers, polishing cups, and prophy paste. The use of adjunctive antimicrobials (e.g., chlorhexidine irrigation and mouth rinse) to mechanical debridement can enhance treatment outcome.

Peri-implantitis

The treatment of peri-implantitis includes nonsurgical and surgical interventions, both of which may be combined with the adjunctive use of antimicrobials. Nonsurgical interventions consist of antimicrobial rinse and irrigation, local antibiotics, ultrasonic debridement, mechanical debridement with air-abrasive devices, and laser therapy. Surgical treatment includes full-thickness flap elevation for access followed by degranulation, surface debridement by laser or mechanical instruments, surface decontamination with laser or antimicrobials, and bone augmentation.

Lang et al. in 2004 gave consensus statements and recommendations for clinical procedures regarding implant survival and complications which included mechanical therapy, adjunctive antimicrobials, photodynamic therapy, local drug delivery, laser, implantoplasty, guided bone regeneration, peri-implant resective therapy, and cumulative interceptive surgical therapy (CIST) as all possible treatment modalities once disease sets in.

CIST protocol has been recommended for the management of the peri-implant lesions. It is not a single procedure, rather a sequence of therapeutic procedures with increasing antibacterial potential and type of therapy based on the severity and extent of the lesion.

Application of the CIST includes the assessment of the following parameters: (1) presence or absence of dental plaque, (2) presence or absence of bleeding on gentle probing, (3) presence or absence of suppuration, (4) peri-implant probing depth, and (5) evidence of radiographic bone loss. This protocol is divided into four stages of treatment sequence as follows:

1. Protocol A (mechanical debridement): In case of implants with evident plaque or calculus deposits adjacent to only slightly inflamed peri-implant tissues (bleeding on probing is positive).
2. Protocol B (antiseptic treatment): It is performed in situation where in addition to plaque and Bleeding on probing (BOP), probing depth in increased up to 4–5 mm. Chlorhexidine digluconate either in the form of daily rinse of 0.1%, 0.12%, or 0.2% or as a gel applied to the site of desired action.
3. Protocol C (antibiotic treatment): When probing depth value of the peri-implant sulcus or pocket increase to 6 mm or more. Beside the protocol A and B, an antibiotic directed at the elimination of gram-negative anaerobic bacteria is administrated.
4. Protocol D (regenerative or resective therapy): Only if infection is controlled successfully by A, B, and C as evidenced by an absence of suppuration and reduced edema. It aimed to restore the bony support of the implant by means of regenerative techniques. (Although protocol D has not been assessed in its entirety, prospective cohort studies have evaluated the treatment modalities A, B, C. The benefits of adding surgical therapy D to the CIST protocol are documented in case series, single case reports, and in a series of animal experiments.)

In 2004, it was modified and called AKUT-concept by Lang et al. The basis of this concept is a regular recall of the implanted patient and repeated assessment of plaque, bleeding, suppuration, pockets, and radiological evidence of bone loss.

Based on two systematic reviews, currently available scientific data is insufficient to suggest which treatment intervention of peri-implantitis is most effective and which antibiotic should be administered locally or systematically. Implant-surface decontamination/disinfection remains challenging especially for implants with roughened surfaces. For some treatment modalities, recurrence of peri-implantitis appears to be high (up to 100%) after 1 or more years of treatment and retreatment may be necessary. Surgical access appears to be necessary to arrest peri-implant bone loss. Surgical treatment may result in gingival recession and compromise esthetics. At sites with high esthetic demands, definitive treatment of peri-implantitis may include the removal of the implant, grafting of the site, and placement of another implant.

Supportive Implant Therapy

Rationale for Supportive Implant Therapy

Although dental implants are not vulnerable to dental caries, they are still susceptible to mechanical complications and peri-implant plaque-induced inflammatory tissue changes. A 10-year retrospective study of 397 fixed-implant reconstructions in 300 patients observed a mechanical complication rate of 24.7%. The most frequent complication was ceramic chipping (20.31%), followed by occlusal screw loosening (2.57%), and loss of retention (2.06%). Although relatively infrequent, occlusal screw loosening can result in a subgingival gap at the implant–abutment junction that retains plaque and stimulates an inflammatory reaction in both the soft and hard tissue.

Biologically, peri-implant plaque accumulation due to inadequate or lack of access for oral hygiene can result in peri-implant mucositis and peri-implantitis. Peri-implant mucositis is characterized by inflammation confined to the soft tissue and is reported to affect up to 80% of patients with dental implants. Peri-implantitis is characterized by peri-implant inflammation with progressive crestal bone loss beyond the initial remodeling. The prevalence of peri-implantitis in patients ranges from 11.2% to 53%. Poor oral hygiene, residual cement, current or history of periodontitis, cigarette smoking, and diabetes mellitus are risk factors for peri-implant diseases.

The relationship between peri-implant mucositis and peri-implantitis is similar to that of gingivitis and periodontitis. Although peri-implant mucositis does not necessarily progress to peri-implantitis, it is likely the precursor to peri-implantitis. The inflammatory response in peri-implant disease appears to be similar to that in periodontal disease. However, severity and rate of disease progression appear to be more pronounced around implants. This, perhaps, is due to the absence of a "self-limiting" process, observed in periodontitis, around implants that separates the inflammatory cell infiltrate from the bone. Experimental models demonstrated that peri-implant mucositis is reversible at the biomarker level [matrix metalloproteinase 8 (MMP-8) and interleukin-1β (IL-1β)]. A review of the literature reported that peri-implant mucositis can be effectively treated with nonsurgical mechanical therapy while such modalities tend to be ineffective against peri-implantitis. Furthermore, results of surgical treatment for peri-implantitis are not predictable. For these reasons, the prevention, early detection, and early treatment of peri-implant diseases are critical. Periodic and well-regimented supportive implant treatment is essential to the long-term success of dental implant therapy.

Methods for Patient Oral Hygiene

The importance of good oral hygiene should be stressed even before implants are placed, and peri-implant oral hygiene for plaque control should begin as early as possible once the implant is exposed to the oral cavity. A cotton tip, cotton gauze, or soft toothbrush can be used to gently remove plaque from healing abutments or provisional restorations during the early postoperative phase of healing. Once implant osseointegration has been achieved and verified, a comprehensive oral hygiene regimen is needed. The research in this area is limited and has not lead to a standard protocol or regimen for implant maintenance. Most recommendations are based on expert opinion, research of natural teeth, and experience. Evidence from a systematic review showed that mechanical plaque control with either a powered or manual toothbrush can be effective in reducing mucositis. However, the experts in different consensus discussions have stressed over a consolidated "Implant-Care Regimen" approach for implant health maintenance, including the use of dentifrices, powered tooth brushes, and oral irrigators.

Dentifrices play a vital role in peri-implant health maintenance by facilitating plaque removal, disrupting biofilms, providing antimicrobial action, and ensuring gentle cleaning without causing damage to the implant or surrounding tissues. Regular and proper oral hygiene practices, including brushing with appropriate dentifrices, are essential for the long-term success and stability of dental implants. Specifically, dentifrices such as Colgate Periogard containing combination of antimicrobial agents, that is, zinc and pyrophosphate, are helpful to reduce the build-up of soft and hard accretions on the implant surface and reduce the risk of biofilm-associated infection and inflammation around the implant site.

Brushing around dental implants should be performed at least twice daily using a gentle but thorough cleaning motion. Patients should be educated on proper brushing techniques. Improvised designs of manual toothbrushes with high dense (6000+) soft & slimmer bristle (0.01mm tip diameter) with flexible neck to reduce the pressure while brushing e.g Colgate Periogard© Gum expert toothbrush provide better access in difficult to reach areas around dental implants e.g subgingival implant abutment interface and offer better cleaning efficiency for these patients. It is suggested that the oscillating/rotating type of powered toothbrush is effective, safe, and comfortable for patients rehabilitated by means of oral implant-supported prostheses. A powered toothbrush confers good brushing technique and appears to enhance the patient's motivation to brush (Fig. 61.6). In a 1-year study by Vanderkerckhove and colleagues, an Oral-B oscillating-rotating electric toothbrush was found to be effective, safe to use, and comfortable for patients with implant-supported fixed prostheses. The safety and acceptability findings were corroborated in a separate 1-year study by Rasperini et al. Truhlar et al. compared a powered toothbrush and a manual toothbrush with respect to reducing plaque and gingivitis around oral implants and found a greater effect with the powered toothbrush. In a group of elderly patients, both a manual toothbrush and an oscillating/rotating powered toothbrush were found to be equally effective.

In addition to regular brushing, patients with dental implants may be advised to use special brushes or devices, such as interdental brushes, proxa brushes, or water flossers, to clean around the implant abutments and prosthetic components thoroughly (Fig. 61.7).

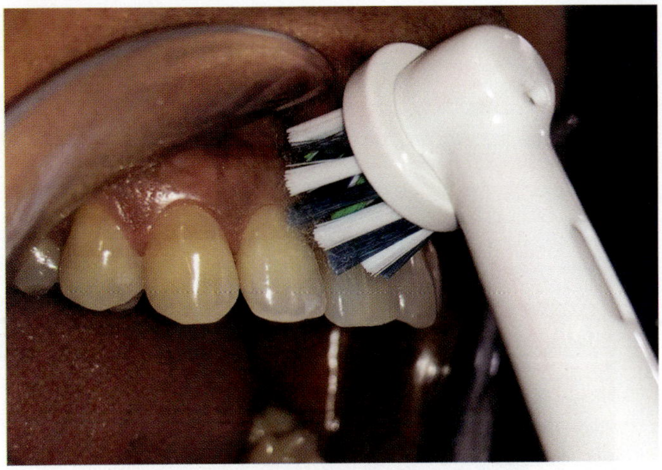

Fig. 61.6 Powered toothbrush.

A powered water flosser has been studied with implants. One study reported subgingival irrigation of 0.06% chlorhexidine gluconate with a Waterpik Water Flosser (Water Pik, Inc., Fort Collins, CO, USA) to be more effective at reducing plaque and mucosal inflammation and produced less stains than rinsing with 0.12% chlorhexidine gluconate once a day (Fig. 61.8). Another randomized controlled study compared a water flosser to string floss over 4 weeks. The water flosser group showed an 81% reduction in bleeding compared to 33% for string floss, which is a 2.45-fold difference. Patients require products that they can easily maneuver around the prosthetic replacement and access areas susceptible to plaque accumulation to prevent peri-implant diseases. A cordless, portable, and rechargeable oral irrigator Colgate Blast with 1600 pulsations per minute, three adjustable pressure modes viz. gentle, regular, pulse, and a nozzle size of 0.55 mm provides a flushing zone to expel the debris and bacteria from the sulcus or pocket with a thin line of water flow around an implant and is reported to be three times more effective than a continuous-stream device (see Chapter 34).

Methods for Professional Recall Maintenance

Professional maintenance consists of the removal of dental plaque and calculus from implant components exposed to the oral environment. Similar to root surfaces, the transmucosal surfaces of implants should be smooth to minimize plaque accumulation and to facilitate oral hygiene practices. As such, at sites with excellent plaque control and peri-implant health, the need for professional instrumentation is minimal and should be limited to prevent iatrogenic damage to implant components that can contribute to plaque and calculus accumulation. In the presence of plaque, calculus, and tenacious deposits, care should be taken to minimize damage to transmucosal implant surfaces. However, priority should be placed on the complete removal of implant surface deposits.

All metal instruments, including metal curettes, scalers, and (ultra)sonic scalers, increase surface roughness of polished titanium. As such, the use of plastic, Teflon-coated, carbon- and gold-coated curettes, and nonmetal ultrasonic tips have been advocated to protect the titanium-implant surface and the titanium abutment from contamination by other metals and to reduce the likelihood of scratching the surface. Unfortunately, the large size and flexibility of nonmetal curettes may not allow effective plaque and calculus removal; and Teflon- and gold-coated curettes cannot be sharpened. Most current implant prostheses are made with gold alloys or

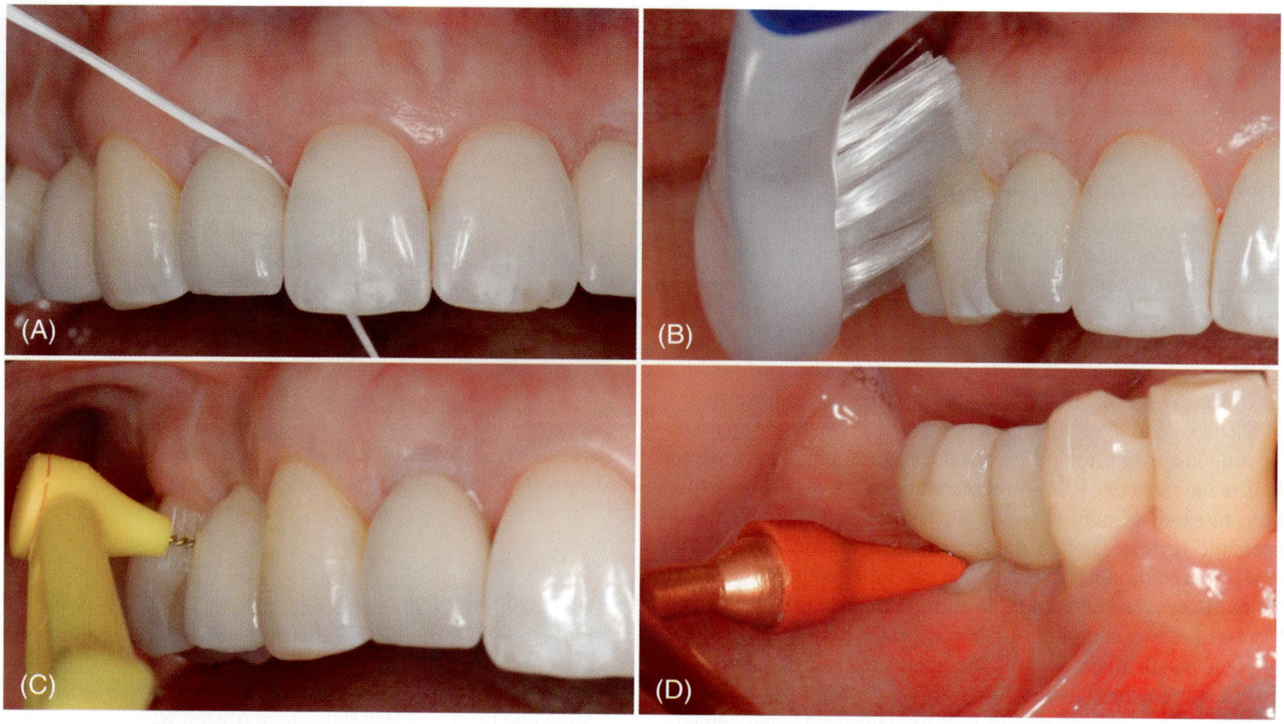

Fig. 61.7 Methods for patient oral hygiene. A, Flossing. B, Bass method of brushing with extrasoft toothbrush. C, Interproximal brushing. D, Removal of plaque with a rubber tip. Note: hygiene is targeted at the removal of plaque along the gingival margin.

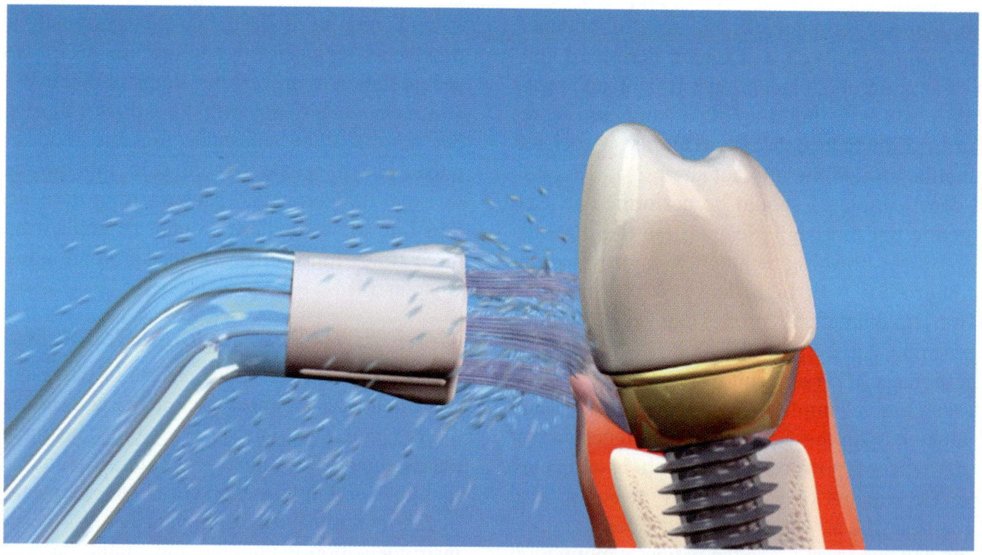

Fig. 61.8 Water flosser tip with three tufts of bristles recommended for implants. *(Courtesy: Water Pik, Inc., Fort Collins, CO, USA.)*

ceramic materials, which are usually identical to the materials used in restorations for the natural dentition. Furthermore, the location of the connection between these restorative materials and the implant is typically below the mucosa and often near the crest of bone; most calculus removal occurs above this level. Thus, the fear of contaminating the titanium implant is unwarranted. The gold alloy or ceramic surfaces can be debrided with most scalers and curettes (plastic, gold-coated, and stainless steel) without damaging the surface. Rubber cups and polishing paste can be used to remove plaque or biofilm and to enhance surface smoothness of machined and polished surfaces. Magnetostrictive and piezoelectric ultrasonic instruments with metal tips (e.g., Cavitron) should be used with caution because of irregularities that can easily be created in the surface.

Referral of Patients to the Periodontist

The guidelines described in this chapter will allow many implant patients to be maintained very well by their primary dental care provider (i.e., general dentists). Referral to a periodontist should be considered if peri-implantitis or peri-implant mucositis is diagnosed and not resolved with improved oral hygiene and professional maintenance care. Early referral is advantageous to stop progression and limit extent of bone loss.

Key points

- Peri-implant mucositis is characterized by inflammation confined to the soft tissue.
- Peri-implantitis is characterized by peri-implant inflammation with progressive crestal bone loss beyond the initial remodeling.
- Mobility of an implant is highly specific for the detection of implant failure or lack of osseointegration.
- Two noninvasive techniques to evaluate implant stability are impact resistance (e.g., Periotest) and resonance frequency analysis (RFA).
- An increase in the RFA value indicates increased implant stability, whereas a decrease indicates loss of stability.
- A solid resonating sound on tapping of an implant usually indicates implant osseointegration, whereas a dull sound may indicate that the implant is fibrous encapsulated.

Suggested Readings

Academy Report: Peri-implant mucositis and peri-implantitis: a current understanding of their diagnoses and clinical implications, *J Periodontol* 84(4):436-443, 2013.

De Bruyn H, Vandeweghe S, Ruyffelaert C, et al: Radiographic evaluation of modern oral implants with emphasis on crestal bone level and relevance to peri-implant health, *Periodontol 2000* 62(1):256-270, 2013.

Esposito M, Grusovin MG, Worthington HV: Interventions for replacing missing teeth: treatment of peri-implantitis, *Cochrane Database Syst Rev* Jan 18(1):CD004970, 2012.

Lang NP, Berglundh T: Working Group 4 of Seventh European Workshop on Periodontology: Peri-implant diseases: where are we now? Consensus of the Seventh European Workshop on Periodontology, *J Clin Periodontol* 38(Suppl 11):178-181, 2010.

Lindhe J, Meyle J: Group D of European Workshop on Periodontology. Peri-implant diseases: Consensus Report of the Sixth European Workshop on Periodontology, *J Clin Periodontol* 35(Suppl 8):282-285, 2008.

Louropoulou A, Slot DE, Van derWeijden FA: Titanium surface alterations following the use of different mechanical instruments: a systematic review, *Clin Oral Implants Res* 23(6):643-658, 2012.

Salvi GE, Aglietta M, Eick S, et al: Reversibility of experimental peri-implant mucositis compared with experimental gingivitis in humans, *Clin Oral Implants Res* 23(2):182-190, 2012.

Satpathy A, Grover V, Kumar A, et al. Indian Society of Periodontology Good Clinical Practice Recommendations for Peri-implant Care. *J Indian Soc Periodontol*. 2024;28(1):6-31. doi: 10.4103/jisp.jisp_124_24

Serino G, Turri A, Lang NP: Probing at implants with peri-implantitis and its relation to clinical peri-implant bone loss, *Clin Oral Implants Res* 24(1):91-95, 2013.

vanWinkelhoff AJ: Antibiotics in the treatment of peri-implantitis, *Eur J Oral Implantol* 5 (Suppl):S43-S50, 2012.

References

References and MCQs with answers for the chapter are available on www.medenact.com.

CHAPTER 62

Digital Implant Workflow: Planning, Placement, and Restoration

D Chao | RJ Crockett | PR Klokkevold | A Jain | V Grover

CHAPTER OUTLINE

In conventional presurgical planning, implant positions are determined with a combination of study models, wax-ups of the proposed dental prosthesis, and diagnostic imaging with a laboratory fabricated acrylic resin radiographic guide. This radiographic guide has limited correlation with the underlying bone and needs to be modified (i.e., open access for drills) to be used as a surgical guide following imaging. The transfer of imaging information correlating the prosthetic plan to the alveolar bone via the radiographic/surgical guide is prone to inaccuracies and offers minimal guidance. As a result, the final position of the implant is determined by the clinician by using the surgical guide along with his or her interpretation of the diagnostic information, clinical experience, and surgical skills to replicate the plan.

Digital technology in implant dentistry is rapidly evolving. The **digital implant workflow** can help clinicians plan more efficiently and execute more accurately. Advances in implant surgical technology include simulation software, static **computer-aided design/computer-aided manufacturing** (CAD/CAM) surgical guides, and **dynamic navigation** for dental implant surgery (Tables 62.1 and 62.2).

- **Virtual surgical planning or implant simulation software** is used preoperatively to simulate implant placement on a virtual patient. The software allows clinicians to interact with three-dimensional (3D) renderings of the patient created from computed tomography (CT) or cone-beam CT (CBCT) scan data.
- **Static CAD/CAM surgical guides** can be designed from the virtual plan and produced with various technologies including milling and 3D printing. Metal drill sleeves or bushings are manually luted to the guide after production in precise locations designed to receive them. In select manufacturing methods, the drill sleeves can be integrated into the guide and manufactured as a single piece, eliminating the need for inserting metal sleeves. Along with drill handles, keys, or integrated drill stops, the sleeves provide static and physical guidance for the osteotomy drills and implants. The drill handles, keys, or integrated drill stops are system-specific based on the manufacturer.
- **Dynamic navigation** employs real-time tracking and visual guidance to execute the virtual surgical plan. The plan is superimposed onto scan data, registered with the patient via **fiducial markers**, and observed interactively during live surgery to aid the surgeon in preparing osteotomy sites and placing dental implants.

This chapter provides an overview of the terminology, technical requirements, and limitations of digitally assisted implant placement surgery.

Data and Image Acquisition

The presurgical workup for digitally assisted implant placement begins with the acquisition of diagnostic data. For partially **edentulous** scenarios, a set of accurate diagnostic casts is needed. This can be accomplished with either conventional impressions or digital impressions via intraoral scanning. If conventional impressions and corresponding diagnostic casts are made, they must be digitized with a desktop or laboratory scanner. These digital scans are commonly exported in the **Standard Tessellation Language (STL)** format to be utilized for virtual planning and fabrication of tooth-supported surgical guides.

Conversely, for fully edentulous scenarios, a set of diagnostic casts is not needed for the presurgical workup. Complete **dentures** or record bases with teeth set in wax are used to convey the necessary information through the dual scan protocol. This protocol involves two CT or CBCT scans: one with patients wearing their dentures with fiducial markers attached and another scan of the denture(s) alone with the fiducial markers still attached (Fig. 62.1). The quality of the complete dentures or record bases with the wax setups are of utmost importance for a successful outcome.

TABLE 62.1 Advantages and Disadvantages of Static CAD/CAM Surgical Guides

Advantages of Static CAD/CAM Surgical Guides

- Implant placement is more accurate compared to the freehand method.
- Flapless surgeries are possible with mucosa-supported surgical guides.
- Less hand-eye coordination is required for implant placement because static surgical guides offer physical guidance.
- A bone-supported alveoloplasty guide can accurately direct the amount of bone removal necessary for the planned prosthesis.
- Static surgical guides can be used to guide the pick-up procedure for an immediately loaded prosthesis.

Disadvantages of Static CAD/CAM Surgical Guides

- Implant placement cannot occur right after imaging because time is required to manufacture the surgical guide.
- It may be difficult to place posterior (second molar) implants and implants in patients with limited mouth opening because the osteotomy drill and handpiece must overcome the height of the surgical sleeve.
- Static surgical guides may not be possible in tight interdental spaces.
- Bone-supported surgical guides are associated with invasive flaps.
- Incorrect guide position that goes unnoticed will result in inaccurate implant placement.
- Cost is associated with guide production (milling, 3D printing, guide sleeve).

CAD/CAM, Computer-aided design/computer-aided manufacturing; *3D*, three-dimensional.

TABLE 62.2 Advantages and Disadvantages of Dynamic Navigation

Advantages of Dynamic Navigation

- Implant placement is more accurate compared to the freehand method.
- Flapless surgeries are possible.
- Implant placement can occur right after imaging.
- It may be less difficult to place posterior (second molar) implants and implants in patients with limited mouth opening.
- Implant placement has the potential to be less invasive because large flaps are not necessary.
- Implant placement in tight interdental spaces is limited only by the diameter of the osteotomy drills.

Disadvantages of Dynamic Navigation

- Hand-eye coordination is needed because dynamic navigation only offers visual guidance.
- Two surgeries are required for completely edentulous patients due to the need to place fiducial markers (bone screws).
- There is no physical guide to guide the pick-up procedure for an immediately loaded prosthesis
- Incorrect patient tracking that goes unnoticed will result in inaccurate implant placement.
- Significant cost may be associated with the dynamic navigation software and hardware.

Simulation is not possible without the acquisition of CT or CBCT scans. Several factors, such as radiation exposure, limitations in accuracy, and scatter due to the presence of metallic restorations, should be considered when utilizing these imaging modalities. CBCT scans are obtained in multiple "slices" in **Digital Imaging and Communications in Medicine (DICOM)** format, which has achieved a near universal level of acceptance among dental simulation software. Clinicians, however, must be cognizant that not all patients should be scanned the same way, and these scans should be prescribed based on how the patient presents at the time dental records are made (see Chapter 58).

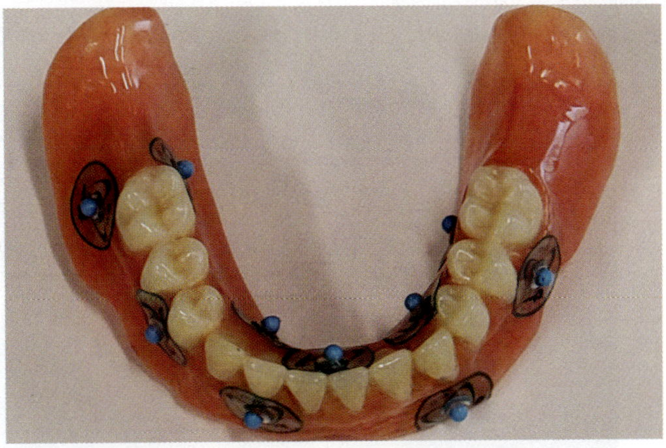

Fig. 62.1 Fiducial markers/stickers are distributed on a mandibular complete denture in preparation for the dual scan protocol.

Virtual Surgical Planning Software and Implant Simulation

The DICOM files are imported into a planning software of choice. These programs are categorized as either open or closed architecture. An open architecture software outputs files in the STL format, which can be manipulated across various CAD/CAM programs. A closed architecture software outputs files in proprietary formats, which can only be manipulated by specific proprietary/authorized programs. Generally, open architecture software is preferred for complex cases because the use of multiple programs may be necessary.

The virtual patient (i.e., 3D surface models of the patient) is derived from the CBCT dataset using gray value **segmentation**. Typically, a gray value is assigned to a specific tissue type due to radiation attenuation, which refers to the process by which the number of particles entering a body of matter is reduced by absorption and scattering. Most simulation software has the option to limit the range of gray value displayed on screen, which enables the segmentation of specific tissue types such as soft tissue and bone. Some programs also permit selective editing of segmentations, which allows structures with different densities to be separated (e.g., separating teeth from alveolar bone). For complex cases, it is good practice to manually remove any scatter artifacts and to separate structures such as the maxillary teeth, mandibular teeth, maxilla, and mandible into independent objects so they can be turned on and off for planning purposes (Fig. 62.2). Segmentation can be especially useful in the prevention of placing guide fixation pins, which may be required in select scenarios, through the roots of teeth to be extracted.

In most simulation software, certain parameters should be set and modified as necessary to achieve the highest quality output and improve the user interface. One of these parameters is patient data orientation or patient coordinate system. When a CBCT scan is imported into a simulation software, the orientation of the virtual patient is dependent on how the scan was taken. For example, if the patient was off-center or had his or her head rotated or titled during the scan, the virtual patient will be created in a similar manner (i.e., deviated). Prior to implant planning, any deviations in roll, yaw, and pitch should be addressed accordingly (Fig. 62.3).

Another important parameter is the panoramic curve. It is defined by drawing a curve based on the patient's maxilla or mandible in the axial view. The shape, position, and width of the curve determine how the patient's anatomy is visualized in the panoramic and sagittal cross-sectional viewing windows in the user interface. The

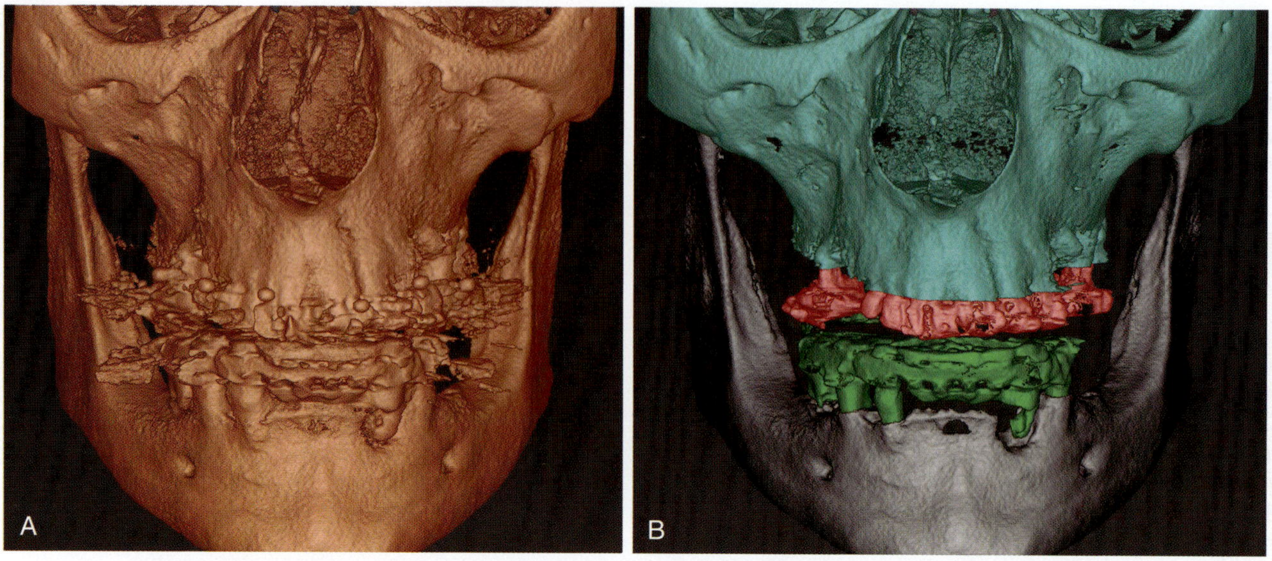

Fig. 62.2 Segmentation of the cone-beam CT (CBCT) scan dataset. A, The patient is reconstructed from CBCT data. B, The maxilla *(teal)*, maxillary teeth *(red)*, mandible *(dark gray)*, and mandibular teeth *(green)* are segmented into independent objects for implant planning.

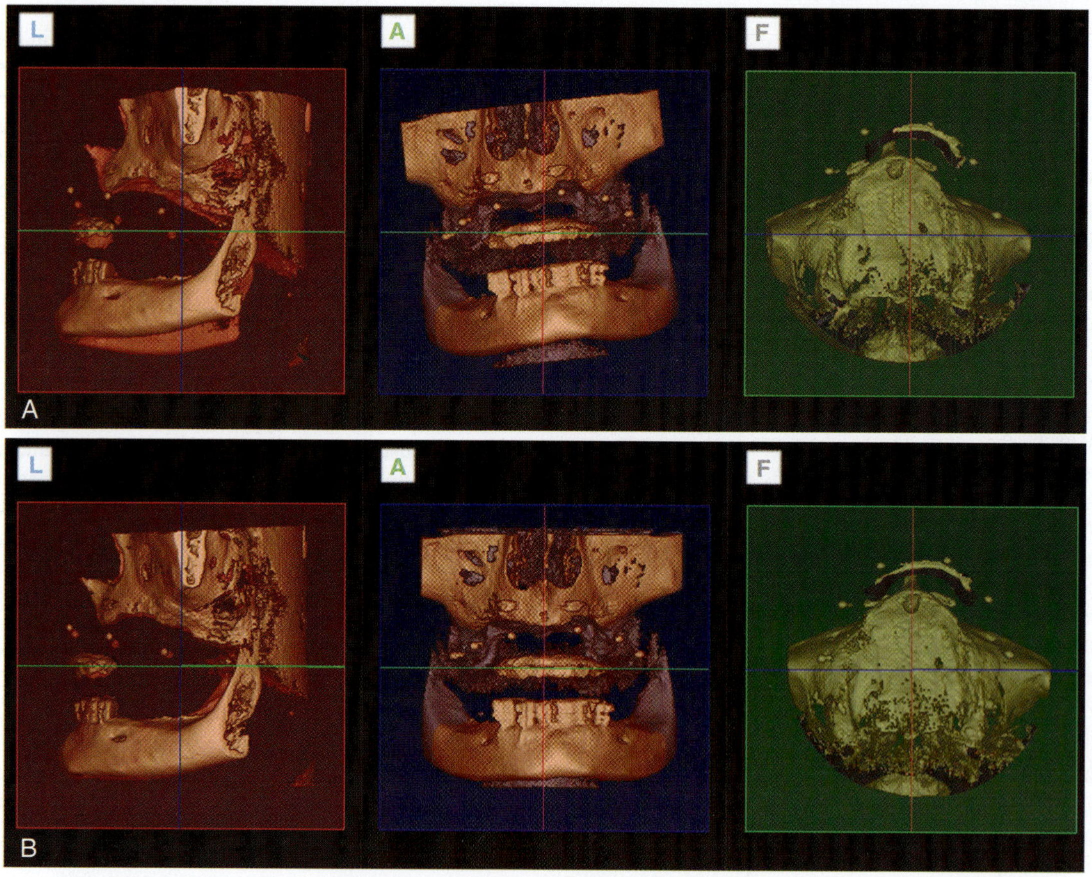

Fig. 62.3 Redefining patient orientation or the patient coordinate system. A, The patient's head was tilted during the cone-beam CT scan which resulted in a cant in the scan data. B, Patient orientation is corrected by modifying the roll, yaw, and pitch accordingly.

defined panoramic view is created from the 3D data that falls within the curve. While this is a useful view to visualize the overall plan and structures, it is important to recognize that the panoramic view is prone to distortion and should not be used as the sole view for implant planning. All planned implants must be evaluated in multiple cross-sectional views and in various directions for accurate assessment. Lastly, unlike a conventional panoramic image, the defined panoramic view generated from the panoramic curve will not show anatomic structures that are not within the panoramic curve. Specifically, vital anatomic structures such as the inferior alveolar nerve will only be visible on the defined panoramic view when it is included in the panoramic curve (Fig. 62.4).

The teeth directly segmented from the CBCT dataset are not accurate enough for tooth-supported surgical guide fabrication, especially if metal-induced scatter is present. To circumvent this problem, **digital diagnostic casts** (with or without analog diagnostic wax-ups) must be imported and aligned prior to the implant planning process. Alignment of the digital diagnostic casts to the CBCT is called **registration**. Registration is accomplished by selecting common reference points between two datasets. In partially edentulous scenarios, the remaining teeth can be used as common points (Fig. 62.5). If the dual scan protocol is utilized, such as in completely edentulous scenarios, the applied fiducial markers are selected as common points (Fig. 62.6). Because the registration between datasets is critical for the accurate transfer of the planned implant position into the surgical guide and in turn, to the intraoral site, the clinician is strongly advised to double-check the registration results. Alignment must be manually corrected if visual deviation is observed (Fig. 62.7).

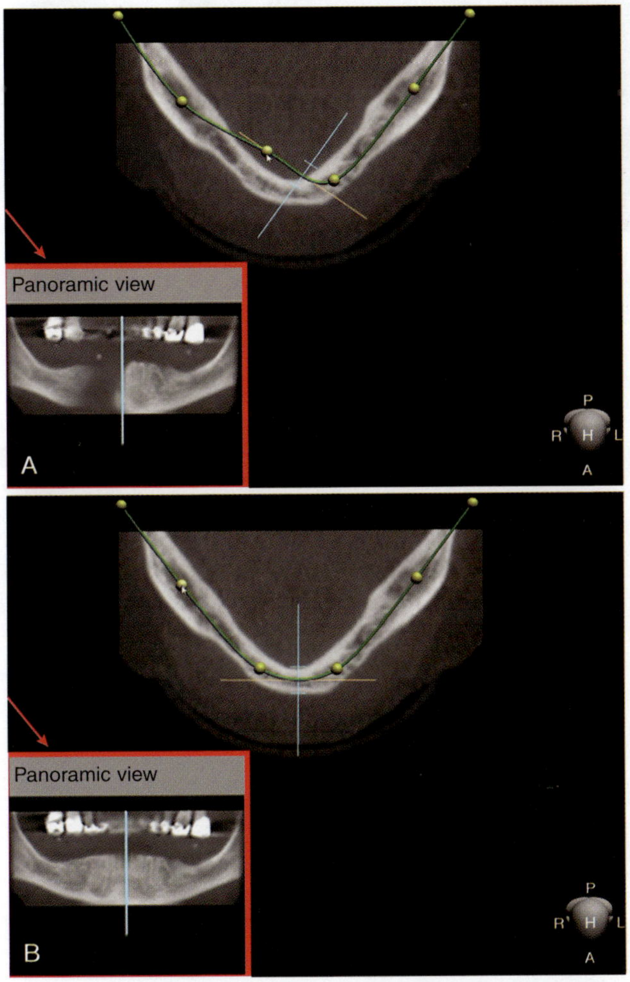

Fig. 62.4 Defining the panoramic curve. A The panoramic curve is defined incorrectly. The mandible appears to be discontinuous because the curve is positioned lingual to the mandible in the symphysis region. B, The panoramic curve is defined properly.

Following registration of datasets, virtual implant planning can begin. Diagnostic wax-ups (manual or digital) remain crucial for the proper positioning of dental implants with the digital workflow. Analog wax-ups must be digitized with diagnostic casts through desktop scanning while digital wax-ups can be directly generated from the simulation software (Fig. 62.8). In cases where the dual scan protocol is utilized, the prosthesis scan itself functions as the diagnostic wax-up. The wax-up of the proposed implant prosthesis must be optimally positioned and take the **emergence profile**, morphology, occlusal, and proximal contacts into consideration.

Virtual implants from a library or database of manufacturer-defined implants are simulated to the virtual patient's jaw and placed in prosthetically driven positions while avoiding vital anatomic structures. Most implant planning software programs have the ability to apply program or user defined safety checks or boundaries (e.g., 2-mm circumferential zone) around the virtual implants that warn users when implants are positioned too close to vital structures such as neighboring implants, adjacent teeth, sinus cavities, and nerves (Fig. 62.9). The planned implant positions can be viewed and adjusted in two-dimensional (2D) cross-sectional images and on the 3D, surface models to ensure these parameters are met.

While prosthetically driven, the proposed implants should be adequately surrounded by bone. If minor bony deficiencies are observed, bone augmentation procedures should be considered. However, if major bony deficiencies not conducive to bone augmentation are observed, the clinician should consider modifying the prosthetic plan.

In scenarios where no (stable) dentition remains, guide fixation is recommended to maximize guide stability. Fixation is achieved with guide fixation pins. They can be brought in from a library and simulated. Similar to virtual implants, virtual fixation pins should not be placed in close proximity to proposed dental implants, teeth, or vital anatomic structures. The pins should be placed in solid bone for stabilization and should avoid existing teeth and sockets of teeth to be extracted (Fig. 62.10). If the implant surgeon is not present

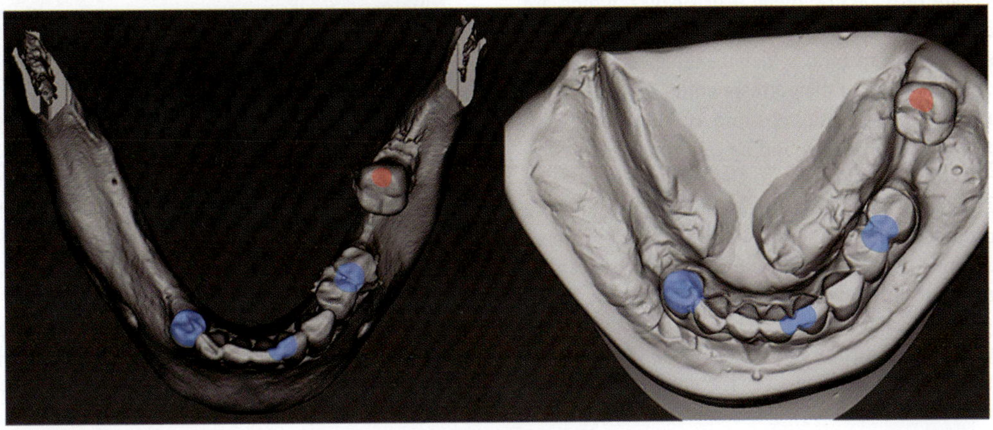

Fig. 62.5 Registration of the cone-beam CT patient dataset with the virtual diagnostic cast in partially edentulous scenarios is accomplished by selecting the remaining dentition as common points.

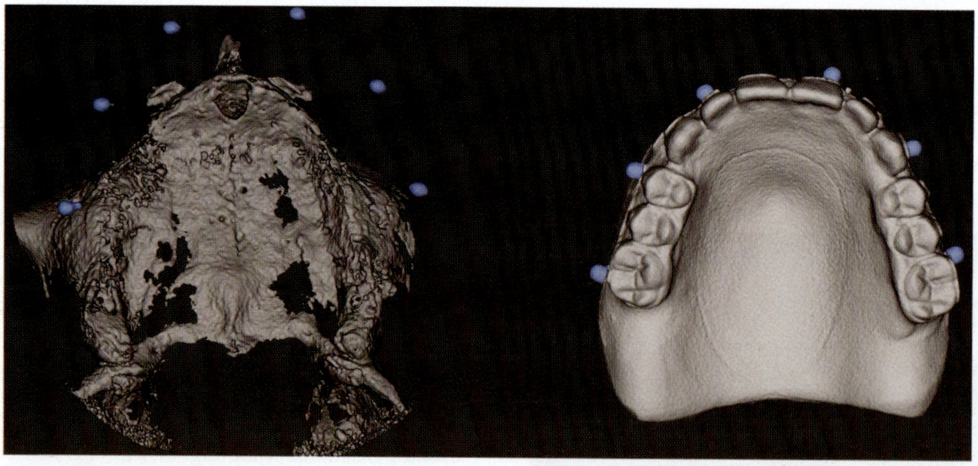

Fig. 62.6 Registration of the cone-beam CT patient dataset with the prosthesis dataset obtained via the dual scan protocol in completely edentulous scenarios is accomplished by selecting fiducial markers as common points.

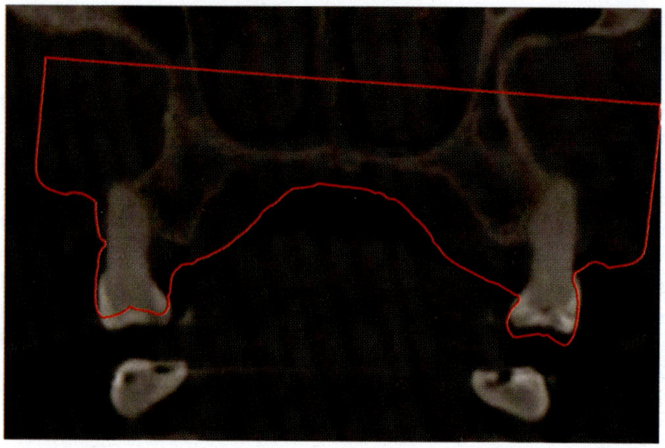

Fig. 62.7 Deviation is observed in the registration process. This must be corrected prior to implant planning and surgical guide design.

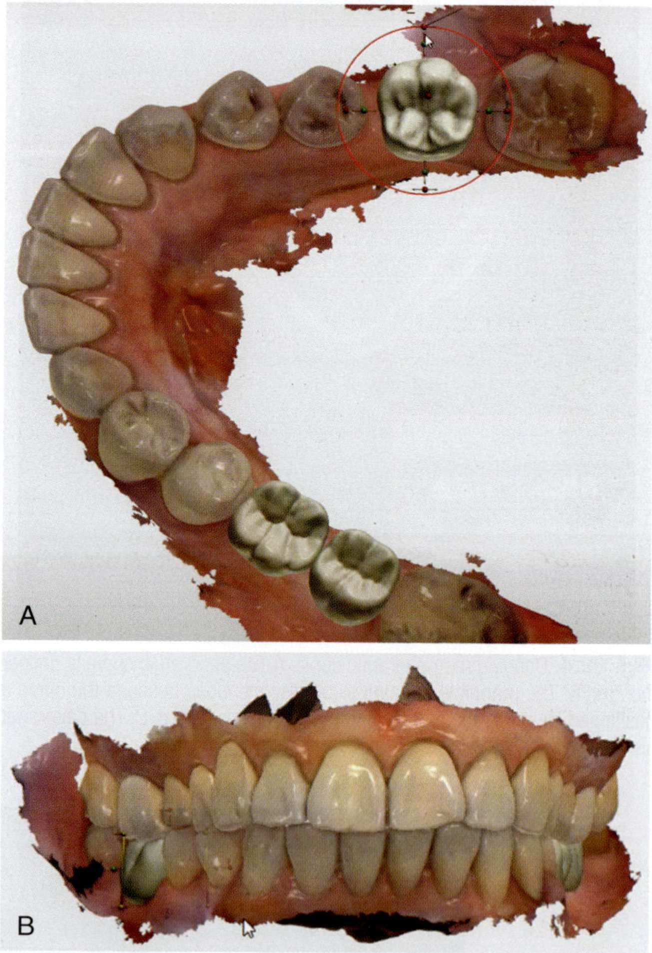

Fig. 62.8 Digital diagnostic wax-ups. A, The proposed implant restorations are digitally waxed up in the simulation software. B, The buccal contour and emergence profile of the proposed restorations can be modified from the frontal view.

during the implant planning, he or she must review and approve the final implant positions and fixation pins prior to surgical guide design and fabrication.

Static CAD/CAM surgical guides can offer pilot guidance, partial guidance, or full guidance. With pilot and partial guidance, only the pilot drill and/or initial twist drill are guided, and all subsequent osteotomy preparations will be performed without the guide. With full guidance, all drills and implants are utilized through the guide. Drill and implant guidance are provided by metal drill sleeves, which are brought in from a library for each proposed implant and fixation pin. The sleeves are implant system specific, which means specific sleeves will only work with surgical kits of the corresponding system.

The buccolingual and mesiodistal position of the metal drill sleeves are based on implant positions and largely fixed. However, the distance from the implant platform to the drill sleeve or the vertical sleeve position (Fig. 62.11) can be modified to create more accessible drilling protocols. Most (but not all) guided systems have several presets available. In general, the vertical sleeve position should be kept to a minimum and as close to the bone (for bone-supported guides) or soft tissue (for mucosa-supported and tooth-supported guides) as possible to maximize access to the surgical site. The consequence of placing drill sleeves too apically, however, is potential interferences with underlying bone or mucosa, which can prevent the complete seating of the guide (Fig. 62.12). In cases where implants are purposely simulated/planned deeper and impediments are inevitable, the underside of the metal sleeves must be manually trimmed prior to surgery, or the interfering bone or soft tissue must be removed during surgery. Following positioning of the drill sleeves, the simulation software will generate a tailored report with drilling protocols specific to the length, diameter, and system of the planned implants (Fig. 62.13).

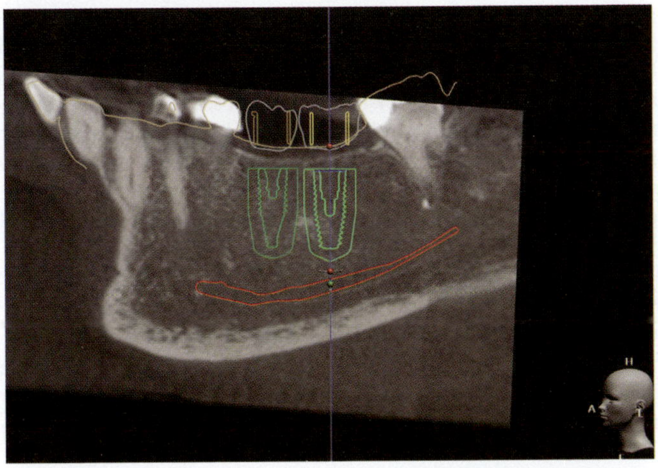

Fig. 62.9 Safety checks or boundaries are available in virtual surgical planning software to prevent potential impingement on vital structures such as adjacent teeth, implants, sinus cavities, and the inferior alveolar nerve.

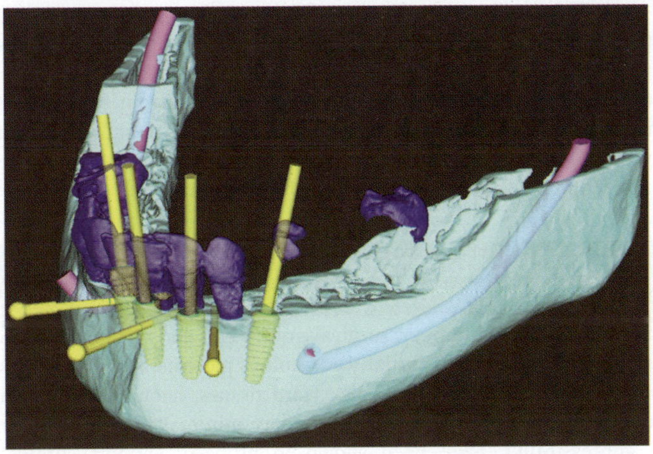

Fig. 62.10 Segmentation of different anatomical structures into independent objects is useful, especially when planning guide fixation pins.

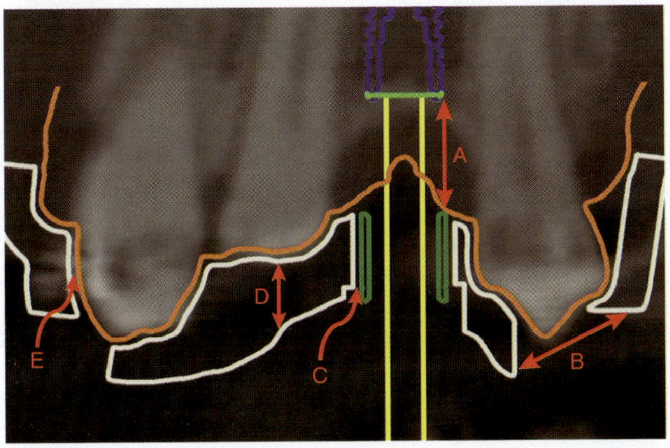

Fig. 62.11 A cross-sectional diagram of a static tooth-supported computer-aided design/computer-aided manufacturing surgical guide. The digital impression of the arch *(orange)* is registered to the cone-beam CT dataset. The surgical guide *(white)* is then designed to be supported by teeth captured in the digital impression. A, Represents the vertical sleeve position. B, Represents an inspection window. C, Represents the sleeve diameter offset. D, Represents the wall thickness. E, Represents guide offset.

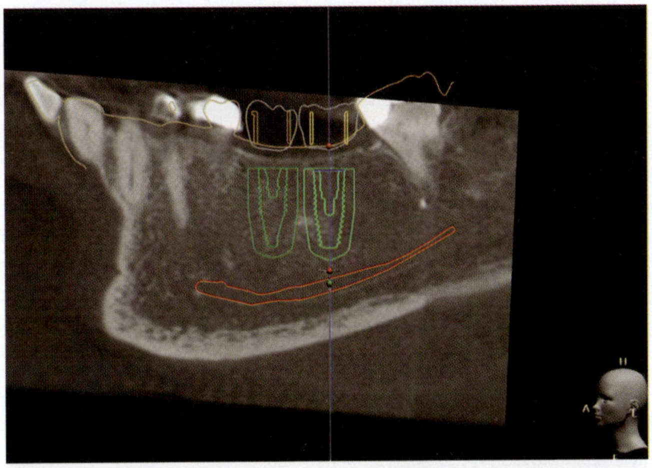

Fig. 62.12 The apical aspect of the drill sleeve intersects with the bony ridge. The surgical guide will not seat fully unless this interference is removed.

Position	Milling cutter	Pilot drill	Guided drill	Guided drill	Guided drill	Profile drill	Tap	Implant	Depth stop
28	ø 3.5	ø 2.2 BLT T1–T3 or dense cortex only =	ø 2.8 BLT T1–T4 =	ø 3.5 BLT T1–T3 or dense cortex only =		ø 4.1 BLT T1–T2 or dense cortex only H4	ø 4.1 BLT T1 H4	021.5310G BLT RC ø 4.1 10 mm SLActive	H4
29	ø 3.5	ø 2.2 BLT T1–T3 or dense cortex only =	ø 2.8 BLT T1–T4 =	ø 3.5 BLT T1–T3 or dense cortex only =		ø 4.1 BLT T1–T2 or dense cortex only H4	ø 4.1 BLT T1 H4	021.5310G BLT RC ø 4.1 10 mm SLActive	H4
30	ø 3.5	ø 2.2 BLT T1–T3 or dense cortex only =	ø 2.8 BLT T1–T4 =	ø 3.5 BLT T1–T3 or dense cortex only =		ø 4.1 BLT T1–T2 or dense cortex only H4	ø 4.1 BLT T1 H4	021.5310G BLT RC ø 4.1 10 mm SLActive	H4

Fig. 62.13 The fully guided drilling protocol is automatically generated by the virtual surgical planning software.

Due to the closed architecture nature of some implant systems, the drilling protocols are only available in the company's own proprietary software. However, some open architecture programs allow the creation of drilling protocols through the custom drill sleeve module. The geometry parameter (diameter and length) and the vertical sleeve position of the third-party drill sleeve(s) to be utilized must be specifically defined for this purpose.

Static Computer-Aided Design/Computer-Aided Manufacturing Surgical Guides

Static CAD/CAM implant surgical guides can derive support from several tissue types. In partially edentulous patients, surgical guides are tooth-supported (Fig. 62.14). Hard tissues, such as teeth with normal **periodontal** support that display minimal mobility and/or compressibility, have been shown to properly support surgical guides for accurate guided implant placement. In completely edentulous patients with sufficient bone volume requiring no alveoloplasty or bone reduction, surgical guides can be mucosa-supported (Fig. 62.15). Mucosa-supported surgical guides enable flapless surgery and can reach similar levels of accuracy in guided implant placement compared to tooth-supported surgical guides, provided the soft tissues are minimally compressible. In completely edentulous patients with limited restorative space requiring alveoloplasty, surgical guides are bone-supported (Fig. 62.16). While bone is a hard tissue without mobility or compressibility, a **systematic review** on the accuracy of guided implant placement based on supporting tissue types demonstrated that bone-supported surgical guides are the least accurate. This inaccuracy could arise from several factors, including the quality of the CBCT scan, the segmentation process, and the guide seating. Complete seating of bone-supported surgical guides requires extensive full thickness flap reflection.

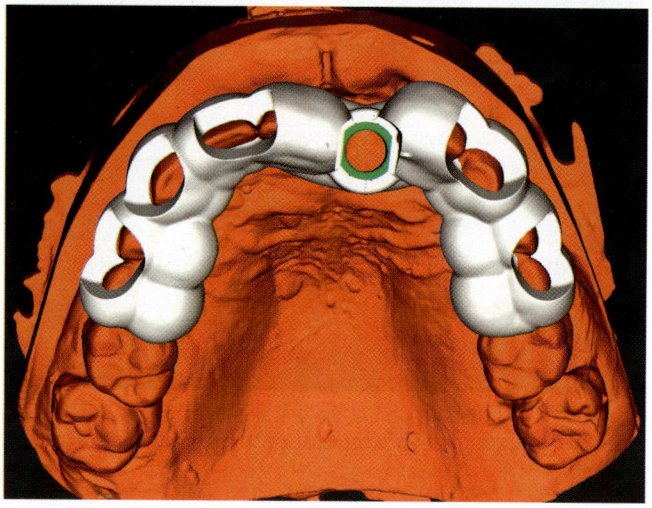

Fig. 62.14 A tooth-supported static computer-aided design/computer-aided manufacturing surgical guide.

Surgical Guide Design Process

Computer-aided design of static guides starts with defining the insertion direction for the guide. For tooth-supported guides, the insertion direction is defined on the digital diagnostic cast. For mucosa-supported guides or any scenarios where dual scans are involved, the insertion direction is defined from the underside of the dual scanned prosthesis or appliance. And for bone-supported guides, the insertion direction is defined on the bone segmentation of the jaw of interest. Defining the insertion direction ensures that the guide will seat passively because all areas underneath the height of contour, as viewed from the defined insertion direction, are blocked out by the software to prevent the guide from engaging any undercuts (Fig. 62.17).

Next, contact surfaces or areas used to index and support the guide are highlighted. In tooth-supported scenarios, teeth immediately adjacent to the edentulous span are selected. However, guide stability can be increased by incorporating additional teeth. In mucosa-supported scenarios, the whole intaglio surface of the dual scanned prosthesis is selected and duplicated into the surgical guide. Because the mucosa-supported guide will fit identically to the dual scanned appliance, it is critical that the prosthesis fit optimally (and relined if fit is suboptimal) prior to any imaging. A bone-supported surgical guide is generally indicated when alveoloplasty is needed. Because the ridge crest will be reduced, support and stability of the surgical guide must be derived elsewhere. In these scenarios, the buccal and lingual or palatal slopes of the alveolar bone apical to the level of the alveoloplasty must be selected. The 3D rendering of the surgical guide is then generated by the software through a digital vacuform-like process over the highlighted areas, and the recesses where the metal drill sleeves will occupy are incorporated automatically.

Before finalizing the design, the addition of **inspection windows** is strongly advised. Inspection windows are openings in the surgical guide which allow the operator to verify guide adaptation via visual

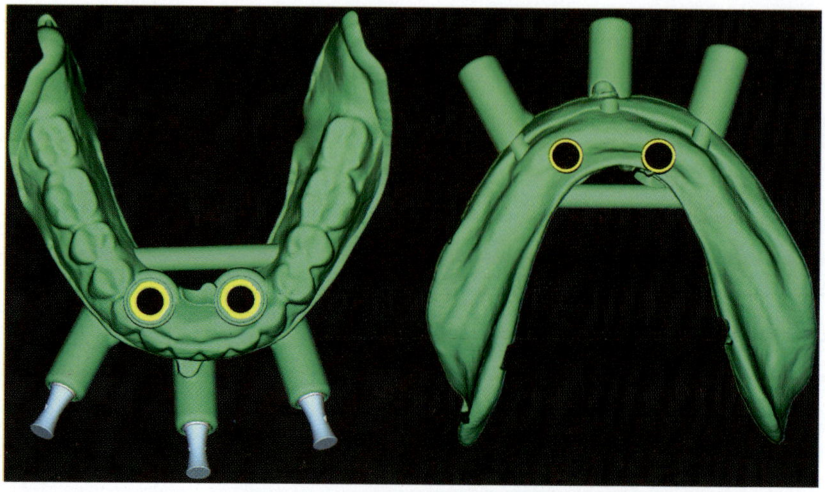

Fig. 62.15 A mucosa-supported static computer-aided design/computer-aided manufacturing surgical guide.

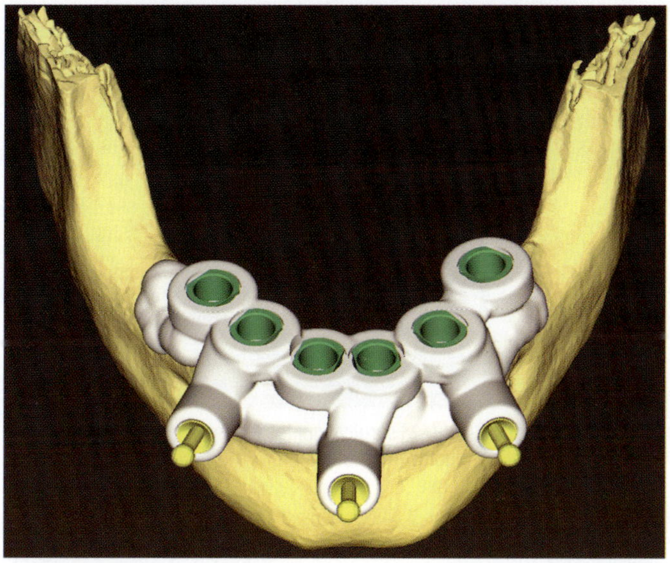

Fig. 62.16 A bone-supported static computer-aided design/computer-aided manufacturing surgical guide.

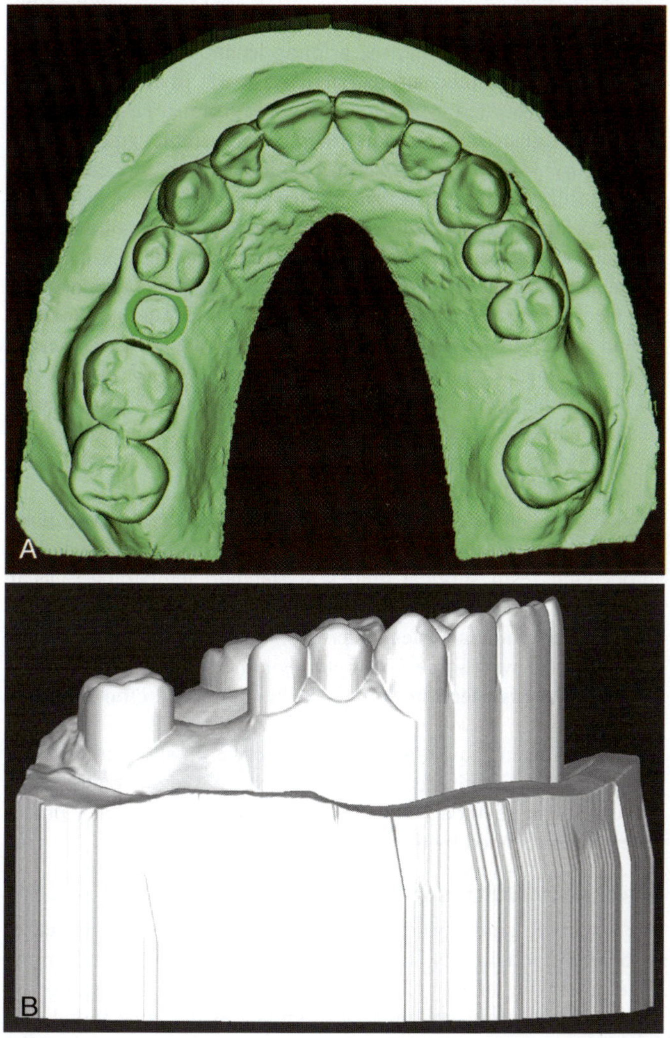

Fig. 62.17 Surgical guide insertion direction. A, The insertion direction for the surgical guide is generally defined from the occlusal direction. B, All undercuts beneath the height of contour as viewed from the defined insertion direction are blocked out.

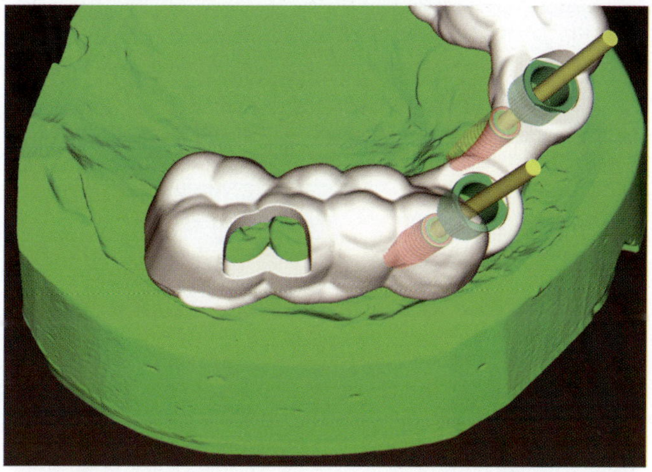

Fig. 62.18 Inspection windows can be created digitally and are essential in confirming that the surgical guide is fully seated.

inspection. These windows are useful regardless of the type of tissue supporting the guide. If a significant amount of space is observed between the surgical guide and the underlying tissues, the guide is likely not seated properly and areas of binding must be adjusted prior to preparing the osteotomies. Inspection windows can be created digitally with a subtraction operation (Fig. 62.18) or manually with a bur following guide production.

Prior to manufacturing, several additional parameters which may affect the static surgical guide should be considered and modified as necessary (see Fig. 62.11):

- **Wall thickness** is correlated with the strength of the surgical guide. Overly thin walls are associated with breakages and fractures while excessively thick walls are associated with bulkiness and difficulties in seating due to potential collisions with soft tissues.
    - Depending on the material, this parameter should be kept as low as possible without compromising the rigidity of the guide. For most resin-based materials, wall thickness of 3–3.5 mm is appropriate. For metal-based materials, thinner dimensions are possible.
- **Guide offset** is the tolerance between the surgical guide and the tissues that support the guide. Little to no guide offset is associated with binding and incomplete seating while large guide offset is associated with loosely fitting guides. This setting is usually applied to the whole intaglio surface of the surgical guide.
    - Guide offset is a fluid setting based on the accuracy of the manufacturing method. Calibration is recommended to determine the optimal guide offset for a specific method. Guides with different offsets should be manufactured to determine the optimal setting for future guides. This is usually in the range of 0.1–0.3 mm.
    - Because bone-supported surgical guides are made directly from the segmentation or 3D reconstruction of the jawbones, the thickness of the CBCT slices may affect the guide offset setting. Thicker slices are associated with a staircase-like appearance (Fig. 62.19) of the reconstructed image and may require additional offset for complete guide seating.
- **Sleeve diameter offset** is the tolerance between the surgical guide and the metal drill sleeve. Like guide offset, calibration is recommended to determine the optimal sleeve diameter offset so metal drill sleeves can fit precisely without additional adjustments. Some software can generate a sleeve calibration matrix which allows the operator to easily identify the best setting.

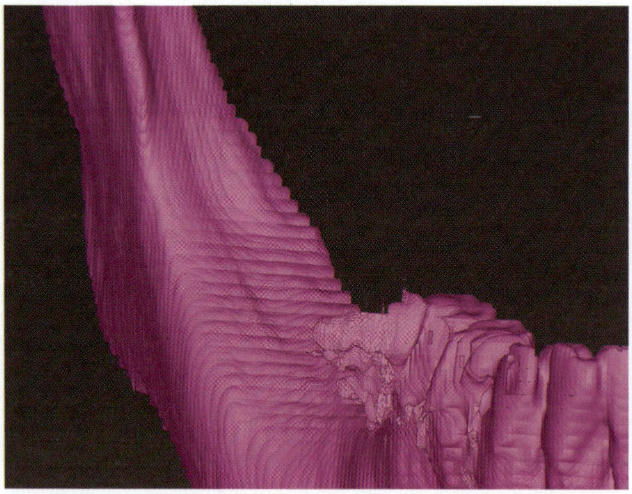

Fig. 62.19 3D reconstructions from thick cone-beam CT slices will have a staircase-like appearance which may necessitate additional guide offset for bone-supported surgical guides.

Surgical Guide Manufacturing Process

The manufacturing of static surgical guides is executed through a central production facility for closed architecture software or by the software operator for open architecture programs. Surgical guides can be produced via subtractive or additive manufacturing processes usually in polymer resins or less commonly, metal alloys.

Subtractive manufacturing techniques such as milling involve grinding and removing stock from a block or disk of material through computer numerical control until the desired shape is obtained (Fig. 62.20). Although milling is arguably the most precise method of manufacturing, with the greatest selection of materials, it is limited by part size, part complexity, tool size, and cost.

- **Part size:** Only objects that fit into the block or disk of material can be milled.
- **Part complexity:** Accurate milling of complex objects is largely dependent on the number of axes available to the milling machine. Parts with internal structures or significant undercuts may not be possible.
- **Tool size:** Internal corners and square edges are often not able to be milled due to the accessibility and angle needed by the mill spindle.
- **Cost:** Cost of implementation is higher compared to additive manufacturing. Subtractive manufacturing is also a more wasteful process because the removed stock is rarely recycled.

Additive manufacturing techniques such as rapid prototyping or 3D printing involve adding material layer by layer until the desired shape is obtained. This method is very popular for surgical guide production because it is relatively accurate, affordable, and not limited by part complexity and tool size. To prevent sagging and distortion, the 3D printed element must be properly supported by resin struts or support material of some kind (Fig. 62.21). However, care must be taken to avoid placing supports on the intaglio surface of surgical guides as to not compromise fit. Other factors, such as the 3D printer and the printing technology, can affect the precision of 3D printed surgical guides as well. In contrast to milling, most 3D printed guides require some form of postprocessing to achieve full strength and final shape. For example, guides manufactured by 3D printers that utilize photochemical processes such as stereolithography (SLA) should have all supporting structures removed after printing, followed by an isopropyl alcohol wash and ultraviolet light-curing process to increase mechanical properties.

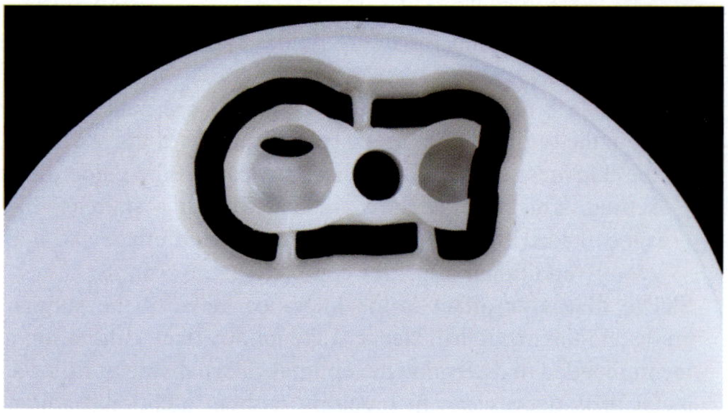

Fig. 62.20 Static CAD/CAM surgical guides can be manufactured by milling (subtractive manufacturing).

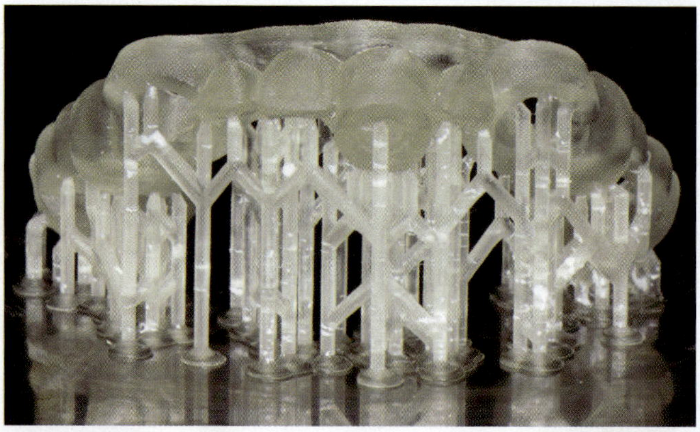

Fig. 62.21 Static CAD/CAM surgical guides are more commonly manufactured via 3D printing (additive manufacturing). The resin supports must be removed prior to clinical use.

After postprocessing, metal drill sleeves are manually inserted. The sleeves must be completely seated (the upper edges of a sleeve should be level with the surgical guide) to ensure accurate transfer of the planned implant positions to the oral cavity. If properly calibrated, the friction between the sleeve and surgical guide should be sufficient to retain the sleeve for drilling. If the sleeve feels loose, cyanoacrylate or other preferred luting cement can be used between the sleeve and surgical guide for retention.

All static surgical guides should be sterilized or at least disinfected prior to live surgery. Manufacturers usually advise against autoclaving resin surgical guides at standard temperatures as to avoid deformation. However, plasma sterilization with hydrogen peroxide and autoclave steam sterilization at 121°C were shown to be compatible with some 3D printed polymers. A common method for chemical **disinfection** is to soak the guide in a **chlorhexidine** gluconate bath; however, soaking the guide in 70% ethanol for 15 min has been proven to be more effective. In short, differences in sterilization or disinfection protocols exist based on materials and manufacturing methods. The clinician should follow proper procedures recommended by the manufacturers.

Stackable Guides

The stackable guide system has been gaining popularity for cases involving alveoloplasty, immediate implant placement, and immediate prosthetic loading. This system involves two guides: a bone-supported alveoloplasty guide, also known as the bone foundation guide (BFG), and a secondary guide which stacks on top of the BFG (Fig. 62.22A–C).

Because the BFG is bone-supported, accurate bone segmentation and registration of the dual scanned prosthesis or wax-up are

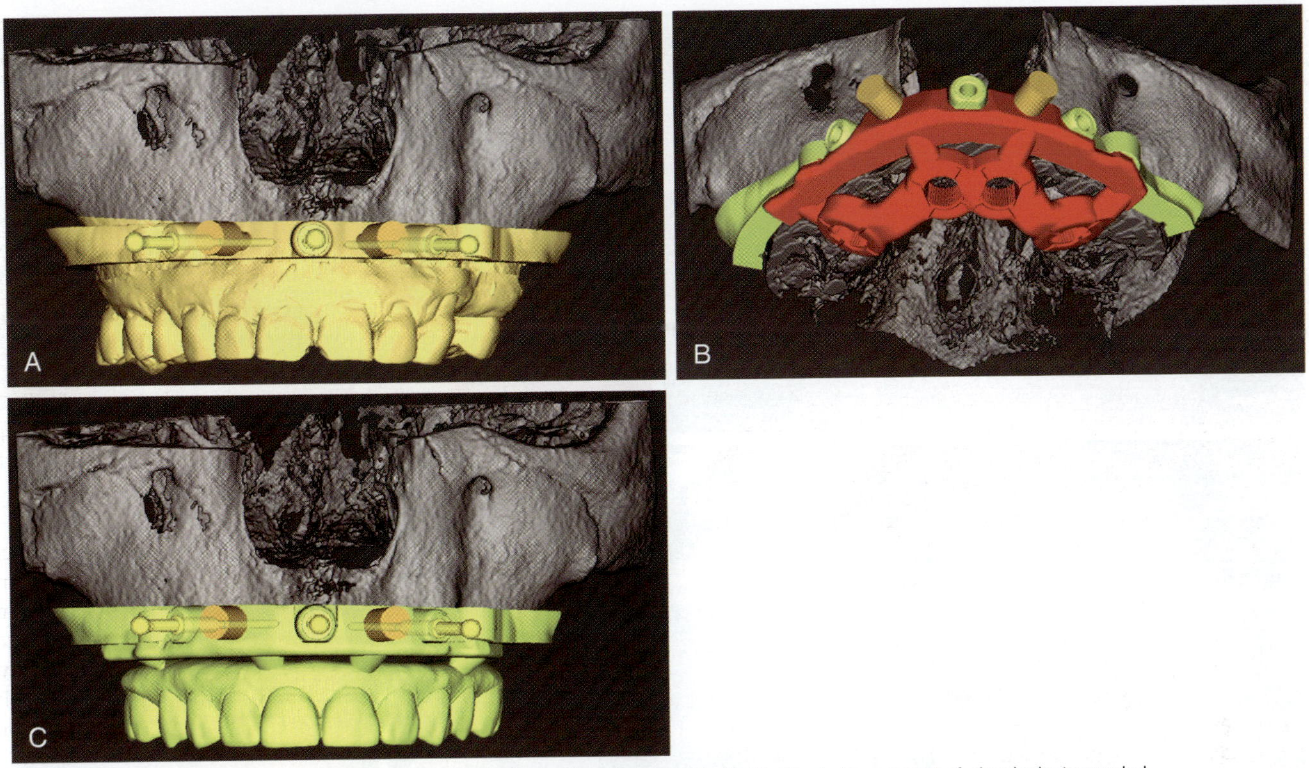

Fig. 62.22 Stackable guides. A, The bone foundation guide (BFG) directs the amount of alveoloplasty needed and serves as the base that all subsequent steps are built upon. B, The secondary guide or implant placement guide stacks on top of the BFG and provides fully guided implant placement. C, The pick-up procedure for the immediately loaded prosthesis can be guided by the BFG.

critical for success. This guide is rigidly fixed to the jawbone via guide fixation pins or screws and directs the amount of bone reduction. Once fixed, it remains in place throughout the entire procedure and serves as the foundation for the secondary guide and prefabricated prosthesis. Because the BFG is the foundation on which everything else is built, it must be seated in the correct position prior to fixation. The BFG can be seated using several different methods. The most common is to simply utilize the bony anatomy such as the buccal and lingual/palatal slopes of the alveolar bone to orient the guide into place. If some teeth remain, they can be used prior to extraction to index a seating jig which in turn can help orient the BFG. If no teeth remain, a seating jig referencing the occlusion established by the prosthesis/prostheses can be employed.

Following guided alveoloplasty, another template with drill sleeves, which stacks on top of the BFG, directs the implant osteotomies and placement. This template can also guide the pick-up procedure for an immediately loaded fixed complete arch prosthesis. When a prosthesis is being stacked onto the BFG for immediate loading, it is crucial that the preoperative records include a precise interocclusal record at the proposed occlusal vertical dimension and centric relation position. If not, the occlusion of the prosthesis will not be correct. Detailed stackable guide design is beyond the scope of this chapter. Some commercial dental laboratories offer services to help clinicians design and execute these cases if proper dental records are provided.

Surgical Implant Placement Using Static CAD/CAM Surgical Guide

Surgical implant placement using a static CAD/CAM surgical guide enables clinicians to accurately place implants in the jaw according to the prosthetically driven implant positions as planned in simulation software. As a result, the implant placement surgery is greatly facilitated in terms of reduced time, less need for checking and validating osteotomy position and direction during surgical preparation, and, ultimately, more accurately placed implants. However, the accuracy and surgical expediency is entirely dependent on the care, attention to details, and avoidance of errors during data collection, planning, and processing of surgical guide, as well as the proper positioning of the surgical guide at the time of implant placement surgery. This final step in the process (proper positioning) is the critical key step. Regardless of how precisely the surgical guide was made to capture the planned implant positions, the translation of that information to the patient will only be accurate if the guide fits the patient's jaw and is seated as it was intended.

As described previously, static CAD/CAM implant surgical guides can be used to place implants for the partially edentulous patient/arch with tooth-supported guides or the fully edentulous patient/arch with either a mucosa-supported or a bone-supported guide. In each case, care must be taken to verify the surgical guide is positioned and seated properly and that it is stable and secure for the procedure (Fig. 62.23A and B).

Partially Edentulous Tooth-Supported Surgical Guide

For a surgical guide that is supported by periodontally stable teeth with good cross arch and anterior-posterior distribution, it will be adequately stabilized by the teeth. However, if there are few remaining teeth that are not well distributed (i.e., unilateral), the guide may not be stable. In this case, it will be advantageous to plan the case with fixation pins. If the guide is designed to be both tooth and mucosa-supported, then an occlusal index may be needed to establish the proper position since the mucosa-supported portion will have resilience and movement.

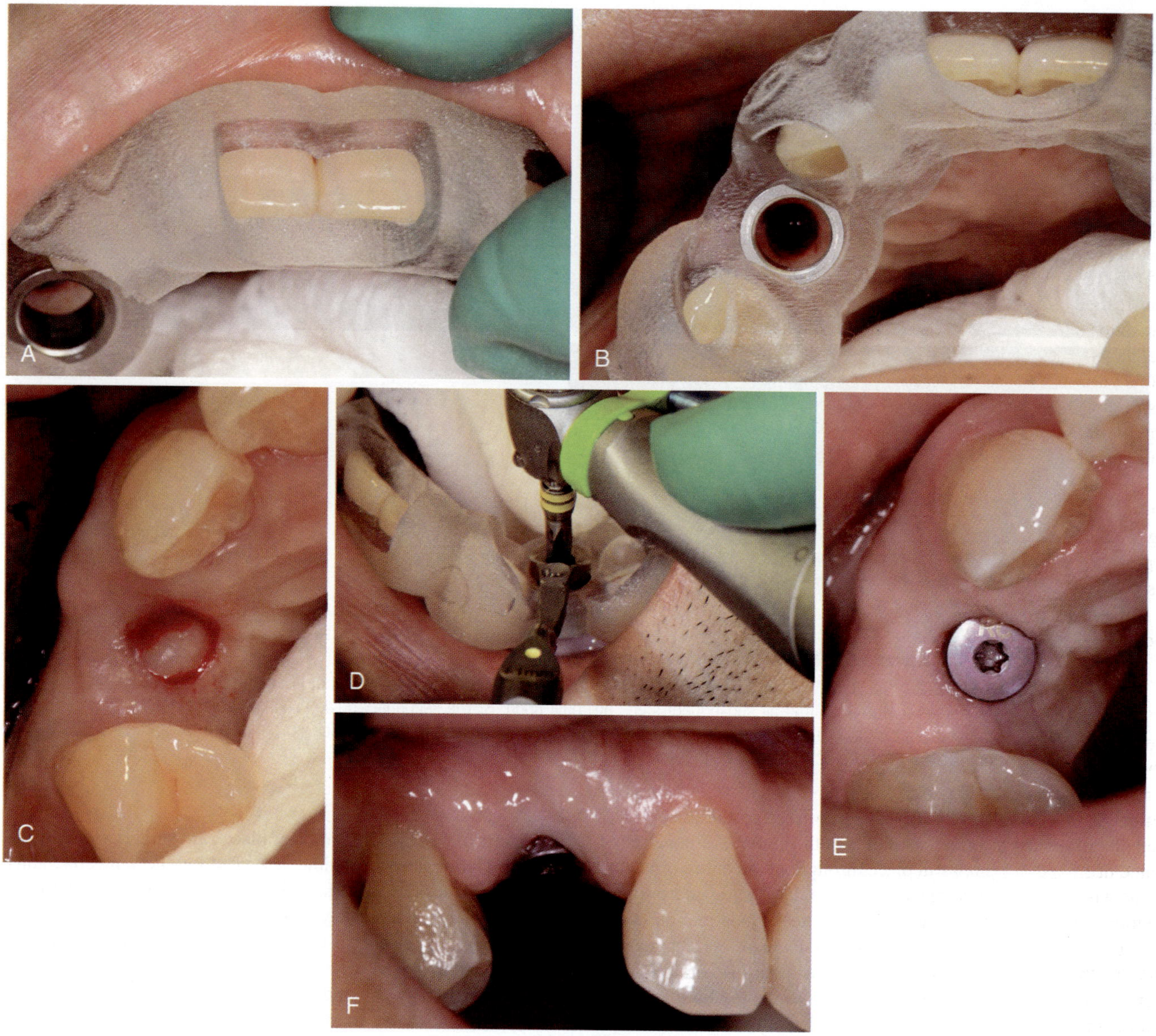

Fig. 62.23 A–D, Static surgical guide designed for implant placement #6 (maxillary right cuspid) with inspection windows that allow clinician to confirm complete seating of the guide. A, The intimacy of the surgical guide with the central incisors as observed through the inspection window. B, Additional inspection windows demonstrate intimate fit of guide with posterior teeth to confirm the guide is properly seated. A tissue punch is used through the guide to remove a circular portion of the **gingival** tissue to allow implant site osteotomy preparation. C, Clinical view without guide of tissue incised with circular punch. D, Preparation of implant site with static surgical guide using handles and following surgical plan. E, Occlusal and F, labial clinical views of healing abutment attached to implant immediately after placement with static surgical guide using a flapless approach.

Fully Edentulous Mucosa-Supported or Bone-Supported Surgical Guide

For a fully edentulous surgical guide supported by mucosa or bone, it will be necessary to plan the case using multiple fixation pins. Most fully edentulous surgical guides will require two to three fixation pins to achieve reliable stability. If the guide is mucosa-supported, an occlusal index should be used to establish the proper position since the mucosa-supported portion will have resilience and movement. An occlusal index can be used to position a bone-supported guide as well, but it may not be required since bone is a rigid tissue.

Fixation pins are secured through the guide using a sleeve that has a specific diameter and length for the pins and planned using the implant simulation software. Once the surgical guide is properly positioned, drills are used to prepare fixation pin osteotomies. The fixation pins are then pushed through the sleeve into the bone to stabilize and secure the surgical guide.

Flap Versus Flapless Procedures

The ability to accurately prepare and place implants in planned locations with a static CAD/CAM surgical guide invites the possibility to perform the procedure without soft tissue flap reflection. When implant osteotomies can be prepared and implants can be placed without soft tissue flap reflection, it saves time and decreases surgical morbidity. Both partially edentulous and fully edentulous cases can be successfully executed using a flapless surgical technique with tooth-supported or mucosa-supported guides, respectively. However, there are circumstances that preclude clinicians from preparing and placing implants using flapless surgery, including a lack of bone volume at the implant site(s) and/or a lack of adequate **keratinized** attached soft tissue at the implant site(s).

If there is a lack of bone volume and a need for bone grafting at the time of implant placement, then a full-thickness flap reflection will be required. This is true regardless of whether the bone deficiency is large or small. Even if the bone deficiency is a minor dehiscence or fenestration, a full-thickness flap reflection should be used because, in addition to the need to graft such defects, if the implant placement is slightly off in the direction of the deficiency, then the deficit of bone surrounding the implant will be significant and the clinician may not recognize the problem without flap reflection. If there is a lack of keratinized attached soft tissue at the implant site such that the soft tissue access incision will be in mobile, unattached mucosa, it is preferable to use a full-thickness flap reflection during implant placement surgery and to manage soft tissue positioning separately. Again, these criteria for adequate bone volume and keratinized attached soft tissue at implant sites apply to both partially edentulous and fully edentulous cases.

The flapless implant placement procedure uses a tissue punch to make a circular incision through the guide at each implant site (see Fig. 62.23B and C). The size of the circular incision is large enough to prepare the osteotomy and place the implant without further soft tissue excision or reflection (see Fig. 62.23D–F). The incised circular soft tissue islands are removed (full thickness) to expose the underlying bone.

Preparing Implant Osteotomy Sites With Static CAD/CAM Surgical Guide

Preparation of implant osteotomy sites are similar regardless of whether the surgical guide is tooth-supported, mucosa-supported, or bone supported. Depending on the implant system, the guide will be designed with drill sleeves that are used with or without drill handles or keys, or the osteotomy drills themselves could have integrated drill stops. Implant osteotomies are prepared with a sequence of increasingly larger diameter drills that are precisely guided in position, direction, and depth by the surgical guide. Some systems will also incorporate timing markers to allow the clinician to specifically align the implant rotation. This may be important for prefabricated prosthesis/crown or to facilitate the use of angled abutments, allowing for predetermined angled abutment selection and positioning. As with all implant site preparations, profuse irrigation should be used to cool drills and flush debris from the osteotomy sites. It is particularly important when using computer-generated surgical guides because much of the drill is covered by the drill sleeve and guide material.

Depending on bone density, the final steps of the implant osteotomy may be to use bone profilers and taps. Both can be done through the surgical guide using system specific keys or handles. Before implant placement, osteotomy sites should be thoroughly irrigated with sterile saline to flush any residual debris. Implants can be placed through the surgical guide. Some systems will use specific mounts with depth indicators to place implants through the guide sleeve, whereas others have timing indicators so implants can be precisely placed in terms of rotation as well as position and depth.

Dynamic Navigation

Dynamically navigated implant placement is a type of computer-assisted surgery that utilizes optical motion tracking. Optical motion tracking systems can be either active or passive. Active system tracker arrays emit infrared light that is tracked by stereo cameras, while passive system tracker arrays use reflective spheres to reflect infrared light emitted from a light source to stereo cameras.

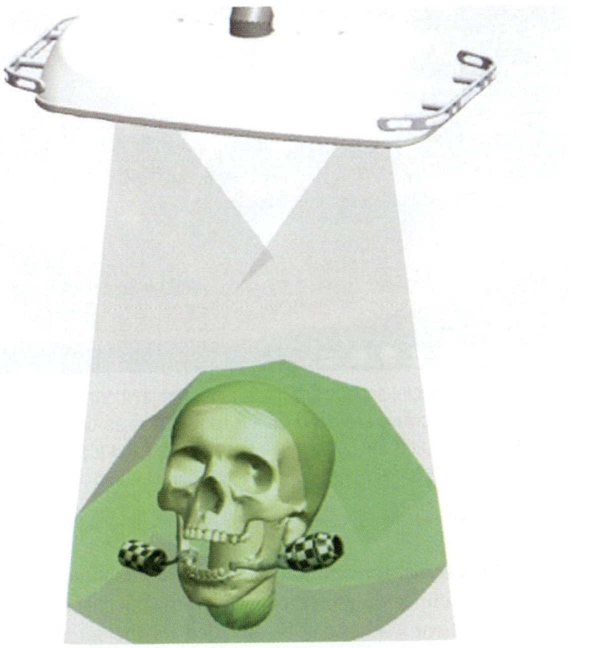

Fig. 62.24 Light is projected inferiorly from a source and reflected off tracking arrays attached to the patient and the surgical instrument. The reflection is captured by stereo cameras above the surgical field so the patient and surgical instrument can be tracked in real-time. *(Courtesy X-Nav Technologies, LLC, Lansdale, PA.)*

Currently, passive tracking systems are more commonly utilized in dentistry. In passively tracked, dynamically navigated implant surgery, a light source above the surgical field projects infrared light down toward the patient. This light is subsequently reflected off tracking arrays attached to both the patient and the surgical handpiece. The reflected light is detected by stereo cameras so the dynamic navigation program can calculate the real-time position of the patient and the handpiece relative to the surgical plan (Fig. 62.24). Following calculation, a virtual image is displayed on screen that provides the implant surgeon with visual guidance.

The sequence of steps to achieve dynamic navigation includes data and image acquisition, virtual surgical planning, calibration, and, finally, executing the dynamically navigated surgery.

Data and Image Acquisition

The acquisition of quality CT or CBCT scans is a prerequisite for successful dynamic navigation. Because the patient, surgical handpiece, and surgical plan must correlate with each other for implant placement, fiducial markers are necessary during image acquisition and live surgery. Similar to the workflow for static CAD/CAM surgical guides, there are important nuances to consider when scans are taken based on patient presentation.

- Partial edentulism
  - A clip with fiducial markers or fiducial clip is utilized for imaging .The clip part of the apparatus functions as an impression tray so a sectional impression of the patient's teeth can be made with a thermoplastic material. This fiducial clip must be properly supported and stabilized by the dentition and indexed back into the same location during the CBCT scan and live surgery. If rocking or instability is detected, the thermoplastic material needs to be reheated so the impression can be remade prior to imaging. Teeth that are mobile should not be used to support the clip. The clip should be placed on the arch of interest in a location that will not interfere with

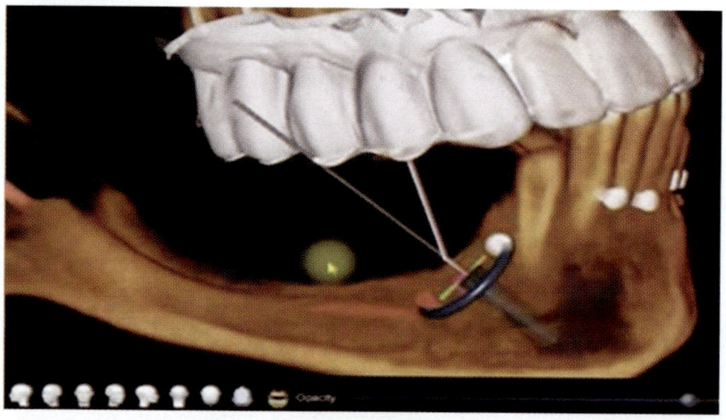

Fig. 62.25 Fiducial screws are fixated into the jawbone of interest prior to imaging. These screws are used during registration as common points between the patient and the cone-beam CT dataset. *(Courtesy X-Nav Technologies, LLC, Lansdale, PA.)*

surgical instrumentation. Finally, the attachment component on the clip should be facing outward (buccal) so an arm with the patient tracker can be attached for the surgery.
    - Although not absolutely required, a set of digital diagnostic casts can be helpful in planning implants in prosthetically driven positions.
- Complete edentulism
    - In edentulous scenarios, fiducial markers come in the form of small bone screws. Four or more screws are placed in the jaw of interest prior to imaging and will not be retrieved until after the implant surgery (Fig. 62.25). They should be well distributed along the arch for optimal triangulation. If alveoloplasty is being considered, the screws must be placed apical to the planned reduction, so they are not accidentally removed when bone is cut. Like the partially edentulous scenario, these fiducial markers need to be rigidly fixed. If movement is detected in a screw, it must be moved to another site. Care should be taken when placing these screws to avoid impingement upon the infraorbital nerve in the maxilla and inferior alveolar nerve in the mandible. Finally, sufficient space is required between the screws for an edentulous fiducial plate to be secured during surgery for the purpose of attaching the patient tracker arm.
    - The dual scan protocol is recommended to aid in planning implants in prosthetically driven positions.

Virtual Surgical Planning

The DICOM files are imported into a planning software specific to the dynamic navigation system of choice. All dynamic navigation planning software is proprietary and must be purchased as a package along with the hardware. All steps involved in the virtual surgical planning process such as segmentation, patient data orientation, panoramic curve, registration of datasets, and implant simulation are identical to the aforementioned steps for static guides.

Simulation of implant positions must be prosthetically driven. The virtual implants should be positioned below the proposed prosthesis and account for proper restorative space and emergence profile mesiodistally as well as buccolingually. As described before, diagnostic wax-ups are crucial for this process. Most dynamic navigation planning software programs can generate individual teeth to be used as wax-ups. Alternatively, analog wax-ups can be performed and converted into the digital realm. For completely edentulous cases, the prosthesis scan obtained from the dual scan protocol is utilized for planning implant positions.

Calibration

The surgical instruments (such as the contra-angle handpiece) and the patient must be calibrated prior to live surgery so proper tracking can occur. (Important: Partially edentulous and completely edentulous patients are calibrated differently.)

- Partial edentulism
    - The handpiece is calibrated by attaching a tracker onto the base of the handpiece. This handpiece and tracker assembly is then placed about 60–80 cm away from the stereo cameras and rotated slowly so the cameras can read and register the patterns on the tracker (Fig. 62.26).
    - The chuck is calibrated by a chuck plate inserted into the handpiece. The plate is spun slowly underneath the cameras for calibration.
    - The partially edentulous patient is calibrated by attaching a tracker onto a patient tracker arm. The fiducial clip (tailored to the patient's dentition) is then secured to the arm. This assembly is rotated underneath the cameras for calibration (Fig. 62.27).
    - Before surgical execution and between every drill change, drill length must be verified. This is achieved by placing an implant drill into the handpiece and positioning the drill perpendicular at the center of a calibration plate (see Fig. 62.26). If this step fails, the chuck calibration step needs to be performed again.
- Complete edentulism
    - The handpiece, chuck, and drill length are calibrated the same way as described above.
    - To calibrate the completely edentulous patient, an edentulous patient probe needs to be calibrated first. This probe is calibrated in a similar manner as the handpiece (Fig. 62.28).
    - An edentulous fiducial plate is secured to the jawbone of interest in an area with no fiducial markers or screws (Fig. 62.29). This plate serves as an attachment mechanism

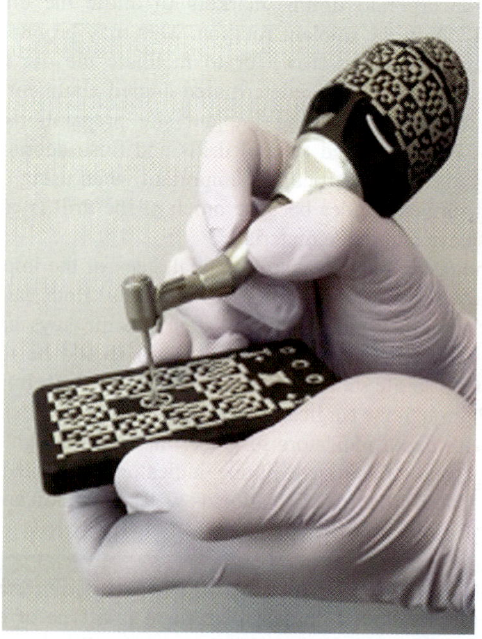

Fig. 62.26 The handpiece is connected to a patterned tracker followed by calibration. Prior to surgical execution, the length of the drill is verified by placing the drill into the calibrated handpiece and positioning the drill at the center of but perpendicular to a calibration plate. *(Courtesy X-Nav Technologies, LLC, Lansdale, PA.)*

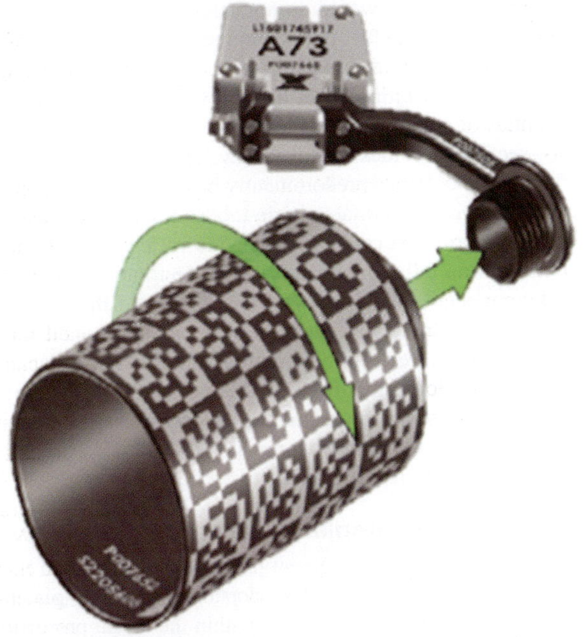

Fig. 62.27 The fiducial clip, patient tracker arm, and tracker are assembled followed by calibration. *(Courtesy X-Nav Technologies, LLC, Lansdale, PA.)*

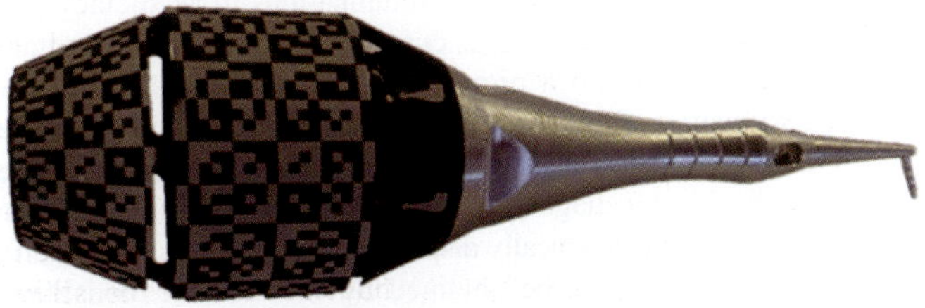

Fig. 62.28 The edentulous patient probe is connected to a patterned tracker and calibrated. *(Courtesy X-Nav Technologies, LLC, Lansdale, PA.)*

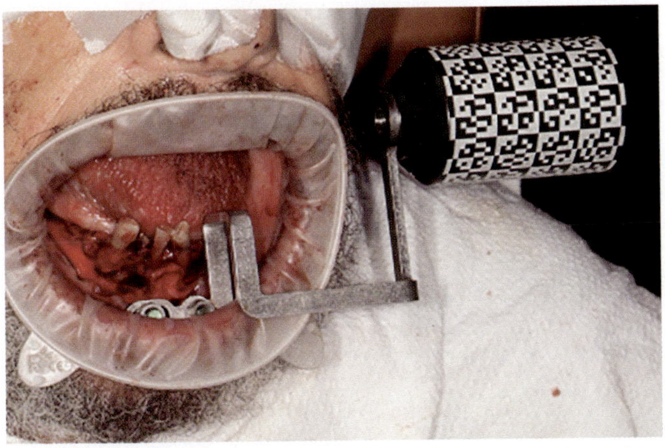

Fig. 62.29 Because completely edentulous or terminal dentition cases do not have teeth suitable for stabilizing the fiducial clip, the fiducial plate serves as the attachment apparatus for the tracker instead. *(Courtesy X-Nav Technologies, LLC, Lansdale, PA.)*

for the tracker arm and tracker assembly. The tracker and fiducial screws are then calibrated to the dynamic navigation system via touching the screws with the previously calibrated probe. The fiducial screws register the patient to the virtual surgical plan while the tracker allows the patient to be tracked in real time.

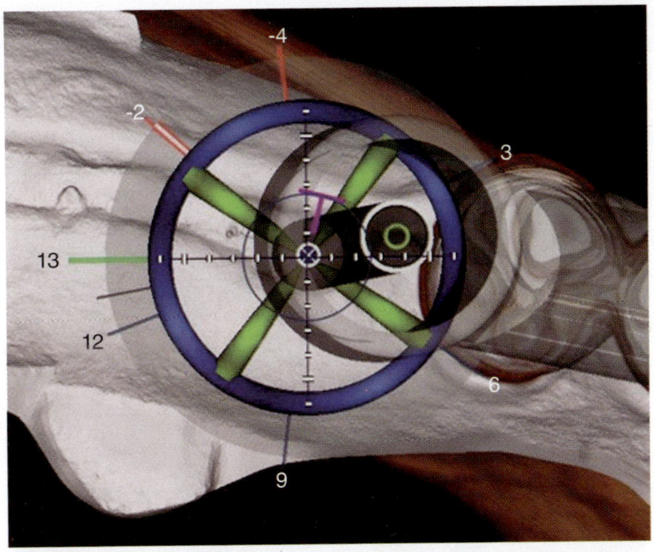

Fig. 62.30 A diagram of the dynamic navigation monitor. The center of the green X represents the center of the implant. The blue dot represents the drill tip which should be placed at the center of the green X. The green circle represents the drill angulation which should be superimposed directly over the blue dot prior to drilling. *(Courtesy X-Nav Technologies, LLC, Lansdale, PA.)*

Surgical Implant Placement Using Dynamic Navigation

In dynamic navigation, the surgeon prepares the osteotomies and places the implants by looking at the computer screen. The navigation screen displays the virtual plan with the target implant sites, virtual drills, and indicators specific for drilling angle, drilling depth, and timing of the planned implants (Fig. 62.30).

The tip of the virtual drill is often indicated by a dot on the screen. This dot should be moved to and centered over the target implant site. A circle is usually directly over the dot and signifies drilling angle. The handpiece should be angulated so the dot is centered in the circle prior to drilling. As drilling occurs, depth is commonly displayed by changes in color of the depth indicator. In a popular dynamic navigation system (X-Nav Technologies, Lansdale, PA), the color of the depth indicator changes from yellow to green and green to red, with red denoting that the proper depth has been reached and the surgeon should stop drilling (Fig. 62.31).

During surgery, system checks should be performed frequently to ensure that the dynamic navigation system is tracking correctly. System checks can be accomplished by touching anatomic landmarks with calibrated surgical instruments. The operator can then confirm that the landmark on the screen correlates with what was touched. Optimal landmarks include adjacent teeth or the alveolar ridge near the planned implant site for partially edentulous cases or fiducial markers (screws) for completely edentulous cases.

Computer-Guided Implant Placement Surgery: A Foundation for Digitally Aided Provisionalization

The foundation upon which most digitally aided implant provisionalization workflows rest is computer-guided implant surgery. However, nonguided options are also available and will be addressed in this chapter. Historically, analog approaches have been the preeminent methodologies for the manufacturing of **transmucosal** provisional implant restorations. Such restorations typically consist of prefabricated interim **abutments** supporting a crown form made of restorative material such as polymethylmethacrylate or bis-acryl composite resin. Implant-supported provisional restorations can be fabricated chairside (direct method) or in a laboratory using a physical model after indexing the implant (indirect method). While such workflows are predictable, they perpetuate a fragmented implant therapy workflow and do not offer the ability to capitalize on the prosthetic benefits that computer-guided surgery offers. Therefore, to better understand the mechanics of digitally aided implant provisionalization, it is first important to understand the fundamentals of computer-guided implant surgery.

This section provides an overview of contemporary digital workflow methodologies predominantly based on computer-guided surgery protocols to facilitate single-tooth implant provisionalization. Digital workflows can support a wide variety of custom healing abutments or full contour provisional restorations. Whether a **coronal** component is present or absent as part of the provisional **prosthesis**, the desired **endpoint** is the same: a peri-implant biologic environment that is free of inflammation, dimensionally stable, and conducive to esthetic contours. With these concepts in mind, it will be easier to understand the relative advantages and limitations of various digitally aided implant provisionalization workflows and their subsequent definitive prosthetic workflows.

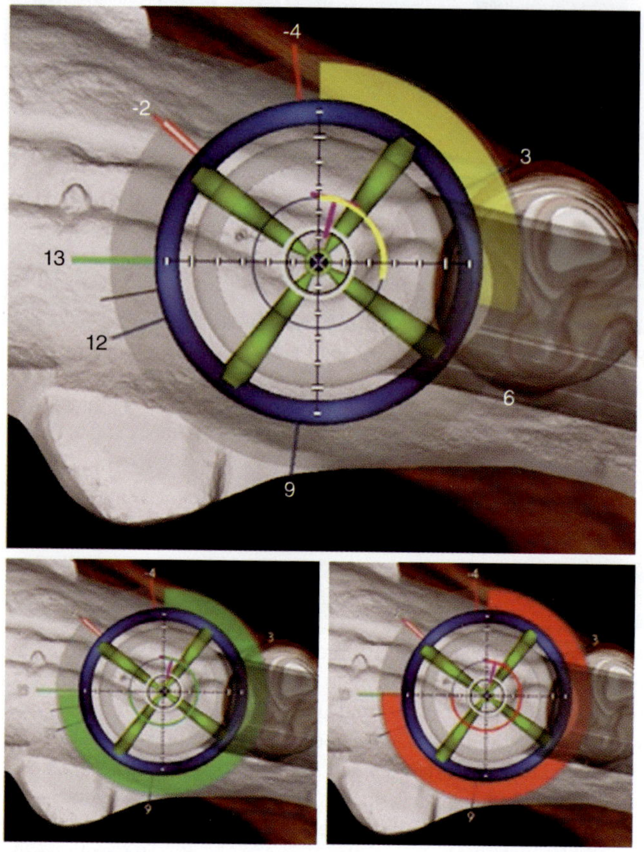

Fig. 62.31 Drilling depth is denoted by an outer ring which can change colors. *Yellow* is a prompt for the operator to start drilling. *Green* denotes the current depth to be 0.5 mm shy of the planned depth while *red* represents that the planned depth has been achieved. *(Courtesy X-Nav Technologies, LLC, Lansdale, PA.)*

Computer-Guided Implant Placement Workflows

Computer-guided implant placement protocols are supported by several planning software platforms. The adoption of computer-guided implant placement has rapidly expanded within the dental profession in recent years, and its use has demonstrably improved implant planning and placement accuracy when compared to free-hand approaches.

Implant planning software often requires the conversion of **DICOM** (Digital Imaging and Communications in Medicine) data files (typically displayed with a .dcm file extension) that contain raw radiographic data to a proprietary file format specific to the planning software before a case can be planned. To facilitate guide design and manufacturing, the proprietary conversion file can be merged with either a diagnostic intraoral scan file or a scan of a diagnostic stone model (typically displayed with an **.stl** file extension).

Surgical guidance can be obtained by two distinct modalities, either *dynamic* or *static* guidance. Both modalities require the patient to undergo a cone-beam computed tomography (CBCT) scan of the involved arch and, as previously mentioned, the use of a proprietary planning software package to virtually plan the implant placement a priori by the **interdisciplinary** team (Fig. 62.32). The distinction between these two forms of guidance is related to the mode of execution of the surgical intervention.

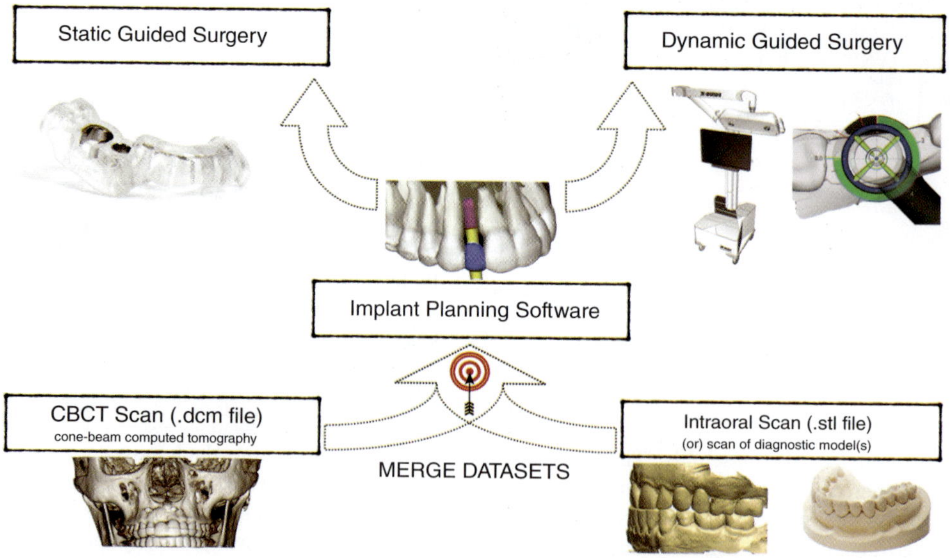

Fig. 62.32 Workflow overview comparing *static* and *dynamic* computer-guided implant placement surgery based on data acquisition.

With **dynamic guidance**, a physical surgical guide (or stent) is not necessary. Instead, the clinician receives both real-time haptic feedback and, through fiduciary markers in the operative field, visual guidance on the position of the **osteotomy** drill and the patient's **alveolar** ridge relative to the a priori surgical plan, as previously designed in the planning software, using imaging tools on a monitor. The clinician can make intraoperative adjustments while performing the osteotomy (e.g., depth and angle) to best match the final implant position in the superimposed virtual plan, as referenced by the planning software.

Comparatively, **static guidance** depends on the additive (stereolithic) or subtractive (computer-aided machining) manufacturing of a surgical guide from the a priori surgical plan, as dictated via the planning software. Such guides can be supported by various intraoral structures, depending on the clinical scenario, including mucosa, bone, or teeth (Fig. 62.33). Recent evidence has demonstrated that tooth-borne static surgical guides fabricated through computer-aided design and computer-aided manufacturing (CAD/CAM) offer superior accuracy when compared to the mucosa or bone-supported static guides, which may be important when considering subsequent restrictive implant provisionalization protocols. Digitally designed and manufactured static surgical guides typically contain embedded metal sleeves that restrict the orientation of the drills during osteotomy preparation (Fig. 62.34). Depending on the level of restriction preferred by the clinician, considering factors such as case complexity, anatomical restrictions, and clinical experience of the operator, guidance may range from pilot-drill guidance, partial guidance, to fully guided surgery (Fig. 62.35).

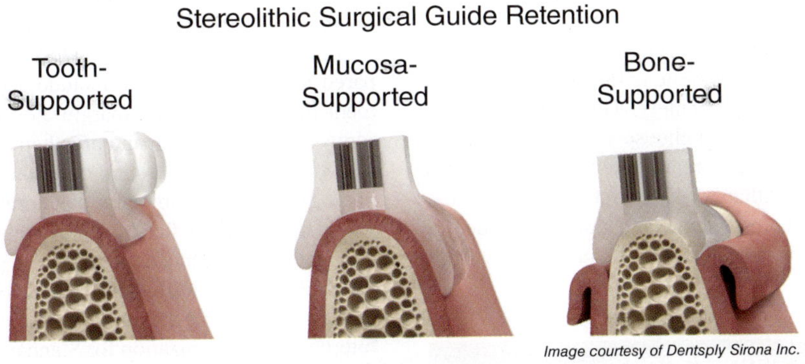

Fig. 62.33 Graphical depiction of retention options for static stereolithic surgical guides, including tooth-supported, mucosa-supported, and bone-supported, depending on the clinical scenario.

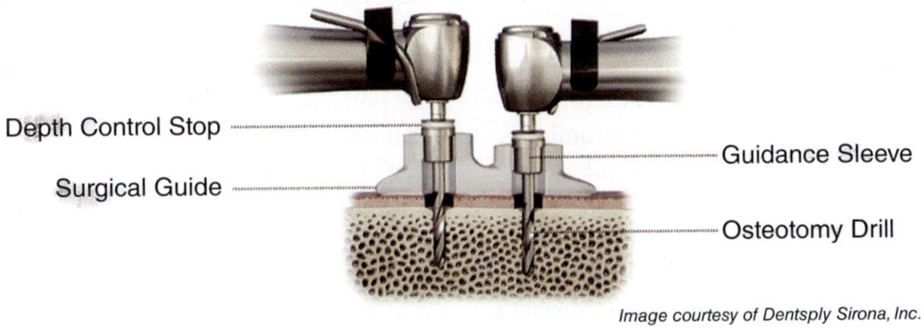

Fig. 62.34 Digital stereolithic surgical guides, manufactured based on computer-guidance software, facilitate osteotomy restriction via the use of specific guidance sleeves and stops, which can either be embedded in the guide, or attached to the osteotomy drill, depending on the manufacturer, and selected protocol.

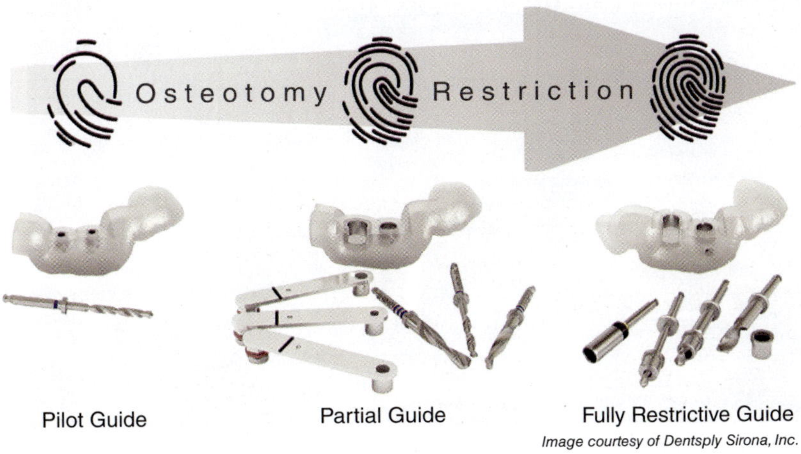

Fig. 62.35 Digitally designed and fabricated surgical guides can vary on the level of surgical restriction, depending on case dynamics, from pilot guidance to full guidance.

Studies evaluating comparative accuracy between these different levels of restrictive guidance have demonstrated a significantly better correlation between planned and placed implants in fully guided protocols, as compared to free-handed and pilot guidance, with mixed outcomes on full versus partial guidance.

When comparing dynamic and static guided implant placement surgery, there are advantages and disadvantages to both modalities. An advantage of dynamic guidance is direct visualization of the surgical field, whereas with static guidance, the clinician's direct line of view of the osteotomy site is temporarily obscured by the guide. This also applies to the surgical assistant, who can directly apply irrigation to the field in dynamic guidance, while indirect irrigation ports are required in static guidance. Conventional surgical osteotomy drills and kits can be used in dynamic guided surgery, while static guidance necessitates protocol-specific kits and drills, aside from the physical surgical guide, increasing costs and componentry necessary to properly execute the procedure. However, the largest consideration for most clinicians contemplating the incorporation of dynamic guidance in their routine is the cost to purchase and space to store the navigation machinery. This factor tends to compel a larger number of clinicians to choose static guided protocols, as guide fabrication costs are relatively inexpensive, and no additional machinery other than drills and kits is necessary. The comparative accuracy of both dynamic and static guidance has been evaluated in clinical trials that have found equivocal levels of precision.

Digital Prosthetic Considerations

Digital technologies have also transformed prosthetic workflows, design (CAD), customization, and manufacturing (CAM) processes. Prior to the adoption of CAD/CAM workflows for fabricating prosthetic components, such as **implant abutments**, framework suprastructures, and coronal restorations, most prosthetic components (whether for interim or definitive restorations) were either prefabricated or customized via labor-intensive and often cost-prohibitive methodologies, such as casting with the lost-wax technique.

Abutment Design and Manufacturing

When considering definitive transmucosal abutments, for instance, prefabricated **titanium** abutments have historically offered clinicians simplicity and cost-effectiveness. However, due to their static emergence design, they are also associated with significant drawbacks when considering clinical situations that exhibit limited restorative space, nonideal implant positioning, and/or compromised soft-tissue esthetics. In contrast, custom abutments designed and fabricated in an analog workflow require castable components that are waxed, invested, and cast by an individual technician, with wide-ranging outcomes. Such castable custom abutments (often referred to as a University of California at Los Angeles [UCLA] abutment) are often associated with compromised biomechanical properties, decreased biocompatibility, increased cost, and elongated fabrication turnaround time.

Additionally, analog workflows prevent detailed communication between the clinician and the technician as to the optimal implant abutment prosthetic features, such as **emergence profile** morphology, **interocclusal** clearance, and axial wall taper, height, and thickness (Fig. 62.36). Consequently, customization of abutment parameters via digital CAD/CAM workflows has increasingly been adopted as an approach to improve clinical outcomes, while the use of stock abutments has declined.

Further advantages of CAD/CAM custom abutments, when compared to stock abutments, include access to removal of excess cement through prosthetic margin elevation, conversion of prosthetic screw-channel location and prosthetic fixation method via angulated screw access (ASA) design, optimizing the emergence profile morphology based on implant positioning and mucosal **phenotype**, which allows to predictably support the peri-implant soft tissue, and duplication of diagnostic information garnered through implant provisionalization. CAD/CAM workflows also make available the opportunity to leverage standardization of manufacturing according to International Organization for Standardization 9000 and good manufacturing practices, CAD-design archiving, and use of abutment design data (via STereoLithography [STL] files) to facilitate expedited design and manufacturing of abutment-supported implant restorations (provisional or definitive) by either the laboratory or clinician. Digital CAD/CAM abutment design technology has also recently been used to design and fabricate custom healing abutments to guide the peri-implant mucosal architecture during nonfunctional loaded healing, contain bone graft materials, and give the restorative clinician the option to move directly to a properly contoured definitive abutment following **osseointegration** without the use of an interim coronal restoration (Fig. 62.37). Given the plethora of advantages (e.g., reduced time and cost, design specificity, and flexibility), CAD/CAM abutments have quickly become a standard of care over the past decade, as well as a therapeutic resource to maximize functional and esthetic outcomes for implant-supported restorations.

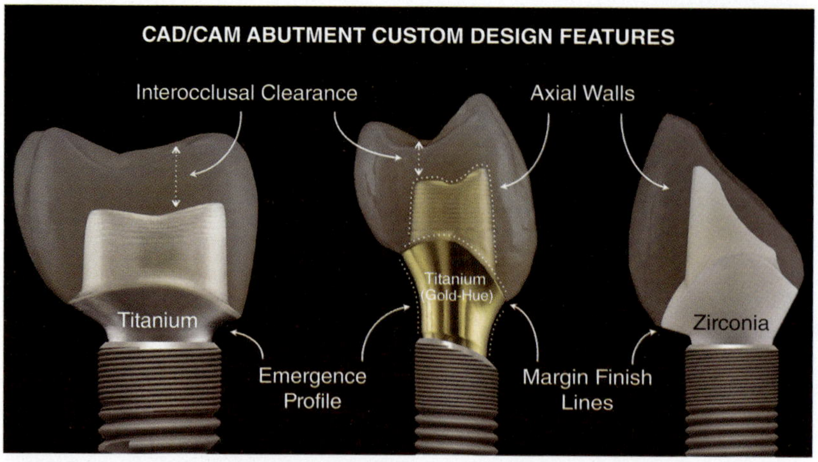

Fig. 62.36 Computer-aided design and computer-aided manufacturing *(CAD/CAM)* prosthetic abutments enable clinicians a full range of parameters for design and fabrication, including biomaterial selection, emergence profile morphology, marginal finish lines, and axial wall taper and interocclusal clearance.

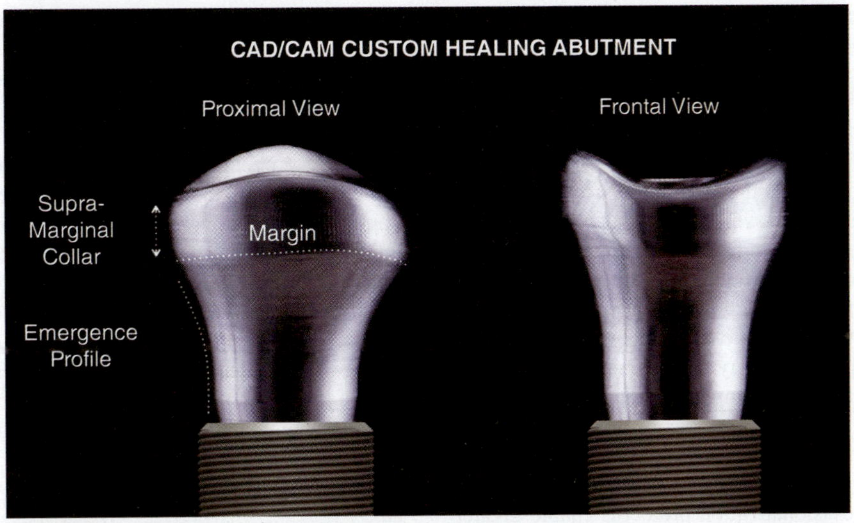

Fig. 62.37 Computer-aided design and computer-aided manufacturing *(CAD/CAM)* custom healing abutments facilitate the development of the peri-implant mucosal architecture and morphology without the need for a coronal component, decreasing chances for occlusal overload in clinical scenarios not suitable for implant provisionalization or in patients that are not compliant with postoperative instructions.

Digitally Aided Implant Provisionalization: A Union of Workflows

By merging the aforementioned advantages that computer-guided surgery and digital prosthetic design and manufacturing offer into a contiguous workflow, robust opportunities for digitally facilitated implant provisionalization have recently emerged and are likely to continue to evolve in the future across different platforms. The following sections will provide a broad overview of various digitally aided provisionalization workflow options, primarily based on the degree of surgical and prosthetic restriction selected. System- and manufacturer-specific workflow variations need to be considered for the selection of a preferred workflow. Referencing general categories based on the level of restrictive constraints, there are three different workflow domains in digitally aided provisionalization (Fig. 62.38).

Nonrestrictive Digitally Aided Provisionalization

In nonrestrictive digitally aided implant provisionalization, both the surgical and prosthetic phases of treatment occur in a nonrestrictive workflow. By selecting a nonrestrictive workflow, surgical and restorative clinicians prioritize having flexibility in both the osteotomy preparation and implant placement, as well as in interim abutment placement and provisional prosthesis coupling to the interim abutment. Such versatility may be preferable in situations where implants are immediately placed into extraction sockets, and/or the integrity or quality of the residual alveolar bone may be in question, but where either immediate (or) delayed provisionalization may be advantageous. Surgically, such nonrestrictive single-tooth implant guides may be designed in various forms and in various digital environments, from laboratory-based design software to chairside intraoral scanners. They can be fabricated by stereolithography using a variety of acrylic and resin materials via 3D printing (additively), or they can be fabricated in subtractive approaches by milling a precured block of resin or acrylic material. Regarding the provisional restorations, such nonrestrictive restorations can similarly be fabricated via different digitally aided additive or subtractive approaches, using both lab and clinical-based software platforms and from a variety of acrylic, resin, or resin-ceramic hybrid materials. A prefabricated abutment is then coupled to the nonrestrictive provisional crown either peri-operatively for immedi-

Provisionalization Workflow	Surgical Restriction (Guidance)	Prosthetic Restriction
Non-Restrictive	No Restriction (or) Pilot-Guide 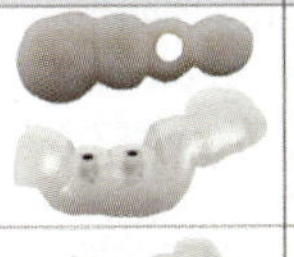	Flexibility to facilitate rotational, apico-coronal, and bodily orientation of interim coronal restoration 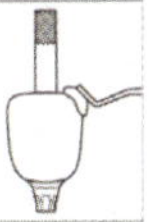
Semi-Restrictive	Partial (or) Full-Guidance 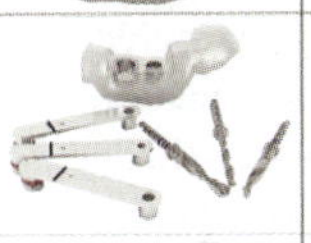	Flexibility to facilitate rotational and apico-coronal, but <u>not</u> bodily orientation of interim coronal restoration 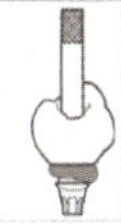
Fully-Restrictive	Full Guidance 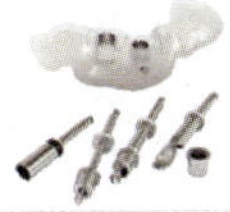	No flexibility for changes in rotation, apico-coronal, or bodily orientation of the interim coronal restoration, components all site-specific 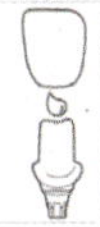

Fig. 62.38 Graphical depiction of the levels of surgical and prosthetic restriction in *digitally aided implant provisionalization.*

ate provisionalization cases or after osseointegration, and full healing has occurred for delayed provisionalization cases.

Semirestrictive Digitally Aided Provisionalization

Utilizing semirestrictive digitally aided implant provisionalization protocols offers more guidance as compared tothe nonrestrictive protocol while still allowing for either the surgeon or restorative clinician, or both, to have control over the implant placement and provisionalization parameters. Semirestrictive protocols provide opportunities for clinicians to make small adjustments to the osteotomy and implant placement parameters, as well as the orientation and mechanism by which the prosthetic components (abutment and crown) are joined. These protocols may be preferentially indicated in situations where more restrictive implant guidance is necessary (e.g., partial guidance) for anatomic, biologic, or functional reasons but where full guidance may be unnecessary or prohibitive to provisionalization. Conversely, even if full restrictive implant guidance is used, semirestrictive provisionalization protocols enable greater prosthetic flexibility and can leverage prefabricated prosthetic components, such as stock provisional abutments. Hence, semirestrictive protocols reduce complexity and cost and offer the clinician carrying out implant provisionalization greater latitude intraoperatively when providing this treatment, as compared to fully restrictive digitally facilitated provisionalization protocols.

Fully Restrictive Digitally Aided Provisionalization

With *nonrestrictive* and *semirestrictive* provisionalization workflows, surgical and prosthetic aspects of care can be executed with varying degrees of flexibility, depending on the nature and degree of adjustments that are required. *Fully restrictive* digitally aided implant provisionalization protocols, in contrast, require complete adherence to full guidance during the surgical and prosthetic phases of treatment, including osteotomy preparation and implant placement and the use of patient and site-specific custom componentry for implant provisionalization. Taken together, this form of provisionalization requires a high degree of coordination during virtual planning of surgery and digital design of the custom prosthetic componentry, as well as between surgical and prosthetic phases during the actual execution of treatment.

The main differentiating factor of fully restrictive digitally aided provisionalization is the use of custom prosthetic componentry, such as custom CAD/CAM abutments and milled or printed provisional crowns. Therefore, this modality requires that implant placement is strictly controlled through the stereolithic guide to constrain implant depth, angulation, and circumferential rotation (sometimes referred to as *timing*) for the site-specific CAD/CAM abutment and provisional crown to fit correctly.

Therefore, with regard to workflow considerations, digital planning typically ensues in two phases. First, implant placement planning must be done in planning software that supports fully restrictive implant guidance. After that, a prosthetic design that predicates the design parameters of the abutment and crown on the aspects of implant positioning and depth established previously can occur. Such prosthetic design factors may include abutment material selection, emergence profile morphology, marginal finish line location, axial wall height and clearance, prosthetic crown form and shade, type of prosthetic fixation, and occlusal scheme. Upon completion of design and manufacture of all relevant components, including the stereolithic surgical guide, the CAD/CAM custom abutment, and the provisional crown, they should be sterilized prior to the execution of therapy.

While the most technically and clinically sophisticated of the three forms of digitally aided implant provisionalization reviewed in this chapter, it is important to note that not all cases will be amenable or even fully benefit from *fully restrictive digitally aided provisionalization*. Several factors determine the suitability of such a workflow, including the timing of implant placement (delayed vs immediate) and the integrity of either the healed ridge or extraction socket, the mucosal phenotype of the implant site, patient compliance, the occlusal status of the patient, and the predictability to accomplish implant placement in the exact a priori planned location to permit implant provisionalization with customized prosthetic components. In clinical scenarios where immediate provisionalization is planned, an additional stipulation must be met: adequate primary stability at the predetermined position to support immediate provisionalization protocols. Therefore, clinician experience, local factors, and patient compliance are variables that must be carefully considered when selecting the modality of implant provisionalization.

Digitally Aided Implant Provisionalization: Alternative Approaches

When clinicians plan implant provisionalization, they may limit their **treatment planning** process to only consider the replacement of coronal form, function, and esthetics as a means of psychosocial support for the patient. However, an important benefit of implant provisionalization, whether digitally aided or analog, is the optimization of peri-implant soft tissue morphology to improve the design of the definitive restorative components and achieve an optimal esthetic outcome. Such treatment objectives can be achieved with digitally designed and manufactured custom healing abutments in clinical scenarios where conventional, full coronal provisionalization may not be feasible or may jeopardize healing and osseointegration of the implant or where patient compliance may be in doubt. Such workflows enable the achievement of an anatomically correct peri-implant sulcus without many of the potential **risk factors** at play in the aforementioned digitally facilitated provisionalization scenarios. The design and fabrication methods for such custom CAD/CAM healing abutments vary between manufacturers but will predominantly be based, as summarized previously for digitally aided coronal provisionalization, on some form of computer-guided surgery.

Conclusion

Digitally assisted implant placement with static CAD/CAM surgical guides has been shown to be more accurate when compared to freehand methods. Likewise, implant placement via dynamic navigation has displayed comparable results. Between static surgical guides and dynamic navigation, however, it is unclear as to which method is superior in terms of accuracy of implant placement. While both methods enable flapless surgeries and are capable of replicating the planned implant position, angulation, and depth, each method has its own set of advantages and disadvantages. At this point in time, the choice between utilizing static guides or dynamic navigation will depend on the operator's personal preference, experience level, and access to required technologies and devices.

Digital approaches and workflows to facilitate implant provisionalization offer the interdisciplinary team flexibility in choosing what level of restriction and customization is appropriate based on their preferences and the presenting clinical scenario(s). As the clinical examples highlight, *digitally aided implant provisionalization* provides the opportunity to customize and accelerate treatment outcomes for patients, providing psychosocial and esthetic benefits while optimizing the peri-implant mucosal architecture. Emerging digital workflows also enable clinicians to provide customized

CAD/CAM transmucosal healing abutments that provide some of the benefits of digitally fabricated provisional restorations without the risk of premature loading.

Key points

- The **digital implant workflow** can help clinicians plan more efficiently and execute more accurately.
- **Static CAD/CAM surgical guides** can be designed from the virtual plan and produced with various technologies including milling and 3D printing.
- **Dynamic navigation** employs real-time tracking and visual guidance to execute the virtual surgical plan.
- Digital technologies have also transformed prosthetic workflows, design (CAD), customization, and manufacturing (CAM) processes.
- By merging the computer-guided surgery and digital prosthetic design and manufacturing provide a contiguous workflow and robust opportunities for digitally facilitated implant provisionalization have recently emerged.

Suggested Readings

Abdel Raheem IM, Hammad IA,Abel Kader SH, Fahmy RA: Fabrication of a CAD-CAM custom healing abutment guided by a conventional dental radiograph for delayed loaded dental implants: a dental technique. *J Prosthet Dent* 127 (1):49–54, 2022.

Barwacz CA, Hernandez M: Maximizing esthetics of fixed interim restorations via direct extrinsic characterization. *JCD* 29:122–131, 2013.

Barwacz CA, Summerwill M, Avila-Ortiz G: Leveraging digital workflows for immediate single-tooth replacement therapy: a case report. *Int J Oral Implantol* 14:321–333, 2021.

Chen P, Nikoyan L: Guided implant surgery: a technique whose time has come. *Dent Clin North Am* 65:67–80, 2021.

Chu Kan JY, Lee EA, et al: Restorative emergence profile for single-tooth implants in healthy periodontal patients: clinical guidelines and decision-making strategies. *Int J Periodontics Restorative Dent* 40:19–29, 2019.

Hartman MJ: A workflow to design and fabricate a customized healing abutment from a dynamic navigation virtual treatment plan. *Compend Contin Educ Dent* 42:86–92, 2021.

Kaewsiri D, Panmekiate S, Subbalekha K, Mattheos N, Pimkhaokham A: The accuracy of static vs. dynamic computer-assisted implant surgery in single tooth space: a randomized controlled trial. *Clin Oral Implants Res* 30:505–514, 2019.

Kernen F, Kramer J, Wanner L, et al: A review of virtual planning software for guided implant surgery – data import and visualization, drill guide design and manufacturing. *BMC Oral Health* 20:251, 2020.

Panchal N, Mahmood L, Retana A, et al: Dynamic navigation for dental implant surgery. *Oral Maxillofac Surg Clin North Am* 31:539–547, 2019.

Putra RH, Yoda N, Astuti ER, Sasaki K. The accuracy of implant placement with computer-guided surgery in partially edentulous patients and possible influencing factors: a systematic review and meta-analysis. *J Prosthodont Res* 2021.

Raico Gallardo YN, da Silva-Olivio IRT, Mukai E, et al: Accuracy comparison of guided surgery for dental implants according to the tissue of support: a systematic review and meta-analysis. *Clin Oral Implants Res* 28:602–612, 2017.

Tahmaseb A, Wismeijer D, Coucke W, et al: Computer technology applications in surgical implant dentistry: a systematic review. *Int J Oral Maxillofac Implants* 29:25, 2014.

Tattan M, Chambrone L, González-Martín O, Avila-Ortiz G: Static computer-aided, partially guided, and free-handed implant placement: a systematic review and meta-analysis of randomized controlled trials. *Clin Oral Implants Res* 31:889–916, 2020.

Van Assche N, Vercruyssen M, Coucke W, Teughels W, Jacobs R, Quirynen M: Accuracy of computer-aided implant placement. *Clin Oral Implants Res* 23 (suppl 6):112–123, 2012.

Varga E, Antal M, Major L, Kiscsatári R, Braunitzer G, Piffkó J: Guidance means accuracy: a randomized clinical trial on freehand versus guided dental implantation. *Clin Oral Impl Res* 31:417–430, 2020.

Younes F, Cosyn J, De Bruyckere T, Cleymaet R, Bouckaert E, Eghbali A: A randomized controlled study on the accuracy of free-handed, pilot-drill guided and fully guided implant surgery in partially edentulous patients. *J Clin Periodontol* 45:721–732, 2018.

Refrences

References and MCQs with answers for the chapter are available on www.medenact.com.

INDEX

G

N

O

P

Q

R

T